Schaffer's
Fifth Edition # Diseases
of the
Newborn

MARY ELLEN AVERY, M.D.

Thomas Morgan Rotch Professor of Pediatrics
Harvard Medical School;
Physician-in-Chief
The Children's Hospital
Boston, Massachusetts

H. WILLIAM TAEUSCH, JR., M.D.

Associate Professor of Pediatrics
Harvard Medical School;
Director, Joint Program in Neonatology,
The Children's Hospital
Brigham and Women's Hospital and
Beth Israel Hospital,
Boston, Massachusetts

W. B. Saunders Company

Philadelphia London Toronto Mexico City Rio de Janeiro Sydney Tokyo

W. B. Saunders Company   West Washington Square
Philadelphia, PA 19105

1 St. Anne's Road
Eastbourne, East Sussex BN21 3UN, England

1 Goldthorne Avenue
Toronto, Ontario M8Z 5T9, Canada

Apartado 26370—Cedro 512
Mexico 4, D.F., Mexico

Rua Coronel Cabrita, 8
Sao Cristovao Caixa Postal 21176
Rio de Janeiro, Brazil

9 Waltham Street
Artarmon, N.S.W. 2064, Australia

Ichibancho, Central Bldg., 22-1 Ichibancho
Chiyoda-Ku, Tokyo 102, Japan

Listed here is the latest translated edition of this book together with the language of the translation and the publisher.

Spanish (*3rd Edition*)—Salvat Editores, S.A., Barcelona, Spain
Portuguese (*4th Edition*)—Editora Interamericana Ltda. Rio de Janeiro, Brazil

Library of Congress Cataloging in Publication Data

Schaffer, Alexander J.
  Schaffer's Diseases of the newborn.

  1. Infants (Newborn)—Diseases.   I. Avery, Mary
Ellen.   II. Taeusch, H. William.   III. Title.
IV. Title: Diseases of the newborn.   [DNLM: 1. Infant,
Newborn, Diseases.   WS 420 S296d]
RJ254.S3   1984   618.92'01   82-48499
ISBN 0-7216-1458-2

RJ254
S3
1984

Schaffer's Diseases of the Newborn   ISBN   0-7216-1458-2

Last digit is the print number: 9   8   7   6   5   4   3

Contributors

CONSTANTINE S. ANAST, M.D.

Professor of Pediatrics, Harvard Medical School, Boston, Massachusetts. Senior Associate in Medicine, Senior Associate in Endocrinology and Director of Endocrine Laboratories, The Children's Hospital, Boston, Massachusetts.

Disorders of Mineral and Bone Metabolism; Disorders of the Adrenal Glands and Sodium Metabolism; Disorders of the Thyroid Gland; Abnormalities of Sexual Differentiation

T. BERRY BRAZELTON, M.D.

Associate Professor of Pediatrics, Harvard Medical School, Boston, Massachusetts. Chief, Child Development Unit, The Children's Hospital, Boston, Massachusetts.

Neonatal Behavior and Its Significance

MICHAEL F. EPSTEIN, M.D.

Assistant Professor of Pediatrics, Harvard Medical School, Boston, Massachusetts. Physician in Charge of Newborn Intensive Care Units, The Children's Hospital and Brigham and Women's Hospital, Boston, Massachusetts.

Resuscitation

NANCY B. ESTERLY, M.D.

Professor of Pediatrics and Dermatology, Northwestern University Medical School, Chicago, Illinois. Head, Division of Dermatology, The Children's Memorial Hospital, Chicago, Illinois.

Congenital and Hereditary Disorders of the Skin; Infections of the Skin; Nevi and Cutaneous Tumors; Miscellaneous Skin Disorders

ELAINE E. FARRELL, M.D.

Assistant Professor of Pediatrics, Northwestern University Medical School, Chicago, Illinois. Attending Neonatologist, Evanston Hospital, Evanston, Illinois.

Infant Nutrition

IVAN D. FRANTZ III, M.D.

Assistant Professor of Pediatrics, Harvard Medical School, Boston, Massachusetts. Associate Chief, Division of Newborn Medicine, The Children's Hospital, Boston, Massachusetts. Senior Pediatrician, Brigham and Women's Hospital, Boston, Massachusetts. Associate in Pediatrics, Beth Israel Hospital, Boston, Massachusetts.

Mechanical Ventilation

F. CLARKE FRASER, Ph.D., M.D., C.M., D.Sc., F.R.S.C.

Professor of Clinical Genetics and Professor of Pediatrics, Memorial University of Newfoundland Faculty of Medicine, Health Sciences Center, St. John's, Newfoundland, Canada. Staff, Department of Medicine, General Hospital, Health Sciences Center, St. John's, Newfoundland, Canada. Staff, Department of Medicine, Janeway Child Health Centre, St. John's, Newfoundland, Canada.

The Branchial Arch Syndromes and Cleft Lip and Cleft Palate; The Chondrodystrophies; Other Congenital Defects Involving Bones; Congenital Defects Involving Joints; Miscellaneous Disorders of the Skeletal System; Gross Chromosomal Aberrations; Some Multiple Malformation Syndromes Not Caused by Gross Chromosomal Aberrations

MICHAEL D. FREED, M.D.

Associate Professor of Pediatrics, Harvard Medical School, Boston, Massachusetts. Senior Associate in Cardiology and Chief of Clinical Cardiology, The Children's Hospital, Boston, Massachusetts.

General Considerations; Congenital Cardiac Malformations; Cardiomyopathies; Cardiac Dysrhythmias

KENNETH H. GABBAY, M.D.

Associate Professor of Pediatrics, Harvard Medical School, Boston, Massachusetts. Director, Diabetes Unit, The Children's Hospital, Boston, Massachusetts.

Disorders of Carbohydrate Metabolism

BERTIL E. GLADER, Ph.D., M.D.

Associate Professor of Pediatrics, Stanford University School of Medicine, Stanford, California. Director, Hematology/Oncology Program, Children's Hospital at Stanford, Palo Alto, California.

Bleeding Disorders in the Newborn Infant; Neonatal Leukocyte Disorders; Erythrocyte Disorders in Infancy

RICHARD J. GRAND, M.D.

Professor of Pediatrics, Tufts University School of Medicine, Boston, Massachusetts. Chief, Division

of Pediatric Gastroenterology and Nutrition, New England Medical Center—The Floating Hospital, Boston Massachusetts.
General Considerations

WILLIAM R. GREEN, M.D.
Professor of Ophthalmology and Associate Professor of Pathology, The Johns Hopkins University School of Medicine, Baltimore, Maryland. Ophthalmologist, Pathologist, and Chief of Eye Pathology Laboratory, The Johns Hopkins Hospital, Baltimore, Maryland.
Tumors of the Eye and Orbit

WARREN E. GRUPE, M.D.
Associate Professor of Pediatrics, Harvard Medical School, Boston, Massachusetts. Associate Professor of Pediatrics and Chief, Division of Nephrology, The Children's Hospital, Boston Massachusetts.
General Considerations; Abnormalities of the Genital Tract; Congenital Malformations of the Genitourinary Tract; Congenital Malformations of the Kidney; Hydronephrosis; Renal Vascular Thrombosis; Hypertension; Differential Diagnosis of the Enlarged Kidney; Nephropathies; Acute Renal Failure

DAVID L. GUYTON, M.D.
Associate Professor of Ophthalmology, The Johns Hopkins University School of Medicine, Baltimore, Maryland. Active Staff, The Johns Hopkins Hospital, Baltimore, Maryland.
Disturbances of Motility

LAWRENCE W. HIRST, M.D., M.P.H.
Assistant Professor of Ophthalmology, The Johns Hopkins University School of Medicine, Baltimore, Maryland. Assistant Director of Corneal Services, The Wilmer Ophthalmological Institute, The Johns Hopkins Hospital, Baltimore, Maryland.
Other Neonatal Disorders of the Eye; Infections of the Eye

SAMUEL A. LATT, M.D., Ph.D.
Professor of Pediatrics, Harvard Medical School, Boston, Massachusetts. Chief, Division of Genetics, The Children's Hospital, Boston, Massachusetts. Director, Cytogenetics Laboratory, Brigham and Women's Hospital, Boston Massachusetts.
Prenatal Genetic Diagnosis

HARVEY L. LEVY, M.D.
Associate Professor of Neurology, Harvard Medical School, Boston, Massachusetts. Senior Associate in Medicine, The Children's Hospital, Boston, Massachusetts. Director, IEM-PKU Program, The Children's Hospital, Boston, Massachusetts. Associate Pediatrician and Assistant in Neurology, Massachusetts General Hospital, Boston, Massachusetts.
Newborn Screening; General Considerations; Inborn Errors of Carbohydrate Metabolism; Inborn Errors of Amino Acid Metabolism; Inborn Errors of Organic Acids; Inborn Errors of Lipid Metabolism; Miscellaneous Inborn Errors of Metabolism

KENNETH McINTOSH, M.D.
Associate Professor of Pediatrics, Harvard Medical School, Boston, Massachusetts. Clinical Chief, Division of Infectious Disease, The Children's Hospital, Boston, Massachusetts.
Bacterial Infections of the Newborn; Other Specific Bacterial Infections; Viral Infections of the Fetus and Newborn; Fungus Infections; Protozoal Infections: Congenital Toxoplasmosis

JOHN H. MENKES, M.D.
Clinical Professor of Pediatrics and Neurology, UCLA School of Medicine, Los Angeles, California. Staff, UCLA Center for the Health Sciences, Cedars-Sinai Medical Center, Los Angeles, California.
Neurologic Evaluation of the Newborn Infant; Perinatal Trauma and Asphyxia; Malformations of the Central Nervous System; Paroxysmal Disorders; Diseases of the Motor Unit; Miscellaneous Neurological Disorders Presenting in the Newborn.

FRANK A. OSKI, M.D.
Professor of Pediatrics and Chairman, Department of Pediatrics, Upstate Medical Center College of Medicine, State University of New York, Syracuse, New York.
General Considerations; Physiologic Jaundice; Unconjugated Hyperbilirubinemia; Kernicterus; Hydrops Fetalis; Obstructive Jaundice Due to Biliary Atresia and Neonatal Hepatitis; Conjugated Hyperbilirubinemia Other Than That Due to Hepatitis and Biliary Atresia; Differential Diagnosis of Jaundice

ROBERTSON PARKMAN, M.D.
Professor of Microbiology and Pediatrics, University of Southern California School of Medicine, Los Angeles, California. Head, Division of Research Immunology and Bone Marrow Transplantation, The Children's Hospital of Los Angeles, Los Angeles, California.
Immunology

ARNALL PATZ, M.D.
William Holland Wilmer Professor and Chairman of Department of Ophthalmology, The Johns Hopkins University School of Medicine, Baltimore, Maryland. Seeing Eye Research Professor, The Wilmer Ophthalmological Institute, The Johns Hopkins Hospital, Baltimore, Maryland.
Tumors of the Eye and Orbit

JOHN W. PAYNE, M.D.
Assistant Professor of Ophthalmology, The Johns Hopkins University School of Medicine, Baltimore, Maryland. Attending Ophthalmologist, The Wilmer Ophthalmological Institute, The Johns Hopkins Hospital and Greater Baltimore Medical Center, Baltimore, Maryland.
Retinopathy of Prematurity

ROBERT J. ROBERTS, M.D., Ph.D.
Professor, Department of Pediatrics and Pharmacology, The University of Iowa College of Medicine, Iowa City, Iowa.
Principles of Neonatal Pharmacology

SAMUEL R. SCHUSTER, M.D.
Associate Professor of Surgery, Harvard Medical School, Boston, Massachusetts. Senior Associate in Surgery, The Children's Hospital, Boston, Massachusetts.
Intestinal Obstruction

ALLEN D. SCHWARTZ, M.D.
Professor of Pediatrics, University of Maryland School of Medicine, Baltimore, Maryland. Professor of Oncology, University of Maryland Cancer Center, Baltimore, Maryland. Chief of Pediatric Hematology and Oncology, University of Maryland Hospital, Baltimore, Maryland.
Congenital Malignant Disorders

MANDEL R. SHER, M.D.
Fellow, Pediatric Rheumatology, The University of Michigan Medical School, Ann Arbor, Michigan.
Rheumatic Disorders

LAWRENCE M. SOLOMON, M.D.
Professor and Head, Department of Dermatology, The Abraham Lincoln School of Medicine, The University of Illinois, Chicago, Illinois.
Congenital and Hereditary Disorders of the Skin; Infections of the Skin; Nevi and Cutaneous Tumors; Miscellaneous Skin Disorders

HARLAND S. WINTER, M.D.
Assistant Professor of Pediatrics, Harvard Medical School, Boston, Massachusetts. Assistant in Gastroenterology, The Children's Hospital, Boston, Massachusetts.
Disorders of the Esophagus; Tracheal Esophageal Fistulas and Atresia; Disorders of Neuromuscular Control of the Esophagus; Hirschsprung's Disease

Foreword

While writing the first edition of *Diseases of the Newborn*, Alexander Schaffer found himself in the 1950s facing a recent "gigantic growth . . . of knowledge concerning the newborn" with "the apparently insurmountable obstacle of [his] own limitation of knowledge." He therefore considered substituting "a collection of essays by eight or ten . . . specialists" for "the less erudite and less detailed" volume he might produce almost alone. He chose the latter course for the characteristically sound reason that "we practitioners of pediatrics are the newborn's first and primary physicians." If in so doing Dr. Schaffer was thereby launching one more subspecialty (*neonatology,* whose name he suggested in 1960), his choice was still correct. Pediatric practitioners, even those drawn into the earlier subspecialties, still have to be the "baby doctors" they always were, and few can or would relinquish all responsibilities for newborn patients.

The accumulated knowledge with which any primary physician now approaches such a patient makes the "gigantic growth" observed during the 1950s seem relatively modest. Yet the work accomplished during that decade was at least a beginning. Many of us can recall the 1930s and 1940s, when physiologic information was so scanty that a skillful delivery, an incubator (with unrestricted oxygen), an experienced nurse, and a "hands-off" policy for the first day or two after premature birth seemed defensible. By the 1950s we recognized, at least, how little was actually known and were seeking, if slowly, to increase our store of information.

Today, many clinical and research workers have brought much new technology and information into that search. Reports of their findings now outnumber the abstracts from any other subsection submitted to the meetings of the American Pediatric and Pediatric Research Societies. The state of the art clearly requires this fifth edition. But although many of the contributors to *Schaffer's Diseases of the Newborn* must now represent even more subspecialties, the editors have wisely continued to direct the fifth edition of this book, as Dr. Schaffer directed the original, toward the practitioners of pediatrics as the newborn patient's first and primary physicians. For them, as in the past, it will be immediately (and often urgently) useful on many occasions. For the house officers, nurses, and neonatologists of all intensive care nurseries, it will continue to be required and repeated reading. Much evidence indicates that the efforts of all will thereby continue to increase the understanding, improve the care, and reduce the morbidity and mortality of newborn infants.

CLEMENT A. SMITH

Preface to the Fifth Edition

The challenge in the revision of a textbook is to preserve the wisdom of the past but reduce the encumbrance and at the same time to incorporate the newest insights and avoid speculation.

We have tried to provide our readers with a synopsis of the current views on the care of newborn infants based on a review of accumulated experiments and experience. When factual evidence exists, we have included it and discussed its limitations. When empiricism dictates practice, we have tried to discuss its strengths and weaknesses. When we do not understand the phenomena we see, we have declared the limits of our knowledge.

No author or group of contributors claims more than a limited perspective on a responsibility so great as that of prescribing the best approaches to the care of newborn infants. All who work with them or undertake to teach others how to care for them are humbled by the challenge.

In this, the fifth edition of *Schaffer's Diseases of the Newborn*, we have tried to combine the experience of professionals devoted to the study of neonatal adaptations and disorders with that of individuals who participate in day-to-day care of infants. The contributors to this volume have an enormous accumulated experience that they have chosen to share with our readers.

The editors are grateful to the 29 individuals who contributed chapters to this work, to Ms. Florence Avitabile for her many editorial contributions, and to the publishers, W. B. Saunders Company, especially Ms. Mary Cowell and Ms. Linda Fitzpatrick, who encouraged all of us to try to say, in 1983, what is known and what has been found helpful on the frontlines of the newborn nurseries. We also most gratefully acknowledge the innumerable contributions of fellows in neonatology, house staff, and nurses who continually remind us that the printed word can be helpful as they pursue their tasks at the bedside.

In particular, many of our colleagues have reviewed sections of this book and offered much appreciated advice. They include Drs. Jason Birnholz, Elizabeth Brown, William Cochran, Thomas Cone, Elaine Farrell, Jonathan Gitlin, Thorne Griscom, Celeste Marx, Trevor McGill, Samuel Schuster, Arthur Rhodes, Barry Smith, Ilene Sosenko, and Marjorie Wilson.

MARY ELLEN AVERY
H. WILLIAM TAEUSCH, JR.

Preface to the First Edition

This book was intended to be an Atlas of Diseases of the Newborn. It was to consist of a large number of illustrations and a minimum number of words. Justifiably or not, we soon found ourselves changing this plan. The chief reason was that many important topics were simply not amenable to photographic treatment. How does one go about handling galactosemia or phenylketonuria pictorially? Of what use to a student or a practitioner would a book on the newborn be which omitted any discussion of an inborn error of metabolism whose early recognition spells the difference between vision and blindness, intelligence and stupidity, longevity and early death?

The second consideration which changed the structure of this book was the gigantic growth within the past decade of the corpus of knowledge concerning the newborn. Pathologists, physiologists of many varieties, radiologists and clinicians have begun to swarm over the newborn in ever-increasing numbers. Much has been learned, even though much still remains to be discovered. We felt that the time was ripe for this new knowledge to be collected and to be integrated with the old into an omnium-gatherum of *Diseases of the Newborn*. This could not be accomplished with pictures alone.

We were then confronted with the apparently insurmountable obstacle of our own limitation of knowledge. Clearly no one man can hope to know as much about disturbances in bodily chemistry *and* endocrinology *and* congenital heart disease *and* the premature infant as do the various subspecialists in these limited fields. Would not a collection of essays written by eight or ten of these specialists constitute a superior kind of volume to this necessarily less erudite and less detailed one? We ventured to guess that, for the purpose we had in mind, it would not be as useful. For we practitioners of pediatrics are the newborn's first and primary physicians. We are the ones who should be aware of genetic predispositions which may dictate laboratory studies even before our newborn becomes ill. In this connection we call to your attention the proper management of babies born in families which contain known sufferers from congenital galactosemia or phenylpyruvic oligophrenia. We are the ones who should not, indeed must not, allow even the most trifling deviations from normal to escape our attention in our original examination. Overlooking a cornea which is larger than it should be may spell the difference between ultimate good vision and blindness. Not noticing, or attaching no significance to, a tiny red spot over the spine may mean that the baby will suffer one or two bouts of staphylococcal meningitis before his dermal sinus is diagnosed and excised. In these situations the ophthalmologist and the neurologic surgeon are of absolutely no help to us until we have made the all-important original observation. Finally we are the ones called when cyanosis, dyspnea, fever or convulsions appear, and we must make rapid decisions as to immediate treatment and further study. We must categorize the illness accurately and ask help, when needed, of the proper subspecialist. We have quoted in the text the unfortunate story of a newborn with dextrocardia for whom the aid of a cardiologist was sought. Both practitioner and cardiologist stood by while the infant died of untreated pneumothorax.

In actuality the situation of the pediatrician practicing neonatology differs but little qualitatively from his everyday posture with respect to older infants and children. Much of his function consists in screening, expediting and directing his patients to other subspecialists. But quantitative differences exist in the neonatal period. When newborns are sick they are often so terribly sick that one is loath to endanger their lives by performing diagnostic procedures that would be sheerest routine in older infants. At the same time physical examination is less rewarding in them. Finally the clinical entities peculiar to their age group are just beginning to be defined and are far from being neatly classified in any fixed nosologic schema. Thus even the simplest decisions, for instance whether cyanosis is caused by a congenital heart defect or by pulmonary or intracranial disorder, can be far from simple in the neonate. We believe the practitioner needs a reference book which brings these matters up to date and which may permit him to make these important decisions more promptly and more accurately. Detailed information about pathologic physiology, pathology and embryology may be obtained from other sources.

This, then, is a book on clinical neonatology, written by a practitioner who is neither pathologist nor physiologist, neither biochemist nor virologist. It will therefore have suffered from lack of detailed knowledge in these fields. It is our hope that it will have gained something by virtue of the author's preoccupation for many busy years with the diagnosis, natural history and treatment of disorders of the sick newborn.

Many acknowledgments are in order, too many to detail in this place. The first must go to my wife, who accepted with extraordinary good grace almost complete withdrawal from social life plus the inconvenience of having been awakened at or before dawn every morning for about five years. The second is directed to Dr. Harry H. Gordon, who stimulated me to begin this work and whose constant interest and affectionate concern were mine throughout its long-drawn-out course. He must not be held responsible for any of its imperfections. Neither must my associate, Dr. Milton Markowitz, who not only wrote the section devoted to cardiac disorders, but also struggled with me over most of the sick infants who formed the basis of such knowledge of neonatology as we may possess. Dr. Anthony Perlman, my former associate, was equally conscientious in the matters of diagnosis and treatment of many of these infants and in the mechanical job of keeping detailed day-by-day records of their progress. Pathologists at three hospitals have cooperated freely at the expense of much of their valuable time. Dr. William J. Lovitt, Dr. Ella Oppenheimer and Dr. Tobias Weinberg of The Hospital for the Women of Maryland, The Johns Hopkins and the Sinai Hospitals of Baltimore, respectively, deserve my thanks. The interpretations placed upon their observations are my own. So do the librarians of the Medical and Chirurgical Faculty of Maryland, chiefly Miss Louise D. C. King and Miss M. Florence Woods, and my own secretary Miss Patricia Lilly. I am obligated deeply to all those physicians and surgeons who have given permission to utilize cases and have supplied me with prints of illustrations which my own files did not contain. In this connection the photographers at the various hospitals must be thanked, especially Mr. Harold A. Thomas at The Sinai Hospital of Baltimore.

I am singularly indebted to three good friends whose financial aid made it possible for me to amass an extensive and expensive collection of prints, lantern slides and color transparencies. They are the Messrs. Alan Wurtzburger, James H. Levi and the late Stuart M. Weiler and their wives. Dr. Markowitz is equally grateful to the Benjamin and Minnie Landsberg Memorial Foundation for their support of his studies in the field of heart disease in infancy and childhood.

I must mention my special feeling of gratitude to my publishers, W. B. Saunders Company. My contacts and correspondence with them were effected largely through the medium of John Dusseau, less often through Robert Rowan. Their help, their encouragement, their sound advice and, not least, their exhilarating senses of humor have carried me over many rough spots.

Finally I must thank the administrators of the aforementioned hospitals, plus those of the Union Memorial, University and Lutheran Hospitals of Baltimore, and the heads of their respective Pediatric and Obstetrical Departments for their permission to utilize their cases to illustrate many of my points.

ALEXANDER J. SCHAFFER

Contents

Introduction 1

Part 1
PERINATOLOGY   7

1 Maternal Conditions and
   Exogenous Influences that
   Affect the Fetus/Newborn 8

2 Prenatal Genetic Diagnosis 24

3 Assessment of Fetal Risk in the
   Third Trimester 36

4 Fetal Growth and Neonatal
   Adaptations 43

Part 2
THE NEWBORN INFANT   53

5 Normal Newborn 54

6 Newborn Screening 60

7 Neonatal Behavior and Its
   Significance 68

8 Prematurity 83

9 Intrauterine Growth Retardation 92

10 Resuscitation 100

Part 3
DISORDERS OF THE RESPIRATORY
SYSTEM   109

11 General Considerations 110

12 Nasal Obstructions 120

13 Stridors in the Newborn 122

14 Aspiration Syndromes 128

15 Hyaline Membrane Disease 133

16 Bronchopulmonary Dysplasia
    and Other Persistent
    Pulmonary Dysfunctions 148

17 Air Leak and Air Trapping 154

18 Persistent Fetal Circulation
    (Pulmonary Hypertension) 161

19 Pneumonia 165

20 Miscellaneous Pulmonary Disorders . . .181

21 Disorders of the Diaphragm 189

22 Disorders of the Chest Wall 197

23 Pulmonary Cysts and Intrathoracic
    Masses 199

24 Chylothorax and Pulmonary
    Hemorrhage .213

25 Mechanical Ventilation 217

Part 4
DISORDERS OF THE CARDIOVASCULAR
SYSTEM   223

26 General Considerations 224

27 Congenital Cardiac Malformations 243

28 Cardiomyopathies 291

29 Cardiac Dysrhythmias 304

Part 5
DISORDERS OF THE GASTROINTESTINAL
TRACT   309

30 General Considerations 310

31 Disorders of the Mouth, Tongue,
    and Neck 318

32 Disorders of the Esophagus 324

33 Tracheal Esophageal Fistulas
    and Atresia 332

34 Disorders of Neuromuscular Control
    of the Esophagus 338

35 Disorders of the Stomach 340

36 Intestinal Obstruction 346

37 Congenital Intestinal Obstruction 351

38 Acquired Intestinal Obstruction 364

39 Hirschsprung's Disease 368

40 Disorders of the Umbilicus 372

41 Congenital Malformations of the Omphalomesenteric (Vitelline) Duct . . . 381

42 Fetal Ascites, Neonatal Ascites, Peritonitis, and Lymphedema 386

Part 6
DISORDERS OF THE GENITOURINARY TRACT   393

43 General Considerations 394

44 Abnormalities of the Genital Tract 401

45 Congenital Malformations of the Genitourinary Tract 411

46 Congenital Malformations of the Kidney 420

47 Hydronephrosis 427

48 Renal Vascular Thrombosis 437

49 Hypertension 441

50 Differential Diagnosis of the Enlarged Kidney 447

51 Nephropathies 451

52 Acute Renal Failure 456

Part 7
DISORDERS OF MINERAL METABOLISM AND THE ENDOCRINE SYSTEM   463

53 Disorders of Mineral and Bone Metabolism 464

54 Disorders of the Adrenal Glands and Sodium Metabolism 479

55 Disorders of the Thyroid Gland 490

56 Abnormalities of Sexual Differentiation 503

57 Disorders of Carbohydrate Metabolism 514

Part 8
INBORN ERRORS OF METABOLISM   525

58 General Considerations 526

59 Inborn Errors of Carbohydrate Metabolism 529

60 Inborn Errors of Amino Acid Metabolism 536

61 Inborn Errors of Organic Acids 549

62 Inborn Errors of Lipid Metabolism 552

63 Miscellaneous Inborn Errors of Metabolism 554

Part 9
DISORDERS OF BLOOD AND BLOOD VESSELS   559

64 Bleeding Disorders in the Newborn Infant 560

65 Neonatal Leukocyte Disorders 575

66 Erythrocyte Disorders in Infancy 581

67 Rheumatic Disorders 615

Part 10
JAUNDICE   621

68 General Considerations 622

69 Physiologic Jaundice 625

70 Unconjugated Hyperbilirubinemia 630

71 Kernicterus 633

72 Hydrops Fetalis 635

73 Obstructive Jaundice Due to Biliary Atresia and Neonatal Hepatitis 637

74 Conjugated Hyperbilirubinemia Other Than That Due to Hepatitis and Biliary Atresia 644

75 Differential Diagnosis of Jaundice 646

Part 11
DISORDERS OF THE NERVOUS SYSTEM 651

76 Neurologic Evaluation of the
    Newborn Infant 652

77 Perinatal Trauma and Asphyxia 661

78 Malformations of the Central
    Nervous System 680

79 Paroxysmal Disorders 702

80 Diseases of the Motor Unit 707

81 Miscellaneous Neurologic Disorders
    Presenting in the Newborn 713

Part 12
INFECTIONS 719

82 Immunology 720

83 Bacterial Infections of the Newborn . . . 729

84 Other Specific Bacterial Infections 748

85 Viral Infections of the Fetus
    and Newborn 754

86 Fungus Infections 769

87 Protozoal Infections: Congenital
    Toxoplasmosis 775

88 Infections with Spirochetal
    Organisms 778

Part 13
DISORDERS OF NUTRITION 783

89 Infant Nutrition 784

90 Disorders of Vitamins and Trace
    Minerals 800

Part 14
DISORDERS OF THE SKELETAL
SYSTEM 815

91 The Branchial Arch Syndromes
    and Cleft Lip and Cleft Palate 816

92 The Chondrodystrophies 820

93 Other Congenital Defects
    Involving Bones 827

94 Congenital Defects Involving Joints . . . 833

95 Miscellaneous Disorders of the
    Skeletal System 839

Part 15
CONSTELLATIONS OF CONGENITAL
MALFORMATIONS (ODD-LOOKING
BABIES) 845

96 Gross Chromosomal Aberrations 846

97 Some Multiple Malformation
    Syndromes Not Caused by
    Gross Chromosomal Aberrations 854

Part 16
DISORDERS OF THE SKIN 867

98 Congenital and Hereditary
    Disorders of the Skin 868

99 Infections of the Skin 879

100 Nevi and Cutaneous Tumors 884

101 Miscellaneous Skin Disorders 897

Part 17
DISORDERS OF THE EYE 905

102 Disturbances of Motility 906

103 Retinopathy of Prematurity 909

104 Other Neonatal Disorders
    of the Eyes 915

105 Infections of the Eye 918

106 Tumors of the Eye and Orbit 924

Part 18

MISCELLANEOUS DISORDERS   927

107 Congenital Malignant Disorders 928

Part 19

NEONATAL PHARMACOLOGY   949

108 Principles of Neonatal
Pharmacology 950

APPENDICES   969

Appendix 1
Pharmacopeia for the Newborn Period 970

Appendix 2
Composition of Frequently Used Formulas . . . 974

Appendix 3
Illustrative Forms and Normal Values 981

Index 995

Introduction

The aim of neonatology is to provide optimal care for newborn infants. Achieving that aim requires the study of events that occur around the time of birth as the basis for understanding methods of promoting successful adjustments to extrauterine existence. With understanding of physiology and pathology comes the obligation to record, teach, and practice in the light of new knowledge. Since the process of acquiring understanding is continuous, all those who care for newborn infants have need of up-to-date information.

The following paragraph written by the late Alexander Schaffer introduced the fourth edition of this text and is still true:

We trust we have been forgiven for coining the words "neonatology" and "neonatologist." The one designates the art and science of diagnosis and treatment of disorders of the newborn infant, the other the physician whose primary concern lies in this specialty. The words follow logically the stem "neonate," in common usage, and seem to be at least as appropriate as the neologisms "geriatrics" and "geriatrist" or "gerontologist." A new subspecialty has emerged in pediatrics, at least as defined by board certification and fellowship training programs. Such a subdivision has, we suspect, as much merit as does adolescent medicine or even pediatric endocrinology and pediatric cardiology. The period of greatest mortality in life is the first day, and a high mortality rate characterizes the entire first month. . . . If we add to these the deaths which take place in the last months of pregnancy and during labor and delivery, the sum total of so-called perinatal deaths adds up to a staggering figure, a figure which has not fallen nearly so rapidly since the dawn of modern medicine as have the mortality rates for any of the other age groups. . . . The perinatal period, therefore, represents [a new] frontier of medicine, territory which has just begun to be cleared of its forests and underbrush in preparation for its eagerly anticipated crops of saved lives. Until such time as a new subspecialty may be established, it behooves the pediatrician and the general practitioner who supervise the growth and development of infants and children to become more adept in diagnosis, therapy, and prevention of the disorders of the newborn infant.

The current emphasis of neonatology is to find ways to prevent the problems that now call for so much attention and resources. Too often we are delivering a high level of medical care, at great expense, to those who have already been imprinted with damage such as birth asphyxia, severe lung disease, and anomalies. We wish in this edition to underscore the importance of prenatal events in an effort to effect care concerned with preventing problems rather than treating them after they occur. As was true for our predecessors, the required answers will probably result from discoveries made not only by those who care for infants but also by those in basic science who we hope will continue to be stimulated by awareness of the problems of newborn infants.

Although we are able to point with pride at diminishing fetal, neonatal, and infant mortality rates, it is necessary for us to admit that neonatology and neonatal intensive care form an "incomplete solution" to many problems of newborn infants. Cost effectiveness, efficiency, availability, and long-term results of neonatal intensive care are topics of continuing concern. Likewise, some of the serious mistakes that physicians may commit when trying to withhold intensive care pose perplexing questions. Partly because of the tension deriving from these sorts of issues, neonatology is emerging as one of the most self-critical subspecialties in medicine.

Ethical Dilemmas in Newborn Medicine

The questions of how to reduce morbidity and mortality in small infants sometimes involve ethical dilemmas. Because all the various strategies for reaching the same goal are difficult and expensive, choices—priorities—have to be made. At present, the choice of a few centralized perinatal centers serving the needs of the many seems a useful compromise. Nevertheless, with the advent of new intensive care services for infants, we keep discovering new and more specific moral questions. Is it possible that attempts to save all newborn infants, those with brain damage for example, should not be made? What is one to do with the 500 gm abortus that makes gasping movements in a unit with the facilities to care for a 600 gm prematurely born infant, especially when there is demand from community hospitals for greater availability of neonatal intensive care beds for their infants? How can one justify extensive and heroic attempts to save an infant whose chances of survival are less than 10 per cent and whose chances of survival without brain damage are less than 2 per cent?

The questions posed in this manner probably appear more difficult to lay people and health care workers who lack direct experience than to physicians and nurses who encounter these situations daily. While this could be construed as an argument for elitism it may, on the other hand, argue for expert opinion in situations requiring firsthand knowledge of the issues. For example, we have come to believe that a neonatologist is a most appropriate consultant to a service in which an abortus may be born who approaches limits of viability. The neonatologist is a logical person to help judge whether the infant is capable of survival with support. Life and death situations regarding respirator support are less difficult to judge on the scene

1

than from an armchair. When the question of whether to persist with life support is unclear, a uniform process for making these difficult choices should be continually sought. There is general agreement that the strenuous support of an anencephalic infant would be absurd and that the comfort of such an infant and the support of the parents at a difficult time are paramount. There is general disagreement about what to do when parents of an infant with Down syndrome refuse to sign an operative permit allowing corrective surgery for congenital heart disease. Few agree on the precise guidelines for starting respiratory support of the tiniest premature infant; few are sure of how long to persist and whether to persist after a massive intracranial hemorrhage has occurred.

Because no one individual is wise enough to know the answers to these questions, an emerging trend is to introduce more people into the medical decision-making process: judges, everybody caring for the infant, or a hospital committee. In our view, the best decisions are made when the final responsibility for choice is given to the attending physician after he or she has conscientiously conferred with all concerned, mainly the parents, nurses, and social workers, and frequently with one or two other physicians who represent other specialties.

As new insights and new technologies become available, yesterday's dilemma is today's certainty. How long to support the life of an infant with an inoperable heart defect is no longer an issue when corrective surgery becomes available. Thus, the guidelines of the 1980s may not be appropriate in the 1990s. We cannot therefore ever expect to become comfortable with crisp mandates for action or inaction. Existence in a gray zone of decision-making is inevitable; equally inevitable are the changing boundaries of the gray zone. Wide acceptance of the necessity to live with uncertainty could do much to alleviate the anxieties of physicians, nurses, parents, and jurists. Allowing freedom of action in these areas (although infrequent in current society) will, ultimately, be of benefit to the infants.

Regionalization

One of the major advances of recent years has been the evolution of perinatal-neonatal intensive care facilities in centers with adequate staff and enough babies who require care to maintain a high level of experience. A model system for regionalization of perinatal health care was outlined in the publication *Toward Improving the Outcome of Pregnancy* (March of Dimes publication, 1977). The establishment of centers has of course necessitated transport of either the mother before delivery or the

infant after birth. Risks of transport for the infant are finite. They can be minimized by insistence on a well-equipped ambulance and an experienced physician-nurse team to accompany each infant during transport.

High-risk infants (or mothers expected to have such infants) are transferred to perinatal centers (level III units) that essentially combine a high-risk obstetric service with a neonatal intensive care unit. Round-the-clock sophisticated medical and ancillary services should be available. The level II unit is a large community hospital (i.e., one in which there are approximately 1000 deliveries per year) that provides intermediate care to infants who have returned from intensive care units for convalescence and growth or to problem newborns who do not require intensive care. Most babies in the United States are born in this sort of hospital. Intermediate care for infants and services relating to the needs of their parents should be most highly developed and best provided in the level II units. For every intensive care bed, there should be 4 to 6 intermediate care beds, with the exact number based on an estimate of length of stay.

Perinatal Statistics

In some respects, modern perinatology began with the careful recording of fetal and neonatal deaths and standardization of definitions. The criterion for prematurity was established at the latest by 1888, when Budin used 2500 gm as a weight that distinguished preterm from term infants. Not until 1935 did the American Academy of Pediatrics adopt the same definition, and it was only in 1950 that the World Health Organization (WHO) endorsed it.

In a 1974 clarification of definitions by WHO, Dr. Peter Dunn wrote, "The perinatal period occupies less than 0.5% of the average life span, yet accounts in many countries for more deaths than the next 30 years. With the reduction in infant and childhood mortality, attention is increasingly being focused on the prevention of perinatal mortality."

The definitions agreed upon by that group for reporting purposes remain appropriate in the 1980s. The perinatal period extends from the twenty-eighth completed week of pregnancy to the seventh day of life. Clearly, some infants survive after only 25 weeks' gestation, and, in the future, recording of these births and deaths will be appropriate in societies that are prepared to provide intensive care for newborns. Of course, infant deaths also occur after 7 days, and in this country neonatal deaths are often defined as deaths that occur within 28 days of birth, or, for local hospital purposes, deaths that occur before discharge from hospital after preterm birth.

A reason to maintain the WHO nomenclature for worldwide comparisons relates to the incomplete records available in some societies for very immature infants. Although infants born before 28 weeks account for fewer than 1 per cent of livebirths, careful recording of births and deaths and inclusion in na-

Table I–1. Neonatal "In-Hospital" Mortality (Beth Israel and Brigham and Women's Hospitals, 1981)

	n*
Extreme prematurity (<1000 gm birthweight)	48
Congenital anomalies	28
Asphyxia-related	8
Meconium aspiration pneumonia	
Asphyxia (primary)	
Persistent fetal circulation	
Sepsis/infection	6
Respiratory distress syndrome (>1000 gm birthweight)	3
Other	3

* n — number of infants who died with the condition.

Table I–2. Incidence of Neonatal Illness at Brigham and Women's Hospital and Beth Israel Hospital for 1981 (10,409 Livebirths)

	Number of Cases per Livebirths
Respiratory distress syndrome	22/1000
Infection	11/1000
Asphyxia	10/1000
Meconium aspiration pneumonia	4/1000
Necrotizing enterocolitis	2/1000

tional statistics penalizes the countries that have the best reporting.

Preterm. Preterm is defined as less than 37 completed weeks, or 259 days. The definition is, of course, arbitrary, but it is based on the greater likelihood of conditions associated with immaturity, such as hyaline membrane disease, in the group of infants born before 259 days. For most developed countries, 37 completed weeks corresponds to 3000 gm birth weight, up from 2500 gm in an earlier era.

Stillbirth and Fetal Death. By definition, early fetal death occurs at less than 20 completed weeks of gestation, intermediate fetal death occurs at more than 20 and less than 28 completed weeks, and late fetal death occurs after 28 weeks. The word "stillbirth" is usually applied to late fetal deaths.

Livebirth. The World Health Organization defines livebirth as "the complete expulsion or extraction from its mother of a product of conception, irrespective of the duration of pregnancy, which, after such separation, breathes or shows any other evi-

Table I–3. Diagnostic and Therapeutic Advances in Perinatology

		Pediatrics	Obstetrics
1950–1960	Infections	Nursery infection control Widespread use of antibiotics	Control of endometritis Near elimination of maternal mortality in childbirth
	Rh disease	Exchange transfusions	Serum antibody testing Amniocentesis for bilirubin pigments
	Surgery	PDA, imperforate anus, TE fistula	Avoidance of midforceps delivery, improved maternal anesthesia
	Toxicology	Chloramphenicol, sulfonamides, oxygen	Thalidomide, diethylstilbestrol
1961–1970	Rh disease/jaundice	Phototherapy	Prevention of isoimmunization
	Regionalization	High-risk infants: neonatal intensive care units, intermediate care units	High-risk mothers: perinatal centers
	Monitoring	Intra-arterial blood gases, blood pressure	Fetal heart rate monitoring, fetal scalp pH
		Continuous heart and respiratory rate monitoring	Maternal estrogen excretion
	Amniotic fluid testing	Improved genetic counseling	Detection of fetal genetic disorders
1971–1983	Infection	Cord blood serologies for detection of chronic fetal infections	Rubella immunization
	Respiratory disease	Ventilator support with continuous distending airway pressure Microtesting of blood samples Transcutaneous O_2 and CO_2 monitoring	Amniotic fluid testing for RDS risk Prenatal glucocorticoids to accelerate fetal lung maturation Improved suctioning techniques for removal of meconium in the upper airway
	Genetics	Neonatal screening: PKU, hypothyroidism, and other metabolic diseases	Heterozygote definition (Tay-Sachs) Fetal diagnosis of hemoglobinopathies
	Imaging	CAT scanning and ultrasonography	Fetal ultrasonography
	Prematurity	Intravenous hyperalimentation Psychological support of parents of ICU infants	Suppression of premature labor

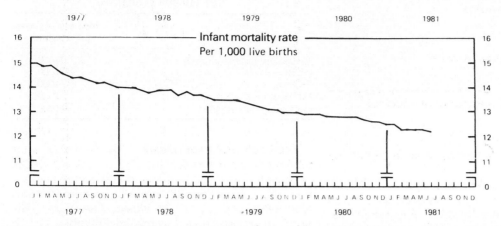

Figure I–1. Infant mortality by months, United States, 1977–1981. Rates are for successive 12-month periods, ending with each month indicated. (Data from National Center for Health Statistics. Figure from Wegman, M. E.: Pediatrics *68*:755, 1981.)

dence of life, such as beating of the heart, pulsation of the umbilical cord, or definite movement of voluntary muscles, whether or not the umbilical cord has been cut or the placenta is attached; each product of such a birth is considered liveborn."

Term.   This defines births that occur from 37 to less than 42 completed weeks, measured from the day of onset of the last normal menstrual period (259 to 293 days, with an average of 280 days).

Post-term.   This refers to births that occur at 42 or more completed weeks (294 days and over).

Early Neonatal Death.   This describes the death of a liveborn infant during the first 7 completed days of life.

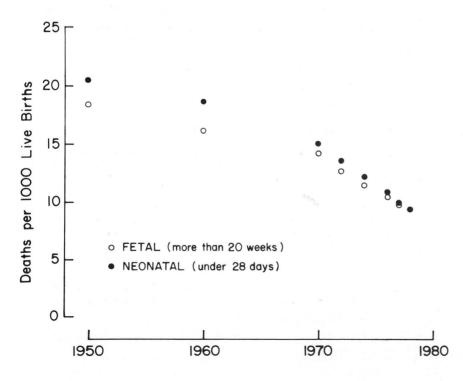

Figure I–2. From Monthly Vital Statistics Report. National Center for Health Statistics, Vol. 29, No. 13, Sept. 17, 1981.

Table I–4. Infant Mortality by Age for Certain Years*

	<1 Year	<28 Days	28 Days to 11 Months
1980(est)	12.5	8.4	4.1
1979(est)	13.0	8.7	4.2
1970	20.0	15.1	4.9
1960	26.0	18.7	7.3
1950	29.2	20.5	8.7
1940	47.0	28.8	18.2
1930	64.6	35.7	29.0

* Data from National Center for Health Statistics and U.S. Bureau of the Census.
(From Wegman, M. E.: Pediatr. *68:* 755, 1981.)

Late Neonatal Death. This refers to the death of a liveborn infant after 7 but before 28 completed days of life.

In-hospital Death. While this term is not included in the WHO system, we have found that it is useful in recent years to record as "in-hospital" neonatal mortality any death that occurs within a hospital period that is continuous from birth. Therefore, infants who die at 3 to 6 months or later and who have been hospitalized continuously from birth because of complications and chronic disease following respiratory distress syndrome, congenital anomalies, and so forth are included in this category.

NEONATAL MORTALITY AND MORBIDITY

Why do newborns die in the 1980s? "In-hospital mortality," which refers to those deaths that occur before discharge, for our hospitals in 1981 is shown in Table I–1. Leading causes of death and relative contributions of various diseases are not different for outborn and inborn infants, and they have been pooled for this analysis. Extreme prematurity, anomalies, and asphyxia lead the list.

Analysis of diseases associated with neonatal death is a rough indicator of admission diagnoses, diseases prevalent in intensive care units, and neonatal disease incidence (Table I–2). The incidence of these diseases obviously depends on stringency of diagnostic criteria.

THE NATIONAL SCENE

The outlook for a successful outcome of pregnancy has improved dramatically over the past five decades.

Table I–6. Survival: Black vs. White (Both Sexes)

Weight (gm)	Black Survival	White Survival	Significance
<1000	43.7% (16)	32.1% (81)	None
1001–1500	80.4% (56)	80.2% (192)	None
1501–2000	95.5% (88)	91.0% (256)	None
2001–2500	94.9% (59)	92.5 (214)	None
Over 2500	88.5% (78)	91.4% (453)	None
Total	87.9% (297)	85.7% (1196)	None

(Data from 1974 to 1981, University of Kentucky. Courtesy of Dr. Douglas Cunningham.)

A rough chronology of major advances is listed in Table I–3. The impact of new knowledge and its application have resulted in an impressive reduction in deaths in the first year of life on the national scene, with a 50 per cent reduction in mortality rates from 1960 (26.0 per 1000 live births) to 1980 (12.5 per 1000 live births) (Figs. I–1 and I–2 and Table I–4).

Those data can be translated into approximate number of lives saved: In the United States in 1968, 56,456 infant deaths were recorded (1.6 per cent of births); in 1978, the number was 31,618 (0.9 per cent of births). The prematurity rate fell from 8.2 per cent of infants with a birth weight under 2.5 kg in 1968 to 7.1 per cent in 1978 (Table I–5). The greatest number of deaths occurred among those of the lowest socioeconomic status, especially nonwhite infants, whose mortality remains nearly double that of white infants. These disturbing differences relate mostly to the greater proportion of premature infants among the nonwhite group. The data from Kentucky in Table I–6 illustrate that lack of differential mortality when comparisons are made on a weight-specific basis.

As shown in Table I–1, the biggest problems in neonatology as indicated by mortality are immaturity, frequently linked with respiratory distress syndrome (RDS) and intracranial hemorrhage, asphyxia, anomalies, and infections. Perelman and coworkers note that the incidence of neonatal deaths from asphyxia and respiratory distress syndrome has de-

Table I–5. Annual U.S. Statistics

Year	Total Births	Total Neonatal Deaths	Deaths (Per Cent)	Live Births Low Birth Weight <2.5 kg	<2.5 kg (Per Cent)
1968	3.50 million	56,456	1.6	286,500	8.2
1978	3.33 million	31,618	.9	236,300	7.1
1981	3.64 million	26,828	.7	247,900	6.8

clined threefold in the last decade. Of note is their finding that deaths from RDS in 1978 approximated 1 in 4000 livebirths in the state of Wisconsin, compared with 1 in 1000 for the national average. Presumably, wide dissemination of the best current practices could be remarkably effective in further lowering neonatal mortality in this country.

Continued efforts on many fronts are required to reduce both mortality and morbidity further. We lack sufficient knowledge to prevent all stillbirths and neonatal deaths; we have clearly not met the challenge of applying all that we know to all pregnancies. We hope the subsequent pages of this text will make a contribution toward the goal of a successful outcome of human pregnancy.

References

Cloherty, J. P., and Stark, A. R. (Eds.): Manual of Neonatal Care. Boston, Little, Brown and Co., 1980.

Committee on Perinatal Health: Toward Improving the Outcome of Pregnancy. National Foundation March of Dimes, 1275 Mamaroneck Ave., White Plains, N. Y., 10605, 1977.

Fost, N.: Ethical issues in the treatment of critically ill newborns. Pediatr. Ann. 10:16, 1981.

Kuhse, H.: Debate: extraordinary means and the sanctity of life. J. Med. Ethics 7:74, 1981.

Modanlou, H., Dorchester, W., Freeman, R., and Rommal, C.: Perinatal transport to a regional perinatal center in a metropolitan area: maternal vs. neonatal transport. Am. J. Obstet. Gynecol. 138:1157, 1980.

Perelman, R., and Farrell, P.: Analysis of causes of neonatal death in the U.S. with specific emphasis on fetal hyaline membrane disease. Pediatrics 70:570, 1982.

Philip, A., Little, G., Polivy, D., and Lucey, J.: Neonatal mortality risk for the eighties: Importance of birthweight/gestational age groups. Pediatrics 68:122, 1981.

Sinclair, J., Torrance, G., Boyle, M., Horwoods, S., Saigal, S., and Sackett, D.: Evaluation of neonatal intensive care programs. N. Engl. J. Med. 305:489, 1981.

Wegman, M.E.: Annual summary of vital statistics—1981. Pediatrics 70:835, 1982.

PART 1 PERINATOLOGY

Maternal Conditions and Exogenous Influences that Affect the Fetus/Newborn

Introduction

A number of maternal conditions and exogenous influences affect fertility, fertilization, embryogenesis, and fetal development. Some toxic influences exert adverse effects throughout development, leading to an array of reproductive wastage; for example, radiation can lead to infertility, abortion, chromosomal damage, teratogenic effects, and organ maldevelopment of the fetus. Other agents, such as thalidomide, are highly specific in dose and timing for teratogenic effect. In this chapter, we review briefly and selectively the wide range of influences that may affect in utero development (Tables 1–1 and 1–2).

For birth defects involving morphogenesis (as opposed to those that are genetic and biochemical defects without visible birth defects, e.g., cystic fibrosis, phenylketonuria), the terminology has been chosen with the recommendations of an international working group in mind (Spranger et al., 1982). The members of this group classify disorders of morphogenesis into four categories.

Malformations are morphologic defects of all or part of one or more organs resulting from the time of embryogenesis. Malformations represent developmental field defects in which altered tissue-tissue interaction occurs in reaction to disrupted chemical or physical influences. Therefore, malformations may include single gene disorders or chromosomal abnormalities or may result from exogenous adverse influences.

Disruptions are defects resulting from an extrinsic "breakdown or interference with an originally normal developmental process." An example is thalidomide syndrome.

Deformations are abnormalities caused by adverse mechanical forces. Examples are amniotic band syndrome and some forms of clubfoot.

Dysplasias are the "process and consequences of dyshistiogenesis." Examples are hemangiomata and osteogenesis imperfecta. These too can be genetic or acquired or both, as in the case of genetic predisposition to the adverse influence of noxious agents (Spranger et al., 1982).

Epidemiology of Malformations

Despite progress in prenatal diagnosis and postnatal management, the proportion of infants being delivered with significant congenital malformations has been largely unchanged in the past several decades and represents about 2 to 3 per cent of all live-births. Prenatal prediction and possible abortion before 20 weeks gestation, genetic counseling, and avoidance of known teratogens represent the only clinical approaches to the problem at the current time. In a 1981 report, Warkany summarizes past progress and urges that indirect approaches be added to mechanistic studies in order to reduce the frequency of birth defects. As he points out, the major protection against the birth of malformed infants is their usual spontaneous abortion during the first 2 trimesters. What recognition signals allow the process of spontaneous abortion to proceed are not understood, but ways of inducing spontaneous abortion of

Table 1–1. Etiology of Serious Malformations in 18,555 Newborns at Boston Hospital for Women, 1972–1974

		Total Malformations	Per Cent of Total	Per Cent of Total Newborns
I.	Multifactorial inheritance	127	40	0.7
II.	Single mutant gene with Mendelian inheritance	67	21	0.4
III.	Chromosomal abnormalities*	28	9	0.2
IV.	Other (includes possible teratogens and unknowns)	95	30	0.5
		317	100	1.8

* Only infants with malformations were karyotyped. (Courtesy of Dr. Lewis B. Holmes.)

Table 1–2. Incidence and Sex Ratio of the
Commoner Malformations in England and Wales

	Incidence per 1000 Live Births	Sex Ratio Male/Female
Anencephaly	2	0.4
Spina bifida	2.5	0.8
Down's syndrome	2	1.0
Pyloric stenosis	3	5.0
Cleft lip	1	1.8
Talipes equinovarus	1	2.0
Congenital hip dislocation	1	0.15
Congenital heart malformations	4	1.0

(From Carter C. O.: Proc. Roy. Soc. Med. *61*: 991, 1968.)

a malformed embryo is an indirect solution worthy of study.

Congenital anomalies, defects, and malformations are responsible for approximately one tenth of the deaths in the first month of life. The deaths represent only a small fraction of the total problem that they cause. McIntosh and coworkers found that 3.6 per cent of consecutive newborns in a large series manifested at least one *major* congenital anomaly, defined by Marden and associates as one that has an adverse effect upon either function or social acceptability. When these babies were followed closely, the percentage of anomalies that must have been present at birth rose to 7.5 per cent by the age of 5 years. Marden and his collaborators found one or more *minor* anomalies in 14.7 per cent of more than 5000 consecutive liveborns. In this volume, congenital malformations will be treated as the highly important segments of the disorders of each organ system, and they will therefore be discussed throughout the book. Multiple congenital defects and disorders not readily classifiable in any one system have been assigned a section of their own (see Chapter 97 and Table 5–1).

Congenital malformations and defects are caused by a variety of diverse pathogenetic agents. These fall into the following main categories:

Gross Chromosomal Aberrations. The pathogenesis of gross chromosomal aberrations and the descriptions of the syndromes that are clearly associated with them are discussed in detail in Chapter 96.

Defective Genes. The malformations and malfunctions in this group are by definition familial and hereditary. Some are transmitted as dominants, some as recessives; some may be sex-linked. Examples include classic achondroplasia, often transmitted as a dominant, and hemophilia A, a sex-linked defect.

The occurrence of major genetic disease in a newborn without a family history usually implies an autosomal recessive disorder or a mutational event. That the latter is not an unusual occurrence is exemplified by the fact that approximately one third of all sex-linked hereditary disorders occur as a consequence of mutation. Significant mutation rates also occur in the dominant genetic disorders; for example, approximately 50 per cent of cases of infant tuberosclerosis, retinoblastoma, and many other dominant disorders are due to sporadic mutations.

Congenital malformations caused by sex-linked inheritance may be particularly important, since prenatal sex determination could assist in their subsequent prevention. Hydrocephalus in some forms, imperforate anus, microphthalmia, anhidrotic ectodermal dysplasia, and certain biochemical disorders represent only a few of the more than 30 syndromes noted in this category.

Multifactorial (polygenic) inheritance reflects the combined effects of several minor gene abnormalities and environmental factors. Neural tube defects (anencephaly, spina bifida) are perhaps the commonest examples in this group, which also includes pyloric stenosis, dislocation of the hips, and cleft lip and palate. Genetic factors (increased frequency in people of Irish extraction) in the neural tube defects combine with recognizable environmental influences that include low socioeconomic classes, more frequent winter and fall births, and geographic location.

Deformations

Growth in utero can be impeded generally (growth retardation) or specifically (club foot) by a variety of uterine conditions. Early amnion rupture is now known to result in band-induced amputation as well as craniofacial defects (Torpin, 1965). Miller and coworkers have enlarged the spectrum of malformations due to amnion rupture to include compression-related limb or body wall deletions. They reported 27 such instances from their own experience and the published literature. They emphasized the sporadic nature of the event, which led to a wide variety of deficiencies. Evidence of amniotic bands was present in 41 per cent of the cases. Postural defects and growth retardation were common. Half the infants were stillborn. Pulmonary hypoplasia was common in the liveborn group.

Multiple fetuses may crowd and malform one another. Fibromata, in utero birth control devices, or uterine anomalies have all been associated with deformations. Reassurance can generally be given to parents that multiple internal anomalies are not present and that recurrence risk is low (Smith, 1982).

Maternal Age

Within limits, maternal age represents a nonspecific influence on fertility, embryogenesis, fetal well-being, time of delivery, and ultimate infant care. The increased number of pregnancies among adolescents in recent years has stimulated much analysis of the salient issues (Fig. 1–1). Since pregnancy among ad-

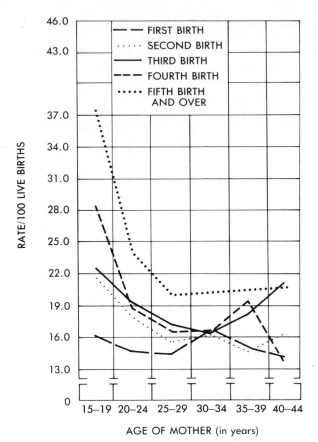

Figure 1–1. Neonatal mortality rates of infants weighing 2500 gm or less, by age of mother for each total-birth order group, United States, early in 1950. (From U. S. National Office of Vital Statistics: Weight at birth and survival of newborn, by age of mother and total-birth order: United States, early 1950. Vital Statistics—Special Reports 47:2, 1958.)

olescents occurs more commonly among mothers of lower socioeconomic status and more often among nonwhites than whites, the problem of assigning relative importance to these and other factors that coexist with young maternal age has been a challenge.

Several reasons are often cited for the rise in teenage pregnancies, principally the growing number of teenagers and the increase in sexual activity. In the United States, over 600,000 teenage women become pregnant each year; of these, 30,000 are 15 years or younger. Adolescent mothers contribute 19 per cent of the births but have 26 per cent of the low birth weight infants. These mothers have increased risks for death in childbirth, toxemia, anemia, and neurologic disorders in their offspring. On the average, infants born to adolescent mothers may be less well nurtured, have greater risk of child abuse, and receive less health supervision as children. Similarly, adolescent mothers who have infants are more prone to marital dissolution and emotional disturbances.

Obviously, causes and effects are difficult to unravel, but there is little doubt that for a young woman between 15 and 19 years, pregnancy may contribute to what Smith in 1980 described as "a dismal future of unemployment, poverty, dropping out of school, family breakdowns, emotional stress, dependency on public health agencies, and health problems for mother and child."

Pregnancy after maternal age 40 years is associated with another set of hazards for the baby. For pregnant women over 40 years, a sharp increase in deaths around the time of birth (perinatal mortality) occurs with each subsequent year of age. After age 40 years, the hazards are greater if it is the woman's first pregnancy rather than a subsequent pregnancy. One of the risks of pregnancy after age 40 years is the approximately 2.6 per cent incidence of Down's syndrome in the baby, compared with an overall incidence of 0.15 per cent. Another problem relates to diminished elasticity of the pelvic structures and difficulties with delivery. Diagnostic amniocentesis for detection of chromosomal abnormalities such as Down's syndrome can alert the mother to that possibility and provide her with the option of abortion. Skillful obstetric management can reduce these hazards around the time of delivery.

Prenatal Care

Numerous studies have documented the higher incidence of prematurity and growth retardation in infants of mothers from a lower socioeconomic group and among the findings is a specific association with lack of prenatal care. In Miller's study of pregnant Kansas women starting in March, 1973, the incidence of prematurity among 120 women with less than three prenatal visits was 17.5 per cent. Among those with more than three prenatal visits, the incidence was 4.4 per cent. If the mother had made 9 to 12 visits, no infants were born prematurely. Although the number of undergrown for gestational age infants was small, an inverse relation to prenatal visits was also noted.

Many confounding factors complicate the interpretation of these and similar findings. Indeed, we do not know what aspects of prenatal care are significant determinants of outcome. It seems reasonable to give much credit to health education. The mothers who want to do what is best for their babies are probably the ones who elect prenatal care. Early detection of risk factors, hypertension, and poor or excessive weight gain surely dictate appropriate interventions, which on the whole improve the outcome of pregnancy.

Maternal Nutrition

In developed countries, the knowledge about adequate diet is so common (or the fetus so well protected) that nutritional supplements during pregnancy have generally not altered fetal growth. The major impact of maternal nutrition may occur during the period of ovulation or implantation, with failure of implantation or subsequent pregnancy wastage the result in suboptimally nourished mothers. In 1947, Smith reported that 50 per cent of Dutch women became amenorrheic and that half the remainder had irregular menses throughout a period of severe food deprivation during World War II. However, in those who carried the pregnancy to term, birth weight averaged only a few hundred grams less than normal. Neither short-term nor long-term disability in these infants has been evident in follow-up studies. In general, increasing caloric intake about 10 to 15 per cent above prepregnancy norms for maternal age and size appears appropriate and results in maternal weight gains of 20 to 30 pounds by term. Sodium restriction and strict monitoring of weight gain during pregnancy for normal mothers are obstetric trends that have waned.

Current attention is directed at the need for micronutrients. Usual obstetric care includes supplementation with vitamins (A, C, D, B_6, B_{12}, folate), calcium, and iron. For a woman who follows a well-balanced diet, convincing evidence of benefits from this supplementation is lacking, and possible harm may result from overzealous use of these agents. Vitamin A is characteristically teratogenic in animals, but has no known teratogenic effects in humans. Excess maternal vitamin D may cause anomalies and hypercalcemia in infants. Iron for supplementation during pregnancy can be poisonous to toddlers in the household who accidentally ingest it.

There is little knowledge concerning food faddism and its effects on outcome of pregnancy, but a vegetarian diet lacking sufficient iron has led to severe maternal anemia in some cases (Gluck, 1981; Moghissi, 1981; Stevenson, 1973; Kaminetzky and Baker, 1981).

Adverse Effects of Exogenous Agents on the Fetus

The probability that a woman's exposure to a drug will produce harm in her fetus depends on the dose, route of administration, stage of gestation, and genotype of mother and embryo. Drugs at nonteratogenic dosage levels can become highly teratogenic in the presence of other drugs or environmental variables such as specific nutritional deficiency, hypoxia, or food and water restriction. Teratogens have their own "critical period," the gestational age at which they are most teratogenic; these periods vary for different teratogens and may precede, by varying lengths of time, the developmental event that they interrupt (Fig. 1–2).

Known specific teratogens in humans are listed in Table 1–3. *Diphenylhydantoin* (phenytoin) and trimethadione are now known to produce defects in offspring, such as cleft lip and palate, microcephaly, and congenital heart disease. Hypoplasia of the nails

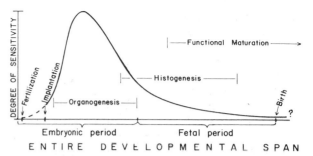

Figure 1–2. Curve approximating the susceptibility to teratogenesis from fertilization throughout intrauterine development. The highest sensitivity, at least to structural deviation, occurs during the period of organogenesis, which in the human is from approximately day 18 through day 60 (ovulation age). (From Wilson, J. G.: Environment and Birth Defects, New York, Academic Press, 1973.)

and digits may occur in one fifth of exposed infants, with one third suffering intellectual impairment (Hansen et al., 1976). The frequency and severity of maternal seizures may dictate continued use of these agents in some pregnancies, even though the "fetal hydantoin syndrome" is a possibility.

Table 1–3. Known Teratogenic Agents in Humans

Radiation
  Therapeutic
  Atomic weapons
  Radioiodine
Infections
  Rubella virus
  Cytomegalovirus
  Herpes virus hominis? I and II
  Toxoplasmosis
  Syphilis
  ?Varicella virus
  Venezuelan equine encephalitis virus
Maternal metabolic imbalance
  Endemic cretinism
  ?Diabetes
  Phenylketonuria
  Virilizing tumors
  Alcoholism
Drugs and environmental chemicals
  Androgenic hormones (testosterone, progestins)
  Aminopterin and methylaminopterin
  Cyclophosphamide
  Busulfan
  Thalidomide
  Mercury
  Chlorobiphenyls
  Diethylstilbestrol
  Diphenylhydantoin and trimethadione
  Coumarin

(From Shepard, T., and Fantel, A.: Teratology of therapeutic agents. *In* Iffy, S., and Kaminetzky, H. [Eds.]: Principles and Practice of Obstetrics and Perinatology. New York, J. Wiley & Sons, 1981.)

The teratogenic effects of *antimetabolites* and folic acid antagonists have been well recognized. One infant reported 14 years ago by the late author, Alexander Schaffer, was born after the failed abortifacient use of methotrexate. Other infants similarly exposed had comparable phenotypic abnormalities. This child, when last seen, had incompletely ossified skull defects, an I.Q. within the normal range, and an extremely small stature. Other anticancer, antimetabolic agents have been used throughout pregnancies in mothers with malignancies or renal transplants with surprisingly good outcomes in some (Barber, 1981). As noted in an excellent recent review by Shepard and Fantel, long-term assessment of cerebral function may reveal increasing morbidity in offspring exposed to these drugs.

Coumarin is known to be associated with nasal hypoplasia, growth retardation, and stippled epiphyses (Conradi syndrome) (Shaul and Hall, 1977). Heparin, probably because of its polarity when given to the mother, does not reach the fetus, and its use is not associated with teratologic effects.

DIETHYLSTILBESTROL (DES)

Between 1 and 10 per cent of pregnant women were treated with DES between 1951 and 1953. Despite little evidence of efficacy in reducing fetal wastage, its practice continued until 1971, when the Food and Drug Administration banned its use following a report documenting the association of adenocarcinoma of the lower genital tract in offspring of treated women (Herbst, 1971). The risk of adenocarcinoma is now estimated to be about 1/1000 in exposed women, but nonmalignant changes of the uterus, cervix, or vagina occur in about 25 per cent of exposed offspring (Herbst, 1981), and genitourinary abnormalities are detectable in male offspring. Several studies have shown increased fetal death, miscarriages, and premature birth in adult women who had fetal exposure to DES, thus indicating risk into the third generation from a woman first exposed to DES (Herbst, 1980).

OTHER EXOGENOUS PROGESTINS AND ESTROGENS

Wilson and Brent reviewed the question of teratogenicity of exogenous progestins and estrogens not related to DES. Exposure to the fetus may occur when a woman using birth control pills finds she is pregnant or when synthetic progestational agents have been used in cases of threatened premature delivery in the third trimester. Other uses of sex steroids during pregnancy (i.e., hormonal pregnancy tests and progestins in the first trimester) are no longer recommended. No non–sex organ teratogenicity is likely to occur in the first trimester after exposure to these sorts of drugs. A major reason may be that sex hormone receptors appear to develop in tissues other than sex organs after the first trimester, if at all. This reasoning argues against the conclusions of both Nara and Rothman and coworkers, who state that birth control pills taken during pregnancy may be associated with increased risk of fetal anomalies. Androgens, or progestins with androgenic activity, may masculinize the fetus, but masculinization does not progress after birth.

MERCURY AND LEAD

Also listed as teratogenic agents in Table 1–3 are heavy metals. Organic mercury poisoning during pregnancy (Minimata disease) disturbs brain development (Kalter and Warkany, 1983). Whether prenatal lead exposure is associated with fetal anomalies in humans is not known. Both increased frequency of stillbirth and congenital malformations were noted in infants of mothers with high lead exposure toward the latter part of the nineteenth century. More recently, attention has focused on neurologic damage in asymptomatic children who have had an increased exposure to lead. Studies of lead-associated hyperactivity in mice and the demonstration of slow learning in sheep with borderline blood-lead levels raise worrisome questions in these suggestive animal models of human disease. Since it is known that lead affects rapidly growing tissues, the observation that increased cord blood lead in infants of mothers in high lead exposure areas (e.g., near expressways) cannot be ignored (Scanlon, 1972).

Table 1–3 also presents relatively nonspecific insults during embryogenesis. Effect of maternal smoking on the fetus is discussed in Chapter 4.

RADIATION

Before organogenesis, radiation in doses as low as 5 rads may cause mortality and resorption. During organogenesis, exposures of 10 to 300 rads may be associated with fetal death, skeletal defects, growth retardation, anencephaly, and microcephaly. In the fetal period, exposure of the mother to radiation has been associated with reports of postnatal increased risk of neoplasia, behavioral effects due to radiosensitivity of developing neurons, and cytogenic alterations. Although this field of study is vast, conclusions concerning effects on human beings are few. One clear conclusion seems to be that as studies become more discriminant, lower and lower doses of radiation are found to have adverse effects on developing organisms (Hoffman, 1981).

The atomic bombs exploded in Japan afforded an unwelcome opportunity to study the wholesale effects of overexposure to radiant energy. Plummer found that 11 pregnant women had been within 1200 meters of the hypocenter at the moment of

Table 1–5. Modified White Classification of Diabetes and Pregnancy

Class A—High fetal survival, no insulin, minimal dietary regulation.
   1. Gestational diabetes—abnormal glucose tolerance test during pregnancy that reverts to normal within a few weeks after delivery.
   2. Prediabetes—normal glucose tolerance test, but family history of diabetes, previous large infants, or unexplained stillbirths.
Class B—Onset of diabetes in adult life after age 20 years, duration less than 10 years, no vascular disease.
Class C—Diabetes of long duration (10–19 years) with onset during adolescence (over 10 years) with minimal vascular disease.
Class D—Diabetes of 20 years or more duration, onset before age 10 years, evidence of vascular disease (i.e., retinitis, albuminuria, hypertension).
Class E—Patients with D plus calcification of pelvic arteries.
Class F—Patients with D plus nephropathy.
Class G—Many pregnancy failures.
Class H—Cardiopathy.
Class R—Proliferating retinopathy.
Class T—Renal transplant.

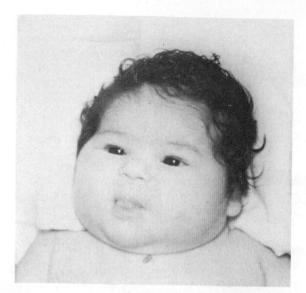

Figure 1–4. Photograph showing the puffy rounded contour suggesting the "cushingoid syndrome," characteristic of some infants of diabetic mothers.

tests are carried out if the nonstress test is nonreactive (see p. 39 for description). If fetal jeopardy is suspected on the basis of these procedures, then amniotic fluid testing for phospholipids to assess fetal lung maturity is performed and interpreted according to norms for diabetics rather than a normal population. Delivery should be carried out as close to term as possible, with maternal euglycemia and oxygenation maintained throughout labor and delivery. With this approach, no fetal deaths and one neonatal death (from congenital anomalies) occurred in 140 consecutive diabetic pregnancies in one recent series, compared with a perinatal mortality rate of 18 per cent in a diabetic population in 1960 (Jorge et al., 1981).

Until the mid 1970s, it was thought that risk of congenital anomalies and fetal death was so great in diabetics with nephropathy that pregnancy should be avoided. More recently, Kitzmiller and others have studied pregnancy outcome in 35 class F diabetic women (proteinuria >400 mg/24 hrs). Rigorous control of both hypertension and blood sugar was maintained throughout pregnancy; timing and route of delivery were individualized. Fetal and neonatal results for this group compared with outcome for a group of less severely affected diabetic women are shown in Table 1–4.

Congenital Anomalies in Offspring of Diabetic Mothers

In a Boston study of 116 diabetic women, those with elevated hemoglobin A_{1C} (indicating poor diabetic control) measured in the first trimester had more infants with anomalies than did those with euglycemic control diabetes (Miller et al., 1981). In over 200 German women, rigorous diabetic control was established before and throughout pregnancy. No offspring were born with congenital anomalies (risk

lower than for a normal population), suggesting that lack of diabetic control in the first trimester is associated with increased risk of congenital anomalies.

Various types of anomalies may be overrepresented in infants of diabetic mothers. These include caudal regression syndrome and vertebral dysplasia, anencephaly and meningocele, congenital heart disease, and microcolon. These studies of women with diabetes during pregnancy indicate that modern obstetric and pediatric management can largely obviate the risk of malformations.

OTHER MATERNAL DISEASES THAT MAY AFFECT THE FETUS

Noninfectious non–pregnancy-related diseases may have transient (myasthenia gravis) or permanent (phenylketonuria) effects on the infant (Table 1–6). These conditions are discussed throughout this volume under the appropriate chapter heading (e.g., for effects of maternal Graves' disease, see Chapter 55). Two excellent reviews of this subject were published by Stevenson in 1973 and by Schulman and Simpson in 1981.

Premature Rupture of the Membranes (Amniorrhexis)

The common management problem to be resolved when amniotic membranes rupture before the onset of labor is to determine whether risk of infection to

mother and fetus is greater than risk of premature birth to the fetus and risk of immediate delivery for the mother. Near term, the frequency of amniorrhexis is 10 per cent. Mechanisms of rupture may relate to infection, cervical dilatation, trauma, or increased intrauterine mass (e.g., polyhydramnios, multiple fetuses). For mothers and fetuses at or near term, current obstetric recommendation is to deliver within 24 to 48 hours in order to obviate risk of maternal and fetal infection.

Perinatal mortality and risk of endometritis double or triple if delivery is delayed more than 48 hours after membrane rupture in term infants. Routine prophylactic antibiotics in this group have not been shown to benefit the fetus, although some studies have suggested that they decrease infections in mothers (Huff, 1979).

If an infant is born near term to a mother with prolonged rupture of the membranes or if there have been no signs of infection in mother or infant, we usually take routine surface cultures and observe the infant in the well-baby nursery without isolation. If the infant remains well, antibiotics are not used in term infants, even if surface cultures are positive for a single organism. Signs of endometritis in the mother or signs of any distress in the infant would prompt us to obtain cultures of cerebrospinal fluid, urine, and blood in addition to surface cultures and blood counts and to administer antibiotics for at least 3 days, pending results of these further studies.

Rupture of membranes presents a more difficult management problem in the preterm mother. Formerly, obstetric management would usually result in delivery of the preterm infant within 48 hours of rupture of membranes. Spontaneous labor is often a concomitant feature of premature rupture of membranes; labor is evident within 72 hours in 95 per cent of women at term and in 70 per cent of women prior to term after rupture of membranes. Currently, obstetric opinion seems to favor cautious management of the mother with preterm premature rupture of the membranes, if risk of delivery of an immature fetus is high. Such a mother may be admitted to a perinatal high risk unit, placed on bed rest, and observed closely for signs of chorioamnionitis. Tocolytic agents and glucocorticoids may be used if amniotic fluid reveals no evidence of infection and if phospholipids are indicative of high risk of respiratory distress syndrome for the infant (Mead and Clapp, 1977). To deliver a 30-week infant by cesarean section because the mother has had rupture of the membranes for 48 hours seems to us to be harmful if there have been no signs of infection. This mother may, with bed rest (and possibly tocolytics and steroids), deliver a more mature fetus vaginally in days to weeks.

Cesarean Section

Declining perinatal mortality rates have been matched by increasing cesarean section rates in the past decade. At Brigham and Women's Hospital, the primary section rate has doubled from less than 10 per cent to more than 20 per cent in the past two decades. Suggested reasons for this trend include referral of high-risk mothers, increased diagnoses of fetal asphyxia with electronic fetal heart rate monitoring, a decline in the use of midforceps and in vaginal breech deliveries, and aggressive management of uterine inertia. The risks of cesarean section to the mother in terms of mortality should be no greater than those associated with vaginal delivery, although maternal disability and cost are clearly high (Gibbs, 1978; Frigoletto et al., 1980).

In a summary of a recent workshop sponsored by the National Institutes of Health, the recommenda-

Table 1–6. Maternal Conditions Related to Perinatal Death and Birth Weight

Condition	White with Condition			Black with Condition		
	Per cent	Perinatal Death Rate*	Birth Weight Rate Below 2501 gm	Per cent	Perinatal Death Rate*	Birth Weight Rate Below 2501 gm
Organic heart disease	1.44	55.2	176.5	1.76	71.4	189.0
Pneumonia during pregnancy	.57	27.8	103.8	.44	56.8	139.5
Bronchial asthma	.93	28.4	105.3	1.42	70.4	159.3
Diabetes	.66	144.0	95.7	.65	139.5	149.1
Convulsions, not eclamptic	.35	30.3	46.9	.21	119.1	194.4
Psychosis or neurosis	4.71	36.0	89.7	1.69	29.6	186.8
Hyperemesis gravidarum	1.64	35.7	66.7	.71	35.5	117.7
Incompetent cervix	.34	323.1	614.0	.36	478.9	679.3
Hydramnios	1.54	137.9	86.5	1.26	99.2	87.9
Placenta previa	.77	176.1	328.2	.56	190.9	529.4
Abruptio placentae	2.39	195.5	263.0	1.90	360.7	476.9
Prolapse of cord	1.10	168.3	118.6	.78	298.0	235.3
All cases	—	35.1	71.4	—	41.9	134.2

* Perinatal deaths include stillbirths and neonatal deaths.
(From Niswander, K., and Gordon, M. [Eds]: The Women and Their Pregnancies. Philadelphia, W. B. Saunders Co., 1972.)

Table 1–7. Liveborn Infants: (500–1000 gm)
University College Hospital, London, 1971 to 1977.

Method of delivery	28-day Survival (%)	(n)*
Vertex, spontaneous	29	(58)
Vertex, forceps	36	(25)
Cesarean section with labor	50	(10)
Cesarean section, elective	76	(17)

* n = total number of infants in each group.
(Data from Fairweather, D.: J. Reprod. Med. 26:387, 1981.)

tion was made for a trial of labor for mothers who had had previous low transverse cesarean sections, since the incision is less likely to result in uterine rupture than vertical uterine incision. By this means, the 25 per cent of cesarean sections that are done solely because the mother had a previous section may be reduced (Kurzel and Cetrulo, 1981). A second approach that may reduce the section rate is external rotation of the fetus in breech position after uterine relaxation (see further on).

Among the possible benefits of cesarean section to the fetus/newborn are (1) avoidance or minimization of asphyxia in cases of abruptio placentae, cord compression, placenta previa, or a prolonged second stage; (2) early delivery in the presence of evidence of a decrease in fetal well-being in conditions such as toxemia, erythroblastosis, or maternal diabetes; and (3) avoidance of birth trauma (e.g., for infants with macrosomia or for those in the breech position).

The possibility that delivery of a very low birth weight infant may represent a new indication for cesarean section has been raised by Stewart and coworkers. They found that for very low birth weight infants (≤1000 gm), survival was 64 per cent after section and 27 per cent after vaginal delivery. More recent data compiled by Fairweather also suggest that very low birth weight infants (excluding those born in breech position) have increased survival at birth if born by cesarean section.

Presumably, the beneficial effect of cesarean section in this group is due to the fact that asphyxia associated with vaginal delivery is avoided. We are not prepared to advocate section for such small in-

fants without careful consideration of all other relevant information. It is important to note, however, that section does not seem to jeopardize these infants.

Hazards to the fetus/newborn from cesarean section have been discussed for years. In earlier editions of this book, Schaffer noted that section was associated with doubling of mortality for term infants and a fivefold increase for premature infants in studies that dated from the 1940s (Schaffer and Avery, 1977). No doubt, much of this high mortality was due to the indications for cesarean section rather than to the procedure itself.

Tachypnea and increased risk of transient tachypnea presumably due to delayed absorption of fetal lung fluid are sometimes associated with cesarean birth. Bland and coworkers, in a 1979 study of rabbits born by section, found higher plasma protein concentrations and lower extravascular lung water in cases in which labor had preceded delivery. These results indicate that processes associated with labor may partially regulate rates of absorption of lung water in the first hours of life. Comparing human newborn infants delivered by cesarean section with and without preceding labor, Sola and Gregory found a 13 per cent higher plasma colloid oncotic pressure in those born by section after labor, suggesting that this latter group may be less susceptible to delayed absorption of lung fluid when other factors are equal.

Debate continues as to whether cesarean section increases risk of respiratory distress in preterm infants. Butler and coworkers found that the risk of respiratory distress syndrome was not increased above that for vaginally delivered infants in cases in which labor had preceded the operation; Hardy and colleagues found no relationship between labor and respiratory distress syndrome. Again, substances associated with labor (glucocorticoids, catecholamines, thyroid hormone) may prepare the lung prenatally for postnatal function.

The questions relating to cesarean section and neonatal respiratory problems therefore are concerned with *when* the cesarean occurs during ges-

Table 1 8. Cesarean Section (vs. Vaginal Delivery) and its Relationship to Neonatal Respiratory Problems

1. *If* done to prevent asphyxia,
    then there will be decreased risk of respiratory distress syndrome, congestive heart failure, and meconium aspiration pneumonia.
2. *If* done for the infants < 1000 gm birth weight,
    then neonatal mortality and asphyxia may be less.
3. *If* done for the infant in the 1500 to 2000 gm birth weight group,
    then respiratory distress syndrome may be increased for two reasons:
        (a) iatrogenic respiratory distress syndrome may occur (mistaken gestation);
        (b) events associated with labor may mature lungs.
4. *If* done at term,
    then increased transient tachypnea due to delayed resorption of fetal alveolar fluid may occur.
5. *If* done with the newborn elevated or with rapid cord clamping or both,
    then hypotension may occur.
6. *If* done without regard to maternal anesthesia, blood pressure, uterine blood flow, and oxygenation,
    then increased risk of neonatal asphyxia may occur.

Table 1–9. Complications Associated with Vaginal Breech Delivery

Prolapsed cord
Prolonged second stage of labor
Fetal/neonatal asphyxia
Aspiration syndromes
Bruising with secondary jaundice
Crush injuries; shock
Other trauma
   Fractured long bones
   Epiphyseal injuries
   Brachial plexus injury
   Hyperextension of neck—cervical fracture and dislocation, spinal cord injury, CNS ischemia from vertebral artery circulation
Ruptured internal organs

tation, *why* it is occurring, and *how* it is performed. Some of these factors are listed in Table 1–8.

Breech Delivery

Breech position of the fetus at the time of delivery occurs in about 8 per cent of women in labor (Dunn, 1976). In about 25 per cent of cases, conditions such as placenta previa, uterine or fetal malformations, prematurity, or twinning may be present. Vaginal delivery of an infant in the breech position is associated with many complications (Tables 1–9 and 1–10). Evaluating all infants born vaginally in a 2-year period, Dunn found that death from central nervous system asphyxia/trauma occurred six times more frequently in the breech group than in the vertex group. When the infant is term and physicians experienced in vaginal delivery of the breech fetus are available, then, in the absence of other factors, neonatal risk appears slightly higher if delivery is vaginal and maternal risk slightly higher if cesarean section is performed (Collea et al., 1978).

The situation for premature delivery of the breech fetus is more clear-cut, with most evidence favoring delivery by section because of the distinctly increased risk associated with vaginal delivery of the preterm

Table 1–10. Comparison of Neonatal Problems: Breech vs. Vertex Vaginal Deliveries

Condition	Breech	Vertex	B/V
Number births	358	4396	.08
Death from central nervous system damage (per cent)	.08	.01	6
Facial nerve palsy (per cent)	.03	.03	1
Erb's palsy (per cent)	.03	.01	3
Fractures (per cent)	.14	.005	28
Testicular trauma (per cent)	.31	0	—

(Data from Dunn, P: Breech delivery: perinatal morbidity and mortality. *In* Rooth, G., and Brattebay, L. [Eds.]: Fifth European Congress of Perinatal Medicine. Stockholm, Almqvist and Wiksell, 1976, p. 57.)

breech fetus. For example, Westgren and Svenningsen found more instances of neonatal mortality, central nervous system hemorrhage, asphyxia, and long-term neurologic disability in a group of 48 breech infants less than 36 weeks gestation born vaginally than in a similar group born by cesarean section.

Amniotic Fluid : Oligohydramnios and Polyhydramnios

The infant at term is surrounded by about 1000 ml of amniotic fluid formed from fetal urine, lung secretions, and transudate from surrounding membranes. Less than 500 ml indicates oligohydramnios, and more than 2000 ml signifies polyhydramnios. Near term, the fetus drinks about 125 ml/kg body weight of amniotic fluid per day (equivalent to postnatal milk intakes). The fluid has a pH of 7.2, which is alkaline with respect to vaginal secretions; therefore, a test for leakage of amniotic fluid is to measure vaginal fluid pH. The changing constituents of amniotic fluid over time, represented by falling osmolarity and protein, rising bilirubin, creatinine, urea, cellular constituents, and phospholipids, all serve as the basis for tests of fetal well-being, gestational age, and lung maturity.

Clinically, oligohydramnios or hydramnios is most commonly present when fetal swallowing or micturition is increased or decreased or in cases of fetal edema (hydrops).

Hydramnios occurs in about 1.5 per cent of livebirths. Many of the conditions listed in Table 1–12 are associated with upper gastrointestinal blockage or central nervous system defects that may impair swallowing. Increased fetal urine output from a glucose-induced osmotic diuresis has been proposed but not proved as a mechanism for hydramnios in some women with diabetes. Postnatal diabetes insipidus, one would reason, should also be associated with hydramnios.

Death of the fetus in utero, tight wrapping of the cord about the neck, anencephaly, and high obstructions of the gastrointestinal tract are major causes of hydramnios (Fig. 1–5). For the pediatrician, it is this last group that lends importance to the phenomenon. Although high intestinal obstructions and anenceph-

Table 1–11. Approximate Constituents of Human Amniotic Fluid Near Term

Volume	1000 ml
pH	7.2
Na	120 meq/l
Ca	3–6 meq/l
Mg	1–4 meq/l
pCO_2	50 torr
Glucose	20 mg/100 ml
K	4 meq/l
Cl	98–140 meq/l
Protein	5 gm/l
Phosphatidyl-choline	3–10 mg/100 ml

From Sandler, M.: Amniotic Fluid and Its Clinical Significance. New York, Marcel Dekker, 1981.

Table 1–12.   Clinical Conditions Associated with Hydramnios

Agnathia (microstomia synotia syndrome)
Aminopterin syndrome
Anencephaly and other central nervous system defects
Arthrogryposis
Beckwith–Wiedemann syndrome
Congenital chylothorax
Conjoined twins
Diaphragmatic hernia
Fetal death
Fetal hydrops
Gastroschisis
Hemangioma
Maternal diabetes
Teratoma (brain, mouth, neck, sacrum)
Trisomies
Tumors (lungs, placenta, ovary)
Umbilical cord compression
Upper gastrointestinal obstruction (e.g., duodenal atresia)
Werdnig–Hoffmann disease

aly are the most common malformations associated with hydramnios, it occurs in nearly one third of the mothers of trisomy infants, even in the absence of intestinal obstruction. In the British Perinatal Study, over one fourth of all deaths of infants with malformations followed a pregnancy complicated by hydramnios. When hydramnios is noted by the obstetrician, the pediatrician must be on the alert for the earliest indications of esophageal or high intestinal obstruction.

In about 1 to 2 per cent of newborns with severe oligohydramnios, pulmonary hypoplasia may be present, despite normal kidneys. Arthrogryposis and deformations (club foot) are reported with prolonged oligohydramnios, indicating that one function of the amniotic fluid is to allow free range of motion and "lebensraum" for the fetus.

Birth Injuries

Abnormal presentations of all sorts are associated with increased risk of asphyxia and trauma at birth.

Shoulder dystocia as well as transverse and face presentations prolong total labor, especially its second stage. To the asphyxial effect of prolongation of labor one may have to add the traumatic results of vigorous manual or instrumental manipulation. Asphyxia with cerebral anoxia or massive aspiration of amniotic sac contents or trauma, either intracranial or peripheral, may follow.

Congenital malformations occur nearly twice as often in breech deliveries. Anencephaly is regularly associated with spontaneous face or brow presentations.

Excessively rapid deliveries appear to be as hazardous as prolonged ones. The most problematic factor in this situation may be quick compression of the skull, caused by its sudden entrance into and passage through the vagina. Having no time in which to mold gently to conform with the contours of the snugly fitting cervix, the head lengthens abruptly in the anteroposterior direction, thereby causing sudden broadening of the bitemporal diameter, which stretches and may tear one or both leaves of the tentorium. Subdural hemorrhage follows, which may be supratentorial, infratentorial, or both. In some instances, the cranial bones override instantaneously and catch bridging veins to the superior longitudinal sinus between them. Other factors, not fully understood, may be operative.

Completion of delivery with low or outlet forceps is an innocuous procedure. The use of midforceps or high forceps, on the other hand, is associated with an increase in neonatal morbidity and mortality. Tightly applied forceps can fracture the skull, although these fractures are rarely depressed. Excessive compression of the skull may lead to intracranial bleeding. Traction on the head applied so as to pull it to one side stretches and can tear the spinal roots of the brachial plexus of the opposite side. In a review of obstetric birth injuries, Rubin found that most were

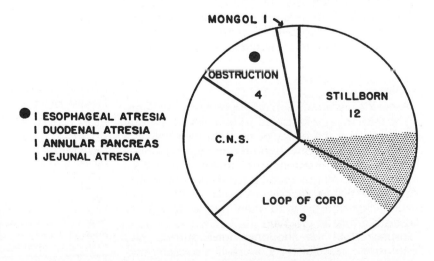

I ESOPHAGEAL ATRESIA
I DUODENAL ATRESIA
I ANNULAR PANCREAS
I JEJUNAL ATRESIA

Figure 1–5. Type of abnormality in 33 abnormal babies born to 76 mothers with hydramnios. (From Lloyd, J. R., and Clatworthy, H. W., Jr.: Pediatrics *21*: 903, 1958.)

Table 1–13. Distribution of Injuries in 15,435 Births

Soft tissue lacerations	
Scalp	1
Eye	3
Face	3
Vagina	1
Buttock	1
Other injuries	
Skull fracture	1
Intracranial	1
Facial nerve	21
Fracture of clavicle	43
Spinal cord	1
Brachial plexus	18
Phrenic nerve	2
Fracture of humerus	7
Amputation of phalanx	1

(Data from Rubin, A.: Hosp. Med. *13*:114, 1977.)

Bell's palsy, fractured clavicle, or brachial plexus injuries.

Placental and Umbilical Cord Problems

The physician caring for the infant in the delivery room may be preoccupied with the newborn by the time the placenta arrives, but inspecting it before leaving may prevent diagnostic dilemmas later. Inspection of the placenta can properly be considered part of the newborn's physical examination. The weight at term (cord and membranes excised 2 cm from insertion) is about 500 gm, with about half the weight representing maternal blood and about 15 per cent composed of fetal blood. The cord may demonstrate one umbilical artery (0.7 per cent), true knots, evidence of vascular rupture, cord compression, tight spirals, hematoma, or edema. In some infants with intrauterine growth retardation, the cord and chorionic plate may be stained dark green and there may be a diminution of Wharton's jelly. The insertion of the cord may be central or marginal or incorporated into the membranes (velamentous), sometimes with vasa praevia (splitting of the vessels in the membranes before insertion into the placenta proper).

Amniotic membranes may show evidence of banding or thickening (associated with infection). In multiple gestations, there may be no membrane between cord insertions (monochorionic, monoamniotic), a thin transparent membrane (diamniotic), or a thick but separable opaque membrane (dichorionic, diamniotic). The first two conditions indicate monozygotic pregnancies, and the third often, but not always, indicates a dizygotic pregnancy.

Inspection of the chorionic (fetal) surface may demonstrate vascular tears, amniotic nodosum, meconium staining, infection, or evidence of cross circulation in multiple births. Culture (with a swab) of the fetal side of the placenta may yield results that are relatively free of contamination with vaginal flora.

The maternal aspect of the placenta may indicate old clot (abruptio placentae) or evidence of premature marginal separation (placenta previa). Infarcts or abscesses may be present and offer evidence of maternal vascular disease or infection.

Histologic evaluation is most useful in cases of repeated premature birth, prolonged rupture of the membranes, or intrauterine growth retardation (Fox, 1978; Philippe and Sauvage, 1981).

TIMING OF UMBILICAL CORD CLAMPING AT BIRTH

Many events at childbirth can determine the relative volumes of blood left in the infant and the placenta after birth. Prenatal asphyxia appears to shift blood from the placenta to the fetus, and, in these cases, because of the frequent need to suction meconium and to resuscitate the infant, no delay in cord clamping would appear useful. In normal infants, if the cord is clamped within 5 seconds of delivery before a contraction compresses the placenta and if the infant is held well above the placenta, then it is reasonable to think that the newborn may be deprived of an adequate supply of blood. If the obstetrician is overly zealous and delays clamping of the cord and "strips" the cord towards the newborn, the placental transfusion predisposes the infant to hyperbilirubinemia, hyperviscosity, and transient tachypnea of the newborn. Despite years of research and debate on the subject, no consensus has yet emerged on optimal timing of cord clamping. Some recent obstetric texts ignore the subject, and this is often obvious in obstetric and pediatric practice in which the timing and nature of separation of the fetus from the placenta are rarely noted (Table 1–14).

Blood volume ranges between 85 and 100 ml/kg body weight in term infants and between 100 and 110 ml/kg in preterm infants. Values are in the lower range with rapid cord clamping and can be 35 per cent higher with delayed clamping. At birth, 75 to 100 ml of fetal blood (20 to 35 ml/kg fetal body

Table 1–14. Factors Determining Neonatal/Placental Blood Volume at Birth

Prenatal drugs (e.g., ergot derivatives)
Maternal disease (preeclampsia)
Fetal asphyxia
Rate of umbilical artery constriction
Gravity effects
Uterine contractions (frequency, amplitude, duration)
Time of cord clamping after delivery
Neonatal cardiac output and venous return
Fetal blood volume (hydrops)
Time of placental separation
Neonatal blood volume greater after first breath
Route of delivery
Cord compression

weight) is available to the newborn from the placenta. Compare this with the size of the "usual" blood transfusion for prematures in the days following birth (10 ml/kg).

Lacking better data, we would recommend performing rapid (0 to 15 seconds) cord clamping of the asphyxiated term infant and allowing 30 to 45 seconds before clamping the cord of the preterm or non-asphyxiated term infant while holding the infant at the level of the placenta. Nasopharyngeal suctioning with a catheter can be performed during this useful period. The significantly preterm (often asphyxiated) newborn poses a difficult problem, but our guess would be that 30 to 45 seconds delay in cord clamping is useful in cases in which there will be multiple iatrogenic demands on the infant's blood volume during the next 12 hours (Sisson, 1978).

Anesthesia During Childbirth

The aims of physicians and others who assist with childbirth should be to make the process as pleasant and safe as possible for the mother and fetus/newborn. The aims of obstetric anesthesia are to minimize both childbirth pain and the amount of anesthetic administered. Risks of asphyxia for the fetus/newborn can occur with either too little or too much anesthesia. Various studies have shown that anxiety and childbirth pain may increase maternal circulating catecholamines and reduce uterine blood flow (Shnider, 1981). Anesthesia can contribute to risk of asphyxia by decreasing maternal blood pressure and uterine blood flow, by causing diffusion hypoxia (N_2O), by leading to maternal hypoventilation or hyperventilation, by slowing labor, or by decreasing respiratory drive in the newborn.

There is no single best approach to these issues, except possibly choosing a skilled and caring anesthesiologist. For most cesarean sections and vaginal deliveries at this time, the preferred approach is caudal or lumbar epidural anesthesia with local anesthetics. Advantages are that maternal respiratory depression is avoided, the mother remains awake and cooperative, and the drug does not reach the fetus to a significant degree. The major complication is maternal hypotension, and care should be taken to obviate vena cava compression (wedge) and to maintain blood volume (intravenous crystalloid). Voluntary or involuntary maternal hyperventilation has been found to decrease uteroplacental blood flow and should be avoided (Shnider and Maya, 1974).

Emergency cesarean section deliveries (e.g., those involving fetal asphyxia, prolapsed cord, placenta previa, abruptio placentae) are routinely performed under general anesthesia. How long it takes to deliver an infant from the time at which the decision is made is one index of the quality of an obstetric service. Risks of general anesthesia are maternal vomiting and aspiration during induction and neonatal depression. Induction is accomplished with fast-acting barbiturates, given intravenously, followed by a muscle relaxant (pancuronium bromide) that does not cross the placenta. Rapid intubation of the mother with a cuffed endotracheal tube is carried out, and N_2O/O_2 mixtures are administered and sometimes supplemented with halothane. Delivery within 10 minutes is associated with minimal neonatal depression from anesthesia. The mother should breathe 50 to 75 per cent oxygen and be positioned in such a way that vena cava compression by the gravid uterus before and during delivery is prevented.

REFERENCES

Abel, E. (Ed.): Fetal Alcohol Syndrome. Vol. II. Human Studies. Boca Raton, CRC Press, 1982.

Barber, H.: Fetal and neonatal effects of cytotoxic agents. Obstet. Gynecol. *58*:41, (Suppl.), 1981.

Benson, R.: Current Obstetric and Gynecologic Diagnosis and Treatment. Los Altos, Calif., Lange Publishers, 1978.

Benirschke, K., and Kim, C. K.: Multiple pregnancy. N. Engl. J. Med. *288*:1276, 1973.

Berry, C. L. (Ed.): Human malformations. Br. Med. Bull. *32*:1–94, 1976.

Bland, R., Bressack, M., and McMillan, D.: Labor decreases the lung water content of newborn rabbits. Am. J. Obstet. Gynecol. *135*:364, 1979.

Bonner, J., MacGilvray, I., and Symonds, E., (Eds.): Pregnancy Hypertension. Baltimore, University Park Press, 1980.

Boston Collaborative Drug Surveillance Program: Diethylstilbestrol in pregnancy. Frequency of exposure and usage patterns. Cancer *31*:573, 1973.

Branstrup, E., Osler, M., and Pedersen, J.: Perinatal mortality in diabetic pregnancy. Acta Endocrinol. *37*:434, 1961.

Brent, R.: Environmental factors: radiation. *In* Brent, R., and Harris, M. (Eds.): Prevention of Embryonic, Fetal, and Perinatal Disease. DHEW Publication No. (NIH) 76-853, 1976, p. 179.

Browne, D.: Congenital deformities of mechanical origin. Arch. Dis. Child. *30*:37, 1955.

Butler, N. R., and Alberman, E. D.: Perinatal Problems. The Second Report of the 1958 British Perinatal Mortality Survey. London, E. & S. Livingstone, Ltd., 1969.

Butler, N. R., and Bonham, D. G.: Perinatal Mortality. The First Report of the 1968 Perinatal Mortality Survey. London, E. & S. Livingstone, Ltd., 1963.

Carter, C. O.: The genetics of congenital malformations. Proc. Roy. Soc. Med. *61*:991, 1968.

Charache, S., Scott, J., Niebyl, J., and Bonds, D.: Management of sickle cell disease in pregnant patients. Obstet. Gynecol. *55*:407, 1980.

Clarren, S., and Smith, D.: Congenital deformities. Pediatr. Clin. North Am. *24*:665, 1977.

Cohlan, S. Q.: Congenital anomalies in the rat produced by excessive intake of vitamin A during pregnancy. Pediatrics, *13*:556, 1954.

Collaborative Trial Group on Antenatal Steroid Therapy: Effect of antenatal dexamethasone administration on the prevention of respiratory distress syndrome. Am. J. Obstet. Gynecol. *141*:276, 1981.

Collea, J., Robin, S., Weghorst, G., et al.: Breech presentation: vaginal delivery vs. c-section. Randomized management of term frank breech presentation. Am. J. Obstet. Gynecol. *131*:186, 1978.

Cornblath, M., and Schwartz, R.: Disorders of Carbohydrate Metabolism in Infancy. 2nd. ed. Philadelphia, W. B. Saunders Company, 1976, p 115.

Cosmi, E.: Obstetric Anesthesia and Perinatology. New York, Appleton-Century-Crofts, 1981.

Daikoku, N., Kaltreider, F., Johnson, T., et al.: Premature rupture of membranes and preterm labor: neonatal infection and perinatal mortality risks. Obstet. Gynecol. 58:417, 1981.

Driscoll, S. G., Benirschke, K., and Curtis, G. W.: Neonatal deaths among infants of diabetic mothers. Am. J. Dis. Child. 100:818, 1960.

Dunn, P.: Breech delivery: perinatal morbidity and mortality. In Rooth, G., and Bratteby, L. (Eds.): Fifth European Congress of Perinatal Medicine. Stockholm, Almqvist and Wiksell, 1976, p. 57.

Dunn, P.: Congenital postural deformities. Br. Med. J. 32:71, 1976.

Ekelund, H., Kullander, S., and Kallen, B.: Major and minor malformations in newborns and infants up to one year of age. Acta Paediat. Scand. 59:297, 1970.

Fairweather, D.: Obstetric management of the very low birth weight infant. J. Reprod. Med. 26:387, 1981.

Fairweather, D., and Eskes, T: Amniotic Fluid: Research and Clinical Application. Amsterdam, Excerpta Medica, 1978.

Farquhar, J. W.: Prognosis for babies born to diabetic mothers in Edinburgh. Arch. Dis. Child. 44:36, 1969.

Fields, G. A., Schwarz, R. H., Dickens, H. O., and Tunnessen, W.: Sacral agenesis in the infant of a gestational diabetic. J. Obstet. Gynecol. 32:778, 1968.

Flaksman, R., Vollman, J., and Benfield, D.: Iatrogenic prematurity due to elective termination of the uncomplicated pregnancy: a major perinatal health care problem. Am. J. Obstet. Gynecol. 132:885, 1978.

Fox, H.: Pathology of the placenta. In Major Problems in Pathology, Vol. VII. Philadelphia, W. B. Saunders, 1978.

Fraser, F.: Prevention of birth defects: How are we doing? Teratology 17:193, 1978.

Fraumeni, J. F., Jr.: Chemicals in human teratogenesis and transplacental carcinogenesis. Pediatrics 53:807, 1974.

Frigoletto, F., Ryan, K., and Philippe, M.: Maternal mortality rate associated with caesarian section: an appraisal. Am. J. Obstet. Gynecol. 136:969, 1980.

Gabbe, S. G.: Congenital malformations in infants of diabetic mothers. Obstet. Gynecol. Surv. 32:125, 1977.

Garite, T., Freeman, R., Linzey, M., et al.: Prospective randomized study of corticosteroids in management of premature rupture of the membranes. Am. J. Obstet. Gynecol. 141:508, 1981.

Gedda, L., Parisi, P., and Nance, W.: Twin Research 3. Proc. Third Internat. Cong. Twin Studies. New York, Alan R. Liss, Inc., 1980.

Gellis, S. S., and Hsia, D. Y.-Y.: The infant of the diabetic mother. A.M.A.J. Dis. Child. 97:1, 1959.

Gibbs, R.: Antibiotic therapy of endometritis following cesarean section. Obstet. Gynecol. 52:50, 1978.

Gluck, L. (Ed.): Obstetrical Decisions and Neonatal Outcome. Report of the 78th Ross Conference. Columbus, Ohio, Ross Laboratories, 1981.

Goldstein, M: Incompetent cervix in offspring of DES treated women. Obstet. Gynecol. 52:735 (Suppl.), 1978.

Hall, J., Pauli, R., and Wilson, K.: Maternal and fetal sequelae of anticoagulation during pregnancy. Am. J. Med. 68:122, 1980.

Hansen, J., Theopoulos, M., Harvey, M., et al.: Risks to offspring of women treated with hydantoin anticonvulsants. J. Pediatr. 89:662, 1976.

Hardy, J. B., Drage J. S., and Jackson, E. C.: The First Year of Life. The Collaborative Perinatal Project of the National Institute of Neurological and Communicative Disorders and Stroke. Baltimore, Johns Hopkins University Press, 1979.

Herbst, A.: Diethylstilbestrol and other sex hormones during pregnancy. Obstet. Gynecol. 58:35S (Suppl.), 1981.

Herbst, A., Hubby, M., Blough, R., et al.: A comparison of pregnancy experience in DES-exposed and DES-unexposed daughters. J. Reprod. Med. 24:62, 1980.

Herbst, A. L., Ulfelder, H., and Poskanzer, D. C.: Adenocarcinoma of the vagina. Association of maternal diethylstilbestrol with tumor appearance in young women. N. Engl. J. Med. 284:878, 1971.

Hill, H.: Drugs in pregnancy. Obstet. Gynecol. Surv. 34:643, 1979.

Hoffman, D., Felten, R., and Cyr, W.: Effects of ionizing radiation on the developing embryo and fetus. U.S. Dept. of Health and Human Services Publ. FDA 81-8170, Washington, D.C., August, 1981.

Holmes, L. B.: Inborn errors of morphogenesis—a review of localized hereditary malformations. N. Engl. J. Med. 291:763, 1974.

Huff, R.: Antibiotic prophylaxis for puerperal endometritis following premature rupture of the membranes. J. Reprod. Med. 19:79, 1979.

Hurley, L.: Developmental Nutrition. Englewood Cliffs, N.J., Prentice-Hall, 1980.

Jones, K., and Smith, D.: Recognition of the fetal alcohol syndrome in early infancy. Lancet 2:999, 1973.

Jones, K., Smith, D., Hall, B. et al.: A pattern of craniofacial and limb defects secondary to aberrant tissue bands. J. Pediatr. 84:90, 1974.

Jones, K. L., Smith, D. W., Streissguth, A. P., et al.: Outcome in offspring of chronic alcoholic women. Lancet 1:1076, 1974.

Jones, K. L., Smith, D. W., Ulleland, C. N., et al.: Pattern of malformation in offspring of chronic alcoholic mothers. Lancet 1:7815, 1973.

Jorge, C., Artal, R., Paul, R. et al.: Antepartum fetal surveillance in diabetic pregnant patients. Am. J. Obstet. Gynecol. 141:641, 1981.

Kaminetzky, H., and Baker, H.: Nutritional needs in pregnancy. In Iffy, L., and Kaminetzky, H. (Eds.): Principles and Practice of Obstetrics and Perinatology. New York, J. Wiley & Sons, 1981, p. 655.

Kitzmiller, J., Brown, E., Philippe, M., et al.: Diabetic nephropathy and perinatal outcome. Am. J. Obstet. Gynecol. 141:741, 1981.

Kurzel, R., and Cetrulo, C.: When to do cesarean section. Perinatology/Neonatology 5:19, 1981.

Lauersen, N., and Hochberg, H.: Clinical Perinatal Biochemical Monitoring. Baltimore, Williams & Wilkins, 1981.

Leck, I., and Record, R. G.: Seasonal incidence of anencephalus. Br. J. Prev. Soc. Med. 20:67, 1966.

Lemoine, P., Harousseau, H., Borteyru, J., et al.: Les enfants de parents alcooliques: anomalies observées à propos de 127 cas. Arch. Fr. Pediatr. 25:830, 1968.

Lenz, W., and Maier, W.: Congenital malformations and maternal diabetes. Lancet 2:1124, 1964.

Levin, D. L.: Effects of inhibition of prostaglandin synthesis on fetal development. Semin. Perinatol. 4:35, 1980.

Lin, C., Lindheimer, M., River, P., and Moawad, A.: Fetal outcome in hypertensive disorders of pregnancy. Am. J. Obstet. Gynecol. 142:255, 1982.

Longo, L.: Environmental pollution and pregnancy. Am. J. Obstet. Gynecol. 137:162, 1980.

Lubs, H. A., and Ruddle, F. H.: Chromosomal abnormalities in the human population: Estimation of rates based on New Haven newborn study. Science 169:495, 1970.

Marden, P. M., Smith, D. W., and McDonald, M. J.: Congenital anomalies in the newborn infant, including minor variations. J. Pediatr. 64:357, 1964.

McIntosh, R., Merritt, K. K., Richards, M. R., Samuels, M. H., and Bellows, M. T.: The incidence of congenital malformations: A study of 5964 pregnancies. Pediatrics 14:505, 1954.

Mead, P. B., and Clapp, J. F.: Betamethasone and timed delivery in management of premature rupture of the membranes in preterm pregnancy. J. Reprod. Med. 19:3, 1977.

Meltzer, H. J.: Congenital anomalies due to attempted abortion with 4-aminopteroglutamic acid. J.A.M.A. 161:1253, 1956.

Mikamo, K.: Anatomic and chromosomal anomalies in spontaneous abortions. Am. J. Obstet. Gynecol. 106:243, 1970.

Miller, P., Smith, D., and Shepard, T.: Maternal hyperthermia as a possible cause of anencephaly. Lancet 1:519, 1978.

Miller, E., Hare, J., Cloherty, J., Dunn, P., et al.: Elevated maternal HbA_{1c} in early pregnancy and major congenital anomalies in infants of diabetic mothers. N. Engl. J. Med. 304:1331, 1981.

Milner, A., Saunders, R., and Hopkin, I.: Effects of delivery by caesarian section on lung mechanics and lung volume in the human neonate. Arch. Dis. Child. *53*:545, 1978.

Milunsky, A., Graef, J., and Gaynor, M.: Methotrexate-induced congenital malformations, with a review of the literature. J. Pediatr. *72*:790, 1968.

Moghissi, K.: Risks and benefits of nutritional supplements during pregnancy. Obstet. Gynecol. *58*:685, 1981.

Monson, R. R., Rosenberg, L., Hartz, S. C., et al.: Diphenylhydantoin and selected congenital malformations. N. Engl. J. Med. *289*:1049, 1973.

Nara, A., and Nara, J.: A syndrome of multiple congenital anomalies associated with teratogenic exposure. Arch. Environ. Health *30*:17, 1975.

Neel, J. V.: A study of major congenital defects in Japanese infants. Am. J. Hum. Genet. *10*:398, 1958.

Nichols, J., and Schrepfer, R.: Polyhydramnios in anencephaly. J.A.M.A. *197*:549, 1966.

Niswander, K., and Gordon, M. (Eds): The Women and Their Pregnancies. Philadelphia, W. B. Saunders, Co., 1972.

Ogata, E., Kitterman, J., Kleinberg, F., et al.: The effects of time of cord clamping and maternal blood pressure on placental transfusion with cesarean section. Am. J. Obstet. Gynecol. *128*:197, 1977.

Osler, M., and Pedersen, J.: The body composition of newborn infants of diabetic mothers. Pediatrics *26*:985, 1960.

Passarge, E., and Lenz, W.: Syndrome of caudal regression in infants of diabetic mothers. Observations of further cases. Pediatrics *37*:672, 1966.

Penrose, L. S., and Smith, G. F.: Down's Anomaly. Boston, Little, Brown and Company, 1966.

Philippe, E., and Sauvage, J.: The placenta and its membranes. *In* Iffy, L., and Kaminetzy, H. (Eds.): Principles and Practice of Obstetrics and Perinatology. New York, J. Wiley & Sons, 1981.

Plummer, G.: Anomalies occurring in children exposed in utero to the atomic bomb in Hiroshima. Pediatrics *10*:687, 1952.

Polani, P. E.: Incidence of developmental and other genetic abnormalities. Proc. Roy. Soc. Med. *66*:1118, 1973.

Rothman, K., Fyler, D., Goldblatt, A., et al.: Exogenous hormones and other drug exposures of children with congenital heart disease. Am. J. Epidemiol. *109*:433, 1979.

Rothman, K. J., and Fyler, D. C.: Seasonal occurrence of complex ventricular septal defect. Lancet *2*:193, 1974.

Rubin, A.: Birth injuries. Hosp. Med. *13*:114, 1977.

Sandler, M.: Amniotic Fluid and Its Clinical Significance. New York, Marcel Dekker, Inc., 1981.

Scanlon, J.: Fetal effects of lead exposure. Pediatrics *49*:145, 1972.

Schaffer, A., and Avery, M. E.: Diseases of the Newborn. 4th ed. Philadelphia, W. B. Saunders Co., 1977, p. 84.

Schardein, J.: Drugs as Teratogens. Cleveland, CRC Press, 1976.

Schulman, J., and Simpson, J.: Genetic Diseases in Pregnancy. Maternal Effects and Fetal Outcome. New York, Academic Press, 1981.

Scott, K., Field, T., and Robertson, E.: Teenage Parents and Their Offspring. New York, Grune & Stratton, 1981.

Sever, J., and White, L. R.: Intrauterine viral infections. Ann. Rev. Med. *19*:471, 1968.

Shaul, W., and Hall, J.: Multiple congenital anomalies associated with oral anticoagulants. Am. J. Obstet. Gynecol. *127*:191, 1977.

Shepard, T., and Fantel, A.: Teratology of therapeutic agents. *In* Iffy, L., and Kaminetzky, H. (Eds.): Principles and Practice of Obstetrics and Perinatology. New York, J. Wiley & Sons, 1981.

Shepard, T. H.: Catalog of Teratogenic Agents. Baltimore, Johns Hopkins University Press, 1973.

Shnider, S.: Choice of anesthesia for labor and delivery. Obstet. Gynecol. *58*:245, 1981.

Shnider, S., and Maya, F. (Eds.): The Anesthesiologist, Mother, and Newborn. Baltimore, Williams and Wilkins, 1974, p. 98.

Sisson, T.: Blood Volume. *In* Stave, U. (Ed.): Perinatal Physiology. New York, Plenum Medical Books, 1978, p. 181.

Smith, C., and Nelson, N.: The Physiology of the Newborn Infant. 4th ed. Springfield, Ill. Charles Thomas, 1976.

Smith, C. A.: Effects of maternal undernutrition upon the newborn infant in Holland (1944–1945). J. Pediatr. *30*:229, 1947.

Smith, C. A.: When should one ligate the umbilical cord? Editorial. Pediatrics *40*:5, 1967.

Smith, D.: Deformations due to in utero compression. Pediatr. Ann. *10*:8, 1981.

Smith, D.: Recognizable Patterns of Human Malformation. 3rd ed. Philadelphia, W. B. Saunders. Co., 1982.

Smith, P., and Mumford, D. (Eds.): Adolescent Pregnancy. Boston, C. K. Hall & Co., 1980, p. 18.

Smith, S., Clarren, S., and Harvey, M.: Hyperthermia as a possible teratogenic agent. J. Pediatr. *92*:878, 1978.

Smithells, R.: Environmental teratogens of man. Br. Med. Bull. *32*:27, 1976.

Sola, A., and Gregory, G.: Colloid osmotic pressure of normal newborns and premature infants. Crit. Care Med. *9*:568, 1981.

Speidel, B. D., and Meadow, S. R.: Maternal epilepsy and abnormalities of the fetus and newborn. Lancet *2*:839, 1972.

Spranger, J., Benirschke, K., Hall, J., Lenz, W., et al.: Errors of morphogenesis: concepts and terms. J. Pediatr. *100*:160, 1982.

Stevenson, R.: The Fetus and Newly Born Infant. Influences of the Prenatal Environment. St. Louis, C. V. Mosby, 1973.

Stewart, A.: Follow-up of preterm infants. *In* Pre-Term Labour. Proceedings of the 5th Study Group of the Royal College of Obstetricians, Gynaecologists, 1977, p. 372.

Streissguth, A., Landesman-Dwyer, S., Martin, J., et al.: Teratogenic effects of alcohol in humans and animals. Science *209*:353, 1980.

Taeusch, H. W., Jr, Frigoletto, F., Kitzmiller, J., et al.: Risk of respiratory distress syndrome after prenatal dexamethasone treatment. Pediatrics *63*:64, 1979.

Torpin, R.: Amniochorionic mesoblastic fibrous strings and amniotic bands: associated constricting fetal malformations or fetal death. Am. J. Obstet. Gynecol. *91*:65, 1965.

Usher, R., McLean, F., and Maughan, G. B.: Respiratory distress syndrome in infants delivered by cesarean section. Am. J. Obstet. Gynecol. *88*:806, 1964.

Usher, R., Shephard, M., and Lind, J.: The blood volume of the newborn infant and the placental transfusion. Acta Paediat. Scand. *52*:497, 1963.

Van Vunakis, H., Langone, J. J., and Milunsky, A.: Nicotine and Cotinine in the amniotic fluid of smokers in the early period of gestation. Am. J. Obstet. Gynecol. *120*:64, 1974.

Warkany, J.: Etiology of congenital malformations. Advances in Pediatrics. Vol. 2. New York, Interscience Publishers, Inc., 1947.

Warkany, J.: Prevention of congenital malformations. Teratology *23*:175, 1981.

Westgren, M., and Svenningsen, N.: Long term follow-up of preterm infants in breech presentation delivered by cesarean section: prospective study. Lancet *2*:172, 1978.

White, P.: Diabetes mellitus in pregnancy. Clinics in Perinatology. Philadelphia, W. B. Saunders Co., 1974, p. 331.

Wilson, J. G.: Environment and Birth Defects. New York, Academic Press, 1973.

Wilson, J. G., and Brent, R.: Are female sex hormones teratogenic? Am. J. Obstet. Gynecol. *141*:567, 1981.

2

Prenatal Genetic Diagnosis

By Samuel A. Latt

Introduction

Prenatal genetic diagnosis is an evolving field that has exploited both the ever-increasing ability to monitor a fetus during gestation and technological advances in cell and molecular biology that permit analysis of fetal material (Milunsky, 1979; Hamerton and Simpson, 1980; Latt and Darlington, 1982). The diagnostic procedures evaluate fetal status typically (but not exclusively) by sampling amniotic fluid components (Table 2–1). Information can be obtained from procedures performed on cells or supernatant of amniotic fluid, acquired transabdominally, customarily between the fifteenth and nineteenth weeks of gestation (menstrual age). Additional information can be provided by analysis of fetal or maternal serum, by ultrasonography (Hobbins et al., 1980), radiography, amniography, or fetoscopy (Mahoney and Hobbins, 1979; Mahoney, 1982).

The risk of amniotic fluid sample acquisition is not precisely known. Most estimates place an upper limit of 0.5 per cent on fetal morbidity and mortality, recorded in centers in which the procedure is regularly performed by highly trained personnel using "state-of-the-art" facilities (reviewed by Simpson et al., 1980). However, the prenatal diagnostic procedure is sufficiently involved that it should be reserved as a secondary test, to be performed after appropriate analysis has identified pregnancies at increased risk for conditions detectable in utero. It should also be realized that the primary option currently available once data are obtained (i.e., pregnancy intervention) falls short of the ultimate goal (i.e., in utero treatment) (Birnholz and Frigoletto, 1981).

The total of all currently accepted indications for prenatal genetic diagnosis involves 5 to 7 per cent of all pregnancies. Hence, acquisition and utilization of information about the indications for prenatal diagnosis are important (Table 2–2). Currently, potential cytogenetic abnormalities constitute the most common indication for prenatal diagnosis (Polani et al., 1979; Golbus et al., 1979a; Milunsky, 1979; Hamerton and Simpson, 1980). A group of conditions known as open neural tube defects constitutes the

Table 2–1. Prenatal Genetic Diagnosis (Simplified Scheme)

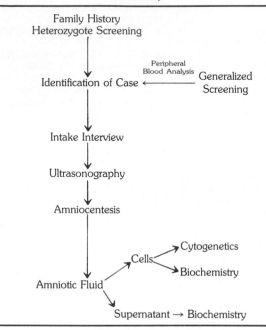

second most common indication for prenatal diagnosis. Diagnosis of these relies heavily on measurements of alpha-fetoprotein (Crandall and Brazier, 1978; Alpha-fetoprotein Conference Proceedings, 1980; Haddow and Miller, 1982). Third in overall importance, but with the greatest potential for increase in risk, is the collection of hereditary "single-gene" defects, each of which has a relatively low incidence. Thousands of these conditions exist (McKusick, 1978), and more than 100 can already be diagnosed in utero (Milunsky, 1979; Grabowski and Desnick, 1982). Indications, procedures, and prospects for advances in each of these categories will be considered in turn.

Table 2–2. Types of Indications for Prenatal Diagnosis

Cytogenetics
 Advanced maternal age
 Previous autosomal trisomy
 Parent who carries a translocation
 Repeated fetal wastage
Neural-Tube–Related
 Family history of open NTD
 Detection of condition by AFP screening program
Biochemical
 Enzyme defect
 X-linked recessive condition
 Detection of condition by DNA studies

MATERNAL AGE

The most common indication for prenatal cytogenetic diagnosis remains advanced maternal age because of its associated increased risk for offspring with autosomal trisomy (Hamerton et al., 1980). The general incidence of chromosomal abnormalities in newborns is approximately 6 per 1000 (Hook and Hamerton, 1976). Of these, approximately 1.4 per 1000 are autosomal trisomies. Virtually all these involve chromosomes 13, 18, or 21. Trisomy 21, resulting in Down syndrome (Fig. 2–1), is the most common autosomal trisomy, occurring in approximately 1 of every 1000 livebirths.

The risk of having live offspring with autosomal trisomy increases with maternal age. Perhaps owing to the use of 5-year cohorts for initial data acquisition, the definition of "advanced" maternal age focuses on 35 years (the start of the 35- to 39-year interval). Semilogarithmic analysis of data on an annual basis reveals an increase in the incidence of trisomy 21 newborns somewhat earlier (Fig. 2–2): By 35 years of age, the risk of autosomal trisomy is as great as the estimated risk associated with the prenatal diagnostic procedure. The incidence of trisomy 21 is approximately 1 per cent at a maternal age of 40 years, and it rises sharply thereafter. Risks for the other autosomal trisomies, while less than that for trisomy 21, show comparable age dependence. Many conceptuses with trisomy 13, 18, or 21 do not survive until birth (Hook, 1978).

The *practical* definition of advanced maternal age may depend on the outcome of legal decisions addressing situations in which prenatal diagnosis was not offered, as well as operational constraints reflecting the case-load capacity of existing prenatal diagnostic facilities. Realizing the circularity and circumstantial nature of such criteria, one would find it reasonable to define 35 years (at conception) as the maternal age at which the option of prenatal diagnosis for the purpose of detecting autosomal trisomy might be routinely mentioned. This would involve approximately 5 per cent of all pregnant women (Hook and Lindsjö, 1978), amounting to more than 150,000 potential cases per year in the United States alone. This number is several times that of the procedures actually performed (Antenatal Diagnosis, 1979) or feasible with existing facilities. However, it would still not include the two thirds of all infants with Down syndrome who are born to mothers less than 35 years of age (Holmes, 1978).

The earliest age at which prenatal cytogenetic procedures employed by individual diagnostic centers are recommended may be slightly higher than 35

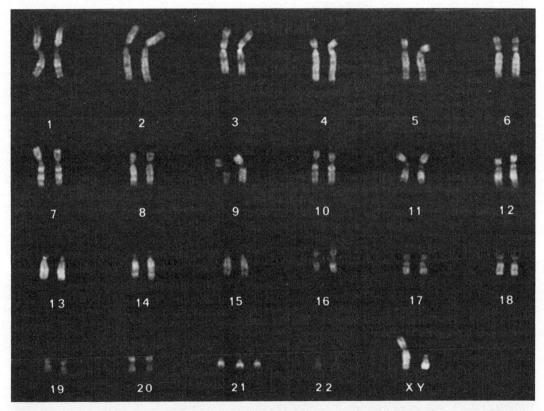

Figure 2–1. Karyotype of a cell from a male fetus with trisomy 21. Amniocentesis was performed because of advanced maternal age (43 yrs. in this case). The chromosomes shown were stained with quinacrine and examined by fluorescence microscopy. (Courtesy of Dr. M. Sandstrom.)

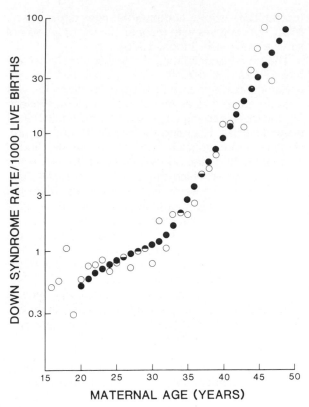

Figure 2–2. Maternal age dependence of Down syndrome. Maternal ages are those at last birthday at time of delivery. The data, obtained over yearly intervals, are those reported by Hook and Lindsjö (1978) and were obtained in America (●) and Sweden (○).

years (Hamerton et al, 1980). Throughout, additional factors relating to family history, personal beliefs, and risk-value emphasis must be recognized in deciding for or against prenatal diagnosis.

FAMILY HISTORY

A related event influencing a decision regarding prenatal cytogenetic diagnosis is the previous incidence of autosomal trisomy in first degree relatives of the couple considering the procedure (i.e., sibs or offspring or both). The average recurrence risk for trisomy 21 is currently estimated to be 0.5 to 1.0 per cent (Milunsky, 1979; Mikkelsen and Stene, 1979). (This probably reflects an aggregate of different causes, each with its own intrinsic recurrence risk.) Based on the high recurrence risk of abortions of infants with autosomal trisomy (Alberman et al., 1976), it is suspected that the occurrence of *any* liveborn infant with autosomal trisomy implies an approximately 1 per cent risk of a similar condition (most commonly trisomy 21) in a subsequent pregnancy.

Not all extra autosomes are of maternal origin. For example, in approximately 25 per cent of trisomy 21 births, the extra 21 comes from the father (Mikkelsen et al., 1976; Magenis et al., 1977). However, it is not yet known whether the parental source of a supernumerary autosome influences its recurrence risk.

Balanced Chromosomal Rearrangement

A less common indication for prenatal diagnostic analysis, which often carries a much greater recurrence risk, is a balanced chromosomal rearrangement in one of the parents. When discernible, this can be indicated by the previous birth of infants in whom there is chromosomal imbalance (including a small fraction of cases clinically identified as Down syndrome) or by a family history of unexplained fetal wastage (e.g., two or more miscarriages without underlying hormonal or anatomic abnormalities). Prenatal diagnosis for this reason should be preceded by a careful cytogenetic analysis of the parents, both to identify those couples and other family members at risk and to characterize the chromosomal rearrangement involved. The latter information can guide subsequent analysis of amniotic fluid chromosome preparations for detection of subtle abnormalities.

Robertsonian Translocations. The most common balanced chromosomal rearrangements, Robertsonian translocations, occur between the centromeric regions of two acrocentric chromosomes. For example, a Robertsonian translocation between chromosomes 21 and 14, that is, t(14q;21q), predisposes one's offspring to Down syndrome: It is possible for a gamete to receive *both* a normal chromosome 21 and the translocation chromosome (containing most of a 21) from the parent with the translocation. Since another chromosome 21 will be provided by the second parent, the conceptus would then be trisomic for most of chromosome 21. The risk for such an outcome is approximately 15 per cent if the mother carries the translocation, but, for unknown reasons, only about 5 per cent if the father carries the translocation (Hamerton, 1980). Unbalanced offspring of parents with other Robertsonian translocations involve more severe chromosomal imbalance and either are not liveborn or have even more serious abnormalities (e.g., trisomy 13). In addition to producing their abnormal offspring, these parents can have phenotypically normal offspring, some of whom will also carry balanced translocations. Other reciprocal non-Robertsonian translocations involving small segments of other chromosomes exist (Fig. 2–3) and can constitute indications for prenatal diagnosis.

Neural Tube Defects

The second disease category for prenatal genetic diagnosis consists of the set of conditions termed neural tube defects (NTDs), which includes anen-

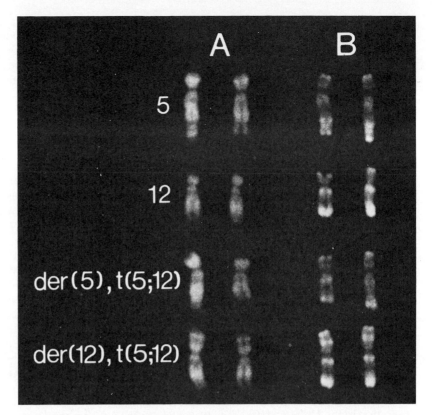

Figure 2–3. Analysis of a reciprocal translocation by quinacrine (*A*) and chromomycin A₃-methyl green (*B*) fluorescence. The chromosomes shown are from cells of a fetus who had a parent with a reciprocal translocation between chromosomes #5 and #12 (i.e., rcp t(5q; 12p). The normal chromosomes are in the top two rows, while the translocation chromosomes are in the last two rows. The fetus had the translocation in a balanced form and was born phenotypically normal. (From Sandstrom M. M., et al: Prenatal cytogenetic diagnosis. *In* Latt, S., and Darlington, G. [Eds.]: Prenatal Diagnosis: Cell Biological Aspects. New York, Academic Press, 1982.)

cephaly and myelomeningocele (Brock, 1977; Haddow and Miller, 1982). The total incidence of severe NTDs in the United States is approximately 2 cases per 1000 births. This incidence depends on ethnic origins, being a few times higher in people of Celtic origin in the United Kingdom and somewhat lower in black populations. The working model for the inheritance of NTDs indicates that it depends on both environmental and multiple genetic determinants (i.e., "multifactorial" inheritance). The birth of one child with an NTD in a family results in a tenfold risk to siblings born subsequently (Wald and Cuckle, 1979). The birth of additional affected children results in even larger risks for future pregnancies. The occurrence of NTDs in more distant family members, particularly in children of maternal aunts (Zackai,

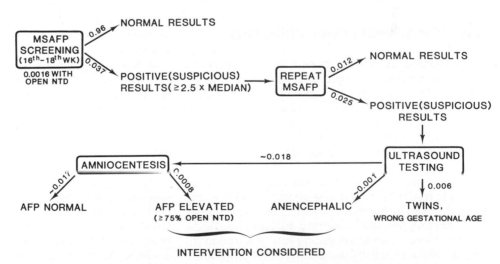

Figure 2–4. Flow chart indicating the diagnostic sequence associated with maternal serum alpha-fetoprotein screening. The numbers shown are approximate and are subject to variation, depending, for example, on the incidence of NTDs in the particular population considered. Addition of acetylcholinesterase analysis (Haddow et al., 1981) further assists evaluation of AFP data. (Adapted from Layde, P. M., et al.: Work group paper: Maternal serum alpha-fetoprotein screening—A cost benefit analysis. *In* Gastel, B., et al. [Eds.]: Maternal Serum Alpha-Fetoprotein. NCHT Conference Proceedings. Supt. Documents, U.S. Government Printing Office, 1980.)

1978), has a lesser but non-negligible impact on future risk estimates.

A positive family history of NTD, as just defined, is sufficient indication for performing amniocentesis to search for biochemical and/or cellular evidence of an open NTD. In addition, it is standard practice to perform alpha-fetoprotein (AFP) analysis on aliquots of amniotic fluid samples obtained for other (typically cytogenetic) purposes. The other option (i.e., cytogenetic analysis of samples obtained primarily because an open NTD is suspected) has less support (Gosden et al., 1981). This latter situation has assumed greater importance with the advent of programs for screening maternal serum alpha-fetoprotein, which are applicable to all pregnancies (Fig. 2–4). Current protocols for such screening programs result in amniocentesis in approximately 2 per cent of all pregnant women screened, out of which perhaps one tenth will eventually be identified as carrying a fetus with an open NTD. The consequences of mass serum AFP screening have been most thoroughly evaluated in the United Kingdom (Wald and Cuckle, 1979), where the overall risk of NTD is higher than that in the United States; the applicability of such a program in the United States is less certain. Factors such as the results of ancillary tests (e.g., ultrasonographic examination) will influence ultimate practice, as will any success of strategies directed primarily at reducing the incidence of NTDs (e.g., vitamin therapy) (Smithells et al., 1980).

Single-gene Disorders

AUTOSOMAL RECESSIVE CONDITIONS

The third class of conditions prompting prenatal diagnosis consists of single-gene disorders and includes a large number of metabolic abnormalities. The prototypic disorder, Tay-Sachs disease, is characterized by a defect in a lysosomal enzyme, hexosaminidase A (Kaback et al., 1977a,b; Kaback, 1981) and results in severe neurologic deficits and death in childhood. Each parent of an offspring affected with this autosomal recessive disorder is heterozygous (i.e., has one normal and one abnormal allele at the hexosaminidase A locus). Detection of heterozygotes is a necessary prelude to prenatal analysis. Tay-Sachs disease is most prevalent among (but not limited to) individuals with an Ashkenazi Jewish background. Within this group, the heterozygote frequency approximates 1 in 30, and large-scale screening procedures are cost-effective (Kaback et al., 1977a,b). In the case of Tay-Sachs disease, heterozygote screening is most effective if initiated before pregnancy, though modified tests of hexosaminidase A are also possible with leukocytes of pregnant females.

As with other autosomal recessive conditions, identification of both parents as heterozygotes implies a 1 in 4 risk for each offspring and serves as the indication for amniocentesis followed by enzyme analysis on cultured cells. This analysis includes both a quantitation of heat-labile and heat-stable hexosaminidase A *plus* an electrophoretic analysis, the latter to check for variant isozymes.

Analogous strategies are theoretically possible with other autosomal recessive conditions (see Grabowski and Desnick, 1982). However, because most of these conditions are not localized in subpopulations with a high risk, mass screening for most of them is not yet practical. In such cases, the indication for prenatal diagnosis is the previous birth of an affected offspring. Particular attention to the development of broad-based screening methods for heterozygotes for multiple autosomal recessive diseases might be given to prospective parents who are related (e.g., first cousins), for whom the risk of a fetus affected with an autosomal recessive disease is significantly increased (Cavalli-Sforza and Bodmer, 1971).

AUTOSOMAL DOMINANT CONDITIONS

Different diagnostic strategies must be employed for conditions with other inheritance modes. For autosomal dominant inheritance, the presence of disease in a parent implies a 50 per cent risk of genetic transmission to a child; occurrence of the disease in a child also depends on the disease penetrance. Alternatively, if the affected family member is a previous child, one must consider the possibility that this child represented a fresh mutation (an event whose likelihood is proportional to the disease lethality) (Cavalli-Sforza and Bodmer, 1971). The metabolic etiology of most autosomal dominant disorders remains obscure, and prenatal diagnosis of autosomal dominant conditions has been relatively infrequent, limited to unusual metabolic diseases, such as acute intermittent porphyria (Kleijer et al. 1980), or to certain connective tissue/skeletal disorders (Omenn et al., 1977; Omenn, 1978). However, increased risk can be expected for certain familial cancers that formally follow autosomal dominant inheritance, such as retinoblastoma (Knudson et al., 1976), Wilms' tumor (Riccardi et al., 1977), and hypernephroma (Cohen et al., 1979), in which chromosomal deletion or rearrangement can imply increased disease risk, and tracing of autosomal dominant inheritance might ultimately become possible for conditions such as Huntington's chorea, in which genetic expression is delayed and phenotypic markers are unavailable but for which different types of genetic linkage analysis might prove of diagnostic use (Botstein et al., 1980).

X-LINKED CONDITIONS

In the case of X-linked disease, most of which follows a recessive inheritance pattern, pedigrees are characterized by affected males related through female carriers. Prototypic conditions include Lesch-Nyhan syndrome, Duchenne's muscular dystrophy, and hemophilia types A and B. In computing risk estimates to guide prenatal testing strategies, one must consider the possibility that either an affected male or a carrier female will reflect a fresh mutation. If the condition is a genetic lethal (i.e., no males reproduce), the former probability can be as high as 1 in 3, while the latter is 1 in 2. Fortunately, for some of these conditions, methods of detecting heterozygotes exist; for example, factor VIII analysis (Klein et al., 1977) and creatine-phosphokinase analysis (Emery, 1969; but see King et al., 1972) help define risk estimates, especially if performed *prior* to pregnancy. Unfortunately, owing in part to the phenomenon of random X-inactivation, none of these methods, which rely on phenotypic expression, is 100 per cent accurate. In view of this and the nearly 50 per cent frequency of mutant heterozygotes in lethal X-linked conditions, family history cannot reveal all heterozygotes. For commoner conditions, mass carrier screening may prove practical.

Once a pregnancy at risk for an X-linked recessive disease is identified, two types of diagnostic strategies are possible. For some conditions, such as Lesch-Nyhan syndrome, direct analysis of fetal cells (in this case for the enzyme HGPRT'ase) can differentiate affected and unaffected fetuses. For other conditions, one can only determine sex by fetal karyotype and subsequently abort male fetuses to eliminate disease risk. This represents a less satisfactory alternative, since it cannot alone determine which male fetuses at risk are actually affected.

Another X-linked condition that is receiving increased attention is a form of familial retardation (Renpenning et al., 1962), at times associated with physical abnormalities, in which the X chromosome of affected individuals and, perhaps, to a much lesser extent, heterozygotes, can exhibit a structural discontinuity near the long arm terminus (at the junction of bands Xq27 and Xq28) (Lubs, 1969; Sutherland, 1979). Techniques for increasing the detection efficiency of this "fragile X," most of which alter thymidine and/or one carbon metabolism (Glover, 1981; Howard-Peebles et al., 1981), are being developed. Thus far, diagnostic analyses have focused on peripheral blood samples of affected individuals and their relatives. However, it seems reasonable to anticipate that the option of screening amniotic fluid samples for the "fragile X" will become available in the near future.

Methodology

Once a decision to perform prenatal genetic diagnosis is reached, standard sample acquisition is followed by tests tailored to the condition in question. Transabdominal withdrawal of 15 to 20 ml of amniotic fluid provides sufficient material for most analyses. Sterile collection conditions must be employed.

Sample syringe and storage conditions should be chosen to maximize successful cell culture (Hoehn and Salk, 1982; Sandstrom et al., 1982). Twin pregnancies require special procedures, such as injection of marker dye after acquisition of the first sample, to ensure that both amniotic sacs are sampled. Detailed procedures for obtaining and processing the resulting materials are available (CDC Brochure, 1981; Hamerton and Simpson, 1980; Sandstrom et al., 1982).

Chromosome analysis requires 2 to 3 weeks. Cells are examined as primary colonies or as dispersed monolayers. Banding analysis (e.g., with quinacrine or Giemsa trypsin or both) of 10 cells plus chromosome counts on at least 15 other cells (sampling multiple colonies) is probably a reasonable standard. Special tests such as replication kinetics, silver staining, C band, R band (e.g., using the combination of chromomycin A_3 and methyl green), or sister chromatid exchange analysis can be performed if indicated (Sandstrom et al., 1982). The overall accuracy of prenatal cytogenetic analyses is greater than 99 per cent.

Alpha-fetoprotein (AFP) measurement is used to screen for neural tube defects. It can be measured in amniotic fluid or maternal blood samples. The former is technically simpler and more reliable. The latter carries less risk to the fetus and serves primarily to identify patients requiring amniotic fluid analysis. AFP in amniotic fluid can be measured by the rocket immunoelectrophoresis technique (Haddow and Miller, 1982). The sample is electrophoresed into a gel containing antibody, and AFP is quantitated by measuring the height of the immunoprecipitate pattern produced. The normal value of amniotic fluid AFP depends markedly on gestational age, being near 20 μg/ml at the fourteenth week of gestation and decreasing thereafter (Fig. 2–5A). The AFP concentration in fetal blood is much higher (in the range of 2 to 3 mg/ml). Detection of values of amniotic fluid AFP greater than 5 standard deviations above normal results in prediction of over 95 per cent of *open* neural tube defects, while giving a false-positive result in 0.2 per cent of unaffected pregnancies (Haddow and Miller, 1982). The incidence of false-positive diag-

Table 2–3. Selected Conditions Associated with Elevated Alpha-Fetoprotein

Maternal:	Hepatocarcinoma and other tumors
	Liver cell regeneration
	Tyrosinemia
	Ataxia-telangiectasia
Fetal:	Tumors, cysts, omphalocele
	Fetal blood in amniotic fluid
	Open neural tube defects, encephalocele, anencephaly
	Nephrosis
	Gastrointestinal obstruction
	Fetal demise or threatened demise

noses decreases as the "a priori" risk of an NTD increases.

Maternal serum AFP measurement by radioimmunoassay allows analysis of the ability of a sample to compete with a standard amount of antigen. The normal value at 14 weeks of gestation is 20 ng/ml, and it *increases* over the next 10 weeks (Fig. *2–5B*). Maternal serum AFP concentrations are typically 0.1 to 1.0 per cent of those found in amniotic fluid. While maternal serum alpha-fetoprotein is somehow de-

rived from fetal alpha-fetoprotein, existing information (N. Wald, personal communication) indicates that measurements of maternal serum and amniotic fluid alpha-fetoprotein are not entirely redundant. That is, even if amniotic fluid AFP is measured, analysis of maternal serum AFP can provide additional information. With two multiples of the median for any gestational age used as the cut-off criterion for maternal serum alpha-fetoprotein, more than 75 per cent of open NTDs can be detected. However, 90 per cent of fetuses in pregnancies scored as positive by this criterion do not have an open NTD.

Additional tests can serve as an adjunct to AFP measurement for evaluating pregnancies in which an

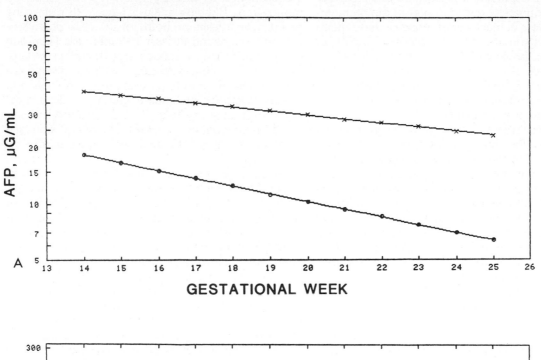

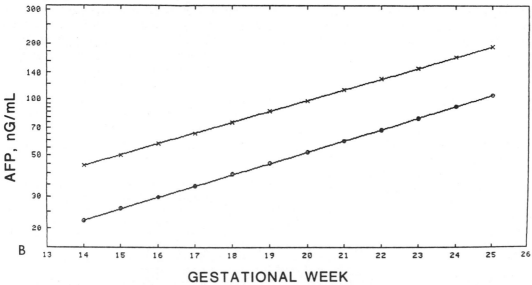

Figure 2–5. Dependence of second trimester alpha-fetoprotein levels in *A*, amniotic fluid (mean: ●——●) and *B*, maternal serum (median: ●——●) as a function of gestational age. Shown in each graph are the cutoff levels (x——x) for concluding that a value is significantly elevated (≥5 standard deviations above the mean in *A*; ≥2 multiples of the median in *B*.) (Data courtesy of Dr. James Haddow.)

open NTD is suspected. Measurement of rapidly adhering cells has been employed to detect cells with unusual morphology (e.g., neural cells) (Gosden et al., 1977). However, interpretation of this test remains difficult. Electrophoretic analysis of amniotic fluid acetylcholinesterase is a more useful corroborative test when elevation of amniotic fluid AFP is suspected to result from fetal blood contamination (Haddow et al., 1981). Ultrasonographic analysis (Fig. 2–6) is useful for ascertaining fetal position, determining gestational age (within 1 to 2 weeks), detecting twins, and, in some cases (e.g., those in which there is anencephaly or a very large spinal defect), corroborating the provisional diagnosis of an open NTD. No one biochemical or physical measurement yet provides a fully reliable NTD diagnosis. However, information from the aforementioned tests and, in some cases, others (e.g., amniography) can be very useful in guiding case management when properly integrated.

The specifics of individual biochemical studies vary too much with the diagnosis in question (Grabowski and Desnick, 1982) to be detailed here. Processing of amniotic fluid cells for enzymatic analysis currently requires 4 to 6 weeks, primarily because of a need for growth of large numbers of cells. Often, one needs to check parents for the presence of enzyme variants that might lead to the erroneous conclusion that a fetal abnormality exists. Recent instrumental developments (Galjaard, 1982), which involve performing some tests on a smaller scale, can reduce the total time required to culture a sufficient number of amniotic fluid cells for some biochemical analyses.

Other prenatal diagnostic tests can be performed directly on fetal blood obtained by fetoscopy (Mahoney and Hobbins, 1979). For example, one can attempt direct measurement of factor VIII activity (Mi-bashan et al., 1979) or immunoreactivity (Firshein et al., 1979) if hemophilia A is suspected. Chronic granulomatous disease can be diagnosed by assaying male polymorphonuclear lymphocytes for nitroblue tetrazolium reduction (Newburger et al., 1979). However, fetoscopy carries up to a 10 per cent fetal mortality risk (Benzie et al., 1980; Mahoney, 1982).

Additional biochemical studies can be performed on DNA isolated from freshly acquired or cultivated amniotic fluid cells (discussed in more detail subsequently). New experimental technologies continually increase the types of diagnostic information obtainable from amniotic fluid samples as well as the ease and speed with which this information can be acquired.

A noninvasive method of sampling amniotic fluid contents would reduce the overall risk of prenatal diagnosis. Herzenberg and associates have demonstrated the use of fluorescence-activated flow sorting to isolate fetal lymphocytes that are present in maternal blood samples (Herzenberg et al., 1979, 1980; Parks et al., 1982). These cells, which compose perhaps 0.02 to 0.1 per cent of the nucleated cell population present (Iverson et al., 1980; Parks et al., 1982), are detected in a flow cytometer following immunofluorescent staining of fetal surface (HLA-A2) antigens that differ from those of the mother. This staining difference is interpreted as a "fluorescent signal" that allows the cells to be sorted into one tube or another. By this same approach, Rh-D–positive fetal erythrocytes can be detected in the circulation of an Rh-D–negative mother. At analysis rates

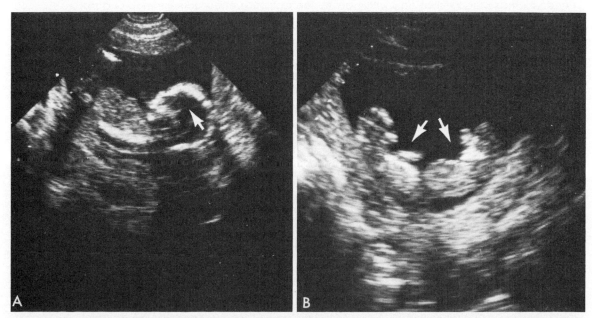

Figure 2–6. Appearance on ultrasonographic examination (B-mode scan, 5.0 M Hz) of *A*, a singleton pregnancy at approximately 4 months gestation and *B*, a twin pregnancy at approximately 12 weeks of gestation. The arrow in *A* points to the fetal cranium. The arrows in *B* indicate the fetuses. (Courtesy of Dr. Jason Birnholz.)

of 2000 to 3000 cells per second, 10^5 cells, up to 10 per cent of which might be of fetal origin, can be obtained by this method in 1 hour. Such a sample is not suitable for most biochemical tests, although it might suffice for chromosomal analysis.

Thus far, it has not been possible to stimulate the sorted fetal cells to divide so that they can be trapped at metaphase. Fetal sexing, based, for example, on quinacrine mustard staining for detection of a bright nuclear spot corresponding to the distal part of the long arm of the Y chromosome, has been successful (Herzenberg et al., 1979; Iverson et al., 1980), encouraging attempts to generalize this approach to allow detection of multiple surface antigens so that it could be used in more cases. Additional work will be

needed to simplify and increase the yield of fetal cell acquisition and to search for a way to stimulate sorted cells to progress to metaphase. It will also be of interest to understand how immunoincompatible fetal cells manage to persist in the maternal circulation and to develop methods capable of differentiating cells from a current pregnancy from those from previous pregnancies. The work done thus far constitutes an elegant demonstration of the possibility of fetal cell analysis in maternal blood, although current methodology is too involved to be practical on a large scale.

Methods of increasing the speed with which prenatal diagnostic results can be obtained would help reduce waiting time and parents' anxiety and might in some cases permit data acquisition in cases diagnosed at a relatively late gestational age. Success in this area has been primarily in biochemical analyses. For example, enzyme activities can be measured

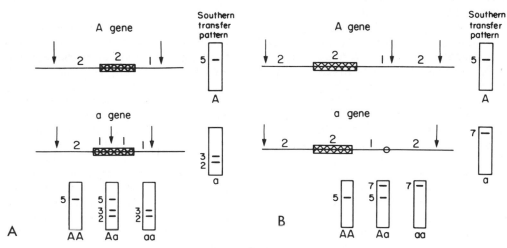

Figure 2–7. Two different ways of detecting genetic variation at the DNA level. *A*, Changes of endonuclease recognition sites within genes. The restriction endonuclease map of a putative wild-type (**A**) gene is shown. Endonuclease recognition sites are designated by arrows. Arabic numbers give distances in kilobases (kb); each kilobase equals 1000 bases. In the example chosen, the **A** gene, which is 2 kb long, has no endonuclease recognition sites within the gene, and is flanked by endonuclease recognition sites 2 kb upstream from the left (5′) side of the gene and 1 kb downstream from the right (3′) side of the gene. After restriction endonuclease digestion, the gene will lie on a single fragment 5 kb long, which would appear as a single band following Southern transfer and in situ hybridization with a radioactive probe specific for the gene.

A mutant allele (**a** gene), resulting from a mutation within the gene that caused the creation of a new endonuclease recognition site, would alter the restriction map as shown. After restriction endonuclease digestion, two fragments containing the gene would be detected following Southern transfer: a 3 kb and a 2 kb piece. Thus, the Southern transfer pattern from a wild-type homozygote (**AA**) would show only a 5 kb fragment; that from a heterozygote (**Aa**) would reveal 5 kb, 3 kb, and 2 kb fragments; and that from an affected homozygote (**aa**) would demonstrate only 3 kb and 2 kb fragments.

B, Changes of recognition sites in flanking sequences. An expanded restriction map of the **A** gene is shown, which demonstrates an additional endonuclease recognition site 2 kb downstream from the site located 1 kb from the right end of the gene. In this case, the mutant **A** gene does not result in the creation of a new recognition site within the gene. However, the mutation is closely linked to a DNA sequence change 1 kb downstream from the right end of the gene, resulting in an altered sequence that no longer functions as a recognition site. As before, a 5 kb fragment would be detected after both endonuclease digestion of DNA containing the **A** gene and subsequent Southern transfer. However, digestion of DNA containing the **a** gene will result in a longer 7 kb fragment. Again, this will allow for distinction between the **AA** (5 kb only), **Aa** (5 kb and 7 kb), and **a** (7 kb only) genotypes. A variation of this approach would involve an alteration in restriction endonuclease sites flanking a second DNA segment, used as a probe, which is closely linked (e.g., ≤1000 kb) to the **A** gene (Botstein et al., 1980; Wyman and White, 1980). (From Kurnit, D., and Hoehn, H.: Annu. Rev. Genet. *13*:235, 1979.)

using small numbers of cells (Galjaard, 1982), while DNA analysis (discussed subsequently) is, in some cases, possible even without cell culture. Attempts at accelerating the proliferation of amniotic fluid cells have employed various growth factors (e.g., those derived from epidermis, fibroblasts, or cartilage) which have been observed to increase cell growth rates (Epstein, 1982). The use of growth factors has not yet been standardized for routine use; more research is expected.

The scope of possible prenatal diagnostic tests can be increased by exploiting the genetic information present in every amniotic fluid cell. In some cases, it is possible to activate these cells to express proteins they do not express normally, for example, to produce human liver-specific proteins by fusing human amniotic fluid cells with rodent hepatoma cells (Darlington, 1982). In an increasing number of other instances, one can analyze the gene content in amniotic fluid cells directly, using specific nucleic acid probes (Orkin et al., 1978; Kan and Dozy, 1978; Kurnit and Hoehn, 1979; Kurnit et al., 1982; Davies, 1981).

Recombinant DNA techniques are providing cloned sequences specific for human genes that can be used, together with restriction endonuclease digestion of amniotic fluid cell DNA followed by Southern blotting (Southern, 1975), to detect the presence (Orkin et al., 1978) of a sequence and the spacing of enzyme recognition sites in DNA around that sequence (Fig. 2–7). In unusual cases, one can identify gene mutations because of a change in the recognition site of a restriction endonuclease (Fig. 2–7A). Recently, Geever and coworkers have described the use of an enzyme (DdeI) that cleaves DNA at the site of the disease-related mutation (e.g., a glu→val codon change in the hemoglobin S mutation), permitting direct identification of a mutant allele. In a few cases, e.g. the sickle cell gene in individuals of West African descent, a change in one restriction endonuclease site is distant (5400 base pairs away) but closely linked in a mendelian sense to the altered allele (Kan and Dozy, 1978) (Fig. 2–7B). The presence of the sickle cell gene is then frequently associated with an increase in the size of the DNA fragment, produced in this case by HpaI digestion, containing the beta globin gene. Alternatively, probes can be chosen (Wyman and White, 1979) that give distinctive restriction digest hybridization patterns that can serve as linkage markers for nearby genes. In both cases, the utility of a particular nucleic acid probe cannot always be assumed, and parental DNA samples should first be analyzed to determine whether the condition in question can be detected (or excluded) by use of this probe (Kazazian et al., 1980; Phillips et al., 1980).

While only a small number of conditions can currently be ascertained prenatally using DNA probes, the scope of the approach is virtually limitless. The number of useful available probes is increasing, as is the number and heterozygosity of individual or clusters of known polymorphic restriction endonuclease digestion sites. The DNA required for an individual test at present can be obtained from fewer than 100,000 cells, an amount often present in uncultured amniotic fluid samples. Alternatively, cultured cells are used. The detection methodology is improving, and results of Southern blot analyses can theoretically be obtained a few days after isolation of the DNA sample. One can safely anticipate that, within the next 5 to 10 years, the number of conditions diagnosable prenatally using Southern blotting or related techniques will be comparable to or exceed that accessible by all other techniques.

Problems

Practical problems in prenatal diagnosis can occur in a number of areas. Technical difficulties include poor cell growth due to (1) improper container or sample handling, (2) mycoplasma infection, (3) a bloody sample, or (4) a predominance of epithelioid cells that grow poorly. Maternal cell contamination of amniotic fluid samples is another problem. Poor cell growth is evident within 2 weeks of sample receipt and necessitates a second amniotic fluid sample. Maternal cell contamination occurs in perhaps 2 to 3 per every 1000 cases (Milunsky, 1979), and, at an average frequency of abnormals of 2 per 100 tests, it will mask an abnormality in nearly 1 of every 10,000 cases. This could be avoided by comparing parental and fetal chromosome polymorphisms or reduced by analyzing amniotic fluid testosterone to detect male fetuses, which would decrease such errors by nearly 50 per cent (Menutti et al., 1977). The cost-effectiveness of these extra steps is uncertain.

Chromosomal mosaicism (or pseudomosaicism) is a complication that reinforces the need to examine multiple cells, preferably from different colonies, before arriving at a cytogenetic diagnosis. Analysis of cells as primary cultures of (presumptive) single colonies is invaluable in distinguishing pseudomosaicism, which occurs in a small percentage of cases, from true mosaicism, which is very rare (Peakman et al., 1979). Twin pregnancies constitute another obvious problem that is readily detectable by prenatal ultrasonographic examination.

Analysis of alpha-fetoprotein data can be confounded in a number of ways, which may, in spite of ancillary tests (e.g., ultrasonography, acetylcholinesterase analyses), lead to erroneous diagnosis. Fetal blood contamination can further complicate the picture. For example, AFP levels in fetal blood are 100 times those in amniotic fluid and often more than 10,000 times those in maternal serum. Amniotic fluid may contain fetal blood, and the release of minute amounts of fetal blood into the maternal circulation during amniocentesis can cause a small increase in maternal serum AFP. Both gross and immunologic detection of fetal hemoglobin can help one estimate such contamination, especially the levels found in amniotic fluid. Also, until recently, availability of reagents for AFP analysis was limited. As various laboratories begin performing AFP measurements, this problem may be replaced by one related to test variation due to lack of interlaboratory standardization.

As mentioned earlier, there are risks associated with acquisition of fetal material. Amniocentesis is associated with a small risk of iatrogenic abortion. Also, Rh-negative patients usually receive Rh-D immune globulin after the procedure (Golbus et al., 1979). Fetoscopy is more difficult than amniocentesis and also entails greater risk. Additional problems relate to laboratory management. Case loads are increasing, while available facilities and trained personnel are limited. Elective taps, performed in women younger than a set minimum maternal age (e.g., 35 years) and without specific indications other than anxiety, may prove difficult to accommodate.

A number of additional practical considerations are important in case management. AFP studies (especially those associated with maternal serum AFP screening) require careful patient counseling and clear-cut criteria regarding cytogenetic analysis. Ascertainment of indications for biochemical studies often requires a pre-tap interview. An intake interview must be conducted to avoid overlooking important secondary indications for specific tests. It is important to maintain close contact with the obstetrician to minimize delay if a repeat sampling is required. Care should be taken in the communication of test results. The family should indicate *prior* to the test whether they wish to be informed about fetal sex. Reports should be sent to the referring physician and to the genetic counseling clinic (if involved).

If the prenatal test results are normal, a laboratory might verbally communicate the information as soon as the result is known, following this with a formal report. It is then important, as a follow-up measure, to ascertain the condition of the child after birth. In contrast, if the prenatal test results are abnormal, one should consult the referring physician about the best means of communicating information to the patient. In some cases, such as those involving prenatal hydrocephalus (Birnholz and Frigoletto, 1981), treatment may be possible. In most others, however, the only form of intervention available is termination of pregnancy. Then it will be important to carry out pathologic, chromosomal, and/or biochemical (if relevant) studies on abortus tissue. Alternatively, if a pregnancy is not terminated, one should attempt to ascertain the condition of the child. In either case, it is important to communicate risk estimates for future pregnancies.

ACKNOWLEDGMENTS

Research in the author's laboratory is supported by funds from the N.I.H., the American Cancer Society, and the National Foundation March of Dimes. The advice of Dr. David Kurnit and other colleagues at Children's Hospital Medical Center and the Brigham and Women's Hospital, as well as the provision of illustrative material by Dr. Kurnit, Dr. Mary Sandstrom, Dr. James Haddow, and Dr. Jason Birnholz, is greatly appreciated.

REFERENCES

Alberman, E., Creasy, M., and Elliott, M.: Maternal factors associated with fetal chromosome anomalies in spontaneous abortions. Br. J. Obstet. Gynecol. *83*:621–627, 1976.

Alpha-fetoprotein: Maternal Serum Alpha-fetoprotein. Proceedings of a July 28–30, 1980 Conference held by the National Center for Health Care Technology and the Food and Drug Administration. Supt. of Documents, U.S. Govt. Printing Office, Washington, D.C., 20402.

Amniotic Fluid Cell Culture Training Manual. U.S. Dept. of Health and Human Services, Center for Disease Control, Atlanta, 1981.

Antenatal Diagnosis. NIH Publication No. 80-1973, 1979.

Benzie, R., Mahoney, M. J., Fairweather, D. V. I., Golbus, M., Hall, P. F., Perry, T., Philip, J., Rodeck, C. H., Scrimgeour, J. B., and Simpson, J. E.: Fetoscopy and fetal tissue sampling. *In* Hamerton, J. L., and Simpson, N. E. (Eds.): Prenatal Diagnosis. New York, John Wiley and Sons, 1980, pp. 29–33.

Birnholz, J. C., and Frigoletto, F. D.: Antenatal treatment of hydrocephalus. N. Engl. J. Med. *303*:1021–1023, 1981.

Botstein, D., White, R. L., Skolnick, M., and Davis, R. W.: Construction of a genetic linkage map in man using restriction fragment length polymorphisms. Am. J. Hum. Genet. *32*:314–331, 1980.

Brock, D. J. H.: Prenatal diagnosis of neural tube defects. Europ. J. Clin. Invest. *7*:465–472, 1977.

Brock, D. J. H.: *In* Steinberg, A. G., Bearn, A. G., Motulsky, A. G., and Childs, B. (Eds.): Progress in Medical Genetics. Vol. II. Philadelphia, W. B. Saunders Co., 1977, pp. 1–37.

Campbell, S., Griffin, D., Little, D., and Allan, L.: Use of ultrasound in the prenatal diagnosis of congenital disorders. *In* Latt, S., and Darlington, G. (Eds.): Prenatal Diagnosis: Cell Biological Aspects. Methods in Cell Biology. Vol. 26. New York, Academic Press, 1982, pp. 181–227.

Cavalli-Sforza, L., and Bodmer, W.: The Genetics of Human Populations. San Francisco, W. H. Freeman and Co., 1971.

CDC Amniotic Fluid Cell Culture Training Manual. 3rd ed. CDC, Atlanta, Georgia, 1981.

Cohen, A. J., Li, F. P., Berg, S., Marchetto, D. J., Tsai, S., Jacobs, S. C., and Brown, R. S.: Hereditary renal-cell carcinoma associated with a chromosomal translocation. N. Engl. J. Med. *301*:592–595, 1979.

Crandall, B. F., and Brazier, M. A. B. (Eds.): Prevention of Neural Tube Defects; The Role of Alpha-fetoprotein. New York, Academic Press, 1978.

Darlington, G. J.: Application of cell fusion techniques to induce amniotic fluid cells to express special functions. *In* Latt, S. A., and Darlington, G. Methods in Cell Biology. Vol. 26. New York, Academic Press, 1982.

Davies, K. E.: The application of DNA recombinant technology to the analysis of the human genome and genetic disease. Hum. Genet. *58*:351–357, 1981.

Emery, A. E. H.: Genetic counseling in X-linked muscular dystrophy. J. Neurol. Sci. *8*:579–587, 1969.

Epstein, C. J.: Uses of growth factors to accelerate amniotic fluid cell proliferation. *In* Latt, S., and Darlington, G. (Eds.): Prenatal Diagnosis: Cell Biological Aspects. Methods in Cell Biology. Vol. 26. New York, Academic Press, 1982, pp. 269–276.

Firshein, S. I., Hoyer, L. W., Sazarchick, J., Hobbins, J. C., Pitlick, F. A., Merkatz, I. R., and Mahoney, M. J.: Prenatal diagnosis of classic hemophilia. N. Engl. J. Med. *300*:937–941, 1979.

Galjaard, H.: Miniaturization of biochemical analysis of cultured (amniotic fluid) cells. *In* Latt, S., and Darlington, G. (Eds.): Prenatal Diagnosis: Cell Biological Aspects. Methods in Cell Biology. Vol. 26. New York, Academic Press, 1982, pp. 241–268.

Gastel, B., Haddow, J. E., Fletcher, J. C., and Neale, A. (Eds.): Maternal Serum Alpha-Fetoprotein. NCHCT Conference Proceedings. Supt. Documents, U.S. Govt. Printing Office, 1980, pp. 99–107.

Geever, R. F., Wilson, L. B., Nallaseth, F. S., Milner, P. F., Bittner, M., and Wilson, J. T.: Direct identification of sickle cell anemia by blot hybridization. Proc. Natl. Acad. Sci. U.S.A. 78:5081–5085, 1981.

Glover, T. W.: FUdR induction of the X chromosome fragile site: Evidence for the mechanism of folic acid and thymidine inhibition. Am. J. Hum. Genet. 33:234–242, 1981.

Golbus, M. S., Loughman, W. D., Epstein, C. J., Halbasch, G., Stephens, J. D., and Hall, B. D.: Prenatal genetic diagnosis in 3000 amniocenteses. N. Engl. J. Med. 300:157–163, 1979a.

Golbus, M. S., Stephens, J. D., Mahoney, M. J., Hobbins, J. C., Maselline, E. P., Caskey, C. T., and Banker, B. Q.: Failure of fetal creatine phosphokinase as a diagnostic indicator of Duchenne muscular dystrophy. N. Engl. J. Med. 300:860–861, 1979b.

Gosden, C., Brock, D. J. H., and Eason, P.: The origin of the rapidly adhering cells found in amniotic fluids from foetuses with neural tube defects. Clin. Genet. 12:193–201, 1972.

Gosden, C., Buckton, K., Fotheringham, Z., and Brock, D. J. H.: Prenatal fetal karyotyping and maternal serum alpha-fetoprotein screening. Br. Med. J. 282:255, 1981.

Grabowski, G. A., and Desnick, R. J.: Prenatal diagnosis of inherited metabolic diseases: principles, pitfalls, and prospects. In Latt, S., and Darlington, G. (Eds.): Prenatal Diagnosis: Cell Biological Aspects. Methods in Cell Biology. Vol. 26. New York, Academic Press, 1982, pp. 95–179.

Haddow, J. E., and Miller, W. A.: Prenatal diagnosis of open neural tube defects. In Latt, S., and Darlington, G. (Eds.): Prenatal Diagnosis: Cell Biological Aspects. Methods in Cell Biology. Vol. 26. New York, Academic Press, 1982, pp. 67–94.

Haddow, J. E., Morin, M. E., Holman, M. S., and Miller, W. A.: Acetylcholinesterase and fetal malformations: Modified qualitative technique for diagnosis of neural tube defects. Clin. Chem. 27:61–63, 1981.

Hamerton, J. L.: Chromosome disease. In Hamerton, J. L., and Simpson, N. E. (Eds.): Prenatal Diagnosis. New York, John Wiley and Sons, 1980, pp. 11–21.

Hamerton, J. L., and Simpson, N. E. (Eds.): Prenatal Diagnosis, Special Issue: Prenatal Diagnosis—Past, Present and Future. New York, J. Wiley, December, 1980.

Hamerton, J. L., and Simpson, N. E. (Eds.): Recommendations and conclusions. In Prenatal Diagnosis. New York, John Wiley and Sons, 1980, pp. 51–57.

Herzenberg, L. A., Bianchi, D. W., Schroder, J., Cann, H. M., and Iverson, G. M.: Fetal cells in the blood of pregnant women: Detection and enrichment by fluorescence-activated cell sorting. Proc. Natl. Acad. Sci. U.S.A. 76:1453–1455, 1979.

Hobbins, J. C., and Winsberg, F.: Ultrasonography in Obstetrics and Gynecology. Baltimore, Williams & Wilkins, Co., 1977.

Hobbins, J. C., Winsberg, F., Blanchett, M., Bennett, M., Boisvert, J., Hunter, A., Melancon, S., Miskin, M., and Whetham, J.: Fetal imaging. In Hamerton, J. L., and Simpson, N. E. (Eds.): Prenatal Diagnosis. New York, John Wiley and Sons, 1980, pp. 35–36.

Hoehn, H., and Salk, D.: Morphological and biochemical heterogeneity of amniotic fluid cells in culture. In Latt, S., and Darlington, G. (Eds.): Prenatal Diagnosis: Cell Biological Aspects. Methods in Cell Biology. Vol. 26. New York, Academic Press, 1982, pp. 12–34.

Holmes, L. B.: Genetic counseling for the older pregnant woman: new data and questions. N. Engl. J. Med. 298:1419–1421, 1978.

Hook, E. B.: Spontaneous deaths of fetuses with chromosomal abnormalities diagnosed prenatally. N. Engl. J. Med. 299:1036–1038, 1978.

Hook, E. B., and Hamerton, J.: The frequency of chromosome abnormalities detected in consecutive newborn studies—differences between studies—results by sex and by severity of phenotypic involvement. In Hook, E. B., and Porter, I. H. (Eds.):

Population Cytogenetics. New York, Academic Press, 1976, pp. 63–80.

Hook, E. B., and Lindsjö, A.: Down syndrome in live births by single year maternal age interval in a Swedish study: comparison with results from a New York State study. Am. J. Hum. Genet. 30:19–27, 1978.

Howard-Peebles, P. N., and Pryor, J. C.: Fragile sites in human chromosomes. I. The effect of methionine on the Xq fragile site. Clin. Genet. 19:228–232, 1981.

Iverson, G. M., Bianchi, D. W., Cann, H. M., and Herzenberg, L. A.: Detection and isolation of fetal cells from maternal blood using the fluorescence activated cell sorter (FACS). Prenatal Diagnosis. 1:61–73, 1980.

Kaback, M. M., Nathan, T. J., and Greenwald, S.: In Kaback, M. M., Rimoin, D. L., and O'Brien, J. S. (Eds.): Tay-Sachs Disease: Screening and Prevention. New York, Alan R. Liss, Inc., 1977a, pp. 13–36.

Kaback, M. M., Rimoin, D. L., and O'Brien, J. S.: In Kaback, M. M., Rimoin, D. L., and O'Brien, J. S. (Eds.): Tay-Sachs Disease: Screening and Prevention. New York, Alan R. Liss, Inc., 1977b.

Kaback, M. M.: In Callahan, J. W., and Lowden, J. A. (Eds.): Lysosomes and Lysosomal Storage Diseases. New York, Raven Press, 1981, pp. 331–342.

Kalter, H., and Warkany, J.: Congenital malformations: etiologic factors and their role in prevention. N. Engl. J. Med.: 308:424, 1983.

Kan, Y. W., and Dozy, A. M.: Antenatal diagnosis of sickle-cell anemia by DNA analysis of amniotic-fluid cells. Lancet 2:910–912, 1978.

Kazazian, H. H., Phillips, J. A., Boehm, C. D., Vik, T. A., Mahoney, M. J., and Ritchey, A. K.: Prenatal diagnosis of β-thalassemias by amniocentesis: linkage analysis using multiple polymorphic restriction endonuclease sites. Blood 56:926–930, 1980.

King, B., Spikesman, A., and Emery, A. E. H.: The effect of pregnancy on serum levels of creatine kinase. Clin. Chem. Acta 36:267–269, 1972.

Kleijer, W. J., Patrick, A. D., Aula, P., Berg, K., Goldman, H., Manutti, M. M., and Potier, M.: Metabolic disorders. In Hamerton, J. L., and Simpson, N. E. (Eds.): Prenatal Diagnosis. New York, John Wiley and Sons, 1980, pp. 39–42.

Klein, H. G., Aledort, L. M., Bouma, B. N., Hoyer, L. W., Zimmerman, T. S., and DeMets, D. L.: A co-operative study for the detection of the carrier state of classic hemophilia. N. Engl. J. Med. 296:959–962, 1977.

Knudson, A. G., Meadows, A. T., Nichols, W. W., and Hill, R.: Chromosomal deletion and retinoblastoma. N. Engl. J. Med. 295: 1120–1123, 1976.

Kurnit, D., and Hoehn, H.: Prenatal diagnosis of human genome variation. Ann. Rev. Genet. 13:235–258, 1979.

Kurnit, D., Orkin, S., and White, R.: Prenatal analysis of human DNA sequence variation. Methods in Cell Biology. Vol. 26. New York, Academic Press, 1980.

Latt, S., and Darlington, G. (Eds.): Prenatal Diagnosis. Cell Biological Aspects. Methods in Cell Biology. Vol. 26. New York, Academic Press, 1982.

Layde, P. M., von Allmen, S. D., and Oakley, G. P., Jr.: Maternal serum alpha-fetoprotein screening—a cost benefit analysis. Am. J. Pub. Health 69:566, 1979.

Lubs, H. A.: A marker X chromosome. Am. J. Hum. Genet. 21:231–244, 1969.

Magenis, R. E., Overton, K. M., Chamberlin, J., Brady, T., and Lovrien, E.: Parental origin of the extra chromosome in Down's syndrome. Hum. Genet. 37:7–16, 1977.

Mahoney, M. J.: Fetoscopy. In Latt, S., and Darlington, G. (Eds.): Prenatal Diagnosis: Cell Biological Aspects. Methods in Cell Biology. Vol. 26. New York, Academic Press, 1982, pp. 229–240.

Mahoney, M. J., and Hobbins, J. C.: Fetoscopy and fetal blood sampling. In Milunsky, A. (Ed.): Genetic Disorders and the Fetus. New York, Plenum Press, 1979.

McKusick, V. M.: Mendelian Inheritance in Man. 5th ed. Baltimore, Johns Hopkins University Press, 1978.

Menutti, M. T., Wu, C. H., Mellman, W. H., and Mikhail, G.: Amniotic fluid testosterone and follicle stimulating hormone levels as indicators of fetal sex during mid-pregnancy. Am. J. Med. Genet. 1:211–216, 1977.

Mibashan, R. S., Rodeck, C. H., Thumpston, J. K., Edwards, R. J., Singer, J. D., White, J. M., and Campbell, S.: Plasma assay of fetal factors VIIIC and IX for prenatal diagnosis of haemophilia. Lancet 1:1309–1311, 1979.

Mikkelsen, M., Hallberg, A., and Poulsen, H.: Maternal and paternal origin of extra chromosome in trisomy 21. Hum. Genet. 32:17–21, 1970.

Mikkelsen, M., and Stene, J.: Previous child with Down-syndrome and other chromosome aberration. In Murken, J. D., Stengel-Rutkowski, S., and Schwinger, E. (Eds.): Prenatal Diagnosis. Stuttgart, F. Enke, 1979, pp. 22–29.

Milunsky, A.: Antenatal diagnosis of genetic disorders. In Schaffer, A. J., and Avery, M. E. (Eds.): Diseases of the Newborn. 4th ed. Philadelphia, W. B. Saunders Co., 1974.

Milunsky, A.: Genetic Disorders and the Fetus. New York, Plenum Press, 1979.

Newburger, P. E., Cohen, H. J., Rothchild, S. B., Hobbins, J. C., Malawista, S. C., and Mahoney, M. J.: Prenatal diagnosis of chronic granulomatous disease. N. Engl. J. Med. 300:178–181, 1979.

Omenn, G. S.: Prenatal diagnosis of genetic disorders. Science 200:952–958, 1978.

Omenn, G. S., Hall, J. G., Graham, C. B., and Karp, L. E.: The use of radiographic visualization for the prenatal diagnosis. Birth Defects Original Article Series XII. 217:229, 1977.

Orkin, S. H., Alter, B. P., Altay, C., Mahoney, M. J., Lazarus, H., Hobbins, J. C., and Nathan, D. G.: Endonuclease mapping to detect globin-gene deletion in prenatal diagnosis of thalassemias. N. Engl. J. Med. 299:166–177, 1978.

Orkin, S. H., and Nathan, D. G.: The molecular genetics of thalassemia. In Harris, H., and Hirschhorn, K. (Eds.): Advances in Human Genetics. Vol. 2. New York, Plenum Press, 1981.

Parks, D. R., and Herzenberg, L. A.: Fetal cells from maternal blood: their selection and prospects for use in prenatal diagnosis. In Latt, S., and Darlington, G. (Eds.): Prenatal Diagnosis: Cell Biological Aspects. Methods in Cell Biology. Vol. 26. New York, Academic Press, 1982, pp. 278–295.

Peakman, D. C., Moreton, M. F., Corn, B. J., and Robinson, A.: Chromosomal mosaicism in amniotic fluid cell cultures. Am. J. Hum. Genet. 31:149–155, 1979.

Phillips, J. A., Panny, S. R., Kazazian, H. H., Boehm, C. D., Scott, A. F., and Smith, K. D.: Prenatal diagnosis of sickle cell anemia by restriction endonuclease analysis: HindIII polymorphisms in γ-globin genes extend test applicability. Proc. Natl. Acad. Sci. U.S.A. 77:2853–2856, 1980.

Polani, P. E., Alberman, E., Alexander, B. J., Benson, P. F., Berry, A. C., Blunt, S., Daker, M. G., Fensom, A. H., Garrett, D. M., McGuire, V. M., Roberts, J. A., Seller, M. J., Singer, J. D.: Sixteen years experience of counselling, diagnosis, and prenatal detection in one genetic centre: Progress, results, and problems. J. Med. Genet. 16:166–175, 1979.

Renpenning, H., Gerrard, J. W., Zaleski, W. A., and Tabata, T.: Familial sex-linked mental retardation. Canad. Med. Assoc. J. 87:954, 1962.

Riccardi, V. M., Sujansky, E., Smith, A. C., and Francke, U.: Chromosomal imbalance in the aniridia-Wilms' tumor association: 11 p interstitial deletion. Pediatrics 61:604–610, 1978.

Sandstrom, M. M., Beauchesne, M. T., Gustashaw, K. M., and Latt, S. A.: Prenatal cytogenetic diagnosis. In Latt, S., and Darlington, G. (Eds.): Prenatal Diagnosis: Cell Biological Aspects. Methods in Cell Biology. Vol. 26. New York, Academic Press, 1982, pp. 35–66.

Simpson, N. E., Turnbull, A. C., Alexander, D., et al.: Genetic amniocentesis. In Hamerton, J. L., and Simpson, N. E. (Eds.): Prenatal Diagnosis. New York, John Wiley and Sons, 1980, pp. 4–10.

Smithells, R. W., Sheppard, S., and Scorach, C. J.: Possible prevention of neural tube defects by preconceptional vitamin supplementation. Lancet 1:339–340, 1980 (addendum p. 647).

Southern, E. M.: Detection of specific sequences among DNA fragments separated by gel electrophoresis. J. Mol. Biol. 98:503–517, 1975.

Stephenson, S., and Weaver, D: Prenatal diagnosis—a compilation of diagnosed conditions. Am. J. Obstet. Gynecol. 141:319, 1981.

Sutherland, G. R.: Heritable fragile sites on human chromosomes. I. Factors affecting expression in lymphocyte culture. Am. J. Hum. Genet. 31:125–135, 1979.

Wald, N. J., and Cuckle, H. S.: Amniotic-fluid alpha-fetoprotein measurement in antenatal diagnosis of anencephaly and open spina bifida in early pregnancy. Second Report of the U.K. Collaborative Study on Alpha-Fetoprotein in Relation to Neural-Tube Defects. Lancet 2:651–662, 1979.

Ward, R. H., Fairweather, D. V., Whyley, G. A., et al.: Four years experience of maternal alpha-fetoprotein screening and its effect on the pattern of antenatal care. Prenatal Diagnosis 1:91–101, 1981.

Wyman, A. R., and White, R.: A highly polymorphic locus in human DNA. Proc. Natl. Acad. Sci. U.S.A. 77:6754–6758, 1980.

Zackai, E. H., Spielman, R. S., Mellman, W. J., Ames, M., and Bodurtha, J.: The risk of neural tube defects to first cousins of affected individuals. In Crandall, B. F., and Brazier, M. A. B. (Eds.): Prevention of Neural Tube Defects. New York, Academic Press, 1978, pp. 99–102.

3

Assessment of Fetal Risk in the Third Trimester

The working relationship between obstetricians and pediatricians continues to grow closer because of new technologies that permit more precise evaluation of fetal growth and well-being. The optimal timing of delivery requires knowledge of the relative risks of prolonged pregnancy versus the outlook for a prematurely delivered infant. Some of the currently available tests are listed in Table 3–1.

Ultrasonographic Assessment of the Fetus

In the second trimester, the fetus can be visualized with ultrasonography (resolution ±2 mm). Tubal pregnancies, molar pregnancies, multiple births,

Table 3–1.   Fetal Assessment

First and second trimester
  Amniotic fluid and cells
  Maternal and fetal blood

Third trimester
  Nonstress, stress tests
  Maternal estriol
  Amniotic fluid phospholipids and bilirubin

Perinatal period
  Continuous fetal heart rate monitoring
  Fetal scalp pH
  Fetal transcutaneous O_2
  Cord blood gases

Throughout pregnancy
  History and physical examination, maternal antibody testing,
    serology, blood pressure, urinalysis, hematocrit
  Dating (last menstrual period, first heart sounds, quickening,
    uterine growth)
  Radiography (fetal anomalies, pelvimetry)
  Ultrasonography (anomalies, growth, function)

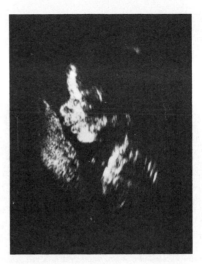

Figure 3–1. Ultrasonographic examination of a 32-week fetus. Note detail of face and thorax. (Courtesy of Drs. Farrell and Birnholz.)

major malformations, and fetal viability can be readily assessed. By 18 to 20 weeks, ultrasonographic examination can provide a complete assessment of fetal size (and of fetal growth with repeat exams), presence or absence of major anomalies, and fetal condition (Table 3–2).

Ultrasonographic examination is important before 20 weeks of pregnancy because it allows for termination of pregnancy if major malformations are detected, and it provides an early point against which fetal growth can be compared.

Ultrasonography for assessment of fetal size and condition and of presence or absence of malforma-

tions becomes simpler as the fetus grows during the third trimester. Resolution of even the lens of the fetal eyes and heart chambers is possible (Figs. 3–1 to 3–3). Instruments can now provide continuous imaging at 30 frames/sec and allow evaluation of fetal respiratory and other movements (Birnholz, 1981).

Gestational age can usually be estimated by ultrasonographic assessment of fetal size before 20 weeks. Thereafter, serial measurements reflect fetal growth and permit an indirect evaluation of the adequacy of the placenta.

Fetal weight can be estimated ultrasonographically with precision, as verified by 132 cases studied within hours of delivery. The birth weights ranged from 500

Table 3–2.   Fetal Abnormalities Diagnosed by Ultrasonography

Hydrocephaly, hydranencephaly, anencephaly,
  myelomeningocele

Conjoined twins

Fetal heart structural abnormalities

Heart rate abnormalities (tachycardia, bradycardia)

Upper gastrointestinal obstruction

Fetal death

Ascites/hydrops

Omphalocele

Diaphragmatic hernia

Multicystic kidneys

Urinary obstruction

Renal agenesis

Skeletal dysplasias (e.g., thanatophoric dwarfism,
  achondroplasia)

Placenta previa, abruptio placentae

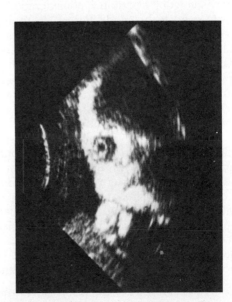

Figure 3–2. Ultrasonographic appearance of a 28-week fetus. Note the large eye with the open eyelid. (Courtesy of Drs. Farrell and Birnholz.)

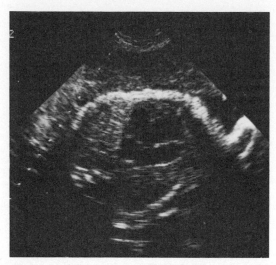

Figure 3–3. Transverse thoracic ultrasonographic view of a 31-week fetus, with the four cardiac chambers clearly visible. (Courtesy of Dr. J. Birnholz.)

Table 3–3. Ultrasonographic Assessment of the Fetus

I. *Size and growth*
    A. Increment since last exam and comparison with obstetric estimate of length of gestation

II. *Physical examination*
    A. UTERUS
        1. Fibroids
        2. Amniotic fluid
        3. Bifid uterus
    B. PLACENTA
        1. Previa
        2. Abruptio
        3. Size
    C. FETUS
        1. Malformations and anatomy (CNS, spine, heart, gut, chest, kidneys, limbs, bladder, skeleton)
        2. Sex, fetal genitalia
        3. Multiple fetuses

III. *Condition*
    A. Limb movements
    B. Heart rate, and reactivity
    C. Eye movements
    D. Swallowing
    E. Respiratory-like movements/diaphragm movement
    F. Amniotic fluid volume
    G. Bladder emptying

to 4000 gm. Correlation coefficient of ultrasonographic estimate with actual birth weight was 0.992, and the standard error was 112 gm. The following formula was used to determine fetal weight:*

Fetal weight (gm)

$$= \frac{0.34255 \, BD^2 \, OFD}{1000} + \frac{2.7093 \, AD^3}{1000} + 156.75$$

Underestimates may occur with oligohydramnios or with macrosomic infants of diabetic mothers, for whom correction factors can be applied.

Diagnosis of anomalies is no doubt easier as fetal size increases, but if abortion is considered, these assessments need to be made before 20 weeks. The onset of some anomalies (e.g., some cases of hydrocephalus) may occur after this time. Evaluation of fetal condition is one of the newest uses of ultrasonography. Limb, eye, or diaphragm movements can be visualized and quantified for their spontaneous occurrence rate or in response to pressure, sound, light, or changes in fetal chemical/hormonal milieu. Associations between movements may be useful; for example, respiratory-like movements without rapid fetal eye movements before 33 weeks may imply fetal central nervous system dysfunction (Birnholz, 1981). A complete ultrasonographic examination is thought to be free of risk to mother and infant and takes approximately 10 minutes. A complete examination is outlined in Table 3–3.

Birnholz has described the development of fetal eye movements in human fetuses, using ultrasonographic visualization. During a 3-minute study period with ultrasonography, Birnholz found that fetal rapid eye movements increase in frequency after 24 weeks. Eye inactivity associated with rhythmic diaphragm movements analogous to postnatal "quiet sleep" was normally seen only after 36 weeks, although two infants, perhaps with precocious central nervous system maturation, demonstrated this finding at earlier weeks of gestation.

Shalev and coworkers report that fetal sex could be determined in 352 of 369 singleton pregnancies after 20 weeks' gestation (95 per cent) and in 24 fetuses of 12 twin pregnancies. Male sex was diagnosed correctly in 186 of 186 singleton pregnancies, and female sex was correctly diagnosed in 163 of 168 pregnancies. All twins were assigned correctly.

DeVore and associates visualized dilatation of the umbilical vein in erythroblastosis by fetal ultrasonography before fetal ascites or elevated optical density measurements on amniotic fluid were present. They suggest that the mechanism is reduction of umbilical venous return due to compression of vessels within the enlarging fetal liver. This finding may help identify those who may need fetal transfusion.

Because of the wealth of information obtained, the negligible rate of "false-positives," the safety, and the relatively modest cost, it is our view that it will soon become reasonable for women with known risk factors to be ultrasonographically assessed at 18 to 20 weeks and again at 30 to 32 weeks as part of routine perinatal care. Eventually, all prenatal visits may include ultrasonographic studies of the fetus as a normal part of the pregnancy evaluation.

With these tools, the obstetrician should be able to

---

* BD = cranial biparietal diameter (mm); OFD = cranial occipitofrontal diameter (mm); AD = average anteroposterior and transverse abdominal diameter (mm) (Birnholz, 1980).

obtain reasonable knowledge about fetal anatomy and gestational age as the pregnancy enters the third trimester, at which stage the major risk to the fetus is premature birth. The combined obstetric/pediatric approach to this problem is discussed in Chapter 8. Other useful tests available to the obstetrician for evaluating the third trimester fetus are listed in Table 3–1.

Maternal Estriol Excretion

The production and excretion of estrogens requires integrity of the fetal-placental unit. Cholesterol from the mother serves as a source for placental production of progesterone and pregnenolone. Pregnenolone is sulfated by fetal tissues and serves as substrate for dehydroepiandrosterone sulfate (DHEA-S) synthesis by the fetal adrenal. In the placenta, DHEA-S from the fetus and DHEA and DHEA-S from the mother are desulfurated and aromatized into estrone and estradiol. Most fetal DHEA-S is hydroxylated in the fetal liver, and this hormone, when aromatized in the placenta, is converted to estriol, which is the predominant estrogen excreted by pregnant women in the third trimester. Estrogen is an important trophic hormone for the uterus and has complex interactions with progesterone for both implantation and maintenance of pregnancy. It is useful as a marker for fetal/placental well-being in the last trimester and has particular value in pregnancies complicated by preeclampsia, intrauterine fetal growth retardation, and prolonged gestation (Table 3–4).

A variety of reasons may explain decreasing maternal estriol excretion. With diminished placental or fetal (liver and/or adrenal) function, estriol production (and maternal excretion) is reduced. Placental size correlates to some degree with estriol production, and, partly for this reason, the fetus of the diabetic mother or the fetus with erythroblastosis (both having relatively large placentas) may be in jeopardy despite normal maternal estriol. With maternal antibiotics altered gut flora may allow decreased reabsorption of estriol and decreased urinary excretion and plasma levels on this basis. Any decrease in fetal adrenal function (diminished ACTH as in anencephaly, or with exogenous glucocorticoids) would decrease substrate (DHEA-S) for maternal estriol.

Measurements of either urinary or plasma estriol

Table 3–4. Causes of Low or Falling Maternal Urinary Estriol Excretion

1. Uteroplacental insufficiency, nonacute.
2. Maternal renal or liver disease.
3. Maternal drugs: ampicillin, neomycin, methenamine mandelate, corticosteroids.
4. Small fetus for gestational age.
5. Fetal adrenal dysfunction: primary hypoplasia; secondary hypoplasia (anencephaly)
6. Placental aromatase or sulfatase deficiency (rare).
7. Errors in pregnancy dating, urine collection, lab measurements.

Table 3–5. Indications for Nonstress/Stress Testing of Fetus

Postmaturity
Intrauterine growth retardation
Decreased fetal movement
Preeclampsia/chronic hypertension
Diabetes mellitus
Premature rupture of membranes/premature labor
Rhesus sensitization
Hydramnios

are used in different centers. Either appears useful, but each has its individual disadvantages. Despite suggestions for many other hormonal tests by which placental/fetal function can be assessed, measurement of estrogen synthesis and secretion remains most useful.

Fetal Heart Rate Monitoring Prior to Labor: Stress and Nonstress Tests

If there are questions about fetal/placental integrity, this form of fetal assessment is indicated. Usual indications include preeclampsia, fetal growth retardation, prolonged pregnancy, and maternal disease (e.g., heart, renal, pulmonary, or diabetes). The nonstress test measures average fetal heart rate (indicated by abdominal ultrasonography) after fetal movements are discerned by the mother. Normally, an increase of 15 or more beats per minute occurs for a few seconds after each movement. At least four of these fetal accelerations should be noted in a 20-minute period. Negative results may occur if the fetus is in quiet sleep or if the mother's blood sugar is low. If no fetal heart rate accelerations occur, the test is called nonreactive, or abnormal (Table 3–5).

If abnormal, the nonstress test may be immediately followed by a *stress test*, the oxytocin challenge test, in which intravenous oxytocin is infused into the mother in order to induce mild uterine contractions (i.e., "stress" the fetus). A normal test would show fetal heart rate accelerations or early decelerations associated with contractions. An abnormal test results in late decelerations (Fig. 3–4).

Fetal Heart Rate Monitoring During Labor

The usefulness of this procedure is based on the fact that fetal asphyxia is regularly followed by fetal heart rate abnormalities. Fetal heart rate may be measured by abdominal phonocardiogram, electrocardiogram, ultrasonography, or auscultation. We prefer ultrasonography because it provides some measure of fetal heart rate, fetal heart rate variability, and uterine contractions. After rupture of membranes, clearer signals may be obtained with an intrauterine pressure probe and a fetal scalp EKG. The latter technique offers information about intensity of contractions and indicates whether uterine hypertonicity may be present, information that is not obtainable with external monitoring (Freeman and Goute, 1981).

Normally, fetal heart rate (FHR) is 120 to 160 beats/min, with marked tachycardia in the range of 180 and marked bradycardia about 100 or less. Tachycardia may be associated with fever, immaturity, asphyxia, and betamimetic and anticholinergic drug administration. Bradycardia is usually associated with more severe asphyxia, but in mild cases it may be an effect of adrenergic blockers.

Fetal heart rate variability ("short term variability") is graded absent or minimal (0 to 5 beats/min) or normal (6 to 25 beats/min). Variability may be eliminated after administration of anticholinergics and tranquillizers (diazepam) and correction of fetal asphyxia or reduced with sedatives and narcotics.

Periodic fetal heart rate patterns are classified as "early," "late," and "variable" (Fig. 3–4).

Early decelerations are benign and represent fetal cardiac slowing mediated by the vagus in response to fetal head compression from uterine contractions. Maternal atropine blocks early fetal heart rate decelerations. Late decelerations are ominous and often associated with fetal asphyxia related to uterine contractions.

When asphyxia is sufficient to be associated with fetal acidemia, then late decelerations are thought to be due to myocardial depression. In less severe cases, decreased oxygen to the fetus may trigger an adrenergic response related to a rise in systemic blood pressure associated with parasympathetic (vagal) heart rate slowing. In a sense, late decelerations are directly analogous to bradycardia in the infant with severe apneic spells. Decelerations that are variable in shape and in relation to uterine contractions are thought to reflect umbilical cord compression. The mechanisms whereby cord compression can cause heart rate slowing include myocardial depression and vagal effects.

If labor is progressing in association with severe repetitive late or variable decelerations, an appropriate response is to administer oxygen to the mother, stop uterine stimulants (oxytocin) if any are being administered, reposition the mother to decompress the abdominal aorta and vena cava, correct hypotension if present, and then consider a fetal scalp pH measurement or immediate delivery if the situation is not corrected.

Much controversy surrounds the use of continuous electronic fetal heart rate monitoring, particularly in normal pregnancies. Critics argue that only 25 per cent of fetal heart rate abnormalities are associated with abnormal fetal outcome and that use of this form of monitoring leads to unnecessary cesarean sections. Lay critics argue that this form of monitoring represents costly and unnecessary biomedical technologic invasiveness urged on women without due regard for their feelings by an unsympathetic medical establishment. Our view is that perinatal asphyxia should be minimized and that any means by which doctors, nurses, and mothers can work together comfortably to this end should be supported wholeheartedly (Wood et al., 1981; Haverkamp et al., 1976; Schifrin

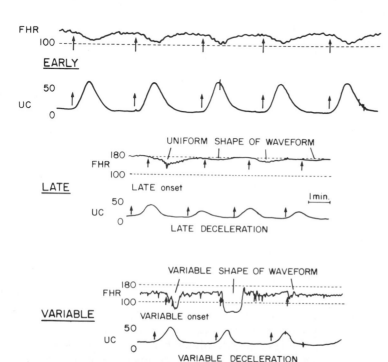

Figure 3–4. Early, late, and variable average fetal heart rate responses are recorded on the ordinate, with time on the abscissa. Uterine contractions (mm Hg) are shown in relation to the heart rate changes. (FHR = fetal heart rate. UC = intrauterine pressure.)

et al., 1979). The most recent review available supports electronic fetal heart rate monitoring for all high-risk patients and urges that it be available to all low-risk patients who desire it. This report offers such stringent ground rules for fetal heart rate monitoring by auscultation that we feel most obstetricians would find electronic monitoring easier and more reliable.

Fetal Scalp pH

Saling first introduced this technique in 1962, and subsequent extensive experience has confirmed its usefulness. With the mother in lateral Sims' position, an endoscope is placed through the cervix on the fetal scalp. After cleansing and application of silicone, a 2 mm incision is made just before a contraction, and capillary blood is drawn into a heparinized tube by gravity. Normal values are as follows: pH $\approx$ 7.25; $PO_2 \approx 18$; $PCO_2 \approx 45$. Rarely, abnormal values may reflect maternal values, a possibility that can be verified by assessment of maternal blood gases. Fetal scalp blood gases and pH are usually evaluated when heart rate monitoring indicates possible asphyxia.

COMPLICATIONS

In rare cases (i.e., in approximately 4 per cent of monitored patients), bleeding or infection can result with internal monitoring and scalp blood collection. We would recommend immediate postnatal scalp inspection and cleansing, if these procedures are used, in such a situation. Maternal herpes infection is a contraindication.

Assessment of Fetal Lung Maturity

Adams, Nelson, Ogawa, and Gluck were the first to suggest that amniotic fluid phospholipids might indicate the ability of the fetal lung to produce surfactant. In 1971, Gluck and colleagues demonstrated that assessment of amniotic fluid phospholipids allowed prediction of risk of respiratory distress syndrome. Various considerations of this subject have been published during the last 10 years. These tests are most useful between 28 and 35 weeks' gestation, since before that time risk of RDS is roughly more than 60 per cent, and after that time less than 12 per cent, at least for women without systemic illness (e.g., preeclampsia and diabetes). With the use of increasingly effective tocolytic agents and glucocorticoids, perinatologists are able to respond to the fetus defined as high-risk on the basis of amniotic fluid phospholipid tests.

The overall complication rate for third trimester amniocentesis, used to obtain amniotic fluid for phospholipid analysis, is about 5 per cent. Induction of labor, fetal or maternal bleeding, fetal injury, placental damage, and rupture of membranes are the most common complications. In 6 of 146 patients in whom

fetal heart rate was monitored after amniocentesis, severe bradycardia or another severe fetal heart rate abnormality appeared within 2 hours of the amniocentesis. All infants were delivered by cesarean section. One of the infants with bradycardia was normal, and at birth the other was in shock due to an umbilical cord hematoma. The other four cases of fetal jeopardy included two cases of premature labor and two of abruptio placentae. In this series, therefore, serious fetal risk following amniocentesis was 4 per cent, and all the fetuses with complications associated with amniocentesis could be diagnosed with fetal heart rate monitoring and managed so that no fetal or neonatal deaths occurred (Klein et al., 1981).

Current Tests for Fetal Surfactant Lipids in Amniotic Fluid

Direct evidence that fetal lung surfactant lipids flow into the amniotic cavity is provided by the microscopic demonstration of lamellar bodies in amniotic fluid (Lee et al., 1980). These are identical with the storage forms of pulmonary surfactant seen in alveoli and alveolar lining cells. Gluck hypothesized that measurement of surfactant lipid in amniotic fluid would allow assessment of risk of hyaline membrane disease should the fetus be delivered soon after amniotic fluid testing. In the years since those observations, discussion has focused on ways of improving the sensitivity and specificity of the test, particularly when amniotic fluid may be contaminated or when it is obtained from women with diabetes. Currently, the lecithin/sphingomyelin ratio is the major test used in most delivery hospitals in North America. A ratio of greater than 2:1, except in diabetic pregnancies, indicates adequate amounts of surfactant. In diabetic pregnancies, for reasons that remain unclear, respiratory distress syndrome may occur when the L/S ratio is above the usual "mature" value. The disadvantages of the L/S ratio are that it requires about 2 hours to perform, may not be available on a 24-hour basis, and is unreliable when blood or excess mucus is present. Direct assay of saturated phosphatidyl choline (SPC) improves the specificity of the test and is preferred in our laboratory (Torday et al., 1979). Measurement of phosphatidyl glycerol and phosphatidyl inositol in addition to phosphatidyl choline has proved useful for Hallman and coworkers, as discussed in their 1976 report.

A simplified assay for surfactant activity in amniotic fluid was proposed by Clements and colleagues in 1972. They called their test of foam stability the "shake test" and showed that it was a good screening test, although for many obstetricians it has been less dependable than the L/S ratio. The test requires addition of 1 ml of ethanol/water (95/5 by volume) to exactly 1 ml of amniotic liquid. The ethanol inhibits

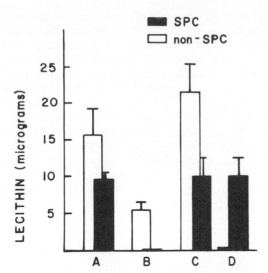

Figure 3–5. *A,* Amniotic fluid contains saturated (SPC) and unsaturated lecithin (non-SPC) in about equal amounts. Only the saturated lecithin is thought to originate as a constituent of fetal lung surfactant. *B,* Meconium and blood, which commonly contaminate amniotic fluid specimens, contain little SPC. *C,* Amniotic fluid (*A*) and contaminant (*B*) have been added together. Note that non-SPC is increased but not SPC. *D,* Amniotic fluid mixed with contaminant (*C*) has been assayed for SPC. Note that this measurement is unaffected by contaminants in amniotic fluid. (Lecithin is the same as phosphatidylcholine.) (Data from Torday, J., et al.: N. Engl. J. Med. *301:*1013, 1979.)

foam formation by constituents other than surface-active phospholipids. Serial dilution in test tubes provides a crude index of the amount of surfactant that is based on the persistence of a ring of stable bubbles at the air-liquid interface.

A modification of Clements' shake test, proposed by Sher and coworkers in 1981, has proved very reliable. Their quantitative foam stability index test required centrifugation of amniotic fluid at 1000 g for 3 minutes. The supernatant was decanted and added to different amounts of 95 per cent ethanol to produce final ethanol fractions between 0.42 and 0.55. The mixture was shaken for 30 seconds, allowed to settle for 15 seconds, and evaluated for an uninterrupted ring of foam at the meniscus. They found no cases of hyaline membrane disease when the index was above 0.48.

CASE 1–1

This infant was born to a 34-year-old mother with preeclampsia. This was her first pregnancy. She was admitted after a normal pregnancy at an estimated 29 weeks of gestation because of hypertension and mild edema. Maternal blood pressure was refractory to bed-rest and an antihypertensive medication. Maternal urinary estriols dropped over the course of 4 days from 5.2 to 1.5 mg for 24 hours. Ultrasonography revealed a fetus of approximately 700 gm without anomalies. An amniocentesis revealed amniotic fluid with an L/S ratio of 1.5 : 1 and a saturated phosphatidylcholine of 215 μg/ dl, which suggest lung immaturity and surfactant deficiency. Because of poor fetal growth and the declining estriols, the mother was given a 48-hour course of dexamethasone phosphate (24 mg total) and was delivered by cesarean section. The infant was a girl with Apgar scores of 6 and 8 and by Dubowitz examination was estimated to be 29 weeks' gestation. The birth weight was 720 gm and the head circumference 23.5 cm, both of which were below the tenth percentile for that gestation. The baby sustained good respirations during the first 2 hours after birth, but because Pa_{CO_2} rose from 40 to 45 torr, the baby was intubated and ventilated. Chest radiograph revealed a normal heart and reticulogranular densities consistent with hyaline membrane disease. The baby was ventilated for 6 days with low rates and pressures and ambient oxygen. During that time, results of several ultrasonographic examinations of heart and head were normal. Thereafter, the hospital course was marked by apnea treated with theophylline, bilirubin that peaked at a total of 6 mg per 100 ml and that was treated with phototherapy, and several episodes of possible necrotizing enterocolitis or sepsis or both that were treated for 3 days with antibiotics, with the signs of infection abating rapidly. Evaluation for other causes of fetal growth retardation was unremarkable, and poor growth was therefore attributed to placental insufficiency associated with preeclampsia. The infant grew according to predicted growth curves, with a weight of 900 gm at 1 month of age and 1500 gm at an approximate age of 2½ months.

This case illustrates the use of ultrasonography, urinary estriol excretion, and amniocentesis as well as prenatal glucocorticoids in a very low birth weight infant with a successful outcome.

REFERENCES

Adams, J., and Fujiwara, T.: Surfactant in fetal lamb tracheal fluid. J. Pediatr. *63:*537, 1963.

Barrett, J., Salzer, S., and Boehm, F.: The non-stress test: an evaluation of 1000 patients. Am. J. Obstet. Gynecol. *141:*153, 1981.

Birnholz, J. C.: Electronic Fetal Monitoring. AMA Council on Scientific Affairs. J.A.M.A. *246:*2370, 1981.

Birnholz, J. C.: The development of human fetal eye movement patterns. Science *213:*679, 1981.

Birnholz, J. C.: Ultrasound characteristics of fetal growth. Ultrasonic Imaging *2:*135, 1980.

Buster, J., Freeman, A., and Hobel, C.: An algorithm for determining gestational age from unconjugated estriol levels. Obstet. Gynecol. *56:*649, 1980.

Caldeyro-Garcia, R., Mendez-Bauer, C., Poseiro, J., et al.: Control of the human fetal heart rate during labor. *In* Cassels, D. (Ed.): The Heart and Circulation in the Newborn Infant. New York, Grune & Stratton, 1966.

Clements, J., Platzker, A., Tierney, D., Hobel, C., et al.: Assessment of the risk of the respiratory distress syndrome by a rapid test for surfactant in amniotic fluid. N. Engl. J. Med. *286:*1077, 1972.

Coyle, M., and Brown, J.: Urinary excretion of oestriol during pregnancy. II. Results in normal and abnormal pregnancies. J. Obstet. Gynaec. Brit. Comm. *70:*225, 1963.

DeVore, G., Mayden, K., Tortora, M., et al.: Dilatation of the fetal umbilical vein in rhesus hemolytic anemia: a predictor of severe disease. Am. J. Obstet. Gynecol. 141:464, 1981.

Evertson, L., Gauthier, R., Schifrin, B., et al.: Antepartum fetal heart testing. I. Evolution of the non-stress test. Am. J. Obstet. Gynecol. 133:29, 1979.

Freeman, R., and Goute, T.: Fetal Heart Rate Monitoring. Baltimore, Williams & Wilkins, 1981.

Freer, D., and Statland, B.: Measurement of amniotic fluid surfactant. Clin. Chem. 27:1629, 1981.

Gluck, L., Kulovich, M., Borer, M., et al.: Diagnosis of RDS by amniocentesis. Am. J. Obstet. Gynecol. 109:440, 1971.

Hallman, M., Kulovich, M., Kirkpatrick, E., et al.: Phosphatidyl-inositol and phosphatidyl glycerol in amniotic fluid: Indices of lung maturity. Am. J. Obstet. Gynecol. 125:613, 1976.

Haverkamp, A., Thompson, H., McFee, J., et al.: The evaluation of continuous fetal heart rate monitoring in high risk pregnancy. Am. J. Obstet. Gynecol. 125:310, 1976.

Klein, S., Young, B., Wilson, S., et al.: Continuous fetal heart rate monitoring following third trimester amniocentesis. Obstet. Gynecol. 58:444, 1981.

Lee, W., Bell, M., and Navy, M.: Pulmonary lamellar bodies in human amniotic fluid. Am. J. Obstet. Gynecol. 136:60, 1980.

Nelson, G.: Relationship between amniotic fluid lecithin concentration and respiratory distress syndrome. Am. J. Obstet. Gynecol. 112:827, 1972.

Ogawa, Y.: Fetal pulmonary surfactant in amniotic fluid of ewes. Tohoku J. Exper. Med. 108:307, 1972.

Patrick, J., Challis, J., Campbell, K., et al.: Circadian rhythms in maternal plasma cortisol and estriol concentrations at 30 to 39 weeks gestational age. Am. J. Obstet. Gynecol. 136:325, 1980.

Paul, R., and Hon, E.: Clinical fetal monitoring: effect on perinatal outcome. Am. J. Obstet. Gynecol. 118:592, 1974.

Sabbagha, R.: Diagnostic Ultrasound Applied to Obstetrics and Gynecology. New York, Harper & Row, 1980.

Saling, E.: A new method for examination of the child during labor: introduction, technique, and principles. Arch. Gynaekol. 197:108, 1962.

Schifrin, B., Foye, G., Amato, J, et al.: Routine fetal heart rate monitoring in the antepartum. Obstet. Gynecol. 54:21, 1979.

Schlueter, M., Phibbs, R., Creasy, R., et al.: Antenatal prediction of graduated risk of hyaline membrane disease by amniotic fluid foam test for surfactant. Am. J. Obstet. Gynecol. 134:761, 1979.

Shalev, E., Weiner, E., and Zuckerman, H.: Ultrasound determination of fetal sex. Am. J. Obstet. Gynecol. 141:582, 1981.

Sher, G., Statland, B. E., Knutzen, V. K.: Evaluation of the small third-trimester fetus using the foam stability index test. Obstet. Gynecol. 58:314, 1981.

Torday, J., Carson, L., and Lawson, E.: Saturated phosphatidyl-choline in amniotic fluid and the prediction of respiratory distress syndrome. N. Engl. J. Med. 301:1013, 1979.

Tulchinsky, D.: The value of estrogens in the high risk pregnancy. In Spellacy, W. N. (Ed.): Management of the High Risk Pregnancy. Baltimore, University Park Press, 1978, pp. 29–47.

Tulchinsky, D., and Ryan, K. J. (Eds.): Maternal-Fetal Endocrinology. Philadelphia, W. B. Saunders Co., 1980.

Wittman, B., Rurak, D., Gruber, N., et al.: Real-time ultrasound observation of breathing and movements in the fetal lamb. Am. J. Obstet. Gynecol. 141:807, 1981.

Wood, C., Renou, P., Oates, J., et al.: A controlled trial of fetal heart rate monitoring in a low risk population. Am. J. Obstet. Gynecol. 141:527, 1981.

Young, B.: Antenatal Diagnosis. Part II. Predictors of Fetal Maturation. Department of Health, Education, and Welfare, National Institutes of Health Publication 79-1973, April 1979, p. 73.

4

Fetal Growth and Neonatal Adaptations

The newborn infant may be born after a shorter than average gestation, in which event he is said to be premature. He may be born of low birth weight for gestational age, either before or at term, in which instance he is undergrown. Such infants are often described as having intrauterine growth retardation, or as being "small for dates." Some babies are the products of a prolonged gestation and are therefore termed postmature. It is the purpose of this chapter to consider fetal growth, variations in the size of the infant, and some of the physiological events at the time of birth.

Size at Term. The length of gestation in the human is variable. "Term" is arbitrarily defined as the duration at which most infants more than 19 inches (48 cm) in length and 6 pounds (2800 gm) in weight are born (Fig. 4–1). Thus, 280 to 284 days after the first day of the last menstrual period is the most likely gestational period, although infants born at any time from the beginning of the thirty-eighth week to the forty-third week have similar characteristics and a low mortality. The average weight of an infant born at term is approximately 7 pounds 8 ounces (3400 gm) for the white male at sea level and 7 pounds (3200 gm) for the white female at sea level. Black infants tend to weigh about ½ pound (200 gm) less than white infants at term. Excessive weight is sometimes encountered, and, according to some reports, there have been infants who have weighed as much as 17 pounds (7700 gm) at term. The usual length of a term infant is 20 inches (51 cm), with a range of 18½ to 23 inches (46 to 57 cm). Head circumference is a remarkably constant 13 to 15 inches (33 to 37 cm). The circumference of the chest is usu-

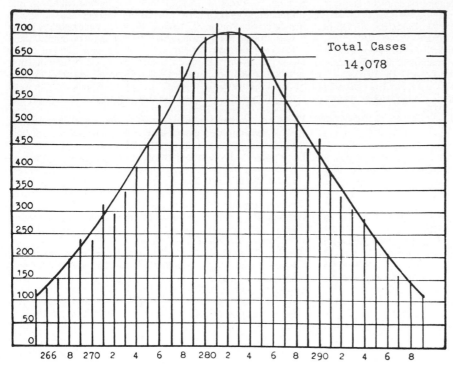

Figure 4–1. Distribution curve of duration of pregnancy (from first day of last menstrual period) in 14,078 cases. The infants were at least 48 cm in length and 2800 gm in weight. Note that the median duration of pregnancy in this series was 282 days. (From Speitkamp.)

ally almost the same as that of the head or a few centimeters smaller. The body segment from crown to symphysis pubis is about 1.7 times the length from pubis to heel.

Prematurity. The former definition of prematurity had been birth weight of or under 5 pounds 8 ounces (2500 gm). The definition was based on the ease and accuracy of the measurement of weight and

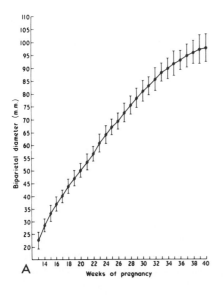

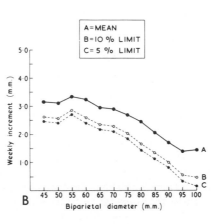

Figure 4–2. *A,* Mean biparietal diameter values (±2 S.D.) for each week of pregnancy from 13 to 40 weeks' menstrual age; 1029 individual readings made during normal pregnancy. This graph is used to assess fetal maturity and size. *B,* Mean weekly increments in the fetal biparietal diameter with lower tolerance limits according to the size of the biparietal diameter; longitudinal data obtained from normal pregnancies. This graph is used to assess the fetal growth rate. (From Campbell, S.: Clin. Perinatol. *1:*512, 1974. Reproduced with permission.)

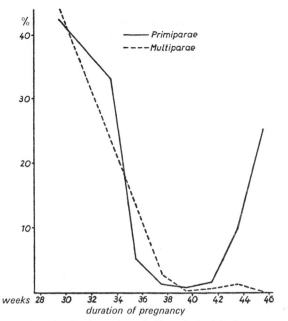

Figure 4–3. Perinatal mortality rate in primiparous and multiparous women. (Kloosterman, G. J.: Aspects of Prematurity and Dysmaturity. Nutricia Symposium. Leiden, H. E. Stenfert Kroese, 1968.)

the difficulty of measuring the length of gestation. More accurately, the word prematurity should not be synonymous with low birth weight, since it is widely recognized that many factors can produce low birth weight in infants born at term. It is nonetheless useful for statistical purposes to report mortality by weight groups, which is done usually in 500-gm but preferably in 100-gm increments.

Infants born before the thirty-seventh week are considered premature, and they are usually of low birth weight. The most common exception is the infant of the diabetic mother, whose size often is large for his gestational age. Perinatal mortality is clearly related to the length of gestation, increasing at either extreme from the lowest mortality of thirty-eight– to forty-two–week pregnancies (Fig. 4–3).

The intrauterine growth charts constructed by Usher and McLean are shown in Figure 4–4. These charts, and others for somewhat different populations, are of great value in assessing the appropriateness of weight for stated gestational age. Some differences exist in the many fetal growth charts that have been constructed in recent years, depending in part on the sorts of infants included and on the region of the world studied. The Denver data of Lubchenco are representative of infants born at an elevation of approximately 1 mile. Infants born at sea level are slightly heavier at a given gestational age. In a detailed study in England, Thomson and coworkers note the significant effects of sex and birth order, the first-born females being lighter at a given gestational age. (See Appendix 3 for table of gestational length and embryonic and fetal bodily dimensions.)

Increasingly, those writing about newborn infants speak of size as "under the tenth percentile" or under

two standard deviations from the mean weight for age when identifying undergrown infants. Note that the period of most rapid weight gain is from 32 to 38 weeks, the gestational period during which the fetus stores both fat and carbohydrate. Infants born before then appear wasted.

Low Birth Weight for Gestational Age. Significant growth retardation is usually considered present in infants below the tenth percentile weight for gestational age. These infants differ in a number of important respects from those of similar size who were born after a gestational interval appropriate for their size. Even the group identified as small for gestational age is a heterogeneous one, since a variety of different events may predispose infants to poor intrauterine weight gain.

The identification of the small-for-dates infant depends on collecting the appropriate facts about family history and clinical information. Growth retardation should be suspected if there is a discrepancy in weight and dates, if any of the conditions cited in Table 9–2 are present, and if physical signs and neurologic findings are present that indicate maturation inappropriate to the low birth weight. Usher and his colleagues have listed some of the important clinical signs that are indices of physical maturation (see Table 9–1).

Perhaps of most value in assessment of gestational age is a careful examination of the nervous system (see Chapter 76).

Genetic Regulation of Growth. *Before birth,* environmental influences have a much stronger influence on fetal size than does the genome. The interactions are, of course, complex, but studies of birth weight as influenced by maternal and fetal factors led Penrose to conclude that intrauterine influences, such as twin pregnancy, were the dominant ones. He calculated the relative magnitude of a number of factors observed in an affluent western European population as shown in Table 4–1.

Although less than half the variations in birth weight at term can be ascribed to the influence of genes, some single genes can affect fetal size. Siblings of individuals with cystic fibrosis, phenylketonuria, or Bloom's disease, for example, are large for gestational age. Chromosomal abnormalities may disturb development and reduce size for age. Autosomal mutations have a more pronounced effect than anomalies of sex chromosomes. In fact, Polani estimates that the effect of chromosomal mutations is so great that they occur in about 40 per cent of all spontaneous abortions, which is in a sense the ultimate adverse effect on growth. Another way of stating the problem is that nearly 97 per cent of autosomally abnormal fetuses are spontaneously aborted.

Body Composition. Important changes in body and organ composition take place during fetal and neonatal life. As Widdowson remarked, "In some respects we can regard birth as an incident in chemical development, which pursues the same steady course if all goes well from conception to maturity, and it matters little whether the organism spends the last few weeks of normal gestation inside or outside the uterus." Among the major trends in maturation are a decrease in body water, from 86 to 90 per cent at 28 weeks to 70 to 74 per cent by 6 months of post-

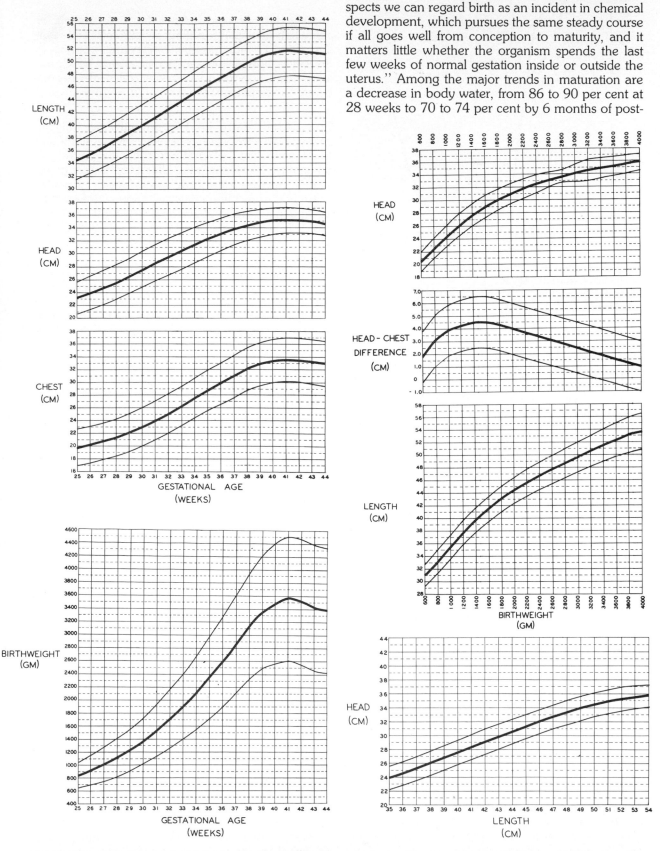

Figure 4–4. Smooth curve values of the mean plus or minus two standard deviations (third and ninety-seventh percentiles). Caucasian infants at sea level (Montreal). (Usher, R., and McLean, F.: J. Pediatr. *74*:901, 1969.)

Table 4–1. Approximate Magnitudes of Hereditary and Environmental Causes of Variation in Birth Weight

	Per Cent
Maternal hereditary constitution	20
Fetal hereditary factors: sex	2
Fetal hereditary factors: remaining constitution	16
Maternal general health and nutrition	16
Maternal health during each particular pregnancy	8
Maternal parity	7
Maternal age	1
Unidentified intrauterine influences, posture, etc.	30

(From L. S. Penrose (Ed.): Recent Advances in Human Genetics. Boston, Little, Brown and Co., 1961.)

natal age (Fig. 4–5). The concentration of nitrogen in fat-free tissues doubles in the last half of pregnancy; in the skin it doubles again by adulthood.

Proteins form about 12 per cent of body weight in babies at term, compared with 15 per cent in the animals studies by Widdowson and Spray. Accumulation of amino acids by the fetus leads to a concentration that is higher on the fetal side of the placenta than on the maternal side. Not all amino acids are elevated in fetal plasma. Cystine, for example, has been shown by Gaull to be transferred from the mother and thus is an "essential" amino acid for the fetus. The regulation of transfer depends on blood flows on either side of the placenta. Young showed in the guinea pig that a 30 per cent reduction in maternal placental blood flow reduced transfer of amino nitrogen by 20 per cent but reduced essential amino acids by 50 per cent. She postulates that fetal growth is critically dependent on maternal uterine circulation. Perhaps this fact is responsible in part for conflicting views on the influence of maternal nutritional supplements on fetal weight gain.

The stores of fat and carbohydrate increase approximately fivefold in the last trimester of pregnancy and are the food reserves for the newborn infant. Protein stores provide very few calories for the starving newborn, only 4 per cent of the total as compared with 20 per cent in the starving adult. This protein-sparing during starvation is a manifestation of the anabolic tendency of the baby.

Minerals are stored in the body during pregnancy. The average term infant is born with 270 mg of iron, approximately 140 to 170 mg of which is in hemoglobin. During the first week of life, in association with decreased erythropoiesis and red cell destruction, some iron is excreted into the intestine. The negative iron balance persists for the first few months of life, at which time there is little utilization of dietary iron as well. Serum iron levels at birth are about 160 µg of iron per 100 ml of serum. The level falls to 50 µg per 100 ml by 24 hours after birth and then rises over the next 2 weeks.

Calcium accumulates in the body approximately linearly from the eighth week to term, when it is about 1.0 gm per 100 gm of fat-free body tissue. The calcium-phosphorus ratio is about 1.75. Magnesium doubles in amount per 100 gm of tissue from the twelfth to the fortieth week of gestation, when it is about 0.2 gm per 100 gm of fat-free tissue (Table 4–2).

Concentrations of sodium tend to fall and those of potassium to rise during fetal life and in the weeks after birth, when intracellular potassium concentrations increase markedly. Despite such significant changes in intracellular and extracellular distribution of ions, their concentrations in blood remain markedly constant. The serum sodium and chloride con-

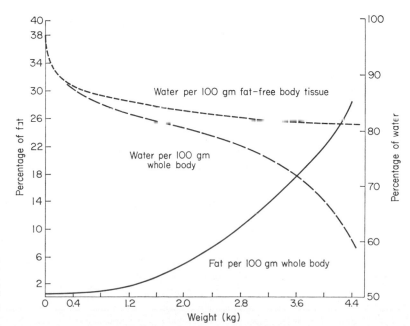

Figure 4–5. Percentage of water and fat in the human fetus in relation to body weight. (Widdowson, E.: In Assali, N. S. [ed.]: Biology of Gestation. Vol. II. New York, Academic Press, 1968. Reproduced with permission.)

centrations are the same in an immature fetus as those in an adult.

The full-term infant has three times the copper content per kilogram (4.5 mg per kilogram) of the adult (1.5 mg per kilogram). The concentration in the liver falls after the second month of postnatal life. Surprisingly, the serum copper is lower at birth than at any other time of life—50 µg per 100 ml, associated with low levels of the copper-protein enzyme, ceruloplasmin. It rises during the first week after birth to 150 µg per 100 ml and then falls to the adult value of 100 µg per 100 ml.

Neonatal Weight Loss. A postnatal weight loss of 5 to 8 per cent of the body weight is a constant feature of the first few days of life. The magnitude of the loss is affected by feeding practices and, to a lesser extent, by the humidity in the environment. Some of the weight is lost in the form of meconium, vernix, and the remnant of the umbilical cord, but most of the loss is in the form of insensible water and urine.

The rise in intracellular fluid that occurs throughout fetal life is temporarily reversed at birth. It is as if the stores of water, particularly in the skin, are released at birth, when the extracellular volume increases at the expense of the intracellular volume. The major changes occur during the first 72 hours, when infants may normally have a variable fluid intake. After several days, a new equilibrium is established, and intracellular water gradually increases with respect to extracellular water throughout childhood.

Infants mobilize and excrete water and electrolytes even in the fasting state. Plasma osmolarity does not change despite urinary sodium losses, suggesting a movement of sodium from intracellular to extracellular space (MacLaurin, 1966). The provision of added water accelerates these losses (Hansen and Smith, 1953). In rabbit pups, there is an inverse correlation between body hydration and fluid intake. Low fluid intake results in retention of cell water, whereas higher intakes speed release (Coulter and Avery, 1980).

The changes are most evident in premature infants who seem gelatinous and puffy at birth with their relatively large extracellular fluid accumulations. After several days, they assume a more wizened look. Significant shifts in electrolyte concentrations between intracellular and extracellular tissues occur, as sodium is lost from cells and intracellular potassium concentrations rise.

Fluid Balance in the Neonate. The general principles governing fluid balance at all ages apply to the newborn infant. Knowledge of daily requirements, assessment of any unusual losses or gains from illness or environmental conditions in the recent past, and prediction and measurement of ongoing water losses or gains allow a rational approach to management.

The special conditions that affect the calculation of water requirements in the newborn include differing needs as a function of gestational age, postnatal age, activity, and the environment (i.e., incubator humidity, respiration, and temperature).

The changes in body composition with gestational age include an increase in mass, a relative increase in the intracellular compartment with a decrease in the extracellular one, and an increase in the proportion of protein and fat. The clinical relevance of these changes would be that the very immature infant has minimal reserves and the greatest need for growth. Thus, prolonged fasting or deprivation of basal caloric needs would seem to be most serious in the undersized infant.

The changes with postnatal age include the shift of intracellular water to the extracellular space and its excretion, which accounts for the 5 to 8 per cent weight loss seen in most infants during the first day of postnatal life. Of course, the degree of postnatal weight loss is influenced by fluid intake; the average values cited are for normal infants. The quantity of solutes excreted is relatively independent of the water intake. Thus, the solutes tend to determine the urine volume rather than the urine volume determining solute excretion.

Water balance between compartments is partly determined by colloid osmotic pressures. The membrane osmometer is now available for direct measurement; excellent correlation with total serum solids has been shown by Wu and associates (1981). Infants under 1 kg have colloid osmotic pressures of about 11 mm Hg; in those over 2.5 kg, the average values

Table 4–2. Total Amounts of Water, Fat, Nitrogen, and Minerals in the Body of the Developing Fetus

Body Weight (gm)	Approximate Fetal Age (Weeks)	Water (gm)	Fat (gm)	N (gm)	Ca (gm)	P (gm)	Mg (gm)	Na (mEq)	K (mEq)	Cl (mEq)	Fe (mg)	Cu (mg)	Zn (mg)
30	13	27	0.2	0.4	0.09	0.09	0.003	3.6	1.4	2.4	—	—	—
100	15	89	0.5	1.0	0.3	0.2	0.01	9	2.6	7	5.1	—	—
200	17	177	1.0	2.8	0.7	0.6	0.03	20	7.9	14	10	0.7	2.6
500	23	440	3.0	7.0	2.2	1.5	0.10	49	22	33	28	2.4	9.4
1000	26	860	10	14	6.0	3.4	0.22	90	41	66	64	3.5	16
1500	31	1270	35	25	10	5.6	0.35	125	60	96	100	5.6	25
2000	33	1620	100	37	15	8.2	0.46	160	84	120	160	8.0	35
2500	35	1940	185	49	20	11	0.58	200	110	130	220	10	43
3000	38	2180	360	55	25	14	0.70	240	130	150	260	12	50
3500	40	2400	560	62	30	17	0.78	280	150	160	280	14	53

(From Widdowson E. In Assali, N. S. (Ed.): Biology of Gestation. Vol. II. New York, Academic Press, 1968.)

are 18.5 mm Hg. Total serum solids are about 3 gm/dl in infants under 1 kg and 5.6 gm/dl at term. These measurements are directly correlated with body weight and with each other.

Environmental influences such as temperature and humidity greatly affect insensible water losses. For example, O'Brien and coworkers estimated that at 30 to 50 per cent relative humidity, the average term infant lost 24 ml of water/kg/day, approximately 60 per cent from the lungs and 40 per cent from the skin. These losses are prevented by breathing air saturated with water vapor at body temperature and in a similar warm and moist incubator. Fanaroff and colleagues found weight losses of 60 gm/kg/day in infants under 1250 grams studied nude in single-walled incubators. They reduced these losses with the addition of a plastic heat shield, which presumably altered patterns of air flow over the skin.

Some of the unusual environmental influences need to be considered for sick infants. For example, the influence of continuous distending airway pressure is to impede venous return to the heart. The effects of a decreased central blood volume are stimulation of antidiuretic hormone production, reduction of urine volume, and promotion of fluid retention. Salt and water requirements are reduced under these circumstances. The degree of reduction differs as a function of the condition of the individual infant and is best ascertained by measuring urine output and daily weight. An accentuation of postnatal water loss is found in infants under phototherapy, who not infrequently have loose stools, and have increased insensible water loss as well. Oh and Karecki found increased respiratory rates and more skin evaporation in term infants under phototherapy. The oral intake of the infants was about 20 per cent greater when under phototherapy.

Lorenz and coworkers studied 88 infants between 750 and 1500 gm birth weight. They found that protocols allowing for different sodium and water intakes in the first week of life had no discernible effects on incidence of intracranial hemorrhage, bronchopulmonary dysplasia, time of diuresis, patent ductus arteriosus, or dehydration *so long as* (1) fluid and sodium intakes allowed a decrease in weight of no more than 5 to 15 per cent of birth weight in the first week, and (2) sodium values in the serum were maintained at 130 to 150 mEq/l. The average birth weight of these infants was about 1200 gm. After the first day, sodium intakes averaged 1 to 3 mEq/kg/day, and fluid intakes ranged from 60 to 140 ml/kg/day. Urine outputs ranged from 70 to 120 ml/kg/day, urine specific gravities were 1.005 to 1.012, and serum sodiums were 138 to 146 mEq/l. Higher fluid intakes resulted in relatively small changes in weight loss and were associated with significantly increased urine outputs. These infants were cared for in high humidity; infants nursed in lower humidity and those with higher insensible water losses would require greater intakes to limit weight loss in the first week to 5 to 15 per cent.

The effectiveness of parenteral fluid therapy requires close monitoring of the infant with respect to intake, output, body weight and urine specific gravity or osmolarity, and blood H$^+$ concentration and electrolytes. Urine specific gravity should be 1.005 to 1.012 (unless glucosuria is present) with a volume of 35 to 100 ml per kilogram per 24 hours. Urine osmolarity of 75 to 300 mOsm per kg indicates appropriate hydration. Higher or lower values indicate stress on the concentrating or diluting mechanisms.

Energy Requirements. Of central importance is the recognition that every infant should be given at least his basal caloric needs each 24 hours. The absence of provision of calories forces the utilization of limited stores or tissue breakdown. The extent of the stress of forcing catabolism on an organism geared for growth has not been studied adequately in the human, but logic dictates that it should be avoided if possible. Total caloric needs cannot be met by 10 per cent dextrose in water. For example, a 1 kg infant requires at least 60 cal/24 hours to sustain life. If the infant receives 100 ml of 10 per cent dextrose in water, he is receiving only 40 cal/24 hours. For the first few days of life, glucose alone may be adequate, but the infant must be put in positive nitrogen balance after that time to prevent tissue breakdown.

The partition of daily caloric expenditure in a typical, growing, premature infant (1.5 to 2.5 kg) is shown in Table 4–3. Very low birth weight infants (under 1300 grams) were studied by indirect calorimetry and nitrogen balance by Reichman and colleagues in Toronto. When the infants were about 3 weeks old and gaining weight at 16.8 ± 1 gm/kg/day, their caloric intake was 148 kcal/kg/day. The energy partition was as follows:

Stool and urine	18.2
Basal metabolic rate	47.0
Cost of activity	4.3
Thermal effect food	11.3
Energy stored in new tissue	67.8

Increased activity or environmental temperature outside the thermoneutral range increased energy expenditure. The energy cost of growth was 4.9 kcal/gm of weight gain. The authors concluded that to maintain growth at a rate equivalent to normal intrauterine growth, a metabolizable energy intake of 60 kcal/kg/day in excess of maintenance 51.3 kcal/kg/day must be provided.

Acid-Base Disturbances. Significant departures from normal hydrogen ion concentrations are common in the neonatal period. Intrauterine asphyxia can result in a severe metabolic acidosis at birth, and postnatal asphyxia adds a respiratory component, so that pH values may be 6.8 to 7.0 in some asphyxiated infants. Adequate ventilation and oxygenation, increased cardiac output, and renal perfusion operate toward rapid correction of the acidemia in the minutes and hours after birth.

Table 4–3. Partition of Daily Caloric Expenditure in a Typical Growing Premature Infant

Item	Cal/kg/24 hr
Resting caloric expenditure	50
Intermittent activity	15
Occasional cold stress	10
Specific dynamic action	8
Fecal loss	12
Growth allowance	25
TOTAL	120

(From Driscoll, J. M. *In* Behrman, R. E. (Ed.): Neonatology, St. Louis, C. V. Mosby Company, 1973.)

In profound asphyxia, intravenous infusion of 5 to 10 ml of 25 mEq per 100 ml sodium bicarbonate in water at a rate of 1 mEq per minute is recommended, concomitant with artificial ventilation to facilitate removal of carbon dioxide. Thereafter, maintenance infusion of 5 to 15 mEq $NaHCO_3$ per 100 ml in 5 to 10 per cent glucose is appropriate, as indicated by serial measurements of pH, P_{CO_2}, and HCO_3^-. If hyponatremia and a hypertonic urine are found, inappropriate ADH secretion is likely, which is a frequent result of severe asphyxia.

The weight of recent evidence supports slow infusions of alkali to correct a metabolic acidosis with a maximum of 6 mEq per kg per 24 hours of $NaHCO_3$. Rapid infusions of hyperosmolar solutions have been associated with hypernatremia and intracranial hemorrhage, according to Simmons and others. In infants requiring intravenous fluids for several days, as in the respiratory distress syndrome, the serum calcium may fall, and supplements are occasionally needed.

Temperature Regulation. A newborn infant (especially of low birth weight) is at a disadvantage in maintaining body temperature chiefly because of a large surface-volume ratio and relatively little insulating subcutaneous tissue. When chilled, the infant's skin becomes pale or blue soon after birth, and the rectal temperature falls, often several degrees below the intrauterine temperature of 37.6°C (99° to 100°F). This phenomenon of a rapid fall in body tem-

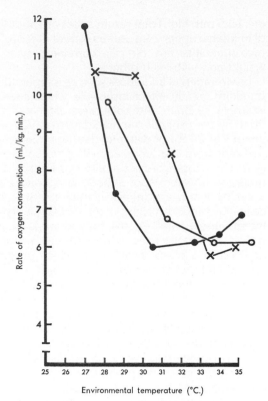

× —— × 2,340-g. baby, 35 weeks' gestation, age 4 days
○ —— ○ 2,430-g. baby, 38 weeks' gestation, age 4 days
● —— ● 3,800-g. baby, 40 weeks' gestation, age 5 days

Figure 4–6. Relation of oxygen consumption rate to environmental temperature in three babies. (Scopes, J. W.: Br. Med. Bull. *22*:88, 1966. Reproduced with permission.)

perature, most pronounced in very small infants, is such a regular occurrence that the concept that infants are poikilothermic became widely accepted. Studies done mostly in the late 1950s and early 1960s have established that the infant is indeed homeothermic and tries to regulate his body temperature, although often he cannot match heat losses in the minutes or hours after birth. The avenues of heat loss in the infant are evaporation (particularly at birth, when he is covered with amniotic liquid), radiation, conduction, and convection. The magnitude of the losses depends upon environmental conditions. The term baby can increase insensible water loss about fourfold in a warm environment by sweating, particularly around the head. Preterm infants have less

Table 4–4. The Mean Temperature Needed to Provide Thermal Neutrality for a Healthy Baby Nursed Naked in Draft-Free Surroundings of Uniform Temperature and Moderate Humidity After Birth

Birth Weight (kg)	Operative Environmental Temperature*						
	35°C		34°C		33°C		32°C
1.0	For 10 days	→	After 10 days	→	After 3 weeks	→	After 5 weeks
1.5	—		For 10 days	→	After 10 days	→	After 4 weeks
2.0	—		For 2 days	→	After 2 days	→	After 3 weeks
>2.5	—		—		For 2 days	→	After 2 days

* To estimate operative temperature in a single-walled incubator, subtract 1°C from incubator air temperature for every 7°C by which this temperature exceeds room temperature.
(From Hey, E.: Br. Med. Bull. *31*:72, 1975.)

ability to sweat, and virtually no sweating is possible before 32 weeks. All infants are at risk of hyperthermia in an overheated environment. The outstanding clinical sign is flushed skin from peripheral vasodilatation. Any bright red infant should be suspected of being overheated.

The sources of heat production are basal metabolism, muscular activity, and chemical thermogenesis mediated through the release of catecholamines. Shivering, an important form of muscular activity that increases heat production 200 to 300 per cent in the adult, is rarely seen in the infant. Chemical thermogenesis appears to be a particularly important mechanism for added heat production in the infant. Skin receptors, presumably concentrated in the face, sense the change in temperature and transmit this information to the central nervous system, which then activates the autonomic nervous system. Sympathetic impulses cause a release of norepinephrine, both from the adrenal and locally at nerve endings in the brown fat. Peripheral vasoconstriction occurs, and the brown fat is activated to break down stores of triglyceride to fatty acids, with the local production of heat. Indeed brown fat—located chiefly in the interscapular area, in the nape of the neck, and around the heart and kidneys—has greater oxidative capacity per milligram of protein than any other organ and has led George Cahill to suggest that fat is not only an insulator but, perhaps, an "electric blanket" as well.

Thermographic studies in infants show the increase in skin heat over brown fat after 30 minutes of cold exposure in about 25 per cent of infants in the first postnatal hour and in all infants between 1 and 14 days of age. This response disappeared by 3 to 6 months of age (Rylander, 1972). At thermoneutrality for the term infant (32°C) the warmest skin is over the central core. Clark and Stothers ascertained with infrared color thermography that upper arm and upper thigh areas are most representative of mean body temperature. The upper abdominal surface and the head are least responsive to changes in environmental temperature, and the distal extremities are the most responsive.

The increase in metabolism that is a consequence of cold stress is measured as an increase in oxygen consumption (Fig. 4–6). The magnitude of the effect is apparent from the many reported studies on infants of differing size and postnatal age. *A fall in environmental temperature of only 2°C, from 33 to 31°C (91.4° to 87.8°F), is a sufficient stimulus to double the oxygen consumption of a normal term infant* (Hill and Rahimtulla, 1965). A change in environmental temperature from 36° to 34°C (96.8° to 93.2°F) will be associated with a similar doubling of oxygen consumption in infants under 1.5 kg (Scopes, 1966). The necessity of increasing oxygen consumption to maintain body temperature requires approximately the same percentage of increase in ventilation. For the normal term infant, this increase in ventilation is usually reached without difficulty. The low birth weight infant, on the other hand, frequently has some pulmonary insufficiency in the first days of life and may

be unable to achieve the appropriate increase in ventilation when chilled. The consequence of increased oxygen needs in the face of pulmonary insufficiency is an oxygen debt, as evidenced by the accumulation of lactate, leading to metabolic acidosis. Importantly, it has also been shown by at least three independent studies that *the survival rate of low birth weight infants is less when the environmental temperature is several degrees below their thermal neutral environment*, defined as that temperature at which oxygen consumption is minimal (Silverman et al., 1966; Buetow and Klein, 1964; Day et al., 1964).

The ability of the infant to increase his oxygen consumption during cold stress is depressed in a low oxygen environment. An arterial oxygen tension of 45 to 55 mm Hg depresses the response, and a P_{O_2} of 30 mm Hg abolishes it. The fall in body temperature in infants with respiratory distress has been used as a rough index of their blood oxygenation.

Clinical Considerations. The difficulties in knowing the optimal thermal environment for a given infant have been discussed by Adamsons and Scopes. Practically, it appears that it is optimal to maintain the skin temperature at 36° to 36.5°C (96.8° to 97.6°F). This can be achieved by servo-incubators or by the use of thermistors to record skin temperature continuously, with judicious adjustment of the incubator to achieve the desired skin temperature. In the absence of servo-incubators, general guidelines for appropriate incubator temperatures were proposed by Hey, as shown in Table 4–4.

REFERENCES

Adamsons, K., Jr.: The role of thermal factors in fetal and neonatal life. Pediatr. Clin. North Am. 13:599, 1966.

Beard, R. W., Morris, E. D., and Clayton, S. C.: pH of foetal capillary blood as an indicator of the condition of the foetus. J. Obstet. Gynaec. Brit. Comm. 74:812, 1967.

Bergstrom, W. H.: Total body water and normal electrolyte composition. Pediatr. Clin. North Am. 6:5, 1959.

Boyd, E.: Origins of the Study of Human Growth. Portland, Oregon, University of Oregon Health Sciences Center Foundation, 1980.

Brück, K.: Temperature regulation in the newborn infant. Biol. Neonatol 3:65, 1961

Buetow, K. C., and Klein, S. W.: Effect of maintenance of "normal" skin temperature on survival of infants of low birth weight. Pediatrics 34:163, 1964.

Cheek, D. B., Maddison, T. G., Malinek, M., and Coldbeck, J. H.: Further observations on the corrected bromide space of the neonate and investigation of water and electrolyte status in infants born of diabetic mothers. Pediatrics 28:861, 1961.

Christie, A., Martin, M., Williams, E. L., Hudson, G., and Lanier, J. C.: The estimation of fetal maturity by roentgen studies of osseous development. Am. J. Obstet. Gynecol. 60:133, 1950.

Clark, R. P., and Stothers, J. K.: Neonatal skin temperature distribution using infra-red colour thermography. J. Physiol (Lond.) 302:323, 1980.

Comline, K. S., Cross, K. W., Dawes, G. S., and Nathamelsz, P. W. (Eds.): Foetal and Neonatal Physiology. Proceedings of The Sir Joseph Barcroft Centenary Symposium. Cambridge University Press, 1973.

Coulter, D. M., and Avery, M. E.: Paradoxical reduction in tissue hydration with weight gain in neonatal rabbit pups. Pediatr. Res. 14:1122, 1980.

Darrow, D. C.: The significance of body size. Am. J. Dis. Child. 98:416, 1959.

Davies, P. A., Robinson, R. J., Scopes, J. W., et al.: Medical Care of Newborn Babies. Philadelphia, J. B. Lippincott Co., 1972.

Davis, J. A., and Dobbing, J. (Eds.): Scientific Foundations of Pediatrics. 2nd ed. London, William Heineman Medical Books, Ltd., 1981.

Dawkins, M. J. R., and Hull, D.: The production of heat by fat. Sci. Amer. 213:62, 1965.

Day, R. L., Caliguiri, L., Kamenski, C., and Ehrlich, F.: Body temperature and survival of premature infants. Pediatrics 34:171, 1964.

Diczfalusy, E.: Endocrine functions of the human foeto-placental unit. Fed. Proc. 23:791–798, 1964.

Drescher, A. M., Barnett, H. L., and Troupkou, V.: Water balance in infants during water deprivation. Am. J. Dis. Child. 104:366, 1962.

Elliott, K., and Knight, J. (Eds.): Size at Birth. Ciba Foundation Symposium 27 (new series), Elsevier-Excerpta Med. North-Holland, 1974.

Fanaroff, A. A., Wald, M., Gruber, H. S., and Klaus, M. H.: Insensible water loss in low birth weight infants. Pediatrics 50:236, 1972.

Foster, K. G., Hey, E. N., and Katz, G.: The response of the sweat glands of the newborn baby to thermal stimuli and to intradermal acetylcholine. J. Physiol. 203:13, 1969.

Gaull, G. E.: Sulphur amino acids, folate and DNA: metabolic interrelationships during fetal development. In Comline, K. S., Cross, K. W., Dawes, G. S., and Nathamelsz, P. W. (Eds.): Foetal and Neonatal Physiology. Proceedings of The Sir Joseph Barcroft Centenary Symposium. Cambridge University Press, 1973, p. 339.

Glass, L., Silverman, W. A., and Sinclair, J. C.: Effect of thermal environment on cold resistance and growth of small infants after the first week of life. Pediatr. 41:1033, 1968.

Hansen, J. D. L., and Smith, C. A.: The effects of withholding fluid in the immediate postnatal period. Pediatrics 12:99, 1953.

Hardy, J. B., Drage, J. S., and Jackson, E. C.: The First Year of Life. The Collaborative Perinatal Project of the National Institute of Neurological and Communicative Disorders and Stroke. Baltimore, Johns Hopkins University Press, 1979.

Heimler, R., Sumner, J. E., Grausz, J. P., Kien, C. L., and Glaspey, J. C.: Thermal environment change in growing premature infants: effect on general somatic growth and subcutaneous fat accumulation. Pediatrics. 68:82, 1981.

Hey, E. N.: Thermal neutrality. Br. Med. Bull. 31:69, 1975.

Hey, E. N., and Katz, G.: The range of thermal insulation in the tissue of the newborn baby. J. Physiol. 207:667, 1970.

Hey, E. N.: The relationship between environmental temperature and oxygen consumption in the newborn baby. J. Physiol. 200:589, 1969.

Hey, E., and Katz, G.: Evaporative water loss in the newborn baby. J. Physiol. 200:605, 1969.

Hey, E. N., and Maurice, N. P.: Effect of humidity on production and loss of heat in the newborn baby. Arch. Dis. Child. 43:166, 1968.

Hill, J. R., and Rahimtulla, K. A.: Heat balance and the metabolic rate of newborn babies in relation to environmental temperature, and the effect of age and weight on basal metabolic rate. J. Physiol. 180:239, 1965.

Hull, D.: Brown adipose tissue. Br. Med. Bull. 22:92, 1966.

Kravath, R., Aharon, A., Abal, G., and Finberg, L.: Clinically significant physiologic changes from rapidly administered hypertonic solutions: Acute osmol poisoning. Pediatrics 46:267, 1970.

Lorenz, J., Kleinman, L., Katagel, U., and Reller, M.: Water balance in very low birth weight infants: relationship to water and sodium intake and effect on outcome. J. Pediatr. 101:423, 1982.

MacLaurin, J. C.: Changes in body water distribution during the first two weeks of life. Arch. Dis. Child. 41:286, 1966.

Mestyan, J., Fekete, M., Bata, O., and Jarai, I.: The basal metabolic rate of premature infants. Biol. Neonatol. 7:11, 1964.

Miller, H. C., and Merritt, T. A.: Fetal Growth in Humans. Chicago, Yearbook Medical Publishers, 1979.

Nervez, C. T., Shott, R. J., Bergstrom, W. H., and Williams, M. L.: Prophylaxis against hypocalcemia in low-birth-weight infants requiring bicarbonate infusion. J. Pediatr. 87:439, 1975.

O'Brien, D., Hansen, J. D. L., and Smith, C. A.: Effect of supersaturated atmospheres on insensible water loss in the newborn infant. Pediatrics 13:126, 1954.

Oh, W., and Karecki, H.: Phototherapy and insensible water loss in the newborn infant. Am. J. Dis. Child. 124:230, 1972.

O'Neill, E. M.: Normal head growth and prediction of head size in infantile hydrocephalus. Arch. Dis. Child. 36:241, 1961.

Perlstein, P. H., Edwards, N. K., and Sutherland, J. M.: Apnoea in premature infants and incubator-air temperature changes. N. Engl. J. Med. 282:461, 1970.

Polani, P. E.: Chromosomal and other genetic influences on birth weight variation. In Elliott, K., and Knight, J. (Eds.): Size at Birth. Ciba Foundation Symposium 27 (new series). Elsevier-North Holland, 1974.

Reichman, B. C., Chessen, P., Putet, G., et al.: Partition of energy metabolism and energy cost of growth in the very low birth weight infant. Pediatrics 69:446, 1982.

Reynolds, D. W., Dweck, H. S., and Cassady, G.: Inappropriate antidiuretic hormone secretion in a neonate with meningitis. Am. J. Dis. Child. 123:251, 1972.

Roy, R. N., and Sinclair, J. C.: Hydration of the low birth weight infant. Clin. Perinatol. 2:393, 1975.

Rylander, E.: Age dependent reactions of rectal and skin temperatures of infants during exposure to cold. Acta Pediatr. Scand. 61:579, 1972.

Scopes, J. W.: Metabolic rate and temperature control in the human baby. Br. Med. Bull. 22:88, 1966.

Siggaard-Andersen, O.: The Acid-Base Status of the Blood. 3rd ed. Baltimore, The Williams & Wilkins Company, 1965.

Silverman, W. A., Sinclair, J. C., and Agate, F. J., Jr.: The oxygen cost of minor changes in heat balance of small newborn infants. Acta Paediatr. 55:294, 1966.

Silverman, W., Zamelis, A., Sinclair, J. C., and Agate, F. J. Jr.: Warm nape of the newborn. Pediatrics 33:984, 1964.

Simmons, M. A., Adcock, E. W., III, Bard, H., and Battaglia, F. C.: Hypernatremia and intracranial hemorrhage in infants. N. Engl. J. Med. 291:6, 1974.

Sinclair, J. C., Driscoll, J. M., Jr., Heird, W. C., and Winters, R. W.: Supportive management of the sick neonate; parenteral calories, water, and electrolytes. Pediatr. Clin. North Am. 17:863, 1970.

Stothers, J. K.: Head insulation and heat loss in the newborn. Arch. Dis. Child. 56:530, 1981.

Taylor, D. C.: The influence of sexual differentiation on growth development and disease. In Davis, J., and Dobbing, J. (Eds.): Scientific Foundations of Pediatrics. London, William Heineman Medical Books, Ltd., 1981.

Thomson, A. M., Billewicz, W. Z., and Hytten, F. E.: The assessment of fetal growth. J. Obstet. Gynaec. Brit. Comm. 75:903, 1968.

Torday, J., Carson, L., and Lawson, E. E.: Saturated phosphatidyl choline in amniotic fluid and prediction of the respiratory distress syndrome. N. Eng. J. Med. 301:1013, 1979.

Usher, R., and McLean, F.: Intrauterine growth of live-born Caucasian infants at sea level. Standards obtained from measurements in 7 dimensions of infants born between 25–44 weeks of gestation. J. Pediatr. 74:901, 1969.

van Assche, F., and Robertson, W. (Eds.): Fetal Growth Retardation. London, Churchill Livingstone, 1981.

Widdowson, E. M., and Spray, C. M.: Chemical development "in utero." Arch. Dis. Child. 26:205, 1951.

World Health Organization Technical Report Series No. 540: Maturation of Fetal Body Systems. Geneva, 1974.

Wu, P. Y. K., Rockwell, G., Chan, L., et al.: Colloid osmotic pressure in newborn infants. Pediatrics 68:814, 1981.

Young, M.: Placental factors and fetal nutrition. Am. J. Clin. Nutr. 34:738, 1981.

Young, M.: Amino acid uptake by the fetus. Placenta (suppl.) 1:125, 1981.

PART 2

THE NEWBORN INFANT

5

Normal Newborn

General Pediatric Assessment of the Newborn: History and Physical Examination

FEATURES OF NEWBORN HISTORY

The assessment of the newborn logically begins with the mother's history and includes that of the pregnancy and delivery. Maternal events and their effects on the newborn have been discussed in Chapter 1 and are summarized in Table 5–1.

Table 5–1. Maternal, Pregnancy, and Perinatal Features of Newborn History

Maternal
  Diseases: diabetes, asthma, tuberculosis, venereal disease
  Drugs: "street drugs," chronic medications such as anti-hypertensives or diuretics
  Trauma/surgery: injury to abdomen, radiography (remote or recent), blood transfusions (blood type and sensitization)
  Prior pregnancies: gestation, birth weights, anomalies, abortions, problems of infancy
  Sociofamilial/educational: future parenting potential
  Familial/genetic: congenital diseases (e.g., cystic fibrosis, phenylketonuria, sickle cell disease)
Present Pregnancy
  Bleeding
  Infections
  Contractions
  Illnesses
  Trauma/surgery
  Medications
  Last menstrual period
  Heart sounds first heard
  Quickening
  Fetal sizes
  Fetal test results
Perinatal Events
  Medications
  Time of rupture of membranes
  Phospholipids, estriols, fetal monitoring
  Duration of labor
  Amniotic fluid (meconium, hydramnios)
  Maternal blood pressure, blood sugar
  Uterine perfusion
  Type of fetal/neonatal suctioning
  Time and events related to cord clamping
  Cord blood gases
  General neonatal assessment, resuscitation, and temperature control

The obstetric history of the current pregnancy needs review—the greater the concern for the newborn, the greater the scrutiny of this aspect of the history. First trimester bleeding occasionally indicates a missed abortion of an infant with chronic intrauterine infection, anomalies, or chromosomal defects. Third trimester bleeding could indicate abnormalities of placentation, impending premature delivery, intrauterine infection, or trauma to the uterus and fetus. Symptoms relating to generalized or localized infection either near or far from the time of delivery could indicate acute or chronic fetal infection. Pregnancy-related diseases such as toxemia suggest risk of growth retardation, perinatal asphyxia, and neonatal effects from maternal medication such as magnesium sulfate. Results of all fetal assessments should be noted (e.g., first trimester amniocentesis for alpha-fetoprotein and chromosomes, third trimester amniocentesis for bilirubin pigments or phospholipid testing, results of ultrasonography, results of estriols, and fetal heart rate monitoring).

Estimates of fetal growth in utero should be derived from the last menstrual period, date of quickening (16 to 18 weeks), and the first appearance of fetal heart sounds (18 to 20 weeks by fetoscope) as well as from growth of the fundus of the uterus (Anderson, 1981). Nägele's rule allows one to estimate the time of term delivery by subtracting 3 calendar months from the first day of the last menstrual period and adding 7 days. The fundus is usually at the umbilicus by the fifth month after the last menstrual period and at the lower rib margin by term.

Occurrences during labor and delivery may have extreme impact on the infant and often are poorly documented owing to the rapid pace of events. The reasons for the timing and route of delivery are of obvious importance to the neonatologist; for example, concern for the infant is very different if delivery is induced at term or if an emergency cesarean section is performed for a fetus of 32 weeks with a persistent heart rate of 80 per minute in a mother with severe preeclampsia. Assessing rapidity of responses to fetal problems as well as prepartum care and medications are important. Were glucocorticoids and beta-adrenergics used for preterm labor? Were membranes ruptured? Did the mother have signs of endometritis? Were antibiotics given? Were cultures taken? Did the mother have a wedge to decompress abdominal large vessels? What was the interval between recogniton of fetal asphyxia and delivery of the infant? Was there too much or too little amniotic fluid? Was bleeding excessive? Were maternal blood pressure and gas exchange adequate? What sort of analgesia/anesthesia was used? These are the questions that occupy the physician who awaits delivery of a potentially high-risk infant.

The immediate postnatal events obviously relate to the condition of the infant at birth, time of cord clamping, rigors of delivery itself, and immediate indications of asphyxia, anomalies, trauma, hypovolemia, or infection. If these indicators and the history are benign, the infant should (when provided with warmth, a clear airway, and a good nurse) rejoin the mother almost instantly and remain with her until a more detailed examination can be performed in the hours ahead.

PHYSICAL EXAMINATION

Various aspects of the newborn examination are discussed elsewhere (e.g., neurological examination, Chapter 76; Apgar examination and delivery room assessment, Chapter 10; gestational age assessment, Chapter 9; behavioral assessment, Chapter 7). Generally speaking, whether the infant is sick or well, whether he is significantly premature or small for gestational age or both, whether he is free of evident major birth defects, and whether he has adapted to the extrauterine environment can be discerned within seconds by inspection. The results of this inspection coupled with the history (Table 5–1) will generally allow an accurate distinction between well infants and infants with real or potential problems.

There are several general considerations that should precede description of the ''physical examination'' as it relates to newborn infants. First, especially in newborns, it is a highly time-dependent exercise—that is, what is normal at 5 minutes of age is not normal at 3 hours (e.g., with regard to respiratory effort and color). For this reason all descriptions, medical and nursing, of all newborn events should be dated and *timed*. Second, it follows that the ''physical examination'' is a running appraisal of findings over time continually combined in a record of nurses' and physicians' observations and laboratory observations. A one-time ''physical'' in the newborn period is worthless except for the most obvious and static of birth defects. Third, the examination, especially when performed by the unskilled on a premature sick infant, can have adverse results. Decreased temperature, decreased skin perfusion, and decreased oxygenation can all be caused by exposure during an examination. Sometimes, failure to palpate both kidneys may favor the infant even if it displeases one's colleagues. Nosocomial infections are one of the results of casual ''baby-to-baby'' examinations performed by nurses or doctors, and Albert and Condie fault us correctly for a ''low level of mysophobia.''

The examination should be performed with the infant completely unclothed in a warm environment and should take no more than a few minutes. A skilled examiner leaves a dressed, warm, contented infant, an event appreciated by the infant, parents, and nurses. Handwashing to the elbows after removal of rings, bracelets, and watches should be performed immediately before and immediately after touching the infant, with no handling of fomites in the period during which the infant is handled. The bell and diaphragm of the stethoscope are cleaned for each infant and should be completely cleaned once a day.

Vital Signs

Required vital signs vary from the admission temperature, weight, length, head circumference, and heart and respiratory rates usually recorded for the term newborn in a well-baby nursery to those that can be obtained more or less continuously from a completely ''instrumented'' infant with, for example, labile persistent fetal circulation in a neonatal intensive care unit: systolic, diastolic, and mean blood pressures from right atrium, pulmonary artery, and descending aorta, upper and lower body transcutaneous P_{CO_2}, P_{O_2}, and skin blood flow, ventilator measures, heart rate, fontanel pressure, carotid blood flow, and so forth.

Temperature. For the normal newborn, some care should be taken with assessment of even routine vital signs. *Temperature* is best measured in the axilla with an electronic thermometer. This method helps prevent occasional rectal bleeding and perforation from trauma, and the measurement obtained correlates with rectal temperature. There are those who believe that a routine rectal temperature should be taken at least once to avoid missing an imperforate anus but we believe inspection and absent or misdirected stool are more direct indicators of this anomaly. It is now trite to say that a normal core temperature does not necessarily indicate an optimal environmental temperature for the infant (Hey, 1975). An infant who is chilled and vasoconstricted after a bath or a small sick premature infant with an inversion of the normal core-skin decrement may have a normal core temperatue but a suboptimal environmental temperature. A premature infant near a cold window may radiate heat despite ''normal'' ambient and core temperatures. Skin sensors are widely used for continuous monitoring and are sometimes coupled with servo-controlled radiant heaters or incubator heaters. In these circumstances, it is essential to have the temperature sensor attached firmly to the skin with porous tape to avoid overheating. The usual site had been the upper abdominal wall, although the upper thigh or arm is preferred as more representative of mean body temperature. A high relative humidity is important in servo-controlled incubators to prevent a paradoxically low core temperature. When radiant heaters are used, the ambient humidity should be at least 40 percent.

Respiratory Rates. For all spontaneously breathing infants, term and premature, *respiratory rates* normally fall to within a range of 40 to 60 breaths per minute by 1 hour of age. Once or twice a year, we see a term infant who has a persisting respiratory rate of 100 on the second day of life, with no evident clinical, radiographic, or laboratory abnormality. These problems have always resolved. Persisting bradypnea is rare and usually seen only in severely ill infants. Apneic pauses of more than 10 seconds, especially if accompanied by cyanosis and bradycardia, are abnormal after 36 weeks postconceptional age, and a cause should be sought before discharge.

Heart Rate. The *heart rate* for newborns is normally between 120 and 180 beats per minute (see also Chapter 26). *Blood pressure* has differing normal values, depending on both postnatal and gestational age. Lower and upper limits of mean blood pressures are 23 and 43 torr for a 1 kg infant and 30 and 50 torr for a 2 kg infant in the first 12 hours of life. Cuff width should be about 50 per cent of the arm circumference, and systolic pressure should be noted when flow is "heard" by Doppler (Lum, 1977; Kirkland, 1972).

Weight, Length, and Head Circumference. Measurements of weight length, and head circumference must be recorded for all newborns. Weight should be measured with care and in grams for greatest accuracy. For infants from 500 to 800 gm birth weight, errors of only 100 gm can change the prognosis by 50 per cent. Too little attention has been given to the importance of a careful measurement of length. The value of the information is well worth the effort required to do it well. A board or box with a sliding panel to bring up to the foot of the infant is invaluable. The tonic neck reflex can be used to straighten the leg. Gently turn the head toward the examiner, and the opposite leg will extend. The length can be read from a centimeter scale attached to the measuring device (Miller and Hassancin, 1971). Measurements of length obtained by one person using a measuring tape on a squirming infant are commonly inaccurate by several centimeters. Head circumference is determined by placing the soft tape measure just above the eyebrows and finding the largest circumference over the occiput. Head circumferences measured at discharge are probably more independent of changes due to molding than those taken at birth.

Anomalies. The most frequent and embarrassing "misses" during physical examination have been posterior cleft palates, minor ear and hand anomalies, dislocated hips, and subtle cardiac anomalies. Because the nursing staff will have already diagnosed the apparent abnormalities, it is wise to concentrate on sites of those that are most likely unsuspected—that is, those that can be detected with the neurologic, cardiac, and abdominal examinations.

Gestational Age Assessment. This evaluation is best performed by recording several estimates (e.g., gestation from last menstrual period, the gestation that matches 50 percentiles for length, weight, and head circumference, and a gestational estimate based on physical characteristics). Usually, these multiple indicators can be summarized as an "obstetric" estimate of gestation and a "pediatric" estimate of gestation. In our minds, the physical assessments of gestation have been overemphasized, because it is clear that both skin and central nervous system features can be affected to some degree by factors other than duration of gestation. The scoring examination that appears simplest to us is the one described by Ballard and coworkers (see Appendix 3).

INSPECTION

General Observations. *Inspection* is the most important aspect of the physical examination and is best performed with the infant quiet and completely nude. Occasionally, the two states are found incompatible by the infant, in which case the infant can usually be quieted by rocking him forwards and backwards while making faces and babbling. This time-honored method usually catches the surprised attention of the infant (and other personnel who happen by).

Next, one takes an overall look at the baby. Does he appear to be sick or well? Is he normally fashioned or not? More specifically, one examines his color, looking for pallor, the pallid cyanosis of shock, cyanosis, and jaundice. If his skin is pale, are his mucous membranes and nail beds also pale? Or is the pallor a grayish sickly color of the skin alone, while nail beds and lips are duskily blue? If the latter is the case, the discoloration is more likely to be the result of shock; if the former is true, discoloration is likely due to anemia. Cyanosis may be generalized, or it may be localized to the distal parts of the extremities, to the head and face, to one side of the body, or to the upper or lower half of the trunk. The significance of these color changes will be discussed later. Does cyanosis disappear in an environment of 100 per cent oxygen? Jaundice may be intense and obvious, or one may have to bring out the yellow color of the milder forms by thumb pressure blanching of the skin.

The extremities should bear a normal relationship to the trunk, and the abdomen should be full, not scaphoid as with some cases of diaphragmatic hernias or protuberant as may be seen with volvulus. Measurements of upper segment/lower segment (using the pubis as the midpoint) or abdominal girth should be taken if these observations are suspicious.

Right and left differences should be noted. Is hemihypertrophy present? Is the left chest prominent, as with some obstructive cardiac lesions? Are the limbs asymmetric in posture or movement, indicating fracture, neurologic damage, infection, or soft tissue injury?

Respirations can be assessed by observation. Apnea, bradypnea, or tachypnea will be noted, as will unusually irregular, periodic, and gasping breathing. Although normally fairly shallow, breaths may be abnormally shallow or deep. Obstruction to the airway will be indicated by retraction of intercostal spaces, suprasternal notch, sternum, and lower ribs in ascending order of degree of obstruction. Stridor during inspiration or expiration or both is significant, as is wheezing or grunting expiration.

The cry should be lusty and angry-sounding with repetitive bursts after a single stimulus. Weak or high-pitched cry, hoarseness, or aphonia call for study.

When undisturbed, the infant should lie quietly. If cold, annoyed, or hurt, he will cry vigorously and move his extremities. If he cries constantly when undisturbed or if he cries not at all when disturbed, his behavior is not normal. Similarly, if he is in constant motion or is unusually still, one has cause for alarm. Violent, anxious overactivity and stupor or coma are especially disturbing. Muscle tonus is normally a bit exaggerated, but true rigidity and its opposite, flaccidity, are frightening, as are signs of cerebral irritation such as muscle twitching and convulsions.

Skin. At birth, the skin is usually covered with white vernix, which is most abundant in premature infants and becomes less prominent toward term. Post-term infants characteristically have no vernix caseosa, and the skin is dry, cracked, and wrinkled. Its texture must be investigated with special reference to dryness, scaliness, flakiness, inelasticity or extraordinary elasticity, and unusual thinness or thickness. Is edema present, and, if so, is it generalized or localized? One looks for tumors, mainly hemangiomas, and for urticarial, pustular, vesicular, nodular, or gangrenous rashes. One looks for dermal sinuses in the midline of the back from occiput to coccyx and in the pilonidal region and near the ears and in the neck. One should look carefully along the midline for dimples, sinuses, small red spots, hirsute areas, or cystic swellings that suggest the presence of congenital cranial dermal sinuses or other defects in the underlying vertebral column.

Ecchymoses may be present and related to birth trauma, and they may also serve as a source for bilirubin. Petechiae may be noted on the face after a difficult vaginal breech or vertex delivery, but generalized and recurring petechiae usually signify more serious infectious or hematologic problems or both. Milia are white papules measuring about 1 mm in diameter that are scattered across the forehead. These and white vesicles with a red macular base (erythema toxicum) are transient and benign and occasionally must be differentiated from pustules. Large dark areas in the posterior lumbar areas (Mongolian spots) are frequently present in black and Oriental infants and often alarm parents. They nearly always resolve by 4 years of age. Flame hemangiomas are common in the nape of the neck (''stork's bite'') and

on the bridge of the nose, forehead, and eyelids. On the face, these usually disappear by a few months, but those on the neck persist.

Jaundice in the first day of life is nearly always abnormal. Usually, jaundice appears on the head and face and becomes more prominent on the trunk and extremities and, lastly, on the sclerae as the bilirubin rises. Reliance on this progression should not take the place of measurement of serum bilirubin.

Head. Molding during descent through the birth canal may obscure significant alterations in head shape that will not become apparent until some days later. At that time, excessive height or length, narrowness or broadness, or bizarre knobbings or depressions may be noted. The commonest abnormalities of the head are caput succedaneum and cephalohematoma. The first is edema of the scalp skin and crosses suture lines; cephalohematomas are subperiosteal and therefore do not cross suture lines. Frequently, the impression of a depressed skull fracture appears when the rim of a cephalohematoma is palpated. This is so common and so rarely indicative of an underlying fracture of any kind that we will not usually take radiographs of the skull in such cases. The fontanels and sutures are also often distorted by molding, so that instead of separations one palpates ridges where cranial bones override others. Again, after a few days one can better estimate the size of fontanels and their flatness, fullness, or tenseness and the width of suture lines (Popich, 1972; Faix, 1982). Absent suture separations are as significant as excessive spreading of the lines, and one should always make a practice of running a fingertip from occiput to nasion along the sagittal and metopic sutures, from one temporal region to the other along the coronal suture, and over the occipitoparietal junctures to define the lambdoidal sutures. Large fontanels and split sutures most often are a normal variant, but they can be associated with increased intracranial pressure or conditions (e.g., hypothyroidism) that impair bone growth. Likewise, small fontanels and overriding sutures are generally of little significance but may be associated with conditions (e.g., microcephalies) in which brain growth has not kept pace with growth of the calvarium.

Eyes. Recent irritation by silver nitrate will make the eye examination no easier, but the eyes will usually open when the infant is held upright. The color of the conjunctiva and the presence of discharge within its sac may or may not indicate irritative response to the antigonorrheal bactericide recently instilled. The size of the eyeball is significant, as is true of apparent proptosis; so is its tension, and estimation of the tension of all eyeballs is recommended so that increase will be appreciated when encountered. Breadth of cornea is of utmost significance. Haziness

Table 5–2. Disorders Sometimes Associated with Abnormal Fontanel Size

Too large:	Skeletal disorders (e.g., hypophosphatasia, osteogenesis imperfecta)
	Chromosomal disorders (e.g., trisomies)
	Other (e.g., hypothyroidism, increased intracranial pressure)
Too small:	Hormonal disorders (e.g., hyperthyroidism)
	Skeletal disorders (e.g., craniosynostosis)
	Other (e.g., microcephaly)

(After Popich, G., and Smith, D.: J. Pediatr. *80*:749, 1972.)

or cloudiness of the cornea or lens or media can be quickly noted, and transient mild corneal haziness is not unusual in the newborn period. Tumors, such as small dermoids and hemangiomas, are easy to see, but one may need tangential illumination to discern the grayish color of retinoblastoma through the dilated, fixed pupil. Squint or ptosis of the upper lids will be obvious, as will inability to close one or both eyes due to peripheral facial nerve palsy. Unusual slanting of the lid slit, whether upward from within outward as in mongolism or downward from within outward as in mandibulofacial dysostosis deserves attention, as does epicanthus. The fundi can usually be seen, fleetingly at least, to provide assurance that a red reflex is present. Flame-shaped and linear hemorrhages in the retina may be seen in approximately one third of all babies born after cephalic deliveries and are of no significance.

Ears. The ears can be grossly malformed, uncommonly large or small, angled abnormally, or set lower on the head than is usual. Very low placement plus unusual size, floppiness, and perpendicularity to the skull suggest renal agenesis or gross chromosomal aberration. Malformations stemming from the first branchial arch often involve the ears, and one must always look carefully for abnormal skin tags, dimples, and deep sinuses, especially in front of and below the tragus. The newborn infant should respond to a loud noise or tone. Although not usually routine, otoscopic examination is important if the infant has been in an infected intrauterine environment.

Mouth. An excess of mucoid secretion in the mouth and pharynx suggests esophageal atresia. Clefts of the lip are obvious. One corner of the lip should not droop, and when the infant is crying both corners should move equally well; it may be necessary to apply a painful stimulus to a toe or the sole of the foot in order to demonstrate this. The alveolar ridges must be inspected for tumors (epignathus, epulis) and for clefts, for retention cysts (which resemble unerupted teeth, but are not), and for the elevated plaques of thrush. The tongue may be too large for the mouth and may tend to fall backward to block the pharynx. If possible, one should get a clear view of the pharynx, but the newborn's tongue is extremely difficult, at times impossible, to depress. One often does better by forcibly depressing the lower jaw and making the baby cry than by using a tongue depressor. During this part of the examination, one is looking for nasopharyngeal teratoma, aberrant thyroid, and thyroglossal duct cysts, among other items. On the palate or gums, one can occasionally see white shiny epithelial "pearls," which are benign and transient. The frenulum may be short, but it should always be left intact in the newborn period.

Jaw. The size of the jaw is of some interest. The small, undersized jaw of micrognathia can be the source of great respiratory and feeding difficulty (Pierre Robin syndrome).

Nose. The nose, too, can be the site of airway obstruction. One can and should assure oneself at the original examination that the posterior choanae are patent so that the newborn can breathe through his nose. This can be accomplished by forcibly holding the mouth closed and watching for evidence of respiratory distress or by listening with the stethoscope to the outrush of air from each naris when the mouth is closed and the other naris is occluded. Inspection up each naris may reveal a tumor or, at times, an encephalocele in the nasal airway.

Neck. Rarely, the neck is unusually short and has limited mobility; these signs suggest that Klippel-Feil syndrome may be present. The neck is the site of important congenital cysts that arise from the branchial arches and of dimples and sinuses that are related to them. Sternomastoid tumor, hygroma, thyroglossal duct cyst, and enlarged thyroid should be sought. Stiffness and retraction are important signs. Webbing caused by abnormal folds of skin running from the mastoid to the acromial area is highly significant. One runs a finger the length of each clavicle to be sure that it has not been fractured.

Chest. The chest deserves primary concern, as it is the site of the majority of troubles, both acquired and inborn, that affect the newborn. By observation, one notes whether it is overfilled with air, whether it moves adequately with respiration, and whether it is symmetric with respect to both size and motion of either side. One assesses the rate, rhythm, and depth of respiration and the presence or absence of retraction and the use of accessory muscles to aid breathing. Percussion and auscultation are not nearly so rewarding as they are in older children, but hyperresonance or dullness, diminution of air entry, rales, rhonchi, bowel sounds, and wheezes may be heard either diffusely or locally. Equally important is determination of the heart size and position and of mediastinal shift by these methods of physical examination. The interpretation of these physical signs is based upon the same principles one utilizes in older patients, aided by the foreknowledge of the statistical incidence of various disorders in the neonate. What is of greatest importance is that one examine every newborn by these methods, gaining assurance from year to year in one's ability to distinguish deviations from the normal. Interpretation will follow naturally.

Size and position of the heart as well as the rate, rhythm, and strength of its sounds are as important as the presence or absence of murmurs, if not more so. Extrathoracic signs such as cyanosis, size of the liver, dilatation of superficial veins, and palpability of femoral and other distal arterial pulsations are equally significant in arriving at diagnoses in the cardiac field.

Abdomen. In the abdomen, one looks for unusual flatness or emptiness (as an aid in diagnosing diaphragmatic hernia) and for abnormal fullness. If distention is present, one must determine by palpation, percussion, and auscultation whether this is due to an excess of air within or outside the bowels, to excess fluid (which might be clear or chylous exudate, purulent or sanguineous), to an enlarged viscus or viscera, or to the presence of a cystic or solid tumor. One determines carefully the size of the liver, the edge of which is normally palpable just below the costal margin, and the size of the kidneys, whose lower poles one can usually barely feel deep in the flanks. The ability to feel many small hard masses throughout the distended, doughy abdomen is highly significant. One also looks for evidence of venous obstruction in the form of dilated veins over the abdominal wall or, when severe, of cyanosis and edema of genitals and legs. Visible gastric or bowel patterns may be considered an almost certain sign of obstruction. The umbilicus will be inspected carefully for signs of infection, bleeding, polyp, granuloma, or abnormal communication with intra-abdominal viscera.

Genital Area. Items one must note in the apparent male include size and formation of the penis, position of the meatus, size of the scrotum and nature of its skin, and descent or nondescent of testes. In the apparent female, one notes the size of the clitoris, the nature of the skin of the labia majora, degree of fusion or nonfusion of the labia, and, if possible, the position of the vaginal and urethral orifices. One should also palpate carefully over the inguinal canals for possible presence of hernias or gonads.

The perineum should be scrutinized for unusual bulging. One must ascertain that the anus is perforate.

Back and Hips. With the baby prone, one examines the posterior part of the chest by percussion and auscultation. This is the time at which one can inspect and feel the occipital region minutely for hemangioma, cephalohematoma, encephalocele, and congenital dermal sinuses. The lumbosacral region and buttocks are inspected and probed for possible teratoma, meningocele, or lipomeningocele. With the baby still prone, one inspects the creases in the two thighs. If these do not match, further observations are in order. With the infant supine again, one attempts to compare the lengths of the two legs and then to abduct the thighs from a position of right-angle flexion laterally and downward to the table top. The significance of these findings is discussed in Chapter 94.

Extremities. Do all four move well and approximately symmetrically, or is one arm limp or one wrist dropped? Unusual resistance to flexion or extension or its converse, excessive malleability, or flaccidity, will be noted. Deep tendon reflexes can be tested in a moment. The distal extremities must be scrutinized for polydactylism or syndactylism, for clubbing, for edema, and for unusual creasing of the palms or soles.

Neurologic Assessment. A fairly complete neurologic examination will have been performed during the general one, since reaction to stimuli, activity, grasping, and character of the cry are readily noted. See Chapters 76 and 7 for details of the neurologic evaluation and the behavioral assessment.

Special Considerations in Examination of the Premature

With the increasing use of transcutaneous oxygen monitoring, it has again become obvious that a strenuous physical examination (especially when repeated) can be a stressful event resulting in severe hypoxemia followed by metabolic acidosis. For a 1000 gm infant who is intubated and receiving ventilatory support, the physical assessment must be continually provided by both nurses and physicians but should not be detrimental. One can perform a rapid gestational assessment using the method of Ballard. Nontraditional continual "vital signs," including transcutaneous O_2 and blood pressure and, occasionally, central venous pressure as well as F_{IO_2} should be evaluated, and respirator settings should be available. In the future, continuous pre- and postductal T_cPo_2, T_cPco_2, and intracranial pressure monitoring may be routine. A screening, top to bottom, for anomalies can be done rapidly. Fontanel pressure and degree of obtundation can be assessed (if the infant has not received muscle relaxants) during ventilator support. Adequacy of ventilation, endotracheal tube patency and position, and degree of leak, as well as presence or absence of intrathoracic air leak, are assessed with the stethoscope, measurements of pH and blood gases and blood pressure, and, often, thoracic transillumination. The abdomen is examined frequently for signs of hepatomegaly and intra-abdominal catastrophies. Nurses' and physicians' comprehensive or selective observations should be recorded sequentially and jointly in nonredundant fashion along with important lab values in a carefully timed and dated log. For an acutely ill infant, the reams of data obtained over days require a high degree of organization for the information to be useful. A variety of data storage and retrieval systems have been used, but, to our minds, they have not yet become sufficiently inexpensive, reliable, and "user-friendly" for widespread use.

Summary

The general pediatric history and examination should take less time than it takes to read this chapter, and the infant should remain no worse for the exercise. A refined judgment should now be possible as to whether the infant is well or sick, normal or abnormal, anomalous or not, and this information should be discussed with the parents. In discussions with them, their questions, whether realistic or not, can be answered while the infant's future home is evaluated and gaps in the history are filled in.

After the first day, daily visits by the physician or nurse practitioner to assess and discuss feeding, activity, jaundice, signs of illness, infant-parent rapport, and postdischarge planning are part of routine care. A brief complete physical examination on the day of discharge is currently performed routinely, followed by a brief discussion with the mother or both parents.

REFERENCES

Albert, R., and Condie, F.: Hand washing patterns in medical intensive care units. N. Engl. J. Med. *304*:1465, 1981.

Anderson, F., Johnson, T., Flora, J., and Borclay, M.: Gestational age assessment. II. Prediction from combined clinical observations. Am. J. Obstet. Gynecol. *140*:770, 1981.

Ballard, J. L., Novak, K. K., and Driver, M.: A simplified score for assessment of fetal maturation of newly born infants. J. Pediatr. *95*:769, 1979.

Crelin, E.: Anatomy of the Newborn—An Atlas. Philadelphia, Lea & Febiger. 1969.

Davies, P. A., Robinson, R. J., Scopes, J. W., et al.: Medical Care of Newborn Infants. Philadelphia, J. B. Lippincott Co., 1972.

Faix, R.: Fontanelle size in black and white newborn infants. J. Pediatr. *100*:304, 1982.

Hey, E.: Thermal neutrality. Br. Med. Bull. *31*:69, 1975.

Kirkland, R., and Kirkland, J.: Systolic blood pressure measurements in the newborn infant with transcutaneous Doppler method. Pediatrics *80*:52, 1972.

Klaus, M., and Fanaroff, A.: Care of the High-Risk Neonate. 2nd ed. Philadelphia, W. B. Saunders Co., 1979.

Lum, L., and Jones, M.: Effect of cuff width on systolic blood pressure measurements in neonates. J. Pediatr. *91*:963, 1977.

Miller, H. C., and Hassancin, K.: Diagnosis of impaired fetal growth in newborn infants. Pediatrics *38*:511, 1971.

Phibbs, R.: Evaluation of the newborn. *In* Rudolph, A. (Ed): Pediatrics. 2nd ed. New York, Appleton Century Crofts, 1982.

Popich, G., and Smith, D.: Fontanels, range of normal size. J. Pediatr. *80*:749, 1972.

Scanlon, J. W.: A System of Newborn Physical Examination. Baltimore, University Park Press, 1979.

Sunshine, P. (Ed.): Regionalization of Perinatal Care. Report of the 66th Ross Conference on Pediatric Research, 1974.

Versmold, H., Kitterman, J., Phibbs, J., et al.: Aortic blood pressure in the first 12 hours of life. Pediatrics *67*:607, 1981.

6

Newborn Screening

By Harvey L. Levy

Many metabolic disorders produce clinical effects postnatally. The clinical disease seems to be a consequence of the biochemical abnormalities that appear once the infant is on his own and no longer protected by the maternal circulation. The infant with phenylketonuria (PKU), for instance, is born with a normal blood phenylalanine level but develops a markedly increased level within the first day of life. If this biochemical abnormality is allowed to continue, the infant begins to show signs of developmental delay by the age of 3 or 4 months and will eventually become mentally retarded. If dietary therapy is ini-

tiated and the blood phenylalanine level thereby controlled during the first weeks of life, however, mental retardation from PKU is prevented.

The benefit of early dietary therapy in PKU was known by the middle 1950s. The challenge was to detect infants with PKU before clinical signs of brain damage appeared. This meant that the method of detection had to be biochemical rather than clinical.

This challenge was met in 1962 when Guthrie developed a simple bacterial inhibition assay for phenylalanine that could be applied to blood impregnated into filter paper. Thus, infants in newborn nurseries could be routinely tested for PKU from blood specimens obtained by sticking the heel with a lancet and blotting a filter paper card with a few drops of the blood. This paper blood specimen could be mailed to a central laboratory for PKU testing. An increased phenylalanine concentration in the blood specimen suggested that the infant had PKU.

By the middle 1960s, many states had begun routine newborn PKU screening programs. Infants with PKU were identified in larger numbers than had been anticipated and were showing normal development while on treatment. The success of PKU screening led to the addition of tests for other metabolic disorders that were similar in principle to PKU. These tests could be applied to the same filter paper specimen that was obtained for PKU screening. Thus, infants in some states were also routinely screened for galactosemia, homocystinuria, and maple syrup urine disease. Most recently, a test for congenital hypothyroidism has been added in most newborn screening programs throughout North America and Europe and in parts of Asia. This has been the most valuable addition since screening began.

Screening Programs

Specimen. The blood specimen is obtained from the heel of the infant, as depicted in Figure 6–1. This simple filter paper blood specimen developed by Guthrie has had an enormous impact on newborn screening. The specimen is not only easily obtained but also inexpensively mailed or otherwise delivered to a central facility for testing. There are no complications in obtaining this specimen from the newborn, contrary to early fears that this procedure would produce problems such as infection of the heel or excessive bleeding. The major considerations are that the specimen is obtained from *every newborn prior to nursery discharge* or by the fourth day of life (whichever is first) and that the circles on the filter paper card are fully saturated with blood.

With the growing practice of earlier nursery discharge, often during the first or second day of life, there is concern that the infant has not ingested sufficient protein for an amino acid elevation to occur when a metabolic disorder is present and that a specimen obtained at that early age will not reflect the disorder. The major fear is missing an infant who has

PKU. Recent information, however, indicates that most if not all neonates with PKU have an elevated blood phenylalanine concentration during the first day of life and should not be overlooked by newborn screening. The markers for congenital hypothyroidism, galactosemia, and maple syrup urine disease should also be present in early blood specimens. It must be emphasized that a blood specimen should be obtained for routine screening from *all neonates* prior to hospital discharge, regardless of when this occurs. A repeat blood specimen should be obtained at 2 to 3 weeks of age from those infants whose initial specimen was obtained within the first 24 hours of life.

Screening Laboratory. Newborn screening tests are usually performed in a centralized state, provincial, or regional laboratory. In the United States, for example, the blood specimen is usually mailed to the state public health laboratory. It may be tested in that laboratory or sent to a neighboring state laboratory that serves as a central testing facility for several states in the region. The screening laboratory performs the basic screening tests and notifies the attending physician (or collaborating state laboratory) of all abnormal test results. Confirmatory testing is also conducted in some screening laboratories.

Screening Tests. The testing procedure begins with the punching of small discs (each ⅛ inch in diameter) from the filter paper specimen. This process may be performed manually with a paper punch (e.g., for the congenital hypothyroidism test) or with a semiautomated punch indexer machine. In the bacterial assays for PKU and other inborn errors of metabolism (galactosemia, homocystinuria, and maple

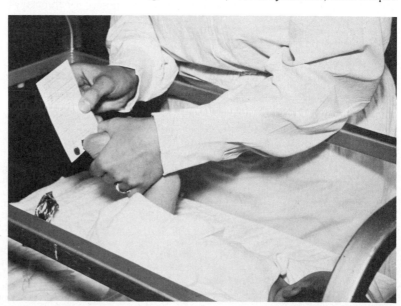

Figure 6–1. Filter paper specimen of blood collected from the heel of a neonate for routine newborn screening.

syrup urine disease), the discs are placed on agar gels that contain bacteria, growth media, and other necessary ingredients. Each bacterial plate is constituted to respond to a particular metabolite, and the amount of bacterial growth around the disc is proportional to the concentration of the metabolite in the blood. In the Guthrie test for PKU, for instance, the disc from the blood specimen of an affected newborn is surrounded by a large zone of bacterial growth (Fig. 6–2). Guthrie and others have developed a number of these bacterial assays, at least five of which are currently used in newborn screening (Table 6–1).

A radioimmunoassay for thyroxine (T_4) is the usual screening test for congenital hypothyroidism (Table 6–1). The disc of blood is placed in a test tube into which is introduced radioactive (^{125}I) T_4, anti-T_4 antibodies, and a chemical to prevent binding by thyroxine binding globulin. T_4 in the blood competes with the ^{125}I-T_4 for binding to antibody. When the T_4 concentration in the blood is low (e.g., in congenital hypothyroidism), more antibody binding sites are occupied by ^{125}I-T_4, and there is less free ^{125}I-T_4. Free and bound T_4 are separated, and the radioactivity in one of the fractions is counted (gamma counting). Following integration by a computing device, a T_4 level is assigned to each blood specimen. Any specimen with a low T_4 value is tested for thyroid stimulating hormone (TSH), also by radioimmunoassay. An elevated TSH concentration combined with a low T_4 level indicates primary hypothyroidism. In several programs, the radioimmunoassay for TSH is used as the primary screening test for hypothyroidism.

Several other screening tests are infrequently used (Table 6–1). Hemoglobin electrophoresis with blood eluted from the filter paper disc is employed for sickle cell disease screening. The Beutler enzyme spot assay for galactose-1-phosphate uridyl transferase is used

Table 6–1. Tests Used in Newborn Screening

Type of Test	Test Marker	Disorder
Bacterial assay	↑ Phenylalanine	Phenylketonuria
	↑ Galactose (-1-P)	Galactosemia
	↑ Methionine	Homocystinuria
	↑ Leucine	Maple syrup urine disease
	↑ Tyrosine	Tyrosinemia
	↑ Histidine	Histidinemia
Radioimmunoassay	↓ T4, ↑ TSH	Congenital hypothyroidism
Hemoglobin electrophoresis	Sickle hemoglobin	Sickle cell disease
Enzyme spot assay	↓ Gal-1-P uridyl transferase	Galactosemia
Fluorometric	↑ Phenylalanine	Phenylketonuria

to screen for galactosemia in some programs. Several programs in North America screen for PKU with a fluorometric assay for phenylalanine.

Confirmatory Tests. An abnormal finding on a newborn screening test is *not diagnostic* of a metabolic disorder. It is only an indication that the infant might have a disorder. Abnormalities in the newborn specimen can also be transient or result from artifacts. *Additional tests* must be performed so that a metabolic disorder is either confirmed or ruled out.

In screening for congenital hypothyroidism, the newborn blood specimen that contains a low T_4 level can be used for the TSH assay, as noted previously. Confirmation of PKU, galactosemia, or other inborn errors of metabolism requires additional specimens, since confirmatory testing for these disorders cannot be performed on the newborn blood specimen. Consequently, a repeat blood specimen (filter paper or plasma) and, often, a urine specimen are necessary for specific testing when the newborn blood specimen has an abnormality of this type. These confirmatory tests include quantitative amino acid analysis, paper or thin-layer chromatography, and enzyme assays.

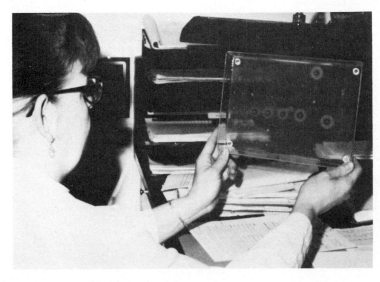

Figure 6–2. Guthrie bacterial assay for phenylalanine to identify PKU in the neonate. Small discs from the filter paper blood specimen are placed on the assay agar gel. Note the large growth around the disc at the upper right, indicating PKU in this infant. The center row of discs are control specimens containing known amounts of phenylalanine. The remaining discs are from normal neonates and are surrounded by little or no bacterial growth, indicating normal concentrations of phenylalanine.

Physician Contact. The pediatrician or other physician of record should be called whenever the newborn blood specimen contains such a striking abnormality that a metabolic disorder is strongly suspected. Thus, as noted in Table 6–1, a very low level of T_4 combined with an elevated TSH concentration indicates congenital hypothyroidism, and a markedly elevated level of phenylalanine, galactose, methionine, or leucine indicates PKU, galactosemia, homocystinuria, or maple syrup urine disease, respectively. If the infant is well, confirmatory testing should be performed, and, if these confirm the disorder, the infant should be evaluated at a metabolic center. If the infant is ill, specimens for confirmatory testing should be obtained, and treatment for the illness should be initiated without delay. If possible, the infant should be transferred to a special care nursery in a center that has a unit with professionals experienced in the diagnosis and treatment of inborn errors of metabolism.

Less striking abnormalities in the newborn blood specimen can be followed up by a letter to the physician that requests a repeat specimen(s). The results of repeat testing should be sent to the physician as soon as possible.

Most infants with a positive screening result, particularly when this result is only mildly or moderately abnormal, do not have a metabolic disorder. Transient or nonspecific abnormalities are quite frequent. Though all infants with an abnormal screening result must have repeat testing, the families should be informed that an initial positive result may have no medical implications. This may alleviate excessive anxiety and prevent unnecessary diagnostic procedures and treatment.

It is important to emphasize that the physician should contact the screening laboratory whenever the results of repeat testing have not been received or when an infant has clinical signs that suggest a metabolic disorder. In the latter instance, the screening laboratory can check the results of the newborn or repeat testing or may be able to perform additional tests on the specimen.

Disorders

Phenylketonuria (PKU). This metabolic disorder should always be identified by newborn blood screening (see Chapter 60). Most neonates with an elevated blood phenylalanine level will either have PKU or a variant such as hyperphenylalaninemia or have a transient elevation. Infants with other metabolic disorders, however, may also have an increased concentration or phenylalanine in blood, especially when they are acutely ill. These disorders include galactosemia and maple syrup urine disease.

Urine screening, either by ferric chloride testing for phenylketone identification or by Guthrie bacterial assay, is *unreliable* for newborn detection of PKU and should never be used for this purpose. The newborn infant, even one with severe PKU, rarely has detectable phenylketones or increased phenylalanine in urine, unlike the older infant or child.

Treatment for PKU should *never* be given on the basis of a positive screening test alone. The dietary therapy is difficult and can be extremely hazardous to an infant who does not have PKU. Only after repeat testing and confirmation of PKU should treatment be given, and then only in conjunction with a metabolic center.

Congenital Hypothyroidism. This is the most frequent of the disorders now identified by routine newborn screening. It occurs in about 1:4000 to 1:5000 screened infants, as compared with the PKU frequency of approximately 1:14,000.

The screening procedure for congenital hypothyroidism is quite reliable for identifying the affected infants, whether the primary screen is for a low T_4 level or for a high TSH concentration. Nevertheless, affected infants are missed in the screening process. This may be due to lack of the "marker" (either low T_4 or high TSH) in the newborn specimen, but it is probably more often due to laboratory error in misreading or overlooking the abnormal result. This type of error is much more likely to occur in radioimmunoassay procedures than, for instance, in the simpler and more easily interpreted Guthrie assay for PKU.

False-positive results are quite frequent in screening for congenital hypothyroidism. When low T_4 is the marker, this frequency may be as high as 3 per cent of all screened neonates. Most of these infants have a normal TSH concentration and are premature. Nevertheless, to avoid missing an infant with congenital hypothyroidism, screening programs usually require a repeat blood specimen from each of these infants.

Infants with a positive screening test should neither be "labeled" as having congenital hypothyroidism nor treated for this disorder until repeat and confirmatory testing is at least in progress. If the newborn blood specimen contains a high TSH concentration as well as a low T_4 level, treatment can be initiated before the results of the confirmatory tests are known. If the TSH concentration in the newborn blood specimen is normal, however, treatment should be withheld until confirmatory test results are available.

Galactosemia. Newborn screening for this disorder is strongly advisable. Without routine newborn screening, many affected infants are not diagnosed until they are terminally ill with sepsis (see Chapter 59), or they are never diagnosed. In addition, other disorders of galactose metabolism, particularly galactokinase deficiency, may not be identified until there are irreversible complications such as cataracts.

An assay for galactose (and galactose-1-phosphate), such as the Paigen *E. coli*-phage assay, is preferable to a specific enzyme assay, such as the Beutler spot test for galactose-1-phosphate uridyl transferase. This is so because the former assay is more reliable for the detection of galactosemia and will also identify other galactose disorders.

The immediate confirmatory test for a positive newborn screening result should be urine testing for reducing substance. This will always be strongly positive in galactosemia and at least moderately positive in galactokinase or epimerase deficiency. If the urine contains reducing substance and the infant has clinical signs of galactosemia, milk feedings (breast or formula) should be discontinued, and blood specimens for confirmatory testing should be obtained. If the urine is negative for reducing substance, the newborn screening result is probably false positive. Nevertheless, repeat blood and urine testing should be performed.

Homocystinuria. The newborn screening marker for this detection is an increased level of methionine in the newborn blood specimen, as identified by the Guthrie assay (Table 6–1). This screening is included in some programs, and affected neonates have been identified. Infants with homocystinuria have also been missed in newborn screening, probably because at that time their blood methionine concentration was not increased. Some of these infants can be identified in a follow-up blood specimen obtained at age 2 to 4 weeks.

Newborn infants frequently have slight increases in the blood methionine concentration as a transient phenomenon. At 3 to 6 weeks of age, these transient increases can be quite marked. To confirm homocystinuria, a repeat blood specimen is required. If the methionine concentration is again increased in the blood, quantitative amino acid analysis of plasma and urine should be performed. In the homocystinuric infant, there will usually be detectable homocystine in plasma and urine, increased methionine in plasma, and little or no cystine.

Newborn screening for methionine elevations will also occasionally identify a rare inborn error known as hypermethioninemia (see Chapter 60). On confirmatory testing, these infants will have markedly increased methionine in plasma but no homocystine in plasma or urine and a normal concentration of plasma cystine.

Maple Syrup Urine Disease. The marker for this disorder is increased leucine in the newborn blood specimen (Table 6–1). Neonates with "classic" maple syrup urine disease (MSUD) will virtually always have a fourfold or greater elevation of leucine. Transient increases in the blood leucine concentration are infrequent and usually no more than double the normal concentration.

MSUD can be a fulminant disease associated with severe metabolic acidosis and profound neurologic effect (see Chapter 60). Consequently, the finding of a substantial increase in the newborn blood leucine level should immediately be reported to the attending physician. If the infant is ill, confirmatory plasma and urine specimens should be obtained and emergency therapy initiated. If the infant has MSUD, the plasma will contain markedly increased concentrations of leucine, isoleucine, and valine (the branched-chain amino acids), and the urine will be strongly positive for ketones and contain huge quantities of the branched-chain ketoacids and amino acids. The characteristic odor reminiscent of maple syrup may not yet be present on the body or in urine of a neonate with MSUD.

Milder variants of MSUD can be missed in newborn screening. The neonate with the intermediate variant may have not yet developed an elevated blood leucine level or may have such a slight increase that it is overlooked. In the intermittent variant, the blood leucine concentration is elevated only during acute metabolic episodes.

Sickle Cell Disease. In a number of state newborn screening programs, notably those in New York and in the southern part of the United States, the newborn blood specimen is tested for hemoglobin abnormalities. The major purpose of this is to identify the infant with sickle cell disease.

When sickle hemoglobin is found, it is important to perform confirmatory testing so that the infant with the disease (homozygous for the sickle hemoglobin gene) is differentiated from the carrier of this gene (heterozygote). Only those who are homozygous should be diagnosed as having sickle cell disease. The much more frequent heterozygous infant should never develop the complications of this disease and should not be followed and stigmatized as an affected individual.

Other Screening

Cord Blood. Umbilical cord blood can be screened for maternal metabolic disorders that may affect the fetus and result in neonatal abnormalities. Paramount among these is maternal PKU (see Chapter 60). Cord serum or plasma contains the increased phenylalanine concentration that has been passively transferred from the maternal circulation. Disorders intrinsic to the infant in which the abnormality is present in erythrocytes can also be screened in cord blood, since this specimen contains the fetal erythrocytes. Among these disorders is galactosemia, in which there is no transferase activity and increased galactose-1-phosphate in cord blood.

Routine cord blood screening was conducted in Massachusetts for over 10 years. A filter paper card was soaked with blood from the umbilical cord at delivery and sent to the state screening laboratory. Initially, this specimen was screened for galactosemia and maternal PKU. Subsequently, galactosemia

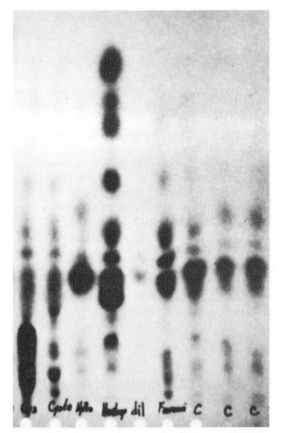

Figure 6–3. A paper chromatogram of newborn urine screening that depicts normal urine (C) and several abnormalities. These include (from left to right) cystinuria, cystathioninuria, hyperglycinuria, Hartnup "disease," and the renal Fanconi syndrome.

screening was discontinued, since this disease was effectively screened in the newborn blood specimen. Screening for maternal metabolic disorders such as maternal PKU and maternal histidinemia continued and yielded much valuable information about these disorders and their relation to the fetus. The information was of only very limited value to the families, however, and cord blood screening has been discontinued.

Urine. Routine newborn urine screening has been conducted in one or two states, in Quebec, and in Australia. This screening identifies infants with disorders that are not identifiable by blood screening. Among these are organic acid disorders such as methylmalonic acidemia (see Chapter 61), certain aminoacidopathies such as several urea cycle disorders (see Chapter 60), and renal transport disorders such as cystinuria and Hartnup disorder.

The specimen for this screening is obtained by the parent when the infant is about 4 weeks old. The usual method of collection is to press a wet portion of the diaper into filter paper that the parent is given upon leaving the hospital with the newborn infant. This filter paper specimen is sent to the screening laboratory, where it is tested by chromatography, either paper or thin-layer method. Figure 6–3 depicts

several abnormalities identified by newborn urine screening.

Specific Issues of Newborn Screening

SPECIMEN COLLECTION

Early Discharge. The identification of PKU and other amino acid disorders in the newborn depends upon an amino acid elevation in the newborn blood specimen. This elevation occurs after birth and results from the intake of protein as well as, probably, other factors, notably the normal postnatal endogenous proteolysis. There is concern that with nursery discharge on the first or second day of life, the neonate with a metabolic disorder such as PKU will not have ingested sufficient protein for the blood amino acid level to increase and that a blood specimen obtained at that time will be normal.

This concern appears to be largely unfounded with regard to the identification of PKU. Recent studies indicate that virtually all infants with PKU have an elevated blood phenylalanine level during the first day of life. This may not be true of infants with mild hyperphenylalaninemia, but this is usually benign and not treated.

An occasional infant with congenital hypothyroidism might be missed in a blood specimen obtained during the first day of life, since the T_4 level in these infants tends to decrease postnatally. Infants with homocystinuria and rare variant forms of other metabolic disorders might also be missed in an early specimen.

The 1982 statement on newborn screening of the American Academy of Pediatrics recommends that a repeat blood specimen be obtained at 2 to 4 weeks of age from every infant who is initially tested before 24 hours of age. Most importantly, a newborn blood specimen should be obtained from every infant prior to nursery discharge, regardless of how early this discharge occurs. A metabolic disorder is far more likely to be missed because a newborn blood specimen was never obtained than because it was obtained too early.

Routine Follow-up (Repeat) Screening. The procedure of obtaining a second blood specimen from all infants at 4 to 6 weeks of age was recommended when newborn screening began and was followed by most screening programs during the 1960s. After several years of this practice, however, it became apparent that very few infants with metabolic disorders, particularly PKU, were identified by this specimen. Thus, most screening programs began to discontinue routine follow-up specimen collection. A survey of this practice within the United States disclosed that only four infants with PKU were identified among over 2.3 million follow-up specimens tested, and at least three of these four infants should have been detected by initial newborn blood screening. By comparison, 290 infants with PKU were identified among 3.4 million initial newborn blood specimens tested in these surveyed states. Routine follow-up screening is not justifiable for PKU detection and is probably unjustified for the detection of other metabolic disorders.

Informed Consent. During the 1970s, there was lively discussion about the need for informed consent for newborn screening. Advocates argued that parents should decide whether newborn screening is to be performed and that public health laws mandating newborn screening or even routine medical practice are unethical. This advocacy has waned during the past few years, primarily because of the virtually insurmountable complications in obtaining truly informed consent from the parents of all newborn infants.

The issue of informed consent has implications that go beyond practicality. A major question is whether specific informed consent should be required for routine newborn screening for metabolic disorders when it is not required for other newborn tests (e.g., serum bilirubin). Is screening for disorders that may cause clinical illness and for which there is preventive treatment less important than testing the newborn when he is ill? An affirmative answer to this question is certainly contrary to the current focus of medicine.

SCREENING PROGRAMS

Central Laboratories. Newborn screening should be consolidated in relatively few large laboratories. This usually means a single state laboratory or a regional laboratory that serves several states. This decreases the costs of screening by virtue of mass analysis. Screening accuracy is enhanced because in a large laboratory there is much greater exposure to and thus familiarity with specimen abnormalities. Perhaps most important, a large central laboratory can include a professional and administrative unit that will continually monitor the process of specimen collection and requested repeat testing.

Missed Cases. Infants with PKU, congenital hypothyroidism, and other screened metabolic disorders have been missed in newborn screening. Laboratory or program error is the usual cause of these missed infants. In some instances, the mistakes occurred because the laboratory had no administrative or professional supervision. In other cases, however, the mistakes were the inevitable result of mass

screening in which very large numbers of specimens and results are processed daily. Thus, physicians must continue to rely upon clinical judgment and not fall into the trap of excluding a diagnosis because an infant has presumably been screened. Specific testing for metabolic disorders should be performed in any infant or child with signs that suggest such a diagnosis, regardless of the presumptive screening result.

Metabolic Disorders not Screened. A frequent error is the assumption that routine newborn screening covers metabolic disorders in general and that a normal result excludes most if not all of these disorders. Actually, most screening programs in North America test only for PKU and congenital hypothyroidism. Other programs in the United States and many in Europe and Japan include screening for galactosemia, homocystinuria, and maple syrup urine disease. Most metabolic disorders are not covered by newborn screening. All infants and children with signs that suggest a metabolic diagnosis should have specific testing, just as previously noted in considering the possibility of a missed infant.

OTHER DISORDERS CONSIDERED FOR SCREENING

Muscular Dystrophy. This disorder can be detected by newborn blood screening. The test is an assay that identifies increased creatine phosphokinase (CPK) activity. Several areas in France and Germany have included this in screening programs. The absence of therapy that will prevent the clinical manifestations of this disease, however, seems to militate against its use in routine newborn screening.

Congenital Adrenal Hyperplasia. Infants with the salt-losing form of this disorder can die precipitously, often without a specific diagnosis. Thus, newborn screening would be a valuable aid in early diagnosis and prompt therapy. A radioimmunoassay that identifies an increased concentration of 17-hydroxyprogesterone in the newborn blood specimen as a marker for this disease has been described. Unfortunately, this assay is more complicated and more costly than the radioimmunoassay for T_4 that is used in screening for congenital hypothyroidism. Whether the frequency of congenital adrenal hyperplasia and the value of newborn screening detection justify the difficulty of this assay remains to be seen. Should a simpler and less expensive detection method become available, this screening would probably be added in a number of programs.

Cystic Fibrosis. The frequency and severity of this disorder have made it prominently considered for routine newborn detection. Several screening tests have been proposed. Most notable among these is one that determines increased albumin in extracts of meconium. The meconium from affected infants will usually contain markedly increased albumin, owing to reduced pancreatic proteolytic enzymes. However, many conditions including prematurity can result in increased meconium albumin. Conversely, the meconium from an occasional infant with cystic fibrosis may contain normal or only slightly increased albumin. Thus, this test lacks the specificity and perhaps also the sensitivity necessary for feasible newborn screening.

Recently, a radioimmunoassay for serum trypsin has been proposed as screening for cystic fibrosis. This assay can be applied to the newborn filter paper blood specimen. It has not yet been used for mass screening, and some infants with cystic fibrosis may not have sufficient serum trypsin to be detected by this assay.

If an effective screening test for cystic fibrosis is developed, there will be controversy over whether it should be employed for early detection of a disease in which there is no preventive therapy. Unlike muscular dystrophy, however, preclinical identification of cystic fibrosis would lead to supportive therapy that might substantially reduce complications and prolong life.

Hyperlipidemia. Screening for the hyperlipidemias, specifically β-lipoproteinemia, seems to have little or no place in newborn screening. Lipids can be measured in the newborn filter paper blood specimen, but the rates of false-positive and false-negative results are unacceptably high. Of equal importance is the serious question about whether there is effective therapy that will consistently reduce the level of lipoprotein and prevent premature atherosclerosis.

Histidinemia. Among the Guthrie bacterial assays that can be applied to the newborn filter paper blood specimen is one for histidine (Table 6–1). This will identify an increased histidine concentration, the marker for histidinemia. This test is included in the New York State screening program and in programs in Austria and Japan. Many infants with histidinemia have been identified, although the frequency of false-negative results seems to be relatively high. However, there seems to be little need for this screening, since histidinemia is probably benign in most if not all individuals (see Chapter 60).

Summary

It is clear that routine newborn screening for a number of metabolic disorders is an effective and desirable health measure. Already the vast majority of newborns within the United States and in many other countries are routinely screened for phenylketonuria. In addition, a growing number are being screened for congenital hypothyroidism, galactosemia, maple syrup urine disease, and several other disorders. However, it is advisable to select carefully the type of error for which screening is performed. For instance, certain inborn errors of metabolism may have strikingly prominent biochemical abnormalities and yet be clinically benign. Screening is unnecessary for such disorders, since no treatment need or should be given. Among disorders that produce clinical abnormalities, the lack of preventive therapy militates against resources being devoted to their screening. Unfortunately, clear decisions regarding the nature and scope of routine newborn screening are currently made with difficulty, since there is, to some extent, a lack of information regarding the clinical consequences of many disorders and also a difference of opinion as to what may or may not constitute "therapy" in several given situations. These questions are under study at the present time, and it is hoped that a clearer picture of proper newborn screening will emerge over the next few years.

REFERENCES

Bickel, H., Bachmann, C., et al.: Neonatal mass screening for metabolic disorders. Summary of recent sessions of the Committee of Experts to Study Inborn Metabolic Diseases, Public Health Committee, Council of Europe. Eur. J. Pediatr. 137:133, 1981.

Bickel, H., Guthrie, R., and Hammersen, G. (Eds.): Neonatal Screening for Inborn Errors of Metabolism. Berlin, Springer-Verlag, 1980.

Committee on Genetics, American Academy of Pediatrics: New issues in newborn screening for phenylketonuria and congenital hypothyroidism. Pediatrics 69:104, 1982.

Committee for the Study of Inborn Errors of Metabolism: Genetic Screening. Programs, Principles, and Research. Washington, National Academy of Sciences, 1975.

Holtzman, N. A.: Hyperlipidemia screening: A search for Heffalumps? Pediatrics 64:270, 1979.

Holtzman, N. A., Leonard, C. O., and Farfel, M. R.: Issues in antenatal and neonatal screening and surveillance for hereditary and congenital disorders. Ann. Rev. Public Health 2:219, 1981.

Levy, H. L.: Genetic Screening for Inborn Errors of Metabolism. Washington, DHEW Publication No. (HSA) 75–5708. U.S. Government Printing Office, 1975.

Levy, H. L., and Hammersen, G.: Newborn screening for galactosemia and other galactose metabolic defects. J. Pediatr. 92:871, 1978.

Levy, H. L., and Mitchell, M. L.: Regional newborn screening for hypothyroidism. Pediatrics 63:340, 1979.

Medical Research Council Steering Committee for the MRC/DHSS Phenylketonuria Register: Routine neonatal screening for phenylketonuria in the United Kingdom 1964–78. Br. Med. J. 282:1680, 1981.

Meryash, D. L., Levy, H. L., et al.: Prospective study of early neonatal screening for phenylketonuria. N. Engl. J. Med. 304:294, 1981.

Naylor, E. W., and Guthrie, R.: Newborn screening for maple syrup urine disease (branched-chain ketoaciduria). Pediatrics 61:262, 1978.

Sepe, S. J., Levy, H. L., and Mount, F. W.: An evaluation of routine follow-up blood screening of infants for phenylketonuria. N. Engl. J. Med. 300:606, 1979.

7

Neonatal Behavior and Its Significance

By T. Berry Brazelton

The newborn infant has been thought of as neurologically insufficient (Flechsig, 1920), subcortical in his behavior (Lorenz, 1970), a blank slate to be written upon by his environment, his world a blooming, buzzing confusion (James, 1890). None of these descriptions fits the kind of predictable, directed responses one sees in a neonate when he is in social interaction with a nurturing adult or as he responds to an attractive auditory or visual stimulus. For, when positive rather than intrusive stimuli are utilized, the neonate has marvelous capacities for alerting and attention, for suppressing interfering reflex responses in order to attend. With very predictable behaviors, he responds to and interacts with his environment from birth. But this predictability requires a knowledge of his ongoing state of consciousness.* When "state" is accounted for, most of his reactions are predictable—to both negative and positive stimuli, from internal as well as external sources. State becomes a matrix for understanding his reactions.

The classic pediatric neurologic assessment of the neonate is based in part on his responses to painful or intrusive stimuli, and, as such, the resulting reflex behavior is, indeed, mediated by the midbrain. But such an examination neglects the available organized behavior that the infant can demonstrate as he suppresses reflexive behavior in order to attend to more "interesting" stimuli—such as the human face or voice, a soft rattle or a light caress:

As a newborn lies undressed and uncovered in the nursery, his color begins to change, with mottled uneven acrocyanosis of his extremities, as he attempts to control loss of body heat. He begins to shiver, then to cry and flail his limbs in jerky thrusting movements in an effort to raise his own temperature. In the face of such enormous demands, as one speaks gently and insistently into one ear, his move-ments become smoother and slower, and he gradually quiets completely. His face softens then brightens, and his eyes move smoothly to the side from which the voice is coming. His head follows with a sudden smooth turn toward the voice, and he searches for the face of the speaker. He fixes on the eyes of the examiner and listens intently for several minutes. If the examiner moves his face slowly to the baby's midline and then across to the other side, the newborn will track him, his head and eyes smoothly turning in an 180° arc.

This complex interaction of visual, auditory, and motor behavior in response to a human stimulus is managed by the neonate despite the enormous physiologic demands of being undressed and unrestrained in a cold, overstimulating nursery. If one ignores the importance of this capacity as he evaluates the neurologic and physiologic integrity of the neonate, he misses the implication of the powerful effect of the cortex on the autonomic and physiologic systems in the neonatal period. As pediatricians, we must be aware of the interactions between physiologic and psychologic mechanisms, as they represent integrity in the neonate and predict the individual differences in developmental outcome.

A pediatrician has tools for assessing the central nervous system of a neonate. A neonate may pass him by unless he pays attention to the baby's capacity to quiet down when spoken to, to alert when picked up and handled, and to lock onto and follow the examiner's face when the eyes are open.

Intrauterine Influences

The neonate's behavioral responses have already been powerfully influenced by intrauterine events and experiences. The extent of intrauterine shaping of behavior can only be guessed. Intrauterine nutrition and infection would be expected to be powerful in determining the DNA and RNA complements of the central nervous system and other organs, such as adrenals and thyroids, which underly neonatal behavior.

Winick suggests that as much as 40 per cent of the expectable DNA content of a neonate's brain may be reduced by prolonged, severe intrauterine malnutrition. We have examined a group of neonates from protein-caloric–deprived Guatemalan women in a nutritional study by Incap (Brazelton et al., 1977). We have found that caloric intake during pregnancy correlates with the behavior of the neonate. Infants with higher birth weight were more vigorous and motorically mature as well as more able to attend to visual and auditory stimuli than were low birth weight

---

* State of consciousness, or "state," of the infant becomes a most important matrix for interpretation of neonatal behavior. The newborn's reactions to all stimuli—internal and external—are dependent on his ongoing state of consciousness. Using "state" as a matrix, one can predict behavioral responses quite accurately. "State" depends on physiologic variables such as hunger, nutrition, degree of hydration, and the timing within the wake-sleep cycle of the infant. Our criteria for state throughout this chapter are based on the descriptions of Prechtl and Beintema.

infants. These infants were the offspring of better nourished mothers.

In addition to the physiologic effects of intrauterine depletion from under-nutrition and infection, we have been impressed with other intrauterine influences—for example, the influence of maternal experience on the behavior of the offspring. Sontag first suggested that in utero conditioning of human fetal behavioral responses might represent a kind of "learning" that would contribute to individual differences seen in neonatal behavior. When the fetal heart rate was monitored by a cardiotachometer placed on the mother's abdomen, the fetal heart responded to auditory stimuli, cigarette smoking, and emotional shocks administered to the mother. As these stimuli were repeated, the fetal heart rate response became diminished and its latency prolonged. In another study, Ando and Hattori demonstrated that infants near an airfield in Okinawa who had been exposed to high noise levels during the first 4 months of gestation were significantly less reactive to loud sounds after birth. Thus, one can expect that all kinds of information and stimulation—both that directly received by the fetus and that received via the neurologic and chemical responses of the mother—might shape infant behavior. But effects may not be seen as linear in the outcome behavior of the neonate. For example, the fetus may respond to anxiety in the mother by becoming more active and reactive (more anxious); or he may "learn" to cope with the stress induced by her anxiety and become quieter—having learned to shut down on his own responses to her signals. At birth, the baby may be intensely driving, overreactive, or he may be quietly able to handle stimulation or he may demonstrate a mixture of both these mechanisms.

Prenatal behavioral organization has been outlined by Hooker, Gesell, and Windle. More recently, the study of prenatal responses has been greatly advanced with ultrasonographic imaging. Distinct movement patterns have been correlated with gestational age (Birnholz et al., 1978; Ianniruberto and Tajani, 1981; Milani-Comparetti, 1981). Observations of eye movements and breathing patterns appear to be sensitive indicators of the functional development of the central nervous system. Birnholz has described eye movements as early as 16 weeks, with more complex movements after 23 weeks. The absence of eye movements was noted in several infants with major malformations of the brain.

PRETERM INFANTS

The greater numbers of low birth weight infants who now survive provide a new challenge to the behaviorists. Evaluation of the responses of these infants in the first days of life is difficult when they are being ventilated and monitored, but even then changes in heart rate and transcutaneous oxygen tensions, for example, can reflect changes in state (Long et al., 1980). Increasingly, we note that the nurses

depend on changes in oxygenation to indicate the need for less vigorous suctioning, for example, and occasionally establish a schedule of adequate rest for an infant who may have been overstressed by procedures. Simply covering the incubator with a blanket during rest periods may be useful.

The intensive care nursery can be a life-saving environment, but it can also be a hostile one. Continuous noise from the incubator motor (80 to 90 decibels), constant light, and procedures that require frequent handling can literally bombard the infant with stimuli that would not have been present in utero (Gottfried, 1981). Surely, some stimuli are useful, but we have little information concerning the appropriate amounts (Gorski et al., 1979). Klaus and Kennell have urged more direct parent contact with the infant, and they have found that the parents' sense of competence in parenting improves with early and frequent interactions (including touching or stroking the infant).

We have translated these findings into a practice that allows, even encourages, parents to visit and touch their infant. As soon as the medical condition permits, we encourage holding the baby and nursing. Parents quickly perceive small signals from the baby, such as eye contact, and even "smiles" at a few weeks of age in infants only 28 to 30 weeks postconceptual age. At least a contented expression is readily elicited.

Organization of Motor Behavior

The organization and quality of the newborn's motor behavior can provide much information on the current state of the newborn. However, one must be constantly aware of the conditions that will influence the infant's performance in a period of observation. These include (1) his state of arousal; (2) environmental factors such as temperature, lighting, and sound levels that influence his arousal state; (3) chemical imbalance such as hypoglycemia or hypercalcemia; (4) state of hydration; (5) state of wellbeing—e.g., illness or other stress; and (6) degree of recovery from perinatal and other stresses. Effective hand-to-mouth activity may be important not only because it signifies the baby's capacity to perform a complex motor feat but also because he may use it for quieting himself in order to attend to his environment or keep himself under control. Then it becomes a significant observation in the neonatal nursery.

Complex behavioral patterns available to the neonate become a way of measuring his integrity. Spontaneous hand-to-mouth efforts as he becomes upset and tries to keep himself under control or hand-to-mouth responses as his cheek is stroked or his palm is touched become a way of seeing his capacity for motor organization. This complex behavioral arc of hand-to-mouth was first described and named by Babkin in 1960.

Defensive reactions are structured motor patterns, and the infant's effectiveness in approaching and removing an obtrusive stimulus becomes a way of testing for motor pathways and their organization. For example, covering the baby's face with a cloth elicits a series of motor maneuvers. First he roots, then twists his head from side to side, stretches his neck backward in active arching, and finally brings each arm up to swipe at the offending cloth. Many newborns effectively push the cloth off the face. These responses (hand-to-mouth, defensive movements, or other sequential motor acts) may be of equal value to elicited reflexes as the examiner assesses the upper extremities for neurologic adequacy.

Motor activity may be observed for other than its value as an assessment of neurologic integrity and maturation. There have been reports in the literature that seem to point to differences in genetic endowment. Geber first described a kind of motor precocity in African neonates that seemed to place them 4 to 6 weeks ahead of a control group of European neonates. Her methodology and findings are under dispute (Warren, 1972), but Super has found that East African mothers stimulate their babies in a way that fosters early motor development. This raises the question as to whether mothers are sensing a kind of motor "excitement" in their babies that they foster in subsequent interactive behavior leading to precocity. This is supported by findings of extremely balanced motor tone and well-organized, smooth movements of Gusii newborns in Kenya (Keefer, 1981).

To assign genetic differences in precocity or motor behavior without seeing this neonatal behavior as an interaction between genetic endowment and intrauterine experience would be naive, for we are becoming more aware of nutritional and chemical effects on motor development in utero. Hence, the reports of genetic differences must be evaluated with intrauterine shaping in mind.

There is little question that the neonate's motor potential and his kind of motor activity react powerfully to the environment around him. For example, an intensely driving motoric neonate can be predicted to be fussy, or "colicky." This kind of infant is easily aroused to intense, driving motor activity. His response to almost any stimulus is a startle, followed by an intense crying state. He thrusts his arms and legs in violent activity. This reaction sets off startles that continue to upset him. Each startle produces more activity and crying. He tends to perpetuate this cyclic, disturbed crying activity for long periods. A parent's upset reaction to this crying contributes more tension, and one sees the anlage for "colic" in the neonatal period. When one assesses such a neonate

and finds this hyperactivity to stimuli not suppressed by him or by reasonable, calming maneuvers, one can predict a "colicky" infant and a period of stress for the parents. With such a prediction, the physician can begin to intervene during the neonatal period, and his role becomes supportive to the neonate's parents. His responsibilities include (1) relieving them of their inevitable upset about having fostered the infant's disturbed behavior and about being unable to find a "magical" solution that will soothe him and suppress his hyperactive, hypersensitive behavior; and (2) predicting for them that a consistent, low-keyed environment will lead to relief from the baby's "colicky" behavior after a few months and eventually, in all likelihood, to a well-organized, rather exciting baby. As a result, careful observation and assessment of the way an infant moves and how he uses his motor capacities may be extremely important as a predictor of his CNS integrity, of his genetic and intrauterine experience, of his perinatal recovery, of his individual temperamental endowment, and of his potential influence on the environment around him.

Sensory Capacities

The newborn is equipped with the capacity for processing complex visual stimulation and showing organized visuomotor behavior. When a bright light is flashed into a neonate's eyes, his pupils constrict, he blinks, his eyelids and whole face contract, he withdraws his head by arching his whole body, often setting off a complete startle as he withdraws, his heart rate and respirations increase, and an evoked response registers on his visual occipital EEG. Repeated stimulation of this nature will induce diminishing responses. For example, in a series of 20 bright-light stimuli presented at 1-minute intervals, we found that the infant rapidly "habituated" out the behavioral responses, and, by the tenth stimulus, not only his observable motor responses had decreased but also his cardiac and respiratory responses had begun to decrease markedly. The latency to evoked responses as measured by EEG tracings was increasing, and, by the fifteenth stimulus, his EEG reflected the induction of a quiet, unresponsive state similar to that seen in sleep (Brazelton, 1961). His capacity to shut out repetitive disturbing visual stimuli protects him from having to respond to visual stimulation and at the same time frees him to save his energy to meet his physiologic demands. The capacity to habituate to visual stimuli is decreased, although present, in immature infants (Hrbek and Mares, 1964) and is depressed by medication such as barbiturates given to mothers as premedication at the time of delivery. This has led Brazier to postulate that the primary focus for this mechanism is in the reticular formation and midbrain. However, the cortical control over this mechanism seems apparent as one observes a neonate who is initially in irregular, light sleep become drowsier with repeated stimulation. He then becomes deeply asleep, with tightened, flexed extremities, little

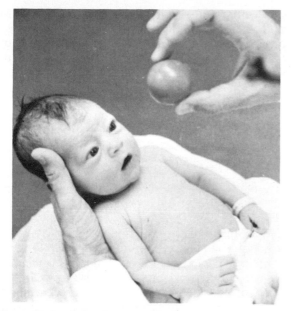

Figure 7–1. Following a red ball.

movement except jerky startles, no eyeblinks, deep, regular respirations, and rapid, regular heart rate. This state seems to resemble a defense against the assaults of the environment, and, upon cessation of the stimulation, the infant almost immediately goes back to his initial state or an even more alert state. One can often see neonates in noisy, brightly lighted neonatal nurseries in this "defensive" sleep state.

Just as he is equipped with the capacity to shut out certain stimuli, he also demonstrates the capacity to alert to and to turn his eyes and head to follow and fix upon a stimulus. Fantz first pointed out neonatal preference for complex visual stimuli. More recently, Goren (1975) showed that immediately after delivery, a human neonate would not only fix upon a drawing that resembled a human face but would also

follow it in 180 degree arcs, with eyes and head turning to follow. A scrambled face did not receive the same kind of attention, nor did the infant follow the distorted face with his eyes and head for the same degree of lateral following.

Extremes of brightness and noise in the environment have been found to interfere with the neonate's capacity to respond. In a noisy, overlighted nursery, the neonate tends to shut down on his capacity to attend, but, in a semidarkened room, a normal neonate in an alert state can be brought to respond to the human face as well as to a red or shiny object. For example, the following description indicates the behaviors of which the infant is capable:

The neonate is held or propped up at a 30° angle. Vestibular responses enhance eye opening and tend to bring him to a more alert state (Korner and Thoman, 1970). His eyes begin to scan the environment with a dull look, wide pupils, and saccadic lateral movements of both eyes.

As a bright red ball is brought into his line of vision and is moved slowly up and down to attract his attention, his pupils contract slightly. As the ball is moved slowly from side to side, his face begins to brighten, his eyes widen, his limbs still, and he stares fixedly at the object, beginning slowly to track the ball from side to side. He maintains the stilled posture in order to attend to the ball. His eyes first track in small arcs that take him off the target, but as he becomes more invested, the eye movements become smoother. As his eyes move laterally, his head begins to turn, and he moves his head from side to side in order to facilitate the tracking of the object. He is able to follow it for as much as 120°, to right and left, and will even make eye and head movements to follow it 30° up or down. Meanwhile, interfering body movement or startles seem to be actively suppressed. He can maintain this intense visual involvement for several minutes before he startles, be-

Figure 7–2. Head turning to follow.

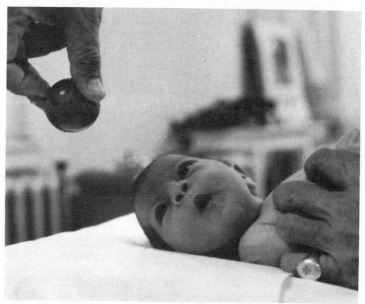

comes upset or dull, and loses the alert state necessary for this kind of visual behavior.

Tronick and Clanton have experimentally demonstrated that these complex patterns of coordination of head and eye movements appear to be very organized, and they suggested that the infant has a cortically controlled visual system at birth that coordinates head and eye for the extraction of information from the environment.

Adamson has demonstrated the importance of vision to the neonate by covering an alert baby's eyes with both an opaque and a clear plastic shield. He swipes at and attempts vigorously to remove the opaque shield, building up to frantic activity to do so and quieting suddenly when it is removed. When the clear shield is substituted, he becomes calm enough to look interestedly through it.

Bower and Tronick have demonstrated that neonates will actively defend themselves from looming visual targets with a defensive reaction to an approaching object. The defense includes head turning and directed arm movements.

Salapatek and Haith have found that the highest points of concentration of fixation in the neonatal period are on the contrasting edges of an object. In the neonate, the eyes or sides of the head seem to be the most compelling features of the face. Thus, the neonate seems to be highly programmed for visual learning from birth. The visual stimuli that are "appropriate" or appealing, such as the human face and eyes or a moving object, seem to be adapted to capture his attention very early. This allows for very

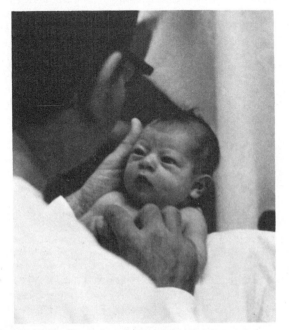

Figure 7–3. Fixation and intense interest in the human face.

early learning about his human caretakers and the world around him. If his physiologic systems are not overwhelmed with demands of too much information or too prolonged a period of attention, he will attend for long alert periods.

When an examiner can produce graded visual and motor responses in a neonate, he can be encouraged to predict a normal, well-integrated nervous system.

AUDITORY

The neonate's auditory responses are specific and well organized. But often assessments are not sensitive to the complexity of newborn behavior. For example, the loud clackers used in the Collaborative Project of The National Institutes of Health for early detection of central nervous system defects were ineffective in loud, noisy nurseries. A large percentage of neonates tested with such a routine were unresponsive and appeared to have shut out or habituated to auditory stimuli. Another approach in these conditions would have been to use a soft rattle. This stimulus would have been more appropriate to the habituated state of these neonates. Hence, a routine test for hearing should include several stimuli—animate as well as inanimate—with careful pairing of the stimulus so that it will break through the neonate's present state of consciousness; for example, a rattle in light sleep, a voice in awake states, and a clap in deep sleep. Respirations and eyeblinks, as well as more obvious behavioral responses, should be monitored for reactions to auditory stimuli.

A pediatrician can test this in the nursery. By speaking softly in a high-pitched voice to one side of the baby's head, the doctor should be able to see the infant become quiet and alert-looking and gradually turn his head toward the voice. As the examiner continues to talk, the infant begins to search for the source of the voice with his eyes, his face intent. This train of behavior is found in intact, normal infants and is a good sign of central nervous system integrity.

The neonate can discriminate sound on the basis of frequency, intensity, and stimulus-dimensionality. A low frequency stimulus tends to have a soothing effect on the neonate, whereas a high frequency stimulus causes an immediate arousal. Kearsley found that a noise of 70 db with a rise time of a few milliseconds shows an immediate response in the form of startle, closing of the eyes, and increase in heart rate. If the same noise is presented at a rise time of 2 seconds, the infant merrily opens his eyes and looks around. Thus, toy makers usually employ the acoustic signals used in behavorial audiometry largely because of their sudden and rapid rise time. There are also more complex than pure tones, and these include high frequency components that have the best arousal value. The noise makers most commonly used are a small bell that produces frequency around 4000 Hz and a plastic rattle with sand inside that produces a sound peak at 1000 Hz. The noise makers, when activated within 3 inches of the baby's ear, produce a sound of 35 db SPL. The aforementioned sound levels and frequencies give the examiner some consistent measured levels that can be replicated.

Noise levels ranging from 80 to 100 db have been measured in the usual nursery. The newborn has been exposed to sounds of 72 db in utero and is therefore accustomed to background noise. Under these circumstances, the ideal environment for testing hearing is a soundproof room, or at least a quiet area. A positive response to a sound stimulus is a definite eye blink immediately following the stimulus or a slight shudder of the whole body. This response must be seen within 2 seconds of the presentation of the stimulus. If positive responses are not elicited by the softer noise makers, other stimuli can be employed (e.g., crushed paper, a voice at 45 db, and, finally, a sudden voice burst at 60 to 70 db).

In sum then, as one defines the neonate's behavioral response to an appropriate sound, one sees a series of regular steps. As the sound is localized cardiac rate first increases (Lipton et al., 1966) and may be accompanied by a mild startle. If the auditory stimulus is attractive to the infant, his face will brighten, his heart rate will decelerate, his breathing will slow, and he will alert and search with his eyes until the source of the sound is localized and in the "en face" midline of the baby. This train of behavior, which occurs as a response to an attractive auditory stimulus such as the human voice, becomes a measure of the neonate's capacity to organize his central nervous system.

OLFACTORY

Engen and coworkers have demonstrated differentiated responses to acetic acid, anise, asafetida, and alcohol in the neonatal period. More recently, MacFarlane has shown that 7-day-old neonates can reliably distinguish their own mothers' breast pads from those of other mothers. They turn their heads toward their own mothers' breast pads with 80 per cent reliability, after controls for laterality are imposed. We have seen that at 3 weeks, infants who are breastfeeding may refuse to accept a formula from their mothers. This refusal seems to be related to the infants' ability to choose the available breast by smell. Yet fathers are successful in giving a bottle to these same babies. Thus, it seems that the neonate does have the capacity to make choices from olfactory stimuli, and that this information too can be used as part of the attachment process.

TASTE

The newborn has fine differential responses to taste. Nelson (Jensen, 1932) observed differentiated sucking responses to sugar, salt, quinine water, and citric acid solutions, with increased sucking to sugar and decreased sucking to the others. More recently, it has been reported that a newborn's differentiation

is expressed in an even more complex fashion. When an infant is fed different fluids through a monitored nipple, his sucking pattern is recorded. With a cow's milk formula he will suck in a rather continuous fashion, pausing at irregular intervals. If breast milk is fed to him in this paradigm, he will register his recognition of the change after a short latency, then suck in bursts, with frequent pauses at regular intervals. The pauses seem to be directly related to breast milk as if he were programmed for other kinds of stimuli (such as social communication) in the pauses.

TACTILE

The sensitivity of the infant to handling and to touch is quite apparent. A mother's first response to an upset baby is to contain him—to shut down on his disturbing motor activity by touching or holding him. Swaddling has been used in many cultures to replace the important constraints offered first by the uterus and then by mothers and caretakers. As a restraining influence on the overreactions of hyperreactive neonates, the supportive control that is offered by placing a steady hand on a baby's abdomen or by holding his arms so that he cannot startle reproduces the swaddling effects of holding or wrapping a neonate. This added control of disturbing motor responses allows the neonate to attend to and interact with his environment (Lipton et al., 1965).

First used for containment, tactile stimuli can be used to rouse or sooth the neonate. A patting motion of three times per minute seems to be soothing, whereas at five or six times a minute he becomes more excited and alert for other kinds of stimuli.

A test of the baby's responsiveness may be to place a hand firmly on his belly when he is beginning to become upset. If he can utilize this tactile pressure to calm himself down, the examiner can feel better about him. Holding onto the arm or arms of a crying, flailing baby will usually break through the cycle of startling and crying to comfort him.

This maneuver can be used when the infant is undressed and beginning to become upset in order to auscultate the heart and lungs.

SUCKING

The awake, hungry newborn exhibits rapid searching movements in response to tactile stimulation in the region around the mouth, and even as far out on the face as the cheek and sides of the jaw and head. This is called the rooting reflex and is present in the premature even before sucking itself is effective (Prechtl, 1956).

The infant sucks in a more or less regular pattern

of bursts and pauses. During nonnutritive sucking, his rate varies around two sucks per second (Wolff, 1966). Bursts seem to occur in packages of 5 to 24 sucks per burst (Kaye, 1967). The pause between bursts has been considered to be a rest and recovery period as well as a period during which cognitive information is being processed by the neonate (Halverson, 1944; Bruner, 1969). Kaye found that the pauses were important ethologically, since they are used by mothers as signals to stimulate the infant to return to sucking. However, the mother's jiggling actually prolongs the pause as the infant responds to the information given to him by his mother.

Bernbaum and colleagues found nonnutritive sucking to enhance maturation of the sucking reflex in preterm infants. Coordinated sucking was usually achieved by 33 to 34 weeks gestation. The use of a pacifier during gavage feeding enhanced the ability to generate normal suction pressures by 39 weeks. In a controlled study, the infants stimulated with a pacifier were able to move to full bottle feedings earlier, and, at the same total milk intake, showed a better weight gain.

Finger sucking is common in the neonatal period, and there is evidence that the insertion of parts of the hand in the mouth occurs commonly in the uterus. The importance of sucking as a regulatory response can be seen in a newborn as he begins to build up from a quiet state to crying. His own attempts to achieve hand-to-mouth contact in order to keep his activity under control are fulfilled when he is able to insert a finger into his mouth, suck on it, and quiet himself. The sense of satisfaction and of gratification at having achieved this self-regulation are apparent. His face softens and alerts as he begins

to concentrate on maintaining this kind of self-regulation. A pacifier can provide this same kind of quieting in an upset baby but may not serve the self-regulatory feedback system as richly as the baby's own maneuver.

The newborn sucks most when highly aroused and is, in general, soothed through the sucking act. Piaget asserts that the first changes in sucking that come about as part of his learning about the world are "the beginning of the infant's psychology." We should add to our neonatal examination a test for CNS integration: (1) Insert a gloved finger into the baby's mouth to produce a sucking response; (2) as soon as he is sucking well, test his hearing and his vision by observing his sucking response to a light and a rattle or a voice; (3) if he responds by a brief cessation of sucking, as he should, repeat the auditory or visual stimulus several times at short intervals. He should gradually lose interest in the stimulus and continue his sucking pattern without interruption. This simple set of maneuvers demonstrates auditory and visual integrity as well as his capacity for complex interactions between systems, and, most important, it shows his ability to shut out repeated nonsignificant information.

Heart Rate as a Measure of Attention and Habituation

The neonate's capacity to attend to external stimuli is coupled with the capacity to habituate or tune them out. In states of alert inactivity, he can be brought to a state of alert attention by many kinds of stimuli. His capacity to discriminate between stimuli, to attend to or to shut out stimuli, is complex and highly organized.

Bridger and Reiser as well as Lipton and colleagues have demonstrated that the prestimulus heart rate is likely to be inversely correlated with the response as well as the magnitude of heart rate response. Most infants have a reliable resting heart rate toward which their poststimulus rate will tend in a cyclic homeostatic curve. If the infant's prestimulus rate is high, a response will bring about relative deceleration; if his prestimulus rate is low, his response will be toward acceleration. Negative or disturbing stimuli produce little or no deceleration; soothing stimuli produce a mild decrease in base rate and a stable low-grade homeostatic response; an attractive or interesting stimulus may bring about marked, brief acceleration followed by a period of observable deceleration.

Habituation to repeated stimuli can be monitored by this technique (Bartoshuk, 1964; Bridger, 1961). Since habituation is generally thought to reflect cortical storage of information about a stimulus, the decrease in heart rate response over repeated trials with a stimulus might reflect the infant's cortical functioning. With an intrusive stimulus, one sees a gradual, diminishing shutdown on the degree of acceleratory cardiac responses to the repetitious stimulus. With an interesting stimulus, the acceleratory component may

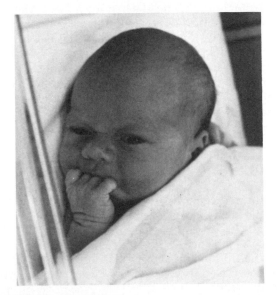

Figure 7–4. Sucking.

decrease slightly, but the deceleratory phase is markedly affected with repeated presentations. This, then, becomes a measure of cortical function. Dishabituation (or recovery of the total response) when the stimulus is changed can be seen in the neonatal period and can be used as another measure of cortical and subcortical function in the neonatal period (Brackbill, 1973; Eisenberg, 1965).

Since these measures are dependent on the integrity of the central nervous system as well as upon the demands on the cardiac system, it is not surprising that stressed infants do not demonstrate this complex behavior. Lester demonstrated a substantial orienting response followed by rapid habituation to auditory signals with dishabituation to changes in tonal frequency in well-nourished infants. But infants who had been undernourished showed an attenuation or complete absence of the orienting response and no dishabituation to changes in tonal frequency. The decrease in these responses seemed highly correlated with the degree of malnutrition to which the infants had been exposed.

Heart rate responses to auditory, visual, tactile, and the kinesthetic stimuli have been underutilized in assessing the cognitive and physiologic status of stressed neonates. We have utilized both negative (bright light, bell) and positive stimuli (soft rattle, touch, human voice) in assessing immature infants and have monitored changes in skin color as we presented the stimuli. One can observe clinically an initial change in skin color followed by recovery to good color when the infant can either habituate to disturbing stimuli or attend to interesting stimuli. When he cannot habituate or attend, his poor color increases and he can be stimulated until he is in cardiovascular collapse (as was observed with repeated visual responses in an anencephalic baby [Brazelton, Scholl, and Robey, 1966]).

State

The matrix of state as a concept for organization in the neonate has become of importance since its use as a background for neurologic behavior in Prechtl's assessment. Within the context of optimal state of alertness, he demonstrated that the newborn's midbrain reflexive behavior improved, and the neurologic exam became a better diagnostic measure.

Sleep states have been recognized and defined since the 1937 study by Wagner. She described some of the behaviors seen in deep or regular sleep—jerky startles and relative unresponsiveness to external stimuli as well as more regulated smooth movements accompanied by responsiveness to stimuli in lighter sleep. Wolff added his observations of deep sleep—regular, deep respirations with sudden spontaneous motor patterns such as sobs, mouthing, and sucking as well as erections that occurred at fairly regular intervals in an otherwise inactive baby. He observed that babies were more responsive to stimuli in light sleep. Aserinsky and Kleitman described cycles of quiet, regular sleep followed by active periods of body movements and rapid eye movements (REMs) under closed lids. Hence, light sleep has come to be designated as REM sleep. At term, active sleep (REM) occupies 45 to 50 per cent of total sleep time, indeterminate sleep occupies 10 per cent, and quiet sleep accounts for 35 to 45 per cent. The predominance of active sleep has led to the hypothesis that REM sleep mechanisms stimulate the growth of the neural systems by cyclic excitation, and it is in REM sleep that much of the differentiation of neuronal structures and neurophysiologic discharge patterns occurs (Anders and Roffwarg, 1973). Quiet sleep seems to serve the purpose of inhibiting CNS activity and is truly a habituated state of rest.

The length of sleep cycles (REM active and quiet sleep) changes with age. At term, they occur in a periodicity of 45 to 50 minutes, but immature babies have even shorter, less well defined cycles. Newborn infants have as much active REM in the first half of the deep period as in the second half. Initial brief, individual sleep and wake patterns coalesce as the environment presses the neonate to develop diurnal patterns of daytime wakefulness and night sleep. Appropriate feeding patterns, diet, absence of excess anxiety, sufficient nurturing stimulation, and a fussing period prior to a long sleep have all been implicated as reinforcing to the CNS maturation necessary to the development of diurnal cycling of sleep and wakefulness. Sleep polygrams, as determined by both EEG and activity monitoring, are proving to be sensitive indicators of neurological maturation and integrity in the neonatal period. Steinschneider has analyzed the occurrence of apnea episodes during sleep as part of a study on the sudden infant death syndrome (SIDS). He found that these episodes are more likely to occur during REM sleep, and has suggested that prolonged apnea, a concomitant of sleep, is part of a final physiological pathway culminating in SIDS.

In our behavioral assessment of neonates, we have utilized the two states of deep, regular and active REM sleep described by Wolff and Prechtl. These states can be reliably determined by observation and without any instrumentation.

1. Deep sleep: regular breathing, eyes closed; spontaneous activity confined to startles, and jerky movements at quite regular intervals. Responses to external stimuli are partially inhibited and any response is likely to be delayed. No eye movements, and state changes are less likely after stimuli or startles than in other states.

2. Active REM sleep: irregular breathing, sucking movements, eyes closed but rapid eye movements can be detected underneath the closed lids. Also characterized by low activity level, irregular smooth

organized movements of extremities and trunk. Startles or startle equivalents as response to external stimuli occur with change of state.

Alert states have been separated into four states for our behavioral assessment:

1. Drowsy: semidozing, eyes may be open or closed, eyelids often fluttering, activity level variable, with interspersed mild startles and slow, smoothly monitored movements of extremities at periodic intervals; reactive to sensory stimuli but with some delay, state change frequently after stimulation.

2. Wide awake: alert bright look; attention focused on sources of auditory or visual stimuli; motor activity suppressed in order to attend to stimuli. Impinging stimuli break through with a delayed response.

3. Active awake: eyes open, considerable motor activity, thrusting movements of extremities, occasional startles set off by activity. Reactive to external stimulation with an increase in startles or motor activity, discrete reactions difficult to distinguish because of general high activity level.

4. Crying: intense crying, jerky motor movements, difficult to break through with stimulation.

The waking states are easily influenced by fatigue, hunger, or other organic needs, and they may last for variable amounts of time. However, in the neonatal period, they are at the mercy of the sleep cycles and surround them in a fairly regular fashion. Waking states are infrequently observed in noisy, overlighted neonatal nurseries, but, in a rooming-in situation or at home, they become a large part of each 4-hour cycle, and the neonate lies in his crib looking around for as much as 20 to 30 minutes at a time. Appropriate stimulation can bring him up to alert state 2. Rocking, gently jiggling, crooning, stroking, setting off vestibular responses by bringing him upright or by rotating him all serve to open his eyes. Then his interest in visual and auditory stimuli helps him to maintain a quiet alert state. In this state, his respirations are regular at a rate of 50 to 60 a minute, his cardiac rate, too, is regular and fairly slow (around 100 to 120/min.), his eyes are wide, shiny, and capable of conjugate movements to scan and to follow with head turning to appropriate objects; his limbs, trunk, and face are relaxed and inactive; the skin is pink and uniform in color. Alert inactive states occur in the first 30 to 60 minutes after delivery but then are likely to decrease in duration and occurrence over the next 48 hours as the infant recovers, but they return after the first 2 days and make up as much as 8 to 16 per cent of total observation time in the first month (Wolff, 1966).

Kleitman talks of wakefulness of "necessity" and of "choice." Wakefulness of necessity is brought about by stimuli such as hunger, cold, and bowel movements or by external stimuli that disturb sleep cycles. Sleep recurs as soon as the response to the disturbing stimuli is completed. Wakefulness of choice is related to neocortical activity and is a late acquisition coinciding with the emergence of voluntary motor actions and a mature capacity to achieve and maintain full consciousness. Absence of hunger and fatigue, bowel and bladder activity, and gross motor activity are necessary components of this state. After a few weeks, this state can accompany gross motor activity as long as the infant is not too active. Pursuit movements of his extremities accompany visual fixation and following as early as 2 to 3 weeks (Brazelton et al., 1974). The occurrence and duration of these quiet inactive states may be highly correlated with intactness and mature organization of the neonate's central nervous system.

A pediatrician can obtain a sense of the infant's state organization from the mother by asking her how long and deeply he sleeps and how much time he spends in wideawake alertness. When the infant is easily disorganized or thrown from either of these states by minor stimuli, one can suspect a hypersensitive central nervous system. Such an infant is difficult for parents, and they will need advice concerning maneuvers that will help the infant to control his reactions (e.g., advice as to swaddling, pacifiers, rocking in order to help him to quiet down to sleep, etc.).

Crying serves many purposes in the neonate—not the least of which is to shut out painful or disturbing stimuli. Hunger and pain are also responded to with crying, which brings the caretaker to him. And there is a kind of fussy crying that occurs periodically throughout the day—usually in a cyclic fashion—that seems to act as a discharge of energy and an organizer of the states that ensue (Brazelton, 1962). After a period of such fussy crying, the neonate may be more alert or he may sleep more deeply. Most parents can distinguish cries of pain, hunger and fussiness by 2 to 3 weeks, and they learn quickly to respond appropriately (Wolff, 1969).

Parents need to be reassured that there is a certain amount of normal crying to be expected—usually at a regular time, at the end of the day. This crying period is predictable and is not a sign of "colic" or internal stress, as it is likely to be interpreted by parents. They feel that they should and must find the right solution to it and it will stop. As their efforts to quiet the baby increase, the crying period can increase from 1½ hours to as much as 6 to 8 hours a day, as the infant begins to reflect the anxiety and unpredictable handling of the frantic parents. By warning new parents in advance that a certain amount of fussiness is normal and by assuring them that there are no magical cures they are missing, a pediatrician can often nip this disturbance in their relationship in the bud and prevent the more severe colic (Brazelton, 1962).

The neonate's cry has been analyzed by some authors (Lind, 1966; Wasz-Hockert et al., 1966), for diagnostic purposes. It is a complex, serially organized acoustic pattern that is directly regulated by the

CNS. Wolff (1969) found that there were three distinct acoustical patterns of cries in normal infants: hunger, anger, and pain. Lind as well as Wasz-Hockert and coworkers found four patterns: birth, hunger, pain, and pleasure.

We have found differences in newborns in their use of states. The difficulty in rousing certain infants from sleep states to alert or crying with disturbing stimuli versus the rapidity with which others go from sleep to crying and down again, the lability that certain newborns demonstrate as they move rapidly from one state to another, the ease with which others are consoled from crying, and the self-quieting efforts on the part of other infants in order to maintain alert or quiet states are all differentiating characteristics that will help to predict in neonates their future individualities. Certainly, these differences will affect the kind of nurturing they will receive from their environments. We reported an infant whose rapidly labile movement from crying to deep sleep left no opportunity for his mother to reach him. She found him such a difficult infant that we correctly predicted profound difficulties in their relationship. Since we had found this difficult state of lability and unreachability in the neonatal period, we were able to support the mother with extra advice, along with a preventive approach to her anxiety. We supported her in maintaining their relationship until the baby could begin to develop more adequate state controls. As his threshold for sensory input became more adequate, he became more reachable by those around him. In this case, neonatal observations served to prevent a serious breakdown in the mother-infant interaction, as we could assure the mother that his lability was not due to her handling of the infant.

Evaluation of the Neonate

As the potential for early intervention increases, it becomes more important to identify at-risk infants as early as possible. Repeated evaluations in the neonatal nursery are necessary in order to record the depth and duration of postdelivery depression. Scanlon has developed an assessment technique that has high reliability among observers and serves to record the depth of the newborn's depression. It seems to be sensitive to the effects of maternal medication and anesthesia as well as to hypoxic events in the immediate paranatal period. This test includes two categories of responses: (1) neuromuscular—body tone, arm recoil, truncal tone, head control, Moro response, root and suck; and (2) adaptive—observations of alertness to auditory and visual stimuli and capacity to shut out such stimuli, including pinprick, Moro, bright light, and loud noises. He follows babies hourly over the first 6 hours with this 5-minute test and can evaluate the effects of paranatal variables on this recovery curve.

Graham was the first to use behavioral measures as part of a predictive neurologic exam. Her techniques included qualitative assessments of tension and motor response measures, tactile responses, irritability ratings, ease of quieting, and visual and auditory responsiveness. She evaluated these measures within the context of state of arousal. Rosenblith established the validity of her assessment as a predictor as well as its day-to-day test-retest reliability, finding correlations between many of the newborn measures and their outcome at 4, 8, and 12 months and at 2 years in the Collaborative Perinatal Research Project.

In order to record and evaluate some of the integrative processes evidenced in neonatal behavior, we have developed a behavioral evaluation scale (Brazelton, 1973) that tests and documents the infant's use of state behavior (state of consciousness) and the response to various kinds of stimulation.

Since the infant's reactions to all stimuli are dependent on his ongoing "state," any interpretation of them must be made with this in mind. His use of state to maintain control of his reactions to environmental and internal stimuli is an important mechanism and reflects his potential for organization. Specifically, our examination tracks the lability and direction of state changes over the course of the examination. The variability of state points to the infant's capacities for self-organization. His ability to quiet himself and his need for stimulation also measure this adequacy.

The behavior examination tests for neurologic adequacy with 20 reflex measures and for 26 behavioral responses to environmental stimuli, including the kind of interpersonal stimuli that mothers use in their handling of the infant as they attempt to help him adapt to the new world. In the examination, there is a graded series of procedures—talking, placing hand on belly, restraining, holding, and rocking—designed to soothe and alert the infant. His responsiveness to animate stimuli, such as voice and face, and to inanimate stimuli, such as rattle, bell, red ball, white light, and temperature change, is assessed. Estimates of vigor and attentional excitement are measured, and motor activity and tone are assessed, as is autonomic responsiveness, as he changes state. With this examination given on successive days, we have been able to outline (1) the initial period of alertness immediately after delivery, presumably the result of stimulation from labor and the new environment after delivery; (2) the period of depression and disorganization that follows and lasts for 24 to 48 hours in infants with uncomplicated deliveries and no medication effects but that lasts for periods of 3 to 4 days if they have been compromised by medication given their mothers during labor; and (3) the curve of recovery to "optimal" function after several days. This third period may be the best single predictor of individual potential function, and it seems to correlate

portant predictor of his future central nervous system organization.

The Neonate as a Social Being

The newborn infant is obviously not prepared to exist outside a matrix of social supports from a responsive care giver. But he is also *not* passive within this matrix. On the contrary, the behavior patterns and sensory capabilities discussed elsewhere in this chapter shape the caretaker's behavior. Moreover, the "feelings of efficacy" that are engendered in the infant and his caretakers by the mutuality that is established becomes a source of energy to each participant (White, 1959).

well with the neonate's retest ability at 30 days. The shape of the curve made by several examinations may be the most important assessment of the basic CNS intactness, of the neonate's ability to integrate CNS and other physiologic recovery mechanisms, and of the strength of his compensatory capacities when there have been compromising insults to him during labor and delivery. Test-retest reliability is greater than .8, and interscorer reliability of 90 per cent can be achieved with training and maintained for at least a year. The examination takes 20 minutes to perform and 10 minutes to score reliably.

This neonatal behavioral examination has been used in cross-cultural studies to outline genetic differences, with prematures to predict their outcome successfully, to document behavioral correlates of intrauterine protein depletion, to determine the effects of rapidly repeated pregnancies, and to assess the influence of medication given the mother during labor, as well as maternal addiction to heroin and methadone.

The behavioral items are as follows:
Response decrement to repeated visual stimuli
Response decrement to repeated auditory stimuli
Response decrement to pinprick
Orienting responses to inanimate visual and auditory stimuli
Orienting responses to the examiner's face and voice
Quality and duration of alert periods
General muscle tone—in resting and in response to being handled (passive and active)
Motor maturity
Traction responses as he is pulled to sit
Responses to being cuddled by the examiner
Defensive reactions to a cloth over his face
Consolability with intervention by examiner
Attempts to console self and control state behavior
Rapidity of build-up to crying state
Peak of excitement and capacity to control himself
Irritability during the examination
General assessment of kind and degree of activity
Tremulousness
Amount of startling
Lability of skin color (measuring autonomic lability)
Lability of states during entire examination
Hand-to mouth activity
In addition to 26 items of behavior, assessed on a 9-point scale, there are 20 reflex responses that are also assessed.

We feel that the behavioral items are tapping in on more important evidences of cortical control and responsiveness, even in the neonatal period. The neonate's capacity to manage and overcome the physiologic demands of this adjustment period in order to attend to, differentiate, and habituate to the complex stimuli of an examiner's maneuvers may be an im-

Moss and Goldberg point to the trigger-like value in setting off mothering activities of the newborn's small size, helpless appearance, and distress cries. Klaus and Kennell have described the kinds of initial contacts mothers make with their newborn infants and the distortions in this behavior when the mother is depressed by abnormalities in the baby, such as prematurity, illness in the neonatal period, and so forth. Eye-to-eye contact, touching, handling, and nursing behavior on the part of the mother may be assessed and judged to predict her ability to relate to the new baby. Changes in these behaviors over time are stressed as indicators of recovery or nonrecovery of maternal capacity to attach to the baby by mothers who have been depressed and unable to function optimally by having produced a sick or deformed infant.

The ability of the baby to precipitate and encourage the mother's attachment and care-taking behavior must be considered. With an unresponsive neonate, the feedback mechanisms necessary to fuel mothering behavior are severely impaired. The possibility of creating or compounding the problems of infants at risk by a distortion of the environment's reactions to them is too important, and our tools for predicting this should be sharpened during the lying-in period. The opportunity for observing the pair together is never again as available, and surely we are missing valuable predictive information when we do not make regular, repeated observations of interactive situations, such as feeding periods, bathing, and "play" periods after feeding.

In the normally competent mother-infant pair, there are preadapted complementary behaviors that guarantee a high level of mutually rewarding experience (Goldberg, 1977). A competent infant is one who roots and sucks efficiently, alerts to stimulation selectively, modulates states of arousal, cries loudly when uncomfortable, and quiets when comforted. Lorenz pointed out that certain features make up a "kewpie doll" face that elicits parenting responses— the short vertical axis and puffed cheeks of the face, the relatively large head to body size, the uncoordinated body movements, the soft fuzzy skin and hair. The fact that the infant prefers and quiets down to human stimuli such as the voice and face are critical to maternal attachment. Fathers report that they begin to develop strong affectional ties only after the infant has begun to look at and smile at them, and many mothers do not feel attachment until the second or third month, when eye-to-eye contact and rhythmic reactive behaviors are firmly established (Robson and Moss, 1970).

In stressed neonates, the responsive behavior that normally exists to feed back to the mother may not be present or satisfying, and the relationship may flounder. If the eliciting stimuli the baby presents to care-givers are not forthcoming or are distorted, parental behavior in turn becomes distorted. Prechtl reports the high incidence of brain-damaged infants who appear normal externally but elicit anger and rejection from their parents, even before an official diagnosis of damage has been made. Klein and Stern report an unexpectedly large number of battered children within a premature population. Klaus and Kennell attribute this in part to the effects on the parents of early separation from their prematures. We would add the effects of maternal depression after the delivery of a sick neonate. And the syndrome of failure to thrive seems to be a sequel to many infants who are small for gestational age at birth (SGA), some of whom are later given up for adoption (Miller and Hassanein, 1973).

We are interested in determining the role of aberrant behavior in the premature or SGA infant that might lend itself to an already adversely influenced maternal attachment. We have found that premature and SGA babies are poorer in interactive behaviors, in alerting responses and in selecting for the female voice and for the human face in auditory and visual responses, in state modulation, and in producing satisfactory motor behavior. Throughout the first year of life, these SGA babies evidence a high incidence of hyperactivity and temperamental and organizational instability. These difficulties are bound to and do result in parental frustrations (Als, 1981).

It is thus apparent that in addition to the physiologic and neurologic problems at-risk newborns have to cope with, they generate by their distorted behavior deficient parenting patterns that, in turn, exacerbate an already compromised start on life. The interactive cyclical nature of this process cannot be overstressed and must be taken into account whenever one deals with other than healthy normal newborns.

We have seen that the infant in the first few weeks requires that the mother adapt her behavior to a cyclic attentional cycle that comes from the infant. When an infant attends to and becomes intensely involved with a familiar adult, he attends to her with a cyclical pattern of attention—withdrawal and recovery—that resembles a homeostatic curve, at a rate of four cycles per minute in a period of intense interaction. A mother or father who is sensitive to the baby's needs reflects this self-regulatory mechanism and regulates affective and cognitive information to the infant's requirements. An insensitive parent overloads the neonate, and their interaction becomes stressed.

In an optimal interaction, the reciprocity that is established on these cycles of attention and recovery becomes the base for affective development and fuel for learning about his environment. This interdependency of rhythms seems to be at the root of both their attachment and their communication (Brazelton, 1974; Chapple, 1970). From this interdependency, the infant learns rules about his environment and about himself. Thus, the quality of the interaction becomes more important in assessing an at-risk pair than does an evaluation of either participant alone. Prevention of future difficulties for the child may well hinge on early identification of failure in this interaction.

A pediatrician can observe and record a lack of synchrony or "fit" between a mother and her baby. When they are unable to achieve a rhythmic period of playing looking or vocal games with each other, he should be alerted to an interaction that may well be at risk for future stress or failure.

Summary

An assessment of the neonate's behavioral responses should be a part of every pediatric examination. Integration of his central and autonomic nervous systems is necessary for him to overcome the physiologic demands of recovery in the immediate period after delivery. This very fact makes such an assessment a valuable opportunity to see and quantitate his stage of well-being. That behavioral responses are dependent on his capacity to regulate his states of consciousness is of primary importance in such an assessment. For his state, behavior marks both his capacity to alert to an interesting or appropriate stimulus and his capacity to shut out a disturbing or inappropriate one. This potential signifies his viability as well as his capacity to adapt to his environment with a potential for learning the information essential to his future progress. It is also involved in his capacity to respond to his care-giver in a way that will connect him or her to the infant in a mutual feedback system that will provide the nurturing necessary for his future affective and cognitive growth.

The pattern of recovery of the infant's potential for behavior becomes the most important way of predicting not only his immediate coping capacity but also his future reactions to stress. Thus, several assessments in the perinatal period become significant.

An important additional reason for a careful assessment of the behavior of a newborn infant in the mother's presence is the benefit to the mother of seeing the skills of her own infant. Widmayer and Field found improved fine motor abilities on the Denver scale at 4 months and significantly higher scores on the Bayley Infant Development examination at

12 months among infants whose mothers were present during the administration of the Brazelton Behavioral Assessment, compared to a carefully matched control group of preterm infants.

REFERENCES

Adamson, L.: Infants response to visual and tactile occlusions. Ph.D. Dissertation, University of California at Berkeley, in preparation, 1976.

Als, H., and Brazelton, T. B.: A new model of assessing the behavioral organization in preterm and full term infants. J. Am. Acad. Child. Psychiatry 20:239, 1981.

Als, H., Lester, B. M., and Brazelton, T. B.: Dynamics of the behavioral organization of the premature infant: a theoretical perspective. In Field, T., Sostek, A., Goldberg, S., and Shuman, H. H. (Eds.): Infants Born at Risk. Jamaica, N.Y., Spectrum Pub., 1979.

Als, H., Lester, B. M., Tronick, E., and Brazelton, T. B.: Towards a systematic assessment of the preterm infant's behavioral development. In Fitzgerald, H. E., Lester, B. M., and Yogman, M. W. (Eds.): Theory and Research in Behavioral Pediatrics. New York, Plenum Press, 1981.

Anders, T. F., and Roffwarg, H.: The effects of selective interruption and total sleep deprivation in the human newborn. Dev. Psychobiol. 6:77, 1973.

Anders, T. F., and Weinstein, P.: Sleep and its disorders in infants and children: A review. Pediatrics 50:312, 1972.

Ando, Y., and Hattori, H.: Effects of intense noise during fetal life upon postnatal adaptability. J. Acoust. Soc. Am. 47:1128, 1970.

Aserinsky, E., and Kleitman, N.: A motility cycle in sleeping infants as manifested by ocular and gross motor activity. J. Appl. Physiol. 8:11, 1955.

Babkin, P. S.: The establishment of reflex activity in early postnatal life. In Central Nervous System and Behavior, 3rd Conference, Princeton, N.J., U.S. Dept. HEW (OTS 62-43772), 24, 1960.

Ball, W., and Tronick, E.: Infant response to impending collision: optical and real. Science 171:818, 1971.

Barnard, K. E.: A program of temporally patterned movement and sound stimulation for premature infants. In Smeriglio, V. L. (Ed.): Newborns and Parents. Hillsdale, N.J., Lawrence Erlbaum Associates, Inc., 1981, p. 31.

Bartoshuk, A. K., and Tennant, J. M.: Human neonatal correlates of sleep wakefulness and neural maturation. J. Psychiat. Res. 2:73, 1964.

Bernbaum, J., Pereira, G. R., and Watkins, J. B.: Nonnutritive sucking (NNS) enhances maturation of the sucking reflex in premature infants. Pediatr. Res. 15:477 (abstr.), 1981.

Birnholz, J. C.: The development of human fetal eye movement patterns. Science 213:679, 1981.

Birnholz, J. C., Stephens, V. C., and Faria, M.: Fetal movement patterns: a possible means of defining neurologic developmental milestones in utero. Am. J. Roentgenol. 130:537, 1978.

Bower, T. G. R.: The determinants of perceptual unity in infancy. Psychon. Sci. 3:323, 1965.

Bowlby, J.: Attachment and Loss, Vol. I: Attachment. New York, Basic Books, 1969.

Brackbill, Y.: Continuous stimulation and arousal level in infants: Additive effects. Proc. 78th Annu. Conv. Am. Psychol. Assoc. 5:271, 1970; and in Stone, L. V., Smith, H. T. and Murphy, L. B. (Eds.): The Competent Infant. New York, Basic Books, 1973, p. 300.

Brazelton, T. B.: Sucking in infancy. Pediatrics 17:400, 1956.

Brazelton, T. B.: Psychophysiologic reactions in the neonate. J. Pediatr. 58:513, 1961.

Brazelton, T. B.: Observations of the neonate. J. Acad. Child Psychol. 1:38, 1962.

Brazelton, T. B.: Infants and Mothers: Differences in Development. New York, Delacorte Press, 1969.

Brazelton, T. B.: Effect of prenatal drugs on the behavior of the neonate. Am. J. Psychiatry 126:95, 1970.

Brazelton, T. B.: Assessment of the infant at risk. Clin. Obstet. Gynecol. 16:361, 1973.

Brazelton, T. B.: Neonatal Behavioral Assessment Scale. National Spastics Foundation. Monograph No. 50. London, William Heinemann Co., 1973.

Brazelton, T. B.: Influence of perinatal drugs on the behavior of the neonate. In Hellmuth, J. (Ed.): Exceptional Infant. Vol. 2. New York, Bruner Mazel, 1971, p. 419.

Brazelton, T. B., Koslowski, B., and Main, M.: Origins of reciprocity. In Lewis, M., and Rosenblum, L. (Eds.): Mother Infant Interaction. New York, J. Wiley & Sons, Inc., 1974, pp. 49–76.

Brazelton, T. B., Koslowski, B., and Tronick, E.: Study of neonatal behavior in Zambian and American neonates. Am. Acad. Child Psychiatry 15:97, 1976.

Brazelton, T. B., Robey, J. S., and Collier, G. A.: Infant development in the Zinacantec Indians of Southern Mexico. Pediatrics 44:274, 1969.

Brazelton, T. B., Scholl, M. L., and Robey, J. S.: Visual responses in the newborn. Pediatrics 37:284, 1966.

Brazelton, T. B., Tronick, E., Lechtig, A., Lasky, R., and Klein, R.: The behavior of nutritionally deprived Guatemalan neonates. Dev. Med. Child Neurol. 19:364, 1977.

Brazier, M. A. B. (Ed.): The central nervous system and behavior. Trans. 2nd Conf., Josiah Macy Fdn., 1959.

Bridger, W. H.: Sensory habituation of discrimination in the human neonate. Am. J. Psychiatry 117:991, 1961.

Bridger, W. H., and Reiser, M. F.: Psychophysiologic studies of the neonate: An approach toward the methodological and theoretical problems involved. Psychosom. Med. 21:265, 1959.

Brigman, T., Haith, M. M., and Mann, L.: Development of eye contact and facial scanning in infants. Paper presented at Soc. Res. Child Devel., Minneapolis, April 1974.

Bruner, J. S.: Eye, hand and mind. In Elkind, D., and Flavell, J. H. (Eds.): Studies in Cognitive Development. New York, Oxford University Press, 1969, p. 223.

Chapple, E.: Experimental production of transients in human interaction. Nature 228:630, 1970.

Clifton, R. K.: Cardiac conditioning and orienting in the human infant. In Obrist, P., Black, A. H., Brener, J., and DiCara, L. (Eds.): Cardiovascular Physiology. Chicago, Aldine Press, 1974, p. 479.

Crook, C. K.: Taste perception in the newborn infant. Infant Behav. Dev. 1:52, 1978.

Dayton, G. O., Jr., Jones, M. H., Aiu, P., Rawson, R. A., Steele, B., and Rose, M.: Developmental study of coordinated eye movements in the human infant. Arch. Ophthalmol. 71:865, 1964.

DeCasper, A. J., and Fifer, W. P.: Of human bonding: newborns prefer their mothers' voices. Science 208:1174, 1980.

Dixon, S., Keefer, C., Tronick, E., and Brazelton, T.B.: Perinatal circumstances and newborn outcome among the Gusii of Kenya. Infant Behav. Dev. 5:11, 1982.

Drage, J. S., Kennedy, C., and Berendes, H.: The 5 minute Apgar scores and 4 year psychological performance. Dev. Med. Child Neurol. 8:141, 1966.

Dreyfus-Brisac, C., Flescher, J., and Plessart, E.: L'électroencephalogramme: critère d'âge conceptionnel du nouveau-né à terme et prématuré. Biol. Neonatol. 4:154, 1962.

Dreyfus-Brisac, C.: The bioelectrical development of the central nervous system during early life. In Falkner, J. (Ed.): Human Development. Philadelphia, W. B. Saunders Co., pp. 286–305, 1966.

Dubowitz, L., and Dubowitz, V.: Clinical assessment of gestational age in the newborn infant. J. Pediatr. 77:1, 1970.

Dubowitz, V., Whittaker, G. F., Brown, B. H., and Robinson, A.: Nerve conduction velocity: An index of neurological maturity of the newborn infant. Dev. Med. Child Neurol. 10:741, 1968.

Eisenberg, R. B.: Auditory behavior in the human neonate: Methodologic problems. J. Aud. Res. 5:159, 1965.

Ellingson, R. V.: Cortical electrical responses to visual stimulation in the human infant. Electroencephalogr. Clin. Neurophysiol. 12:663, 1960.

Engen, T., Lipsett, L. P., and Kaye, H.: Olfactory responses and adaptation in the human neonate. J. Comp. Physiol. Psychol. 56:73, 1963.

Fantz, R. L.: Visual perception from birth as shown by pattern selectivity. Ann. N.Y. Acad. Sci. 118:793, 1965.

Farr, V., Mitchell, R. G., Nelligan, G. A., and Parkin, V. M.: The definition of some external characteristics used in the assessment of gestational age in the newborn infant. Dev. Med. Child Neurol. 8:507, 1966.

Fischelli, V., and Karelitz, S.: The cry latencies of normal infants and those with brain damage. Pediatrics 62:724, 1963.

Flechsig, P. E.: Anatomie des menschlichen Gehirns und Ruckenmarks auf myelogenetischer Grundlage. Leipzig, Georg Thieme, 1920.

Freedman, D. C., and Freedman, N · Behavioral differences between Chinese American and American newborns. Nature 224:227, 1969.

Geber, M., and Dean, R. F. A.: The state of development of newborn African children. Lancet 272:1216, 1957.

Gesell, A.: The Embryology of Behavior. New York, Harper, 1945.

Goldberg, S.: Social competence in infancy: A model of parent-infant interaction. Merrill Palmer Quart. 23:163, 1977.

Goldberg, S.: Premature birth: consequences for the parent-infant relationship. Am. Sci. 67:214, 1979.

Goren, C., Sarty, M., and Wu, P.: Visual following and pattern discrimination of face-like stimuli by newborn infants. Pediatrics 56:544, 1975.

Gorman, J. J., Cogan, D. G., and Gillis, S. S.: An apparatus for grading the visual acuity of infants on the basis of opticokinetic nystagmus. Pediatrics 19:1088, 1957.

Gorski, P. A., Davidson, M. F., and Brazelton, T. B.: Stages of behavioral organization in the high risk neonate. Semin. Perinatol. 3:61, 1979.

Gottfried, A. W.: Behavioral issues and environmental engineering in special care units. In Smeriglio, V. L. (Ed.): Parent Infant Contact and Newborn Sensory Stimulation. Hillsdale, N.J., Lawrence Erlbaum Associates, Inc., 1981, p. 55.

Graham, F. K., and Clifton, R. K.: Heart rate change as a component of the orienting response. Psychol. Bull. 65:305, 1966.

Graham, F. K., Matarazzo, R. G., and Caldwell, B. M.: Behavioral differences between normal and traumatized newborns. Psychol. Monogr. 70:427, 1956.

Graziano, L. J., Weitzman, E. D., and Velasco, M. S. A.: Neurologic maturation and auditory evoked responses in low birth weight infants. Pediatrics 41:483, 1968.

Gryboski, J. D.: The swallowing mechanism of the neonate: esophageal and gastric motility. Pediatrics 35:445, 1965.

Haith, M. M., Kessen, W., and Collins, D.: Response of the human infant to level of complexity of intermittent visual movement. J. Exp. Child Psychol. 7:52, 1969.

Halverson, H. M.: Mechanisms of early feeding. J. Genet. Psychol. 64:185, 1944.

Haynes, H., White, B. L., and Held, R.: Visual accommodation in human infants. Science 148:528, 1965.

Hershenson, M.: Visual discrimination in the human newborn. J. Comp. Physiol. Psychol. 58:270, 1964.

Hooker, D.: The Prenatal Origin of Behavior. 3rd ed. New York, Hafner Publishing Co., 1969.

Horowitz, F. D., Self, P. A., Paden, L. N., Culp, R., Laub, K., Boyd, E., and Mann, M. E.: Newborn and four week retest on a normative population using the Brazelton Newborn Assessment Procedure. Paper presented at Soc. Res. Child Devel. Meetings, Minneapolis, 1971.

Hrbek, A., and Mares, P.: Cortical evoked responses to visual stimulation in full term and premature infants. EEG Clin. Neurophysiol. 16:575, 1964.

Humphry, J.: Postnatal repetition of human prenatal activity sequences with some suggestions of their neuro-anatomical basis. In Robinson, R. J. (Ed.): Brain and Early Behavior. London, Academic Press, 43, 1969.

Hutt, C., and Ounsted, C.: The biological significance of gaze aversion with particular reference to the syndrome of infantile autism. Behav. Sci. 11:346, 1966.

Ianniruberto, A., and Tajani, E.: Ultrasonographic study of fetal movements. Semin. Perinatol. 5:175, 1981.

Illingsworth, R.: Crying in infants and children. Br. Med. J. 1:75, 1955.

James, L. S.: The effect of pain relief for labor and delivery of the fetus and newborn. Anesthesiology 21:405, 1960.

James, W.: The principles of psychology. New York, Henry Holt, 1890, p. 488.

Jensen, K.: Differential reactions to taste and temperature stimuli in newborn infants. Genet. Psychol. Monogr. 12:361, 1932.

Kaplan, S. L., et al.: Correlations between scores on the Brazelton Neonatal Assessment Scale, measures of newborn sucking behavior, and birthweight in infants born to narcotic addicted mothers. In Ellis, N. R. (Ed.): Aberrant Development in Infancy. Hillsdale, N.J., Lawrence Erlbaum Associates, Inc., 1975.

Karelitz, S., and Fischelli, V.: The cry thresholds of normal infants and those with brain damage. J. Pediatr. 61:679, 1962.

Kaye, H.: Infant sucking and its modification. In Lipsitt, L. P., and Spiker, C. C. (Eds.): Advances in Child Development and Behavior. Vol III. New York, Academic Press, 1967, p. 1.

Kaye, K., and Brazelton, T. B.: The orthological significance of the burst-pause pattern in infant sucking. Paper given at Soc. Res. Child Dev., Minneapolis, April, 1971.

Kearsley, R., Snider, M., Richie, R., and Talbot, N.: Study of relations between psychologic environment and child behavior. Am. J. Dis. Child. 104:12, 1962.

Keeley, K.: Prenatal influence on the behavior of offspring of crowded mice. Science 135:44, 1962.

Kessen, W., Haith, M. M., and Salapatek, P. H.: Human infancy: A bibliography and guide. In Mussen, P. (Ed.): Carmichael's Manual of Child Psychology. Vol 1. New York, J. Wiley & Sons, Inc., 1970, p. 287.

Klaus, M. H., and Kennell, J. H.: Mothers separated from their newborn infants. Pediatr. Clin. North Am. 17:1015, 1970.

Klein, M., and Stern, L.: Low birthweight and the battered child syndrome. Am. J. Dis. Child. 122:15, 1971.

Korner, A. F.: Intervention with preterm infants. In Smeriglio, V. L. (Ed.): Newborns and Parents. Hillsdale, N.J., Lawrence Erlbaum Associates, Inc., 1981, p. 13.

Korner, A. F., and Thoman, E. B.: Visual alertness in neonates as evoked by maternal care. J. Exp. Child Psychol. 10:67, 1970.

Kron, R. E., Stein, M., and Goddard, K. E.: A method of measuring sucking behavior of newborn infants. Psychosom. Med. 25:181, 1963.

Lester, B. M.: Cardiac habituation of the orienting response to an auditory signal in infants of varying nutritional status. Dev. Psychol. 11:432, 1975.

Lewis, M., Bartels, B., Campbell, H. and Goldberg, S.: Individual differences in attention. Am. J. Dis. Child. 112:461, 1967.

Lieberman, M. W.: Early developmental stress and later behavior. Science 141:824, 1963.

Lind, J., Wasz-Hockert, O., Vuorenkoski, F., Partanen, T., Theorell, K., and Valanne, E.: Vocal responses to painful stimuli in newborn and young infants. Ann. Paediatr. Fenn. 12:55, 1966.

Lipsitt, L. P.: Learning in the human infant. In Stevenson, H. W., Rheingold, M. D., and Hess, E. (Eds.): Early Behavior: Comparative and Behavioral Approaches. New York, J. Wiley & Sons, Inc., 1967, pp. 225–247.

Lipton, E. L., Steinschneider, A., and Richmond, J.: Auditory sensitivity in the infant: Effect of intensity on cardiac and motor responsivity. Child Dev. 37:233, 1966.

Lipton, E. L., Steinschneider, A., and Richmond, J.: Swaddling—a child care practice: Historical, cultural and experimental observations. Monogr. Pediatr. 35:521, 1965.

Long, J. G., Lucey, J. F., and Philip, A. G. S.: Noise and hypoxemia in the intensive care nursery. Pediatrics 65:143, 1980.

Long, J. G., Philip, A. G. S., and Lucey, J. F.: Excessive handling as a cause of hypoxemia. Pediatrics 65:203, 1980.

Lorenz, K.: Die angeborenen Formen möglicher Erfahrung. *In* Nash, J. (Ed.): Developmental Psychology: A Psychobiological Approach. Englewood, N.J., Prentice-Hall, 1970.

Lubchenco, L. O., Bard, H., Goldman, A. L., Coyer, W. E., McIntyre, C., and Smith, D.: Newborn intensive care and long-term prognosis. Dev. Med. Child Neurol. *16*:421, 1974.

Lubchenco, L. O., Hansman, C., Dressler, M., and Boyd, E.: Intrauterine growth estimated from liveborn, birthweight data at 24 to 42 weeks of gestation. Pediatrics *32*:793, 1963.

MacFarlane, A.: Olfaction in the development of preferences in the human neonate. *In* Parent-Infant Evaluation. Ciba Foundation Symposium 33. New York, American Elsevier Publishers, Inc., 1975, pp. 103–119.

Marzullo, G., and Hine, B.: Of human bonding: Newborns prefer their mothers' voices. Science *208*:1174, 1980.

Michaelis, R., Parmelee, A., Stern, E., and Haber, A.: Activity states in premature and term infants. Dev. Psychobiol. *6*:209, 1973.

Michaelis, R., Schulte, F. J., and Nolte, R.: Motor behavior of small for gestational age newborn infants. J. Pediatr. *76*:208, 1970.

Milani-Comparetti, A.: The neurophysiologic and clinical implications of studies on fetal motor behavior. Semin. Perinatol. *5*:183, 1981.

Miller, H. and Hassanein, K.: Fetal malnutrition in white newborn infants: Maternal factors. Pediatrics *52*:504, 1973.

Moss, H. A.: Methodological issues in studying mother-infant interaction. Am. J. Orthopsychiatry *35*:482, 1965.

Osofsky, J., and Danzger, B.: Relationships between neonatal characteristics and mother-infant interaction. Dev. Psychol. *10*:124, 1974.

Parmelee, A.: Infant crying and neurologic diagnosis. J. Pediatr. *61*:801, 1962.

Parmelee, A. H., and Michaelis, R.: Neurologic examination of the newborn. *In* Hellmuth, J. (Ed.): Exceptional Infant. Vol. II. New York, Bruner Mazel, 1971, pp. 3–24.

Parmelee, A. H., Jr., Schulte, F. J., Akiyama, Y., Wenner, W. H., Schultz, M. A., and Stern, E.: Maturation of EEG activity during sleep in premature infants. Electroencephalogr. Clin. Neurophysiol. *24*:319, 1968.

Partanen, J., Wasz-Hockert, O., Vuroenkoski, V., Theorell, K., Valann, E., and Lind, J.: Auditory identification of pain cry signals of young infants in pathological conditions and its spectrographic basis. Ann. Paediatr. Fenn. *13*:56, 1967.

Porzes, S. W.: Indices of newborn attentional responsivity. Merrill Palmer Quart. *20*:231, 1974.

Pratt, K. C.: The effects of repeated visual stimulation upon the activity of newborn infants. J. Genet. Psychol. *44*:117, 1934.

Prechtl, H. F. R.: The directed head turning response and allied movements of the human baby. Behavior *13*:212, 1956.

Prechtl, H., and Beintema, D.: The neurological examination of the full term newborn infant. Clin. Dev. Med., National Spastics Monograph No. 12. London, W. M. Heinemann and Sons, 1964.

Robinson, R. J.: Assessment of gestational age by neurological examination. Arch. Dis. Child. *41*:437, 1966.

Robson, K. S., and Moss, H. A.: Patterns and determinants of maternal attachment. J. Pediatr. *77*:976, 1970.

Rosenblith, J. F.: Prognostic value of behavioral assessment of neonates. Biol. Neonatol. *6*:76, 1964.

Salapatek, P. H., and Kessen, W.: Visual scanning of triangles by the human newborn. J. Exp. Child Psychol. *3*:155, 1966.

Sameroff, A. J.: The components of sucking in the human newborn. J. Exp. Child Psychol. *6*:607, 1968.

Scanlon, J. W., Brown, W. V., Weiss, J. B., and Alper, N. H.: Neurobehavioral responses of newborns after maternal epidural anesthesia. Anesthesiology *40*:121, 1974.

Scarr, S., and Williams, M.: The effects of early stimulation on low birthweight infants. Child Dev. *44*:94, 1973.

Schulte, F. J., Michaelis, R., Linke, I., and Nolte, R.: Motor nerve conduction velocity in term, preterm, and small for dates newborn infants. Dev. Psychobiol. *1*:41, 1968.

Sontag, L. W., and Richardo, T. W.: Studies in fetal behavior: Fetal heart rate as a behavioral indicator. Monogr. Soc. Res. Child Dev. *3*:(4), 1938.

Soule, A. B., Standley, K., Copans, S. A., and Davis, M.: Clinical uses of the Brazelton Neonatal Scale. Pediatrics *54*:583, 1974.

Stechler, G., and Latz, E.: Some observations on attention and arousal in the human infant. J. Acad. Child Psych. *5*:517, 1966.

Super, C. M.: Cross environmental effects on motor development: the case of African motor precocity. Devel. Med. Child Neurol. *18*:561, 1976.

Tronick, E., Wise, S., Als, H., Adamson, L., Scanlon, J., and Brazelton, T. B.: The effects of regional obstetric anesthesia on newborn behavior over the first ten days of life. Pediatrics *58*:94, 1977.

Truby, H. M., Bosma, J. F., and Lind, J.: Newborn infant cry. Acta Paediatr. Scand. Suppl. *163*, 1965.

Wagner, I. F.: The establishment of a criterion of depth of sleep in the newborn infant. J. Genet. Psychol. *51*:17, 1937.

Warkany, J., Monroe, B., and Sutherland, B.: Intrauterine growth retardation. Am. J. Dis. Child. *102*:127, 1961.

Warren, N.: Reevaluation of motor precocity in African children. Personal Communication, 1972.

Wasz-Hockert, O., Lind, J., Vuorenkoski, V., Partanen, T., and Valanne, E.: The infant cry. Clin. Dev. Med. *29*, 1968.

Weitzman, E. D., Fishbein, W., and Graziani, D.: Auditory evoked responses obtained from the scalp EEG of the full term infant during sleep. Pediatrics *35*:458, 1965.

White, R. W.: Motivation reconsidered: The concept of competence. Psychol. Rev. *66*:297, 1959.

Widmayer, S. M., and Field, T. M.: Effects of Brazelton demonstrations for mothers on the development of preterm infants. Pediatrics *67*:711, 1981.

Winick, M.: Malnutrition and brain development, J. Pediatr. *74*:667, 1969.

Winick, M.: Nucleic acid and protein content during growth of human brain. Pediatr. Res. *2*:352, 1968.

Wolff, P.: The causes, controls, and organization of behavior in the neonate. Psychol. Monogr. *5*:(17), 1966.

Wolff, P.: The natural history of crying and other vocalizations in early infancy. *In* Foss, B. W. (Ed.): Determinants of Infant Behavior. IV. London, Methuen & Co., 1969, p. 81.

Wurtman, R., and Wiesel, J.: Effects of light on premature infant. Endocrinology *85*:1218, 1969.

Prematurity

In earlier editions of this book, we attempted to discuss the medical problems of low birth weight infants in the chapter of this title rather than include them within the discussions of relevant organ systems. Such a distinction now seems unwarranted, since considerations of diagnosis and treatment of hyperbilirubinemia or patent ductus arteriosus, for example, are a part of the spectrum of disorders discussed more fully in terms of the organ system. Aspects of temperature regulation, feeding, and infectious diseases are presented in other chapters. We have elected in this chapter to focus on some aspects of etiology of premature birth, changing outlook for survival, and follow-up studies of low birth weight infants.

On the basis of both severity and frequency, the greatest risk to an unborn fetus after the twentieth week of gestation is premature birth. Perinatal and neonatal mortality rates are linked closely with the frequency of prematurity and very low birth weight rates.

Incidence

The incidence of premature birth depends on the number of women with risk factors predictive of premature labor. In the general population in the United States, the risk of premature birth is estimated as approximately 6 to 7 per cent (with prematurity defined as birth weight less than 2500 gm). Risk of extreme prematurity (birth weight less than 1250 gm) is a more useful risk measure, since most morbidity and mortality associated with prematurity falls within this group. The risk of extreme prematurity in the general population is estimated at about 0.6 to 1.0 per cent of all live births. Table 8–1 lists the major epidemiologic factors usually associated with spontaneous premature birth. With these factors, various risk-prediction scores have been devised that allow improved prediction; for example, by classification of about 10 per cent of pregnant women as high risk on the basis of the features listed in Table 8–1, about 60 per cent of preterm deliveries can be predicted.

Pathophysiology

Although the mechanisms that trigger the onset of labor have received well-deserved attention in recent years, the precise sequence of events remains a mystery. Some of the changes that occur with the onset of labor are shown in Figure 8–1. However, no abrupt changes in circulating hormones such as progesterone or estrogen occur when labor begins, nor

does cortisol appear to have as significant a role in the human as it has in sheep and goats. Oxytocin and prostaglandins are clearly important, although it is not known whether they are a cause or a result of uterine contractions. The concentration of oxytocin receptors reaches a maximum in early labor. Fuchs and coworkers postulate that the stimulus for prostaglandin release may be oxytocin. Alternately, a (possibly) local decrease in progesterone from the aging placenta may allow destabilization of decidual lysosomes containing phospholipase A_2. Its release sets up a reaction allowing for prostaglandin release in myometrium, inducing myometrial contractility. Trauma, stretch, infection, or premature senescence of the placenta might similarly trigger this chain of events, resulting in premature labor.

The treatment of preterm labor has been based on interventions that block various pathways shown in Figure 8–1. For example, ethanol has been used to block oxytocin release, indomethacin to block prostaglandin synthetase, progesterone to prevent lysosome destabilization, and control of infection and beta-adrenergics to suppress uterine contractility more directly. Efficacy of these treatments depends on the endpoint being used, that is, suppression of labor for a few days or until term.

Table 8–1. Events Associated with Spontaneous Premature Birth

Maternal Factors
History of previous premature birth
Malnutrition
Uterine abnormalities
Uterine stretch (hydramnios)
Age less than 16 years or over 35 years
Cyanotic heart disease and other chronic diseases
Short interval between births
Infection
Trauma
Hypertension
Diethylstilbestrol exposure
Fetal factors
Malformations
Multiple births
Premature rupture of membranes
Environmental effects
Lower socioeconomic class
Habits
Smoking
Fatigue/activity

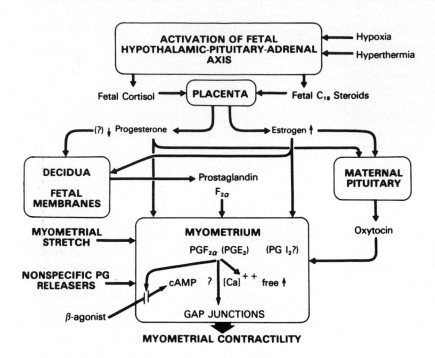

Figure 8–1. A general schematic illustration of mechanisms thought to play a role in the onset of human parturition. The final common pathway involves prostaglandin release at the myometrium. The usual primary "timer" that triggers the onset of these mechanisms may lie in the mother, the placenta, or the fetus (From Challis, J.: Perinat. Dev. Med. *15*:8, 1979.)

Delay of labor, even for several days, may allow for transfer of a high-risk mother to a prenatal center and use of prenatal glucocorticoids to reduce risk of respiratory distress syndrome. Complications and relative merits of labor suppressants (tocolytic agents) are listed in Table 8–2.

Potential neonatal toxicity of tocolytic therapy is indicated in Table 8–2, and dosage regimens are shown in Table 8–3. Beta-adrenergics, with increasing specificity for suppressing uterine contractility (β_2), are becoming the most widely used form of tocolytic therapy. In our institution, the only evident complication in newborns after administration of ritodrine to mothers has been hypoglycemia that has been relatively easy to control and a small price to pay for delaying premature birth by days or weeks.

Beta-adrenergic agents are thought to cross the placenta freely, and the obvious question concerns whether these agents have any effects on fetal lung maturation in a manner analogous to glucocorticoids.

Table 8–2.   Drugs Used to Stop Labor

Tocolytic	Advantages	Disadvantages
Ethanol		Low efficacy
		Possible fetal toxicity
		Neonatal hypoglycemia
		Maternal inebriation and aspiration
Progestins	Maternal safety	Prophylaxis not treatment for preterm labor
		Possible fetal risks
Indomethacin	Efficacious	Neonatal persistent fetal circulation
		Closure of fetal patent ductus arteriosus
Magnesium sulfate		Low efficacy
		Maternal toxicity
		Neonatal hypotonia
Isoxsuprine	Large clinical experience	Maternal and fetal cardiac effects at high dosage
		Additional side effects as for terbutaline and ritodrine
Terbutaline	Selective uterine action (B_2 stimulator)	High doses → maternal myocardial ischemia
Ritodrine	Stimulates fetal pulmonary surfactant	Rarely, pulmonary edema when used with steroids
		Neonatal hypoglycemia

Table 8–3. Tocolytic Drugs

	Ritodrine	Terbutaline	Isoxsuprine	Magnesium Sulfate
Initial dose	50–100 μg/min	10 μg/min	0.2 mg/min	4 gm (10% solution)
Incremental dose until contractions cease	50 μg/min every 10 min	5 μg/min every 10 min	10–25 mg/min every 10 min	2 gm/hr maintenance infusion (2% solution)
Maximum dose	350 μg/min	25 μg/min	1 mg/min	2 gm/hr
Duration of infusion	12 hours	12 hours	12 hours	12 hours
Oral maintenance	10 mg 30 min before stopping infusion, then 10–20 mg every 4–6 hours	2.5 mg 30 min before stopping infusion, then 2.5–5.0 mg every 4–6 hours	10 mg 30 min before stopping infusion, then 10–20 mg every 4–6 hours	May be followed by any of the oral tocolytic drugs

(From Bowes, W. A.: Delivery of the very low birth weight infant. Symposium on Difficult Labor and Delivery. Clin. Perinatol. *8*:183, 1981.)

While much evidence from animal studies suggests that adrenergic drugs increase fetal pulmonary production and release of surfactant, no well-controlled clinical studies have yet reported diminution of risk from respiratory distress syndrome after treating the mother with adrenergics. One group, with a well-designed trial, revealed a slightly increased risk of neonatal respiratory distress after maternal ritodrine treatment (Kristofferson and Hansen, 1979). Another trial, in which various protocols were used, showed that risk of RDS was almost halved in the group exposed to ritodrine (Merkatz et al., 1980).

Robertson and coworkers have suggested that isoxsuprine may be associated with less severe maternal cardiovascular complications than terbutaline. In their series, maternal pulmonary edema or myocardial ischemia occurred in about 5 per cent of treated women. High beta-adrenergic infusion rates, fluid overload, and concomitant glucocorticoid therapy were not associated with the cardiovascular complications. These problems did appear to be associated with adrenergic tocolytic therapy for mothers with twins.

Table 8–4. Presenting Problems of Pregnant Women Admitted at Risk of Delivery Between 20 and 37 Weeks Gestation
(4 Months in 1977, Brigham & Women's Hospital)
(n = 209)

	Per Cent
Labor, intact membranes, cervix < 5 cm	25
Labor, intact membranes, cervix > 5 cm	10
No labor, membranes ruptured	19
Labor, membranes ruptured	15
Vaginal bleeding	13
Maternal illness (Rh diabetes, toxemia)	14
Fetal death	3

(Unpublished data of P. Stubblefield and E. Nicolls.)

The potential impact of tocolytic therapy for reduction of prematurity can be assessed by analysis of presenting complaints of women admitted at risk of delivery of a very low birth weight infant (Table 8–4). At least 50 per cent of these women would potentially benefit from measures taken to delay parturition. Women at risk of delivering a very low birth weight infant who do not receive tocolytic therapy (if they have no contraindications) are receiving poor medical care, as illustrated in the following case history.

CASE 8–1

B.B.F. was born at 760 gm and 25 weeks gestation 12 hours after the mother entered the hospital with premature contractions. Membranes were ruptured when the cervical os was found to be 6 cm dilated because it was thought that the mother was delivering a previable infant. The infant, after vaginal delivery, had Apgar scores of 6 and 5 and needed intubation in the delivery room for cyanosis and poor respiratory efforts. The infant was transferred to a neonatal intensive care unit, where he received ventilator therapy for 3 days without improvement. Ultrasonographic examination at that time revealed a massive intracranial hemorrhage. The infant died on the third day.

One year later the mother became pregnant again, and weekly exams starting at 24 weeks revealed a dilating cervical os. At 26 weeks, she was admitted to a perinatal center with occasional uterine contractions and cervical dilation of 4 cm. Nonstress tests, blood pressure, and estriol excretion were normal, as was fetal and placental assessment by ultrasonography. She was placed on bed rest and 0.25 mg terbutaline administered subcutaneously every hour until the contractions ceased (6 hours), then 5 mg by mouth every 4 hours for 48 hours, then 5 mg daily. Cervical circlage was considered but ruled out on the basis of the risks of inducing labor, rupture of membranes, and infections, which are associated with the procedure at this gestation. After 1 week she was discharged home, where she remained on bed rest until 36 weeks, when terbutaline was withdrawn and labor started within 48 hours. Fetal heart rate monitoring throughout labor was normal, and she delivered a 2600 gm male who was normal in all respects.

Mortality Associated with Premature Birth

Premature birth occurs more commonly towards term, whereas the problems associated with premature birth occur with greatest frequency in the most immature infants.

To illustrate, Figure 8–2 shows the percentage of live births of different birth weights in Brigham and Women's Hospital (formerly Boston Lying-in, Boston Hospital for Women) and The Beth Israel Hospital since 1977. Long-term trends for low birth weight mortality and survival are illustrated in various ways in Figs. 8–2 to 8–4. From all data, it appears unequivocal that smaller and more immature infants have increased chances of survival in recent years.

Nonetheless, liveborn babies of very low birth weight (≤1500 gm birth weight) are relatively rare (4.5 per cent of livebirths) but account for a disproportionate share of cost, medical resources, mortality (90 per cent of neonatal deaths), morbidity, and poor outcome associated with prematurity.

In our institution, the approximate birth weight and gestation with which (on the average) half the infants would be discharged alive and half would die is 740

gm and about 26 weeks gestation (Fig. 8–3). The corresponding weight was about 1300 gm 20 years ago, and about 1100 gm 10 years ago.

All these data illustrate the need for health professionals to have access to current data on outcome to ensure good management of perinatal problems that may occur. The following case history illustrates how an obstetrician and a physician-father, using outdated information, nearly precipitated a tragic situation.

CASE 8–2

B.B.G. was born at estimated 26 weeks gestation after spontaneous rupture of membranes occurred in a 29-year-old, gravida 2, para 1 mother whose first child was now a normal 3-year-old born after premature labor at 34 weeks gestation. Because the obstetrician and the father believed that a 26-week infant was previable (or, if viable, would be brain damaged), oxytocin was used to induce labor one day after rupture of membranes occurred to end the pregnancy. No amniocentesis for phospholipids, ultrasonography, tocolytic therapy, or glucocorticoids were used. The 810 gm female infant was born with Apgar scores of 5 and 7, and, because of the father's wishes, was placed in 40 per cent oxygen with no further intervention. Twelve hours later, in the morning, a neonatologist was consulted because the infant remained alive. The infant was transferred to a neonatal intensive care unit, where the course over the next 3 months was relatively benign, except for septic thrombophlebitis from a peripheral venous catheter, apnea, and occasional mild feeding intolerance. At 18 months, the infant appears normal, except for skin discoloration at sites on which transcutaneous O_2 electrodes had been placed.

This infant was fortunate in being relatively mature at birth for her gestation, and fortunate in not suffering evident harm from misguided medical care—possible iatrogenic early delivery and unmonitored oxygen administration in the first hours of life.

Limits of Viability

Surely one of the smallest reported survivors was an infant born in 1973 at 27 weeks with a weight of 450 gm that fell to 360 gm (Lelek et al., 1973). It seems probable that most very low birth weight infants who live are undersized for gestational age. We know of surviving infants born at 25 weeks who have weighed over 600 gm but of none born before 24 weeks who have been discharged from the nursery. In our program over the past 6 years, from a base of about 65,000 livebirths, approximately 30 liveborn infants were delivered with birth weights between 500 and 600 gm. None has survived the first year of life. In offspring of approximately 50,000 pregnant women studied during the period from 1959 to 1965, the three smallest infants surviving to 1 year were all black females (birth weights 727, 822, 879 gm) (Hardy et al., 1979).

With the limits of viability decreasing over the past 20 years for very low birth weight infants, it is logical

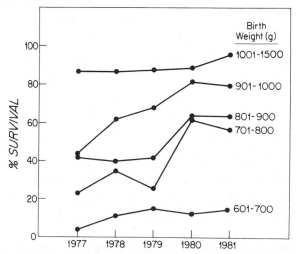

Figure 8–2. Percentage of low birth weight infants who survive is plotted on the ordinate, and the years from which the data were obtained is plotted on the abscissa. Data are from births that occurred at Brigham and Women's and Beth Israel Hospitals in Boston.

LOW BIRTH WEIGHT SURVIVAL

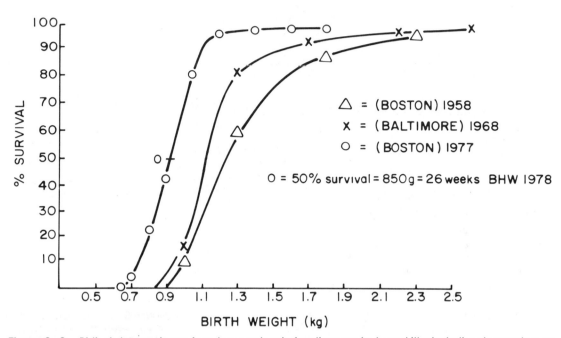

Figure 8–3. Birth data are shown from two centers in four time periods and illustrate the dependency of survival on birth weight. Note that a difference of 300 g (approximately 1½ weeks gestation) in 1977 could alter chances of survival from less than 5 per cent to more than 95 per cent.

to wonder where the limits will eventually be. A danger of guessing at these limits is that the estimate of the limits of viability could be formalized into absolutes. The question is, "When can one reasonably expect newborn infants to have brains and, particularly, lungs capable of functioning in a manner that allows for extrauterine life with conventional support for reasonable periods of time?" The lungs are, before 24 weeks, a largely canalicular organ incapable of alveolar-capillary gas exchange, and the brain has not, to a large degree, differentiated sufficiently to allow for regular respiration. Granted the conceptual possibility of raising an extrauterine fetus attached to an artificial placenta in a fluid environment, the technical, scientific, and ethical questions relating to this approach have not been carefully considered. Therefore, our belief is that current limits of viability, without major changes in our approach to care, will remain unchanged from those of the present in the next few years.

Exact estimation of fetal weight and gestation can be critical in determining whether a woman should (for example) be delivered by cesarean section when fetal weight is between 400 and 900 gm and gestation is between 22 and 27 weeks. As seen in Figures 8–

2 and 8–4 and in Table 8–5, a difference of 1 to 2 weeks gestation and 200 to 300 gm fetal weight can mean the difference between 100 per cent mortality risk versus 20 per cent mortality. Unfortunately, the usual predelivery evaluations may underestimate gestation and birth weight (in as many as 35 per cent of cases), and, if this should occur, mortality risks may be doubled if management is not carried out with the belief that a viable infant is the probable outcome (Paul, 1979).

Using the data summarized above, we have outlined our current perinatal approach to the threatened delivery of a very low birth weight infant in Table 8–6.

Long-Term Outcome of Low Birth Weight Infants

PERINATAL FACTORS

The most serious problems for low birth weight infants who survive relate to the number and severity of perinatal problems, for example, CNS is-

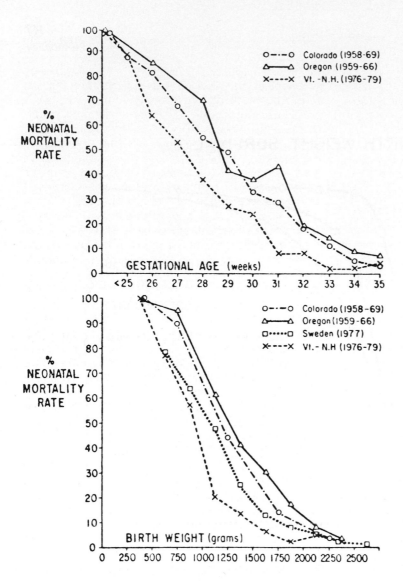

Figure 8—4. Studies from different centers have been summarized by Bowes. The best and most recent data in this figure indicate a 50 per cent mortality for the 900 to 1000 g birthweight group. This "LD-50" for prematurity has since decreased to 700 to 800 g (Table 8–5). (From Bowes, W.: Clin. Perinatol. *8*:183, 1981.)

Table 8–5. Perinatal Mortality (501 to 1500 gm) at the University of Colorado Health Sciences Center from January 1975 to December 1979

Birth Weight (gm)	Total Births	Fetal Deaths	Neonatal Deaths	Perinatal Mortality (Per Cent)	Neonatal Mortality (Per Cent)	Neonatal Survival (Per Cent)
501–600	25	8	16	96	94	6
601–700	42	9	19	67	58	42
701–800	50	8	26	68	62	38
801–900	34	7	12	56	44	56
901–1000	56	5	16	38	31	69
1001–1100	60	10	11	35	22	78
1101–1200	64	2	12	22	19	81
1201–1300	64	1	10	17	16	84
1301–1400	57	2	4	11	7	93
1401–1500	69	3	3	9	5	95
501–1000	207	37	89	61	52	48
1001–1500	314	18	40	18	14	86
501–1500	521	55	129	35	28	72

(From Bowes, W. A.: Delivery of the very low birth weight infant. Symposium on Difficult Labor and Delivery. Clin. Perinatol. *8*:183, 1981.)

Table 8–6.

I. Maternal/Fetal Care
When Premature Birth Threatens

A. Careful dating of gestation.
B. Admission and bed rest, history and physical.
C. One cervical exam for assessment of effacement, dilatation, status of membranes, and culture.
D. Ultrasonographic examination of fetus to assess size, physical status, function, and placentation.
E. Consultation with neonatologist.
F. If fetus is over 600 gms, maternal and fetal management as for 34-week pregnancy (i.e., cesarean section on fetal indication, etc.).
G. Bed rest, labor suppressants.
H. Glucocorticoids if less than 32 weeks gestation and/or if amniotic fluid examination indicates pulmonary immaturity of the fetus.
I. Elective delivery in perinatal center with intramural intensive care.

II. Neonatal Care

A. Neonatologist present before and at delivery.
B. Measurement of arterial cord blood gases.
C. Resuscitation and stabilization in intramural intensive care unit.
D. Continuous assessment of viability in the neonatal period.
E. Detailed communication with parents anticipating the next set of problems confronting the infant.
F. Withdrawal of respirator support if parents, physicians, and nurses agree that the infant is nonviable.

chemia/asphyxia, intraventricular hemorrhage, respiratory distress syndrome, bronchopulmonary dysplasia, retrolental fibroplasia, infectious and metabolic problems (e.g., acidosis, hypoglycemia, hyperbilirubinemia, and rickets). Since these problems occur more frequently with decreasing gestation (Fig. 8–5), it is obvious that low birth weight infants, on the average, may have problems with cognitive, auditory, visual, and motor CNS functions and with diseases such as hydrocephalus, cerebral palsy, and chronic lung disease. Nonetheless, it is reassuring to parents to be told that if a very low birth weight infant escapes most or all of the aforementioned acute

problems in the neonatal period, then the prognosis should be excellent; that is, not immaturity per se but problems associated with immaturity lead to later difficulty. This concept is useful because it is testable, and it removes the mystique from an approach to the question, "How do we know if our infant will be normal?" Therefore, prognosis, we believe, requires an integration of prognoses of the (usually several) problems occurring in the neonatal period.

For all infants, a number of studies have indicated that degree of immaturity at birth as well as socioeconomic and educational levels of the parents are the most important determinants of a newborn's chances of well-being in later childhood (Hardy et al., 1979). A group of women can be defined who are at special risk of contributing to perinatal and infant mortality and morbidity, that is, those who have previously had premature infants, fetal, neonatal, and infant deaths, and children with damage relating to the fetal/infancy period. The women in this group of mothers are often young, impoverished, minimally educated, and in poor health.

Shapiro reviewed data gathered in 1975 from eight perinatal centers in different regions of the United States that included about 6 per cent of total U.S. births. Morbidity data at 1 year were collected from a random sample household survey of nearly 5000 infants. Birth weight was a discriminating variable not only for neonatal and postnatal death but also for congenital anomalies. Nearly one third of infants weighing less than 1500 gm at birth were hospitalized for a wide range of morbidities after discharge from neonatal care. Maternal age corresponded with infant risk in mothers at both ends of the age spectrum (i.e., those under 18 years and over 35 years) but only as it affected birth weight. The highest incidence of anomalies was found among infants of older mothers. In contrast, postneonatal death and significant

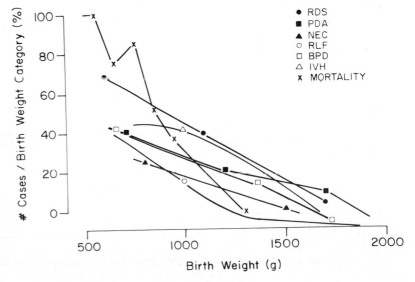

Figure 8–5. Morbidity as well as mortality increases with decreasing birthweight and gestational age. In this figure, rough incidences for various diseases are contrasted with mortality. The denominator is the number of live births per each birthweight category. Data are from a variety of reports in the literature. RDS = respiratory distress syndrome; PDA = patent ductus arteriosus; NEC = necrotizing enterocolitis; RLF = retrolental fibroplasia; BPD = bronchopulmonary dysplasia; IVH = intraventricular hemorrhage.

illness were more common among infants of mothers under 18 years. Maternal education was one of the most important variables. The proportion of low birth weight infants is inversely related to maternal educational attainment.

Cesarean section may be associated with lower mortality rates among very small infants, as reported by Stewart and coworkers. Others have found that overall mortality was higher among infants delivered by section, probably because of the many serious problems that dictate section. In general, risk factors for perinatal deaths significantly parallel those for morbidities in the first year of life. The magnitude of the morbidity is substantial, since 28 per cent of infants of mothers with perinatal risk factors had conditions that presented problems of consequence in the first year of life.

Drillien has been a long-time student of the impact of perinatal events on later life. She studied survivors from a group of low birth weight infants delivered from 1966 to 1970 at an average age of 6 years, 8 months. This group included small for gestational age infants and infants who had varying degrees of in- and ex-utero problems. A 94 per cent follow-up rate was obtained for those alive at time of follow-up. An "impairment score" was constructed, and children with a score of 0 to 1 were progressing well in school, those with a score of 2 were having mild learning problems, and those with a score of 3 were having considerable problems and required special education. Infants of low birth weight who were neurologically normal in the first year of life were indistinguishable from control infants at 6 to 7 years of age.

Hearing loss occurred in 9 per cent of 111 infants under 1500 gm birth weight between 1966 and 1972 at University College Hospital, London (Abramovich et al., 1979). Only 4 per cent were seriously handicapped by their sensory neural hearing loss. Predisposing factors in addition to prematurity were apneic spells, with some additional insult from hyperbilirubinemia. No relation to duration of stay in an incubator or evidence of noise toxicity was found.

Studying an inborn population of infants less than 1250 gm birth weight, Kumar and others found a 55 per cent mortality rate. Follow-up data were available on 80 per cent of the survivors, and 14 per cent of them had major handicaps.

Among infants at risk for later handicap are those of less than 1000 gm birth weight who require ventilator support. Ruiz and coworkers (1981) followed 38 of 40 infants with birth weights of less than 1000 gm. They were evaluated between 8 and 15 months of age. Twenty-eight (74 per cent) of the infants were normal or had mild problems. Most of the disabilities were multiple and were present in survivors who needed ventilator support. The need for ventilatory support no doubt defines those in this birth weight group with more significant disease. Thirty per cent of the ventilated group survived, 20 per cent with severe retrolental fibroplasia, 75 per cent with bronchopulmonary dysplasia, and 45 per cent with severe neurologic handicaps.

In another study, Britton and colleagues studied 37 infants at 18 months (post-term) who were born with birth weights less than 801 gm and who were transferred to a neonatal intensive care unit. In retrospect, it is evident that in this study chances of survival were enhanced by cesarean section, absence of asphyxia, and relatively advanced gestation within the group. Handicap among the survivors related only to sepsis/meningitis and birth weight and not to the need for ventilatory support. Forty-nine per cent of the group had significant neurodevelopmental abnormalities at follow-up, and all the infants weighing less than 700 gm had significant handicap.

The prognostic significance of head circumference was underscored by Lipper and colleagues from Albert Einstein College of Medicine. An abnormal neurobehavioral outcome was seen more than twice as often among infants whose head circumference was less than the tenth percentile for gestational age when compared with those of appropriate head circumferences.

The report entitled *The Cost and Effectiveness of Neonatal Care* is perhaps one of the most comprehensive reviews of morbidity and mortality associated with neonatal intensive care of low birth weight infants. In this 1981 study, Budette and coworkers estimate that about 350 infants weighing less than 1500 gm at birth (who would not have lived in 1960) survive in the United States every year with severe handicaps. This figure can be contrasted with approximately 16,000 infants in this group who now survive without handicaps.

Table 8–7.   Outcome of Low Birth Weight Infants at 6 to 7 Years

	Controls (≥2000 gm birth weight)				Low Birth Weight (≤2000 gm birth weight)			
Social grade*	1	2	3	4	1	2	3	4
Average I.Q.	120	109	103	94	110	105	98	91
Per cent with impairment score ≥3	0	0	9	17	5	6	18	32
Number of children	18	16	54	23	36	54	101	89

* 1 = high; 4 = low.

(Data from Drillien, C., et al.: Low birth weight children at early school age. Dev. Med. Child. Neurol. 22:26, 1980.)

None of these studies emphasizes the strain on the parents of living with an infant who may be in an intensive care unit for 3 months at high risk of death. During and after this time, appropriate anxieties about chronic illness and handicap must be considered. Reports of increased risk of child abuse and other familial pathology for families such as these attest to the occasional results of this strain and, in our view, represent the most prevalent adverse outcome after the birth of a very immature infant. Strategies that add support to parents during this time need increased emphasis. Primary nurses, doctors, and social workers who will relate to the parents at least weekly in meetings throughout the infant's stay and afterwards are useful in our nurseries. Anticipatory counseling concerning the most likely steps to follow next for care of the infant and the usual prophylactic or therapeutic approach greatly help the parents cope. Permitting time for the parents to ask all their questions without being intimidated by the intensive care setting and personnel is clearly important.

REFERENCES

Abramovich, S. J., Gregory, S., Slemick, M., and Stewart, A.: Hearing loss in very low birthweight infants treated with neonatal intensive care. Arch. Dis. Child. 54:421, 1979.

Barden, T., Peter, J., and Merkatz, I.: Ritodrine: a beta-mimetic agent for use in preterm labor. I. Pharmacology, clinical history, administration, side effects, and safety. Obstet. Gynecol. 56:1, 1980.

Bowes, W.: Delivery of the very low birth weight infant. Clin. Perinatol. 8:183, 1981.

Brazy, J., and Pipkin, M.: Effect of maternal isoxsuprine administration on preterm infants. J. Pediatr. 94:444, 1979.

Britton, S., Fitzhardinge, P., and Ashby, S.: Is intensive care justified for infants weighing less than 801 g at birth? J. Pediatr. 99:937, 1981.

Budette, P., McManus, P., Barrand, N., et al.: The Costs and Effectiveness of Neonatal Intensive Care. Case Study #10, Background Paper #2. Case Studies of Medical Technology. Office of Technology Assessment, August, 1981.

Caputo, D., Goldstern, K., and Taub, H.: The development of prematurely born children through middle childhood. In Field, T. (Ed.): Infants Born at Risk: Behavior and Development. New York, SP Medical and Scientific Books, 1979.

Caritis, S., Edelstone, D., and Mueller-Meubach, E.: Pharmacologic inhibition of preterm labor. Am. J. Obstet. Gynecol. 133:557, 1979.

Challis, J.: Endocrinology of parturition. In Premature Labor. Mead Johnson Symp. Perinat. Dev. Med. 15:8, 1979.

Challis, J., and Mitchell, B.: Hormonal control of preterm and term parturition. Semin. Perinatol. 5:191, 1981.

Cordero, L., Backes, C., and Zuspan, F.: Very low birth weight infants. I. Influence of place of birth on survival. Am. J. Obstet. Gynecol. 143:533, 1982.

Creasy, R., Gummer, B., and Liggins, G.: A system for predicting spontaneous preterm birth. Obstet. Gynecol. 55:692, 1980.

Creasy, R., and Herron, M.: Prevention of premature birth. Semin. Perinatol. 5:295, 1981.

Creasy, R., and Liggins, G.: Aetiology and management of preterm labour. Rec. Adv. Obstet. Gynecol. 13:21, 1979.

Csapo, H., and Herczeg, J.: Arrest of premature labor by isoxsuprine. Am. J. Obstet. Gynecol. 129:482, 1977.

Drillien, C., Thomson, A., and Burgoyne, K.: Low birthweight children at early school age. Dev. Med. Child. Neurol. 22:26, 1980.

Elder, M. G., and Hendricks, C. H. (Eds.): Preterm Labor. Butterworth's International Medical Reviews, London, Butterworth & Co., 1981.

Epstein, M., Nicolls, E., and Stubblefield, P.: Neonatal hyperglycemia after beta sympathomimetic tocolytic therapy. J. Pediatr. 94:449, 1979.

Fuchs, A. R., Fuchs, F., Hysslein, P. et al.: Oxytocin receptors and human parturition: a dual role for oxytocin in the initiation of labor. Science 215:1396, 1982.

Fuchs, F.: Prevention of prematurity. Am. J. Obstet. Gynecol. 126:809, 1976.

Gluck, L. (Ed.): Obstetrical Decisions and Neonatal Outcome. Report of the 78th Ross Conference on Pediatric Research, 1981.

Hack, M., Faneroff, A., and Merkatz, I.: Low birthweight infant. Evolution of a changing outlook. N. Engl. J. Med. 301:1162, 1979.

Hardy, J. B., Drage, J. S., and Jackson, E. C.: The First Year of Life. The Collaborative Perinatal Project of the National Institute of Neurological and Communicative Disorders and Stroke. Baltimore, Johns Hopkins University Press, 1979.

Hein, H.: Evaluation of a rural perinatal care system. Pediatrics 66:540, 1980.

Hoskins, E., Elliot, E., Shennan, A.: Outcome of very low birth weight infants born at a perinatal center. Am. J. Obstet. Gynecol. 145:135, 1983.

Ingemarson, I.: Effect of terbutaline on premature labor. Am. J. Obstet. Gynecol. 125:520, 1976.

Johnson, J., Lee, P., Zachery, A., et al.: High risk prematurity, progestin treatment and steroid studies. Obstet. Gynecol. 54:412, 1979.

Jones, R., Cummins, M., and Davies, P.: Infants of very low birth weight—a fifteen year analysis. Lancet 2:1332, 1979.

Kristofferson, K., and Kern Hansen, M.: The foetus and infant in cases treated with ritodrine. Dan. Med. Bull. 26:121, 1979.

Kumar, S., Anday, E., Sacks, L., et al.: Follow-up studies of very low birthweight infants (1250 g and less) born and treated within a perinatal center. Pediatrics 66:438, 1980.

Lear, M.: Heartsounds. New York, Simon and Schuster, 1981.

Lelek, K., Limanowski, J., and Hager-Malecka, B.: A three-month-old infant with birth weight 450 g. Pediatr. Pol. 48:221, 1973.

Lipper, E., Gartner, L. M., and Grellong, B.: Determinants of neurobehavioral outcome in low-birth-weight infants. Pediatrics 67:502, 1981.

Martin, A.: Severe unwanted effects associated with beta sympathomimetics when used in the treatment of premature labor. Br. J. Clin. Pract. 35:325, 1981.

Merkatz, I., Peter, J., and Barden, T.: Ritodrine hydrochloride. II. Evidence of efficacy. Obstet. Gynecol. 56:7, 1980.

Niebyl, J.: Prostaglandin synthetase inhibitors (for premature labor). Semin. Perinatol. 5:274, 1981.

Paul, R., Koh, K., and Monfared, A.: Obstetric factors influencing outcome in infants weighing from 1001 1500 g. Am. J. Obstet Gynecol. 133:503, 1979.

Petrie, R.: Stopping premature labor with magnesium sulfate. Contemp. Obstet. Gynecol. 11:187, 1978.

Philip, A. G. S., Little, G. A., Polivy, D. R., et al.: Neonatal mortality risk for the 80's: the importance of birth weight/gestational age groups. Pediatrics 68:122, 1981.

Robertson, P., Herron, M., Katz, M., et al.: Maternal morbidity associated with isoxsuprine and terbutaline tocolysis. Eur. J. Obstet. Gynecol. Reprod. Biol. 11:371, 1981.

Ross, G.: Parental responses to infants in intensive care. Clin. Perinatol. 7:47, 1980.

Ruiz, M., LeFever, J., Hakanson, D., et al.: Early development of infants of birthweight less than 1000 g with reference to mechanical ventilation in the newborn period. Pediatrics 68:330, 1981.

Shapiro, S., McCormick, M. C., Starfield, B. H., et al.: Relevance of correlates of infant deaths for significant morbidity at 1 year of age. Am. J. Obstet. Gynecol. *136*:363, 1980.

Stubblefield, P. G.: Pulmonary edema occurring after therapy with dexamethasone and terbutaline for premature labor. Am. J. Obstet. Gynecol. *132*:341, 1978.

Taeusch, H. W., Jr., and Avery, M. E.: Neonatal intensive care: incomplete solutions. Harv. Med. Alum. Bull. *53*:27, 1978.

Taeusch, H. W., and Tulchinsky, D.: Obstetric factors affecting risk of respiratory distress syndrome in premature labor. *In* Premature Labor. Mead Johnson Symp. Perinat. Dev. Med. *15*:48, 1979.

Tulchinsky, D., and Ryan, K. J.: Maternal-Fetal Endocrinology. Philadelphia, W. B. Saunders Co., 1980.

Wallace, R., Caldwell, D., Ansbacher, R., et al.: Inhibition of premature labor with terbutaline. Obstet. Gynecol. *15*:387, 1978.

Zuckerman, H., Reiss, U., and Rubinstein, I.: Inhibition of human premature labor by indomethacin. Obstet. Gynecol. *44*:787, 1974.

9

Intrauterine Growth Retardation

Although pediatricians have been concerned with undersized infants for many years, much clarification and definition remains for the future. We have witnessed construction of intrauterine growth charts from many sources. They relate gestational age to measurements made at the time of birth with consideration of some of the important influences on this relationship. Separate charts for males and females indicate that the male is slightly heavier at any given gestational age. Usually, but not always, ethnicity is documented. The somewhat lighter black infant may, of course, reflect genetic effects and may also demonstrate the impact of socioeconomic class. Altitude does have some small effect on intrauterine growth—a fact that should be kept in mind when one refers to the widely used growth chart of Lubchenco, which is based on newborn measurements obtained in mile-high Denver. The comparatively low weights at the tenth percentile of that chart may reflect the effect of altitude (Fig. 9–1).

Miller has noted that birth weight is affected significantly by five intrinsic factors: gestational age (which is the abscissa in most charts), ethnic group (which has usually but not always been considered), and parity, height, and prepregnancy weight of the mother (which have rarely been evaluated). Few of the existing growth charts have considered more than several of the approximately 30 factors that can affect weight.

Given the extent of interaction of genetic and environmental influences on size at birth, the definition of "normal" must be arbitrary. Whether one uses the lower tenth percentile, fifth percentile, or 2 standard deviations from the mean is a matter of choice. In a given pregnancy, careful documentation of history and assessment of known influences on fetal growth will allow useful description of the infant and direct subsequent interventions.

Diagnosis. The main screening method for the obstetrician is evaluation of both obstetric history and fundal height. If fundal height lags, repeated sonography and endocrinologic studies are indicated.

Ultrasonography. Fetal size can be estimated on the basis of serial biparietal diameters, head-body ratio, and total intrauterine volume. About 80 per cent of growth-retarded infants will have biparietal diameters below the third percentile for age. The accuracy of this measurement is higher before 24 weeks than later. When head and body do not grow in concordance or when both are small, growth retardation should be suspected. Serial studies will establish whether the fetus is on an appropriate or inappropriate trajectory for growth.

Endocrine evaluation. Estriol levels in maternal plasma or 24-hour urine collections are low when fetal growth retardation is present. Presumably, reduced trophoblastic surface of the placenta limits conversion of dihydroepiandrosterone sulfate into estriol. However, as many as 30 per cent of mothers whose fetuses are growth-retarded will have normal estriol values.

Human placental lactogen (HPL) correlates with placental weight. As with estriol, about 30 per cent of women with growth-retarded fetuses will have normal values.

Timing of delivery. Among the considerations that should be shared by obstetrician and pediatrician is the knowledge that up to 10 per cent of growth-retarded fetuses will have major congenital anomalies. Repeated ultrasonographic studies and, possibly, amniocentesis should be considered. With falling

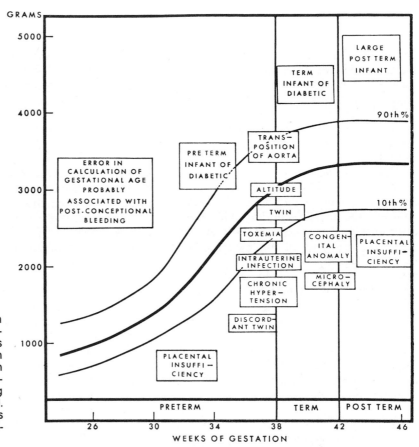

Figure 9–1. Graphic representation of conditions associated with deviations of intrauterine growth. The boxes symbolize the approximate birth weight and gestational age at which the condition is likely to occur. (Lubchenco, L. D., et al.: Factors influencing fetal growth. *In* Jonxis, J. H. P., Visser, H. K. A., and Troelstra, J. A. [Eds.]: Aspects of Praematurity and Dysmaturity. Leiden, H. G. Stenfert Kroese, 1968.)

estriol values, fetal heart monitoring should be performed to ascertain fetal distress. If delivery is contemplated, performing amniocentesis to measure the lecithin/sphingomyelin ratio is in order, and, if it is low, 48 hours of prenatal dexamethasone should be given to the mother if her condition permits.

Delivery should be planned in a setting that can provide neonatal intensive care, since intrapartum deaths are 5- to 6-fold higher among these infants and because risk of meconium aspiration is increased after fetal distress.

Physical Examination. The general appearance of the undersized for gestational age infant provides the first insight into etiology. The infant may appear wasted, as if suffering from intrauterine malnutrition. Subcutaneous fat is diminished, and skin and appendages resemble those in term infants more closely than those in preterm infants (see criteria of Usher, Table 9–1). The neurologic assessment (in the absence of disease of the nervous system) marks chronologic development relatively independent of weight. The Dubowitz scoring system takes note of the maturation of the nervous system.

If the infant is relatively long for weight (low ponderal index), the insult to growth is more likely to

have come from inadequate intrauterine support in the last trimester. Such infants are susceptible to asphyxia. Other infants are symmetrically undergrown and do not appear wasted. According to Miller, low birth weight for gestational age infants are divided approximately equally into these two categories. The symmetrically undergrown, or "skeletal," type of growth delay may coexist with soft-tissue wasting. The short infants are thought to represent a more adverse chronic intrauterine environment, such as that which occurs with maternal cigarette smoking.

A useful approach to the clinical assessment of gestational age is a modified and simplified adaptation of the Dubowitz scales (see Appendix). A useful approach to evaluation of muscle tone in upper and lower extremities is that of Amiel-Tison (Fig. 9–2). The state of arousal of the infant must be noted during any of these examinations.

Etiology. Many adverse conditions can impair intrauterine growth. Some of them are listed in Table 9–2 and Figure 9–1. It is at once obvious that the causes of fetal growth failure are multiple, and the inescapable conclusion is that studies of body composition, diseases, and prognosis that are based on the fact of intrauterine growth retardation alone, without regard to etiology, are likely to give variable and conflicting results. For example, some cite the improved chances for survival in infants who are over 37 weeks' gestation but undersized compared with the changes in infants of similar and appropriate size but under 37 weeks' gestation. Statistics may support such a conclusion if the cause of fetal growth retardation is maternal toxemia or cigarette smoking. If, on the other hand, a rubella epidemic had occurred, the small-for-dates infants would have a higher mortality than true prematures of comparable birth weight.

Placental Factors. Placental growth is essential to fetal growth. Normal placentas show a linear increase in size until about 36 weeks. Both human placental lactogen (HPL) and human chorionic gonadotropin (HCG) are required. HPL is secreted by the syncytiotrophoblast of the placenta as early as 5 weeks of gestation. HCG comes from the corpus luteum of pregnancy early in gestation and is thought to promote natural immunologic tolerance in the fetus.

Placental deficiencies can sometimes be appreciated on inspection at birth. The umbilical cord may be of reduced caliber, and the placenta itself may be thin. More detailed studies have shown a reduction in cell number, protein, and glycogen in placentas of small-for-dates infants.

Hormones. Fetal growth hormone can be detected from the fifth week of pregnancy and increases until the twenty-fourth week. Although the effect of growth hormone on fetal growth is small, its absence is associated with a reduction in cell number and modest reduction in body length. Thyroid hormone also has a limited but important role in determining fetal growth. Athyroid infants show a decrease in body length, a reduction in skeletal ossification, and reduced neural maturation. The kidneys, heart, liver, spleen, and muscle are all delayed in growth in the absence of thyroxin.

Insulin is the essential growth factor for the fetus. Deficiency of beta cells in the islets leads to profound growth retardation, as found in congenital absence of the pancreas. Higher insulin levels are found in cord blood of larger infants, and depressed levels appear in undergrown babies. Infant's sex does not influence the levels.

Maternal Smoking. One of the most important determinants of fetal size (and well-being) relates to maternal cigarette smoking. Meyer and coworkers analyzed the outcome of pregnancy in the Ontario Perinatal Mortality Study of some 50,000 births and found that 1300 deaths occurred in this group during 1960 and 1961. They found the relative risk of an infant of under 2500 gm nearly double in the smokers, and the effect was more pronounced the more the mother smoked. In a prospective study, Rush and Kass identified 86 per cent excess mortality among infants of black smokers compared with that among babies of black nonsmokers. The difference among the white population was only 11 per cent excess among smokers. The authors pointed out the pow-

Table 9–1.   Clinical Criteria for Classification of Low Birth Weight Infants: Premature vs. Dysmature ("Small for Dates")*

Criteria	36 Weeks (Premature)	37–38 Weeks (Borderline Premature)	39 Weeks (Full Term)
Creases on sole of foot	One or two transverse creases running anteriorly, smooth posterior ¾ of foot	More creases appear anteriorly, heel remains smooth	Creases extend throughout soles, prominent deep clefts
Size of breast nodule (large nodules, full term; but small ones may be found in premature or small for dates)	Not palpable before 33 wks; rarely exceeds 3 mm by 36 weeks	Average is 4 mm	Average is 7 mm, sizable mass readily seen
Hair on head	Cotton wool quality, difficult to distinguish one strand from another	Same, with some progression toward 38 weeks characteristic	Silky texture because of thickening of hair; each strand of hair can be distinguished
Cartilaginous development of earlobe	Shapeless, pliable with little cartilaginous support		Rigid earlobe, stiffened with cartilage; folds of helix and anthelix prominent (distinct ridges)
Testicular descent and scrotal changes	Small scrotum with rugae on its inferior aspect limited to a small area; testes at junction of inguinal canal and superior aspect of scrotum not completely descended	Gradual descent with scrotal enlargement	Enlarged scrotum with fully descended testes, pendulous in appearance; inferior surface of scrotum completely covered with rugae

* Modified from Usher, R., et al.: Pediatr. Clin. North Am. *13*:835, 1966.

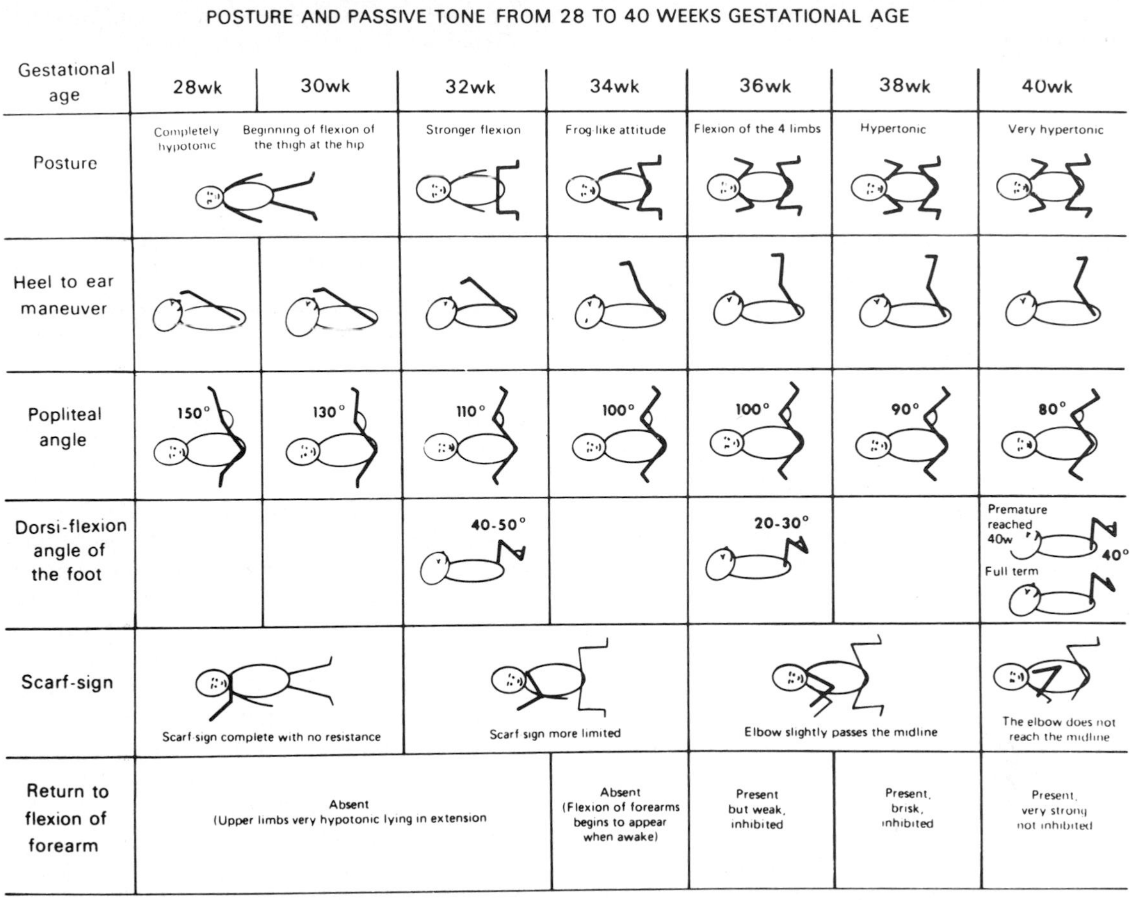

Gestational age	28wk	30wk	32wk	34wk	36wk	38wk	40wk
Posture	Completely hypotonic	Beginning of flexion of the thigh at the hip	Stronger flexion	Frog like attitude	Flexion of the 4 limbs	Hypertonic	Very hypertonic
Heel to ear maneuver							
Popliteal angle	150°	130°	110°	100°	100°	90°	80°
Dorsi-flexion angle of the foot			40-50°		20-30°		Premature reached 40w 40° / Full term
Scarf-sign	Scarf sign complete with no resistance		Scarf sign more limited		Elbow slightly passes the midline		The elbow does not reach the midline
Return to flexion of forearm	Absent (Upper limbs very hypotonic lying in extension			Absent (Flexion of forearms begins to appear when awake)	Present but weak, inhibited	Present, brisk, inhibited	Present, very strong not inhibited

Figure 9–2. Posture and passive tone from 28 to 40 weeks of gestation, indicating increasing muscle tone in upper and lower extremities, which develops with increasing gestational age. (From Amiel-Tison, C.: *In* Rudolph, A. M., Barnett, H. L., and Einhorn, A. H. [Eds.]: Pediatrics. 16th ed. New York, Appleton-Century-Crofts, 1977. Reprinted with permission.)

Table 9–2. Some Findings Associated with Intrauterine Growth Retardation

Maternal factors
    Infections such as rubella, cytomegalovirus, toxoplasmosis, syphilis
    Toxemia or chronic hypertension
    Cyanotic heart disease
    Short stature (height less than 150 cm)
    Primiparity
    Severe malnutrition
    Cigarette smoking
    Narcotic usage
    Low maternal age
    Previous baby 2.5 kg or less
Environmental factors
    Residence at high altitude
    Radiation
    Exposure to teratogens
Placental factors
    Infarcts
    Thrombosis of fetal vessels
    Single umbilical artery
    Premature partial separation
    Twin-twin transfusion
Fetal factors
    Twins (multiple pregnancy)
    Chromosomal abnormalities
    Other congenital malformations
    Inborn errors of metabolism
    Insulin deficiency

erful interaction among smoking, race, and social class.

The placentas of smoking mothers are, on the average, 10 per cent heavier than those of nonsmokers. Presumably, chronic hypoxia from increased levels of carboxyhemoglobin produces the physiologic equivalent of residence at altitude. Blood flow to the placenta is affected during smoking, as indicated by thermograms. Placental "aging," as indicated by calcification and subchorionic fibrin deposits, has been described by Christianson. All these events may promote undergrowth for gestational age in some infants, and in others they may result in premature birth from abruptio placentae or placental aging.

Altitude. Infants born to mothers who reside at high altitude are of lower average birth weight than those born at sea level. In a study of infants born at 4300 meters (14,000 feet) in the Peruvian Andes, Saco-Pollitt observed lighter and shorter infants who did not differ from sea-level contemporaries in head circumference or skin-fold thickness. She noted consistent evidence of behavioral immaturity, as determined by the Brazelton assessment score. It seems probable that chronic exposure to reduced oxygen tensions at altitude compromises oxygen supply to the fetus. Some compensation is possible by an increase in placental size. However, the fetus tends to have relative growth retardation in altitude-induced hypoxia, as is the case with both maternal cyanotic heart disease and maternal cigarette smoking.

Multiple Pregnancy. Fetal size is, on the average, lower when there is more than one fetus per pregnancy. Monozygotic twins weigh less than dizygotic twins for unknown reasons. Premature birth is partly responsible for low birth weight among infants in multiple pregnancy, but other factors are operative. Abnormal placentation may occur, and twin-twin transfusion can promote major discrepancies in size among monochorionic twins. The donor twin has reduced cytoplasmic mass, as in other instances of intrauterine deprivation, such as extensive placental infarction (Benirschke and Kim, 1973).

Pathology. The findings at autopsy of undersized infants have been described in detail by Gruenwald and are summarized in Table 9–3. Organ maturation proceeds even though the expected increase in body size does not occur. The small size of the thymus and adrenal has been cited as evidence of chronic intrauterine stress.

Course. The likelihood of some postnatal problems such as the respiratory distress syndrome and hyperbilirubinemia is reduced with increasing gestational age. In low birth weight infants, the risk of hypoglycemia and pulmonary hemorrhage is substantially increased. The possibility of fetal infection, chromosomal abnormalities, and other congenital malformations is greater in such infants, since those events are etiologic in the production of growth retardation.

The possibility that growth retardation may predispose an infant to congenital malformations by increasing his susceptibility to another insult

Table 9–3. Pathologic Findings in Intrauterine Growth Retardation

Placenta: Findings are variable. Occasionally the placenta is small; microinfarcts and occlusion of vessels in small villous systems may be present.
Organs that tend to be heavier than expected for weight:
  Brain
  Heart
  Spleen
Organs that tend to be lighter than expected for weight:
  Lungs
  Liver
  Thymus
  Adrenals
Gross findings:
  More convolutions in brain than expected for weight
  Greater glomerular development than expected
  Alveolar development appropriate for gestational age rather than weight
  Scant extramedullary erythropoiesis

Table 9–4. Perinatal Mortality and Selected Pregnancy Complications by Maternal Cigarette Smoking

Outcome	Nonsmokers	Smokers	
		<1 pack/day	>1 pack/day
	n = 28,358	n = 15,328	n = 6,581
Perinatal mortality	23.3	28.0	28.9
Abruptio placentae	16.1	20.6	28.9
Bleeding during pregnancy	116.5	141.6	180.1

(Data from Meyer, M. B., and Tonascia, J. A.: Am. J. Obstet. Gynecol. *128*:494, 1977.)

was proposed by Spiers, based on epidemiologic considerations.

Management. Recognition of the significant risk of symptomatic hypoglycemia makes serial measurements of blood glucose advisable (see Chapter 57). We attempt to determine blood glucose by the glucose oxidase method on capillary blood by 1 hour of age and frequently thereafter. Prevention of hypoglycemia seems warranted and is achieved by the early institution of oral feedings if the infant is vigorous or by the intravenous route if he is depressed. We aim to give glucose and water in some form to undersized infants no later than 1 hour of postnatal age and often earlier.

Undersized infants have been shown by Sinclair, Scopes, and Silverman to have a greater oxygen consumption per kilogram of body weight than true premature infants. This evidence of "hypermetabolism" probably relates to the percentage of body weight contributed by visceral organs with relatively large oxygen consumptions per unit size. The practical point to emerge from measurements of metabolism is that fluid and caloric needs of undersized infants are somewhat increased when calculated per kilogram of body weight. We try to individualize the requirements of each infant. Some, who seem hungry, may reach full oral feedings by 3 days of age; others tolerate only those amounts that would be accepted by the true premature. When offered formula early, the infants show less postnatal weight loss than true premature infants and may gain weight more rapidly.

Screening for occult intrauterine infection with cord IgM levels would seem appropriate in these undersized infants.

Prognosis. The long-term outcome of intrauterine growth retardation of unknown etiology remains under active study.

In a longitudinal study of preterm infants and those small for gestational age, Cruise found that infants of 28 to 32 weeks gestation "caught up" about as fast as others of 33 to 36 weeks. By 1 year of age, they averaged 9.3 kg and 9.6 kg, respectively, compared with 10.2 kg in term infants. Lengths were 72.3 cm and 74 cm, respectively, compared with a length of 76.5 cm in term infants. Small for gestational age infants weighed a little less than preterm infants at 1 year, but they had caught up to infants of similar birth weight by 3 years. We do not have systematic longitudinal data for infants born before 28 weeks.

Few serial measurements from large groups of infants exist. Most growth charts reflect cross-sectional measurements. When Garn and Shaw analyzed the 20,000 clinically normal participants in the Collaborative Perinatal Project, they found size at birth the best predictor of size at 7 years (even better than maternal size or social class). They note that birthsize–specific growth charts would be helpful. Meanwhile, knowledge that a third-percentile baby will probably be a third-percentile 7-year-old child is useful and is well known to pediatricians. These observations pertain to length and head circumference as well as to weight.

The reports of Fitzhardinge and Steven suggest that some children remain undersized, while others show complete catch-up growth. The best predictor of later growth is the growth rate in the first 12 months of life. Cerebral palsy was rare among these infants, but minimal cerebral dysfunction was present in 25 per cent. Speech problems were noted in one third of the boys and in one fourth of the girls. Poor performance in school was a common problem, present in one half of the boys and in more than one third of the girls.

School achievement among infants whose birth weights were under the tenth percentile for gestational age was evaluated by Parkinson and coworkers. When intrauterine head growth retardation had begun before 26 weeks gestation, the children had problems with reading, writing, drawing, and concentrating. Slow head growth that started between 27 and 34 weeks was not as serious. The girls had less difficulty than the boys with similar delay in head growth.

In the British Perinatal Study, Butler compared the long-term effects of birth weight under the tenth percentile (Table 9–5).

Future Directions. Since it is apparent that many adverse events can affect fetal growth, it is important that prognosis at birth be made in light of differing etiologies. For example, the infant whose growth was stunted by intrauterine infection may have an outlook very different from that of one with a small infarcted placenta or of one born to a preeclamptic mother. Even in the absence of known predisposing events, the tall, thin infant appears to have a greater capacity for catch-up growth than the symmetrically undergrown one. Careful attention to crown-heel length and to weight should be a routine consideration in assessing the newborn infant.

Prolonged Gestation (Postmaturity)

Some infants are born appearing normal after a gestation of 300 days or longer; others appear to have suffered intrauterine weight loss, have macerated and wrinkled skins, and may die in the first days of life. This latter group of infants may be designated as "postmature" (Clifford, 1954).

Incidence. Kunstadter and Schnitz found that 247 of 2877 infants had gestational ages of 42 weeks or over; 132 of these were over 43 weeks. This incidence of 4.59 per cent is lower than Sjöstedt's 9.5 per cent but agrees with the findings of Clifford and most other observers.

Etiology. Until the mechanisms of the initiation of normal labor are more clearly understood, it seems unlikely that the etiology of prolonged gestation will be evident. The reports of Liggins on pregnant ewes suggest that the fetal pituitary-adrenal axis may be central to the initiation of labor. Whether or not this is true in the human remains to be established.

Diagnosis. The salient features of the postmature infant are the apparently recent weight loss, an appearance of unusual alertness, or a wide-eyed look, absence of vernix caseosa, dry skin, and, often, a

Table 9–5. Long-Term Effects of Birth Weight Under the Tenth Percentile

	Birth Weight < Tenth Percentile (Per Cent)	Birth Weight > Tenth Percentile (Per Cent)	P
Physical and multiple handicap	2.5	1.4	<0.01
Educational handicap	3.3	1.5	<0.001
Maladjustment	4.4	2.8	<0.01
Poor copying of designs	15.1	10.3	<0.001
Poor physical coordination	15.6	12.3	<0.01
Poor hand control	26.3	19.0	<0.001
Unintelligible speech	13.9	9.8	<0.001
Suboptimal reading	33.4	24.1	<0.001
Enuresis	13.2	10.7	<0.05
Impaired hearing	4.6	4.6	NS
Impaired vision (6/24 or worse, one eye)	16.6	13.5	<0.01

(From Butler, N.: Risk factors in human intrauterine growth retardation. *In* Elliott, K., and Knight, J. [Eds.]: Size at Birth. Ciba Foundation Symposium. New York, Elsevier North-Holland, 1974.)

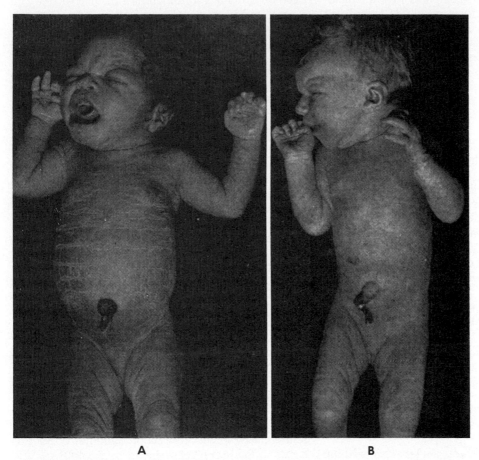

A   B

Figure 9–3. *A*, First stage of postmaturity (placental dysfunction syndrome). Gestational age, 310 days; birth weight, 6 pounds 12 ounces. Relatively long and thin. Dry, cracking, collodionlike skin. No staining. Notable loss of subcutaneous tissue. *B*, Third stage of postmaturity (placental dysfunction). Gestational age, 290 days. Yellow-stained skin and greenish-yellow cord and membranes. Generalized desquamation. Long, thin, wasted muscles and subcutaneous tissue. (Clifford, S. H.: J. Pediat. *44*:1, 1954.)

greenish color of the umbilical cord and skin (Fig. 9–3). The skull is well calcified and feels harder than normal. Resuscitative efforts will often have been required in the delivery room. Aspiration of meconium and squames is common, and pulmonary hemorrhage has been noted in this group of infants. Hypoglycemia may be more common among these infants.

Treatment. Increasingly, pregnancy is monitored carefully and sometimes artificially terminated if it lasts longer than 42 weeks because of the danger of intrauterine asphyxia to the fetus. Ultrasonography will permit assessment of fetal growth. If growth slows or stops, consideration of stimulating labor is appropriate. Serial estriol levels are indicated. Many post-

mature infants require no special treatment. If they seem hungry, it is our practice to feed them full-strength formula as early as 4 hours. If they are depressed, intravenous fluids with 10 per cent dextrose are indicated prophylaxis for hypoglycemia. Neonatal mortality in postmature infants is much greater if the interval between the previous pregnancy and the present one has been on the order of ten years.

REFERENCES

Antonov, A. N.: Children born during the siege of Leningrad in 1942. J. Pediatr. *30*:250, 1947.
Avery, M. E.: Considerations on the definition of viability. N. Engl. J. Med. *292*:206, 1975.
Babson, S. G., Kangas, J., Young, N., and Bramhall, J. I.: Growth

and development of twins of dissimilar size at birth. Pediatrics 33:327, 1964.

Battaglia, F. C., Frazier, T., and Hellegers, A. E.: Obstetric and pediatric complications of juvenile pregnancy. Pediatrics 32:902, 1963.

Beard, A. G., Panos, T. C., Marasigan, B. V., Eminians, J., Kennedy, H. F., and Lamb, J.: Perinatal stress and the premature neonate. II. Effect of fluid and calorie deprivation on blood glucose. J. Pediatr. 68:329, 1966.

Bennett, F. C., Chandler, L. S., Robinson, N. M., and Sells, C. J.: Spastic diplegia in premature infants. Am. J. Dis. Child. 135:732, 1981.

Benirschke, K., and Kim, C. K.: Multiple pregnancy (Part I). N. Engl. J. Med. 288:1276, 1973.

Chernick, V., Heldrich, F., and Avery, M. E.: Periodic breathing of premature infants. J. Pediatr. 64:330, 1964.

Christianson, R. E.: Gross differences observed in the placentas of smokers and nonsmokers. Am. J. Epidemiol. 110:178, 1979.

Clifford, S. H.: Postmaturity—with placental dysfunction; clinical syndrome and pathologic findings. J. Pediatr. 44:1, 1954.

Cruise, M. O.: A longitudinal study of the growth of low-birthweight infants. Pediatrics 51:620, 1973.

Dallman, P. R.: Iron, vitamin E and folate in the preterm infant. J. Pediatr. 85:742, 1974.

Davidson, M., Levine, S. Z., Bauer, C. H., and Dann, M.: Feeding studies in low-birth-weight infants. J. Pediatr. 70:695, 1967.

Davies, P. A., and Stewart, A. L.: Low-birth-weight infants: Neurological sequelae and later intelligence. Brit. Med. Bull. 31:85, 1975.

Davies, P., and Tizard, J. P. M.: Very low birth weight and subsequent neurological defect. Dev. Med. Child Neurol. 17:3, 1975.

Drillien, C. M.: Growth and development in a group of children of very low birth weight. Arch. Dis. Child. 33:10, 1958.

Dubowitz, L. M. S., Dubowitz, V., and Goldberg, C.: Clinical assessment of gestational age in the newborn infant. J. Pediatr. 77:1, 1970.

Evans, T. N., Koeff, S. T., and Morley, G. W.: Fetal effects of prolonged pregnancy. Am. J. Obstet. Gynecol. 85:701, 1963.

Falkner, F.: Maternal nutrition and fetal growth. Am. J. Clin. Nutr. 34:769, 1981.

Fitzhardinge, P. M.: Early growth and development in low-birthweight infants following treatment in an intensive care nursery. Pediatrics 56:162, 1975.

Fitzhardinge, P. M., and Steven, E. M.: The small-for-date infant. I. Later growth patterns. Pediatrics 49:67, 1972.

Fitzhardinge, P., and Steven, E.: The small-for-date infant: II. Neurological and intellectual sequelae. Pediatrics 50:50, 1972.

Fomon, S. J.: Infant Nutrition. 2nd ed. Philadelphia, W. B. Saunders Co., 1974.

Garn, S. M., and Shaw, H. A.: Birth size and growth appraisal. J. Pediatr. 90:1049, 1977.

Gordon, H. H., and Levine, S. Z.: The metabolic basis for the individualized feeding of infants, premature and full-term. J. Pediatr. 25:464, 1944.

Gordon, H. H., Levine, S. Z., and McNamara, W.: The feeding of premature infants, a comparison of human and cow's milk. Am. J. Dis. Child. 73:442, 1947.

Gruenwald, P.: Abnormalities of placental vascularity in relation to intrauterine deprivation and retardation of fetal growth: Significance of avascular chorionic villi. N.Y. State J. Med. 61:1508, 1961.

Gruenwald, P.: Chronic fetal distress and placental insufficiency. Biol. Neonat. 5:215, 1963.

Gruenwald, P., and Minh, H. N.: Evaluation of body and organ weights in perinatal pathology. Am. J. Obstet. Gynecol. 82:312, 1961.

Hanson, J. W., Jones, K. L., and Smith, D. W.: The fetal alcohol syndrome. J.A.M.A. 235:1458, 1976.

Hardy, J. B., Drage, J. S., and Jackson, E. C.: The First Year of Life. The Collaborative Perinatal Project of the National Institute of Neurological and Communicative Disorders and Stroke. Baltimore, Johns Hopkins University Press, 1979.

Harper, P. A., Fischer, L., and Rider, R.: Neurological and intellectual status of prematures at three to five years of age. J. Pediatr. 55:679, 1959.

Iyengar, L.: Chemical composition of placenta in pregnancies with small-for-dates infants. Am. J. Obstet. Gynecol. 116:66, 1973.

Johnson, L., Schaffer, D., and Boggs, T. R.: The premature infant, vitamin E deficiency and retrolental fibroplasia. Am. J. Clin. Nutr. 27:1158, 1974.

Jones, K. L., and Smith, D. W.: Recognition of the fetal alcohol syndrome in early infancy. Lancet 2:999, 1973.

Jonsen, A. R., Phibbs, R. H., Tooley, W. H., and Garland, M. J.: Critical issues in newborn intensive care: A conference report and policy proposal. Pediatrics. 55:756, 1975.

Jonxis, J. H. P., Visser, H. K. A., and Troelstra, J. A. (Eds.): Aspects of Praematurity and Dysmaturity. Nutricia Symposium. Leiden, H. E. Stenfert Kroese, 1968.

Knobloch, H., Rider, R., Harper, P., and Pasamanick, B.: Neuropsychiatric sequelae of prematurity. J.A.M.A. 161:581, 1956.

Liggins, G. C.: Premature delivery of fetal lambs infused with glucocorticoids. J. Endocrinol. 45:515, 1969.

Longo, L. D.: Carbon monoxide: effects on oxygenation of the fetus in utero. Science 194:523, 1976.

Lubchenco, L., Delivoria-Papadopoulos, M., and Searls, D.: Long-term follow-up studies of prematurely born infants. II. Influence of birth weight and gestational age on sequelae. J. Pediatr. 80:509, 1972.

Lubchenco, L. O., Bard, H., Goldman, A. L., Coyer, W. E, McIntyre, C., and Smith, D. M.: Newborn intensive care and long-term prognosis. Dev. Med. Child. Neurol. 16:421, 1974.

Lubchenco, L. O., Hansman, C., Dressler, M., and Boyd, E.: Intrauterine growth as estimated from liveborn birth-weight data at 24 to 42 weeks of gestation. Pediatrics 32:793, 1963.

Mamunes, P., et al.: Intellectual deficits after transient tyrosinemia in the term neonate. Pediatrics 57:675, 1976.

Meyer, M. B., and Tonascia, J. A.: Maternal smoking, pregnancy complications, and perinatal mortality. Am. J. Obstet. Gynecol. 128:494, 1977.

Meyer, M. B., Jonas, B. S., and Tonascia, J. A.: Perinatal events associated with maternal smoking during pregnancy. Am. J. Epidemiol. 103:464, 1976.

Miller, H. C.: Intrauterine growth retardation. An unmet challenge. Am. J. Dis. Child. 135:944, 1981.

Miller, H. C., and Merritt, T. A.: Fetal Growth in Humans. Chicago, Yearbook Medical Publishers, 1979.

Neims, A. H., Warner, M., et al.: Relative deficiency in the elimination of hexachlorophene by neonatal rodents. In Marselli, P. L., et al. (Eds.): Basic and Therapeutic Aspects of Perinatal Pharmacology. New York, Raven Press, 1975.

Nyhan, W. L., and Fousek, M. D.: Septicemia of the newborn, Pediatrics 22:268, 1958.

Ouellette, E. M., Rosett, H. L., Rosman, N. P. et al.: Adverse effects on offspring of maternal alcohol abuse during pregnancy. N. Engl. J. Med. 297:528, 1977.

Parkinson, C. E., Wallis, S., and Harvey, D.: School achievement and behaviour of children who were small-for-dates at birth Dev. Med. Child Neurol. 23:41, 1981.

Pincus, J. B., Gittleman, Z. F., Saito, M., and Sobel, A. E.: Study of plasma values of sodium, potassium, chloride, carbon dioxide, carbon dioxide tension, sugar, urea and the protein base-binding power, pH and hematocrit in prematures on the first day of life. Pediatrics 18:39, 1956.

Radde, I. C., et al.: Growth and mineral metabolism in very low birth weight infants. I. Comparison of two modes of $NaHCO_3$ treatment of late metabolic acidosis. Pediatr. Res. 9:564, 1975.

Rawlings, G., Reynolds, E. O. R., Stewart, A., and Strang, L. B.: Changing prognosis for infants of very low birth weight. Lancet 1:516, 1971.

Rush, D., and Kass, E. H.: Maternal smoking: a reassessment of the association with perinatal mortality. Am. J. Epidemiol. 96:183, 1972.

Saco-Pollitt, C.: Birth in the Peruvian Andes: Physical and behavioral consequences in the neonate. Child Dev. 52:839, 1981.

Scott, K. E., and Usher, R.: Fetal malnutrition. Its incidence, causes and effects. Am. J. Obstet. Gynecol. 94:951, 1966.

Silverman, W. A., and Sinclair, J. C.: Evaluation of precautions before entering a neonatal unit. Pediatrics 40:900, 1967.

Sinclair, J. C., Scopes, J. M., and Silverman, W. A.: Metabolic reference standards for the neonate. Pediatrics 39:724, 1967.

Sjöstedt, S., Engleson, G., and Rooth, G.: Dysmaturity. Arch. Dis. Child. 33:123, 1958.

Spiers, P. S.: Does growth retardation predispose the fetus to congenital malformation? Lancet 1:312, 1982.

Stiehm, E. R.: Fetal defense mechanisms. Am. J. Dis. Child. 129:438, 1975.

Thomson, A. M., Billewicz, W. Z., and Hytten, F. E.: The assessment of fetal growth. J. Obstet. Gynaec. Brit. Comm. 75:903, 1968.

Usher, R., McLean, F., and Scott, K. E.: Judgment of fetal age. II. Clinical significance of gestational age and an objective method of its assessment. Pediatr. Clin. North Am. 13:835, 1966.

Van den Berg, B. J., and Yerushalmy, J.: The relationship of the rate of intrauterine growth of infants of low birth weight to mortality, morbidity, and congenital anomalies. J. Pediatr. 69:531, 1966.

Wennberg, R. P., Schwartz, R., and Sweet, A. Y.: Early versus delayed feeding of low birth weight infants: Effects on physiologic jaundice. J. Pediatr. 68:860, 1966.

Widdowson, E. M.: Changes in the composition of the body at birth and their bearing on function and food requirements. In Jonxis, J. H. P., Visser, H. K. A., and Troelstra, J. A. (Eds.): The Adaptation of the Newborn Infant to Extra-uterine Life. Leiden, H. E. Stenfert Kroese, 1964.

Widdowson, E. M.: The relation between the nature of the fat in the diet of young babies and their absorption of calcium. Biol. Neonatol. 9:279, 1966.

Wu, P. Y. K., Teilman, P., Gabler, M., Vaughan, M., and Metcoff, J.: "Early" versus "late" feeding of low birth weight neonates: Effect on serum bilirubin, blood sugar, and responses to glucagon and epinephrine tolerance tests. Pediatrics 39:733, 1967.

10

Resuscitation

By Michael F. Epstein

The improvement in perinatal mortality in the United States during the past two decades is largely due to improved methods of assessing the condition of the fetus and newborn during the critical phase of transition that surrounds delivery. In contrast, the actual practice of delivery room resuscitation of the newborn is not significantly different from the suggested practices of 20 years ago. The change is in the dynamic approach based on the expectation that every woman who is admitted in labor in the third trimester will be delivered of a live newborn who will reach the intensive care nursery with the potential for normal survival.

That expectation has led to marked changes in the monitoring and management of labor as well as to an increased emphasis on the assessment and immediate care of the newborn infant. Both the American College of Obstetrics and Gynecology and the American Academy of Pediatrics have stated that someone in the delivery room must have primary responsibility for and be skilled in infant resuscitation (Brann and Cefalo, 1979). This may have had little practical effect on pediatricians in medical centers with delivery rooms often crowded with anesthesiologists and neonatologists; however, for those physicians practicing in smaller, less heavily staffed hospitals, it means that the responsibility for the safe arrival of the infant into the nursery begins during and even before delivery.

Advances in fetal assessment now permit the obstetrician to anticipate many instances of potential perinatal asphyxia and allow time for prenatal consultation with the responsible pediatrician. With ultrasonographic evaluation (fetal weight, proportional or disproportional growth retardation, position of fetus and placenta, and presence of significant congenital malformations) and biophysical and biochemical evaluation (oxytocin-stimulated and nonstress testing of fetal heart rate variability and responsiveness, urinary or serum estriols, amniotic fluid optical density, phospholipid concentrations, or bacterial culture), the obstetrician and pediatrician can best jointly plan for the optimal timing and mode of delivery. Such prenatal consultation allows maximal preparation for the infant's care, in both the delivery room (where the specimens of the placenta, blood, and amniotic fluid may be obtained for early diagnosis) and the Neonatal Intensive Care Unit. Moreover, the early anticipation of significant risks for the newborn may allow transfer of the mother to a tertiary care facility before delivery.

Resuscitation of the newborn has frequently been viewed with foreboding, because of both the small size of the patient and the focus placed on the mechanics of intubation, umbilical vein catheterization, and administration of drugs, in which skills become rusty with infrequent practice. These procedures are not inherently difficult but do require frequent renewal. In addition, fewer than 5 per cent of newborns need to be intubated, and fewer than 0.5 per cent need administration of drugs via an umbilical catheter. These numbers can be decreased even further by prompt and proper attention to earlier steps in assessment and treatment of the mildly to moderately asphyxiated infant.

Many useful reviews of resuscitation of the newborn have been directed at pediatricians, neonatologists, and anesthesiologists. This chapter will try to place their concepts in a perspective of basic physiology and make them relevant to the immediate assessment and care of the baby in the delivery room.

Physiology

The immediate transition from fetus to newborn at delivery involves fundamental changes in respiratory and circulatory functions. During fetal life, cardiorespiratory function is directed at supporting the placenta's primary role in gas exchange. In contrast, at birth that role is transferred to the newborn's lungs by a series of alterations in lung inflation and perfusion.

There are two major cardiorespiratory differences between the fetus and the newborn. First, the fetal lungs are filled with fluid and do not function as organs of gas exchange. Second, the fetal circulation is arranged so that most blood bypasses the nonventilated lungs to travel more directly to and from the placenta for gas exchange and delivery of oxygenated blood to fetal tissues. The bypasses are two right-to-left shunts, one through the ductus arteriosus and the other through the foramen ovale.

LUNGS

At birth, the fluid-filled and minimally perfused lungs must be promptly altered for independent existence. Although these alterations in ventilation and perfusion are essentially simultaneous, description will be aided if clearance of the lung liquid is considered before the changes of circulation.

The lungs in the fetus are not metabolically inert tissues merely enlarging through gestation in preparation for postdelivery inflation. Instead, through complicated parenchymal and mesenchymal interaction coordinated with vascular development (Inselman and Mellins, 1981) they form, during the 40 weeks of gestation, thousands of alveolar sacs lined with surface active material in close apposition to a rich capillary bed. Although an organ thus adapted for large volume gas exchange, the lungs at delivery are filled with pulmonary fluid. This is not amniotic fluid aspirated by fetal breathing movement but a combination of filtered plasma and phospholipids, proteins, and other compounds secreted actively by lung parenchyma to a volume approximating that of the newborn's residual lung capacity to be achieved after several hours of air breathing (i.e., approximately 30 ml/kg body weight). Thus, the term baby has 100–120 ml of fluid in the lungs before delivery.

This fluid must be either expelled from the nose or mouth by the pressure of the vaginal walls or the uterus and maternal abdominal wall at delivery or driven down the trachea and bronchi into the alveoli and thence into the pulmonary capillary bed and the circulation. Karlberg and coworkers (1962) showed that the force needed to move this air-liquid meniscus down the tracheobronchial tree with the first breath may well reach pressures greater than 30 to 50 cm H_2O (ten times greater than those pressures with which the resting newborn of several hours of age breathes) (Karlberg et al., 1962).

Clearance of the lung liquid is followed quickly by achievement of a functional residual volume in the lung that allows efficient and effective breathing (Boon et al., 1979). That, in turn, requires stabilization of the alveoli at the end of each expiration by surfactant. This group of compounds (primarily saturated phosphatidylcholine or lecithin, phosphatidylglycerol, and a lung-specific protein) reduces the surface tension at the air/tissue interface and allows for maintenance of alveolar patency throughout the respiratory cycle. A deficiency of surfactant results in hyaline membrane disease or respiratory distress syndrome of the premature.

This orderly process of replacement of lung liquid with air, establishment of a residual lung capacity, and maintenance of efficient and effective breathing can be disrupted by many other conditions of fetal or neonatal origin from physical blockage of the airway (e.g., meconium aspiration) to inadequate respiratory effort (e.g., neuromuscular disease or extreme prematurity). Whatever the cause of disruption of this orderly process, without effective inflation of the lungs and continued ventilation, fetal to neonatal transition will fail.

CIRCULATORY SYSTEM

Conversion of the circulatory system is the second critical adaptation experienced by the infant at delivery. In the fetus, blood is routed through the ductus arteriosus and the foramen ovale from right to left past the lungs so as to provide the blood most enriched with oxygen directly from the placenta to vital organs and to avoid a useless passage through the lungs. At delivery, when respiratory function switches from the placenta to the lungs, blood flow must similarly change to provide the lungs with perfusion.

Dawes described a transitional neonatal circulation in which the ductus arteriosus remains partially or intermittently open, maybe persisting for hours or days before complete closure and conversion ultimately occur (Dawes, 1968). As long as the ductus remains open, the direction of blood flow in and around the heart and great vessels is determined by the relationship between pulmonary (PVR) and systemic (SVR) vascular resistance. The fetal and therefore neonatal pulmonary arterial bed is rich in muscle, and the resistance in these vessels is very responsive to hypoxia and acidosis. Rudolph and Yuan (1966) described the marked increases in PVR in newborn calves in response to a lowering of Po_2 or pH or both (Rudolph and Yuan, 1966). The fetus with its baseline Po_2 of 25 to 28 torr maintains its pulmonary resistance vessels in a state of tonic vasoconstriction resulting in a high PVR. At the same time, with 40 per cent of the fetal cardiac output flowing to the placental bed, the SVR in the fetus is quite low. The resultant gradient between high PVR and low SVR leads to shunting of nearly all the right ventricular output to the aorta via the ductus arteriosus. The small amount of blood that does reach the pulmonary circulation and returns to the left atrium exerts far less pressure than is measured in the right atrium, which receives the venous return from the superior vena cava as well as the umbilical venous return via the ductus venosus and inferior vena cava. This imbalance in right and left atrial returns keeps open the flap valve on the foramen ovale located in the atrial septum. The consequent right-to-left shunt at the foramen ovale completes the fetal circulation.

At delivery, with the first effective breath and the constriction of the umbilical arteries (either spontaneously or by cord clamping) the circulation begins to change. Inflation of the lung with air decreases physical compression of the pulmonary vessels, and local diffusion of oxygen begins to relieve the vasoconstriction. While PVR begins to decrease, removal of the placenta from the systemic circulation and cooling of the skin capillary bed results in an increase in SVR. These combined alterations in resistance diminish and ultimately close the right-to-left shunt through the ductus arteriosus. Right ventricular output goes to the lungs, and the blood is oxygenated and returns to the left atrium. Left and right atrial pressures are equalized, and the foramen ovale closes, leaving an intact atrial septum. Once the fetal shunts have thus closed, ongoing maintenance of oxygenation normally results in continuation of their closure, and as the fetal (or neonatal) becomes the adult circulation, the ducti arteriosus and venosus fibrose and remain as vestigial reminders of fetal life.

However, in its initial stages, this transition remains tentative and reversible: A compromise of oxygenation or severe respiratory or metabolic acidosis may result in so marked an increase in pulmonary vascular resistance that the pattern of fetal circulation recurs. This so-called persistent fetal circulation (PFC), or persistent pulmonary hypertension, most commonly seen in the term or post-term baby with severe meconium aspiration pneumonia or perinatal asphyxia or both, is associated with a high mortality rate. Its treatment is frustrating because the pulmonary arterial bed may remain so tightly constricted that perfusion of the lungs is sometimes impossible, despite the eventual achievement of adequate ventilation.

Right-to-left shunting may also continue into the newborn period when a low systemic blood pressure results from blood loss, sepsis, or the myocardial injury of asphyxia. This condition is commonly less severe than persistent pulmonary hypertension and is more easily diagnosed, since systemic blood pressure is measured more easily than pulmonary pressure.

Asphyxia present before delivery may cause significant impairment in the ability of the fetus to accomplish these postnatal transitions. Antenatal asphyxia may also cause ischemic-hypoxic damage to the CNS and other critical organs, and thus fetal death, if extreme, as with catastrophic cord or placental accidents such as a prolapsed cord, vasa praevia, or abruptio placentae. Less acute asphyxial conditions in utero may be diagnosed and treatment begun before delivery.

The obstetrician may be alerted to impending fetal compromise by monitoring the fetal heart rate and the pH of capillary blood obtained from the fetal scalp. Newer methods allow continuous transcutaneous monitoring of fetal Po_2 and Pco_2. Severe compromise should lead to immediate delivery by cesarean section or per vagina if cervical dilatation and the station of the fetal head allow. If fetal heart rate or scalp pH measurements indicate less severe asphyxia, several measures may offer "treatment" of the fetal asphyxia in utero. These measures are designed to improve the delivery of oxygen to the fetus and include turning the mother onto her left side to relieve vena caval obstruction, maintaining a normal maternal blood pressure by administering fluid intravenously or by using pressors such as ephedrine (especially if hypotension is secondary to regional block anesthesia), and administering oxygen to the mother. The use of beta-adrenergic drugs for in utero resuscitation has been described in Europe but has not received wide acceptance in the United States. Careful maintenance of euglycemia may also be important in view of several animal studies that describe worsening of fetal or neonatal acidemia in hypoxia accompanied by hyperglycemia (Meyers and Meyers, 1979; Haynes and Shelley, 1976). Close monitoring of fetal heart rate variability and decelerations as well as fetal scalp pH must accompany any attempted therapeutic interventions so that delivery can be speedily accomplished should there be any deterioration in fetal condition.

Successful cardiorespiratory adaptations at delivery can be most succinctly summarized in two words: adequate oxygenation. Once this is established by initiation and maintenance of adequate breathing through a patent airway, the circulatory adjustments will follow. Appreciation of the central role of initiation and continued maintenance of adequate breathing will provide the proper focus for the assessment and management of every baby in the delivery room.

Assessment of the Newborn

Nowhere in medicine does treatment precede assessment or diagnosis, and the delivery room is no exception. Errors in resuscitation stem from inaccurate or inadequate assessment of the baby's condition and include errors of commission as well as omission. Both types of mistakes may result in a worse situation than if correct assessment had indicated a proper approach.

Assessment of the newborn in the delivery room is best accomplished by the Apgar score originated by a wise and observant anesthesiologist over a quarter century ago (Apgar, 1953). In a setting in which laboratory tests, radiographs, and prolonged observation are all impossible, immediate and repeated Apgar scoring provides a rapid but dependable measurement of physiologic status. Based on a simple assignment of 0, 1, or 2 points for vital functions (such as color, respiratory effort, and heart rate) and for central nervous system oxygenation (such as tone and reflex irritability) the components of the Apgar score correlate well with how smoothly the transition from fetal to newborn life is made (Table 10–1). Dawes and colleagues correlated the hypoxia, hypercarbia, and acidemia that accompanies the failure to initiate respiration at delivery in the monkey with the gasping and ultimately absent respiratory efforts and the rapid fall in heart rate. The correlation between cord blood pH as a measure of asphyxia and 1-minute Apgar score has been similarly demonstrated in human infants.

The Apgar scoring system is perhaps most hampered by the ease with which it can be assigned and,

consequently, by the lack of rigor in its current application. Although most babies will in fact have scores of ≥8 at and beyond 1 minute, the value of assigning the Apgar score carefully and conscientiously to each and every baby is that one can confidently recognize, for example, that a score of 6 means all is not well and should be acted upon rather than simply observed or disregarded. Diagnostic skills in the delivery room are only as good as our care and attention in forming good habits for using them.

Routine scoring at 1 minute and 5 minutes after delivery has become the usual practice. The 1-minute score correlates closely with the pH of umbilical cord arterial blood, while the 5-minute score may most closely correlate with later neurologic outcome (Macdonald et al., 1980). However, the Apgar score is most useful when used in a continuous manner, rather than only at 1 and 5 minutes, as a guide to selecting resuscitation measures specific to the changing situation of an individual baby.

A first Apgar score can be easily assigned within 20 to 30 seconds of delivery, as color, respiratory effort, and tone are all either recognized immediately by the physician or evaluated while he holds the infant during the brief walk from delivery bed to warming table. Upon reaching the warming table, the physician's right hand can use the bulb syringe to suction out the mouth and nose, either eliciting a reflex response or failing to do so, while the left hand reaches down to the umbilical cord stump and palpates the baby's heart to determine whether the rate is fast (>100), slow (<100), or absent. Thus, within 20 to 30 seconds of delivery, the physician can assign the first of a continuous series of assessments, each of which will determine what course of action to follow with that baby.

One exception to the interpretation of the Apgar score is encountered in infants of very low birth weight. Those infants of <1500 gm and/or <32 weeks gestational age may have low Apgar scores in the absence of asphyxia, as shown by Tooley and coworkers and by Simmons and Bowes. They may have low scores simply on the basis of prematurity alone. Inadequate respiratory effort, poor color and tone, absent reflex responsiveness, and rapid onset of bradycardia are all characteristics consistent with prematurity alone and may not indicate asphyxia. This observation does not argue for a less aggressive approach to these babies. Rather, it should encourage a more rapid and vigorous resuscitative effort since these babies may not suffer from asphyxia and may be easily resuscitated with early attention to adequate ventilation. Certainly, the aggressive management of these babies in the delivery room and neonatal intensive care unit has resulted in improved survival and outcome (Table 10–2).

Table 10–1. Apgar Scoring System

Features Evaluated	0 points	1 point	2 points
Heart rate	0	<100	>100
Respiratory effort	Apnea	Irregular, shallow, or gasping respirations	Vigorous and crying
Color	Pale, blue	Pale or blue extremities	Pink
Muscle tone	Absent	Weak, passive tone	Active movement
Reflex irritability	Absent	Grimace	Active avoidance

Table 10–2. Birth-weight Specific Neonatal Mortality Statistics for Babies Born at Brigham and Women's and Beth Israel Hospitals, 1980.

Weight in Grams	Liveborn	Discharged Alive	Survival (Per Cent)
601–700	10	2	20
701–800	25	14	56
801–900	19	13	68
901–1000	26	20	77
1001–1500	159	143	90
1501–2000	182	177	97

Treatment

The delivery room treatment of the newborn infant is based on the physician's assessment of how successfully the baby is accomplishing the changeover from fetus to newborn. As stated previously, with modern obstetric management, nearly 90 per cent of babies will accomplish this transition without difficulty or help from the medical profession. The identification of the 10 per cent in need of specialized assistance requires careful, continuous observation within the framework of the Apgar score.

Table 10–3 provides a flow sheet describing a step-by-step approach based on Apgar score, and Table 10–4 lists the equipment and medications that should be available in the delivery room. A few additional points should be emphasized.

First: The suctioning of all babies, except those with thick meconium (see further on), should be done with a bulb syringe and not a suction catheter. Cordero and Hon found significant arrhythmia or apneic episodes in 14 per cent of babies suctioned with catheters immediately after delivery but none in a second group suctioned immediately with a bulb syringe (Cordero and Hon, 1971). However, when a suction catheter was used 5 minutes after delivery, none of the babies developed problems, probably because of the greater vagal response to laryngeal stimulation during the relative asphyxia of all babies immediately after delivery. Whatever the explanation, the risk of inducing apnea or bradycardia in an otherwise healthy newborn can be avoided by using the bulb syringe during the first postnatal minutes. Emptying of the stomach via a nasal catheter is not routinely indicated, but when a gastric aspirate is needed for diagnostic studies (e.g., foam stability shake test for lung maturity or Gram stain and culture when there is a question of infection) or when there has been thick meconium passed into the amniotic fluid, gastric contents should be aspirated only after achievement of adequate oxygenation as indicated by Apgar score of ≥8 at or beyond 5 minutes after delivery.

Second: The administration of unwarmed oxygen if blown into the newborn's face at a high flow rate may result in the slowing of respiration and heart (Brown et al., 1976). Therefore, when oxygen treatment is indicated by an Apgar score in the 5 to 7 range, low-flow, "blow-by" oxygen (if possible, warmed and humidified) accompanied by gentle stimulation should be carefully administered to the mildly depressed infant. Routine oxygen administration is not indicated for all babies.

Third: In an asphyxiated infant who does not respond to stimulation, blow-by oxygen, or bag and mask ventilation, rapid endotracheal intubation should be performed. Recent studies have indicated that after intubation of an infant, the most efficacious way of achieving a residual lung volume is by a prolonged initial inspiration (Vyas et al., 1981). By using a water-filled esophageal catheter to measure transpulmonary pressures, Vyas and associates found that prolonged inspiration with a 3- 5-second plateau produced a larger initial inflation volume and an earlier achievement of FRC than did ventilation with the standard 1-second square wave inspirations. The shape of the initial inspiration (i.e., square wave or slow-rise) did not appear to be significant.

If a severely asphyxiated infant fails to respond to ventilation with 100 per cent oxygen, the commonest remediable cause is displacement of the endotracheal tube from the trachea. A brief pause in cardiac massage to ensure that chest motion (not lower rib cage over the stomach) is adequate with good breath sounds bilaterally (auscultated in the axillae, not over the sternum) is warranted every 30 seconds. If endotracheal tube placement is in doubt, direct visualization of the tube passing through the vocal cords is essential. Cardiac massage, umbilical venous catheters, and drugs are all useless unless a secure airway and adequate ventilation with 100 per cent oxygen are first achieved. This most fundamental of all lessons is the one most frequently neglected by the "occasional resuscitator" and is the one that most needs emphasis. "Airway + Breathing must precede Cardiac output + Drugs," a lesson known to all lay people who have graduated from CPR workshops and courses, is just as critical in the delivery room.

Fourth: The administration of sodium bicarbonate (HCO_3^-) remains a controversial management issue. The efforts of Finberg and numerous others have effectively and appropriately eliminated the routine administration of rapidly infused hypertonic HCO_3^- solutions to the small premature baby in the intensive care nursery (Finberg, 1977). However, the need for rapid correction of severe metabolic acidosis in the severely asphyxiated newborn remains, and the use of hypertonic HCO_3^- remains the best choice now available. The increased incidence of intracranial hemorrhage reported in newborn beagle pups who were asphyxiated and then given intravenous bicarbonate is of concern (Edwards et al., 1982), but in a similar study in newborn sheep, HCO_3^- administration was associated with improved survival, and there was no evidence of such bleeding (Wheeler et al., 1979). Perhaps the best guideline is to use HCO_3^- only when a base deficit > 10 to 12 mEq/l indicates that severe metabolic acidosis is present. This can be inferred without blood gas measurement when bradycardia has been present for more than several minutes after delivery. However, if the newborn's heart rate has increased with initial ventilation and other supportive measures,

the decision to administer bicarbonate should be based on the arterial or capillary blood pH and P_{CO_2}. If these measurements indicate a metabolic or mixed acidosis with a base deficit in excess of 10 to 12 mEq/l, then bicarbonate administration is appropriate. One

Table 10–3

Apgar Score	Management
A. 8, 9, or 10 = no asphyxia	Pink, active, responsive, crying baby with rapid heart rate: 1. Gently suction airway, including nares, with bulb syringe. 2. Dry thoroughly, including head. 3. Maintain body temperature. 4. Perform brief physical examination. 5. Assign 5-min Apgar score. 6. Unite baby with parents.
B. 5, 6, or 7 = mild asphyxia	Slightly cyanotic, moving with decreased muscle tone, breathing shallowly or periodically, heart rate >100: 1. Repeat steps 1, 2, 3 for management outlined in part A in rapid succession. 2. Stimulate to breathe more frequently by gentle but forceful slapping of soles of feet or rubbing of spine or sternum. 3. Provide enriched oxygen ambient atmosphere via anesthesia bag and mask held by baby's face. 4. If improving, complete steps 4, 5, 6 outlined in part A when Apgar score reaches 8. 5. If heart rate falls to <100, Apgar score is ≤4. 6. Administer Narcan 0.01 mg/kg I.M. if mother has received a narcotic analgesic during labor.
C. 3 or 4 = moderate asphyxia	Cyanotic, poor tone, weak respiratory efforts, slowing heart rate (<100): 1. Repeat steps 1, 2, 3 from part A and call for additional personnel to continuously monitor heart rate, manage airway, provide cardiac massage, etc. Resuscitation for the moderately to severely asphyxiated infant is a three-person job. 2. Provide brief trial of stimulation plus O_2 by mask. If there is no improvement by 1 minute, follow step 3. 3. Ventilate with bag and mask, using 100 per cent oxygen and pressure adequate to move the chest. Continue bagging until heart rate >100, color is pink, and spontaneous respirations have begun. If the chest cannot be adequately moved with bag and mask ventilation, intubate. 4. If heart rate <60, intubate and begin cardiac massage at rate of 2 compressions/second, using fingers wrapped around back and thumbs over the sternum (Todres et al., 1975).
D. 0, 1, or 2 = severe asphyxia	Deeply cyanotic, no muscle tone, absent respiratory effort or periodic gasps, heart rate slow or absent: 1. Proceed directly to intubation and bag ventilation with 100 per cent O_2 at 40 to 60 breaths/min at pressures great enough to move the upper chest wall. 2. Perform cardiac massage. 3. If heart rate is not >100 despite 2 minutes of adequate ventilation with 100 per cent O_2 and cardiac massage, insert umbilical venous catheter and administer drugs. Insertion of the catheter is facilitated by cutting the cord at a point ≤1 to 2 cm from the abdominal wall. The catheter is most safely inserted only 2 to 3 cm to avoid administering hypertonic solutions directly into a small hepatic vein. All solutions must be flushed through the catheter to ensure their reaching the central circulation. Delivery room drug treatment is directed at improving myocardial contractility and rate by initially correcting metabolic acidosis (2 to 4 mEq $NaHCO_3$/kg body weight) and by providing carbohydrate substrate (equal volume of 50 per cent dextrose). This combined $NaHCO_3$-dextrose solution can be infused over 3 to 5 minutes. Next, epinephrine (0.5 to 1.0 ml, 1:10,000) or atropine (0.1 ml/kg) can be injected to reverse bradycardia. Finally, a slow infusion of 1.0 to 2.0 ml/kg of calcium gluconate may provide for further enhancement of cardiac output. None of these drugs is effective unless adequate ventilation with oxygen has been achieved. If the heart rate >100 and adequate ventilation is achieved either spontaneously or via assisted ventilation, the use of drugs is not necessary in the delivery room, and the baby should be moved to the nursery. There, measurement of vital signs (including heart rate, respiratory rate, blood pressure, and temperature), arterial or capillary blood gases (Pa_{O_2}, Pa_{CO_2}, and pH), and a chest radiograph allow a rational basis for further care. The administration of hypertonic $NaHCO_3$, cardiotonic drugs, or volume expanders all carry risk. Their use should be withheld pending specific documentation of their need by the above studies if adequate ventilation and heart rate >100 can be achieved in the delivery room.

must also remember that bicarbonate is buffered by the formation of carbonic acid and, ultimately, CO_2 and H_2O, so the ventilation must be adequate to dispose of the newly generated CO_2. Otherwise, the administration of HCO_3^- for a respiratory acidosis or in the face of inadequate ventilation (i.e., $P_{CO_2} > 45$ torr) may result in a more severe acidemia (Steichen and Kleinman, 1977).

Fifth: Another area of uncertainty surrounding the treatment of the asphyxiated infant relates to the use of glucose. The early studies of Dawes, Adamsons, and others indicated that resuscitation was aided by administering glucose to the asphyxiated newborn animal. Other animal studies have shown survival in neonatal asphyxia to be related to cardiac glycogen content and that pretreatment of the fetus (via the mother) with glucose prolongs cardiac contractility during postnatal asphyxia. In contrast, the work of Myers, Haynes and coworkers, and Epstein and associates has indicated that when fetal or neonatal hypoxia is accompanied by an elevated blood glucose concentration, the metabolic acidemia is worsened

and survival time is shortened. Perhaps the best way to apply the evidence from these studies to the newborn in the delivery room would be to ensure that hypoxia has been treated before administering glucose. This should be accomplished by the establishment of an airway and effective ventilation with 100 per cent oxygen. If bradycardia should persist despite this attention to ventilation, glucose administration may be needed to provide substrate for improved cardiac contractility.

Sixth: Another controversy in the pharmacologic approach to resuscitation involves the use of atropine. Advocated by many authors as a treatment for bradycardia, the use of atropine has been criticized because its vagolytic action may only relieve the bradycardia that is a valuable clinical indicator of hypoxia and fail to correct the main effect of bradycardia, poor cardiac output. Cohn and coworkers have shown that atropine increased the heart rate of severely hypoxic fetal sheep, but the effective cardiac output was unchanged. Thus, the major indication of hypoxia in the newborn, bradycardia, may be abolished without treating its cause or reversing its effect. Others object to the use of atropine because it may interfere with the theoretical benefits of the dive reflex, which shunts the blood in diving mam-

---

Table 10–4.   Equipment Needed for Newborn Resuscitation

1. Well-lit, flat, stable, and heated area for observation and management of the infant. Modern radiant warming tables provide an ideal setting. Standard infant care bassinets are inadequate for access to the baby.

2. Oxygen source with adjustable flow meter. Ideally, this gas should be warmed and humidified.

3. Suction. Bulb syringe should be available for all babies. Wall suction with adjustable vacuum and #8 to #12 catheters provide ideal means for clearing the oropharynx and nares of thick meconium. If that is not available, deLee suction traps are adequate.

4. Flow-through anesthesia bag with adjustable pressure valve. These bags can provide 100 per cent oxygen and allow the resuscitator to vary inspiratory and expiratory pressure without adjusting the liter flow at the wall outlet or the mask's seal on the baby's face. Ambu bags are not acceptable, since they cannot deliver more than 40 per cent oxygen, cannot provide continuous oxygen flow out the mask, and cannot produce pressures greater than a preset pop-off valve allows (usually 25 to 35 cm H_2O).

5. Masks of assorted sizes and configurations.

6. Laryngoscope with Miller 1 and Miller 0 blades. The former are necessary only in the larger, term baby of >3.5 kg. The 0 blade allows visualization of the vocal cords in all smaller babies.

7. Endotracheal tubes of 3.5, 3.0, and 2.5 mm diameter. Both flanged (Cole) and unflanged tubes should be available. The former have advantages of being stiffer and maintaining a curve similar to that of the posterior pharynx, allowing easier placement. Moreover, the flange makes it less likely that the tube will be placed too far down the trachea and into the right main stem bronchus, a common error. The unflanged tube is sometimes easier to insert in the <1000-gm infant.

8. Umbilical catheters of 3.5 and 5.0 Fr size, with umbilical tape for securing the stump.

9. Syringes and needles.

10. Medications: $NaHCO_3$ 0.9 mEq/ml or 0.45 mEq/ml.
    Dextrose 50 per cent and 10 per cent
    Epinephrine 1:10,000
    Atropine 0.4 mg/0.5 ml
    Calcium gluconate 9 per cent
    Narcan .02 mg/ml (neonatal solution)
    Albumin 5 per cent

○⊖ packed red blood cells should be available in the blood bank for emergency use.

mals from the splanchnic bed and skin to the brain, heart, and adrenals. If this reflex is operative in the asphyxiated newborn, atropine may further compromise the hypoxic cerebral vascular bed with an added ischemic insult. On the other hand, some anesthesiologists recommend atropine to prevent the reflex vagal bradycardia that may accompany laryngoscopy. Therefore, in the baby who is to undergo laryngoscopy and tracheal suction for meconium in the amniotic fluid but who is not bradycardic atropine may be an appropriate preventive measure.

This controversy and significant questions about the dosage, route of administration, and proper indications for bicarbonate and glucose remain important topics for future research.

Finally, resuscitation is not a solo performance. Although both the American College of Obstetrics and Gynecology and the American Academy of Pediatrics place responsibility for resuscitation of the newborn with an individual, the principles and procedures involved must be understood by all personnel working in the labor and delivery room area. Treatment of the moderately to severely depressed newborn calls for a coordinated team approach. One member skilled in management of the airway and ventilation is ordinarily the coordinator for the remaining members of the team. The latter may be nurses, anesthetists, or other physicians, but all must be skilled in assignment of Apgar score (especially monitoring of the heart rate by auscultation or palpation), positioning of the baby to facilitate intubation, closed cardiac massage, and administration of drugs via an umbilical venous catheter. The latter is facilitated by posting of a list of drugs and dosages in all delivery rooms in view of those participating in a resuscitation.

Practice of the actual resuscitative procedures of bag and mask ventilation, intubation, and catheterization of the umbilical vein is an important program for all hospitals in which babies are delivered. Bag and mask ventilation is perhaps best learned by applying the technique to a resuscitation doll, several of which are available commercially. This allows the operator to achieve dexterity in the application of the mask to a baby's face while adjusting oxygen flow and pressure applied to the bag with the other hand. Facility in the intubation of the newborn can be aided by the experimental use of kittens anesthetized intramuscularly with ketamine, a short-acting hypnotic drug (Jennings et al., 1974). The pharyngeal and laryngeal anatomy of the kitten is quite similar to that of the human newborn, and several practice sessions per year for the delivery room staff responsible for resuscitation serve to maintain otherwise infrequently used skills. The same applies to umbilical vein cannulation, which can be practiced with any placenta with an attached cord and should be frequently practiced by the relevant staff. Full-scale practice resuscitations in the delivery room with the actual use of warming table, oxygen, equipment, drugs, and umbilical vein cannulation are valuable exercises for all delivery services.

Special Situations

While the aforementioned guidelines for assessment and treatment in the delivery room apply to all babies, two special situations that may arise call for modification of the standard approaches. These are (1) the presence of meconium-stained amniotic fluid, and (2) pallor and shock-like appearances indicating pre- or intrapartum hemorrhage.

Approximately 9 to 15 per cent of all fetuses pass meconium into the amniotic fluid before delivery and thus risk aspiration of this thick, viscid material into the mouth, pharynx, trachea, and bronchi either before, during, or after delivery. Meconium aspiration in utero probably occurs from fetal gasping, and it now appears that many babies who die with meconium aspiration syndrome (MAS) and persistent fetal circulation (PFC) have chronic pulmonary vascular changes that antedate their intrapartum asphyxia and aspiration (Murphy et al., 1981). Nevertheless, most babies who have passed meconium in utero can be aided by several therapeutic maneuvers taken to minimize the risk of further or initial aspiration after delivery. The removal of all or most of the meconium from the nasopharynx and the trachea before the first breath or before the physician initiates positive pressure ventilation has reduced the incidence of severe pneumonitis, atelectasis, and the air-leak phenomena of meconium aspiration syndrome.

The combined obstetric and pediatric approach recommended by Carson and coworkers calls for the obstetrician to suction the mouth and nares thoroughly before the delivery of the shoulders and thorax. They recommended using a suction catheter, and Gage and colleagues have used an animal model and radiolabeled meconium solution to demonstrate that a catheter is superior to a bulb syringe for the evacuation of meconium. Clearing of the upper airway before delivery of the thorax may be critical, since a net change of intrathoracic pressure of several cm H_2O occurs from decompression of the chest during vaginal delivery (Karlberg et al., 1962).

After delivery, the cord should be expeditiously clamped and cut and the baby immediately handed to the resuscitator who intubates the trachea. Direct suction applied to the end of the orotracheal tube by the resuscitator's mouth or the use of a suction catheter should be equally efficacious in removing meconium from the trachea, and it should be repeated until no more meconium is obtained or until the newborn's heart rate slows to <40 beats/min. The most concerted effort should be made in large term or post-term babies with thick meconium and intrapartum asphyxia, since these babies continue to have a 25 to 30 per cent case-fatality rate from severe meconium aspiration. Prevention is the best hope, and access to the trachea for suctioning ensures a ready route for ventilation once suctioning is completed. Use of this approach at the Brigham and Women's Hospital has resulted in reduction of the incidence of MAS from 5 per every 1000 births in 1975 to 1.1 per every 1000 births in the period ranging from 1978 to 1980; however, there continue to be 2 to 3 babies every year (total deliveries 7500 per year) who die from MAS and PFC.

The second group of infants with specialized needs are those with significant pre- or intrapartum hemorrhage. These infants present with pallor and shock in the delivery room caused by intrapartum blood loss from placental separation, fetal-placental or fetal-maternal hemorrhage, avulsion of the umbilical cord from the placenta, vasa or placenta previa, incision through an anterior placenta at cesarean section, twin-twin transfusion, or rupture of an abdominal viscus (liver or spleen) during a difficult delivery. These infants will be tachycardic (over 180 beats/min), tachypneic, and hypotensive with poor capillary filling and weak pulses. Keep in mind that a peripheral or central hematocrit immediately after delivery may be normal despite a major intrapartum hemorrhage. After stabilization of respiration and heart rate, immediate transfusion with O-negative packed red blood cells and fresh frozen plasma may be necessary, and a volume of 20 ml/kg can be given over several minutes through an umbilical venous catheter. If clinical improvement is not seen, causes of further blood loss should be sought, and more vigorous blood and colloid replacement should be continued. If blood is not immediately available in the hospital, autologous cord blood from the placenta may be used (Golden et al., 1980). A 20-ml syringe rinsed with 50U of heparin and filled from the povidone-iodine–prepared umbilical vein provides a suitably anticoagulated specimen. Although there is a risk of bacterial contamination, the provision of such blood transfusion may be life-saving in certain circumstances.

REFERENCES

Adamsons, K., Behrman, R., Dawes, G. S., Dawkins, M. J. R., James, L. S., and Ross, B. B.: The treatment of acidosis with alkali and glucose during asphyxia in foetal rhesus monkeys. J. Physiol. *169*: 679, 1963.

Apgar, V.: A proposal for new method of evaluation of the newborn infant. Anesth. Analg. *32*:260, 1953.

Boon, A. W., Milner, A. D., and Hopkin, I. E.: Lung expansion, tidal volume, and formation of the functional residual capacity during resuscitation of asphyxiated newborns. J. Pediatr. *95*:1031, 1979.

Brann, A. W., and Cefalo, R. C.: Care of the newborn in the delivery room. Pediatrics *64*:970, 1979.

Brown, W. U., Ostheimer, G. W., Bell, G. C., and Datta, S. S.: Newborn response to oxygen blown over the face. Anesthesiology *44*:535, 1976.

Carson, B. S., Lasey, B. W., Bowes, W. A., and Simmons, M. A.: Combined obstetric and pediatric approach to prevent meconium aspiration syndrome. Am. J. Obstet. Gynecol. *126*:712, 1976.

Cohn, H. E., Piasecki, G. J., and Jackson, B. T.: The effect of fetal heart rate on cardiovascular function during hypoxemia. Am. J. Obstet. Gynecol. *138*:1190, 1980.

Cordero, L., and Hon, E. H.: Neonatal bradycardia following nasopharyngeal stimulation. J. Pediatr. *78*:441, 1971.

Dawes, G. S.: Foetal and Neonatal Physiology. Chicago, Year Book Medical Publishers, 1968.

Dawes, G. S., Jacobson, H. N., Mott, J. C., Shelley, H. I., and Stafford, A.: The treatment of asphyxiated mature foetal lambs and rhesus monkeys with intravenous glucose and sodium carbonate. J. Physiol. *169*:167, 1963.

Edwards, W., Nattie, E., and Marin-Padialla, M.: The pathogenesis of intracranial hemorrhage in the newborn dog. Pediatr. Res. *16*:286A, 1982.

Epstein, M. E., Hartig-Beecken, I., and Loo, S. W.: Effect of maternal diabetes on response to hypoxia in the newborn rabbit. Biol. Neonate *40*:56, 1981.

Finberg, L.: The relationship of intravenous infusions and intracranial hemorrhage—a commentary. J. Pediatr. *91*:777, 1977.

Gage, J. G., Taeusch, H. W., Treves, S., and Caldecott, W.: Suctioning of upper airway meconium in newborn infants. J.A.M.A. *246*:2590, 1981.

Golden, S. M., O'Brien, W. F., Lissner, C., Cefalo, R. C., Schumacher, H., and Stass, S.: Hematologic and bacteriologic assessment of autologous cord blood for neonatal transfusions. J. Pediatr. *97*:810, 1980.

Haynes, P. J., and Shelley, H. J.: Relationships between plasma glucose, lactate and pH in well oxygenated and hypoxic chronically catheterized fetal lambs. Br. J. Obstet. Gynecol. *83*:330, 1976.

Inselman, L. S., and Mellins. R. B.: Growth and development of the lung. J. Pediatr. *98*:1, 1981.

James, L. S., Weisbrot, I. M., Prince, C. E., Holaday, D. A., and Apgar, V.: Acid base studies of human infants in relation to birth asphyxia and onset of respiration. J. Pediatr. *52*:379, 1958.

Jennings, P. B., Alden, E. R., and Brenz, R. W.: A teaching model for pediatric intubation utilizing ketamine sedated kittens. Pediatrics *53*:283, 1974.

Karlberg, P., Cherry, R. B., Escardo, F. E., and Koch, G.: Pulmonary ventilation and mechanics of breathing in the first minutes of life, including the onset of respiration. Acta Paediatr. *51*:121, 1962.

MacDonald, H. M., Mulligan, J. C., Allen, A. C., and Taylor, P. M.: Neonatal Asphyxia I: Relationship of obstetric and neonatal complications to neonatal mortality in 38,405 consecutive deliveries. J. Pediatr. *96*:898, 1980.

Murphy, J. D., Rabinovitch, M., Goldstein, J. D., and Reid, L. M.: Structural basis of persistent hypertension of the newborn. J. Pediatr. *98*:962, 1981.

Myers, R. E., and Myers, S. E.: Use of sedative analgesic and anesthetic drugs during labor, delivery: bane or boon. Am. J. Obstet. Gynecol. *133*:83, 1979.

Rudolph, A. M., and Yuan, S.: Response of the pulmonary vasculature to hypoxia and H^+ ion concentration changes. J. Clin. Invest. *45*:399, 1966.

Simmons, M. A., and Bowes, W. A.: Apgar scores in infants less than 1500 grams. Pediatr. Res. *12*(abst):534, 1978.

Steichen, J. J., and Kleinman, L. I.: Studies on acid-base balance: I. Effect of alkali therapy in newborn dogs with mechanically fixed ventilation. J. Pediatr. *91*:287, 1977.

Tooley, W. H., Phibbs, R. H., and Schlueter, M. A.: Intrauterine Asphyxia and the Developing Fetal Brain. Chicago, Year Book Medical Publishers, 1977, pp. 251–261.

Vyas, H., Milner, H. O., Hopkin, I. E., and Boon, A. W.: Physiologic responses to prolonged and slow-rise inflation in the resuscitation of the asphyxiated newborn infant. J. Pediatr. *99*:635, 1981.

Wheeler, A. S., Sadri, S., Gutsche, B. B., DeVore, J. S., David-Mian, Z., and Latyshevsky, H.: Intracranial hemorrhage following intravenous administration of sodium bicarbonate or saline solution in the newborn lamb asphyxiated in utero. Anesthesiology *51*:517, 1979.

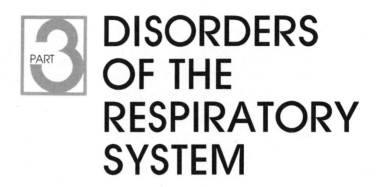

PART 3

DISORDERS OF THE RESPIRATORY SYSTEM

11

General Considerations

An understanding of the disorders of respiration in the neonatal period demands a clear understanding of the physiology of respiration in the fetus and in the neonate, and of the alterations that accompany the precipitous changeover from the aquatic state to the air-breathing state.

It is hardly surprising that any adjustment of such magnitude does not always proceed normally. Sometimes, the problem relates to poor lung development, chest wall or diaphragmatic defects, or deficiencies in the central nervous system regulatory apparatus. Other times, problems with perfusion impair gas exchange, and, of course, aspiration and infection can occur. The following sections will highlight some of the salient aspects of developmental physiology and lung disorders around the time of birth.

The Fetal Lung

The fetal lung does not function as an organ of gas exchange, but it must develop in such a way that it can assume this role as soon as the placental circulation is interrupted at birth. In fetal life, only 4 per cent of the cardiac output perfuses the pulmonary vascular bed; after birth, the whole of the cardiac output must go through the lung. The vascular bed must develop the capacity to accept this enormous increase in perfusion. Similarly, the airways and terminal air spaces are distended with liquid in fetal life; after birth, they must adapt to a gaseous environment and remain inflated at end-expiration. Rapid, irregular respiratory movements are present some of the time in utero; after birth, the central respiratory regulatory apparatus not only must initiate the forceful respirations needed to inflate the airless lung but also must sustain rhythmic breathing. Such major physiologic adjustments in the circulatory, respiratory, and central nervous systems are not required at any other time of life; it is thus not surprising that they sometimes fail to function perfectly. The remarkable fact is that they so often succeed so perfectly and that cardiorespiratory function is nearly normal within hours of the moment of birth.

The fetal lung contains liquid that in the normal state is the product of the lung itself. Its volume, estimated on the basis of studies in animals, is about 40 to 60 ml; its composition differs from amniotic liquid in being somewhat more acid (pH 6.43, compared with 7.07 of amniotic liquid), with a CO_2 level of 4.4 mEq per liter, compared with 18.4 mEq per liter of amniotic liquid. Fetal lung liquid contains acid mucopolysaccharides, mucoproteins, and surface-active lipoproteins, and it has a variable total protein content averaging 300 mg per cent.

Strang and colleagues in London have studied lung liquid formation in the fetal lamb with the aid of labeled molecules injected into the circulation or mixed with lung liquid. They found that macromolecules measuring up to 11 nm crossed lung capillary walls and appeared in lymph. Alveolar walls were impermeable to large polar molecules. No transfer of molecules larger than inulin moved from lung liquid to lymph. The authors deduced the presence of active ion transport of chloride and potassium from plasma to lung liquid. The chloride pump probably provides the distribution of molecules that produces the volume flow of lung liquid by osmotic forces and the negative electrical potential on the inner side of the pulmonary epithelium. Strang and his coworkers measured lung liquid secretion rate as 68.5 ml/24 hr/kg fetal weight. Little is known of the control of lung liquid formation except that epinephrine will inhibit tracheal efflux for as long as 24 hours after infusion. Since the effect is blocked by propanolol, it is assumed that it depends on β-adrenergic receptors.

Occasionally, there is admixture of the fetal lung liquid with amniotic liquid, presumably from gasping in utero. Squamous epithelial cells from the infant's skin have been identified in lungs of some infants who died weeks after birth from nonpulmonary causes. They are not regularly present in the lungs of all infants, however, and the weight of the evidence at hand suggests that the fetal lung, as well as the kidney, is the normal source of amniotic liquid rather than that the amniotic liquid is aspirated and distends the fetal lung. In the lamb, over 100 ml per day of lung liquid is produced. Fetal swallowing also occurs, on the average of 100 ml/kg/day.

Effects of lung liquid on lung growth have been studied in fetal lambs by tracheal ligation or tracheal drainage in utero at 105 to 110 days (term = 147 days). After 3 to 4 weeks of ligation, the lungs were large but relatively immature. The drained lungs were only half the expected size but had abundant Type II cells. (Alcorn et al., 1977).

The gaseous environment of the fetus is maintained by the placenta. Studies in monkeys with catheters placed in fetal vessels reveal the arterial oxygen saturation to be between 80 and 95 per cent, Po_2 between 30 and 40 mm of mercury, pH 7.37 to 7.40, and Pco_2 approximately 35 to 40 mm of mercury.

Measurements of capillary blood from the human fetal scalp during labor show a pH of approximately 7.30, standard bicarbonate of 19 mEq per liter, P_{CO_2} of 44 mm of mercury, and P_{O_2} of approximately 20 to 25 mm of mercury. It can be safely assumed that fetal arterial blood before labor would have a slightly higher pH and P_{O_2} and a lower P_{CO_2}. Sampling of fetal scalp blood, plus comparison with maternal capillary blood, has become a useful tool in the detection of stress in the fetus.

Fetal Breathing

Breathing is practiced by the fetus, but only about half the time, and then with rapid, irregular movements that do not shift more than a few milliliters of liquid along the tracheobronchial tree. Most breathing movements occur during active, or REM, sleep states. Fetal breathing is stimulated by maternal inhalation of carbon dioxide and, in the lamb at least, by adrenergic and cholinergic compounds and inhibitors of prostaglandin synthesis. Cessation of fetal breathing occurs with the onset of labor. It is depressed or absent during hypoxia and hypoglycemia and after maternal smoking. Tracheal fluid flow is negligible during periods of fetal breathing.

Deeper breaths, gasps, can be elicited by combined hypoxic and hypercarbic stimuli, but these are not sustained.

Indirect evidence supports the idea that fetal breathing is a prerequisite for normal lung growth. When phrenic innervation is absent or when there is high cervical cord transection, the lungs are hypoplastic.

One of the most puzzling problems concerns why sustained fetal respiratory movements are absent for periods of many hours and why the regular breathing on which life depends persists after birth. Although many explanations have been proposed (e.g., a fetal respiratory inhibitor that could arise from the placenta, endorphins, prostaglandins—or other substances available to the fetus but not the neonate—phasic changes in gas tensions when the lung instead of the placenta is the organ of gas exchange, postnatal increases in oxygenation) no single explanation is universally accepted.

The First Breath of Air

The introduction of air into the airless lung requires higher pressure than that needed at any other time of life. Actual measurements of the forces applied by the infant range from 10 to 70 cm of water for intervals lasting 0.5 to 1.0 second. The first expiration is usually associated with a positive pressure of 20 to 30 cm of water (Vyas et al., 1981). These pressures should be interpreted in the context of the 4 cm of water required on the average for normal breathing in the infant after the first few breaths, as in the adult.

The reason higher pressures are required at birth is the necessity to overcome the opposing forces of the viscosity of liquid in the airways (some 100 times that of air) and of surface tension, whose effect is maximal in the airways of smallest caliber. Associated with the introduction of the 50 or so milliliters of air that is usual with the first breath is the necessity that some of it, usually 20 to 30 ml, remain behind to establish the functional residual capacity. At the same time, the liquid that was in the air spaces must be removed. Some of it is aspirated from the oropharynx or expelled by the infant; most of it is removed by the pulmonary circulation, which increases manyfold at birth. The proteins in the lung liquid, and as much as one third of the total volume, are removed through the rich lymphatic network of the lung.

The stimuli that initiate breathing at birth are multiple. Uncertainty persists as to their relative importance. The changes in blood gases after interruption of the placental circulation are predictable, namely, a fall in oxygen tension and pH and a rise in P_{CO_2}. These changes at first stimulate respiration, although they can quickly become so profound as to depress it. Very low oxygen tensions suppress the responsiveness of the central nervous system, just as high CO_2 tensions can be narcotizing. Nonchemical stimuli, such as a change in temperature and tactile input, enhance "neuronal traffic" through the medulla and increase the discharge of the central respiratory neurons. It seems possible that added neural stimuli are associated with changes in the distribution of blood flow after the umbilical cord is clamped. In the exteriorized fetal animal, the most reliable stimulus to the initiation of breathing is clamping the cord. In the human, the first breath may precede clamping the cord, although interruption of the umbilical circulation in the course of delivery may have the same physiologic consequences.

Evaluation of the Newborn

The most widely used method of assessing the infant at one and five minutes of age is the Apgar score, introduced in 1950. Apgar assigned a figure of 0, 1, or 2 to five objective signs determined 1 minute after delivery, the sum constituting the infant's score. Thus (1) a heart rate of 100 to 140 rates a score of 2, no heart beat, of 0, less than 100, of 1; (2) respiratory effort is rated 2 if the infant breathes promptly and cries lustily, 0 if apneic or if only one or two gasps are made, and 1 for anything in between; (3) reflex irritability is rated 2 if good, 0 if there is no response to stimulation, 1 for anything between; (4) muscle tone is assigned 0 for flaccidity, 2 for good tone, 1 for intermediate tone or for hypertonus; and (5) color is rated 2 if the entire body is pink, 0 if all blue, 1 if anything between. In Apgar's own series, score of 0,

1, or 2 presaged a 14 per cent mortality, scores of 3, 4, 5, 6, or 7, 1.1 per cent, and those of 8, 9, and 10, 0.13 per cent. Apgar scoring has been universally accepted as a useful procedure. Its correlation with mortality in the first 28 days is greater with the 5-minute score than that obtained at 1 minute, and scoring at both times seems appropriate.

In a longitudinal study of 49,000 infants enrolled in a collaborative project undertaken by the National Institutes of Health and followed to age 7 years, little relationship was found between the score at 5 minutes and later cerebral palsy (Nelson and Ellenberg, 1981). Of those children with cerebral palsy, 73 per cent had a good score of 7 or over at 5 minutes of age. Of those children with very low scores (less than 3), who must have been the most depressed at birth,

80 per cent were free of any major handicap at age 7 years.

The major value of the score is to monitor perinatal events and designate infants most in need of immediate assistance.

A great variety of disorders cause the neonate to breathe with excessive effort. Some are listed in Table 11–1.

Frequency of Disorders of Respiration

The frequency of any given cause of respiratory distress will depend on the gestational age of the infant under consideration, the condition of the mother, and the environment. Table 11–1 lists some causes of respiratory distress.

The differential diagnosis of the many causes of dyspnea in the newborn infant appears throughout

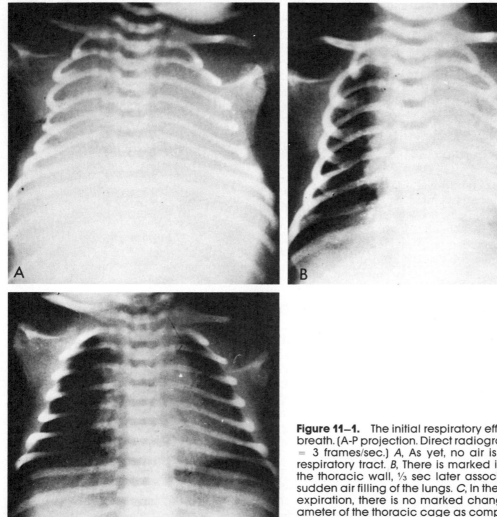

Figure 11–1. The initial respiratory effort of the first breath. (A-P projection. Direct radiography; speed = 3 frames/sec.) *A,* As yet, no air is seen in the respiratory tract. *B,* There is marked indrawing of the thoracic wall, ⅓ sec later associated with a sudden air filling of the lungs. *C,* In the subsequent expiration, there is no marked change in the diameter of the thoracic cage as compared to that illustrated in *A,* despite the good air filling of the lungs. (From Lind, J., Stern, L., and Wegelius, C.: The Human Foetal and Neonatal Circulation. Springfield, Ill., Charles C Thomas, 1964.)

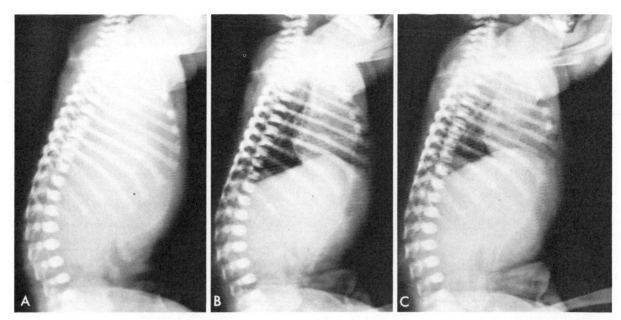

Figure 11–2. Lateral views of airways and lungs with the first breath. *A*, Air now outlines the entire oral cavity as well as the epipharynx and mesopharynx. *B*, The posterior portion of the tongue and the palate have moved dorsocephalad, and the tongue, palate, and posterior pharyngeal wall are in proximity. The hyoid has moved ventrad. The mandible is essentially unchanged in position. Increase in intrapharyngeal pressure is indicated by diminution of the retropharyngeal space. Air is present in the lung. *C*, The hyoid and mandible have moved slightly cephalad. The tongue, palate, and wall of the epipharynx are in tight closure. The posterior wall of the epipharynx is displaced farther ventrad than that of the mesopharynx. The lungs are well aerated, and the epigastrium is protruded. (From Bosma, J. F., Lind, J., and Gentz, N.: Motions of the pharynx of the newborn. Acta Paediatr. *48*:200, 1959.)

Table 11–1. Causes of Respiratory Distress

I. Obstruction of the airway
   A. Choanal atresia
   B. Congenital stridors
   C. Tracheal stenosis
   D. Bronchial stenosis
II. Lung parenchymal disease
   A. Aspiration syndromes
   B. Atelectasis
   C. Hyperinflation
   D. Pneumomediastinum and pneumothorax
   E. Idiopathic lobar emphysema
   F. Congenital pulmonary lymphangiectasis
   G. Wilson-Mikity syndrome
   H. Hyaline membrane disease
   I. Pneumonia
   J. Retained lung liquid (transient tachypnea of the newborn)

III. Nonpulmonary causes
   A. Heart failure
   B. Intracranial lesions
   C. Salicylism
   D. Metabolic acidosis
IV. Miscellaneous
   A. Pulmonary agenesis
   B. Disorders of the diaphragm and chest wall
   C. Tracheoesophageal fistula
   D. Pulmonary cysts
   E. Intrathoracic tumors and cysts
   F. Pulmonary sequestration
   G. Pleural effusions
   H. Pulmonary hemorrhage

the text. Some useful clues to diagnosis are included in Table 11–2.

Breathing Patterns

Irregularities in respiratory patterns occur in all newborn infants, increasingly so in the more premature ones. When the pattern is characterized by a ventilatory burst followed by an apneic pause of 5 to 15 seconds, repetitively, it is called "periodic breathing." More sporadic and prolonged apneic intervals are called "apneic spells." Breathing patterns are influenced greatly by state of consciousness; deep sleep is associated with reasonably regular patterns, rapid eye movement (REM) sleep by periodic breathing, and wakefulness by grossly irregular breathing associated with muscle movement, sucking, and crying. Inspiratory gasps are frequent, occasionally characterized by a second inspiration imposed on the first to achieve a doubling or more of tidal volume.

Some of the characteristics of periodic breathing may be summarized as follows:

1. Periods of apnea of 5 to 10 seconds; periods of ventilation of 10 to 15 seconds; average rate 30 to 40 per minute; rate during ventilatory interval 50 to 60 per minute.

2. It is most common in most premature infants, but it is rarely seen in first few days of life.

3. It is more common during REM sleep.

4. It persists intermittently until infants are about 36 weeks of gestational age, regardless of time of birth.

5. It is more common at altitude than at sea level.

6. It can be abolished with increased inspired oxygen and increased carbon dioxide.

7. Its net effect is slight hyperventilation.

8. An increase in lung volume tends to reduce its amount.

9. No significant changes in heart rate occur during the apneic interval.

10. No prognostic significance is associated with it.

Table 11–2. Clues to Diagnosis of Types of Respiratory Distress

Information from Maternal History	Most Likely Condition in Infant
Prematurity	Hyaline membrane disease
Diabetes	Hyaline membrane disease
Hemorrhage in the days before premature delivery	Hyaline membrane disease
Infection	Pneumonia
Premature rupture of membranes	Pneumonia
Prolonged labor	Pneumonia
Meconium-stained amniotic fluid	Meconium aspiration
Hydramnios	Tracheoesophageal fistula
Excessive medications	Central nervous system depression
Reserpine	Stuffy nose
Traumatic or breech delivery	Central nervous system hemorrhage
	Phrenic nerve paralysis
Fetal tachycardia or bradycardia	Asphyxia
Prolapsed cord or cord entanglements	Asphyxia
Postmaturity	Aspiration

Signs in the Baby	Most Likely Associated Condition
Single umbilical artery	Congenital anomalies
Other congenital anomalies	Associated cardiopulmonary anomalies
Scaphoid abdomen	Diaphragmatic hernia
Erb's palsy	Phrenic nerve palsy
Inability to breathe with mouth closed	Choanal atresia
	Stuffy nose
Gasping with little air exchange	Upper airway obstruction
Overdistention of lungs	Aspiration, lobar emphysema, or pneumothorax
Shift of apical pulse	Pneumothorax
	Chylothorax
	Hypoplastic lung
Fever or rise in temperature in a constant temperature environment	Pneumonia
Shrill cry, hypertonia, or flaccidity	Central nervous system disorder
Atonia	Trauma, myasthenia, poliomyelitis, amyotonia
Frothy blood from larynx	Pulmonary hemorrhage
Extension of head in the absence of neurologic findings	Laryngeal obstruction or vascular rings
Choking after feedings	Tracheoesophageal fistula or pharyngeal incoordination

(From Avery, M. E., Fletcher, B. D., and Williams, R. G.: The Lung and Its Disorders in the Newborn Infant. 4th ed. Philadelphia, W. B. Saunders Co., 1981.)

In contrast with periodic breathing, apneic spells are associated with other illnesses, such as sepsis, pneumonia, meningitis, hypoglycemia, and intracranial hemorrhage. They may also occur in very premature infants in the absence of recognized pathology. Much recent study has been directed toward understanding the etiology and evaluating the therapy of apneic spells, in part because they may carry a poor prognosis and sometimes, if unrecognized, can be fatal. The overrepresentation of low birth weight among infants who die suddenly and unexpectedly at several months of age further stimulates interest and study of apneic spells as observed in the nursery.

Infants likely to have apneic spells may be moderately depressed from other causes. Unlike most of those with periodic breathing, they can have some carbon dioxide retention, with Pa_{CO_2} of 40 to 60 mm Hg. Occasionally, periodic breathing may precede a series of apneic spells, and the same infants can, and often do, display both types of respiratory patterns.

Apneic spells may accompany other illness, such as sepsis or hypoglycemia, or can be associated with a number of conditions.

Factors associated with apneic spells:
1. Prematurity.
2. Hypoxia.
3. Active (REM) sleep.
4. Absence of core-skin temperature difference.
5. Upper airway obstruction.
6. Possible inadequate nutrition.
7. Gastroesophageal reflux.
8. Fatigue.

Factors that reduce the frequency of apneic spells:
1. Maturity.
2. Normoxia.
3. Quiet sleep or wakefulness.
4. Increased afferent input.
   (a) Presence of core-skin temperature difference.
   (b) Presence of cutaneous stimulation.
5. Increased lung volume.
6. Good nutrition.
7. Methylxanthines.

Extensive studies have helped delineate types of apnea. In general, it is thought of as obstructive or central or a combination of the two (mixed). Obstructive apnea can be demonstrated experimentally in infant animals who, after submersion, fail to institute or sustain respiratory efforts. In human infants, neck flexion can produce apnea without arousal. Sometimes, loss of electrical stimuli from brain can be associated with apnea that is only secondarily obstructive. Tonic and phasic activity of the genioglossus muscle established its role as a muscle of respiration that maintains patency of the airway at the level of the pharynx. One of the effects of arousal is activation of the genioglossus muscle, which pulls the tongue forward and opens the pharyngeal airway (Brouillette and Thach, 1980).

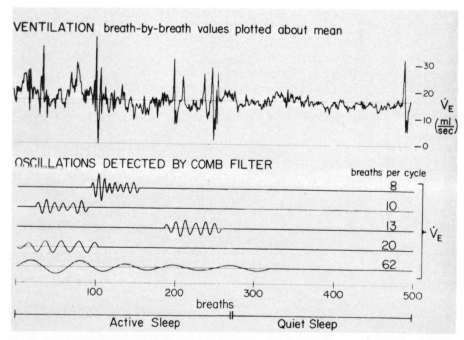

Figure 11–3. Instantaneous minute ventilation is shown in the top line during active and quiet sleep. Oscillations can be found in the patterns, which when of high amplitude result in apnea. (From Waggener, T., et al.: J. Appl. Physiol. *52*:1289, 1982).

Sleep state affects respiratory patterns. Most serious apneic spells occur during active, or rapid-eye-movement, sleep (see Table 11–3). During active sleep, spinal motoneuron reflexes are diminished, CO_2 responsiveness is depressed, and thoracic gas volume is reduced, as is arterial oxygen tension. The respiratory centers show more marked oscillation in infants prone to apneic spells, as if one aspect of immaturity is an underdamped respiratory control mechanism. Any increase in stimuli, such as rocking, recruiting more lung volume (and presumably stretch receptors), thermal stimuli, and stimulant drugs such as caffeine, will tend to stabilize the system and reduce the tendency for minute ventilation to demonstrate oscillations (Fig. 11–3).

The relationship between apneic spells in premature infants and sudden infant death syndrome (SIDS) remains unclear. Although premature infants are overrepresented among victims of SIDS, many infants with recurrent apneic spells do very well in later months and years, and not all victims of SIDS have had documented apneic spells. The finding of abnormalities in the pulmonary vessels of SIDS victims suggests many more had underventilated chronically or had had unnoticed apneic spells in the past.

Decreased ventilatory responses to hypoxia have been described among "near miss" victims as well as in some infants who subsequently became victims (Hunt et al., 1981).

Treatment. The experience with theophylline has been extensive ever since the first report of its efficiency in treating apneic spells in 1973 (Kuzemko and Paala, 1973). When a serum level is 10 to 15 mg/l, the frequency of apneic spells decreases, and the response to inspired carbon dioxide increases. Theophylline has other actions that might be useful in premature infants prone to apnea. For example, it increases the efficiency of diaphragmatic contractions, and it is also a well-known bronchodilator (Aubier et al., 1981).

The half-life of the drug differs sufficiently between infants that monitoring of blood levels is desirable.

At the very least, careful monitoring of heart rate is essential, since tachycardia is an early sign of toxicity.

The usual dose of caffeine citrate intravenously or orally is 10 to 20 mg/kg/dose one to three times daily. Sometimes, lower doses are adequate. As little as 2 mg/kg/day of theophylline has been found effective (Myers et al., 1980).

A reasonable approach to treatment of apneic spells in immature infants is as follows:

1. Search for and treat underlying disease.
2. Establish 0.5°C skin-core temperature gradient.
3. Place infant in prone position to increase oxygenation.
4. Keep arterial P_{O_2} in the 50 to 80 mm Hg range.
5. Rock the infant gently.
6. Administer theophylline 2 mg/kg/day to bring blood levels to 3 to 4 mg/liter. Alternately, caffeine citrate, 10 to 20 mg/kg/dose, can be given one to three times daily to bring blood levels to about 10 mg/liter. Dose can be monitored by heart rate. Do not repeat if heart rate is above baseline.
7. Provide continuous distending airway pressure or mechanical ventilation.

FAILURE OF AUTOMATIC CONTROL OF VENTILATION (ONDINE'S CURSE)

Some infants exhibit hypoventilation and cyanosis as a result of failure of the automatic control of ventilation. Described by Mellins and coworkers in 1970 as "Ondine's curse," this rare but very serious disorder has been recognized in the first hours of life. Hypotonia, apnea, and cyanosis responsive to stimulation are the usual symptoms in these infants who initially have normal heart and lungs. After time, the recurrent episodic hypoxia results in pulmonary vascular changes and right heart failure.

The cause of this condition is not known. It can be described as defective integration of ventilatory stimuli during sleep. Characteristically, rhythmic respiration is normal in the awake state. The hypoxic drive during hypoventilation keeps the infants alive for at least some months. Since the pulmonary vascular changes are so serious, most infants in whom this condition has been recognized have been tracheostomized and maintained on ventilators during sleep (Guilleminault et al., 1982).

Table 11–3. Number of Apneic Spells of Different Durations in Relation to Different Sleep States*,†

| Sleep state | Apneic spells (N) | | | | $\dfrac{\text{Actual}}{\text{Estimated}}$ – ratio of a.sp. | Records (N) |
	Total	<20 sec	20–39 sec	≥40 sec		
AS	390	294	74	22	1.29 ± 0.17 S.D.	19
QS	29	25	4	—	0.42 ± 0.22 S.D.	11
UDS	74	51	13	10	1.03 ± 0.46 S.D.	15

* Data of Gabriel et al., 1976.
† Abbreviations: AS, active sleep; QS, quiet sleep; UDS, undifferentiated sleep; a.sp., apneic spell.
(From Schulte, F. J.: In Human Growth. Vol. 3. Falkner, F., and Tanner, J. M. [Eds]: New York, Plenum Publishing Corp., 1979.)

SIDS remains one of the most threatening of events for all parents, but especially for those of infants born prematurely. The overall risk in the United States is about 2.0/1000 live births. Orientals have the lowest reported risk (0.5/1000), and others in a lower socioeconomic class have a higher risk. This latter observation is difficult to interpret if the population is considered according to ethnic group, since poor blacks are at risk with a rate of 5/1000. In Tasmania, the rate among the Maori is twice that of whites (Grice and McGlashan, 1978). In their 1975 attempt to isolate risk by race as compared with social class, McWeeney and Emery failed to find an association between class and SIDS.

General agreement among epidemiologists exists for the association between SIDS and the following factors:

1. Mothers less than 20 years old, unmarried and poor.
2. Short interpregnancy interval.
3. Previous fetal loss.
4. Cigarette smoking.
5. Methadone addiction.
6. Preterm birth.
7. Low birth weight for gestational age.
8. Second or third in birth order.
9. Multiple pregnancy.
10. Gender of infant is male (males are affected more frequently than females).
11. Sibling with SIDS (some families have had three or more infants with SIDS).

This latter association is, of course, very alarming to parents of victims. The risk is about 2 per cent in subsequent siblings and 4 per cent in a surviving twin (Shannon and Kelly, 1981).

Among the findings at autopsy that may relate to pathogenesis are an abnormal peripheral extension of smooth muscle in the pulmonary arteries, astrogliosis of the brain stem, and a decrease in myelinated fibers in the vagus nerve. These findings support the concept that recurrent or chronic hypoxia may have been present. If the infant is relatively less responsive to irritant receptors in the airways, for example, afferent input to the respiratory centers in the brain stem may decrease output to the genioglossus and other muscles whose tonic contraction is essential to upper airway patency. At least it is known that after death, relaxation of upper airway muscles leads to passive occlusion (Wilson et al., 1980).

By definition of sudden and unexpected death, studies during life cannot be carried out. However, some of the infants have apneic spells from which they are successfully resuscitated, which are considered "near miss" sudden infant deaths (NSID). Since a few such infants have had another "spell" from which they could not be resuscitated, the group as a whole may reasonably be considered at risk of SIDS or near miss SIDS.

Physiologic studies support some of the morphologic ones that suggest recurrent or chronic hypoventilation and may be central to the pathogenesis of SIDS. Shannon and colleagues (1977) found diminished ventilatory responsiveness to 5 per cent CO_2 in inspired air, and Hunt and coworkers (1981) found a diminished response to inhalation of 15 per cent oxygen. A number of individuals have focused on the possibility of abnormalities in the respiratory pattern and control. The observation that death usually occurs quietly during the night, especially in winter months, in infants between 1 and 4 months of age suggests that some aspect of the development of respiratory control during that age is unstable. It is known that the skeletal muscle changes associated with active sleep can promote relaxation of the upper airway muscles, with the possibility of obstruction. Why this is less common in the first month of life than between 1 and 4 months remains a mystery.

Although many longitudinal recordings of respiratory patterns and heart rate have been made and some statistical differences have been demonstrated between the infants who have been resuscitated from a near-SID event and those who are normal, no single measurement made during life has been found to be predictive of subsequent sudden death.

It is not surprising that a problem of such severe and tragic consequences has prompted innumerable investigations and the generation of a large number of hypotheses with respect to etiology. It seems probable that there may be a number of events such as nasopharyngitis, gastric reflux, aspiration, and so forth that can trigger profound apnea with failure to respond in some infants. It seems quite clear that no single event accounts for all episodes of sudden death. Rather, one is left with the feeling that some infants have a vulnerable respiratory control mechanism that, on some occasions, is unresponsive to the usual arousal stimuli.

Diagnosis and Treatment. By definition, if the fatality is sudden and unexpected there can be no treatment. However, there is an ever-growing group of infants labeled "near-SIDS," and that group has become the subject of extensive investigation and evaluation of different approaches to management. Another group that can be identified from epidemiologic factors consists of those infants born prematurely with chronic pulmonary disease (Werthammer et al., 1981) and infants of methadone-addicted mothers, as well as siblings of victims. In all these circumstances, it seems appropriate to evaluate the given infant, both to learn more about the risk factors that can be assessed during life and to ascertain whether it seems appropriate in a given circumstance to advocate monitoring during sleep.

No uniformity of opinion exists on these matters, but many advocate the careful evaluation of each such infant. For example, infants who have had prolonged intubation may have some partial upper airway obstruction that could worsen during sleep. Others may have aberrant vessels that could compress the trachea and further compromise an airway. Those who do not hyperventilate appropriately with added ventilatory loads or who show CO_2 retention during sleep can be treated with stimulants. Some advise the use of a pH probe in the lower esophagus to see whether acid reflux is present. If so, some advocate gastric plication.

Theophylline. Theophylline has come into wide use as a means of lessening the frequency and duration of apneic spells and periodic breathing. First used extensively in preterm infants, it is now recommended for infants who at a later age continue to have episodic apneic spells. The maintenance of a theophylline blood level of 10 to 15 mg/l has been tolerated well by infants so treated, and has been associated with fewer spells. The mechanism of action of theophylline is probably complex, but it includes an increase in responsiveness of the respiratory centers to elevations in arterial CO_2. It also apparently improves the efficiency of diaphragmatic contraction and has well-known effects as a bronchodilator. All these mechanisms are beneficial, depending on the relative contribution of the several likely pathogenetic events.

Monitors. The use of monitors of heart rate or ventilatory rate have become widely accepted for some infants who are viewed as high-risk SIDS candidates. Home monitoring is not without its own problems, but these can be lessened if a program is worked out with the appropriate support personnel from both medical and psychosocial backgrounds. Currently, impedance monitoring is most widely used in the home. An alarm is usually set on a 20-second delay, so that it will sound if no ventilatory effort is recorded during that period. The problem is that with obstructive apnea there may be continued respiratory effort, and cardiac monitoring therefore makes sense. A fall in heart rate to less than 100 can be used to trigger the alarm.

Summary. There is no documentation to date that either theophylline or monitoring of any sort will eliminate some episodes of SIDS. Both interventions seem rational when risks are known to be high and parental anxiety great.

REFERENCES

Adams, F. H.: Functional development of the fetal lung. J. Pediatr. *68*:794, 1966.

Alcorn, D., Adamson, T. M., Lambert, T. F., et al.: Morphological effects of chronic tracheal ligation and drainage in fetal lamb lung. J. Anat. *123*:649, 1977.

Apgar, V.: A proposal for a new method of evaluation of the newborn infant. Anesth. Analg. *32*:260, 1953.

Apgar, V., Holaday, D. A., James, L. S., et al.: Evaluation of the newborn infant—Second report. J.A.M.A. *168*:1985, 1958.

Aubier, M., De Troyer, A., Sampson, M., et al.: Aminophylline improves diaphragmatic contractility. N. Engl. J. Med. *305*:249, 1981.

Avery, M. E., Chernick, V., and Young, M.: Fetal respiratory movements in response to rapid changes of CO_2 in the carotid artery. J. Appl. Physiol. *20*:225, 1965.

Avery, M. E., Fletcher, B. D., and Williams, R. G.: The Lung and Its Disorders in the Newborn Infant. 4th ed. Philadelphia, W. B. Saunders Co., 1981.

Band, D. M., Cameron, I. R., and Semple, S. J. G.: Effects of different methods of CO_2 administration on oscillations of arterial pH in the cat. J. Appl. Physiol. *26*:268, 1969.

Bland, R. D., McMillan, D. D., Bressack, M. A., and Dong, L.: Clearance of liquid from lungs of newborn rabbits. J. Appl. Physiol. *49*:171, 1980.

Barcroft, J.: Fetal circulation and respiration. Physiol. Rev. *16*:103, 1936.

Barcroft, J., and Barron, D. H.: The genesis of respiratory movements in the foetus of the sheep. Physiology *88*:56, 1936–7.

Brouillette, R. T., and Thach, B. T.: Control of genioglossus muscle inspiratory activity. J. Appl. Physiol. *49*:801, 1980.

Brown, E. R., Lawson, E. E., Jansen, A., Russell, B., Chernick, V., and Taeusch, H. W.: Regular fetal breathing induced by pilocarpine infusion in the near term fetal lamb, J. Appl. Physiol. *50*:1348, 1981.

Burns, B. D.: The central control of respiratory movements. Br. Med. Bull. *19*:7, 1963.

Chernick, V., Heldrich, F., and Avery, M. E.: Periodic breathing of premature infants. J. Pediatr. *64*:330, 1964.

Daily, W. J. R., Klaus, M., and Meyer, H. B.: Apnea in premature infants. Monitoring incidence, heart rate changes, and an effect of environmental temperature. Pediatrics *43*:510, 1969.

Dawes, G. S., Fox, H. E., Leduc, B. M., et al.: Respiratory movements and rapid eye movement sleep in the foetal lamb. J. Physiol. *220*:119, 1972.

DeReuck, A. V. S., and Porter, R. (Eds): Development of the Lung. Ciba Foundation Symposium. London, J. & A. Churchill, Ltd., 1967.

Drage, J. S., Kennedy, C., and Schwarz, B. K.: The Apgar Score as an index of neonatal mortality. A report from the Collaborative Study of Cerebral Palsy. Obstet. Gynecol. *24*:222, 1964.

Farber, S., and Sweet, L. K.: Amniotic sac contents in lungs of infants. Am. J. Dis. Child. *42*:1372, 1931.

Fenner, A., Schalk, U., Hoenicke, H., et al.: Periodic breathing in premature and neonatal babies. Pediatr. Res. *7*:174, 1973.

Fewell, J. E., Lee, C. C., and Kitterman, J. A.: Effects of phrenic nerve section on the respiratory system of fetal lambs. J. Appl. Physiol. *51*:293, 1981.

Fleming, B. J., Bryan, A. C., and Bryan, M. H.: Functional immaturity of pulmonary irritant receptors and apnea in newborn preterm infants. Pediatrics *61*:515, 1978.

Gabriel, M., Albani, M., and Schulte, F. J.: Apneic spells and sleep states in preterm infants. Pediatrics *57*:142, 1976.

Grice, A. C., and McGlashan, N. D.: Sudden death in infancy in Tasmania. Med. J. Aust. *2*:177, 1978.

Guilleminault, C., McQuitty, J., Ariagno, R. L., et al.: Congenital central alveolar ventilation syndrome in six infants. Pediatrics *70*:684, 1982.

Guilleminault, C., Peraita, R., Soquet, M., and Dement, W. C.: Apneas during sleep in infants: possible relationship with sudden infant death syndrome. Science *190*:677, 1975.

Henderson-Smart, D., Pettigrew, A., and Campbell, D.: Clinical apnea and brain-stem neural function in preterm infants. N. Engl. J. Med. *308*:353, 1983.

Hoppenbrouwers, T., Hodgman, T. E., Arakawa, K., et al.: Respiration during the first six months of life in normal infants. III. Computer identification of breathing pauses. Pediatr. Res. *13*:1230, 1980.

Hunt, C. E., McCullock, K., and Brouillette, R. T.: Diminished hypoxic ventilatory responses in near-miss sudden infant death syndrome. J. Appl. Physiol. *50*:1313, 1981.

Jansen, A. H., and Chernick, V.: Cardiorespiratory response to central cyanide in fetal sheep. J. Appl. Physiol. *37*:18, 1974.

Karlberg, P.: The adaptive changes in the immediate postnatal period, with particular reference to respiration. J. Pediatr. *56*:585, 1960.

Kitterman, J. A., Liggins, G. C., and Campos, G. A.: Prepartum maturation of the lung in fetal sheep: relation to cortisol. J. Appl. Physiol. *51*:384, 1981.

Kitterman, J. A., Liggins, G. C., Clements, J. A., and Tooley, W. H.: Stimulation of breathing movements in fetal sheep by inhibitors of prostaglandin synthesis. J. Develop. Physiol. *1*:452, 1979.

Korner, A. F., Guilleminault, C., Hoed, J. V., and Baldwin, R. B.: Reduction of sleep apnea and bradycardia in preterm infants on oscillating water beds: a controlled polygraphic study. Pediatrics *61*:528, 1978.

Kuzemko, J. A., and Paala, J.: Apnoeic attacks in the newborn treated with aminophylline. Arch. Dis. Child *48*:404, 1973.

Lawson, E. E., Brown, E. R., Torday, J. S., et al.: The effect of epinephrine on tracheal fluid flow and surfactant efflux in fetal sheep. Am. Rev. Resp. Dis. *118*:1023, 1978.

Lewak, N., van den Berg, B. J., and Beckwith, J. B.: Sudden infant death syndrome risk factors. Prospective data review. Clin. Pediatr. *18*:404, 1979.

McWeeney, P. M., and Emery, J. L.: Unexpected post-neonatal deaths (cot deaths) due to recognizable disease. Arch. Dis. Child. *80*:191, 1975.

Mellins, R. B., Balfour, H. H., Turino, G. M., et al.: Failure of automatic control of ventilation (Ondine's curse). Medicine *49*:487, 1970.

Miller, H. C., Behrle, F. C., and Snull, N. W.: Apnea and irregular respiratory rhythms among premature infants. Pediatrics *23*:676, 1959.

Myers, T. F., Milsap, R. L., Krauss, A. N., et al.: Low-dose theophylline therapy in idiopathic apnea of prematurity. J. Pediatr. *96*:99, 1980.

Naeye, R. L.: Pulmonary arterial abnormalities in the sudden infant death syndrome. N. Engl. J. Med. *289*:1167, 1973.

Naeye, R. L., Whalen, P., Ryser, M., and Fisher, R.: Cardiac and other abnormalities in the sudden infant death syndrome. Am. J. Pathol. *82*:1, 1976.

Nelson, K. B., and Ellenberg, J. H.: Apgar scores as predictors of chronic neurologic disability. Pediatrics *68*:36, 1981.

Oliver, T. K. (Ed.): Neonatal Respiratory Adaptation. Bethesda, Md., U.S. Department of Health, Education, and Welfare, 1964.

Olver, R. E., and Strang, L. B.: Ion fluxes across the pulmonary epithelium and secretion of lung liquid in the foetal lamb. J. Physiol. *241*:327, 1974.

Perlstein, P. H., Edwards, N. K., and Sutherland, J. M.: Apnea in premature infants and incubator-air-temperature changes. N. Engl. J. Med. *282*:461, 1970.

Phillipson, E. A.: Control of breathing during sleep. Am. Rev. Resp. Dis. *118*:909, 1978.

Phillipson, E. A., Bowes, G., Townsend, E. R., Duffin, J., and Cooper, J. D.: Carotid chemoreceptors in ventilatory responses to changes in venous CO_2 load. J. Appl. Physiol. *51*:1398, 1981.

Phillipson, E. A., Duffin, J., and Cooper, J. D.: Critical dependence of respiratory rhythmicity on metabolic CO_2 load. J. Appl. Physiol. *50*:45, 1981.

Rigatto, H., and Brady, J. P.: Periodic breathing and apnea in preterm infant. I. Evidence for hypoventilation possibly due to central respiratory depression. Pediatrics *50*:202, 1972.

Rigatto, H., Verdazco, R., and Cates, D. B.: Effects of O_2 on the ventilatory response to CO_2 in preterm infants. J. Appl. Physiol. *39*:896, 1975.

Sachis, P. N., Armstrong, D. L., Becker, I. E., and Bryan, A. C.: The vagus nerve and sudden infant death syndrome: a morphometric study. J. Pediatr. *98*:278, 1981.

Saunders, R. A., and Milner, A. D.: Pulmonary pressure/volume relationships during the last phase of delivery and the first postnatal breaths in human subjects. J. Pediatr. *93*:667, 1978.

Scarpelli, E. M., and Auld, P. A. M.: Pulmonary Physiology of the Fetus, Newborn, and Child. Philadelphia, Lea and Febiger, 1975.

Schulte, F. J.: Developmental aspects of the neuronal control of breathing. *In* Falkner, F., and Tanner, J. M. (Eds.): Human Growth. Vol. 3. New York, Plenum Publishing Corp., 1979.

Shannon, D. C., Gotay, F., Stein, I. M., et al.: Prevention of apnea and bradycardia in low-birth-weight infants. Pediatrics *55*:589, 1975.

Shannon, D. C., Kelly, D. H., and O'Connell, K.: Impaired regulation of alveolar ventilation and sudden infant death syndrome. Science *197*:367, 1977.

Shannon, D. C., Kelly, D. H., and O'Connell, K.: Abnormal regulation of ventilation in infants at risk of sudden infant death syndrome. N. Engl. J. Med. *297*:747, 1977.

Shannon, D. C., and Kelly, D. H.: SIDS and near SIDS. N. Engl. J. Med. *306*:959, 1982.

Stark, A. R., and Thach, B. T.: Recovery of airway patency after obstruction in normal infants. Am. Rev. Resp. Dis. *123*:961, 1981.

Stein, I. M., White, A., Kennedy, J. L., et al.: Apnea recordings of healthy infants at 40, 44, and 52 weeks post conception. Pediatrics *63*:724, 1979.

Strang, L. B.: The lungs at birth. Arch. Dis. Child. *40*:575, 1965.

Strang, L. B.: Uptake of liquid from the lungs at the start of breathing. *In* De Reuck, A. V. S., and Porter, R. (Eds.): Development of the Lung. Ciba Foundation Symposium. London, J. & A. Churchill, 1967.

Strang, L. B.: Pulmonary circulation at birth. *In* Neonatal Respiration. Physiological and Clinical Studies. Oxford, Blackwell Scientific Publications, 1977.

Sultan, C., Migeon, B. R., Rothwell, S. W., et al.: Androgen receptors and metabolism in cultured human fetal fibroblasts. Pediatr. Res. *13*:67, 1980.

Thach, B. T., and Stark, A. R.: Spontaneous neck flexion and airway obstruction during apneic spells in preterm infants. J. Pediatr. *94*:275, 1979.

Thach, B. T., and Taeusch, H. W.: Sighing in newborn human infants: role of inflation augmenting reflex. J. Appl. Physiol. *41*:502, 1976.

Valdes-Dapena, M. A.: Sudden infant death syndrome. A review of the medical literature 1974–79. Pediatrics *66*:597, 1980.

Vyas, H., Miller, A. D., and Hopkin, I. E.: Intrathoracic pressure and volume changes during the spontaneous onset of respiration in babies born by cesarean section and by vaginal delivery. J. Pediatr. *99*:787, 1981.

Waggener, T. B., Frantz, I. D., Stark, A. R., and Kronauer, R. E.: Oscillatory breathing patterns leading to apneic spells in infants. J. Appl. Physiol. *52*:1288, 1982.

Werthammer, J., Brown, E. R., Neff, R., and Taeusch, H. W., Jr.: Sudden infant death syndrome (SIDS) in infants with bronchopulmonary dysplasia. Pediatrics *69*:301, 1982.

Williams, A., Vawter, G., and Reid, L.: Increased muscularity of the pulmonary circulation in victims of sudden infant death syndrome. Pediatrics *63*:18, 1979.

Wilson, S. L., Thach, B. T., Brouillette, R. T., and Abu-Osba, Y. K.: Upper airway patency in the human infant: influence of airway pressure and posture. J. Appl. Physiol. *48*:500, 1980.

Yamamoto, W. S., and Edwards, M. W., Jr.: Homeostasis of carbon dioxide during intravenous infusion of carbon dioxide. J. Appl. Physiol. *15*:807, 1960.

12

Nasal Obstructions

Nasal obstruction in a newborn infant can be a very serious, even life-threatening, event if not recognized as a cause of marked difficulty breathing. Complete obstruction demands the establishment of an alternate airway with urgency. Once the oral airway is in place, careful inspection of the nares and nasopharynx can be undertaken to establish the cause of obstruction.

Choanal atresia is the most common cause of total nasal obstruction. The obstructing element is most commonly a bony plate $\frac{1}{8}$ to $\frac{1}{4}$ inch thick, but it may be only a thin membrane. Obstruction may be unilateral and partial or bilateral and complete. Symptomatology varies considerably in these two varieties. Associated congenital defects include Treacher Collins syndrome, palatal abnormalities, colobomas, tracheoesophageal fistula, and congenital heart disease, according to the series of Flake and Ferguson.

Hall noted small ears in 13 of 17 infants with choanal atresia and some degree of mental retardation in 11 of them. Although some authors have reported a female preponderance, others have not found a difference in incidence between sexes. The estimated frequency of 1 in every 8000 births may be low, since unilateral lesions may be unrecognized.

Etiology and Pathogenesis. The familial tendency to choanal atresia is evident in most large series reported, including McGovern's cases as well as those of Phelps. The inheritance pattern appears multifactorial, hence, the risk to siblings would be less than 5 per cent.

The mouth and nares develop from invaginations that deepen caudad in the embryonic head, while the primitive foregut and its offshoot, the trachea, grow cephalad. Normally, these canals meet in the region of the pharynx and fuse into the widely patent foodway and airway. Rarely, the embryologic septum separating nares from foregut fails to disappear, leaving the foodway intact but the airway obstructed. The septum may remain membranous, but commonly it becomes converted into bone.

Diagnosis

Bilateral Choanal Atresia. Symptoms may or may not be manifest immediately after birth. Two of our four infants cried and breathed within seconds after delivery, but one was described as "limp and cyanotic at birth," while another did not breathe immediately or well and was said to have become "full of mucus" very shortly. All had breathing difficulty within a few hours. In some this was episodic and associated with attempts to feed; in others, it was constant.

The diagnosis is suspected when an infant has marked retractions and is mouth-breathing. If the nostrils are occluded, no adverse effect is noted; if the mouth is occluded, the infant may struggle and become cyanotic and limp. The inability to pass a feeding tube through the nostril suggests the diagnosis. Direct inspection of the nares with an otoscope allows definitive diagnosis of obstruction. A few drops of methylene blue may be instilled into the nostril; if the dye enters the pharynx, choanal atresia is not present. Failure of the dye to penetrate to the pharynx could be due to edema as well as choanal atresia. A CT scan will permit delineation of the extent of obstruction (Fig. 12–1).

Unilateral Choanal Atresia. When congenital obstruction is limited to one side, which is the case in about 20 per cent of infants, the diagnosis is seldom made in the neonatal period. In four cases with which we are acquainted, the diagnosis was not made until the ages of 3, 6, 10, and 38 years. In all these cases, the retrospective story was that of inability to breathe through one side of the nose since birth, unilateral nasal discharge, and frequently recurrent upper respiratory tract infections.

Other forms of nasal obstruction, usually partial, may be associated with other craniofacial anomalies, as in Crouzon's or Apert's syndrome or with the Treacher Collins malformation. These infants may have intermittent obstruction in association with upper respiratory tract infections. The diagnosis is made on direct inspection of the choanae with an otoscope.

Treatment. Once the presence of nasal obstruction is established and an oral airway is in place, the infant still requires meticulous nursing care. For example, the infant must be gavage-fed as long as there is an oral airway or until a satisfactory nasal airway is established.

The treatment of choice for membranous obstructions, or those with less than a millimeter of bone, is transnasal resection with the CO_2 laser. This technique, pioneered by Healy, has been successful in more than 20 patients, some of whom were less than 24 hours of age. When the bony plate is thicker, it can be perforated with the laser, but it should be excised with a microrongeur. (The laser beam results in overheating the bone with possible sequestration and scarring.)

If the laser technique is not available or if the obstructing bone is too thick for transnasal excision, definitive surgical repair should be undertaken when the infant is a few weeks old. There will be the need for stenting of the air passages with plastic tubes for some weeks thereafter, so throughout that period continuous, meticulous attention to maintenance of the oral airway as well as nutrition through gavage feeding is required.

We should note that the early definitive repair represents a change in philosphy from that of a decade ago, when many infants were allowed to wait 12 to 18 months for further growth of the nose before the definitive repair was undertaken. The earlier operation clearly is a difficult one but is associated with excellent results in experienced hands. Skilled nursing care is essential.

CASE 12–1

A 3300-gm female was noted to have slight cyanosis after delivery by cesarean section. She was resuscitated by suctioning and placed in an incubator. The baby continued to have difficulty breathing, which was initially attributed to nasal congestion. When feeding was first attempted, the baby became cyanotic with increasing sternal retraction. After cessation of feeding, an oral airway was inserted and secured to the cheeks with tape. This relieved the respiratory distress. The child was transferred to Children's Hospital Medical Center, oral airway in place, and a diagnosis of possible bilateral choanal atresia was made.

The choanal atresia was confirmed by failure to pass a No. 6 French catheter through the nasal cavity into the oropharynx. Excellent visualization of the atresia plate was achieved by means of an otoscope. The atresia plate was palpated by a No. 20 suction tip, and a bilateral bony atresia was confirmed.

The oral airway was kept in place and gavage feedings continued. Detailed physical examination failed to reveal any additional congenital anomaly.

On the fifth day of life, the baby was taken to the operating room, and a microsurgical resection of the bilateral choanal atresia was performed with a CO$_2$

laser. A 3.00 mm polyvinyl tubing stent was placed in each nostril to keep the newly crested choanal opening patent. Oral feedings were possible on the first postoperative day, and the baby did not experience any respiratory difficulty. The parents were instructed in the use of nasal suctioning to keep the stent tube open, and the baby was discharged on the sixth postoperative day.

The baby did well with normal feeding and gained weight. The stents were removed 4 weeks postoperatively. At age 3 months, the infant developed increasing nasal secretions and required more frequent nasal suctioning. After admission to hospital, examination revealed stenosis of both choanal openings that required dilatation and reinsertion of nasal stent under general anesthesia. The stents were removed after 3 weeks with resumption of normal nasal respiration. At 6 and 9 months, the choanal openings required dilatation without stenting. The child is now 3 years of age, and both openings are patent with normal nasal function.

REFERENCES

Cohen, H. J., and Witchell, I. S.: Bilateral congenital choanal atresia in newborn. A.M.A. Am. J. Dis. Child. *83*:328, 1952.

Fearon, B., and Dickson, J.: Bilateral choanal atresia in the newborn. Plan of action. Laryngoscope 9:1487, 1968.

Ferguson, C. F., and Kendig, E. L.: Pediatric Otolaryngology, 2nd ed. Philadelphia, W. B. Saunders Co., 1972, pp. 1002–1112.

Flake, C. G., and Ferguson, C. E.: Congenital choanal atresia in infants and children. Ann. Otol. Rhinol. Laryngol. *73*:458, 1964.

Grahne, B., and Kaltiokallio, K.: Congenital choanal atresia and its heredity. Acta Otolaryngol. *62*:193, 1966.

Hall, B. D.: Choanal atresia and associated multiple anomalies. J. Pediatr. *95*:395, 1979.

Healy, G., McGill, T., Jako, G. J., Strong, M. S., and Vaughan, C. W.: Management of choanal atresia with the carbon dioxide laser. Ann. Otol. Rhinol. Laryngol. *87*:658, 1978.

McGovern, F. H.: Congenital choanal atresia. Laryngoscope *60*:815, 1950.

Phelps, K. A.: Congenital occlusion of choanae. Ann. Otol. Rhinol. Laryngol. *35*:143, 1926.

Strome, M.: Differential Diagnosis in Pediatric Otolaryngology. Boston, Little, Brown and Co., 1975.

13

Stridors in the Newborn

The term stridor is used to include all cases in which a stridulous or crowing noise is made from birth or begins within a few weeks after birth. Stridor is produced when the glottis or trachea is narrowed or deformed, when neighboring structures intrude upon the glottic opening or trachea, or when the vocal cords move abnormally. The primary cause may lie within or near the larynx, within the chest, or within the central nervous system. A suggested system of classification is outlined in Table 13–1.

Simple Congenital Laryngeal Stridor

We use this term to designate those instances of stridor in which, because of various clinical characteristics, no serious laryngeal or extralaryngeal lesions are suspected, or in which, if studies are performed, only minor alterations in laryngeal structure or function are discovered.

Incidence. The condition is common. Holinger and associates were able to report on 305 cases gathered in a period of 7 years. Every pediatrician encounters one every few months in the course of a practice of average size.

Etiology. There is no complete unanimity of opinion as to the cause of simple congenital stridor. Laryngoscopy generally reveals a larynx that is softer than usual, which collapses abnormally with inspiration. At times, the epiglottis seems at fault, being overlong, curved, even tube-shaped, and drawn into the glottic opening with the indrawn breath. At other times, the arytenoids may be loose and flabby or the aryepiglottic folds redundant, and these tissues may sag into the glottis with inspiration. For these reasons, the disorder has also been called "laryngomalacia," "congenital flaccid larynx," and "inspiratory laryngeal collapse."

The condition occurs in males twice as often as in females. It may be associated with pectus excavatum.

Diagnosis. The onset of noisy respiration is commonly stated to be noted at birth or shortly thereafter. In our experience, stridor is rarely heard in the newborn nursery, and, when it is heard that early in life, it is more likely to be one of the more serious varieties

of the disorder. Simple stridor is usually brought to the attention of the pediatrician at the first monthly checkup, not too infrequently at the second, and, occasionally, as late as four months. The noise is unlike the pharyngeal moist snore. It may at times have the quality of a dry, high-pitched crowing inspiration, though more often it is lower pitched and vibratory or fluttering. The noise is generally confined to the inspiratory phase, but rarely, in severe examples, expiration may also be noisy.

These points are of importance in distinguishing simple stridor from the more serious varieties. Phonation is unimpaired; voice and cry are strong. It is commonly intermittent rather than constant, increasing with excitement and physical activity, diminishing and often disappearing when the infant is at complete rest. It is altered by change of position, being intensified when the infant is supine, ameliorated when prone. Most important of all, although the parents are greatly disturbed by the extraordinarily noisy breathing, the infant himself seems not bothered by it at all. His color remains good, his appetite unimpaired, and, usually, his weight curve rises steadily. Occasionally, feeding difficulties are sufficient to slow weight gain. This is true in spite of the observation that during the periods in which stridor is at its height, there is usually retraction with inspiration of the suprasternal notch and intercostal spaces and even of the sternum itself. This type of stridor has been convincingly demonstrated radiographically by Dunbar. With the infant in the supine position, horizontal beam lateral views of the neck are made with high-speed cinerecording. When stridor is present, antero-inferior displacement and vibration of the aryepiglottic folds can be seen on inspiration.

Prognosis. Simple congenital stridor usually disappears between 6 and 18 months. It may last longer. The disorder does not carry with it any strong predilection for either upper or lower respiratory tract infections.

Treatment. No specific treatment is required or indicated. The appearance of stridor within the first month or so demands a leisurely detailed discussion of the problem with the parents. It must be explained that most of these infants suffer from no great abnormality but that a few of them do. If the child fails to feed properly, if weight does not rise satisfactorily, if his color becomes poor either constantly or in attacks, if his voice does not remain strong, or if he appears restless or unhappy, studies should then be made to rule out more serious causes of stridor. Some parents will prefer that such studies be made immediately; these include radiographs of neck and chest with cinefluoroscopy. Direct laryngoscopy will confirm the diagnosis.

Congenital Laryngeal and Tracheal Stenoses

Under this all-inclusive term are grouped the various anatomic lesions in the glottis and subglottic areas that may produce stridor at or shortly after birth. They are thrown into this heterogeneous group because the pediatrician cannot hope to differentiate one from the other by simple physical examination owing to the similarity of their symptoms and signs. Differentiation and therapy lie in the domain of the otolaryngologist. The pediatrician should, however, be aware of the various possibilities.

Nabarro has reported a remarkable instance of stridor from birth in which there was extensive calcification of laryngeal and tracheal cartilages.

LARYNGEAL WEBS

Webs are usually glottic in location; that is, they obstruct at the level of the true vocal cords, but they may be supraglottic or subglottic. They may be small, connecting only the anterior ends of the cords, or they may cover the entire glottic chink. In the first instance, symptoms may be lacking; in the second, respiratory difficulty is great.

Etiology. Webs arise in the seventh to tenth week of gestation. At this time, the larynx is developing from the floor of the pharynx and from outgrowths of the third, fourth, and fifth branchial arches, around the stem of the trachea. Like many other embryologic lumens, the stoma that originally opens from the floor of the pharynx into the trachea becomes fused by epithelial ingrowth. After a few weeks, this obliteration is dissolved and the lumen is re-established. Incomplete recanalization of the primitive laryngeal airway results in web formation.

Incidence. Laryngeal webs are well recognized. Holinger has reported 32 in a series of 866 patients with laryngeal abnormalities; however, his experience is that of a laryngologist to whom those patients were referred. A pediatrician rarely sees one, since they occur approximately once in 10,000 births.

Diagnosis. Symptoms are usually present at birth, and the degree of symptomatology depends upon the extent of the web. If it is complete, a few gasps may occur before death. If it is partial, in addition to the stridor the cry will be weak or hoarse, and respirations will be labored. Definitive diagnosis depends on direct laryngoscopy.

Treatment. Perforation of an obstructing web may be lifesaving. Partial webs may be incised or dilated;

Table 13–1. Anatomic Classification of Congenital Anomalies of the Larynx

Supraglottic:	A. Congenital flaccid larynx—laryngomalacia
	B. Bifid epiglottis with subglottic stenosis and congenital cysts
	C. Absence of epiglottis with associated subglottic stenosis
	D. Overdeveloped elongated epiglottis with broad base
	E. Internal thyroglossal duct cysts
	F. Webs
	G. Cysts
	H. Laryngocele
	(1) Ventricular
	(2) Arytenoid and aryepiglottic fold
	I. Hemangioma
Glottic:	A. Webs
	B. Atresia
	C. Cysts
	D. Laryngeal paralysis
	E. Cri-du-Chat
	F. Arytenoid displacement (Birth trauma)
	G. Papilloma
	H. Vocal cord sulcus
Subglottic:	A. Stenosis
	B. Webs
	C. Atresia
	D. Hemangioma
	E. Lymphangioma
	F. Chondroma
	G. Laryngeal cleft

(From Tucker, G. F. *In* Healy, G. B., and McGill, T. J. I. [Eds.]: Laryngo-tracheal problems in the pediatric patient. Springfield, Ill. Charles C Thomas, 1979.)

tracheostomy may be needed during these procedures until dilatation is adequate.

CONGENITAL ATRESIA OF THE LARYNX

A few cases of complete obstruction to the airway at birth have been reported. In Holinger's case the entire glottis was encased in a thick fibrous sheet, almost cartilaginous in consistency.

These are of importance only because someone in the delivery room—obstetrician, anesthetist, or nurse—must recognize immediately that violent inspiratory effort without resultant air entry distinguishes them from the run-of-the-mill asphyxias of the newborn. Unless an airway can be established immediately, either by producing an aperture in the membrane or by tracheotomy, death in a few minutes is inevitable.

The few reported survivors had a tracheoesophageal fistula that permitted some gas exchange until the laryngeal obstruction could be relieved.

CONGENITAL SUBGLOTTIC STENOSIS

This group also is rare. Pathologically, this condition is extremely variable and difficult to evaluate, consisting as it does of nonspecific thickening of any of the structures beneath the glottis. Obstruction is usually maximal 2 to 3 mm beneath the glottic chink and is almost never inflammatory. In two of Holinger's cases, the cricoid cartilage was deformed, its anteroposterior measurement increased so that it protruded into the airway.

There is stridor from birth unless the stenosis is minimal. In this instance, stridor may only follow respiratory infection, the children having repeated attacks of "croup," often with superimposed laryngotracheobronchitis. Since the narrowing is subglottic, the voice is unaffected. Direct laryngoscopy will confirm the diagnosis.

Tracheotomy is often required for more severe degrees of stenosis or during inflammatory episodes in the milder ones. Growth of the larynx with advancing age ameliorates the condition when narrowing is slight, but more advanced stenosis demands repeated dilatations. Cricoid reconstruction with costal cartilage is sometimes required. Cotton and Seid have reported success with anterior cricoid split.

ACQUIRED SUBGLOTTIC STENOSIS

As more infants survive prolonged intubation and mechanical ventilation, it is hardly surprising that some infants will have injury to the vocal cords or the cricoid cartilage. The incidence of this complication may differ between centers as a function of the duration of intubation, frequency of changes of endotracheal tubes, and, perhaps, the fit of the tube. It has been noted in about 10 per cent of intubated infants, although it should be less common with soft (not cuffed) endotracheal tubes. The diagnosis may not be evident in the nursery in the absence of hoarseness or stridor. A few months after discharge, sometimes in association with a mild infection, stridor becomes evident and may persist (Papsidero and Pashley, 1980).

Couriel and Phelan described three infants born at 26 to 28 weeks gestation who received prolonged endotracheal intubation in the neonatal period. At intervals from 15 weeks to 2 years later, stridor was noted with intercurrent infection. On bronchoscopy, smooth-walled cysts, 2 to 3 mm in diameter, were noted below the cords. They were ruptured by the bronchoscope and eventually disappeared or left some granulation tissue. When granulation tissue persists, laser dissection is useful in removing it without further inflammation.

TRACHEAL STENOSIS

Narrowing of the trachea may be either intrinsic or extrinsic. A few cases are on record of extreme congenital hypoplastic narrowing of the trachea. They are suspected because of persistent inspiratory difficulty with stridor, present from birth until death. Laryngeal stenosis can be differentiated by the fact that the voice is unimpaired. Diagnosis can be made only by bronchoscopy or tracheography and bronchography. Both because of its extreme rarity and because no definitive treatment is available for this lethal congenital defect, we shall not describe it in detail.

TRACHEAL COMPRESSION BY NEIGHBORING STRUCTURES

Both the larynx and the trachea may be narrowed by extrinsic masses. These include tumors of the neck and mediastinal cysts and tumors, which are discussed elsewhere (see Chapter 23). Perhaps the most common form of compression of the airway is that produced by a blood vessel that pursues an abnormal course through the mediastinum. Because these are not exceedingly rare and because diagnosis can now be arrived at fairly early in life and definitive treatment may be lifesaving, these are considered in some detail in the following pages.

BRONCHIAL STENOSIS

Acquired bronchial stenosis is very rare, but it has been described in infants who were intubated prematures requiring frequent suctioning. Presumably, the catheter tip was inserted into a bronchus and caused local injury. In one infant who died, nodular granulations and squamous metaplasia were found in the distal trachea and bronchi.

Anomalies of the Great Vessels

Maldevelopment of the aortic arch and malposition of one or more of the great vessels arising from the arch produce important and recognizable clinical syndromes in the infant. Early recognition is of considerable importance, since early surgical correction saves lives and eliminates much serious morbidity. Many minor deviations from the normal in origin and course of intrathoracic arteries go unnoticed because in their anomalous locations they do not impinge upon either the trachea or the esophagus. Neuhauser classified the group as follows:

I. Right aortic arch
   A. With situs inversus viscerum
   B. Without inversion
      1. Anterior type
      2. Posterior type
II. Double aortic arch
III. Anomalous right subclavian artery
IV. Patent ductus arteriosus
V. Coarctation of the aorta

Patent ductus arteriosus and coarctation of the aorta are described in Chapter 27. The first two conditions listed are discussed here because the symptom-complex they induce is more closely identified with the respiratory and gastrointestinal systems than with the cardiovascular system. Rarer anomalies such as left-sided right subclavian artery, anomalous left common carotid artery, anomalous innominate artery, and aberrant, or right-sided, patent ductus will not be discussed individually.

In addition to the obstructive disorders that arise from anomalies of the aortic arch or one of its branches, occasional instances in which similar trouble is engendered by aberrant pulmonary arteries are encountered.

Etiology. The development of the aortic arch is effected by a complicated series of evolutions of the primitive paired aortic arches.

Incidence. The total number of anomalies in this category is large, but only a minority produce symptoms. In the symptomatic group, double aortic arch is the commonest malformation. Right aortic arch is also not at all uncommon, but an even larger proportion of these cases produce no symptoms. They are symptomatic only when a ductus arteriosus or ligamentum arteriosum and another anomalously placed vessel complete the encircling ring.

Diagnosis. The symptoms and signs produced depend upon the location of the aberrant vessel or vessels and the degree to which they compromise the esophagus and airway. A combination of respiratory and digestive signs is to be expected in double aortic arch, although respiratory symptoms are distinctly more prominent. Dyspnea is present from birth or appears within several weeks. Respirations are stridulous in the majority, although in many expiratory wheezing rather than inspiratory stridor is heard. Stridor often persists during sleep and is increased by crying. Cyanosis may be constant or episodic. Feeding is likely to initiate or accentuate stridor and to produce or deepen dyspnea and cyanosis. Food offered by nipple is often taken poorly and may be regurgitated. Vomitus may contain fresh or altered blood. Feeding may also stimulate paroxysmal cough. All signs are aggravated by the respiratory infections that repeatedly plague these infants. During these infections, breathing may be extremely difficult and "croupy," suggesting that caused by acute laryngotracheobronchitis. *Severely affected babies prefer to lie with the head sharply retracted, and flexion of the neck exaggerates dyspnea.* The cough is characteristically brassy or bitonal.

Right aortic arch per se produces no or few symptoms. Rarely, as it turns to the right instead of the left, it may impinge upon the trachea or it may compress the bronchi to any of the right lung lobes. Compression then results in either atelectasis or emphysema or a combination of these. Trouble most often arises when it forms one limb of a complete vascular ring, the others composed of a patent ductus arteriosus or ligamentum arteriosum and a pulmonary artery or an anomalous left carotid or left subclavian artery. When a constricting vascular ring is present, it is clinically indistinguishable from double aortic arch.

The most common anomaly in the course of a single vessel involves the left subclavian, which arises from the right side of the arch and crosses to the left. Usually, it courses behind the esophagus; infrequently, it is found between the esophagus and the trachea or, rarely indeed, in front of the trachea. Symptoms, if present, are apt to be restricted to dysphagia, but if one of the two less usual courses is followed, respiration may also be involved.

Respiratory symptoms in the absence of esophageal symptoms should suggest compression of the trachea by an anomalous innominate artery. Signs and symptoms may not be present at birth, but they may become more severe in the first months of life and subside thereafter. Episodic apnea, limpness, and cyanosis may occur in this condition, as in other forms of tracheal compression from aberrant vessels.

Radiographic Diagnosis. Localized atelectasis or emphysema in the newborn, if persistent, should make one consider vascular compression of a major bronchus as a possible cause. Visualization of the trachea in plain posteroanterior and lateral films at times reveals narrowing above the carina plus displacement in either the sagittal or horizontal plane. The most fruitful diagnostic procedure is the barium swallow cineradiographic examination, which demonstrates abnormalities in esophageal contour. High kilovoltage films will improve the contrast between air and soft tissues and aid in identification of tracheal compression.

A right aortic arch might be suspected in the plain anteroposterior film if the aortic arch is observed to lie to the right, if the "knob" on the left is absent, and if the trachea is deviated to the left. Esophagram reveals a rounded indentation into the right border of the esophagus but none on the left or on the anterior or posterior face. Double aortic arch is characterized by narrowing and anterior displacement of the trachea, seen in the plain lateral film. When the esophagus is filled with barium, it is seen to be displaced forward by a rounded, pulsating mass. Spot films show constriction from both sides and, in the lateral view, deep indentation both in front and in back. An anomalous right subclavian artery taking its usual course from left to right produces an oblique defect in the posterior aspect of the esophagus about 0.5 cm wide and 3 to 4 cm long.

Contrast tracheograms and angiograms are indicated in those instances in which plain films and esophagrams have not sufficed to establish the suspected diagnosis. They are also useful to the surgeon by indicating whether the anterior or the posterior arch is the smaller one, hence the one he will wish to ligate. His choice of incision may be determined by this information.

Prognosis. The outlook varies with the degree of tracheal obstruction, the nature of the anomaly, and the treatment given. Infants symptomatic early must be observed carefully, since tightness of the ring often increases with growth. Sudden death may occur. Lower respiratory tract infections are common, and some are pneumonic, most resembling severe laryngotracheobronchitis. After operative correction, stridor is expected to persist for many months, even though dyspnea has been relieved promptly.

Treatment. Successful surgical correction, pioneered by Gross, has been accomplished in all types of vascular ring anomalies. Operative risk is still not inconsiderable, especially for double aortic arch. In selecting the proper time for operation, this risk must be balanced against the degree of respiratory difficulty. If this is severe from the start, surgery is indicated in the neonatal period. If one can wait, one does, but each respiratory infection must be treated with antimicrobial agents both early and vigorously.

The most common problem in the postoperative period is the persistence of respiratory distress after division of the obstructing vessel. The failure of the trachea to resume normal dimensions may result from hypoplastic segments of trachea, and these may require further operative intervention. Vasko and

Ahn have reported the use of autologous rib as a tracheal splint for symptomatic tracheomalacia. Tracheostomy may be necessary in some situations.

Cysts and Neoplasms of the Larynx

Cysts arise either from one of the three branchial arches concerned in the development of the larynx or, as retention cysts, from its lining mucous membrane. Laryngoceles may simulate true cysts in both appearance and symptomatology, but these are encountered only rarely in infancy.

The presenting signs of cyst are hoarseness, muffled voice or aphonia, and stridor. Onset is usually at birth, but it may be delayed weeks or months. Severity of dyspnea depends upon the size of the cyst. Diagnosis rests upon laryngoscopy.

Treatment is carried out through the laryngoscope and consists of either aspiration or resection. The laser seems promising for such lesions. Tracheotomy is indicated for some patients until respiratory obstruction can be controlled. External operative approach is seldom required.

Subglottic cysts may follow prolonged intubation, presumably from obstruction of the excretory ducts of the mucous glands by squamous metaplasia (Couriel and Phelan, 1981).

A limited variety of *tumors* has been discovered to involve the larynx. The angioma group, including hemangioma, lymphangioma, and hemangioendothelioma, has supplied the greatest number. Some of the hemangiomas have been limited to the larynx, but in others laryngeal tumor was part of a widespread angiomatous involvement of the face, neck, and pharynx. Fibrosarcomas of the larynx and trachea have been reported, as has a neurofibroma that at autopsy proved to be but one of many such new growths scattered throughout the body.

Tumors of neighboring structures such as cystic hygroma of the neck, thyroglossal duct cyst or aberrant thyroid at the base of the tongue, and congenital goiter often produce dyspnea but seldom cause stridor.

Treatment of laryngeal tumor depends upon its histologic characteristics. Remarkable regression in cutaneous hemangiomas occurs after 1 to 2 weeks of steroid therapy, in the dose range of prednisone, 2 to 3 mg/kg/day. Laryngeal hemangiomas sometimes respond to oral corticosteroid therapy within a few days, and usually by 10 days. Tracheostomy may be necessary for control of dyspnea until these definitive measures are undertaken. Promising results with the CO_2 laser have been reported for benign lesions of the larynx, including hemangioma (Simpson et al., 1979; Healy et al., 1980).

Neurogenic Stridor

It has been suspected for a long time that certain examples of stridor might be initiated by some aberration in nervous control of the larynx. Thus, Schwartz wrote of an "overzealous reflex of laryngeal closure during the threatening experience of regurgitation." Allen, Towsley, and Wilson elaborated on this problem in a beautifully comprehensive study of the literature plus a careful investigation of four instructive case histories of their own. They came to the conclusion, impossible to gainsay from the evidence presented, that episodes of stridor coupled with apnea and cyanosis, often hazardous to life, may be precipitated by a neurogenic mechanism. This differs from idiopathic epilepsy by the fact that the stimulus is an identifiable, localizable trigger mechanism, such as nipple feeding, regurgitation, or tactile stimulation of the esophagus or larynx. In one of their cases carotid sinus pressure induced heart block. This child was greatly improved after administration of atropine. In their first patient, in whom attacks of stridor, apnea, and cyanosis precipitated by bottle feeding were at times followed by convulsion, the electroencephalogram was distinctly abnormal. Anticonvulsant therapy (phenytoin and phenobarbital) not only put an end to attacks but also quickly improved the electroencephalographic tracing.

This syndrome is particularly frequent after repair of tracheoesophageal stricture. We have encountered one infant in whom bougienage for stricture subsequent to this operation induced complete heart stoppage. The two mechanisms must not be dissimilar.

Allen and coworkers concluded that avoidance of esophageal stimulation at the one end (gavage rather than nipple feeding), depression of the cerebrum at the other (anticonvulsive therapy), or breaking the reflex arc at the level of the vagus nerve (atropine) are effective methods of combatting attacks of neurogenic stridor.

Paralysis of Vocal Cords

Incidence. The literature abounds with reports of vocal cord paralysis in adults, but few cases have been reported in the newborn. That it is not an extreme rarity is attested to by the fact that we saw two such cases within 2 years.

Etiology. Paralysis may be bilateral or unilateral. When bilateral, it is almost invariably central in origin and nature, producing spastic palsy. In the newborn, birth trauma involving the brain stem seems to be the only important etiologic factor.

Unilateral palsies are peripheral and flaccid and are almost always left-sided, although a few right-sided ones are met. The left-sided variety predominates for two reasons: (1) because the recurrent laryngeal nerve on that side arises lower in the neck and its course is therefore longer, and (2) because it loops around the aorta from front to back before ascending alongside the trachea. It is thus susceptible to injury by dilatation of the aorta or by this vessel's displacement by enlargement of the conus or of nearby chambers of the heart. A few cases are caused by pressure upon the nerves by mediastinal tumors.

Diagnosis. Hoarseness or aphonia is present, depending upon the type and degree of paralysis. Stridor almost invariably is heard, inspiratory in time, and often associated with deep thoracic retraction. Laryngoscopic inspection is required in order to differentiate the stridor of vocal cord paralysis from that due to laryngeal stenosis. Concomitant signs of congenital heart disease or mediastinal tumor may or may not be elicited.

Prognosis. The outcome depends entirely upon the basic disorder. Central paralyses commonly disappear with the subsidence of edema or absorption of blood within the cranial cavity. Palsies caused by pressure will persist until pressure is relieved.

Treatment. This is directed toward discovery and, if possible, relief of the basic disorder. The finding of unilateral vocal cord paralysis calls for careful study of the mediastinal contents and includes fluoroscopy, x-ray films, barium swallow films, and, often, angiocardiography.

REFERENCES

Allen, R. J., Towsley, H. A., and Wilson, J. L.: Neurogenic stridor in infancy. A.M.A. Am. J. Dis. Child. *87*:179, 1954.

Ardran, G. M., and Kemp, F. H.: The mechanism of changes in form of the cervical airway in infancy. Med. Radiogr. Photogr. *44*:26, 1968.

Baker, D. C., Jr.: Congenital disorders of the larynx. N.Y.J. Med. *54*:2458, 1954.

Berdan, W. E., Baker, D. H., et al.: Innominate artery compression of the trachea in infants with stridor and apnea. Radiology *92*:272, 1969.

Blumenthal, S., and Ravitch, M. M.: Seminar on aortic vascular rings and other anomalies of the aortic arch. Pediatrics *20*:896, 1957.

Bradham, R. R., Sealy, W. C., and Young, W. G.: Respiratory distress associated with anomalies of the aortic arch. Surg. Gynecol. Obstet. *126.9*, 1968.

Butz, R. O.: Length and cross-section growth patterns in the human trachea. Pediatrics *42*:336, 1968.

Campbell, J. S., Wiglesworth, F. W., Latorroca, R., et al.: Congenital subglottic hemangiomas of larynx and trachea. Pediatrics *22*:727, 1958.

Clerf, L. H.: Unilateral vocal cord paralysis. J.A.M.A. *151*:900, 1953.

Cotton, R. T., and Richardson, M. A.: Congenital laryngeal anomalies. Otol. Clin. North Am. *14*:203, 1981.

Cotton, R. T., and Seid, A. B.: Management of the extubation problem in the premature child: anterior cricoid split as an alternative to tracheotomy. Ann. Otol. *89*:508, 1980.

Couriel, J. M., and Phelan, P. D.: Subglottic cysts: a complication of neonatal endotracheal intubation? Pediatrics *68*:103, 1981.

Dunbar, J. S.: Upper respiratory tract obstruction in infants and children. Am. J. Roentgenol. *109*:227, 1970.

Fearon, B., and Shortreed, R.: Tracheobronchial compression by congenital cardiovascular anomalies in children. Syndrome of apnea. Ann. Otol. Rhinol. Laryngol. *72*:949, 1963.

Ferguson, C. F.: Congenital abnormalities of the infant larynx. Otol. Clin. North Am. 3:185, 1970.

Fost, N. C., and Esterly, N.: Successful treatment of juvenile hemangiomas with prednisone. J. Pediatr. 72:351, 1968.

Gross, R. E., and Neuhauser, E. B. D.: Compression of the trachea or esophagus by vascular anomalies: Surgical therapy in 40 cases. Pediatrics 7:69, 1951.

Healy, G. B., Fearon, B., French, R., and McGill, T.: Treatment of subglottic hemangioma with the carbon dioxide laser. Laryngoscope 90:809, 1980.

Holinger, P. H., Johnston, K. C., and Schiller, F.: Congenital anomalies of the larynx. Ann. Otol. Rhinol. Laryngol. 63:581, 1954.

Holinger, P. H., Johnston, K. C., and Zoss, A. R.: Tracheal and bronchial obstruction due to congenital cardiovascular anomalies. Ann. Otol. Rhinol. Laryngol. 57:808, 1948.

Holinger, P. H., Schild, J. A., and Weprin, L.: Pediatric laryngology. Otol. Clin. North Am. 3:625, 1970.

Holinger, P. H., Slaughter, D. P., and Novak, F. J., III: Unusual tumors obstructing the lower respiratory tract of infants and children. Trans. Am. Acad. Ophthal. 54:223, 1949–50.

Hudson, P.: Congenital web of larynx. A.M.A. Am. J. Dis. Child. 81:545, 1951.

Keleman, G.: Congenital laryngeal stridor. A.M.A. Arch. Otolaryngol. 58:245, 1953.

Jones, R., Bodnar, A., Roan, Y., and Johnson, D.: Subglottic ste-

nosis in newborn intensive care graduates. Am. J. Dis. Child. 135:367, 1981.

Loeb, W. J., and Smith, E. E.: Airway obstruction in a newborn by pedunculated pharyngeal dermoid. Pediatrics 40:20, 1967.

Mercer, R. D.: Laryngeal stridor with temporary cardiac and respiratory arrest. Am. J. Dis. Child. 70:336, 1945.

Morrison, L. F.: Recurrent laryngeal nerve paralysis; A revised conception based on the dissection of one hundred cadavers. Ann. Otol. Rhinol. Laryngol. 61:567, 1952.

Nabarro, S.: Calcification of the laryngeal and tracheal cartilages associated with congenital stridor in an infant. Arch. Dis. Child. 27:185, 1952.

Neuhauser, E. B. D.: The roentgen diagnosis of double aortic arch and other anomalies of the great vessels. Am. J. Roentgenol. 56:1, 1946.

Papsidero, M. J., and Pashley, N. R. T.: Acquired stenosis of the upper airway in neonates: an increasing problem. Ann. Otol. 89:512, 1980.

Sayre, J. W., and Hall, E. G.: Anomalies of larynx associated with tracheo-esophageal fistula. Pediatrics 13:150, 1954.

Schwartz, A. B.: Functional disorders of the larynx in early infancy. J. Pediatr. 42:457, 1953.

Simpson, G. T., McGill, T., Healy, G. B., et al.: Benign tumors and lesions of the larynx in children. Ann. Otol. Rhinol. Laryngol. 88:479, 1979.

Suchs, O. W., and Powell, D. B.: Congenital cysts of the larynx in infants. Laryngoscope 77:654, 1967.

Vasko, J. S., and Ahn, C.: Surgical management of secondary tracheomalacia. Ann. Thorac. Surg. 6:269, 1968.

Welsh, T. M., and Munro, J. B.: Congenital stridor caused by aberrant pulmonary artery. Arch. Dis. Child. 29:101, 1954.

Wilson, T. G.: Some observations on the anatomy of the infantile larynx. Acta Otolaryngol. 43:95, 1953.

14

Aspiration Syndromes

Aspiration can occur either before or after birth, in insignificant or lethal quantities. Since many of the circumstances that provoke aspiration are preventable, it is important to describe past experiences, most of which we hope will never be repeated. The recent reduction in deaths of term infants is, to a considerable extent, the result of better monitoring of the fetus before birth with delivery at the first signs of distress (by section if necessary) and prompt attention to the infant at birth if aspiration has occurred. With appropriate use of ventilators and other supportive measures, many infants can be saved from what was formerly considered lethal aspiration. Schaffer noted in previous editions of this text, "By both clinical and pathological evidence, aspiration is one of the most common accidents that affect the lungs of newborn infants." That sentence no longer

applies, since modern obstetrics has made it possible to consider aspiration a preventable condition.

Incidence. Considering the many possible times that aspiration may occur, it is not surprising that it remains among the most common causes of respiratory distress in infants. Meconium was seen in the trachea of 0.5 per cent of infants examined prospectively by Gregory and coworkers; 20 per cent of their group of meconium-stained infants had pulmonary disease. In our Boston nurseries, one to three infants per 1000 live births have meconium aspiration pneumonia. Second-born twins or infants delivered by vaginal breech extraction are at risk for aspiration.

Pathology. The lungs of fetuses or infants who have aspirated before or during delivery are firm and poorly aerated and sink in the fixing solution. The bronchi contain fluid or thin mucus. Cut surfaces exude fluid. Under the microscope (Fig. 14–1) many alveoli are collapsed, but others are overexpanded, filled with fluid and, in some instances, squamae and other recognizable amniotic debris. In many, congestion, edema, and hemorrhage are prominent. Segments or patches of atelectasis or areas of emphysema or both are seen. In a number of the lungs, simple emphysema has progressed to one of its more advanced stages. Pleural fluid is found occasionally.

In many lungs, overfilling and distention of pulmonary capillaries are visible, and, in a few, this finding is striking. Dilatation of the right side of the heart may be obvious.

Pathophysiology: Aspiration in Utero.

Rapid shallow respiratory movements are a normal feature of fetal life. The movements, which occur only about half the time, are of such frequency and depth that only about a milliliter of lung fluid moves along the tracheobronchial tree. The net direction of liquid movement in the lung is from alveoli to the amniotic fluid. Even the occasional sigh or gasp that can be observed before birth does not allow entry of amniotic sac contents into the lungs.

Experimentally induced asphyxia in lambs, at least, induces a series of sustained deep breaths that can result in massive aspiration (Dawes, 1972). We assume that in the human events that impair fetal gas exchange across the placenta, such as infarcts, premature separation, cord occlusion, or maternal hypotension, can stimulate sufficiently vigorous fetal respiratory efforts to permit entry of either normal or contaminated amniotic liquid. The effects on the infant obviously will depend on the quantity aspirated and its contents, such as squamous cells, blood, vernix, or meconium.

Examination of lungs of stillborn infants occasionally reveals extensive aspiration of squamous debris. Evidence of nonfatal disease from squamous cells has not been recognized. Jose and colleagues subjected adult rabbits to 4 to 6 ml/kg of amniotic fluid with cell counts up to 2300 cells/ml and could not demonstrate any adverse effects compared with equal volumes of clear fluid. More gross contamination with blood or pus would be indistinguishable from pneumonia. Excessive aspiration of clear amniotic liquid would presumably be a cause of transient tachypnea of the newborn (see Chapter 20).

Meconium Aspiration.

Passage of meconium before birth usually indicates some measure of fetal distress. Some infants escape any aspiration and are simply meconium stained. It is estimated that this event occurs in nearly 10 per cent of all deliveries. In about half the cases in which thick meconium is present, some meconium is found in the trachea. The symptoms are sometimes mild, only tachypnea lasting for a day or so. Other times, the material obstructs either the upper or the lower airways and is occasionally associated with profound pulmonary vasoconstriction (see also discussion of persistent fetal circulation, Chapter 18).

The importance of direct visualization of the larynx and prompt suctioning of any visible meconium cannot be overemphasized. Deep tracheal suction may be required; lavage is not helpful. Carson and coworkers reported in 1976 that this vigorous approach to suctioning of the trachea reduced mortality and morbidity to the extent of no deaths among a series of 273 meconium-stained infants.

Although it is clear that meconium aspiration should usually be prevented, when it occurs the question concerns the best approach to treatment. If the infant is having significant respiratory distress after aspiration of the upper airway, one should first note that air leak is a common complication of significant meconium aspiration. Madansky and coworkers found it present in 13 of 32 infants. Chest radiographs and transillumination of the chest are important measures in following such infants. Some may require ventilatory assistance and increased inspired oxygen. When the oxygen requirements are very

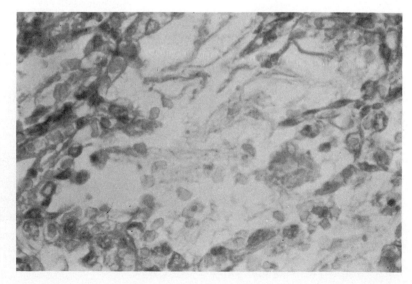

Figure 14–1. Section of lung of a full-term infant weighing 7 pounds 8 ounces (3400 gm) who died 15 minutes after birth after having gasped only a few times. Prolonged labor, uterine inertia, stimulation of labor by a Pitocin drip, and, finally, midforceps extraction characterized his delivery. The microscopic section shows much fluid, debris, and many squamae within dilated terminal air spaces. Virtually every section from both lungs looked like this one.

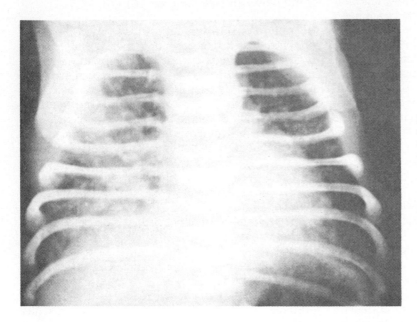

Figure 14—2. Anteroposterior view of chest made at ten hours of age in a male infant weighing 8 pounds 8 ounces (3855 gm), born ten days after his E.D.C. and an uncomplicated labor and delivery. He was covered with thick meconium at birth. He was tachypneic and dyspneic for two days, better on the third day, and well on the fourth day.

Note the intense patchy opacification almost filling the right hemithorax, maximal about the heart shadow, but extending to the periphery in the right middle zone. Some, but much less, is seen on the left side.

great, the probability of a component of pulmonary vasoconstriction should be considered. In this event, as much as 100 per cent oxygen may be required with a ventilator. The role of hyperventilation should be considered in such instances, but with the caution that the high applied pressures may aggravate pneumothorax or interstitial emphysema. We advocate antibiotics for all these infants, since infection has fre-

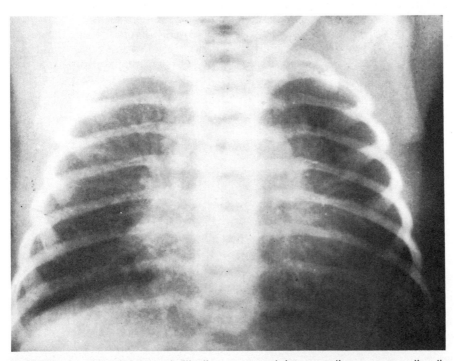

Figure 14—3. There is intense infiltration, some patchy, some linear, surrounding the heart and obliterating its normally sharp silhouette. The opacification extends outward and downward a short distance on the left side and toward the right base, but it involves the entire right upper lobe heavily.

quently been the initial reason for fetal distress, and infectious pneumonia may coexist with meconium aspiration.

Other forms of treatment that have been suggested, such as corticosteroids and ultrasonic mist, have not been established as effective.

Aspiration After Birth. Depression of laryngeal reflexes may allow aspiration of oropharyngeal contents. The fetal lamb appears to have a reflex that limits entry of water or cow's milk into the lung. Sheep's milk, on the other hand, can be aspirated (Johnson, 1973). Although similar reflexes have not been found in the human, some infants seem prone to aspiration, particularly during the first hours of life. Perhaps the fact that human milk is present in very small quantities during the first days after birth is a protective mechanism that prevents overfeeding when swallowing may not be well coordinated.

Postnatal aspiration may occur in depressed infants after gavage feeding, after overfeeding, sometimes in association with swallowing excessive amounts of air, and with intestinal obstruction. Infants of low gestational age and birth weight seem particularly prone to aspiration after feedings, and that has been the principal argument for use of intravenous alimentation until they can tolerate gavage feedings without regurgitation.

In the event of recurrent aspiration or whenever coughing or choking occurs with feedings, the possibility of an anatomic defect should be considered. The most common of these is tracheoesophageal fistula, but posterior laryngeal clefts can produce similar symptoms.

A functional cause of recurrent aspiration was described by DeCarlo and others in 1952 and was later labeled "pharyngeal incoordination of infancy." Apparently, 10 to 15 per cent of all infants aspirate somewhat during the first days of life but rarely there-

after. The diagnosis is made by the demonstration of oily contrast medium entering the trachea as well as the esophagus. When pharyngeal incoordination persists, the diagnosis of dysautonomia should be considered. Some infants may have difficulty swallowing for weeks, but they seem to recover fully. Formula should be given by gastric tube. Water may occasionally be offered by mouth to see if swallowing has improved.

Radiographic Features. Coarse, irregular densities usually follow the distribution of the bronchial tree. Focal areas of hyperinflation are common, and the domes of the diaphragm are occasionally flattened. Some clearing is usually evident by 24 hours. The lesion is not pathognomonic for aspiration and is indistinguishable from pneumonia and hemorrhage. Persistent air trapping and even pneumatocele formation may be evident for several months.

Treatment. Once it is recognized that aspiration has occurred, prompt suctioning of the oropharynx is mandatory. Inspection of the larynx and deep tracheal suction may be required, depending, of course, on the infant's condition. Vigorous respiratory efforts without movement of air are the hallmarks of recent airway obstruction. If the obstruction is total, apnea will follow a minute or two of intensive respiratory effort.

CASE 14–1

A 21-year-old mother had a normal pregnancy until 30 weeks, when she noticed onset of brisk vaginal bleeding and abdominal pain, and the diagnosis of

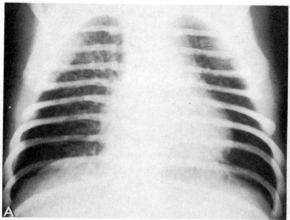 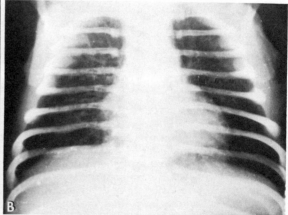

Figure 14–4. A, Anteroposterior view of the chest taken on the first day of life. Noteworthy are the heavy patchy infiltration of both lungs, more intense in the upper lung fields, and the overaeration of the lower lobes. The opacification appears soft, not granular. Note, too, the blurring of the normally sharp cardiac silhouette. B, Radiograph taken on the third day. There has been some clearing of the opacification, although a moderate amount is still visible, especially in the right upper lobe and hugging the heart shadow. The emphysema appears to have increased somewhat.

abruptio placentae was made. The infant was delivered by emergency cesarean section with a weight of 1.52 kg. Apgar score at 1 minute was 5, and at 5 minutes it was 8. The infant was cyanotic and given 100 per cent oxygen in the delivery room. When intubated, fresh blood was aspirated from the trachea. Blood-tinged material was also removed from the gastric aspirate, and the baby subsequently had clotted blood in the stools. An Apt test on the material from the gastric aspirate revealed maternal hemoglobin.

The baby's hematocrit was 62. The infant remained cyanotic and had greatly diminished air exchange with crepitant breath sounds. He required mechanical ventilation with 100 per cent oxygen and was given pancuronium for muscle relaxation to facilitate mechanical ventilation. The pressures required reached a peak pressure of 35 cm of water and end-expiratory pressure of 7 cm of water. Over the next 2 days the infant improved; he was extubated and then maintained on 30 to 35 per cent oxygen.

The initial chest film showed opacified lungs bilaterally, but after intubation with muscle relaxation the lungs could be reasonably well aerated. A diffuse reticular granular pattern, consistent with hyaline membrane disease, was evident bilaterally. After extubation with less end-expiratory pressure, the lung fields appeared hazier than they had when the infant was on the ventilator. Retractions were present, but the infant was able to maintain adequate gas exchange without further ventilatory assistance.

Comment. This infant, delivered by emergency cesarean section because of maternal hemorrhage, clearly had hyaline membrane disease. The aspiration of blood from the trachea and the crepitant breath sounds are both consistent with aspiration of maternal blood and the hyaline membrane disease. Clearing was reasonably prompt, and the infant had no subsequent bleeding, thus ruling out pulmonary hemorrhage and pulmonary hypertension as the underlying problem. The positive test for maternal hemoglobin further supports this diagnosis of aspiration of blood-stained amniotic fluid superimposed on hyaline membrane disease.

CASE 14–2

A 3.2 kg male infant was born to a gravida 2, para 1, 27-year-old woman after 41 weeks of pregnancy. The mother presented to the hospital on the day of delivery in labor with a moderate amount of vaginal bleeding. Ultrasonography revealed an anterior placenta previa. A cesarean section was performed and the membranes were ruptured during the delivery. At this time, thick meconium was noted in the amniotic fluid, and a large retroplacental clot was observed. The infant was suctioned vigorously with a catheter after delivery of the head and then again below the vocal cords after complete delivery and before breathing. Approximately 2 ml of thick meconium was aspirated from below the

cords, with 10 ml from the oropharynx and another 10 ml from the stomach. Grunting, flaring, and retracting respirations occurred soon after birth. The Apgars were 2 and 7. An umbilical artery line was placed.

The physical examination revealed an infant who was well nourished, active, jittery, and hypertonic. The nails and umbilical cord were meconium stained. The pulse was 140, the breaths were spontaneous and shallow and the respiratory rate was 100, systolic blood pressure was 87, and temperature was 37° C with an incubator temperature of 36° C.

After stabilization, the infant was transferred to the neonatal intensive care unit at approximately 3 hours of life. At that time, the baby was intubated, and intermittent mandatory ventilation was started. The infant was treated with hyperventilation and vigorous blood volume support (initial hematocrit was 42 per cent). The aim was to keep Pa_{O_2} between 90 and 110 torr, Pa_{CO_2} between 25 and 30 torr, and pH >7.4 in order to promote pulmonary vasodilation. Arterial oxygenation diminished at about 8 hours of life, when the infant was noted to be breathing out of phase with the ventilator and apparently fighting ventilator support. Morphine was administered without evident effect, and the infant was then paralyzed with pancuronium. Thereafter, blood gases improved with only minor changes in ventilator support. The infant was weaned from the respirator within 3 days with no complications.

Comment. This infant had classic meconium aspiration syndrome, presumably associated with intrauterine asphyxia due to placenta previa and abruptio placentae. Delivery room suctioning appeared to be adequate. The infant avoided development of severe persistent fetal circulation despite two periods of poor arterial oxygenation in the first 8 hours of life—the first associated with insufficient ambient oxygen during transport (later corrected with intubation), and the second with the infant "fighting" the ventilator (no response to morphine, corrected with pancuronium). This infant was treated with hyperventilation, vigorous blood volume support, and liberal ambient oxygen. Paralysis made it impossible to assess central nervous system signs of asphyxia except by electroencephalogram.

Prognosis. As the case histories demonstrate, most infants who have been presumed to aspirate amniotic or vaginal contents do well. Some are doubtless included with those infants considered to have transient tachypnea. They recover clinically after 2 or 3 days, radiologically after 5 to 7 days.

Most infants with meconium aspiration have mild symptoms that resolve by 24 hours, especially in hospitals in which there is a vigorous approach to monitoring and responding to fetal distress with a smooth plan for combined obstetric/pediatric removal of meconium from the airway. In infants who are more severely ill, lung disease may be overshadowed by asphyxial damage to other organs. Severe meconium aspiration pneumonia requiring intensive care may be associated with a mortality rate as high as 50 per cent. The major pulmonary risks associated with meconium aspiration are air leak, persistent fetal circulation, and, rarely (in the survivors with the most severe disease), a chronic lung disease identical with bronchopulmonary dysplasia. Virtually all infants with meconium aspiration needing ventilation for more than 2 days have associated persistent fetal circulation. It is useful to know that air leak, if it occurs, is usually seen during the first 24 hours with meconium aspiration.

With a very conservative approach to gastric feeding of the sick or immature newborn, aspiration of milk and gastric contents during the newborn period is rarer and usually mild (risk estimate 2/1000 ICU patients). Presumably in the more severe cases, complications would be similar to those seen with meconium aspiration.

REFERENCES

Baghdassarian, O. H., and Gatewood, W. M.: Barium swallow in evaluation of chronic or recurrent pneumonias in infancy and childhood. Md. State Med. J. *14*:51, 1965

Bryan, C. S.: Enhancement of bacterial infection by meconium. Johns Hopkins Med. J. *121*:9, 1967.

Carson, B. S., Losey, R. W., Bowes, W. A., and Simmons, M. A.: Combined obstetric and pediatric approach to prevent meconium aspiration syndrome. Am. J. Obstet. Gynecol. *126*:712, 1976.

Case records of Massachusetts General Hospital. N. Engl. J. Med. *227*:516, 1942.

Cordero, L., and Hon, E.: Neonatal bradycardia following nasopharyngeal stimulation. J. Pediatr. *78*:441, 1971.

DeCarlo, J., Tramer, A., and Startzman, H. H.: Iodized oil aspiration in the newborn. Am. J. Dis. Child. *84*:442, 1952.

Farber, S., and Wilson, J. L.: Atelectasis of the newborn: A study and critical review. Am. J. Dis. Child. *46*:572, 1933.

Fletcher, B. D., Outerbridge, E. W., and Dunbar, J. S.: Pulmonary interstitial emphysema in the newborn. J. Can. Assoc. Radiol. *21*:273, 1970.

Gage, J., Taeusch, H. W., Treves, S., and Caldicott, W.: Suctioning of upper airway meconium in newborn infants. J. Am. Med. Assoc. *246*:2590, 1981.

Gregory, G. A., Gooding, C. A., Phibbs, R. H., et al.: Meconium aspiration in infants—A prospective study. J. Pediatr. *85*:848, 1974.

Johnson, P., Robinson, J. S., and Salisbury, D.: The onset and control of breathing after birth. *In* Foetal and Neonatal Physiology. Proceedings of The Sir Joseph Barcroft Centenary Symposium. Cambridge, Cambridge University Press, 1973, p. 217.

Jose, J., Schreiner, R., Mirkin, L., Lemons, J., and Gresham, E.: Non-association of cell content with respiratory distress in adult rabbits aspirating human amniotic fluid. Pediatr. Res. *15*:1672 (abstract), 1981.

Madansky, D. L., Lawson, E. E., Chernick, V., and Taeusch, H. W.: Pneumothorax and other forms of pulmonary air leak in newborns. Am. Rev. Resp. Dis. *120*:729, 1979.

Marshall, R., Tyrala, E., McAlister, W., and Sheehan, M.: Meconium aspiration syndrome. Neonatal and follow-up study. Am. J. Obstet. Gynecol. *131*:672, 1978.

Ting, P., and Brady, J.: Tracheal suction in meconium aspiration. Am. J. Obstet. Gynecol. *122*:767, 1975.

Vidyasagar, D., Yeh, T., Harris, V., and Pildes, R.: Assisted ventilation in infants with meconium aspiration syndrome. Pediatrics *56*:208, 1975.

15

Hyaline Membrane Disease

Hyaline membrane disease, sometimes referred to as respiratory distress syndrome, occurs after the onset of breathing in infants with lung immaturity and deficiency of pulmonary surfactants.

Epidemiology. Although there is no universal agreement on clinical or pathologic diagnostic criteria, the almost complete accord between investigators allows assessment of incidence and mortality rates. Described in all populations of the world, hyaline membrane disease appears to be somewhat more common in prematurely born white than black infants and nearly twice as common in males as in females, with a familial likelihood of recurrence in a subsequent prematurely born infant. The incidence of respiratory distress syndrome in the United States is estimated to be 1 per cent of all livebirths. The disorder over the past decade has accounted for about 7000 deaths per year in the United States, with few deaths among infants over 1.5 kg but an increasing proportion the more immature the infant. Hyaline membrane disease is the leading cause of death of liveborn infants, responsible for nearly 20 per cent of neonatal deaths. Age at death is nearly always 72 hours or less, except in some infants who die of complications of the disease or its treatment later in the first few weeks of life.

Infants at special risk are those delivered prematurely, with the incidence increasing with degree of prematurity. Precipitous delivery after maternal hemorrhage or asphyxia is associated with a greater likelihood of hyaline membrane disease. The second-born twin is at greater risk than the firstborn. Some maternal conditions are thought to have a sparing effect, namely, conditions associated with chronic intrauterine distress that lead to undersized infants, maternal steroid treatment, and, in some instances, prolonged labor following rupture of the membranes (Table 15–2).

Table 15–1. Neonatal Deaths from Hyaline Membrane Disease: United States

| Year | Neonatal Deaths | | Live Births $\times 10^3$ | | |
	HMD	All Causes	Total	<2.5 kg	<2.5 kg (Per Cent)
1968	8273	56,456	3502.	286.	8.2
1970	9767	57,279	3137.	294.	9.4
1972	8962	44,432	3258.	249.	7.6
1974	8242	38,738	3146.	234.	7.4
1976	6836	34,587	3168.	229.	7.2
1978	5536	31,618	3333.	236.	7.1

(From Perelman and Farrell: Pediatrics 70:570, 1982.)

Table 15–2. Categorization of Observations in Hyaline Membrane Disease*†

Established	Probable	Possible
Epidemiology		
Worldwide	Second-born twin at greater risk	Maternal diabetes predisposes
Prematurity predisposes	PROM spares	Maternal hemorrhage predisposes
C-Section without labor predisposes	IUGR spares	Familial predisposition
Perinatal asphyxia predisposes	Maternal toxemia spares	Prenatal corticoids spare
Male mortality >female		Maternal heroin addiction spares
		Late pulmonary sequelae
Clinical signs		
Onset near the time of birth	Fine inspiratory rales	Pulmonary edema
Retractions and tachypnea	Hypothermia	PDA murmur
Expiratory grunt	Peripheral edema	
Cyanosis		
Systematic hypotension		
Characteristic chest radiograph		
Course to death or recovery lasts 3 to 5 days		
Pathophysiology		
Reduced lung compliance	Poor peripheral perfusion	Myocardial malconduction
Reduced FRC	Poor renal perfusion	
Poor lung distensibility		
Poor alveolar stability		
Right-to-left shunts		
Reduced effective pulmonary blood flow		
Pathobiochemistry		
Respiratory acidosis	Hyperbilirubinemia	Hyperkalemia
Metabolic acidosis	Decreased total serum proteins	Pepsinogen in lung
Decreased saturated P-lipids	Decreased fibrinolysins	
Preceded by low AF L/S ratio		
Preceded by low AF surfactant titer		
Pathology		
Atelectasis	Osmiophilic lamellar bodies decreased early, increased later	Small adrenal glands
Injury to epithelial cells		Intracranial hemorrhage
Membrane contains fibrin and cellular products		
Etiology		
Surfactant deficiency during disease	Primary surfactant deficiency (in utero)	Absent corticoid stimulus (in utero)
		DPL synthesis impaired and/or destruction increased
		Autonomic dysfunction
		Primary pulmonary hypoperfusion
		Hypovolemia

* From Farrell, P., and Avery, M. E.: Am. Rev. Resp. Dis. 111:657, 1975.

† The following abbreviations are used in this table: PROM—prolonged rupture of membranes (>16 hours); IUGR—intrauterine growth retardation; PDA—patent ductus arteriosus; FRC—functional residual capacity; AF—amniotic fluid; L/S—lecithin-sphingomyelin ratio; DPL—dipalmitoyl lecithin.

Cesarean Section. Infants delivered by cesarean section are at risk for hyaline membrane disease. Since the reasons for operative delivery may in themselves be related to lung immaturity, it is not possible to assign a causal role to mode of delivery. About 4 per cent of all infants delivered by section will have hyaline membrane disease (Hardy et al., 1979). In the British Perinatal Study, infants delivered before the onset of labor were at greater risk than those whose mothers had begun labor. This observation, also reported by Worthington and colleagues, was interesting because of the possibility that the increase in maternal glucocorticoids that occurs near term could promote lung maturation. Section before labor might deprive the infant of the physiologic hormonal stimulus to maturation. The Collaborative Perinatal Study of babies born between 1959 and 1966 confirmed the association of hyaline membrane disease and section but did not show any relationship between the disease and labor. The Perinatal Study did confirm the relationship between hyaline membrane disease and breech delivery. Respiratory distress syndrome was reported in 5.8 per cent of white babies and 7.8 per cent of black babies delivered by the breech method. They were of low birth weight, and, consequently, immaturity rather than presentation at delivery was probably an important confounding factor.

Maternal Diabetes. A relationship between maternal diabetes and hyaline membrane disease has been documented since the 1950s, when hyaline membrane disease was noted to be the outstanding finding at autopsy in infants of diabetic mothers (Driscoll et al., 1960). At that time, physicians delivered most infants of diabetic mothers by section between the thirty-sixth and thirty-seventh weeks of pregnancy without any means of assessing the degree of lung maturity.

During the past 20 years, dramatic reductions in mortality have been associated with newer approaches to monitoring fetal well-being, performing more vaginal deliveries close to term, and developing improved neonatal intensive care. In a 1978 review of 10 years of experience with insulin-dependent diabetic women, Kitzmiller and coworkers found that the perinatal mortality was 3.4 per cent and the incidence of severe respiratory distress was 7 per cent, and they reported only two deaths due to hyaline membrane disease among 147 infants. Similar benefits of improved perinatal care were reported by Lemons and coworkers in 1981.

Nonetheless, an association between maternal diabetes and hyaline membrane disease remains established, as reported by Robert and colleagues in 1976. In a retrospective review, they controlled for the confounding factors of gestational age, route of delivery, sex, and maternal complications other than diabetes, and they noted the relative risk of respiratory distress to be 5.6 times higher in infants of diabetic mothers.

Subsequently, it has become evident that indices of fetal lung maturity, such as the lecithin-sphingomyelin ratio, or concentration of saturated phosphatidylcholine in amniotic fluid, may be within the normal range, and the infant still may have severe respiratory distress syndrome when maternal diabetes is present. According to some authors, using measures of amniotic fluid phosphatidylglycerol and disaturated lecithins can reduce the frequency of false-positive tests.

In an effort to understand these phenomena, Sosenko and coworkers carried out a series of studies in rabbits made diabetic by treatment with alloxan before mating. Blood glucose concentrations were elevated to 200 to 400 mg/dl throughout pregnancy. The fetuses were delivered before term and compared with the controls, normal rabbits. In this study, no differences were found in the quantities of surface-active lipids in the lungs, even though the lungs of the pups of diabetic rabbits were less stable as measured by pressure-volume relationships and less mature histologically. Others have suggested that surfactant lipids are altered in the lungs of offspring of "diabetic" mothers. Prenatal glucocorticoids were effective in normalizing (but not enhancing) lung maturation in these animals, just as they may be in infants of human diabetic mothers.

The reasons for the disturbed lung function in the infant of the diabetic mother remain unexplained. What is certain is that rigorous control of maternal hyperglycemia improves the outlook for the pregnancy and minimizes the pulmonary complications in the newborn infant.

Pathology. On gross examination, the lungs are voluminous and liver-like, and they generally sink in water or formalin. Under the microscope, much of the lung appears solid, owing to the tight apposition of most of the alveolar walls. Scattered throughout are dilated air spaces, respiratory bronchioles, alveolar ducts, and a few alveoli, some of whose walls are lined with pink-staining "hyaline" material containing fibrin and cellular debris. The capillaries are strikingly congested, and there may be pulmonary edema and lymphatic distention (Figs. 15–1 and 15–2).

Epithelial necrosis in the terminal bronchioles at sites underlying the membrane suggests that a reaction to injury has taken place. Hypersecretion is evident, and reparative phenomena such as a proliferation of type II cells are evident in infants who die in the second or third day of life.

The most striking abnormality at autopsy is that it is impossible to inflate the lungs, even with pressures in excess of those applied during life. On deflation, the lungs become airless. This phenomenon is in contrast to the behavior of lungs of infants without surfactant deficiency. Although they may also be airless and liver-like after death, inflation with air is possible, and air is retained on deflation to atmospheric pressures.

Pathogenesis. Although numerous explanations concerning pathogenesis have been proposed since the first clinical description of this condition in 1949, the weight of evidence supports the central role of immaturity of the lung, particularly with respect to surfactant synthesis or suppression of synthesis adequate to meet postnatal demands, as, for example, by asphyxia. The observations that support the role of surfactant deficiency include (1) the epidemiologic finding of a higher incidence in more immature infants; (2) the postmortem biochemical observations of lungs of infants who die with the disorder; (3) the high order of predictability of this disease in the presence of low levels of lecithin (especially disaturated phosphatidylcholine) in amniotic liquid; (4) the reduced likelihood of the disease following events that accelerate lung maturation, such as intrauterine stress in association with intrauterine growth retardation, maternal heroin addiction, or prenatal glucocorticoid therapy; and (5) the increased likelihood of the disease in the presence of maternal diabetes in which fetal insulin production can oppose the lung-matur-

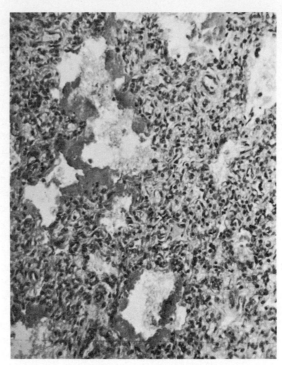

Figure 15–2. Photomicrograph of section of lung of a premature infant weighing 5 pounds (2270 gm) at birth whose dyspnea was first noticed at eight hours and who died after steadily increasing respiratory difficulty at 27 hours. The appearance of the section of lung is in all respects similar to that in Figure 15–1.

ation effect of corticoid. The 3-day course of mild to moderate hyaline membrane disease is also consistent with postnatal induction of enzyme activity with respect to surfactant synthesis.

Surfactant deficiency interferes with lung function by preventing the formation of a functional residual capacity of air by failing to stabilize small air spaces at end-expiration. Each new inspiration requires the application of sufficient transpulmonary pressure to reinflate atelectatic air spaces. High frequencies and large applied pressures are employed to maintain alveolar ventilation. Uneven distribution of inspired air and perfusion of atelectatic air spaces result in poor gas exchange, characterized chiefly by hypoxemia. The infant grunts in an attempt to prolong inspiration, a pattern of breathing that can be shown experimentally to improve alveolar ventilation.

Pulmonary vascular resistance may be raised in some infants by vasoconstriction aggravated by hypoxia, increasing right-to-left shunts through the persistent fetal vascular pathways, ductus arteriosus and foramen ovale. Some blood perfuses airless parts of lung, further contributing to the hypoxemia. As much as 80 per cent of the cardiac output may be shunted past airless lung.

Wasted ventilation and perfusion initiate a series of events that accounts for most of the findings in hyaline membrane disease. For example; reduced oxygenation to the heart impairs cardiac output, which in turn means reduced perfusion of organs

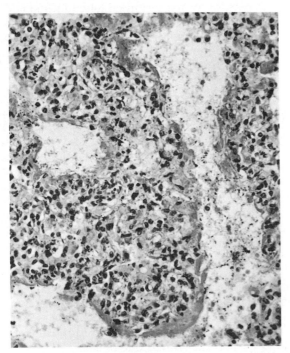

Figure 15–1. Photomicrograph of section of lung of an infant born in the thirty-second week of gestation weighing 3 pounds 10 ounces (1640 gm). He seemed well for one hour; then dyspnea appeared and gradually increased with deepening sternal and costal retraction. He died at 22 hours of age. One sees unexpanded lung, with dilated air spaces lined with thick, homogeneously staining membrane.

Table 15–3. Differential Diagnosis of Hyaline Membrane Disease

Condition	Comment
Pneumonia, especially group B streptococcus	More likely if mother has infection. Sometimes indistinguishable from HMD by radiograph.
Spontaneous pneumothorax	More common in term or post-term infants, especially with meconium aspiration.
Transient tachypnea of newborn	More common in term infants and resolves more quickly than HMD.
Congenital cyanotic heart disease, especially anomalous venous return	Other signs of heart disease should be demonstrable by radiograph, ultrasonography, or EKG.
Respiratory tract anomalies, such as hypoplastic lungs with or without diaphragmatic hernia	Should be identified by radiographs.
Neurologic problems	Intracranial hemorrhage may be associated with depression of respiration. Retractions are uncommon in this circumstance, and other signs of CNS dysfunction are usually present.
	Phrenic nerve injury or other causes of diaphragmatic dysfunction should be considered when heart and lungs are normal but respiratory distress is present.

such as the kidney, whose ability to maintain acid-base homeostasis is compromised. Poor perfusion of peripheral tissues contributes to lactic acidemia and a profound metabolic acidosis. The association of intraventricular hemorrhage with hyaline membrane disease may be related to cerebral hypoxia and ischemia or to intravascular coagulation, which is seen in some seriously ill infants.

Elevations of cerebral arterial or venous pressures have been associated with intraventricular hemorrhage in premature infants. Rapid or bolus injections of sodium bicarbonate, blood, or plasma should be avoided in these infants.

Diagnosis. The onset of symptoms occurs within minutes of birth, but often they are not recognized as significant for some hours. Duskiness, tachypnea, grunting, and significant retractions are characteristic. Increasing cyanosis, often relatively unresponsive to increased inspired oxygen concentrations, is a necessary feature of the disease. Air exchange may be reduced; rales may or may not be present. Sometimes, the upper sternum seems prominent as the lower sternum is sucked in with each inspiratory effort.

Rarely, an infant will have normal respirations for as long as 12 to 18 hours of age and then develop increasing respiratory distress. This variant, which we call "late onset respiratory distress syndrome," may relate to consumption of surfactant in the presence of an inability to synthesize or secrete adequate amounts.

Death is most likely to occur within the first 24 hours but may be much later with use of ventilators and other life-support interventions.

CASE 15–1

The infant was a 1070-gm boy of 28 weeks gestation, born vaginally with Pitocin augmentation of labor because of white cell count and temperature elevation in the mother. Rupture of membranes had occurred 12 hours before delivery, and terbutaline and dexamethasone had been started. Apgar scores were 8 at 1 and 5 minutes. Mild flaring and grunting occurred in the first hour. With an inspired oxygen concentration of 40 per cent, transcutaneous O_2 was approximately 120 torr. Because his condition was stable, an umbilical artery catheter was withdrawn after 20 hours, and feedings were started. The initial chest radiograph was read as normal. Respiratory signs and need for ambient oxygen had disappeared by 1 to 2 hours of age.

By 24 hours, the infant had transcutaneous O_2 readings of 50 to 60 torr and was placed in 25 per cent O_2 with a good response. Radiographic changes are shown

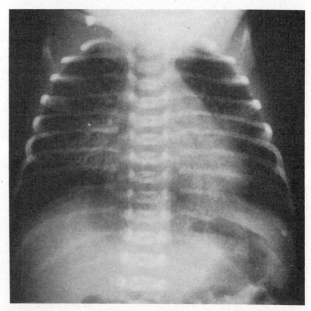

Figure 15–3. Initial radiograph at about 4 hours of age was normal. On the second day of life, evidence of moderate hyaline membrane disease was present on the film shown here. Follow-up radiograph at 9 days of age showed clearing of reticulogranular infiltrates.

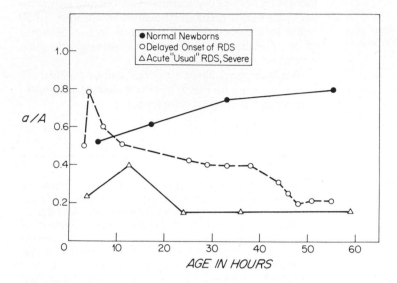

Figure 15–4. Arterial/alveolar oxygen tension is plotted against the postnatal age of the infant whose radiograph is illustrated in Figure 15–3 (○——○). These measurements are contrasted with those from normal infants (●——●) and with those from an infant with severe "classic" hyaline membrane disease, or RDS (△——△).

in Figure 15–3. Respirations increased at this time to 60 to 70/min with mild retractions. The subsequent course is illustrated in Figure 15–4, which shows that the a/A ratios (arterial P_{O_2}/alveolar P_{O_2}) for this infant contrasted with those from normal infants and with those from an infant with classic hyaline membrane disease. Oxygen requirements and symptoms in-creased, and from days 3 to 7 of life the infant had moderately severe respiratory distress with a consistent chest radiograph and was finally transferred to an intensive care unit, where after a week of respirator support he was weaned and did well.

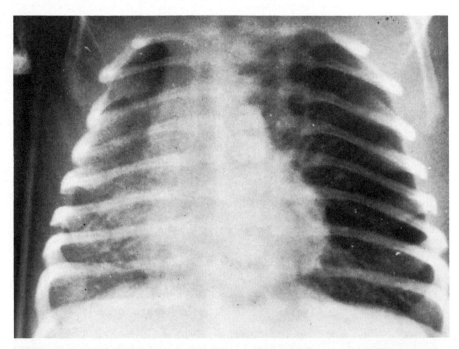

Figure 15–5. Anteroposterior view of chest of a premature infant with typical hyaline membrane disease on the second day of life. Fine reticulogranular markings can still be seen at the left base. They have disappeared from view in the remainder of the left lung, which has become markedly emphysematous. They have become coarser and more crowded in the right lung as it has become more atelectatic.

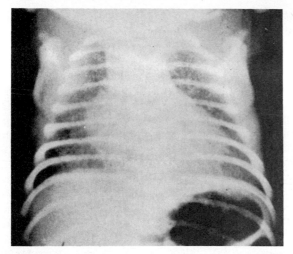

Figure 15–6. Anteroposterior view of thorax taken on the second day of life. Note the universal symmetrical, finely reticulogranular appearance of both lung fields.

Comment. With the clear chest radiograph, no increased oxygen requirement, and no respiratory signs from 2 to 18 hours of life, this infant, in whom no infection could be proved, appears to illustrate delayed onset respiratory distress. Whether this illness represents a slow depletion of alveolar surfactant with gradual appearance of increased alveolar fluid or atelectasis or both is unclear. It is not known whether this disease follows particular dose/duration effects of adrenergics and steroids.

The usual differential diagnosis is summarized in Table 15–3.

Radiographic Findings. The earliest findings are a fine miliary mottling of the lungs, with central consolidation. The air-filled tracheobronchial tree stands out in relief against the opacified hila, which often obscure the cardiothymic silhouette. The radiographic appearance may change minute to minute, depending on the recent lung-volume history. For example, a good cry can aerate both lungs, and a deep inspiratory effort may show minimal disease. Expiration, particularly after oxygen breathing, can lead to gas-freeing of lungs and a virtual "white-out" of the thorax.

The miliary reticulogranularity of the lung parenchyma is usually present within minutes of birth. Occasionally, the changes are more prominent in the right than in the left hemithorax, and they are sometimes more evident in lower lobes than in upper lobes (Figs. 15–5, 15–6, and 15–7).

During the course of the disease, the radiograph may show a number of changes, including interstitial emphysema, pneumomediastinum, and pneumothorax. In some infants, recovery is slow, and complex radiologic changes occur over subsequent months (see Chapter 16).

Prenatal Diagnosis. Recognition that a deficiency of alveolar surfactant is an essential aspect of hyaline membrane disease and knowledge that lung liquids contribute to amniotic liquid led to a search for components of the surfactant in amniotic liquid. Gluck and coworkers first established the relationship between a low lecithin-sphingomyelin ratio and clinical respiratory distress, establishing the ability to predict with a greater than 90 per cent accuracy which infant was at risk (Figs. 15–8 and 15–9).

Other approaches to prenatal diagnosis, such as the foam stability test of Clements, have subsequently found wide use among obstetricians. Since the phospholipids that are most surface-active are saturated, a measure of the concentration of disaturated phosphatidylcholine allows greater accuracy in studies on amniotic fluid, even in the presence of

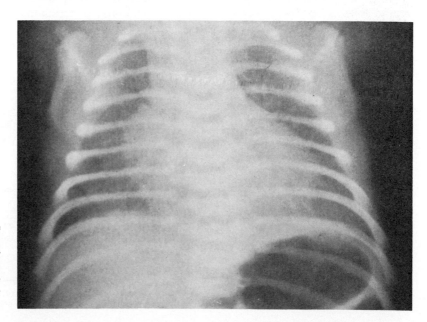

Figure 15–7. Anteroposterior view of chest of a prematurely born twin. Tachypnea began immediately after birth and was followed by increasing dyspnea. One sees the fine reticulogranular opacities scattered homogeneously throughout both lungs.

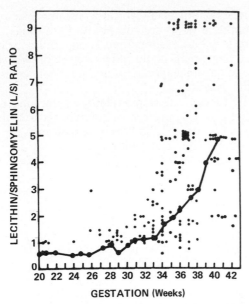

Figure 15–8. Note the wide variation among individuals of the same gestational age. The lecithin-sphingomyelin ratio is a better index of lung "maturity" than is gestational age. (Data of L. Gluck et al.) (From Farrell, P. M., and Avery, M. E.: Am. Rev. Resp. Dis. *111*:657, 1975.)

blood or mucus. Torday and colleagues introduced this test, which we use routinely when prediction of lung maturity is to be made from amniotic fluid samples.

Treatment

Mechanical Ventilation. Over the past 20 years, more experience with ever smaller babies and constantly improving equipment have made the outlook increasingly positive for infants who require mechanical ventilation, or, as it used to be called, "artificial respiration." For example, during the 1960s many questioned the wisdom of even trying to ventilate a baby whose birth weight was under 1 kg. Now the majority of such small infants are given assistance with their breathing from the first minutes after birth. In general, the infants are ventilated when they are not breathing regularly on their own (i.e., when they are having apneic spells) or when it is evident, from measurements of the oxygen and carbon dioxide in their blood, that they are not maintaining adequate gas exchange. In general, when the infant cannot maintain an arterial partial pressure of oxygen of 50 mm Hg when breathing 100 per cent oxygen or when the carbon dioxide tension in the blood is greater than 65 mm Hg, the consequences to the infant are predictably devastating unless mechanical ventilation is employed.

Our usual criterion for mechanical ventilation is a Pa_{CO_2} of about 50 mm Hg that is rising on repeat 15-minute checks. We would be slower to start ven-

tilation for an infant of over 1750 gm than for a smaller infant (1000 gm).

Ventilators are designed with settings that allow adjustment of rate, the inspiratory and expiratory durations, and adjustment of peak inspiratory pressure and end-expiratory pressure. The peak inspiratory pressure is the pressure required to move an adequate volume of air into the lungs, and the end-expiratory pressure is the pressure maintained at the end of expiration to prevent the lungs from going to too small a volume. Typical initial respirator settings would be peak inspiratory 25 cm H_2O, end-expiratory pressure 5 cm H_2O, inspiratory duration 1 sec, rate 25/min. Currently, almost all infants are intubated. We prefer nasotracheal intubation to orotracheal intubation because we believe that the nasotracheal tube, owing to its smaller diameter, is associated with a smaller risk of subglottic stenosis. Sometimes, the infants are given muscle relaxants such as pancuronium so that they do not fight the ventilator, but of course they then become totally ventilator-dependent. In very small infants, orotracheal intubation may be the only feasible route.

Because fixed tidal volume breathing, whether spontaneous or supplied by a respirator, leads to progressive atelectasis, some provision must be made for "sighing." Either the infant takes occasional large breaths spontaneously (crying while intubated) or sighs can be provided by suctioning and bagging intermittently (1 to 3 hours, depending on secretions and Pa_{O_2} lability during the procedure) or by having the ventilator provide sighs every 5 to 10 minutes (see Chapter 10).

During the recovery phase of the respiratory distress syndrome, many infants become dependent on intermittent mandatory ventilation (IMV). The infants breathe spontaneously, but about ten times per minute their inspiratory effort can trigger an assist from a ventilator that accomplishes a tidal volume two to three times as great as that which would be achieved spontaneously.

Infants breathing spontaneously show a "breath-upon-a-breath" phenomenon, or an inflation aug-

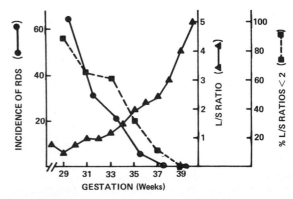

Figure 15–9. Comparison of incidence figures for RDS with average values of lecithin/sphingomyelin in amniotic liquid. Each value is plotted as a function of gestational age. (From Farrell, P. M., and Avery, M. E.: Am. Rev. Resp. Dis. *111*:657, 1975.)

mentation reflex. These gasps are more frequent on the first and third days of life and accomplish an increase in the functional residual capacity of the baby (Thach and Taeusch, 1976). Intermittent mandatory ventilation does, in effect, the same thing. During many hours of observation with IMV, it was noted that infants did not have any spontaneous sighs. This observation supports the thesis that the sigh in a normal infant is triggered by low lung volume, presumably through stretch receptors, and the maintenance of a normal functional residual capacity with a ventilator eliminates the necessity for a sigh.

Complications of mechanical ventilation are unfortunately all too frequent. It is worth noting that the need for mechanical ventilation immediately determines that an infant has disease of significant severity, and many "ventilator complications" are therefore attributable to the disease and not to the ventilator. Major air leaks (pneumothorax or interstitial emphysema) occur in approximately 25 per cent of the infants who require mechanical ventilation (Madansky et al., 1979). Ultrasonographic examination may reveal some evidence of intraventricular hemorrhage in as many as 40 per cent of these ba-

bies, although it is not clear that that event is associated with use of the ventilator. It may well be a consequence of being very premature and having circulatory problems associated with asphyxia during or shortly after birth. Nonetheless, there is an association between bleeding into the ventricles of the brain and the requirement of mechanical ventilation. Lazzara and coworkers found that 68 of their 98 infants with intraventricular hemorrhage seen on CT scan had been ventilated or maintained on continuous distending airway pressure. Not all hemorrhages are of clinical significance.

These observations have stimulated a search for ways to promote gas exchange more effectively at lower pressures. The introduction of very high frequency ventilation (over 300 breaths/minute) or oscillator respirators is promising. Preliminary studies by the Toronto group on animals established the possibility of maintaining normal gas exchange with tidal volumes less than the dead space and with mean pressures lower than those required with conventional ventilators. The method represents a new approach to mechanical ventilation based on enhanced diffusion of gases produced by the turbulence associated with very high frequency oscillations (Bohn et al., 1980). Frantz and colleagues in Boston have successfully ventilated infants whose course of hyaline membrane disease was complicated by interstitial emphysema with ventilatory rates of 600/min (10 Hz) and lower peak pressures than required by conventional ventilators (25 cm H_2O instead of 45 cm H_2O). Marchak and coworkers from Toronto have preliminary encouraging results.

Infants who survive the first week or so of illness may become ventilator- and oxygen-dependent. Typically, they undergo a series of changes in their lungs characterized by air-trapping, atelectasis, fibrosis, cyst formation, and basilar emphysema. Originally described by Northway and Rosan in 1968 as "bronchopulmonary dysplasia," this condition is now well known to everyone caring for premature infants. The course is chronic, sometimes lasting for months or years, with complete recovery a possibility, although death from intercurrent illness is a constant threat. At autopsy, the lungs are heavy, hypercellular, and fibrotic, with squamous metaplasia of even smaller airways. Since the cilia are gone, it is not surprising that secretions pool; either atelectasis or lobular emphysema is common.

Increasingly, as the number of survivors of mechanical ventilation grows, we note atelectasis of the right upper lobe after extubation (Finer, 1979). Even when extubation occurs at 2 to 3 cm H_2O continuous distending pressure, lobar atelectasis may occur in as many as 40 to 50 per cent of infants. We position the infants on their left side to allow maximal pleural pressures to be applied on the right side. Gentle chest vibration, advocated by Finer, may be useful.

Table 15–4. Priorities in Initial Evaluation of Infant with Respiratory Distress

Assess	Response
Ventilation	Provide oxygen as indicated by cyanosis. Ventilate by mask and bag or through endotracheal tube if infant is unable to move sufficient air.
Circulation	Listen to heart, measure blood pressure, pulse, hematocrit. Provide blood or other volume expander if infant is in shock or anemic.
Temperature	Provide sufficient heat to bring axillary temperature to 37.5°C and to prevent peripheral vasoconstriction.
Cause of respiratory distress	Locate cardiac impulse. Transilluminate. Obtain chest radiograph.
Level of maturity	Estimate gestational age by appearance and responses. Weigh infant.
Possibility of infection	Obtain cultures of blood, amniotic fluid, blood count. Administer antibiotics.
Metabolic status	Measure pH, blood gases, blood glucose, and treat according to findings.
History	Review with parents events of pregnancy and family history, and keep them informed realistically of the changing status of the infant.

The very compliant chest walls of small premature infants, whose resting end-expiratory pressure may be only 1 to 2 cm H_2O below atmospheric pressure, makes them prone to atelectasis. The weak gag reflex and ineffective coughing make these infants dependent on frequent suctioning to clear secretions. Frequent changes of position, with preference for the prone position, should help prevent this problem. (Lung volume is higher when the infant is prone than when he is supine because of the position of the diaphragm.)

Bronchopulmonary dysplasia, a chronic lung disorder in premature infants who have been ventilated, is less common when the duration of high concentrations of inspired oxygen is reduced by continuous distending airway pressure or prolonged inspiratory-expiratory ratios. The similarity of the lesion to that of chronic oxygen toxicity is striking, and it may be related to oxygen alone. The contribution of high applied airway pressures to the pathogenesis of the lesion remains a possibility, supported by the experimental production of lung injury by barotrauma in

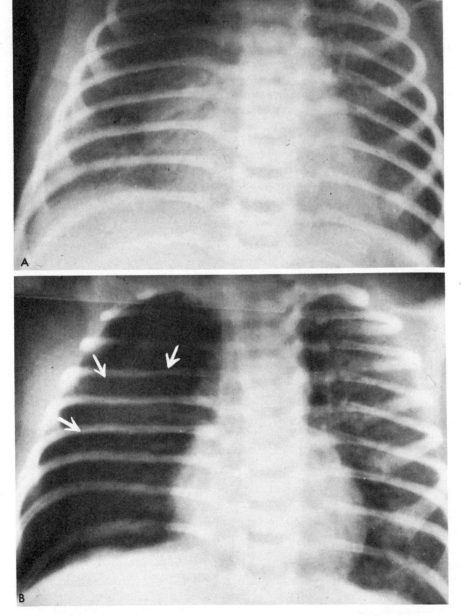

Figure 15–10. *A*, Film taken at eight hours of age shows the reticulogranular pattern in the left lung and right base, while the right upper lobe is distinctly hyperinflated. *B*, Six hours later. Now rupture has occurred on the right side, and a large pneumothorax can be seen surrounding the collapsed right lung.

prematurely delivered rabbits (Nilsson et al., 1978) (see Chapter 16).

Surfactant Replacement. Ever since it was realized that hyaline membrane disease was the consequence of surfactant deficiency, attempts have been made to replace this substance by aerosol to deliver some surface-active constituents of the alveolar lining layer to the lung. Preliminary reports in humans by Chu and coworkers in 1967 and by Ivey and colleagues in 1976 with dipalmitoyl lecithin either alone or with phosphatidylglycerol were not impressive enough to justify further investigation. Meanwhile, some success in rabbits and lambs with homologous surfactant seemed encouraging (Enhorning and Robertson, 1972; Adams et al., 1978; Metcalfe et al., 1982).

The most impressive result was described by Fujiwara and coworkers, who modified minced cow's lung by extraction with acetone and addition of surface-active phospholipids. They instilled the mixture into the endotracheal tube and positioned the infants so as to promote spreading. Dramatic improvement in blood gases occurred within 20 minutes to 3 hours.

The duration of surface activity after instillation of labeled natural surfactant into premature lambs was only about 3 hours in the studies of Ikegami and colleagues. They postulate the presence of a protein leak that inhibits surface active properties.

These preliminary observations will surely stimulate further efforts to find an "ideal" surfactant for use in all surfactant deficiency states.

Other Supportive Measures. Nutritional support of the sick low birth weight infant is essential to recovery from disease as well as to growth. Experience teaches us that aspiration is more likely to occur with high respiratory rates and respiratory distress. For this reason, intravenous fluids are begun early in the course of the disease. If metabolic acidosis is present on the first day of life, 10 per cent glucose with $NaHCO_3$ (5 to 15 mEq per 100 ml solution) is appropriate in a volume of 60 to 120 ml/kg body weight. If the infant is breathing air saturated with water vapor in a fully saturated environment, water needs may be closer to 50 ml/kg; in a dry environment and with high respiratory rates without a respirator, approximately 100 to 150 ml/kg or more may be more appropriate. Fluid and electrolyte balance may be difficult to achieve in a small, sick infant on a ventilator. Requirements may change precipitously and, sometimes, unpredictably. Serial determinations of serum sodium, administered as often as every 4 hours, may be required in the first days of life. Over the following days it seems important to keep infants in positive balance with respect to calories, nitrogen, and glucose. The addition of amino acid mixtures and lipid emulsions to intravenous therapy seems to be a major advance in management. Although many details remain to be evaluated, it now appears that there is little excuse to impose starvation upon sick premature infants.

Temperature Regulation. Maintenance of a thermal-neutral environment (defined as that thermal environment in which oxygen consumption is at a minimum) seems to improve survival of sick low birth weight infants. Even a few degrees can change oxygen consumption and, hence, metabolic demands and, in turn, ventilatory requirements. The goal is to keep the infant in a thermal neutral state, with skin temperature about 36.5° C and core temperature at 37° C. We use a servo-controlled heating system that responds to a sensor applied to the skin over the upper abdominal wall. Very small infants do best under a plastic shell that serves as a heat shield to reduce losses by convection. Peripheral vasoconstriction is a sign of an adverse thermal environment and can be used to indicate whether or not incubator temperatures are appropriate.

Persistent Patent Ductus Arteriosus (see also p. 278). With increasing survival of low birth weight infants, we are seeing a growing number of infants with symptomatic patent ductus arteriosus. Many are convalescing from their respiratory distress when a systolic or continuous murmur becomes evident, respiratory effort increases, the heart enlarges, and, sometimes, a bounding pulse appears. Pulmonary edema can be detected by the appearance of rales and further opacification of the lung fields on radiographs. Echocardiograms are very useful in visualizing left atrial enlargement. If the ratio between left atrial and aortic diameters exceeds 1.87, a significant left-to-right shunt exists. Serial measurements are most useful in assessing whether pharmacologic or surgical intervention is indicated.

Some infants can be managed with fluid restriction and diuretics such as furosemide, 1 mg/kg/dose as needed. Digitalis is indicated in the presence of congestive failure, although it may not be effective if the duct remains widely patent. We use intravenous digoxin, 30 μg/kg over 12 to 24 hours. A maintenance dose of 10 to 15 μg/kg/day rarely results in toxicity. Oral feedings should be withheld during the acute phase of congestive failure.

The ductus can sometimes close with arterial oxygen tensions at 60 to 80 torr. When it remains patent, the next intervention is indomethacin, a prostaglandin inhibitor first proposed by Friedman and coworkers. Subsequent extensive experience, including a controlled prospective clinical trial, established the usefulness of this agent and, importantly, the lack of any serious toxicity. The dose used in the Collaborative Controlled Trial was 0.2 mg/kg, administered intravenously. Impaired renal function is the only recognized contraindication. No long-term morbidity was found in the study reported by Merritt and colleagues.

Some infants do not respond to pharmacologic interventions and require surgical ligation. Excellent results have been reported from centers in which cardiac surgeons are experienced with this operation. Improvement is immediate once the ductus is closed.

Prevention. Very soon after the initial observation that glucocorticoids accelerated lung maturation in the fetal lamb, Liggins and Howie undertook a prospective controlled clinical trial, first reported in 1972 and later with follow-up studies in 1977 (Howie and Liggins, 1977). Their findings of a significant reduction in the respiratory distress syndrome when betamethasone was given at least 24 hours before birth in infants under 32 weeks' gestation have been widely confirmed. In the dozen published controlled trials, respiratory distress occurred in the controls about three times as often as in the treated patients, and mortality was correspondingly reduced (Caspi, 1976; Block et al., 1977; Papageorgiou et al., 1979; Ballard et al., 1979; Taeusch et al., 1979). Betamethasone or dexamethasone has been given intramuscularly to the mother, usually in 6-mg doses every 12 hours for 2 days before birth. Hydrocortisone was used by Dluholucky and colleagues in 1976 in a single 100-mg dose intramuscularly and by Morrison and coworkers in 1978 in 500-mg doses administered intravenously every 12 hours, with a total of four doses. Liggins recommends repeat doses if delivery does not occur in 7 days. Studies of lambs conducted by Taeusch and colleagues in 1981 support the need for repeat treatment, since the effect on surfactant production may not be sustained. The Collaborative Group trial of antenatal dexamethasone (5 mg I.M. every 12 hours, up to 4 doses) was a prospective controlled clinical trial that showed a reduction of respiratory distress syndrome in treated infants. An important finding in this trial was that the benefit was restricted to the female infants. No significant complications were noted among the mothers or the infants. At follow-up at 40 weeks postconceptual age, the infants whose mothers received dexamethasone performed as well as their placebo-treated controls on the Prechtl neurologic assessment. A 4-year follow-up of infants of mothers who were treated with betamethasone antenatally, reported from New Zealand, showed that no adverse effects could be demonstrated by the detailed psychologic tests administered to 144 infants of treated mothers compared with 114 control patients (MacArthur et al., 1981).

Concern about possible short- or long-term complications of glucocorticoids given prenatally has delayed wide acceptance of this intervention. A number of studies in animals with shorter gestation periods and in monkeys, reviewed by Taeusch in 1975, establish the occurrence of significant and sometimes lethal effects on the fetus. In 1973, Carson and coworkers noted a 12 per cent reduction in lung weight and cell number in rabbits after prenatal administration of glucocorticoid, which Kotas and associates found reversible by about 3 weeks of age. In the monkey, no change in lung size occurs, although remarkable enhancement of distensibility follows prenatal administration of betamethasone (Mintzer et al., 1979). The same authors have alerted us to possible reductions in placenta, thymus, adrenal weights, and head circumference in monkeys after prenatal administration of glucocorticoids.

Contrasting with these worrisome observations in animals is the larger human experience with maternal glucocorticoid administration, often prescribed throughout pregnancy in therapeutic doses because of maternal illness. In 1977, Koppe and coworkers reviewed the experience with treated mothers in Holland and found no adverse effects on the fetus. In a study of infants in the New Zealand clinical trial of Liggins and Howie, which included over 300 treated infants, Howie reported no differences at 4 years of age between treated and control infants (Howie, 1977).

The response to betamethasone is greater among female than among male fetuses, as shown in the Collaborative Group trial. It remains to be seen whether this results from the differences in lung maturation known to exist between the sexes, as described in rabbits by Kotas and Avery in 1980, or represents some type of hormonal antagonism. Evidence of hormonal effects comes from studies on rabbits. Nielsen and coworkers have inhibited normal lung maturation in fetal female rabbit pups by injecting the pregnant doe with testosterone. They also noted that male fetal rabbits with male neighbors in the uterine horn have the least mature lungs, that females with male neighbors come next, and that the most mature lungs are found in females with female neighbors. They postulate that a hormonal influence from the male delays lung maturation.

The effects of maternal betamethasone on steroid and growth hormone levels in premature infants were studied by Ballard and colleagues in 1980. In the doses used by Liggins and Howie in 1972, betamethasone resulted in lower levels of cortisol and growth hormone in cord blood. Betamethasone levels in cord blood had about the same glucocorticoid potency as that found in normal infants from endogenous cortisol. By 2 days of age, infants of mothers who received betamethasone who were exposed to neonatal stress achieved levels of cortisol similar to those in untreated controls. Growth hormone levels were above those in controls by 2 to 4 postnatal days. In our view, glucocorticoids are indicated if the mother's health permits, if delivery can be delayed at least 24 hours, and if fetal lung immaturity is likely. A lecithin-sphingomyelin ratio for amniotic fluid or some other measure of surfactant adequacy in the fetal lung is helpful but not always available, especially in infants under 32 weeks. We have too little experience with infants under 28 weeks to be confident that these drugs will be of benefit to them. In animal studies, the effect is greater just before normal maturation of surfactant synthesis. Thus, in the human, the effect may be less in very immature infants. Neither maternal toxemia nor diabetes necessarily contraindicates the use of prenatal glucocorticoids, although careful attention to blood pressure and blood glucose is mandatory.

Future directions will surely include evaluation of other means of accelerating lung maturation. Thyroid hormones can also stimulate lung development by a different mechanism than that of glucocorticoids (Hitchcock, 1979). Smith has evidence from studies in tissue culture that the fibroblasts may be the major target cells for glucocorticoids, and T_3 sensitizes the Type II alveolar cells to a fibroblast pneumonocyte factor.

Ballard and coworkers have found that a synthetic analogue of thyroxin accelerates lung maturation in fetal lambs. These promising animal studies will surely stimulate development of clinical trials in which efforts will be made to reduce the incidence of respiratory distress syndrome further.

Prognosis. The chances of survival of infants with hyaline membrane disease who require ventilation are directly related to their birth weights. Those who are born after 34 weeks gestation and who need ventilation in the first hours of life have more than 90 per cent chance of surviving. Those born between 28 and 33 weeks have at least a 75 per cent chance of survival, and those between 26 and 28 weeks have, on the average, about a 50 per cent chance of survival. For infants whose birth weight is less than 1.0 kg, the chances of survival are improving every year but depend very much on the gestational age of the infant: The more mature the infant, the better the outlook. Rarely does an infant of less than 600 gm birth weight survive.

Follow-up of infants who have recovered from the disease shows that the majority have no further respiratory dysfunction. Increasingly, in recent years, reports of recurrent lower respiratory tract disease among survivors have suggested that either the disease or some features of its therapy, such as oxygen or respirators, may have left the lungs unusually susceptible to bronchiolitis.

In 1968, Lewis reported respirator infection requiring hospitalization in 17.5 per cent of 63 survivors, and, in the same year, Shepard and coworkers described bronchiolitis and bronchopneumonia in 33 per cent of nonventilated survivors and in 26 per cent of those who were on respirators.

In a 1977 study of children up to 10 years after their previous respiratory distress syndrome, Coates and colleagues found evidence of an increase in both large and small airway resistance in the surviving infants. Lung volumes and arterial oxygen tensions in the surviving infants with respiratory distress did not differ from those in the premature infants without the disease.

Neurologic sequelae are found in surviving small premature infants, although they are not more frequent among survivors who recovered from respiratory distress than among other infants of similar

birth weight (Robertson and Crichton, 1969; Outerbridge et al., 1974). In 1976, during a 2-year follow-up of 73 infants who presumably would have died without ventilatory assistance, Fitzhardinge and colleagues noted that 16 were significantly handicapped by hydrocephaly, hemiplegia, spastic diplegia, or quadriplegia. A strong correlation was found between major neurologic deficits and a history of seizures or intracranial hemorrhage in the neonatal period. Morbidity was greater in boys than in girls. Lower respiratory tract infections occurred in the first year of life in 24 per cent of the group.

Continual monitoring of the outcome of low birth weight infants, correlated with perinatal interventions, seems mandatory, given the degree of morbidity noted by Fitzhardinge and colleagues in a setting in which all the infants were transported from other hospitals. Whether the results of intramural intensive care of very low birth weight infants will improve remains to be seen.

REFERENCES

Ablow, R. C., and Orzalesi, M. M.: Localized roentgenographic pattern of hyaline membrane disease. Evidence that the upper lobes of human lung mature earlier than the lower lobes. Am. J. Roentgenol. *112*:23, 1971.

Adams, F. H., et al.: Effects of tracheal instillation of natural surfactant in premature lambs. I. Clinical and autopsy findings. Pediatr. Res. *12*:841, 1978.

Auld, P. A. M., Bhangananda, P., and Mehta, S.: The influence of an early caloric intake with I-V glucose on catabolism of premature infants. Pediatrics *37*:592, 1966.

Avery, M. E.: Pharmacological approaches to acceleration of fetal lung maturation. Br. Med. Bull. *31*:131, 1975.

Avery, M. E., Fletcher, B. D., and Williams, R. G.: The Lung and Its Disorders in the Newborn Infant. 4th ed. Philadelphia, W. B. Saunders Company, 1981.

Avery, M. E., and Mead, J.: Surface properties in relation to atelectasis and hyaline membrane disease. Am. J. Dis. Child. *97*:517, 1959.

Ballard, P. L., Ballard, R. A., Granberg, J. P., Sniderman, S., Gluckman, P. D., Kaplan, S. L., and Grumbach, M. M.: Fetal sex and prenatal betamethasone therapy. J. Pediatr. *97*:451, 1980.

Ballard, P. L., Benson, B. J., Brehier, A., Carter, J. P., Kriz, B. M., and Jorgensen, E. C.: Transplacental stimulation of lung development in the fetal rabbit by 3,5-dimethyl-3'-isopropyl-L-thyronine. J. Clin. Invest. *65*:1407, 1980.

Ballard, P. L., Gluckman, P. D., Liggins, G. C., Kaplan, S. L., and Grumbach, M. M.: Steroid and growth hormone levels in premature infants after prenatal betamethasone therapy to prevent respiratory distress syndrome. Pediatrics *14*:122, 1980.

Ballard, R. A., Ballard, P. L., Granberg, J. P., and Sniderman, S.: Prenatal administration of betamethasone for prevention of respiratory distress syndrome. J. Pediatr. *94*:97, 1979.

Bancalari, E., Garcia, O. L., and Jesse, M. J.: Effects of continuous negative pressure on lung mechanisms in idiopathic respiratory distress syndrome. Pediatrics *51*:485, 1973.

Block, M. F., Kling, O. R., and Crosby, W. M.: Antenatal glucocorticoid therapy for the prevention of respiratory distress syndrome in the premature infant. Obstet. Gynecol. *50*:186, 1977.

Blystad, W., Landing, B. H., and Smith, C. A.: Pulmonary hyaline membranes in newborn infants. Pediatrics *8*:5, 1951.

Bohn, D. J., Miyasaka, K., Marchak, B. E., et al.: Ventilation by high frequency oscillation. J. Appl. Physiol. 48:710, 1980.

Brumley, G. W., Hodson, W. A., and Avery, M. E.: Lung phospholipids and surface tension correlations in infants with and without hyaline membrane disease and in adults. Pediatrics 40:13, 1967.

Carson, S., Taeusch, H. W., Jr., and Avery, M. E.: The effects of cortisol injection on lung growth in fetal rabbits. J. Appl. Physiol. 34:660, 1973.

Caspi, E., Schreyer, P., Weinraub, Z., Reif, R., Levi, I., and Mundel, G.: Prevention of respiratory distress syndrome in premature infants by antepartum glucocorticoid therapy. Br. J. Obstet. Gynecol. 83:187, 1976.

Chu, J., Clements, J. A., Cotton, E. K., et al.: Neonatal pulmonary ischemia. Pediatrics 40:709, 1967.

Clements, J. A., Platzker, A. C. G., Tierney, D. F., et al.: Assessment of the risk of the respiratory distress syndrome by a rapid test for surfactant in amniotic fluid. N. Engl. J. Med. 286:1077, 1972.

Coates, A. L., Bergsteinsson, H., Desmond, K., Outerbridge, E. W., and Beaudry, P. H.: Long-term pulmonary sequelae of premature birth with and without idiopathic respiratory distress syndrome. J. Pediatr. 90:611, 1977.

Collaborative Group of Antenatal Steroid Therapy: Effect of antenatal dexamethasone administration on the prevention of respiratory distress syndrome. Am. J. Obstet. Gynecol. 141:276, 1981.

Davies, P. A., Robinson, R. J., Scopes, J. W., et al.: Medical Care of Newborn Babies. Philadelphia, J. B. Lippincott Co., 1972.

DeLemos, R. A., Shermeta, D. W., Knelson, J. H., et al.: Acceleration of appearance of pulmonary surfactant in the fetal lamb by administration of corticosteroids. Am. Rev. Resp. Dis. 102:459, 1970.

DeReuck, A. V. S., and Porter, R. (Eds.): Ciba Foundation Symposium: Development of the Lung. London, J. & A. Churchill, Ltd., 1967.

Dluholucky, S., Babic, J., and Taufer, I.: Reduction of incidence and mortality by RDS by administration of hydrocortisone to mother. Arch. Dis. Child. 51:420, 1976.

Driscoll, S. G., Benirschke, K., and Curtis, G. W.: Neonatal deaths among infants of diabetic mothers. Am. J. Dis. Child. 100:818, 1960.

Edmunds, L. H., Gregory, G. A., Heymann, M. A., et al.: Surgical closure of ductus arteriosus in premature infants. Circulation 48:856, 1973.

Enhorning, G., and Robertson, B.: Lung expansion in the premature rabbit fetus after tracheal deposition of surfactant. Pediatrics 50:58, 1972.

Evans, J. J.: Prediction of respiratory distress syndrome by shake test on newborn gastric aspirate. N. Engl. J. Med. 292:1113, 1975.

Fanaroff, A. A., Cha, C. C., Sosa, R., et al.: A controlled trial of continuous negative external pressure in the treatment of severe respiratory distress syndrome. J. Pediatr. 82:921, 1973.

Farrell, P. M., and Avery, M. E.: Hyaline membrane disease. State of the art. Am. Rev. Resp. Dis. 111:657, 1975.

Fencl, M., and Tulchinsky, D.: Total cortisol in amniotic fluid and fetal lung maturation. N. Engl. J. Med. 292:133, 1975.

Finer, N. N., Moriartey, R. R., Boyd, J., et al.: Postextubation atelectasis: A retrospective study and a prospective controlled study. J. Pediatr. 94:110, 1979.

Fisch, R. O., Gravem, H. J., and Engle, R. R.: Neurological status of survivors of neonatal respiratory distress syndrome. J. Pediatr. 73:395, 1968.

Fitzhardinge, P. M., Pape, K., Arstikaitis, M., et al.: Mechanical ventilation of infants of less than 1,501 gm. birth weight: health, growth and neurologic sequelae. J. Pediatr. 88:531, 1976.

Frantz, I. D., Stark, A. R., and Dorkin, H. L.: Ventilation of infants at frequencies up to 1800/min. Pediatr. Res. 14:642 (abstract), 1980.

Friedman, W. F., et al.: Pharmacologic closure of patent ductus arteriosus in the premature infant. N. Engl. J. Med. 295:526, 1976.

Fujiwara, T., Maeta, H., Chida, S., Morita, T., Watabe, Y., and Abe, T.: Artificial surfactant therapy in hyaline membrane disease. Lancet 1:55, 1980.

Gandy, G., Jacobson, W., and Gairdner, D.: Hyaline membrane disease. 1. Cellular changes. Arch. Dis. Child. 45:289, 1970.

Gluck, L., and Kulovich, N. V.: Lecithin-sphingomyelin ratios in amniotic fluid in normal and abnormal pregnancy. Am. J. Obstet. Gynecol. 115:539, 1973.

Graven, S. N., and Misenheimer, H. R.: Respiratory distress syndrome and the high risk mother. Am. J. Dis. Child. 109:489, 1965.

Gregory, G. A., Kitterman, J. A., Phibbs, R. H., et al.: Treatment of idiopathic respiratory distress syndrome with continuous positive airway pressure. N. Engl. J. Med. 284:1333, 1971.

Hardy, J. B., Drage, J. S., and Jackson, E. C.: The First Year of Life. The Collaborative Perinatal Project of the National Institute of Neurological and Communicative Disorders and Stroke. Baltimore, Johns Hopkins University Press, 1979.

Harrison, V. C., Heese, H. de V., and Klein, M.: The significance of grunting in hyaline membrane disease. Pediatrics 41:549, 1968.

Heymann, M. A., Rudolph, A. M., and Silverman, N. H.: Closure of the ductus arteriosus in premature infants by inhibition of prostaglandin synthesis. N. Engl. J. Med. 295:530, 1976.

Hitchcock, K. R.: Hormones and the lung. I. Thyroid hormones and glucocorticoids in lung development. Anat. Rec. 194:15, 1979.

Howie, R. N.: Clinical trial of antepartum betamethasone therapy for prevention of respiratory distress syndrome in pre-term infants. In Pre-Term Labour, Proceedings of the 5th Study Group of Royal College of Obstetricians and Gynaecologists, The Royal College, 27 Sussex Place, Regent's Park, London, 1977, p. 281.

Huch, R., Lübbers, D., and Huch, A.: Reliability of transcutaneous monitoring of arterial PO_2 in newborn infants. Arch. Dis. Child. 49:213, 1974.

Ikegami, M., Jobe, A., and Glatz, T.: Surface activity following natural surfactant treatment in premature lambs. J. Appl. Physiol. 51:306, 1981.

Ivey, H. H., Roth, S., and Kattwinkel, J.: Use of nebulized surfactants in treatment of the respiratory distress syndrome of infancy. Pediatr. Res. 10(abstr.):462, 1976.

Kitzmiller, J. L., Cloherty, J. P., Younger, M. D., et al.: Diabetic pregnancy and perinatal morbidity. Am. J. Obstet. Gynecol. 131:560, 1978.

Klaus, M. H., and Fanaroff, A. A.: Care of the High-Risk Neonate. 2nd ed. Philadelphia, W. B. Saunders Company, 1979.

Knelson, J. H., and Avery, M. E.: Site of blood sampling. Letter to editor. Pediatrics 43:638, 1969.

Knelson, J. H., Howatt, W. F., and DeMuth, G. R.: The physiologic significance of grunting respiration. Pediatrics 44:393, 1969.

Koppe, J. G., Smolder-de Haas, H., and Kloosterman, G. J.: Effects of glucocorticoids during pregnancy on the outcome of the children directly after birth and in the long run. Eur. J. Obstet. Gynecol. Reprod. Biol. 7:293, 1977.

Kotas, R. V., and Avery, M. E.: The influence of sex on fetal rabbit lung maturation and on the response to glucocorticoid. Am. Rev. Resp. Dis. 121:377, 1980.

Kotas, R. V., Mims, L. C., and Hart, L. K.: Reversible inhibition of lung cell number after glucocorticoid injection into fetal rabbits to enhance surfactant appearance. Pediatrics 53:358, 1974.

Krouskop, R. W., Brown, E. G., and Sweet, A. Y.: The early use of continuous positive airway pressure in the treatment of idiopathic respiratory distress syndrome. J. Pediatr. 87:263, 1975.

Landing, B. H.: Pulmonary lesions of newborn infants: A statistical study. Pediatrics 19:217, 1957.

Lazzara, A., Ahmann, P., Dykes, F., Brann, A. W., Jr., and Schwartz, J.: Clinical predictability of intraventricular hemorrhage in preterm infants. Pediatrics 65:30, 1980.

Lemons, J. A., Vargas, P., and Delaney, J. J.: Infant of the diabetic mother: review of 225 cases. Obstet. Gynecol. 57:187, 1981.

Lewis, S.: A follow up study of the respiratory distress syndrome. Proc. Soc. Med. 61:771, 1968.

Liggins, G. C., and Howie, R. N.: A controlled trial of antepartum glucocorticoid treatment for prevention of the respiratory distress syndrome in premature infants. Pediatrics 50:515, 1972.

MacArthur, B. A., Howie, R. N., Dezoete, J. A., and Elkins, J.: Cognitive and psychosocial development of 4-year-old children whose mothers were treated antenatally with betamethasone. Pediatrics 68:638, 1981.

Madansky, D. L., Lawson, E. E., Chernick, V., and Taeusch, H. W., Jr.: Pneumothorax and other forms of pulmonary air leak in newborns. Am. Rev. Resp. Dis. 120:729, 1979.

Marchak, B.E., Thompson, W. K., Duffty, P. et al.: Treatment of RDS by high-frequency oscillatory ventilation: a preliminary report. J. Pediatr. 99:287, 1981.

Merritt, T. A., White, C. L., Jaco, J., Kurlinski, J., Martin, J., DiSessa, T. G., Edwards, D., Friedman, W. F., and Gluck, L.: Patent ductus arteriosus treated with ligation or indomethacin: a follow-up study. J. Pediatr. 95:588, 1979.

Metcalfe, I. L., Pototschnik, R., Burgoyne, R., and Enhorning, G.: Lung expansion and survival in rabbit neonates treated with surfactant extract. J. Appl. Physiol. 53:838, 1982.

Miller, H. C., and Hamilton, T. R.: The pathogenesis of the "vernix membrane": relation to aspiration pneumonia in stillborn and newborn infants. Pediatrics 3:735, 1949.

Mintzer, W., Johnson, J. W. C., Scott, R., London, W. R., and Palmer, W. E.: Effect of betamethasone on pressure-volume relationship of fetal rhesus monkey lung. J. Appl. Physiol. 47:377, 1979.

Mockrin, L. D., and Bancalari, E. H.: Early versus delayed initiation of continuous negative pressure in infants with hyaline membrane disease. J. Pediatr. 87:596, 1975.

Morrison, J. C., Whybrew, W. D., Bucovaz, E. T., et al.: Injection of corticosteroids into mother to prevent neonatal respiratory distress syndrome. Am. J. Obstet. Gynecol. 131:358, 1978.

Moss, A. J., Duffie, E. R., Jr., and Fagan, L. M.: Respiratory distress syndrome in newborn: study on association of cord clamping and pathogenesis of distress. J.A.M.A. 184:48, 1963.

Nielsen, H. C., Zinman, H. M., and Torday, J. S.: Dihydrotestosterone inhibits fetal rabbit pulmonary surfactant production. J. Clin. Invest. 69:611, 1982.

Nilsson, R., Grossmann, G., and Robertson, B.: Lung surfactant and the pathogenesis of neonatal bronchiolar lesions induced by artificial ventilation. Pediatr. Res. 12:249, 1978.

Northway, W. H., and Rosan, R. C.: Radiographic features of pulmonary oxygen toxicity in the newborn: Bronchopulmonary dysplasia. Radiology 91:49, 1968.

Outerbridge, E. W., and Stern, L.: Developmental follow-up of survivors of neonatal respiratory failure. Crit. Care Med. 2:23, 1974.

Papageorgiou, A. N., Desgranges, M. F., Masson, M., Colle, E., Shatz, R., and Gelfand, M. M.: The antenatal use of betamethasone in the prevention of respiratory distress syndrome: a controlled double blind trial. Pediatrics 63:73, 1979.

Perelman, R. H., and Farrell, P. M.: Analysis of causes of neonatal death in the United States with specific emphasis on fatal hyaline membrane disease. Pediatrics 70:570, 1982.

Reynolds, E. O. R.: Management of hyaline membrane disease. Br. Med. Bull. 31:18, 1975.

Rhodes, P. G., Hall, R. T., and Leonidas, J. C.: Chronic pulmonary disease in neonates with assisted ventilation. Pediatrics 55:788, 1975.

Robert, M. F., Neff, R. K., Hubbell, J. P., Taeusch, H. W., and Avery, M. E.: Association between maternal diabetes and the respiratory distress syndrome in the newborn. N. Engl. J. Med. 294:357, 1976.

Robertson, A. M., and Crichton, J. U.: Neurological sequelae in children with neonatal respiratory distress. Am. J. Dis. Child. 117:271, 1969.

Robertson, B., Tunell, R., and Rudhe, U.: Late stages of pulmonary hyaline membranes of the newborn. Acta Paediatr. 53:433, 1964.

Rokos, J., Vaeusorn, O., Nachman, R., et al.: Hyaline membrane disease in twins. Pediatrics 42:204, 1968.

Shanklin, D. R.: The sex of premature infants with HMD. South. Med. J. 56:1018, 1963.

Shepard, F. M., Johnston, R. B., Klatte, E. C., et al.: Residual pulmonary findings in clinical hyaline membrane disease. N. Engl. J. Med. 279:1063, 1968.

Singer, A. D., Thibeault, D. W., Hobel, C. J., and Heiner, D. C.: Alpha-1-antitrypsin in amniotic fluid and cord blood of preterm infants with the respiratory distress syndrome. J. Pediatr. 88:87, 1976.

Smith, B. T., and Sabry, K.: Synergistic effects of glucocorticoids and thyroid hormones on lung maturation; role of fibroblast pneumonocyte factor. (abstr.): Pediatr. Res. 16:362A, 1982.

Sosenko, I. R. S., Hartig-Beecken, I., and Frantz, I. D., III: Cortisol reversal of functional delay of lung maturation in fetuses of diabetic rabbits. J. Appl. Physiol. 49:971, 1980.

Stark, A. R., Bascom, R., and Frantz, I. D., III: Muscle relaxation in mechanically ventilated infants. J. Pediatr. 94:439, 1979.

Taeusch, H. W., Jr., Brown, E., Torday, J. S., and Nielsen, H. C.: Magnitude and duration of lung response to dexamethasone in fetal sheep. Am. J. Obstet. Gynecol. 140:452, 1981.

Taeusch, H. W., Jr., Frigoletto, F., Kitzmiller, J., Avery, M. E., Hehre, A., Fromm, B., Lawson, E., and Neff, R. K.: Risk of respiratory distress syndrome after prenatal dexamethasone treatment. Pediatrics 63:64, 1979.

Taghizadeh, A., and Reynolds, E. O. R.: Pathogenesis of bronchopulmonary dysplasia following hyaline membrane disease. Am. J. Pathol. 82:241, 1976.

Tanswell, A. K., Clubb, R. A., Smith, B. T., and Boston, R. W.: Individualized continuous distending pressure applied within six hours of delivery in infants with respiratory distress syndrome. Arch. Dis. Child. 55:33, 1980.

Tchou, C. S., Fletcher, B. D., Branke, P., et al.: Asymmetric distribution of the roentgen pattern in hyaline membrane disease. J. Can. Assoc. Radiol. 23:85, 1972.

Thach, B. T., and Taeusch, H. W.: Sighing in newborn human infants: role of inflation-augmenting reflex. J. Appl. Physiol. 41:502, 1976.

Thibeault, D. W., Emmanouilides, G. C., Nelson, R. J., et al.: Patent ductus arteriosus complicating the respiratory distress syndrome in preterm infants. J. Pediatr. 86:120, 1975.

Torday, J., Carson, L., and Lawson, E. E.: Saturated phosphatidylcholine in amniotic fluid and prediction of the respiratory distress syndrome. N. Engl. J. Med. 301:1013, 1979.

Worthington, D., Maloney, G. H. A., and Smith, B. T.: Fetal lung maturation. I. Mode of onset of premature labor; influence of premature rupture of membranes. Obstet. Gynecol. 49:275, 1977.

16

Bronchopulmonary Dysplasia and Other Persistent Pulmonary Dysfunctions

Some premature infants have chronic pulmonary dysfunction with persisting oxygen dependency, reduced lung compliance, and elevated respiratory rates. These findings have been described under various names, by Wilson and Mikity in 1960, by Burnard and colleagues in 1965, by Northway and coworkers in 1967, and by Krauss and associates in 1975. Although there is no reason to consider the pathophysiology of these conditions to be the same in all instances, we have considered them in this one chapter because they have enough features in common and share the same differential diagnosis.

Bronchopulmonary Dysplasia

Low birth weight infants who require high concentrations of oxygen and ventilatory support may show persisting, chronic pulmonary dysfunction, named by Northway and coworkers "bronchopulmonary dysplasia."

Incidence. This problem occurs only in neonatal intensive care centers among infants who have required vigorous therapy to sustain life. It normally follows hyaline membrane disease, but it may occur after use of ventilators and high inspired-oxygen mixtures for other conditions such as persistent pulmonary hypertension.

The less mature the infant the greater the risk. In one center during 1979, Bancalari and coworkers reported the condition in 14.5 per cent of infants who survived 30 days and were ventilated more than 3 days. Prolonged oxygen and ventilator dependence occurs in about 20 per cent of infants under 1000 gm who survive the first few days of life.

Diagnosis. Persistent pulmonary insufficiency after apparent improvement from the respiratory distress syndrome raises the possibility of bronchopulmonary dysplasia. In the first week or two of life, a persistent patent ductus arteriosus can produce similar symptoms, and it is often associated with bronchopulmonary dysplasia. The infants often fail to grow, remain hypoxic in room air, may have apneic spells, and often require continuous or intermittent mandatory ventilation for weeks or even months.

Radiographic Findings. Four distinct, gradually progressive stages have been defined. Initially, the films are indistinguishable from those of severe hyaline membrane disease. From 4 to 10 days (stage II), the lungs become more consolidated. From 10 to 20 days (stage III), numerous cystic areas of varying size appear, resembling Wilson-Mikity disease or even pulmonary interstitial emphysema (Fig. 16–1). Lung volume is increased. In stage IV, generalized emphysema with strandlike densities or areas of atelectasis appear. The heart may enlarge, and eventually cor pulmonale can develop. The appearance of the infant and the radiograph can change rapidly, presumably in association with changes in position of the endotracheal tube, pooled secretions that obstruct airways, or loculated air. In 1979, Edwards noted that the pathologic stage of the disease was more advanced than appreciated radiographically more than half the time.

Pathogenesis. The disorder may represent the result of lung injury from hyaline membrane disease, oxygen toxicity, or stresses from mechanical ventilation. DeLemos and associates produced similar lung changes in newborn lambs breathing 95+ per cent oxygen with or without a respirator, and Robinson and colleagues documented chronic proliferative pulmonary lesions, with squamous metaplasia in adult monkey lungs on prolonged exposure to high oxygen. However, in a review of the experience at University College Hospital, London, Reynolds found the form of mechanical ventilation to be more critical than the amount of oxygen. When he changed the ventilatory pattern to a rate of 30 cycles/minute and a 2–3 : 1 inspiratory-expiratory ratio (with a peak pressure no higher than 25 cm H_2O), he greatly reduced the problem in his nursery.

In addition to injury from hyperoxia and barotrauma on an immature lung, excess fluid intake and congestive heart failure in association with a patent ductus arteriosus may contribute to the changes seen in bronchopulmonary dysplasia. It is tempting to speculate that chronic pulmonary edema from whatever cause in the immature lung may interfere with postnatal lung growth (Brown et al., 1978).

Treatment. Optimal nutrition, oxygenation, and general supportive care to encourage growth and de-

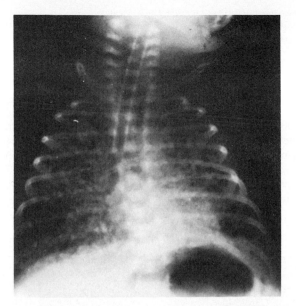

Figure 16–1. This 1450-gm infant had hyaline membrane disease and required high ventilator pressures and 100 per cent oxygen. This film at 3 months of age shows the multicystic changes of bronchopulmonary dysplasia. The infant remains intubated and respirator-dependent.

ically with digitalis, and there was subsequent improvement; however, there were continued failure to gain weight, apneic episodes, and intermittent dependence on a respirator. By 5 months of age, the infant had grown to a weight of 2900 grams and was discharged home. There were several subsequent admissions, however, for increasing cyanosis and labored respirations, usually associated with new pulmonary infiltrates. The chest film never cleared completely and, when the infant was 8 months of age, showed persistent scarring in the right upper lobe and the left lower lobe (Fig. 16–2C). By 11 months of age, the infant had been readmitted to the hospital requiring intubation, artificial ventilation, and 40 to 50 per cent oxygen. Because she was too weak to suck well, she had failed to gain weight sufficiently so that at 1 year of age she weighed only 4.1 kg. For this reason, a gastrostomy was inserted for nutritional support with slow, subsequent weight gain. However, during this period there was an increase in cardiomegaly and persistent right heart failure refractory to oxygen and diuretics (Fig. 16–2D). The infant died of respiratory failure at 13 months of age.

velopment is all we have to offer. Although glucocorticoids have been tried, no success has been recorded, and the hazards of reducing host defenses against infection and growth suppression would seem to contraindicate them. Antibiotics are appropriate for intercurrent infections. Chest physical therapy may help if atelectasis is present. Diuretics or fluid restriction should be considered if rales are prominent and pulmonary edema thought to be present. Increased inspired oxygen sufficient to keep the arterial level at about 60 mm Hg and maintenance of a hematocrit of over 30 to 35 to provide adequate oxygen-carrying capacity would seem appropriate. Some infants do well with indwelling nasal cannulae to provide continuous administration of increased inspired oxygen.

CASE 16–1

The female infant was delivered by a 21-year-old mother after the spontaneous onset of labor at a presumed gestational age of 37 weeks with a weight of 1600 grams. On physical examination, the infant had characteristics more consistent with 33 weeks of development. Immediately after birth, there was grunting respiration with tachypnea and retractions (Fig. 16–2A and B). The infant required 60 to 80 per cent oxygen for the first 3 days of life but gradually was able to tolerate 40 to 50 per cent over the next several days. During this first week of life, the infant was ventilated with positive pressure and continuous end-expiratory pressure through an endotracheal tube. Dependence on the respirator persisted through the first month of life, but the baby was successfully extubated at 1 month of age. However, shortly thereafter there was evidence of increasing respiratory difficulty in association with a large patent ductus arteriosus. This was managed med-

Prognosis. The course and prognosis of bronchopulmonary dysplasia are variable. Since the problem has increased in recent years with increasing survival of ventilated infants, we are now following more infants with persistent but usually asymptomatic evidence of pulmonary dysfunction. Sustained elevated respiratory rates, intermittent (or persistent) wheezes, repeated hospitalizations for bronchiolitic episodes, and right ventricular hypertrophy are found in the first year and, with less frequency, in the second year. In a study of nine children between 7.2 and 9.6 years of age with a history of severe bronchopulmonary dysplasia, Smyth and coworkers from Toronto found evidence of pulmonary dysfunction in seven of them. All were attending school and participating in normal play activities, although with limited exercise tolerance. On testing, the children had evidence of lower airway obstructive disease and bronchial hyperreactivity. Radiographically, most had hyperinflation. Right ventricular hypertrophy was seen by EKG and echocardiography.

Developmental prognosis relates to the severity and duration of the respiratory symptoms, which in turn depend on the perinatal and neonatal events. In a 2-year follow-up of 20 infants, Markestad and Fitzhardinge found that the average weights were in the third to tenth percentiles and that the heights were slightly better. Five of the 20 infants were below normal (<85) on the Bayley scales at 18 months after term.

Wilson-Mikity Syndrome

As more attention has been focused on premature infants and more chest films obtained, it is not surprising that new syndromes have been identified. One of these was first reported in 1960 by Wilson and Mikity and in recent years has borne their names.

Incidence. The disorder has been reported in widely separated centers in Europe and North America. Mikity and coworkers estimate the incidence at 1:450 live births of premature infants. Apparently, the condition is restricted to infants of less than 36 weeks' gestational age and appears to be more fre-

quent in those of very low birth weight. It has been noted in black and white infants of both sexes.

We cannot know for certain whether this syndrome is sporadic or on the decrease. Certainly, we do not often use the label to describe most infants with chronic pulmonary changes. In some infants with late onset pulmonary insufficiency, the condition would probably be called Type II respiratory distress in some centers, CPIP (chronic pulmonary insufficiency of prematurity) in others, or even chronic aspiration pneumonia by some radiologists. We admit to confusion of nomenclature and know of no means of clarifying it at this time. We have chosen to describe the conditions as they were originally delineated and

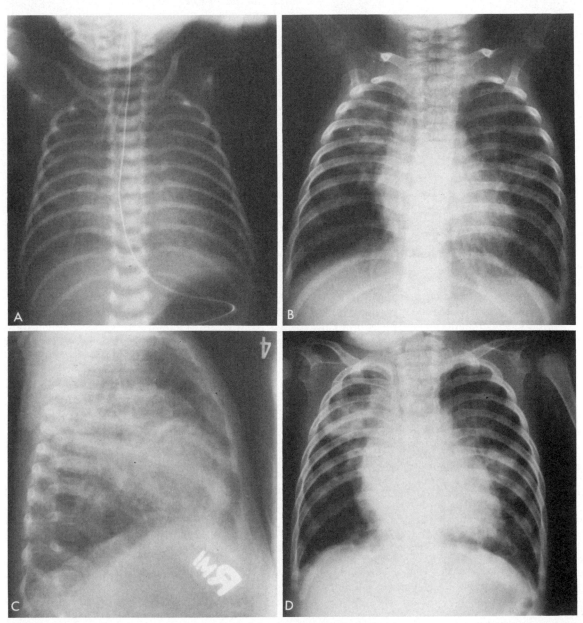

Figure 16–2. *A*, Film on first day of life of 1600-gm infant with respiratory distress. A feeding tube and an endotracheal tube are in place. A diffuse reticulogranular pattern is present in both lungs. *B* and *C*, The same infant, age 5 months, with areas of infiltration and hyperaeration. *D*, Age 11 months. The infant continued to need intermittent artificial respiration and 25 to 30 per cent oxygen. The heart is enlarged, with ECG evidence of right ventricular enlargement.

to perpetuate the labels with full awareness that increased insight into pathogenesis will doubtless make redefinition desirable.

Clinical Findings. No consistent abnormalities of pregnancy have been noted. The infants may have some respiratory distress at birth, occasionally severe and thought to be hyaline membrane disease. Others may have no respiratory symptoms and receive no added oxygen, but some weeks later they may have the insidious onset of cyanosis and a rapid respiratory rate. Even those with early respiratory distress usually improve for a week or more before cyanosis and retractions reappear. On the whole, the symptoms increase over a 2- to 6-week interval and may persist for several months. The infants characteristically appear in good general condition, gain weight, and are active. Their symptomatology is restricted to the lung and is characterized by a striking oxygen dependency. Fine rales and, sometimes, wheezing have been noted, but, more commonly, breath sounds have a grating, sandpaper quality to them.

An associated finding of interest in several reported series is a fractured rib. The etiology of the rib fracture has not been determined, and fractures in other bones have not been reported.

Laboratory Findings. Exhaustive attempts to define an etiologic agent by laboratory studies during life and examination of the lungs post mortem have failed to unearth a causative organism. The association of ECHO type 19 virus was noted in one infant but has not been found in others. Serologic studies for respiratory viruses, routine blood studies, and sweat chloride determinations have all been negative. Definite abnormalities of pulmonary function have been documented, mostly by Swyer and co-workers, who report CO_2 retention, substantial right-to-left shunts, a reduction in lung compliance, and an increase in airway resistance. Cardiovascular function is usually normal, except very late in the illness, when cor pulmonale may occur.

Radiographic Findings. In the first weeks of life, the chest film is usually normal. Early abnormalities are a bilateral, coarse, streaky infiltrate, and, later, cystic lesions in both lungs. The walls of the cysts average 0.5 to 1 mm in thickness, and the cysts themselves measure 1 to 4 mm in diameter. Later, the cysts enlarge and coalesce, and overexpanded hyperlucent lungs are seen. Resolution of these changes lags behind clinical improvement; complete radiographic clearing may not occur until 2 years of age (Mikity et al., 1967). (Fig. 16–3).

Pathologic Findings. A similarity to interstitial fibrosis was noted by Wilson and Mikity in their original article, but since then major differences have become apparent. The excised lung, inflated, has a characteristic hobnail appearance on the surface, as if terminal air spaces were overdistended and restricting fibrous septa were prominent. The lung contains more air per gram of tissue than would be expected, unlike interstitial fibrosis. Histologically, there are no pathognomonic features. Some of the alveolar septa appear thick; however, no increase in fibrotic tissue is found.

Electron microscopic studies have not uncovered any characteristic lesion (Swyer et al., 1965). It is believed that an arrest in lung development may have occurred, with an inadequate alveolar-capillary interface to support gas exchange in the growing infant.

Treatment. Only supportive measures can be rec-

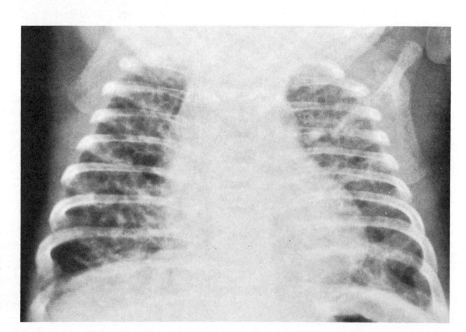

Figure 16–3. Posteroanterior view of chest shows a lacy network of linear opacifications throughout both lungs. Many round dark areas are seen. (Baghdassarian, O., Avery, M. E., and Neuhauser, E. B.: Am. J. Roentgenol. *89*:1020, 1963.)

ommended at this time. It is of critical importance to use only as much added oxygen as needed to overcome cyanosis or to keep the arterial blood tensions in a safe range, presumably 60 to 80 mm Hg. Attempts to alter the course of the disease by digitalization and with the use of steroids and antibiotics have been fruitless.

Prognosis.   In one study of five children conducted 8 to 10 years after they had had Wilson-Mikity syndrome, Coates and associates found a reduction in airflow rates compared with those of infants of similar birth weight with chronic pulmonary disease (weights 750 to 1446 gm). Some of the children studied had had episodes of bronchiolitis during the first year of life, but none was symptomatic at the time of study.

Other Chronic Pulmonary Problems of Preterm Infants

PERSISTENT PULMONARY DYSFUNCTION

Some infants of low birth weight may have normal respiratory function for some days or even weeks and then show a number of signs of deterioration. Blood gases worsen, and radiographic findings of streaking and atelectasis may occur and persist for several months and then recover spontaneously.

In serial studies on these infants, Burnard and colleagues described a loss of lung volume and reduction in compliance. Resistance to airflow was elevated. They improved over a period of months. Burnard thought that the changes were a reflection of immature airways and chest wall; the lungs could be subjected to regional pressure differences during respiration in a way that would produce collapse of some of the very compliant airways.

CHRONIC PULMONARY INSUFFICIENCY OF PREMATURITY (CPIP)

A syndrome of delayed onset respiratory distress in infants under 1250 gm was first described by Krauss and associates in eight infants studied at the New York Hospital between 1968 and 1973.

The infants had no respiratory distress for the first few days of life, but at about 4 to 7 days of age they required supplemental oxygen and had apneic spells. The infants had normal radiographs except for low lung volume. By the third to fourth weeks of life, the infants gradually improved, and most were well by 2 months of age without any specific interventions.

The course of the New York infants was like that seen in Wilson-Mikity syndrome, but the absence of

characteristic radiographic findings of "bubbly lungs" distinguished the CPIP babies. Krauss and coworkers gave the important warning to neonatologists that reassurance with respect to neonatal lung function should not be offered until 1 week of age or later when an infant has a very low birth weight.

Comment.   We have become increasingly familiar with the spectrum of relatively late onset pulmonary insufficiency, as more infants of very low birth weight are living longer. In fact this problem, still poorly understood, is one of the most prominent in intensive care nurseries of the 1980s.

Typically, the infants establish normal ventilation in the first hours of life and may have clear lung fields by examination and radiographs at that time. Blood gases may be normal with room air or with modest increased oxygen concentrations (25 to 30 per cent).

Several days later, color changes and apneic spells may be noted, and carbon dioxide tensions may slowly rise. Lung compliance decreases. More often than not, radiographic changes are present (Fig. 16–4). Sometimes, lung volume is decreased; at other times, it is normal with a hazy appearance. We suspect pulmonary edema in some infants in the absence of evidence of hemodynamic changes. Rarely do we now see the evolution of multicystic changes, or "bubbly lung," that is the hallmark of Wilson-Mikity syndrome. Maybe one reason is that the changes just described usually dictate intubation with continuous distending airway pressure and even mechanical ventilation. The subsequent course of events may be altered by these interventions. If high pressures and high oxygen concentrations become necessary,

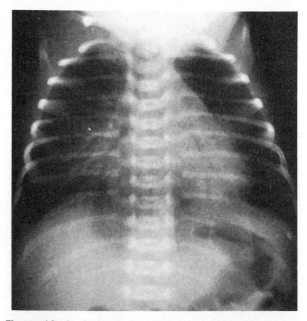

Figure 16–4. Late onset respiratory distress. This 1.1-kg infant had a clear chest film at 2 hours of age. An air bronchogram obtained at age 28 hours, shown here, reveals bilateral infiltrates. No evidence of infection was found. The infant required mechanical ventilation for three days, then recovered.

the later changes of bronchopulmonary dysplasia may follow, just as they do after the same interventions in infants with hyaline membrane disease.

Possible Mechanisms. We would like to suggest several possible but unproved explanations for the sequence of events in delayed pulmonary insufficiency, assuming absence of infection.

One explanation for the secondary low lung volume seen in the infants described by Krauss could be secondary surfactant deficiency. Large volume excursions can deplete surfactant stores, particularly when the functional residual capacity is low, as it may be in the presence of a very compliant chest wall. If the balance between synthesis of surfactant and its consumption or turnover is upset, a deficiency state could occur and persist until further lung maturation takes place (Wyszogrodski et al., 1975).

Another explanation, related to the first, is exhaustion of the muscles of respiration. Perhaps the infant at birth is in a relatively better nutritional state than after a few days, and muscle weakness increases to the extent that respiratory failure occurs. For whatever reason, muscle exhaustion can occur even in normal infants if there is distention of the rib cage, as in REM sleep. Muller and colleagues in Toronto measured diaphragmatic EMG from surface electrodes in infants being weaned from ventilators. When muscle fatigue was present, the infants had apneic spells, which were followed by reduced rib cage distortion from an increase in intercostal muscle activity.

The consequences of recurrent muscle exhaustion could be reduced lung volume, atelectasis, and a progressive mismatch of ventilation and perfusion. It seems probable that this sequence of events was present in some of the infants described by Krauss.

A third explanation, particularly applicable to infants with hazy lung fields on radiograph, is the possibility of persistent secretion of lung liquid, or "persistent fetal lung." The fetal lung secretes liquid into the potential airways and is a source of amniotic liquid (Strang, 1977). The regulation of flow of lung liquid is not well understood, but it is known that epinephrine has a powerful inhibiting effect, which in the lamb lasts for nearly 24 hours (Lawson, et al., 1978; Walters and Olver, 1978). Presumably, the secreting process or, perhaps, cell permeability is under beta-adrenergic control. Glucocorticoids have also been found to reduce tracheal effluent in the chronically intubated fetal lamb.

Since birth is characterized by an outpouring of epinephrine and glucocorticoids, the lung liquid secretory process is arrested. In most infants, this arrest is permanent, but we wonder whether it could be temporary in some very immature infants and whether the hazy lungs on radiographs and the deteriorated function could represent continuing secretion of fetal lung liquid. Continuous distending airway pressure would be a useful intervention in such a circumstance. One would also have to postulate adrenergic depletion or exhaustion in these infants.

REFERENCES

Bancalari, E., Abdenour, G. E., Feller, R., and Gannon, J.: Bronchopulmonary dysplasia: Clinical presentation. J. Pediatr. 95:819, 1979.

Brown, E. R.: Increased risk of bronchopulmonary dysplasia in infants with patent ductus arteriosus. J. Pediatr. 95:865, 1979.

Brown, E. R., Stark, A., Lawson, E., and Avery, M. E.: Bronchopulmonary dysplasia: Possible relationship to pulmonary edema. J. Pediatr. 92:982, 1978.

Burnard, E. D., Grattan-Smith, P., Picton-Warlow, C. G., and Grauaug, A.: Pulmonary insufficiency in prematurity. Austr. Paediat. J. 1:12, 1965.

Coates, A. L., Bergsteinsson, H., Desmond K., et al.: Long-term pulmonary sequelae of the Wilson-Mikity syndrome. J. Pediatr. 92:247, 1978.

Dahms, B. B., Krauss, A. N., and Auld, P. A. M.: Pulmonary function in dysmature infants. J. Pediatr. 84:434, 1974.

DeLemos, R., Wolfsdorf, J., Nachman, R., Block, A. J., Leiby, G., Wilkinson, H., Allen, T., Haller, J. A., Morgan, W., and Avery, M. E.: Lung injury from oxygen in lambs. Anesthesiology 30:609, 1969.

Edwards, D. K.: Radiographic aspects of bronchopulmonary dysplasia. J. Pediatr. 95:823, 1979.

Edwards, D. K., Colby, T. V., and Northway, W. H., Jr.: Radiographic-pathologic correlation in bronchopulmonary dysplasia. J. Pediatr. 95:834, 1979.

Grossman, H., Levin, A. R., Winchester, P. H., and Auld, P. A. M.: Pulmonary hypertension in the Wilson-Mikity syndrome. Am. J. Roentgenol. 114:293, 1972.

Kafer, E. R.: Pulmonary oxygen toxicity. A review of the evidence for acute and chronic oxygen toxicity in man. Br. J. Anaesth. 43:687, 1971.

Krauss, A. N., Klain, D. B., and Auld, P. A. M.: Chronic pulmonary insufficiency of the premature (CPIP). Pediatrics 55:55, 1975.

Lawson, E. E., Brown, E. R., Torday, J. S., Madansky, D. L., and Taeusch, H. W., Jr.: The effect of epinephrine on tracheal fluid flow and surfactant efflux in fetal sheep. Am. Rev. Resp. Dis. 118:1023, 1978.

Markestad, T., and Fitzhardinge, P. M.: Growth and development in children recovering from bronchopulmonary dysplasia. J. Pediatr. 98:597, 1981.

Mikity, V., Hodgman, J. E., and Tatter, D.: The radiological findings in delayed pulmonary maturation in premature infants. Progr. Pediatr. Radiol. 1:149, 1967.

Muller, N., Gulston, G., Cade, D., et al.: Diaphragmatic muscle fatigue in the newborn. J. Appl. Physiol. 46:688, 1979.

Northway, W. H., Jr., and Rosan, R. C.: Radiographic features of pulmonary oxygen toxicity in the newborn. Radiology 91:49, 1968.

Northway, W. H., Jr., Rosan, R. C., and Porter D. Y.: Pulmonary disease following respirator therapy. N. Engl. J. Med. 276:357, 1967.

Reynolds, E. O. R., and Taghizadeh, A.: Improved prognosis of infants mechanically ventilated for hyaline membrane disease. Arch. Dis. Child. 49:505, 1974.

Rhodes, P. G., Hall, R. T., and Leonidas, J. C.: Chronic pulmonary disease in neonates with assisted ventilation. Pediatrics 55:788, 1975.

Robinson, R. F., Harper, D. T., Thomas, A. S., et al.: Proliferative pulmonary lesions in monkeys exposed to high concentrations of oxygen. Aerosp. Med. 38:481, 1967.

Smyth, J. A., Tabachnik, E., Duncan, W. J., Reilly, B. J., and Levison, H.: Pulmonary function and bronchial hyperreactivity in long-term survivors of bronchopulmonary dysplasia. Pediatrics 68:336, 1981.

Strang, L. B.: Neonatal Respiration. Physiological and Clinical Studies. Oxford, Blackwell Scientific Publication, 1977.

Swyer, P. R., Delivoria-Papadopoulos, M., Levison, H., Reilly, B. J., and Balis, J. U.: The pulmonary syndrome of Wilson and Mikity. Pediatrics *36*:374, 1965.

Taghizadeh, A., and Reynolds, E. O. R.: Pathogenesis of bronchopulmonary dysplasia following hyaline membrane disease. Am. J. Pathol. *82*:241, 1976.

Walters, D. V., and Olver, R. E.: The role of catecholamines in lung liquid absorption at birth. Pediatr. Res. *12*:239, 1978.

Wilson, M. G., and Mikity, V. G.: A new form of respiratory disease in premature infants. Am. J. Dis. Child. *99*:489, 1960.

Wung, J. T., Koons, A. H., Driscoll, J. M., Jr., and James, S.: Changing incidence of bronchopulmonary dysplasia. J. Pediatr. *95*:845, 1979.

Wyszogrodski, I., Kyei-Aboagye, K., Taeusch, H. W., Jr., and Avery, M. E.: Surfactant inactivation by hyperventilation: Conservation by end-expiratory pressure. J. Appl. Physiol. *38*:461, 1975.

17

Air Leak and Air Trapping

The lung of the newborn infant becomes hyperaerated with great frequency. Both lungs in their entirety or one lung or a lobe or a segment of a lung may be so affected. *Simple hyperaeration* (overdistention of terminal air spaces) may progress to *interstitial emphysema*, in which septa are broken and air escapes into interstitial tissue. Collection of this air into bullae or blebs may permit rupture into the pleural space either directly or after being carried down the sheaths of blood and lymph vessels to the mediastinum.

Pathogenesis. The only basic causes of hyperinflation are (1) some obstructive process that permits ingress of air into the terminal air spaces but impedes egress, (2) expansion of a segment of lung by the normally negative intrathoracic pressure to compensate for loss of volume in another lobe, or (3) overgrowth of a portion of lung.

Some immediate causes of hyperinflation are:

1. Intrinsic partial obstruction by
   a. Mucus
   b. Meconium or squamous cells
   c. Inflammatory exudate
2. Extrinsic compression by
   a. Bronchogenic cyst
   b. Aberrant vessel
3. Idiopathic unilobar emphysema
4. Compensatory hyperinflation in presence of
   a. Atelectasis
   b. Pulmonary agenesis or hyperplasia
5. Iatrogenic

Diagnosis. Many of the infants suffering from emphysema will have been born after some abnormality of pregnancy or labor. Postmaturity, toxemia, placental bleeding, cord accidents, maternal hypotension, vigorous instrumental extraction, breech delivery, and other problems figure prominently in the histories. Many will have been ill at birth, with breathing and crying time delayed, and positive pressure insufflation will have been attempted. Within a few minutes or hours after spontaneous respiration has become established, the signs of emphysema become noticeable. These may begin and remain relatively mild. They may progress over the course of 12 to 48 hours to severer forms or they may strike catastrophically with the first few breaths.

When obstructive emphysema is fully developed, the diagnosis can be made by physical examination with relative ease. The chest is visibly hyperinflated. Respirations are rapid and shallow, with some retraction, and the chest fails to deflate completely upon expiration. Percussion reveals hyperresonance, depressed diaphragm, and contracted area of cardiac dullness. Breath sounds are diminished in intensity. Rales are not usually heard. A wheeze may be heard during expiration. Lesser degrees of emphysema and the emphysema that coexists with patchy atelectasis may not produce such characteristic signs and may be diagnosable only by radiograph.

Mediastinal emphysema may also not be recognizable by its signs. When there is great accumulation of air in the mediastinum, the sternum is thrust forward, the percussion note over it and for a short distance to either side is strikingly hyperresonant, and, rarely, a clicking or crunching noise may be heard synchronous with the heart beat. Heart sounds may appear to be distant. These infants, too, are extremely ill, and cyanosis may become intense.

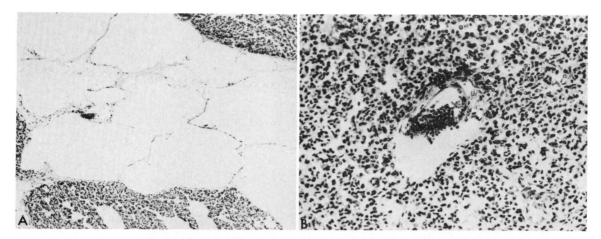

Figure 17–1. *A,* Photomicrograph of lung of an infant who died of emphysema and bilateral pneumothorax. The alveoli in the center show much distention, their septa thinned. Some of the septa have ruptured. In the periphery, the lung is atelectatic. *B,* Higher-power view showing a blood vessel in cross section. The vessel is compressed by a surrounding collar of air that has filled and ballooned the perivascular space.

Pneumothorax

The most common cause of increased intrathoracic tension is pneumothorax, with or without associated pneumomediastinum and interstitial emphysema. Spontaneous pneumothorax is more common in the first days of life than at any other time of childhood.

Incidence. When radiographs have been taken on consecutive infants, small asymptomatic pneumothoraces have been detected in about 1 or 2 per cent of them. Symptomatic pneumothoraces are rarer, occurring about once in a thousand live births. A higher incidence than that would suggest overzealous resuscitative efforts in the delivery room.

In infants who require mechanical ventilation, air leak occurs with much greater frequency. In several reviews of this subject, the incidence of alveolar rupture in infants on ventilators has been between 20 and 40 per cent, with the higher proportion in those who were treated with positive end-expiratory pressure (Ogata et al., 1976; Madansky et al., 1979).

Pathogenesis. Clearly, the lung can be ruptured by the application of excessive pressure during resuscitation. Equally clearly, pneumothorax can occur in the absence of artificial ventilation. It is associated with postmaturity and meconium staining, suggesting that aspirated materials may partially obstruct portions of the lung and allow excessive pressure to be applied to the previously aerated alveoli by the descent of the diaphragm. This hypothesis explaining the reasons for the predisposition to pneumothorax

in the first hours of life was proposed by Chernick and Avery in 1963 after studies on the mechanism of inflation of the airless lung. The serial opening of the terminal ventilatory units would allow shearing forces to be applied to those that are open when others are obstructed. There seems to be no need to consider congenital defects in these lungs, since recurrences after an episode in infancy have not been reported.

Spontaneous pneumothorax has been described by Lubchenco in premature infants, occurring in the first weeks of life. We also have seen it under those

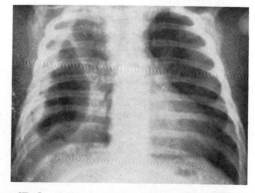

Figure 17–2. Anteroposterior view of the chest taken at 33 hours of age. Emphysema of the left lung predominates, with ribs widely spread and slight herniation of the upper lobe into the mediastinum. There is patchy atelectasis in the right lung. The mass in the right upper section is almost surely the thymus, slightly dislocated to the right.

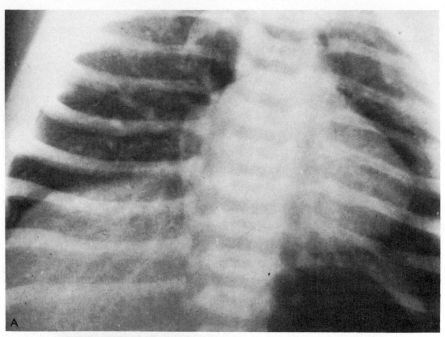

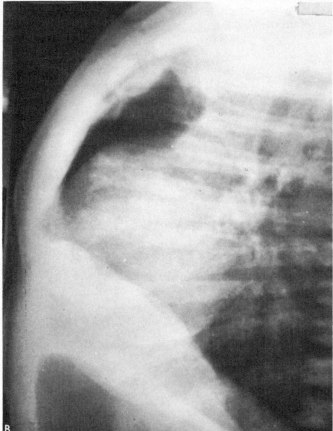

Figure 17–3. *A*, Two large bubbles of air are visible in the right upper mediastinum. One of them appears to be lifting the thymus outward and upward. *B*, Lateral view showing the large collection of air in the anterior mediastinum.

circumstances and have noted it in a number of infants with hyaline membrane disease. Nevertheless, it seems to be overwhelmingly a problem of the mature or postmature infant. Indeed, Adler and Wyszogrodski have demonstrated that the more mature lung ruptures at lower transpulmonary pressures than the less mature lung.

Symptoms. Any sudden change in vital signs should alert the physician to possible air leak. Infants with significant accumulation of air in the pleural space are usually tachypneic and often cyanotic, and they may have asymmetric chests. Hyperresonance is often evident, but the expected decrease in breath sounds on the affected side may be absent, since breath sounds are so widely transmitted in infants. Irritability is usually prominent. The cardiac impulses may be shifted; indeed, careful following of the point of maximal impulse is a useful guide to the possibility of increase or decrease in the pneumothorax.

Among infants on ventilators, pneumothorax should be suspected when the chest is observed to be overdistended or when oxygen requirements increase.

Diagnosis and Treatment. If the infant is critically ill and the chest is found to be hyperresonant, a needle should be inserted immediately, preferably attached via a three-way stopcock to a syringe. The removal of air under tension should give prompt relief. When the situation is less critical, a chest film is indicated. Large collections of air in the pleural space are readily recognizable on chest films by identification of the visceral pleural line, mediastinal shift or a hyperlucent hemithorax. Since air tends to accumulate in the uppermost regions of the thorax, it may

be overlooked on an anteroposterior view of the thorax of a supine infant. A lateral view with a horizontal beam may demonstrate air in the retrosternal space. Kuhns and colleagues have used fiberoptic transillumination to identify and follow pneumothoraces, and we have found this technique very useful. The decision to remove the air by needle aspiration, closed-suction drainage, or oxygen breathing depends on the clinical state. If the child is not severely ill, close observation over the subsequent hours should reveal whether he is getting better or worse. Often, complete resolution occurs without any intervention. Occasionally, removal of the air by a simple aspiration is satisfactory. In the absence of continuing leak, administration of 40 to 50 per cent oxygen will greatly facilitate removal of the loculated air on the basis of nitrogen washout, as demonstrated by Chernick and Avery. If air continues to accumulate, water-seal drainage for a few days may be indicated.

Mediastinal Air. The presence of significant amounts of mediastinal air is indicated by elevation of the thymus as seen on the anteroposterior and lateral chest films (Fig. 17–3). Occasionally, a halo of air, often with indistinct margins, is seen adjacent to the borders of the heart. Air in that location and subcutaneous and interstitial air are, of course, difficult to aspirate. Oxygen breathing (even 100 per cent oxygen for a few hours) will hasten removal of air from those locations. High oxygen mixtures should not be given unless symptoms are severe, and they then should be withdrawn as soon as the infant has improved.

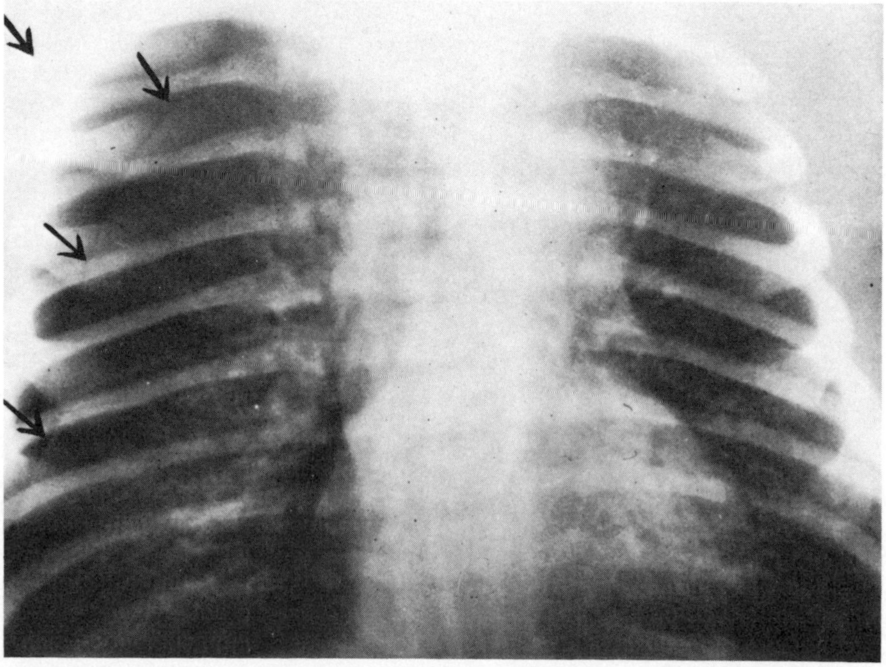

Figure 17–4. Marked pneumothorax is visible on the right.

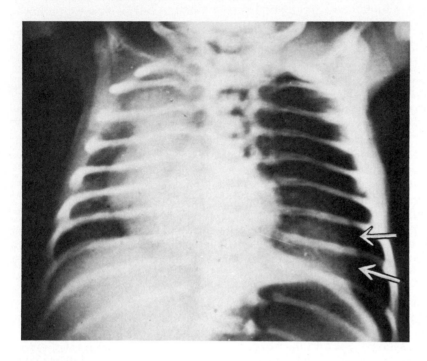

Figure 17–5. Anteroposterior view of chest of infant 3 hours old. Respiratory distress began, for no known reason, a few minutes after birth, shortly after the original cry. One sees left pneumothorax, the collapsed left lung, shift of the heart and mediastinum to the right, and atelectasis of the right upper lobe.

Interstitial Emphysema

This form of air leak, characterized by collections of air trapped in the interstitial tissues, has become much more commonly recognized in recent years as a complication of mechanical ventilation. The ma-

jority of cases appear in premature infants during the course of respiratory distress syndrome.

The radiologic findings are voluminous lungs with multiple cyst-like radiolucencies, sometimes localized to one lobe but more commonly bilateral. Nearly half of these infants will later develop pneumothoraces.

Treatment. The diffuse type of interstitial emphysema is often fatal. Very careful adjustment of ventilator settings with a close eye on a continuous oxygen monitor will allow the physician to optimize ventilation with the most appropriate pressures. Very high frequency ventilation (600 to 800 times/min) was shown by Frantz and Stark to be life-saving for a few infants. Further experience with this approach, which requires lower peak airway pressures, is surely warranted.

The collections of trapped air may persist for weeks or even months before spontaneous resolution. Sometimes, when the loculated air is localized, intubation of the normal lung and ventilation with 100 per cent oxygen will promote resorption of trapped gas in the emphysematous lung.

Pneumopericardium

Pneumopericardium is one of the most critical emergencies occurring in neonatal intensive care units. It appears occasionally after the onset of pulmonary interstitial emphysema or other air leak. Until a decade ago, this complication was nearly always fatal. In a review of air leak in a population of ap-

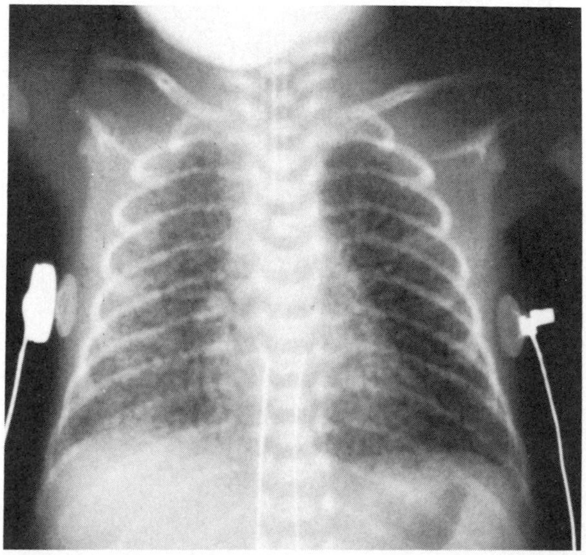

Figure 17–6. Chest radiograph of an 860 gm infant with respiratory distress syndrome on the third day of life. This 28-week gestation infant (a first-born twin) developed severe pulmonary interstitial emphysema on the second day of life. The infant died on the fourth day of life because of progressive respiratory insufficiency.

proximately 11,000 deliveries in 1975 to 1976, Madansky and coworkers found three cases. Pneumopericardium is limited to infants who are being ventilated for severe respiratory disease, usually in the first week of life. In a retrospective review of 13 cases of pneumopericardium, Baumgart and coworkers found peak inspiratory pressures increased from 30 to 42 torr (average) in the 24-hour period prior to the discovery of pneumopericardium. No other ventilator settings were found, on the average, to change significantly during this period. The authors conclude that pneumopericardium is associated with the increase in peak airway pressure that occurs as an attempt to maintain alveolar ventilation as respiratory disease worsens.

The diagnosis should be suspected whenever a severly ill infant on a ventilator shows a sudden deterioration (i.e., one that occurs within seconds) (Fig. 17–7). Blood pressure drops to shock levels as cardiac tamponade occurs from intrapericardial air, with rapid drops in Pa_{O_2}. Death may occur within minutes if corrective measures are not instituted. The differential diagnosis includes other kinds of air leak: tension pneumothorax, pulmonary interstitial emphysema, and other catastrophies (intraventricular hemorrhage, blocked airway, cardiac arrhythmias, intrabdominal organ rupture, and shock from hypovolemia, vascular collapse, or cardiac failure).

Current management approaches have been reviewed by Lawson and coworkers. Usually, we perform needle aspirations of the pericardial space once or twice, and, if air recurs, a pericardial suction tube is placed. Rarely, when the situation could not be managed with these procedures, we have asked thoracic surgeons to place a large pericardial tube in conjunction with opening a pericardial window. Occasionally, pericardial air may be seen on chest radiograph with no clinical signs of cardiac tamponade. In these cases, removal of air is probably unnecessary. Complications of pericardial drainage are ventricular perforation and infection. Pneumopericardium may be a frequent unrecognized terminal event in the intensive care setting (Fig. 17–7). With aggressive management, the rate of survival is now about 50 per cent in these very ill infants.

Lobar Emphysema

This syndrome has also been called "congenital lobar emphysema," "unilobar obstructive emphysema," "localized hypertrophic emphysema," and "infantile lobar emphysema." In our present confused state of knowledge about causation, it would appear to be wise to use the simplest descriptive term without qualifying adjectives that may be apposite for some but not for all. The syndrome is characterized by emphysematous expansion of one lobe. Dyspnea and cyanosis are produced, and these progress slowly or rapidly until serious respiratory difficulty develops.

Incidence. The syndrome has been recognized only in the past 40 years. Up until 1960, about 30 cases had been reported. It is therefore rare, but the rate at which reports have been accruing in the past few years makes it reasonable to believe that it is not the extreme rarity it was once thought to be. Leape and Longino, for example, reported 21 additional cases in 1964, and Lincoln and coworkers added 28 in 1971.

Pathology and Pathogenesis. At operation or autopsy, one lobe (usually an upper, less often the right middle, rarely a lower) is ballooned to many times its normal size. It is usually pink and spongy in appearance, resembling, according to one author, a pink soufflé. When excised, it retains its overinflated appearance. Under the microscope, most of the alveoli are distended, many have coalesced because of rupture of the septa, and subpleural blebs may have been formed. Careful postmortem studies by Reid and her colleagues have illuminated the variety of findings in this condition. In some infants, the tissue is normal with respect to alveolar and airway numbers but simply overdistended, as by a mucous plug. In others, the numbers of airways and alveoli are

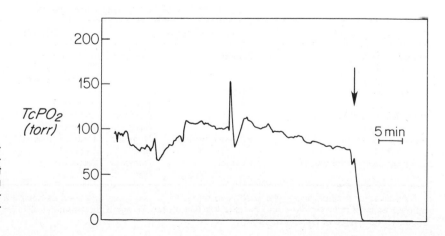

Figure 17–7. Transcutaneous oxygen trace from an infant weighing 2500 gm with severe persistent fetal circulation. The infant had a sudden deterioration (arrow) leading to death from a tension pneumopericardium.

reduced (a hypoplastic overdistended lobe). Radiographically, they are unusually translucent but not overdistended. Rarely, a lobe may show normal airways but an excess of alveoli, the so-called "polyalveolar lobe." Finally, atresia of a bronchus can permit overdistention of some segments but poor egress of air, leading to radiolucency of segments of lung.

In many lungs, lesions have been alleged to have been found to account for the progressive hyperinflation. Bronchial alterations have been described: namely, mucosal folds; diminution, absence, or flaccidity of bronchial cartilage; and stenoses due to inflammation, cysts, or mucous plugs. Deficient cartilage was found in 22 of 28 resected lobes in the series reported by Lincoln and colleagues in 1971. Extrabronchial compression by aberrant blood vessels, chiefly the ductus arteriosus or its residual fibrous cord, has been found in a few. A pathologic classification of lobar emphysema has been proposed by Dr. Lynne Reid (Table 17–1).

Diagnosis. First symptoms are noted at birth in a few cases, during the first week in a few more, between 1 week and 1 month in the majority. In a scattered minority, the original signs of illness make their appearance between 1 and 6 months of age. It is therefore by and large a neonatal disease.

Spells of dyspnea with cyanosis ordinarily usher in the disorder, and these signs soon become persistent and severe. Wheezing expiration is noted not too infrequently. Vomiting and cough are encountered rarely.

On examination, dyspnea, with labored inspiration accompanied by retraction of variable degree, and grunting or prolonged wheezing expiration are the rule. An area of hyperresonance involving one upper lobe or one entire lung is discovered, and over this area air entry is diminished. The heart and mediastinum are dislocated away from the hyperresonant side.

Radiographic Findings. One lobe, usually the right or left upper or the right middle, is voluminous and radiolucent. It often can be seen crossing the midline anterior to the heart. Adjacent lobes are atelectatic. The heart is shifted to the side opposite the overexpanded lobe and can usually be seen to be pressed posteriorly by the herniated lung.

Treatment. If the infant is in severe respiratory distress, immediate intervention is indicated. After a chest film, we prefer to invite a pediatric surgeon and an otolaryngologist to work with us, the latter to perform endoscopy on the operating table, with the surgeon prepared to do an immediate thoracotomy if necessary. Occasionally, an obstructing mucous plug may be removed by suction, and thoracotomy will not be required. If immediate relief is not forthcoming, thoracotomy is in order. The operative mortality has been very low. It was zero in 21 cases reported by Leape and Longino in 1964. During the same interval, 3 infants died who were symptomatic in the newborn period and not operated upon.

In asymptomatic infants in whom lobar overdistention is discovered incidentally, bronchoscopy is indicated. We have elected to follow some such infants without operation, and they have remained asymptomatic. Occasionally the overdistended lobe returns to normal volume, as noted by Roghair in 1972.

Prognosis. The outlook after operation is usually excellent. Few functional evaluations have been made, but DeMuth and Sloan in 1966 did note some persistent reduction in midexpiratory flow rates in two children, suggesting that the disease is not always limited to the most obviously involved lobes.

McBride and colleagues described pulmonary function in 15 subjects who had had lobar resections for emphysema in infancy. They were between 8 and 30 years of age, and all were clinically well. Lung volume was normal, which suggested compensatory tissue growth, and perfusion was equally distributed between the normal and operated side. Low expiratory flows were the only persistent abnormality. Four subjects showed a reversible response to iso-

Table 17–1. Types of Childhood Lobar Emphysema

Type	No. of Airways	Alveoli	
Polyalveolar lobe	Normal	*Number:*	Increased
		Size:	May or may not be increased (i.e. emphysema)
Overinflation	Normal	*Number:*	Normal*
		Size:	Increased
Hypoplastic emphysema	Decreased	*Number:*	Decreased
		Size:	Increased
Atresia of bronchus	Probably normal	*Number:*	Probably normal*
		Size:	Increased
Compensatory emphysema	Normal	*Number:*	Normal*
		Size:	Increased

* As alveolar multiplication after birth is so rapid, these two types described as having a normal alveolar number at birth may rapidly come to have too few alveoli for age if the postnatal alveolar multiplication is impaired. (Courtesy of Dr. Lynne Reid.)

proterenol. The authors proposed that airway growth was not commensurate with alveolar growth to account for the reduced specific airway conductance.

REFERENCES

Adler, S. M., and Wyszogrodski, I.: Pneumothorax as a function of gestational age: Clinical and experimental studies. J. Pediatr. 87:771, 1975.

Aranda, J. V., Stern, L., and Dunbar, J. S.: Pneumothorax with pneumoperitoneum in a newborn infant. Am. J. Dis. Child 123:163, 1972.

Baumgart, S., Cohen, D., Borian, F., and Stephenson, L.: Peak inflation pressures vs. positive end expiratory pressure in pneumopericardium. Pediatr. Res. 16:277A, 1982.

Boland, R. B., Schneider, A. F., and Boggs, J. D.: Infantile lobar emphysema; Etiological concept. A.M.A. Arch Pathol. 61:289, 1956.

Brooks, J. G., Bustamante, S. A., Koops, B. L., Hilton, S., Cooper, D., Wesenberg, R. L., and Simmons, M. A.: Selective bronchial intubation for the treatment of severe localized pulmonary interstitial emphysema in newborn infants. J. Pediatr. 91:648, 1977.

Campbell, P. E.: Congenital lobar emphysema: Etiologic studies. Aust. Paediatr. J. 5:226, 1969.

Campbell, R. E.: Intrapulmonary interstitial emphysema: A complication of hyaline membrane disease. Am. J. Roentgenol. 110:449, 1970.

Chernick, V., and Avery, M. E.: Spontaneous alveolar rupture in newborn infants. Pediatrics 32:816, 1963.

Day, R., Goodfellow, A. M., Apgar, V., et al.: Pressure-time relation in the safe correction of atelectasis in animal lungs. Pediatrics 10:593, 1952.

DeMuth, G. R., and Sloan, H.: Congenital lobar emphysema: Long-term effects and sequelae in treated cases. Surgery 59:601, 1966.

Donahoe, P. K., et al.: Pneumoperitoneum secondary to pulmonary air leak. J. Pediatr. 81:797, 1972.

Emery, J. L.: Interstitial emphysema, pneumothorax and "airblock" in the newborn. Lancet 1:405, 1956.

Fischer, H. W., Potts, W. J., and Holinger, P. H.: Lobar emphysema in infants and children. J. Pediatr. 41:403, 1952.

Gregoire, R., Yulish, B., Martin, R., Fletcher, B., and Fanaroff, A.: Natural history of pulmonary interstitial emphysema in the preterm infant. Pediatr. Res. 13:495, 1979.

Hislop, A., and Reid, L.: Growth and development of the respiratory system—Anatomical development. In Davis, J. A., and Dobbing, J. (Eds.): Scientific Foundations of Paediatrics. Philadelphia, W. B. Saunders Co., 1974.

Holzel, A., Bennett, E., and Vaughan, B. F.: Congenital lobar emphysema. Arch. Dis. Child. 31:216, 1956.

Kuhns, L. R., Bednarek, F. J., Wyman, M. L., et al.: Diagnosis of pneumothorax or pneumomediastinum in the neonate by transillumination. Pediatrics 56:355, 1975.

Lawson, E. E., Gould, J. B., and Taeusch, H. W.: Neonatal pneumopericardium: Current management. J. Pediatr. Surg. 15:181, 1980.

Leape, L. L., and Longino, L. A.: Infantile lobar emphysema. Pediatrics 34:246, 1964.

Lincoln, J. C. R., Stark, J., Subramanian, S., et al.: Congenital lobar emphysema. Ann. Surg. 173:55, 1971.

Lubchenco, L. O.: Recognition of spontaneous pneumothorax in premature infants. Pediatrics 24:996, 1959.

Madansky, D. L., Lawson, E. E., Chernick, V., and Taeusch, H. W., Jr.: Pneumothorax and other forms of pulmonary air leak in newborns. Am. Rev. Resp. Dis. 120:729, 1979.

McBride, J. T., Wohl, M. E., Strieder, D. J., et al.: Lung growth and airway function after lobectomy in infancy for congenital lobar emphysema. J. Clin. Invest. 66:962, 1980.

Nelson, T.: Tension emphysema in infants. Arch. Dis. Child. 32:38, 1957.

Ogata, E. S., Gregory, G. A., Kitterman, J. A., Phibbs, R. H., and Tooley, W. H.: Pneumothorax in the respiratory distress syndrome: Incidence and effect on vital signs, blood gases, and pH. Pediatrics 58:177, 1976.

Patterson, W. H., and Fawcitt, J.: Non-traumatic mediastinal emphysema in childhood. Arch. Dis. Child. 29:451, 1954.

Roghair, G. D.: Non-operative management of lobar emphysema. Long-term follow-up. Radiology 102:125, 1972.

Shaw, R. R.: Localized hypertrophic emphysema. Pediatrics 9:220, 1952.

Stocker, J. T., and Madewell, J. E.: Persistent interstitial pulmonary emphysema: Another complication of the respiratory distress syndrome. Pediatrics 59:847, 1977.

Strunge, P.: Infantile lobar emphysema with lobar agenesis and congenital heart disease. Acta Paediatr. Scand. 61:209, 1972.

Thompson, J., and Forfar, J. O.: Regional obstructive emphysema in infancy. Arch. Dis. Child. 33:97, 1958.

18

Persistent Fetal Circulation (Pulmonary Hypertension)

In recent years, a number of reports have appeared describing newborns who, shortly after birth, develop tachypnea, cyanosis, cardiomegaly, and, sometimes, heart failure, and who therefore closely mimic infants with cyanotic congenital heart disease. Studies of these infants have revealed pulmonary hypertension and large right-to-left shunts through fetal channels but otherwise anatomically normal hearts and without evidence of pulmonary parenchymal disease.

Various terms other than persistent fetal circulation have been used to describe this clinical syndrome: "persistent pulmonary hypertension," "persistence of fetal cardiopulmonary circulation," "pulmonary vascular obstruction," and "progressive pulmonary hypertension." The incidence of this syndrome is not known, but it is probably more common than generally appreciated (Gersony et al., 1969; Fox, 1977; Rowe et al., 1981.)

Etiology. As more attention has been given to this phenomenon, the wide spectrum of its occurrence has become clearer. Most commonly seen in post-asphyxial states, it can also occur in the course of severe respiratory distress syndrome, in hydrops fetalis, and in association with pneumonia among both term and preterm infants. This syndrome has been described in infants with hypoglycemia not associated with maternal diabetes (Beard et al., 1971). It also has been recognized in newborns with polycythemia and hyperviscosity (Gatti et al., 1966; Gross et al., 1973). In another series, Roberton and associates found a high incidence of perinatal asphyxia, suggesting that intrauterine stress with hypoxia may be an important precipitating factor. It is likely that there are a number of different factors that retard the normal changes in pulmonary vasculature either by pulmonary vasoconstriction or because of developmental abnormalities. The pathogenic mechanisms are still not known, nor is it clear whether the disease in some of these infants who have a protracted clinical course bears any relationship to primary pulmonary vascular disease of older children (Burnell et al., 1972; Levin et al., 1975).

In a series of experimental studies, Murphy and colleagues found chronic exposure of rats to hypoxia produced new muscularization of small pulmonary arteries. To produce the severity of change seen in the infants who died of persistent fetal circulation, 10 to 14 days were required. Examination of lungs of infants who died with meconium aspiration shows similar muscularization of the pulmonary arteries. It seems probable that those infants who die have been subjected to prolonged intrauterine asphyxia. Presumably, the more acute episodes of meconium aspiration are treated with suction and, sometimes, with mechanical ventilation.

Pathophysiology. In normal newborns, the pulmonary vascular resistance decreases rapidly after birth. Hemodynamic studies on infants with persistent pulmonary hypertension have consistently shown an abnormally high pulmonary vascular resistance along with arterial unsaturation at the ductal or atrial level or both, indicative of right-to-left shunting. Cineangiographic and autopsy studies have revealed no evidence of other anatomic cardiac defects, nor has there been evidence of pulmonary parenchymal disease. However, medial hypertrophy of the pulmonary arterioles, as well as extension of the musculature into more peripheral vessels, has been a common finding (Haworth and Reid, 1976) (Figs. 18–1 and 18–2).

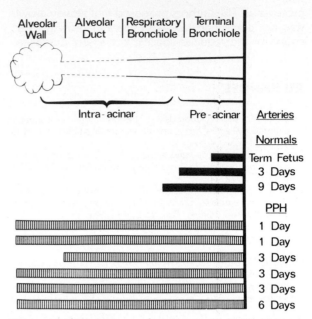

Figure 18–1. Diagrammatic location of muscle in the walls of the intra-acinar arteries. In normal infants who are less than 1 week of age, no muscular arteries are found within the acinus. All the patients with persistent pulmonary hypertension had "extension" of muscle into the small intra-acinar arteries. (From Reid, L: J. Pediatr. 98:962, 1981.)

Pulmonary hypertension may develop after several months in very premature infants. One such infant is described in the following case history (reported by Rendas et al., 1980).

CASE 18–1

A 610-gm female infant was born after 34 weeks gestation to a 17-year-old black mother. The pregnancy was complicated by toxemia for 2 months before delivery. Amniotic fluid was meconium-stained and foul-smelling. The infant had Apgar scores of 5 at 1 and 5 minutes of age. The infant was the size of an infant of 22 weeks gestation, functioned at a level of 28 weeks according to Dubowitz score, and was 34 weeks by menstrual history. She had only mild respiratory distress and was weaned to room air at 3 days of age. Her chest film was normal. She went home at 5 months of age and appeared normal but had a slow rate of growth. She was readmitted at 10 months of age, well below the third percentile for height and weight (2.86 kg). On radiograph, she had borderline enlargement of the heart. EKG showed right axis deviation and strain, and echocardiography showed a large right ventricle and pulmonary artery. At cardiac catheterization, pulmonary artery pressure was 100/40, systemic 80/40, with normal pulmonary wedge pressure. She died shortly after the procedure.

At autopsy, the heart was enlarged, with the right ventricular wall thicker than the left. Quantitative morphology of the pulmonary vessels showed an increase in muscle wall thickness and abnormal peripheral extension of muscle into small arteries. The artery number was significantly reduced to levels below that of a normal newborn.

Comment. The mild course in the newborn period suggests the absence of significant pulmonary hypertension at that time. We suspect that the hypoplasia of the pulmonary vascular bed limited subsequent growth and resulted in suprasystemic pressures in the later part of her first year of life. Whether the problem was the consequence of prolonged fetal distress at a critical stage in the development of the pulmonary vascular bed remains conjectural. At least precocious induction of the surfactant system must have occurred to explain the excellent pulmonary function in the early days of life.

Clinical Features. The likelihood of persistent fetal circulation may be suspected in an infant of a post-term mother when fetal heart rate decelerations are present (Type II dips; see Chapter 3). Artificial rupture of membranes may reveal meconium-stained amniotic fluid. Emergency cesarean section is indicated under these circumstances to prevent further fetal asphyxia. The infant may require intubation, suction of the contaminated fluid from the airway, and mechanical ventilation. Some become deeply cyanotic despite increased inspired oxygen. Another group of infants may not have aspirated but breathe rapidly and have intermittent or persistent severe cyanosis shortly after birth. There are usually neither severe retractions nor grunting. Except for harsh bronchiolar breath sounds, the lung fields are clear to auscultation. A soft ejection systolic murmur is often present. Hepatomegaly is common, suggesting the presence of congestive heart failure. The peripheral circulation is usually normal.

Roentgenogram of the chest shows a mild to moderate degree of cardiac enlargement with normal pulmonary vasculature. The electrocardiogram may show a greater right ventricular preponderance than normal for the newborn, but the findings are often inconclusive. The blood gases reveal a decrease in arterial oxygen tension, often strikingly low, with only slight abnormalities of arterial pH and P_{CO_2}.

The clinical course is variable. Infants who are going to survive usually improve rapidly within 3 to 6 days. Persistent cyanosis of the first week is a poor prognostic sign. However, the patient reported by Levin and his associates survived after a prolonged course. The prognosis in newborns with persistent fetal circulation associated with hypoglycemia or polycythemia is generally good, and the cardiopulmonary manifestations improve following treatment for the underlying condition.

Diagnosis. The clinical manifestations of persistent pulmonary hypertension must be distinguished from those of congenital heart disease and parenchymal lung disease. The occurrence in full-term infants, the degree of cyanosis without severe respiratory retractions, the lack of improvement with adequate oxygenation, and the absence of radiographic evidence of pulmonary disease should alert the physician to the diagnosis.

The distinction from cyanotic forms of congenital heart disease is often very difficult. Murmurs are rarely prominent in persistent pulmonary hypertension syndrome, but they may also be absent in congenital heart disease. Infants with cardiac defects of sufficient severity to cause tachypnea and cyanosis shortly after birth often develop frank congestive

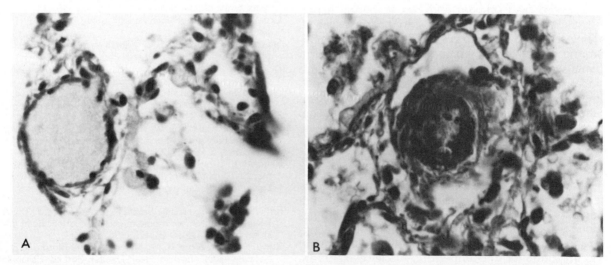

Figure 18–2. Photomicrographs of alveolar wall arteries distended with the barium gelatin suspension from A, a 3-day-old infant with normal lungs and B, a 3-day-old infant with persistent pulmonary hypertension. The normal artery (A) is nonmuscular with a single endothelial cell lining surrounded by a thin layer of connective tissue. In section (B), the artery wall is composed of smooth muscle (darkly stained) two-cell-layers thick surrounded by a thick connective tissue sheath enclosing a dilated lymphatic (located superiorly). (Elastin-van Gieson stain × 250.) (Courtesy Dr. John Murphy.)

heart failure earlier. They are also more likely to have more distinctive electrocardiographic and radiographic findings than infants with persistent pulmonary hypertension. Echocardiography to rule out other anatomic lesions has become an essential aid to diagnosis. Occasionally, cardiac catheterization is needed to clarify the diagnosis and to ascertain the site of right-to-left shunt. Blood sugar and hematocrit should be determined in all infants with cardiopulmonary disease of uncertain etiology. It should be recognized, however, that hypoglycemia is not uncommon in infants with failure from congenital heart disease. Patients with either hypoglycemia or polycythemia can present with central nervous system manifestations. Cyanosis may precede these manifestations. Cyanosis and signs of cardiac failure in a plethoric newborn should strongly suggest persistent fetal circulation associated with polycythemia and hyperviscosity.

Treatment. If the primary diagnosis is hypoglycemia, glucose should be administered to maintain normoglycemic levels. In infants with polycythemia, either a partial exchange transfusion, replacing whole blood with plasma, or a phlebotomy is indicated.

The treatment of infants with persistent pulmonary hypertension in whom no underlying disease process can be identified is much less satisfactory. Oxygen therapy should be maintained and the concentration adjusted depending on the arterial oxygen tension. Since many of these infants are first suspected of having congenital heart disease, digitalis and diuretics are often administered, although there is no evidence that they influence the course of the disease.

Intubation and mechanical ventilation have been advocated by Peckham and Fox to permit hyperventilation and to enhance pulmonary vasodilation. They studied a series of infants with continuous monitoring of pulmonary artery pressure. When the infants were hyperventilated to reduce P_{CO_2} from a mean of 49 mm Hg to 28 mm Hg, the mean pulmonary artery pressure fell by 36 mm Hg. Oxygenation improved at the same inspired concentration. We aim to keep arterial oxygen tensions in the 90 to 110 torr range. The efficacy of this approach to management can be monitored with transcutaneous oxygen electrodes. One problem is the high ventilator pressures required to achieve significant hyperventilation in some of these infants. Continuous distending airway pressure may be needed if aspiration has been significant, but it may be harmful if the lungs are well aerated or even overinflated. We know of no substitute for trial and error. Muscle relaxants are often required to permit adequate gas exchange at reasonable pressures. Some infants respond promptly and recover within a day or two. Others (we presume those who have been victims of pro-

longed intrauterine distress and who have increased musculature in the walls of their small pulmonary arteries) will not respond to oxygenation and hypocapnea.

The published experience with vasodilators is inconclusive. Peckham reviewed 21 clinical research reports and noted that none were controlled randomized trials. Few studies reported pulmonary artery pressures. The outcome was viewed as favorable on occasion but by no means predictable. Only 54 per cent of 314 infants survived. In general, we prefer to support the infant with mechanical ventilation sufficient to produce a respiratory alkalosis and provide adequate oxygenation rather than risk systemic hypotension from vasodilators reaching the systemic vascular bed. In desperate situations, we will infuse an alpha-adrenergic antagonist such as tolazoline, 1 mg/kg over a 10 to 30 minute period. Careful monitoring of systemic blood pressure and circulatory support with plasma or other colloid are usually required. Dopamine is a useful pressor agent when hypotension is persistent. Since responses to all these agents are unpredictable, therapy must be monitored and individualized (Drummond et al., 1981).

REFERENCES

Beard, A., et al.: Neonatal hypoglycemia: Discussion. J. Pediatr. 79:314, 1971.

Burnell, R. H., et al.: Progressive pulmonary hypertension in newborn infants. Am. J. Dis. Child. 123:167, 1972.

Drummond, W. H., Gregory, G. A., Heymann, M. A., and Phibbs, R. A.: The independent effects of hyperventilation, tolazoline, and dopamine on infants with persistent pulmonary hypertension. J. Pediatr. 98:603, 1981.

Fox, W. W., Gewitz, M. H., Dinwiddie, R., Drummond, W. H., et al.: Pulmonary hypertension in the perinatal aspiration syndromes. Pediatrics 59:205, 1977.

Gatti, R. A.: Neonatal polycythemia with transient cyanosis and cardiorespiratory abnormalities. J. Pediatr. 69:1063, 1966.

Gersony, W. M., Duc, G. V., and Sinclair, J. C.: "PFC" syndrome (persistence of fetal circulation). Circulation 40:111, 1969.

Gross, G. P., et al.: Hyperviscosity in the neonate. J. Pediatr. 82:1004, 1973.

Haworth, S. G., and Reid, L.: Persistent fetal circulation. Newly recognized structural features. J. Pediatr. 88:614, 1976.

Levin, D. L., et al.: Persistence of the fetal cardiopulmonary circulatory pathway. Pediatrics 56:58, 1975.

Murphy, J.D., Rabinowitz, M., Goldstein, J. D., and Reid, L.M.: The structural basis of persistent pulmonary hypertension of the newborn infant. J. Pediatr. 98:962, 1981.

Peckham, G. J., and Fox, W. W.: Physiologic factors affecting pulmonary artery pressure in infants with persistent pulmonary hypertension. J. Pediatr. 93:1005, 1978.

Rendas, A., Brown, E. R., Avery, M. E., and Reid, L. M.: Prematurity, hypoplasia of the vascular bed, and hypertension: fatal outcome in a ten-month-old infant. Am. Rev. Resp. Dis. 121:873, 1980.

Roberton, N. R. C., Hallidie-Smith, K. A., and Davis, J. A.: Severe respiratory distress syndrome mimicking cyanotic heart disease in term babies. Lancet 2:1108, 1967.

Rowe, R. D., Freedom, R. M., Mehrizi, A., and Bloom, K. R.: The Neonate with Congenital Heart Disease. 2nd ed. Philadelphia, W. B. Saunders Co., 1981.

Rudolph, A. M.: High pulmonary vascular resistance after birth. Clin. Pediatr. 19:585, 1980.

Siassi, B., et al.: Persistent pulmonary vascular obstruction in newborn infants. J. Pediatr. 78:610, 1971.

19

Pneumonia

Pneumonia of infectious etiology, acquired before, during, after birth as an isolated manifestation of infection or, more commonly, in association with generalized infection remains an important problem. Since infections and their treatment are discussed in detail in terms of etiology in Part 12, in this chapter we will focus on some aspects of incidence, pathogenesis, diagnosis, and course of pneumonia as seen in the perinatal period.

Incidence. In a review published in 1955, Schaffer and colleagues reported pneumonia in 35 per cent of 76 autopsies and believed it to be the cause of death in 8 per cent of those infants. The Collaborative Perinatal Project reported on 37,288 liveborn infants seen in the twelve participating university-based neonatal services between 1959 and 1966. Pneumonia was diagnosed in 75 white (0.42 per cent) and 101 black (0.52 per cent) babies on the basis of stringent diagnostic criteria. In 1974, we diagnosed pneumonia in 24 infants among 4000 newborns (0.6 per cent), and 9 of the 24 died.

Premature infants are at special risk of intrauterine infection. Probably the acquisition of infection contributes to the events that trigger premature birth. Bernstein and Wang in a review of 55 fatal cases of pneumonia found that nearly half the infants were born preterm.

Pneumonia may be acquired (1) before the beginning of labor, that is, in utero, (2) during the course of labor, (3) at the moment of delivery, or (4) after birth.

In the Collaborative Perinatal Study, labor was strongly associated with risk of pneumonia. Only 2 of 368 black babies delivered by cesarean section before the onset of labor had pneumonia.

Intrauterine Pneumonia

Intrauterine pneumonia may produce death of the fetus in utero, or live infants may be born with fully developed pneumonia that originated within the uterus. Many of these infants die within the first 2 or 3 days. The pathologic picture of intrauterine pneumonia differs considerably from that of the postnatally acquired disease. The clinical picture is no less different. The prognosis is poor but not hopeless.

Pathology. Gross examination of the lungs is unrewarding. There are no distinct areas of consolidation or pleurisy, no abscess formation, and little or no exudate in the bronchi. Characteristic is the diffuseness of the involvement on microscopic examination, practically all the alveoli in all portions of the lungs being affected. These are filled with exudate in which are found polymorphonuclear cells, some mononuclears, and often red blood cells. Fibrin is striking by its absence. In some lungs, amniotic debris is virtually absent (Fig. 19–1); in others, large amounts are present in distended alveoli (Fig. 19–2). One assumes that in the latter instance, intrauterine aspiration caused pneumonitis, whereas the former appearance suggests that pneumonitis was hematogenous in origin.

Pathogenesis. From studies of stillborns whose sole cause of death was pneumonia, determined by postmortem examination, and of newborns who lived only a few hours or days and in whom no other cause of death was discovered at autopsy, one concludes that intrauterine pneumonia develops under two different circumstances:

1. Pneumonia may follow prolonged membrane rupture. Amniotic fluids become contaminated by ascending vaginal organisms in increasing numbers the longer the membranes remain ruptured before delivery. If labor is active while membranes are ruptured, such contamination proceeds more rapidly, so that 100 per cent of fluids are infected by the end of 24 hours. Since all fetuses continually swallow amniotic fluid, the oropharynx and the gastrointestinal tract are the most common portals of entry for fetal infection. But since the fetus is induced to gasp as a result of any asphyxial insult, massive aspiration of contaminated amniotic fluid undoubtedly plays a role in pathogenesis.

Kjessler and Pryles and coworkers have confirmed the importance of prolonged membrane rupture time in the causation of pneumonitis and sepsis, while Blanc described in detail the possible routes of ascending fetal infection under the title "amniotic infection syndrome." Less commonly, infection may ascend through intact, unruptured membrane.

Gastric aspirates from infants from infected environments often show swallowed polymorphonuclear leukocytes. Evidence from identification of Y chromosome fluorescence established that, in most instances, the polymorphonuclear cells were of maternal origin and thus need not imply fetal infection (Vasan et al., 1977).

Shubeck has reported the results of a prospective study of more than 30,000 infants born consecutively and included in the Collaborative Perinatal Mortality Study. As membrane rupture time increased from 0 to 72 hours, amnionitis increased in linear fashion to about 50 per cent, funisitis to about 25 per cent, and documented infection of the fetus or the newborn infant to about 8 per cent.

The importance of the ascending route of infection was underscored by a study of 170 consecutive twin placentas. In 17 cases, the twin nearest the cervix was infected, and in six cases both twins were infected. The second twin was never the only one infected (Bernischke, 1960).

2. Fetal pneumonia may result from transmission of microorganisms across the placental barrier to the fetal circulation and thence to the lungs. These organisms may be carried to the placenta by maternal blood. A number of cases of intrauterine pneumococcal pneumonia have developed while the mother suffered from pneumococcal septicemia. That other organisms, including viruses, may cross the placenta

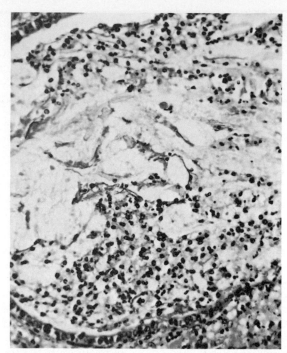

Figure 19–2. Microscopic section of lung (× 300) of a full-term infant who lived for two days. The membranes had ruptured 26 hours before delivery, and the cord was wrapped tightly about the baby's neck. Resuscitated with difficulty, she had tachypnea and low-grade fever throughout life. Note the large amount of amniotic aspirate overfilling alveoli in the center, while the surrounding areas are the sites of intense inflammation, most of the cells being polymorphonuclears.

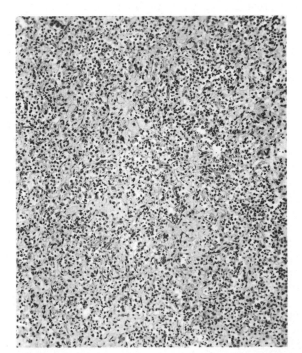

Figure 19–1. Microscopic section of lung (× 150) of a stillborn infant weighing 8 pounds 5 ounces (3770 gm). The mother's membranes had ruptured 48 hours before delivery. No treatment had been given. Note the diffuse pneumonitis, with fluid and inflammatory cells, mostly polymorphonuclears, homogeneously and heavily infiltrating interstitial tissue as well as the potential air spaces. A little amniotic debris is visible.

in similar fashion appears certain. Placental transmission of viruses is well documented, although the impact of fetal viremia is usually more devastating to the central nervous system, liver, and spleen than it is to the lung (Fig. 19–3). Cytomegalovirus, rubella, varicella, and herpes are all capable of producing fetal pneumonia. Phelan and Campbell described seven infants with interstitial pneumonia caused by rubella, six of whom died of their pneumonia.

Diagnosis. A history of obstetric difficulty is usually obtained. Prolonged ruptured membrane time, especially when this interval has exceeded 12 hours, is highly suggestive. So is maternal antepartum or intrapartum fever or urinary tract infection (Fig. 19–4). Obstetric accidents or prolonged labor leading to fetal asphyxia and vigorous manipulation during delivery, if coupled with prolonged membrane rupture, makes the possibility of intrauterine pneumonia a strong probability.

Examination of the tracheal aspirate by smear and culture is useful in diagnosis, especially if it can be obtained within the infant's first 8 hours of life. Sherman and colleagues obtained material by direct aspiration or immediately after intubation in 320 newborns with respiratory distress and one or more perinatal risk factors for infection. Bacteria were evident on the smear of the aspirates from 25 of these infants. The same organism was isolated from blood in 14 of the 25 newborns. In another group of 25 newborns with normal smears, there were three infants with positive cultures of aspirate and three with positive blood cultures. Thus, examination of both aspirates and blood cultures is necessary.

The infant may be asphyxiated at birth. The first cry is delayed 2 to 10 minutes or longer, and spontaneous respirations are not established quickly. These infants will have required resuscitative efforts immediately after birth. A falling Apgar score should suggest the possibility of pneumonia.

When respirations become established, they are rapid. Tachypnea may be accompanied by slight or moderate, never severe, retraction. Expiration is often grunting. Fever is present at times in the full-term infant. Often, this is low in degree, but occasionally it may reach 40°C (104°F) or more. Premature infants with pneumonia do not ordinarily become febrile, but they often manifest wide fluctuations of temperature below the normal line. There is no cough.

Physical signs are variable. Occasionally, localized dullness and rales may be heard over several areas of the lung fields on the first examination. Usually, the appearance of these signs is delayed for 12 to 48 hours, and at times they can never be elicited through the entire course of the disease. Breath sounds may be diminished over one or more areas or may be generally reduced in intensity, or in places they may be unduly harsh. Seldom does one hear classic tubular breathing.

The white blood cell count in some cases has been in the neighborhood of 30,000, with 75 per cent or more polymorphonuclears, while in a few the count is definitely leukopenic, 4000 per cu ml or less. In the majority, the white cell count is within normal limits for the newborn (5000 to 25,000), and the polymorphonuclear percentage is not high. In our experience, blood cultures have been only rarely positive, and cultures from the throat and nasopharynx have revealed a mixture of the usual vaginal flora. Gastric aspirate obtained in the first hours of life may contain polymorphonuclear cells and bacteria visible with Gram stain (Fig. 19–5). If the pneumonia progresses, and no organism has been demonstrated from the placenta or gastric aspirate, needle

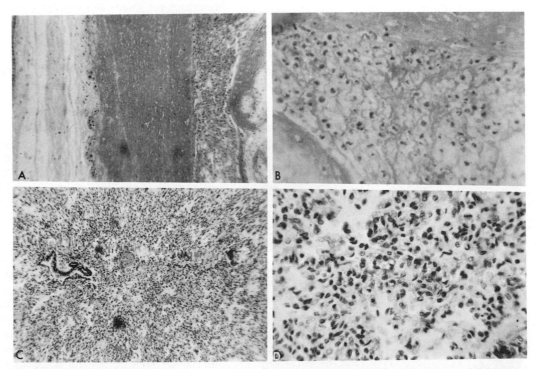

Figure 19–3. *A*, Microscopic section of placenta showing ascending fetal infection leading to intrauterine pneumonia. *B*, High-power view of the subchorionic region. *C*, Low-power view of section of lung to show dense homogeneous exudation and leukocytic infiltration. No amniotic debris is visible. *D*, Higher-power view of same.

The infant was one whose mother's labor was induced, because of Rh incompatibility, two weeks before term. Manual stripping of the membranes did not succeed on one day and was repeated the following day. The infant was promptly exchange-transfused, but died, for unknown reasons, in the midst of the procedure. The findings of placentitis and pneumonitis were unexpected.

(This case was presented by Dr. Peter Gruenwald at a Johns Hopkins Fetal Mortality Clinic. The photographs are reprinted with his kind permission.)

aspiration of the lung may be indicated. The quick insertion and withdrawal of a #23 needle attached to a syringe with about 0.5 ml saline can contaminate the needle with the offending organism, which may then be cultured. The saline allows the contents of the needle to be flushed into the culture medium.

Virus isolation, demonstration of rising titers of specific antibody, and serum IgM and IgA levels are increasingly available and of essential help in diagnosis of viral infections.

Neurologic abnormalities appear in the course of the disease with unexpected frequency. The infant who was flaccid at birth may remain flaccid for days. Other infants become hypertonic, even rigid. Some have muscular twitchings, some frank convulsions. These phenomena are encountered when the disease is severe, and these infants usually do poorly. At autopsy, no gross intracranial lesion may be discovered.

Several of our infants with extensive early neonatal pneumonia have had heart failure, signaled by cardiac enlargement, poor, rapid heart sounds, and sudden increase in size of the liver.

Radiographic Findings. Radiograms supply the supporting evidence for the diagnosis of pneumonia of the newborn. They yield positive evidence in almost all cases in which the clinical picture fits the aforementioned pattern. Patches of consolidation

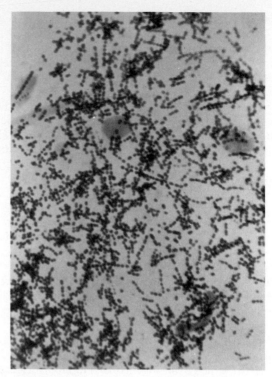

Figure 19–5. Gram-stain of gastric aspirate of infant described in legend of Figure 19–4. Note the myriad of streptococci evident on this smear. (Courtesy of Dr. William Cochran, Boston Hospital for Women.)

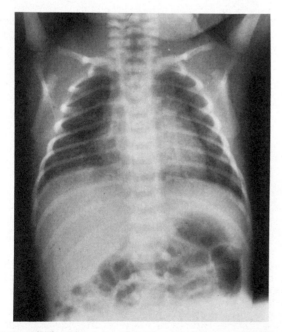

Figure 19–4. Film of an infant, age 4 hours, with moderate tachypnea, born of a mother with Group B streptococcal urinary tract infection. Although the infiltrates appear only moderate, the infant died of septicemia and pneumonia at 20 hours of age.

may not become obvious until the second or even the third day. This is analogous to the situation in older patients, in whom pneumonic areas may not become radiopaque for a number of days after the onset.

We feel that there are several radiographic patterns of congenital pneumonia. The first is one of bilateral homogeneous opacification involving the major portions of both lungs (Figs. 19–6 and 19–7). This pattern is rarely seen and must be confined to those cases in which pneumonia developed in the fetus many days before delivery. The second pattern is similar to diffuse bronchopneumonia at any age. It consists of coarse irregular opacities heavily clustered about the hilus and extending fanwise in diminishing amounts toward the periphery on both sides. Often it is ill defined on the first day of life, becoming more opaque as well as more extensive on the second and third days. In a few examples we have seen recently, there is linear, hard-looking opacification extending fanwise from the hilus on one side, while on the other there is an area or several areas of soft-appearing homogeneous density. Peribronchial thickening as a part of the bronchopneumonic process will appear as tiny ring-like densities in the perihilar areas when the bronchi are seen on end. Air bronchograms may also be present as the air-filled bronchi are contrasted against airless alveoli.

Prognosis. The more seriously ill infants are likely to die in utero or within the first day or two of life,

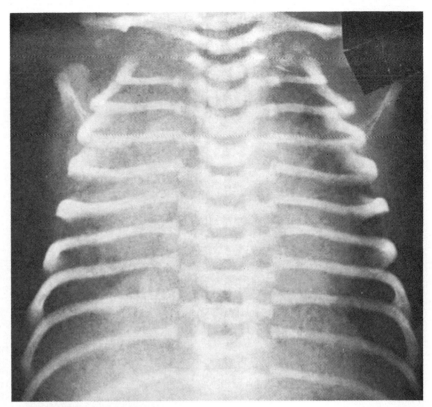

Figure 19-6. Anteroposterior view of chest taken at 16 hours of age. The lungs appear to be almost completely consolidated, the periphery of the left lung and the extreme right base alone containing air. The opacification is homogeneous and dense.

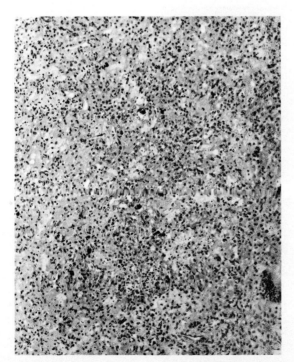

Figure 19-7. Microscopic section of lung shows widespread homogeneous exudation and leukocytic infiltration. Alveoli, bronchi, and interstitial tissue are all equally involved.

regardless of the quality of treatment. They may die from widespread encroachment of the pneumonic process upon functioning lung tissue alone or "cerebral deaths" with rigidity and convulsions, or from associated heart failure.

Treatment. When the diagnosis of intrauterine pneumonia can be made with a fair degree of certainty, treatment must be prompt and vigorous. When pneumonia is suspected, antibiotics should be ordered as soon as blood and oropharyngeal cultures and gastric aspirate are collected.

If the organism is unknown, choice of antibiotics depends on the historical experience of those working in the nursery and the antimicrobial sensitivities of bacteria recently isolated from sick and healthy infants. Initially, we prefer ampicillin in combination with an aminoglycoside, either kanamycin or gentamicin. Once the pathogen is identified, the most effective and least toxic drug or combination of drugs is appropriate. Tobramycin or amikacin should be reserved for organisms known to be resistant to kanamycin or gentamicin to reduce emergence of more resistant organisms.

General supportive measures for the infant with pneumonia are as essential as appropriate antibiotics.

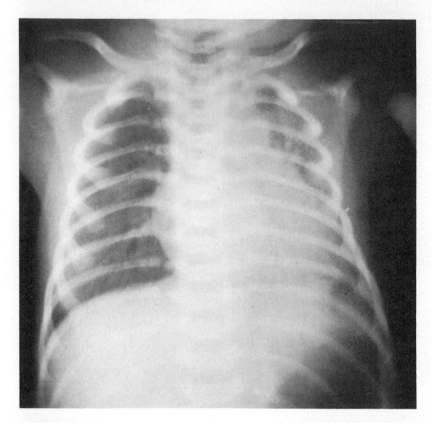

Figure 19–8. There is soft linear infiltration spreading outward fanwise from the right hilus. The left lung is almost entirely opacified by confluent areas of homogeneous density. This infant, whose weight was 4 pounds 5 ounces (1956 gm), was born 11½ hours after membranes had been ruptured. Amniotic fluid was meconium stained; Apgar score was 2 at one minute. Tachypnea and dyspnea were followed by apneic spells and then convulsions; he died at 25 hours of age.

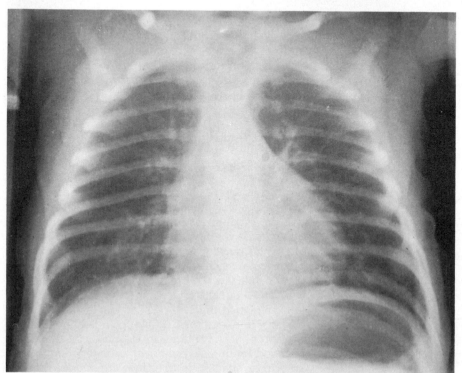

Figure 19–9. Anteroposterior view of chest of an infant who was born 36 hours after membrane rupture and demonstrated fever and tachypnea with mild retraction for five days. He undoubtedly had intrauterine pneumonia.

Many of these infants have diffuse disease that impairs ventilation. Close attention to blood gases is important to assess the need for mechanical ventilation. Premature infants in particular may tire from the added work required to ventilate a stiff lung. Venous admixture is common, and in some infants right-to-left shunting of blood through a persistent patent ductus will occur. Increased inspired oxygen concentrations are most always needed.

Meticulous attention must be paid to thermal requirements to keep the infants in a "thermal neutral" range, that is, the body temperature at which energy requirements are minimized (see pp. 50 and 51).

Water balance and nutritional requirements must be considered with the same care as for any sick neonate. Intravenous fluids are appropriate, since gastric distention is common in association with infection, and the risk of aspiration, which would aggravate the pneumonia, is ever present.

Prevention. Opinion is still divided as to the efficacy of maternal therapy prior to delivery in preventing fetal infection when the membranes have ruptured prematurely. No one any longer advocates treating a mother with full doses of antibiotics for weeks or months. But since concomitant labor seems to hasten upward spread of infection from vagina to fetus, one might logically attempt to prevent ascent by treatment during this critical period. This might be accomplished by beginning vigorous antibiotic therapy a few weeks before the expected date of confinement, continuing it for 2 or 3 days, and then inducing labor. In any event, one might give the mother antibiotics from the moment labor begins. A broad-spectrum antibacterial agent such as ampicillin must be used.

The next question is whether one should treat babies routinely who have been born after prolonged membrane rupture time or after asphyxia-producing obstetric accidents that predispose the infant to neonatal pneumonia. No controlled studies to date have

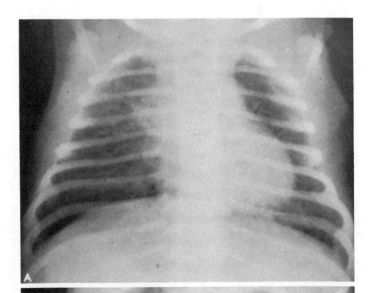

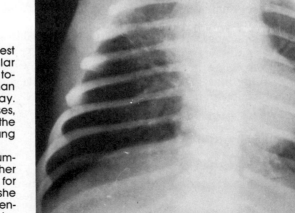

Figure 19–10. *A,* Anteroposterior view of chest made on the first day. One sees patchy irregular infiltration, maximal about the hili, diminishing toward the periphery, and greater on the right than on the left side. *B,* Film taken the following day. Now there is definite emphysema of both bases, probably involving both lower lobes and the right middle lobe. Infiltration in the upper lung fields is still heavy.

This was a full-term infant with meconium-stained foul-smelling amniotic fluid but no other obstetrical abnormalities. She was dyspneic for eight days and febrile for most of that time; she then made a perfect recovery, treated with penicillin, streptomycin, and erythromycin. An alpha streptococcus and a hemolytic staphylococcus were grown from the nasopharynx.

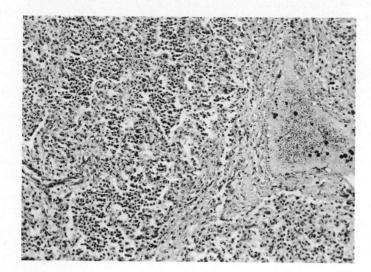

Figure 19–11. Microscopic section of lung. Widespread homogeneous pneumonitis with little or no amniotic aspirate is seen.

shown that babies so treated suffer less mortality or morbidity than those from whom treatment is withheld until indicated by appropriate signs or symptoms. But these infants must be monitored assiduously, and vigorous treatment must be instituted at the first sign of respiratory trouble.

Pneumonia Acquired During Birth

Some infants acquire pathogens during vaginal delivery. Symptoms will not occur until after the appropriate incubation period. Often, colonization may occur with no subsequent manifestations of disease, as in the case of cytomegalovirus. With other organisms such as Type 2 (genital) herpes, infants most often acquire infection during vaginal delivery and manifest illness at 5 to 10 days of age, after discharge from the nursery as well babies. Skin lesions are the usual first manifestations. Systemic disease involves liver, central nervous system, and other organs as well as lung. The pneumonic symptoms are apneic spells followed by respiratory rales and, finally, evidence of pulmonary insufficiency.

As soon as the diagnosis is established, the infant should receive adenine arabinoside (vidarabine) 15 mg/kg/day intravenously over a 12-hour period for at least 10 days. If the disease does not involve the central nervous system, the prognosis is excellent (see Chapter 83).

Neonatal varicella is most often acquired near the time of birth. In a review, Gershon found reports of 50 cases in the literature, apparently acquired from maternal infection at or near term. The incubation period is between 10 and 21 days. In the absence of passively transferred maternal antibody, the infant is at risk of systemic illness. Pneumonia is then only one manifestation of generalized disease (see Chapter 83).

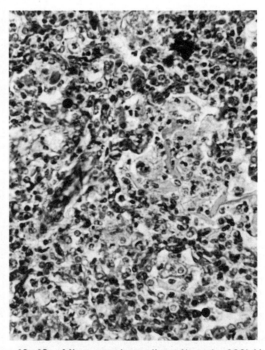

Figure 19–12. Microscopic section of lung (× 300). Note the areas of poor staining interspersed throughout unexpanded lung in which the alveoli are lined by cuboidal epithelium. Throughout is a myriad of inflammatory cells, mostly polymorphonuclear cells. The lighter-stained areas seem to be made up of necrotic cells plus aspirate.

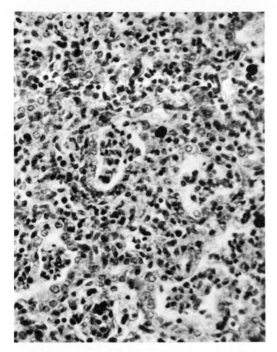

Figure 19–13. Microscopic section of lung of a premature infant. Here no aspirate or necrotic cells are seen, but the whole is a mass of unexpanded lung, the alveoli composed of cuboidal cells, all infiltrated by inflammatory blood cells.

Postnatally Acquired Pneumonia: Aspiration of Gastric Contents

One of the commoner forms of neonatal pneumonia is that due to aspiration of food, gastric contents, or oronasopharyngeal secretions. Predisposing causes are obstructive lesions anywhere in the gastrointestinal tract, such as esophageal atresia, with or without tracheoesophageal fistula, intestinal atresia,

Table 19–1. Incidence of Prematurity Among Stillborns with Pneumonia Versus Liveborns Who Died of Pneumonia in the First Three Days

	No.	Prematures	Full Term	Prematures (Per Cent)
Stillborns	28	4	24	14
Liveborns	23	14	9	60

and imperforate anus. Aspiration pneumonia does occur, however, in the absence of organic obstruction, especially in premature or feeble infants, who are prone to regurgitate ingested liquids. It also jeopardizes those infants who experience difficulty in swallowing for various other reasons, such as autonomic dysfunction and thrush esophagitis. The insertion of a nasogastric or orogastric tube to decompress the stomach is essential whenever aspiration due to mechanical reasons is probable.

Whenever an infant is tachypneic or has gastric or abdominal distention, oral feeding should be discontinued. The infant should receive fluid requirements intravenously. If the need to withhold feedings persists for more than 24 hours, intravenous alimentation should be considered.

Some infants whose problem is regurgitation or swallowing dysfunction may be fed by a slow infusion into a catheter inserted from nose to stomach (see Chapter 89).

Pathology. The distribution of aspiration pneumonia is similar to that of other bronchopneumonias.

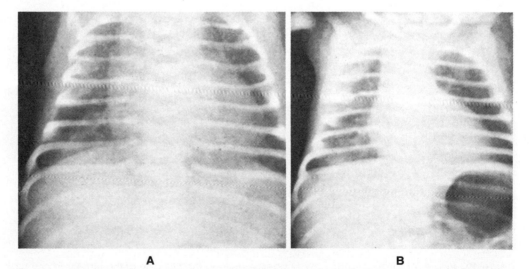

A　　　　　　　　　　**B**

Figure 19–14. *A,* Anteroposterior view of chest made on the third day of life. Patchy infiltration of both lungs is seen, somewhat greater at the right base. *B,* Four days later. The infiltration is more extensive, and the individual patches seem somewhat larger. The left lower lobe may be a trifle hyperinflated.

Its cellular reaction differs in that macrophages, often fat-filled if milk has been fed, are present in large numbers. In addition, mononuclear cells and polymorphonuclears are usually found. Scattered patches may be actually necrotic, possibly because of aspiration of gastric digestive juices. These areas often swarm with bacteria of all varieties.

Associated ulcerative lesions of the lower esophagus are not rare.

Staphylococcal Pneumonia

Incidence. Staphylococcal infections of all varieties are a distressing problem in newborn nurseries. They occur sporadically and in epidemics. They were rare until the mid-1940s and became much more frequent in the succeeding 10 or 15 years, but they now appear to have declined in numbers throughout most of the United States. Phage group I *Staphylococcus aureus* was the most common offending agent in the 1950s.

It is easy to underestimate the frequency of serious staphylococcal complication, especially in large communities in which more than one hospital cares for sick babies. Infants discharged from nurseries with skin or conjunctival infection apparently cured are likely to turn up at another hospital when osteomyelitis, lung abscess, or pneumonia supervenes days or weeks later. True incidence can be determined only by painstaking follow-up study.

In the 1960s, when hexachlorophene-containing soaps were widely used in nurseries, staphylococcal epidemics were rare. When it became known that even 3 per cent solutions of hexachlorophene would give measurable blood levels, and some white matter lesions could be found associated with hexachlorophene toxicity, routine use of such soaps was abandoned, with the consequence of several outbreaks of staphylococcal infection. A reasonable approach would seem to be to recognize the efficacy of hexachlorophene-containing soaps in the face of a high prevalence of staphylococci but to avoid routine bathing of all infants with a potentially toxic substance. Using these soaps occasionally for bathing infected infants and for handwashing by adults should break the chain of spread of staphylococci in nurseries.

Etiology. The offending organism in recent years has been phage group II *Staphylococcus aureus*. Coagulase-negative staphylococci can be pathogenic and are frequently but not always associated with indwelling catheters.

Control of an Epidemic. In the event of an epidemic, it is useful to culture the anterior nares of all infants at the time of discharge from the nursery in order to monitor the frequency of colonization and the phage types of the organisms. A colonization rate of about 4 per cent is usual; up to 10 per cent may not be alarming. Any sudden change in the patterns of colonization or the types of organisms should lead to a search for the source and improvement in techniques.

Pathogenesis. Staphylococcal pneumonias fall into two groups. The primary (bronchogenic) form originates in the infant's nasopharynx and spreads downward. The secondary (septic) variety originates in skin or umbilical cord stump, possibly also in the conjunctiva or nasopharynx, and spreads to lung,

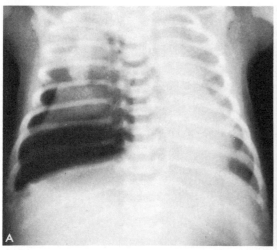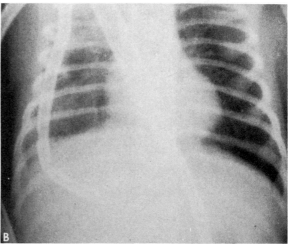

Figure 19–15. *A,* Anteroposterior view of chest made on the first day of the illness, about eight hours after the first symptom had been noted. Air under tension can be seen to collapse the right lung, flatten the diaphragm, and displace the heart and mediastinum far to the left. *B,* Film taken 24 hours later, after air and pus had been suctioned continuously from the pleural cavity. The right lung has re-expanded, the left is overaerated. Diffuse patchy infiltration can be seen in both lungs now.

bone, meninges, or other viscera via the blood stream.

The infecting agent may be recovered in the course of a nursery epidemic from the surfaces of the walls, floors, and cribs, and from bed linens and infants' clothing. It may also be recovered from the nares and skin of a significant number of the adults who constitute the working personnel of the nursery: physicians, nurses, and nurses' aides. From all these sources, a pool of pathogenic staphylococci is built up in each nursery. Newborn infants admitted to such nurseries become contaminated first externally, that is, on the skin and umbilical cord stump, and from here the organisms are carried to effect nasal colonization. Staphylococcal disease may or may not follow colonization, depending upon variables such as dosage, degree of pathogenicity, and individual immunologic states.

One of the outstanding virtues of "rooming-in" is the comparative freedom of these relatively isolated babies from staphylococcal infections.

Staphylococcal pulmonary infection eventually complicates almost all cases of cystic fibrosis of the pancreas. Neonates are not immune to this complication, although in this age group it is rare. The discovery of staphylococcal infection of the lung demands a sweat test to rule out cystic fibrosis.

Pathology. A few cases are fulminating and cause death in 1 or 2 days. In these cases, the lungs are massively consolidated, and with the intense, predominantly polymorphonuclear infiltration one finds equally intense hemorrhagic alteration.

Most cases are less explosive in onset and, if fatal, are less rapidly so. These show patchy infiltration, with clusters of abscesses about the smaller bronchi, especially in the periphery. Pleurisy and empyema are common, as is pyopneumothorax produced by

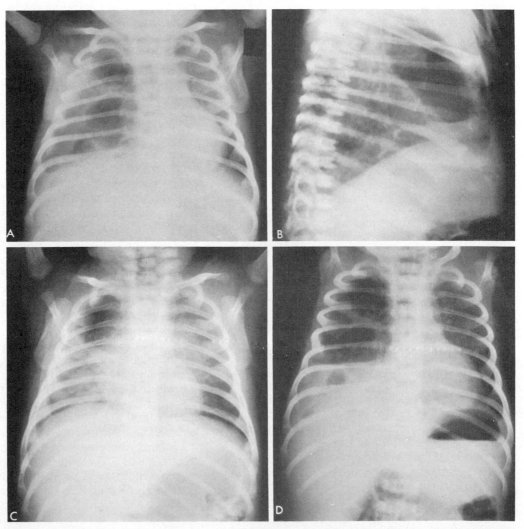

Figure 19–16. *A, C,* and *D,* Anteroposterior projections made at various times throughout the patient's long course. *B,* Lateral view taken at the same time as *A.* They show differing degrees of infiltration, pleural thickening, and pneumatocele formation.

rupture of superficial abscesses into the pleural cavity. Interstitial emphysema, mediastinal emphysema, and pneumothorax are frequently discovered, resulting from extravasation of air into perivascular sheaths and its progression along the blood vessels to the mediastinum (see Chapter 17). Subpleural blebs, or pneumatoceles, are a hallmark of the disease.

Diagnosis. The onset is apt to be mild, with low-grade fever, irritability, and, usually, upper respiratory tract symptoms. These are not invariably present, and, not too infrequently, vomiting and diarrhea usher in the disease. At times, the onset is catastrophic, owing either to the fact that the disease is of the fulminating variety or, as is more likely, to the development of an unheralded pneumothorax. We might point out here that pneumothorax that appears in the first few days of life is apt to be the result of obstructive emphysema, while that which develops in the second week or later is almost always the result of staphylococcal disease.

After 1 to 4 days of mild prodromata, fever rises and respirations become rapid and, frequently, labored, and they are accompanied by expiratory grunt. At this stage, areas of dullness and fine crepitant rales may be discovered. Later, the signs of pleural effusion, pneumothorax, or hydropneumothorax frequently supervene. Distention is often distressing and intractable. Fever may be absent or low-grade or high and sustained throughout. Scattered pustules may be discovered over the trunk or extremities.

Laboratory Findings. By far, the majority of these babies show a polymorphonuclear leukocytosis. A few show a normal or leukopenic count, but the widespread notion that leukopenia is characteristic of staphylococcal infection is undoubtedly incorrect. Kanof and colleagues found granulocytosis in 38 of their 41 reported cases.

Staphylococcus can be grown regularly and readily from pleural exudate and abscess contents. It is almost invariably the predominant organism in throat and nasopharyngeal cultures. In a large percentage of cases it can be cultivated from the blood. Phage typing and sensitivities will usually demonstrate that the organism belongs to one of several phage types that seem to be particularly pathogenic and that it is insensitive to penicillin and many other antibiotics.

A moderate to severe anemia develops in the course of the disease, and small transfusions may be required.

Radiographic Findings. Kanof and coworkers found infiltrations indistinguishable from other forms of bronchopneumonia in all their patients. In addition, empyema was noted in 57 per cent, multiple abscesses in 48 per cent, pneumothorax in 38 per cent, and pleural blebs, or pneumatoceles, in 25 per cent (Figs. 19–15 and 19–16).

Prognosis. Before the antibiotic era, nearly all neonates with this infection died. Since the advent of various antimicrobial agents, there has been a succession of periods of favorable and unfavorable prognosis corresponding to the times during which staphylococci were sensitive, then insensitive, to each new drug. But with the great variety of drugs now available, one can usually be found that will control the infection.

Treatment. Oxacillin or methicillin is the drug of choice for penicillinase-resistant organisms. All the young babies in the series of Klein and associates who were treated with oxacillin recovered. If the infection is from coagulase-negative staphylococci, vancomycin is the drug of choice (Schaad et al., 1980). Methicillin or oxacillin may be substituted if the organism is sensitive in vitro.

The prognosis depends partly on control of the pneumonitis and partly on the location of metastatic infections secondary to septicemia. Meningitis, pericarditis, peritonitis, renal abscess, brain abscess, and osteomyelitis are some of the complications to be expected, and the presence of one or more of these may reduce chances for recovery.

Group B Streptococcal Infections

Increasingly, Group B streptococcal infections are recognized as a significant cause of pneumonia and suppurative meningitis. Some infants have respiratory distress at the time of delivery, whereas others are considered normal at birth and suddenly deteriorate in the first day or two of life. Clinically, they may be indistinguishable from infants with hyaline membrane disease.

The early onset of fulminant forms may be fatal, even with prompt and appropriate antibiotic therapy. The infection is presumably acquired in utero in some infants (Baker, 1978).

Menke and coworkers contrasted the clinical and laboratory findings of infants with Group B streptococcal pneumonia with those of infants with hyaline membrane disease. The significant differences were a lower initial white blood count in the infants with pneumonia and a marked fall in white count to 2900 ± 189 (800 to 6400 range) in the second 12 hours of life. The absolute neutrophil count was lower in the infants with pneumonia. Hypotension was more frequent in the infected infants. Both groups of infants required mechanical ventilation with similar peak inspiratory pressures. The only diagnostic test that can definitively distinguish these conditions is recovery of gram-positive cocci in gastric aspirate. Rapid, specific diagnosis is possible with counterimmunoelectrophoresis.

Radiographic findings in premature infants are the

same as those seen in hyaline membrane disease, namely diffuse reticulogranular infiltrates with an air bronchogram. As the disease worsens, the opacification of the lungs progresses. The lungs of infants born at term with Group B streptococcal pneumonia have more localized consolidations. Pleural effusions are common and help distinguish infants with pneumonia from those with hyaline membrane disease.

One of the problems in recognition of this illness is that hospital laboratories may not report Group B hemolytic streptococci by that name, since grouping by the precipitin method is not always available. They can be suspected by colony morphology and type of hemolysis, and may be bacitracin-resistant. Apparently most beta-hemolytic streptococci isolated from the vagina will be Group B.

Treatment.   Treatment should begin as soon as the disease is suspected and cultures have been taken. Aqueous penicillin, 200,000 to 300,000 units/kg/day intravenously, is appropriate.

Prevention is achievable by culture of the vagina, and of the husband's urethra if streptococci are recovered from the vagina. Franciosi et al. recommend 1.2 M units parenteral benzathine penicillin be given to the parents.

Chlamydia Trachomatis

Incidence.   First described as a cause of infection in infants in 1975, this intracellular bacterium-like parasite is widely distributed. It has been identified in the vagina in 2 to 13 per cent of women. It is transmitted from mother to infant at the time of vaginal delivery. About 20 per cent of infected infants have pneumonia.

Clinical Features.   Pneumonia usually occurs at 4 weeks to 3 months of age, sometimes but not always preceded by conjunctivitis, which most commonly appears at 5 to 14 days. Cough is usually present and sometimes is paroxysmal. Rales are often heard. Radiographs may be disproportionally severe in some infants with mild symptoms. There are no pathognomonic signs. Diagnosis depends on recovery of the organism from conjunctiva or nasopharyngeal aspirate. A rise in serum antibodies confirms the diagnosis.

Treatment.   It is not clear to what extent treatment alters the course of the disease. The agent is sensitive to a number of microbial agents, including erythromycin. Current recommendations are to give 40 to 60 mg/kg/day for 2 to 3 weeks (Beem et al., 1979). Complete recovery follows between 2 weeks and 2 months.

Nosocomial Infections

Acquisition of infection from organisms not usually considered pathogenic has long been a problem, especially in intensive care nurseries in which incubators, humidifiers, sinks, and other equipment can become reservoirs for "water bugs." Drug-resistant Enterobacteriaceae, including *Klebsiella pneumoniae*, *Enterobacter*, and *Serratia marcescens*, have been associated with sepsis and meningitis, and they have also aggravated the course of infants with chronic lung disease by superimposition of pneumonia.

Klebsiella-Aerobacter Pneumonia

(see Chapter 83)

It has become customary to regard *Klebsiella pneumoniae* and *Aerobacter aerogenes* as members of the same group in which a great number (77 at last count) of strains are distinguishable on the basis of specific capsular antigens. Within recent decades, *Klebsiella* has become a not uncommon infecting pathogenic organism in the newborn period.

The infants most at risk are the long-term residents of neonatal intensive care units. The majority of infants colonized do not become ill, but those who do may shed the organism for months, despite antibiotic therapy.

Several nursery outbreaks have been reported in recent years. We give it brief mention here in order to re-emphasize the point that almost any disorder that involves older persons may attack the newborn. In addition, certain characteristics of its clinicopathologic course are unique.

Klebsiella pneumoniae gives rise to two forms of illness: a lobar form that is indistinguishable on clinical and radiologic grounds from pneumococcal pneumonia and a chronic type that is characterized by an insidious onset or that may follow partial subsidence of the acute form. Progression is marked by pulmonary necrosis, abscess formation, sloughing, and cavitation, and if healing sets in, by fibrosis. Before the antibiotic era, the mortality rate was greater than 80 per cent.

The choice of antibiotic depends on the organism's sensitivities. Kanamycin, 15 mg/kg/day, or gentamicin, 5 to 7.5 mg/kg/day, is often effective. Resistance to antibiotics may develop during treatment.

Pseudomonas Pneumonia

Incidence.   The *Pseudomonas* group of bacilli, like staphylococci and some fungi, have benefited by the widespread use of antibiotics. In the last 25 years, their importance as pathogens has increased. This increase in morbidity and mortality is most notable in nurseries and infants' wards.

Etiology. *Pseudomonas* is a group of organisms of low pathogenicity. It is, in fact, practically nonpathogenic for a mature, healthy person unless ingested or inoculated in overwhelming dosage or unless its growth potential is artificially increased by the destruction of its normal antagonists, the gram-positive cocci. This effect is successfully achieved by the prolonged use of penicillin.

Pathology. *Pseudomonas* is almost unique in that it calls forth no inflammatory response in invaded tissues. Infected areas of lung or intestine are killed by its toxin, but few polymorphonuclear or mononuclear cells wander into the devastated areas. The resultant lesions have been called "necrobiotic." In addition, it stimulates no leukocytosis of the peripheral blood. In many instances, indeed, it appears to suppress leukocytes, causing profound leukopenia and granulocytopenia as well as platelet production. Suppression of platelet production is responsible for intractable bleeding that may complicate the late stages of the disease and that, at times, may constitute the presenting sign at its onset.

Pathogenesis. Most infections are acquired in the hospital, either in the premature or full-term nurseries or in the wards for sick infants. As is the case with the *Staphylococcus* infection, *Pseudomonas* pneumonia may be primary, that is, a direct result of infection of the upper respiratory tract by extension downward, or secondary, as a metastatic infection from generalized septicemia. These originate in some instances from a primary focus in the gastrointestinal tract, in others from an accidental or operative wound in either skin or mucous membrane.

Once having gained a foothold in a nursery or ward, *Pseudomonas* is difficult to eradicate. It can be cultivated from walls and floors, furniture and linens, and even from basins of many conventional antiseptic solutions. This ubiquity renders it a constant potential hazard, not to the healthy newborn so much as to the premature infant or the one enfeebled by other disease. It is particularly prone to gain entrance to the blood stream by invading operative wounds. Prolonged use of penicillin in any child, in prophylactic or therapeutic dosage, makes him more liable to *Pseudomonas* infection, and its continued use is apt to make that infection more hazardous. In a series of eight cases reported from the Brooke General Hospital, including gangrenous infections of the skin, gastroenteritis, and respiratory infections and ranging in patient age from 5 days to 9 years, penicillin had been given for various reasons and varying periods to every child.

Diagnosis. The rare case of primary pneumonia due to *Pseudomonas aeruginosa* differs in no rec-ognizable way, clinically or radiologically, from pneumonia of the newborn caused by many other organisms. Diagnosis depends entirely upon recovery of the organism from the nose or throat. The diagnosis of secondary *Pseudomonas* pneumonia may be made more easily if other signs, particularly characteristic skin lesions, are present. These will be discussed fully in the section on infections of the newborn.

Treatment. As indicated earlier, there is no regularity of response of various strains of *Pseudomonas* to the antimicrobial agents. Most are killed in vitro by polymyxin B, but the clinical response to this drug is not so striking as its performance in vitro. A combination of polymyxin B in small dosage (1.0 mg/kg/day) with streptomycin (20 to 40 mg/kg/day) or colistin (2 to 5 mg/kg/day) is often effective. Polymyxin B and colistin have a similar spectrum of activity, and both can be toxic to the kidneys. Daily urinalyses are indicated. Gentamicin 5 mg/kg/day or carbenicillin is useful.

The usual supportive measures will be utilized. Multiple small transfusions may be required if granulopenia and thrombocytopenia ensue, but the appearance of these hematologic complications makes the prognosis extremely grave.

Prevention. The ubiquitous "water bugs," as they have been labeled, depend on moist surfaces for growth. Prevention depends on meticulous cleansing and drying of incubators and inhalation therapy equipment. A 0.25 per cent solution of acetic acid in incubators or nebulizers has been shown by Edmondson and others to reduce contamination. A regimen of gas sterilization or autoclaving of all nebulizers and suction equipment every 48 hours is recommended.

Viral Pneumonias

Respiratory syncytial virus pneumonia may occur in epidemic form in intensive care nurseries. The initial symptoms are coryza, cough, and, later, dyspnea. Chest films may show minimal changes or extensive consolidation.

In a prospective study in Rochester among infants hospitalized for 6 or more days, Hall found that 35 per cent were infected between January and March of 1977. Two thirds of this group had respiratory symptoms, and the remainder demonstrated their illness by apneic spells, lethargy, irritability, or poor feeding.

Infected infants should be isolated from noninfected ones, although control of infection during an epidemic has proved very difficult. Infants can shed virus as long as 22 days after the onset of symptoms. Adults with any kind of upper or lower respiratory tract symptoms should excuse themselves from the care of infants during an epidemic of respiratory syncytial virus disease.

Pneumocystis carinii Pneumonia

Pneumocystis carinii pneumonia is rare in newborn nurseries in this country, although it has been noted in epidemics in Europe. It occurs most commonly in infants of several months or years of age with other debilitating disease, such as immune deficiency states and malignancies.

Incidence. First described in nursery epidemics in Europe during the 1940s, *Pneumocystis carinii* pneumonia has been recognized with greater frequency in this country in later years. The largest experience has been in immunosuppressed hosts. The advent of counterimmunoelectrophoresis has made detection more possible. Stagno and coworkers found it in 10 of 27 infants with pneumonia, suggesting that the diagnosis has been overlooked in the past.

Etiology and Pathology. The offending organism, *Pneumocystis carinii*, has not been classified with certainty. It is believed to belong to the family of protozoa by most, of fungi by some. The organism is widely distributed among animals, including rats, mice, dogs, cats, sheep, and goats, and it has been identified in all parts of the world. It is found, often with difficulty, in Giemsa-stained sections of involved lungs. These are voluminous, emphysematous, inelastic, and firm, and under the microscope heavy interstitial fibrous proliferation and cellular infiltration are seen. In the European form, most of these cells are plasma cells, whereas elsewhere in the world, when hypogammaglobulinemia is the underlying predisposing disorder, as it often is, lymphocytes and macrophages make up the infiltrate. The alveoli are distended with foamy, lacy, honeycombed exudate in which the cysts may be found.

Diagnosis. In its epidemic form, the disease begins within the second month of life or a bit later. A short period of loss of appetite and failure to gain weight is followed by duskiness and tachypnea. Cyanosis deepens gradually, and mild to severe dyspnea may appear. The lungs seem normal to percussion and auscultation, but radiographs characteristically show a prominent interstitial infiltration. Bilateral central opacification occurs 5 to 8 days after the onset of cough or apneic spells. Pneumothorax is common in these infants. There is little or no fever. The white blood count may be normal or elevated.

The diagnosis depends on seeing the organism. Occasionally, it can be recovered from tracheal aspirates. More commonly, a lung aspirate is required. Smear of the aspirated cells, and Giemsa stain, may reveal the encysted organism. Circulating antigens can be detected by counterimmunoelectrophoresis (CIE).

In its sporadic form, as seen in the United States, the disease strikes later, usually from 4 months to 2 years, and involves infants or children who have impaired immunologic responses. A few others debili-

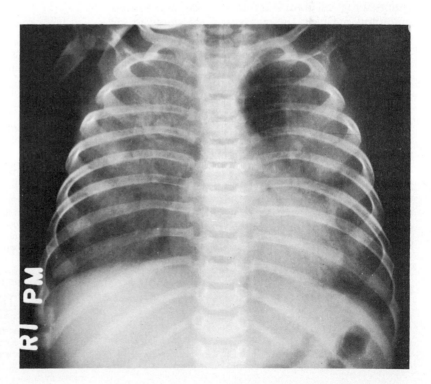

Figure 19–17. Chest film of a white male infant, 6 months of age, who had a cough and some cyanosis, with severe respiratory distress. No rales were heard, despite the extensive homogeneous infiltrates on the film. He had no measurable gamma globulins. *Pneumocystis carinii* was seen on the smear of a lung aspirate.

tated by advanced malignancy or after prolonged steroid therapy have been reported (Hughes et al., 1978). Since reduction of gamma globulin is associated with sparsity or absence of plasma cells, it is understandable that these cells are not found in the pneumonitis of these children. In other respects, the sporadic disease is similar to the epidemic form.

Treatment. Trimethoprim-sulfamethoxazole administered in a combination of 20 mg/kg trimethoprim and 100 mg/kg/day sulfamethoxazole is the treatment of choice. The drug should be given for at least 2 weeks. The infants require general supportive therapy and may need mechanical ventilation. If coughing interferes with nutrition, intravenous alimentation may be required.

Pneumonia Associated with More Than One Pathogen

The coexistence of several pathogens in pneumonias of infancy is probably not surprising, particularly when the premature infants are compromised with respect to their resistance. The most common agents found together are *Chlamydia, Pneumocystis,* and *Ureaplasma.* Stagno and colleagues found that of 65 infants from whom an identifiable infectious agent could be recovered, 74 per cent were infected with a single pathogen, but 13 were infected with two and 4 patients with three microorganisms. All these infants were less than 3 months of age, and all had pneumonia. Cytomegalovirus was recovered in 20 per cent, *Pneumocystis* in 18 per cent, *Chlamydia* in 25 per cent, and *Ureaplasma urealyticum* in 21 per cent. Other viruses were identified among these infants in association with some of the aforementioned organisms. These findings, reported from Birmingham, Alabama and from Memphis, Tennessee, may not be duplicated in other parts of the country. Nonetheless, it becomes evident that, in particular, premature babies who have pneumonia in the first months of life may well harbor more than one organism. Unfortunately, the pneumonias associated with many of the more common microorganisms are clinically indistinguishable from each other; hence, specific laboratory tests must be used to establish the diagnosis.

REFERENCES

Adams, J. M.: Congenital pneumonitis in newborn infants. Am. J. Dis. Child. 75:544, 1948.

Alford, C. A., Stagno, S., and Reynolds, D. W.: Diagnosis of chronic perinatal infections. Am. J. Dis. Child. 129:455, 1975.

Baker, C. J.: Early onset group B streptococcal disease. J. Pediatr. 93:124, 1978.

Baker, C. J., Barrett, F. F., Gordon, R. C., et al.: Suppurative meningitis due to streptococci of Lancefield group B: A study of 33 infants. J. Pediatr. 82:724, 1973.

Beem, M. O., Saxon, E., and Tipple, M. A.: Treatment of chlamydial pneumonia in infancy. Pediatrics 63:198, 1979.

Benirschke, K.: Routes and types of infection in the fetus and newborn. Am. J. Dis. Child 99:714, 1960.

Bernstein, J., and Wang, J.: The pathology of neonatal pneumonia. Am. J. Dis. Child. 101:350, 1961.

Blanc, W. A.: Amniotic infection syndrome: Pathogenesis, morphology and significance in circumnatal mortality. Clin. Obstet. Gynecol. 2:705, 1959.

Bloomer, W. E., Giammona, S., Lindskog, G. E., et al.: Staphylococcal pneumonia and empyema in infancy. J. Thorac. Surg. 30:265, 1955.

Calkins, L. A.: Premature spontaneous rupture of the membranes. Am. J. Obstet. Gynecol. 64:871, 1952.

Ceruti, E., Contreras, J., and Neira, M.: Staphylococcal pneumonia in childhood. Am. J. Dis. Child. 122:386, 1971.

Ciba Foundation Symposium 10 (new series): Intrauterine Infections. Elsevier, Excerpta Medica, North Holland, 1973.

Davies, P. A., and Aherne, W.: Congenital pneumonia. Arch. Dis. Child. 38:598, 1963.

Edmondson, E. B., Reinarz, J. A., Pierce, A. K., et al.: Nebulization equipment: A potential source of infection in gram-negative pneumonias. Am. J. Dis. Child. 111:357, 1966.

Franciosi, R. A., Knostman, J. D., and Zimmerman, R. A.: Group B streptococcal infections. J. Pediatr. 82:707, 1973.

Frommell, G. T., Rothenberg, R., Wang, S. P., and McIntosh, K.: Chlamydial infections of mothers and infants. J. Pediatr. 95:28, 1979.

Gajdusek, D. C.: Pneumocystis carinii—Etiologic agent of plasma cell pneumonia of premature and young infants. Pediatrics. 19:543, 1957.

Geppert, L. J., Baker, H. J., Copple, B. I., et al.: Pseudomonas infections in infants and children. J. Pediatr. 4:555, 1952.

Gershon, A. A.: Varicella in mother and infant: problems old and new. *In* Krugman, S., and Gershon, A. A. (Eds.): Infections of the Fetus and the Newborn Infant. New York, Alan R. Liss, Inc., 1975, pp. 79–95.

Goldmann, D. A., Leclair, J., and Macone, A.: Bacterial colonization of neonates admitted to an intensive care environment. J. Pediatr. 93:288, 1978.

Hall, C. B., Kopelman, A. E., Douglas, R. G., et al.: Neonatal respiratory syncytial virus infection. N. Engl. J. Med. 300:393, 1979.

Hammerschlag, M.: Chlamydial pneumonia in infants. N. Engl. J. Med. 298:1083, 1978.

Hanshaw, J. B., and Dudgeon, J. A.: Viral Diseases of the Fetus and Newborn. Philadelphia, W. B. Saunders Co., 1978.

Helwig, F. C.: Congenital aspiration pneumonia in stillborn and newborn infants. Am. J. Obstet. Gynecol. 26:849, 1933.

Hess Thaysen, T. E.: Die akuten nichtspezifischen Pneumonien der ersten Lebenstag. Jahrb. Kinderh. 79:140, 1914.

Hook, H., and Katz, K.: Über angeborene nichtspezifische Pneumonie und Pneumonie der ersten Lebenstage nach Aspiration innerhalb der Geburtswege. Virchow's Arch. Pathol. Anat. 267:571, 1928.

Hughes, W. T.: Pneumocystis pneumonia: a plague of the immunosuppressed. Johns Hopkins Med. J. 143:184, 1978.

Kanof, A., Epstein, B. S., Kramer, B., et al.: Staphylococcal pneumonia and empyema. Pediatrics 11:385, 1953.

Kjessler, A.: The time factor in rupture of the membranes and its influence on perinatal mortality. Acta Obstet. Gynecol. 35:495, 1956.

Klein, J. O.: Diagnostic lung puncture in the pneumonias of infants and children. 44:486, 1969.

Light, I., Sutherland, J. M., and Schott, J. E.: Control of a staphylococcal outbreak in a nursery: Use of bacterial interference. J.A.M.A. 193:699, 1965.

Menke, J. A., Giacoia, G. P., and Jockin, H.: Group B betahemolytic streptococcal sepsis and the idiopathic respiratory distress syndrome: a comparison. J. Pediatr. 94:467, 1979.

Miller, B. W., Orris, H. W., and Taus, H. H.: Friedländer's pneumonia in infancy. J. Pediatr. 31:521, 1947.

Moran, T. J.: Milk aspiration pneumonia in human and animal subjects. Arch. Pathol. *55*:286, 1953.

Naeye, R. L., Dellinger, W. S., and Blanc, W. A.: Fetal and maternal features of antenatal bacterial infections. J. Pediatr. *69*:733, 1971.

Nahmias, A. J., Josey, W. E., Naib, Z., et al.: Perinatal risk associated with maternal herpes simplex virus infection. Am. J. Obstet. Gynecol. *110*:825, 1971.

Neter, E., and Weintraub, D. H.: An epidemiologic study of Pseudomonas aeruginosa (B. Pyocyanes) in premature infants in the presence and absence of infection. J. Pediatr. *46*:280, 1955.

Olsen, M.: The benign effects on rabbits' lungs of the aspiration of water compared with 5% glucose and milk. Pediatrics *46*:538, 1970.

Overall, J., and Glasgow, L.: Virus infections of the fetus and newborn infant. J. Pediatr. *77*:315, 1970.

Penner, D. W., and McInnis, A. C.: Intrauterine and neonatal pneumonia. Am. J. Obstet. Gynecol. *69*:147, 1955.

Phelan, P., and Campbell, P.: Pulmonary complications of rubella embryopathy. J. Pediatr. *75*:202, 1969.

Potter, E. L.: Pathology of the Fetus and Newborn. Chicago, Year Book Medical Publishers, Inc., 1952.

Potter, E. L., and Adair, F. L.: Fetal and Neonatal Death. 2nd ed. Chicago, University of Chicago Press, 1949.

Pryles, C. V., Steg, N. L., Nair, S., et al.: A controlled study of the incidence of prolonged premature rupture of the amniotic membranes. Pediatrics *31*:608, 1963.

Robbins, J. B.: Pneumocystis carinii pneumonitis: A review. Pediatr. Res. *1*:131, 1967.

Sano, T., Niitsu, I., and Nakagawa, I.: Newborn virus pneumonitis (Type Sendai). I. Report: Clinical observation of a new virus pneumonitis of the newborn. Yokohama Med. Bull. *4*:199, 1953.

Schaad, U. B., McCracken, G. H., and Nelson, J. D.: Clinical pharmacology and efficacy of vancomycin in pediatric patients. J. Pediatr. *96*:119, 1980.

Schachter, J.: Chlamydial infections. N. Engl. J. Med. *298*:540, 1978.

Schaffer, A. J., Markowitz, M., and Perlman, A.: Pneumonia of newborn infants. J.A.M.A. *159*:663, 1955.

Sherman, M. P., Goetzman, B. W., Ahlfors, C. E., and Wennberg, R. P.: Tracheal aspiration and its clinical correlates in the diagnosis of congenital pneumonia. Pediatrics *65*:258, 1980.

Shinefield, H. R., Wilsey, J. D., Kibble, J. C., et al.: Interactions of staphylococcal colonization. Am. J. Dis. Child. *111*:11, 1966.

Shubeck, F., Benson, R. C., Clark, W. W., et al.: Fetal hazard after rupture of the membranes. A report from the collaborative project. Pediatrics *37*:672, 1966.

Smith, J. A. M., Jennison, R. F., and Langley, F. A.: Perinatal infection and perinatal death: clinical aspects. Lancet *2*:903, 1956.

Smith, R. M., Brumley, G. W., and Stannard, M. W.: Neonatal pneumonia associated with medium-chain triglyceride feeding supplement. J. Pediatr. *92*:801, 1978.

Stagno, S., Brasfield, D. M., Brown, M. B. et al.: Infant pneumonitis associated with cytomegalovirus, *Chlamydia, Pneumocystis,* and *Ureaplasma*: a prospective study. Pediatrics *68*:322, 1981.

Stagno, S., Pifer, L. L., Hughes, W. T. et al.: *Pneumocystis carinii* pneumonitis in young immunocompetent infants. Pediatrics *66*:56, 1980.

Thaler, M. M.: Klebsiella-Aerobacter pneumonia in infants: A review of the literature and report of a case. Pediatrics *30*:206, 1962.

Vasan, U., Lim, D., Greenstein, R. W., and Raye, J. R.: Origin of gastric aspirate polymorphonuclear leukocytes in infants born after prolonged rupture of membranes. J. Pediatr. *91*:69, 1977.

Vessal, K., Post, C., Dutz, W., et al.: Roentgenographic changes in infantile pneumocystis carinii pneumonia. Am. J. Roentgenol. *120*:254, 1974.

Warren, W. S., and Stool, S.: Otitis media in low-birthweight infants. J. Pediatr. *79*:740, 1971.

20

Miscellaneous Pulmonary Disorders

Transient Tachypnea of the Newborn*

Transient tachypnea was first described as a syndrome in 1966 on the basis of eight infants with very similar signs and clinical course. The pathogenesis is unknown, and the diagnosis is one of exclusion of other known causes of respiratory distress (Avery et al., 1969). "Transient respiratory distress of the newborn" and "wet-lung disease" have been offered as alternative names for this syndrome; a number of the babies in whom it occurred, however, had birth asphyxia.

The infants are usually born at term and have no specific antenatal events in common. In the first hours of life, they exhibit elevated respiratory rates, up to 120/min, in the absence of significant retractions or rales. They may be minimally cyanotic, but alveolar ventilation is normal as measured by blood pH and Pco_2. No cardiovascular abnormalities have been found. Sundell and colleagues reported 36 infants with problems similar to those described by Avery and coworkers. They used the name "type II respiratory distress" to designate their infants, most of whom were of low birth weight, although late in gestation. Mild depression at birth was common in the

---

* This section adapted from Avery, M. E., Fletcher, B. D., and Williams, R.: The Lung and Its Disorders in the Newborn Infant. Philadelphia, W. B. Saunders Co., 1981.

series described by Sundell. Prompt increase in oxygenation on administration of oxygen distinguished these infants from those with hyaline membrane disease. A benign course was emphasized by both groups reporting on this disorder.

Some infants have a more prolonged course and may require added inspired oxygen for several days. Echocardiography reveals abnormalities in systolic time intervals consistent with generalized myocardial failure. Halliday and associates used echocardiography to distinguish ''classic'' mild transient tachypnea with evidence of left ventricular overload from the ''severe'' form with involvement of both ventricles and pulmonary hypertension.

The chest radiographs show prominent, ill-defined vascular markings, edematous interlobar septa, and pleural effusions in the costophrenic angles and interlobar fissures, typical of interstitial edema. Occasionally alveolar edema may be present. The lungs tend to be slightly hyperaerated. Clearing of the lungs is usually evident the next day, although complete clearing may require 3 to 7 days (Fig. 20–1).

One suggested mechanism for the tachypnea is a delay in resorption of fetal lung liquid. The prominent perihilar streaking may represent engorgement of the periarterial lymphatics, which have been shown to participate in clearance of alveolar liquid with the initiation of air breathing. Fletcher and associates tested the possibility that delayed clearance of lung liquid could account for the findings by sequential chest films in newborn lambs. When lung water content was elevated and radiographic abnormalities were present, the respiratory rates were increased.

Elevated central venous pressure from whatever cause, including placental transfusion, may delay clearance of lung liquid through the thoracic duct.

Sequential films in asymptomatic newborn infants sometimes show vascular engorgement in the first 2 hours of life. Northway as well as Steele and Copeland pointed out that the vascular engorgement was not always associated with tachypnea.

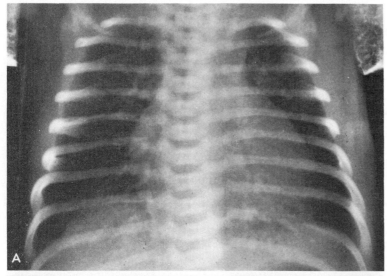

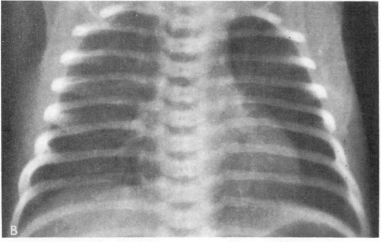

Figure 20–1. The large cardiovascular silhouette, air bronchogram, and streaky lung fields were seen at 2 hours of age (*A*) but had cleared by 24 hours of age (*B*), typical of transient tachypnea of the newborn or delayed clearance of lung liquid via the lymphatics after birth.

The process is self-limited, and infants followed for as long as 1 year had no recurrence of tachypnea or other evidence of pulmonary dysfunction.

Persistent Liquid-Filled Lung

Animal experiments involving fetal tracheal ligation established the fetal lung as a secretory organ in which liquid could accumulate (Jost and Policard, 1948; Lanman et al., 1971). It is hardly surprising, then, that bronchial occlusion in utero can promote liquid accumulation in the affected lobe. Griscom and coworkers reported two infants in whom bronchial obstruction was present with a space-occupying radiopaque mass noted on roentgenogram. At operation, liquid-filled lung distal to the obstruction was noted. With removal of the obstruction, aeration occurred in one infant; in the other, normal lung was resected.

Agenesis

All gradations of underdevelopment of the lung are encountered, ranging from hypoplasia of one segment or lobe to complete absence of both lungs.

Incidence. The condition is extremely rare. Olcott and Dooley reported the first case found at autopsy in the New York Hospital in more than 10,000 postmortem examinations. In 1953, Oyamada and coworkers were able to find, in an exhaustive survey of the world literature, 109 reported cases of all varieties. Fifty of these were right-sided defects, 59 left-sided.

Etiology. Agenesis, aplasia, and hypoplasia are all congenital defects. They represent failure of development of the primitive lung bud in slightly different stages of ontogeny.

Diagnosis. The time of onset of symptoms is remarkably variable. Some infants are in great difficulty at birth and survive only one or two gasping respirations. Levy's 49-year-old patient, on the other hand, complained of only occasional slight dyspnea, while the 40-year-old woman reported by Nesbit and colleagues stated merely that she never had had the reserve strength of her associates, her activity having been limited somewhat by dyspnea.

The presenting symptom is, at times, tachypnea without cyanosis; tachypnea occurs with cyanosis only upon undue exertion. More often, the presenting complaint has been repeated attacks of lower respiratory tract infection, described as bronchitis, asthmatic bronchitis, or pneumonia. A few infants have been noted to have had "stertorous breathing" or to have made "gurgling sounds" from birth. Wheezing respirations, either in attacks or present constantly, have been reported.

Physical examination reveals characteristic signs. The affected hemithorax may be slightly flattened, but usually little difference can be made out in the size of the two sides. One side, however, moves less well than the other. On this side, the percussion note is at first flat from top to bottom, front and back, but later some resonance appears over the upper part of the chest in front where the emphysematous normal lung has herniated across the midline. Breath sounds follow the same pattern, completely absent over one lung at first, later present but diminished over the upper lobe in front. The heart and mediastinum are found, by percussion and auscultation and by observation and palpation of the apex beat, to have shifted far to the affected side. The note on the good side is resonant or hyperresonant, the breath sounds are stronger, and no adventitious sounds are heard.

Differential Diagnosis. Clinically, there is no possible method of differentiating complete agenesis from massive atelectasis involving one entire lung. Atelectasis of this degree is much less frequently encountered than is agenesis, rare as the latter is. On only one occasion has almost complete collapse of one lung, caused by anomalous vascular compression of the main bronchus, confused us in this manner. It is at times difficult to be certain that there is no lesion on one side that dislocates the heart and mediastinal contents in the opposite direction, but the complete normality of physical signs on that side is usually distinction enough. Solid tumor or fluid-filled cyst or pleural effusion should be appreciated easily by percussion changes. Air-filled cyst and pneumothorax should produce hyperresonance bordering upon tympany, and, in all these conditions, breath sounds are commonly diminished to a considerable degree.

Radiographic Findings. Anteroposterior films show almost complete opacity of the affected side. If the agenesis is of the left lung, the right border of the heart and mediastinum is seen as a sharp perpendicular line at or within the left border of the sternum. The left border, when agenesis is right-sided, is found well to the right of the sternum, the entire cardiac shadow often being continuous with that of the liver. The trachea deviates toward the affected side. As the infant grows older, the good lung can be seen to overexpand across the midline until a sizable amount of aerated lung lies within the opposite upper hemithorax. In the lateral film, this herniated lung can be seen just beneath the sternum, pressing the heart and great vessels posteriorly. If aerated lung is visible anywhere, either far laterally or toward the base, the disorder is not complete agenesis; it is either incomplete atelectasis or hypoplasia of one lung.

Bronchoscopy. Often, no carina is seen through the bronchoscope. The single main bronchus appears continuous with the trachea. In aplasia, a narrow bronchus may be seen that terminates completely after a course of a few centimeters, or the bronchus may be represented only by a dimple in the tracheal wall. The remaining normal bronchus turns sharply toward the side that contains normal lung.

Bronchography. Bronchogram shows the absent or rudimentary main bronchus. Films of the well-developed lung are usually normal, with the exception of deviation of the bronchial tree toward the opposite side and the demonstration of herniated lung in the anterior mediastinum and the upper portion of the opposite hemithorax.

Prognosis. Half of all the reported patients die either at birth or within the first 5 years of life. Nearly half the patients have other congenital anomalies that may be the cause of death (Maltz and Nadas, 1968). The majority die in the course of one of their repeated lower respiratory tract infections.

Persons with agenesis of the left lung have a longer life expectancy than do those with agenesis of the right lung (Fig. 20–2). This statement is based upon an analysis of the cases compiled by Oyamada and colleagues. Beginning with 50 right-sided and 59 left-sided instances of agenesis, the authors found that only 16 of the former versus 35 of the latter patients survived the first year of life, while the figures for 5 years were 9 versus 32, for 10 years 8 versus 26, and for 20 years 7 versus 20. No significant difference was found in the percentage of associated congenital malformations. We are forced to assume, therefore, that right-sided agenesis is more hazardous than left-sided agenesis. The only reason for this discrepancy that comes to mind is that the shift of mediastinal contents is greater when agenesis is right-sided. Thus, there is more lateral deviation of great vessels and large bronchi, and these may actually become kinked or compressed in the process. The prominence of lower respiratory tract disease in the histories of the patients suggests that malposition of the larger bronchi is the fact of greater importance. McCormick and Kuhns described tracheal compression caused by a normal but deviated aortic arch in an infant with right pulmonary agenesis.

CASE 20–1

A black female infant whose birth weight was 5 pounds 1 ounce (2300 gm) was born spontaneously after a long first stage but short second stage of labor. Pregnancy had been complicated by laparotomy at the second month of gestation for abdominal pain, when nothing abnormal was found, and an episode of pyuria in the sixth month. She cried spontaneously but soon became cyanotic, making regular but not vigorous respiratory efforts. On examination shortly after birth, the right hemithorax was flat to percussion, and the left was dull. Heart sounds were loudest to the right of the sternum. With positive pressure oxygen followed by high environmental oxygen, there was improvement. On the second day, her color in oxygen was good except for cyanosis of the hands and feet. Breath sounds were now loud over the left hemithorax and inaudible over the

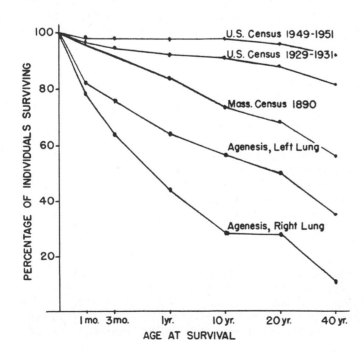

Figure 20–2. Comparative survival curves of patients with agenesis of a lung are contrasted with those of the total population, 1949 to 1951 (topmost curve), with those of the total population, 1929 to 1931 (second from top), and with those of the population of the state of Massachusetts at the end of the nineteenth century. It is clear that survival with agenesis of either lung is poorer than that of the general population and that survival with agenesis of the right lung is significantly worse than when the left lung is missing from birth. (Schaffer, A. J., and Rider, R. V.: Trans. Am. Climatol. Assoc. *68*:25, 1956.)

right. Fluoroscopy and x-ray study revealed a homogeneously dense right hemithorax (Fig. 20–3). There was slow improvement, but feeding remained difficult, and cyanosis reappeared when she was removed from the incubator.

Bronchoscopy on the fifth day of life showed no excess mucus in the airway. The rest of this examination was unsatisfactory.

For the next 3 weeks, the infant ate better and gained slowly. At 4 weeks, her temperature began to rise, reaching 40.5°C (105°F) a few days later. Death occurred on the thirty-fifth day.

At autopsy, the right lung was represented by a fleshy mass 3 × 3 × 1 cm in size. This lay posteriorly and was connected to the mediastinum by a tiny bronchus and a small artery. The right ventricle was large and dilated, the ductus arteriosus was patent, and no right pulmonary artery was seen. Under the microscope the hypoplastic lung was almost completely atelectatic but did contain a little air in some sections, while the left lung was patchily consolidated, with mononuclear infiltration and edema.

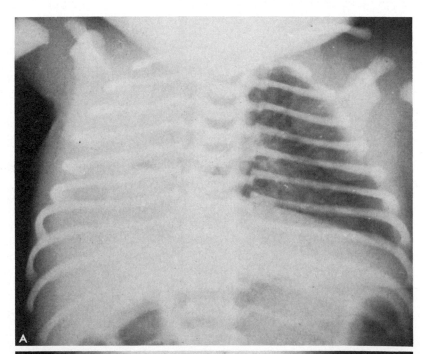

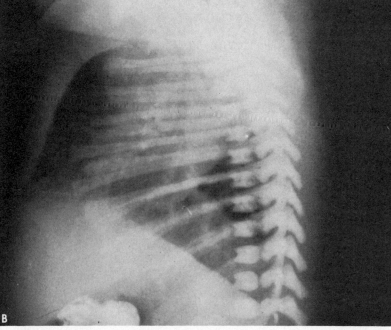

Figure 20–3. *A,* Anteroposterior view of chest made on the second day of life. There is complete opacity of the right hemithorax except for a small bubble of air in midchest. The heart and mediastinal contents are displaced entirely into the right side. The left lung is somewhat emphysematous, the ribs on that side are more widely spread, and the diaphragm is flattened. *B,* Lateral view. The anterior mediastinum is deep, and there is a broad band of translucency between sternum and heart. This indicates herniation of the left upper lobe toward the right.

each bronchus may lead to a normal number of mature alveoli.

Comment. In this case, cyanosis was prominent, dyspnea not great, almost immediately after birth. Signs suggested complete absence of the right lung, with mediastinal shift to that side. Bronchoscopy was not helpful, as it frequently is not in such small infants. X-ray film showed virtual absence of the right lung and emphysema of the left, the lateral view in particular revealing herniation of lung into the anterior mediastinum. At autopsy, the right lung was represented by a small hypoplastic mass. Death was due to pneumonia of the remaining lung.

Hypoplastic Lungs

Hypoplastic lungs are most often associated with other congenital malformations such as diaphragmatic hernia, renal agenesis, anomalous vertebrae, or absent phrenic nerves.

ASSOCIATED CONDITIONS

Diaphragmatic Hernia (see also Chapter 21)

In this situation, the degree of failure of lung growth relates to the degree of compromise of thoracic space from herniated viscera. With a moderate degree of herniation, the lung may be mature but small. With severe restriction of volume from early gestation, the number of bronchial branches is reduced, although

Oligohydramnios

Lung hypoplasia is associated with oligohydramnios in the case of renal agenesis (Potter's syndrome) (see Chapter 46). Abundant evidence links oligohydramnios with lung hypoplasia. In a pair of identical twins, one with renal agenesis had normal lungs, presumably because there was adequate amniotic fluid from the other twin's urine production (Maurer et al., 1974). However, lung hypoplasia may be sufficiently profound to antedate the time of fetal urine production (Hislop et al., 1979).

Lack of fetal lung fluid, induced experimentally by tracheal drainage in lambs, led to a reduction in lung size and a delay in thinning of alveolar walls (Alcorn et al., 1977). An association between prolonged leakage of amniotic liquid and lung size was noted in the human by Perlman and colleagues. Alveoli were reduced in number.

Absent Phrenic Nerves

A single infant was reported by Goldstein and coworkers to have absent phrenic nerves, absent diaphragmatic musculature, and profound pulmonary hypoplasia. This case suggests the possibility that fetal respiratory movements and diaphragmatic tone must be important in providing suitable thoracic space for lung growth.

Studies by Wigglesworth in rabbits support this view. He proposed that situations in which thoracic

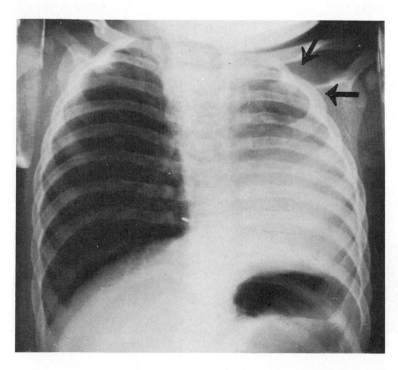

Figure 20–4. Anteroposterior view of chest was made when patient was 3 weeks old. The right hemithorax is expanded, the left contracted. The right lung is emphysematous, and its upper lobe has herniated across the midline to fill almost completely the left upper hemithorax. The heart is displaced far to the left and downward. There may be a small segment of aerated lung tissue in the left costophrenic angle.

volume is compromised, as in diaphragmatic hernia or absent phrenic nerves, will primarily restrict lung growth but not maturation. Fewell and coworkers found that phrenic nerve section in fetal lambs (116 to 121 days, term 147 days) eliminated fetal breathing movements and decreased airway fluid volume, lung weight, and total lung DNA. Tracheal fluid production and the concentration of saturated phosphatidylcholine in it were not affected.

Congenital Pulmonary Lymphangiectasis

Congenital pulmonary lymphangiectasis is a rare disorder first described over 100 years ago by Virchow. It is usually lethal in infancy and diagnosed only on postmortem examination; sometimes, however, it is compatible with longer life and may even be asymptomatic.

Pathogenesis. Dilatation of pulmonary parenchymal lymphatics can occur from failure of normal formation of connections to the lymphatic ducts, as part of generalized lymphangiectasis, or secondary to pulmonary venous obstruction. Noonan and coworkers reviewed 45 patients described in the literature. Isolated pulmonary lymphangiectasis was present in 30 of the 45 patients. The disorder is not known to be familial.

Clinical Manifestations. In the majority of infants reported, respiratory distress was noted at birth, and cyanosis was marked and persistent. The duration of life in such infants has ranged from 30 minutes to 30 days. Very rarely, symptoms abate and survivals up to 4 years are known in infants who were sympto-

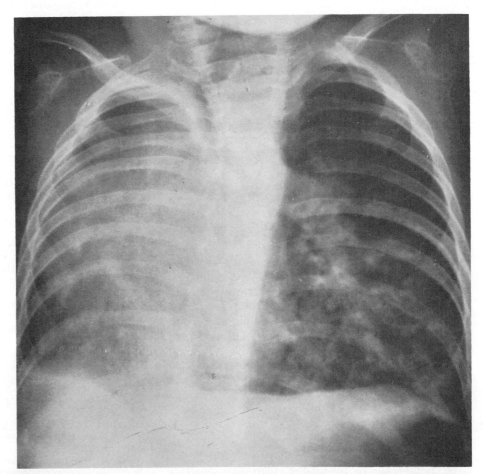

Figure 20–5. Anteroposterior view of chest shows heart shifted far to right, trachea also dislocated to right, moderate emphysema of left lung, and diminution in size of the right hemithorax. Note the great increase of vascular shadows on the left.

The infant was well at birth, but respirations were rapid from the start, and a loud systolic murmur was heard on the original examination. He improved but suffered numerous respiratory infections throughout infancy.

His mother and brother have hypoplastic right lungs, eventration of the right diaphragm, and anomalous venous return. This infant almost surely has the same defects without the eventration. (We are indebted to Dr. Olga M. Baghdassarian for this film.)

matic in infancy. Those children with asymptomatic pulmonary lymphangiectasis have usually had associated malformations of the lymphatic system, such as lymphangiomas of the extremities or intestinal lymphangiectasis. The pulmonary lesion has occasionally been recognized only after a routine chest film was taken. The condition has been reported twice as commonly in males as in females and usually after term birth. Other congenital malformations, particularly of the cardiovascular system, have been noted in over half the cases coming to autopsy.

Radiographic Features. The lungs are usually diffusely involved with a reticular pattern, and sometimes the fissures are prominent. Hyperaeration is regularly noted and helps to distinguish the condition from hyaline membrane disease, with which it may be confused.

Pathology. Grossly, the lungs show both thin-walled vesicles on their surfaces and thickened, interlobular septa; they tend to be heavy and airless. The cut surface reveals a honeycomb pattern of irregularly shaped, fluid-filled cysts, which on microscopic examination are dilated lymphatic vessels lined by a thin layer of elongated epithelial cells. The surrounding connective tissue is loose and embryonal, and the pulmonary parenchyma is airless and underdeveloped.

Pulmonary Alveolar Proteinosis

A very rare cause of widespread alveolar infiltrations is pulmonary alveolar proteinosis. The infant reported by Coleman and coworkers was symptomatic at birth. Tachypnea, cyanosis, and diffuse infiltrates evident on chest film persisted throughout the 1 year of this infant's life. A granular eosinophilic material, positive to periodic acid–Schiff stain, was found in the alveolar spaces. Other infants with the disease have died at several months of age.

Teja and colleagues studied five reported affected siblings. An association with thymic alymphoplasia has been noted.

Immotile Cilia Syndrome

Bronchiectasis in association with situs inversus (Kartagener's syndrome) is well known in adults but has rarely been recognized as a cause of respiratory distress in infants. Whitelaw and associates reported six infants with the onset of respiratory distress within 24 hours of birth. Four of these infants also had chronic otitis media. Early recognition of the presence of situs inversus and physiotherapy led to a good response in these infants.

REFERENCES

Alcorn, D., Adamson, T. M., Lambert, T. F., et al.: Morphological effects of chronic tracheal ligation and drainage in fetal lamb lung. J. Anat. 123:649, 1977.

Areechon, W., and Reid, L.: Hypoplasia of lung with congenital diaphragmatic hernia. Br. Med. J. 1:230, 1963.

Avery, M. E., Gatewood, O. B., and Brumley, G.: Transient tachypnea of the newborn. Am. J. Dis. Child. 117:710, 1969.

Coleman, M., Dehner, L. P., Sibley, R. K., Burke, B. A., L'Heureux, P. R., and Thompson, T. R.: Pulmonary alveolar proteinosis: an uncommon cause of chronic neonatal respiratory distress. Am. Rev. Resp. Dis. 121:583, 1980.

deLormier, A. A., Tierney, D. F., and Parker, H. R.: Hypoplastic lungs in fetal lambs with surgically produced congenital diaphragmatic hernia. Surgery 62:12, 1967.

De Weese, E. R., and Howard, J. C., Jr.: Congenital absence of a lung diagnosed before death. Radiology 42:389, 1944.

Ekelund, H., Palmstierna, S., Østberg, G.: Congenital pulmonary lymphangiectasis. Acta Paediatr. Scand. 55:121, 1966.

Fewell, J. E., Lee, C. C., and Kitterman, J. A.: Effects of phrenic nerve section on the respiratory system of fetal lambs. J. Appl. Physiol. 51:293, 1981.

Field, C. E.: Pulmonary agenesis and hypoplasia. Arch. Dis. Child. 21:61, 1946.

Fletcher, B. D., Sachs, B. F., and Kotas, R. V.: Radiologic demonstration of post-natal liquid in the lungs of newborn lambs. Pediatrics 46:252, 1970.

Giammalvo, J. T.: Congenital lymphangiectasis of the lung: A form of cystic disease. Lab. Invest. 4:450, 1955.

Goldstein, J. D., and Reid, L. M.: Pulmonary hypoplasia resulting from phrenic nerve agenesis and diaphragmatic amyoplasia. J. Pediatr. 97:282, 1980.

Griscom, N. T., Harris, G. B. C., Wohl, M. E. B., Vawter, G. F., and Eraklis, A. J.: Fluid-filled lung due to airway obstruction in the newborn. Pediatrics 43:383, 1969.

Halliday, H. L., McClure, G., and McCreid, M.: Transient tachypnea of the newborn: two distinct clinical entities. Arch. Dis. Child. 56:322, 1981.

Hislop, A., Hey, E., and Reid, L.: The lungs in congenital bilateral renal agenesis and dysplasia. Arch. Dis. Child. 54:32, 1979.

Javett, S. N., Webster, I., and Braudo, J. L.: Congenital dilatation of the pulmonary lymphatics. Pediatrics 31:416, 1963.

Jost, A., and Policard, A.: Contribution expérimentale à l'étude du dévelopment du poumon chez le lapin. Arch. Anat. Microsc. 37:323, 1948.

Klein, Z. L.: An accessory lobe of lung in a newborn. Pediatrics 45:118, 1970.

Lanman, J. H., Schaffer, A., Herod, L., Ogawa, Y., and Castellanos, R.: Distensibility of the fetal lung with fluid in sheep. Pediatr. Res. 5:586, 1971.

Laurence, K. M.: Congenital pulmonary cystic lymphangiectasis. J. Pathol. 70:325, 1955.

Levy, C. S.: Congenital absence of one lung. Am. J. Med. Sci. 159:237, 1920.

Maltz, D. L., and Nadas, A. S.: Agenesis of the lung: Presentation of eight new cases and review of the literature. Pediatrics 42:175, 1968.

Maurer, S. M., Dobrin, R. S., and Vernier, R. L.: Unilateral and bilateral renal agenesis in monoamniotic twins. J. Pediatr. 84:236, 1974.

McCormick, T. L., and Kuhns, L. R.: Tracheal compression by a normal aorta associated with right lung agenesis. Radiology 130:659, 1979.

Neill, C. A., Ferencz, C., Sabiston, D. C., and Sheldon, H.: The familial occurrence of hypoplastic right lung with systemic arterial supply and venous drainage "scimitar syndrome." Bull. Johns Hopkins Hosp. 107:1, 1960.

Nesbit, W. M., Paul, K. W., and Middleton, W. S.: Congenital aplasia of the lung: a case report. Am. J. Roentgenol. 57:446, 1947.

Noonan, J. A., Walters, L. R., and Reeves, J. T.: Congenital pulmonary lymphangiectasis. Am. J. Dis. Child. 120:314, 1970.

Northway, W. H., Jr., Daily, W. J. R., Parker, B. R., Hackel, A., Bensch, K. G., Vosti, K. L., and Sunshine, P.: Perinatal pulmonary study. Invest. Radiol. 6:354, 1971.

O'Connor, J. F., Shapiro, J. H., and Ingall, D.: Erythrocythemia as a cause of respiratory distress in the newborn: radiologic findings. Radiology 90:333, 1968.

Olcott, C. T., and Dooley, S. W.: Agenesis of lung in an infant. Am. J. Dis. Child. 65:777, 1943.

Olver R. E.: Of labor and the lungs. Arch. Dis. Child. 56:659, 1981.

Oyamada, A., Gasul, B. M., and Holinger, P. H.: Agenesis of the lung. Am. J. Dis. Child. 85:182, 1953.

Pearl, M.: Sequestration of the lung. Am. J. Dis. Child. 124:706, 1972.

Perlman, M., Williams, J., and Hirsch, M.:Neonatal pulmonary hypoplasia after prolonged leakage of amniotic fluids. Arch. Dis. Child. 51:349, 1976.

Roe, B. B., and Stephens, J. B.: Congenital diaphragmatic hernia and hypoplastic lung. J. Thorac. Surg. 32:279, 1956.

Saigal, S., Wilson, R., and Usher, R.: Radiological findings in symptomatic neonatal plethora resulting from placental transfusion. Radiology 125:185, 1977.

Steele, R. W., and Copeland, G. A.: Delayed resorption of pulmonary alveolar fluid in the neonate. Radiology 103:637, 1972.

Swischuk, L. E., Richardson, C. J., Nichols, M. M., and Ingman, M. J.: Primary pulmonary hypoplasia in the neonate. J. Pediatr. 95:573, 1979.

Teja, K., Cooper, P. H., Squires, J. E., et al.: Pulmonary alveolar proteinosis in five siblings. N. Engl. J. Med. 305:1390, 1981.

Thomas, L. B., and Boyden, E. A.: Agenesis of the right lung: report of 3 cases. Surgery 31:429, 1952.

Thurlbeck, W. M.: Postnatal growth and development of the lung. Am. Rev. Resp. Dis. 111:803, 1975.

Tsang, R. C., Chen, I., Hayes, W., et al.: Neonatal hypocalcemia in infants with birth asphyxia. J. Pediatr. 84:428, 1974.

Valle, A. R., and Graham, E. A.: Agenesis of the lung. J. Thorac. Surg. 13:345, 1944.

Wexels, P.: Agenesis of the lung. Thorax 6:171, 1951.

Whitelaw, A., Evans, A., and Corrin, B.: Immotile cilia syndrome: a new cause of neonatal respiratory distress. Arch. Dis. Child. 56:432, 1981.

Wigglesworth, J. S., Desai, R., and Guerrini, P.: Fetal lung hypoplasia: biochemical and structural variations and their possible significance. Arch. Dis. Child. 56:606, 1981.

21

Disorders of the Diaphragm

Congenital Diaphragmatic Hernia

Congenital diaphragmatic hernia is characterized by the presence of abdominal viscera in the thoracic cavity, above one or both diaphragms. Usually, the abnormally placed viscera are the hollow ones, stomach or small or large bowel, but spleen and liver may also be present. Herniation ordinarily occurs through the left diaphragm. The proportion of left-sided to right-sided hernias varies in reported series from four to one to eight to one. They are rarely bilateral.

Incidence.   It is difficult to compute a firm figure for the frequency of diaphragmatic hernia. In the British Perinatal Survey of March 1958, diaphragmatic hernias were found in 1.4 per cent of all postmortems, and once in every 2200 total births.

The Collaborative Perinatal Project in the United States (1959 to 1966) found only 15 diaphragmatic defects, or 1 per 2500 livebirths.

Etiology.   The muscular portion of the diaphragm derives myoblasts from two sources. The costal part arises from myoblasts in the lateral body walls, while the crural part arises from the dorsal mesentery of the esophagus. These two portions differ in muscle fiber composition and innervation. De Troyer and coworkers recently described the different actions of these muscles on the chest wall. In instances in which the muscles do not come together in development, the defect permits hernia of abdominal viscera into the chest cavity. The most common abnormality is incomplete closure of the pleuroperitoneal sinus (foramen of Bochdalek), situated in the posterolateral aspect of the diaphragm. Less common are herniations through the substernal sinus (of Morgagni or Larrey) and through the esophageal hiatus. Thoracic stomach with short esophagus is a different type of defect that will be discussed with diseases of the gastrointestinal tract (see p. 340).

The hernias are usually "false"; that is, not covered by a peritoneal sac. Rarely, a sac is present, indicating that migration of abdominal contents took place a little later in embryologic life, after rather than before the peritoneal lining was completed. It is of no clinical importance except that the sac may confuse diagnosis because it simulates diaphragm, as it did on one occasion in our own experience.

Diagnosis.   The diagnostic criteria of congenital diaphragmatic hernia vary with the volume of viscera herniated and, perhaps because of this, with the time of onset of symptoms. Infants may be seriously ill at the moment of birth; others may become ill at any time during infancy, childhood, or even adult life. Indeed, some hernias remain completely asymptomatic and are discovered only in the course of routine radiographic examination of the chest.

If the volume of intrathoracic abdominal viscera is great, symptoms are apt to appear immediately after birth. The symptoms are entirely respiratory at this stage. The commonly repeated dictum that the diagnosis of diaphragmatic hernia is suggested by a combination of respiratory and gastrointestinal symptoms is true only for those that manifest themselves later. Usually the baby, born after normal pregnancy and labor, breathes or gasps once and is then seen to be in great trouble. He may make no further respiratory effort until resuscitative measures have been taken. Cyanosis develops. When spontaneous respirations are established, they are deep and labored, often gasping and irregular, and associated with deep sternal and costal retraction. Cyanosis may or may not clear in high concentrations of oxygen.

In other instances, difficulty does not become manifest until some hours or days after birth. Tachypnea may be the first sign, followed by a variable degree of retraction. Attempts at feeding may initiate vomiting, but this is not common. Rarely, the first intimation that hernia is present is supplied by the signs of intestinal obstruction produced by strangulation of intrathoracic bowel.

Physical signs are variable, depending not only on the quantity of displaced viscera but also on their consistency. Observation may yield the valuable information that the chest, especially the left hemithorax, is overfilled, while the abdomen is flat or sca-

phoid. Air-filled bowel produces a tympanitic note on percussion, but over empty bowel, liver, and spleen the note is flat. In our experience with large hernias, the combination of flatness over one portion of the hemithorax and tympany over another was almost always discovered. Tinkling peristaltic sounds may be heard after air has penetrated thoracic bowel. The heart is displaced to the side opposite the lesion, usually to the right. Part of the adjacent and opposite lung is invariably atelectatic; therefore, over these areas the percussion note is dull, and fine crackling rales may be heard. Rarely, one hears bronchial breath sounds over such collapsed areas.

Differential diagnosis is not too difficult. In lobar atelectasis, difficult respiration begins some hours after birth. The heart is shifted toward the affected side, and the lung of the side opposite the shift appears normal or emphysematous. Physical examination alone may not be sufficient to differentiate from hernia all the other lesions that dislocate the heart and mediastinal structures toward the opposite side. Tympany could signify pneumothorax, lobar emphysema, or air-containing cyst as well as air-filled hollow viscus. Dullness or flatness might indicate tumor, fluid-filled cyst, or pleural effusion as well as solid abdominal viscus. A combination of tympany over one portion of the affected hemithorax and flatness over another is strongly suggestive of diaphragmatic hernia. An overfilled chest and concave abdomen constitute strong evidence for this diagnosis. Peristaltic sounds heard in the chest are pathognomonic.

Plain radiographs, anteroposterior and lateral, should resolve any residual doubt. It is unwise to rely entirely upon fluoroscopy. The variety of pictures produced by congenital diaphragmatic hernia is consistent with the variation in quantity and type of abdominal viscera that may be displaced. Rather than

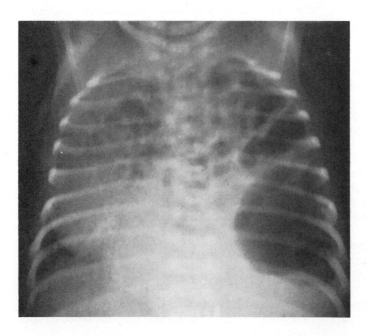

Figure 21–1. Anteroposterior view of chest taken on the second day of life. The chest is overexpanded and barrel-shaped. Round translucencies of varying size fill the left hemithorax and part of the right. The heart occupies the lower lateral corner of the right hemithorax. Both diaphragms are depressed, the left more than the right. The translucency in the left lower hemithorax resembles stomach, one or two above it looks like large bowel, while the remainder appear to be loops of small bowel.

describe all possible combinations and permutations, a number of examples are reproduced. If there is any doubt about whether the air-containing shadows in the chest are stomach or bowel, a barium meal x-ray series may be made (Figs. 21–1 to 21–3).

Treatment. *Once the diagnosis is suspected, a feeding tube should be inserted into the stomach, and, with continuous suction, air and gastric contents should be aspirated.* The only treatment available is replacement of the displaced viscera into the abdominal cavity and surgical correction of the congenital defect. It is imperative that this be effected immediately, that is, as soon as the diagnosis is established

and proper resuscitation and preoperative preparation has been completed. The hazards of delay are sudden death, probably due to dislocation of mediastinal contents, and the supervention of pneumonia. The newborn within the first day or two of life tolerates protracted procedures as well as or better than he does later. Nothing is gained and much may be lost by waiting.

Persistent pulmonary hypertension may be responsible for continued respiratory distress postop-

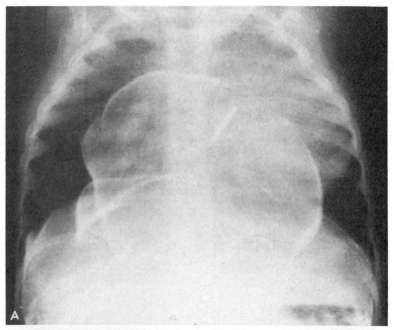

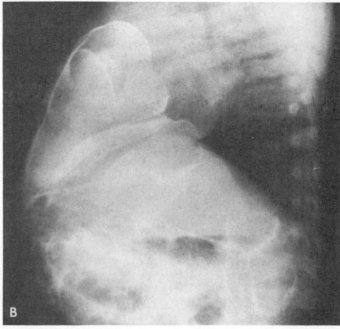

Figure 21–2. Hernias of the foramen of Morgagni frequently present as a mass, contiguous with the right heart margin. Water soluble contrast medium injected into the peritoneal cavity outlines the mass. (From Oh, K. S., et al.: Radiology *108*:647, 1973.)

eratively (Dibbins and Weiner, 1974). Pharmacologic approaches to lowering pulmonary artery pressures are sometimes effective. Intravenous tolazoline administered 1 to 5 mg/kg/hr, with an occasional bolus of 2 mg/kg, may improve oxygenation. Bloss and colleagues found it helpful in about one third of their patients. When the infant does not become better oxygenated with vasodilators, it is probable that the ductal shunt right-to-left is distributing the drug to the systemic circulation. Peripheral blood pressures must be closely monitored under these circumstances. Maintenance of blood volume and pressures is essential. Isoproterenol or dopamine or both may be required in some instances.

The choice of surgical approach, whether thoracic, abdominal, or both, is a moot question that the pediatrician fortunately does not have to answer. The abdominal approach would appear to be superior for several reasons. It is likely, however, that prognosis depends less upon the approach than upon the skill of the surgeon. He will no doubt get the best results by utilizing the method in which he has become adept. Gastrostomy is a useful device for minimizing

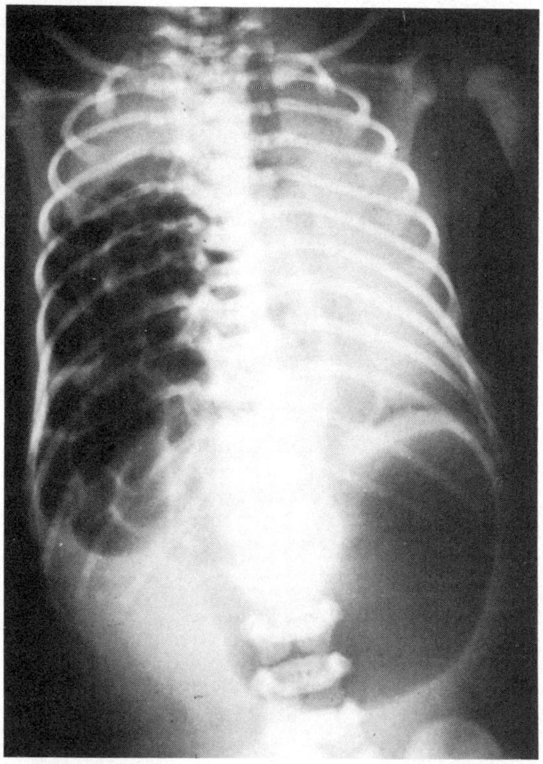

Figure 21–3. Right-sided diaphragmatic hernia. This infant was resuscitated by mask and bag without intubation. The consequence was disastrous overdistention of stomach and bowel. When lungs resist insufflation, intubation is mandatory to prevent this kind of complication.

distention and improving postoperative respiratory exchange.

Prognosis. The percentage of cure varies directly with (1) the promptness with which diagnosis is made and operation is performed, (2) the experience and skill of the operator, (3) the excellence of preoperative and postoperative care, and (4) the degree of hypoplasia of the compressed lung.

Infants with posterolateral diaphragmatic hernias operated on before 24 hours of age have survival rates of only 40 to 70 per cent. Infants with herniations of less severity or shorter duration who can survive the first day of life are excellent candidates for successful repair, with a cure rate greater than 90 per cent. Postoperatively, pneumothorax is common. Gentle catheter suction of the ipsilateral thorax is appropriate, and concern for rupture of the contralateral lung is important.

The prognosis may depend as well on the presence of other anomalies. In nearly half the infants in the British Perinatal Study, other major anomalies were present and severe enough to account for death. These included anencephaly, Arnold-Chiari malformation, hydrocephaly, and iniencephaly. Congenital heart disease and urogenital anomalies may also coexist with diaphragmatic hernias.

Several long-term follow-up studies indicate an optimistic outlook. Wohl and coworkers examined 19 patients aged 6 to 18 years. The patients were asymptomatic. On study, however, reduced blood volume and blood flow on the side of the hernia persisted. Reid and Hutcherson in Australia had similar findings in their 30 patients followed 5 to 21 years. In addition, they noted one child with hypoplasia of the soft tissues of the whole left chest wall, including the breast.

Diaphragmatic Paralysis

Unilateral paralysis of the diaphragm is encountered rarely in the newborn. Approximately three fourths of the cases are associated with Erb's palsy of the arm of the same side. Most are right-sided.

Incidence. France was able to discover only 39 reported cases up to 1954, when he added another of his own. By 1957, Richard and colleagues identified 64 cases and added 10 new ones. Paralysis was on the right in 58 cases and on the left in only 16. It is probable that many mild instances of the disorder have been overlooked because of failure to perform fluoroscopic or ultrasonographic examination on all dyspneic newborns.

Etiology. Most cases follow difficult breech deliveries. Lateral hyperextension of the neck causes overstretching of the nerves of the brachial plexus and avulsion of the anterior roots supplying the phrenic nerve. In France's case, there was complete avulsion of the anterior roots of C 3, C 4, and C 5.

Iatrogenic paralysis of the diaphragm may complicate negative pressure respiratory therapy. Apparently, the seal around the neck can injure the phrenic nerve (Wexler and Poole, 1976). Paralysis of the phrenic nerve has been described in Werdnig-Hoffmann disease by Mellins and associates.

Diagnosis. How frequently the diagnosis of diaphragmatic paralysis is missed is exemplified by Schifrin's experience, reported in 1952. He described in detail the histories of four infants. In none of these was the diagnosis made before the age of 6 weeks. Three had been discharged from the nursery at the end of the first week in spite of the fact that all were tachypneic. Two had had radiographic examination, none had had fluoroscopy. The fourth infant remained in the hospital with tachypnea and bouts of cyanosis as well as two episodes of pneumonia, but he was 3 months old before the right diaphragm was noted to be elevated. Many radiographs had been made prior to this one, but there is no report of his having been studied by fluoroscopy.

Many of the infants are flaccid and make poor respiratory effort immediately after birth. This initial difficulty may be ascribed to the prolonged and difficult labor and instrumental delivery rather than to the diaphragmatic palsy. After resuscitation (if needed) and the establishment of spontaneous respiration, the infants are tachypneic or dyspneic. Dyspnea may subside within a few days to be followed by persistent tachypnea. Episodes of transient cyanosis may occur. The situation may deteriorate and terminate in death within the first few months, or improvement may begin as early as the second week or as late as the fifth month and total recovery ensue.

Physical examination shows diminished respiratory excursion on the affected side, which after several weeks may appear flattened. There are dullness and diminished breath sounds over the affected base and often signs of atelectasis over the lung above. Later, these findings may be confused with the signs of complicating pneumonia. The heart may or may not be shifted toward the side opposite the lesion. Diaphragmatic movement or its absence can at times be appreciated by deep palpation of the upper part of the abdomen just beneath the ribs.

Radiographic Findings and Fluoroscopy. Within the first few days only slight elevation of the affected diaphragm may be seen on the radiograph, and this may be so minor that its significance is overlooked. Later the diaphragm rises higher, the heart and mediastinal contents are displaced, and areas of atelectasis may be seen to abut the elevated diaphragm as well as the displaced heart.

The only certain way to clinch the diagnosis early in the course of the disorder is by fluoroscopy or ultrasonography. Characteristic paradoxical movement can be seen, the paralyzed diaphragm rising with inspiration and descending with expiration, while its normal mate moves simultaneously in the opposite direction.

Prognosis. France's compilation of 40 reported cases revealed an overall mortality rate of 22.5 per cent (nine deaths). He pointed out, however, that prognosis was much better if there was no associated Erb's palsy (one of 11, or 9 percent) than if brachial palsy was also present (eight of 29, or 27.6 per cent).

Recovery is often accomplished by gradual restoration of power and movement to the affected diaphragm. However, in Schifrin's case IV this was never completed, even at the age of 17 months. It is likely that some patients recover clinically, though their diaphragms never regain movement. These may account for cases diagnosed later as eventration of the diaphragm.

Treatment. Placing the infant in an environment with increased oxygen concentration usually suffices to tide him over the first hazardous days. Whether movement of the diaphragm will return depends upon the degree of avulsion of the roots and the possibility of reestablishment of continuity of the torn tissue. It is unlikely that measures such as faradic stimulation will have any effect on the ultimate outcome, although this has been attempted. Faradic stimulation may be used, however, as a prognostic test, since absence of any response indicates complete phrenic nerve degeneration. If after 3 or 4 months electrical stimulation produces no diaphragmatic movement, and if serious symptoms persist or increase, one might consider operative intervention. The operation of choice is plication of the paralyzed diaphragm (see following discussion).

Eventration of the Diaphragm

When one leaf of the diaphragm balloons abnormally high in the chest yet is attached normally to the chest wall and is intact, the condition is called *eventration.*

Incidence. The disorder has been discovered in mass radiographic surveys of adults approximately once in 10,000 films. Only within the past 20 years has it been realized that it may cause serious trouble in young infants, including the newborn.

Etiology. Most cases of eventration appear to be due to congenital insufficiency of muscle. A few follow phrenic nerve paralysis, and, in at least one instance, eventration was associated with bilateral absence of phrenic nerves and hypoplastic lungs (Goldstein and Reid, 1980).

Diagnosis. Many of the adults in whom eventration was discovered by routine radiographic examination had been completely symptom-free. In the newborn, the symptoms and signs may duplicate those of congenital diaphragmatic hernia. After prompt initial respiration, tachypnea, dyspnea, and intermittent cyanosis appear. Dullness and absent breath sounds over the lower half or two thirds of one hemithorax are the only consistent abnormal physical findings. The heart may be displaced toward the opposite side.

Anteroposterior and lateral films show the greatly elevated diaphragm and the displaced heart and mediastinum. Under the fluoroscope, the excursion of the elevated diaphragm is at first diminished but in the proper direction; later, it may become paradoxical.

Prognosis. Some of the reported patients have died. Judging from the comparatively large number of cases discovered in adults, it is evident that many patients survive the neonatal period. We cannot be sure that all these were symptom-free as newborns.

Treatment. Undoubtedly, many patients recover with the aid of simple supportive measures. When, in spite of these, dyspnea persists and serious episodes of cyanosis either do not diminish or increase in frequency and severity, transthoracic plication of the diaphragm is indicated.

A black male infant was born after a normal pregnancy and delivery, his birth weight 7 pounds (3175 gm). He was kept in an incubator because of "weakness" for 3 days, but was sent home at the usual time. He was said to have had a "cold" continuously since birth. Feeding was well supervised, and milk, Pablum, and egg yolk as well as adequate amounts of vitamins A, C, and D had been taken. When he was 3 months old, his "cold" became worse and wheezing was noted. He was irritable, ran a low-grade fever, and was treated with penicillin. A few days later he was diagnosed as having left-sided pneumonia. He was then hospitalized locally, and a diagnosis of eventration of the left diaphragm was made. He was referred to the Johns Hopkins Hospital. Neither cyanosis nor dyspnea had ever been noted.

Admission examination (age 3½ months) showed a temperature of 37.4° C., pulse 144, respirations 52, weight 6.24 kg. (13 pounds 12 ounces). Nutrition was fair. His abdomen appeared small. The heart was slightly displaced to the right. Percussion note over the left hemithorax was flat, and over this area no breath sounds were heard. The radiograph shows elevation of the left diaphragm. Gas-filled structures are seen within the thorax beneath it. The heart is displaced to the right (Fig. 21-5). Fluoroscopy on the same day revealed good motion of both leaves of the diaphragm. Operation was performed. The stomach, duodenum, left lobe of the liver, and the spleen lay within the left hemithorax beneath a saccular structure that terminated in lateral ridges of muscle. The sac was later found to contain a few muscle fibers. It was removed, and the ridges of muscle were sewn tightly together. The central portion of this diaphragm was a sac almost devoid of muscle. Whether this was a congenital defect or the late result of diaphragmatic paralysis one cannot say.

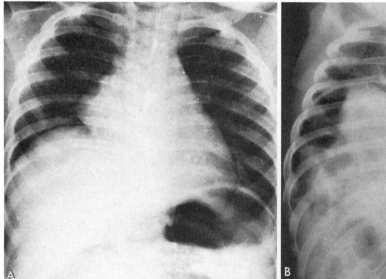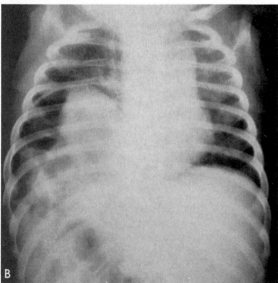

Figure 21-4. *A,* Anteroposterior view of chest showing a moderately elevated right diaphragm. This case history is not summarized in the text because the infant was completely asymptomatic, the x-ray picture having been taken because a sibling had tuberculosis. There had been no difficulty in labor and no respiratory trouble in the neonate. The probable diagnosis is eventration of the diaphragm. *B,* Diaphragmatic paralysis has the same appearance. On fluoroscopy, paradoxical diaphragmatic movement would indicate paralysis.

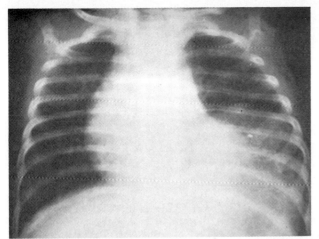

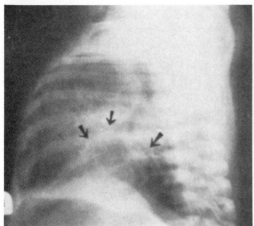

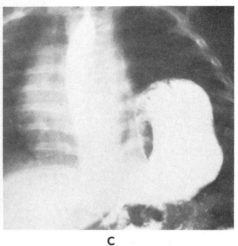

Figure 21–5. *A*, Anteroposterior view of chest made at 3½ months of age. The left diaphragm is elevated to the level of the fourth rib. The heart is displaced a little to the right. *B*, Lateral view on same date. The left diaphragm can be seen considerably higher in the chest than the right. Arrows point to the domed diaphragm. *C*, With barium in the esophagus and stomach, the stomach can be seen to lie largely within the thorax. It is inverted. The esophagus is displaced toward the right.

Figure 21–6. Anteroposterior view of chest made when patient was 3 weeks old.

Labor had been difficult and prolonged because of shoulder dystocia; delivery was completed by forceps extraction. Right-sided Erb's palsy, tachypnea, and dyspnea were noted, and there was one severe bout of pneumonitis at 4 weeks. All finally cleared at 2½ months of age.

The right diaphragm is elevated to the level of the fourth rib. The right lung contains patches of increased density. The heart is displaced a little toward the left. The left lung is moderately emphysematous, its diaphragm flattened and depressed.

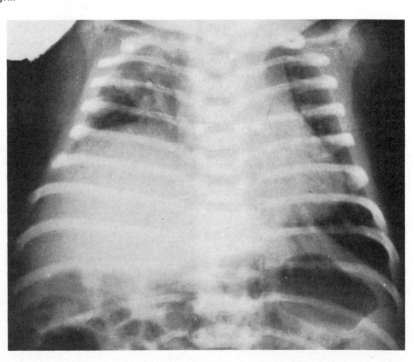

Comment. The birth of this infant was said to have been easy, and he was not unusually large. There is little evidence to make one suspect paralysis of the diaphragm due to brachial plexus trauma. He was neither tachypneic nor dyspneic and did not demonstrate paradoxical movement at any time. The likelihood, then, is that the weak, elevated diaphragm containing very little muscle tissue represents a congenital defect, or a true eventration. Operation successfully restored the proper anatomic relationships.

Accessory Diaphragm

This extremely rare anomaly consists of a supernumerary membranous and muscular structure that divides the hemithorax into two compartments. Four cases have been reported in the past three or four decades. Hashida and Sherman state that "pressure at the hiatus and disturbed mechanics due to . . . interference with function, especially of the contents of the inferior compartment" are responsible for the signs and symptoms. Anomalies of vascular supply and of lobulation may coexist. Their own infant was mildly cyanotic from birth, became more deeply so steadily, and developed grunting and radiographic evidence of pneumothorax. The left hemithorax moved poorly, and breath sounds over it were absent. He died at 5 hours of age.

The left hemithorax was divided into two unequal compartments by an accessory diaphragm. A semicircular orifice through which bronchi and vessels passed divided the upper from the lower compartment.

Agenesis of Diaphragm

A very rare anomaly is the complete absence of the diaphragm, with only a rim of tissue attached to the chest wall. In one set of identical twins, the anomaly was present in one twin only. Eichelberger and colleagues repaired the defect in one infant with dacron mesh sutured to the persisting rim. The infant survived 8½ months before dying from bronchopulmonary dysplasia.

REFERENCES

Allen, M. S., and Thomson, S. A.: Congenital diaphragmatic hernia in children under one year of age: a 24 year review. J. Pediatr. Surg. 1:157, 1966.

Baran, E. M., Houston, H. E., Lynn, H. B., et al.: Foramen of Morgagni hernias in children. Surgery 62:1076, 1967.

Bishop, H. C., and Koop, C. E.: Acquired eventration of the diaphragm in infancy. Pediatrics 22:1088, 1958.

Bloss, R. S., Aranda, J. V., and Beardmore, H. E.: Vasodilator response and prediction of survival in congenital diaphragmatic hernia. J. Pediatr. Surg. 16:118, 1981.

Bowers, V. M., Jr., McElin, T. W., and Dorsey, J. M.: Diaphragmatic hernia in the newborn; diagnostic responsibility of the obstetrician. Obstet. Gynecol. 6:262, 1955.

Butler, N., and Claireaux, A. E.: Congenital diaphragmatic hernia as a cause of perinatal mortality. Lancet 1:659, 1962.

Comer, T. P., and Clagett, O. T.: Surgical treatment of hernia of the foramen of Morgagni. J. Thoracic Cardiovasc. Surg. 52:461, 1966.

DeTroyer, A., Sampson, M., Sigrist, S., and Macklem, P. T.: The diaphragm: two muscles. Science 213:237, 1981.

Dibbins, A. W., and Weiner, E. S.: Mortality from neonatal diaphragmatic hernia. J. Pediatr. Surg. 9:653, 1974.

Eichelberger, M. R., Kettrick, R. G., Hoelzer, D. T., Swedlow, D. B., and Schnaufer, L.: Agenesis of the left diaphragm: Surgical repair and physiological consequences. J. Pediatr. Surg. 15:395, 1980.

France, N. E.: Unilateral diaphragmatic paralysis and Erb's palsy in the newborn. Arch. Dis. Child. 29:357, 1954.

Goldstein, J. D., and Reid, L. M.: Pulmonary hypoplasia resulting from phrenic nerve agenesis and diaphragmatic amyoplasia. J. Pediatr. 97:282, 1980.

Hashida, Y., and Sherman, F. E.: Accessory diaphragm associated with neonatal respiratory distress. J. Pediatr. 59:529, 1961.

Johnson, D. G., Deaner, R. M., and Koop, C. E.: Diaphragmatic hernia in infancy: factors affecting the mortality rate. Surgery 62:1082, 1967.

Laxdal, O. E., McDougall, H. A., and Mellin, G. W.: Congenital eventration of the diaphragm. N. Engl. J. Med. 250:401, 1954.

Levy, J. L., Jr., Guynes, W. A., Jr., Louis, J. E., et al.: Bilateral congenital diaphragmatic hernias through the foramina of Bochdalek. J. Pediatr. Surg. 4:557, 1969.

Longino, L. A., and Jewett, T. C.: Congenital bifid sternum. Surgery 38:610, 1955.

McNamara, J. J., Eraklis, A. J., and Gross, R. E.: Congenital posterolateral diaphragmatic hernia in the newborn. J. Thorac. Cardiovasc. Surg. 55:55, 1968.

Mellins, R. B., Hays, A. P., Gold, A. P., Berdon, W. E., and Bowdler, J. D.: Respiratory distress as the initial manifestation of Werdnig-Hoffmann disease. Pediatrics 53:33, 1974.

Perinatal Mortality: The First Report of the British Perinatal Mortality Survey. Edinburgh and London, E. & S. Livingstone, Ltd., 1963.

Philipp, E. E., and Skelton, M. O.: Congenital diaphragmatic hernia in siblings. Br. Med. J. 1:1283, 1952.

Reid, I. S., and Hutcherson, R. J.: Long term follow-up of patients with congenital diaphragmatic hernia. J. Pediatr. Surg. 11:939, 1976.

Richard, J., et al.: Diaphragmatic obstetric paralysis. Report of 10 cases. Arch. Franç. Pediatr. 14:563, 1957.

Rickham, P. P.: Strangulated diaphragmatic hernia in the neonatal period. Thorax 10:104, 1955.

Schifrin, N.: Unilateral paralysis of the diaphragm in the newborn infant due to phrenic nerve injury, with and without associated brachial palsy. Pediatrics 9:69, 1952.

Smith, B. T.: Isolated phrenic nerve palsy in the newborn. Pediatrics 49:449, 1972.

Wayne, E. R., Campbell, J. B., Burrington, J. D., and Davis, W. D.: Eventration of the diaphragm in the newborn. J. Pediatr. Surg. 9:643, 1974.

Wexler, H. A., and Poole, C. A.: Neonatal diaphragmatic dysfunction. Am. J. Roentgenol. 127:617, 1976.

Wohl, M. E. B., Griscom, N. T., Strieder, D. J., Schuster, S. R., Treves, S., and Zwerdling, R. G.: The lung following repair of congenital diaphragmatic hernia. J. Pediatr. 90:405, 1977.

22

Disorders of the Chest Wall

Abnormalities of bone and muscle of the chest wall may occur and be a mechanical hindrance to ventilation. Although bony abnormalities are rare, they may be recognized immediately and are sometimes amenable to operative correction.

Defects in the fusion of the sternum are uncommon, but numerous instances have been described since 1947, when Burton reported two cases in which successful operative repair was accomplished. *Complete separation of the sternum* allows protrusion of cardiovascular structures (ectopia cordis). Lethal malformations of the heart are commonly associated with this condition. *Upper sternal clefts* are more common. Early operation is advised in order to shield the underlying structures from injury and because of the greater ease of approximating the separated parts in the first days of life than later.

The most common of the sternal defects is *pectus excavatum*, sometimes associated with the Pierre Robin syndrome and Marfan's syndrome. A similar deformity is commonly seen in premature infants with respiratory distress that commonly resolves in time. Rarely is it a fixed or severe deformity until several months of postnatal age. A family history of some type of anterior thoracic deformity was found in 37 per cent of patients, according to Welch. The indications for operative correction are debatable. In our opinion, correction should not be undertaken until several years of age and then only in those few children in whom the deformity appears to be progressing. Serial photographs are the best way to document changes in pectus excavatum. Periodic evaluation of cardiovascular status with ultrasonography and EKG and assessment of pulmonary function is appropriate in the presence of progressive deformity. Results of operative correction are often excellent in over 80 per cent of patients and almost always lead to improvement. Recurrences may occur during later active growth.

A rare deformity of the thoracic cage, *asphyxiating thoracic dystrophy*, is part of a serious generalized chondrodystrophy. It was first described by Jeune in 1954. The ribs are broad and short and the thorax rigid. Some degree of lung hypoplasia may be present. Renal cystic dysplasia may be present and lead to hypertension and renal failure.

About 60 cases have been reported. Oberklaid and coworkers studied 10 of them and noted that only two patients were alive at the time of the report. One of the two was in excellent health at 15 years of age. The more severely affected infants had respiratory distress from birth. Three patients have been described in one family. The expectation is occurrence in one of four siblings. No parent-child occurrence has been described.

Deficiency of pectoral muscles on one side (Poland's syndrome) may also be associated with abnormal ribs (2 to 4) and hypoplasia of the breast. Breathing may be paradoxical and the cardiac impulse easily observed through the soft tissues. No operative intervention is required in infancy, although mammoplasty may later be desirable in affected girls after puberty.

Other causes of thoracic dysfunction are diseases of the muscles, including myasthenia gravis, poliomyelitis, amyotonia congenita, muscular dystrophy, glycogen storage disease, and spinal cord injury or tumor. Such conditions are usually recognized in the context of the associated systemic muscular weakness or paralysis. They should be suspected in any infant in whom hypoventilation is present when the chest film shows normal heart and lungs.

Table 22–1. Surgical Correction of Anterior Chest Wall Deformities in Patients at The Children's Hospital, Boston, 1952 to 1982

Type of Deformity	No. of Cases	
Pectus excavatum	970	M, 775
		F, 195
Pectus carinatum	138	M, 95
		F, 43
Recurrent pectus excavatum	14	
Poland's syndrome	12	
Vertebral and rib anomalies	7	
Lower cleft	7	
Upper cleft	5	
Ectopia cordis	3	
Total	1156	

(Courtesy of Dr. Kenneth Welch.)

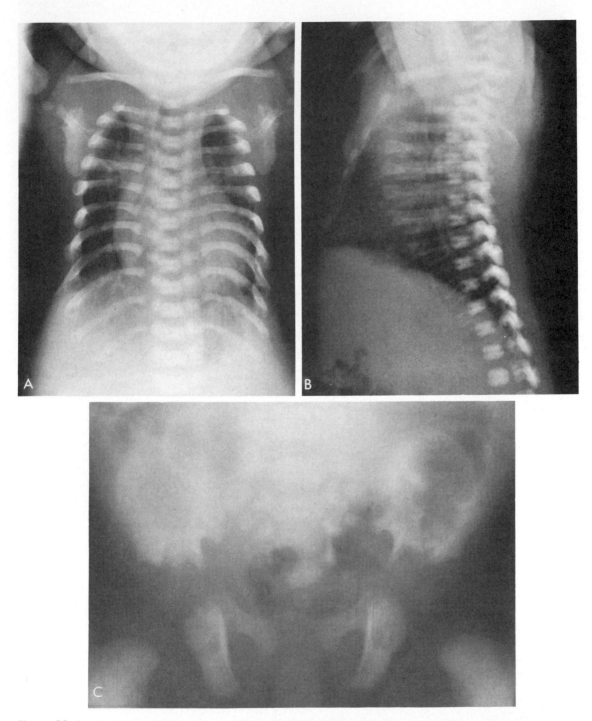

Figure 22–1. *A,* Anteroposterior film of infant with asphyxiating thoracic dystrophy. The thoracic circumference is reduced as compared with the abdominal circumference, and the liver and spleen are displaced downward. *B,* Lateral projection of the same infant further demonstrates the reduced thoracic volume. (*A* and *B,* Courtesy of Dr. John Kirkpatrick.) *C,* The film of the pelvis shows flaring of the iliac crest and irregular calcification of the triradiate cartilage with typical bony protrusions. (*C,* From Avery, M. E., Fletcher, B. D., and Williams, R. G.: The Lung and Its Disorders in the Newborn Infant. 4th ed. Philadelphia, W. B. Saunders Co., 1981.)

Gyllesward, A.: Pectus excavatum. A clinical study with long term postoperative follow-up. Acta Pediatr. Scand. *255*:1(suppl.), 1975.

Jeune, N., Carron, R., Berand, C., et al.: Polychondrodystrophie avec blocage thoracique d'évolution fatale. Pédiatrie *9*:390, 1954.

Kohler, E., and Babbitt, D. P.: Dystrophic thoraces and infantile asphyxia. Radiology *94*:55, 1970.

Langer, L. O.: Thoracic-pelvic-phalangeal dystrophy. Radiology *91*:447, 1968.

Maier, H. C., and Bortone, F.: Complete failure of sternal fusion with herniation of pericardium. J. Thorac. Surg. *18*:851, 1949.

Oberklaid, F., Danks, D. M., Mayne, V., and Campbell, P.: Asphyxiating thoracic dysplasia: clinical radiological and pathological information on 10 patients. Arch. Dis. Child. *52*:758, 1977.

Ravitch, M. M.: Congenital Deformities of the Chest Wall and Their Operative Correction. Philadelphia, W. B. Saunders Co., 1977.

Sabiston, D. C.: The surgical management of congenital bifid sternum with partial ectopia cordis. J. Thorac. Surg. *35*:118, 1958.

Welch, K. J.: Chest wall deformities. *In* Holder, T. M., and Ashcraft, K. W. (Eds.): Pediatric Surgery. Philadelphia, W. B. Saunders Co., 1980, p. 162.

23

Pulmonary Cysts and Intrathoracic Masses

Air-containing cysts within the lung are not encountered frequently, but cysts are present in such a variety of forms that they constitute an interesting diagnostic and therapeutic problem in the neonatal period. They may be single or multiple, unilateral or bilateral, filled with air or fluid, or both. They may be infected or clean, and the air within them may or may not be under tension. They may be congenital or acquired. At times, conservative measures of treatment are proper, but, occasionally, immediate surgical intervention is required.

Incidence. By 1933, Anspach and Wolman were able to find 150 cases in the medical literature, and the number has surely doubled since then. Cooke and Blades stated that one asymptomatic case per 20,000 was found in mass surveys and that one admission to the Walter Reed Hospital in every 2400 was for pulmonary cyst. In spite of these low figures, they concluded that the disease was "relatively common." Few of the total make their presence known during the first month of life.

Classification. Cooke and Blades proposed the following simple classification:
I. Congenital pulmonary cysts
   A. Bronchogenic cell type
      1. Solitary
      2. Multiple (synonyms: congenital or fetal bronchiectasis)
   B. Alveolar cell type
      1. Solitary (synonyms: balloon cyst, pneumatocele)
      2. Multiple
   C. Combination of A and B
II. Acquired pulmonary cysts
   A. Bullous emphysema
   B. Subpleural blebs

Pathology and Pathogenesis. Congenital cysts form when there is a developmental error in the ontogeny of the lung in the region of the medium-sized bronchi (*bronchogenic* cell type) or just proximal to the alveoli (*alveolar* cell type). These defects may be single or multiple. If multiple, they usually involve several segments of one lobe, more rarely of two or three contiguous lobes, but fortunately they are almost never bilateral. Characteristics of the congenital variety are said to be a wall containing smooth muscle and bits of cartilage. Being lined by epithelium is no proof of congenital origin, since epithelial cells have been found to grow over and line a resected surface. In the bronchogenic cell type, the lining cells are cuboidal or columnar and ciliated; in the alveolar type, they are squamous. Caffey doubts the specificity of these pathologic alterations, maintaining that acquired cysts may present the same picture.

Congenital cysts usually have a connection with the bronchial tree. Often, this is a minute tortuous passage to a small bronchiole. Acquired cysts, however, connect freely with adjacent bronchioles in many places.

The circumstance of their being in free communication with the tracheobronchial tree is responsible for almost all the trouble lung cysts cause. Infection spreads readily from bronchi into the interior of cysts, where, once established, it may be difficult to eradicate. Besides this, free egress of inspired air may be impeded by check-valve action at the communicating channel, resulting in increased tension. Without infection or tension most pulmonary cysts go unnoticed, only to be discovered on radiographs taken for some other reason.

Emphysematous bullae and subpleural blebs are produced by either obstruction or infection (see pp. 148 and 176).

Diagnosis. Newborns who become ill with cystic disease of the lungs usually suffer from the effects of

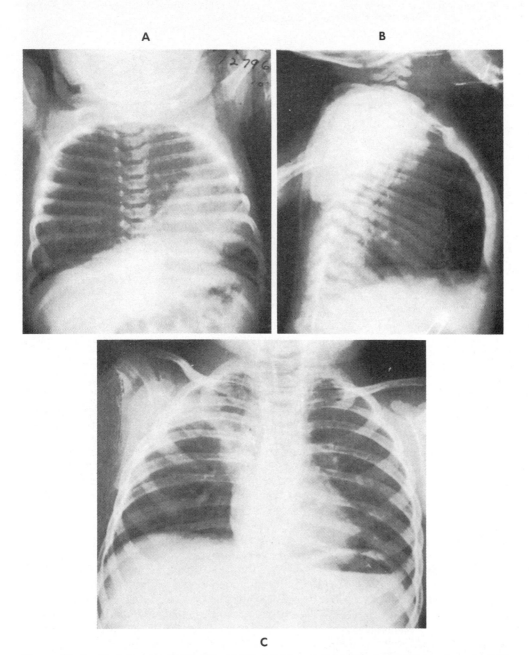

A   B

C

Figure 23–1. *A,* Anteroposterior film of chest taken at 1 month of age. A number of cystic shadows can be made out within the right lung field. The right lung herniates across the midline to half fill the left upper part of the chest. The heart is displaced far to the left. *B,* Lateral view, same time. The sternum is thrust forward, and the heart is dislocated posteriorly by herniated lung in the anterior mediastinum. Rounded cystic shadows can again be seen. *C,* Two years after operation. Aside from pleural thickening at the right upper lobe and overaeration of the right lower lobe, the lungs appear quite normal. (Fischer, C. C., Tropea, F., Jr., and Bailey, C. P.: J. Pediatr. *23:*219, 1943.)

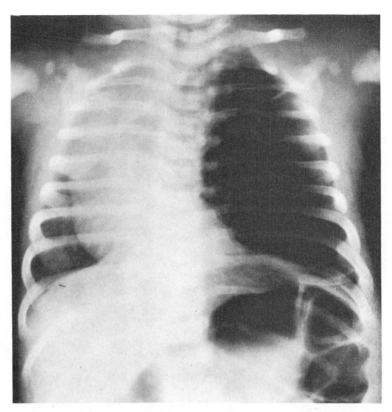

Figure 23–2. Anteroposterior film of chest made at 8 weeks of age. Note the shift of heart and mediastinum far to the right, herniation of left lung into right hemithorax, and deviation of trachea to the right. The overfilled, overaerated left hemithorax suggests the appearance of tension cyst rather than pneumothorax because the left hilus is empty and the lower border is curved. No collapsed lung can be seen. (Hill, L. F.: J. Pediatr. *38*:511, 1951.)

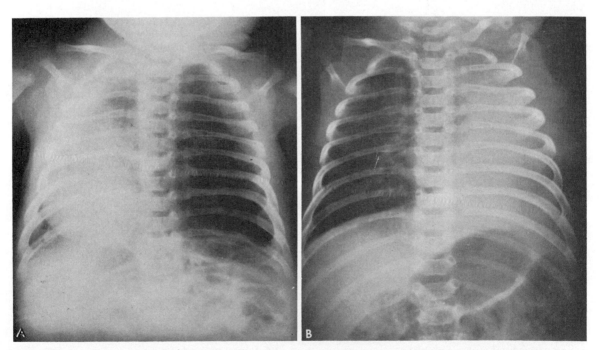

Figure 23–3. *A*, Preoperative anteroposterior film of chest made at 7 weeks of age. This shows the left hemithorax overexpanded by a huge translucent mass. Pneumothorax can be ruled out because the lower border is rounded, there is no shadow of collapsed lung, and fine trabecular markings are visible throughout most of the translucent area. The left upper lobe is herniated into the right upper hemithorax, and the heart and mediastinum are dislocated far to the right. *B*, Postoperative film shows the heart now displaced to the left, homogeneous opacification of the entire left hemithorax, probably due to thickened pleura, and compensatory emphysema of the right lung. (Leahy, L. J., and Butsch, W. L.: Arch. Surg. *59*:466, 1949.)

rapid expansion of the cysts. Tachypnea or dyspnea may begin at birth or at any time thereafter. Dyspnea may progress rapidly or slowly. In the first instance, the infant's condition can become critical within hours; in the latter, it may remain almost static for weeks or months.

A minority of neonates demonstrate the effects of infection rather than of increased tension. In these, persistent or repeated exacerbations of pneumonitis are the presenting symptom. When this is so, it is often difficult to decide whether infection came first and produced emphysematous bullae and subpleural

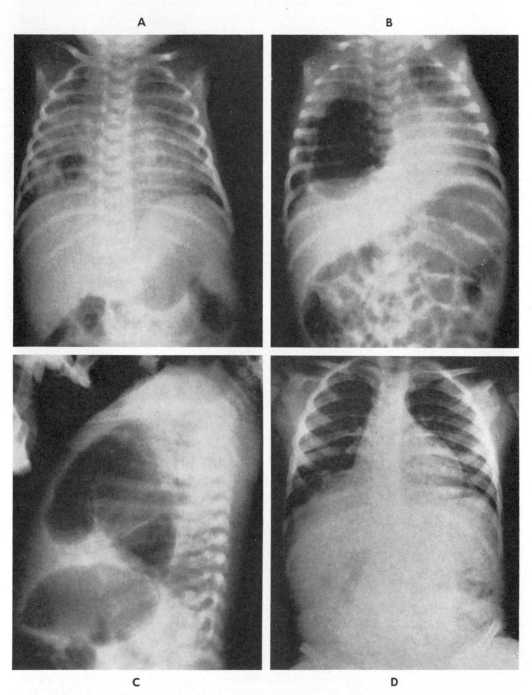

A

B

C

D

Figure 23–4. *A,* Anteroposterior view of chest taken on the twenty-first day of life. An air-filled cyst can be seen in the right lower part of the chest. *B* and *C,* Thirty days later, showing great increase in size of cyst and dislocation of heart toward the left axilla. *D,* Anteroposterior view at the age of 3 years. The lungs appear essentially normal. (Swan, H., and Aragon, G. E.: Pediatrics *14*:651, 1954.)

blebs or whether the cystic areas were true congenital cysts that became secondarily infected.

When cysts are solitary and large, they are discoverable by flatness of the percussion note if pus-filled, or, if they are air-filled (as is more commonly the case), they are indicated by hyperresonance or tympany. Breath sounds are diminished to absent over them. The heart is shifted away from the affected side unless a cyst lying adjacent to a bronchus has completely occluded it and has produced atelectasis of the distal segment of lung. Rales may be heard, owing to compression of contiguous lobes. Even when multiple cysts are present, the physical signs may be exactly the same, since the condition of the largest of the cysts dominates the clinical picture.

Radiographic Findings. Large balloon cysts filled with air under tension are often mistaken for tension pneumothorax. One hemithorax is overfilled, the diaphragm flattened or even concave, the mediastinum and heart pushed to or beyond the midline. Points that may distinguish balloon cysts from pneumothorax are (1) a delicate linear pattern within the

translucent area denoting their fine trabeculation, (2) the presence of compressed lung at the apex and at the costophrenic and cardiohepatic angles, often demarcated from the cyst by a curving line visible in one or another projection, and (3) the absence of all hilar shadows. In pneumothorax, the collapsed lung is often visible as a dense shadow projecting from the hilar region or upward from the diaphragm.

Multiple cysts are visualized as a collection of round or oval translucent areas within the hemithorax. If similar shadows are present in both sides of the chest, they are more likely to represent emphysematous bullae or blebs, but unilaterality does not rule out the latter possibility.

The round or oval areas of translucency produced by intrathoracic bowel may offer difficulty at times. When one is in doubt about the possibility of diaphragmatic hernia, a barium meal gastrointestinal series must be performed.

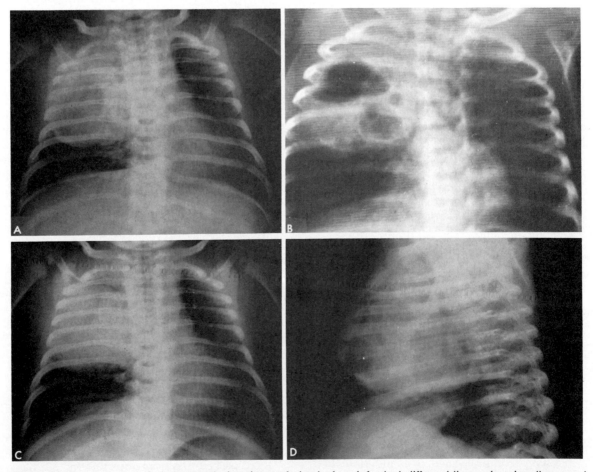

Figure 23–5. *A, B,* and *C,* Anteroposterior views of chest of an infant at different times showing the great variability in appearance of the same cystic lung. Differences in appearance depend upon whether one or all of the component cysts are air-filled or fluid-filled at that particular time. *D,* Lateral view made on the same day that *C* was taken.

Large cysts containing both air and fluid are hard to differentiate from hydropneumothorax or pyopneumothorax. Here again, visualization of a curved concave border between the cyst and compressed lung at the apex or base is the important differentiating feature.

Prognosis. Since many cystic lesions of the lung are completely asymptomatic and are discovered accidentally on chest films, it is safe to assume that a good many of those that might be discovered in this way in the neonatal period will never cause trouble. Once symptoms have developed, whether of increasing tension or of infection, the outlook becomes more serious. It is nevertheless true that most cystic-appearing lung lesions disappear with no surgical treatment.

Treatment. The absolute indication for immediate surgical treatment is increasing air tension within the cyst. This indication is unequivocal, and, what is more, radical intervention is called for. Repeated aspirations of air by needle and syringe or constant suction through an introduced catheter gives no more than temporary relief. They should be used, if at all, only for that reason, to tide the infant over a critical period until definitive operative measures can be taken. Operation should then consist of removal of as small a portion of the lung as is necessary, either a segment of a lobe or one or two lobes or the entire lung.

Infection within the cyst cavity constitutes the second indication for lobectomy or pneumonectomy. When there is pus, with or without air, within the cyst cavity, operation may be delayed until antibiotic and supportive therapy has improved the infant's general condition.

Cystic lesions subsequent to obstruction or infection are seldom lethal in themselves, and only treatment directed toward the underlying condition is indicated. If, after a waiting period of months, improvement has not occurred or if growth and development are retarded by persistent or repeated respiratory infection, it may be necessary to perform lobectomy or pneumonectomy.

Cystic Adenomatoid Malformation of the Lung

A rare form of congenital cystic disease of the lung, characterized by a mass of cysts lined by proliferating bronchial or cuboidal epithelium, has been described now in several hundred infants. In an extensive review, Stocker and others concluded that cystic adenomatoid malformations can be considered in three classes. According to their report, Type I is characterized by multiple large cysts, Type II is distinguished by evenly spaced cysts not more than 1.2 cm in diameter, and Type III is a bulky, firm mass with evenly spaced small cysts.

Onset and Symptoms. The onset of symptoms usually occurs during the first week of life, although it may be overlooked until much later in childhood if asymptomatic. About 10 per cent of cases present after age 1 year (Wexler and Valdes-Dapena, 1978). The disorder has occurred in all lobes of the lung but has rarely been bilateral. There is no suggestion of a familial predisposition to this malformation, and males and females are equally affected. Associated congenital anomalies were present in nearly 20 per cent of the infants described by Stocker and colleagues.

Radiographic Findings. In most cases, the lesion presents in an expansile, multicystic pattern and occasionally results in a mediastinal shift. Usually, only one lobe is involved.

Pathology. The affected lobe may be much increased in size and weight, and lobular septation is usually deficient. The epithelium is polypoid. Aberrant vessels are not a feature of this syndrome as they are in a sequestered lobe. Gottschalk and Abramson noted placental edema and fetal hydrops with cystic adenomatoid malformation, presumably on the basis of obstructed venous return. Merenstein found that 14 of 47 patients had anasarca.

Treatment. The infants who present with respiratory distress constitute a surgical emergency, since many of these cysts may enlarge with subsequent air breathing. If they are only detected incidentally at a later age, there is obviously no emergency. In all instances, however, resection seems the appropriate treatment (Nishibayashi et al., 1981).

Intrathoracic Tumors and Fluid-Filled Cysts

A large variety of solid tumors and fluid-filled cysts, in addition to the air-filled cysts just described, are encountered in the thoraces of adults. Many of these have already been observed in newborns, and we have no doubt that others will be recorded. Those that result from congenital maldevelopment, such as intrathoracic cysts of gastrointestinal origin and dermoid cysts, or teratomatous tumors, are more common in the neonatal period than are neoplasms and lymphomas. This last group, so common in adults as to account for up to 40 per cent of most series of mediastinal tumors, is of small numerical importance in the young infant. Too few neonatal cases have accumulated up to the present to warrant detailed classification.

Hope and Koop believe that intrathoracic mass lesions are best subdivided into those that arise in the posterior, middle, and anterior mediastinal spaces. A few others arise within the substance of the lung itself. In the posterior space, neurogenic tumors, duplications of the foregut, and neurenteric and bronchogenic cysts are most commonly encountered in the neonate. The middle mediastinum is the site almost exclusively of vascular lesions, while enlarged thymus and teratomas are masses most often seen in the anterior mediastinal space.

Thymus

The thymus occupies the upper anterior mediastinum, and it is more prominent in the newborn period than at any time of life. It may be so large as to reach the diaphragm or obscure both cardiac borders on radiographs. The normal thymus can be distinguished from an abnormal mass by the absence of tracheal deviation or compression. It changes in position with respiration and is less prominent with deep inspiration. It also involutes with stress as well as with corticosteroid therapy. Absence of the thymic shadow in an infant should alert one to the possibility of thymic agenesis and subacute combined immunodeficiency.

The cardiothymic-thoracic ratio provides an index of thymic size. Fletcher as well as Gewolb and colleagues noted that a large ratio is present on the first day in infants at risk for hyaline membrane disease, presumably because of less than normal levels of glucocorticoids before birth.

Thymic cysts have been reported in infants but rarely in newborns. Thompson and Love described a persistent cervical thymoma in a newborn infant that presented as an outpouch in the sternal notch with crying.

Mediastinal Neuroblastoma

Neuroblastoma, the most common solid tumor in the mediastinum of infants, arises from neural tissue,

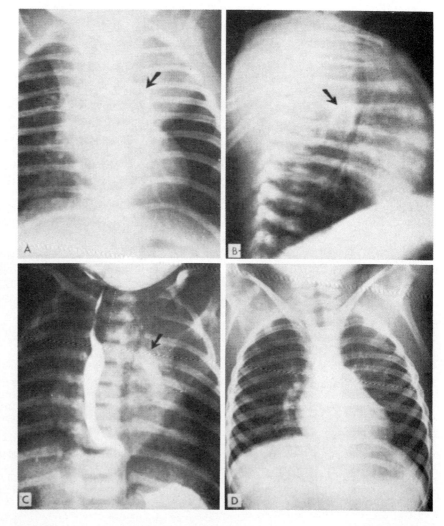

Figure 23–6. A 7-week-old male infant entered the hospital for repair of an inguinal hernia and was found to have a lymph node in the left cervical region. This finding prompted a roentgen examination of the chest. *A,* Anteroposterior roentgenogram showing a large area of density in the left upper hemithorax. Within the homogeneous density, a curvilinear calcification is present (arrow). *B,* Lateral roentgenogram showing the mass lesion to be in the posterior mediastinum with some anterior deviation of the trachea. The calcification appears to be in the shape of a horseshoe (arrow). *C,* Anteroposterior view of barium-filled esophagus showing the large size of the mass lesion more graphically. The calcification is more clearly visualized (arrow). At operation, the lesion proved to be a neuroblastoma. It was entirely excised. *D,* Posteroanterior roentgenogram 5 years later showing a normal chest. (Hope, J. W., and Koop, C. E.: Pediatr. Clin. North Am. 6:379, 1959.)

either intercostal or sympathetic nerves for the most part. Because it typically lies in the thoracic gutter, it is almost always posterior in location, and it may involve superior, mid-, or inferior mediastinum. From here it may extend to either side and invade one or both lungs. Extension through a vertebral foramen may result in neurologic manifestations.

Diagnosis is suggested by the discovery of an intrathoracic mass. It may follow roentgenography of the chest because of lower respiratory tract infection. Such infections afflict these infants more commonly than others because the growing tumor compresses bronchi. Alternatively, radiographs may be taken because of increasing dyspnea coupled with the physical signs of a solid intrathoracic mass.

Differentiation from other posterior mediastinal masses may be impossible before exploration. Neuroblastoma is not likely to be so sharply demarcated or to have so smooth and round a lower border as does a mediastinal cyst. Invasion of neighboring lung parenchyma strongly supports a diagnosis of neuroblastoma. Elevated urinary vanillylmandelic acid (VMA) may be present. Its absence does not rule out neuroblastoma.

Treatment. Exploration is indicated for any intrathoracic mass. If the tumor proves to be neuroblastoma, as much of it should be excised as is feasible surgically. The tumor should be staged according to the system of Evans, and subsequent therapy should be dictated by the stage (see Chapter 107).

Prognosis. The outlook for neuroblastomas in extra-adrenal locations is better than that for their suprarenal counterparts (Young et al., 1970). If the lesion can be completely removed and if no distant metastases are present, the probable survival rate is better than 75 per cent.

Bronchogenic Cysts

Fluid-filled cysts of tracheobronchogenous origin are distinguished with difficulty from those of gastroenterogenous origin.

Incidence. In several series of cases of neoplasms and cysts of the mediastinum among patients of all ages reported from various clinics, bronchogenic cysts outnumber those of gastric or enteric derivation. Most observers comment upon the fact that the distribution differs in young infants and children, so that gastroenterogenous and enterogenous ones outnumber the bronchogenic. In a 20-year experience

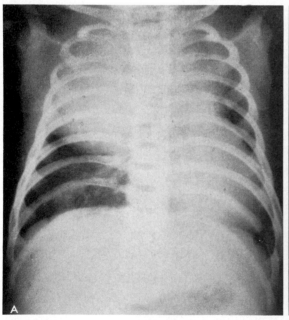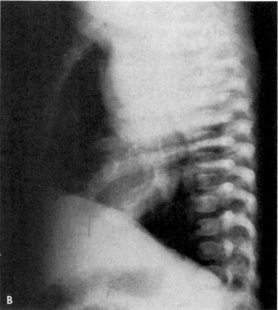

Figure 23–7. *A,* Anteroposterior view of chest of a 7-week-old infant admitted because of a severe respiratory infection. An opacity is seen filling the upper half of the right hemithorax and extending beyond the midline halfway to the left axilla. Its lower and left borders are rounded. The heart is displaced to the left and downward. The opacity gives the appearance of a solid tumor. *B,* Lateral view. The opaque mass juts forward from the posterior chest wall, from clavicle halfway down the chest to abut on the heart. Its outline is round.

At operation, a tumor was seen in the mediastinum that invaded all adjacent structures, including the left upper lobe. Biopsy revealed neuroblastoma. No excision was attempted. Radiotherapy was ineffective. Aminopterin was begun 2 months later and was followed by rapid improvement. Two years later, the patient appeared perfectly well, and no tumor was visualized on x-ray films. (Case 7 of Dr. Gladys Boyd, abstracted with her kind permission.)

and review of the literature, deParedes and associates found 68 cases and added 12 of their own. In the neonate, bronchogenic cysts are encountered infrequently.

Pathology. Bronchogenic cysts seldom attain large size. They contain clear fluid and are lined with columnar, cuboidal, or pseudostratified epithelium, and their walls generally contain smooth muscle and cartilage. They may, but do not always, communicate with the tracheobronchial tree. They tend to lie in the posterior mediastinum, but some have been found in the anterior space.

Diagnosis. Lying as they do, near the carina, these cysts commonly produce signs of respiratory embarrassment from birth or soon after. Generally, their size is not such that they can be discovered by percussion or auscultation, but physical signs are likely to reveal their secondary effects, emphysema or atelectasis, rather than the tumor itself. Opsahl and Berman reported a case that showed emphysema on the left, followed by clearing, then equally notable emphysema on the right.

Radiographic examination often shows a mass projecting forward from the superior mediastinal

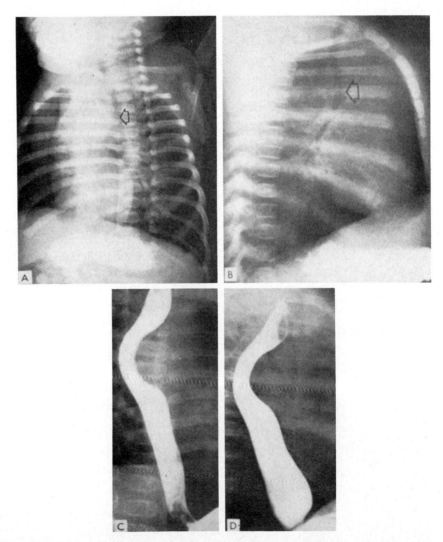

Figure 23–8. A 10-week-old male infant with dyspnea since birth. *A,* Left anterior oblique roentgenogram showing a mass lesion just below the carina (arrow). *B,* Lateral roentgenogram showing anterior deviation of the trachea (arrow). *C,* Anteroposterior view of barium-filled esophagus showing extreme deviation of the esophagus to the right just above the level of the carina. *D,* Lateral view of barium-filled esophagus showing posterior deviation of the esophagus just above the level of the carina. A bronchogenic cyst was removed at operation. (Hope, J. W., and Koop, C. E.: Pediatr. Clin. North Am. *6:*379, 1959.)

shadow, not large and not necessarily rounded. Ultrasonography can help localize the lesion.

Barium swallow may reveal indentation of the esophagus from an anterior direction.

Bronchoscopy reveals compression of the trachea and often of one major bronchus.

Treatment. Immediate excision should be performed.

Esophageal, Gastrogenic, and Enterogenous Cysts

These three varieties of intrathoracic fluid-filled cysts are discussed together, since they are indistinguishable on clinical grounds.

Incidence. Together they constitute a large group of mediastinal masses found in the neonatal period. Although they are not encountered frequently, they are far from uncommon.

Pathology and Etiology. These cysts are duplicated segments of gut that have become partially or completely detached from the parent viscus. They lie in or near the posterior mediastinum but, with increasing size, may project far into one or the other hemithorax. Their walls are composed of a mucosal layer characteristic of that of their site of origin and of one or more muscular layers. They contain fluid that is also similar to the secretion normally manu-

factured in their parent locus. The material within gastrogenic cysts contains pepsin, protein, and inorganic salts in roughly the same concentrations as are present in gastric juice.

The foregut becomes duplicated in the course of embryonic development by failure of complete resorption of occluding epithelium, resulting in the formation of a supernumerary wall. The high percentage of vertebral malformations coincident with gastroenterogenous cysts led Veeneklaas to suggest that the primary embryonic defect lies in abnormal persistence of the primitive adherence of notochord to foregut. When foregut descends from its early position in the region of the neck, this adhesion causes anomalies in vertebral bodies derived from notochord and pinches off a portion of the foregut and prevents its descent.

Diagnosis. Symptoms depend upon the size and location of the cyst. Since the cysts are all posterior and lie close to the trachea, esophagus, and great vessels, they are seldom symptomless. Cyanosis, tachypnea, and dyspnea are often present from birth. Swallowing difficulty and vomiting are less frequent. Recurrent lower respiratory tract infections characterize a few. Hemorrhage, from either the mouth or nose, from lungs or stomach, or in the form of melena, is not at all uncommon. In most instances, hemorrhage indicates that the cyst is of gastrogenic origin, since the fluid within these cysts contains pepsin and is capable of eroding through the cyst wall to break down adjacent blood vessels. Technetium scans should be useful in delineating cysts lined with gastric mucosa.

Radiographs of the chest show abnormal shadows that are often difficult to distinguish from unusual cardiac contours. Lateral and oblique films may be needed in order to make the differentiation with cer-

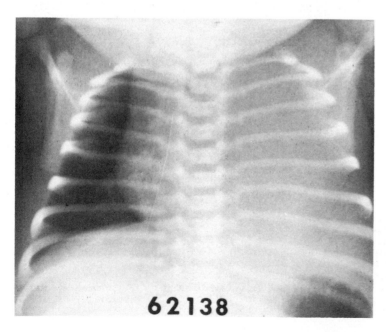

Figure 23–9. Air within the stomach shows the level of the left hemidiaphragm. The ribs on the left are separated, and the mediastinal structures are displaced slightly to the right. At thoracotomy, the left lung was large and engorged. During operation, the lung became aerated, presumably as bronchial obstruction was relieved, and a bronchogenic cyst was removed. (Griscom, N. T., et al.: Pediatrics 43:383, 1969.)

62138

tainty. In one or another projection, the rounded border of the cyst contiguous to the heart should be able to be visualized. Barium swallow commonly shows displacement of the esophagus. Bronchiogenic cysts may either partially or totally compress the bronchus, with consequent overdistention or atelectasis. Sometimes, the symptoms are intermittent as the cyst enlarges or empties.

Bronchoscopy and esophagoscopy are not ordinarily required in order to clinch the diagnosis. When performed, they may show compression of one or

both structures from without. Cyst puncture should not be performed.

Treatment. Operation is indicated as soon as the diagnosis of mediastinal mass is made. It is neither necessary nor wise to delay exploration until a specific diagnosis has been made.

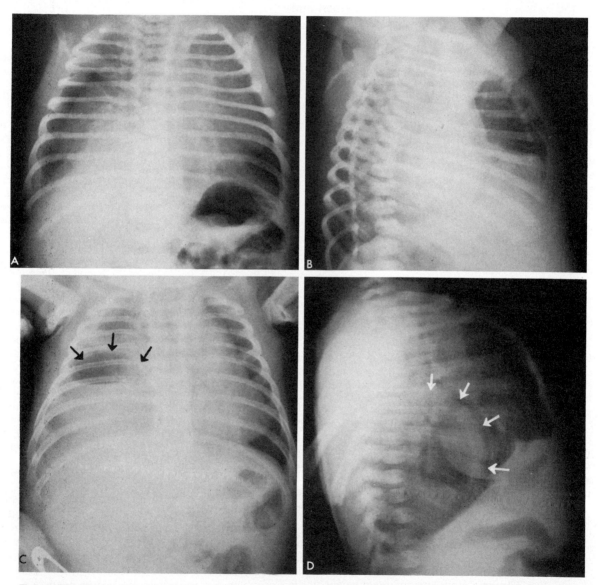

Figure 23–10. *A,* Anteroposterior view of chest taken within the first week of life, interpreted as showing atelectasis of right upper and lower lobes. The left border of the heart almost touches the left axillary wall, while its right border appears to be almost as far in the right hemithorax. It is difficult to tell whether this shadow is that of a hugely enlarged heart or whether it is composed of more than one element. *B,* Lateral view. In this view, the opacity filling the lower half of the chest is also difficult to diagnose, but it almost surely is not all heart. *C,* Anteroposterior view taken 4 weeks later. In the interim, fluid had been withdrawn six times, and in the process air had been introduced into the right hemithorax. Now one can see a mass in the right middle and lower hemithorax containing a bubble of air that delineates its rounded upper border. Removal of fluid has permitted the heart to return to a position more nearly normal. *D,* Lateral view, same day. Here the rounded margin of almost the entire cyst can be visualized. (Leahy, L. J., and Butsch, W. L.: Arch. Surg. *59:*466, 1949.)

Mediastinal Teratomas

The shadow of the enlarged thymus is the most common radiopaque mass visualized in the anterior mediastinum of the newborn. The enlarged thymus, however, appears to cause little if any trouble in the neonatal period. Thymoma has not been reported. When an anterior mediastinal mass is associated with respiratory distress in the newborn, the strong likelihood is that the lesion is a teratoma. Seibert and coworkers reported one infant with tracheal compression from a teratoma. Normal thymus should not compress the trachea or great vessels. All other anterior masses (lymphomas, lymphangiomas, substernal thyroids, etc.) occur with the utmost infrequency in this age period.

Fibrosarcoma of the Lung

An unusual solid tumor of the lung in a newborn was reported to us in a personal communication from Sir Douglas Robb, of Auckland, New Zealand. As far as we can determine, this is the only fibrosarcoma of the lung thus far identified in a newborn.

CASE 23–1

(Case of Douglas Robb, from the Thoracic Surgical Unit, Green Lane Hospital, Auckland, N. Z. Personal communication to the author.)

"A male child, birth weight 8 lb., 5 oz. (3770 gm) was found to have his heart beat in the right chest and dullness over the left hemithorax. X-ray showed radiopacity of the left chest and heart displaced to the right. Barium swallow showed the cardia and stomach to lie below a normally placed left diaphragm, thus suggesting that the mass was of thoracic origin.

"On the second day of life a left thoracotomy displayed a yellowish spherical tumor occupying most of the lower lobe of the left lung, with fringes of lung tissue around. No adhesions, . . . no pleural fluid, . . . the hilar structures were normal and not infiltrated and showed no enlarged glands. Left lower lobectomy was performed, recovery was uneventful and progress subsequently was good."

The specimen was examined by Dr. Stephen Williams, Pathologist. Sections showed the 6.5 by 6.0 cm tumor to be composed of poorly differentiated round and spindle cells arranged in sheets lying in various planes. Van Giesen's stain showed collagenous fibrils in some areas. Diagnosis was sarcoma, probably of fibroblastic origin.

Comment. The findings of dullness in one hemithorax with shift of the heart and mediastinum to the opposite side led to radiographic investigation. Identical signs might have been elicited from various solid tumors or fluid-filled cysts or even from pleural effusion or chylothorax. The radiographic shadow indicated that a tumor was present, and this was immediately removed. This assured the infant the maximum opportunity for complete cure.

Hamartoma of Lung

Hamartoma is not a true neoplasm. It is a mass composed of the normal elements that make up an organ, combined in an abnormal manner. In the lung it is usually encapsulated and firm and ordinarily does not attain a great size. Under the microscope, varying amounts of mesenchymal and epithelial elements are seen, often surrounding bits of cartilage. An abstract of one example in infancy follows.

CASE 23–2

(Case of Graham and Singleton, abstracted with permission of the authors.)

A white female infant born at term after normal pregnancy and labor, birth weight 7 pounds 4 ounces (3290 gm), seemed well during her 3-day nursery stay. At 6 weeks deep sternal retraction was seen. The time of onset of this symptom was not known.

Examination revealed shifting of the heart far to the right. There were no respiratory distress, no cyanosis, no murmurs, no abnormal heart sounds. A diagnosis of dextrocardia was made. On the following day the temperature rose to 103° F; cough appeared and later became severe and persistent. The infant began to vomit some feedings and to be mildly dyspneic. Breath sounds decreased on the left, and coarse and fine rales became audible on this side. X-ray study showed a homogeneous density filling the left hemithorax with mediastinal and cardiac shift to the right. The mass was anterior. With penicillin, oxygen, and a transfusion she promptly became afebrile. Operation at 7½ weeks revealed a firm, rubbery left upper lobe and several large hilar nodes. Left upper lobectomy was done. The specimen was a firm mass with some aerated lung about the periphery. Under the microscope the septa were thick and cellular; the alveolar spaces were dilated and lined by tall cuboidal or columnar epithelium. Many spaces resembled bronchioles of an immature type. The diagnosis was hamartoma.

Comment. In this instance, dyspnea appeared first, evidence of cardiac dislocation next, and pneumonitis supervened a bit later. The radiograph revealed an intrathoracic mass. Despite its benign nature, immediate excision was imperative because its very size was producing pressure effects and infection, either of which might have caused early death.

Accessory and Sequestered Lobes

More than 300 cases of pulmonary sequestration have been reported in the literature; these were reviewed by Carter in 1969 and by Landing in 1979.

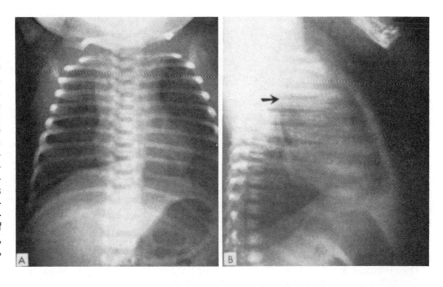

Figure 23–11. An 11-day-old male infant with severe respiratory distress and cyanosis since 2 days of age. *A,* Anteroposterior roentgenogram showing extreme hyperaeration of both lung fields and a wide superior mediastinum. *B,* Lateral roentgenogram showing extreme hyperaeration of the lungs and a mass filling the anterior mediastinum producing posterior deviation and compression of the trachea (arrow). The tumor was excised and proved to be a benign teratoma lying behind a normal thymus gland and in front of the trachea. (Hope, J. W., and Koop, C. E.: Pediatr. Clin. North Am. *6:*379, 1959.)

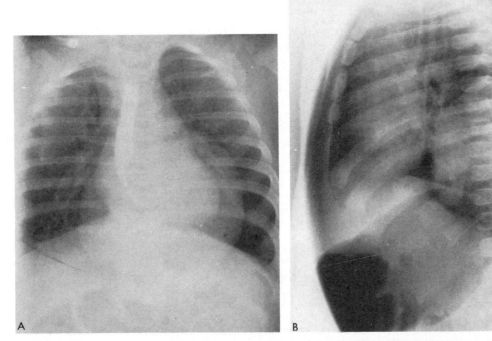

Figure 23–12. *A,* Anteroposterior view shows a homogeneous circular shadow surrounding the heart shadow. The heart appears normal, the lungs clear. *B,* In the lateral view, the mass is seen to be disc-shaped and to lie in the posterior mediastinum. This proved to be an accessory lobe.

They have rarely produced symptoms in newborn infants and have usually been detected on chest films taken for other reasons. A sequestered lobe sometimes manifests itself in children or young adults by repeated infections in a fluid-filled cyst. The lesion should be suspected in infants with cystic lesions, especially in the lower lobes.

The malformation is slightly more common in males and is distinctly more likely on the left side. Approximately two thirds of the cases involve the left lower lobe. Connections with the foregut may occur. Anomalous arteries from the aorta (above or below the diaphragm) usually enter the sequestered lobe, which does not receive pulmonary blood flow. Venous drainage is by the pulmonary veins or the azygos system. Complex congenital malformations coexist with extralobar sequestered lobes in 15 to 40 per cent of cases. Associated malformations are rare with intralobar sequestrations. Anomalous venous drainage, eventration of the diaphragm, and foregut duplications are among the more frequently associated conditions.

Usually, the sequestered lobe does not communicate with the tracheobronchial tree. This may occur, however, as in the infant reported by Bozic who also had atelectasis and hyaline membranes in all lobes except the sequestered one, which was perfused solely by the systemic circulation.

The most useful aid in diagnosis is a chest radiograph. It is helpful to have an angiographic study preoperatively to alert the surgeon as to the position of anomalous vessels.

The treatment is resection because repeated infections are the rule.

Accessory lobes differ from sequestered ones in that they derive their blood supply from the pulmonary vascular system.

REFERENCES

Abell, M. R.: Mediastinal cysts. A.M.A. Arch. Pathol. 61:360, 1956.
Anspach, W. E., and Wolman, I. J.: Large pulmonary air cysts of infancy, with special reference to pathogenesis and diagnosis. Surg. Gynecol. Obstet. 56:634, 1933.
Bates, M.: Total unilateral pulmonary sequestration. Thorax 23:311, 1968.
Boyd, G. L.: Solid intrathoracic masses in children. Pediatrics 19:142, 1957.
Bozic, C.: Pulmonary hyaline membranes and vascular anomalies of the lung. Description of a case. Pediatrics 32:1094, 1963.
Buntain, W. L., Isaacs, H., Payne, V. C., et al.: Lobar emphysema, cystic adenomatoid malformation, pulmonary sequestration and bronchogenic cyst in infancy and childhood: A clinical group. J. Pediatr. Surg. 9:85, 1974.
Burnett, W. E., and Caswell, H. T.: Lobectomy for pulmonary cysts in a fifteen-day-old infant with recovery. Surgery 23:84, 1948.
Caffey, J.: On the natural regression of pulmonary cysts during early infancy. Pediatrics 11:48, 1953.
Carter, R.: Pulmonary sequestration—collective review. Ann. Thorac. Surg. 7:68, 1969.
Clark, N. S., Nairn, R. C., and Gowar, F. J. S.: Cystic disease of the lung in the newborn treated by pneumonectomy. Arch. Dis. Child. 31:358, 1956.
Cooke, F. N., and Blades, B. B.: Cystic disease of the lungs. J. Thorac. Surg. 23:546, 1952.
de Paredes, C. G., Pierce, W. S., Johnson, D. G., et al.: Pulmonary sequestration in infants and children. A 20-year experience and review of the literature. J. Pediatr. Surg. 5:136, 1970.
Ellis, F. H., Jr., Kirklin, J. W., Hodgson, et al.: Surgical implications of the mediastinal shadow in thoracic roentgenograms of infants and children. Surg. Gynecol. Obstet. 100:532, 1955.
Eraklis, A. J., Griscom, N. T., and McGovern, J. B.: Bronchogenic cyst of the mediastinum. N. Engl. J. Med. 281:1150, 1969.
Evans, A. E., D'Angio, G. J., and Randolph, J.: A proposed staging for children with neuroblastoma. Cancer 27:324, 1971.
Ferguson, C. C., Young, L. N., Sutherland, J. B., and Macpherson, R. I.: Intrathoracic gastrogenic cyst—preoperative diagnosis by technetium pertechnetate scan. J. Pediatr. Surg. 8:827, 1973.
Fischer, C. C., Tropea, F., Jr., and Bailey, C. P.: Congenital pulmonary cysts; report of an infant treated by lobectomy with recovery. J. Pediatr. 23:219, 1943.
Fletcher, B. D., Masson, M., Lisbona, A., et al.: Thymic response to endogenous and exogenous steroids in premature infants. J. Pediatr. 95:111, 1979.
Gerle, R. D., Jaretski, A., Ashley, C. A., et al.: Congenital bronchopulmonary foregut malformation. Pulmonary sequestration communicating with the gastrointestinal tract. N. Engl. J. Med. 278:1413, 1968.
Gewolb, I. H., Lebowitz, R. L., and Taeusch, H. W.: Thymic size and its relationship to the respiratory distress syndrome. J. Pediatr. 95:108, 1979.
Gottschalk, W., and Abramson, D.: Placental edema and fetal hydrops. Obstet. Gynecol. 10:626, 1957.
Graham, G. G., and Singleton, J. W.: Diffuse hamartoma of the upper lobe in an infant: Report of successful surgical removal. A.M.A. J. Dis. Child. 89:609, 1955.
Gross, R. E.: Congenital cystic lung: Successful pneumonectomy in a three-week-old baby. Ann. Surg. 123:229, 1946.
Hill, L. F.: Conference at Raymond Blank Memorial Hospital for Children, Des Moines, Iowa. J. Pediatr. 38:511, 1951.
Holder, T. M., and Christy, M. G.: Cystic adenomatoid malformation of the lung. J. Thorac. Cardiovasc. Surg. 47:590, 1964.
Hope, J. W., and Koop, C. E.: Differential diagnosis of mediastinal masses. Pediatr. Clin. N. Amer. 6:379, 1959.
Izzo, C., and Rickham, P. P.: Neonatal pulmonary hamartoma. J. Pediatr. Surg. 3:77, 1968.
Kafka, V., and Beco, V.: Simultaneous intra- and extrapulmonary sequestration. Arch. Dis. Child. 35:51, 1960.
Kwittken, J., and Reiner, L.: Congenital cystic adenomatoid malformation of the lung. Pediatrics 30:759, 1962.
Landing, B. H.: Congenital malformations and genetic disorders of the respiratory tract (larynx, trachea, bronchi and lungs). Am. Rev. Resp. Dis. 120:151, 1979.
Leahy, L. J., and Butsch, W. L.: Surgical management of respiratory emergencies during the first few weeks of life. Arch. Surg. 59:466, 1949.
Merenstein, G. B.: Congenital cystic adenomatoid malformation of the lung. Am. J. Dis. Child. 118:772, 1969.
Nishibayashi, S. W., Andrassy, R. J., and Woolley, M. M.: Congenital cystic adenomatoid malformation: a 30-year experience. J. Pediatr. Surg. 16:704, 1981.
Opsahl, T., and Berman, E. J.: Bronchogenic mediastinal cysts in infants: Case report and review of the literature. Pediatrics 30:372, 1962.
Sabiston, D. C., Jr., and Scott, H. W., Jr.: Primary neoplasms and cysts of the mediastinum. Ann. Surg. 136:777, 1952.
Seibert, J. J., Marvin, W. J., and Schieker, R. M.: Mediastinal teratoma: a rare cause of severe respiratory distress in the newborn. J. Pediatr. Surg. 11:253, 1976.
Spock, A., Schneider, S., and Baylin, G. J.: Mediastinal gastric cysts: A case report and review of the English literature. Am. Rev. Resp. Dis. 94:97, 1966.

Stocker, J. T., Drake, R. M., and Madewell, J. E.: Cystic and congenital lung disease in the newborn. Perspect. Pediat. Path. 4:93, 1978.

Swan, H., and Aragon, G. E.: Surgical treatment of pulmonary cysts in infancy. Pediatrics 14:651, 1954.

Thompson, R. E., and Love, W. G.: Persistent cervical thymoma, apparent with crying. Am. J. Dis. Child. 124:761, 1972.

Veeneklaas, G. M. H.: Pathogenesis of intrathoracic gastrogenic cysts. Am. J. Dis. Child. 83:500, 1952.

Wexler, H. A., and Valdes-Dapena, M.: Congenital cystic adeno-

matoid malformation: a report of three unusual cases. Radiology 126:737, 1978.

Young, L. W., Rubin, P., and Hanson, R. E.: The extra-adrenal neuroblastoma: high radiocurability and diagnostic accuracy. Am. J. Roentgenol. 108:75, 1970.

24

Chylothorax and Pulmonary Hemorrhage

Incidence. Chylothorax is relatively rare in the neonatal period. Spontaneous effusions occur in males twice as often as in females.

Etiology. Spontaneous chylothorax may be the result of anomalous lymphatic channels or failure of normal ones to drain into the lymphatic duct. More often than not, no single lesion can be demonstrated on surgical exploration.

Recently, we have seen acquired chylothorax in the postoperative period after cardiac surgery. Interference with lymphatic drainage is usually temporary under these circumstances. Acquired chylothorax may follow obstruction of the superior vena cava. A cause of this problem is thrombosis at the site of a central venous catheter.

Diagnosis. Respiratory distress may be noted shortly after birth or any time up to a few weeks of age. Tachypnea and retractions are usually noted, and cyanosis may be present. A mediastinal shift away from the area of dullness suggests an effusion. The effusions are most common on the right side and are rarely bilateral.

Radiographs will show pleural effusions and mediastinal shifts. The most consistent diagnostic feature is the presence of several thousand white cells, over 90 per cent mononuclear, in the pleural fluid.

If the infant has been fed milk, the fluid will be chylous and have a milky opalescent appearance. In the absence of milk feeds, it will be clear pale yellow. On the average, the fluid contains about 4 per cent protein.

Prognosis. One can never be sure how an infant will respond. Janet's infant recovered after one aspiration, Sakula's after two, Wessel's after 13. Three of the reported examples ceased pouring out pleural fluid after severe bouts of diarrhea. The association, if any, is unclear. There were three deaths in the series, one at 20 days, another at 21 days. In this latter instance, a leakage point was discovered in the posterior mediastinum. A third death occurred after 42 taps had been performed over a 2-month period. In this case, no thoracic duct or cisterna chyli was found. The majority of infants have recovered after single or multiple thoracenteses. Usually, there are no associated problems and no recurrences.

Treatment. Thoracenteses, repeated as often and as long as required, lead to eventual cure in most instances. If, after a reasonable period, continued tapping every 3 to 4 days does not seem to improve the infant, one is justified in considering exploration. A reparable tear in the thoracic duct might be found. We are not certain exactly what constitutes a reasonable period, but we suggest that 2 months and 12 to 20 taps might be an adequate period of trial.

Curci and Dibbins found that a partial pleurectomy resulted in immediate clearing of chylothorax in a 1.6-kg infant who had spontaneous bilateral pneumothorax. The right side cleared with thoracentesis, but the left drained an average of 240 ml of fluid per day for 3 weeks. Surgical exploration at that time did not reveal a single site of leakage. Partial pleurectomy was carried out with an impressive cure.

Continuous drainage via a chest tube can lead to protein depletion, inanition, lymphocyte depletion, and impaired host defenses. If such treatment is needed to relieve symptoms, careful attention to nutrition is imperative.

Medium-chain-triglyceride formulas are useful in reducing chyle formation, hence the volume of chyle in the thorax.

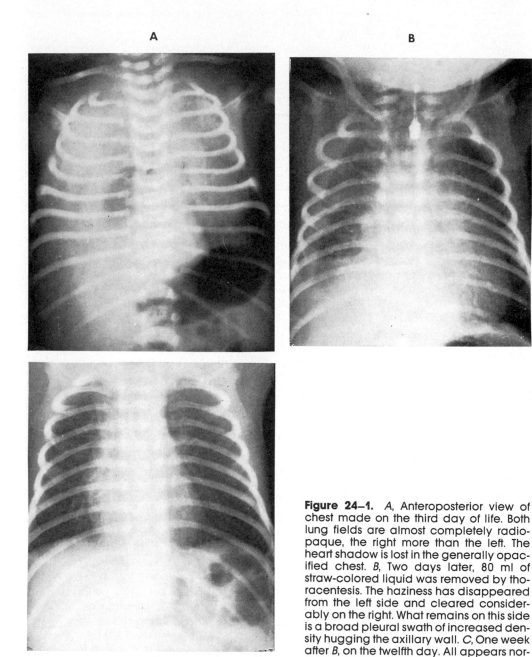

Figure 24–1. *A*, Anteroposterior view of chest made on the third day of life. Both lung fields are almost completely radiopaque, the right more than the left. The heart shadow is lost in the generally opacified chest. *B*, Two days later, 80 ml of straw-colored liquid was removed by thoracentesis. The haziness has disappeared from the left side and cleared considerably on the right. What remains on this side is a broad pleural swath of increased density hugging the axillary wall. *C*, One week after *B*, on the twelfth day. All appears normal.

Pulmonary Hemorrhage

Among the many disorders afflicting the newborn in which pathogenesis is poorly understood, diagnosis difficult or impossible, and therapy thoroughly unsatisfactory, pulmonary hemorrhage unquestionably deserves first rank.

Incidence. Landing discovered pulmonary hemorrhage, described as extravasated red blood cells in air spaces or septa, or both, in 68 per cent of lungs of 125 consecutive infants who died within the first week of life. Massive pulmonary hemorrhage was found in 17.8 per cent of autopsies (0.38 per cent of live births) at The Johns Hopkins Hospital by Esterly and Oppenheimer. From 1961 to 1968, DeSa and MacLean reported only 0.21 cases per 1000 live-births in a series from Oxford. In practice, one currently sees only a few newborns who die with extensive pulmonary hemorrhage as the outstanding pathologic lesion.

Etiology and Pathogenesis. Pulmonary hemorrhage is more common in infants of low birth size than in those of average size, and it is particularly common in infants of low birth weight for gestational age.

At times, it is associated with evidence of bleeding elsewhere. In these cases, it may be noted that puncture wounds made either for venipuncture or for subcutaneous or intramuscular injections continue to ooze for hours. No specific clotting defect is found in the blood of these infants, nor do they generally cease bleeding in response to transfusion of citrated or unmodified blood. Pulmonary hemorrhage may prove to be the cause of death in severe hemolytic anemia of the newborn or in infants born of diabetic mothers. In none of these conditions do we understand the cause of bleeding into the lungs.

Rothman pointed out that pulmonary hemorrhage may follow labors during which uterine contractions are extremely vigorous. He believed that this may lead to increased blood volume in the fetus, producing capillary engorgement and rupture.

The finding of a low hematocrit on bloody fluid aspirated from the respiratory tract led Adamson and associates to suggest that the fluid was a filtrate from pulmonary capillaries and indicative of their engorgement. Presumably, asphyxia may lead to acute left ventricular failure in some infants.

Landing's aforementioned statistical analysis uncovers the fact that pulmonary hemorrhage is found more frequently in association with evidences of acute infection than with any other pulmonary lesion. It has long been contended that hemorrhage constitutes one of the early signs of pneumonia in the newborn. The literature contains many references to this so-called hemorrhagic pneumonia. In a review of 40 infants with cytomegalovirus disease, Smith and colleagues found that 35 per cent had interstitial pneumonia. Several had a hemorrhagic component with recovery of iron-laden macrophages.

Aspiration of maternal blood can surely occur, as proved by the presence of maternal sickle cells in the alveoli but not in the vascular bed of an infant reported by Ceballos.

Evidence of increased intracranial pressure and anoxic brain injury was noted in association with pulmonary hemorrhage by McAdams. Intracranial hemorrhage may coexist with pulmonary hemorrhage.

We have encountered pulmonary hemorrhage, along with hemorrhage from other sites, in *E. coli* sepsis with extensive intravascular thrombosis, and once with intravascular thrombosis without any evidence of sepsis.

Pulmonary hemosiderosis has been reported in newborn infants. In the case report of Livingstone and Boczarow, the term infant was well until 1 week of age, when hypothermia and edema developed. Hemosiderin was identified in macrophages, although no hemoptysis was noted. It is not clear how to relate this infant to the others identified as patients with pulmonary hemorrhage of unknown origin. The infant died at 5 weeks of age of heart failure in association with pulmonary hypertension.

Diagnosis. There is only one characteristic sign that distinguishes pulmonary hemorrhage from other disorders producing dyspnea in the newborn, and it is only present in half the proved cases. This is coughing up or regurgitating material containing blood from the mouth or nose or both. It may be brown and mixed with mucus or may resemble unmixed fresh blood. The infants usually have respiratory distress immediately after birth, but it may be delayed 3 days or more. They may or may not bleed excessively from venipuncture wounds. Physical examination reveals nothing diagnostic. Emphysema or atelectasis or both may be found, and medium to coarse rales are sometimes heard. Roentgenographic changes vary from massive consolidation to minimal streaking or patchy lesions.

Treatment. No therapeutic methods appear to be effective. We have utilized transfusions of citrated blood in several and direct transfusion in one without altering the downhill course of the disorder. The prognosis is extremely grave (The cases cited subsequently are from an earlier era, before ventilators were available.)

CASE 24–1

A full-term white male infant, birth weight 6 pounds 2 ounces (2780 gm), was born with a loop of cord wrapped tightly about his neck. Cry was spontaneous, but dyspnea and cyanosis were noted after respirations had become established. Examination revealed multiple petechiae of the face and tachypnea with retractions but nothing else. Rapid irregular respirations continued, color remained dusky, and the infant frequently coughed up brownish mucoid material. Blood studies were not revealing. An electrocardiogram showed "T wave changes suggestive of myocardial ischemia," but was otherwise normal. The chest radiograph showed infiltration of both upper lobes and hyperaeration of both lower lobes. At 46 hours of age, apnea, cyanosis, and flaccidity developed. The trachea was suctioned, some reddish-brown material was aspirated, and oxygen under positive pressure was given, but the infant died 1 hour later.

Autopsy showed little more than massive hemorrhage throughout the lungs and into air spaces and septa.

Comment. This example was impossible to distinguish from a massive aspiration, with patchy atelectasis and emphysema as sequelae. The one suggestive difference was that brownish material was brought up from the lungs. Is it possible that the tightly wrapped cord about the neck induced increased blood flow through the pulmonary arteries and led to overfilling and rupture of capillaries?

CASE 24–2

A white male infant was born at the Women's Hospital of Maryland after a spontaneous delivery at the thirtieth week of gestation. Pregnancy and labor had been apparently normal in all respects. Amniotic fluid was clear, birth weight was 3 pounds 14 ounces (1760 gm), and crying time was less than 5 minutes. For a short time there was cyanosis of the face and head; respirations were 40 to 50 per minute. In the incubator, with the routine care for premature infants, all went well until the evening of the fourth day. At this time, long periods of apnea began, during which the color became livid then ashen. Examination showed nothing except a tendency to hold the head sharply retracted. Between spells, color was fair while the infant was in oxygen and very dusky when he was taken out. Jaundice had been noted on the fourth day and became intense by the seventh day. On this day he suddenly vomited large amounts of bright red blood mixed with formula and after this became apneic, ashen, and limp. After resuscitation, respirations recommenced but were irregular and gasping, and the heart rate was slow. Endotracheal suction produced blood-stained material. Substernal retractions were noted after this procedure. A transfusion of 15 ml of type O Rh-negative blood was given, and the infant improved briefly. Apneic spells recurred, regurgitation of fresh blood continued, color deteriorated, and he died.

Autopsy showed massive pulmonary hemorrhage and moderate-sized subarachnoid hemorrhage.

Comment. This example seems to fall into an entirely different category from the first one cited. In the first case, the cord wrapped tightly around the neck; in this one, prematurity and deep physiologic icterus were the possibly pathogenic abnormalities. In the first, respiratory difficulty was apparent shortly after birth; in this case, it made its appearance on the fourth day. In the former, the difficulty consisted of dyspnea with retraction; in the latter, the problem was apneic spells. Evidences of massive aspiration were clear-cut in the first case, absent in the second. The only facts of which we can be certain are that the lung may be the site of massive bleeding in the neonatal period for a variety of reasons and that the disorder may manifest itself in a variety of ways.

REFERENCES

Adamson, T. M., Boyd, R. D. H., Normand, I. C. S., et al.: Hemorrhagic pulmonary oedema in the newborn. Lancet 1:494, 1969.

Brodman, R. F., Zavelson, T. M., and Schiebler, G. L.: Treatment of congenital chylothorax. J. Pediatr. 85:516, 1974.

Ceballos, R.: Aspiration of maternal blood in the etiology of massive pulmonary hemorrhage in the newborn infant. J. Pediatr. 72:390, 1968.

Chernick, V., and Reed, M. H.: Pneumothorax and chylothorax in the neonatal period. J. Pediatr. 76:624, 1970.

Cole, V. A., et al.: Pathogenesis of hemorrhagic pulmonary edema and massive pulmonary hemorrhage in the newborn. Pediatrics 51:175, 1973.

Curci, M. R., and Dibbins, A. W.: Bilateral chylothorax in a newborn. J. Pediatr. Surg. 15:663, 1980.

DeSa, D. J., and MacLean, B. S.: An analysis of massive pulmonary hemorrhage in Oxford 1948–68. J. Obstet. Gynaecol. Br. Commonw. 77:158, 1970.

Esterly, J. R., and Oppenheimer, E. H.: Massive pulmonary hemorrhage in the newborn. I. Pathologic considerations. J. Pediatr. 69:3, 1966.

Gershanik, J. J., Jonsson, H. T., Riopel, D. A., et al.: Dietary management of neonatal chylothorax. Pediatrics 53:400, 1974.

Gwinn, J. L.: Radiological case of the month. Chylothorax in the newborn. Am. J. Dis. Child. 115:59, 1968.

Hashim, S., A., Rohott, H. B., Babayan, V. K., et al.: Treatment of chyluria and chylothorax with medium chain triglyceride. N. Engl. J. Med. 270:756, 1964.

Janet, quoted by Sakula (vide infra).

Landing, B. H.: Pulmonary lesions of newborn infants: A statistical study. Pediatrics 19:217, 1957.

Livingstone, C. S., and Boczarow, B.: Idiopathic pulmonary hemosiderosis in a newborn. Arch. Dis. Child. 42:543, 1967.

McAdams, A. J.: Pulmonary hemorrhage in the newborn. Am. J. Dis. Child. 113:255, 1967.

McKendry, J. B., Lindsay, W. K., and Gerstein, M. C.: Congenital defects of the lymphatics in infancy. Pediatrics 19:21, 1957.

Perry, R. E., Hodgman, J., and Cass, A. B.: Pleural effusion in the neonatal period. J. Pediatr. 62:838, 1963.

Randolph, J. G., and Gross, R. E.: Congenital chylothorax, A.M.A. Arch. Surg. 74:405, 1957.

Rothman, P. E.: Intense uterine contractions, with special reference to massive pulmonary hemorrhage of the newborn. West. J. Surg. 65:308, 1957.

Rowe, S., and Avery, M. E.: Massive pulmonary hemorrhage in the newborn. II. Clinical considerations. J. Pediatr. 69:12, 1966.

Sakula, J.: Chylothorax in the newborn. Arch. Dis. Child. 25:340, 1950.

Smith, S. D., Cho, C. T., Brahmacupta, N., and Lenahan, M. F.: Pulmonary involvement with cytomegalovirus infections in children. Arch. Dis. Child. 52:441, 1977.

Stewart, C. A., and Linner, H. P.: Chylothorax in the newborn infant. Am. J. Dis. Child. 31:654, 1926.

Stirlacci, J. R.: Spontaneous chylothorax in a newborn infant. J. Pediatr. 46:581, 1955.

Trompeter, R., Yu, V. Y. H., Aynsley-Green, A., and Roberton, N. R. C.: Massive pulmonary hemorrhage in the newborn infant. Arch. Dis. Child. 50:123, 1975.

Vain, N. E., Swarner, O. W., and Cha, C. C.: Neonatal chylothorax: a report and discussion of nine consecutive cases. J. Pediatr. Surg. 15:261, 1980.

Wessel, M. A.: Chylothorax in a two-week-old infant with spontaneous recovery. J. Pediatr. 25:201, 1944.

25

Mechanical Ventilation

By Ivan D. Frantz III

As knowledge of respiratory physiology of infants has increased along with knowledge of the pathophysiology of their particular disease states our ability to apply techniques of mechanical ventilation successfully has improved. Since more newborn infants are ventilated because of hyaline membrane disease (HMD, or the respiratory distress syndrome, RDS) than for any other cause, this chapter will be devoted particularly to the problems associated with this disease. Modifications for infants with other lung disturbances or with normal lungs will be considered where indicated. Discussion here will be confined to respiration; other aspects of overall management during ventilator care, such as thermal control, fluid and electrolyte balance, and nutrition are discussed elsewhere in this book.

Oxygen Therapy

As in any other form of therapy, mechanical ventilation of infants should increase the rate of survival while reducing risks of complications. In practical terms, this means improvement of oxygenation and elimination of carbon dioxide at the lowest possible concentration of inspired oxygen (F_{IO_2}) and least airway pressure. The initial treatment of any infant with RDS will require administration of oxygen in a concentration adequate to maintain arterial oxygen tension in the range of 50 to 80 torr. During such treatment, F_{IO_2} and P_{O_2} must be measured and recorded. Transcutaneous or capillary estimates may be acceptable, but it should be remembered that neither may be reliable in the first hours of life. When oxygen is administered, it must be both heated and humidified to prevent thermal stress to the infant and drying of the respiratory mucosa.

Continuous Distending Airway Pressure (CDAP)

Since the publication of the observations of Gregory and coworkers in 1971, the early use of continuous distending airway pressure (CDAP) has been widely advocated for the treatment of RDS. Not all agree, however, on what constitutes early. Tanswell and colleagues found that CDAP initiated at a time earlier than 6 hours of life resulted in lower oxygen requirements when this group of infants with RDS was compared with a group for whom CDAP was started after 6 hours of life. Other investigators initiated CDAP as soon as the infant required 40 per cent oxygen, and they also found that elevated F_{IO_2} was needed for shorter periods of time and that there was less need for mechanical ventilation (Gerard et al., 1975; Krouskop et al., 1975). The level of CDAP required by any given infant varies with the severity of his disease and its time course. The optimal level of CDAP has been defined as that amount that is just transmitted to the mediastinum (Fig. 25–1). Tanswell has shown that the amount of pressure administered that results in an increase in esophageal pressure correlates well with an increase in arterial P_{O_2}. The optimal level of distending pressure may be determined by placing the infant on a moderate pressure (4 to 5 cm H_2O) initially and, while observing transcutaneous oxygen level, increasing CDAP by 1 to 2 cm H_2O until an increment in P_{O_2} is seen. Further increases should be avoided, since they may reduce venous return to the heart. As the disease progresses, the amount of pressure needed may increase, and during resolution it will diminish.

The reason for the amelioration of RDS with early CDAP is not entirely understood. Since the alveolar to arterial gradient for oxygen is decreased with CDAP and the oxygen requirement is diminished, it

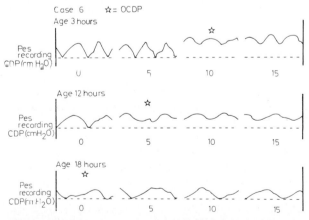

Figure 25–1. In the top tracing of esophageal pressure (recorded at 3 hours of age), optimal CDAP, defined as that level at which pressure is just transmitted to the mediastinum, is 10 cm H_2O. With increasing age (middle and lower tracings) the optimal level of CPAP decreases. (From Tanswell, A. F., et al.: Arch. Dis. Child. 55:33, 1980.)

is possible that there is less oxygen toxicity to the lung. Animal studies by Wyszogrodski and associates have demonstrated that surfactant is conserved by the use of CDAP. It is possible that early CDAP may conserve marginal surfactant stores until full production begins.

CDAP may be administered by a variety of methods. Use of either a negative pressure box around the thorax or a positive pressure box around the head obviates the need for an endotracheal tube, but both methods have proved cumbersome. Administration of positive pressure via nasal prongs or a nasopharyngeal tube seems more satisfactory. In large infants or in those who do not keep their mouths closed, these techniques may also fail, and one may have to resort to endotracheal intubation.

Techniques of Mechanical Ventilation

If apnea ensues, or Pco_2 rises over 55 to 60 torr, or the infant requires over 70 per cent oxygen, mechanical ventilation must be instituted (Stark, 1980). Two principal types of ventilators are available. The volume-limited ventilator has the advantage of delivering the same minute ventilation despite changes in pulmonary compliance. Its disadvantages are its high cost and its complexity and the fact that the preset tidal volume is largely dissipated in circuit compliance and endotracheal tube leak. These disadvantages have led the majority of neonatologists to favor the constant-flow, pressure-limited ventilator, a relatively simple device that allows for easy application of intermittent mandatory ventilation.

Initial ventilator settings can be based on observation of chest wall excursion and auscultation of breath sounds with simultaneous notation of the pressure required in manual ventilation with an anesthesia bag. If transcutaneous oxygen and carbon dioxide monitors are available, appropriate Fi_{O_2}, inspiratory and end-expiratory pressures, and frequency may be quickly chosen. An arbitrary starting point of 25 cm H_2O inspiratory pressure, 5 cm H_2O expiratory pressure, 25 breaths per minute, and the same Fi_{O_2} as that required before will serve in most cases.

Adjustments of ventilator settings are best based on the general principles that changes in mean airway pressure (MAP) will affect oxygenation and changes in minute ventilation will affect Pco_2. Both Reynolds and Boros have shown that Po_2 correlates well with mean airway pressure, regardless of what combination of peak-inspiratory pressure (PIP), positive end-expiratory pressure (PEEP), and inspiratory time (T_I) is chosen to achieve a given level of pressure and regardless of what combination of settings is cho-

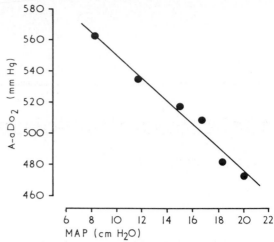

Figure 25–2. Relationship between alveolar and arterial gradient for oxygen and mean airway pressure. (From Herman, S. and Reynolds, E. O. R.: Arch. Dis. Child. *48*:612, 1973.)

sen to achieve a given mean airway pressure (Fig. 25–2). If increased oxygenation is required, the choice of ventilator manipulation may be based on the desired concomitant effect on Pco_2. If Pco_2 should remain unchanged, mean airway pressure should be increased without affecting minute ventilation (Fig. 25–3). This may be accomplished by increasing T_I and shortening expiratory time (T_E) so that rate is unchanged. T_I should not be prolonged over 1.5 sec in order to avoid compromising cardiac output. If overventilation requires increase of Pco_2 while increasing mean airway pressure, positive end-expiratory pressure should be increased. The decrease in minute ventilation will result from a decrease in tidal volume (Fig. 25–4). Alternatively, an increase in both mean airway pressure and ventilation can be achieved by increasing inspiratory pressure (Fig. 25–4).

Muscle relaxants are useful adjuncts to the mechanical ventilation of severely diseased infants. Without them, the infant's own respiratory efforts, when out of phase with the ventilator, may increase transpulmonary pressures (Stark, 1979) and thus the risk of pneumothorax and the "barotrauma" leading to bronchopulmonary dysplasia (Pollitzer et al., 1981). Several investigators have noted improvement in oxygenation with their use (Crone and Favorito, 1980; Finer and Tomney, 1981). Finer also observed fewer periods of increased intracranial pressure during muscle relaxation. We administer muscle relaxants (pancuronium bromide, 0.1 mg/kg/dose) to infants who require ventilator pressures of greater than 30 cm H_2O.

Some clinicians have attempted to minimize peak airway pressure by using respirator rates that are more rapid than the standard ones. With rates of 60 or more breaths per minute, Heicher and others reported adequate gas exchange with a lower occurrence of pneumothorax and maintenance of the relationship of oxygenation to mean airway pressure.

Ventilation with an oscillator ventilator can be

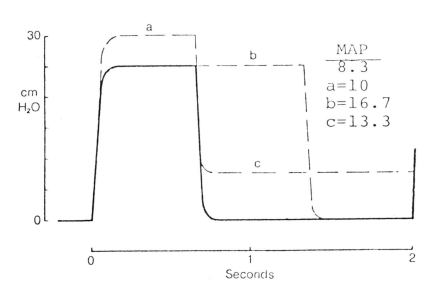

Figure 25–3. Effects of changes in ventilator settings on mean airway pressure. The solid line (P_I = 25 cm H_2O, CDAP = 0 cm H_2O, T_I = 0.75 sec, T_E = 1.25 sec) results in a MAP of 8.3 cm H_2O. Increasing P_I to 30 cm H_2O (curve a) increases MAP to 10 cm H_2O and also increases ventilation. Doubling T_I (curve b) increases MAP to 16.7 cm H_2O, with no effect on ventilation. Adding CDAP (curve c) results in a MAP of 13.3 cm H_2O, with a decrease in ventilation. (Modified from Reynolds, E. O. R. *In* Keuskamp, D. H. G. (Ed.): Neonatal and Pediatric Ventilation. Boston, Little, Brown and Company, 1974.)

achieved at much higher frequencies (up to 1800/min) with tidal volumes less than that of the dead space and lower mean airway pressures than those obtained with conventional ventilators. This new approach to enhancing gas exchange by increased turbulence in the airways is useful in conditions such as interstitial emphysema. Its ultimate role in neonatal respiratory care awaits further study. (Frantz et al., 1980, 1981; Marchak et al., 1982).

Chest physiotherapy is sometimes an important adjunct to mechanical ventilation (Fox et al., 1978). The frequency of physiotherapy, including saline instillation, sighing, chest vibration, and suctioning, should vary with the needs and tolerance of the in-

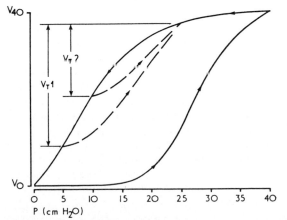

Figure 25–4. Pressure volume curve of the lungs demonstrating the effect of increasing CPAP on tidal volume. As CPAP is increased from 5 to 10 cm H_2O, there is a major decrease in tidal volume (V_t). Increasing peak inspiratory pressure by 5 cm H_2O does not fully compensate for this because of the flat nature of the pressure volume curve at higher pressure and volume. (From Herman, S., and Reynolds, E. O. R.: Arch. Dis. Child. *48*:612, 1973.)

fant. Physiotherapy may be important in preventing the lobar collapse that is frequently seen postextubation (Finer and Boyd, 1978).

Weaning from the Ventilator

As the infant's condition improves, the process of weaning begins. Since high peak inspiratory pressure and high oxygen concentration appear to be the factors most harmful to the lung, these should be decreased first. After pressure has been lowered to 25 to 30 cm H_2O and F_{IO_2} to 40 per cent, the rate may be lowered. If a ventilator with the capability for intermittent mandatory ventilation is used, the process of weaning becomes greatly simplified because, as rate is lowered, the infant is able to increase the amount of ventilation supplied by his own efforts. During weaning, the infant's requirement for PEEP is diminishing, and this should be gradually decreased to 2 to 3 cm H_2O. Ultimately, the rate can be decreased to the point at which the infant is breathing entirely on his own, with 2 to 3 cm H_2O CDAP. When the infant has tolerated this condition for several hours, he may be extubated. It is not desirable to bring the child to 0 cm H_2O CDAP because this results in a decrease in functional residual capacity below normal and a fall in oxygenation (Fox et al., 1977). It appears that the extubated infant uses his glottis to supply the equivalent of 2 to 3 cm H_2O "natural" CDAP. Following extubation, the infant should be placed in an ambient F_{IO_2} 5 to 10 per cent higher than that maintained with CDAP. When the infant is stable in less than 40 per cent oxygen, the arterial catheter may be removed, and transcutaneous and capillary sampling may be used for blood gas measurements. The weaning process may occasionally

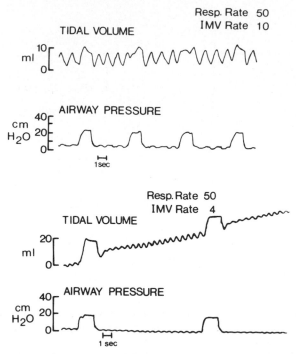

Figure 25–5. On the top half of the figure, the infant's own respiratory rate is 50 breaths/min, whereas the intermittent mandatory ventilation (IMV) rate is 10 breaths/min. Note that the infant's spontaneous breaths are similar in size to those of the respirator (which correspond to the large excursions of airway pressure); thus, the infant provides a large fraction of his own ventilation. In the lower half of the illustration, the infant's spontaneous breaths are much smaller than those of the ventilator and provide only about one third of the total ventilation.

fail, owing to underestimation of the proportion of the total ventilation supplied by the respirator. Even at very low rates (5 to 8 breaths per minute), the respirator may be providing half the ventilation of an infant whose own breaths are ineffectual (Fig. 25–5). In other cases, postextubation atelectasis may necessitate reintubation for lung expansion and physiotherapy.

Complications

Any infant who suddenly deteriorates during mechanical ventilation should be carefully examined for a dislodged or blocked endotracheal tube or pneumothorax. Endotracheal tube position can best be assessed through direct visualization with a laryngoscope, and a blocked tube can be diagnosed by attempting to pass a suction catheter through it. Retrospective surveys of infants ventilated for RDS have indicated a 20 to 25 per cent incidence of pneumothorax (Madansky et al., 1979). Transillumination of the chest with a high-intensity light provides instant confirmation of pneumothorax, which should be fol-

lowed by rapid treatment. The pneumothorax may be temporarily relieved by either inserting a scalp vein needle and aspirating with a syringe and stopcock or placing the end of the tubing under water while preparations for chest tube placement are being made.

The major chronic pulmonary complication attributed to treatment of RDS is bronchopulmonary dysplasia. Bronchopulmonary dysplasia, thought to be related at least in part to high respirator pressure and inspired oxygen, occurs in 10 to 15 per cent of ventilated infants (Taghizadeh and Reynolds, 1976). Its relationship to such entities as Wilson-Mikity syndrome and chronic pulmonary insufficiency of prematurity, both of which occur in infants who have had no underlying lung disease or ventilator treatment, is unclear. Efforts to lower both peak inspiratory pressure and inspired oxygen concentration have met with some success in decreasing the incidence of bronchopulmonary dysplasia. Although initially promising, administration of vitamin E, an antioxidant, has not proved efficacious (Ehrenkranz et al., 1979).

Considerations in Infants with Disorders Other Than RDS

Infants who require mechanical ventilation for problems other than RDS require special consideration. Those with neuromuscular disorders or congenital heart disease but relatively normal lungs require lower peak-inspiratory and end-expiratory pressures. An end-expiratory pressure that is too high may impede cardiac output, and an inspiratory pressure that is too great may result in pneumothorax. In meconium aspiration syndrome, airway obstruction plays an important part in the pathophysiology of the disease (Vidyasagar et al., 1975). Meconium may be cleared from large airways by suctioning in the delivery room. Migration of meconium to smaller airways may cause either partial or complete obstruction. Partial obstruction predisposes the infant to pneumothorax because a check-valve phenomenon may occur, with air trapping on expiration. Atelectasis may occur with complete obstruction and predispose the newborn to pneumothorax because of overexpansion of relatively normal areas. Inspiratory pressure, PEEP, and inspiratory time should all be kept to a minimum because of the possibility of pneumothorax. Infants with congenital pneumonia generally have more compliant lungs than those with RDS and thus will require less pressure. They may also be predisposed to pneumothorax because of uneven aeration.

REFERENCES

Boros, S. J.: Variations in inspiratory:expiratory ratio and airway pressure wave form during mechanical ventilation: The significance of mean airway pressure. J. Pediatr. *94*:114, 1979.

Crone, R. K., and Favorito, J.: The effects of pancuronium bromide on infants with hyaline membrane disease. J. Pediatr. *97*:991, 1980.

Ehrenkranz, R. A., Ablow, R. C., and Warshaw, J. B.: Prevention of bronchopulmonary dysplasia with vitamin E administration during the acute stages of respiratory distress syndrome. J. Pediatr. *95*.873, 1979.

Finer, N. N., and Boyd, J.: Chest physiotherapy in the neonate: a controlled study. Pediatrics *61*:282, 1978.

Finer, N. N., and Tomney, P. M.: Controlled evaluation of muscle relaxation in the ventilated neonate. Pediatrics *67*:641, 1981.

Fox, W. W., Berman, L. S., Dinwiddie, R., and Shaffer, T. H.: Tracheal extubation of the neonate at 2 to 3 cm H_2O continuous positive airway pressure. Pediatrics *59*:257, 1977.

Fox, W. W., Schwartz, J. G., and Shaffer, T. H.: Pulmonary physiotherapy in neonates: physiologic changes and respiratory management. J. Pediatr. *92*:977, 1978.

Frantz, I. D., Stark, A. R., and Dorkin, H. L.: Ventilation of infants at frequencies up to 1800/min. Pediatr. Res. *14*:642, 1980.

Frantz, I. D., Stark, A. R., and Werthammer, J. W.: Improvement in pulmonary interstitial emphysema with high frequency ventilation. Pediatr. Res. *15*:719, 1981.

Gerard, P., Fox, W. W., Outerbridge, E. W., Beaudry, P. H., and Stern, L.: Early versus late introduction of continuous negative pressure in the management of idiopathic respiratory distress syndrome. J. Pediatr. *87*:591, 1975.

Gregory, G. A., Gooding, C. A., Phibbs, R. H., et al.: Treatment of the idiopathic respiratory distress syndrome with continuous positive airway pressure. N. Engl. J. Med. *284*:1333, 1971.

Heicher, D. A., Kasting, D. S., and Harrod, J. R.: Prospective clinical comparison of two methods for mechanical ventilation of neonates: rapid rate and short inspiratory time versus slow rate and long inspiratory time. J. Pediatr. *98*:957, 1981.

Herman, S., and Reynolds, E. O. R.: Methods for improving oxygenation in infants mechanically ventilated for severe hyaline membrane disease. Arch. Dis. Child. *48*:612, 1973.

Krouskop, R. W., Brown, E. G., and Sweet, A. Y.: The early use of continuous positive airway pressure in the treatment of idiopathic respiratory distress syndrome. J. Pediatr. *87*:263, 1975.

Madansky, D. L., Lawson, E. E., Chernick, V., and Taeusch, H. W.: Pneumothorax and other forms of pulmonary air leak in newborns. Am. Rev. Resp. Dis. *120*:729, 1979.

Marchak, B. E., Thompson, W. K., Duffty, P., Miyaki, T., Bryan, M. II., Bryan, A. C., and Froese, A. B.: Treatment of RDS by high frequency oscillatory ventilation: a preliminary report. J. Pediatr. *99*:287, 1981.

Muller, N., Gulston, G., Cade, D., Whitton, J., Froese, A. B., Bryan, M. H., and Bryan, A. C.: Diaphragmatic muscle fatigue in the newborn. J. Appl. Physiol. *46*:688, 1979.

Pollitzer, M. J., Reynolds, E. O. R., Shaw, D. G., and Thomas R. M.: Pancuronium during mechanical ventilation speeds recovery of lungs of infants with hyaline membrane disease. Lancet *1*:346, 1981.

Reynolds, E.O.R.: Pressure waveform and ventilator settings for mechanical ventilation in severe hyaline membrane disease. *In* Keuskamp, D. H. G. (Ed.): Neonatal and Pediatric Ventilation. Boston, Little, Brown and Company, 1974, pp. 259–280.

Stark, A. R.: Hyaline membrane disease. *In* Cloherty, J. P., and Stark, A. R. (Eds.): Manual of Neonatal Care. Boston, Little, Brown and Company, 1980, pp. 131–138.

Stark, A. R., Bascom, R., and Frantz, I. D.: Muscle relaxation in mechanically ventilated infants. J. Pediatr. *94*:439, 1979.

Taghizadeh, A., and Reynolds, E. O. R.: Pathogenesis of bronchopulmonary dysplasia following hyaline membrane disease. Am. J. Pathol. *82*:241, 1976.

Tanswell, A. K., Clubb, R. A., Smith, B. T., and Boston, R. W.: Individualised continuous distending pressure applied within 6 hours of delivery in infants with respiratory distress syndrome. Arch. Dis. Child. *55*:33, 1980.

Vidyasagar, D., Yeh, T. F., Harris, V., and Pildes, R. S.: Assisted ventilation in infant with meconium aspiration syndrome. Pediatrics *56*:208, 1975.

Wyszogrodski, I, Kyei-Aboagye, K., Taeusch, H. W., and Avery, M. E.: Surfactant inactivation by hyperventilation: Conservation by end-expiratory pressure. J. Appl. Physiol. *38*:461, 1975.

PART 4 DISORDERS OF THE CARDIOVASCULAR SYSTEM

26

General Considerations

By Michael D. Freed

Introduction

Much progress has been made in the diagnosis and treatment of neonatal cardiac conditions. A better understanding of the physiology of the neonate as well as technical improvements in angiography, echocardiography, and radionuclide imaging have allowed for a more complete diagnosis to be made without undue risk. Advances in cardiovascular surgery in the neonate, especially the introduction of deep hypothermia (20°C) with circulatory arrest, have permitted total correction of some forms of congenital heart disease (e.g., ventricular septal defect, tetralogy of Fallot, and transposition of the great arteries) during the neonatal period in some centers. Even repair of one of the most complex cardiac conditions, aortic and mitral valve atresia with a hypoplastic left ventricle, has yielded to a physiologic correction (Norwood et al., 1983).

Despite this evidence of progress, at present more than 50 per cent of children who present with critical congenital heart disease in the first month of life are dead before their first birthday (Fyler et al., 1980).

Neonates with critical heart disease rarely get better on their own and frequently deteriorate over a short period of time. Much of the recent progress results from more prompt recognition and referral to major centers with staffs skilled in cardiology and cardiovascular surgery. The chapters that follow are an attempt to describe the "state-of-the-art" early in 1983. The certainty that these chapters will be outdated within a few years remains one of the most exciting aspects of neonatal cardiology.

The Fetal Circulation

Although some research has been done with human fetuses (Lind and Wegelius, 1954; Lind et al., 1964), most of our understanding of the in utero circulation is from work on fetal lambs (Dawes, 1968; Rudolph, 1970; Heymann and Rudolph, 1972; Rudolph, 1974).

The fetal circulation is arranged in parallel rather than in series, with mixing between the streams at the atrial and great vessel level (Fig. 26–1). These adaptations allowing diversion of blood from the immature lungs to the placenta for oxygen exchange permit fetal survival with a variety of cardiac lesions.

Normally, blood returning from the placenta passes either into the portal system of the liver and then into the inferior vena cava (IVC) or into the ductus venosus and inferior vena cava directly. In the right atrium, the IVC blood is diverted into two streams by the crista dividens. The smaller stream is diverted across the foramen ovale into the left atrium, where it mixes with pulmonary venous return and

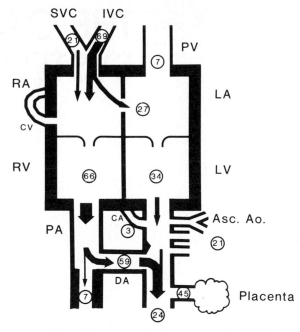

Figure 26–1. The course of the circulation in the late gestation fetal lamb. The numbers within the circles represent percentage of combined ventricular output. Some of the return from the inferior vena cava (IVC) is diverted by the crista dividens in the right atrium (RA) through the foramen ovale into the left atrium (LA), where it meets the pulmonary venous (PV) return and passes into the left ventricle (LV) and is pumped into the ascending aorta (Asc Ao). Most of the aortic flow goes to the coronary artery (CA) and subclavian and carotid arteries with only 10 per cent of combined ventricular output passing through the aortic arch into the descending aorta. The remainder of the inferior vena cava flow mixes with return from the superior vena cava (SVC) and coronary veins (CV) and passes into the right atrium and right ventricle (RV) and is pumped into the pulmonary artery (PA). Because of the high pulmonary resistance, only 7 per cent passes into the lungs, with the rest going into the ductus arteriosus (DA) and then to the descending aorta to the placenta and lower half of the body. (Modified from Rudolph, A. M.: Congenital Disease of the Heart. Chicago, Year Book Medical Publishers, Inc., 1974.)

passes through the mitral valve into the left ventricle. This blood is pumped out into the ascending aorta, where it supplies the coronary, carotid, and subclavian arteries with only 10 per cent of combined ventricular output passing through the aortic arch into the descending aorta.

The majority of blood from the IVC is diverted into the right atrium, where it joins the superior vena caval (SVC) drainage and coronary sinus return before passing through the tricuspid valve into the right ventricle and pulmonary artery. Since the fluid-filled lungs and constricted pulmonary arterioles offer a high resistance to flow, most of the blood in the main pulmonary artery goes through the ductus arteriosus into the low-resistance descending aorta and placenta.

The oxygen content of blood in the fetus is considerably lower than that in the neonate or child (Fig. 26–2). Since the placenta is the organ of oxygen exchange, umbilical venous blood has the highest Po_2 (32 to 35 torr, oxygen saturation 70 per cent, with the mother breathing room air). The blood destined for the left side of the heart mixes with the less saturated inferior vena caval and pulmonary venous return, lowering the Po_2 to about 26 to 28 torr (oxygen saturation about 65 per cent) before passing into the left ventricle and ascending aorta.

The umbilical venous return destined for the right

ventricle mixes with the SVC return (Po_2 12 to 14 torr, oxygen saturation 40 per cent), reducing the oxygen in the blood destined to go to the right ventricle, pulmonary artery, descending aorta, and placenta to 20 to 22 torr (oxygen saturation 50 to 55 per cent). Thus, the blood with the highest oxygen content is diverted to the coronary arteries and brain, and that with the lowest oxygen content is diverted to the placenta. An additional fetal adaptation to oxygen transport at low oxygen saturation is the presence of high levels of fetal hemoglobin, which has a high oxygen affinity and, consequently, a low P 50 (partial pressure of oxygen at 50 per cent hemoglobin saturation) of approximately 18 or 19 torr. This leftward shift of the oxygen dissociation curve facilitates oxygen uptake at the placenta.

The wide communication between the atria allows for equalization of pressures in the atrium; similarly, the patency of the ductus arteriosus results in equalization of pressures in the aorta and pulmonary artery.

Since atrial and great vessel pressures are equal on both sides of the heart, in the absence of pulmonary or aortic stenosis the ventricular pressures are also equal, with the systolic pressure about 70 mm Hg and the amniotic pressure considered zero.

Fetal hemodynamics have significant consequences in the neonate with congenital heart disease:

1. The parallel circulation with connections at the atrial and great vessel level allows a wide variety of structural cardiac problems to occur while still normally transporting blood to the placenta and fetal organs for gas exchange.

2. The right ventricle does approximately two thirds of the cardiac work before birth. This is reflected in the size and thickness of the right ventricle before and after birth and may explain why left-sided heart defects are tolerated more poorly after birth than are right-sided lesions.

3. The normal flow across the preductal aortic arch is small (10 per cent of CVO), particularly when compared with the flow across the ductus arteriosus (60 per cent of CVO), with most of the descending aortic flow derived from the pulmonary artery. This makes the aortic isthmus especially vulnerable to small changes in blood flow and may explain the high incidence of coarctation of the aorta and interruption in this region in association with other congenital cardiac lesions.

4. Since pulmonary blood flow in utero accounts for a small proportion of the necessary flow after birth, anomalies that prevent normal pulmonary venous return (such as total anomalous pulmonary venous return or mitral stenosis) may be masked in utero when pulmonary venous return is minimal.

5. The low levels of circulating oxygen before birth (Po_2 26 to 28 torr in the ascending aorta and Po_2 20 to 22 torr in the descending aorta) may account

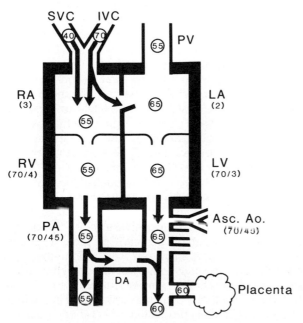

Figure 26–2. The oxygen saturation (represented by the encircled numbers) and pressures (shown in parentheses) in the late gestation fetal lamb. The oxygen saturation is the highest in the inferior vena cava, representing flow that is primarily from the placenta. The saturation of the blood in the heart is slightly higher on the left side than on the right side. Since large communications between the atrium and great vessels are present, the pressures on both sides of the heart are virtually identical. The abbreviations in this diagram are the same as those in Figure 26–1. (Modified from Rudolph, A. M.: Congenital Disease of the Heart. Chicago, Year Book Medical Publishers, Inc., 1974.)

for the relative postnatal comfort of infants with cyanotic congenital heart disease, who may be quite active and feed well with an arterial P_{O_2} of 25, a level that would lead to cerebral and cardiac anoxia, acidosis, and death within a few minutes in the older child or adult.

Transitional Circulation

Soon after the neonate begins to breathe air, the low-resistance placenta is removed from the circulation, and systemic resistance increases. At the same time, the onset of air breathing expands the lung and brings oxygen to the pulmonary alveoli. Although some drop in pulmonary resistance can be explained by simple physical expansion, most of this decrease results from chemoreflex vasodilatation of the pulmonary arteries, which is caused by the high level of oxygen in the alveolar gas.

Both the increase in systemic vascular resistance due to clamping of the umbilical cord and the approximately 80 per cent drop in pulmonary vascular

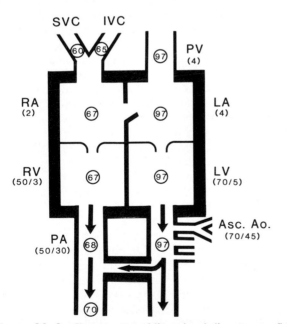

Figure 26–3. The course of the circulation soon after birth. The numbers within the circles represent oxygen saturation in per cent, and the numbers within the parentheses signify pressures in mm Hg. The circulation is now arranged in series rather than in parallel with blood traversing the right side of the heart to get to the lungs for oxygenation and then the left side of the heart for delivery to the body. There is still minimal shunting from aorta to pulmonary artery through the constricting ductus arteriosus. The right-sided pressures have dropped below left-sided pressures and will drop further over the next 48 hours of life. The abbreviations in this diagram are the same as those used in Figure 26–1. (Modified from Rudolph, A. M.: Congenital Disease of the Heart. Chicago, Year Book Medical Publishers, Inc., 1974.)

resistance that occurs with the onset of respiration cause increased pulmonary flow and decreased ductal flow. Before birth, the relative pulmonary and systemic resistances cause 90 per cent of right ventricular blood to go through the ductus to the descending aorta; by a few minutes after birth, 90 per cent goes to the pulmonary arteries.

The rapid drop in systemic venous return to the IVC as the umbilical venous flow is cut off and the increase in pulmonary venous return as the pulmonary blood flow increases cause the left atrial pressure to increase and exceed right atrial pressure, resulting in apposition of the valve of the foramen ovale against the edge of the crista dividens with functional closure of the foramen ovale. Thus, within moments, the pulmonary and systemic circulations have changed from a parallel to a series arrangement (Fig. 26–3).

The ductus arteriosus usually remains patent for several hours or days after birth. Initially, the pulmonary vascular resistance may exceed systemic, resulting in a small right-to-left (pulmonary artery-to-aorta) shunt with some systemic desaturation in the lower half of the body (Fig. 26–4). Anything that increases pulmonary vascular resistance or prevents postnatal decrease in it (e.g., acidosis, hypoxemia, polycythemia, lung disease, or cesarean section) may exacerbate or prolong this normally transient right-to-left shunt.

Within a few hours of life, the pulmonary vascular resistance normally falls lower than systemic resistance, resulting in a small "physiologic" left-to-right (aorta-to-pulmonary artery) shunt. Normally, within 10 to 15 hours after birth, the ductus arteriosus closes, although permanent structural closure may not take place for another 2 to 3 weeks. The mechanism of ductal closure is still not completely understood, although it has been clear for some time that oxygen plays a role. Prostaglandins of the E series seem to be responsible for maintaining patency of the ductus arteriosus during fetal life (Coceani and Olley, 1973). It has been possible to keep the ductus open for days or weeks in infants with congenital heart disease by infusion of exogenous PGE_1 or PGE_2 (Freed et al., 1981), and it has been possible to close the ductus arteriosus in about 80 per cent of preterm infants weighing less than 1750 gm with indomethacin, a nonselective prostaglandin-synthesis inhibitor. It remains unclear whether normal ductal closure is due to reduced synthesis or increased removal in the lung of E prostaglandins, production of another prostanoic acid (possibly thromboxane) with constrictor properties, or a lack of local responsiveness of all prostaglandin receptors that is due to an increase in oxygen with active ductal constriction (Coceani and Olley, 1980).

Although some hypoxemia is present soon after birth, the normal arterial P_{O_2} gradually increases (P_{O_2} 50 at 10 minutes, 62 at 1 hour, and 75 to 83 between 3 hours and 2 days) over the first hours of life, with continued pulmonary vasodilatation and improved ventilation-perfusion ratios. In addition, the pulmo-

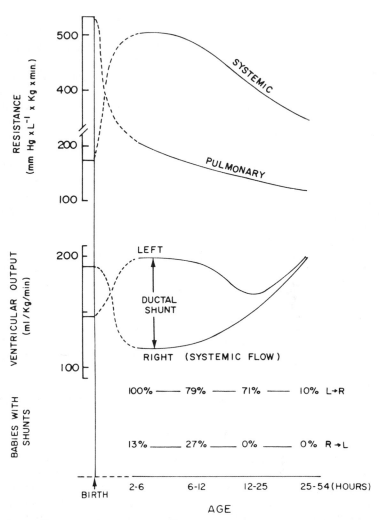

Figure 26–4. Hemodynamics of the cardio-respiratory conversion in the newborn. The pulmonary and systemic vascular resistance are shown on top, the ventricular outputs in the middle, and the percentage of babies with left-to-right and right-to-left shunts in the bottom panel. Before birth, the pulmonary resistance exceeds the systemic resistance, so shunting through the ductus is from the right side of the heart (pulmonary artery) to the left side of the heart (aorta).

Soon after birth, the pulmonary resistance falls secondary to arteriolar vasodilatation, and the systemic resistance increases as the low resistance placenta is excluded from the systemic circulation. When the systemic resistance exceeds pulmonary resistance within a few moments of birth, shunting through the ductus reverses, going from the higher resistance aorta (left) to the lower resistance pulmonary artery (right). By 12 to 24 hours of age, the ductus has closed. Anything that increases pulmonary resistance (e.g., hypoxemia, acidosis, or hypoglycemia) will cause the right-to-left shunt to persist or temporarily reduce left-to-right shunting. (From Nelson, N. M.: Respiration and circulation after birth. *In* Smith, C. A., and Nelson, N. M.: The Physiology of the Newborn Infant. 4th ed. Springfield Ill., Charles C Thomas, Publisher, 1976. Reproduced with permission.)

nary pressure gradually falls to about 30 torr systolic within about 48 hours (Emmanouilides et al., 1964). Although the pulmonary vascular resistance will continue to decrease for several weeks, the transition to the adult circulation is virtually complete by 2 days of age.

Evaluation of the Cardiovascular System in the Neonate

History. The age at which symptoms or murmurs presented may be helpful; for example, heart failure at birth suggests an intrauterine arrhythmia such as supraventricular tachycardia, or an arteriovenous fistula. Murmurs of semilunar valve obstruction or atrioventricular regurgitation are usually present soon after birth, whereas the murmur of a ventricular septal defect or patent ductus arteriosus is usually not audible until later, since the magnitude of the left-to-right shunt depends on the decline in pulmonary vascular resistance over the first days and weeks of life.

A good feeding history is essential. Neonates with congestive heart failure may tire with feeding and be able to ingest only 1 or 2 ounces before becoming exhausted and falling asleep. These infants remain quite hungry and irritable and frequently exhibit poor weight gain, partly because their caloric intake is reduced.

Infants with congestive failure are often tachypneic and dyspneic. Parents or nurses may report rapid respiratory rates that occur while the infant is sleeping or subcostal and intercostal retractions. Excessive perspiration, most obvious on the head while the infant is feeding, is another sign of congestive failure.

The history should include questions regarding cyanosis. Acrocyanosis of the hands and feet, a benign manifestation of increased extraction of oxygen in the peripheral capillary beds, can be quite marked in the first few days or weeks of life. It is usually most noticeable when the extremities are cold and improves or disappears with warming. True cyanosis of the mucous membranes beyond 2 to 3 hours of age is abnormal. It is highly suggestive of (but does not necessarily prove the existence of) pulmonary, central nervous system, and congenital heart disease (see further on). A history of illnesses during pregnancy should be obtained whenever possible because of the association of congenital heart disease with maternal diabetes, congenital heart block with maternal lupus erythematosus, and patent ductus arteriosus with maternal rubella during the first trimester. Finally, a careful family history is important because the recurrence rate for congenital heart disease is higher in affected families.

Physical Examination. A thorough physical examination of the neonate begins with observation. The chromosomal anomalies and such syndromes as Holt-Oram and Williams have obvious stigmata and are associated with heart disease in a large number of cases.

The vital signs should be checked, preferably with the infant resting or asleep. Heart rates above 160 to 180 beats/minute may be seen with agitation but may also indicate congestive failure or a tachyarrhythmia. Bradycardia may be normal as a manifestation of increased vagal tone but may be due to complete heart block. A respiratory rate of greater than 60 per minute in the neonatal period and more than 45 thereafter is probably abnormal. While there are many causes, most of them pulmonary, congenital heart disease must be considered.

The blood pressure in both arms and a leg should be taken in all neonates suspected of having congenital heart disease. We have found the Doppler to be an excellent method for measuring blood pressures in neonates, although palpation can also be used successfully. The flush method is probably outdated. One must be sure to use a large cuff (preferably the 2-inch size), placing it over the forearm if the upper arm is too small. In coarctation of the aorta, the blood pressure is increased in both arms compared with that in the legs, although the left arm pressure may be low if the coarctation involves the origin of the left subclavian, and the right arm may be low if the right subclavian arises anomalously below the coarctation.

The infant should be weighed and measured. Normally, the neonate loses 5 to 10 per cent of his birth weight in the first few days of life but regains birth weight by 7 to 10 days. Thereafter, he should gain about 28 gm (1 oz) every day for the remainder of the first month. Infants who have not gained 350 to 450 gm (12 to 16 ounces) by the end of the first month are failing to thrive.

The color of the skin and mucous membranes should then be evaluated, and evidence of acrocyanosis or true cyanosis should be recorded. Occasionally, the lower body is more cyanotic than the upper (differential cyanosis), which suggests right-to-left shunting of venous blood through the ductus arteriosus. This finding may be present in coarctation of the aorta, interrupted aortic arch, or the persistent fetal circulation syndrome but may be normal in the first hours of life.

Observation of the thorax can sometimes reveal anomalies in the neonate. Occasionally, the heart is hyperactive and the cardiac impulse is visible on the left side of the chest. Subcostal or intercostal retractions suggest respiratory distress. The precordium should then be palpated. Volume overload lesions such as a ventricular septal defect, atrioventricular valve regurgitation, and arteriovenous fistula will give a tapping or even rocking impulse. Rarely, stenosis of a semilunar valve, regurgitation of an atrioventricular valve, or a large left-to-right shunt through a ventricular septal defect or patent ductus arteriosus will cause a thrill.

Auscultation remains the most important part of the examination of the neonate but is in danger of being neglected with the advent of more complicated technical tools. The first heart sound (S_1) is loudest at the apex. It represents mitral and tricuspid closure and is narrowly split (phonocardiographically) but is usually heard as a single sound. A split S_1 suggests delayed tricuspid closure and is occasionally present in Ebstein's anomaly. An accentuated S_1 suggests an atrial septal defect, or a short P–R interval; a diminished S_1 suggests a prolonged P–R interval, or congestive heart failure.

The second heart sound (S_2), heard best at the left upper sternal border, has two components representing aortic and pulmonic valve closure. Normally, S_2 is split during inspiration (when increased right heart volume delays right ventricular ejection) and single during expiration. The rapid heart rates make appreciation of the splitting difficult, which is unfortunate because it is one of the most helpful signs in the clinical evaluation of the neonate. Wide splitting of S_2 is seen with an atrial septal defect or anomalous pulmonary venous return or when there is a delay in right ventricular ejection because of either a conduction delay (e.g., right bundle-branch block) or an obstruction to right ventricular ejection (e.g., pulmonic stenosis).

The pulmonary component of S_2 is loud in the presence of pulmonary hypertension and soft or inaudible in the presence of pulmonic stenosis, either isolated or in association with a ventricular septal defect, single ventricle, or tricuspid atresia. Obviously, S_2 is single in the presence of pulmonary or aortic atresia.

Third and fourth heart sounds (S_3 and S_4) are infrequently heard. They may be present in infants with congestive cardiac failure, but the rapid heart rates associated with failure make appreciation on auscultation difficult.

Systolic ejection clicks, early in systole, result from dilatation of the great vessels. Aortic ejection clicks, constant through the respiratory cycle and loudest at the apex, are usually found in association with valvular aortic stenosis. Variable ejection clicks are soft or inaudible during inspiration and loudest along the left sternal border, and they are noted in association with pulmonary valve stenosis.

Heart murmurs may be audible during systole or diastole or may be continuous. A systolic murmur is classified as either an ejection or a regurgitant type.

Ejection murmurs are caused by turbulence of blood as it leaves the heart through a narrowed orifice. The murmur is crescendo-decrescendo, or diamond-shaped, and begins a fraction of a second after S_1, the delay caused by the isovolumic contraction phase between closing of the atrioventricular valves and opening of the semilunar valves. Ejection murmurs are characteristic of aortic or pulmonic valve, or subvalvular, stenosis.

Regurgitant murmurs are pansystolic; that is, they start with S_1 and last until S_2. Regurgitant murmurs are even in intensity through systole and are characteristic of atrioventricular valve regurgitation (either mitral or tricuspid) or a ventricular septal defect. The presence of a regurgitant murmur in the first day or two of life suggests A-V valve regurgitation, since the normal elevation of pulmonary vascular resistance usually prevents the murmurs of a ventricular defect from being audible until later in the first week of life.

Diastolic murmurs may represent regurgitation through one of the semilunar valves or stenosis across an atrioventricular valve. Murmurs of aortic or pulmonary regurgitation tend to occur early in diastole and are uncommon in neonates. Infants with tetralogy of Fallot with an absent pulmonary valve, however, may have loud systolic and low-pitched diastolic murmurs generated by stenosis and regurgitation at the pulmonary valve annulus. Mid- and late-diastolic murmurs usually represent murmurs across one of the atrioventricular valves. Occasionally, these are due to anatomic narrowing, either mitral or tricuspid stenosis, but they more frequently result from relative stenosis from a large flow across a structurally normal valve. For example, a large left-to-right shunt through a ventricular septal defect often causes a mid-diastolic mitral flow rumble at the apex, and total anomalous pulmonary venous return without pulmonary venous obstruction is likely to cause a tricuspid flow rumble along the left sternal border.

Continuous murmurs heard throughout systole and diastole result from flow between a high pressure vessel and a low pressure vessel throughout the cardiac cycle, usually the aorta and pulmonary artery with a patent ductus arteriosus. Occasionally, an arteriovenous fistula may cause a continuous murmur over the head or liver. A continuous murmur in a cyanotic neonate in the first week of life is almost always due to collateral vessels from aorta to pulmonary artery in infants with a ventricular septal defect and pulmonary atresia.

The liver is usually palpable 3 cm (at most) below the costal margin in the right midclavicular line. It may be larger in cases of congestive heart failure, hemolytic disease, and a variety of liver diseases, and it may be downwardly displaced without hepatomeg-

aly with hyperexpansion of the lung. A midline or left-sided liver suggests the heterotaxy syndrome.

Peripheral edema is rarely due to heart disease, but it may be seen during the early postnatal period in infants with in utero supraventricular tachycardia.

Finally, the peripheral pulses should be evaluated. Asymmetric pulses between the arm and legs suggest coarctation of the aorta or interrupted aortic arch with a closing ductus arteriosus. Symmetrically decreased pulses suggest congestive heart failure or cardiogenic shock. Increased pulses are present when there is a diastolic "run-off" from the aorta seen in patent ductus arteriosus, aorticopulmonary window—truncus arteriosus, and arteriovenous fistula.

Electrocardiography. Although most of the methods used in the cardiac evaluation of the neonate are helpful in assessing the child's current status, electrocardiography in great part reflects the abnormal hemodynamic burdens placed on the heart in utero For example, in the normal fetus the right ventricle does most of the cardiac work before birth; therefore, the presence of left ventricular hypertrophy on the electrocardiogram in a newborn suggests either the increased left ventricular work in utero that is seen with aortic stenosis or the decreased right ventricular work in utero that appears with tricuspid atresia and a hypoplastic right ventricle.

Some electrocardiographic patterns are virtually diagnostic of specific cardiac lesions; these will be discussed in more detail in Chapters 27 and 28.

Electrocardiography can be used to assess severity of disease by determining the degree of atrial or ventricular hypertrophy or by revealing changes in the S–T segments or T waves, which suggest myocardial ischemia. Electrocardiography is also the major diagnostic method of evaluating dysrhythmias (see Chapter 29) and electrolyte imbalances of potassium or calcium.

The Normal Electrocardiogram in the Term Infant. Before electrocardiography can be used successfully in the management of infants with congenital heart disease, the ranges of normal must be appreciated. The rest of this section, dealing primarily with the normal electrocardiogram, is based on the classic work of Ziegler (1951), Cassels and Ziegler (1966), and Davignon and coworkers (1980).

HEART RATE. The average resting heart rate for a neonate in the first week of life is about 125 to 130 beats per minute, but rates as low as 85 or 90 beats per minute with sleep or as high as 190 to 200 with crying or agitation may be seen. In general, the normal resting rate gradually increases over the first month of life so that the mean value at 30 days is about 150 beats per minute (Table 26–1).

RHYTHM. Normal sinus rhythm with a P wave preceding each QRS complex predominates. A sinus

Table 26–1.   Electrocardiographic Standards in Neonates

Parameter	Age in days			
	0–1	1–3	3–7	7–30
Number of patients	189	179	181	119
Heart rate (beats/min)	122 (99–147)	123 (97–148)	128 (100–160)	148 (114–177)
QRS axis (degrees)	135 (91–185)	134 (93–188)	133 (92–185)	108 (78–152)
P–R duration II (msec)	107 (82–138)	108 (85–132)	103 (78–130)	101 (75–128)
QRS duration V_5 (msec)	50 (26–69)	48 (27–61)	49 (26–63)	53 (27–75)
Q–T duration V_5 (msec)	290 (220–360)	280 (235–330)	272 (272–315)	258 (230–290)
P amplitude II (mvolts)	0.16 (0.07–0.25)	0.16 (0.05–0.25)	0.17 (0.08–0.27)	0.19 (0.09–0.29)
R amplitude V_{3R} (mvolts)	1.05 (0.40–1.79)	1.19 (0.52–1.95)	1.02 (0.18–1.80)	0.82 (0.30–1.50)
R amplitude V_1 (mvolts)	1.35 (0.65–2.37)	1.48 (0.70–2.42)	1.28 (0.50–2.15)	1.05 (0.45–1.81)
R amplitude V_5 (mvolts)	1.0 (0.25–1.85)	1.1 (0.48–1.95)	1.3 (0.48–1.95)	1.45 (0.60–2.1)
R amplitude V_6 (mvolts)	0.45 (0.05–0.95)	0.48 (0.05–0.95)	0.51 (0.10–1.05)	0.76 (0.26–1.35)
S amplitude V_{3R} (mvolts)	0.43 (0.07–1.18)	0.5 (0.05–1.2)	0.36 (0.05–0.8)	0.20 (0.05–0.64)
S amplitude V_1 (mvolts)	0.85 (0.10–1.85)	0.95 (0.15–1.90)	0.68 (0.10–1.50)	0.4 (0.05–0.97)
S amplitude V_5 (mvolts)	0.99 (0.38–1.79)	0.98 (0.20–1.59)	0.95 (0.38–1.63)	0.8 (0.24–1.38)
S amplitude V_6 (mvolts)	0.35 (0.02–0.79)	0.32 (0.02–0.76)	0.37 (0.02–0.80)	0.32 (0.02–0.82)
R/S amplitude V_{3R}	1.5 (0.2–4.8)	1.6 (0.2–4.2)	1.8 (0.2–5.8)	1.9 (0.2–2.5)
R/S amplitude V_1	2.2 (0.4–7.0)	2.0 (6.4–5.4)	2.8 (0.05–7.2)	2.9 (1.1–6.3)
R/S amplitude V_5	0.7 (0–7.0)	1.0 (0–5.0)	1.5 (0–5.0)	2.0 (0–5.1)
R/S amplitude V_6	2 (0–8)	3 (0–9)	2 (0–8)	4 (0–9)
Mean (5 and 95 per cent values)				

(From Davignon, A., Rautaharju, P., Boiselle, E., Soumis, F., Megelas, M., and Choquette, A.: Normal ECG standards for infants and children. Pediatr. Cardiol. *1*:123, 1979–1980.)

arrhythmia with each QRS preceded by a P wave but slight variation in the interval between P waves (P–P interval) is not uncommon, especially with careful monitoring and 24-hour recordings.

P WAVE.   The P-wave duration varies but is usually between 0.04 and 0.08 second. Although a prolonged P wave suggests left atrial hypertrophy in the older child or adult, this sign is not as helpful in diagnosis of the neonate. The amplitude of the P wave is best appreciated in lead II and should be less than 3 mm (0.3 mv) in height; taller P waves suggest right atrial hypertrophy. The P-wave axis is usually between 0 and +90 degrees (upright in leads I and aV$_F$), averaging +60 degrees; an abnormal P-wave axis suggests an ectopic atrial pacemaker or abnormal position of the atria.

P–R INTERVAL.   The normal P–R interval is 0.08 to 0.14 second (mean = 0.10) (Table 26–1). A short P–R interval suggests a nodal pacemaker, rapid conduction through a bypass tract (as in Wolff-Parkinson-White syndrome), or facilitated conduction in glycogen storage disease. A prolonged P–R interval (first-degree heart block) is frequently benign but may be a manifestation of conduction system disease (see p. 306).

QRS COMPLEX.   The QRS duration is usually 0.03 to 0.07 second (Table 26–1). A longer interval suggests an interventricular conduction delay. The QRS axis is usually +90 to +180 degrees (negative in lead I, positive in aV$_F$) with a mean of about 135 degrees during the first week of life, but it shifts leftward so that by 1 month of age the mean value is about 105 degrees (range 75 to 150). An axis that is shifted abnormally leftward (0 to 60 degrees) suggests the right ventricular hypoplasia that is seen in pulmonary atresia and an intact ventricular septum. A superior leftward axis of −30 to −90 degrees suggests either tricuspid atresia or an endocardial cushion defect (see p. 281).

The amplitude of the QRS complexes varies considerably (Table 26–1). Since the right ventricle predominates in utero, is anterior in the chest, and benefits from its proximity to the electrodes, right ventricular hypertrophy is the rule.

Although there is still some controversy concerning diagnosis of right, left, and combined ventricular hypertrophy in the neonate, some guidelines based on the 1980 data of Davignon and coworkers are listed in Table 26–2.

T WAVE.   There are marked shifts in the T waves on the surface electrocardiogram that represent ventricular repolarization changes over the first few minutes, hours, and days of life.

The T waves are usually upright in the right chest

Table 26–2. Criteria for Ventricular Overload in Newborn Infants

1. Right ventricular
   qR in V_{4R} or V_1
   $RV_{3R} > 18$ mm
   $RV_1 > 25$ mm
   $SV_6 > 10$ mm
   R/S ratio V_{4R}, $V_1 > 7$
   TV_1 positive after day 4
2. Left ventricular
   $SV_{3R} > 15$ mm
   $SV_1 > 20$ mm
   $RV_6 > 12$ mm (15 at 1 month)
   R/S $V_6 > 8$ mm
   $QV_6 > 3$ mm
3. Combined
   Signs of LV and RV
   Signs of RV plus:
   a. Q > 2 mm in left chest
   b. Normal LV forces in V_6

leads (V_{3R} to V_2) for the first 6 to 24 hours of life. They become inverted during the first or second day in virtually all neonates; persistently upright T waves in leads V_{4R} or V_1 beyond 4 days suggest elevated right ventricular pressure. The T waves may be inverted in V_6 and V_7 soon after birth but are usually upright by 8 hours of age; persistence of inverted T waves beyond 48 hours is definitely abnormal and suggests left ventricular strain.

Q–T INTERVAL. The Q–T interval usually decreases over the first month of life. At birth, it averages 0.28 to 0.30 seconds but may vary considerably (ninety-fifth percentile values range from 0.22 to 0.36 seconds). By 1 day of age, the average has fallen to 0.26 seconds. Since the Q–T interval is closely correlated with heart rate, the corrected ($Q–T_c$) interval is usually calculated (Q–T/R–R interval). This is quite constant over the first month, averaging 0.40 seconds. A prolonged $Q–T_c$ interval is associated with hypocalcemia; hypercalcemia shortens the $Q–T_c$ interval.

Electrocardiogram in the Premature Infant. Premature infants tend to have a slightly higher resting heart rate with a greater variation; rates of 70 beats per minute may be seen during sleep, and rates of up to 210 with crying are not unusual. The P waves tend to be of shorter duration, with a slight leftward shift in the P-wave axis to about +40 degrees. The P–R and QRS intervals for the premature infant are shorter than those for the term infant, averaging 0.10 and 0.04 second, respectively. The QRS amplitudes tend to be lower, and there is less right ventricular predominance and a more rapid shift to the adult pattern, with the initial R/S ratio in V_1 often less than 1.

Chest Radiograph. The chest radiograph provides useful and often unique information about the cardiovascular system in the newborn (Swischuk, 1979). However, it is frequently either not helpful or frankly misleading because of variations in technique (underexposure, overexposure, expiratory or rotated film) that make interpretation difficult. Although the hazards of excess radiation should not be underestimated, the dosage from a standard chest radiograph is minimal, about 9 mrad (approximating the radiation in Denver over a 3-week period), and thus poor studies should be repeated to obtain precise information. Data concerning the cardiac size, contour, and position as well as the status of the pulmonary vascular markings may give important clues about the differential diagnosis and hemodynamic status of the neonate with congenital heart disease. We have found that the oblique films have little diagnostic value and now use only anteroposterior and lateral projections. Fluoroscopy for cardiac diagnosis except as a part of cardiac catheterization is now only used in cases in which a vascular ring must be excluded.

Cardiac Size. Some noncardiac factors influence the size of the cardiac silhouette. The most common is radiographing the heart during the expiratory phase of respiration. Also, a large thymus in the anterior mediastinum may obscure the heart border on the anteroposterior projection, but with the stress of cardiac disease the thymus often involutes, making evaluation of the heart size more accurate in the sick neonate. Rarely, a pericardial effusion may enlarge the cardiac silhouette when the heart is not enlarged, but an echocardiogram will usually clarify such findings. Cardiac size depends primarily on the volume of blood within the chambers rather than on the thickness of the muscle. Thus, events that tend to increase intravascular volume (e.g., stripping the umbilical cord at birth and overhydration) tend to increase the heart size.

Normally, the cardiothoracic ratio in the neonate should be less than 0.60. Cardiac enlargement may appear with left-to-right shunts, atrioventricular or semilunar valve regurgitation, or ventricular failure. Specific chamber size is often very difficult to evaluate, but occasionally the right atrial dilatation with Ebstein's disease of the tricuspid valve or with pulmonary atresia and an intact ventricular septum and tricuspid regurgitation may be evident.

Cardiac Position. The heart may be in the right or left thorax or present as a midline structure. Malpositioning may be secondary to hypoplasia of one of the lungs, atelectasis, tension pneumothorax, or diaphragmatic hernia. Primary malpositions are frequently associated with heart disease. Dextrocardia (heart in the right chest), is associated with a very high incidence of intracardiac anomalies unless there is associated situs inversus of the viscera (stomach on the right, liver on the left, etc.). Similarly, levocardia (heart in the left chest) is frequently associated with major anomalies if there is situs inversus of the viscera. Both these situations suggest the heterotaxy syndromes (see p. 265).

Pulmonary Vascularity. The assessment of pulmonary vascularity is one of the most important parts of the cardiac evaluation of the neonate, since it may be helpful in the differential diagnosis of neonatal heart disease.

In the posteroanterior film of the normal infant, the right pulmonary artery and the primary branches are usually visible in the right hilum. The left pulmonary artery and its primary branches may be hidden behind the heart. The vessels seen gradually taper peripherally and are usually too small to be seen in the distal third of the lung fields (Fig. 26–5A).

Four abnormal patterns can be distinguished. If the pulmonary blood flow is decreased (Fig. 26–5B), as is seen with most cyanotic heart disease, the lungs appear dark, the pulmonary vessels in the hilum are decreased in size, and no vessels are seen in the middle third of the lung fields. If the pulmonary blood flow is increased, as is seen with all significant left-to-right shunts, the hilar vessels are enlarged, the middle third of the lung fields has vessels larger than normal, and vessels may often be seen out to the distal third of the lung (Fig. 26–5C).

The third pattern is associated with pulmonary

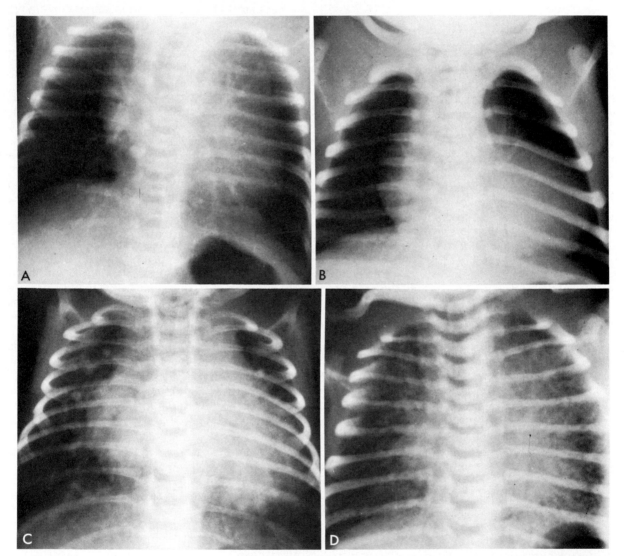

Figure 26–5. *A,* Chest radiograph in a normal newborn infant. The cardiothoracic silhouette is increased in size, especially in the superior mediastinum, probably because of an enlarged thymus. The pulmonary vascularity is visible in the middle third of the lung field, but no large vessels are seen distally. *B,* Chest radiograph in a child with Ebstein's disease of the tricuspid valve with right-to-left shunting at the atrial level. The heart is enlarged secondary to tricuspid regurgitation. The lung fields are dark, with no pulmonary vessels visible in the middle third of the lung field, findings that reflect diminished pulmonary vascularity. *C,* Chest radiograph in an infant with a large ventricular septal defect. The heart is enlarged, and the distal pulmonary vessels are engorged because of the large left-to-right shunt. *D,* Chest radiograph in a child with total anomalous pulmonary venous return with obstruction. The pulmonary vessels are indistinct, and the lung fields are hazy, indicating increased pulmonary venous pressure.

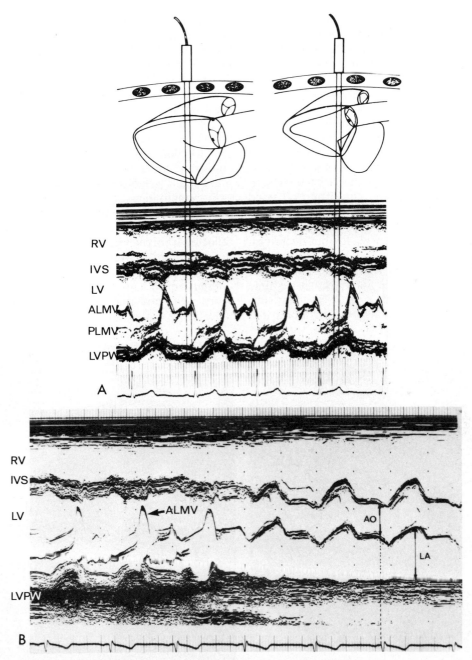

Figure 26–6. *A,* A normal M-mode echocardiogram with the ultrasonographic beam traversing the chest wall, right ventricle (RV), interventricular septum (IVS), left ventricular cavity (LV), and left ventricular posterior wall (LVPW). On the left, the anterior leaflet of the mitral valve (ALMV) and posterior leaflet of the mitral valve are imaged in diastole when the leaflets are open. On the right side of the slide, the imaging is in systole when the valve is closed. *B,* Starting from the same transducer position as in *A* (the first two complexes), the beam has been gradually rotated superiorly so the anterior leaflet of the mitral valve is seen to be continuous with the posterior portion of the aortic root (AO). At this level, the left atrium (LA) is posterior to the aorta. (From Williams, R. G., and Tucker, C. R.: Echocardiographic Diagnosis of Congenital Heart Disease. Boston, Little, Brown and Company, 1977. Reproduced with permission.)

venous hypertension. The hila are prominent owing to dilation of the pulmonary veins, and the peripheral pulmonary arteries are indistinct because the elevated pulmonary venous pressure causes an increase in interstitial fluid, diminishing the contrast between the air-filled alveoli and the fluid-filled arteries (Fig. 26–5D). The entire lung field may be hazy. Pulmonary redistribution with vessels that are larger in the upper lung fields than in the lower, Kerley's B lines, and the "butterfly" pattern of pulmonary edema are characteristic of older children and adults with pulmonary venous hypertension and are not seen in the neonate. Pulmonary venous congestion may be seen with total anomalous pulmonary venous return with obstruction, the hypoplastic left heart syndrome, or any lesion causing significant left-sided heart failure.

The last pattern, infrequently seen, is pulmonary plethora in the peripheral lung fields but decreased central and hilar vessels. This pattern is occasionally seen with tetralogy of Fallot with pulmonary atresia, in which the central pulmonary arteries may be quite hypoplastic or atretic with pulmonary blood flow supplied by large collateral vessels from the aorta that enter the lung distally and anastomose to the peripheral pulmonary arteries.

Echocardiography. Echocardiography is a valuable method of diagnosing neonatal congenital heart disease. One should not underestimate the usefulness of the M-mode examination and the more recent two-dimensional method in the differentiation of congenital heart disease from other abnormalities (e.g., sepsis, persistent fetal circulation) and in the distinction among the various forms of congenital heart disease. Ultrasonography appeals to clinicians because it is noninvasive, painless, and, with the equipment now available, associated with no adverse effects. It must be emphasized, however, that echocardiography should not be used alone but with physical examination, electrocardiography, and chest radiography to plan effectively for future studies (usually cardiac catheterization and angiography) and to make intelligent diagnostic and prognostic decisions.

In modern ultrasonography, sound waves are generated by a piezoelectric crystal at a frequency of 5 to 7.5 MHz (million cycles/second). The sounds are reflected from the interfaces of different density (e.g., the boundary between blood and muscle) back to the crystal, which then reconverts them to electrical energy, which can then be displayed on an oscilloscope or permanently recorded. Since the angle of reflection is equal to the angle of incidence, only ul-

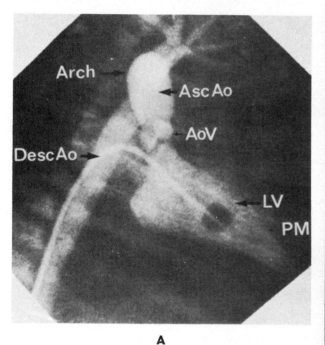

A

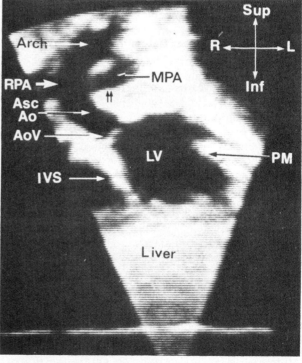

B

Figure 26–7. Normal left ventricle. A, Right anterior oblique cineangiogram. B, Longitudinal, subxiphoid, two-dimensional echocardiogram. The aorta terminates at the proximal transverse arch. The main pulmonary artery (MPA) is seen in cross section to the left of the ascending aorta (Asc Ao) and gives rise to the right pulmonary artery (RPA), indicated by parallel arrows in the center. Arch = transverse arch; Desc Ao = descending aorta; AoV = aortic valve; LV = left ventricle; PM = papillary muscle; IVS = interventricular septum. (From Bierman, F. Z., and Williams, R. G.: Prospective diagnosis of d-transposition of the great arteries in neonates by subxiphoid two-dimensional echocardiography. Circulation 60:1496, 1979. Reproduced with permission.)

trasounds from an interface almost perfectly perpendicular to the beam are received by the small transducer (Fig. 26–6).

Two-dimensional images are quite similar in principle but have either multiple piezoelectric crystals to develop multiple images (phased array) or a rotating beam so that multiple images can be obtained with a single crystal (mechanical sector scanner). The major advantage of the two-dimensional scanner is that it allows one to view a large part of the heart in real time and to modify the view of the heart (much as one would angle the child to obtain an angiocardiogram), depending on the position of the heart in the chest and the diagnosis found (Fig. 26–7). By viewing the heart in long-axial, short-axial, apical, subxiphoid (4-chamber), and suprasternal views, one can determine the relationships among the atria, ventricles, great vessels, and semilunar and atrioventricular valves.

Recent technologic advances are currently making the M-mode obsolete. At present, we use it for visualization of chamber size and function, but it is quite likely that even for these functions the M-mode will be supplanted by two-dimensional studies within the next few years.

M-mode echocardiographic values for normal neonates are listed in Table 26–3. Brief descriptions of the pertinent echocardiographic findings in specific types of congenital heart disease are listed in the discussions of the individual lesions in Chapter 27. Those interested in a more comprehensive review of the principles and techniques of ultrasonography are referred to the text of either Williams and Tucker (1977) or Meyer (1977) for discussions of M-mode echocardiography and to the writings of Goldberg and coworkers (1980), Tajik (1978) or Silverman and Snider (1982) for information about two-dimensional studies.

Cardiac Catheterization and Angiocardiography. Over the past decade, the increased use of noninvasive or semi-invasive studies such as echocardiography and radionuclide studies has improved the diagnostic acumen of the cardiologist. Although these studies have occasionally obviated the need for catheterization (as in aortic atresia or Ebstein's disease of the tricuspid valve in which the diagnosis is unmistakable on echocardiogram) we continue to depend on catheterization for definitive anatomic and physiologic information.

At present, we catheterize all infants critically ill with cyanotic congenital heart disease, those with congestive heart failure (except the premature with an obvious patent ductus arteriosus or the neonate with paroxysmal supraventricular tachycardia), and those doing poorly after cardiac surgery if there is a possibility that a significant residual problem is present.

Infants with heart disease are often critically ill, and careful monitoring during the procedure is necessary. We continuously evaluate body temperature with a rectal probe, pulse rate and rhythm with an oscilloscope, arterial blood pressure through an umbilical artery or femoral artery cannula, and Po_2 with a transcutaneous oxygen monitor. In addition, every 15 to 30 minutes we obtain arterial blood gases and replace blood loss. Meticulous monitoring will minimize complications. We do not routinely sedate the

Table 26–3. Echocardiographic Values for Normal Newborns

Weight	Premature* Left atrial dimension (cm)	Left ventricular end diastolic dimension (cm)
600–900	0.60 (0.5–0.7)	1.07 (0.9–1.2)
901–1200	0.65 (0.5–0.8)	1.08 (0.9–1.3)
1201–1500	0.69 (0.5–0.9)	1.18 (1.0–1.3)
1501–1800	0.79 (0.6–1.0)	1.37 (1.2–1.5)
1801–2200	0.88 (0.7–1.1) mean (± 2 SD)	1.39 (1.1–1.6)

Full-term†	
Number	200
Weight (lbs)	7.6 (6–10)
Aortic root diameter (mm)	10.0 (8.1–12.0)
Left atrial diameter (mm)	7.0 (5.0–10.0)
Pulmonary artery diameter (mm)	11.1 (9.4–13.0)
Interventricular septal thickness (mm)	2.7 (1.8–4.0)
LV end systolic dimension (mm)	13.3 (8.0–18.6)
LV end diastolic dimension (mm)	18.7 (12.0–23.3)
LV end systolic wall thickness (mm)	4.3 (2.5–6.0)
LV end diastolic wall thickness (mm)	2.6 (1.6–3.7)
RV end diastolic dimension (mm)	11.4 (6.1–15.0)
Mean (± 2 SD)	

* Adapted from Meyer, R. A.: Pediatric Echocardiography. Philadelphia, Lea and Febiger, 1977.
† Adapted from Hagan, A. D., et al.: Echocardiographic criteria for normal newborn infants. Circulation 48:1221, 1973.

neonate, but if he remains unconsolable after receiving a pacifier dipped in glucose water, we administer morphine (0.05 mg/kg I.V.) judiciously.

Methods. The techniques of catheterization vary widely depending upon local customs. For the purpose of simplicity, only our methodology will be considered here. Those interested in other approaches should read the excellent chapters in Rudolph (1974) or Moller and Neal (1981).

In the first week of life we prefer to use the umbilical vessels when patent. If access to the heart is not possible after the umbilical vein and ductus venosus are probed, we use the femoral vein. Catheterization of the femoral vein is almost always performed percutaneously. A #21 needle is introduced into the vessel, and a 0.021-inch guide wire is inserted through the needle. The needle is then removed, and a dilator and sheath are advanced over the wire. Once the sheath is in place, the wire and dilator are removed and a catheter is inserted. Alternatively, the femoral vein or artery or both may be surgically isolated by cutdown, and the catheter can be inserted through a hole made with small scissors or a scalpel blade. Although many types of catheters have been used over the years, we prefer the balloon-tipped, flow-directed variety. They seem easier to use and cause less cardiac trauma, and, at least in our experience, they are associated with a lower incidence of cardiac perforation with catheter manipulation or angiography. A #5 French catheter (external circumference 5 mm, external diameter 1.6 mm) is used almost exclusively on the venous side, since this is large enough for good pressure measurement and angiography but still small enough to be flexible and fit a newborn's femoral vein comfortably.

If the arterial study can be performed using the umbilical artery, a #5 umbilical artery catheter is usually used, but a #4 French or #5 French angiographic catheter may be substituted if angiography is necessary. After 1 week of age, the umbilical artery may not be accessible. We then percutaneously place a #21 or #22 Teflon cannula into the femoral artery for pressure monitoring and blood-gas sampling. If a retrograde arterial study is necessary, we exchange the cannula for a #4 French or, more recently, a #3.2 French pigtail-shaped angiographic catheter. At the end of the study, the catheters are removed unless needed for monitoring. If the vessels were entered percutaneously, pressure is applied to the site for 10 minutes. If a cutdown was performed, the vessels are repaired and the skin is closed.

DATA COLLECTION AND ANALYSIS. Information at catheterization is provided by one or more of the following: catheter course, oxygen data, pressure data, and angiography.

Catheter Course. Normally, the catheter course is predictable: the venous catheter can be advanced from the vena cava to the right atrium and ventricle and then into the pulmonary artery, and the arterial catheter can be advanced retrograde from the aorta into the left ventricle. Occasionally, the catheter will take an anomalous course. If the catheter can be passed from the right to the left atrium, it suggests a patent foramen ovale or atrial septal defect. If it passes from the pulmonary artery into the descending aorta, it suggests an aortopulmonary window or a patent ductus arteriosus. These unusual catheter positions often provide helpful information regarding the nature of the underlying anomaly.

Oxygen Data. In the normal infant, the oxygen saturation in the superior vena cava is about 70 per cent, with no changes as the venous blood goes through the right atrium, right ventricle, and into the main and peripheral pulmonary arteries. Similarly, the oxygen saturation of the pulmonary veins, normally 95 to 98 per cent, should not change in the passage through the left heart to the peripheral arteries. Any significant increase in the oxygen saturation as the blood goes through the right heart chambers suggests contamination with blood from the left heart, a left-to-right shunt. This "step-up" may occur (1) at the atrial level in the presence of an atrial septal defect, a partial anomalous pulmonary venous return, endocardial cushion defect, or a ventricular septal defect with tricuspid regurgitation; (2) at the ventricular level with a ventricular septal defect or single ventricle; or (3) at the great-vessel level in aortico-pulmonary window or patent ductus arteriosus. Some variation in saturation is usually present because of incomplete mixing, and the step-up should be at least 10 per cent at the atrial level, 7 per cent at the ventricular level, or 5 per cent at the great-vessel level to be considered significant if only one sample is obtained.

The oxygen saturation in the pulmonary veins should be about 95 per cent. Lung disease may reduce the pulmonary venous oxygen content, and inhomogeneous lung disease may lead to different saturations in the individual pulmonary veins. A drop in saturation between pulmonary veins and left atrium, a right-to-left shunt, suggests tricuspid atresia, pulmonary atresia, or right ventricular dysfunction. Right-to-left shunting at the ventricular level is seen with a ventricular septal defect and pulmonary stenosis or in a single ventricle. Right-to-left shunting at the great vessel level may be seen in truncus arteriosus or tetralogy of Fallot.

Pressure Data. The normal intracardiac pressures beyond 3 days of age are listed in Table 26–4. The atrial mean pressures are elevated in the presence of congestive heart failure or atrioventricular-valve stenosis. If the latter is present, the ventricular end diastolic pressure will be normal; with heart failure, the end diastolic pressures are increased as well. Increased V waves in the atrium suggest atrioventricular-valve regurgitation (mitral or tricuspid), and elevated A waves suggest atrioventricular-valve stenosis.

The pulmonary artery pressure is elevated for the first 8 to 72 hours of life. Persistently elevated pul-

Table 26–4. Normal Intracardiac Pressures in the Infant (Older Than 72 Hours)

Right atrium	a = 5–7 v = 3–5 m = 0–2	Left atrium	a = 3–5 v = 5–8 m = 3–6
Right ventricle	$\dfrac{15-25}{5-7}$	Left ventricle	$\dfrac{65-80}{3-5}$
Pulmonary artery	$\dfrac{15-25}{8-12}$ m = 10–16	Aorta	$\dfrac{65-80}{45-60}$ m = 60–65

monary artery pressure may be seen with active pulmonary arteriolar vasoconstriction in the presence of lung disease and hypoxia. The pulmonary artery pressure will also be elevated when there is obstruction to the egress of pulmonary venous blood seen with mitral stenosis or atresia, or total anomalous pulmonary venous return, or when the pulmonary arteries are indirectly connected to the left ventricle in neonates with a large ventricular septal defect or single ventricle or with a large connection at the great-vessel level (e.g., a large patent ductus, aorticopulmonary window, or truncus arteriosus).

Right ventricular systolic hypertension occurs with increased pulmonary artery pressure and also, if there is obstruction to right ventricular egress secondary to pulmonic stenosis or atresia, with normal pulmonary artery pressure.

Systemic hypertension in the ascending aorta is seen in neonates with coarctation of the aorta and, rarely, in those with catastrophic renal vascular disease. In the latter, the ascending aorta and descending aorta pressures are equal. In the former, there is a gradient from obstruction at the site of the coarctation.

Left ventricular systolic pressures are increased whenever the aortic pressures are increased and in valvular aortic stenosis when the aortic pressures are normal or low.

Angiocardiography. Angiocardiography remains the mainstay of the anatomic delineation of the various forms of congenital heart disease. Over the past few years, we have switched from "all purpose" catheters to special catheters for angiocardiography in the hope of increasing the information obtained while reducing the complications. On the venous side, we use a #5 French balloon-tipped angiography catheter with multiple side holes proximal to the balloon. In those situations that require an arterial study, we prefer a specially designed #3.2 French thin-walled catheter with a "pigtail" at the end to minimize recoil. Any one of the commercially available contrast materials may be used, but we prefer Renovist (except when the sodium load is a concern, in which case we use Hypaque). Each angiocardiogram is performed with 1 ml/kg of contrast material injected within about ½ second, unless a large left-to-right shunt is present, in which case 1.5 or even 2.0 ml/kg is necessary. We rarely inject more than 4 ml/kg during the entire study.

Filming is done on cine film at 64 frames/second, with simultaneous video taping of the television image so that the pictures can be reviewed immediately, before the angiocardiograms are developed. Biplane filming is usually preferred, since it gives much more information without significantly increased risks.

A major advance in angiocardiography during the past decade is the recognition that the heart does not lie in the anteroposterior projection in the chest and that rotation of the x-ray beam or the patient or both reveals previously hidden anatomic details (Bargeron et al., 1977; Elliot et al., 1977; Fellows et al., 1977) (Table 26–5). It is occasionally hard to position the patient, but the advantages of these views more than compensate for difficulties encountered.

Complications. Complications of cardiac catheterization may arise from the procedure itself or from the precarious nature of these critically ill neonates.

In 1968, a cooperative study on catheterization re-

Table 26–5. Angled Views in the Cineangiography of Congenital Heart Disease

1. *Cranial 45°, left oblique 30°*
   ("Hepatoclavicular," or "4-chamber," view of Bargeron; with vertical (frontal) intensifier, patient's thorax is elevated 45° to sitting position and his left shoulder is rotated 45° anteriorly while his body is slanted to the right 10°–15° in the horizontal plane.)
   General advantage: Distinguishes the four chambers of the heart and demonstrates the posterior aspect of the ventricular septum.
   Specific advantage in:
     Defects in endocardial cushion, A–V canal
     LV-to-RA shunt
     VSD of A–V canal type
     Left coronary artery distribution
     Overriding A–V valves
2. *Cranial 20°, left oblique 70°*
   ("Long axial oblique" view of Bargeron; with horizontal or lateral intensifier, the patient's right shoulder is elevated 15° to 20° and his body is slanted 15° to 20° away from the intensifier.)
   General advantage: Demonstrates left ventricular outflow tract and most of the interventricular septum.
   Specific advantage in:
     VSD (muscular and membranous)
     Subaortic stenosis
     Subpulmonic stenosis in transposition
     Asymmetric septal hypertrophy
     Prolapse, anterior leaflet of mitral valve
     Overriding tricuspid valve
3. *Cranial 45° (± right or left oblique 10° to 15°)*
   ("Sitting" view of Bargeron; with the vertical intensifier, the patient's thorax is elevated 45°.)
   General advantage: Provides superior view of extracardiac mediastinal vessels.
   Specific advantage in:
     Bifurcation of pulmonary artery
     Supravalvular PS, pulmonary artery band
     Pulmonary arteries in pseudotruncus
     Pulmonary arteries in truncus
     Vascular rings and slings

(Courtesy of Dr. K. Fellows, Children's Hospital Medical Center, Boston.)

viewed the complications of 325 studies on infants less than 1 month of age between November 1, 1963 and October 31, 1965 (Braunwald and Swan, 1968). In this group, there were 50 neonates (15 per cent) with major complications and 20 deaths (6 per cent), six from perforation of the heart or great vessels, five from cardiac arrhythmias, four resulting from deterioration during the procedure, and five due to decline following the procedure.

In 1974, Stanger and coworkers reviewed their experience from 1970 to 1972 with 218 neonates in San Francisco. There were 20 deaths (9 per cent), two during the catheterization, and 18 within 24 hours of the study. Almost all the deaths were in children with irreparable heart disease and were believed to be the result of progressive clinical deterioration rather than a specific incident leading to demise. In only two infants (1 per cent) was there reason to believe that the catheterization was causally related to death.

Our review of the data from New England Regional Infant Cardiac Program for the year 1979 revealed two deaths among 300 neonates. Findings of this group support those of Stanger and colleagues. With balloon-tipped catheters for manipulation and either balloon or "pigtail" catheters for angiography, myocardial perforation and intramyocardial injection of contrast rarely occur. Arrhythmias (primarily atrial tachycardia and complete atrioventricular dissociation) still occur, but the judicious use of drugs, cardioversion, and pacing have made these complications less feared than previously. Umbilical and percutaneous femoral catheterizations have made infections at the site of catheter insertion less common, and infusion of prostaglandin E_1 to maintain the ductal patency has reduced the incidence of cyanotic spells and progressive deterioration from hypoxia and acidosis.

Manifestations of Cardiac Disease in the Neonate

Fortunately, there are only a limited number of ways that neonates with cardiovascular problems present to the pediatrician or neonatologist (Rowe et al., 1981). A cardiac disorder should be suspected in the presence of any one or more of the following: (1) congestive heart failure, (2) cyanosis, (3) heart murmurs, and (4) dysrhythmias. The first three of these cardinal manifestations of heart disease will subsequently be reviewed in more detail. Dysrhythmias will be discussed in Chapter 29.

Congestive Heart Failure. Congestive heart failure (CHF) is a clinical syndrome in which the heart is unable to perform its pump function to meet the metabolic demands of the body. CHF may be the result of either increased demands on the heart, usually due to structural alterations that impose a volume or a pressure load, or a diminished ability of the heart to meet the normal metabolic demands of the tissues, usually secondary to inflammatory disease or metabolic abnormalities. Occasionally, both factors may coexist. Compared with the older child or adult, the neonate seems particularly susceptible to congestive failure. Part of this tendency is undoubtedly due to the complex structural abnormalities that affect the newborn, but other factors may also be important. For example, the ventricular myocardium has fewer contractile elements per unit mass compared with that in older children (Sheldon et al., 1976). In addition, the heavy demands placed on the left ventricle at birth undoubtedly reduce the cardiac reserve.

In congestive failure, a number of compensatory mechanisms become operational. Chronic volume overload causes cardiac dilatation, which by the Frank-Starling mechanism permits ejection of a larger stroke volume, albeit at a higher wall tension and increased myocardial oxygen requirements. The increased wall tension, by an as yet unknown mechanism, stimulates protein synthesis, resulting in myocardial hypertrophy. There is also an increase in the release of catecholamines, especially norepinephrine, which increases both the heart rate and the velocity of ejection. As CHF progresses and cardiac output diminishes, blood is redistributed by vasoconstriction away from the periphery to other organs with greater metabolic needs. Reduction in renal blood flow stimulates release of aldosterone and renin, leading to sodium and water retention. Finally, tissue oxygenation is facilitated by release of 2,3-diphosphoglycerates, which increases the P 50 and shifts the oxygen dissociation curve to the right.

Unfortunately, the infant is less able to take advantage of many of these compensatory mechanisms than is the older child or adult. For example, heart failure develops and progresses too rapidly for RNA synthesis and myocardial hypertrophy to be of much benefit. In addition, the adrenergic receptors are only partially innervated at birth, and the norepinephrine stores are reduced, so the neonate derives less benefit than does the older child from the release of catecholamines (Friedman et al., 1968). Finally, neonates have predominantly fetal hemoglobin in the red cells, which tightly binds oxygen, negating the beneficial effects on tissue oxygenation of 2,3-diphosphoglycerate.

Clinical Manifestations. The signs and symptoms of heart failure are related to impaired myocardial performance as well as to pulmonary and systemic venous congestion and include tachycardia, tachypnea, hepatomegaly, diaphoresis, feeding difficulties, cardiomegaly, and occasionally peripheral edema or rales.

Normally, the heart rate of the neonate will increase to 180 to 200 with crying as a result of adrenergic stimulation, but persistent heart rates at this level when the neonate is quiet suggest increased autonomic activity that occurs to compensate for a failing myocardium. An early sign of left-sided failure is an increase in the respiratory rate above 50 to 60 per minute, usually without an increase in depth of respiration. At first, the baby is not distressed; grunting, flaring of the alae nasi, and intercostal retractions are unusual unless there is associated pulmonary disease or frank pulmonary edema. The tachypnea is probably associated with increased stiffness of the lung secondary to increased interstitial fluid from elevated pulmonary venous pressure (Rushmer, 1976).

Although neck vein distention is usually not discernible in the neonate, elevated systemic venous pressure results in enlargement of the liver beyond 3 cm below the right costal margin in the midclavicular line. However, other signs of systemic venous congestion in the older child and adult, edema and ascites, are unusual in the neonate. Hepatomegaly is not specific for CHF and may also be present in the neonate with a blood dyscrasia or congenital infection. A palpable liver without true hepatomegaly may also be seen with hyperinflated lungs when the liver is displaced inferiorly.

A fairly constant feature of heart failure in the neonate is difficult feeding. Although the normal infant will take an appropriate volume of formula for age and size within 15 to 20 minutes, the term neonate with heart failure will often take 45 to 60 minutes to consume 1 or 2 ounces. Occasionally, the child becomes dyspneic with the exertion required, but frequently he tires and falls asleep after a minimal effort. Diaphoresis, especially of the head with feeding, is a common finding that is probably a manifestation of increased adrenergic activity.

Cardiac enlargement on physical examination or, more commonly, on chest radiograph is one of the most consistent signs of impaired cardiac function and congestive failure. Rales over both lung fields may occasionally be heard, a result of a pulmonary venous congestion. As left heart failure progresses, the transudate may reach the level of the bronchioles, making wheezing or rhonchi more prominent.

Heart failure may progress very rapidly, with cardiovascular collapse and cardiogenic shock being the first manifestations. These infants have no pulses, mottled and cool extremities, rapid or gasping respirations, hypothermia, indistinct heart sounds, and usually no murmurs. The liver and spleen are usually very large. This picture simulates that of the infant with septicemia or meningitis; the very large liver and cardiomegaly on radiograph should indicate heart disease as the cause.

Pharmacologic Management

DIGITALIS (see also Chapter 108). Digitalis has been used to treat congestive heart failure for almost 200 years. Digoxin is the most widely used preparation in neonates, infants, and older children because of its excellent bioavailability (oral absorption is rapid, with peak levels occurring within 1 hour) and its relatively rapid excretion rate. Both factors allow for adjustments of dosage to meet individual demands. Although the mechanism of action is still not completely clear, digoxin appears to inhibit Na + ,K + - ATPase in the sodium pump, thereby increasing sodium and, secondarily, calcium transport to the contractile proteins, resulting in a greater force of contraction (Akera and Brody, 1977). Digoxin may be given orally, intravenously, or, rarely, intramuscularly. Absorption from the gastrointestinal tract is relatively rapid, with peak plasma levels and onset of action occurring within 30 to 60 minutes (Wettrell and Anderson, 1977). Oral absorption is somewhat variable, but usually 75 per cent is absorbed, with the rest lost in the feces (Wettrell and Anderson, 1977). In cases in which more rapid action is necessary, the intravenous preparation may be used, with the onset of action occurring within 5 to 30 minutes and the peak effect appearing within 2 hours. The half-life of digoxin is about 37 hours in the small full-term newborn and 57 hours in the premature (Lang and Von Bernuth, 1977), with approximately one fourth of the body stores metabolized daily. Therefore, after digitalization to fill the body stores, the maintenance dose is about one fourth of the total digitalizing dose and is usually given in two divided doses. Digoxin is excreted primarily by the kidney. Decreased renal function reduces the dose of digoxin required. In adults, the percentage of digoxin lost per day equals 14 + creatine clearance in ml/min/5. This probably applies to children as well. To calculate an approximate value for the daily dosage, multiply the percentage lost per day by the total digitalizing dose.

Several points should be emphasized. First, digitalization is an individual titration; there are wide variations in the responses, and each child must be watched carefully for signs of toxicity. This is especially true of infants with inflammatory disease of the myocardium, in which enhanced sensitivity to the drug is common. Secondly, the dose calculation should be done in duplicate and preferably by two physicians. Explicit instructions must then be given with the dosage in milligrams as well as milliliters to the person administering the digoxin. Although it might seem unnecessary to emphasize these details, the toxic—therapeutic range is narrow, and the authors have personally seen a few tragedies because of dosage errors with digitalis in infants.

The starting dose for digitalization has been a source of controversy for many years. Although infants may tolerate higher serum concentrations before manifesting toxicity, there is little evidence that they substantially benefit from the higher level. At present, we tend to be conservative and recommend a total oral digitalizing dose of 0.02 mg/kg in the preterm infant and 0.04 mg/kg in the term infant. Parenteral administration requires only 70 per cent of the oral dose because of more complete absorption.

Digitalis toxicity is an all too frequent occurrence

because of the narrow gap between therapeutic and toxic levels and frequent abnormalities of electrolytes and renal function in the critically ill infant. Serum levels greater than 3.5 mg/ml indicate toxicity. The most common manifestations of digitalis toxicity in the neonate are poor feeding and vomiting, symptoms for which there are many other causes. Dysrhythmias, especially sinus bradycardia, second and third degree heart block, and supraventricular arrhythmias are the usual manifestations, but virtually any dysrhythmia may be seen. It is probably safest to consider any arrhythmia (except possibly atrial fibrillation) a manifestation of digoxin toxicity especially if the drug is being given parenterally. Serum digoxin concentrations are especially helpful in questionable situations, but withholding digoxin while awaiting the laboratory report is prudent. Prolongation of the P–R interval, sagging S–T segments, and T-wave inversion on the electrocardiogram are signs of digoxin effect and do not imply toxicity; no dosage changes are required for these EKG changes alone.

The treatment of digitalis toxicity is to stop the drug. This is usually sufficient. If potassium levels are low, supplemental potassium should be supplied. Life-threatening ectopic arrhythmias should be suppressed; phenytoin (diphenylhydantoin) and lidocaine may be especially helpful. For serious bradyarrhythmias, a pacemaker may be required. Digitalis-specific antibody has been used in a few cases of suicidal ingestion of digoxin in adults and may play a future role in digitalis toxicity in the neonate (Smith et al., 1976).

DIURETICS (see also Chapter 108). Diminished renal blood flow secondary to congestive heart failure results in sodium and fluid retention. Diuretics act directly on the kidney to inhibit solute and water reabsorption and thus increase urine volume. A wide variety of diuretics have been used, but only furosemide (Lasix), ethacrynic acid (Edacrin), and, occasionally, chlorothiazide (Diuril) and spironolactone (Aldactone) are used with any frequency in infants. Furosemide and ethacrynic acid, the most potent of the diuretics, act by inhibiting chloride transport in the ascending limb of Henle and thereby moving the gradient for water movement from the medullary ducts into the renal interstitium (Grantham and Chonko, 1978). The thiazide diuretics reduce the permeability of the distal convoluted tubule to sodium, chloride, and potassium and thereby increase excretion of these ions as well as water. Spironolactone is a weak diuretic when used alone, but when it is used in conjunction with one of the other three diuretics, it contributes to an antialdosterone effect that promotes retention of potassium. We currently use furosemide (1 mg/kg I.V.) for acute diuresis with chlorothiazide (10 to 20 mg/kg/day) and spironolactone (1 to 2 mg/kg/day) as maintenance therapy. Abnormalities of electrolyte balance are not uncommon, and serum sodium, potassium, and chloride must be monitored during vigorous diuresis.

OTHER INOTROPIC AGENTS (see also Chapter 108). Other inotropic agents may be necessary in severe congestive heart failure and cardiogenic shock. The beta-adrenergic agonists, isoproterenol and dopamine, have been the most commonly used. Isoproterenol will improve tissue perfusion primarily by its positive inotropic effects on contractility, but, unfortunately, its chronotropic effects increase heart rate excessively, limiting its clinical usefulness. Dopamine, the immediate precursor of norepinephrine, appears to have much the same inotropic effects but less chronotropic effect and also selectively increases renal, mesenteric, cerebral, and myocardial blood flow without increasing flow to the skeletal muscle bed (Driscoll et al., 1978; Lang et al., 1980). The dosages of these inotropic agents are discussed further in Chapter 108.

Afterload Reduction. It has been recognized for some time that myocardial performance is a function of the preload (atrial filling pressures), contractility, and afterload (systemic vascular resistance). Children and adults with congestive failure have increased levels of circulating catecholamines that cause peripheral vasoconstriction, which increases the systemic vascular resistance. Although this helps maintain systemic blood pressure in the presence of a low cardiac output (blood pressure = cardiac output × systemic vascular resistance), the increased afterload adversely affects myocardial performance. It has been found that in children and adults with elevated systemic vascular resistance, the use of vasodilators to reduce afterload may result in such an improvement in cardiac output that the blood pressure remains stable. Sodium nitroprusside is the most widely used vasodilator in adults and probably in children as well, but there is currently little information concerning its use in neonates. It would seem more useful in newborns with myocardial disease than in those with shunts or obstructive lesions. Arterial blood pressure and atrial pressures must be carefully monitored. The starting dose is usually 0.1 μg/kg/min, with the dose titrated up to 5 μg/kg/min, depending on the response. Hydralazine may be used as an oral preparation.

Other Therapeutic Measures. Using a modified neonatal chair or tilting the incubator or radiant heater to 15 to 45 degrees maintains the lower extremities dependent and permits some peripheral pooling, which seems to reduce pulmonary congestion and ease the work of breathing by lessening pressure on the diaphragm. Since virtually all the infants with congestive failure have some pulmonary venous desaturation secondary to ventilation perfusion imbalance, they may benefit from 30 to 35 per cent oxygen either in the incubator or by mask. An occasional child will be relatively anemic; slow transfusion of packed red blood cells should be given to increase the hematocrit to 45 to 55 per cent to improve the oxygen-carrying capacity of the blood.

If severe pulmonary edema and congestive heart

failure exhaust the neonate so that he develops respiratory failure (e.g., $PCO_2 > 45$ torr), nasotracheal intubation with respirator-assisted ventilation may be necessary. By utilizing positive end-expiratory pressure, one may improve pulmonary congestion, facilitating further diagnostic studies and therapeutic measures.

Finally, attention should be given to a proper diet. Although breast milk and usual infant formulas may be adequate for growth of a normal newborn, they contain excessive sodium and insufficient solute for the neonate with congestive heart failure. We usually recommend a low-sodium formula (Similac PM 60/40 or SMA) and slowly increase the caloric content from 2 calories/3 ml (20 calories/ounce) to 1 calorie/ml with glucose polymers and medium chain triglycerides if such a diet can be tolerated without diarrhea. By providing frequent small feedings of 45 to 75 ml, we are frequently able to maintain the neonate's caloric intake at 125 to 150 calories/kg/day, enough for normal or slightly below normal growth. We have found this far more efficacious than fluid restriction, which almost inevitably slowly deprives the neonate of necessary caloric intake.

Cyanosis. It is now commonly accepted that the clinical perception of cyanosis is determined not by the percentage of hemoglobin attached to oxygen (percentage of oxygen saturation) but by the absolute amount of reduced hemoglobin in the arterial and capillary beds (Lees, 1970). The critical amount of reduced hemoglobin necessary for recognition depends on the clinical experience of the observer and the lighting but is probably about 4 gm per 100 ml in the neonate and slightly less in the older child. In patients with a normal hematocrit and hemoglobin, this corresponds to an arterial saturation of about 78 to 80 per cent. However, if the neonate is polycythemic (hemoglobin 25 gm), cyanosis may be recognized at an arterial saturation of 84 per cent; if he is anemic (hemoglobin 10 gm), it will not be noticeable until the arterial saturation is 60 per cent or less.

Central cyanosis involves the trunk and mucous membranes as well as the extremities and is caused by an increase of reduced hemoglobin in the arterial blood because of an abnormality of oxygen transport originating in the heart, lung, or blood. Central cyanosis may be caused by one of five pathophysiologic mechanisms: (1) right-to-left shunting, (2) alveolar hypoventilation, (3) diffusion impairment in the lung, (4) ventilation perfusion imbalance, and (5) abnormalities in hemoglobin transport of oxygen. Diffusion abnormalities seem not to play a role in central cyanosis of the infant.

Diagnosis. The differentiation of central cyanosis of a cardiac origin due to right-to-left shunts from central cyanosis caused by other factors can almost always be made without cardiac catheterization.

One of the most helpful signs is the breathing pattern. Infants with cardiac cyanosis may be tachypneic but are seldom in significant distress. They rarely exhibit intercostal retractions, flaring of the alae nasi, or grunting. The latter signs suggest primary pulmonary pathology. Stridor suggests mechanical interference with ventilation and is seen with vascular rings, Pierre Robin syndrome, tracheomalacia, and other conditions in which there is obstruction of the airway during inspiration. Cyanosis due to central nervous system disease usually is episodic and associated with periodic breathing, bradypnea, or apnea.

The chest radiograph of infants with cyanotic congenital heart disease usually shows decreased pulmonary blood flow, although the flow may be normal in transposition of the great arteries. With pulmonary disease, the vascular markings of the lungs are normal. The pulmonary causes of cyanosis, including respiratory distress syndrome, pneumonia, pneumothorax, diaphragmatic hernia, and hypoplasia or agenesis of the lungs, reveal characteristic patterns on radiograph that are usually not difficult to distinguish from heart disease. However, it may be difficult to distinguish infants with severe heart failure and pulmonary edema from those with lung disease. The signs and symptoms of heart failure and the massive cardiac enlargement on radiograph should allow differentiation in difficult cases.

The arterial blood gases in room air and in 100 per cent oxygen may be helpful in differentiating the cyanosis from hypoventilation, from ventilation/perfusion ($\dot{V}/\dot{Q}$) imbalance, and from right-to-left shunting. In all three situations, the Pa_{O_2} is decreased in room air. However, with alveolar hypoventilation the Pa_{CO_2} is usually increased to 50 torr or greater, whereas with $\dot{V}/\dot{Q}$ abnormalities or intracardiac shunts the Pa_{CO_2} is normal. When the infant with alveolar hypoventilation or $\dot{V}/\dot{Q}$ abnormality is placed in 100 per cent oxygen for 10 minutes, the increased O_2 concentration in the alveoli will raise the pulmonary venous P_{O_2} and therefore the Pa_{O_2} to more than 150 torr. By contrast, those with right-to-left intracardiac shunt under similar conditions will increase the pulmonary venous P_{O_2}, but because of the intracardiac shunting of hypoxemic blood to the aorta, the Pa_{O_2} will not change significantly. A rise of greater than 30 torr is highly suggestive of lung disease. Occasionally, however, intracardiac shunting may be present with lung disease (persistent fetal circulation syndrome), and hypoventilation and ventilation/perfusion imbalances may be found with pulmonary edema secondary to structural heart disease. One should be careful to avoid exposing the premature infants to even transient hyperoxemia. Differentiation of causes of cyanosis can be inferred from alveolar-arterial differences at any known inspired concentration.

Infants with methemoglobinemia have an alarming lavender hue to their skin but are rarely in any distress. On arterial blood gases, the Pa_{O_2} is normal and increases to greater than 200 torr in 100 per cent oxygen. Confirmation of the diagnosis is by spectroscopy and by the rapid response to I.V. methylene blue (1 mg/kg).

If history, physical examination, chest radiograph, and arterial blood gases do not distinguish primary pulmonary from cardiac disease, the two-dimensional echocardiogram can virtually always determine whether the heart, great vessels, and pulmonary venous return are normal. A cardiac catheterization diagnosis of "structurally normal heart" should be quite uncommon in the future.

Heart Murmurs. Heart murmurs are the auditory manifestations of turbulence within the heart or great vessels that is transmitted to the chest wall. As pointed out by others, soft murmurs are not uncommon during the transitional circulation as the branch pulmonary arteries increase their flow from 7 per cent to 50 per cent of combined ventricular output, causing physiologic peripheral pulmonary stenosis (Danilowicz et al., 1965), and the ductus arteriosus closes. In 1961, Braudo and Rowe serially examined a group of 80 newborn infants and found that 48 (60 per cent) had murmurs audible in the first 24 hours of life. Nevertheless, loud murmurs heard in the first day or so of life usually represent stenosis of one of the semilunar valves or regurgitation through one of the atrioventricular valves, since the high pulmonary vascular resistance in the first day or two of life usually prevents enough shunting in the presence of communications between the left and right side of the heart to cause a loud murmur. Murmurs of a ventricular septal defect or patent ductus arteriosus may be heard on discharge from the hospital, but with the increasing tendency to discharge on the second or third day of life the murmurs are often now being heard for the first time at 4- to 6-week well-baby checkup. Murmurs of pulmonic stenosis are usually loudest at the left upper sternal border and may be associated with an ejection click early in systole that diminishes in intensity or disappears during inspiration. Murmurs of aortic stenosis may be audible at the left upper sternal border, but they are usually loudest at the right upper sternal border and are associated with a constant ejection click. The murmur of a ventricular septal defect is pansystolic (see p. 277) and loudest along the left lower sternal border. Unfortunately, wide radiation of the murmurs over the entire precordium is the rule in infancy, and it may be difficult to localize the point of maximum intensity. The minimum evaluation of a heart murmur that is loud or that persists for 24 hours consists of a chest radiograph and an electrocardiogram. If these tests are normal and there is no evidence of cyanosis or congestive heart failure, elective referral to a pediatric cardiologist is sufficient.

REFERENCES

Akera, T., and Brody, T. M.: The role of Na +,K + -ATPase in the inotropic action of digitalis. Pharmacol. Rev. 29:187, 1977.

Bargeron, L. M., Jr., Elliott, L. P., Soto, B., Bream, P. R., and Curry, G. C.: Axial cineangiography in congenital heart disease, Section I: Concept, technical and anatomic considerations. Circulation 56:1075, 1977.

Braudo, M., and Rowe, R. D.: Auscultation of the heart in the early neonatal period. Am. J. Dis. Child. 101:575, 1961.

Braunwald, E., and Swan, H. J. C. (Eds.): Cooperative study on cardiac catheterization. Circulation 37–38 (suppl. III), 1968.

Cassels, D. E., and Ziegler, R. F. (Eds.): Electrocardiography in Infants and Children. New York, Grune and Stratton, 1966.

Coceani, F., and Olley, P. M.: The response of the ductus arteriosus to prostaglandins. Can. J. Physiol. Pharmacol. 51:220, 1973.

Coceani, F., and Olley, P. M.: Role of prostaglandins, prostacyclin, and thromboxanes in the control of prenatal patency and postnatal closure of the ductus arteriosus. Semin. Perinatol. 4:109, 1980.

Danilowicz, D., Rudolph, A. M., and Hoffman, J. I. E.: Vascular resistance in the large pulmonary arteries in infancy. Circulation 31–32 (suppl. II) 74, 1965.

Davignon, A., Rautaharju, P., Boiselle, E., Soumis, F., Megelas, M., and Choquette, A.: Normal ECG standards for infants and children. Pediatr. Cardiol. 1:123, 1979–1980.

Dawes, G. S.: Foetal and Neonatal Physiology. Chicago, Year Book Medical Publishers, Inc., 1968.

Driscoll, D. J., Gillette, P. C., and McNamara, D. G.: The use of dopamine in children. J. Pediatr. 92:309, 1978.

Elliott, L. P., Bargeron, L. M., Jr., Bream, P. R., Soto, B., and Curry, G. C.: Axial cineangiography in congenital heart disease, Section II: Specific lesions. Circulation 56:1084, 1977.

Emmanouilides, G. C., Moss, A. J., Duffie, E. R., Jr., and Adams, F. H.: Pulmonary arterial pressure changes in human newborn infants from birth to 3 days of age. J. Pediatr. 65:327, 1964.

Fellows, K. E., Keane, J. F., and Freed, M. D.: Angled views in cineangiocardiography of congenital heart disease. Circulation 56:485, 1977.

Freed, M. D., Heymann, M. A., Lewis, A. B., Roehl, S. L., and Kensey, R. C.: Prostaglandin E-1 in infants with ductus arteriosus dependent congenital heart disease. Circulation 64:899, 1981.

Friedman, W. F., Pool, P. E., Jacobowitz, D., Seagren, S. C., and Braunwald, E.: Sympathetic innervation of the developing rabbit heart. Circ. Res. 23:25, 1968.

Fyler, D. C., Buckley, L. P., Hellenbrand, W. E., and Cohn, H. E.: Report of the New England Regional Infant Cardiac Program. Pediatrics 65(suppl.):375, 1980.

Goldberg, S. J., Allen, H. D., and Sahn, D. J.: Pediatric and Adolescent Echocardiography. 2nd ed. Chicago, Year Book Medical Publishers, Inc., 1980.

Grantham, J. J., and Chonko, A. M.: The physiological basis and clinical use of diuretics. In Brenner, B. M., and Stein, J. H. (Eds.): Sodium and Water Homeostasis, Volume 1. New York, Churchill-Livingstone, 1978, p. 178.

Hagan, A. D., Deeley, W. J., Sahn, D., and Friedman, W. F.: Echocardiographic criteria for normal newborn infants. Circulation 48:1221, 1973.

Heymann, M. A., and Rudolph, A. M.: Effects of congenital heart disease on fetal and neonatal circulations. Prog. Cardiovasc. Dis. 15:115, 1972.

Lang, D., and Von Bernuth, G.: Serum concentration and serum half-life of Digoxin in premature and mature newborns. Pediatrics 59:902, 1977.

Lang, P., Williams, R. G., Norwood, W. I., and Castaneda, A. R.: The hemodynamic effects of dopamine in infants after corrective cardiac surgery. J. Pediatr. 96:630, 1980.

Lees, M. H.: Cyanosis of the newborn infant. Recognition and clinical evaluation. J. Pediatr. 77:484, 1970.

Lind, J., Stern, L., and Wegelius, C.: Human Foetal and Neonatal Circulation. Springfield, Ill., Charles C Thomas, 1964.

Lind, J., and Wegelius, C.: Human fetal circulation: changes in the cardiovascular system at birth and disturbances in the post-natal closure of the foramen ovale and ductus arteriosus. Cold Spring Harbor Symp. Quant. Biol. *19*:109, 1954.

Meyer, R. A.: Pediatric Echocardiography. Philadelphia, Lea and Febiger, 1977.

Moller, J. I I., and Neal, W. A.: Heart Disease in Infancy. New York, Appleton-Century-Crofts, 1981.

Norwood, W. I., Lang, P., and Hansen, D. D.: Physiologic repair of aortic atresia—hypoplastic left heart syndrome. N. Engl. J. Med. *308*:23, 1983.

Rowe, R. D., Freedom, R. M., Mehrizi, A., and Bloom, K. R.: The Neonate with Congenital Heart Disease. 2nd ed. Philadelphia, W. B. Saunders Company, 1981.

Rudolph, A. M.: The changes in the circulation after birth. Their importance in congenital heart disease. Circulation *41*:343, 1970.

Rudolph, A. M.: Congenital Diseases of the Heart. Chicago, Year Book Medical Publishers, Inc., 1974.

Rushmer, R. F.: Cardiac compensation, hypertrophy, myopathy, and congestive heart failure. *In* Rushmer, R. F. (Eds.): Cardiovascular Dynamics. Philadelphia, W. B. Saunders Co., 1976.

Sheldon, C. A., Friedman, W. F., and Sybers, H. D.: Scanning electron microscopy of fetal and neonatal lamb cardiac cells. J. Mol. Cell Cardiol. *8*:853, 1976.

Silverman, N. H., and Snider, A. R.: Two Dimensional Echocardiography in Congenital Heart Disease. Norwalk, Conn., Appleton-Century-Crofts, 1982.

Smith, T. W., Haber, E., Yeatman, L., and Butler, V. P., Jr.: Reversal of advanced digoxin intoxication with Fab fragments of digoxin specific antibodies. N. Engl. J. Med. *294*:797, 1976.

Stanger, P., Heymann, M. A., Tarnoff, H., Hoffman, J. I. E., and Rudolph, A. M.: Complications of cardiac catheterization of neonates, infants, and children. A three-year study. Circulation *50*:595, 1974.

Swischuk, L. E.: Plain Film Interpretation in Congenital Heart Disease 2nd ed. Baltimore, The Williams and Wilkins Co., 1979.

Tajik, A. J., Seward, J. B., Hagler, D. J., Mair, D. D., and Lie, J. T.: Two-dimensional realtime ultrasonic imaging of the heart and great vessels. Technique, image orientation, structure identification, and validation. Mayo Clin. Proc. *53*:271, 1978.

Wettrell, G., and Andersson, K. E.: Clinical pharmacokinetics of digoxin in infants. Clin. Pharmacokinet. *2*:17, 1977.

Williams, R. G., and Tucker, C. R.: Echocardiographic Diagnosis of Congenital Heart Disease. Boston, Little, Brown and Company, 1977.

Ziegler, R. F.: Electrocardiographic Studies in Normal Infants and Children. Springfield, Ill., Charles C Thomas, 1951.

27

Congenital Cardiac Malformations

By Michael D. Freed

In this chapter, the incidence, etiology, and embryology of congenital heart disease will be discussed, and the current status of some common cardiac problems presenting in the first month of life will subsequently be reviewed. The discussion of each cardiac malformation will understandably be brief; those readers interested in a more comprehensive consideration of this subject are encouraged to consult one of three textbooks on newborn heart disease by Godman and Marquis (1979), Moller and Neal (1981), and Rowe and coworkers (1981).

Incidence. Congenital malformations of the heart occur in about eight of every 1000 livebirths and represent about 10 per cent of all congenital malformations. It is difficult to obtain precise incidence data for all congenital heart disease, since signs and symptoms of heart disease may be absent at birth and not be evident until years or, as in the case of a bicuspid aortic valve, decades later. In addition, some neonates with murmurs at birth do not have significant disease; the murmurs are due to normal turbulence of the closing ductus arteriosus or physiologic turbulence in the pulmonary artery.

The New England Regional Infant Cardiac Program (NERICP) provides valuable information on the incidence of specific lesions (Fyler et al., 1980). Between July, 1968 and July, 1974, careful data were kept on all the infants in the region who were sick enough to require cardiac catheterization or surgery or who died from their congenital heart disease. During the 6-year period, there were 2251 infants with *critical* heart disease among 1,083,083 births, an incidence of 2.08/1000 livebirths. The incidence is much lower than the aforementioned overall incidence of 8/1000, since those with trivial ventricular defects, atrial defects, or other milder forms of heart disease are not included. Since this chapter deals with critical heart disease, however, these data are relevant.

The relative frequency of the different diagnoses are listed in Table 27–1. Ventricular septal defects, the most common type of heart disease in older children, are the most common type of heart disease in neonates as well. In contrast, neonates with atrial defects are rarely symptomatic and thus represent a small percentage of this group, although they represent a large proportion of older children with heart disease.

In the NERICP study, 58 per cent (1310/2251) of infants with congenital heart disease were seen in the first 4 weeks of life and 896 (40 per cent) were seen in the first week. The most common diagnosis found in each age group (during the first, second, third, and fourth weeks of life) is listed in Table 27–2.

Transposition of the great arteries is the most common lesion seen in the first week of life, coarctation is the most common malformation seen during the second week, and ventricular septal defects are the most common abnormalities observed in the third and fourth weeks of life.

Etiology. Although a topic of great interest over the past two decades, there is as yet no clear understanding of the etiology of most congenital heart disease. In about 8 per cent of children with heart disease, there are clear genetic causes (Nora, 1977). Most of these are associated with obvious chromosomal anomalies. Down syndrome (trisomy 21) is associated with congenital heart disease in 50 per cent of cases, trisomy 18 and 13 in more than 90 per cent, and the deletion syndromes of chromosomes 18, 13, 5, and 4, in 25 to 50 per cent.

Congenital heart disease is also associated with many of the single mutant gene syndromes. Autosomal dominant syndromes associated with heart disease include Holt-Oram (atrial defects), Alport (ventricular defects), leopard (pulmonary stenosis), Noonan (pulmonary stenosis), and tuberous sclerosis (myocardial rhabdomyoma). Autosomal recessive syndromes associated with heart disease include Ellis–van Creveld (single atrium) as well as Friedreich ataxia and Laurence-Moon-Biedl (ventricular defects). In total, however, the single gene syndromes account for only about 3 per cent of all congenital heart disease.

Environmental factors may play an important role in the etiology of congenital cardiac malformations. Maternal ingestion of drugs such as thalidomide, the antimetabolites, and Coumadin have been shown to be associated with a high incidence of cardiac malformations, and recent interest has focused on congenital malformations associated with the maternal ingestion of alcohol. Several viral infections have been shown to be associated with congenital cardiac malformations, but only congenital rubella, which results in peripheral pulmonic stenosis and patent ductus arteriosus, is known to be clinically significant. In total, however, environmental factors account for no more than 2 per cent of all cases of congenital heart disease.

In more than 85 per cent of children with congenital heart disease, the etiology is unclear. The best explanation seems to be a multifactorial type of inheritance in which a hereditary predisposition for cardiac anomalies in concert with an environmental "trigger" at a vulnerable period during cardiac morphogenesis causes the congenital anomaly (Nora, 1977). This model allows calculation of risk of recurrence among other children in an affected family. For most congenital heart disease, the recurrence risk is between 1 and 5 per cent, with the more common abnormalities falling in the higher end of the range. Several large studies of the families of children with congenital heart disease have confirmed these approximations, although in 1982 Whittemore and coworkers found a much higher recurrence rate, 14.2 per cent, in children born of mothers with congenital heart disease.

Children with congenital heart disease frequently

Table 27–1. Diagnostic Frequencies of Infants*

Diagnosis	Infants		1969–1974, No./1000 livebirths	Number of livebirths/ affected
	(No.)	(Per Cent)		
Ventricular septal defect	374	15.7	0.345	2896
D-transposition of great arteries	236	9.9	0.218	4589
Tetralogy of Fallot	212	8.9	0.196	5109
Coarctation of aorta	179	7.5	0.165	6051
Hypoplastic left heart syndrome	177	7.4	0.163	6119
Patent ductus arteriosus	146	6.1	0.135	7418
Endocardial cushion defect	119	5.0	0.110	9101
Heterotaxias (dextro-, meso-, levo-, asplenia)	95	4.0	0.088	11401
Pulmonary stenosis	79	3.3	0.073	13710
Pulmonary atresia with intact ventricular septum	75	3.1	0.069	14441
Atrial septal defect secundum	70	2.9	0.065	15473
Total anomalous pulmonary venous return	63	2.6	0.058	17192
Myocardial disease	61	2.6	0.056	17755
Tricuspid atresia	61	2.6	0.056	17755
Single ventricle	58	2.4	0.054	18674
Aortic stenosis	45	1.9	0.041	24069
Double outlet right ventricle	35	1.5	0.032	30945
Truncus arteriosus	33	1.4	0.030	32820
L-transposition of great arteries	16	0.7	0.015	67693
Other heart disease	117	4.9	0.108	9257
TOTAL	2251	94.4	2.08	

* The diagnostic frequency of infants with congenital heart disease severe enough to require cardiac catheterization or cardiac surgery or to cause death in the New England Regional Infant Cardiac Program, 1968 through 1974. The group with coarctation of the aorta contains 21 infants with an interrupted aortic arch.

(Adapted from Fyler, D. C., et al. Pediatrics 65[suppl.]:375, 1980.)

have associated extracardiac anomalies (Fyler et al., 1980) that involve the skeletal, gastrointestinal, or genitourinary system. Such findings suggest that the environmental trigger may affect several organs undergoing morphogenesis at the same time.

Embryology. Although knowledge about the embryologic development of the heart is helpful in understanding diagnosis and management of children with congenital heart disease, the subject is complex, incompletely understood, and, for the most part, beyond the scope of this chapter (Hamilton and Mossman, 1972; Langman, 1981).

The heart appears on the eighteenth day after conception and is normally complete by the fortieth day, when the embryo is approximately 15mm (3/4 in) long. Initially, the heart is a straight tube ventral to the gut and consists of, from cephalad to caudad, the truncus arteriosus, bulbus cordis (later right ventricle), primitive ventricle (later left ventricle), and atrium. Soon after the initiation of the heart beat at 20 days, the heart tube normally loops to the right so that the bulbus cordis lies to the right of the primitive ventricle. During the fourth week after conception, the heart continues to twist and bend so that the atrium lies above the primitive ventricles. During the fifth week, the ventricular septum forms, and the aorta and pulmonary artery are septated from the truncus arteriosus, with the conus muscle under the aorta being resorbed so that the aorta comes into continuity with the left ventricle. The endocardial tissue in the central portion of the heart differentiates into separate mitral and tricuspid valves, and the ostium primum closes, separating the right and left atrium. Thus, by the end of the fifth week, the "in series" circulation of the primitive cardiac tube is exchanged for the "in parallel" circulation characteristic of later fetal life. During the sixth week after conception, the membranous septum closes and anatomic cardiac development is completed, the first organ system to do so.

The vessels leading to and exiting from the heart develop at about the same time. By the third week of gestation, a total of six pairs of aortic arches have formed, although not all are present at the same time. Over the next 3 weeks the first, second, and fifth pairs disappear. The third arch becomes the right and left internal carotid artery, the left fourth arch the ascending aorta, and the right fourth becomes the innominate and part of the right subclavian artery. The pulmonary arteries arise from the sixth arch, with the sixth right becoming disconnected from the aorta to become the right pulmonary artery, and the left from the left sixth forming the ductus arteriosus and left pulmonary artery.

Congenital anomalies may be due to any one or more of the following developmental errors:

1. *Aplasia or agenesis (failure of development).*
2. *Hypoplasia (incomplete or defective development).*
3. *Dysplasia (abnormal development).*
4. *Malposition.*
5. *Failure of fusion of adjoining parts.*
6. *Abnormal fusion.*
7. *Incomplete resorption.*
8. *Abnormal persistence of a vessel.*
9. *Early obliteration of a vessel.*

The multitude of things that can go wrong during cardiac morphogenesis reflects the complexity of the embryogenesis of the heart.

Cyanotic Congenital Heart Disease

COMPLETE TRANSPOSITION OF THE GREAT ARTERIES

Anatomy. In transposition of the great arteries (TGA), the position of the great arteries is reversed; that is, the aorta arises anteriorly from the right ventricle and the pulmonary artery posteriorly from the left ventricle. The pulmonary and systemic circulations are therefore arranged in parallel rather than in

Table 27–2. Diagnosis of Infants at Selected Ages*

0–6 days (n = 896)		7–13 days (n = 210)		14–20 days (n = 116)		21–27 days (n = 88)		0–28 days (n = 1310)	
(Per Cent)		*(Per Cent)*		*(Per Cent)*		*(Per Cent)*		*(Per Cent)*	
TGA	17	CoA	19	VSD	20	VSD	21	TGA	14
HLH	12	VSD	15	TGA	17	TGA	9	HLH	11
Lung	10	HLH	11	CoA	16	TOF	8	VSD	9
TOF	9	TGA	9	TOF	8	CoA	8	CoA	9
CoA	7	TOF	6	ECD	6	TAPVR	8	TOF	8
PA	7	Truncus	4	Hetero	6	PDA	7	Lung	7
Hetero	6	Hetero	4	PDA	4	TA	6	PA	5
VSD	7	SV	4	Lung	4	ECD	5	Hetero	5
PDA	4	TAPVR	3	TAPVR	3	SV	3	TA	3
						Lung	3	ECD	3

* Diagnostic frequency of infants less than 4 weeks of age. *Abbreviations:* AS = aortic stenosis, CoA = coarctation of the aorta, ECD = endocardial cushion defect, Hetero = heterotaxy syndrome, HLH = hypoplastic left heart syndrome, Lung = primary lung disease, PA = pulmonary atresia with an intact ventricular septum, PDA = patent ductus arteriosus, SV = single ventricle, TA = tricuspid atresia, TAPVR = total anomalous pulmonary venous return, TGA = transposition of the great arteries, TOF = tetralogy of Fallot, Truncus = truncus arteriosus, VSD = ventricular septal defect.
(Adapted from Fyler, D. C., et al.: Pediatrics 65[suppl.]:375, 1980.)

series, with the systemic venous blood passing through the right heart chambers and then back out to the body and pulmonary venous blood traversing the left heart and returning to the lungs (Fig. 27–1). Survival after birth depends on mixing between the circuits.

The prefixes "D" and "L" are used to denote whether the aorta arises to the right (dextro) or to the left (levo) of the pulmonary artery.

TGA in the neonate is often an isolated defect, but other associated malformations involving defects of the atrial or ventricular septum, stenosis or atresia of the pulmonic valve, and anomalies of the atrioventricular valves are not uncommon and may alter the physiology considerably. Interestingly, extracardiac anomalies are unusual in neonates with TGA.

The embryology of this condition is still not completely understood. Although it was once thought that this anomaly was due to failure of spiraling of the truncal septum, Van Praagh and Van Praagh noted in 1966 that during cardiac development both great vessels are initially elevated by muscular tissue (conus), and they suggested that differential resorption of the subpulmonary rather than subaortic conus allows the pulmonic valve rather than aortic to be inferior and posterior and therefore in continuity with the left ventricle, with the aortic valve superior and anterior in continuity with the right ventricle, with the rest of the heart unaffected.

Incidence.   TGA occurs in slightly more than one per 5000 livebirths (0.218 per 1000) and was the most common form of cyanotic congenital heart dis-

ease in the New England Regional Infant Cardiac Program. Of infants presenting in the region with critical heart disease in the first week of life, 17 per cent had TGA.

Hemodynamics.   In transposition, the pulmonary and systemic circulations are arranged in parallel rather than in series, with the aorta arising from the right ventricle and the pulmonary artery from the left. In utero, there is little disruption in fetal hemodynamics (Fig. 27–2), since blood returning from the systemic and pulmonary veins passes unimpeded into the atrium and ventricles in the normal fashion. Blood from the right ventricle is pumped into the ascending aorta and then to the systemic arteries and placenta. Blood from the left ventricle passes into the pulmonary artery, and then, because of the high pulmonary resistance, most is diverted into the ductus arteriosus and descending aorta. The only variation from the normal fetal circulation is that the slightly less saturated blood from the superior vena cava is preferentially shunted to the head vessels rather than through the ductus arteriosus, and the more saturated blood from the inferior vena cava is shunted to the lungs rather than to the cerebral circulation. In spite of these differences, in utero development appears normal, and thus far no major extrauterine abnormalities have been identified.

After birth, newborns completely depend on mixing between pulmonary and systemic circulations for survival. For a while the fetal pathways, the ductus arteriosus and foramen ovale, suffice. By a few hours of age, the pulmonary resistance is significantly lower than the systemic, so shunting of hypoxemic blood from the aorta to the pulmonary artery is facilitated. Since the pulmonary circuit cannot be overloaded, obligatory shunting of pulmonary venous return from

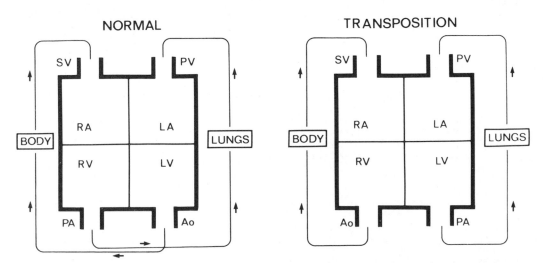

Figure 27–1.   A schematic diagram of the circulation in the normal neonate and the neonate with transposition of the great arteries. In the normal neonate, the circulation is arranged in series; that is, venous blood goes through the right heart chambers to the lungs for oxygenation and then through the left side of the heart to be delivered to the body. In the neonate with transposition, the circulation is arranged in parallel with venous blood passing through the right side of the heart to the aorta and body and oxygenated blood passing through the left side of the heart to the lungs. Mixing between the circuits is necessary for survival after birth. Ao = aorta; LA = left atrium; LV = left ventricle; PA = pulmonary artery; PV = pulmonary vein; RA = right atrium; RV = right ventricle; SV = systemic veins.

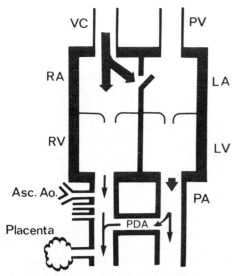

Figure 27–2. Schematic diagram of the fetal circulation in transposition of the great arteries. Venous blood returning to the heart via the vena cava passes either into the right atrium, right ventricle, and aorta or through the foramen ovale to the left atrium, left ventricle, and pulmonary artery. As in the normal fetus, most of the blood entering the main pulmonary artery is diverted through the ductus arteriosus into the descending aorta and placenta because of the high pulmonary vascular resistance. Asc Ao = ascending aorta; LA = left atrium; LV = left ventricle; PA = pulmonary artery; PDA = patent ductus arteriosus; PV = pulmonary vein; RA = right atrium; RV = right ventricle; VC = vena cava.

left atrium to right atrium occurs. This bidirectional shunting from aorta to pulmonary artery and left atrium to right atrium improves mixing and prevents severe cyanosis. As the ductus arteriosus closes, however, the obligatory shunting is eliminated and the only site of mixing is the foramen ovale. Although some bidirectional shunting may occur allowing deoxygenated blood to get to the lungs and oxygenated blood to the systemic circulation, this is usually inadequate, and severe systemic hypoxemia (Po$_2$, 15 to 40 torr; O$_2$ saturation, 30 to 60) results. Occasionally, a small ventricular defect may be present, slightly ameliorating the hypoxemia.

Clinical Manifestations. There is a strong sex predilection in TGA, with males outnumbering females by almost 2:1. Infants are usually cyanotic within the first 12 to 24 hours after birth. In the New England Regional Infant Cardiac Program, 59 per cent of infants with TGA were seen at a cardiac center within the first 2 days of life, and 79 per cent were observed by the end of the second week.

The physical examination is usually unrewarding except for generalized cyanosis. Although peripheral pulses may be somewhat bounding and the right ventricular impulse slightly hyperactive, the heart sounds are usually normal, with physiologic splitting of the second sound present about half the time. Prominent heart murmurs are uncommon, although there may be a short grade 2/6 systolic murmur along the left sternal border. A loud murmur should alert one to the possibility of associated heart disease (e.g., a ven-

tricular septal defect). Signs of congestive failure are usually absent, although tachypnea may be present, probably as a compensatory mechanism for the hypoxemia.

Since there is little disturbance in the intrauterine blood flow, the electrocardiogram is usually normal showing right axis deviation and right ventricular hypertrophy that is within the normal limits for age.

The chest radiograph is also usually normal for a newborn, although the relative anterior-posterior position of the great vessels and the usual (although unexplained) absence of a thymic shadow give the narrow appearance of the superior mediastinum frequently described as an "egg-on-side" appearance (Fig. 27–3). The pulmonary blood flow is rarely increased in the first few days of life, although it may be increased in infants who present later.

With the recent development of echocardiography, the diagnosis of TGA can usually be made with certainty before cardiac catheterization. Since in D transposition the posterior great vessel arising from the left ventricle is the pulmonary artery rather than the aorta, one can establish the diagnosis with two-dimensional echocardiography by identifying the posterior great vessel and tracing it to its bifurcation into right and left branches or by tracing the anterior great vessel to the innominate, carotid, or subclavian branches (Fig. 27–4). Even with M-mode echocardiography, one can recognize TGA by finding the

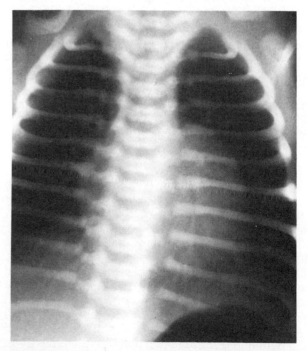

Figure 27–3. Chest radiograph in the anteroposterior projection in a neonate with transposition of the great arteries and an intact ventricular septum. The upper mediastinum is narrowed because of the anteroposterior relationship of the aorta and pulmonary artery. The heart is not enlarged. The pulmonary blood flow is not decreased.

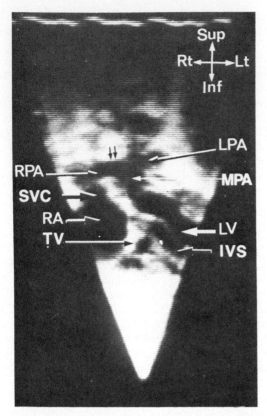

Figure 27–4. *A,* Right anterior oblique angiogram that shows d-transposition of the great arteries. *B,* Longitudinal subxiphoid two-dimensional echocardiogram that shows d-transposition of the great arteries. The main pulmonary artery (MPA) arises from the left ventricle (LV) and bifurcates into the right pulmonary artery (RPA) and left pulmonary artery (LPA). SVC = superior vena cava; RA = right atrium; TV = tricuspid valve; IVS = interventricular septum; IVS = MPA-RPA junction. (From Bierman, F. Z., and Williams, R. G.: Prospective diagnosis of d-transposition of the great arteries in neonates by subxiphoid two-dimensional echocardiography. *Circulation 60*:1496, 1979. Reproduced with permission.)

anterior semilunar valve (aortic) to the right of the posterior semilunar valve (Aziz et al., 1982) rather than to left (as seen with normally related great arteries).

Cardiac catheterization and angiography confirm the diagnosis. Saturations on the right side of the heart are often very low (<40 per cent), with a slight increase between vena cava and right atrium. The saturation in the aorta is about the same as the right ventricle. Saturations in the pulmonary veins and left heart chambers are normal or slightly increased, and the pulmonary artery (when entered) often has a saturation of 92 to 95 per cent. The atrial pressures are usually normal and equal. Any difference between right and left atrial pressure suggests a significant shunt at the ventricular or ductal level. The left ventricular pressure is usually less than simultaneous sys-

temic arterial pressure; TGA is the only heart disease in which this is true. Angiography confirms that the aorta arises from the right ventricle and the pulmonary artery arises from the left ventricle (Fig. 27–4). A balloon atrial septostomy (see discussion of treatment further on) is usually performed.

Diagnosis.   Transposition of the great arteries should be strongly suspected in any cyanotic newborn showing normal-to-increased pulmonary blood flow on the radiograph and right ventricular hypertrophy on the electrocardiogram. Indeed, a severely hypoxemic infant breathing comfortably with a normal physical examination, chest radiograph, and electrocardiogram almost invariably has transposition. All other types of cyanotic congenital heart disease are associated with diminished or congested pulmonary vascular markings on the radiograph and a single second heart sound. Persistent fetal circulation can usually be distinguished by echocardiography.

Treatment.   Untreated, TGA in infants is associated with a dismal prognosis, since 30 per cent die in the first week and 50 per cent succumb in the first months of life (Liebman et al., 1969). Improved survival depends on early recognition and transfer to a cardiac center. The management involves three phases: rapid correction of metabolic derangements, palliation, and later correction. If the infant is acidotic with a pH of less than 7.25 when first seen, sodium bicarbonate should be given to correct the base deficit.

In those who are severely acidotic or in whom further palliation must be delayed, prostaglandin E_1 has been employed to open the ductus arteriosus and improve mixing and oxygenation (Lang et al., 1979).

The palliation of choice is balloon atrial septostomy, developed and described by Rashkind and Miller in 1966. A specially made balloon catheter is inserted into the femoral or umbilical vein and advanced through the foramen ovale into the left atrium and then inflated. The catheter is quickly withdrawn from left to right, tearing the fibrous tissue of the fossa ovalis. This iatrogenic atrial septal defect often increases the mixing between the systemic and pulmonary circulations to such an extent that the Pa_{O_2} rises into the 30s and the saturation elevates into the 70s. Frequently, this improvement is sustained until corrective surgery can be undertaken, but if the Pa_{O_2} drops back into the mid-20s, as it occasionally does, surgical septectomy or correction is required.

"Corrective" surgery is usually performed at about 6 months of age but is being done earlier at many centers, including our own, should palliation fail. Although earlier attempts to correct TGA anatomically with an arterial switch operation (reversing the aorta and pulmonary artery) were unsuccessful, recently there has been a revived interest in this technique (Jatene et al., 1976; Yacob et al., 1980). However, its place in the management of the neonate remains controversial. The more standard approach is to insert a baffle in the atrium to divert systemic venous blood through the mitral valve, left ventricle, and pulmonary artery to the lungs and pulmonary venous blood through the tricuspid valve and right ventricle to the aorta (Mustard et al., 1964; Senning, 1959). This physiologically corrects the circulation, although anatomically the right ventricle remains the systemic ventricle and the left ventricle pumps blood to the lungs.

Prognosis. Although it is difficult to assess long-term prognosis in a time of rapid advances, several studies in the mid-1970s (Gutgesell et al., 1979; Paul, 1977) based on patients operated on in the late 1960s show a 4- to 5-year survival of 60 to 70 per cent. The 1983 review by Marx and coworkers showed a 6-year cumulative survival rate of 78 per cent for children operated on between 1972 and 1978 and a 2-year survival rate of 93 per cent for those operated on between 1978 and 1980. With further advances, these data will undoubtedly continue to improve. Long-term sequelae have involved pulmonary or systemic venous obstruction at the site of the interatrial baffle, atrial arrhythmias, and right (systemic) ventricular dysfunction.

TETRALOGY OF FALLOT

Anatomy. In 1888, Etienne Fallot described a series of cyanotic patients with a ventricular septal defect, pulmonary stenosis, right ventricular hypertrophy, and an aorta that appeared to be over the ventricular septum. For many years, it has been appreciated that the latter two manifestations are secondary to the former two lesions.

The ventricular septal defect location is quite predictably high in ventricular septum; additional defects are present in 15 per cent of the patients. The degree of pulmonic obstruction at the infundibulum (sub-valvular) or secondarily at the pulmonary valve or peripheral pulmonary arteries is quite variable, ranging from mild stenosis to complete atresia, and accounts for the variability of presentation. Associated anomalies include atrial septal defects, right aortic arch (25 per cent), and anomalies of the coronary arteries (5 per cent).

Incidence. Tetralogy of Fallot (TOF) occurred slightly less frequently than transposition in the New England experience (0.196 per 1000, or 1 of every 5000, livebirths) and accounted for 9 per cent of infants presenting in the first week of life.

Hemodynamics. In utero, there does not seem to be any major hemodynamic disturbance, and consequently, newborns with tetralogy are well developed at birth. During fetal life, the aorta carries an increased percentage of combined ventricular output, with the exact proportion a function of the degree of pulmonic stenosis (Fig. 27–5). The ductus arteriosus is smaller than normal, since its flow is di-

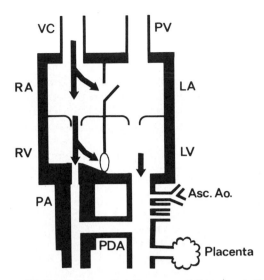

Figure 27–5. Schematic diagram of the circulation in the fetus with tetralogy of Fallot. Because of the right ventricular outflow obstruction, some of the right ventricular output passes across the ventricular septal defect into the left ventricle and out the aorta. If the pulmonary stenosis is severe, pulmonary blood flow may be augmented by blood from the aorta passing through the ductus arteriosus. Blood flow to the placenta is unimpeded. The abbreviations in this diagram are the same as those used in Figure 27–2.

minished, and it may be quite tortuous. Since there is no volume or pressure overload within the heart, the ventricles and atrioventricular valves usually develop normally.

After birth, the degree of shunting depends on the severity of the pulmonary stenosis and the relative pulmonary and systemic arteriolar resistance. In the newborn with severe pulmonary stenosis, the resistance to blood passing out the right ventricular outflow tract is very high, and desaturated venous blood preferentially passes through the ventricular septal defect into the aorta, resulting in arterial hypoxemia and cyanosis. If the pulmonary stenosis is mild, there may be little resistance to blood passing out the pulmonary artery; infants with this condition may behave like those with a ventricular septal defect, with increasing left-to-right shunt and heart failure as the pulmonary arteriolar resistance drops over the first weeks of life. The usual hallmarks of tetralogy of Fallot, arterial hypoxemia and cyanosis, may be completely absent in this group at first. Occasionally, mild-to-moderate pulmonary stenosis may occur in a balanced situation in which pulmonary and systemic resistances are equal and little shunt in either direction occurs; often these infants will shunt right-to-left with crying.

Clinical Manifestations. The presentation of infants with tetralogy is a function of the degree of pulmonary stenosis. Those with severe obstruction usually present in the first days with extreme cyanosis as the ductus arteriosus closes. Those with lesser degrees of pulmonary stenosis may be only mildly cyanotic and present with a systolic ejection murmur along the left sternal border in the delivery room or in the nursery. The pulmonary component of the second heart sound is diminished or inaudible. Signs of congestive heart failure are absent except in a small group with an absent pulmonary valve who present with a to-and-fro murmur at the left upper sternal border due to pulmonary stenosis and regurgitation.

Tetralogy "spells," attacks of paroxysmal dyspnea associated with irritability, extreme cyanosis, and loss of the systolic murmur are an emergency, since cerebral hypoxemia may lead to convulsions, coma, and death. Spells are fortunately unusual in the first months of life.

Since the right ventricle receives normal flow in utero, the electrocardiogram of the newborn is normal, showing right axis deviation and right ventricular hypertrophy.

The heart size on the chest radiograph is usually normal, since neither of the atria or the ventricles is exposed to a volume overload. In those who are very hypoxemic, the pulmonary blood flow is decreased, since venous blood is being diverted away from the lungs to the systemic circuit. The main pulmonary artery segment is often diminished, giving the classic "coeur-en-sabot" appearance (Fig. 27–6). A right aortic arch is present in one fourth of the cases.

On M-mode echocardiography, the anterior wall

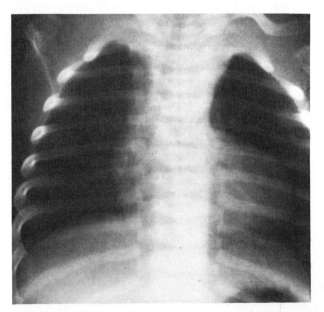

Figure 27–6. Plain anteroposterior roentgenogram from a newborn with tetralogy of Fallot. Note the absent main pulmonary artery segment and uplifted apex (coeur-en-sabot). The pulmonary blood flow is decreased.

of the aorta can be seen anterior to the right septal surface (overriding). The ventricular septal defect can often be appreciated by a drop-out of septal echoes under the aorta (Tajik et al., 1973). The two-dimensional study shows the anatomy quite clearly, especially from the subxiphoid view (Sanders et al., 1982).

Cardiac catheterization and angiography are indicated if the two-dimensional echocardiogram is equivocal or if surgical intervention is contemplated.

A right ventricular angiogram with the baby "sitting" to obtain 40 degrees of cranial angulation will allow one to visualize the infundibular, valvular, and peripheral pulmonary stenosis (Fig. 27–7), and a left ventricular angiogram in the left anterior oblique with axial angulation or hepatoclavicular view will outline the ventricular septal defect(s) and the coronary arteries. Occasionally, an aortic angiogram in the left anterior oblique is necessary to outline the origin and course of the anterior descending coronary artery. This is important, since it occasionally arises as the first branch of the right rather than left coronary artery and traverses the external surface of the right ventricular infundibulum to reach the interventricular groove. Its presence prevents easy patching of the subpulmonic stenosis at surgical repair; since division of this large vessel is almost invariably fatal, a conduit to bridge over this vessel may be necessary.

Diagnosis. The cyanotic infant with decreased pulmonary blood flow and a normal heart size on the chest radiograph, right axis deviation and right ventricular hypertrophy on the electrocardiogram, and a systolic ejection murmur on examination, usually has tetralogy of Fallot (see Differential Diagnosis, p. 285).

Infants with a systolic murmur without cyanosis may be confused with patients with isolated valvular pulmonary stenosis or even those with a ventricular septal defect. More complicated lesions with a physiology similar to that of tetralogy of Fallot, ventricular defect, and pulmonary stenosis must be differentiated by echocardiography or angiocardiography. Examples are double outlet ventricle with pulmonary stenosis, single ventricle with pulmonary stenosis, and transposition (either D or L).

Treatment. We have reserved treatment for those who are profoundly cyanotic with arterial saturations of less than 75 per cent and those who are having "spells." Garson and coworkers recommend propranolol, 2 to 6 mg/kg/day, for palliation of infants having hypoxic spells, but we have usually resorted to surgery in infants with true spells. In the past, the surgical approach to these infants has been an aortopulmonary shunt between the ascending aorta and right pulmonary artery (Waterston) or between the descending aorta and left pulmonary artery (Potts). More recently, as cardiovascular surgeons have transferred the skills in dealing with small vessels in coronary artery surgery to the neonate with congenital heart disease, the Blalock-Taussig shunt between the subclavian and pulmonary artery on the side opposite the aortic arch has become popular (Arciniegas et al., 1982). Some centers, including our own, have started to perform primary correction on neonates rather than the two-stage palliation and later correction. Although it is still too early to tell, it appears this approach will become increasingly popular in the future (Murphy et al., 1980).

Prognosis. Among the 64 infants in the Regional Infant Cardiac Program with tetralogy of Fallot who were treated medically, there was a 17 per cent mortality rate. Of 102 infants sick enough to require surgery, 30 (29 per cent) died (Fyler et al., 1980). More recently, using total repair within the first year of life in 40 infants, we have had a 10 per cent mortality (Murphy et al., 1980). In those who survive to 1 year without an operation, surgery can be performed with a mortality of less than 5 per cent.

TETRALOGY OF FALLOT WITH PULMONARY ATRESIA

Anatomy. This is the severest form of tetralogy of Fallot, with the deviated parietal band of the infundibulum completely occluding the right ventricular outflow tract. Since there is no antegrade flow through the pulmonic valve, development of the pulmonary arteries depends on flow from the embryologic intersegmental or bronchial arteries. If these insert into the pulmonary arteries proximally, the mediastinal portion of the right and left pulmonary arteries may be of good size. If, however, the collaterals insert well within the hilum of the lungs, the

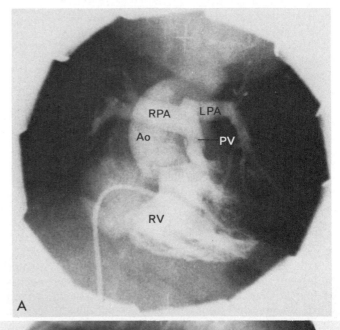

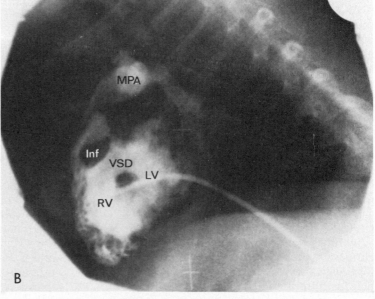

Figure 27–7. The cranially angulated (40 degrees) anteroposterior (*A*) and lateral (*B*) projections of a right ventricular angiogram in a neonate with tetralogy of Fallot. The subpulmonic area (infundibulum) and pulmonary valve are narrowed. The ventricular septal defect is seen on the lateral projection with filling of the left ventricle. Ao = aorta; Inf = infundibulum of the right ventricle; LV = left ventricle; LPA = left pulmonary artery; MPA = main pulmonary artery; PV = pulmonary valve; RPA = right pulmonary artery; RV = right ventricle; VSD = ventricular septal defect.

mediastinal portions may be hypoplastic or even atretic. The postnatal presentation and prognosis of these infants are in great part a function of the intrauterine pulmonary artery development. The ventricular septal defect is invariably large.

Incidence. In the New England Regional Infant Cardiac Program, 46 of 2251 infants seen between 1969 and 1974 had tetralogy of Fallot with pulmonary atresia, representing an incidence of one of every 25,000 births in the region (Fyler et al., 1980).

Hemodynamics. This lesion does not seem to influence the fetal circulation adversely, since in utero pulmonary blood flow is only about 7 per cent of combined ventricular output, a minimal volume that is easily accomodated by a left-to-right shunt through the ductus arteriosus. Since there is no antegrade flow through the pulmonary valve, the combined ventricular output exits the heart through the aorta, which is usually quite dilated.

After birth, flow to the pulmonary arteries continues to be through the ductus arteriosus and collateral vessels. As the ductus usually closes in the first few days of life, the infant depends on flow through the collateral channels. If they are small, hypoxemia may be profound. If the collaterals are huge, pulmonary flow may be large and cyanosis minimal, with congestive heart failure from a torrential left-to-right shunt occasionally being present.

Clinical Features. In the neonate with inadequate collaterals, cyanosis is prominent and increases as the ductus arteriosus constricts. Heart murmurs are frequently absent, although a continuous murmur over the back from the aortopulmonary collaterals may be heard. The second heart sound is single, and a systolic ejection click (presumably from a large aorta) is often present. As in tetralogy of Fallot with pulmonary stenosis, the heart is normal in size, with a concavity in the area of the main pulmonary artery apparent on the radiograph if this region is not obscured by the thymus. The pulmonary flow is usually quite reduced, especially when arterial hypoxemia is profound, and a right aortic arch may be present. The electrocardiogram is usually normal, with a QRS axis of +90 to 180 degrees and a normal degree of right ventricular hypertrophy. On the M-mode echocardiogram, there is overriding of the ventricular septum by the aorta with a small left atrium reflecting diminished pulmonary venous return. The two-dimensional echocardiogram shows the ventricular septal defect and the atretic right ventricular outflow tract.

In the 10 per cent of neonates with large collaterals, congestive heart failure may be the presenting symptom, with cyanosis mild or even absent. Loud continuous murmurs over the chest and back are com-

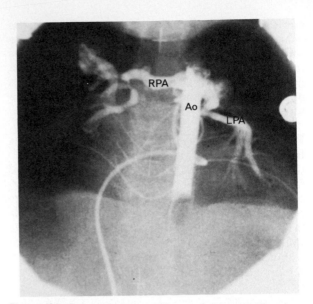

Figure 27–8. Aortogram with cranial angulation in a neonate with tetralogy of Fallot with pulmonary atresia. Both right pulmonary artery (RPA) and left pulmonary artery (LPA) fill from collateral vessels arising from the aorta (Ao).

mon. The cardiac silhouette on radiographs is increased, and the pulmonary vessels are prominent because of the increased blood flow. The cardiogram is usually normal, although some infants have more left ventricular forces than usual because of the left ventricular volume overload. On the M-mode echocardiogram, the aorta overrides the ventricular septum, and the left atrial size is normal or increased.

In all neonates with tetralogy of Fallot with pulmonary atresia, cardiac catheterization demonstrates arterial hypoxemia due to right-to-left shunting at the ventricular level and equal systolic pressure in both ventricles. Visualization of the pulmonary arteries, necessary for treatment, is best accomplished with an aortogram with the patient positioned so that the camera is angled cranially about 40 degrees to allow visualization of the pulmonary arteries filled through the ductus arteriosus or aortopulmonary collaterals (Fig. 27–8).

Diagnosis. A cyanotic infant showing decreased pulmonary blood flow on the radiograph, right ventricular hypertrophy on the EKG, and no murmur or a continuous murmur usually has tetralogy of Fallot with pulmonary atresia (see Differential Diagnosis, p. 286). Neonates with transposition and an intact ventricular septum have no murmurs and may be just as cyanotic but have normal or increased pulmonary blood flow visible on chest radiographs. Infants with total anomalous pulmonary venous return usually show a pulmonary venous congestion pattern on the chest radiographs. More complicated lesions simulating tetralogy of Fallot with pulmonary atresia (e.g., D or L transposition with a ventricular septal defect and pulmonary atresia or single ventricle with pulmonary atresia) must be distinguished by two-dimensional echocardiogram or angiography.

Those infants with large collaterals and congestive heart failure can usually be distinguished from infants with a ventricular septal defect, patent ductus arteriosus, or aortopulmonary window on the basis of their arterial hypoxemia as well as from those with truncus arteriosus and transposition with a ventricular septal defect on the basis of the continuous murmurs.

Treatment. If the collateral vessels are adequate to ensure a systemic saturation of greater than 75 per cent, a conservative approach is warranted in the neonatal period. If the infant becomes progressively cyanotic or acidotic, prostaglandin E_1 will usually improve arterial hypoxemia by maintaining patency of the ductus arteriosus (Olley et al., 1976; Freed et al., 1981). Palliative surgery to ensure patency of the ductus arteriosus by formalin infiltration or construction of an aortopulmonary shunt (Waterston, Potts, Blalock-Taussig) are necessary if oxygenation is inadequate without prostaglandin E_1. Corrective surgery has not yet gained favor among those treating neonates because of the need for a Dacron conduit from right ventricle to pulmonary artery and the certainty of having to replace the conduit as the infant grows. This may be considered the palliation of choice in the future, however. In their 1983 review, Puga and coworkers reported 16 children in whom repair of nonconfluent right and left pulmonary arteries was accomplished with bifurcating conduits. There was no operative mortality.

Prognosis. The prognosis of these infants depends primarily on the size of the pulmonary arteries. If these structures are small, palliative and corrective surgery are quite hazardous. If they are near normal size, the prognosis is improved. Of 46 infants seen in the Regional Infant Cardiac Program between 1969 and 1974, the 1-year mortality was 44 per cent (Fyler et al., 1980).

PULMONARY ATRESIA WITH AN INTACT VENTRICULAR SEPTUM

Anatomy. In pulmonary atresia (PA) with an intact ventricular septum (IVS), the pulmonary valve is an imperforate membrane. In more than 80 per cent of the newborn patients, the right ventricle is moderately or severely hypoplastic, often having a volume of only 1 or 2 ml at birth (Van Praagh et al., 1976). The tricuspid valve annulus is also hypoplastic, corresponding to the size of the right ventricle, and the valve may be stenotic owing to fusion of the chordae. The right atrium is invariably enlarged and hypertrophied and may be enormous in infants with severe tricuspid regurgitation. The high pressure within the right ventricular cavity causes dilation of the normal myocardial sinusoids, and connections are often present between the sinusoids and coronary arteries with flow going from right ventricle to ascending aorta. In contrast to patients with tetralogy of Fallot

associated with pulmonary atresia, the infants with PA and an IVS almost invariably have normal pulmonary arteries.

Incidence. In the Regional Infant Cardiac Program (Fyler et al., 1980), there were 75 infants with PA and an IVS (1 per 14,000 livebirths) 85 per cent of whom were seen by a cardiologist within the first week of life. They represent 7 per cent of infants presenting with heart disease in the first week.

Hemodynamics. Prenatally, egress of blood from the right ventricle is prevented by the pulmonary atresia (Fig. 27–9). All the venous blood returning to the right atrium must pass through the foramen ovale to the left atrium, left ventricle, and ascending aorta; these chambers are dilated compared with those in the normal fetus. Conversely, since flow to the right ventricle is minimal, this chamber is usually quite hypoplastic. The pulmonary blood flow in utero is derived entirely from the aorta via a small, usually quite tortuous, ductus arteriosus. This physiologic arrangement does not disrupt the normal growth and development during fetal life. After birth, there is a continuation of the fetal pattern; the pulmonary blood flow continues to be totally dependent on the small ductus arteriosus. As this closes in the first hours or days of life, the minimal pulmonary blood flow diminishes further, and severe hypoxemia and acidosis follow.

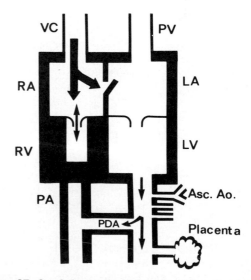

Figure 27–9. Schematic diagram of the circulation in the fetus with pulmonary atresia and an intact ventricular septum. All the systemic venous return from the vena cava passes across the foramen ovale into the left atrium. Pulmonary blood flow before and after birth is derived from the aorta via the ductus arteriosus. Since right ventricular flow is minimal, the chamber remains quite small. The abbreviations in this diagram are the same as those used in Figure 27–2.

Clinical Manifestations. Infants with pulmonary atresia are mildly cyanotic soon after birth but are often intensely cyanotic by 24 hours of age as the ductus arteriosus constricts. On physical examination, the second heart sound is single. A continuous murmur, from left-to-right shunting through the ductus arteriosus, or a systolic regurgitant murmur along the left sternal border secondary to tricuspid regurgitation, may be heard; however, in about 20 per cent of infants no murmur is audible. The liver is enlarged if tricuspid regurgitation is severe and the foramen ovale is restrictive.

On chest radiographs, the cardiothoracic ratio is increased because of dilation of the right atrium and left ventricle, and the pulmonary vascular markings are invariably reduced. The aortic arch is to the left of the trachea in almost all infants.

The EKG is characteristic and extremely helpful in the differential diagnosis (Fig. 27–10). Because of the right ventricular hypoplasia and low volume of blood in the right ventricle and large left ventricle in utero, there is a left ventricular predominance in the precordial leads, with a QRS axis of +30 to +120 degrees. Right atrial hypertrophy is also often seen.

The M-mode echocardiogram can identify the small right ventricle and large aorta, and the two-dimensional study will, in addition, frequently differentiate severe pulmonary stenosis from atresia.

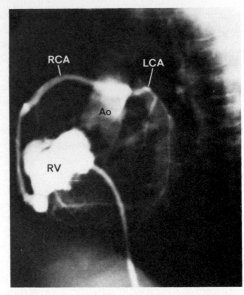

Figure 27–11. Right ventricular angiogram in the lateral position in a neonate with pulmonary atresia and an intact ventricular septum. The right ventricular cavity is small. The right and left coronary arteries and the aorta fill from a right ventricular sinusoid. No ventricular septal defect is present. Ao = aorta; LCA = left coronary artery; RCA = right coronary artery; RV = right ventricle.

Cardiac catheterization will confirm the right-to-left shunt at the atrial level with a normal pulmonary venous saturation but marked desaturation in the left atrium, left ventricle, and aorta. The right ventricular systolic pressure usually exceeds the left ventricular

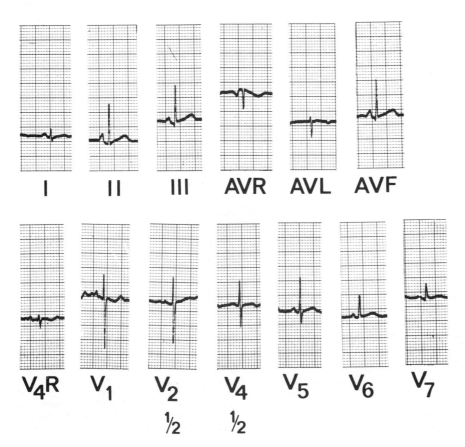

Figure 27–10. Electrocardiogram from a 3-day-old newborn with pulmonary atresia and an intact ventricular septum. Note the leftward QRS axis (+75 degrees) and the left ventricular predominance for age. The P waves are tall and peaked in II, suggesting right atrial hypertrophy.

pressure. Right ventricular angiography is useful in demonstrating the size of the right ventricle, the magnitude of the tricuspid regurgitation, and any right ventricular sinusoidal–coronary artery fistulas (Fig. 27–11). An angiogram in the left ventricle or aorta will allow one to visualize the ductus arteriosus and the pulmonary arteries.

Diagnosis. A very cyanotic newborn with pulmonary atresia and intact ventricular septum can usually be distinguished from an infant with transposition of the great arteries with an intact ventricular septum, since the latter child has a split second heart sound, increased pulmonary flow on the radiograph, right ventricular hypertrophy on the electrocardiogram, and a characteristic echocardiogram. Infants with tricuspid atresia and a hypoplastic right ventricle show decreased pulmonary flow on the radiograph and left ventricular predominance on electrocardiogram, but they almost invariably have a QRS axis of -30 to -90 degrees on the EKG, whereas infants with PA have a QRS axis of $+30$ to $+120$ degrees. Infants with pulmonary stenosis and a hypoplastic right ventricle may be hard to distinguish from those with pulmonary atresia before angiography but usually have a pulmonary ejection murmur rather than a regurgitant murmur and a valve that can be seen on two-dimensional echocardiography.

Treatment. The initial treatment must be directed at correcting the metabolic acidosis with oxygen and bicarbonate. The use of prostaglandin E_1 to dilate the ductus arteriosus, increase pulmonary blood flow, and improve oxygenation has been well demonstrated (Olley et al., 1976; Freed et al, 1981) and is useful in allowing time for stabilization of the infants prior to initiation of surgery.

In the few infants with mild right ventricular hypoplasia and a nonobstructive tricuspid valve, pulmonary valvotomy has been quite effective. Some hypoxemia almost invariably persists even after a good valvotomy, but this usually decreases as the pulmonary vascular resistance drops over the first or second week of life. If extreme hypoxemia persists (arterial saturation less than 60 per cent) after 2 weeks of age, a systemic-to-pulmonary artery shunt may be necessary.

In the presence of severe hypoplasia of the right ventricle and tricuspid valve, it is recognized that pulmonary valvotomy alone is insufficient. The proper initial palliation of these infants is still to be determined, with some favoring shunt alone (ascending aorta to right pulmonary artery or subclavian to pulmonary artery), shunt plus atrial septectomy, shunt plus pulmonary valvotomy, or, more recently, shunt plus right ventricular outflow tract reconstruction and pericardial patching. It appears that eventually some modification of the Fontan operation (Fontan and Baudet, 1971) attaching the right atrium to the pulmonary artery with or without a conduit may be possible in older children if the right ventricle remains hypoplastic, so that the operation that is the least

deforming to the pulmonary arteries and that is associated with the smallest risk of pulmonary vascular disease would seem the most appealing.

Prognosis. Unfortunately, the prognosis for patients with this lesion remains poor, with 77 per cent dying by their first birthday in the Regional Infant Cardiac Program (Fyler et al., 1980). In the group of infants with a good-sized right ventricle, the mortality was 50 per cent. Trusler and coworkers reported a 76 per cent survival (28/37), and Laks and coworkers found an 82 per cent survival (9/11) after initial palliation of this group of neonates.

PULMONARY STENOSIS WITH AN INTACT VENTRICULAR SEPTUM

Anatomy. In this lesion, the pulmonary valve has a narrowed orifice that is usually due to fusion of the three pulmonary commissures. The size of the right ventricular cavity can be normal but is usually somewhat hypoplastic in those infants who present with cyanosis in the first month of life (Freed et al., 1973). The size of the chamber is rarely, if ever, as small as that seen in infants with pulmonary atresia and an intact ventricular septum, and abnormalities of the tricuspid valve and right ventricular sinusoidal–coronary artery fistulas are less common. The main and peripheral pulmonary arteries are usually normal.

Incidence. In the Regional Infant Cardiac Program, there were 79 infants classified as having pulmonary stenosis (1 per 14,000 livebirths); 40 per cent presented in the first week of life (Fyler et al., 1980).

Hemodynamics. In utero, the obstruction at the pulmonary valve results in hypertrophy as well as a loss of compliance of the right ventricle. This leads to diversion of an increased proportion of venous return through the foramen ovale to the left side of the heart and ascending aorta. If the stenosis appears early in gestation and is severe, significant hypoplasia of the right ventricle with corresponding enlargement of the left ventricle occurs, resembling that seen in pulmonary atresia and an intact ventricular septum. If the stenosis is milder and occurs later in gestation, the right ventricle can be normal or near normal in size (Rudolph, 1974).

After birth, the degree of right-to-left shunting at the atrial level and thus arterial hypoxemia depends on the degree of pulmonary stenosis and right ventricular hypoplasia. If the stenosis is severe, right-to-left shunting at the atrial level may be massive and adequate pulmonary blood flow dependent on left-to-right shunting through the ductus arteriosus. If the stenosis is milder, with most of the pulmonary blood flow through the pulmonary valve, there may be little effect from ductal closure. As the pulmonary arteriolar resistance (in series with the pulmonary valve resistance) decreases over the first few weeks of life, the right-to-left shunt at the atrial level and, thus, the systemic hypoxemia may decrease.

Clinical Features. In mild pulmonary stenosis, a loud systolic ejection murmur at the left upper sternal border may be the only finding. In moderate or severe stenosis, the murmur is less prominent but cyanosis is present, increasing as the ductus arteriosus constricts. There is a prominent "a" wave in the jugular venous pulse reflecting reduced right ventricular compliance, and the liver is often enlarged and may even be pulsatile. The pulmonary component of the second heart sound is delayed and diminished and may be inaudible.

On chest radiographs, there is mild cardiomegaly due to an enlarged right atrium and diminished pulmonary blood flow. Poststenotic dilatation in the main pulmonary artery in the newborn is unusual.

The electrocardiogram is normal if the pulmonary stenosis is mild or moderate. With severe pulmonary stenosis and a diminutive right ventricle, the EKG usually demonstrates right atrial enlargement and left ventricular predominance with a QRS axis of $+30$ to $+120$ degrees, similar to that seen in pulmonary atresia with an intact ventricular septum (Fig. 27–10).

M-mode echocardiography may be helpful in assessing the size of the right ventricle, and the two-dimensional study can evaluate the tricuspid valve, right ventricle, and pulmonary arteries.

At cardiac catheterization, the right ventricular systolic pressure is elevated and usually exceeds left ventricular pressure. If the stenosis is severe, right-to-left shunting at the atrial level is common, with the degree of arterial hypoxemia a function of the degree of obstruction and hypoplasia of the right ventricle. On angiograms, the pulmonary valve is domed, thickened, and immobile, and the right ventricle is hypertrophied, with muscle bundles crossing and compromising the cavity size.

Diagnosis. With severe obstruction and right ventricular hypoplasia, pulmonary stenosis can be confused with pulmonary atresia with an intact septum. Usually, an ejection rather than regurgitant murmur at the left upper sternal border will allow one to differentiate these conditions, but, occasionally, echocardiography, angiography, or even surgical inspection is necessary to make the diagnosis with certainty. Neonates with tricuspid atresia usually have a superior axis (-90 to -30 degrees) on the electrocardiogram, and those with transposition rarely have a loud murmur and have normal or increased flow on the chest radiograph. If the right ventricle is not diminutive, the EKG will have right ventricular predominance, and it may be difficult to differentiate

pulmonary stenosis with an intact septum from pulmonary stenosis with a ventricular septal defect (tetralogy of Fallot). Echocardiography will usually detect the latter because of the overriding aorta and absence of echoes in the area of the ventricular septum.

The murmur of mild valvular pulmonary stenosis can be confused with the murmur of a ventricular septal defect, atrial septal defect, or peripheral pulmonary stenosis.

Treatment. The treatment of the cyanotic neonate with critical pulmonary stenosis is surgical. In those who are severely hypoxemic and acidotic, oxygen, bicarbonate, and prostaglandin E_1 are useful in initial stabilization before operation.

Pulmonary valvotomy can be performed via the right ventricle (Brock procedure) or via the pulmonary artery using cardiopulmonary bypass or systemic venous inflow occlusion. We prefer the latter, since it allows direct visualization and, in our experience, good long-term results (Freed et al, 1973; Litwin et al., 1973). Postoperatively, some cyanosis is usually present for a few days or weeks but gradually diminishes, presumably as the right ventricular compliance improves and the pulmonary vascular resistance drops. An occasional infant with severe hypoplasia of the right ventricle will remain quite cyanotic after adequate valvotomy and will require long-term prostaglandin E_1 or systemic-to-pulmonary artery shunt.

Infants with pulmonary stenosis but no cyanosis are usually managed conservatively in the neonatal period, and, if the stenosis appears severe, a catheterization is suggested at 6 to 12 months of age, with surgery recommended if the right ventricular systolic pressure exceeds systemic.

Prognosis. These infants usually do very well. In our experience, the survival is more than 90 per cent (Freed et al., 1973). In the Regional Infant Cardiac Program, 1-year survival was 79 per cent (Fyler et al., 1980). Occasionally, a repeat valvotomy is necessary later in childhood owing to a lack of growth of the pulmonary valve or incomplete relief at the initial operation.

TRICUSPID ATRESIA

Anatomy. In tricuspid atresia, there is a failure of development of the right atrioventricular valve; therefore, an intra-atrial communication, usually a patent foramen ovale, is necessary for survival. There is usually a ventricular septal defect connecting a large left ventricular cavity with a hypoplastic chamber that represents the infundibulum or outflow portion of the right ventricle. The great arteries may be either normally related (Type I) or transposed (Type II), and there may be pulmonary atresia (a), pulmonary stenosis (b), or no pulmonary stenosis (c) (Edwards and Burchell, 1949; Keith et al., 1958). About 70 per cent of infants with tricuspid atresia have Type I, with three fourths of these having pulmonary stenosis (b). In contrast, of the 30 per cent who have Type II (transposition), more than three fourths have no pulmonary stenosis (c) (Dick et al., 1975). The presentation of neonates with tricuspid atresia depends on the anatomy. Those with severe pulmonary stenosis or atresia present with cyanosis in the first few days of life. Infants with a large ventricular septal defect and no pulmonary stenosis present with congestive heart failure, usually late in the first or during the second month as the pulmonary vascular resistance falls.

Incidence.   In the Regional Infant Cardiac Program, there were 61 infants with tricuspid atresia, an incidence of 1 per 18,000 livebirths (Fyler et al., 1980). They represented less than 5 per cent of infants presenting in the first month of life with serious congenital heart disease.

Hemodynamics.   The presence of tricuspid atresia in utero must be compatible with a relatively normal intrauterine circulation, since growth and development proceed normally. Since the tricuspid valve is atretic, all systemic venous return is diverted across the foramen ovale into left atrium and left ventricle (Fig. 27–12). If the great arteries are normally related and the ventricular septum is intact or if the pulmonary valve is atretic, all the left ventricular output passes through the aorta, and pulmonary blood flow is via the ductus arteriosus. If the ventricular septal defect is large, some of the left ventricular ouput passes through the VSD into the hypoplastic right ventricle, exiting the pulmonary artery if the vessels are normally related and the aorta if transposition is present. Either way, there is antegrade flow through the pulmonary artery and ductus arteriosus.

After birth, there is little change in the circulation, but the normal postnatal alterations impose significant handicaps. The neonates with pulmonary atresia or severe pulmonary stenosis continue to depend on the ductus arteriosus for pulmonary blood flow. When the ductus begins to close, severe hypoxemia, acidosis, and, eventually, death follow.

In those infants with a large ventricular septal defect and no pulmonary stenosis, the pulmonary blood flow increases as the pulmonary arteriolar resistance drops and congestive heart failure ensues, usually within the first month of life. Infants with transposition in whom the aorta arises from the hypoplastic right ventricle may develop obstruction physiologically comparable to subaortic stenosis in the infant with normally related great arteries if the ventricular defect is small.

Clinical Features.   Infants with pulmonary stenosis or atresia (a,b) are usually cyanotic soon after birth, with the cyanosis increasing as the ductus arteriosus closes. Those with pulmonary stenosis usually have a loud systolic ejection murmur along the left sternal border; those with pulmonary atresia may have no murmur at all or a continuous murmur from the ductus arteriosus. Infants with type c (no pulmonary stenosis) may have minimal cyanosis with an ejection murmur and heart failure as the major manifestions of heart disease. The heart size and the pulmonary blood flow visible on the radiographs are determined by the degree of pulmonary stenosis. Infants with pulmonary atresia or stenosis have a small heart with decreased pulmonary blood flow; those without pulmonary stenosis have a large heart with increased pulmonary flow. A right aortic arch is occasionally present.

The electrocardiogram is usually very helpful (Fig. 27–13). Because of the right ventricular hypoplasia and increased left ventricular flow in utero, left ventricular predominance with diminished right ventricular forces is almost universal. The QRS axis is almost always superior (0 to −90 degrees) in Type I (Dick et al., 1975), probably owing in large part to early origin of the left bundle of the conducting system and the resultant abnormal depolarization sequence. Right atrial hypertrophy is frequently present.

On the M-mode echocardiogram, tricuspid valve echoes are absent, the right ventricle is hypoplastic, and the aorta is enlarged. A two-dimensional study will demonstrate the imperforate tricuspid membrane, the size of the right ventricle, the ventricular septal defect, and the relationship between the great arteries.

The diagnosis can be confirmed at cardiac catheterization by demonstration of a right-to-left shunt at the atrial level with desaturation in the left atrium

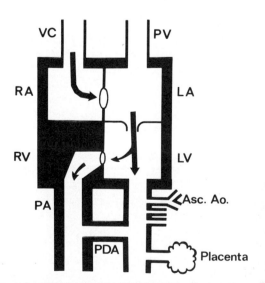

Figure 27–12. Schematic diagram of the circulation in the fetus with tricuspid atresia. All the venous return from the vena cava passes across the atrial septum into the left atrium and ventricle. Pulmonary blood flow before (and after) birth is via a ventricular septal defect or through the ductus arteriosus. Blood flow to the placenta for oxygenation is unimpeded. The abbreviations in this diagram are the same as those used in Figure 27–2.

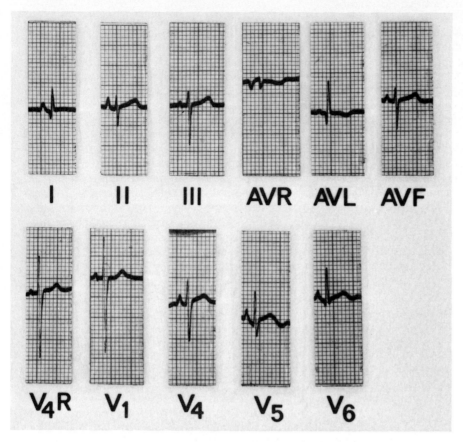

I   II   III   AVR   AVL   AVF

V₄R   V₁   V₄   V₅   V₆

Figure 27–13. An electrocardiogram from a 5-day-old newborn with tricuspid atresia. The QRS axis is superior (−50 degrees). The P waves are peaked in leads II and V₄ to V₆, suggesting right atrial hypertrophy. There is left ventricular predominance for age with a predominant S wave in V₄R and V₁ and a qRS in V₆.

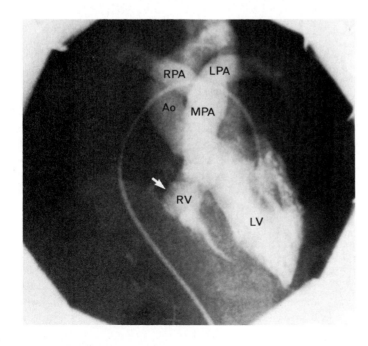

Figure 27–14. Left ventricular angiogram in the hepatoclavicular "4 chamber" position in a newborn with tricuspid atresia. The hypoplastic right ventricle fills through a ventricular septal defect. The arrow points to the atretic tricuspid valve. Ao = aorta; LPA = left pulmonary artery; LV = left ventricle; MPA = main pulmonary artery; RPA = right pulmonary artery; RV = right ventricle.

and a normal saturation in the pulmonary veins and an elevated right atrial pressure (especially the "a" wave) slightly higher than left atrial pressure. Also helpful in confirming the diagnosis is the injection of contrast medium into the right atrium. Dye spills across the atrial septum and fills the left atrium and left ventricle, revealing a characteristically unopacified defect along the left border of the right atrium, where the tricuspid valve and right ventricle are usually seen. Angiocardiography in the left ventricle using 40 degrees of left anterior obliquity and 40 degrees of cranial angulation (hepatoclavicular, or 4-chambered, view) will outline the ventricular defect(s) and demonstrate the size of the right ventricle as well as the degree and location of pulmonary stenosis (Fig. 27–14). Although others have advocated balloon septostomy to enlarge the atrial defect, we have rarely found this necessary.

Diagnosis. In the cyanotic infant, tricuspid atresia can be differentiated from transposition, tetralogy of Fallot, and Ebstein's disease of the tricuspid valve by the demonstration of left ventricular predominance on the electrocardiogram and from pulmonary atresia or stenosis with a diminutive right ventricle on the basis of the superior QRS axis.

In the minimally cyanotic infant, tricuspid atresia can be differentiated from the atrioventricular canal type of ventricular septal defect by electrocardiography or echocardiography and from the more complicated types of acyanotic heart disease by the presence of arterial hypoxemia, which is especially evident while the infant is crying.

Treatment. In the severely hypoxic infant, the primary treatment is oxygen, bicarbonate, and prostaglandin E_1 to maintain patency of the ductus arteriosus (Olley et al., 1976; Freed et al., 1981) followed by a systemic-to-pulmonary artery shunt. Although the Waterston (ascending aorta-to-right pulmonary artery) and Potts (descending aorta-to-left pulmonary artery) shunts are easier to construct, they are difficult to size and often lead to markedly increased pulmonary blood flow, heart failure, and early pulmonary vascular disease. For these reasons as well as other technical advances, the Blalock-Taussig shunt (subclavian-to-pulmonary artery), long the choice in the older child, has recently become more popular in the neonate (Arciniegas et al., 1982).

Children with a large ventricular septal defect and little pulmonary stenosis require pulmonary artery banding to restrict pulmonary blood flow so that congestive heart failure can be controlled and pulmonary vascular disease can be prevented.

Prior to 1971, there was no "corrective" surgery for tricuspid atresia. Over the past decade, many have followed the suggestions of Fontan and Baudet and of Kreutzer and coworkers, who recommend connecting the right atrium with either the right ventricular outflow tract or the pulmonary artery, depending on systemic venous pressure and right atrial contraction to force blood through the lungs. In se-

lected children older than 3 years with low pulmonary artery, left ventricular end-diastolic pressure and normal pulmonary arterial anatomy, this approach has shown great promise and can be performed with a short-term survival of greater than 80 per cent (Sanders et al., 1982). It seems unlikely that this approach will be feasible in the neonate, since it seems to require very low pulmonary vascular resistance, normally not present until 3 to 6 months of age.

Prognosis. When Dick and coworkers reviewed the experience of children with tricuspid atresia at Children's Hospital in Boston between 1941 and 1973, the 1-year survival was 50 per cent, and the 20-year survival was 30 percent. In data from the Regional Infant Cardiac Program that were collected between 1969 and 1974 (Fyler et al., 1980), the 1-year survival of those requiring surgery was 63 per cent. With improvement of surgical techniques on small infants and the application of the Fontan principle to older children, we expect that these rather dismal results will be improved.

EBSTEIN'S ANOMALY OF THE TRICUSPID VALVE

Anatomy. In 1866, Ebstein described the heart of a 19-year-old male patient with cyanosis and palpitations who died of heart failure with an anomaly of the tricuspid valve. The lesion, now known as Ebstein's anomaly of the tricuspid valve, is represented by redundancy and dysplasia of the tricuspid valve with adherence of a variable portion of the septal and, often, posterior leaflets to the right ventricular wall so that the free portion of the leaflets is displaced downward, away from the normal atrioventricular ring. Thus, the atrium and ventricle are divided in three segments: a normal right atrium, a portion of the atrium above the displaced valve that is partly ventricular myocardium, and the true right ventricle. The tricuspid valve is usually regurgitant and, at least in the newborn, quite stenotic. The right atrium is often very large, in part owing to the muscularized segment but primarily because of the tricuspid stenosis and regurgitation; the right ventricle is correspondingly small. An atrial septal defect (or patent foramen ovale) is almost always present in the newborn, and pulmonary stenosis and atresia are not uncommon. Other associated lesions such as ventricular septal defects, coarctation, and transposition are rarely seen.

Incidence. Ebstein's disease is rare in the neonate. There were only 18 infants in the Regional Infant Cardiac Program over 5 years, an incidence of 1 per 80,000 livebirths (Fyler et al., 1980).

Hemodynamics. In utero, the incompetent or stenotic tricuspid valve diverts systemic venous return through the foramen ovale into the left heart, resulting in increased left atrial and ventricular flow. The tricuspid regurgitation into the right atrium leads to severe right atrial dilatation and hypertrophy before birth and may cause in utero heart failure with edema or anasarca.

After birth, the degree of hypoxemia is a function of the right-to-left shunting at the atrial level. This depends on the degree of difficulty with which blood passes through the right ventricle and pulmonary artery into the lungs. With high pulmonary vascular resistance of the neonate increasing right ventricular afterload, the tricuspid regurgitation may be exacerbated and the right-to-left shunting at the atrial level massive. These severely hypoxic infants may depend on the ductus arteriosus for most of their pulmonary blood flow, and, when the ductus closes, the hypoxemia may be very severe and acidosis may develop. If the foramen ovale is restrictive, preventing decompensation of the right atrium, right heart failure with hepatomegaly may be prominent.

If the tricuspid stenosis and regurgitation is less severe, right-to-left shunting and, therefore, cyanosis may be less prominent. In either case, as the pulmonary vascular resistance drops over the first few days and weeks of life, reducing right ventricular afterload and tricuspid regurgitation, dramatic improvements in arterial saturation and congestive heart failure may be seen.

Clinical Manifestations. The infants with Ebstein's disease who present during the neonatal period are almost invariably cyanotic (Kumar et al., 1971). Right-sided congestive heart failure with hepatomegaly due to severe tricuspid regurgitation is frequently present. On auscultation, there may be a quadruple rhythm composed of a loud first sound, single second sound, and loud third and fourth sounds. A pansystolic murmur of tricuspid regurgitation is often audible (Kumar et al., 1971).

On chest radiographs, the cardiac silhouette is usually enlarged because of massive dilatation of the right atrium (Fig. 27–15). The largest hearts in infants with congenital disease are seen in this condition. Often it is difficult for one to see enough lung field to note the diminished pulmonary flow.

The P waves on the electrocardiogram are often tall and peaked, suggesting right atrial hypertrophy. Right ventricular conduction abnormalities prolonging the QRS duration are common, although they are not seen as frequently in the neonate as in the older child. Wolff-Parkinson-White syndrome with a short P–R interval and a delta wave may be seen in as many as 20 per cent of children (Kumar et al., 1971), and atrial tachycardias and flutter are not uncommon.

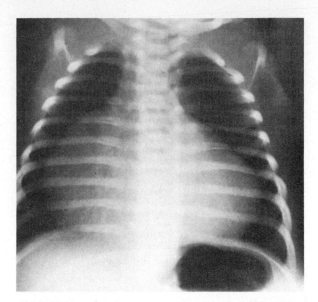

Figure 27–15. Chest radiograph in anteroposterior projection in a newborn with Ebstein's disease. The right atrium is markedly enlarged, and the pulmonary blood flow is reduced.

In 1973, Tajik and coworkers and Lundstrom published the earliest descriptions of the now classic M-mode echocardiographic features of delayed tricuspid valve closure and increased excursion of the anterior leaflet of the tricuspid valve.

The two-dimensional study is usually diagnostic, with the right atrial dilatation and displaced anterior leaflet visible from the apical view. At cardiac catheterization, demonstration of normal pulmonary venous oxygen saturation but desaturation in the left atrium, left ventricle, and aorta confirms the presence of right-to-left shunting at the atrial level. It may be difficult to pass the catheter into the right ventricle because of its small size (especially compared with that of the right atrium) and the tricuspid regurgitation. The right ventricular pressure is usually normal but may be elevated if there is associated pulmonary stenosis or atresia.

Angiography in the right ventricle in the anteroposterior projection shows a double notch, one at the site of the normal tricuspid annulus and another where the displaced anterior leaflet inserts. Atrial arrhythmias are quite common during catheterization, but the dangers of catheterization have probably been exaggerated, and catheterization in infants with this condition is probably no more hazardous than in other cyanotic neonates (Kumar et al., 1971).

Diagnosis. On chest radiographs, the hearts of children with Ebstein's disease are larger than those of children with any other form of congenital heart disease. In the minimally distressed infant with cyanosis, a murmur along the left sternal border, right ventricular hypertrophy on the electrocardiogram, and massive cardiomegaly, the diagnosis is almost certain (see Differential Diagnosis, p. 285).

Patients with pulmonary atresia with an intact ventricular septum or tricuspid atresia may have cyanosis and cardiac enlargement, but they usually have left rather than right ventricular hypertrophy on the electrocardiogram, and the tricuspid valve is hypoplastic or atretic on echocardiogram, rather than large and redundant as in Ebstein's disease. Infants with transposition of the great arteries or tetralogy of Fallot may be just as cyanotic, but the former have increased pulmonary vascularity, and the latter rarely show cardiac enlargement on chest radiographs.

Treatment. Treatment of this condition in the neonate is based on two premises: (1) many infants improve markedly over the first weeks of life, presumably as the pulmonary vascular resistance drops, and (2) surgical approaches to treating the critically ill neonate have thus far been almost uniformly unsuccessful. Anticongestives including digoxin and diuretics may prove useful. Prostaglandin E_1 has been helpful in improving oxygenation in the severely cyanotic infant, presumably by maintaining patency of the ductus arteriosus while the pulmonary vascular resistance falls (Freed et al., 1981).

Tricuspid annuloplasty, or valve replacement, is occasionally successful in the older child but has not been successful in the neonate, and palliative shunts have only occasionally been successful for reasons that remain unclear. Older children have been successfully palliated by either a Glenn (superior vena cava–to–right pulmonary artery) or a Fontan (right atrium–to–main pulmonary artery) procedure, but these operations seem contraindicated in newborn patients because of the high pulmonary vascular resistance in neonates. A corrective operation has been successful in a small group of older children and adults but has not been reported in infants (Danielson et al., 1979).

Prognosis. The prognosis is poor for patients presenting in the newborn period. In an international collaborative study (Watson, 1974), 29 of 35 infants died—15 from heart failure, eight from surgery, five from catheterization, and one suddenly, presumably from an arrhythmia. More recently, there were 12 deaths of 23 patients at the Hospital for Sick Children in Toronto (Rowe et al., 1981), and in the Regional Infant Cardiac Program there were three deaths among 13 patients catheterized or operated on in the first year of life (Fyler et al., 1980).

TRUNCUS ARTERIOSUS

Anatomy. Truncus arteriosus has been defined as the cardiac defect in which a single great artery arises from the base of the heart supplying the coronary, pulmonary, and systemic arteries (Lev and Saphir, 1942). It was previously classified according to the site of origin of the pulmonary arteries and aortopulmonary septum (Collett and Edwards, 1949; Van Praagh and Van Praagh, 1965), but this practice has largely been abandoned because it is often difficult to differentiate a single pulmonary trunk from sep-

arate but closely related left and right pulmonary arteries, even when pathologic specimens are available.

Embryologically, this defect is thought to result from failure of septation of the truncus arteriosus (Edwards, 1976), although Van Praagh and Van Praagh believe that it is closely related to tetralogy of Fallot with atresia rather than hypoplasia of the subpulmonary infundibulum, partial or complete absence of the pulmonary valve, and an aortopulmonary septal defect. This theory is attractive, since both lesions are almost invariably associated with a ventricular septal defect and overriding of the aorta and because a right aortic arch is frequently present in both.

The truncal valve usually resembles a normal aortic valve. In the series of 79 necropsy cases reported in 1976 by Calder and coworkers, the truncal valve was tricuspid in 61 per cent, quadricuspid in 31 per cent, and bicuspid in 8 per cent. Truncal valve thickening was seen in two thirds of the patients, with truncal stenosis in 11 per cent and truncal regurgitation in 15 per cent.

Incidence. Thirty-three cases of truncus arteriosus were seen in the Regional Infant Cardiac Program, representing an incidence of one per 33,000 live births (Fyler et al., 1980); they represent about 2 per cent of infants with congenital heart disease seen in the first year of life.

Hemodynamics. In utero, the main consequence of truncus arteriosus is complete mixing of the systemic and pulmonary venous return above the truncal valve. The truncus is usually quite large, and the ductus arteriosus arising from the pulmonary arteries may be smaller than normal. Since blood flow through the heart is normal, the atrium and ventricles develop normally.

After birth, the flow to the pulmonary arteries and systemic arteries is a function of the relative resistances in the two circuits. Initially, the pulmonary resistance is high, and pulmonary flow will equal or slightly exceed systemic flow. Over the first hours or days of life, however, the pulmonary arteriolar resistance decreases and pulmonary blood flow increases. As the pulmonary venous return increases, the left ventricle must eject an increasing volume load, which eventually leads to congestive failure. Since there is common mixing of systemic and pulmonary venous blood above the truncal valve, the degree of hypoxemia decreases as the pulmonary flow increases so that these infants are only mildly cyanotic until left heart failure and pulmonary edema interfere with oxygen exchange and pulmonary venous desaturation ensues.

In some infants, the pulmonary arteries are hypoplastic or stenotic at their origin; in these patients, the pulmonary blood flow is restricted, and cyanosis rather than congestive failure may be the presenting symptom.

Clinical Manifestations. Children with truncus arteriosus usually present in the first month (and often in the first week) with predominantly left heart failure. Tachypnea, poor feeding, increased perspiration, and intermittent cyanosis are usually prominent, and hepatomegaly is occasionally present. On physical examination, the cardiac impulse is hyperactive, and the pulses are usually bounding secondary to the diastolic run-off from the aorta. On auscultation, the second heart sound is single, although the phonocardiogram can often detect multiple components, presumably from the abnormal truncal valve cusps. Commonly, a systolic ejection click is audible. Although a continuous murmur is often thought to be characteristic of truncus, it is actually quite unusual, since pulmonary hypertension is the rule. Systolic ejection murmurs of moderate intensity (grade 2 or 3/6) due to relative truncal stenosis are common, and a mid-diastolic flow rumble across the mitral valve is often present.

The heart is enlarged on the chest radiograph because of dilatation of the left atrium and ventricle. The pulmonary vascular markings are increased, and pulmonary venous congestion is frequently seen. A right aortic arch is present in about one fourth of cases. The QRS axis is usually normal, with biventricular hypertrophy present in about 60 per cent of infants, left ventricular hypertrophy in 20 per cent, and pure right ventricular hypertrophy in the remainder.

On the M-mode echocardiogram, the condition resembles tetralogy of Fallot, with a large artery and semilunar valve overriding a ventricular septal defect. The presence of a dilated left atrium and ventricle and multiple echoes from the semilunar valve should usually allow one to differentiate the two.

On the two-dimensional echocardiogram, the truncal valve and pulmonary arteries arising from the side of the aorta can usually be visualized.

At cardiac catheterization, the pressures in the two ventricles are identical, and the pulse pressure in the aorta is increased, usually to more than 40 mm Hg. There is often a gradient between the aorta and pulmonary arteries, presumably from the torrential pulmonary flow with relative stenosis at the origin of the pulmonary arteries.

Angiocardiography in the left ventricle in the left anterior oblique projection with some axial angulation will outline the ventricular septal defect(s), and an angiocardiogram above the truncal valve with cranial angulation will outline the truncal valve and pulmonary arteries and rule out truncal regurgitation (Fig. 27–16).

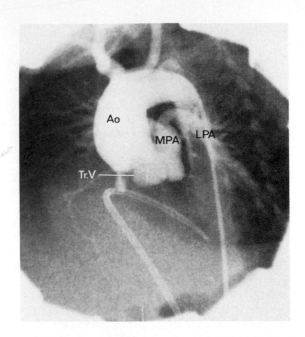

Figure 27–16. Hepatoclavicular view (40 degrees left anterior oblique, 40 degrees cranial angulation) in a newborn with truncus arteriosus. The aorta and main pulmonary artery arise above the truncal valve. Ao = aorta; LPA = left pulmonary artery; MPA = main pulmonary artery; TrV = truncal valve.

Diagnosis. A neonate with mild cyanosis, congestive heart failure, and bounding pulses probably has truncus arteriosus (see Differential Diagnosis, p. 285).

Infants with a ventricular septal defect, patent ductus arteriosus, aortopulmonary window, A-V fistula, or coarctation of the aorta are not cyanotic and infants with tetralogy of Fallot and pulmonary atresia and large collaterals who may have cyanosis and heart failure have loud continuous murmurs. In infants with tricuspid atresia and a large ventricular septal defect, the electrocardiogram shows a superior axis and left ventricular hypertrophy, and infants with transposition and a large ventricular septal defect do not usually have bounding pulses.

Treatment. For the neonate with congestive heart failure, digoxin and diuretics should be tried, but they rarely suffice. Pulmonary artery banding, either single in the rare case of one pulmonary trunk or, more commonly, bilaterally for those with separate origins of the right and left pulmonary artery was formerly the procedure of choice. Unfortunately, banding of these small pulmonary arteries has been associated with a high risk (50 per cent) in most series (Poirier et al., 1975) and frequently deforms the pulmonary arteries so that later correction is impossible.

Recently, several centers have tried surgical repair in infancy by removing the origin of the pulmonary arteries with a cuff of aorta, closing the aorta with a patch, attaching the cuff of the aorta to a valve-bearing conduit that is then attached to the right ventricle, and, finally, closing the ventricular septal defect with the left ventricle in continuity with the truncal valve.

In his 1983 review, Ebert reported a series of 77 patients under 6 months of age who underwent this physiologic correction, and the mortality rate was only 9 per cent.

Prognosis. Untreated, infants with this anomaly have a dismal prognosis. In one series, the median age of death was 5 weeks (Calder et al., 1976). In the Regional Infant Cardiac Program covering the early 1970s, 77 per cent of the 33 infants with this lesion died before their first birthday (Fyler et al., 1980). The long-term results of more innovative surgical approaches are awaited.

TOTAL ANOMALOUS PULMONARY VENOUS RETURN

Anatomy. In this anomaly, the pulmonary veins have no connection with the left atrium and drain either directly or, more commonly, indirectly into the right atrium via one of the normal embryonic channels. The embryologic defect seems to be a failure of development of the common pulmonary vein normally connecting the developing pulmonary venous plexus with the posterior aspect of the left atrium. As a consequence, one or more of the normal anastomotic channels between the pulmonary venous plexus of the lung buds and the cardinal or umbilicovitelline vein persists, allowing drainage of the pulmonary blood flow into the systemic venous atrium (Delisle et al., 1976). If the connection to the left common cardinal system persists, postnatal drainage is to the left innominate vein (35 per cent of cases) or to the coronary sinus (19 per cent). Other pathways that may persist include the right common cardinal system (drainage to right superior vena cava or azygos, 11 per cent of cases) and the umbilicovitelline system (ductus venosus or portal system, 21 per cent). Alternatively, the pulmonary veins may drain directly into the right atrium (4 per cent). In 10 per cent of cases, there is mixed drainage (Gathman and Nadas, 1970). The presence of an interatrial communication, either a patent foramen ovale or a true atrial septal defect, is necessary to sustain life after birth.

The postnatal presentation depends on the degree of obstruction to pulmonary venous drainage. If obstruction is severe (almost invariable with drainage into the umbilicovitelline system, and frequent with drainage into the right superior vena cava or innominate vein), the children present within the first week of life. If obstruction is mild or absent, presentation is usually during the second half of the first year or later. The remainder of this discussion will deal only with the former group, infants with obstruction to the pulmonary venous return.

Incidence. In the New England Regional Infant Cardiac Program, 63 among 2251 infants under 1 year with critical heart disease seen between 1969

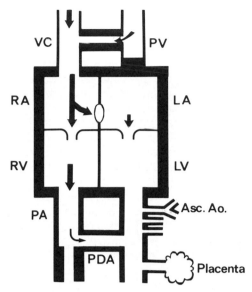

Figure 27–17. Schematic diagram of the circulation in a fetus with total anomalous pulmonary venous return. The intracardiac circulation is normal. Pulmonary venous return is to the anomalous channel connecting with one of the systemic veins. In utero, there is no hemodynamic embarrassment, since pulmonary blood flow is minimal. After birth, if the anomalous channel restricts egress of blood from the pulmonary veins, pulmonary venous hypertension and pulmonary edema follow. The abbreviations are the same as those used in Figure 27–2.

and 1974 had total anomalous pulmonary venous return (TAPVR), representing an incidence of one per 17,000 livebirths.

Hemodynamics. In utero, there is little hemodynamic disruption from TAPVR, since before birth the pulmonary blood flow represents only 5 to 10 per cent of combined ventricular output, an amount that can be handled by the anomalous systemic venous connection (Fig. 27–17). The drainage of pulmonary venous blood to the right side of the heart rather than the left causes no apparent sequelae; the newborns are normal in size and development.

After birth, the fetal pathways persist. The pulmonary venous return continues to drain to the right atrium via one of the systemic venous channels, where it mixes with the normal systemic venous return. A portion of the totally mixed pulmonary and systemic venous return passes into the left atrium, left ventricle, and aorta, and the rest passes into the right ventricle and pulmonary artery. As the pulmonary arteriolar resistance drops, the pulmonary blood flow increases, and, if there is obstruction to the increased pulmonary venous flow, pulmonary edema follows.

The pulmonary venous obstruction increases the pulmonary vascular resistance above systemic, diverting blood from the pulmonary artery into the descending aorta as long as the ductus arteriosus remains open. When the ductus begins to close, the increased pulmonary resistance elevates right ventricular and right atrial pressure and leads to increasing right-to-left shunting at the atrial level. The increased pulmonary resistance secondary to the obstruction reduces pulmonary flow and the pulmonary edema reduces the oxygen content of the blood that is not obstructed, resulting in arterial hypoxemia and, eventually, acidosis and death.

Clinical Manifestations. In infants with severe pulmonary venous obstruction, the predominant finding is cyanosis. The heart is not hyperactive, and other than experiencing tachypnea, the child is usually quite comfortable, at least initially. The second heart sound is single or narrowly split and accentuated. Often, no murmurs are audible.

In neonates with lesser degrees of pulmonary venous obstruction, cyanosis may be less impressive and the signs and symptoms of heart failure—tachypnea, dyspnea, and feeding difficulties—may predominate. In these infants, the right ventricular impulse will be hyperdynamic, and the second heart sound will be widely split, with the pulmonary component increased. A systolic ejection murmur at the left upper sternal border and a mid-diastolic murmur at the left lower sternal border secondary to increased blood flow across the pulmonary and tricuspid valves may be audible.

In infants with severe obstruction, the heart is normal in size on the chest radiograph, and pulmonary venous congestion is obvious. (Fig. 27–18). Those with milder obstruction have right ventricular dilatation and increased pulmonary blood flow. Occasionally, the dilated accessory venous channels to the left or right superior vena cava can be seen on the anteroposterior projection.

The electrocardiogram almost invariably shows right axis deviation and right ventricular hypertrophy (Gathman and Nadas, 1970). In the first week, this may be difficult to distinguish from normal, but in those who present the second week, the right ventricular hypertrophy becomes more obvious and may be associated with right atrial hypertrophy. On the M-mode echocardiogram, the right ventricle and pulmonary artery are dilated, and the left atrium is often small. On two-dimensional study, the posterior wall of the left atrium is bare, and the anomalous channel can be seen connecting the dilated common pulmonary vein behind the left atrium with the left or right superior vena cava, the coronary sinus, or the right atrium, or it may be seen dipping below the diaphragm to connect with the portal system.

On catheterization, the oxygen saturation is nearly identical in both atria, ventricles, and great arteries, reflecting common mixing at the right atrial level. Oc-

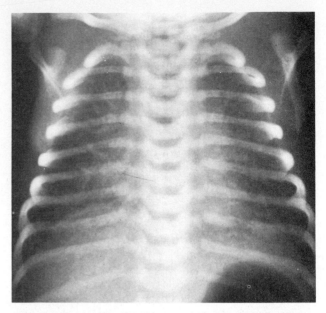

Figure 27–18. Chest radiograph in anteroposterior projection in a newborn with total anomalous venous return to the portal system. The pulmonary vessels are indistinct, reflecting increased interstitial fluid from pulmonary venous congestion. The heart is not enlarged.

casionally, the common pulmonary vein can be entered where the oxygen saturation is higher. The pulmonary artery pressure is elevated and may be above systemic if the ductus arteriosus is closed. The pulmonary artery "wedge" pressure reflecting pulmonary venous pressure is increased, and right atrial exceeds the left atrial pressure.

Angiocardiography, either in the common pulmonary vein entered from the systemic venous connection or in the pulmonary artery with usual long filming will outline the site or sites of pulmonary venous drainage except when the obstruction is almost complete (Fig. 27–19).

Diagnosis. In the infant with severe cyanosis that is unresponsive to oxygen and a small heart and pulmonary venous congestion visible on the radiographs, the diagnosis is usually clear. It is occasionally difficult to distinguish infants with total anomalous pulmonary venous return from those with persistent fetal circulation with or without primary lung disease because (1) both groups of patients demonstrate tachypnea, dyspnea, and cyanosis on physical examination as well as haziness of the lung fields on radiographs, and (2) both may transiently improve with 100 per cent oxygen, since a perfusion imbalance may occur in either condition. In preterm infants, lung disease is more common, but in the term infant, the index of suspicion must be high for total anomalous pulmonary venous return. Echocardiography or even catheterization may occasionally be necessary to distinguish the two with certainty.

The hypoplastic left heart syndrome may also be associated with pulmonary edema on radiographs, but there is usually extreme cardiac enlargement with

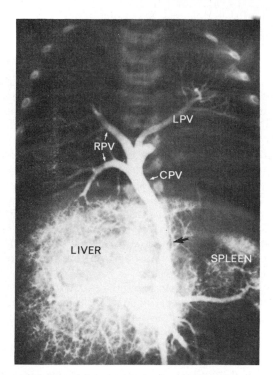

Figure 27–19. A postmortem angiogram in a neonate who died with total anomalous pulmonary venous return into the portal system. The right and left pulmonary veins drain into a common trunk that descends below the diaphragm to join the portal system. Note the discrete narrowing in the pulmonary vein (arrow) that probably occurs as it pierces the diaphragm. CPV = common pulmonary vein; LPV = left pulmonary vein; RPV = right pulmonary vein.

increased pulmonary blood flow visible on the films and severe circulatory collapse.

Treatment. The treatment of TAPVR with obstruction is surgical. Although some authors have advocated balloon atrial septostomy at the time of diagnostic catheterization followed by observation, we have not found this to be a safe approach and now recommend surgery soon after diagnosis.

The surgical technique consists of anastomosis of the horizontal pulmonary venous confluence to the posterior wall of the left atrium and ligation of the anomalous systemic venous channel.

Prognosis. In the Regional Infant Cardiac Program between 1969 and 1974 there were only six survivors among 30 infants who had operations in the first year of life. More recently, with earlier diagnosis and referral to a cardiac center, improved surgical techniques including deep-hypothermic circulatory arrest, and (possibly most important) better postoperative care of these small critically ill infants, the surgical results have improved tremendously. There were only three deaths among 26 children (12 per cent) ranging in age from 2 days to 8 months (median 44 days) operated on at Boston Children's Hospital between September 1973 and the end of 1978 (Norwood et al., 1980).

HETEROTAXY SYNDROMES

The heterotaxy syndromes are characterized by positional abnormalities of the abdominal viscera (midline liver, stomach on the right, malrotation of the gut) splenic abnormalities (absence of spleen or multiple tiny splenules), and complex, usually cyanotic, congenital heart disease. For convenience, they have been classified as asplenia and polysplenia, although the disease associated with asplenia may be present with a normal spleen and polysplenia heart disease may exist with no spleen, many splenules, or a normal spleen.

Asplenia

Anatomy. The liver tends to be midline, with right and left lobes equal in size. Both lungs are trilobed with epiarterial bronchi (bronchus over the pulmonary artery) similar to the bronchus seen in the normal right lung. There is often no rotation or reverse rotation of the midgut loop, with abnormal mesenteric attachments. Often the entire small bowel is on one side of the abdomen and the large intestine on the other. Cardiac malformations usually include bilateral superior vena cava, inferior cava either to the right or left of the spine, common atrium, complete atrioventricular canal, single ventricle, and total anomalous pulmonary venous return. Transposition of the great arteries is common, and severe pulmonary stenosis or atresia is almost invariably present (Van Mierop et al., 1972; Rose et al., 1975).

A helpful pathognomonic feature of asplenia, demonstrable by echocardiography, catheter passage, or angiocardiography, is the finding of the abdominal aorta and inferior vena cava on the same side of the spine.

Incidence. In the Regional Infant Cardiac Program, infants with asplenia and polysplenia were not considered separately. There was a combined incidence of one per 20,000 livebirths (Fyler et al., 1980). In other series, virtually all pathologic in origin, these conditions account for about 1 per cent of all congenital heart disease.

Hemodynamics. The infants are usually normal at birth, a finding that suggests relatively normal intrauterine development. This is not surprising because virtual common mixing of systemic venous and pulmonary venous blood normally occurs before birth, and the pulmonary stenosis or atresia and total anomalous pulmonary venous drainage are less important in utero, since pulmonary blood flow is minimal.

After birth, the presentation is usually similar to that of neonates with a large ventricular septal defect and severe pulmonary stenosis or atresia—profound cyanosis, especially as the ductus arteriosus closes.

Clinical Manifestations. As already noted, cyanosis is usually the presenting symptom. If the infant has pulmonary stenosis rather than atresia, a systolic murmur will be audible along the left sternal border. The second heart sound is single. The asplenia syndrome may be diagnosed by the plain chest radiograph (Fig. 27–20). The liver is midline and symmetric, and the stomach is found in the midline or on the right or left side of the abdomen. If the chest film is of good quality, the bilateral epiarterial bronchi are visible. The heart may be in the right chest (dextrocardia), midline (mesocardia), or in the left chest (levocardia) and is usually normal in size with reduced pulmonary vascularity. The electrocardiogram is variable. There is often a superior QRS axis (0 to −120 degrees) with a counterclockwise loop in the frontal plane typical of an endocardial cushion defect. The configuration of the QRS complex depends on the position of the heart in the chest and the presence or absence of a ventricular septum. The P-wave axis is usually inferior and anterior with a normal P–R interval.

If a single ventricle is present, only one ventricular chamber and one A-V valve is present on the M-mode echocardiograpm. On two-dimensional study, the complexity of the cardiovascular arrangement can usually be appreciated and most of the abnormalities sorted out.

At cardiac catheterization the catheter can be passed into all the heart chambers, but the total anomalous pulmonary venous return causes similar saturations in each chamber, and the large atrial and ventricular defects result in equal pressures in both atria and both ventricles, making chamber localization difficult. Angiocardiography in the ventricle(s), systemic veins, pulmonary veins, and ductus arteriosus is often necessary for outlining of the structures.

Differential Diagnosis. Infants with asplenia must be differentiated from those with large ventricular septal defect and pulmonary stenosis or atresia (tetralogy of Fallot). The characteristic picture of abdominal heterotaxy with bilateral epiarterial bronchi on chest radiographs should alert one to the probability of the asplenia syndrome. Finding the inferior vena cava and abdominal aorta on the same side of the spine seems to be pathognomonic.

It is often more difficult to differentiate between asplenia and polysplenia. In general, the heart disease is more complex with asplenia; the lungs are trilobed, the bronchi epiarterial, the P-wave axis normal, and the inferior vena cava present on the same side as the abdominal aorta. In the polysplenia syndrome, the lungs are bilobed, the bronchi hyparterial (bronchus beneath the pulmonary artery), the inferior vena cava absent, and the P-wave axis superior. Severe pulmonary stenosis is frequent in infants with asplenia and less common in polysplenia.

Treatment. The majority of children with asplenia have heart disease that is uncorrectable by present techniques.

Temporary infusion of prostaglandin E_1 will help those who depend on the ductus arteriosus for pulmonary blood flow (Freed et al., 1981), but the increased pulmonary blood flow may unmask latent pulmonary venous obstruction from the total anomalous pulmonary venous return (Freedom et al., 1978). Palliation in the form of systemic-to-pulmonary artery shunts (Blalock-Taussig, Waterston) has been somewhat successful, except in those with severe obstruction of pulmonary venous return.

Since children without spleens have a high risk of sepsis and, at least in our experience, a higher mortality from sepsis than from their heart disease, we feel that pneumococcal vaccine and prophylactic antibiotics should be administered to all asplenic patients who survive beyond the neonatal period (Waldman et al., 1977).

Prognosis. For the symptomatic neonate, the prognosis remains grim. In the Regional Infant Car-

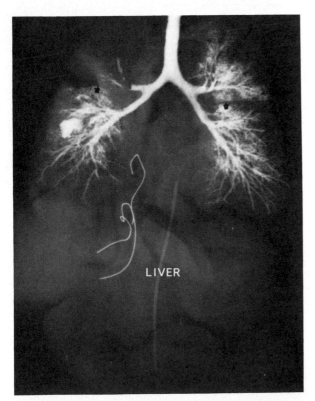

Figure 27–20. A postmortem tracheobronchogram from a newborn who died with the asplenia syndrome. The bronchial pattern is symmetric with the angulation, suggesting bilateral right lungs. The black arrows outline the minor fissure in each lung. The liver is midline and symmetric. (From Rowe, R. D.: The Neonate with Congenital Heart Disease. 2nd ed. Philadelphia, W. B. Saunders Co., 1981.)

LIVER

were dead by 1 year of age; other reports have not been much more positive. Survivors have been reported into adulthood; however, these children almost invariably have just the right amount of pulmonary stenosis to restrict pulmonary blood flow and prevent heart failure but not enough to cause severe hypoxemia.

Polysplenia

Anatomy. In polysplenia there is "bilateral leftsidedness." Multiple splenules are usually present, with the mass of splenic tissue approximating that in the normal spleen. The lungs are usually bilobed, with bilateral hyparterial bronchi (bronchus beneath the pulmonary artery) present in about two thirds of the cases. The liver is often midline, and, in most infants, the stomach is on the right side (Van Mierop et al., 1972). The heart disease may be as complex as that in the infants with asplenia but often is limited to abnormalities of pulmonary venous and systemic venous return. Absence of the renal to hepatic portion of the inferior vena cava is very common, with the hepatic veins draining directly into the right atrium and the lower inferior vena cava into the right or left superior vena cava via an azygos or hemiazygos connection. The superior vena cava is frequently bilateral, and the pulmonary veins often enter separately into both atria, with the right and left veins draining into the ipsilateral atrium. Large atrial septal defects are common, and a common atrium is not unusual. Other cardiac anomalies less frequently seen include pulmonary stenosis, double outlet right ventricle, and endocardial cushion defects. Infants with transposition of the great arteries and single ventricle are uncommon (Van Mierop et al., 1972).

Incidence. (See discussion of asplenia.)

Hemodynamics. The prenatal and postnatal hemodynamics depend on the lesions present. If only abnormalities of pulmonary venous and systemic venous return are present, the children are rarely symptomatic as neonates. If an endocardial cushion type of ventricular septal defect without pulmonary stenosis is present, congestive failure may occur as the pulmonary vascular resistance drops. Less commonly, the pulmonary stenosis is severe, and cyanosis from a right-to-left shunt predominates.

Clinical Manifestations. The clinical findings depend on the associated lesions present. Cyanosis may be present if there is pulmonary stenosis or atresia; congestive failure predominates if there is an endocardial cushion defect without pulmonary obstruction.

The most distinctive feature of the electrocardiogram is the superior P-wave axis, usually known as a "coronary sinus rhythm," with a negative P wave in leads II, III, and AVF (Freedom and Ellison, 1973).

If an endocardial cushion defect is present, the QRS axis will often be superior (0 to -90 degrees) with a counterclockwise loop in the frontal plane.

The chest radiograph is also often distinctive, with a transverse midline liver, right-sided stomach, and absence of the inferior vena cava shadow above the diaphragm in the lateral projection. If the technique is optimal, the bilateral hyparterial bronchi can often be seen.

M-mode and two-dimensional echocardiography are usually helpful in defining the status of the venous return, A-V valves, and ventricular chambers.

Diagnosis. (See discussion of asplenia.)

Treatment and Prognosis. The precise defect will determine the treatment. Those with atrial anomalies alone rarely require treatment in the neonatal period. In infants with more complex anatomy, congestive failure may be prominent and pulmonary artery banding may be necessary to reduce pulmonary blood flow. In the rare child with severe pulmonary stenosis and cyanosis, a palliative shunt to increase pulmonary flow may be beneficial.

The prognosis of these infants depends on the lesions present but is overall somewhat better than that associated with asplenia, since the heart disease is rarely as complex.

Acyanotic Congenital Heart Disease

COARCTATION OF THE AORTA

Anatomy. The sine qua non of this anomaly is the presence of a constriction in the aorta distal to the left subclavian artery, usually at the site of insertion of the ductus arteriosus. There may be, in addition, tubular hypoplasia of the aortic arch and intracardiac anomalies. Coarctation of the aorta formerly was classified as infantile, or preductal, usually with tubular hypoplasia, or adult, or postductal, without tubular hypoplasia. This seems to be an oversimplification, since the preductal type can be seen in older children and a discrete juxtaductal or postductal obstruction can appear in some infants. We prefer the anatomic-physiologic classification suggested in 1972 by Rudolph and coworkers of aortic isthmus narrowing including complete interruption and discrete juxtaductal aortic obstruction. Infants with the former usually have intracardiac defects such as ventricular septal defect, double outlet right ventricle, or tricuspid atresia, and it seems quite likely that the tubular hypoplasia is due to decreased flow through the aortic arch in utero. The etiology of the discrete juxtaductal coarctation is probably different, since the arch is otherwise normal and there are rarely other cardiac anomalies.

One theory is that muscular tissue from the ductus arteriosus extends into the aorta, and, when the ductus closes after birth, the aorta is constricted by this ductal muscle (Ho and Anderson, 1979). Although many still adhere to this theory, histologically the obstruction appears to be on the posterior wall of the aorta, the side opposite to ductal insertion. More recently, it has been suggested that some abnormality of fetal flow or direct injury before birth causes a proliferation of smooth muscle cells and fibrous tissue on the posterior wall of the aorta, resulting in the formation of a shelf of tissue (Rudolph et al., 1972; Talner and Berman, 1975). While the ductus is open in utero or after birth, this shelf is nonobstructive, but when the ductus arteriosus closes, obstruction results.

Incidence. There were 158 cases of infants with coarctation as their primary lesion in the Regional Infant Cardiac Program, representing an incidence of one per 7000 livebirths. Only 35 (17 per cent) of these had juxtaductal coarctation alone; another 35 had coarctation with a ductus arteriosus. There were 73 with a ventricular septal defect with or without a ductus arteriosus, with the remaining 15 having more complex anomalies associated with coarctation. An additional 51 infants had coarctation as a secondary lesion, that is, associated with more complex congenital disease (e.g., single ventricle, transposition of the great arteries, hypoplastic left heart syndrome). Coarctation is the most common congenital heart disease presenting in the second week of life.

Hemodynamics. Since there is normally little flow across the aortic isthmus in utero, the tubular hypoplasia of the arch does not affect fetal growth and development. In the presence of a posterior shelf there is also no significant hemodynamic difficulty, since the flow is small and the large ductus arteriosus allows ample room for it to bypass the narrowing (Fig. 27–21).

After birth, the constriction in the aorta increases left ventricular afterload. In the presence of a ventricular septal defect, this increased systemic resistance leads to a large left-to-right shunt. As the pulmonary vascular resistance falls, the left-to-right shunt increases, resulting in a volume as well as a pressure overload of the left ventricle. In addition to congestive heart failure, there is failure of the blood to pass from ascending to descending aorta if the coarctation is severe. The results are tissue hypoxia, lactic acidosis, and eventual death after the ductus arteriosus closes.

Those infants with a juxtaductal coarctation but no associated anomalies have a slightly different hemodynamic picture. In these neonates, closure of the ductus arteriosus leads to an acute increase in afterload to the left ventricle, as blood must be pumped through the narrowed segment. Since no obstruction

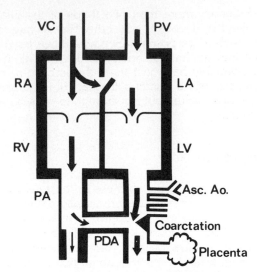

Figure 27–21. Schematic representation of the circulation in a fetus with coarctation of the aorta. The intracardiac blood flow is relatively normal. In utero, the constriction in the aorta is of no physiologic significance, since the open ductus arteriosus allows blood to go around the obstruction. After birth, when the ductus closes, the narrowing is manifest. The abbreviations are the same as those used in Figure 27–2.

was present in utero, no collateral vessels have developed. Owing in part to a reduced number of sympathetic receptors, the neonatal myocardium is not able to respond to increased work as well as the left ventricle of an older child or adult can. Consequently, congestive heart failure, with elevation of left ventricular end-diastolic, left atrial, and pulmonary venous pressures follows. Occasionally, the acute left atrial dilatation causes the septum primum to become incompetent, resulting in an atrial left-to-right shunt. If the coarctation is not too severe, congestive failure may be mild, and there may be time for compensatory mechanisms (e.g., left ventricular hypertrophy or collateral vessels that bypass the obstruction) to develop.

Clinical Features. The neonate with coarctation of the aorta presents with the usual signs and symptoms of congestive heart failure: dyspnea, tachypnea, tachycardia, hepatomegaly, poor feeding, and increased perspiration. A careful examination of the peripheral pulses will demonstrate that pulses and blood pressure (by Doppler or flush method) in the legs are diminished compared with those in the arms. Blood pressure in both arms must be measured, since it may be diminished in the left arm if the coarctation involves the origin of the left subclavian artery and may be decreased in the right arm in the rare situation in which the right subclavian arises anomalously below the coarctation as the last vessel of the aortic arch rather than as the first branch of the innominate. Occasionally, the pulses in the legs will "wax and wane" as the ductus arteriosus opens and closes. In the neonate with an isolated juxtaductal coarctation, there may be no murmur or, occasionally, a short systolic ejection murmur in the axilla or back. In neo nates with tubular hypoplasia and a ventricular septal defect, there is usually a harsh pansystolic murmur at the left lower sternal border, but its absence does not rule out a ventricular defect.

In the absence of complex intracardiac anomalies, there is right axis deviation and right ventricular hypertrophy on the electrocardiogram reflecting normal intrauterine blood flow. On the chest radiograph, the heart is enlarged with the pulmonary vascularity congested and, if a left-to-right shunt is present from a stretched foramen ovale, actively engorged. Poststenotic dilatation in the descending aorta and rib notching, usually present in older children with coarctation, are not seen in neonates.

The left atrium, the ventricle, and, often, the right ventricle are dilated on the M-mode echocardiogram. The two-dimensional study using a subxiphoid or suprasternal view will usually demonstrate the site of obstruction and allows one to estimate the size of the aortic arch. However, some care must be taken, since the isthmus normally is small compared with the ascending and descending aorta in neonates.

Cardiac catheterization and angiocardiography can define the site of obstruction and the size of the aortic arch and document the presence of associated cardiac anomalies, if any. In the neonate with isolated juxtaductal coarctation, there is usually no intracardiac shunting, although a left-to-right shunt at the atrial level may be found. A difference in systolic pressure between the left ventricle or ascending aorta and descending aorta will be found. Angiocardiography in the left ventricle, after insertion of a venous catheter through the foramen ovale, will demonstrate the site of obstruction (Fig. 27–22). In those with more complex disease, the catheterization findings depend on the anomalies present. There is often a left-to-right shunt at the ventricular level, so the pulmonary artery is opacified on a left ventricular injection, making it difficult to visualize the aortic arch. A retrograde study from the umbilical or femoral artery may be necessary to see the coarctation, but we have occasionally been able to show the aortic isthmus from an angiocardiogram done through a #23 indwelling cannula in the radial or brachial artery.

Diagnosis. The diagnosis of coarctation of the aorta is obvious if there is a marked discrepancy in blood pressure between the arms and legs. As already mentioned, however, in some neonates the pulses will "wax and wane," presumably as the ductus arteriosus closes. One must therefore check the pulses and blood pressure more than once if there is any possibility of coarctation.

Coarctation of the aorta must be differentiated from other causes of congestive heart failure in the first or second week of life (see Differential Diagnosis, p. 285). The hypoplastic left heart syndrome usually causes a symmetric decrease in pulses with equal blood pressures in the arms and legs and severe right ventricular hypertrophy on EKG. Aortic stenosis also causes a symmetric decrease in pulses but is usually

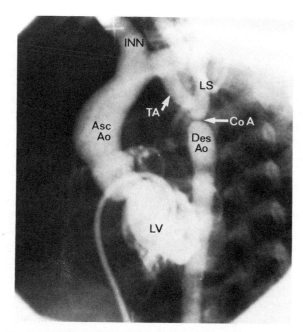

Figure 27–22. Lateral left ventricular angiogram in a newborn with coarctation of the aorta without a ventricular septal defect. There is a discrete narrowing in the aorta just distal to the origin of the left subclavian artery. The transverse aortic arch between the innominate artery and the left subclavian is moderately hypoplastic. Asc Ao = ascending aorta; Co A = coarctation of the aorta; Des Ao = descending aorta; INN = innominate artery; LS = left subclavian artery; LV = left ventricle; TA = transverse aortic arch.

associated with left ventricular hypertrophy and ST–T changes on the electrocardiogram. Echocardiography or catheterization may be necessary to differentiate these lesions if no difference in pulses or blood pressure is apparent.

Treatment. The medical treatment of a neonate with congestive failure from coarctation of the aorta includes digitalis and diuretics and, if acidosis or low outut is present, prostaglandin E_1 to dilate the ductus arteriosus (Freed et al., 1981). Neonates who present later in the first month with a juxtaductal coarctation and no other associated anomalies can occasionally be managed with anticongestives only. In this group, we have postponed surgery until later in the first year of life if heart failure can be controlled and an adequate weight gain sustained. Most neonates who present with coarctation of the aorta, however, have tubular hypoplasia and associated cardiac anomalies. In these infants, heart failure can rarely be controlled, and surgery is eventually mandatory. The most widely used surgical approach has been resection of the abnormal segment of aorta and end-to-end anastomosis of the noninvolved area. Long-term follow-up has demonstrated a relatively high incidence of residual obstruction at the anastomotic site that is due to either incomplete initial relief or, more likely, inadequate growth of the aorta at the anastomotic site through childhood. The subclavian patch plasty has gained favor (Waldhausen et al., 1964) because it avoids a circumferential suture line. With a left thoracotomy, the left subclavian artery is divided, opened lengthwise, turned down, and applied as a patch across the area of obstruction. The initial results of this operation are gratifying, and, in a few reports of long-term follow-up, the good results seem sustained.

Some controversy remains about how to deal with the associated anomalies. If the intracardiac anatomy is complex (single ventricle, transposition with a ventricular defect, etc.) and associated with pulmonary hypertension and a large left-to-right shunt, we place a band around the pulmonary artery to increase pulmonary resistance and reduce pulmonary blood flow at the time of coarctation repair. If the intracardiac anatomy is more straightforward (e.g., a ventricular septal defect or atrioventricular canal), we repair the coarctation using the left thoracotomy and do not band the pulmonary artery. If congestive heart failure cannot be controlled in the postoperative period or if the child cannot be weaned from the respirator, our surgeons will repair the intracardiac defect from a midline approach using deep-hypothermic circulatory arrest. Many surgeons, however, would choose to band these latter infants as well at the time of coarctation repair and postpone definitive repair until later in infancy.

Prognosis. In the New England Regional Infant Cardiac Program extending from 1969 to 1974, only 74 per cent of infants with simple juxtaductal coarctation of the aorta survived to their first birthday. For those with more complex anomalies, the prognosis was even poorer, with less than 50 per cent of infants surviving to 1 year. Surgery in the first week was especially hazardous, with 15 of 17 (88 per cent) neonates dying. Late mortality, usually due to the associated cardiac anomaly, was not uncommon.

More recently, there has been a significant improvement that is due to better preoperative care with prostaglandins, improved surgery, and better perioperative and postoperative management. In 1981, Kamau and coworkers reported a series of 34 children under 6 months of age (20 under 1 month) who underwent surgery; among these patients, there was only one early and one late death. In their 1983 report, Hesslein and coworkers reported a 10-year experience with symptomatic coarctation in infancy. Ten patients without associated lesions had no mortality. Of 87 with associated anomalies, the overall 8-year survival rate was 62 per cent, with most of the deaths occurring in the first 6 months of life. Our experience has been similar over the past few years.

INTERRUPTED AORTIC ARCH

Anatomy. Infants with an interrupted aortic arch have a discontinuity between the ascending and descending aorta. Celoria and Patton classified children with an interrupted aortic arch according to the site of the discontinuity: Type A, distal to the left subclavian artery (42 per cent of cases); Type B, distal to the left common carotid artery (53 per cent of cases); and Type C, distal to the innominate artery (4 per cent of cases) (Van Praagh et al., 1971). Almost any cardiac anomaly can be associated with interrupted aortic arch, but a patent ductus arteriosus and a ventricular septal defect are almost invariably present, and aortic stenosis, double outlet right ventricle, truncus arteriosus, and single ventricle are not uncommon.

The embryologic defect in interrupted aortic arch is not known, but Van Praagh and coworkers suggest that a leftward shift of the crista supraventricularis in the developing heart obstructs the subaortic region, reducing antegrade flow through the aortic valve and diverting flow away from the ascending aorta (arches 3 and 4) and toward the pulmonary artery (arch 6). This results in inappropriate involution of a portion of the transverse arch.

Incidence. In the New England Regional Infant Cardiac Program, there were 21 infants with interrupted aortic arch, an incidence of one per 50,000 livebirths; these infants represent about 1 per cent of critically ill infants with congenital heart disease.

Hemodynamics. In the normal fetus, the left ventricle supplies the ascending aorta and the right ventricle supplies the descending aorta through the ductus arteriosus, with only 10 per cent of combined ventricular output passing through the arch of the aorta from ascending to descending aorta (Rudolph et al., 1974). In the fetus with an interrupted aortic arch, no blood passes through the aortic isthmus, but this results in no major observable hemodynamic abnormalities (Fig. 27–23). After birth, however, the descending aorta continues to depend on the ductus arteriosus to provide systemic output. When the ductus begins to close, flow to the descending aorta diminishes, and tissue hypoxia, acidosis, and death follow. Rarely, the ductus arteriosus remains open. In these infants, congestive heart failure occurs as the pulmonary vascular resistance falls over the first weeks of life and pulmonary blood flow increases.

Clinical Manifestations. The clinical presentations of the various types of interruption are similar. As the pulmonary vascular resistance falls, the neonates develop the signs and symptoms of congestive heart failure: respiratory distress, tachypnea, tachycardia, hepatomegaly, poor feeding, and increased perspiration. As the ductus arteriosus closes, the pulses and perfusion in the lower body diminish and mottling appears. Although differential cyanosis should be observable, since the upper body receives

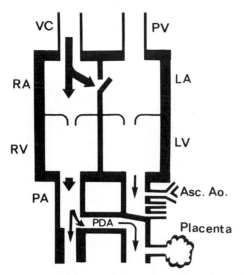

Figure 27-23. Schematic diagram of the circulation in a fetus with an interrupted aortic arch. The intracardiac flow is normal. Blood from the right atrium passes through the right ventricle, pulmonary artery, and ductus arteriosus to the descending aorta and placenta. Flow to the ascending aorta is derived from blood passing through the foramen ovale and left heart chambers. No blood crosses from ascending to descending aorta. After birth, when the ductus arteriosus constricts, blood supply to the lower half of the body is compromised. The abbreviations are the same as those used in Figure 27-2.

suprasternal views as well as outlining the intracardiac structures. However, care must be taken because the aortic isthmus normally narrows significantly.

At cardiac catheterization, the systolic pressures in both ventricles, ascending aorta, and main pulmonary artery are equal because of the large ventricular septal defect. Frequently, there is a gradient between the main pulmonary artery and descending aorta reflecting the closing ductus arteriosus. Although anatomically there is often evidence of subaortic narrowing secondary to the leftward shift of the crista supraventricularis, we have rarely measured a gradient between left ventricle and ascending aorta at catheterization, probably because of reduced antegrade flow.

Angiocardiography in the left and right ventricle usually outlines the site of the interruption, but occasionally an axillary cutdown with injection in the axillary artery or ascending aorta may be necessary (Fig. 27-24).

Diagnosis. The diagnosis of interrupted aortic arch is difficult but should be suspected in any neonate with early congestive heart failure. The finding of differential blood pressures between the arms and legs suggests either coarctation of the aorta or interruption; differences in the pulse between the right and

fully saturated blood from the left ventricle and the lower body receives desaturated venous blood from the pulmonary artery, it is rarely clinically apparent because a large left-to-right shunt through a ventricular septal defect tends to increase the pulmonary artery oxygen saturation, and pulmonary venous desaturation from pulmonary edema lowers the aortic saturation, making the differences minimal and not clinically visible, even to the experienced observer. The presence of strong pulses in the left carotid but not in the left subclavian artery or in the right carotid but not left carotid artery can often localize the site of the interruption. Heart murmurs are rarely impressive in these infants, but a systolic murmur can sometimes be heard along the left sternal border, presumably from the ventricular septal defect. The second sound is usually loud and single.

Since intrauterine flows are normal, the electrocardiogram is rarely helpful at birth; there is usually right axis deviation and right ventricular hypertrophy that is normal for age. No specific anomalies are present on the chest radiograph other than generalized cardiac enlargement and increased pulmonary vascular markings often associated with pulmonary venous congestion.

If only a ventricular septal defect and ductus arteriosus are present, the M-mode echocardiogram will have left atrial and ventricular dilatation and right ventricular hypertrophy. We have been reasonably successful at visualizing the site of the interruption on two-dimensional echocardiography by subxiphoid or

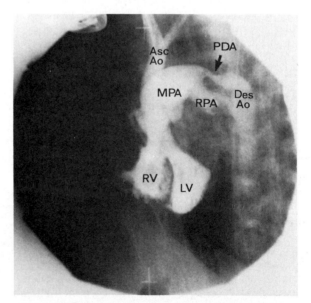

Figure 27-24. Lateral left ventricular angiogram of a neonate with an interrupted aortic arch. There is no connection between the ascending and descending aorta; blood flow to the descending aorta is derived from the pulmonary artery through a closing ductus arteriosus. A ventricular septal defect connecting the right and left ventricle is present. Asc Ao = ascending aorta; Des Ao = descending aorta; LV = left ventricle; MPA = main pulmonary artery; PDA = patent ductus arteriosus; RPA = right pulmonary artery; RV = right ventricle.

left carotid make the latter condition more probable. The distinction between a Type A interruption (distal to the left subclavian) and coarctation is angiocardiographic. Other acyanotic heart diseases in the neonate in which congestive heart failure occurs (e.g., aortic stenosis and hypoplastic left heart syndrome) can usually be excluded by the differential pulses in interrupted aortic arch or by the electrocardiographic finding of left ventricular hypertrophy and strain in aortic stenosis and the echocardiographic demonstration of a small ascending aorta in the hypoplastic left heart syndrome.

Treatment. Although the initial treatment of neonates with an interrupted arch is medical (digoxin, diuretics, and prostaglandin E_1 to dilate the ductus arteriosus), the prognosis is grim without surgical intervention. Initial attempts at palliation with a conduit from pulmonary artery to descending aorta to create a permanent ductus arteriosus and bilateral pulmonary artery banding to reduce pulmonary blood flow (Litwin et al., 1972) were not very successful at our hospital. We prefer total correction of infants with an interrupted aortic arch and a ventricular septal defect (Collins-Nakai et al., 1976).

From a left thoracotomy, a Dacron conduit is attached to the descending aorta. The left thoracotomy is closed and from a midline sternotomy the proximal part of the conduit is attached to the ascending aorta, the patent ductus arteriosus is ligated, and the ventricular septal defect is closed using deep-hypothermic circulatory arrest. Initial results of this complex undertaking have been quite promising, with eight survivors among the last 10 reported neonates (William Norwood, personal communication). For infants with interrupted aortic arch associated with more complex intracardiac anatomy, repair of the aortic arch, and pulmonary artery banding are probably the procedures of choice.

Prognosis. In the Regional Infant Cardiac Program, the prognosis for this group was poor (Collins-Nakai et al., 1976). Of nine patients who were treated medically, eight died at a median age of 4 days. Of the 21 treated surgically, one third had a ventricular septal defect, one third had a ventricular defect and left ventricular outflow obstruction, and one third had complex intracardiac anomalies. The overall mortality was 76 per cent. It remains to be demonstrated how much progress can be expected with earlier diagnosis, better medical management (including prostaglandin E_1 to maintain ductal patency), and improved surgical techniques.

AORTIC STENOSIS

Anatomy. Although left ventricular outflow obstruction in childhood may occur below or above the valve, for all practical purposes only valvular aortic stenosis causes severe symptoms in the neonatal period. The valve is usually unicommissural and unicuspid (Moller et al., 1966), and the tissue is thickened, nodular, and severely deformed. The myocardium is always very hypertrophied, but the left ventricular cavity varies in size. It may be quite dilated, normal, or hypoplastic; when small, the defect gradually becomes a part of the hypoplastic left heart syndrome. In many infants, the left ventricular endocardium is thickened and covered with a gray layer of fibrous and elastic tissue that may involve the papillary muscles, resulting in mitral regurgitation. This "endocardial fibroelastosis" is probably secondary to myocardial hypoxia from the very thick myocardium, which, in the presence of high intracavitary pressures, cannot be adequately perfused in the endocardial layers.

Associated lesions such as coarctation of the aorta and ventricular or atrial septal defects are occasionally seen.

Incidence. In the Regional Infant Cardiac Program there were 45 cases of infants with aortic stenosis, representing an incidence of one per 24,000 livebirths. They represented 2 per cent of infants seen with critical heart disease.

Hemodynamics. In utero, the presence of left ventricular outflow obstruction imposes a pressure load on the left ventricle. If the stenosis occurs early in gestation and is severe, the afterload will reduce flow through the ventricle, and left ventricular hypoplasia and hypoplastic left heart syndrome may result (Rudolph, 1974). If the stenosis is less severe, the left ventricular size will be normal, but the myocardium will be very hypertrophied and fibroelastosis from inadequate endocardial perfusion may be present.

After birth, the left ventricular output normally must increase by about 50 per cent with the switch from a parallel to an in series circulation. In the presence of severe aortic obstruction, the marginally compensated left ventricle may be unable to handle increased volume load. If the foramen ovale is closed, the left atrial pressure will rapidly increase, leading to pulmonary edema. Occasionally, left atrial dilatation makes the septum primum incompetent, allowing the left atrium to decompress through the foramen ovale. This left-to-right shunt at the atrial level may exacerbate the congestive heart failure.

Clinical Manifestations. The infant with critical aortic stenosis is usually normal at birth. A systolic murmur is invariably audible along the left sternal border with radiation to the right upper sternal border but may be only grade 2 or 3/6. The symptoms of congestive heart failure—respiratory distress, poor feeding, and tachypnea—may be delayed by hours to weeks, but once symptoms occur, they may progress very rapidly, leading to a low output state with cool, mottled extremities, very diminished pulses, and a murmur that is barely audible.

The murmur is rarely associated with a thrill, even when output is adequate, but a systolic ejection click at the apex may be present. In stark contrast with its radiographically visible enlargement, the heart is rarely hyperactive on palpation.

The most frequent electrocardiographic pattern is left ventricular hypertrophy with inverted T waves over the left precordium, suggesting left ventricular ischemia (Fig. 27–25). Occasionally, right ventricular hypertrophy may be seen, but in our experience (Keane et al., 1975), this is associated with at least some hypoplasia of the left ventricle. Even in those with right ventricular predominance, inverted T waves over the left precordium are common.

In infants with congestive heart failure, the heart is invariably enlarged on chest radiographs and may be quite massive. The pulmonary vessels are indistinct owing to pulmonary venous congestion and may also be actively engorged if there is a large left-to-right shunt at the atrial level from a stretched foramen ovale.

On the M-mode echocardiogram, there is dilatation of the left atrium and ventricle and increased thickness of the septum and posterior wall. The aortic valve closure is often eccentric within the aortic root, and the valve may show multiple diastolic echoes. The two-dimensional echocardiogram confirms the M-mode findings and allows better visualization of the aortic valve.

At cardiac catheterization, the left ventricle can usually be approached through the foramen ovale, but occasionally a retrograde study across the aortic valve or even a transatrial septal puncture may be necessary. There is usually a pressure gradient of greater than 40 mm Hg between the left ventricle and ascending aorta, with the left ventricular systolic pressure exceeding 120 mm Hg, but occasionally in children with severe congestive heart failure the left ventricle cannot generate such a high pressure, and the gradient may be less. The left ventricular end-diastolic pressure is invariably elevated and has been observed to be as high as 35 mm Hg. If the foramen ovale is incompetent, a left-to-right shunt at the atrial level may be present, with the pulmonary flow–to–systemic flow ratio occasionally exceeding 3 : 1. A left ventricular angiocardiogram in the left anterior oblique projection will outline the domed and thickened aortic valve.

Diagnosis. Aortic stenosis must be differentiated from other causes of heart failure in the first month of life. With aortic atresia and the hypoplastic left heart syndrome, there is congestive failure but no left ventricular hypertrophy on the electrocardiogram. In

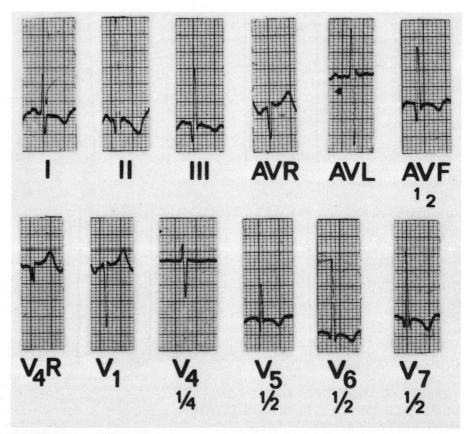

Figure 27–25. Electrocardiogram in a neonate with aortic stenosis. There is left ventricular hypertrophy for age. The inverted T waves in the left precordium suggest left ventricular strain (ischemia).

coarctation of the aorta with or without a ventricular septal defect, the pulses are weak or absent in the legs but are usually palpable in the arms and carotids, and left ventricular strain on the EKG is usually not present. The murmur of aortic stenosis is loudest at the right or left upper sternal borders, whereas in infants with coarctation the murmur is louder at the lower left sternal border or into the axilla. Finally, aortic stenosis is associated with an ejection click that is rarely present in the newborn with coarctation of the aorta.

With acyanotic lesions causing congestive heart failure such as ventricular septal defects, atrioventricular canal defects, and patent ductus arteriosus, there is usually a very hyperactive precordium associated with the large left-to-right shunts. In tricuspid atresia, truncus arteriosus, and single ventricle, there is usually cyanosis with crying.

Treatment. These infants are usually quite sick when first seen, and the usual medical management with digoxin, diuretics, and correction of acidosis must be accomplished without delay. Because a progressive downhill course is almost inevitable once an infant becomes symptomatic, prompt catheterization and surgery are indicated. Aortic valvotomy, under inflow occlusion or cardiopulmonary bypass, is the procedure of choice. The operative risk remains high, in part owing to hypoplasia of the ventricle and aortic annulus or coexisting fibroelastosis, and repeat surgery is not infrequently necessary because of inadequate relief or restenosis (Keane et al., 1975).

Prognosis. In the Regional Infant Cardiac Program, the overall survival rate to the first birthday was only 22 of 45 infants, or 49 per cent (Fyler et al., 1980), with a 68 per cent mortality rate among infants undergoing surgery prior to 2 months of age. Of 18 infants surviving surgery who were followed by Keane and coworkers, residual abnormalities were present in most, and six required repeat operation to relieve residual stenosis or regurgitation. In 1981, Edmunds and coworkers reported a 50 per cent mortality among 14 neonates undergoing aortic valvotomy. They correlated the angiocardiographically determined left ventricular size with operative risk and found that seven of eight newborns with a normally sized ventricle survived valvotomy, with six remaining alive 1½ to 6½ years after operation. Of six patients with a small left ventricle (end-diastolic volume of less than 30 ml/m^2) all succumbed.

HYPOPLASTIC LEFT HEART SYNDROME: AORTIC OR MITRAL ATRESIA OR SEVERE STENOSIS WITH A HYPOPLASTIC LEFT VENTRICLE

Anatomy. On gross pathologic examination, the hearts of children with "hypoplastic left heart syndrome" (Noonan and Nadas, 1958) are all similar, with severe hypoplasia of the left ventricle and ascending aorta and a dilated right ventricle and pulmonary artery. The aortic valve may be atretic with a complete absence of any recognizable valve tissue or may be fused and domed with an eccentric pinhole orifice. The mitral valve is atretic in one fourth of the cases and hypoplastic in the rest. The left ventricle may be slit-like if both mitral and aortic valves are atretic but is somewhat more developed when there is some flow through the mitral valve. The ascending aorta is hypoplastic between the coronaries and the innominate artery, and a coarctation of the aorta may be present. Ventricular septal defects are uncommon.

Incidence. In the New England Regional Infant Cardiac Program there were 177 cases of infants with hypoplastic left heart syndrome reported between 1969 and 1974, representing an incidence of one per 6000 livebirths. The syndrome is the fifth most common form of all congenital heart diseases, the second most common heart disease presenting in the first week of life (after transposition), and the third most common appearing in the second week of life (following coarctation of the aorta and ventricular septal defect).

Hemodynamics. In a fetus with a hypoplastic left heart, the right ventricle must support the entire circulation (Fig. 27–26). Almost all the systemic venous return that enters the right atrium passes into the right

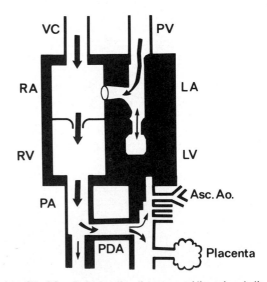

Figure 27–26. Schematic diagram of the circulation in a fetus with hypoplastic left heart syndrome. There is aortic atresia and hypoplasia of the left ventricle, left atrium, and mitral valve. The systemic venous return from the vena cava passes through the right heart chambers into the ductus arteriosus and then to the descending aorta and placenta as well as the ascending aorta. The pulmonary venous return goes through a foramen ovale into the right atrium. After birth, the foramen may be obstructive as pulmonary flow increases. When the ductus arteriosus constricts, flow to the systemic circulation is reduced, and low output shock and death follow. The abbreviations are the same as those used in Figure 27–2.

ventricle and is ejected into the pulmonary artery. A small portion of blood may pass through the foramen ovale, but with mitral or aortic atresia this is minimal. Since the pulmonary resistance is high, virtually all the blood entering the pulmonary artery is diverted through the ductus arteriosus into the aorta rather than passing into the lungs. Most goes to the descending aorta and placenta, but some goes retrograde into the aortic arch and ascending aorta to the subclavian, carotid, and coronary arteries. The ascending aorta is small because the coronary arteries are the only continuation after the takeoff of the innominate artery.

After birth, the pulmonary vascular resistance falls and the systemic resistance increases so that an increasing proportion of blood from the single pulmonary trunk goes to the lungs rather than through the ductus arteriosus. The increased pulmonary blood flow leads to an increase in pulmonary venous return that cannot freely exit from the left atrium because of hypoplasia of the left atrium and foramen ovale and results in pulmonary venous hypertension and pulmonary edema. As the ductus arteriosus begins to close at 12 to 48 hours of age, the perfusion to the systemic circulation is reduced, resulting in systemic and coronary ischemia. Understandably, neonates with this disease are the sickest patients seen by the pediatric cardiologist, with the median age of death 4½ days in untreated infants (Watson and Rowe, 1962).

Clinical Features. The infants are usually normal at birth, but tachypnea and dyspnea soon develop as the pulmonary blood flow increases. Cyanosis is rarely prominent, despite the total mixing of the systemic and pulmonary circulations, since the pulmonary blood flow is so increased. Congestive heart failure with tachypnea, hepatomegaly, and poor feeding are usually present by 24 to 48 hours of age. Finally, as the ductus arteriosus begins to close, the signs of low output—mottling, grayness of the skin, and markedly diminished pulses—follow. Auscultation is rarely helpful because prominent murmurs are unusual and the second heart sound is single.

The electrocardiogram reflects the intrauterine circulation, showing right axis deviation and right ventricular predominance that may be normal for age. Occasionally, diminished left-sided forces due to left ventricular hypoplasia can be appreciated. Right atrial hypertrophy is seen in about two thirds of the infants. Coronary ischemia frequently results in ST–T wave changes.

The heart is markedly enlarged on chest radiographs, with both increased pulmonary blood flow and pulmonary venous congestion prominent.

M-mode echocardiography may be diagnostic. There are a large anterior ventricle and tricuspid valve with a small mitral valve and aortic root. With two-dimensional study, these findings are often better visualized.

Cardiac catheterization may be performed to confirm the clinical and echocardiographic findings and to rule out correctable heart disease if the echocar-

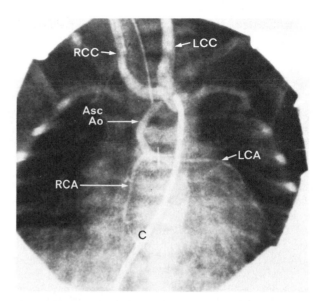

Figure 27–27. Angiogram in the aorta in a child with the hypoplastic left heart syndrome with aortic atresia. There is no antegrade flow through the aortic valve. Blood flow to the hypoplastic ascending aorta is retrograde from the ductus arteriosus. Asc Ao = ascending aorta; C = catheter; LCA = left coronary artery; LCC = left common carotid artery; RCA = right coronary artery; RCC = right common carotid artery.

diogram is equivocal. The pulmonary venous and left atrial pressures are elevated. The right ventricular and pulmonary artery pressures are increased and often exceed the systolic pressure in the aorta, reflecting the gradient across the closing ductus arteriosus. There is a large increase in oxygen saturation between vena cava and right atrium that is due to the torrential flow of pulmonary venous return from the left to the right atrium.

An angiocardiogram in the right ventricle, pulmonary artery, or aorta is usually diagnostic (Fig. 27–27). The ascending aorta is opacified retrograde from the ductus arteriosus and is extremely hypoplastic with little, if any, flow of unopacified blood through the aortic valve. In the presence of mitral stenosis rather than atresia, a left atrial injection will demonstrate the size of the left ventricle.

Diagnosis. Infants with the hypoplastic left heart syndrome must be differentiated from those with other causes of respiratory distress in the first month of life.

In the early stages the tachypnea may suggest lung disease, but the appearance of congestive heart failure with tachycardia, hepatomegaly, and cardiac enlargement on radiographs should allow the two to be differentiated.

After the onset of congestive heart failure, hypoplastic left heart must be differentiated from the two other common causes of failure early in the first week of life: aortic stenosis and the coarctation syndrome. There is usually left ventricular hypertrophy on EKG in the former, and a difference in pulses and blood pressure between the upper and lower extremities is normally present in the latter.

The differentation of low output shock, secondary to hypoplastic left heart syndrome, from the other causes of shock in the neonate is usually straightforward if the index of suspicion of heart disease is high.

Treatment.   Since the hypoplastic left heart syndrome has been uniformly fatal, treatment has usually been terminated at the time of definitive diagnosis. Recently, some centers have suggested palliative operations in an attempt to improve the poor prognosis. In infants for whom palliative procedures are being considered, congestive failure should be treated with digoxin and diuretics. Prostaglandin E_1 infusion will often dilate the ductus arteriosus (Freed et al., 1981) and improve perfusion. Bicarbonate should be given to treat the metabolic acidosis, but the quantity of sodium given must be carefully monitored so as not to create a hyperosmolar state.

Several surgical procedures have been suggested. A palliative procedure involving a pulmonary artery–to–descending aorta conduit, banding the distal pulmonary artery and atrial septectomy (similar to the palliative operation for interrupted aortic arch), has been suggested (Litwin et al., 1972) but has failed to gain favor because of the absence of any definitive procedures. The success of the Fontan and Baudet procedure for tricuspid atresia in demonstrating that a ventricle may not be needed for pumping on the right side of the heart has prompted Norwood and coworkers as well as Behrendt and Rocchini to undertake a two-stage procedure of early palliation (and later Fontan) that potentially may offer long-term survival.

In their 1983 review, Norwood and coworkers reported a survivor of the second stage in whom physiologic correction of this lesion was accomplished for the first time.

The optimal treatment of this disease remains an unanswered question.

Prognosis.   All 86 infants with aortic atresia in the New England Regional Infant Cardiac Program were dead by their first birthday. Of those with mitral atresia and hypoplasia of the left ventricle, only 10 of 60 (17 per cent) survived to their first birthday. How newer surgical innovations will alter the prognosis remains to be seen.

VENTRICULAR SEPTAL DEFECTS

Anatomy.   Ventricular septal defects (VSD) may be isolated, part of a more complex cardiac anomaly such as tetralogy of Fallot, or associated with other congenital cardiac defects such as coarctation of the aorta with a ventricular defect. In this section, only the isolated defect will be considered; the more complicated types are discussed further on in the chapter. Ventricular defects have been classified according to their location in the ventricular septum. The most common site is the membranous portion of the septum that lies between the crista supraventricularis and the papillary muscle of the conus when the heart is viewed from the right ventricular side. Less common sites are the area above crista (subpulmonary), the muscular portion of the septum below the tricuspid valve (atrioventricular canal), and the anterior trabecular portion of the ventricular septum near the apex of the right ventricle. The size of ventricular septal defects varies: They can be as small as a pinhole or large enough to make the ventricular septum almost completely absent. In about 10 per cent of infants, multiple defects are present.

Incidence.   Ventricular septal defects are the most common congenital cardiac anomaly. Rowe and coworkers found 20 neonates with VSD among 13,653 livebirths in New Zealand between 1960 and 1963. In the New England Regional Infant Cardiac Program, there were 374 cases of infants with *large* ventricular defects among slightly more than 1,000,000 livebirths in the six New England states between 1969 and 1974, representing an incidence of one per 3000 livebirths.

Hemodynamics.   Since the right and left sides of the heart are arranged in parallel before birth, the presence of a large communication at the ventricular level in addition to the normal ductus connection at the great vessel level does not significantly alter the fetal circulation. After birth, the hemodynamics depend on the size of the defect and the pulmonary and systemic vascular resistances. If the defect is large (>1 cm^2/m^2 body size or equal to at least half the size of the aortic valve), it offers no resistance to flow. The systolic pressures in both ventricles and both great vessels are approximately equal, and the degree of intracardiac shunting is determined by the systemic and pulmonary vascular resistances. For the first few hours of life, the resistances are about equal, and little shunting (left-to-right or right-to-left) occurs. Over the following hours, days, and weeks, the pulmonary vascular resistance gradually falls, increasing the proportion of blood ejected by the left ventricle that goes through the VSD into the pulmonary artery. When the pulmonary blood flow is about three times greater than the systemic flow, the left ventricle can no longer accommodate the volume load, and signs and symptoms of congestive heart failure develop. In full-term infants with an isolated ventricular defect, this usually occurs late in the first or during the second month of life, but failure is occasionally seen earlier, sometimes in the first week, presumably owing to a more rapid fall in the pulmonary vascular resistance. The left-to-right shunting at the ventricular level results in increased flow in the pulmonary artery, pulmonary vein, left atrium, and left ventricle, with the latter chamber ejecting blood directly into the pulmonary artery. The right atrium and right ventricle are not volume overloaded, but in the presence of a large defect the right ventricle must generate pressures equal to those of the left ventricle, so there is usually right ventricular hypertrophy without significant dilation.

If the ventricular defect is small, it does offer resistance to flow, and the pressures in the two ventricles may differ. These infants are a heterogeneous group, with the hemodynamics depending on the size of the hole rather than the pulmonary vascular resistance. If the defect is very small, the right ventricular and pulmonary artery pressures may be normal and the pulmonary blood flow less than twice the systemic flow. These infants are rarely symptomatic, and a murmur is usually the sole indication of heart disease. If the defect is larger, the right heart pressures may be close to systemic pressures, with flow ratios exceeding 3:1. These infants may have congestive heart failure.

Clinical Features. Newborns with a small ventricular septal defect have a grade 2 or 3/6 high-pitched, pansystolic murmur along the left sternal border and are asymptomatic.

Even if the defect is large, the elevated pulmonary resistance prevents significant shunting in the first few days and weeks of life, so heart failure is unusual. Later, as the left-to-right shunt increases, signs and symptoms of congestive failure—tachypnea, tiring with feeding, poor weight gain, diaphoresis, and hepatomegaly—develop.

On physical examination, the cardiac impulse is usually hyperactive and the apex is displaced laterally. A systolic thrill and grade 4/6 pansystolic murmur can be appreciated along the left sternal border. If the left-to-right shunt is large, a mid-diastolic rumble is audible at the apex from the increased flow across a structurally normal mitral valve. If the pulmonary artery pressure is increased, the pulmonary component of the second heart sound will be single or narrowly split and accentuated.

Although the electrocardiogram is usually an accurate tool for assessing the hemodynamics in older children with a VSD, it is less valuable in the neonate because the normal pattern of right ventricular predominance masks the typical changes. A normal progression from right to left ventricular predominance over the first month is usual for a small VSD, and an increase in both right and left ventricular forces over the first month of life is typical of a large ventricular defect with pulmonary hypertension.

The chest film is a better tool than the electrocardiogram in the evaluation of a neonate with a ventricular defect. If the heart is normal in size and the pulmonary vascular markings are normal, the left-to-right shunt is small. With large shunts, the cardiac silhouette is enlarged, and the pulmonary vascular markings are increased and, if there is an elevated pulmonary venous pressure, indistinct (Fig. 27–28).

The M-mode echocardiogram may be helpful in assessing the size of the left-to-right shunt because

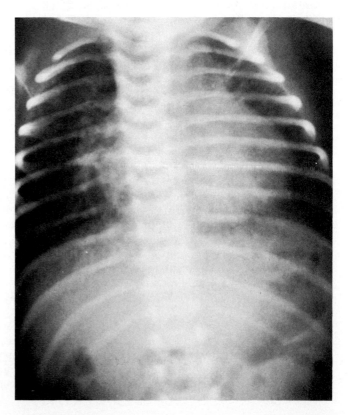

Figure 27–28. Plain anteroposterior chest radiograph in a newborn with a large ventricular septal defect. The heart is enlarged, and the pulmonary blood flow is increased.

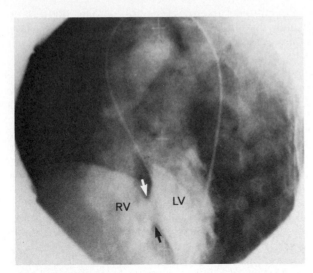

Figure 27–29. Left ventricular angiogram in the hepatoclavicular "4 chamber" projection using 40 degrees of left anterior obliquity and 40 degrees of cranial angulation. A large midmuscular ventricular septal defect is outlined by the arrows. LV = left ventricle; RV = right ventricle.

the left atrium dilates with increasing pulmonary venous return. The two-dimensional echocardiogram can usually visualize defects that are larger than 3 mm and rule out associated cardiac anomalies (Bierman et al., 1980).

Cardiac catheterization is unnecessary in asymptomatic neonates. In symptomatic infants, we defer catheterization until surgery is contemplated if the VSD has been localized and more complicated disease ruled out on two-dimensional echocardiogram. The purposes of the catheterization are to measure the magnitude of the left-to-right shunt and pulmonary artery pressure, to locate the position and number of the ventricular defect(s), and to exclude other anomalies. There is a large increase in saturation between the superior vena cava and pulmonary artery that is usually located between the right atrium and ventricle but occasionally seen between the vena cava and right atrium if an atrial septal defect or stretched foramen ovale is present. Angiocardiography in the left ventricle in the left anterior oblique position with cranial angulation (axial oblique) will outline most of the membranous ventricular septum and the four-chamber, or hepatoclavicular, view will outline the posterior septum (Fig. 27–29). An aortogram is necessary to exclude a coexisting patent ductus arteriosus if the pulmonary artery pressure is elevated.

Diagnosis. As emphasized by Rowe and coworkers, a baby who has congestive heart failure and a systolic murmur in the first 2 weeks of life is not likely to have an isolated ventricular defect. If cyanosis is absent, coarctation (with or without a ventricular defect), critical aortic stenosis, or the hypoplastic left heart syndrome is more likely. They can usually be differentiated by the absence of femoral pulses in coarctation, the presence of left ventricular hypertrophy with strain on the electrocardiogram in aortic stenosis, and the appearance of a shock-like picture in the hypoplastic left heart syndrome. If cyanosis is present, truncus arteriosus, tricuspid atresia, or tetralogy of Fallot must be considered. In the asymptomatic neonate with a murmur, mild aortic stenosis, valvular or peripheral pulmonary stenosis, and tetralogy of Fallot can be confused, especially if the lesions are mild.

Treatment. One must treat neonates with a ventricular septal defect with the knowledge that many, if not most, of small defects will close spontaneously and that up to 20 per cent of large defects will also get much smaller or close (Mesko et al., 1973; Fyler et al., 1980).

Neonates with a small or moderate size ventricular septal defect often require no treatment. For those with mild heart failure, digoxin and diuretics and the usual anticongestive measures often suffice. Occasionally, a child with a large defect will respond poorly to anticongestive measures with continued severe heart failure and poor weight gain in spite of maximal medical management. The procedure of choice has been pulmonary artery banding, a palliative operation in which an iatrogenic obstruction is placed above the pulmonary valve to increase pulmonary resistance and reduce the left-to-right shunt. More recently, we have switched to primary repair using deep-hypothermic circulatory arrest with gratifying results and risks similar to or less than what we used to have with banding alone (Rein et al., 1977). Over the next decade, it seems clear that the trend will be toward early primary repair for the small group of infants with a ventricular defect in whom surgery is necessary.

Prognosis. The prognosis for the neonate with a small VSD is excellent. In one study of 50 children, it was predicted from actuarial analysis that 75 per cent of the defects would close by 10 years of age (Alpert et al., 1979). Many of the large defects that present during the first weeks of life will also become significantly smaller, and some of these will close. Even for the large defect that requires surgical closure, the results have dramatically improved in the past few years, so that correction can be accomplished with risks of 5 per cent or less (Rein et al., 1977).

PATENT DUCTUS ARTERIOSUS

Anatomy. Embryologically, the ductus arteriosus represents a persistence of the left sixth aortic arch. In utero, it serves to divert blood away from the fluid-filled lungs toward the descending aorta and placenta, where oxygen exchange occurs. Histologically, it is composed of more circumferential smooth muscle and less elastic tissue than either the pulmonary artery or the aorta. Although research efforts have been directed over the past decade at the mechanisms involved with patency during fetal life and closure soon after birth, the precise pathways are not yet completely understood.

It seems quite likely, however, that E prostaglandins actively dilate the ductus before birth (Coceani and Olley, 1973). With the onset of respiration and increase in circulating oxygen on the ductal tissue the ductus closes, but it remains unclear whether the response to oxygen is due to a decrease in the local production or increased removal of prostaglandin E or other prostaglandins, an increase in production of other prostanoids with constriction properties, or an end-organ loss of responsiveness to the dilatory properties of all prostaglandins, with active vasoconstriction. In the normal infant, the ductus arteriosus is physiologically closed within the first day or so of life, with permanent anatomic closure complete by 5 to 7 days.

Persistent patency of the ductus may be seen in three different groups of patients: full-term infants who are otherwise normal, premature infants, and infants with heart disease. Only the first two groups will be discussed here; the ductus in infants with other structural cardiac anomalies will be reviewed in discussions of the specific lesions. Persistent patency of the ductus arteriosus is rarely a problem in the term infant, with the diagnosis and management relatively straightforward and the prognosis excellent. Conversely, in the premature infant with lung disease, the diagnosis may be difficult, the management is controversial, and the prognosis, influenced by the accompanying lung disease, is still unclear.

Incidence. In the Regional Infant Cardiac Program, there were 136 cases of infants with a significant patent ductus arteriosus (PDA), representing an incidence of one per 7000 livebirths. About one third of the infants with a PDA were less than 36 weeks gestation, reducing the incidence of hemodynamically significant patent ductus in *term* infants to about one per 10000 livebirths. Premature infants have a much higher incidence of PDA. In one collaborative study involving patent ductus arteriosus in premature infants, 21 per cent of neonates under 1750 gm had clinical or laboratory evidence of a large, hemodynamically significant PDA (Nadas et al., personal communication). The incidence was correlated with birth weight; 40 per cent of infants less than 1000 gm at birth had a clinically significant PDA, compared with 9 per cent of those greater than 1500 gm.

Hemodynamics. As with most left-to-right shunts, the two major factors that influence the hemodynamics are the size of the connection between left and right sides of the circulation and the pulmonary and systemic resistances. In preterm infants with a patent ductus arteriosus, one must also consider the infant's ability to handle the increased volume load.

In infants with a small ductus arteriosus, one that has almost completely closed, the degree of shunting is limited by the cross sectional area of the connection; these patients usually do quite well. With a ductus that has only minimally constricted, the structure itself offers little restriction flow, and the magnitude of the left-to-right shunt is determined by the relative pulmonary and systemic resistances. In term infants, the normal fall in pulmonary resistance is gradual, and the compensatory mechanisms that deal with increased left-sided volumes are relatively well developed. These infants rarely have severe congestive heart failure in the first month.

In the preterm infant without lung disease, however, the pulmonary resistance falls much more rapidly, probably owing to a lack of muscular development in the resistance vessels of the lung, the pulmonary arterioles. This leads to a rapid increase in the magnitude of the left-to-right shunt. In addition, recent studies have demonstrated that the myocardium of the preterm infant has little ability to increase contractility to handle the increased volume load because of a decrease in sympathetic innervation of the immature heart. This rapid fall in resistance and subsequent increasing left-to-right shunt in combination with the lack of compensatory mechanisms available to the premature may lead to significant heart failure in the first 1 or 2 weeks of life.

In the premature neonate with respiratory distress syndrome and hypoxia, the pulmonary vascular resistance may initially exceed systemic vascular resistance, leading to a right-to-left (pulmonary artery–to–aorta) shunt through the ductus arteriosus and a Pa_{O_2} in the descending aorta that is lower than that in the ascending aorta. As the lung disease improves and the pulmonary vascular resistance falls, the shunt reverses and becomes primarily or exclusively left-to-right (aorta–to–pulmonary artery). The more rapid the improvement in lung disease and decrease in pulmonary vascular resistance, the more rapid the increase in pulmonary blood flow, left ventricular volume overload, and congestive failure. Babies with this condition often remain dependent on the respirator, and those who have already been weaned may tire and again need ventilatory support. Since the signs and symptoms of respiratory and cardiac disease are similar, it is frequently difficult in this group to distinguish the pulmonary from the cardiac conditions, and therefore management decisions are often problematic.

Clinical Manifestations. If the ductus arteriosus is small, a continuous murmur will be present that is virtually diagnostic. In the term infant with a large ductus arteriosus, the signs and symptoms of congestive failure—tachycardia, poor intake of milk with slow weight gain, increased perspiration, and hepatomegaly—may occur late in the first month. The heart is usually hyperactive, with a thrill at the left upper sternal border. The heart murmur may be continuous if the pulmonary artery pressure is low but more often is systolic, with some spill into diastole. Occasionally, multiple clicks that sound like "rolling dice" will be present, allowing differentiation of the murmur from that of a ventricular defect. A mid-diastolic rumble at the apex from increased flow across the mitral valve is often audible. The peripheral pulses are bounding with a rapid diastolic drop due to "run off" of blood from the aorta into the pulmonary circuit after aortic valve closure. Cyanosis is absent.

In the preterm infant recovering from respiratory distress syndrome, the clinical manifestations are more difficult to evaluate and distinguish from the overlapping signs and symptoms of the lung disease. Murmurs are frequently present, but the majority are systolic rather than continuous, and in about 10 per cent the murmur is absent in spite of a hemodynamically significant ductus arteriosus ("silent ductus"). The left ventricular impulse is often increased and the peripheral pulses are usually brisk, but mid-diastolic rumbles are infrequently heard.

The electrocardiogram is normal early in the disease, with right ventricular hypertrophy predominating, reflecting normal in utero hemodynamics. In term infants seen later in the first month, the increased left ventricular volume overload may be reflected in left ventricular hypertrophy.

The chest radiograph usually shows cardiac enlargement, increased pulmonary vascular markings, and, in those with congestive heart failure, pulmonary edema. In the preterm infant with respiratory distress syndrome, these findings may be more difficult to assess and distinguish from those of the lung disease present.

The echocardiogram has been quite helpful in evaluating term and preterm infants with a ductus arteriosus (Silverman et al., 1974). Normally, the left atrium and aorta are about the same size. In the presence of a large left-to-right shunt with increased pulmonary venous return to the left atrium, the more distensible left atrium dilates, increasing the left atrial diameter–to–aortic diameter ratio. Large LA:Ao ratio (>1.3) or a serial increase over time is useful confirmatory evidence of a hemodynamically significant ductus.

We have used radionuclide angiocardiography to assess the size of the left-to-right shunt in preterm infants (Treves et al., 1980). A small bolus of technetium is injected into a peripheral vein. A window over the lungs is identified, and a time-activity curve generated by computer. If no left-to-right shunt is present, there will be a single high peak. If a left-to-right shunt is present, there will be a second "bump" on the curve from recirculation of the isotope through the ductus back into the lung. By computer enhancement of the area under the curves, an estimate of the pulmonary-systemic flow ratio may be obtained.

Cardiac catheterization is rarely necessary in the preterm infant but is occasionally necessary in the term infant to differentiate a large patent ductus arteriosus from a ventricular septal defect. In most cases, the catheter can be advanced from the main pulmonary artery into the descending aorta through the ductus arteriosus, even if it is small. The atrial pressures may be elevated if congestive heart failure is present, and, if the ductus is large, the pulmonary artery pressure will be increased to systemic levels. On oximetry, there is a large step-up between the right ventricle and pulmonary artery. An angiocardiogram in the left ventricle (usually via a patent foramen ovale) will confirm the diagnosis and rule out an associated ventricular septal defect.

Diagnosis. In the acyanotic term infant who develops a continuous murmur during the first month of life and has bounding pulses, there is little doubt about the diagnosis. Continuous murmurs may also be seen in infants with pulmonary atresia and a ventricular septal defect from collateral vessels, but these infants are usually cyanotic and have loud continuous murmurs over the right and left precordium and also in the back.

Neonates with a large PDA who have only a systolic murmur and bounding pulses must be differentiated from those who have an aortopulmonary window or truncus arteriosus. The latter are usually cyanotic, but echocardiogram and catheterization are often necessary to distinguish the neonate with a large PDA from the one with an aortopulmonary window.

As mentioned previously, it may be difficult to evaluate the significance of the ductus arteriosus in neonates recovering from respiratory distress syndrome. This problem was considered by authors from 13 centers in a collaborative study of the efficacy of indomethacin, a prostaglandin synthetase inhibitor, in closing the PDA in premature infants. For diagnosis of a "clinically significant" PDA, a series of clinical, ventilatory, and echocardiographic parameters were derived (Table 27–3). These guidelines are considered not definitive statements but only reasonable criteria that were agreed upon by the neonatologists and cardiologists at 13 major centers (Ellison et al., 1983).

In the presence of a continuous murmur, constant need for ventilatory support for more than 96 hours or reinstitution of ventilatory support, or three clinical parameters (two from group A, one from group B; see Table 27–3), or one clinical parameter plus echographic or radiographic findings, or no clinical parameters but both radiographic and echographic findings were considered diagnostic of a hemodynamically significant PDA.

If only a systolic murmur was present, the criteria were slightly more stringent. In these infants, four

Table 27–3.   Criteria for Hemodynamically Significant Ductus Arteriosus

1. Clinical criteria:

A	B
Heart rate > 170 beats/minute	Hyperdynamic LV impulse
Respiratory rate > 70/minute	Pulse pressure > 35 mm Hg or bounding pulses clinically
Hepatomegaly > 3 cm below costal margin	> 96 hours on continuous positive airway pressure (> 4 cm H₂O)

2. Radiographic criteria:
    Pulmonary plethora
    Plus: Cardiothoracic ratio > .60 or
    Cardiothoracic ratio increase > .05 or
    Moderate or marked cardiomegaly

3. Echocardiographic criteria:
    LA:Ao ratio > 1.15 or increase > 0.3 from previous echocardiogram

clinical findings, or two clinical findings and a positive radiograph or echocardiogram, or no clinical findings but a positive radiograph and echocardiogram were considered diagnostic. If no heart murmur was present, it was still possible to diagnose a "silent" ductus if there was continued need for ventilatory support as well as radiographic and echocardiographic criteria, or either radiographic or echocardiographic criteria if the pulse pressure criteria were also met.

Treatment.   In the term infant with a hemodynamically significant ductus arteriosus, we recommend surgical ligation and division. In the asymptomatic term infant, we usually wait until the infants are 6 to 12 months old, but arguments could be made for operating earlier or later.

It has been recognized for some time that indomethacin can constrict and close the ductus arteriosus in some preterm infants with a hemodynamically significant PDA (Friedman et al., 1976; Heymann et al., 1976). In the aforementioned collaborative study among 13 centers, three doses of intravenous indomethacin (0.2 to 0.3 mg/kg) administered 8 to 12 hours apart closed the ductus arteriosus in 71 per cent of preterm infants with a hemodynamically significant ductus; in a group of infants who were given a placebo, there was a 35 per cent incidence of spontaneous closure (Nadas et al., personal communication, 1981). It did not seem to affect the closure rate if indomethacin was given as initial treatment or after a delay for usual medical management, nor did age, birth weight, or gestational age affect the ductus closure rate. The complications of indomethacin in this study appeared minimal. For those infants who failed to close with the indomethacin trial, surgical closure was performed, also with a very low risk. We now recommend a trial of indomethacin in preterm infants with a clinically significant ductus arteriosus unless contraindicated by poor renal function, platelet count below 50,000, evidence of intracranial or other bleeding, or necrotizing enterocolitis. If indomethacin is contraindicated or fails to close the ductus, we recommend surgical closure. Preliminary reports favor use of indomethacin as soon as the patent ductus is recognized, before signs of heart failure develop or even prophylactically in low birth weight infants (Mahony et al., 1982).

Prognosis.   In the term infant the prognosis is excellent. Surgery carries a negligible risk, with a cure rate of virtually 100 per cent.

For the preterm infant, the prognosis depends on the other problems present before and after ductal closure. In the aforementioned collaborative study, there was a 16 per cent hospital mortality. Bronchopulmonary dysplasia, intracranial hemorrhage, necrotizing enterocolitis, sepsis, and renal dysfunction were equally distributed in the groups receiving indomethacin and having surgical closure of their PDA. Minor bleeding problems were slightly more frequent in the group that received indomethacin. Retrolental fibroplasia was more common in the group that had surgical closure. Pneumothoraces and prolonged hospital stays also were more common in the surgically managed group.

ENDOCARDIAL CUSHION DEFECTS

Anatomy.   The endocardial cushion is a mass of embryonic mesenchymal tissue that forms the structures in the middle portion of the heart: the lower portion of the atrial septum, the upper portion of the ventricular septum, and the septal portions of the mitral and tricuspid valves. Any one or all of the components may be abnormal in an endocardial cushion defect, with the spectrum of abnormalities ranging from an isolated cleft in the mitral or tricuspid valve to a complete atrioventricular canal with a huge deficiency of the atrial and ventricular septum and a common atrioventricular valve (Piccoli et al., 1979 A, 1979 B). A variety of classifications have been proposed, but the tremendous spectrum of variations make sharp distinctions difficult, and we prefer a description of the anomalies: atrial septal defect of the ostium primum type, ventricular septal defect of the A-V canal type, clefts of the mitral or tricuspid valve, single atrioventricular valve, and complete atrioventricular canal. Endocardial cushion defects are the most common type of heart disease present in Down syndrome. In Fyler's 1980 series, 45 per cent of infants with endocardial cushion defects had trisomy 21. Other cardiac anomalies are often present in association with endocardial cushion defects. Heterotaxy syndromes, single ventricle, double outlet right ventricle, transposition and pulmonary stenosis are the most common.

Incidence.   There were 119 infants with endocardial cushion defects in the Regional Infant Cardiac

Program, an incidence of one per 9000 livebirths. Infants with endocardial cushion defects represented about 5 per cent of infants with heart disease.

Hemodynamics. The hemodynamics of endocardial cushion defects may be quite complex. In 1974, Rudolph noted that shunting in these infants may be dependent or obligatory. Dependent shunting through either an atrial or ventricular septal defect is a function of the pulmonary and systemic vascular resistance. In the newborn period, when the pulmonary vascular resistance is high, little left-to-right shunt may be present. As the pulmonary resistance drops over the first days and weeks of life, the pulmonary blood flow will increase, eventually leading to congestive heart failure as the left ventricle becomes overloaded. Obligatory shunting occurs from a high pressure chamber to a low pressure chamber, usually from ventricle to atrium, and is independent of resistance. In endocardial cushion defects, obligatory shunting is usually from left ventricle through the mitral portion of the A-V valve into the left atrium and across the atrial defect into the right atrium or, less frequently, directly into the right atrium. This left-to-right shunt due to A-V valve regurgitation is independent of the status of the pulmonary vasculature and may occur even with the high pulmonary vascular resistance seen in the newborn period.

The degree of intracardiac shunting at any given time is the result of a complex interplay between the pulmonary and systemic resistances affecting the dependent shunting and the obligatory shunting. In the first weeks of life, however, when the pulmonary vascular resistance tends to be high, the neonates who present with congestive failure tend to have obligatory shunts due to A-V valve regurgitation.

Clinical Manifestations. When there is only an ostium primum atrial defect present, the children rarely, if ever, are seen in the neonatal period. Infants with an isolated ventricular defect present similarly to the previously described neonates with membranous or muscular ventricular defects (see p. 276).

The age at presentation of infants with a complete A-V canal is related to the presence of A-V valve regurgitation; if severe, the infants may present in the first 1 or 2 weeks of life with the usual manifestations of heart failure, tachycardia, tachypnea, feeding dif-

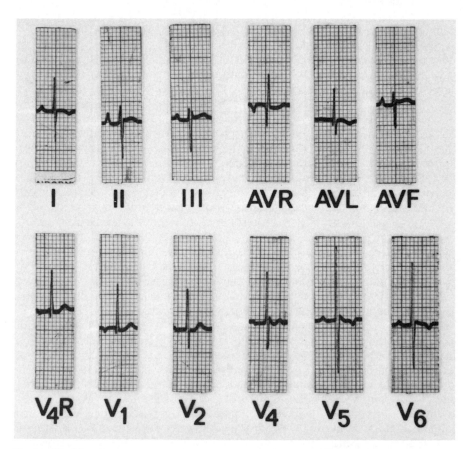

Figure 27–30. Electrocardiogram of a 1-week-old newborn with a complete atrioventricular canal. The QRS axis is −90 degrees with a predominant negative deflection in leads II, III, and AVF. The tall peaked P wave in lead II reflects right atrial hypertrophy, and the upright T waves in V₄R and V₁ suggest right ventricular hypertrophy. There is also first degree heart block with a P-R interval of 0.17 seconds.

ficulties, and sweating. If the atrioventricular valves are competent, infants present later in the first month or even in the second month of life. The precordium is usually hyperactive on palpation, with the maximal impulse displaced laterally and inferiorly. A thrill at the left lower sternal border is often present. If there is significant atrial shunting, the first heart sound is accentuated. In the usual case with pulmonary hypertension, the pulmonary component of the second heart sound is loud. Heart murmurs may be quite variable, but usually there is a loud pansystolic murmur at the lower left sternal border and a flow rumble across the mitral valve best heard at the apex. In the presence of mitral regurgitation, a pansystolic murmur at the apex is audible, but it may be hard to distinguish from the murmur of the ventricular septal defect.

The electrocardiographic features in infants with endocardial cushion defects are very characteristic. Because of posterior displacement of the atrioventricular node, His bundle, and distal left bundle as well as hypoplasia of the anterior portion of the left fascicle and an early origin of the left bundle, there is a characteristic superior QRS axis (0 to −150 degrees) that on vectorcardiogram is inscribed counterclockwise in the frontal plane (Feldt and Titus, 1976). These children also have a prolonged P–R interval, biatrial hypertrophy, and biventricular hypertrophy (Fig. 27–30).

The heart is almost invariably enlarged on the chest radiograph, and the pulmonary blood flow is increased and often congested. The size of the cardiac silhouette is often out of proportion with the increased pulmonary blood flow, presumably owing to the A-V valve regurgitation.

The characteristic features of complete A-V canal on the M-mode echocardiogram are diastolic apposition of the anterior leaflet of the mitral valve to the interventricular septum and apparent continuity of the mitral and tricuspid valves across the ventricular septum. The two-dimensional study is helpful in evaluating the atrial and ventricular component of the defect, the mitral, tricuspid, or common atrioventricular valve, and the size of the ventricles.

At cardiac catheterization, there is a great step-up in saturation between the vena cava and the right atrium that is due to the left-to-right shunt at the atrial level; an additional step-up at the ventricular level is often present. The right and left atrial pressures are equal, as are the right and left ventricular pressures. In the absence of pulmonary stenosis, the systolic pressures in the pulmonary artery and aorta are equal, but the diastolic pressure in the pulmonary artery may be lower because of increased compliance of the pulmonary bed. In the past, we have used the right and left anterior oblique projections for our left ventricular angiocardiogram. More recently, we have switched to the hepatoclavicular, or four-chambered, view because this allows optimal visualization of the atrioventricular valve(s), ventricular septum, and degree of regurgitation (Soto et al., 1981) (Fig. 27–31).

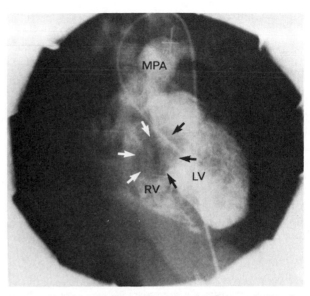

Figure 27–31. A left ventricular angiogram in the hepatoclavicular "4 chamber" projection in a newborn with a complete atrioventricular canal. The ventricular defect allows dye to enter the right ventricle. During atrial systole, unopacified blood is pumped into the ventricles, outlining the common atrioventricular valve (arrows) straddling the ventricular septum. LV = left ventricle; MPA = main pulmonary artery; RV = right ventricle.

Diagnosis. Endocardial cushion defects should be considered in all children who show congestive heart failure, a left-to-right shunt, and a superior axis on the electrocardiogram. Infants with tricuspid atresia without significant pulmonary stenosis may also demonstrate a large heart with increased pulmonary blood flow on the radiograph and a superior axis on the electrocardiogram, but they are desaturated and almost invariably reveal pure left ventricular hypertrophy on the EKG, as opposed to the right or biventricular hypertrophy seen in infants with atrioventricular canal defects. Echocardiography can resolve any remaining questions.

Treatment. When congestive failure is present, the usual medical management consisting of digoxin, diuretics, and high-calorie formula should be started. In some infants, this will suffice for many months, but frequently surgery will be required because of persistent congestive heart failure and failure to thrive. Banding of the pulmonary artery to increase pulmonary resistance and thus decrease pulmonary flow has been the procedure of choice but has remained quite risky, with an associated mortality rate of approximately 30 to 40 per cent (Epstein et al., 1979). The continued high risk is probably due to the fact that the band is excellent palliation for dependent shunting but has no benefit and, in fact, may be detrimental if there is obligatory shunting. More recently, some have attempted to repair infants with A-V canal as a primary operation by dividing the atrioventricular valve, closing the atrial and ventricular portions of the defect, and suspending the reconstructed mitral and tricuspid valves on the patch. Although, this remains a significant undertaking, especially in the neonate, the risks (current mortality rate, about 20 per cent) seem better than those associated with banding (Chin et al., 1982).

Prognosis.   In 1980, Fyler and coworkers reported that in the Regional Infant Cardiac Program (1969 to 1974) the 1-year survival rate for all patients with endocardial cushion defects was 58 per cent. For those with an atrioventricular canal, the 1-year survival rate was only 44 per cent. If the infants with Down syndrome are excluded, the survival rates are only slightly better (65 per cent for those with endocardial cushion defects and 50 per cent for those with atrioventricular canal). The high mortality is probably partly due to the high incidence of severe extracardiac anomalies present in this group of neonates. Recent advances in surgical techniques will undoubtedly increase the survival rates.

ARTERIOVENOUS FISTULAS

Anatomy.   Arteriovenous fistulas are a rare cause of congestive heart failure in the neonate. There are two types of fistulous connections: a direct communication between an artery and vein bypassing the capillary bed and, less commonly in the neonate, an angioma with multiple arterial and venous supply. Although A-V fistulas causing heart failure have been described in the subclavian, internal mammary, and vertebral arteries and hemangiomas may be found in the skin, pelvis, and coronary arteries, most of the neonates with heart failure have either a cerebral A-V fistula or a hemangioma of the liver (Quero Jimenez et al., 1977).

Incidence.   In the Regional Infant Cardiac Program there were 11 arteriovenous fistulas, representing an incidence of one per 100,000 livebirths. There were eight cerebral A-V fistulas and three systemic fistulas, one in the arm, one in the neck, and one in the liver (Fyler et al., 1980).

Hemodynamics.   Atrioventricular fistulas are present in utero but do not seem to cause significant hemodynamic embarrassment. At birth, the babies are well developed without evidence of heart failure, but profound heart failure may develop within a few hours. This dramatic change is a result of the shift from the parallel to the in series circulation after birth. In utero, the systemic venous return including the A-V fistula is divided into two streams. Part of the venous return goes through the right heart chambers into the pulmonary artery and the rest goes through the foramen ovale to the left heart chambers. After birth, the entire systemic return including return from the fistula must pass through the right heart as well as the pulmonary arteries and then to the left heart and aorta. In addition, the removal of the low resistance placenta circuit after birth increases the systemic resistance and forces more blood through the A-V fistula. These changes occurring with the transitional circulation suddenly impart a large volume overload to the right and left sides of the heart. The neonatal heart is unable to tolerate the increased venous return, and heart failure and circulatory collapse result.

Clinical Manifestations.   Congestive heart failure with tachypnea, dyspnea, and feeding difficulties are usually present within the first few days of life. Cyanosis is occasionally seen secondary to pulmonary venous desaturation and right-to-left shunting at the atrial or ductal levels (Cumming, 1980). The peripheral pulses are generally diminished but may be increased in the arteries feeding the fistula. Infants with a cerebral A-V fistula may have dilated veins in the neck. Cardiac enlargement with a hyperdynamic cardiac impulse is present on palpation, and a soft systolic ejection murmur over the semilunar valves or a diastolic flow murmur across the atrioventricular valves may be audible on auscultation. Occasionally, a continuous bruit may be heard over the fistula.

Right axis deviation, right ventricular hypertrophy, and ST–T wave changes are usually present on the electrocardiogram.

On the chest radiograph, there is generalized cardiac enlargement with increased pulmonary blood flow and pulmonary venous congestion. In infants with a cerebral A-V fistula, the superior mediastinum is often widened because of dilatation of the ascending aorta, carotid arteries, jugular vein, and superior vena cava. All cardiac chambers are enlarged on M-mode echocardiogram, and the two-dimensional study will demonstrate the enlarged vessels in the superior mediastinum of an infant with a cerebral A-V fistula or in the liver of an infant with a hepatic hemangioma.

At catheterization, the oximetry data demonstrate a high saturation in the vessels returning from the fistula. The pulmonary artery pressure may be elevated, often above systemic levels. Because of the large aortic run-off, the pulse pressure is usually widened. A very high systemic venous saturation in the superior vena cava with a widened pulse pressure and normal pulmonary venous return to the left atrium is diagnostic of a cerebral A-V fistula. Rather than wasting an angiocardiogram in the left ventricle to confirm the diagnosis, one should immediately perform cerebral angiography in the hope of finding a surgically responsive lesion (Holden et al., 1972) (Fig. 27–32).

Diagnosis. The presence of vascular collapse and congestive heart failure in the first week of life suggests myocarditis or a left-sided obstructive lesion such as hypoplastic left heart, coarctation of the aorta, or aortic stenosis. If there is a bruit over the head with normal or brisk pulses in the head vessels and dilated veins in the neck, a fistula is likely. Occasionally, the clinical diagnosis remains unclear, and echocardiography or catheterization is necessary.

Treatment. For the neonate with circulatory collapse, the usual treatment of congestive heart failure, including correction of acidosis and administration of digoxin and diuretics followed rapidly by diagnostic study, is mandatory. For neonates with cerebral A-V fistulas, there has been limited success with clipping the afferent vessels (Holden et al., 1972), but most infants die from congestive heart failure or neurologic complications or as a result of surgery. The treatment of infants with hepatic hemangioendothelioma is also a challenge. There have been some successes with hepatic arterial ligation, hepatic lobectomy, radiation, and steroids, but no one method appears superior in all cases and individualization is necessary.

Prognosis. In 1972, Holden and coworkers reviewed the literature published prior to 1970 and found only one survivor among 26 patients with cerebral A-V fistula. Of the 11 infants with A-V fistulas in the Regional Infant Cardiac Program, six with cerebral A-V fistulas were admitted in the first 3 days of life. Three of these six infants survived, two with neurosurgery and one without. It remains to be seen whether there will be any major impact from earlier diagnosis and referral, more efficient evaluation with echocardiography or computerized tomography, and improved neurosurgical techniques.

Differential Diagnosis of Heart Disease in the Neonate

The principal characteristics of common congenital and acquired diseases of the heart have been reviewed in preceding discussions and are also considered in the next chapter. In this section, the distinctive features of each condition are used to arrive at the correct diagnosis. Since most of the readers of this book are pediatricians or neonatologists rather than pediatric cardiologists, the differential diagnosis is based on the tools available to the noncardiologist in a hospital setting (i.e., history, physical examination, chest radiograph, electrocardiogram, and arterial blood gases).

Differential diagnosis is difficult in some respects. One problem is the considerable overlap in the clinical manifestations of congenital and acquired heart disease in the neonate. Also, common diseases occasionally present with uncommon manifestations, and features of uncommon diseases may mimic the typical characteristics of their more common counterparts. Nevertheless, it is still worthwhile to attempt some distinctions without specialized tests, since the management of the neonate with, for example, a small ventricular septal defect differs so greatly from that of the infant with transposition. It must be remembered, however, that several studies have confirmed that even experienced pediatric cardiologists diagnose correctly in only 60 to 70 per cent of cases

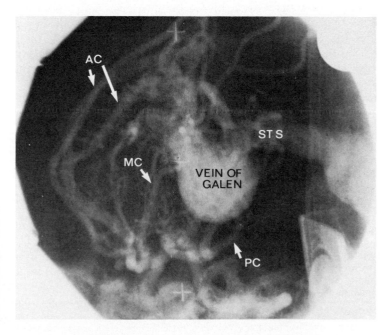

Figure 27–32. A lateral view of the head in a newborn with a cerebral A-V fistula. The dye was injected in the aortic arch. Large branches of the anterior, middle, and cerebral arteries drain into a dilated vein of Galen and then into the straight sinus. Both the number and the size of the arteries are abnormal. AC = anterior cerebral arteries; MC = middle cerebral arteries; PC = posterior cerebral arteries; STS = straight sinus.

in which neither echocardiography nor cardiac catheterization is used.

As mentioned in Chapter 26, infants with heart disease present with heart murmurs, dysrhythmias, cyanosis, or congestive heart failure. In the absence of one or more of the latter manifestations of heart disease, heart murmurs do not indicate medical emergencies, although a persistent murmur probably warrants further studies, including chest radiography, electrocardiography, and elective referral to a pediatric cardiologist.

It is easy for one to auscultate a significant dysrhythmia using a stethoscope. Symptomatic dysrhythmias are usually tachyarrhythmias (supraventricular tachycardia) or bradyarrhythmias (heart block) and are reviewed in Chapter 29.

The diagnostic dilemmas in neonatal heart disease involve the infant with profound cyanosis or congestive failure. Neonates with profound cyanosis rarely have significant heart failure, and newborns with congestive heart failure are rarely profoundly cyanotic, although they may have some arterial hypoxemia. Each group will be reviewed separately.

CYANOSIS

"Profound cyanosis" by definition involves a Pa_{O_2} of less than 50 torr in both room air and 100 per cent O_2. A schema for the differential diagnosis of cyanotic neonates, based on findings obtained from chest radiographs, electrocardiograms, and physical examination, is presented in Table 27–4. Neonates with heart disease may be profoundly cyanotic because of either right-to-left intracardiac shunting or transposition of the great arteries with poor mixing between the systemic and pulmonary circuits. In the former case, the pulmonary blood flow will be markedly reduced because of shunting away from the lungs; in the latter situation, pulmonary blood flow will be normal or increased. Thus, a neonate who is profoundly cyanotic but who shows normal or increased pulmonary blood flow on radiographs almost certainly has *transposition of the great arteries with an intact ventricular septum.* Another virtually pathognomonic pattern of the chest radiograph in a profoundly cyanotic neonate is pulmonary venous congestion (see Figs. 26–5 and 27–18), that suggests *total anomalous pulmonary venous return with obstruction.* The remainder of neonates with severe cyanosis have decreased pulmonary vascular markings on chest radiographs. If the heart is massively enlarged on the radiograph and the degree of right ventricular hypertrophy on the electrocardiogram is normal, the neonate probably has *Ebstein's disease* with severe tricuspid regurgitation (see Fig. 26–5B). Left ventricular hypertrophy on the electrocardiogram in the newborn with cyanosis and diminished pulmonary blood flow on the radiograph suggests a hypoplastic right ventricle. If the QRS is superior (-0 to -90 degrees) in the standard limb leads, *tricuspid atresia* is probably present. If the QRS axis is inferior ($+30$ to 90 degrees), *pulmonary stenosis* with an intact ventricular septum (IVS) is the most likely diagnosis if the child has an ejection murmur at the left upper sternal border. *Pulmonary atresia with an intact ventricular septum* is the most probable diagnosis if there is no murmur or only a regurgitant murmur of tricuspid incompetence along the left lower sternal border.

If the cyanotic infant with decreased pulmonary blood flow has right ventricular predominance on the electrocardiogram and cardiac enlargement on the radiograph, pulmonary stenosis without right ventricular hypoplasia is usually present. If cardiac size is normal, *tetralogy of Fallot (ventricular septal defect and pulmonary stenosis)* is the most likely diagnosis if there is an ejection murmur. *Ventricular septal defect with pulmonary atresia* is the most likely diagnosis if there are no murmurs or continuous murmurs from aortopulmonary collaterals.

This schema will not differentiate the rare and more complex forms of cyanotic heart disease, such as single ventricle, L or D transposition, or endocardial

Table 27–4. Cyanotic Congenital Heart Disease ($Pa_{O_2} < 50$ torr, $F_{I_{O_2}}$ 0.21, 1.0)

Disease	Radiograph Pulmonary Blood Flow	Heart Size	Electrocardiogram Ventricular Predominance	QRS Axis	Murmurs
Transposition with IVS	Normal or increased				
TAPVR	Congested				
Ebstein's	Decreased	Massive	RVH		
Tricuspid atresia	Decreased	Normal	LVH	0 to −90	
Pulmonary atresia, IVS	Decreased	Increased	LVH	30 to +90	Regurgitant
Pulmonary stenosis, IVS	Decreased	Increased	RVH	30 to +90	Ejection
Tetralogy of Fallot, VSD, and pulmonary stenosis	Decreased	Normal	RVH	>90	Ejection
Tetralogy of Fallot with pulmonary atresia	Decreased	Normal	RVH	>90	None or continuous

Abbreviations: IVS = intact ventricular septum, LVH = left ventricular hypertrophy, RVH = right ventricular hypertrophy, TAPVR = total anomalous pulmonary venous return, VSD = ventricular septal defect.

Table 27–5. Causes of Congestive Heart Failure in the First Week of Life

Disease	History	Pulses	EKG	Precordium
Transient myocardial ischemia	+			
Dysrhythmias	±			
Arteriovenous fistula	—	Increased		
Coarctation of the aorta (interrupted aortic arch)	—	Asymmetric		
Aortic stenosis	—	Decreased	LVH	
Hypoplastic left heart syndrome	—	Decreased	RVH	Hyperactive
Myocarditis	—	Decreased	RVH	Decreased

cushion defects with pulmonary stenosis or atresia. One must employ either echocardiography or angiography in order to distinguish these conditions.

CONGESTIVE HEART FAILURE

Myocardial dysfunction, pressure overload, and obligatory volume overload lesions are usually observed during the first week of life; dependent volume overload lesions are not usually seen until the second to fourth weeks, when the pulmonary vascular resistance has dropped enough to allow significant left-to-right shunting. The most common causes of congestive heart failure during the first week of life are listed in Table 27–5.

Neonates with *transient myocardial ischemia* almost invariably have a history of prenatal or perinatal distress. They often have low Apgar scores and very early onset of respiratory distress. The newborn with in utero *dysrhythmias*, usually supraventricular tachycardia or complete heart block, may have heart failure before or immediately after birth; these infants are distinguished by a very rapid or slow pulse. Neonates with cerebral or, less commonly, hepatic *arteriovenous fistulas* usually have a wide pulse pressure and bounding pulses, especially in the arteries feeding the fistula, in contrast with the diminished pulses expected in a newborn with severe heart failure and low cardiac output. In the infant with *coarctation of the aorta* or *interrupted aortic arch*, the pulses are usually asymmetric; that is, they may be normal or increased in the right arm proximal to the obstruction and diminished in the legs. The pulse in the left arm is variable, since the left subclavian artery may be proximal or distal to the obstruction. Neonates with aortic stenosis, hypoplastic left heart syndrome, and myocarditis have diminished pulses throughout. Those with *aortic stenosis* and a normal-sized left ventricle usually have left ventricular hypertrophy with strain on the electrocardiogram, whereas those with the hypoplastic left heart syndrome or myocarditis have the normal right ventricular predominance for age. One can usually distinguish these latter two lesions on the basis of precordial features. In the infant with *hypoplastic left heart syn-* drome, there is a hyperactive precordium, which reflects increased pulmonary blood flow; in the neonate with *myocarditis*, the precordium is quiet. If doubt remains, the M-mode echocardiogram demonstrates a dilated, minimally contractile left ventricle in myocarditis and hypoplasia of the ascending aorta in the hypoplastic left heart syndrome.

The differential diagnosis of the infant with congestive heart failure between the second and fourth weeks of life is quite complex, since in addition to the previously discussed lesions that occasionally are first seen late, there are many cases of dependent left-to-right intracardiac shunting that present as the pulmonary resistance falls over the first month. One helpful way of distinguishing these conditions is to separate those patients with left-to-right or no shunting (who are acyanotic) from those with intracardiac right-to-left shunting who have some degree of arterial hypoxemia. If the neonates in the former group are placed in 100 per cent oxygen for 10 minutes, the Pa_{O_2} will increase considerably, usually above 150 to 200 torr. In those infants with right-to-left intracardiac shunting, the Pa_{O_2} may increase little with the increase in dissolved oxygen in the pulmonary veins, but the mixture of pulmonary venous with systemic venous blood will prevent the Pa_{O_2} from exceeding 150 torr.

Acyanotic neonates (Table 27–6) may have car-

Table 27–6. Causes of Congestive Heart Failure During the Second Through Fourth Weeks of Life

Acyanotic ($Pa_{O_2} > 150$ torr in 100 per cent O_2)
  Coarctation of the aorta
  Aortic stenosis
  Myocarditis
  Endocardial fibroelastosis
  Patent ductus arteriosus
  Aortopulmonary window
  Arteriovenous fistula
  Ventricular septal defect
  Endocardial cushion defect

Cyanotic ($Pa_{O_2} < 150$ torr in 100 per cent O_2)
  Hypoplastic left heart syndrome
  Total anomalous pulmonary venous return
  Truncus arteriosus
  Transposition and a ventricular septal defect
  Tricuspid atresia and a ventricular septal defect
  Single ventricle

diac failure with pressure overload (coarctation of the aorta, aortic stenosis), myocardial dysfunction (myocarditis, endocardial fibroelastosis), or volume overload (patent ductus arteriosus, aortopulmonary window ventricular septal defect, endocardial cushion defect, arteriovenous fistula). Occasionally, a lesion causes both a volume and pressure overload, as is seen in coarctation of the aorta with a ventricular septal defect.

Children with isolated pressure overload or cardiomyopathies show cardiac enlargement with pulmonary venous congestion on radiographs but do not usually have increased pulmonary blood flow. Those with isolated *coarctation of the aorta* have differential pulses and blood pressure between the arms and legs. Neonates with *aortic stenosis* show a systolic ejection murmur at the right upper sternal border, a systolic click at the apex, and left ventricular hypertrophy with strain on the electrocardiogram. Often, one may need to initiate anticongestive measures in order to improve cardiac output enough for the murmur to be audible. Neonates with cardiomyopathies have symmetric pulses and no murmurs or, rarely, a murmur of mitral regurgitation. Those infants with *myocarditis* usually have diminished QRS voltages with ST–T wave changes, whereas those with *endocardial fibroelastosis* have increased QRS voltages, especially across the left precordium.

Left-to-right shunting is the most common cause of heart failure late in the first month of life. Characteristically, there is increased pulmonary blood flow with cardiomegaly on the chest radiograph (see Fig. 26–5C). The shunting is usually at the great vessel or ventricular level, since the relative ventricular compliances prevent a large shunt at the atrial level in this age range. Great vessel shunts are characterized by left ventricular volume overload, with enlargement of the left atrium and left ventricle and bounding pulses due to run-off from the aorta in diastole. Differentiation between *patent ductus arteriosus* and *aortopulmonary window* is accomplished with echocardiography or angiography, although even in full-term neonates, the incidence of patent ductus arteriosus is more than 16 times greater than that of aortopulmonary window. Infants with arteriovenous fistulas usually have a bruit over the head or liver.

Neonates with ventricular level shunts show cardiomegaly and increased blood flow on radiographs, with normal or symmetrically diminished pulses. Those infants with a ventricular septal defect usually have a rightward QRS axis (+90 to +180 degrees), whereas those with an endocardial cushion defect have a superior counterclockwise loop in the frontal plane, with a QRS axis of −30 to −120 degrees.

The differential diagnosis of the remaining lesions, those that present with arterial hypoxemia ($Po_2 < 150$ in 100 per cent oxygen) and congestive failure later in the first month of life (Table 27–6), is especially difficult because the signs and symptoms are remarkably similar and exact diagnosis is usually impossible without echocardiography and, frequently, angiocardiography.

Both *hypoplastic left heart syndrome and total anomalous pulmonary venous return* present with pulmonary venous obstruction on the chest radiograph and right ventricular predominance on the electrocardiogram. Infants with hypoplastic left heart syndrome often are grayish and have diminished pulses throughout as the ductus arteriosus constricts and consequently obstructs systemic blood flow. One may use either M-mode or two-dimensional echocardiography in determining the diagnosis.

One can usually discriminate neonates with *truncus arteriosus* on the basis of the mild cyanosis, bounding pulses, and increased pulmonary blood flow visible on chest radiographs. Infants who present with a clinical picture similar to that of a large ventricular septal defect (with gradually increasing congestive heart failure, a hyperactive precordium, and cardiomegaly) and who, on the hyperoxia test demonstrate that they are cyanotic, usually have (1) *transposition of the great arteries with a ventricular septal defect* if the electrocardiogram shows right ventricular hypertrophy, (2) *tricuspid atresia* if the electrocardiogram reveals left ventricular hypertrophy with a superior QRS axis (0 to −90 degrees), or (3) a *single ventricle* of the left ventricular type if there is left ventricular hypertrophy and an inferior QRS axis (+90 to +180 degrees).

REFERENCES

Alpert, B. S., Cook, D. H., Varghese, P. J., and Rowe, R. D.: Spontaneous closure of small ventricular septal defects: ten year follow up. Pediatrics 63:204, 1979.

Anderson, C., Edmonds, L., and Erickson, J.: Patent ductus arteriosus and ventricular septal defect: trends in reported frequency. Am. J. Epidemiol. 107:281, 1978.

Arciniegas, E., Farooki, Z. Q., Hakimi, M., Perry, B. L., and Green, E. W.: Classic shunting operations for congenital cyanotic heart defects. J. Thorac. Cardiovasc. Surg. 84:88, 1982.

Aziz, K. U., FlorCruz, R. A., Paul, M. H., Cole, R. B., Idriss, F. S., Wessel, H. V., and Muster, A. J.: M-mode echocardiographic assessment of D-transposition of the great arteries and associated defects. Pediatr. Cardiol. 2:131, 1982.

Behrendt, D. M., and Rocchini, A.: An operation for the hypoplastic left heart syndrome; preliminary report. Ann. Thorac. Surg. 32:284, 1981.

Bierman, F. Z., Fellows, K., and Williams, R. G.: Prospective identification of ventricular septal defects in infancy using subxiphoid two-dimensional echocardiography. Circulation 62:807, 1980.

Calder, L., Van Praagh, R., Van Praagh, S., Sears, W. P., Corwin, R., Levy, A., Keith, J. D., and Paul, M. H.: Truncus arteriosus communis. Clinical, angiocardiographic and pathologic findings in 100 patients. Am. Heart J. 92:23, 1976.

Celoria, G. C., and Patton, R. B.: Congential absence of the aortic arch. Am. Heart J. 58:407, 1959.

Chin, A. J., Keane, J. F., Norwood, W. I., and Castaneda, A. R.: Repair of complete atrioventricular canal in infancy. J. Thorac. Cardiovasc. Surg. 84:437, 1982.

Coceani, F., and Olley, P. M.: The response of the ductus arteriosus to prostaglandins. J. Physiol. Pharmacol. 51:220, 1973.

Collett, R. W., and Edwards, J. E.: Persistent truncus arteriosus: a classification according to anatomic types. Surg. Clin. North Am. 29:1245, 1949.

Collins-Nakai, R. L., Dick, M., Parisi-Buckley, L., Fyler, D. C., and Castaneda, A. R.: Interrupted aortic arch in infancy. J. Pediatr. 88:959, 1976.

Cumming, G. R.: Circulation in neonates with intracranial arteriovenous fistula and cardiac failure. Am. J. Cardiol. 45:1019, 1980.

Danielson, G. K., Maloney, J. D., and Devloo, R. A. E.: Surgical repair of Ebstein's anomaly. Mayo Clin. Proc. 54:185, 1979.

Delisle, G., Ando, M., Calder, A. L., et al.: Total anomalous pulmonary venous connection: report of 93 autopsied cases with emphasis on diagnostic and surgical considerations. Am. Heart J. 91:99, 1976.

Dick, M., Fyler, D. C., and Nadas, A. S.: Tricuspid atresia: clinical course in 101 patients. Am. J. Cardiol. 36:327, 1975.

Ebstein, W.: Über einen sehr seltenen Fall von Insufficienz der Valvula Tricuspidalis, bedingt durch eine angeborene hochgradige Missbildung derselben. Arch. Anat. Physiol. Wissensch. Med. 238, 1866.

Ebert, P. A: Truncus arteriosus. In Glenn, W. W. L. (Ed.): Thoracic and Cardiovascular Surgery. 4th ed. Norwalk, Conn., Appleton-Century-Crofts, 1983.

Edmunds, L. H., Wagner, H. R., and Heymann, M. A.: Aortic valvulotomy in neonates. Circulation 61:421, 1981.

Edwards, J. E.: Persistent truncus arteriosus. Am. Heart J. 92:1, 1976.

Edwards, J. E., and Burchell, H. B.: Congenital tricuspid atresia. A classification. Med. Clin. North Am. 33:1177, 1949.

Ellison, R. C., Peckham, G. J., Lang, P., et al.: Evaluation of the preterm infant for ductus arteriosus. Pediatrics 71:364, 1983.

Epstein, M. L., Moller, J. H., Amplatz, K., and Nicoloff, D. M.: Pulmonary artery banding in infants with complete atrioventricular canal. J. Thorac. Cardiovasc. Surg. 78:28, 1979.

Feldt, R. H., and Titus, J. L.: The conduction system in persistent common atrio-ventricular canal. In Feldt, R. H. (Ed.): Atrio-Ventricular Canal Defects. Philadelphia, W. B. Saunders Co., 1976, p. 36.

Ferrer, P. L.: Arrhythmias in the neonate. In Roberts, N. K., and Gelband, H. (Eds.): Cardiac Arrhythmias in the Neonate, Infant, and Child. New York, Appleton-Century-Crofts, 1977.

Fontan, F., and Baudet, E.: Surgical repair of tricuspid atresia. Thorax 26:240, 1971.

Freed, M. D., Heymann, M. A., Lewis, A. B., Roehl, S. L., and Kensey, R. C.: Prostaglandin E₁ in infants with ductus arteriosus dependent congenital heart disease. Circulation 64:899, 1981.

Freed, M. D., Rosenthal, A., Bernhard, W. F., Litwin, S. B., and Nadas, A. S.: Critical pulmonary stenosis with a diminutive right ventricle in neonates. Circulation 48:875, 1973.

Freedom, R. M., and Ellison, R. C.: Coronary sinus rhythm in the polysplenia syndrome. Chest 63:952, 1973.

Freedom, R. M., Olley, P. M., Coceani, F., and Rowe, R. D.: The prostaglandin challenge test to unmask obstructed total anomalous pulmonary venous connections in asplenia syndrome. Br. Heart J. 40:91, 1978.

Friedman, W. F., Hirschklau, M. J., Printz, M. P., Pitlick, P. T., and Kirkpatrick, S. E.: Pharmacologic closure of patent ductus in the premature infant. N. Engl. J. Med. 295:526, 1976.

Fyler, D. C., Buckley, L. P., Hellenbrand, W. et al.: Report of the New England Regional Infant Cardiac Program. Pediatrics 65(suppl.):375, 1980.

Garson, A., Gillette, P. C., and McNamara, D. G.: Propranolol: preferred palliation for tetralogy of Fallot. Am. J. Cardiol. 47:1098, 1981.

Gathman, G. E., and Nadas, A.S.: Total anomalous pulmonary venous connection. Clinical and physiologic observations of 75 pediatric patients. Circulation 42:143, 1970.

Godman, M. J., and Marquis, R. M.: Pediatric Cardiology. Vol. 2. Heart Disease in the Newborn. Edinburgh, Churchill-Livingstone, 1979.

Gutgesell, H. P., Garson, A., and Mc Namara, D. G.: Prognosis for the newborn with transposition of the great arteries. Am. J. Cardiol. 44:96, 1979.

Hamilton,, W. J., and Mossman, H. W.: Hamilton, Boyd, and Mossman's Human Embryology: Prenatal development of form and function. 4th ed. Baltimore, Williams and Wilkins Co., 1972.

Hesslein, P. S., Gutgesell, H. P., and McNamara, D. G.: Prognosis of symptomatic coarctation of the aorta in infancy. Am. J. Cardiol. 52:299, 1983.

Heymann, M. A., Rudolph, A. M., and Silverman, N. H.: Closure of the ductus arteriosus in premature infants by inhibitor of prostaglandin synthesis. N. Engl. J. Med. 295:530, 1976.

Ho, S. Y., and Anderson, R. H.: Coarctation, tubular hypoplasia and the ductus arteriosus. Histologic study of 35 specimens. Br. Heart J. 41:268, 1979.

Holden, A. M., Fyler, D. C., Shillito, J., Jr., and Nadas, A. S.: Congestive heart failure from intracranial arterio-venous fistula in infancy. Pediatrics 49:30, 1972.

Jatene, A. D., Fontes, V. F., Paulista, P. P., Souza, L. C. B., Neger, F., Galantier, M., Sousa, J. E. M., and Zerbini, E. J.: Anatomic correction of transposition of the great arteries. J. Thorac. Cardiovasc. Surg. 72:364, 1976.

Kamau, P., Miles, V., Toews, W., Kelminson, L., Friesen, R., Lockhart, C., Bulterfield, J., Hernandez, J., Hawes, C. R., and Pappas, G.: Surgical repair of coarctation of the aorta in infants less than six months of age: including the question of pulmonary artery banding. J. Thorac. Cardiovasc. Surg. 81:171, 1981.

Keane, J. F., Bernhard, W. F., and Nadas, A. S.: Aortic stenosis surgery in infants. Circulation 52:1138, 1975.

Keith, J. D., Rowe, R. D., and Vlad, P.: Heart Disease in Infancy and Childhood. New York, The Macmillan Co., 1958.

Kreutzer, G., Galindez, E., Bono, H., Depalma, C., and Laura, J. P.: An operation for the correction of tricuspid atresia. J. Thorac. Cardiovasc. Surg. 66:613, 1973.

Kumar, A. E., Fyler, D. C., Miettinen, O. S., and Nadas, A. S.: Ebstein's anomaly: clinical profile and natural history. Am. J. Cardiol. 28:84, 1971.

Laks, H., Hellenbrand, W., Stansel, H. C., Jr., Pennell, R., Kleinman, C., Lister, G., Kopf, G., and Talner, N.: Improved results in the treatment of pulmonary atresia with an intact ventricular septum. Circulation 64(suppl.):30, 1981.

Lang, P., Freed, M. D., Bierman, F. Z., Norwood, W. I., and Nadas, A. S.: Use of prostaglandin E₁ in infants with d-transposition of the great arteries and intact ventricular septum. Am. J. Cardiol. 44:76, 1979.

Langman, J.: Medical Embryology. 4th ed. Baltimore, Williams & Wilkins Co., 1981.

Lev, M., and Saphir, O.: Truncus arteriosus communis persistens. J. Pediatr. 20:74, 1942.

Liebman, J., Cullum, L., and Belloc, N. B.: Natural history of transposition of the great arteries. Anatomy and birth and death characteristics. Circulation 40:237, 1969.

Litwin, S. B., Van Praagh, R., and Bernhard, W. F.: A palliative operation for certain infants with aortic arch interruption. Ann. Thorac. Surg. 14:369, 1972.

Litwin, S. B., Williams, W. W., Freed, M. D., and Bernhard, W. F.: Critical pulmonary stenosis in infants: a surgical emergency. Surgery 74:880, 1973.

Lundstrom, N. R.: Echocardiography in the diagnosis of Ebstein's anomaly of the tricuspid valve. Circulation 47:597, 1973.

Mahony, L., Carhero, V., Heymann, M. A., and Clyman, R. I.: Prophylactic indomethacin in very low birth weight infants. N. Engl. J. Med. 306:506, 1982.

Marx, G. R., Hougen, T. J., Norwood, W. I., Fyler, D. C., Castaneda, A. R., and Nadas, A. S.: Transposition of the great arteries with an intact ventricular septum: results with Mustard and Senning operations in 123 consecutive patients. J. Am. Coll. Cardiol. 1:476, 1983.

Mesko, Z. G., Jones, J. E., and Nadas, A. S.: Diminution and closure of large ventricular septal defects after pulmonary artery banding. Circulation 43:847, 1973.

Moller, J. H., Nakib, A., Eliot, R. S., and Edwards, J. E.: Symptomatic congenital aortic stenosis in the first year of life. J. Pediatr. 69:728, 1966.

Moller, J. H., and Neal, W. A.: Heart Disease in Infancy. New York, Appleton-Century-Crofts, 1981.

Murphy, J. D., Freed, M. D., Keane, J. F., Norwood, W. I., and Castaneda, A. S.: Hemodynamic results after intracardiac repair of tetralogy of Fallot by deep-hypothermia and cardiopulmonary bypass. Circulation 62(suppl.):168, 1980.

Mustard, W. T., Keith, J. D., Trusler, G. A., Fowler, R., and Kidd, L.: The surgical management of transposition of the great vessels. J. Thorac. Cardiovasc. Surg. 48:953, 1964.

Noonan, J. A., and Nadas, A. S.: The hypoplastic left heart syndrome. Pediatr. Clin. North Am. 5:1029, 1958.

Nora, J. J.: Etiologic aspects of congenital heart disease. In Moss, A. J., Adams, R. H., and Emmanouilides, G. C. (Eds.): Heart Disease in Infants, Children, and Adolescents. 2nd ed. Baltimore, The Williams and Wilkins Co., 1977, p. 3.

Norwood, W. I., Hougen, T. J., and Castaneda, A. R.: Total anomalous pulmonary venous connection: surgical considerations. In Engle, M. E. (Ed.): Pediatric Cardiovascular Disease. Cardiovascular Clinics, Philadelphia, F. A. Davis Co., 1980.

Norwood, W. I., Lang, P., Castaneda, A. R., and Campbell, D. N.: Experience with operations for hypoplastic left heart syndrome. J. Thorac. Cardiovasc. Surg. 82:511, 1981.

Norwood, W. J., Lang, P., and Hansen, D. D.: Physiologic repair of aortic atresia hypoplastic left heart syndrome. N. Engl. J. Med. 308:23, 1983.

Olley, P. M., Coceani, F., and Bodach, E.: E type prostaglandins: a new emergency therapy for certain cyanotic congenital heart malformations. Circulation 53:728, 1976.

Paul, M. H.: D-transposition of the great arteries. In Moss, A. J., Adams, F. H., and Emmanouilides, G. S. (Eds.): Heart Disease in Infants, Children, and Adolescents. Baltimore, The Williams and Wilkins Co., 1977, p. 103.

Piccoli, G. P., Gerlis, L. M., Wilkinson, J. L., Lozadi, K., Macartney, F. J., and Anderson, R. H.: Morphology and classification of atrioventricular defects. Br. Heart J. 42:621, 1979 A.

Piccoli, G. P., Wilkinson, J. L., Macartney, F. J., Gerlis, L. M., and Anderson, R. H.: Morphology and classification of complete atrioventricular defects. Br. Heart J. 42:633, 1979 B.

Poirier, R. A., Berman, M. A., and Stansel, H. C., Jr.: Current status of the surgical treatment of truncus arteriosus. J. Thorac. Cardiovas. Surg. 69:169, 1975.

Puga, F. J., McGoon, D. C., Julsrud, P. R., Danielson, G. K., and Mair, D. D.: Complete repair of pulmonary atresia with non-confluent pulmonary arteries. Ann. Thorac. Surg. 35:36, 1983.

Quero Jimenez, M., Acerete Guillen, F., and Castro Guissoni, M. C.: Arterio-venous fistulas. In Moss, A. J., Adams, F. H., and Emmanouilides, G. C. (Eds.): Heart Disease in Infants, Children, and Adolescents. Baltimore, The Williams and Wilkins Co., 1977, p. 470.

Rashkind, W. J., and Miller, W. W.: Creation of an atrial septal defect without thoracotomy: a palliative approach to complete transposition of the great arteries. J.A.M.A. 196:991, 1966.

Rein, J. G., Freed, M. D., Norwood, W. I., and Castaneda, A. R.: Early and late results of closure of ventricular septal defects in infancy. Ann. Thorac. Surg. 24:19, 1977.

Rose, V., Izukawa, T., and Moes, C. A. F.: Syndromes of asplenia and polysplenia: a review of cardiac and non-cardiac malformations in 60 cases with special reference to diagnosis and prognosis. Br. Heart J. 37:840, 1975.

Rowe, R. D., Freedom, R. M., Mehrizi, A., and Bloom, K. R.: The Neonate with Congenital Heart Disease. 2nd ed. Philadelphia, W. B. Saunders Co., 1981.

Rudolph, A. M.: Congenital Diseases of the Heart. Chicago, Year Book Medical Publishers, 1974.

Rudolph, A. M., Heymann, M. A., and Spitznas, U.: Hemodynamic considerations in the development of narrowing of the aorta. Am. J. Cardiol. 30:514, 1972.

Sanders, S. P., Bierman, F. Z., and Williams, R. G.: Conotruncal malformations: diagnosis in infancy using two-dimensional echocardiography. Am. J. Cardiol. 50:1361, 1982.

Sanders, S. P., Wright, G. B., Keane, J. F., Norwood, W. I., and Castaneda, A. R.: Clinical and hemodynamic results of the Fontan operation for tricuspid atresia. Am. J. Cardiol. 49:1733, 1982.

Senning, A.: Surgical correction of transposition of the great vessels. Surgery 45:966, 1959.

Silverman, N. H., Lewis, A. B., Heymann, M. A., and Rudolph, A. M.: Echocardiographic assessment of ductus arteriosus shunt in premature infants. Circulation 50:821, 1974.

Soto, B., Bargeron, L. M., Jr., Pacifico, A. D., Vanini, V., and Kirklin, J. W.: Angiography of the atrio-ventricular canal defects. Am. J. Cardiol. 48:492, 1981.

Tajik, A. J.: Echocardiogram in tetralogy of Fallot. Chest 69:107, 1973.

Tajik, A. J., Gau, G. T., Giuliani, E. R., Ritter, D. G., and Schattenberg, T. T.: Echocardiogram in Ebstein's anomaly with Wolff-Parkinson-White pre-excitation syndrome type B. Circulation 47:813, 1973.

Talner, N. S., and Berman, M. A.: Postnatal development of obstruction in coarctation of the aorta: role of the ductus arteriosus. Pediatrics 56:562, 1975.

Treves, S., Fogle, R., and Lang, P.: Radionuclide angiography in congenital heart disease. Am. J. Cardiol. 46:1247, 1980.

Trusler, G. A., Freedom, R. M., Patel, R., and Williams, W. G.: The surgical management of pulmonary atresia with intact ventricular septum. In Godman, M. J., and Marquis, R. M. (Eds.): Pediatric Cardiology. Vol. 2. Heart Disease in the Newborn. Edinburgh, Churchill-Livingstone, 1979.

Van Mierop, L. H. S., Gessner, I. H., and Schiebler, G. L.: Asplenia and polysplenia syndrome. Birth Defects 8:36, 1972.

Van Praagh, R., Ando, M., Van Praagh, S., Senno, A., Hougen, T. J., Novak, G., and Hastreiter, A. R.: Pulmonary atresia: anatomic considerations. In Kidd, B. S. L., and Rowe, R. D. (Eds.): The Child with Congenital Heart Disease after Surgery. Mt. Kisco, N.Y., Futura Publishers, Inc., 1976, p. 103.

Van Praagh, R., Bernhard, W. F., Rosenthal, A., Parisi, L. F., and Fyler, D. C.: Interrupted aortic arch: surgical treatment. Am. J. Cardiol. 27:200, 1971.

Van Praagh, R., and Van Praagh, S.: The anatomy of common aortopulmonary trunk (truncus arteriosus communis) and its embryologic implications. A study of 57 necropsy cases. Am. J. Cardiol. 16:406, 1965.

Van Praagh, R., and Van Praagh, S.: Isolated ventricular inversion: consideration of the morphogenesis, definition and diagnosis of non-transposed and transposed great arteries. Am. J. Cardiol. 17:395, 1966.

Waldhausen, J. A., Nahrwold, D. L., Lurie, P. R., and Shumaker, H. B., Jr.: Management of coarctation in infancy. J.A.M.A. 187:270, 1964.

Waldman, J. D., Rosenthal, A., Smith, A. L., Shurin, S., and Nadas, A. S.: Sepsis and congenital asplenia. J. Pediatr. 90:555, 1977.

Watson, D. G., and Rowe, R. D.: Aortic-valve atresia. Report of 43 cases. J.A.M.A. 179:14, 1962.

Watson, H.: Natural history of Ebstein's anomaly of the tricuspid valve in children and adolescents: an international cooperative study of 505 cases. Br. Heart J. 36:417, 1974.

Whittemore, R., Hobbins, J. C., and Engle, M. A.: Pregnancy and its outcome with and without surgical treatment of congenital heart diseases. Am. J. Cardiol. 50:641, 1982.

Yacoub, M., Bernhard, A., Lange, P., Radley-Smith, R., Keck, E., Stephan, E., and Heintzen, P.: Clinical and hemodynamic results of two-stage anatomic correction of simple transposition of the great arteries. Circulation 62(suppl.):190, 1980.

By Michael D. Freed[*]

There are several diseases of the newborn in which the myocardium is affected without primary abnormalities of the valves, great vessels, or septum. The heart may be affected by hypoxia and acidosis (transient myocardial ischemia), infection with virus, bacteria, or toxoplasmosis (myocarditis), infiltrative diseases (e.g., glycogen storage disease), tumor (rhabdomyoma, fibroma), or diseases of uncertain etiology (e.g., endocardial fibroelastosis, diabetic myopathy). Although none of the diseases are common, cumulatively they do account for a significant proportion of the heart disease in the neonate. Each will be briefly reviewed in this chapter.

Transient Myocardial Ischemia

Over the past few years, it has been recognized that a number of newborns suffer a form of myocardial ischemia that frequently is transient but that may be associated with significant cardiovascular symptoms and even death (Rowe et al., 1979). In some of these infants, the signs of respiratory distress and congestive heart failure or shock are predominant (Rowe and Hoffman, 1972); in others, myocardial dysfunction and tricuspid regurgitation are the presenting symptoms (Boucek et al., 1976; Bucciarelli et al., 1977).

Pathologic examination of the most severely affected neonates reveals dilated hearts and, frequently, anoxic petechial hemorrhages. On histologic examination, there is often smudging and edema of the myocardial fibers throughout the heart in those infants dying early in their disease and areas of focal myocardial necrosis in those surviving for 3 or 4 days (Rowe et al., 1979).

Since the disease is frequently self-limited and many of these newborns can be saved with careful management, it is important to recognize these infants and institute prompt treatment.

Clinical Features. The infants are usually born at term by a delivery complicated by hypoxic stress that occurs before or during birth. The Apgar score is usually less than 6 at 1 minute. Respiratory distress and cyanosis are frequently present soon after birth, with the neonates developing the signs and symptoms of congestive heart failure (tachypnea, tachycardia, hepatomegaly, and a gallop rhythm) within a few hours. Some will go on to develop hypotension and cardiovascular collapse and shock. About half the neonates will have systolic heart murmurs. In most, the murmur is at the left lower sternal border and suggests tricuspid regurgitation, but in a few the murmur is loudest at the apex and sounds like mitral regurgitation.

The chest radiograph invariably shows cardiomegaly. The pulmonary vascular markings are variable; they have been described as increased, normal, or, rarely, diminished. Pulmonary venous congestion may be apparent, but the indistinctness of the pulmonary vessels may be confused with the "wet" lungs seen with transient tachypnea of the newborn with retained fetal fluid.

The electrocardiogram shows right ventricular predominance that is normal for age and right atrial hypertrophy in the majority. Diffuse ST–T changes are usually present, with the most common pattern being ST depression in the midprecordium and persistent T-wave inversion over the left precordium.

On M-mode and two-dimensional echocardiograms the cardiac structures are normal, but decreased left ventricular contractions, especially of the left ventricular posterior wall, may be seen.

A few neonates with transient myocardial ischemia have been catheterized. In some of these infants, there is persistent pulmonary hypertension with right-to-left shunting through the fetal pathways, the ductus arteriosus, and foramen ovale. The ventricular end diastolic pressures are usually elevated, reflecting ventricular dysfunction (Rowe et al., 1979). In another subgroup, tricuspid regurgitation predominates (Boucek et al., 1976; Bucciarelli et al., 1977). In these neonates the pulmonary artery pressure is only mildly increased, but there is severe tricuspid regurgitation evident on angiocardiogram with right-to-left shunting at the atrial level. In both groups, arterial hypoxemia is almost invariably present but is rarely severe.

Diagnosis. Transient myocardial ischemia should be suspected in all neonates who experience a traumatic birth involving hypoxia and who have respiratory distress, cyanosis, or signs of congestive failure soon after birth. Since this picture may occasionally be seen in neonates with congenital heart disease, echocardiography is essential if congestive failure or cyanosis is prominent. Echocardiography is also help-

---

[*] This chapter, written by Dr. Milton Markowitz in previous editions, has been revised and updated with new material.

ful in distinguishing infants who have tricuspid regurgitation associated with transient ischemia from those who have tricuspid regurgitation caused by Ebstein's disease of the tricuspid valve or critical pulmonary stenosis or pulmonary atresia with an intact ventricular septum.

Treatment. The treatment is symptomatic. Digitalis and diuretics should be given for congestive failure, and the metabolic abnormalities of hypoglycemia and acidosis should be corrected promptly. Those with severe respiratory distress may need intubation and assisted ventilation; those with cardiovascular collapse may benefit from inotropic support with isoproterenol or dopamine. Afterload reduction with nitroprusside should be reserved for the most severely affected.

Prognosis. In the infants without cardiogenic shock, the prognosis is quite good. In the series of Bucciarelli and coworkers and of Boucek and colleagues involving only patients with severe tricuspid regurgitation, 16 of 18 neonates survived, usually with disappearance of the murmur within a couple of weeks and resolution of the electrocardiographic abnormalities within a few months. Five of the 16 survivors had cardiac catheterization 4½ months to 5 years later, with hemodynamics subsequently returning to normal.

In those who are first seen with severe acidosis and cardiogenic shock, the prognosis remains grim, with death likely occurring from heart failure, low output, or failure of a necessary organ system.

Myocarditis

Myocarditis occurs in all age groups, but there is higher frequency in the first month than in any other period of life. It is a well-recognized entity with a clinical pattern sufficiently distinctive for one to make an antemortem diagnosis. Although often a fulminant disease, it is not invariably fatal, and early recognition and prompt treatment may alter the outcome.

Incidence. For the 50 years following Fiedler's original description of primary myocarditis, only a few isolated cases had been reported in the first month of life. Since 1950, there has been a striking increase in the number of reported cases, particularly among newborn infants. Recent nursery outbreaks have been reported (Hall and Miller, 1969; Drew, 1973). In the Regional Infant Cardiac Program reviewing critical heart disease in New England between 1969 and 1974, there were 13 infants with myocarditis, an incidence of 1 of every 80,000 livebirths (Fyler et al., 1980).

Etiology. Any infective agent can cause myocarditis, although the enteroviruses, particularly Coxsackie B and ECHO viruses, are the most common (Lerner et al., 1975). In 1961, Kibrick reported 54 cases in the neonatal period that were due to group B Coxsackie viruses. Of this group, 28 were infected during nursery outbreaks, with the mother as the original source of the infection in many instances. Among the 26 sporadic cases, there were a significant number in whom the infant's illness was associated with a febrile illness in the mother. There is some evidence that in a few patients the infection was acquired in utero, but the majority appear to have been acquired postnatally. Asymptomatic infants in the nursery may also be a source of infection (Brightman et al., 1966).

Neonatal myocarditis may be caused by viruses other than Coxsackie B. Herpes simplex virus has been isolated from the heart of a newborn infant dying of disseminated disease (Wright and Miller, 1965). Myocarditis may be caused by the rubella virus, although this agent has never been isolated from the heart. It has been suggested that rubella myocarditis occurs in utero and may progress after birth, leaving myocardial damage (Ainger et al., 1966; Harris and Nghiem, 1972).

Pathology. On gross examination, the heart is enlarged and dilated. The cardiac muscle feels flabby and is often pale or nutmeg-like in color. Microscopic examination reveals a multicellular infiltration of the myocardium (Fig. 28–1). Lymphocytes, large mononuclear cells, eosinophils, and polymorphonuclear leukocytes are present in varying numbers with either patchy or diffuse distribution. Necrosis and fragmentation of muscle fibers may be present (Burch et al., 1968). Although rare in patients with primary myocarditis, involvement of the endocardium and pericardium may occur. When the Coxsackie virus is the etiologic agent, involvement of other organs, particularly the central nervous system, is common. Involvement of multiple organs is even more common with rubella and herpes viruses.

Clinical Findings. The clinical course of young infants with myocarditis is variable. The initial symptoms may be mild and include lethargy, failure to feed, vomiting, or diarrhea. Jaundice may be present, and evidence of a mild upper respiratory tract infection is sometimes noted. In the milder forms of the disease, clinical manifestations may be limited to slight tachypnea, tachycardia, and poor heart sounds. Frequently, there are no premonitory symptoms whatsoever. The infant becomes seriously ill very suddenly. Respirations increase, become labored, and are often accompanied by a grunt. The infant appears restless and anxious. The skin is pale, mottled, and mildly cyanotic. The temperature may be slightly or greatly elevated or subnormal. The pulse rate is usually rapid, between 150 and 200, and weak. Occasionally, bradycardia is present. The percussion note over the chest may be normal or hyperresonant. Dullness is uncommon. The breath sounds are usually harsh, and rales may be heard at the bases. Although there is always some degree of cardiac enlargement, it is often difficult to detect clinically. The heart sounds are mushy, particularly the first sound, and a gallop rhythm may be present. The liver is almost invariably enlarged. Edema is an uncommon finding, and venous engorgement is almost never detected. There may be signs referable to central nervous system involvement.

Chest radiographs show generalized cardiac enlargement as well as haziness of the lung fields. At times, it is not possible to make the distinction between congestion and pneumonia (Fig. 28–2). Electrocardiograms will often show abnormalities. Low-voltage QRS complexes and either low, isoelectric or inverted T waves are the most frequent findings. There may also be significant disturbances in conduction such as heart block, extrasystoles, and ventricular or atrial tachycardia (Fig. 28–3). The electrocardiographic abnormalities are frequently transient. Although usually not helpful in the acute stage, viral studies should be carried out.

The echocardiogram is helpful in ruling out associated structural heart disease and assessing myocardial function. In infants in whom neither conges-

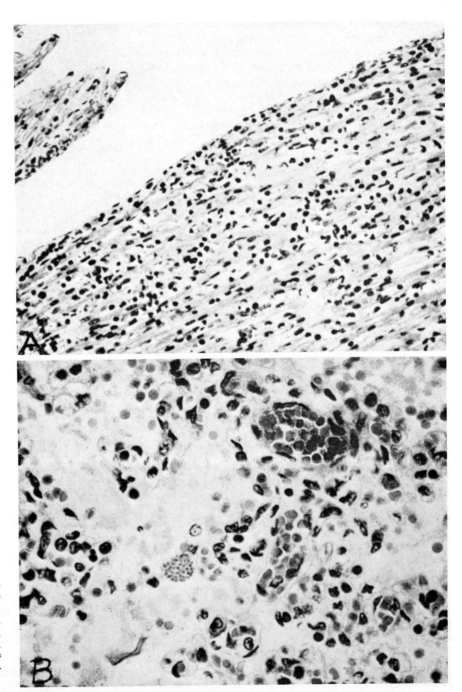

Figure 28–1. *A,* Low-power microscopic view of section of the heart in a patient with myocarditis showing diffuse cellular infiltration in the myocardium. *B,* Higher-power microscopic view of section of myocardium showing cellular infiltration and toxoplasma.

tive failure nor cardiac enlargement appears on the chest radiograph, the echocardiogram is usually normal. When cardiac enlargement does appear on the radiograph, the left atrium and left ventricle are usually dilated, with little change in left ventricular dimensions between systole and diastole, findings that reflect poor ventricular function.

Diagnosis. The diagnosis of myocarditis should be suspected in any neonate with congestive heart failure in whom structural heart disease has been excluded by two-dimensional echocardiogram. The suspicion should be heightened if there is a known respiratory infection in the mother or proved viral illness in other nursery infants. The diagnosis can be confirmed by the recovery of virus from the nasopharynx and the stool or by the development of neutralizing antibodies.

The acute form of myocarditis is commonly mistaken for overwhelming *sepsis* or a *severe lower respiratory tract infection*. This is especially true for the latter, since cyanosis and respiratory distress may initially suggest pneumonia. Myocarditis should be suspected if there are an inordinate tachycardia, poor heart sounds with or without gallop rhythm, a degree of dyspnea disproportionate with the pulmonary findings, and radiographic evidence of cardiac enlargement.

Myocarditis must also be differentiated from other cardiac conditions that may occur in the neonatal period: congenital heart disease with congestive failure precipitated by infection, the acute form of endocardial fibroelastosis, and paroxysmal tachycardia.

Congenital Heart Disease. The absence of heart murmurs does not rule out this possibility. Occasionally, infants with a large left-to-right shunt have

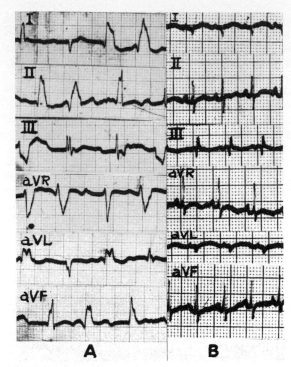

Figure 28–3. *A,* Standard and unipolar limb leads showing conduction disturbances with variable atrioventricular block, bundle branch block, and multifocal ventricular complexes in a child with myocarditis. *B,* Standard and unipolar limb leads showing return to normal rhythm 24 hours later.

an insignificant murmur in the neonatal period. Coarctation of the aorta, a not uncommon cause of heart failure in the neonate, must always be excluded by careful evaluation of the arm-leg pulses and blood pressure.

Endocardial Fibroelastosis. In this condition, there is usually left ventricular hypertrophy indicated in electrocardiographic tracings by high-voltage R waves in precordial leads taken over the left side of

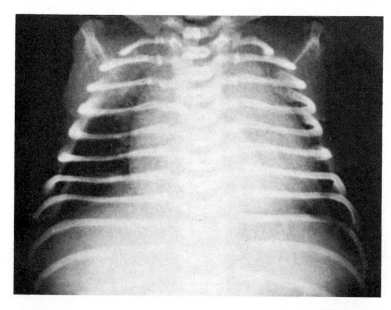

Figure 28–2. Generalized cardiac enlargement caused by myocarditis.

the heart. However, the left ventricular pattern may not be as striking in the first few days or weeks of life. In myocarditis, low-voltage complexes are characteristic and are the result of severe disturbances in myocardial function. Occasionally, infants with endocardial fibroelastosis in severe failure may have low voltage temporarily.

Paroxysmal Tachycardia. Congestive heart failure is frequently present, but in this condition the heart rate is usually much more rapid than in myocarditis.

Mild forms of myocarditis are particularly difficult to recognize. Signs of heart failure may not be prominent or may be absent entirely. The clinical manifestations may include pallor, slight increase in the respiratory rate, tachycardia, and poor heart sounds. Such findings in an infant who has signs of infection and who appears to have a disproportionate degree of cardiac embarrassment should suggest the possibility of myocarditis. Although electrocardiographic studies may aid in the diagnosis, there is no specific pattern, nor does a normal tracing rule out the disorder.

Treatment. Young infants with myocarditis may become critically ill with such rapidity that treatment should be instituted as soon as the diagnosis is suspected. Minimal handling is essential, since restlessness and agitation seem to worsen the cardiac involvement.

Oxygen therapy and digitalization should be started at once with the usual anticongestive measures. We usually prefer diuretics to digoxin in milder cases, since patients with myocarditis may be unusually sensitive to digitalis.

Since the efficiency of the heart muscle is weakened by the infection, recent efforts have been directed at reducing the work of the heart. It has been found that since cardiac work is a function of the volume of blood ejected during systole and the pressure that the heart must generate, reducing systemic resistance and arterial pressure will allow a higher cardiac output to be maintained. Vasodilators such as nitroprusside (0.1 to 5 µg/kg/min) and hydralazine have been found to reduce the "afterload" of the heart and to improve peripheral perfusion in the most severely affected neonates. Inotrophic support with isoproterenol or dopamine may improve cardiac contractility and increase cardiac output in those who are most critically ill.

Although the etiologic agent in myocarditis is frequently viral, bacterial infections of the lung are common, and antibiotics should be given. After the initial digitalization, the patient should be maintained on digitalis until the heart has returned to normal size and the pulse is within normal limits.

Prevention. The fact that viral and bacterial agents may cause neonatal myocarditis emphasizes the need for preventive measures in carrying out nursery routine. The Coxsackie virus may cause minor or inapparent illnesses in adults and yet lead to serious, often fatal disease in newborn infants. Reports of outbreaks in nurseries suggest the infectious nature of this disorder. For these reasons, stress must be placed on the absolute necessity for careful isolation of the mother and the newborn during the course of even mild respiratory infections.

Prognosis. The prognosis for infants with fulminating disease is poor. Patients are occasionally victims of "crib deaths" or arrive at the hospital moribund. Among the 54 cases reported by Kibrick, 12 patients survived. Undoubtedly, milder forms of the disease occur, and the recovery rate in this group is high, although more recent studies continue to show a high mortality, approximately 50 per cent (Rowe et al., 1981). In a study of children 13 years after each had suffered an attack of neonatal myocarditis, no clinical or laboratory abnormalities were found. It is possible that, as the awareness of neonatal myocarditis as a clinical entity increases, earlier diagnosis and more vigorous supportive treatment will improve the overall mortality rate.

Endocardial Fibroelastosis

Endocardial fibroelastosis may occur as an isolated or primary condition or in association with a variety of congenital and acquired cardiac lesions. In the latter groups, the clinical entity is that of the underlying cardiac disease, and the fibroelastosis is a secondary finding on postmortem examination. The description that follows is limited mainly to infants with the primary or isolated form of endocardial fibroelastosis.

Etiology. The cause of primary endocardial fibroelastosis is not known. However, evidence has been presented suggesting that in utero Coxsackie B or other virus infections may play a role (Fruhling et al., 1962; Hastreiter and Miller, 1964; Hutchins and Vie, 1972). This evidence is still inconclusive.

Anderson and Kelly presented fairly convincing evidence that the endocardial thickening seen in association with other congenital cardiac defects is due to abnormal currents of intracardiac blood under increased pressure. Nevertheless, this hypothesis cannot account for its presence in the isolated form.

Incidence. The reports on incidence are confusing because of the inclusion of large numbers of cases with the secondary form of this disease. The 1956 study by Kelly and Anderson makes this distinction clear. In their series from the Babies Hospital, there were 17 instances among 237 necropsy patients with congenital heart disease, an incidence of 7 per cent. Family occurrences were noted in three of the 17 cases. There are several additional reports that record the disease among multiple births and siblings.

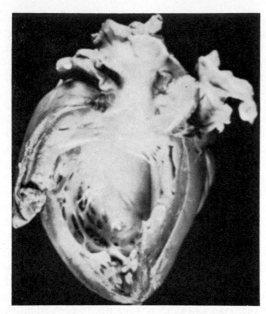

Figure 28–4. Endocardial fibroelastosis in an infant who died at the age of 9 days. The endocardium of both ventricles is thickened and porcelain-white in appearance.

Primary endocardial fibroelastosis may be becoming rarer. Mitchell and coworkers found an incidence of 1 in every 5000 to 6000 births in a prospective national collaborative study during the early 1960s; in the New England Regional Infant Cardiac Program during the early 1970s, endocardial fibroelastosis occurred in only 14 of 1,000,000 livebirths, an incidence of 1 of 70,000 livebirths (Fyler et al., 1980). There does not appear to be any relation to birth weight, sex, or race.

Pathology. Gross enlargement of the heart is a constant finding. The weight is increased, and there are hypertrophy and dilatation of one or more chambers. This is especially true of the left ventricle, which is the most frequent site of endocardial thickening. Involvement of the left atrium is fairly common, but less than half have an additional lesion of the right ventricle and right atrium. Fibroelastosis confined to the right side of the heart is rare. On gross examination the endocardium is diffusely thickened and smooth and has a porcelain-white appearance (Fig. 28–4). About half the cases show involvement of one or more valves, the mitral more commonly than the others. In contrast to the usual pattern of congenital abnormalities, there is a striking absence of other malformations.

Microscopic examination shows an increase in the fibrous and elastic tissue within the endocardium with some extension into the myocardium. When the valves are involved, the picture is similar to that of the endocardium. There is no evidence of inflammation in the heart. Pneumonia and signs of congestive failure are commonly associated autopsy findings.

Clinical Course. The majority of infants have their initial symptoms between the first and sixth months of life. A significant percentage show some difficulty from birth, and a case of heart failure in utero has been reported (Harris and Nghiem, 1973). In a series of 85 collected cases in which the age of onset was noted, 19 patients had difficulty within the first month, and in 13 of these cases signs or symptoms began at birth (Anderson and Kelly).

The clinical pattern of the disease falls into two fairly distinct types, acute and chronic. The mode of onset, symptomatology and course vary with each. In its most fulminant form the infant, previously well, may be discovered dead in his crib. The more typical acute case begins with the nonspecific symptoms of listlessness, failure to feed, vomiting or a mild cold. These are soon followed by onset of labored breathing. The physical findings are variable. Fever may be present, but it is rarely high. The cardiac rate is variable. It may be slow if there is an associated heart block (Fig. 28–5). In two reported cases, heart block was present in utero (Anderson and Kelly, 1956). On the other hand, there may be an extreme tachycardia due to a paroxysmal atrial rhythm (Hung and Walsh, 1962). The heart sounds are often unusually forceful. Although the heart is always enlarged, clinical detection of enlargement may be difficult in the early

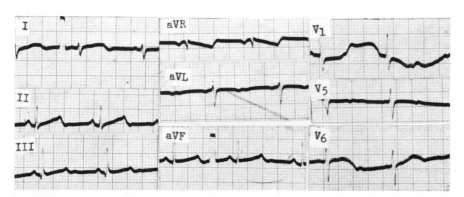

Figure 28–5. Electrocardiogram of an infant with endocardial fibroelastosis, taken at age 6 days, showing a 2:1 heart block.

stages. Signs of heart failure may not be prominent at the onset, but they are almost always present at some time during the course of the disease.

The chronic form of the disease is the more common of the two types. The initial symptom is labored or wheezy breathing. *This may be present from birth.* Failure to gain weight and bouts of irritability are common. There may be intermittent cyanosis. The physical findings are those of a young infant in heart failure. Respirations are increased and grunting. There is flaring of the alae nasi and some intercostal retraction. Cyanosis is minimal or absent except as a terminal event. There may be abnormalities in the cardiac rhythm, as has already been noted. The heart is always enlarged. The heart sounds are of good quality and become muffled only when heart failure is advanced. A murmur is present in about one third of the patients, systolic, and soft and nondescript in quality. The presence of a loud murmur should lead to suspicion of fibroelastic valvular involvement or an associated congenital defect. The liver is enlarged in the presence of heart failure. The blood pressure is either normal or low.

Laboratory Findings. Blood and urine examinations show no abnormality that can be related to the primary disease. The electrocardiogram is often of considerable diagnostic help in the chronic form of the disease. As might be anticipated from the pathology, evidence of left ventricular hypertrophy is common. Features that indicate hypertrophy are noted in the precordial leads over the left side of the chest (V_5 and V_6) and consist of abnormally tall R waves, prominent Q waves, prolonged intrinsicoid deflection, and inverted T waves (Lambert et al., 1953). Supraventricular or nodal tachycardia and partial and complete heart block have been recorded (Fig. 28–5).

Radiographic examination of the heart reveals enlargement, especially of the left ventricle. In many of these infants, left atrial prominence can be demonstrated on the esophagram (Fig. 28–6).

On the echocardiogram, there is often an increase in left atrial and left ventricular dimensions with normal wall thickness. The left ventricular chamber changes little between systole and diastole, reflecting poor ventricular function.

At cardiac catheterization, the left atrial and left ventricular end diastolic pressures are elevated, and, on the angiocardiogram, the left ventricle is dilated and rounded with poor contractility.

Diagnosis. Endocardial fibroelastosis should be suspected in the neonate if abnormalities of cardiac rhythm (e.g., heart block, atrial tachycardia) are present. In the most acute form, diagnosis is difficult. These infants often resemble patients with sepsis or pneumonia. The presence of tachycardia, cardiomegaly, and hepatomegaly should lead to the suspicion of heart failure due to primary heart disease. Differentiation from primary myocarditis may be particularly difficult. The findings in both conditions are remarkably similar. One distinguishing feature is the strikingly low voltage noted on the electrocardiogram in severe myocarditis, but this may occasionally occur in endocardial fibroelastosis. The left ventricular pat-

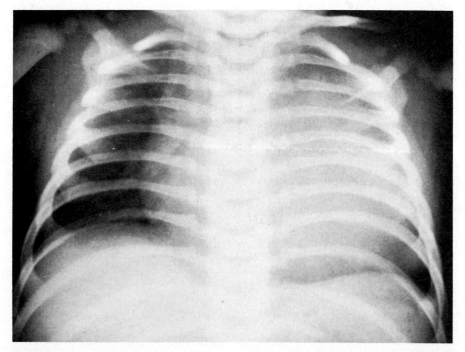

Figure 28–6. Endocardial fibroelastosis in a 6-week-old infant. The heart is diffusely enlarged.

tern commonly found in endocardial fibroelastosis may be slight or absent in the patient less than 1 week old with an acute case.

The chronic form of the disease may cause symptoms from birth, but the diagnosis is rarely suspected until the signs of heart failure are fairly well developed. At times, the wheezing or labored respirations are wrongly interpreted as signs of asthma, an enlarged thymus, or some other obstructive abnormality. The diagnosis should be suspected in any young infant with an enlarged heart, particularly when there is little or no cyanosis and no audible heart murmurs. Absence of the latter signs should exclude most other forms of congenital heart disease. The presence of palpable femoral pulsations eliminates coarctation of the aorta. Infants with anomalous origin of the left coronary artery may have a similar clinical and radiographic picture. The electrocardiogram in this condition is often distinctive, however, and shows a pattern of coronary insufficiency with inverted T waves in leads I and II plus a prominent Q wave in lead I.

Glycogen storage disease of the heart is a rare cause of cardiac enlargement in infancy. Here the enlargement is usually globular, without specific chamber enlargement. The electrocardiographic pattern is more bizarre in glycogen storage disease, and a short P–R interval is often present. A specific diagnosis can be made by analysis of the glycogen content of skeletal muscle.

Treatment. This is directed toward the control of heart failure. Oxygen therapy is indicated. Digitalization should be started immediately. If the patient is extremely ill, one of the more rapid-acting digitalis preparations should be used. The prolonged use of digitalis has been recommended as an important aspect of therapy.

Diuretics should be reserved for infants who have clinical evidence of edema or who fail to respond to oxygen and digitalis. More complete details on the dosage of anticongestive drugs are presented elsewhere.

In the critically ill neonate, reducing the work of the heart by decreasing afterload with nitroprusside or hydralazine may be helpful.

Prognosis. A small number of patients fail to respond to all measures and die within 1 day to 2 weeks after onset of the illness. In a larger group, the response to anticongestive treatment is good, even dramatic at times. Of 19 patients with symptoms before 1 month of life, ten lived from 3 months to 3 years (Kelly and Anderson, 1956). In general, the earlier the onset, the worse the prognosis. Symptoms recur intermittently until death. The terminal illness is usually brief and is the result of heart failure often complicated by pneumonia. The prognosis in infants with the familial type of endocardial fibroelastosis is generally poor.

It is still not certain that endocardial fibroelastosis is an invariably fatal disease. Linde and Adams described 17 patients in whom a presumptive diagnosis of primary endocardial fibroelastosis was made. Of these, four have had completely normal findings over a period of 3 to 10 years. Further observations will be necessary before the overall prognosis in this condition is known. In the meantime, early recognition and vigorous treatment make a favorable outcome possible in some patients.

Hypertrophic Cardiomyopathy of the Infant of the Diabetic Mother

Since the widespread availability of M-mode echocardiography, it has become evident that many large for gestational age infants born to diabetic mothers have an asymmetric hypertrophic cardiomyopathy involving primarily the ventricular septum (Way et al., 1975; Poland et al., 1975; Gutgesell et al., 1976). In 1980, Breitweser and coworkers found an excellent correlation between the degree of neonatal hypoglycemia and the thickness of the interventricular septum on echocardiogram in 18 infants of diabetic mothers and in one infant of a nondiabetic mother with nesidioblastosis (ductoinsular cell proliferation), and they have postulated that fetal hyperinsulinemia contributes directly to the observed septal hypertrophy. The exact mechanism of the cardiac hypertrophy and the reason that the hypertrophy primarily affects the ventricular septum remain a matter of conjecture.

This syndrome does not affect all infants of diabetic mothers. Only 3 of 23 asymptomatic infants had disproportionate thickening of the septum, compared with 10 of 26 symptomatic infants in one study (Gutgesell et al., 1980).

Clinical Features. The involved infants present with the signs and symptoms of congestive heart failure: tachypnea, tachycardia, and hepatomegaly. They usually have respiratory distress and frequently cyanosis from birth. Systolic ejection murmurs are common and, at least according to one study, seem to be correlated with the degree of obstruction to left ventricular ejection by the septal hypertrophy (Way et al., 1979).

Cardiac enlargement on the chest radiograph is almost universal, and pulmonary venous congestion is seen in most symptomatic patients (Way et al., 1979). These abnormalities, however, do not correlate with the echocardiographic findings of wall or septal thickness (Gutgesell et al., 1980).

The electrocardiographic findings are quite variable. Among 24 symptomatic infants studied in 1980 by Gutgesell and coworkers, the electrocardiogram was normal in 12, showed right ventricular hypertrophy in seven, and demonstrated biventricular hypertrophy in five. Although all five neonates who had significant left ventricular outflow obstruction had an abnormal electrocardiogram, there was no consistent pattern between the electrocardiographic evidence of hypertrophy and the echocardiographic measurements of wall thickness.

On echocardiographic evaluation of symptomatic infants, the right ventricular anterior wall, the ventricular septum, and the left ventricular posterior wall are thickened, but the septal wall is disproportionately hypertrophied so that the septal wall—to—left-ventricular-posterior-wall ratio is increased above normal in about one half (Gutgesell, 1980). The internal dimensions of the right and left ventricle were normal, as was the percentage of dimensional change, a measure of cardiac function in this study. In five of the 24 infants, there was evidence of left ventricular outflow tract obstruction due to apposition of the anterior leaflet of the mitral valve to the hypertrophied interventricular septum during systole.

Only a few neonates have undergone cardiac catheterization. Three of five neonates catheterized within the first 2 weeks of life by Way and coworkers in 1979 had a gradient between the left ventricle and the aorta, ranging from 20 to 74 mm Hg. In one, the gradient increased from 20 to 80 mm Hg between catheterization performed at 1 day and 3 weeks of age. Left ventricular angiograms in these infants showed hypertrophy of the papillary muscles, interventricular septum, and left ventricular posterior wall with complete emptying and obliteration of the left ventricular cavity, as frequently seen in older children with the familial form of the disease.

Diagnosis. The echocardiogram is diagnostic and should be performed on all infants of diabetic mothers with signs or symptoms of respiratory distress or congestive heart failure. Other forms of heart disease must be excluded, since the incidence of congenital heart disease in infants of diabetic mothers is five times that of the normal population (Rowland et al., 1973).

Treatment. The treatment is symptomatic. Hypoglycemia and hypocalcemia should be corrected, and maintenance fluids should be provided intravenously if oral intake is not possible. Occasionally, increasing respiratory distress requires intubation and assisted ventilation. Unless severely depressed myocardial contractibility can be demonstrated on echocardiogram, digitalis and other inotropic agents are contraindicated, since they may lead to increased left ventricular outflow obstruction (Rowe et al., 1981).

Prognosis. In contrast to the outlook for neonates, older children, and adults with the progressive familial form of hypertrophic cardiomyopathy with asymmetric hypertrophy, the prognosis in this group of neonates is excellent. Of 11 symptomatic infants reported by Way and colleagues in 1979, all were asymptomatic by 1 month of age, with the radiograph in all, and the electrocardiogram in 10, returning to normal. Echocardiograms showed regression of sep-

tal thickness in all the patients, and repeat cardiac catheterizations in two of the 11 have shown normal hemodynamics with elimination of gradients of 30 and 74 mm Hg between left ventricle and aorta. The findings of Gutgesell and coworkers are similar.

Glycogen Storage Disease of the Heart

Glycogen storage disease of the heart is a rare condition that may manifest symptoms from birth. It is one of 8 types or subtypes of glycogenoses (type II), and it is the only type in which involvement of the heart is a major feature. It is transmitted through a single recessive autosomal gene. The defect is due to the congenital absence of alpha 1,4 glycosidase from intracellular lysosomes (Hers, 1963). This results in the accumulation of normal glycogen in lysosomal sacs, where it cannot be degraded by glycolytic enzymes.

Pathology. The heart is always enlarged, often to enormous proportions. The walls of both ventricles are thick, but the atria are normal. Microscopic examination shows infiltration of the muscle fibers with large vacuoles of glycogen. Varying amounts of glycogen deposition are also found in the skeletal muscles, liver, kidneys, and central nervous system (Fig. 28–7).

Clinical Features. Symptoms were noted from birth in about one fourth of the 54 cases summarized by Ehlers and coworkers. Frequently, the infant appears normal at birth but goes on to have a history of poor feeding, lassitude, and failure to gain weight. Hypotonia may be striking, and the tongue may appear thick. Cardiac enlargement is the rule. A systolic heart murmur may be noted, but it is often soft and variable. The liver is not usually enlarged.

The usual parameters for glycogen metabolism are normal, including glucose tolerance and response to epinephrine and glucagon. These infants do not suffer from hypoglycemia. Radiologic examination shows gross generalized cardiomegaly, although the heart need not be enlarged at birth (Fig. 28–8). The electrocardiogram may show abnormalities at birth or after a period of some weeks. Unusually high voltage of the QRS complexes and the T waves is characteristic. There is evidence of left ventricular hypertrophy. However, a short P–R interval is the most distinctive electrocardiographic feature of glycogen storage disease (Caddell and Whittemore, 1962) (Fig. 28–9).

On echocardiogram, Bloom and coworkers discovered thickening of the left ventricular free wall disproportionate to the thickness of the interventricular septum.

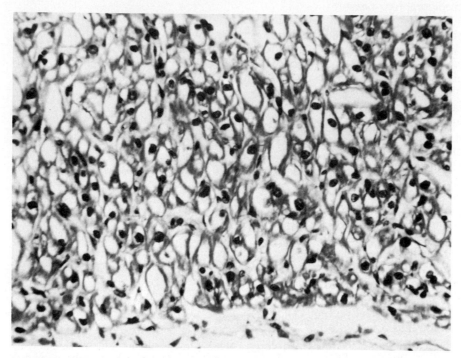

Figure 28–7. Microscopic section of the myocardium of an infant with glycogen storage disease of the heart. Note the vacuolization among the myofibers. These vacuoles were filled with glycogen when appropriately stained.

Diagnosis. The diagnosis is rarely made in the neonatal period unless there is a family history of the disease. The early symptoms are ill-defined and, with the exception of intermittent episodes of dyspnea, do not suggest a cardiac abnormality. The patient is more likely to be several weeks or months old before the cardiac enlargement is detected. The diagnosis should be suspected in any infant with an enlarged heart, especially if the enlargement is great. Muscle weakness is an important additional clue. Macroglossia is often present and may be confused with cretinism or Down syndrome.

This condition must be distinguished from other causes of cardiac enlargement in early infancy. The absence of cyanosis and significant murmurs will exclude many of the congenital defects. *Endocardial fibroelastosis* and *anomalous left coronary artery* are the two conditions that most frequently enter into the

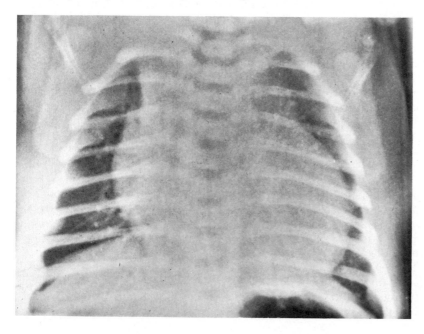

Figure 28–8. X-ray film of the chest of a 12-hour-old infant with glycogen storage disease of the heart. There is considerable cardiac enlargement.

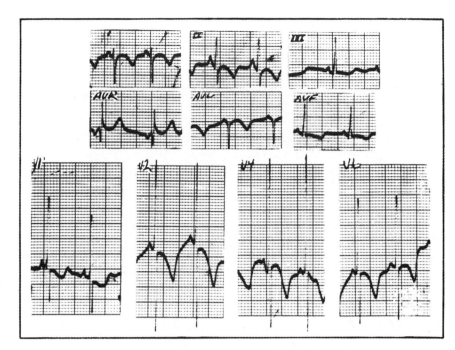

Figure 28–9. Electrocardiogram of a 1-day-old infant with glycogen storage disease of the heart. Note the short P-R interval, increased voltage, and deeply inverted T waves in leads I, II, aV₁, and V_2–V_6.

differential diagnosis. The left ventricular component in the radiograph is more striking in both the aforementioned conditions, whereas the heart in glycogen storage disease is larger and more globular. All three entities may show a left ventricular pattern and striking T-wave changes in the electrocardiogram. In the anomalous left coronary artery the electrocardiographic changes resemble more closely those seen with a posterior infarct. In endocardial fibroelastosis, the T-wave changes are restricted to the left side of the precordium, whereas they are often present in all leads in glycogen storage disease. A short P–R interval does not occur in endocardial fibroelastosis or with an anomalous coronary artery.

The diagnosis of glycogen storage disease can be confirmed by demonstration of increased glycogen in a biopsy of skeletal muscle. It can be more readily confirmed by examination of blood lymphocytes for glycogen content (Nihill et al., 1970).

Prognosis. Death due to heart failure almost always occurs before the end of the first year. Among 54 cases proved at autopsy and reviewed by Keith and Sass-Kortsak, 10 patients died in the first 2 months of life.

Treatment. There is no satisfactory treatment for this condition. Anticongestive therapy and treatment of intercurrent infection may be instituted in an attempt to prolong life.

Tumors of the Heart

Cardiac tumors are very rare entities, but when they do occur, manifestations of heart disease are not infrequently present in the neonatal period. Several types of tumors have been described. Rhabdomyomas are the most common (Bigelow et al., 1954; Nadas and Ellison, 1968; Williams et al., 1972). They consist of numerous nodular areas that contain glycogen (Fig. 28–10). They may occur in association with tuberous sclerosis. An intramural fibroma is less common but has been reported in the neonatal period (Bigelow et al., 1954). Although tumors are almost invariably present within the myocardium, they may occasionally project into the cardiac lumen and cause obstruction (Shaher et al., 1972; Van der Hauwaert, 1971). Myomas and sarcomas are extremely rare.

The *clinical picture* is extremely variable. Arrhyth-

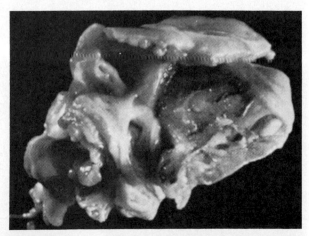

Figure 28–10. Age 1 month. Multiple rhabdomyomas. Gross specimen of the opened heart shows numerous nodular masses within the walls of the ventricle and protruding into the chamber of the heart.

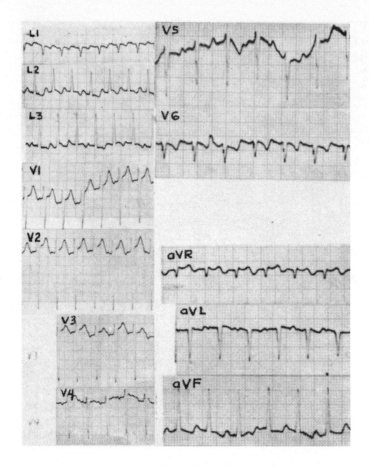

Figure 28–11. Age 7 weeks. Multiple rhabdomyomas of the heart. The electrocardiogram is abnormal. There is T-wave inversion in the limb leads and over the left side of the precordium. The S waves are abnormally deep over the right and left sides of the precordium. The over-all pattern is bizarre.

mias are common with rhabdomyomas. Heart murmurs are usually not present unless the tumor projects into the cardiac cavity, obstructing blood flow. Heart failure is common, and its onset is often very sudden. On the chest radiograph, the heart may be normal or enlarged. Occasionally, bizarre prominences distort the cardiac contour. The electrocardiographic findings are extremely variable. Right, left, or combined ventricular hypertrophy may be seen, with arrythmias frequently present. Often, evidence of abnormal repolarization with inverted T waves may be seen (Fig. 28–11).

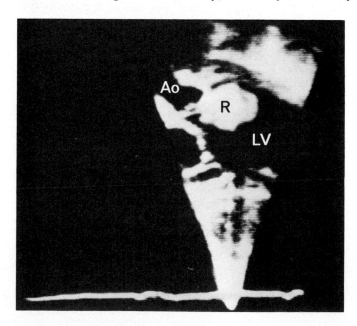

Figure 28–12. A subxiphoid view on two-dimensional echocardiogram of the left ventricle (LV) and aorta (Ao) in a 1-week-old child with tuberous sclerosis. Note the rhabdomyoma (R) that is arising just below the aortic valve and that projects into the lumen of the left ventricle, causing subaortic stenosis. Compare this with Figure 26–2, a normal view of the LV and Ao on two-dimensional echocardiogram. (Courtesy of Roberta G. Williams, M.D.)

With the advent of two-dimensional echocardiography, the diagnosis is more frequently being made during life (Fig. 28–12). It should be suspected in any infant with tuberous sclerosis who shows evidence of cardiac disease, especially if a cardiac arrhythmia is present. The sudden onset of intractable heart failure in a previously well infant should suggest a cardiac tumor if the more common causes such as myocarditis and endocardial fibroelastosis can be excluded.

There is no satisfactory medical treatment for cardiac tumors. Successful surgical removal can be accomplished when the tumors are hemodynamically significant. (Van der Hauwaert, 1971; Williams et al., 1972; Shaher et al., 1972).

REFERENCES

Ainger, L. E., et al.: Neonatal rubella myocarditis. Br. Heart J. 28:691, 1966.

Anderson, D. H., and Kelly, J.: Endocardial fibroelastosis associated with congenital malformations of the heart. Pediatrics 18:513, 1956.

Bigelow, N. H., Klinger, S., and Wright, A. W.: Primary tumors of the heart in infancy and childhood. Cancer 7:549, 1954.

Bloom, K. R., Hug, G., Schubert, W. K., and Kaplan, S.: Pompe's disease and the heart. Circulation, 50(Suppl. III):56, 1974.

Boucek, R. J., Graham, T. P., Jr., Morgan, J. P., Atwood, G. F., and Boerth, R. C.: Spontaneous resolution of massive congenital tricuspid insufficiency. Circulation 54:795, 1976.

Breitweser, J. A., Meyer, R. A., Sperling, M. A., Tsang, R. C., and Kaplan, S.: Cardiac septal hypertrophy in hyperinsulinemic infants. J. Pediatr. 96:535, 1980.

Brightman, V. J., Scott, T. F., Westphal, M., and Boggs, T. R.: An outbreak of Coxsackie B-5 virus infection in a newborn nursery. J. Pediatr. 69:179, 1966.

Bucciarelli, R. L., Nelson, R. M., Eagan, E. A., II, Eitzman, D. V., and Gessner, I. H.: Transient tricuspid insufficiency of the newborn: a form of myocardial dysfunction in stressed newborns. Pediatrics 59:330, 1977.

Burch, G. E., Sun, S., Chu, K., Sohal, R. S., and Colcolough, H. L.: Interstitial and coxsackievirus B myocarditis in infants and children. J.A.M.A. 203:1, 1968.

Caddell, J., and Whittemore, R.: Observations on generalized glycogenesis with emphasis on electrocardiographic changes. Pediatrics 29:743, 1962.

Di Sant'Agnese, P., Anderson, D. H., and Mason, H. H.: Glycogen storage disease of the heart. Pediatrics 6:607, 1950.

Drew, J. H.: ECHO II virus outbreak in a nursery associated with myocarditis. Aust. Pediatr. J. 9:90, 1973.

Ehlers, K. H., Hagstrom, J. W., Lukas, D. S., Redo, S. F., and Engle, M. A.: Glycogen-storage disease of the myocardium with obstruction to left ventricular outflow. Circulation 25:96, 1962.

Fiedler, A.: Ueber akute interstitielle Myocarditis. Zendtralbl. inn. Med. 21:212, 1900.

Fruhling, L., et al.: Chronic fibroelastic myoendocarditis of the newborn and the infant (fibroelastosis). Ann. Anat. Path. (Paris) 7:227, 1962.

Fyler, D. C., Buckley, L. P., Hellenbrand, W., et al.: Report of the New England Regional Infant Cardiac Program. Pediatrics 65(suppl.):375, 1980.

Gutgesell, H. P., et al.: Transient hypertrophic subaortic stenosis in infants of diabetic mothers. J. Pediatr. 89:120, 1976.

Gutgesell, H. P., Speer, M. E., and Rosenberg, H. S.: Characterization of the cardiomyopathy in infants of diabetic mothers. Circulation 61:441, 1980.

Hall, C. B., and Miller, D. G.: The detection of silent Coxsackie B-5 virus perinatal infection. J. Pediatr. 75:124, 1969.

Harris, L. C., and Nghiem, Q. X.: Cardiomyopathies in infants and children. Prog. Cardiovasc. Dis. 15:255, 1972.

Hastreiter, A. R., and Miller, R. A.: Management of primary endomyocardial disease. Pediatr. Clin. North Am. 11:401, 1964.

Hers, H. G.: Alpha glucosidase deficiency in generalized glycogen storage disease (Pompe's disease). Biochem. J. 86:11, 1963.

Hung, W., and Walsh, B. J.: Congenital auricular fibrillation in a newborn infant with endocardial fibroelastosis. J. Pediatr. 61:65, 1962.

Hutchins, G. M., and Vie, S. A.: The progression of interstitial myocarditis to idiopathic endocardial fibroelastosis. Am. J. Pathol. 66:483, 1972.

Keith, J. D., and Sass-Kortsak, A.: Glycogen storage disease of the heart. In Keith, J. D., Rowe, R. D., and Vlad, P.: Heart Disease in Infancy and Childhood. 3rd ed. New York, Macmillan Publishing Co., 1978.

Kelly, J., and Anderson, D. H.: Congenital endocardial fibroelastosis. II. A clinical and pathologic investigation of those cases without associated cardiac malformations, including report of two familial instances. Pediatrics 18:539, 1956.

Kibrick, S.: Viral infections of the fetus and newborn. In Pollard, M. (Ed.): Perspectives in Virology. Vol. II. Minneapolis, Burgess Publishing Co., 1961, pp. 140–157.

Lambert, E. C., Shumway, C. N., and Terplan, K.: Clinical diagnosis of endocardial fibrosis. Analysis of literature with report of four new cases. Pediatrics 11:255, 1953.

Lerner, A. M., Wilson, F. M., and Reyes, M. P.: Enteroviruses and the heart: epidemiological and experimental studies. I. Mod. Concepts Cardiovasc. Dis. 44:7, 1975.

Linde, L. M., and Adams, F. H.: Prognosis in endocardial fibroelastosis. Am. J. Dis. Child. 105:329, 1963.

Mitchell, S. C., Forehlich, L. A., Banas, J. S., and Gilkerson, M. R.: An epidemiologic assessment of primary endocardial fibroelastosis. Am. J. Cardiol. 18:859, 1966.

Nadas, A. S., and Ellison, R. C.: Cardiac tumors in infancy. Am. J. Cardiol. 21:363, 1968.

Nihill, M. R., et al.: Generalized glycogenosis type II (Pompe's disease). Arch. Dis. Child. 45:122, 1970.

Poland, R. L., Walther, L. T., and Chang, C.: Hypertrophic cardiomyopathy in infants of diabetic mothers. Pediatr. Res. 9:269, 1975.

Rowe, R. D., Finley, J. P., Gilday, D. L., Dische, M. R., Jiminez, C. L., and Chance, G. W.: Myocardial ischaemia in the newborn. In Godman, M. J., and Marquis, R. M. (Eds.): Pediatric Cardiology. Vol. 2. Heart Disease in the Newborn. Edinburgh, Churchill-Livingstone, 1979.

Rowe, R. D., Freedom, R. M., Mehrizi, A., and Bloom, K. R.: The Neonate with Congenital Heart Disease. Philadelphia, W.B. Saunders Co., 1981.

Rowe, R. D., and Hoffman, T.: Transient myocardial ischemia of the newborn infant. A form of severe cardio-respiratory distress in full-term infants. J. Pediatr. 81:243, 1972.

Rowland, T. W., Hubbell, J. P., and Nadas, A. S.: Congenital heart disease in infants of diabetic mothers. J. Pediatr. 83:815, 1973.

Shaher, R. M., Mintzer, J., Farina, M., Alley, R., and Bishop, M.: Clinical presentation of rhabdomyoma of the heart in infancy and childhood. Am. J. Cardiol. 30:95, 1972.

Van der Hauwaert, L. G.: Cardiac tumors in infancy and childhood. Br. Heart J. 33:125, 1971.

Way, G. L., Wolfe, R. R., Pettet, G., Merenstein, G., Simmons, M., Spangler, R., and Nora, J.: Echocardiographic assessments of ventricular dimensions and myocardial function in infants of diabetic mothers. Pediatr. Res. 9:273, 1975.

Way, G. L., Wolff, R. R., Eshaghpour, E., Bender, R. L., Jaffe, R. B., and Ruttenberg, H. D.: The natural history of hypertrophic cardiomyopathy of infants of diabetic mothers. J. Pediatr. 95:1020, 1979.

Williams, W. G., Trusler, G. A., Fowler, R. S., Scott, M. R., and Mustard, W. T.: Left ventricular myocardial fibroma: case report and review of cardiac tumors in children. J. Pediatr. Surg. 7:324, 1972.

Wright, H. T., and Miller, A.: Fatal infection in a newborn infant due to herpes simplex virus. J. Pediatr. 67:130, 1965.

29

Cardiac Dysrhythmias

By Michael D. Freed

Cardiac dysrhythmias are not uncommon in the neonate, accompanying the significant changes in circulatory hemodynamics and gas exchange that occur with the switch from the in utero to extrauterine circulations. In a recent review of more then 3000 apparently normal newborns (Southall et al., 1981), about 1 per cent revealed dsyrhythmias on a routine 10-second electrocardiogram prior to discharge. The vast majority of these dysrhythmias were of little significance, but life-threatening arrhythmias may occur on rare occasions. Two excellent reviews of this topic have recently been published (Ferrer, 1977; Losekoot and Lubbers, 1979).

Sinus Arrhythmia, Sinus Tachycardia, Sinus Bradycardia

Sinus arrhythmia is a phasic variation of the sinus node discharge that may occur either in cycle with respiration or independent of it. It is quite common and, as far as can be determined, is of no clinical significance. On electrocardiogram, the P–P interval is irregular, with the P wave, P–Q interval, and QRS complexes normal.

Sinus tachycardia can be defined as a heart rate that exceeds the upper range of normal, usually 175 to 190 beats/minute in a full-term infant and 195 in

a premature. The P–P interval is short, but the P wave, P–Q interval, and QRS complexes are normal. It is usually a manifestation of increased adrenergic activity that may be the result of crying, feeding, or blood letting, but it may also be secondary to congestive heart failure, shock, anemia, or fever. No treatment is necessary if the secondary causes of the tachycardia can be ruled out.

Sinus bradycardia is a heart rate that falls below what is generally accepted as normal (i.e., below 90 to 100 beats/minute), with a normal P wave preceding each QRS. Occasionally, the sinus mechanism is so depressed that the junctional tissue depolarizes first, resulting in a junctional escape rhythm. Sinus bradycardia has been associated with defecation, hiccupping, yawning, and nasopharyngeal stimulation, probably as a result of parasympathetic stimulation, and is frequently seen with prolonged apnea. Occasionally, otherwise normal infants have a sinus bradycardia of 80 to 90 beats/minute in the absence of other findings, probably because of immaturity of the autonomic nervous system and increased vagal tone. No treatment is necessary.

Ectopic Beats: Supraventricular and Ventricular

Although during routine predischarge screening in one series the incidence of ectopic beats was less than 1 per cent (Southall et al., 1981), continuous monitoring of healthy newborns shows that the incidence of ectopic beats is much greater, as high as 13 per cent according to one report (Ferrer et al., 1977).

Supraventricular ectopic beats are usually preceded by a P wave with an abnormal contour, have

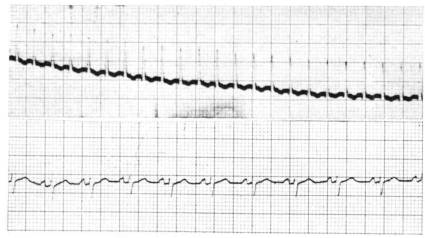

Figure 29–1. The upper tracing is lead III in a 7-day-old infant during a paroxysm of supraventricular tachycardia. The lower tracing (lead I) is in the same infant after the attack.

a normal-appearing QRS, and are followed by an incomplete compensatory pause before the next P wave. Ventricular ectopic beats usually have a wide abnormal QRS, a tall T wave in the opposite direction from the QRS, and a full compensatory pause.

These arrhythmias may be seen with metabolic abnormalities, hypoxia, or digoxin toxicity or following cardiac surgery, but they are also frequently seen in otherwise normal neonates.

Treatment includes correction of the predisposing factors when possible; in otherwise normal infants no treatment is necessary, since the prognosis is excellent, with almost all ectopy disappearing within the first month of life.

Paroxysmal Supraventricular Tachycardia

Paroxysmal supraventricular tachycardia (SVT) is one of the most common serious dysrhythmias occurring in the fetus and neonate. Although precise incidence data are not available, the generally accepted frequency is approximately 1 of every 25,000 children. Although usually relatively benign in the older child, the dysrhythmias may be life-threatening in the fetus or neonate, who generally has a higher ventricular rate and is less able to rely on other mechanisms for support of a failing circulation.

On electrocardiogram there is a rapid regular rhythm, usually 230 to 320 beats/minute, that originates in the atria or junctional region with either normal, abnormal, or inapparent P waves, a normal or slightly widened QRS, and ST segments that are normal or slightly depressed (Fig. 29–1). Several mechanisms play a part in the genesis of supraventricular tachycardias, but a rapid ectopic pacemaker or a circus type of re-entry secondary to different refractory periods of adjacent conducting bundles is the most common. Wolff-Parkinson-White syndrome, in which there is a direct muscular connection between the atrium and ventricle that allows re-entry, is recognizable on the electrocardiogram by a short P–Q interval and slow initial ventricular depolarization (delta wave) and is present in about 50 per cent of the cases (Fig. 29–2).

Clinical Manifestations. Supraventricular tachycardia (SVT) may occur in the fetus (Newburger and Keane, 1979). It may not cause symptoms before birth, but occasionally the rapid rate may lead to in utero congestive heart failure with fetal edema or hydrops and fetal death. Rarely, the fetal SVT is intermittent, and we have observed infants with hydrops born with normal EKGs who subsequently manifest recurrent SVT.

The neonate with SVT presents with signs and symptoms of low cardiac output and congestive heart failure; fussiness, refusal to feed, vomiting, tachypnea, and hepatomegaly are common. At first, the infants have some duskiness or cyanosis of the skin, but later their skin turns ashen grey and their extremities become cool owing to extreme peripheral vasoconstriction. Cardiac examination usually reveals no problem other than tachycardia. Underlying heart disease may be difficult to detect, even if present, because of the rapid heart rate.

At first, the chest radiograph may be normal, but, by the time symptoms occur, there is usually cardiac enlargement, often with pulmonary venous congestion. The echocardiogram is helpful in ruling out associated heart disease.

Diagnosis. SVT is diagnosed electrocardiographically. Occasionally, normal neonates with increased adrenergic activity may have heart rates exceeding 200 beats/minute, but these infants do not have congestive failure and the rate slows down when they are quiet. Occasionally, however, it may be difficult to distinguish neonates with a tachycardia associated with severe congestive failure caused by myocarditis or congenital heart disease from those with SVT. Rates of 220 or more in the neonate are rarely, if ever, of sinus origin and thus require treatment. Rates of 220 or less in the neonate usually represent sinus rhythm. The presence of heart failure with a rate of 200 to 220 suggests underlying heart disease, since this rate alone is rarely rapid enough to cause significant congestive heart failure in the neonate. Another helpful electrocardiographic sign is that SVT is

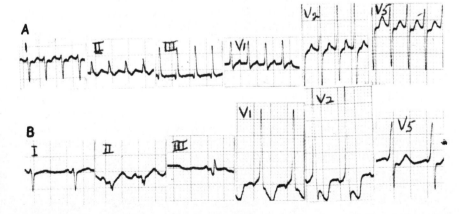

Figure 29–2. Electrocardiogram in a 4-day-old infant. A, Supraventricular tachycardia. B, Tracing after the tachycardia stopped shows a typical Wolff-Parkinson-White pattern with a short P–R interval and a wide QRS. The delta waves can be seen just before the upstroke of the R waves in the precordial leads.

almost always very regular, with variation in heart rate of more than 1 to 2 beats/minute unusual. Therefore, any variation in rate with crying or feeding is likely to signify a sinus mechanism. Rarely, a therapeutic trial of digoxin may be necessary to sort out the underlying mechanism.

Treatment. Supraventricular tachycardia in a neonate represents an emergency, and treatment should not be delayed. Vagal stimulation including gagging, carotid sinus massage, or ice compresses to the head should be tried but are rarely effective. For those infants who are not critically ill, we continue to try digoxin with half the total digitalizing dose of 0.04 mg/kg given stat and the rest in divided doses over the next 12 to 18 hours. If the neonate is sicker, three fourths of the total digitalizing dose can be given immediately intravenously, with the remainder administered within 4 to 8 hours. Other regimens that can be used in an emergency include DC cardioversion (0.25 to 1 joule/kg), propranolol (0.01 to 0.1 mg/kg I.V.), phenylephrine (0.01 to 0.1 mg/kg I.V.), edrophonium (0.2 mg/kg I.V.), or overdrive atrial pacing (Garson, 1981). Verapamil, a slow channel calcium blocker, has been used extensively in Europe. In 1982, it was approved for use in the United States, but there is little published information on its use in newborns. After conversion of SVT, we usually continue administering digoxin for about 1 year. If "breakthroughs" occur, we add propranolol unless contraindicated by underlying congenital heart disease.

Prognosis. The long-term prognosis is quite good. Recurrences occur in about 25 per cent of the infants, but these are usually easily controlled with drug therapy. Rarely, surgery is necessary to interrupt a bypass tract that is facilitating a re-entry tachycardia.

Atrial Flutter

Atrial flutter is a relatively rare dysrhythmia in the neonatal period. The atrial rate ranges between 360 and 480 beats/minute, with the ventricular response one half or, less commonly, one third of that. The atrial activity is best seen as a saw-toothed pattern of the P waves in leads II and V_{4R} to V_2. Neonates with atrial flutter may have congestive heart failure from the tachycardia, but more commonly the 2:1 or 3:1 block reduces the ventricular rate so that the dysrhythmia is well tolerated (Fig. 29–3).

The treatment involves digitalization and, if this fails to revert the rhythm to sinus, cardioversion. The prognosis is not as favorable as with atrial tachycardia, since recurrences are more common, but most infants without associated structural heart disease usually do well.

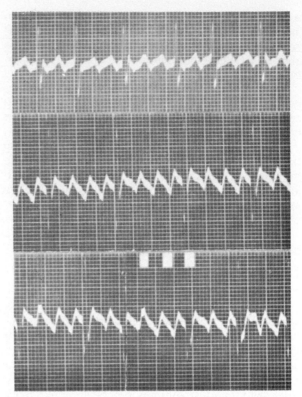

Figure 29–3. Standard limb leads during an attack of atrial flutter.

Ventricular Tachycardia

Ventricular tachycardia in the neonate is uncommon. When it does occur, it is usually in association with structural heart disease and is triggered by cardiac catheterization, surgery, anesthesia, metabolic abnormalities, or digitalis toxicity. The QRS complexes are wide and tall, and the T waves are directed opposite to the QRS complex. The rate is usually less than 200, but higher rates have been reported. The initial treatment should be lidocaine or cardioversion. Other drugs that may occasionally be useful include phenytoin (diphenylhydantoin), procainamide, quinidine, and propranolol. In the idiopathic variety, echocardiography and angiocardiography should be performed to rule out the possibility that a resectable tumor is the source of the tachycardia. Treatment must be individualized, with the long-term prognosis depending primarily on the underlying cardiac problem.

Atrioventricular Block

First and Second Degree Heart Block. First degree heart block is a prolongation of the P–R interval beyond the normal limits, 0.14 second. It is of no hemodynamic significance by itself and requires no treatment. In second degree heart block, there is an intermittent failure of impulse transmission from atria to ventricles. It may manifest as a progressive prolongation of the P–R interval in successive cycles followed by an unconducted atrial impulse (Wenkebach or Mobitz type I) or failure of atrial impulse transmission with dropped ventricular beats and no progressive prolongation of the P–R interval (Mobitz type II). Both type I and type II may be manifestations of infection or digitalis toxicity. Neither type needs treatment, but both should be watched carefully, since either may lead to third degree or complete heart block.

Third Degree Heart Block. In complete heart block (CHB) there is complete failure of the atrial impulse to lead to a ventricular response; the atria and ventricles beat independently, with the latter having a slower rate. On the surface EKG, there is no fixed relationship between the P waves and the QRS complex (Fig. 29–4). CHB is a relatively common problem in the neonate, occurring in 1 of every 15,000 to 20,000 livebirths.

Histologically, there may be an absence of a connection between the atrial conduction tissue and the atrioventricular node, absence or degeneration of the connection between the A–V node tissue and the distal conducting tissue, or a lesion beyond the A–V node that interrupts the bundle of His (Lev, 1972). Intracardiac electrophysiologic studies obtained during cardiac catheterization on 24 older children with congenital complete heart block demonstrated block above or in the A–V node in 79 per cent, within the bundle of His in 13 per cent, and more distal in the conducting system in 4 per cent. The site of block could not be determined in 4 per cent (Karpawich et al., 1981).

Approximately 40 per cent of infants with congenital complete heart block have associated structural heart disease (Michaelsson and Engle, 1972), with corrected transposition of the great arteries, single ventricle, and the heterotaxy syndrome the most common, although virtually any type of heart disease can occasionally be found.

Recently, there have been several reports confirming the association of congenital heart block in the fetus with the presence or later development of maternal lupus erythematosus (McCue et al., 1977).

Clinical Manifestations. The block is often suspected or diagnosed in utero during the third trimester or during labor because of the persistent slow heart rate of the fetus, about 50 to 80 beats/minute. More than half the babies are delivered by emergency cesarean section owing to the mistaken belief that the bradycardia represents fetal distress (Esscher and Michaelsson, 1979). The majority of neonates are symptom-free; those neonates with associated structural congenital heart disease or ventricular rates of less than 50 are the most likely to have the symptoms of heart failure.

In the child without associated structural heart disease or heart failure, the large stroke volume often results in soft systolic flow murmurs across the aortic or pulmonary valves, and the atrioventricular dissociation with variable flow across the A–V valves may produce a variable first heart sound and intermittent flow rumble across the mitral or tricuspid valves. On the radiograph, the heart may be slightly enlarged, but the pulmonary vascular markings are normal and pulmonary venous congestion is absent.

In the neonate with heart failure, the usual manifestations are usually present, with dyspnea, tachypnea, hepatomegaly, and feeding difficulties com-

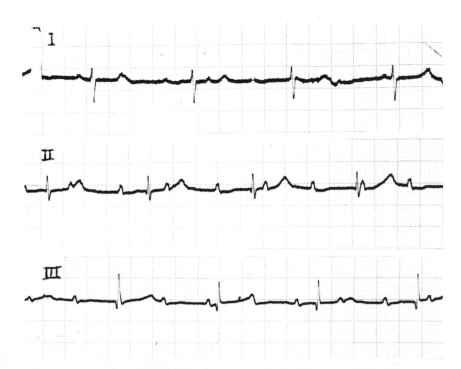

Figure 29–4. Age 4 days. Standard limb leads. Complete heart block is present. The ventricular rate is 90, the atrial rate 120.

mon. The findings on physical examination and radiographs usually depend on the associated cardiac lesions.

Treatment.   Most newborns without structural heart disease are asymptomatic; for these, careful observation will suffice. For the rare child without associated anomalies in whom bradycardia causes heart failure unresponsive to diuretics, a pacemaker is necessary. Isoproterenol may be of temporary help. Although temporary pacing can usually be established by a transvenous catheter route, the possibility of cardiac perforation, emboli from the catheter, and the difficulties encountered with linear growth of the child make epicardial pacing desirable after a thoracotomy for placement of the wires. For neonates with symptoms due to CHB accompanying structural heart disease, treatment usually involves palliation or correction of the underlying cardiac anomaly with epicardial pacing.

Prognosis.   The prognosis greatly depends on the presence and nature of associated structural heart disease. In a group of 118 neonates with complete heart block but without structural heart disease followed for a median interval of 9 years, there were 21 deaths (18 per cent), 15 of them occurring before 2 weeks of age and the remainder before 5 years of age. Thirteen required permanent pacemakers (Esscher and Michaelsson, 1979). In contrast, of 80 neonates with CHB diagnosed soon after birth who had associated heart disease, 34 (43 per cent) died, almost all in the first week of life (Michaelsson and Engle, 1972).

Most of the available data reflect management in the 1960s and early 1970s; with better corrective and palliative surgery as well as microcircuitry and miniaturization of pacemakers, results will likely improve in the next decade.

REFERENCES

Esscher, E., and Michaelsson, M.: Assessment and management of complete heart block. *In* Godman, M. J., and Marquis, R. M. (Eds.): Pediatric Cardiology. Vol 2. Heart Disease in the Newborn. Edinburgh, Churchill-Livingstone, 1979.

Ferrer, P. L.: Arrhythmias in the neonate. *In* Roberts, N. K., and Gelband, H. (Eds.): Cardiac arrhythmias in the neonate, infant, and child. New York, Appleton-Century-Crofts, 1977.

Ferrer, P. L., Gelband, H., Garcia, O. I., Tamer, D. M., and Jesse, M. J.: Occurrence of arrhythmias in the newborn period. Clin. Res. 25:64A, 1977.

Garson, A., Jr.: Supraventricular tachycardia. *In* Gillette, P. C., and Garson, A., Jr. (Eds.): Pediatric Cardiac Dysrhythmias. New York, Grune and Stratton, 1981.

Karpawich, P. P., Gilette, P. C., Garson, A., Hesslein, P. S., Porter, C., and McNamara, D. C.: Congenital complete atrio-ventricular predictors of need for pacemaker insertion. Am. J. Cardiol. 48:1098, 1981.

Lev, M.: Pathogenesis of congenital atrio-ventricular block. Prog. Cardiovasc. Dis. 15:145, 1972.

Losekoot, T. G., and Lubbers, W. J.: Arrhythmias in the neonate. *In* Godman, M. J., and Marquis, R. M. (Eds.): Pediatric Cardiology. Vol 2. Heart Disease in the Newborn. Edinburgh, Churchill-Livingstone, 1979.

McCue, C. M., Mantakas, M. E., Tingelstad, J. B., and Ruddy, S.: Congenital heart block in newborns of mothers with connective tissue disease. Circulation 56:82, 1977.

Michaelsson, M., and Engle, M. A.: Congenital complete heart block: an international study of the natural history. *In* Engle, M. A. (Ed.): Pediatric Cardiology, Cardiovascular Clinics. Philadelphia, F. A. Davis Co., 1972.

Newburger, J. W., and Keane, J. F.: Intrauterine supraventricular tachycardia. J. Pediatr. 95:780, 1979.

Southall, D. P., Johnson, A. M., Shinebourne, E. A., Johnston, P. G., and Vulliamy, D. G.: Frequency and outcome of disorders of cardiac rhythm and conduction in a population of newborn infants. Pediatrics 68:58, 1981.

PART 5

DISORDERS OF THE GASTROINTESTINAL TRACT

30

General Considerations

Revised by Richard J. Grand

The gastrointestinal tract is, with the respiratory epithelium, the major interface between host and environment. At the time of full-term delivery, the normal newborn demonstrates nearly complete morphologic gastrointestinal development. However, contrary to previous teaching, there is considerable postnatal maturation of gastrointestinal, pancreatic, and hepatic function, which is of greater significance for neonatal nutrition in the premature than in the term infant.

Table 30–1 summarizes the intrauterine developmental sequence of structure and function of the digestive organs. Despite considerable knowledge of many of the processes reviewed, significant details remain to be elucidated.

At the time of birth, the newborn has had considerable experience swallowing. Fetal swallowing begins at approximately 16 to 17 weeks of gestation and matures rapidly, so that at term the fetus swallows approximately 20 ml per hr of amniotic fluid. The normal newborn sucks vigorously and swallows almost perfectly, the coordination of sucking, breathing, and swallowing being tightly regulated. Approximately 10 per cent of newborns will show incoordination of swallowing, which normalizes by 2 weeks of age.

Esophageal Function

Esophageal function undergoes important postnatal maturation. The normal newborn under 12 hr of age shows poorly coordinated responses to deglutition, with an extremely rapid peristaltic rate and, often, nonperistaltic, simultaneous contractions along the entire length of the esophagus. As infants grow older, peristalsis becomes more coordinated, the peristaltic rate slows, and simultaneous contractions decrease in frequency, the latter occurring in only 10 per cent of children over 2 years of age. Lower esophageal sphincter pressure is normally low at birth and rises over the first 6 weeks of life toward adult levels (15 to 30 mm Hg). Many normal newborns, however, will demonstrate delayed development of LES pressure, which leads to the syndrome known

Table 30–1. Development of the Human Gastrointestinal Tract

Age (wk)	Crown-rump length (mm)	Stage of development
2.5	1.5	Gut not distinct from yolk sac.
3.5	2.5	Fore- and hindgut present; liver bud present; yolk sac broadly attached to midgut.
4	5	Esophagus short; stomach spindle-shaped; intestine present as a simple tube; liver cords, ducts, and gallbladder form; pancreatic buds appear as outpouching of gut.
	7.5	Esophagus differentiated well from stomach.
5	8	Intestine lengthens into loop.
6	12	Stomach rotates; intestinal loop undergoes torsion; parotid and submandibular buds appear.
7	17	Stomach attaining final position; circular muscle layer present; duodenum temporarily occluded (?); intestine herniates into cord.
	19	Villi begin to develop.
8	23	Taste buds appear; gastric pits in fundus and body; villi lined by single layer of cells.
9	30	Pancreatic cell buds present; Auerbach's plexus appears.
10	40	Gastric pits in pylorus and cardia; intestine reenters coelomic cavity; crypts of Lieberkuhn begin to develop; active transport of glucose present; dipeptidases present.
12	56	Parietal cells detectable; intestinal muscle layers present; active transport of amino acids; alkaline phosphatase and disaccharidase detectable; colonic haustrations appear; enterochromaffin cells appear; pancreatic islets appear; bile secreted.
	78	Circular folds appear.
14		Cytoplasmic vesicles detectable.
16	112	Gastric and intestinal glands proliferating; meconium developing.
	120	Glucose transport in jejunum increasing; dipeptidase and disaccharidase activities increase.
20	160	Peyer's patches present in intestine; muscularis mucosa present.
24	203	Ascending colon recognizable; Paneth cells appear.
28	242	Esophageal glands appear.
32	277	Circular folds present.
38	350	Maturity achieved.

From Grand, R. J., Watkins, J. B., and Torti, F. M.: Development of the human gastrointestinal tract. Gastroenterology 70: 790, 1976.

as chalasia, or postprandial regurgitation. This is a normal maturational phenomenon that usually clears by 9 months of age, is not accompanied by any other clinical symptoms, and is not to be confused with pathologic gastroesophageal reflux (see Esophagus, Chapter 32).

Gastric Function

Gastric acidity increases in the first 24 hours of life. The stomach at birth is filled with a greenish-yellow opalescent fluid of pH 6.0 that consists of endogenous gastric secretions, amniotic fluid, and saliva. When this fluid is aspirated and gastric drainage is performed during the next few hours, it can be shown that the pH of the gastric aspirate falls from 5.7 in the first hour to 4.0 at 8 hours.

Despite the increase in acidity, the rate of gastric acid secretion is lower in the newborn on day 1 than in the older infant. Measurement of basal and pentagastrin-stimulated gastric acid secretion in 1- and 2-day-old newborns suggests either that gastric acid secretion in the newborn is maximal under basal conditions or that the parietal cells are unresponsive to pentagastrin at this age.

By 3 months of age, acid output approaches the lower limits of normal for adults with a clear correlation between increasing acid output, age, body weight, and surface area (Table 30–2).

Intrinsic factor secretion rises slowly and can be readily detected by day 10 or 11 (15 to 60 μg/ml, adult normal 15 to 98 μg/ml). Secretion of intrinsic factor after stimulation parallels acid production in the newborn, rising to levels that are approximately 50 per cent of adult values by 10 to 14 days and reaching mature levels by 3 months of age.

It is very clear that the mean pH achieved during feeding in the newborn exceeds the pH optimum for pepsin activity (1.8 to 3.5). Although it has been suggested that the small premature infant may thus be compromised in its ability to utilize dietary protein, data supporting such a contention are scanty. Lowered proteolytic function in the stomach of the newborn might lead to the facilitation of absorption of intact antibody protein from colostrum and breast milk.

Recently, gastrin levels have been measured in cord blood and in plasma of the human newborn. At term, cord serum contains concentrations of gastrin 2- to 3-fold higher than those in maternal serum studied simultaneously. The levels in newborns are also significantly higher than those in random normal adults. Venous and arterial samples from the umbilical cord are almost identical, suggesting that gastrin is produced by the fetus but fails, to some extent, to cross the placenta into the maternal circulation. Plasma gastrin levels rise on the fourth day of life to a value twice that in cord plasma. Values in older babies have not yet been obtained.

Air enters the stomach of the newborn immediately after birth and fills the small intestine in 2 to 12 hrs and the large bowel within approximately 24 hours. Failure of this pattern suggests mechanical obstruction to the flow of intraluminal contents.

Postnatal Intestinal Development in the Term Infant

Even the normal term infant demonstrates delayed maturation of intestinal function when carefully studied. For example, the capacity for glucose absorption rises markedly after the infancy period, and the apparent K_m for glucose absorption has been calculated to be approximately 5.8 mM in infants and 20 mM or more for adults.

Very little is known about the mucosal capacity for amino acid absorption. Except for the specific disorders of amino acid absorption, no quantification of amino acid or protein absorptive capacity is available in the newborn.

To a certain extent, full-term infants absorb lipid inefficiently. Weijers and coworkers have demonstrated that a majority of infants fed cow's milk formula have a coefficient of fat absorption ranging from 80 to 95 per cent, a defect that is not fully corrected until 1 year of age. Analysis of fecal lipids in the first 2 weeks of life from infants fed modified cow's milk formula has shown that a greater percentage of total fecal lipids exists as glycerides than that which can be found in infants 23 to 72 days of age. Interestingly,

Table 30–2. Postnatal Development of Gastric Acid Secretion and Intrinsic Factor in the Human

Mean age	Mean wt (kg)	Volume (ml/hr)	H^+ concentration (mEq/L)	H^+ output (mEq/hr)	H^+ output (mEq/hr/kg)	IF output (ng B_{12}/hr/kg)
1 day	3.4	3.3	8.1	0.03	0.01	7.1
28 days	3.9	3.1	26.4	0.08	0.02	31.2
12 wk	4.9	13.4	34.8	0.47	0.10	90.0
14 wk	9.2	41.0	18.5	0.77	0.08	
16 wk	11.8	44.0	41.6	1.83	0.17	
24 wk	13.0	64.0	49.2	3.15	0.24	
4–9 yr		42.5	114.2	4.88		
11 yr	25.3			5.25	0.20	
Adult	70.0	143.2	91.2	13.06	0.19	118.4

a considerable proportion of the lipid detected in the stools is triglyceride, strongly suggesting reduced lipolysis during digestion of dietary fat. Indeed, studies of pancreatic secretory function demonstrate a reduction in maximal lipase secretion even at 1 month of age. Furthermore, amylase activity initiated by pancreatic stimulation rises several-hundred–fold after the first month of life; another 10-fold rise can be achieved by one month of age by increasing the quantity of ingested starch.

In addition to reduced lipolytic activity, intraluminal bile acid concentrations are low in term infants and bile acid synthesis and pool size are approximately one-half the values found in normal adults. Thus, the aforementioned lipolytic defect is further compromised by reduced micellar concentrations and decreased solubilization of the products of lipolysis. For reasons that are not yet completely clear, serum primary bile salt levels are higher at birth than after 1 to 2 months of age, a phenomenon termed "physiologic cholestasis."

The efficiency of the intraluminal phase of fat absorption is affected by the composition of dietary lipid. In comparison to the data presented previously concerning the coefficient of fat absorption for term infants fed cow's milk, Weijers and associates have shown that breast milk fat is absorbed with normal efficiency, the coefficient of fat absorption being at or above 95 per cent. The configuration of fatty acids in breast milk triglycerides may explain this improved absorption, although the recently described breast milk and lingual lipases certainly contribute to the efficiency of fat absorption.

Under normal circumstances, none of the aforementioned deficits in digestive or absorptive function have significant nutritional impact on neonatal growth and development. However, these defects are magnified in the premature infant and in the normal term infant during stress or illness. Under such circumstances, clinically significant malnutrition may appear.

Postnatal Intestinal Development in The Premature Infant

The prematurely born human infant is at grave risk for nutritional failure, a danger that increases in severity as birth weight falls. There is ample evidence that intrauterine growth between 24 and 36 weeks of gestation increases exponentially and that severe weight loss that occurs immediately after birth adds an additional challenge to the nutritional support of such infants. Even when a 10 per cent dextrose so-

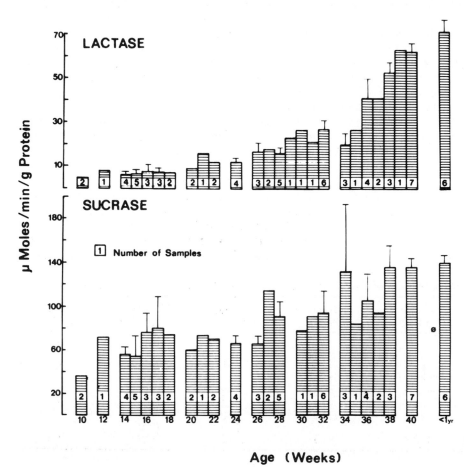

Figure 30–1. Developmental patterns of jejunal lactase and sucrase activities in human fetuses. (Data are mean ± SD and were kindly provided by Dr. Irena Antonowicz, Children's Hospital Medical Center, Boston.)

lution is infused, 3.5 per cent of body protein may be lost in the first 48 hours of life. The need for adequate nutrition as soon after birth as possible is complicated in the premature infant by the immature digestive-absorptive capacity of the gastrointestinal organs.

A consequence of the smaller mucosal surface area in the premature infant may be reduction of the number of glucose transport sites. However, studies of transport are unavailable. Nevertheless, some useful information can be obtained from studies of intestinal disaccharidases. As shown by Antonowicz and associates (Fig. 30–1), sucrase has reached normal postnatal levels by the twenty-eighth week of gestation. In contrast, lactase activity only begins to rise after the thirtieth week of gestation, reaching a maximal level at term. Clearly, very low birth weight infants (born at 28 to 32 weeks) may be lactose intolerant, and some may benefit from an alteration in the carbohydrate component of commercial formulas (i.e., substitution of sucrose for lactose). Nevertheless, many low birth weight infants appear to tolerate the high concentrations of lactose in breast milk without obvious morbidity.

Careful studies of amino acid absorption have not been performed in premature infants. Nevertheless, high concentrations of dietary protein invariably lead to elevated plasma amino acid and ammonia levels in low birth weight infants, suggesting that the absorptive capacity of the intestine may exceed the ability of the liver to handle the amino acid load. A correlation between plasma amino acid levels and dietary protein intake has been demonstrated.

Dietary fat is absorbed even more inefficiently in the preterm infant than in the term newborn. As in the term newborn, the degree of fat malabsorption in the premature is dependent on the quantity and composition of dietary lipid. As expected, the mean coefficient of fat absorption in premature infants who are fed human milk is higher (75 ± 6%) than that in comparable infants who are fed cow's milk (60 ± 11%). In addition, fat absorption improves in the premature infant with advancing age. Figure 30–2 sum-

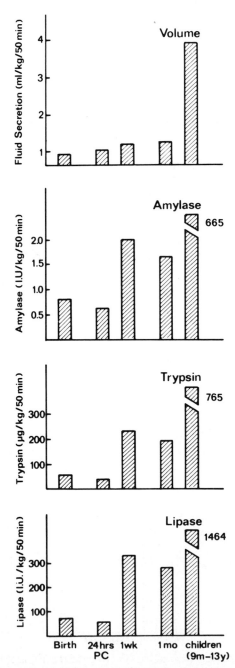

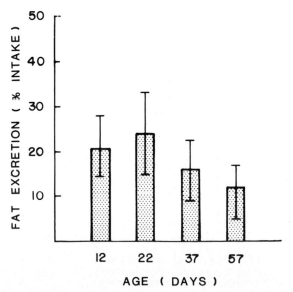

Figure 30–2. Fecal fat excretion in premature infants (<1300 gm birth weight) at various ages after birth. (Data are mean ± SD adapted from Katz and Hamilton, 1974.)

Figure 30–3. Pancreatic secretory response to pancreozymin-cholecystokinin (2 μg/kg, I.V.) and secretin (1 μg/kg, I.V.) administration in infants born at 32 to 34 weeks compared to older infants. (Data drawn from Zoppi et al., 1972, and represent mean values.)

marizes data obtained in such infants who were fed a commercial cow's milk–based formula in which the distribution of lipid closely mimicked that of human breast milk. Although the infants demonstrated marked steatorrhea in the first 12 days of life, fat absorption was nearly normal by the age of 2 months.

Recent studies of intraluminal fat digestion in preterm infants have identified defects in both the lipolytic and micellar phases. Zoppi and coworkers demonstrated reduced responsiveness of the pancreas to stimulation by secretin and pancreozymin (cholecystokinin); the output of digestive enzymes was very low after administration of these hormones (Fig. 30–3). While secretory function increased during the first months of life, levels were considerably lower than those found in infants over 9 months of age. Confirming the presence of reduced lipolysis, Katz and Hamilton described increased concentrations of duodenal triglycerides in very low birth weight infants in the first 2 weeks of life but not thereafter.

In many premature infants, duodenal bile acid concentrations are well below the critical micellar concentration during feeding with breast milk or commercially available breast milk–like formulas. This marked deficit in intraluminal bile acid content in the preterm infant is a result of reductions in bile acid pool size and synthesis rates to levels that are one third to one half (Fig. 30–4).

The nutritional impact of this immaturity of lipolytic and micellar function may be lessened by alterations in the composition of dietary lipid. As discussed previously, steatorrhea is most marked when infants received unprocessed cow's milk, and it is significantly reduced by the use of breast milk or breast milk–like commercial formulas. Interestingly, Roy and colleagues have shown that substitution of medium-chain triglycerides for long-chain triglycerides in formulas fed to preterm infants produces a marked increase in fat absorption, weight gain, and nitrogen retention. Hamosh has also demonstrated that addition of breast milk to commercial formula leads to a marked increase in fat absorption, owing to, at least in part, the effects of breast milk lipases.

Colonic Function

Peristaltic waves and motility of the colon have been observed in the eighth fetal week, and teniae appear, together with the formation of haustra, by the eleventh or twelfth fetal week. Meissner's and Auerbach's plexuses are present by the eighth week and twelfth week, respectively, and there is a cranial to caudal migration of the neuroblasts between the fifth and twelfth weeks of gestation. The distribution of ganglion cells has been well studied in premature and full-term infants, and, aside from the well-described area of hypoganglionosis present in the first 10 mm above the anal valve, a normal distribution of ganglion cells exists in the premature infant as young as 24 weeks and in the full-term infant.

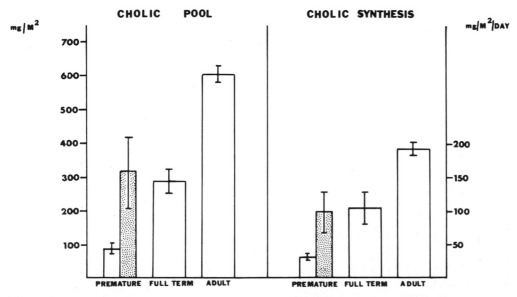

Figure 30–4. Comparison of bile acid pool size and synthesis rate in premature infants, full-term infants, and adults, corrected for body surface area. Shaded bars refer to premature infants whose mothers had received prenatal treatment with dexamethasone or phenobarbital. (Data are mean ± SE. Values for premature infants are from Watkins et al., 1975; those for term infants are from Watkins et al., 1973, and those for adults are from Vlahcevic et al.: Gastroenterology 61:85, 1971. Figure kindly provided by Dr. John B. Watkins, Children's Hospital, Philadelphia.)

Symptoms of Gastrointestinal Disorders

Vomiting

Regurgitation of the first few feedings offered may take place during the first day or two of life without arousing undue alarm. The newborn infant who vomits should, of course, be observed frequently and examined scrupulously for evidences of organic disease. In a fair number of cases, no signs will be discovered to support such a diagnosis, and vomiting ceases on the third or fourth day. Ordinarily, the withholding of milk constitutes adequate treatment, small quantities of water being substituted for milk for one or two feedings. Exactly why these infants vomit is not known. One of a variety of factors may be operative, including minimal intracranial injury, maternal medication, and the swallowing of bloody or purulent amniotic fluid. If the last is suspected, lavage is indicated. The immaturity of the lower esophageal sphincter mechanism may play an important part in this first-week vomiting.

Signs that suggest that vomiting may stem from organic disease are many and varied. Fever points toward parenteral or enteral infection. Failure to pass the first meconium stool within 24 hours suggests intestinal obstruction, especially Hirschsprung's disease. The converse is not true; that is, *the passage of one or more meconium stools does not rule out complete intestinal obstruction.* This is especially true if the obstruction is high in the gastrointestinal tract. Abdominal distention points toward organic obstruction also. Again, the converse is not true. *Complete obstruction, especially at the level of the duodenum or higher, may be present without distention.* Anorexia plus repeated vomiting may completely prevent the development of distention. The development of visible intestinal patterns upon the abdominal wall argues strongly in favor of organic obstruction, but it is not absolutely pathognomonic.

Visible peristaltic waves moving from the left costal margin toward the midline indicate that the point of blockage is at or near the pylorus. When waves move from right to left, they arise in the bowel distal to the duodenum and, hence, point to obstruction in the jejunum, ileum, or colon. One small, palpable, firm mass, deep and just to the right of and either above or below the umbilicus, may represent the hypertrophic pyloric musculature of pyloric stenosis. Multiple firm masses scattered throughout a distended doughy abdomen characterize meconium ileus. A large palpable mass in one or the other flank suggests a malformed, hydronephrotic, or infected kidney that might be the basis of vomiting. Spherical masses of cystic consistency may be cysts or duplications of the stomach or bowel. Rigidity of abdominal muscles is occasionally present in instances of peritonitis, but this sign, useful in older patients, is unfortunately often lacking in the newborn.

The nature of the material regurgitated furnishes useful clues to the location of obstruction. Pure mucus or a mixture of mucus and saliva alone denotes obstruction proximal to the stomach and suggests esophageal stenosis or atresia, rarely cardiospasm or esophageal diverticulum. Unaltered or coagulated milk, unstained with bile, suggests lax esophagus or obstruction of the pylorus or in the duodenum proximal to the ampulla of Vater. Bile-stained vomitus suggests narrowing or closure of the intestinal lumen distal to the ampulla. The presence of bile in vomitus is not absolutely diagnostic but strongly suggests organic obstruction. Fecal vomitus indicates obstruction low in the intestinal tract.

When blood is mixed with the vomitus, it may be difficult to ascertain its source. It must never be forgotten that such blood may be maternal in origin, ingested with the amniotic fluid after placental hemorrhage or ingested with the milk when the nipple is cracked and bleeding. With the Apt test (discussed shortly), we are able to differentiate fetal from maternal blood, since fetal red cells resist alkali denaturation.

Causes of vomiting in the newborn include, therefore, ill-defined ones that are self-limited in the first few days of life and a great variety of organic lesions causing obstruction at any point from the upper portion of the esophagus to the anus. These will be discussed in detail shortly. In addition, there are numerous others. Intracranial lesions, chiefly subdural hemorrhage and hydrocephalus, commonly produce vomiting. Infections of almost any system may be ushered in with vomiting, and, in some of these, such as peritonitis, meningitis, pyelonephritis, and hepatitis, vomiting may continue until the infection is controlled. Uninfected lesions of the genitourinary tract, mainly those that produce hydronephrosis, may in the newborn as well as in the older patient precipitate vomiting. Certain metabolic disorders, such as galactosemia, hereditary fructose intolerance, tyrosinemia, and adrenal cortical hyperplasia, often cause vomiting. The list might be prolonged indefinitely. Our purpose in this paragraph is to point out that vomiting in the newborn may be a sign of disease in the gastrointestinal tract, but it may also, as in the older infant and the child, suggest disease almost anywhere else in the body.

Constipation

The first meconium stool is passed by 69 per cent of normal infants within 12 hours, by 94 per cent within 24 hours, and by 99.8 per cent within 48 hours (Sherry and Kramer, 1955). In 1973, Mangurten and Slade found no significant differences in their more recent study of preterm infants and could discover "no relationship among birth weight, gestational age, Apgar score, or age at first feeding and age at first stool." Failure to pass a stool within the first 24 hours must be regarded with suspicion. This may be the earliest sign of Hirschsprung disease (see p. 368).

After the first two days during which pure meconium is passed, the newborn's stools consist of part meconium and part fecal matter for another day or two, after which they become entirely fecal. The number of stools passed by the normal infant is extremely variable, for some being as few as one every second or third day, for some as many as 10 every 24 hours. In general, the stools of the breast-fed infant are more frequent and more liquid than those of the artificially fed infant. However, it is not too uncommon, nor is it abnormal, for a breast-fed infant to have stools at long intervals, every 24 or 48 hours or even longer. This does not represent constipation unless the stools then passed are hard and dry. At times, this is the result of insufficient intake, but at other times even this is not the case. When intake is adequate and the nature of stool is not abnormal, infrequency of bowel movement may be completely ignored.

In some small newborns, especially prematures, constipation may become a real problem. Stools not only are passed at long intervals but also, when passed, are small, hard, and dry. Constipation in these tiny infants may produce anorexia, distention, and vomiting, and it should not be ignored. Rarely, such constipation is so pronounced that true intestinal obstruction is produced. Laxative medication should be avoided, but a small saline enema when indicated is permissible and often effective. The exact cause of the constipation is not known, but one suspects that weakness of intestinal and abdominal musculature may play an important role in its production. Infants of eclamptic mothers who may be hypermagnesemic are lethargic and flaccid, and their passing of meconium may be delayed.

A most serious form of constipation in the newborn is that associated with cystic fibrosis, so-called "meconium ileus." In this condition, dry, inspissated or thick, gluey meconium may produce total obstruction at the time of birth or even in utero. This latter situation may lead to meconium peritonitis.

Diarrhea

Diarrhea is usually defined as the passage of numerous loose stools. This definition requires several qualifying statements. The breast-fed infant may pass as many as 10 or 12 loose movements in the course of 24 hours yet eat well, gain well, and behave perfectly normally. This is not a disease state and should not be termed diarrhea. Other infants, however, may have but one or two loose movements in a day yet look ill and become dehydrated and acidotic with great rapidity. A large quantity of fluid and electrolytes may become pooled within the intestinal lumen, where it represents a loss of body water and salts as complete as though it had been passed to the outside. Such a situation constitutes diarrhea and may be as hazardous as the passage of 15 or 20 loose stools in a day.

Diarrhea in the newborn is often due to enteral infection, although at times it may represent the intestinal response to parenteral infection. Rarely, it is caused by disaccharidase deficiency, and, even more rarely, it may be the result of deficiency of monosaccharide absorption. (Table 30–3).

Table 30–3. Conditions Associated with Diarrhea from the Time of Birth

Absorptive disorders (symptoms brought on by feeding)
  Glucose-galactose malabsorption
  Sucrase-isomaltase deficiency
  Lactase deficiency (?)
  Enterokinase deficiency
  Cystic fibrosis
Secretory disorders
  Congenital chloridorrhea
  Tumors
    Ganglioneuroma
    Neuroblastoma
Other
  Neonatal necrotizing enterocolitis
  Hirschsprung's disease
  Intractable diarrhea of infancy
  Familial enteropathy

Hematemesis and Melena

The vomiting of blood or blood-stained gastric contents and the passage of bloody stools are not infrequent occurrences in the neonatal period. As mentioned earlier, the physician's first task is to determine whether this blood is maternal in origin or whether the infant is bleeding internally. As little as 3.0 ml of blood ingested by the infant may produce one or more bloody stools that appear 7 to 17 hours after ingestion. By a simple test (the Apt test), maternal blood may be distinguished from the infant's. This test is based on the low percentage of fetal hemoglobin (hemoglobin F) in the former and its high concentration in the latter. The Apt test for the differentiation of fetal from adult hemoglobin is performed as follows:

Mix the specimen under study with an equal quantity of tap water. Either centrifuge the mixture or strain it through filter paper. If the supernate or the filtrate is pink, hemoglobin may be present. To 5 parts of this supernate or filtrate add 1 part of 0.25 per cent sodium hydroxide. The pink color should deepen and persist for more than 2 minutes if hemoglobin F is present. If it turns yellow within 2 minutes, it is hemoglobin A.

Fetal blood indicates one of a variety of lesions, and its source may be difficult, at times impossible, to determine. From retrospective pathologic evidence, we know that bloody vomitus may be due to esophagitis. Peptic ulcer of the stomach or duodenum occurs in the newborn. Since it may not be readily recognizable on physical examination or even radiographic contrast studies, diagnosis rests on exclusion of other causes of bleeding. These include deficiencies in the clotting mechanism and the group of generalized infections. Rarely, the newborn bleeds from peptic ulcers in unusual locations, such as Meckel's diverticulum or gastrogenic cysts within the abdomen or thorax. Duplications of bowel often bleed. More uncommon is hemorrhage from the bowel due to intussusception, which occurs, but with the utmost infrequency, in the neonatal period. Single or multiple polyps and hemangiomas of the bowel might conceivably do the same, but thus far they have not been reported at this early age. Multiple telangiectasia characteristically exhibit no symptoms until late in childhood. Pulmonary hemorrhage is often signaled by the issuance of blood from the mouth or nares or both, and, unless the material is frothy, it is difficult to distinguish from gastric bleeding.

Anorexia

Some newborns eat poorly for a number of days for any one of a great variety of reasons. The reason in any particular case usually becomes obvious as one follows the course of the illness. An occasional newborn refuses to eat for an indefinite time, with no indication of underlying disease. This is not a matter of being unable to swallow but seems rather to be due to a complete lack of the sensation of hunger. Severe brain defect such as hydranencephaly commonly causes this. So do less well-defined brain disorders. Choanal atresia may present with poor feeding because of the inability of the infant to breathe while feeding, when oral breathing is impossible. In one child in our experience, feeding had to be carried out by gavage for 3 months, after which appetite gradually became normal. However, this child subsequently developed psychomotor retardation.

REFERENCES

Abramson, S., Treves, S., Teele, R.: The infant with possible biliary atresia. Evaluation by ultrasound and nuclear medicine. Pediatr. Radiol. *12*:1, 1982.

Agunod, M., Yamaguchi, N., Lopez, R., Luhby, A. L., and Glass, G. B. J.: Correlative study of hydrochloric acid, pepsin and intrinsic factor secretion in newborns and infants. Am. J. Digest. Dis. *14*:400, 1969.

Antonowicz, I., Chang, S. K., and Grand, R. J.: Development and distribution of lysosomal enzymes and disaccharidases in human fetal intestine. Gastroenterology *67*:51, 1974.

Avery, G. B., Randolph, J. G., and Weaver, T.: Gastric acidity in the first day of life. Pediatrics *37*:1005, 1966.

Balistreri, W.: Neonatal cholestasis. *In* Lebenthal, E. (Ed.): Textbook of Gastroenterology and Nutrition in Infancy. New York, Raven Press, 1981, p. 1084.

Ballard, R. A., Vinocour, B., Reynolds, J. W., Wennberg, R. P., Merritt, A., Sweetman, L., and Nyhan, W.: Transient hyperammonemia of the preterm infant. N. Engl. J. Med. *299*:920, 1978.

Berquist, W., Rachelefsky, G., Kadden, M., et al.: Gastroesophageal reflux-associated recurrent pneumonia and chronic asthma in children. Pediatrics *68*:29, 1981.

Borgstrom, B., Lindquist, B., and Lundh, G.: Enzyme concentration and absorption of protein and glucose in duodenum of premature infants. Am. J. Dis. Child. *99*:338, 1960.

Boswell, D., and Lebenthal, E.: Gastroesophageal reflux. *In* Lebenthal, E. (Ed.): Textbook of Gastroenterology and Nutrition in Infancy. New York, Raven Press, 1981, p. 911.

Brown, E., and Sweet, A.: Neonatal Necrotizing Enterocolitis. New York, Grune and Stratton, 1980.

DeCarlo., J., Jr., Tramer, A., and Startzman, H. H., Jr.: Iodized oil aspiration in the newborn. A.M.A. J. Dis. Child. *84*:442, 1952.

Dienstag, J.: Non-A, non-B hepatitis. Adv. Intern. Med. *26*:187, 1980.

Euler, A. R., Ament, M. E., and Walsh, J. H.: Human newborn hypergastrinemia: an investigation of prenatal and perinatal factors and their effects on gastrin. Pediatr. Res. *12*:652, 1978.

Euler, A. R., Byrne, W. J., Cousins, L. M., Ament, M. E., Leake, R. D., and Walsh, J. H.: Increased serum gastrin concentrations and gastric acid hypersecretion in the immediate newborn period. Gastroenterology *72*:1271, 1977.

Euler, A. R., Byrne, W. J., Meis, P. J., Leake, R. D., and Ament, M. E.: Basal and pentagastrin stimulated acid secretion in newborn human infants. Pediatr. Res. *13*:36, 1979.

Frank, M. M., and Gatewood, O. M. B.: Transient pharyngeal incoordination in the newborn. Am. J. Dis. Child. *111*:178, 1966.

Fredrikzon, B., Hernell, O., Bläckberg, L., and Olivecrona, T.: Bile salt–stimulated lipase in human milk. Evidence of activity in vivo and of a role in the digeston of milk retinol esters. Pediatr. Res. *12*:1048, 1978.

Grand, R. J., Watkins, J. B., and Torti, F. M.: Development of the human gastrointestinal tract. Gastroenterolgy *70*:790, 1976.

Gryboski, J. D.: Gastrointestinal Problems in the Infant, Philadelphia, W. B. Saunders Co., 1975.

Gryboski, J. D., Thayer, W. R., and Spiro, H. M.: Esophageal motility in infants and children. Pediatrics *31*:382, 1963.

Haller, J., and Schneider, M.: Pediatric Ultrasound. Chicago, Year Book Medical Publishers, 1980, p. 23.

Hamosh, M.: A review. Fat digestion in the newborn: role of lingual lipase and preduodenal digestion. Pediatr. Res. *13*:615, 1979.

Harries, J. T., and Fraser, A. J.: The acidity of the gastric contents of premature babies during the first 14 days of life. Biol. Neonat. *12*:186, 1968.

Herbst, J. J.: Gastroesophageal reflux. J. Pediatr. *98*:859, 1981.

Illingworth, R. S.: Sucking and swallowing difficulties in infancy: Diagnostic problem of dysphagia. Arch. Dis. Child. *44*:655, 1969.

Jensen, R. G., Hagerty, M. M., and McMahon, K. E.: Lipids of human milk and infant formulas: a review. Am. J. Clin. Nutr. *31*:990, 1978.

Katz, L., and Hamilton, J. R.: Fat absorption in infants of birth weight less than 1,300 gm. J. Pediatr. *85*:608, 1974.

Lebenthal, E., and Lee, P. C.: Development of functional response in human exocrine pancreas. Pediatrics *66*:556, 1980.

Lev, R., and Orlic, D.: Histochemical and radioautographic studies of normal human fetal colon. Histochemistry 39:301, 1974.

Mangurten, H. H., and Slade, C. I.: First stool in the preterm, low birthweight infant. J. Pediatr. 82:1033, 1973.

Rogers, I. M., Davidson, D. C., and Lawrence, J.: Neonatal secretion of gastrin and glucagon. Arch. Dis. Child. 49:796, 1974.

Roy, C. C., Ste-Marie, M., Chartrand, R. T., Weber, A., Bard, H., and Doray, B.: Correction of the malabsorption of the preterm infant with a medium-chain triglyceride formula. J. Pediatr. 86:446, 1975.

Sherry, S. N., and Kramer, I.: The time of passage of the first stool and the first urine by the newborn infant. J. Pediatr. 46:158, 1955.

Signer, E., Murphy, G. M., Edkins, S., and Anderson, C. M.: Role of bile salts in fat malabsorption of premature infants. Arch. Dis. Child. 49:174, 1974.

Sokal, M. M., Koenigsberger, M. R., Rose, J. S., Berdon, W. E., and Santulli, T. V.: Neonatal hypermagnesemia and the meconium plug syndrome. N. Engl. J. Med. 286:823, 1972.

Suchy, F. J. Balistreri, W. F., Heubi, J. E., Searcy, J. E., and Levin, R. S.: Physiologic cholestasis: elevation of the primary serum bile acid concentrations in normal infants. Gastroenterology 80:1037, 1981.

Utian, H. L., and Thomas, R. G.: Cricopharyngeal incoordination in infancy. Pediatrics 43:402, 1969.

Walker, W. A.: Intestinal transport of macromolecules. In Johnson, L. R. (Ed.): Physiology of the Gastrointestinal Tract. New York, Raven Press, 1981, pp. 1271–1289.

Watkins, J. B.: Bile salt metabolism in the newborn. N. Engl. J. Med. 288:431, 1973.

Watkins, J. B., Bliss, M., Donaldson, R. M., and Lester, R.: Characterization of newborn fecal lipid. Pediatrics 53:511, 1974.

Watkins, J., Klein, P., Schoeller, D., et al.: Diagnosis and differentiation of fat malabsorption in children using ^{13}C labelled lipids: triactanoin, triolein, and palmitic acid breath tests. Gastroenterology 82:911, 1982.

Watkins, J. B., Szczepanik, P., Gould, J. B., Klein, P. D., and Lester, R.: Bile salt metabolism in the human premature infant. Gastroenterology 69:706, 1975.

Weijers, H. A., Drion, E. F., and van de Kamer, J. H.: Analysis and interpretation of the fat absorption coefficient. Acta Paediatr. Scand. 49:615, 1960.

Werlin, S. L., Grand, R. J., and Drum, D. E.: Congenital hypertrophic pyloric stenosis: the role of gastrin re-evaluated. Pediatrics 61:883, 1978.

Wolff, P.: The serial organization of sucking in the young infant. Pediatrics 42:943, 1968.

Younoszai, M. K.: Jejunal absorption of hexose in infants and children. J. Pediatr. 85:446, 1974.

Zoppi, G., Andreotti, G., Pajno-Ferrara, F., Njai, D. M., and Gaburro, D.: Exocrine pancreas function in premature and full term neonates. Pediatr. Res. 6:880, 1972.

31

Disorders of the Mouth, Tongue, and Neck

Several minor disorders of the oral cavity may be disposed of briefly. Oral moniliasis will be discussed under Infections (see Chapter 86).

Tongue tie, that universal condition of past generations, has been relegated to its proper place. The frenum binding the tongue to the floor of the mouth is recognized now to be short and not too elastic in the normal newborn. The tongue need not be protruded far from the mouth in the course of the usual activities of the newborn infant, and shortness of the frenum does not hinder proper sucking and deglutition. The short frenum can be expected to lengthen over the course of the years. It need not be cut.

Infants may be born with one or more erupted teeth, commonly called natal teeth, or one or more may erupt during the first month and are hence known as neonatal teeth, usually the lower incisors of the deciduous set. Reported incidence figures range from 1:5000 to 1:10,000 in most series. The abnormality is often transmitted as an autosomal dominant trait. Since only their crowns are calcified, while their roots are imperfectly formed, these teeth are almost always loose. They should be extracted.

Cysts large enough to be visible to the naked eye may be discovered in the mouths of 80 per cent of newborns. In decreasing frequency these "*Epstein's pearls*" or "*Bohn's nodules*" are present along the median palatal raphe, the maxillary alveolar ridge, and the mandibular alveolar ridge. They may be ignored.

Ranula is a retention cyst of the sublingual salivary gland. It presents as a pea- to marble-sized mass on the anterior floor of the mouth filled with clear or yellow contents, pushing the tongue upward. Most will disappear in time; a few may have to be resected.

Congenital Fusions

In *ankyloglossia superior* the tongue is fused to the hard palate and the gums. Other anomalies are associated.

A few infants have been born with partial or complete *fusion of the gums*, without other congenital anomalies. Snijman and Prinsloo's infant did well after a simple operative procedure.

Epignathus

Epignathus is an extremely rare disorder. It defines any kind of growth arising from the upper jaw or palate and projecting from the mouth. The tumors may be polyps, hairy polyps, dermoids, or teratomas. These are believed to arise from embryonal tissue rests, although some still consider them incomplete twins (sphenopagus or palatopagus).

Because of their location and size, some being as large as an orange or small grapefruit, they may cause respiratory difficulty and inability to take food. Most are benign (Fig. 31–1).

Treatment must be directed first toward relief of dyspnea. An introduced airway may be adequate for short periods, but tracheostomy may be required if definitive attempts at cure are delayed. Feeding is best carried out by nasal catheter. Removal of the tumor is not difficult if the attachment is small, as in polyps, but may be practically impossible when the base is broad, as in some teratomas. Nevertheless, surgical removal offers the only hope for cure.

Congenital Epulis

This misnamed tumor arises from the upper or lower jaw, and its projection into the mouth may make closure difficult and sucking impossible. It is misnamed because in none of the reported cases has it arisen from the bone itself as in true epulis of older patients, but from the tissue overlying the bone. Langley and Davson found 23 cases in the literature, of which 15 arose from the maxilla and eight from the mandible. All but three of the patients were newborns, and all but three in whom the sex was known were females. The authors added three cases of their own.

The tumors were similar in appearance. They were covered with squamous epithelium and packed with vascular connective tissue in which were encountered many large polyhedral or round cells with granular cytoplasm and a few elongated or spindle-shaped cells. In spite of the fact that myofibrils have never been seen in these cells, they have generally been assumed to represent myoblasts. The authors doubt that myoblastoma is their proper designation. In no instance has there been either local recurrence, invasion, or metastasis.

Immediate surgical excision is indicated. The results are uniformly satisfactory.

Nasopharyngeal Tumors

Loeb and Smith estimate that at least 50 cases of nasopharyngeal tumors were recorded in the world literature up to 1967. Less than 10, discovered in the newborn period, have been successfully removed. Most of these have been simple hairy polyps or dermoids, a few more highly developed teratomas. Some have thin pedicles, but the rare teratoma may be broadly based far back on the palate or on the posterior pharyngeal wall, from where it may project out of the mouth or upward into the nasopharynx or both. These tumors arise from the midline or near it.

Diagnosis of dermoids not projecting externally may be made by careful examination of the pharynx. The tumor may be visible or palpable as a small sausage-shaped mass. Commonly freely movable, it may cause respiratory obstruction intermittently at

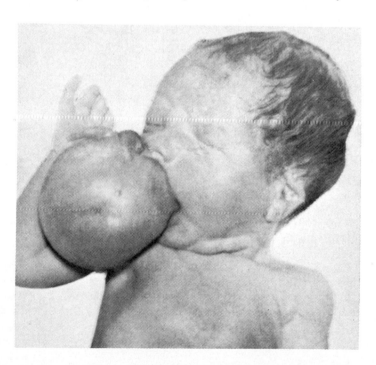

Figure 31–1. Infant with epignathus. The orange-sized mass attached to the maxilla protrudes grotesquely from the mouth. (Wynn, S. K., Waxman, S., Ritchie, G., and Askotsky, M.: A.M.A. J. Dis. Child. *91:*495, 1956. Reprinted with the permission of the authors.)

those moments when it has become caught behind the soft palate, whereas its extrusion into the oropharynx may be accompanied by relief from dyspnea. In the example described by Dieter and coworkers, only feeding difficulty was present from birth until the sixth day, at which time acute episodic respiratory distress began.

Treatment consists in immediate removal. Those dermoids with a thin pedicle may be removed easily with a snare. Those teratomas with a broad base, which are considerably less common, need to be shelled out surgically. The procedure is delicate and time-consuming, and tracheostomy prior to anesthesia is indicated.

Aglossia Congenita

An extremely rare congenital anomaly is absence, or almost complete absence, of the tongue. In Ardran and Kemp's example, the floor of the mouth was covered with filiform mucosa resembling that of the tongue, and there were two lateral ridges and a small pyramidal mass in the midline of the posterior floor that contained some muscle. In addition, there were micrognathia and syndactyly of the left hand.

The infant fed poorly at first but learned to feed after a time with the aid of gravity, suction by depression of the floor of the mouth and jaw, and compression of the nipple by elevation of the floor of the mouth. Swallowing, visualized by cineradiography, was thereafter normal.

Taste is normal, and these children learn to speak with only a few sounds imperfectly formed.

Congenital Macroglossia

Slight enlargement of the tongue may be noted at birth in some otherwise normal newborns, especially in those of short, stocky, muscular body build. For a few months, the tongue may protrude slightly from a mouth not quite capacious enough to contain it. This is not true macroglossia.

Etiology. Moderate enlargement is seen in Down syndrome, in cretinism, and in glycogen storage disease of the heart. In none of these is it sufficiently large to cause trouble in breathing or swallowing

Huge thickening and overgrowth of the tongue to the point that it protrudes from a constantly open mouth, making feeding difficult and respiration noisy and partially obstructed, constitutes true macroglossia. Some of these symptoms are associated with macrosomia and omphalocele and a variety of other congenital defects, and these may accompany symptomatic neonatal hypoglycemia. They fit into the category of Beckwith's syndrome. The rest fall into two large pathologic groups, lymphangioma being the more common and muscular hypertrophy characterizing the remainder. In this latter variety, the individual muscle fibers have been reported to be four or five times as thick as average ones.

Diagnosis. Down syndrome and cretinism will be ruled in or out in the usual fashion. The infant with glycogen disease will probably be limp and flaccid, and a radiograph will show cardiomegaly. Biopsy of skeletal muscle will reveal excess of glycogen in these babies. Macroglossia that is not symmetric but that is localized to one portion of the tongue is almost surely lymphangiomatous, and it may be associated with hygroma of the neck. Biopsy of the tongue should determine whether lymphangioma or muscle hypertrophy is the basic lesion.

Treatment. Plastic surgery is the appropriate treatment for the lymphangiomatous form. Recurrences are common and may necessitate further operations. Bronstein and associates preferred to wait out their case with muscular hypertrophy. Their patience was rewarded by a gradual shrinking in size of the tongue, which, along with growth of the mandible, made disproportion less and less obvious. Koop and Moschakis have seen three newborns among their eight cases of capillary lymphangioma of the tongue, all in association with nearby hygroma. They resected all and performed tracheotomy when needed. They point out that these tongues are liable to a vesicular, hemorrhagic glossitis that they treat by electrodesiccation.

Beckwith's Syndrome

The presence of macroglossia in association with an omphalocele or other umbilical abnormalities and severe hypoglycemia was first described by Beckwith in 1964. This constellation of abnormalities, subsequently noted by a number of authors, is sufficiently characteristic to deserve the appellation of syndrome.

A repetition among sibships has been described in some instances, suggesting that it is an autosomal recessive trait. It has been noted in both white and black infants.

The infants may be born at term or prematurely, and they may be oversized for gestational age. Severe, symptomatic hypoglycemia may be present in the first days of life and persist for several months. The tongue is very large and persists that way, but it becomes less apparent with postnatal growth of the face. There is a midfacial recession and tendency toward exophthalmos. With increasing age, gigantism becomes apparent, and occasionally hemihypertrophy ensues.

A late complication is the tendency toward development of malignant neoplasms; adrenal carcinoma, Wilms' tumor, and bilateral nephroblastomas have been reported.

Pathology. The brain is below expected weight; other organs are similar to predicted weight. Hyperplastic phenomena are noted in the kidneys and the islet cells and acini of the pancreas. The fetal zone of the adrenal cortex is prominent with cytomegaly and cortical cysts.

Treatment. Early recognition of the hypoglycemia and its correction with corticosteroids and glucose may improve the prognosis in this syndrome. The initial descriptions were of autopsied patients; the full clinical spectrum of the syndrome awaits further delineation.

Lingual and Sublingual Thyroid

Rarely, thyroid tissue may persist as solid or cystic tissue in the posterior midline of the tongue or under it. It is rarely recognized in the newborn period. Since it represents failure of migration, often no other thyroid tissue exists, as determined by radioscans.

The treatment consists of excision and appropriate replacement therapy. The ectopic tissue is subject to abnormal function, adenoma, and even carcinoma.

Pharyngeal Diverticulum and Pseudodiverticulum

Congenital diverticula of the hypopharynx, running down into the mediastinum behind the esophagus and clinically simulating esophageal atresia with tracheoesophageal fistula, have been described. More recently, pseudodiverticula, resulting from digital or instrumental trauma to the posterior pharyngeal wall during or after delivery, have also been reported.

In both conditions, the anomalous tracts have been visualized after barium swallow.

Diverticula must be excised surgically. Pseudodiverticula may heal spontaneously, but they too may have to be repaired operatively.

Sialadonitis (Inflammation of the Salivary Glands)

SUPPURATIVE NEONATAL PAROTITIS

Suppurative parotitis strikes the newborn infant very rarely. Until 1970, 62 cases had been reported in the world literature, to which number Leake and Leake added 10. These had been encountered in the Boston Children's Hospital Medical Center in the preceding 25 years.

As a rule, normal pregnancies and labors had preceded birth, and premature infants were involved a bit more often than expected. Swelling of one or both parotids, usually one, appears at any time from the first to the twenty-fifth day. Some babies have been quite well prior to the appearance of swelling, but the majority have suffered some illness: respiratory distress, dehydration, hyperbilirubinemia, pneumonitis, or sepsis. It is widely believed that the dehydration, with cessation of flow from Stensen's duct, permits ascent of organisms from the mouth.

The offending organism is most often the *Staphylococcus aureus*, although *Escherichia coli* and other coliforms have been responsible. Sepsis is not too uncommonly associated.

The parotid gland becomes swollen and the skin over it reddened, and there is usually low fever. Pressure over the gland forces purulent material from the orifice of Stensen's duct. Not infrequently, infection spreads to involve the other parotid or a submaxillary gland. Oxacillin should be used until the organism is identified, and incision and drainage should be resorted to at the first sign of fluctuation.

Prognosis is good for uncomplicated cases.

SUPPURATION OF THE SUBMAXILLARY GLANDS

Several examples of suppuration of a submaxillary gland have been reported, not secondary to infection of the parotid gland. Swelling appeared beneath, in the region of the submaxillary gland, and pus could be expressed from the orifice of Wharton's duct beneath the tip of the tongue. In all other respects it behaves like suppurative parotitis.

Congenital Branchiogenous Anomalies

Anomalous developments of the branchial arches may manifest themselves in a great variety of forms. The most obvious of these are (1) skin tags, (2) pits, (3) fistulas and (4) cysts. They are located for the most part in two sites, the preauricular region and anywhere along the anterior border of the sternocleidomastoid muscle, from mastoid to manubrium.

Skin tags should be removed for cosmetic reasons. Pits may be ignored. Fistulas may discharge mucoid or purulent material; they may penetrate deep in the neck to terminate near the pharynx and rarely may open into the pharynx. Cysts usually lie at the angle of the mandible but may be found low, just above the clavicle. Fistulas should be removed by careful, thorough dissection. Cysts should be extirpated early because they are prone to infection.

Miscellaneous Lesions of Mouth and Neck

Micrognathus is discussed under the First Arch Syndrome, as are *cleft palate* and *harelip* (see Chapter 91).

The *Klippel-Feil syndrome* is discussed in Chapter 95.

The neck is the site of diverse tumorous swellings, either present at birth or becoming manifest within the first few weeks of life.

Sternomastoid tumor can be seen and palpated within the body of the sternocleidomastoid muscle as a firm, smooth, generally ovoid mass. It does not usually appear until on or after the tenth day; it grows for a few months, then recedes spontaneously within another 4 to 8 months. It may be accompanied or followed by torticollis, at times with cranial and facial asymmetry, oculomotor imbalance and high scoliosis. Its cause is not known and there is no general agreement as to correct treatment. Electromyography may be useful in deciding whether or not to excise the mass surgically.

Torticollis unassociated with a palpable sterno-cleidomastoid tumor may be associated with hiatus

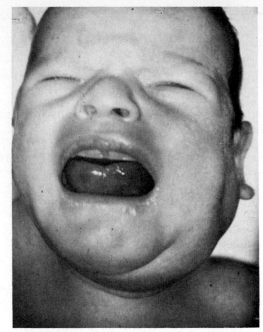

Figure 31–2. Hygroma, neck and tongue.

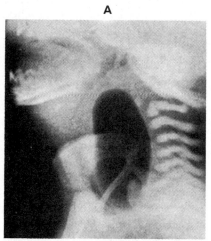

A

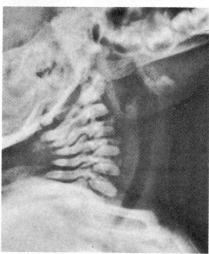

B

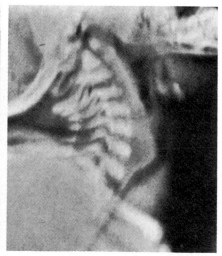

C

Figure 31–3. *A*, Lateral radiograph of the neck shows an air-containing cyst displacing the air passages and esophagus forward. *B*, Lateral view of the neck with patient quiet, demonstrating straight, unobstructed tracheal air column. *C*, Lateral view of neck with patient crying demonstrates mass lesion between the manubrium and the trachea displacing the lower cervical trachea backwards and moderately narrowing this portion of the trachea. (From Thompson, R. E., and Love, W. G.: Persistent cervical thymoma apparent with crying. Am. J. Dis. Child. *124*:761, 1972.)

hernia (Sandifer's syndrome) or cervical spine abnormalities. Often, complete correction can be achieved by gentle stretching exercises. Placing the infant in a position that requires turning the head to see the environment has been helpful. If a full range of motion is not achieved by 1 year, operative division of the muscle is warranted.

Goiter may be visible and palpable at birth as a trilobed enlargement of the thyroid isthmus and its lateral lobes. The enlarged gland may be hypothyroid, euthyroid, or hyperthyroid.

The neck is the favorite site for *cystic hygroma*, although identical cavernous lymphangiomata may arise in many other parts of the body. Its soft, "bag-of-worms" feel and its usual location external to the sternomastoid muscle on one side, between the mastoid and the acromial process, readily differentiate it from other cervical tumors (Fig. 31–2).

Teratomas are found not infrequently in the neck. Most often they are midline, as most teratomata tend to be, arising in or adjacent to the thyroid isthmus. Their very firm, cystic conformation may differentiate them from cystic hygroma, but definitive diagnosis may be impossible prior to operation. The percentage of malignancy is small.

Branchial cysts (also called branchiogenic, lateral cervical, or cervical thymic cysts), arise in the embryo from either the branchial groove, the thymic stalk, or the pharyngeal pouch. They may be present at birth of may appear suddenly at any age. They lie beneath the sternomastoid muscle, but their anterior edge may bulge out from the muscle's anterior margin. They manifest a strong tendency to become infected and pus-filled. Sinniah and Somasundaran reported an extraordinary example in a baby, well at birth, who at 40 hours of age suddenly developed a large swelling on the left side of the neck along with respiratory distress and cyanosis. The radiograph showed a large air-containing cyst that displaced the air passages and esophagus forward (Fig. 31–2). Excision resulted in cure.

We are apt to forget that the *thymus* is one of the organs that arises high in the embryo and must travel caudad before its two lateral buds join in the anterior mediastinum. Their descent may become arrested at any point in the journey. Most present as unilateral, soft, fleshy masses somewhere below the angle of the mandible along the anterior edge of the sternomastoid. Some descend much farther and fuse at a point more caudad than is normal. Thompson and Love reported one such newborn in whom the mass made its appearance as an outpouching in the midline into the sternal notch, but only when the infant cried (Fig. 31–3).

The spherical mass of thyroglossal duct cyst lies in the midline deep in the neck and may extend backward to the base of the tongue, just above the larynx. It usually is cystic but may be solid and consist of thyroid tissue. Indeed, it may represent all the thyroid tissue that the baby possesses. It is difficult to differentiate from teratoma. Very rarely, the submental

gland becomes enlarged, usually as a result of infection, and may present diagnostic difficulty; however, this gland lies anterior to the preferred site of thyroglossal duct cyst. Before surgical intervention, one must make sure by radioiodine uptake studies that the baby has other functioning thyroid tissue.

REFERENCES

Ardran, G. M., and Kemp, F. H.: Aglossia congenita. Arch. Dis. Child. *31*:400, 1956.

Baxter, C. F., Johnson, E. W., Lloyd, J. R., and Clatworthy, W., Jr.: Prognostic significance of electromyography in congenital torticollis. Pediatrics *28*:442, 1961.

Beckwith, J. B.: Extreme cytomegaly of the adrenal fetal cortex, omphalocele, hyperplasia of kidneys and pancreas, and Leydig-cell hyperplasia. Another syndrome? Presented to Western Society for Pediatric Research, November 11, 1963. Abstract read by title, American Pediatric Society, *41*:56, 1964.

Beckwith, J. B.: Macroglossia, omphalocele, adrenal cytomegaly, gigantism, and hyperplastic visceromegaly. Birth Defects: Original Article Series, *5*:188, 1969.

Bell, H. G., and Miller, R. G.: Congenital macroglossia: Report of two cases. Surgery *24*:125, 1948.

Bodenhoff, J., and Gorlin, R. J.: Natal and neonatal teeth. Pediatrics *32*:1087, 1963.

Brintnall, E. S., and Kridelbaugh, W. W.: Congenital diverticulum of posterior hypopharynx simulating atresia of esophagus. Ann. Surg. *131*:564, 1950.

Bronstein, J. P., Abelson, S. M., Jaffé, E. H., and von Bonin, G.: Macroglossia in children. Am. J. Dis. Child. *54*:1328, 1937.

Cataldo, E., and Berkman, M. D.: Cysts of the oral mucosa in newborns. Am. J. Dis. Child. *116*:44, 1968.

Cohen, M. M.: Congenital, genetic and endocrinologic influences on dental occlusion. Dent. Clin. North Am. *19*:499, 1975.

Combs, J. T., et al.: New syndrome of neonatal hypoglycemia. N. Engl. J. Med. *275*:236, 1966.

David, R. B., and O'Connell, E. J.: Suppurative parotitis in children. Am. J. Dis. Child. *119*:332, 1970.

Dieter, R. A., Jr., Holinger, P. H., and Maurizi, D. G.: Angiofibromatous polyp of the pharynx. Am. J. Dis. Child. *119*:91, 1970.

Edson, B., and Holinger, P. H.: Traumatic pharyngeal pseudodiverticulum in the newborn infant. J. Pediatr. *82*:483, 1973.

Filippi, G., and McKusick, V. A.: The Beckwith-Wiedemann syndrome. Medicine *49*:279, 1970.

Foster, J. H.: Congenital dermoid tumor of the nasopharynx. Ann. Otol. Rhinol. Laryngol. *53*:578, 1944.

Gellis, S., and Feingold, M.: Picture of the month. Am. J. Dis. Child. *115*:349, 1968.

Gifford, G. H., Jr., and MacCollum, D.: Facial teratoma in the newborn. Plast. Reconstr. Surg. *49*:616, 1972.

Girdany, B. R., Sieber, W. K., and Ozman, M. Z.: Traumatic pseudodiverticula of the pharynx in newborn infants. N. Engl. J. Med. *280*:237, 1969.

Hajdu, S. I., Faruque, A. A., et al.: Teratoma of the neck in infants. Am. J. Dis. Child. *111*:412, 1970.

Hankey, G. T.: Congenital epulis (granular-cell myoblastoma or fibroblastoma) in a ten-weeks premature infant. Proc. Roy. Soc. Med. *48*:1015, 1955.

Hung, W.: Lingual and sublingual thyroid glands in euthyroid children. Pediatrics *38*:637, 1966.

Irving, I.: Exomphalos with macroglossia: A study of 11 cases. J. Pediatr. Surg. *2*:499, 1967.

Jacobs, P. H., Shafer, S. C., and Higdon, R. S.: Congential branchiogenous anomalies. J.A.M.A. *169*:90, 1959.

Kesson, C. W.: Asphyxia neonatorum due to nasopharyngeal teratoma. Arch. Dis. Child. 29:254, 1954.

Koop, C. E., and Moschakis, E. A.: Capillary lymphangioma of the tongue complicated by glossitis. Pediatrics 27:800, 1961.

Ladd, W. E., and Gross, R. W.: Congenital branchiogenic anomalies. Report of 82 cases. Am. J. Surg. 39:234, 1938.

Langley, F. A., and Davson, J.: Epulis in the newborn. Arch. Dis. Child. 25:89, 1950.

Leake, D., and Leake, R.: Neonatal suppurative parotitis. Pediatrics 46:203, 1970.

Loeb, W. J., and Smith, E. E.: Airway obstruction in a newborn by pedunculated pharyngeal dermoid. Pediatrics 40:20, 1967.

Lofgren, R. H.: Respiratory distress from congenital lingual cysts. Am. J. Dis. Child. 106:610, 1963.

Murphy W. J., Jr., and Gellis, S. S.: Torticollis with hiatus hernia in infancy: Sandifer's syndrome Am. J. Dis. Child. 131:564, 1977.

Ochsner, A., and Ayers, W. B.: Case of epignathus. Surgery 30:560, 1951.

Pannullo, J. N.: Congenital macroglossia, report of a case. Obstet. Gynecol. 7:97, 1956.

Sinniah, D., and Somasundaran, K.: Lateral cervical cyst: a cause of respiratory distress in the newborn. Am. J. Dis. Child. 124:582, 1972.

Smith, C. A.: Physiology of the Newborn Infant. 3rd ed. Springfield, Ill., Charles C Thomas, 1959.

Snijman, P. C., and Prinsloo, J. G.: Congenital fusion of the gums. Am. J. Dis. Child. 112:593, 1966.

Thompson, R. E., and Love, W. G.: Persistent cervical thymoma, apparent with crying. Am. J. Dis. Child. 124:761, 1972.

Wells, D. H.: Suppuration of the submandibular salivary glands in the neonate. Am. J. Dis. Child. 129:628, 1975.

Wynn, S. K., Waxman, S., Ritchie, G., and Askotzky, M.: Epignathus; survey. A.M.A. J. Dis. Child. 91:495, 1956.

32

Disorders of the Esophagus

Revised by Harland S. Winter

The following classification of disorders of the esophagus that are encountered in the neonatal period is a modification of one suggested by Holinger, Johnston, and Potts.

 I. Congenital malformations of the esophagus
 A. Absence
 B. Atresia
 1. With tracheoesophageal fistula
 2. Without tracheoesophageal fistula
 C. Stenosis
 1. Fibrous stricture
 2. Web
 3. External pressure
 D. Duplication
 II. Acquired lesions
 A. Gastroesophageal acid reflux
 1. With hiatus hernia
 B. Erosions
 C. Rupture
 III. Abnormalities in neuromuscular control
 A. Cricopharyngeal incoordination
 B. Achalasia
 C. Familial dysautonomia and other neurologic diseases
 IV. Compression or dislocation by neighboring structures

Absence of Esophagus

Several cases have been reported in which the entire esophagus, from hypopharynx to cardia, has been missing. Since this condition is incompatible with life and is at present uncorrectable, we shall not discuss it further.

Congenital Anomalies of the Esophagus

Esophageal anomalies can be classified according to their relative incidence. Esophageal atresia with distal tracheoesophageal fistula accounts for about 90 per cent of the total. Atresia without fistula and fistula without atresia account for most of the remainder. (These conditions are also discussed in Chapter 33).

Stenosis of Esophagus

The lumen of the esophagus may be narrowed but not completely atretic. Narrowing results in the main from (a) congenital strictures, (b) webs, (c) external pressure, and (d) acquired stenosis. The first two types are discussed together, since their etiology is roughly the same, as is their symptomatology.

Etiology.　Both congenital strictures and webs in the neonate stem from imperfect evolution of the primitive foregut into the mature esophagus. In the complicated process of formation of the esophagus, usually at the point at which the primitive trachea and larynx bud off from the foregut, imperfect recanalization may take place. In some instances, this failure was sharply limited to one point, and a weblike structure persists. In others, the defect encompasses a length of 1 cm or more.

Stenoses are not limited to the junction of the mid-

dle and upper thirds of the esophagus. A number have been reported involving some or all of the lower third. A few are found at or just above the cardia. Some of these are acquired fibrotic narrowings that presumably have resulted from reflux peptic esoph-

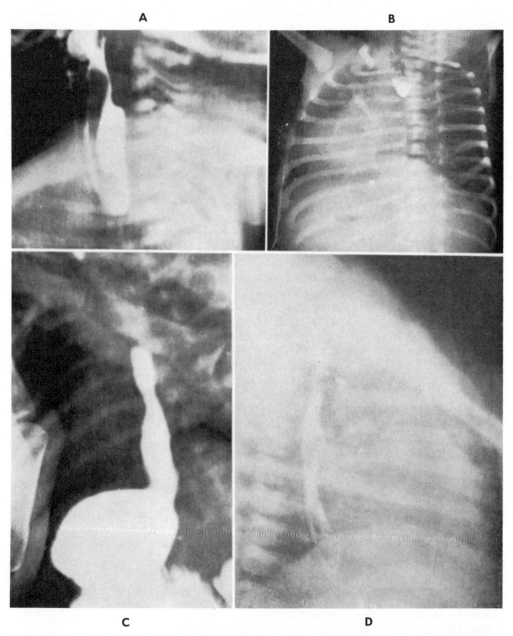

Figure 32–1. *A,* Esophagram recorded at 3 weeks of life, after increasing regurgitation since age of 2 weeks. Decided stenosis of esophagus is seen at about the junction of the upper and middle thirds. The esophagus proximal to the stenotic point is a little dilated. *B,* One week later, showing complete obstruction at the level of the stenosis. *C,* Preoperative regurgitation barium esophagram shows the lower limit of the stenotic area and a normal distal esophagus. At 5 weeks of age, after attempted dilatations from above and below via gastrostomy, the stenosis was relieved by longitudinal incision followed by transverse closure. *D,* Postoperative barium esophagram at 6 weeks of age shows an adequate passageway. At the age of almost 1 year, the patient was eating normally, and the esophagram was still normal. (Case of Dr. Richard H. Segnitz, Milwaukee, Wis. Reprinted with the kind permission of Dr. Segnitz, from Wisc. M. J. *55:*447, 1956.)

agitis. The time it takes for stricture to form depends on the quantity of the acid that is refluxed, the time of acid clearance, and the duration of the reflux. As most neonates do not have disordered esophageal motility, it is rare for an acquired peptic stricture to present in the neonatal period. Nevertheless, infants who vomit from birth and fail to grow may develop esophageal strictures. They usually require surgical repair with a fundoplication. Careful demonstration of both the presence of delayed acid clearance by pH probe study and normal esophageal peristaltic activity by manometric study will avoid surgical intervention in children with congenital esophageal rings or primary motility disorders.

Diagnosis. The prime sign of esophageal stenosis is vomiting. The nature of esophageal vomiting is distinctive. It usually takes place during the feeding, after a few ounces or less of fluid have been ingested, or at the termination of a small meal. It may be repeated several times during the same meal, since it is unaccompanied by nausea and the hungry infant is willing and eager to attempt to eat again after his esophagus has been emptied. The returned material is completely unaltered in appearance except perhaps for an admixture of mucus from the oropharynx or, if ulceration has occurred, an admixture of fresh or old blood. The amount regurgitated is never great, although later, as dilatation progresses, it may exceed in volume the capacity of the normal esophagus.

The time of onset of vomiting is extremely variable and appears to depend almost entirely on the degree of narrowing. Some infants with esophageal stenosis begin to vomit immediately after birth, after, that is, the institution of oral feeding. Some begin to vomit after a few weeks. A great many, perhaps the majority, do not begin to vomit until the attempt is made to add solids to the diet. Others can swallow both liquids and the thin purées commonly added first to the infant's diet, but they cannot manage to swallow small lumps of food. In still others, the onset of vomiting may be delayed for years until an unusually large object (for example, a large lump of meat, a coin, or a marble) that would pass through the normal esophagus becomes plugged in the stenotic stoma.

In many, the vomiting is not at all constant, several meals entering the stomach with no difficulty, followed by some that cannot be swallowed. In a few, vomiting becomes intractable, and swallowing of any type of food is completely impossible. Some older children make pathetic efforts to help push the food into the stomach by introducing a hand deep into the pharynx.

The only other symptom may be pain. In infants and young children, this may be expressed by unusual facial expressions or posturing of the head and neck.

Sandifer's syndrome, in which children hold themselves in a Degas-like fashion, is associated with gastroesophageal acid reflux and esophagitis. In older children, the pain may be localized substernally.

Failure to gain is frequent, and actual loss of weight may be sustained in periods of intractable vomiting. As is to be expected, the smaller infants may rapidly become dehydrated and acidotic when obstruction is nearly complete.

The appearance of blood in the vomitus is due to the development of esophagitis with ulceration. This may be of the superficial variety, or frank ulcers that are deep and linear may develop.

The diagnosis is suggested by the nature of the vomiting. It must be verified by fluoroscopic and radiographic studies.

The etiology of the stenosis must be defined before therapeutic intervention. Gastroesophageal reflux with stricture can be confirmed by pH probe study and esophageal biopsy. Histologic changes, noted in young children, are frequently lacking in neonates with acid reflux. In the absence of acid reflux, cartilaginous rings or hamartomatous lesions should be considered. These may not be demonstrable if the biopsy is too superficial.

Rarely, newborn infants may suffer with strictures from ingestion of lye or other destructive chemicals, and their management should be the same as that for older infants.

Radiographic Findings. Fluoroscopy must be performed carefully to avoid missing minor grades of narrowing. A thin barium mixture may be used, but, if this flows into the stomach rapidly, it should be followed by a thicker paste. The barium column may be seen to stop or hesitate, then to pass through the narrowed point in a thin stream or in narrow jets. Spot films will show, in the fibrous rings, symmetric funneling to a narrow line followed by gradual widening of the opaque column. When a web is present, it may be visualized as a sharp shelf at the point of obstruction. The segment of esophagus proximal to the narrowed point soon becomes dilated.

Treatment. Therapy depends on the etiology of the stenosis. If reflux and esophagitis are present in an infant, the response to antacid medical intervention usually is not successful over a prolonged period of time. Fundoplication is then needed if there is no evidence of a primary motility disorder. Bougienage may be useful if the stenosis is from a hamartomatous, fibrous, or cartilaginous ring. Esophageal resection is rarely required.

Compression of Esophagus by Neighboring Structures

Other mediastinal masses, cystic or solid, may produce narrowing or dislocation of the esophagus. In addition to esophageal duplications, gastrogenic or enterogenic cysts, dermoids, and anterior myelomeningoceles inter alia are included in this group. More common, although still rare, causes of esophageal compression are anomalous blood vessels, such as right aortic arch, double aortic arch, anomalous subclavian arteries, and others. Since the symptomatology of all these is apt to be more closely related to the respiratory than to the gastrointestinal system, these are discussed in the section devoted to the former (see p. 125).

Esophageal Duplications

Spherical or sausage-shaped cysts may be found in the mediastinum. Some have walls composed of mucosa, submucosa, and muscular layers, and they are obviously duplications of some portion of the gastrointestinal tract. The histologic characteristics of a few of this latter group suggest an esophageal origin. Most represent misplaced duplications of stomach or bowel.

The symptoms and signs are indistinguishable from those of other types of posterior mediastinal tumors. These are largely respiratory in nature, although dysphagia, vomiting, and hematemesis may make up part of the clinical picture. Because of the preponderance of respiratory symptoms, this group has been described under Mediastinal Cysts and Tumors on pp. 208 and 209.

Acquired Lesions of the Esophagus

GASTROESOPHAGEAL ACID REFLUX AND HIATUS HERNIA

To separate our consideration of hiatus hernia from the previous discussion of gastroesophageal reflux

and esophageal stricture is somewhat misleading. Hiatus hernia has been associated with congenital short esophagus, but this concept needs to be reevaluated with the newer diagnostic techniques for acid reflux.

Between the fourth and seventh weeks of gestation the esophagus elongates, and the stomach migrates rapidly in a caudal direction. Failure of complete elongation and migration leaves the esophagus short and the stomach completely or partially trapped above the diaphragm. Supradiaphragmatic stomach may be tubular and recognizable during esophagoscopy in the radiograph by the characteristic longitudinal rugal folds of its mucosa, separated from the esophagus above by a more or less well-defined area of narrowing. More often, the portion of intrathoracic stomach below the tubular esophagus and the hiatal constriction is tented and conical in shape. This mechanism may be relevant in the rare cases of diaphragmatic hernia, but most infants with hiatus hernia and a shortened esophagus have severe gastroesophageal reflux and esophagitis. Radiographic studies alone are no longer sufficient to define the pathophysiology. Studies of the duration of esophageal acid clearance and the frequency of intraesophageal acid reflux by continuous pH probe monitoring, manometric determination of the lower esophageal sphincter pressure, and scintigraphic measurement of gastric emptying time can all be fea-

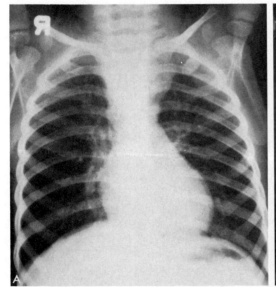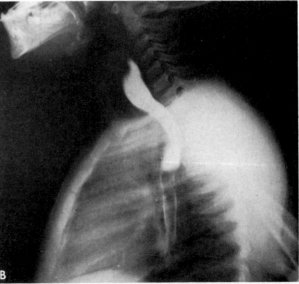

Figure 32–2. *A,* Anteroposterior view of chest shows a triangular shadow in the left upper lung field and deviation of the trachea to the right. *B,* Lateral view with barium in esophagus shows posterior displacement of the esophagus by a round mass. This proved at operation to be a cystic duplication of the esophagus.
This case is not abstracted in the text because the patient was not a newborn. She was a 2-year-old white infant who had had recurrent respiratory infections and respiratory distress since the age of 8 months. A soft mass could be seen in the left side of the neck when she strained or coughed. Cyanosis and dyspnea were marked. (Case of H. T. Langston, W. M. Tuttle, and T. B. Patton. Prints reproduced with kind permission of Dr. Langston, from Arch. Surg. *61*:949, 1950.)

sibly completed in neonates. They provide a physiologic basis for explaining the mechanism of the putative esophageal injury. The angle of His and the anatomy of the gastroesophageal junction provide an important mechanical barrier for reflux in the older child and adult.

The major barrier to gastroesophageal acid reflux in the neonate is the intrinsic pressure of the lower esophageal sphincter. Although some studies have reported that the sphincter pressure increases with age, it is more commonly accepted that the sphincter pressure is highest in the neonate and decreases to adult levels in early childhood. Although this controversy remains, the infant with a poorly developed anatomic or mechanical advantage from the angle of His would seem to require a higher intrinsic pressure to prevent acid reflux. As the stomach grows and the anatomic valvelike mechanism develops, a high pressure may not be required.

Incidence. The difference in apparent incidence of partial thoracic stomach, whether this be due to congenital short esophagus or to sliding hernia, in England as opposed to the United States, is hard to understand. Here the disorder is considered rare. We ourselves encounter no more than one every few years, despite the fact that we have been making exhaustive efforts to discover examples. Yet Carré and his coworkers found 18 cases a year in Birmingham alone, and Thomson observed 48 cases from 1949 to 1955. Friedland and colleagues in California confirmed a higher incidence after the introduction of the criteria of the British radiologists, suggesting that the diagnosis may have been missed in the United States.

Etiology. Congenital short esophagus was at one time believed to make up a large proportion of the hiatus hernia group. There followed a period when short esophagus was considered to have resulted almost always from fibrosing esophagitis. Botha, in 1958, after an exhaustive study of the anatomy of the normal newborn hiatus and a review of the pathology of partial intrathoracic stomach in young infants, reverted to the original position. He concludes that sliding hiatal hernia in adults is an acquired degenerative phenomenon, but in infants it is due to congenital short esophagus or underdeveloped diaphragm. There is no way, he believes, to distinguish these latter two. We believe that the overall evidence suggests that intrathoracic stomach is based on congenitally short esophagus rarely, and on fibrosis secondary to incompetent hiatus much more often.

The children in whom the lower esophageal sphincter is very weak or the esophageal motility is inadequate to clear refluxed acid rapidly may develop esophagitis with resultant esophageal shortening and hiatus hernia.

Botha completely re-examined the questions of the anatomy and physiology of the diaphragmatic hiatus in the neonatal period. He found that it differs in many important respects from the hiatus of adults. In the young infant, the hiatus is small and fits the narrowed portion of esophagus snugly. It is generally composed of encircling fibers of two limbs of the right diaphragmatic crus that surround the esophagus and overlap to produce a constricted oblique tunnel. The muscle ring is firmly attached to the lower esophagus and cardia by a strong phrenoesophageal membrane.

Diagnosis. It is possible to make the diagnosis of hiatus hernia within the neonatal period. The primary symptom is *vomiting*. The infants may begin to vomit from their first feedings, or the onset may be delayed

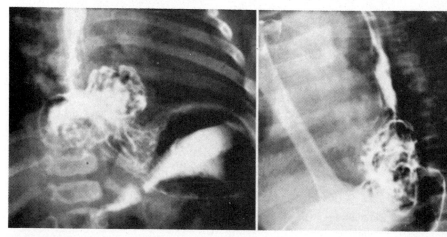

Figure 32–3. Views of esophagus and stomach taken at 1 week of age with patient in the Trendelenburg position. Both show the esophagus narrowing sharply as it enters the stomach, whose distinctive rugal pattern can be seen to lie well above the left diaphragm.

This infant began to vomit immediately after the institution of oral feeding. She was maintained in the semi-erect position for 7 weeks, by which time vomiting had ceased and weight gain commenced. At 1 year of age, she seemed perfectly well.

weeks or months. Some babies regurgitate every meal; others do so intermittently. Only small quantities are brought back. Appetite remains strikingly good, so that refeedings are taken eagerly immediately after regurgitation. The formula is either unchanged or mixed with small quantities of mucus or blood. It is never coagulated, nor does it ever contain bile. Blood admixture may or may not appear early, but, if vomiting persists for weeks or months, it is almost sure to appear. Weight gain may be slow or absent, and some babies lose weight and become dehydrated. The second symptom of importance, present in a large proportion of cases, is *anemia*, at times occult, in that bloodstained vomiting either has not occurred or has not been mentioned. *No anemia of undetermined origin with occult blood in the stool has been investigated completely unless the lower esophagus and cardia have been well visualized by radiography.* The third highly suggestive symptom is *persistent or recurrent lower respiratory infection*, again with or without overt vomiting. In infants suspected of having pathologic reflux, the pH probe is the most sensitive and specific test. With radiography, the incidence of false-positive and false-negative results is high when compared with that of continuous intraesophageal pH probe monitoring.

Most babies who are regurgitating do not require a contrast study or a pH probe study. Unexplained anemia, recurrent pulmonary infections, and failure to gain weight are indications for evaluation. If the vomiting persists after 12 to 15 months of age a work-up is indicated, as the development of esophagitis may be insidious and occur over decades.

Physical examination is unrewarding. The waves of hypertrophic pyloric stenosis have been seen and

its tumor palpated in a fair number of these infants, but, when this is true, pyloric stenosis is a coexisting disorder, not an integral part of this clinical picture.

Esophagoscopy. Esophagoscopy is now applicable to neonates, and the inspection of the esophageal mucosa may be important. However, gross observation is of little value, and there is frequently poor correlation between the endoscopist's impression and the histologic confirmation. Therefore, if one is seeking information only about the status of the esophageal mucosa, suction biopsies are more reliable and much simpler than endoscopy. If one is searching for a source of gastrointestinal blood loss, gross inspection may be advantageous.

Fluoroscopy and Radiographic Examination. Definitive diagnosis of lower esophageal disorders can be made in vivo only by fluoroscopy and radiographic study. These examinations must be conducted with scrupulous care and a foreknowledge of the pitfalls. A simple barium meal with the infant supine often does not suffice. It has been suggested that at first a thin barium mixture be given (weight to volume ratio of 1:2). If this enters the stomach without hesitation, the stomach should be filled with it, and this should be followed by several swallows of a thicker paste (weight to volume ratio of 1:1). Multiple spot films or, better, a cineradiographic strip should be taken in the erect, supine, and Trendelen-

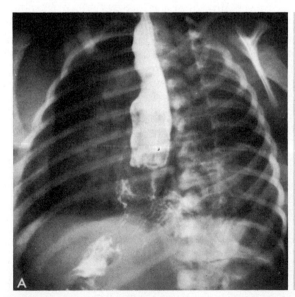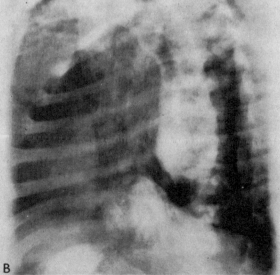

Figure 32–4. *A,* Supine film taken at 1 week of age after a barium meal. The greatly dilated esophagus narrows sharply several centimeters above the level of the diaphragm. *B,* Film taken with patient in the Trendelenburg position with abdominal pressure. The stenotic portion of the esophagus is about 1 cm long. Below it, but well above the diaphragm, lies a large pouch of the stomach.
This infant had multiple malformations, including cyanotic heart disease. She vomited intermittently from the second day of life until her death at 8 weeks of age. Esophagoscopy showed a stricture of the lower esophagus.

burg positions to determine whether reflux is present. Observations should then be made while gentle abdominal pressure is applied.

Stenotic areas in the esophagus will be visualized and the degree of narrowing and dilatation above ascertained. Unusual tightness or laxness at the physiologic cardia, a point 2 or 3 cm above the superior margin of the stomach, will be recognized. Unusual ballooning of the lower esophagus may be found, and spot films will show, by the rugal pattern, whether the dilated structure is lower esophagus or stomach. Irregularities in the mucosal pattern may indicate ulceration.

Cine-esophagography permits careful study of the films at leisure and often demonstrates behavior of the barium column not appreciated at the moment of swallowing.

Prognosis. The course of newborns with hiatus hernia is extremely variable. The rate of development of the sequelae—esophagitis, stricture, hiatus hernia—depends on the amount of acid reflux (competency of the acid barrier) and the rate of acid clearance (esophageal motility). The presence of hematemesis, occult blood loss, or failure to thrive signals more severe gastroesophageal acid reflux. The observation that some neonates and young infants remain asymptomatic is not reassuring, as the esophagitis may continue to progress and serious sequelae develop years later. Close re-evaluation of children with gastroesophageal acid reflux is mandatory.

Treatment. All early cases, and this would obviously include all cases diagnosed in the neonatal period, should be treated at first medically and conservatively. The prime consideration should be the prevention of reflux, for, if this can be accomplished, esophagitis and fibrosis will not follow. Reflux can best be obviated by maintaining the infant in the semi-upright position throughout the day and night. This can be accomplished by elevating the head of the crib 6 to 9 inches or by tilting the mattress. If the infant can change position, pillows are often helpful in restraining movement. Vomiting usually ceases promptly upon change of position, but in some infants the feeding mixture will have to be thickened by the addition of cereal in order to stop regurgitation completely.

Antacids may be useful in the older child, and may be advantageous in the neonate if there is evidence for esophagitis. If an infant is believed to be at high risk for development of a stricture because of esophageal motility problems or central nervous system impairment, administration of antacids should be considered as a prophylactic measure. Newer medications, such as bethanechol or metoclopramide, which have been used in older children for gas-

troesophageal reflux have had limited use in the neonate. Bethanechol chloride, a parasympathomimetic, increases gastric acid secretion and raises lower esophageal sphincter pressure. Metoclopramide acts mainly on gastrointestinal smooth muscle and potentiates gastric emptying as well as increases lower esophageal sphincter pressure. Thus, metaclopramide may be of specific use in the infant with delayed gastric emptying and reflux. These medications will require more clinical trials before becoming generally acceptable.

In the minority in whom simple medical management fails to relieve reflux and regurgitation, operative intervention will have to be considered. This is especially true if admixture of blood with the vomitus indicates esophagitis or if this condition is seen to be present by esophagoscopy and confirmed histologically. The surgeon will attempt to mobilize the esophagus and wrap part of the stomach around the esophagus to construct an anatomic barrier to reflux. Various types of gastric wraps are more effective in preventing acid reflux than gastropexy, which was used previously.

The most difficult sequel of hiatal hernia to treat is the stricture that forms secondarily. This is not an important consideration in the neonatal period, since time is required for a tight stricture to develop. Nevertheless, several authors have commented upon the rapidity with which stricture can form, and full-blown cases have been reported in infants as young as 4 and 6 weeks. After fundoplication, an attempt may be made to handle these by postural therapy and repeated dilatations. The hazard of perforation dictates the value of performing bougienage under direct esophagoscopic vision. Mercury-filled bougies may not be passed blindly until preliminary dilatation has been successfully accomplished. Dilatation in any event is not a long-term solution to the problem, and definitive operative intervention must be advised if the stricture returns and the infant has ongoing acid reflux.

In conclusion, postural treatment often suffices to relieve symptoms of regurgitation; hematemesis, melena, anemia, and obstructive symptoms should make one think seriously of operative intervention; and simple fundoplication is well tolerated by infants and children and can be expected to "give good results in the few infants who require it.

ESOPHAGEAL EROSIONS

The frequency of esophageal erosions at autopsy of infants was noted by Merriam and Benirschke, who found microscopic evidence of necrosis in 30 per cent of infants. It was most commonly associated with hyaline membrane disease but was also noted in stillbirths. Instrumentation was not thought to be a factor in pathogenesis. More gross evidence of esophagitis in stressed infants had previously been described by Gruenwald. He found ulceration and hemorrhage in some instances and felt that all these changes were manifestations of shock.

RUPTURE OF THE ESOPHAGUS

Five newborns have by now been reported with rupture of the esophagus not produced by passage of a tube. In one instance, rupture took place just proximal to a stenosing web, but in the other four, ruptures were spontaneous and unexplained.

In the example of Hohf and coworkers, spitting up of bright red blood at 13 hours of age was the initial sign. This was followed by hydropneumothorax, treated by aspiration, then water-seal drainage. Diagnosis was indicated by passage of ingested milk through the drainage tube and verified by Lipiodol esophagram. The tear was repaired and the patient recovered, but he later had a stricture that required repeated dilatations.

REFERENCES

Astley, R.: Oesophageal "spasm" in infancy. Proc. Roy. Soc. Med. *48*:1045, 1955.
Behar, J., and Ramsby, G.: Gastric emptying and antral motility in reflux esophagitis. Gastroenterology *74*:253, 1978.
Boix-Ochoa, J., Lafuente, J. M., and Gil-Vernet, J. M.: Twenty-four hour esophageal pH monitoring in gastroesophageal reflux. J. Pediatr. Surg. *15*:74, 1980.
Botha, G. S. M.: The gastro-esophageal region in infants: Observations in the anatomy, with special reference to the closing mechanism and partial thoracic stomach, Arch. Dis. Child. *33*:78, 1958.
Carré, I. J., Astley, R., and Smellie, J. M.: Minor degrees of partial thoracic stomach in childhood. Lancet *2*:1150, 1952.
Euler, A. R.: Use of bethanechol for the treatment of gastroesophageal reflux. J. Pediatr. *96*:321, 1980.
Euler, A. R., and Ament, M. E.: Value of esophageal manometric studies in the gastroesophageal reflux of infancy. Pediatrics *59*:58, 1977.
Euler, A. R., Byrne, W. J., Ament, M. E., Fonkalsrud, E. W., Strobel, C. T., Siegel, S. C., Katz, R. M., and Rachelefsky, G. S.: Recurrent pulmonary disease in children: a complication of gastroesophageal reflux. Pediatrics *63*:47, 1979.
Fleischner, F. G.: Hiatal hernia complex. J.A.M.A. *162*:183, 1956.
Foglia, R. P., Fonkalsrud, E. W., Ament, M. E., Byrne, W. J., Berquist, W., Siegel, S. C., Katz, R. M., and Rachelefsky, G. S.: Gastroesophageal fundoplication for the management of chronic pulmonary disease in children. Am. J. Surg. *140*:72, 1980.
Friedland, G. W., Dodds, W. J., Sunshine, P., and Zboralski, F. F.: Apparent disparity in incidence of hiatal hernias in infants and children in Britain and the United States. Am. J. Roentgenol. Rad. Ther. Nucl. Med. *120*:305, 1974.
Goyal, R. K., and Cobb, B. W.: Motility of the pharynx, esophagus, and esophageal sphincters. Physiol. Gastro. Tract. pp. 359, 1981.
Grunwald, P.: Asphyxia, trauma and shock at birth. Arch. Pediatr. *67*:103, 1950.
Hohf, R. P., Kimball, E. R., and Ballenger, J. J.: Rupture of the esophagus in the neonate. J.A.M.A. *181*:939, 1962.
Holder, J. M., and Ashcraft, K. W.: Esophageal atresia and tracheoesophageal fistula. (Collective Review.) Ann. Thorac. Surg. *9*:445, 1970.
Holinger, P. H., Johnston, K. C., and Potts, W. J.: Congenital anomalies of the esophagus. Acta Otolaryngol. Supp. 100, 100, 1951.
Humphreys, G. H., Wiedel, P. D., Baker, D. H., and Berdon, W. E.: Esophageal hiatus hernia in infancy and childhood. Pediatrics *36*:351, 1965.
Jolley, S. G., Herbst, J. J., Johnson, D. G., Matlak, M. E., Book, L. S., and Pena, A.: Postcibal gastroesophageal reflux in children. J. Pediatr. Surg. *16*:487, 1981.
Koch, A., and Gass, R.: Continuous 20–24 hr esophageal pH-monitoring in infancy. J. Pediatr. Surg. *16*:109, 1981.
Mahour, G. H., Woolley, M. M., and Gwinn, J. L.: Elongation of the upper pouch and delayed anatomic reconstruction in esophageal atresia. J. Pediatr. Surg. *9*:373, 1974.
Martin, L. W.: Management of esophageal anomalies. Pediatrics *36*:342, 1965.
McCallum, R. W., Ippoliti, A. F., Cooney, C., and Sturdevant, R. A. L.: A controlled trial of metoclopramide in symptomatic gastroesophageal reflux. N. Engl. J. Med. *296*:354, 1977.
Merriam, J. C., Jr., and Benirschke, K.: Esophageal erosions in the newborn. Lab. Invest. *8*:39, 1959.
Moroz, S. P., Espinoza, J., Cumming, W. A., and Diamanti, N. E.: Lower esophageal sphincter function in children with and without gastroesophageal reflux. Gastroenterology *71*:236, 1976.
Rotch, T. M.: Three types of occlusion of the esophagus in early life. Am. J. Dis. Child. *6*:1, 1913.
Roviralta, E.: The natural evolution of hiatal hernias. Arch. Dis. Child. *39*:143, 1964.
Schatzlein, M. H., Ballantine, T. V. N., Thirunavukkarasu, S., Fitzgerald, J. F., and Grosfeld, J. L.: Gastroesophageal reflux in infants and children. Arch. Surg. *114*:505, 1979.
Sondheimer, J. M., and Morris, B. A.: Gastroesophageal reflux among severely retarded children. J. Pediatr. *94*:710, 1979.
Vanderhoof, J. A., Rapoport, P. J., and Paxson, C. L.: Manometric diagnosis of lower esophageal sphincter incompetence in infants: Use of a small, single-lumen perfused catheter. Pediatrics *62*:805, 1978.
Werlin, S. L., Dodds, W. J., Hogan, W. J., and Arndorfer, R. C.: Mechanisms of gastroesophageal reflux in children. J. Pediatr. *97*:244, 1980.
Winter, H. S., and Grand, R. J.: Gastroesophageal reflux. Pediatrics *68*:132, 1981.

33

Tracheoesphageal Fistulas and Esophageal Atresia

Revised by Harland S. Winter

In 1940, Lanman reported 32 infants, all of whom died with esophageal atresia. On November 28, 1939, Ladd performed a gastrostomy in an infant with esophageal atresia who eventually was able to swallow through an antethoracic skin-lined tube extending from the cervical esophagus to the stomach. In 1941, Haight and Townsley performed the first primary anastomosis, and, in the next decade, Gross and the surgeons at The Children's Hospital Medical Center in Boston reported a 50 per cent survival rate.

Both esophageal atresia and tracheoesophageal fistula are encountered as separate congenital defects. Each alone is extremely rare. More commonly, one finds the two associated in a compound defect. The possible varieties are (1) esophageal atresia alone, (2) esophageal atresia with (*a*) upper fistula, (*b*) lower fistula, or (*c*) double fistula and (3) tracheoesophageal fistula alone. Diagrammatically, the principal types are shown in Figure 33–1.

Tracheoesophageal Fistula With Esophageal Atresia

Incidence. Esophageal atresia with tracheoesophageal fistula is by no means rare. There are probably local differences in its frequency depending upon the varying genetic constitution of populations. In the Collaborative Project, in which babies born in the United States between 1959 and 1966 were studied, tracheoesophageal fistulas were reported in only 1 in 10,000 livebirths. Previous reports had cited the incidence as closer to 1 in 2500 livebirths. In a recent series of 150 cases, 87 were males and 63 females. Approximately 85 per cent of the reported cases consist of esophageal atresia with a fistulous connection between the lower esophageal pouch and the trachea.

Although premature births account for 8 per cent of children born in the United States, 34 per cent of infants with esophageal atresia weigh less than 2.5 kg. The proportion of low birth weight infants with esophageal atresia who are undersize for gestational age is not certain.

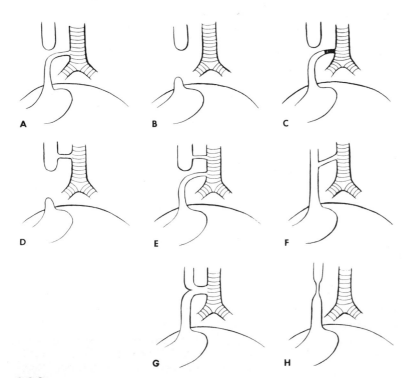

Figure 33–1. Types of tracheoesophageal fistulas. The type labeled A is overwhelmingly the most common, accounting for over 85 per cent of esophageal malformations. Type B is next most common and can be distinguished from type A by the absence of air in the intestinal tract on roentgenogram. All the other types have been noted sporadically. (From Avery, M. E. et al.: The Lung and Its Disorders in the Newborn Infant. 4th ed. Philadelphia, W. B. Saunders Co., 1981.)

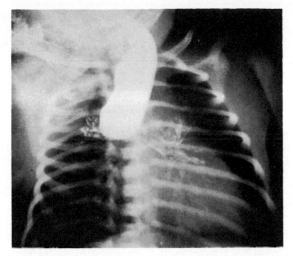

Figure 33–2. Anteroposterior view of chest made on the second day of life, after a Lipiodol swallow. A large, dilated upper esophageal pouch ending blindly in midchest can be seen. There is no air in the abdomen, a fact suggesting either that there is no fistula or that, if one is present, it is an upper one. Some Lipiodol has seeped into the lungs, and one can actually see the outlines of a broad fistulous tract coursing to the left of the lower end of the pouch.

Now that infants who were operated on for esophageal atresia are old enough to have their own children, several reports of vertical transmission of the lesion have appeared. Occurrences in siblings and twins have been known for years, but the first case in a mother and daughter was reported by Engel and colleagues in 1970. In two subsequent reports, the mother had had the same anomaly (Ericksen et al., 1981).

Etiology. The disorder is due to an error in ontogenic development that occurs before the eighth week of gestation. It results from the embryologic fact that the trachea develops as an outgrowth from that portion of the foregut that is destined to become the esophagus. During this complex series of evolutions, incomplete separation of the primitive tubes and imperfect recanalization of the esophageal column may occur.

Associated malformations, most commonly cardiovascular and gastrointestinal-anal atresia, pyloric stenosis, duodenal obstruction, and malrotation, are present in about one half of the infants. Cardiovascular malformations are most frequent when other extracardiac anomalies are present. Isolated ventricular septal defect and patent ductus arteriosus are most commonly found among infants with only esophageal atresia or tracheoesophageal fistula or both. Tetralogy of Fallot, atrial septal defect, and coarctation of the aorta are less frequent. Among infants with other gastrointestinal anomalies, tetralogy of Fallot or atrial septal defect or both occur in over half the infants, whereas ventricular septal defect is less common. Renal agenesis and hydronephrosis are found in the genitourinary tract. Some of the anomalies occur in clusters. One group, named the VATER Syndrome by Quan and Smith,

includes vertebral, anal, tracheoesophageal, radial, and renal malformations. Although the complete set of anomalies is rarely found, the presence of one should stimulate a search for the others.

Diagnosis. The diagnosis of esophageal atresia, with or without a fistula, should be suspected in any infant of a mother with hydramnios. Since the term infant normally swallows about 500 ml of amniotic fluid per day, the fetus clearly has a role in the regulation of amniotic fluid volume. Obstruction at some level of the upper gastrointestinal tract is also associated with hydramnios. Infants born of mothers with excessive amounts of amniotic fluid should have a tube inserted very carefully into the stomach to test for obstruction.

In most cases, the newborn infant cries immediately, breathes spontaneously, and acquires a healthy pink color. After minutes or a few hours, it is noted that inordinate quantities of mucus are accumulating in the pharynx, and these may overflow from the nose and mouth onto bed linen or may be regurgitated. Eventually, because of mucus accumulation, varying degrees of respiratory difficulty become evident. There may be only mild duskiness with rasping inspiration or expiration, or deep cyanosis may supervene with labored inspiration or expiration. Pharyngeal suction commonly ameliorates this situation for a time. Attempted feeding causes an exacerbation of respiratory difficulty and is followed by prompt regurgitation of the ingested fluid mixed with much thick mucus. After feedings, a previously clear chest may become full of coarse rales and rhonchi.

As one listens to the lungs of some of these infants, great variations in air entry may be heard. First one major bronchus and then another becomes plugged, and breath sounds diminish and vanish over large areas for shorter or longer periods. Vigorous pharyngeal or endotracheal suction may reopen the airways. Atelectasis, of the right upper lobe especially, may develop and persist.

The combination of signs, consisting of (1) excessive accumulation of mucus, (2) respiratory difficulty, either persistent or in spells, and (3) regurgitation of all ingested fluids, is pathognomonic of esophageal atresia.

If the abdomen remains flat and gasless, one can usually be certain that no fistula connects the trachea with the lower esophageal pouch. There may be no fistula at all, or the fistula may run from the upper pouch to the trachea, or, very rarely, the fistula may be so small that air has not entered the stomach. In the latter instance, respiratory difficulty and cough, especially after attempts to feed, are apt to be considerably greater.

If, however, the abdomen rapidly becomes distended and the intestine fills with air promptly, one can be certain that the defect is the usual one, that

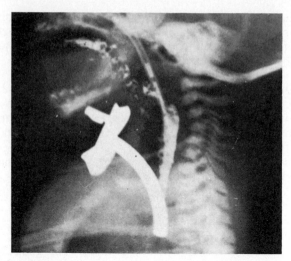

Figure 33–3. Lateral view of chest taken on the fourth day of life after Iodochloral had been instilled by nasal catheter into the esophagus. A tracheostomy tube is in place because of unusually severe dyspnea. Dye fills an upper segment that ends blindly about the level of the carina.

is, esophageal atresia with a fistula connecting the trachea and lower esophageal pouch. Rarely, there may also be a fistula from the upper pouch to the trachea.

Infants with tracheoesophageal fistula without esophageal atresia may not have the regurgitation and mucus accumulation found in patients with the other anatomic variations. Although they have an esophageal motility disorder, the main presenting problem is pneumonia, which most often occurs early. In some children, the diagnosis is not made until school age.

Diagnosis can be confirmed in several ways. A catheter may be passed into the esophagus, where it will meet obstruction a few inches from the mouth. Rarely, one may be misled by its easy passage far enough to have reached the stomach, when actually it is coiling in the blind upper pouch. Simultaneous fluoroscopy clarifies this point.

Further confirmation by radiograph is advisable. A plain film may demonstrate clearly the air-filled upper pouch. Instillation of 0.5 cc of contrast medium demarcates the pouch more sharply, and may reveal the fistula itself.

Careful radiographic studies are frequently required to demonstrate fistulas without atresia. Video-imaging with radiopaque material injected through a tube at different levels of the esophagus should be performed if the diagnosis is anticipated. The most common site for such lesions is above the apex of the pleural cavity. Identification of the aortic arch is necessary, since, if it is right-sided, surgical repair is difficult through a standard left thoracotomy. Occasionally, vascular rings are present in association with tracheoesophageal fistulas.

Treatment. Treatment should begin with insertion of a sump suction catheter into the upper pouch for continuous evacuation of salivary secretions. In addition, it is helpful to keep the patient in a semi-upright position to help avoid regurgitation of acid gastric contents through the fistula into the lungs prior to the establishment of a gastrostomy. Repair of the fistula and esophagus should be undertaken whenever the infant's general condition permits it. Pneumonia, which was once a major cause of death, should be minimal and reversible when the period of gross infection is brief.

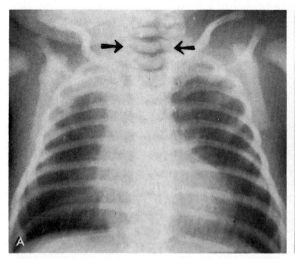
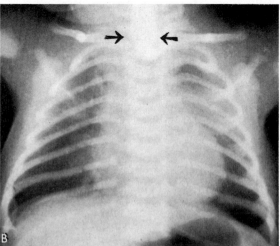

Figure 33–4. *A,* Anteroposterior view of chest taken on the first day of life. One can see clearly the blind upper esophageal pouch sharply outlined by its air content. Air within the abdomen bespeaks lower tracheoesophageal fistula. *B,* After instillation of Lipiodol, the upper esophageal pouch stands out clearly.
This case is not abstracted in the text. It is included only to point out again that diagnosis may often be made on the basis of plain films alone, without Lipiodol instillation.

The operation of choice is division of the fistula and end-to-end anastomosis of the esophageal ends. The upper pouch may be lengthened by creating one or two circumferential myotomies in it. This usually provides sufficient length in the usual type of atresia with fistula; however, in the isolated atresia, the gap between the two ends of the esophagus is usually too great. Some surgeons have recommended lengthening of the upper pouch by bougienage or magnets, but it appears that these maneuvers will produce no more than a 3-cm increase and possibly do no more than would have occurred by waiting. Therefore, these patients often become candidates for some type of "neoesophagus" to bridge the gap. This is usually created at 12 to 18 months of age, and if necessary the child is fed via the gastrostomy tube, and an upper pouch cervical salivary fistula is created.

Postoperative care consists of adequate antibiotic treatment directed toward the pulmonary infection and careful protection of the anastomotic site. This means that nothing is to be taken by mouth for approximately 7 to 10 days. Hydration, proper electrolyte balance, and caloric intake can be maintained by gastrostomy feedings, supplemented at first by intravenous fluids.

Most authorities agree that it is safer to err a little on the side of underhydration rather than of overhydration. A daily total quota of 75 ml per kilogram of body weight of intravenous fluids should suffice.

The infant with atresia may require prolonged parenteral alimentation because the microgastria will not permit large volumes of fluid. After gastrostomy, a contrast study should be obtained via the gastrostomy tube to ensure that there are no distal obstructions. After feeding for about 3 weeks, the infant should have a normal-sized stomach.

Prognosis. Prognosis depends on several factors. Prematures do less well than large, mature infants. Babies diagnosed and operated upon early do better than those who come to surgery late. This difference results from the better state of hydration and blood chemical balance of the younger infant as well as from the fact that pulmonary infection is less deeply seated. There is little excuse with our present knowledge for gastrostomy to be delayed beyond the second day of life. Emergency gastrostomy is a vital first step; definitive repair can be delayed until the infant's condition improves. The survival rate for infants over 2500 gm without pneumonia or associated anomalies should be 95 per cent. Infants who are premature have done less well in the past, but the outlook is much better when neonatal intensive care is available (Holder and Ashcraft, 1980).

Almost all the infants who die have widespread bronchial pneumonia. Leakage from the anastomotic site is responsible for mediastinitis and a stormy postoperative course in a high percentage of the unsuccessful cases. Most of these problems can be managed by prolonged tube drainage of the thorax and nutritional support with intravenous alimentation. By

far, the most common complication is the development of stricture at the operative site. When this is severe, one may be forced to resort to bougienage, but there is general agreement that the hazards of instrumental dilatation warrant great care with this procedure.

These strictures have been attributed in the past to the surgical anastomosis, but recent evidence supports a multifactorial etiology. Children with tracheoesophageal fistula, including those infants without esophageal atresia, have disordered esophageal motility. Although this may result in delayed feeding in infancy, it is rarely of clinical importance in the older child who learns to chew food well, eat slowly, and drink during meals. Initially, conservative management includes thickened feeds, water after feeds, semi-upright position for 1 or 2 hours after eating, and no eating or drinking 2 hours before going to bed. The motility disorder does cause delayed clearance of refluxed gastric contents, and, although the frequency of acid reflux is not increased in these children, the delayed time of acid clearance over many years may result in peptic injury and stricture formation. Esophagitis and Barrett's epithelium have been noted in those infants whose acid clearance is markedly impaired. In the child with recurrent stricture, evaluation of acid clearance from the distal esophagus by continuous overnight intraesophageal pH monitoring will determine the severity of the impairment of the acid clearance. Esophageal manometry is useful in measuring both the extent of the motility disorder and the lower esophageal sphincter pressure. Esophageal biopsies are performed to assess the severity as well as the duration of acid injury; if the results are abnormal, vigorous medical antireflux therapy should be initiated. Some infants also have delayed gastric emptying, determined by ^{99m}Tc radionuclide study. These patients may benefit from a clinical trial of metoclopramide hydrochloride. All these factors may play a role in development of esophageal dysfunction and stricture formation. In the child with recurrent problems, a systematic evaluation to define each aspect should provide the basis for rational therapeutic intervention. It is unusual to continue esophageal dilatation beyond puberty, and the frequency of dilatation usually diminishes after infancy.

Tracheoesophageal Fistula Without Esophageal Atresia

The defect of single or multiple fistulas alone is rare indeed. Only 3 to 4 per cent of fistulas are unassociated with esophageal atresia. Gross found the compound defect to be 60 times, Haight 30 times, as frequent as the solitary one. Although most of the fistulas are somewhere near the carina, a few have been reported in the neck. Multiple fistulas without atresia are very rare but reported by Rehbein in 1964 and by Eckstein and Somasundaram in 1966. Robb described an 11-year-old boy who had experienced attacks of choking from birth and who was found to have an interesting variant of the previously described congenital developmental defects involving the trachea and esophagus together. There was a fistulous connection between foodway and airway, and instead of an atretic esophagus, there was a large diverticulum at the same level. The defect was clearly a congenital one. Careful attention to pulmonary symptoms in infancy avoids delay in diagnosis. Kluth has published an atlas of types of esophageal atresia to which the reader is referred.

Diagnosis. In 1951, Helmsworth and Pryles felt that the clinical picture was so conclusive that surgical treatment could be undertaken without radiographic confirmation. As slightly modified by Herweg and Ogura, the criteria include (1) coughing, choking, and cyanosis immediately after ingesting fluids, (2) no difficulty in swallowing, the distress occurring a few sec-

onds later, (3) clear lung fields becoming full of coarse rales and rhonchi after swallowing, (4) absence of symptoms after gavage feeding, and (5) gastric distention after crying, straining, and coughing.

We insist on confirmation of the diagnosis by cineradiographic studies or endoscopy before surgery is undertaken. The contrast material should be injected through a feeding tube inserted into the esophagus at different levels to permit filling of a small fistula, which often attaches to the trachea cephalad to its level in the esophagus.

Treatment. Once the diagnosis has been made, surgery offers the only possibility of cure. The operation is comparatively simple, exposure and ligation of the fistulous tract being all that is required. The approach is usually through the neck; thoracotomy is rarely indicated.

Laryngotracheoesophageal Cleft

A midline communication between the posterior laryngeal wall and the esophagus presents with the same symptoms as an H-type tracheoesophageal fistula. This rare congenital defect may be very difficult to diagnose by either direct vision or radiography, but careful endoscopy and repeated contrast studies may reveal the cleft. According to Burroughs and

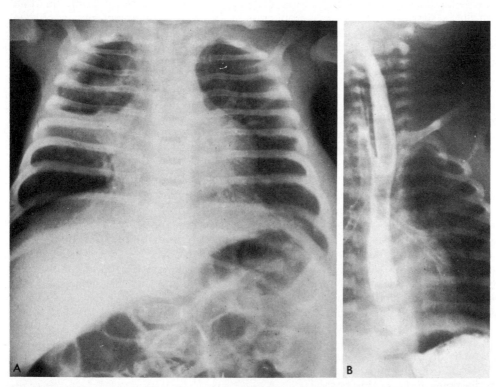

Figure 33–5. *A,* Anteroposterior view of chest of an infant 6 months old. There is atelectasis of the right middle lobe, hyperinflation of the right lower lobe, and some patchy opacification elsewhere. *B,* Spot film taken after barium swallow outlines the esophagus and a fistula of large caliber coursing from it upward toward the trachea. A faint bronchogram is visible. There is no atresia or stenosis of the esophagus.

A tracheoesophageal fistula without esophageal atresia was found at autopsy. (The films were obtained for us by Dr. Thomas D. Michael of Baltimore.)

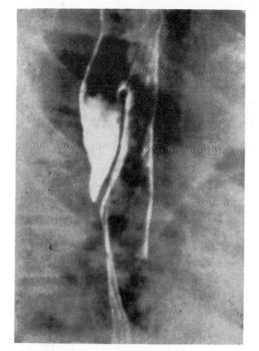

Figure 33–6. Roentgenogram after barium swallow, showing diverticulum before operation. The fistula is not demonstrated. (Robb, D.: Austr. N. Zeal. J. Surg. *22*:120, 1952.)

Leape, 34 such infants had been described in the literature by 1974, with nine survivors, all of whom had had operative repair with tracheostomy. One patient with a cleft survived without operation, requiring nasogastric tube feedings to prevent aspiration for the first 3 months of life. Thereafter, he had no difficulty with swallowing, aspiration, or phonation. A more severe form of this rare anomaly is a persistent esophagotrachea, such as described by Griscom, which is not compatible with life.

Although usually sporadic in occurrence, midline clefts were reported by Phelan and coworkers in two sibships of double first cousins.

REFERENCES

Andrassy, R. J., and Mahour, G. H.: Gastrointestinal anomalies associated with esophageal atresia or tracheoesophageal fistula. Arch. Surg. *114*:1125, 1979.

Avery, M. E., Fletcher, B. D. and Williams, R.: The Lung and Its Disorders in the Newborn Infant. 4th ed. Philadelphia, W. B. Saunders Co., 1981.

Barry, J. E., and Auldist, A. W.: The VATER association: one end of a spectrum of anomalies. Am. J. Dis. Child. *128*:769, 1974.

Benjamin, B., Cohen, D., and Glasson, M.: Tracheomalacia in association with congenital tracheoesophageal fistula. Surgery *79*:504, 1976.

Blumberg, J. B., Stevenson, J. K., Lemire, R. J., and Boyden, E. A.: Laryngotracheoesophageal cleft, the embryologic implications: Review of the literature. Surgery *57*:559, 1965.

Bond-Taylor, W., Starer, F., and Atwell, J. D.: Vertebral anomalies associated with esophageal atresia and tracheoesophageal fistula with reference to the initial operative mortality. J. Pediatr. Surg. *8*:9, 1973.

Burroughs, N., and Leape, L. L.: Laryngotracheoesophageal cleft: report of a case successfully treated and review of the literature. Pediatrics *53*:516, 1974.

Clatworthy, H. W., Jr.: Esophageal atresia; importance of early diagnosis and adequate treatment illustrated by a series of patients. Pediatrics *16*:122, 1955.

Colten, D. H., Middleton, B. W., and Fletcher, J.: Gastric tube esophagoplasty. J. Pediatr. Surg. *9*:451, 1974.

Dudley, N. E. and Phelan, P. D.: Respiratory complications in long-term survival of oesophageal atresia. Arch. Dis. Child. *51*:279, 1976.

Eckstein, H. B., and Somasundaram, K.: Multiple tracheoesophageal fistulas without atresia. Report of a case. J. Pediatr. Surg. *1*:381, 1966.

Engel, P., Vos, L., and Kuiller, P. J.: Esophageal atresia with tracheoesophageal fistula in mother and child. J. Pediatr, Surg, *5*:564, 1970.

Ericksen, C., Hauge, M., Madsen, C. M., et al.: Two generation transmission of oesophageal atresia with tracheo-oesophageal fistula. Acta Pediatr. Scand. *70*:253, 1981.

Ferguson, C. C.: Replacement of the esophagus by colon in infants and children. Can. J. Surg. *13*:396, 1970.

Greenwood, R. D., and Rosenthal, A.: Cardiovascular malformations associated with tracheoesophageal fistula and esophageal atresia. Pediatrics *57*:87, 1976.

Griscom, N. T.: Persistent esophagotrachea: The most severe form of laryngotracheoesophageal cleft. Am. J. Roentgenol. *97*:211, 1966.

Gross, R. E., and Firestone, F. N.: Colonic reconstruction of the esophagus in infants and children. Surgery *61*:995, 1967.

Haight, C., and Townsley, H. A.: Congenital atresia of the esophagus with tracheoesophageal fistula; extrapleural ligation of fistula and end-to-end anastomosis of esophageal segments. Surg. Gynecol. Obstet. *76*:672, 1943.

Helmsworth, J. A., and Pryles, C. V.: Congenital tracheoesophageal fistula without esophageal atresia. J. Pediatr. *38*:610, 1951.

Herweg, J. C., and Ogura, J. H.: Congenital tracheoesophageal fistula without esophageal atresia; endoscopic diagnostic technique. J. Pediatr. *47*:293, 1955.

Hodge, G. B., and Johnson, G. D.: Congenital esophageal atresia with tracheoesophageal fistula. Am. Surg. *19*:569, 1953.

Holder, T. M., and Ashcraft, K. W.: Esophageal atresia and tracheoesophageal fistula. (Collective review.) Ann. Thorac. Surg. *9*:445, 1970.

Holder, T. M., Cloud, D. T., Lewis, J. E., Jr., et al.: Esophageal atresia and tracheoesophageal fistula. Pediatrics *34*:542, 1964.

Holder, T. M., and Ashcraft, K. W.: Pediatric Surgery. Philadelphia, W. B. Saunders Co., 1980.

Kappelman, W. M., Dorst, J., Haller, A., et al.: H-Type tracheoesophageal fistula. Am. J. Dis. Child, *118*:568, 1969.

Kluth, D.: Atlas of Esophageal Atresia. J. Pediatr. Surg. *11*:901, 1976.

Ladd, W. E.: The surgical treatment of esophageal atresia and tracheoesophageal fistulas. N. Engl. J. Med. *230*:625, 1944.

Lanman, T. H.: Congenital atresia of esophagus: study of thirty-two cases. Arch. Surg. *41*:1060, 1940.

Mahour, G. H., Woolley, M. M., and Gwinn, J. L.: Elongation of the upper pouch and delayed anatomic reconstruction in esophageal atresia. J. Pediatr. Surg. *9*:373, 1974.

Milligan, D. W. A., and Levison, H.: Lung function in children following repair of tracheoesophageal fistula. J. Pediatr. *95*:24, 1979.

Orringer, M. B., Kirsch, M. M., and Sloan, H.: Long-term esophageal function following repair of esophageal atresia. Ann. Surg. *186*:436, 1977.

Phelan, P. D., Stocks, J. G., Williams, H. E., and Danks, D. M.: Familial occurrence of congenital laryngeal clefts. Arch. Dis. Child. *48*:275, 1973.

Putnam, T. C.: Esophageal atresia: Critical analysis of 39 cases. Arch. Surg. *114*:288, 1979.

Quan, L., and Smith, D. W.: The VATER association: vertebral defects, anal atresia, T-E fistula with esophageal atresia, radial and renal dysplasia. A spectrum of associated defects. J. Pediatr. *104*:7, 1973.

Rehbein, F.: Esophageal atresia with double tracheoesophageal fistula. Arch. Dis. Child. *39*:138, 1964.

Rickham, P. P.: Infants with esophageal atresia weighing under 3 pounds. J. Pediatr. Surg. *16*:595, 1981.

Robb, D.: Congenital tracheo-esophageal fistula without atresia but with a large esophageal diverticulum. Aust. N. Z. J. Surg. *22*:120, 1952.

Strodel, W. E., Coran, A. G., Kirsh, M. M., et al.: Esophageal atresia—a 41-year experience. Arch. Surg. *114*:523, 1979.

Waterston, D. J., Bonham Carter, R. E., and Aberdeen, E.: Congenital tracheo-esophageal fistula in association with oesophageal atresia. Lancet *2*:55, 1963.

Whitington, P. F., Shermeta, D. W., Seto, D. S. Y., et al.: Role of lower esophageal sphincter incompetence in recurrent pneumonia after repair of esophageal atresia. J. Pediatr. *9*:550, 1977.

Winter, H. S., Madara, J. L., Statford, R. J., et al.: Delayed acid clearance and esophagitis after repair of esophageal atresia. Gastroenterology *80*:1317, 1981.

Woolley, M. M.: Esophageal atresia and tracheoesophageal fistula 1939 to 1979. Am. J. Surg. *39*:771, 1980.

34

Disorders of Neuromuscular Control of the Esophagus

Revised by Harland S. Winter

Fleischner has summarized succinctly and persuasively the controversial problem of the physiology of the lower end of the esophagus. The anatomic cardia at the cardiac incisura probably has no sphincter function. This is reserved for that distal 2- to 4-cm portion of the esophagus just at and extending from 1 to 2 cm above to 1 to 2 cm below the diaphragm. Although no true sphincter exists here in human beings, the muscular layers are specialized and exhibit a "sphincteric capacity," which is especially strong in very young infants. This "internal sphincter" is reinforced by the pinchcock action of the diaphragm and crura, which act as an "external sphincter" (Fig. 34–1).

Cricopharyngeal Incoordination

We have already noted that not all newborn infants can swallow without at times aspirating some of the fluid into their tracheobronchial trees and that in some infants this pharyngeal incoordination leads to recurrent pneumonitis. This is usually of little clinical significance when the incoordination is limited to the pharynx. In children with severe aspiration and pneumonia, a diffuse esophageal motility disorder should be anticipated. This is most commonly observed in children with central nervous system impairment but

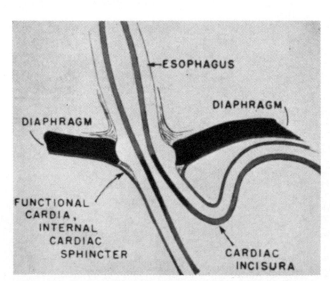

Figure 34–1. Diagram of a normal cardiac region. Esophagus is anchored to rim of esophageal hiatus of diaphragm by fibers of phrenoesophageal ligament. Incisura cardiaca (right lower arrow) indicates site of "anatomic cardia." Diaphragm forms external sphincter of "functional cardia" (lower left arrow). Internal cardiac sphincter is indicated by the diagrammatically exaggerated swelling of muscularis propria of esophagus. Variable zone of transition from esophageal to gastric mucosa is in black. (From Fleischner, F. G.: J.A.M.A. *162*:183, 1956.)

may also be noted in infants with familial dysautonomia or myasthenia gravis.

In 1972, Blank and Silbiger found a variant of this condition in another newborn with a similar history. Her barium-swallow radiograms showed "a ringlike band at the entrance of the cervical esophagus, suggesting a fixed mechanical obstruction. At esophagoscopy, a transverse submucosal bar was seen that was indistinguishable from a normal cricopharyngeal muscle." They termed the condition *cricopharyngeal achalasia.* Motility studies are needed now to define the presumed motor abnormalities in these rare instances.

Achalasia

Achalasia is an idiopathic primary motility disorder of the esophagus that has been described in families but that is usually sporadic.

Achalasia may present with repeated vomiting, which at times is not a conspicuous feature. The diagnosis is suspected because recurrent pneumonitis has called for a chest radiograph. An air-fluid level in the esophagus and an absence of gas in the stomach are frequently noted. On barium esophagram, symmetric beaklike narrowing is seen at the gastroesophageal junction, with moderate to advanced dilatation above the stenotic point.

Esophageal pressure and motility studies reveal that there is increased tone of the lower esophageal sphincter and that relaxation of the sphincter following a swallow is absent or incomplete. In addition, motility in the body of the esophagus is abnormal with either low amplitude aperistaltic activity or spasm consisting of simultaneous contractions. These two criteria—the failure of relaxation of the lower esophageal sphincter and the lack of peristaltic activity in the body of the esophagus—are the hallmarks of this primary motility disorder. Because of its diffuse involvement of denervation in the esophagus, it has been compared with Hirschsprung's disease. The result is dilatation of the esophagus, at times to such a point that the term "megaesophagus" is justified.

Megaesophagus is a frequent complication of Chagas' disease, caused by infection with *Trypanosoma cruzi.* In this condition, microscopic sections show loss of ganglion cells of the intrinsic neural plexus. Similar sparsity or absence of ganglion cells has been reported in idiopathic achalasia in some but not all affected adults.

Fewer than 20 infants with congenital achalasia have been reported, but the motility disorder, when properly defined, appears identical with that observed in older children and adults. There is no therapy at the present time to alter the aperistaltic activity. The goal of therapeutic intervention is to allow adequate drainage of the esophagus. This may be achieved successfully in many adults by pneumatic dilatation, but routine bougienage is rarely of long-term benefit. In infants, surgery is required because pneumatic dilators are not available in the appropri-

ate size, and myotomy provides a permanent solution to the distal esophageal obstruction.

The major complication resulting from myotomy is the development of gastroesophageal acid reflux, which may cause stricture formation at an accelerated rate because of the motility dysfunction in the body of the esophagus. The effectiveness of the myotomy depends on the length that the incision is extended along the lesser curve of the stomach. If the myotomy is too long, gastroesophageal reflux will result from the incompetent acid barrier. One usually treats this conservatively by administering antacids and cimetidine, by positioning the patient comfortably, and by establishing an appropriate diet; however, on rare occasions, a patient is so debilitated that fundoplication is eventually required.

Achalasia is most commonly an isolated finding, but it may be associated with a generalized neuropathic form of chronic idiopathic intestinal pseudo-obstruction syndrome. This is a diffuse motility disorder in which the patients may have bacterial overgrowth from small intestinal stasis and severe constipation with megacolon.

Familial Dysautonomia

Linde and Westover have called attention to the esophageal abnormalities one may expect in familial dysautonomia. Severe swallowing difficulties and recurrent pneumonitis, probably from aspiration, characterize many of these infants from birth. These observers noted, in addition to pharyngeal incoordination, weak peristaltic action that delayed esophageal emptying *in the supine position.* In the erect position, gravity facilitated passage of food into the stomach. They found it necessary to feed each swallow to one of their infants in the supine position, so that milk could reach the hypopharynx, then to sit him up so that it could traverse the esophagus.

REFERENCES

Asch, M. J., Liebman, W., Lachman, R. S., and Moore, T. C.: Esophageal achalasia: Diagnosis and cardiomyotomy in a newborn infant. J. Pediatr. Surg. *9:*911, 1974.

Astley, R.: Oesophageal "spasm" in infancy. Proc. Roy. Soc. Med. *48:*1045, 1955.

Azizkhan, R. G., Tapper, D., and Eraklis, A.: Achalasia in childhood: a 20-year experience. J. Pediatr. Surg. *15:*452, 1980.

Badrawy, R., and Abou-Bieh, A.: Congenital achalasia of the oesophagus in children. J. Laryngol. Otol. *89:*697, 1975.

Berenberg, W., and Neuhauser, E. B. D.: Cardioesophageal relaxation (chalasia) as a cause of vomiting in infants. Pediatrics *5:*414, 1950.

Blank, R. H., and Silbiger, M.: Cricopharyngeal achalasia as a cause of respiratory distress in infancy. J. Pediatr. *81:*95, 1972.

Botha, G. G. M.: The gastro-esophageal region in infants: Observations on the anatomy, with special reference to the closing mechanism and partial thoracic stomach. Arch. Dis. Child. *33*:78, 1958.

Dumars, K. W., Williams, J. J., and Steele-Sandlin, C.: Achalasia and microcephaly. Am. J. Med. Genet. *6*:309, 1980.

Fleischner, F. G.: Hiatal hernia complex. J.A.M.A. *162*:183, 1956.

Forshall, I.: The cardio-oesophageal syndrome in childhood. Arch. Dis. Child. *30*:46, 1955.

Gruenbaum, M.: Radiologic manifestations of familial dysautonomia. Am. J. Dis. Child. *128*:176, 1974.

Ingelfinger, F. J.: The esophagus, March 1961 to February 1963. Gastroenterology *45*:241, 1963.

Linde, L. M., and Westover, J. L.: Esophageal and gastric abnormalities in dysautonomia. Pediatrics *29*:303, 1962.

London, F. A., Raab, D. E., Fuller, J., and Olsen, A. M.: Achalasia in three siblings: A rare occurrence. Mayo Clin. Proc. *52*:97, 1977.

Mackler, D., and Schneider, R.: Achalasia in father and son. Digest. Dis. *23*:1042, 1978.

Matsaniotis, M., Karpouzas, J., et al.: Aspiration due to difficulty in swallowing. Arch. Dis. Child. *46*:788, 1971.

Moazam, F., and Rodgers, B. M.: Infantile achalasia. J. Thorac. Cardiovasc. Surg. *72*:809, 1976.

Neuhauser, E. B. D., and Berenberg, W.: Cardioesophageal relaxation as a cause of vomiting in infants. Radiology *48*:480, 1947.

Vantrappen, G., and Hellemans, J.: Treatment of achalasia and related motor disorders. Gastroenterology *79*:144, 1980.

35

Disorders of the Stomach

Those disorders of the stomach that have clinical importance in the neonatal period may be classified as follows:

I. Congenital anatomic defects
   A. Hypoplasia
   B. Diverticulum
   C. Duplication
   D. Atresia
II. Disorders of the pylorus
   A. Pylorospasm
   B. Hypertrophic stenosis of the pylorus
III. Peptic ulcer
IV. Gastric perforation

Hypoplasia of the Stomach (Congenital Microgastria)

In two of our cases of esophageal atresia with tracheoesophageal fistula (see p. 332, Fig. 33–1), not only was the lower esophageal segment completely atretic but also the stomach itself was hypoplastic. The surgeon described them as "tiny and undeveloped." In these cases, direct esophageal anastomosis was impossible because of the great length of atretic segment, and gastrostomy was performed as a preliminary to further plastic correction. The infants died after this procedure. It is probable that the small size and poor functional capacity of the hypoplastic stomach contributed to the failure of the gastrostomy and hence to death.

In 1973, Blank and Chisolm reported a fascinating case of hypoplasia, without T-E fistula, which they termed congenital microgastria, in which the stomach was small and tubular, the duodenum maldeveloped, and the cecum malpositioned and attached by bands to the abdominal wall and undersurface of the liver. Swallowed barium refluxed not only into the esophagus but also into biliary radicles in both lobes of the liver. At about 1 year of age, when the infant weighed 12¾ pounds (5.8 kg), the bands were cut and a gastrojejunostomy was performed. She improved slowly on frequent small pureed feedings, and at 27 years was the small but healthy mother of three normal daughters.

Dide had described a very similar case in 1894, and Caffey included one in the 1956 edition of his textbook. Two more examples were added to the literature in 1971. Malrotation and other congenital defects were present in most. The value of surgical intervention seems to depend more on these associated anomalies than on the gastric hypoplasia.

Gastric Duplication (Gastrogenic Cyst)

Any portion of the gastrointestinal tract may be duplicated in the course of its ontogenic development. Duplications may be spherical or tubular, contiguous or distant, their lumens communicating or not with the nearby gastrointestinal tract.

The stomach is subject to duplication, but it is one of the less common sites. Some of the cysts produced by its duplication are left behind in the thorax (see p. 208) in the course of the stomach's normal caudad migration. A few arrive within the abdominal cavity. A few remain in both locations, the intrathoracic and abdominal cysts connected by a fistulous tract, which may or may not penetrate the diaphragm.

Symptoms and *signs* may be minimal. The only finding may be a palpable cystic mass in the upper portion of the abdomen. Gastric duplications may produce intestinal obstruction, but they present in this way considerably less frequently than do duplications of the small bowel. Rarely, too, they may undergo peptic ulceration, and, if they communicate, hematemesis and melena may signal their presence.

Radiographic study and *fluoroscopy* may show no abnormality in the absence of obstruction. Barium mixtures rarely fill the cavity of the duplication, even when this communicates with the stomach. Occasionally, however, one may be clearly seen in an upper gastrointestinal series study by a pressure defect involving stomach and bowel, as Figure 35–1 shows. Ultrasonography should prove useful in diagnosis.

Differentiation from mesenteric cyst is difficult in uncomplicated cases, but obstruction renders the likelihood of the latter quite small, and hematemesis or melena points definitely toward duplication.

Treatment. Operative intervention and complete removal are indicated. Extensive resection of the stomach may be necessary if the duplication is tightly adherent. In spite of this, incomplete measures, such as marsupialization, cannot be countenanced.

Intrinsic Obstruction of the Stomach (Pyloric Atresia)

Until 1971, the world literature contained 29 reports of congenital obstruction of the stomach due to atresia. In 19 of these cases, a membrane completely occluded the prepyloric region, in three a fibrous cord joined the blind pyloric and duodenal ends, and in seven the blind ends were discontinuous. One infant of the first group had a membranous partition proximal to the pylorus and a second in the duodenum a few centimeters distal to the pylorus. All the cases presented with signs of high obstruction, but in this last one a visible and palpable cystic mass developed in the epigastrium on the second day of life. The sequestered portion of lower stomach and upper duodenum had become distended with accumulated secretions, and at operation resembled a tight cyst 5 cm in diameter occupying the pyloric portion of the stomach! Atresia of the pylorus occurs in less than 1 per cent of all intestinal atresias.

Diagnosis can be made only after exploration because of intractable vomiting from birth plus epigastric distention.

Treatment consists of excision of, or multiple radial incisions in, the membranous diaphragm. In some of

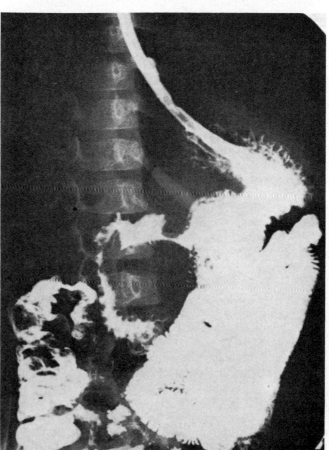

Figure 35–1. Film of a 3-year-old boy who had been well until 4 weeks before admission. Since then, he had bouts of vomiting and abdominal pain alternating with episodes of diarrhea. A vague, tender mass was palpable in the epigastrium. A gastric duplication half the size of the normal stomach was found attached to the greater curvature. (From Gwinn, J. L., and Barnes, G. R.: Am. J. Dis. Child. *113*:581, 1967.)

these, gastroenterostomy may have to be performed because of obstructing edema. In the blind obstructions, a shunt operation will surely have to be performed. Gastroduodenostomy is preferable to gastrojejunostomy.

Delay in Gastric Emptying

Delay in gastric emptying manifests itself by vomiting. Its onset is usually early, sooner than the usual onset of hypertrophic pyloric stenosis. It may begin after the first fluids have been offered or may be delayed until the end of the first week. It is usually intermittent but may follow every feeding. It may be forceful but is seldom projectile. Associated with vomiting is a definite diminution in capacity. A few infants seem unable to accept more than 1½ or 2 ounces at a time, a larger quantity causing discomfort and regurgitation. The pattern of a gastric bubble may appear in the left upper quadrant as one watches the abdomen during feeding, but this moves either not at all or sluggishly toward the midline.

Fluoroscopic examination may demonstrate a short delay in peristaltic activity and initial emptying of the stomach, but in some peristalsis is extremely active, and emptying may be completed unusually rapidly. No lengthening or narrowing of the pyloric canal can be demonstrated.

Treatment.   Response to antispasmodics is generally excellent. Atropine has been our own drug of choice. One may begin with a dose of one drop of a 1:1000 solution of atropine sulfate 10 or 15 minutes before each feeding, increase by one drop each day until flushing appears, and revert to the previous day's dosage as the permanent one. Vomiting usually ceases within a few days, and capacity increases. After a week or two, seldom longer, the antispasmodic drug can ordinarily be discontinued without recurrence of symptoms. Antihistaminics have been used with success. Frequent small feedings, followed by placement of the infant in the semi-upright position, will facilitate burping and lessen gastric distention.

One should investigate carefully the possibility that pylorospasm may have been initiated or perpetuated by unfavorable environmental conditions. Relaxing the parents may effectively relax the infant's pylorus.

Hypertrophic Pyloric Stenosis

Incidence.   It is probable that the frequency of this disorder varies considerably from country to country and, perhaps, within different geographic sections of the same country. An incidence of 1 to 3 per every 1000 livebirths would appear to represent an approximate over-all average.

Males are affected three to four times as often as females. Firstborns account for roughly half the cases; all other births constitute the remaining half. Blacks are decidedly less at risk than whites. Premature infants have pyloric stenosis about as frequently as do full-term babies.

Etiology.   Considerable doubt still exists about the cause of hypertrophic stenosis of the pylorus. A genetic predisposition is thoroughly documented.

Hicks and coworkers have estimated the risk to sons of individuals with pyloric stenosis to be 5 to 20 per cent and the risk to daughters to be 2.5 to 7 per cent. The risk for sons and daughters of affected females is three to four times greater than that for those with affected fathers. In about two thirds of the cases of identical twins born to individuals with pyloric stenosis, both infants are affected.

Rintoul and Kirkman, after studying 38 biopsy specimens and many controls, observed that the myenteric plexus in the pylorus of the infant with hypertrophic stenosis contains no or sparse type I (Dogiel) cells. They were not certain whether this represented a congenital defect or whether it resulted from prolonged autonomic overstimulation, although they inclined toward the former hypothesis.

Diagnosis.   The cardinal signs of pyloric stenosis are vomiting, constipation, gastric peristaltic waves, and pyloric tumor. Vomiting appears first and is followed within a shorter or longer time by the other signs.

Vomiting may begin at any time from birth to the eighth week of life or later. Most infants begin to vomit in the third, fourth, or fifth weeks. We have seen a few who regurgitated their first few feedings while still in the newborn nursery, although days or weeks were to elapse before the diagnosis became certain. Onset beyond the sixth week is rare and becomes progressively rarer with the passage of time, but authentic cases have been reported in the second and third years of life. In premature infants, the onset follows the same pattern postnatally, bearing no relation to true postconceptual age.

At first, vomiting follows feeding infrequently, but within days or weeks it increases in frequency until it follows virtually all feedings. Early it may not be forceful, but it increases steadily in force until many vomits are projectile. Vomitus never contains bile. Rarely, fresh or altered blood appears.

Stools begin to diminish in number when vomiting commences. Soon they become infrequent and dry, firm and scanty.

Gastric patterning becomes visible over the upper portion of the abdomen, and as the observer watches, preferably in strong light that strikes the infant obliquely from above, definite waves may be seen to march in slow, steady progression from the extreme left upper quadrant toward the midline. As one wave reaches the neighborhood of the umbilicus, another forms slowly beneath the far left costal margin and makes its leisurely way toward the right. At times, the gastric pattern may be accentuated and its movement initiated by feeding the infant an ounce or so of glucose solution or milk and then flicking the epigastrium sharply a few times with the fingernail.

In most instances of hypertrophic stenosis, a definite tumor can be felt. Depending on the degree of gastric dilatation, which in the fully developed case may be great indeed, the tumor will be felt either just at the umbilicus or well to its right, at its level, or above or below. It is best felt with the left hand pressing the right flank firmly upward while the right hand presses downward toward it. In this fashion the firm mass, which has the shape of an olive, may be caught and rolled beween the two hands.

Jaundice may be a problem in an occasional infant with pyloric stenosis. There is elevation of indirect bilirubin, which is thought to relate to impaired liver metabolism in the presence of starvation. The jaundice recedes during the days following pyloromyotomy.

Differential Diagnosis. Hypertrophic pyloric stenosis must be distinguished from congenital atresia or stenosis of the upper third of the duodenum, from cardiochalasia, and from pylorospasm. *Atresia* or *stricture of the duodenum* distal to the ampulla of Vater permits bile to appear in the vomitus, a fact that effectively rules out pyloric stenosis. Complete atresia causes severe vomiting almost from the moment of birth. *Stenosis* proximal to the ampulla may be produced, but rarely, by annular pancreas or by external bands, usually in association with malrotation or by intrinsic incomplete stricture. In these conditions, the onset of vomiting may be delayed until the time at which that of pyloric stenosis usually begins. In all there may be coexistent constipation, gastric patterning, and left-to-right peristalsis. But in only one is a tumor to be felt. Further differentiation is afforded by roentgenography.

Ultrasonography and Radiology. Most instances of pyloric stenosis can be diagnosed by history and physical examination. When the pyloric tumor, or "olive," escapes manual detection, ultrasonography may provide definitive evidence of its existence. If it is not seen, further radiographic studies are appropriate for investigation of the causes of delayed gastric emptying. In pyloric stenosis, a thin streak of barium in the pyloric region (the "string sign") clinches the diagnosis. We frequently omit ultrasonographic study because radiographs are so highly accurate in diagnosing this condition.

Treatment. If the infant is dehydrated or has been sick for many days, it is essential to correct the coexisting metabolic alkalosis. Initially, a nasogastric tube should be inserted to decompress the stomach, and nothing should be given by mouth. Intravenous fluids should be started to restore fluid and electrolyte losses and to provide some glucose. If the deficits are

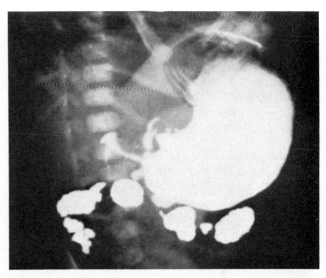

Figure 35–2. Oblique view of abdomen 30 minutes after ingestion of a barium meal. The stomach is still full, and only a little opaque material has escaped into the small bowel. A narrow line replaces the pyloric antrum and the first portion of the duodenum. This represents strikingly narrowed lumen and is a beautiful example of the "string sign" of hypertrophic pyloric stenosis.

severe, several days may be needed to restore the balance. With milder metabolic derangements, frequent small feedings of oral electrolyte solutions may be tolerated.

The treatment of pyloric stenosis is pyloromyotomy. The usual procedure consists of incision of the transverse skin followed by vertical splitting of the rectus. The muscle fibers of the hypertrophied pylorus are then split. The mucosa may be injured in the process, and if so it can be readily repaired.

Postoperatively, one withholds oral feeding for a short time, then offers glucose solution after 8 or 12 hours, in ½-ounce quantities, increasing the amount slowly and changing to breast-feeding or formula 24 hours after operation. Continued vomiting for a day or two is not unusual and need not cause alarm unless it persists into the third or fourth day.

In the unusual cases in which surgery is not an option, such as in remote parts of the world or in the presence of parental objections, medical management can be undertaken. Frequent small feedings, upright position, and, sometimes, intravenous fluids and antispasmodics have been reported to tide the infant over the several months required for spontaneous resolution of the hypertrophy.

Prognosis. Mortality in hypertrophic pyloric stenosis is now almost negligible, largely because of improved skills in management of the small infant with respect to preoperative fluid and electrolyte therapy, to anesthesia, and to control of postoperative infection.

Peptic Ulcer

Gastric or duodenal ulcers of the peptic type identical with those discovered in adults are encountered in the newborn. They are round or oval, sharply circumscribed, and deeply punched out, with clean or rolled edges. Inflammatory reaction is absent or minimal. They may involve mucosa plus submucosa and muscular layers, and they may even perforate serosa.

Incidence. Ulcer is not common in infancy, but many more are found after death than have been suspected in vivo. Lee and Wells encountered a peptic ulcer that had developed in the fetus in utero. Between 1949 and 1969, Seagram and colleagues found an average of five children per year admitted to the Hospital for Sick Children in Toronto with peptic ulcers. The lesion is rare in the first few years of life.

Etiology. Ulcer may develop in gastric mucosa wherever this might be found, in its normal location or in ectopic locations. In this latter category are included Meckel's diverticulum and gastrogenic cysts of either the thorax or abdomen as well as intrathoracic portions of herniated stomach. It also may develop in nongastric mucosa that is bathed by gastric secretions, such as the proximal duodenum, the lower part of the esophagus of infants subject to reflux because of cardiochalasia or hiatus hernia, and near the stomata of surgical gastroenterostomies.

Why ulcer forms in the otherwise normal pyloric antrum or upper part of the duodenum, which is the most common site, is not known. In the newborn, those conditions are not met that have been suggested as precursors and possible instigators of ulcer in the older child or the adult, except that gastric juice is highly acid after the first few hours of life. The opinion has become widespread that ulcer strikes more newborns who have suffered stormy deliveries and who have evidenced postnatal asphyxia than those delivered easily. No convincing proof of this contention has been gathered.

An occasional gastric ulcer results from erosion by the tip of an indwelling catheter.

Diagnosis. In the neonatal period, ulcer is recognized only by the presence of one of or both its disastrous complications, hemorrhage and perforation.

Hemorrhage is manifested by vomiting of fresh or altered blood or by passage of fresh or altered blood by rectum. At times, the loss of blood is considerable, causing rapid development of shock and a precipitous fall in the hematocrit level. At other times, bleeding is more gradual and is recognized only by vomiting of dark brown-stained fluid or by the passage of tarry stools. Most newborns who bleed into the stomach or duodenum lose blood by both routes; that is, by vomiting and by passage of blood by rectum.

Death may occur quickly from blood loss, or, if bleeding is not too massive and if replacement is prompt and adequate, recovery may take place. Hemorrhage may continue for 2 to 4 days, after which it commonly ceases, although at least one infant in our experience continued to bleed for 7 days. Benzidine-positive stools may be passed for 3 or 4 days more, but this does not necessarily indicate continuation of bleeding.

Perforation may occur without prior bleeding or may follow hematemesis and melena. Most often, without premonitory signs of any kind, the newborn suddenly goes into profound shock. The abdomen rapidly distends and becomes full and tight. If shock is not too profound, the abdominal musculature becomes rigid, but this sign is often absent. Percussion reveals a tympanitic note throughout, tympany obscuring the normal area of liver dullness. If death does not occur immediately, signs of peritonitis soon develop.

Gastric and duodenal ulcers can be recognized by radiographic examination in the neonatal period only rarely. We have made many attempts to demonstrate them in newborns with hematemesis and melena and have rarely succeeded.

Perforation is readily demonstrable by radiographic study. Large amounts of free air can be visualized in the peritoneal cavity and over the dome of the liver when films are taken in the erect posture.

Gastroscopy is the most accurate means of diagnosis. Fiberoptic gastroscopes permit inspection of the mucosa in even the smallest of infants (Ament and Christie, 1977).

Treatment. In the presence of hematemesis, no food should be given by mouth until bleeding ceases. Lavage and instillation of antacids are appropriate. Fluids should be administered parenterally as needed. Blood lost should be replaced by transfusion repeated as often as necessary to keep the hematocrit level up to 35 to 40 per cent. Transfusions of 10 ml per kilogram may be given daily or as often as three times in 24 hours if absolutely necessary.

These infants should be watched assiduously for the first sign of perforation. If this occurs, with or without preliminary bleeding, immediate operation is imperative. Closure of the tear in the stomach or duodenum, if performed early, is simple and effective.

Gastric Perforation

We cannot stress too strongly the importance of this disorder. Given a high enough index of suspicion, gastric perforation can be diagnosed promptly enough so that operative intervention will almost always be lifesaving.

Incidence. By 1963, Reams and colleagues were able to find more than 100 cases in the literature, and by 1965 this number had risen to more than 150 (Shaw et al., 1965). A great many have not been recorded.

Etiology. Many perforations are complications of peptic ulcer. Others have been attributed to birth trauma and a few to the ulceration caused by indwelling catheters. Some have been thought to follow rapid overdistention with gas in the course of positive pressure resuscitation, and some have been believed to be due to the overdistention caused by obstructions distal to the stomach. Most of the remainder have been attributed to the rupture of weak points in the gastric wall where muscle was said to be congenitally deficient. Shaw and his collaborators demonstrated in 1965 that all stomachs have potential points of weakness between the interlacing bundles of the muscularis externa and that, after overdistention with air, rupture occurs at one or more of the weak points. The thin edge of the perforation will then show under the microscope only mucosa and submucosa, whereas the muscular layer will be found to have retracted 2 to 10 cm from the mucosal edge. It appears then that this is not a congenital defect and that the stomachs of all newborns are liable to rupture if intragastric pressure rises sufficiently. Since the supine position effectively seals air entrapped within the stomach, continued swallowing of more air may allow intragastric pressure to rise to dangerous heights.

Diagnosis. Low birth weight infants are more prone to gastric perforation than are term ones (58 of 90 in Reams' series, six of eight in Shaw's). Ordinarily, pregnancy, labor, and delivery have not been complicated, and the babies seem quite well at the outset. Symptoms appear usually on the third or fourth day but may present as early as the second or as late as the eighth. Refusal of food, vomiting, respiratory distress, and cyanosis may mark the onset, followed quickly by rapidly progressing abdominal distention.

Physical examination reveals moderate to extreme abdominal distention. The percussion note is usually tympanitic in the upper two thirds of the abdomen, obscuring normal liver dullness, but flat, and shifting with change of position, in the lower third. Often, the distention is of such degree that respiration is embarrassed and cyanosis results. Pitting edema of the skin of the abdomen has been seen in several cases. There may be air filling the scrotal sac.

Flat films of the abdomen show excessive fluid and air within the peritoneal cavity. *One of the films must be taken with a horizontal beam.* Much of the air can be recognized to be free, that is, not within the gastrointestinal lumen. A large air bubble will be seen above the dome of the liver, but below the diaphragm, with the infant in the erect position. When high obstruction coexists, the stomach may be seen to be dilated, or the characteristic double bubble of duodenal obstruction may be visualized.

Treatment. Operative intervention and closure of the rent must be performed immediately; otherwise, bacterial peritonitis will supervene and add a serious complication to an already sufficiently hazardous situation. When the most obvious tear has been repaired, others must be searched for meticulously, since they are not infrequently multiple. Then the surgeon must explore further for a basic defect, and, if this is found, he must correct it at the same time. Failure to follow through in this way led to the death of one baby whom we saw some years ago. One perforation was closed, but upon reoperation 2 days later two more were discovered, and the duodenal atresia that had been responsible for all three was then bypassed. Unfortunately, it was then too late, and the patient did not recover.

In the series of Reams and associates, the chance for survival was about 50 per cent if the patient was operated on within 12 hours of onset and 25 per cent if operated on later.

Gastric Teratoma

Three instances of teratoma arising from the stomach have been reported in very young infants. None has been recognized in the neonatal period; indeed, all patients were 4 months old or slightly older. Since the tumors are undoubtedly congenital, it would appear to be only a matter of time before one is found within the first month.

All these were benign and were removed along with a portion of the stomach wall to which they were broadly attached. All patients did well after removal of the tumor.

REFERENCES

Ament, M., and Christie, D. L.: Upper gastrointestinal fiberoptic endoscopy in pediatric patients. Gastroenterology *72*:1244, 1977.

Benson, C. D., and Coury, J. J.: Congenital intrinsic obstruction of the stomach and duodenum in the newborn. A.M.A. Arch. Surg. *62*:856, 1951.

Blank, E., and Chisolm, A. J.: Congenital microgastria: A case report with a 26-year follow-up. Pediatrics *51*:1037, 1973.

Bronsther, B., Nadeau, M. R., and Abrams, M. W.: Congenital pyloric atresia: A report of three cases and a review of the literature. Surgery *69*:130, 1971.

Caffey, J.: Pediatric X-Ray Diagnosis. 7th ed. Chicago, Year Book Medical Publishers, 1978.

Dide, M.: Sur un estomac d'adulte à type foetal. Bull. Soc. Anat. Paris *66*:669, 1894.

Ducharme, J. C., and Bensoussan, A. L.: Pyloric atresia. J. Pediatr. Surg. *10*:149, 1975.

Euler, A. R., Byrne, W. J. Cousins, L. M., et al.: Increased serum gastrin concentrations and gastric acid hypersecretions in the immediate newborn period. Gastroenterology *72*:1271, 1977.

Grosfeld, J. L., Shipley, F., Fitzgerald, J. F., and Ballantyne, T. V.

N.: Acute peptic ulcer in infancy and childhood. Ann. Surg. 44:13, 1978.

Gross, R. E., Holcomb, G. W., Jr., and Farber, S.: Duplication of the stomach. J. Pediatr. 9:449, 1952.

Handelsman, J. C., Rienhoff, W. F., III, and Ward, G. E.: Benign teratoma of stomach in an infant. A.M.A. J. Dis. Child. 90:196, 1955.

Hicks, L. M., Morgan, A., and Anderson, M. R.: Pyloric stenosis—a report of triplet females and notes on its inheritance. J. Pediatr. Surg. 16:739, 1981.

Holt, L. E.: Duodenal ulcers in infancy. Am. J. Dis. Child. 6:381, 1913.

Kellogg, H. G., Abelson, S. M., and Cornwell, F. A.: Perforation of the stomach in the newborn infant. J. Pediatr. 39:357, 1951.

Lee, W. E., and Wells, J. R.: Perforation in utero of a gastric ulcer. Ann. Surg. 78:36, 1923.

Lloyd, J. R.: Etiology of gastrointestinal perforations in newborn. J. Pediatr. Surg. 4:77, 1969.

McCutcheon, G. T., and Josey, R. B.: Reduplication of the stomach. J. Pediatr. 39:216, 1951.

Meiselas, L. E., and Russakoff, A. H.: Bleeding peptic ulcer in infancy. Am. J. Dis. Child. 67:384, 1944.

Mellish, R. W. P., and Koop, C. E.: Clinical manifestations of duplications of the bowel. Pediatrics 27:397, 1961.

Ogur, G. L., and Kolarsick, A. J.: Gastric diverticula in infancy. J. Pediatr. 39:723, 1951.

Parker, B. C., Guthrie, J., France, N. E., and Atwell, J. D.: Gastric duplication in infancy. J. Pediatr. Surg. 7:294, 1972.

Ravitch, M. M.: The story of pyloric stenosis. Surgery 48:1117, 1960.

Reams, G. B., Dunaway, J. B., and Walls, W. L.: Neonatal gastric perforation with survival. Pediatrics 31:97, 1963.

Rintoul, J. R., and Kirkman, N. F.: The myenteric plexus in infantile hypertrophic pyloric stenosis. Arch. Dis. Child. 36:474, 1961.

Rozenfeld, I. H., and McGrath, J. R.: Melena in the newborn infant. J. Pediatr. 40:180, 1952.

Seagram, C. G. F., Stephens, C. A., and Cummings, W. A.: Peptic ulceration at The Hospital for Sick Children, Toronto, during the 20 year period 1949–1969. J. Pediatr. Surg. 8:407, 1973.

Shaker, I. J., et al.: Aerophagia, a mechanism for spontaneous rupture of the stomach of the newborn. Am. Surg. 39:619, 1973.

Shaw, A., Blanc, W. A., Santulli, T. V., and Kaiser, G.: Spontaneous rupture of the stomach: a clinical and experimental study. Surgery 58:561, 1965.

Tudor, R. B.: Gastric and duodenal ulcers in children. Gastroenterology 62:823, 1972.

Woolley, M. M., Felsher, B. F., Asch, M. J., et al.: Jaundice, pyloric stenosis, and hepatic glucuronyl transferase. J. Pediatr. Surg. 9:359, 1974.

36

Intestinal Obstruction

Revised with the assistance
of Samuel R. Schuster

Complete or partial obstruction somewhere in the gastrointestinal tract from the first portion of the duodenum to the anus is not unusual in the neonatal period. Indeed, the bowel obstructs with surprising frequency even during the period of gestation. A variety of causes produce an identical clinical result. Success or failure in salvage depends not nearly so much on discovering the exact pathogenic mechanism or the precise localization of the obstruction as upon the promptness with which the symptomatic diagnosis is made and operative intervention instituted. However, a futile laparotomy is to be avoided if one can possibly do so.

Among the varieties of obstruction, atresias are the most common. They are encountered approximately twice as frequently as stenoses. The favorite sites of atresia in order of frequency are the ileum, the duodenum, the jejunum, and the colon. This last locus is involved rarely. Multiple atresias are fairly common. Errors in rotation and meconium ileus are the next most common causes. Aganglionosis, annular pancreas, intussusception, incarcerated hernias, and a variety of other miscellaneous disorders are met, but rarely, in every large series.

Classification. The classification suggested by Santulli may be utilized. A free modification of his suggested schema follows:

Causes of Intestinal Obstruction in
the Newborn Infant
I. Mechanical
  A. Congenital.
    1. Intrinsic
      a. Atresia, stenosis, webs
      b. Meconium ileus
      c. Duplications
      d. Imperforate anus
    2. Extrinsic
      a. Peritoneal bands
      b. Midgut volvulus associated with malrotation
      c. Volvulus around omphalomesenteric remnant
      d. Annular pancreas

e. Mesenteric cysts or other tumors
f. Incarcerated hernias
g. Preduodenal portal vein
B. Acquired
1. Necrotizing enterocolitis
2. Intussusception
3. Adhesions secondary to prenatal perforation
4. Mesenteric thrombosis
5. Meconium plug syndrome
II. Functional
A. Hirschsprung's disease
B. Ileus
1. Peritonitis
2. Gastric perforation, cecal perforation
3. Necrotizing enterocolitis
C. Segmental colonic dilatation

Etiology. *Intrinsic Obstructions.* Atresia and intrinsic stenosis have been attributed to failure of proper ontogenic development, but only in the duodenum does this seem a likely mechanism. Between the fourth and tenth weeks of gestation, the entire primitive gut, from proximal esophagus to distal colon, becomes occluded by ingrowth of epithelium that nearly closes the lumen. Subsequently, a continuous lumen develops. Failure of the lumen to reconstitute completely leaves a residue of intraluminal tissue that, if sharply localized, ends as a weblike diaphragm.

In the remainder of the intestine, intrinsic obstructions represent the end results of some accident to the bowel in the latter part of gestation. Louw has produced atresias in animals after vascular insults to the intestine during development. These experiments have clearly demonstrated that atresias identical with those commonly found in neonates can be produced experimentally by compromising the blood supply to a segment of bowel early in fetal life. Accidents include incarceration of the physiologic umbilical hernia, localized volvulus or intussusception, focal peritonitis, and band formation. That such accidents occur in utero is well known; that they may account for single or multiple atresias, abnormalities of the mesentery, and peritoneal bands seems likely from the evidence available.

Meconium ileus is a major cause of obstruction. This earliest manifestation of the syndrome of cystic fibrosis, or mucoviscidosis, occurring in 15 to 20 per cent of patients with cystic fibrosis, is caused by accumulation of abnormally viscid meconium within the small intestinal lumen. Whether meconium is abnormally thick because of absence of pancreatic enzymes throughout fetal life or whether it is just one of many abnormally viscid secretions produced throughout the body in this disease state is still a moot question. Regardless of its pathogenesis, such abnormal meconium acts as an impenetrable barrier to propulsion of air and fluids through the intestinal tract and as a predisposing factor to perforation and meconium peritonitis. Oppenheimer and Esterly believe that intrauterine meconium obstruction may interfere

with mesenteric blood supply, which in turn accounts for the large proportion of congenital anatomic defects found among these infants. These include intestinal atresia, volvulus, mesenteric defects and fibrous bands. Bernstein has further demonstrated that in some instances there is a transmural migration of meconium through the wall of the bowel into the peritoneal cavity. This produces a meconium peritonitis that may further compromise the bowel and increase the likelihood of obstruction.

Meconium plugs may present as transient obstructions. Suppositories or a small saline enema may dislodge the white inspissated mucus, and normal evacuation of meconium may follow. Very small premature infants and some infants of diabetic mothers and those treated with magnesium sulfate are especially likely to have the "meconium-plug syndrome."

Intraluminal cysts are an infrequent cause of intrinsic obstruction in the newborn. They may be of two varieties, duplications of the bowel or retention cysts.

Extrinsic Obstructions. The chief cause of extrinsic obstruction lies in an error in rotation of the bowel. These are of three kinds: nonrotation, malrotation, and reversed rotation.

Briefly summarized, the normal ontogenic sequence is as follows:

By about the fifth week of gestation, the gastrointestinal tract is divided into a primitive foregut, which terminates just distal to the pylorus, the midgut, which ends a little distance beyond the ileocecal junction, and the hindgut. The midgut, which is to form the duodenum, jejunum, ileum, and part of the ascending colon, is extruded into the umbilical cord, forced out by the intestine, which grows more rapidly than the abdominal cavity itself. The mesentery fixes firmly the lower end of the foregut and upper end of the hindgut at points on the posterior abdominal wall that are near one another. This leaves the developing midgut suspended, as it were, by a narrow stalk, the duodenocolic isthmus. By about the tenth week, the midgut begins to reenter the abdominal cavity, completing its return in the short space of a week. The sequence of return is normally from proximal to distal, the most cephalad portion re-entering first, to the right of the superior mesenteric artery, and displacing the hindgut to the left, backward, then upward. The cecum and adjacent colon are reduced last. The cecum migrates counterclockwise from its point of entry in the left lower quadrant to the left, upward, then across to the right upper quadrant. From the eleventh week onward, the cecum gradually descends into the right lower quadrant and becomes fixed by fusion of its mesentery with the posterior parietal peritoneum. In its final position, the midgut has rotated 270 degrees in a counterclockwise direction about the axis of the superior mesenteric ar-

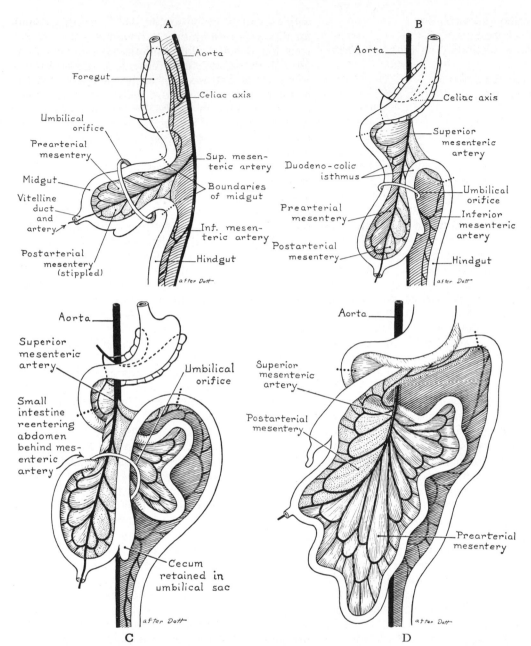

Figure 36–1. Diagrammatic drawings showing normal rotation of alimentary tract. *A,* Fifth week of intrauterine life (lateral view). The foregut, midgut, and hindgut are shown with their individual blood supply supported by the common dorsal mesentery in the sagittal plane. The midgut loop has been extruded into the umbilical cord. *B,* Eighth week of intrauterine life (anteroposterior view). The first stage of rotation is being completed. Note the narrow duodenocolic isthmus from which the midgut loop depends and the right-sided position of the small intestine and left-sided position of the colon. Maintenance of this position within the abdomen after birth is spoken of as nonrotation. *C,* About the tenth week of intrauterine life, during the second stage of rotation (anteroposterior view). The bowel in the temporary umbilical hernia is in the process of reduction, the most proximal part of the prearterial segment entering the abdomen to the right of the superior mesenteric artery first, and the remainder of the bowel following in orderly sequence. The superior mesenteric artery is held forward close to the cecum and ascending colon, permitting the bowel to pass under it. As the coils of small intestine collect within the abdomen, the hindgut is displaced to the left and upward. *D,* Eleventh week of intrauterine life at the end of the second stage of rotation. From its original sagittal position, the midgut has rotated 270 degrees in a counterclockwise direction about the origin of the superior mesenteric artery. The essentials of the permanent disposition of the viscera have been attained. (From Gardner, C. E., Jr., and Hart, D.: Arch. Surg. *29:*942, 1934.)

tery from its original sagittal position within the umbilical cord, the duodenum being fixed behind and the transverse colon coursing over and in front of it (Fig. 36–1).

Nonrotation signifies that there has been no change in position of the bowel after its re-entry into the abdominal cavity. The duodenum descends sharply to the right of the superior mesenteric artery, and the small bowel remains in the right side, the large bowel in the left. The cecum lies to the left of the midline. In *malrotation,* there are irregular defects of rotation and fixation. In *reversed rotation,* the distal midgut re-enters the abdominal cavity first and performs a 90-degree clockwise instead of the usual 270-degree counterclockwise rotation. In this condition, the transverse colon passes behind the duodenum and superior mesenteric artery rather than in front of them.

Abnormal rotation of itself is not responsible for obstruction. This depends upon one of two coincidental factors: (1) The nonrotated midgut lies freely within the abdominal cavity, fixed only at the duodenum and proximal colon. The unattached cecum and small bowel are at liberty to swing in a wide arc in either direction, and, stimulated by the active peristalsis that follows the first ingestion of food, they often rotate in this fashion. The midgut may twist only a few degrees or may make as many as four complete turns. Obstruction depends not upon the amount of twisting, but upon the degree of kinking and vascular obstruction the twisting produces. Midgut volvulus is almost always due to a clockwise twist of the involved bowel and usually obstructs the bowel at or near the duodenojejunal junction. (2) In malrotation, misdirected efforts at fixation of dislocated segments of bowel may lead to the formation of ectopic mesenteric bands. Obstruction, often partial, may be produced by these bands in loops of bowel over which they course. The most frequently seen obstruction resulting from these bands occurs in the second part of the duodenum distal to the ampulla of Vater. This is usually a partial obstruction due to duodenal compression caused by bands stretching from an abnormally positioned cecum across the second portion of the duodenum to the right posterior parietal peritoneum.

Congenital hernias may become incarcerated or strangulated in the noeonatal period exactly as in later life. These hernias may be inguinal, diaphragmatic, or internal. Rarely, an umbilical hernia becomes the site of obstruction.

Annular pancreas may produce partial or complete obstruction at the second portion of the duodenum and may be impossible to differentiate from duodenal web or obstruction at this site due to malrotation associated with "Ladd's bands." It arises from a developmental anomaly. Normally, the pancreas develops from three anlagen, a dorsal and two ventral pancreatic buds that form contiguous to the duodenum. The large dorsal anlage grows into the tail, body, and superior portion of the head. Lecco believes that annular pancreas results when the left ven-

tral bud becomes tightly attached to the duodenum, where, instead of rotating clockwise to meet the dorsal bud, it must stretch around the circumference of the bowel loop. Baldwin agrees but suggests that the right bud also persists and completes the encirclement.

Duplications of the stomach or any part of the bowel may produce large cystic masses that, when filled, may compress adjacent loops to cause obstruction.

Intussusception is rare but far from unknown in the first month of life. A few cases are initiated by an identifiable lead point, such as an intraluminal mass or abnormal fixation of a segment of bowel, but, as in older infants, no initiating mechanism can be discovered in most instances.

Neurogenic Obstructions. As far back as 1901 Tittel pointed out the paucity or absence of ganglion cells of the myenteric plexus in some portions of the large bowel in several cases of megacolon. It was not until 1948 that this observation was confirmed by Zuelzer and Wilson and by Whitehouse and Kernohan. After this, Swenson and his collaborators verified the etiologic role of aganglionosis in Hirschsprung's disease by demonstrating (1) the failure of normal progression of peristaltic waves from splenic flexure to anus; (2) the absence of ganglion cells of the plexus of Auerbach in these same persons; and (3) the permanent cure of megacolon by excision of the aganglionic segment. Congenital aganglionosis, often familial in its distribution, is an important, if rare, cause of intestinal obstruction in the neonate. Since the colon does not become typically dilated and hypertrophied for several weeks or months after birth, the typical roentgenographic features may not be present in the neonate. This is especially true in those bizarre instances in which aganglionosis does not involve the usual site, the rectosigmoid colon, but extends proximally to involve a larger part of the colon or even part or all of the small bowel.

Diagnosis. Usually, the correct diagnosis of intestinal obstruction can be made without too much difficulty. Vomiting and abdominal distention are strongly suggestive, and if bile-stained vomiting is present in the newborn, the presence of intestinal obstruction should be assumed until proved otherwise. Nevertheless, the intensity of these signs and their time of appearance vary according to the location and the completeness of the obstruction. Before discussing in detail the clinical pictures of particular lesions, some general comments might be in order. The problem with a vomiting, possibly distended, newborn is multifaceted. The pediatrician must decide whether the illness may be due to intestinal obstruction. If obstruction appears to be a strong possibility, then the pediatrician and the pediatric surgeon must work together to elucidate the site and cause of obstruction further and proceed with appropriate therapy. *One of the most important single measures for the pediatrician is to insert a nasogastric tube to decompress the stomach and prevent vomiting and aspiration.*

The suspicion that intestinal obstruction exists should arise in one's mind whenever vomiting, constipation, or distention, or any combination of these signs, develops. *Vomiting* begins soon after delivery when an obstruction is high and complete, but it may be delayed some days if it is low or incomplete. Vomitus contains bile if the obstruction is distal to the ampulla of Vater, none if it is proximal to it. Bile-stained vomitus is not an infallible sign of intestinal obstruction, but when it is present in a neonate the burden of proof is on the individual who says that the patient is *not* obstructed. Not infrequently, blood is mixed with vomitus, especially when the obstruction is high, but the presence of blood is not of itself a strong indication of obstruction. Occasional sporadic vomiting is less characteristic than vomiting after every feedings and may be seen in patients with partial obstruction, such as a patient with malrotation and partial obstruction of the duodenum due to "Ladd's bands." If the infant regurgitates continually between feedings, the probability of obstruction is increased. Vomiting may or may not be forceful. It is almost never projectile except in instances of gastric outlet obstruction. Effortless regurgitation alone is not at all uncommon.

Abdominal distention, when present, is an extremely valuable sign. It may be noted at the time of delivery, but, when considerable at that time, it more often indicates that perforation of the bowel had taken place before birth or that the fetus has ascites or a tumor. Ordinarily, distention becomes apparent some hours after birth, reaching its maximum within 24 to 48 hours. The longer abdominal distention persists, the more likely it is that intestinal patterning will be seen through the abdominal wall. Such patterns, with visible peristaltic waves, are an almost certain indication of obstruction. In duodenal—or the rare gastric—obstruction, distention may be limited to the epigastrium, with or without a visible gastric pattern, or it may be absent entirely. This absence of distention is caused by continuous emptying of the stomach by repeated vomiting.

Failure to pass meconium is also a dependable sign. The normal newborn will pass a meconium stool within 12 hours and almost never fails to do so by 24 hours. If he does not, obstruction must be suspected. On the other hand, the newborn with high obstruction almost invariably passes his normal complement of meconium stools. Even when obstruction is low in the ileum, the bowels usually move several times within the first day of life, unless the obstruction is due to a developmental defect such as intestinal

atresia. In these cases, there is no meconium distal to the atresia and therefore no meconium stools.

Additional evidence can sometimes be gained by palpation of the abdomen. Distended, hypertrophied hollow viscera may sometimes be felt as vague, ill-defined tubular masses that can be rolled under the hand. Masses of hard or doughy consistency can often be felt scattered throughout the abdomen in meconium ileus, almost never in other forms of obstruction. A solid or cystic mass may occasionally be the tumor responsible for obstruction.

Radiography is the most useful ancillary diagnostic aid. Films should be taken in three positions: supine posteroanterior, erect posteroanterior, and prone cross-table lateral. *No contrast medium should be used unless plain films have failed to substantiate the diagnosis. If doubt still exists, a barium enema series may be obtained, and only if the diagnosis is still uncertain should a contrast medium mixture be given by mouth.* Specific radiographic alterations will be described with each type of obstruction discussed later, but certain general deviations from the normal will be listed here. Normally, air enters and fills the stomach immediately after birth, the small bowel within 2 to 12 hours, and the colon within 18 to 24 hours. When obstruction exists, the air pattern may be seen to stop abruptly at one point, leaving the remainder of the bowel airless. The stomach and a loop or loops of intestine proximal to the point of obstruction may be dilated and, in the erect position, will show horizontal air-fluid levels. If the obstruction is low, a series of such dilated, air- and fluid-filled coils of intestine, each with its own fluid level, one above the other, makes a characteristic stepladder design. Obstruction at the pylorus produces one large bubble outlining the dilated stomach, whereas obstruction in the duodenum often produces a double-bubble picture, one bubble outlining the dilated stomach, the other the dilated loop of duodenum proximal to the obstruction.

When obstruction is incomplete (that is, in the stenoses or volvulus) dilated viscera may be seen above one point, and a trickle of gas may be visible below.

Barium enema may show the colon distal to the locus of complete obstruction to be narrow and not readily distensible by the injected contrast mixture—so-called "microcolon." The form of obstruction most commonly associated with a microcolon is a small bowel atresia. The other major value of the barium enema is to determine whether or not the cecum is normally located in the right lower quadrant. This finding usually rules out the presence of a malrotation, although this is not absolute and one cannot be certain that some degree of malrotation or at least malfixation is not present. Obviously, the injected fluid does not progress cephalad beyond the obstructed segment.

Upper gastrointestinal series with contrast medium, performed only after the two foregoing studies have failed to supply a certain answer, may show moderate dilatation proximal to a locus of narrowing and a trickle of opaque liquid entering the bowel distal to the stenotic segment.

REFERENCES

Baldwin, cited by R. E. Gross and T. C. Chisholm.

Bennington, J. L., and Huber, S. L.: The embryologic significance of undifferentiated intestinal tract. J. Pediatr. *64*:735, 1964.

Clatworthy, H. W., Jr., Howard, W. H. R., and Lloyd, J.: The meconium plug syndrome. Surgery *39*:131, 1956.

DeLorimier, A., Fonkalsrud, E., and Hays, D.: Congenital atresia and stenosis of jejunum and ileum. Surgery *65*:819, 1969.

Dickinson, S. J.: Origin of intestinal atresia of the newborn. J.A.M.A. *190*:119, 1964.

Duhamel, B.: Retrorectal and transanal pull-through for treatment of Hirschsprung's disease. Dis. Colon Rectum *7*:455, 1964.

Emery, J. L.: The tryptic activity and presence of cornified squames in meconium as diagnostic aid in congenital intestinal obstruction. Arch. Dis. Child. *27*:67, 1952.

Evans, cited by D. C. Benson and I. J. Coury: Arch. Surg. *62*:856, 1951.

Gardner, C. E., Jr., and Hart, D.: Anomalies of intestinal rotation as a cause of intestinal obstruction. Arch. Surg. *29*:942, 1934.

Glover, D. M., and Barry, F. M.: Intestinal obstruction in the newborn. Ann. Surg. *130*:480, 1949.

Grosfeld, J., Schreiner, R., Franken, E., et al.: Changing pattern of gastrointestinal bezoars in infants and children. Surgery *88*:425, 1980.

Gross, R. E., and Chisholm, T. C.: Annular pancreas producing duodenal obstruction. Ann. Surg. *119*:759, 1944.

Gruenwald, P.: Asphyxia, trauma and shock at birth. Arch. Pediatr. *67*:103, 1950.

Holder, T. M., and Leape, L. L.: The acute surgical abdomen in the neonate. N. Engl. J. Med. *278*:605, 1968.

Hutchinson, I. Olayiwola, B., and Young, T.: Intussusception in infancy and childhood. Br. J. Surg. *67*.209, 1980.

Jones, T. W., and Schutt, R. P.: Alimentary tract obstruction in the newborn infant; a review and analysis of 132 cases. Pediatrics *20*:881, 1957.

Lecco, cited by R. E. Gross and T. C. Chisholm.

Lemoh, J., and Brooke, O.: Frequency and weight of normal stools in infancy. Arch. Dis. Child. *54*:719, 1979.

Louw, J. H.: Jejunoileal atresia and stenosis. J. Pediatr. Surg. *1*:8, 1966.

Morikawa, Y., Donahoe, P., and Hendren, H.: Manometry and histochemistry in diagnosis of Hirschsprung's disease. Pediatrics *63*:865, 1979.

Oppenheimer, E. H., and Esterly, J. R.: Observations in cystic fibrosis of the pancreas. II. Neonatal intestinal obstruction. Bull. Johns Hopkins Hosp. *111*:1, 1962.

Preis, O., and Rudolph, N.: Abdominal distention in newborn infants on phototherapy: role of eye occlusion. J. Pediatr. *94*:816, 1979.

Rack, F. J., and Crouch, W. L.: Functional intestinal obstruction in the premature infant. J. Pediatr. *40*:579, 1952.

Santulli, T. V.: Intestinal obstruction in the newborn infant. J. Pediatr. *44*:317, 1954.

Swenson, O., Neuhauser, E. B. D., and Pickett, L. K.: New concepts of the etiology, diagnosis and treatment of congenital megacolon (Hirschsprung's disease). Pediatrics *4*:201, 1949.

Tittel, K.: Ueber eine angeborene Missbildung des Dickdarmes. Wien. klin. Wchnschr. *14*:903, 1901.

Whitehouse, F. R., and Kernohan, J. W.: Myenteric plexus in congenital megacolon. Arch. Intern. Med. *82*:75, 1948.

Zuelzer, W. W., and Wilson, J. L.: Functional intestinal obstruction on congenital neurogenic basis in infancy. Am. J. Dis. Child. *75*:40, 1948.

37

Congenital Intestinal Obstruction

Duodenal Atresia

Atresia is complete obstruction of the lumen of the bowel and should be distinguished from stenosis, which indicates narrowing of the lumen. Atresias occur about twice as often as stenoses.

Incidence. Atresias account for about one third of all intestinal obstructions in the newborn and are the most common cause of congenital obstruction. They occur in about 1 of every 2700 livebirths. Duodenal atresia accounts for about 40 per cent of all intestinal atresias.

Diagnosis. The diagnosis of duodenal atresia is not difficult. Hydramnios is present in about half the cases. Vomiting begins within a few hours after birth, before ingestion of any fluids. The vomited material consists of pharyngeal, gastric, and duodenal secretions. Most atresias involve the second or third portion of the duodenum, so that vomitus almost always

contains bile. Until feedings are begun, vomiting takes the form of repeated regurgitations of small amounts. After a feeding, the amount vomited may be large and moderately forceful, but this episode is followed by frequent, almost continual, regurgitations of small quantities. Distention, if present, is limited to the epigastrium, while the lower half of the abdomen remains flat and even scaphoid. The infant ordinarily passes one to three or more meconium stools in the first 24 to 36 hours. Thereafter, bowel movements cease, although small quantities of thick mucus may continue to be passed from the rectum.

The association of other, often severe congenital malformations with duodenal atresia is noteworthy.

In a series of 157 neonates with duodenal obstruction, Young and Wilkinson reported other abnormalities in 70 per cent. In order of frequency, they were Down syndrome (21 per cent), annular pancreas, cardiovascular anomalies, malrotation, esophageal atresia, small bowel anomaly, and anorectal lesions. Marked jaundice developed in about one third, and a few had biliary atresia. Many of the babies are born prematurely.

The familial occurrence of congenital duodenal atresia has been noted a small but significant number of times. Hyde, for instance, reported one family in which four siblings were born with the identical lesion. Mishalany and colleagues report a concurrence highly suggestive of an autosomal recessive type of inheritance. The parents of each of the affected babies in this remarkable family were first cousins, and all of the four parents descended from one great-grandfather and two great-grandmothers who were themselves sisters.

Radiographs of the abdomen show air in the upper half and complete airlessness elsewhere. No small or large bowel patterns are visible. Usually, the air outlines two dilated hollow structures, the stomach and the upper duodenum, which are readily distinguished in the erect anteroposterior projection and even more clearly outlined in the erect lateral position. At times, this double bubble cannot be discerned. Rarely, there will be insufficient air in the stomach, because of continual regurgitation, to define its outlines clearly. Under these circumstances, it is permissible to inject 10 to 20 cc of air through a gastric tube or to instill through the tube an effervescent mixture. This simple procedure may suffice to clarify an uncertain situation.

Neither barium enema nor upper gastrointestinal radiographs should be needed to diagnose duodenal atresia.

Treatment. Preoperative decompression with a nasogastric tube is imperative. Immediate operation, after restoration of fluids and achievement of good blood chemical values, is essential. The operation of choice is side-to-side duodenoduodenostomy, or if this is not possible, a duodenojejunostomy.

Prognosis. The mortality from operation on duodenal atresia has dropped substantially in recent years from nearly 30 per cent in 1969 to 9 per cent in the period ranging from 1970 to 1978 at Yale–New Haven Hospital (Touloukian, 1980). Most deaths are due to related major anomalies in association with prematurity.

Duodenal Stenosis

Partial obstruction of the duodenum can be produced by intrinsic stenosis, webs, annular pancreas, aberrant peritoneal bands either with or without malrotation, or duodenal kinking (Chamberlain, 1966). In a few cases, an aberrant superior mesenteric artery has been the cause of the obstruction, and in even fewer a preduodenal portal vein. It is comparatively simple to localize the site of the narrowing, but differentiation between these various causes before operation is often impossible.

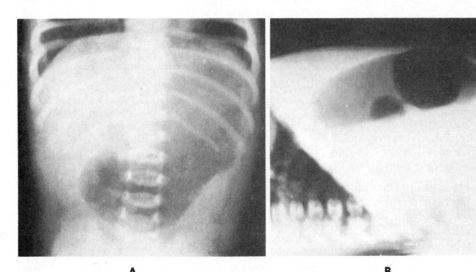

A   **B**

Figure 37–1. *A,* Anteroposterior view in the supine position shows the distended stomach. If one looks carefully, one can see a second air bubble adjacent to the stomach above and to the right of the pyloric antrum. The rest of the bowel is completely airless. *B,* In the supine lateral position, the large gastric bubble is seen, and within it two darker bubbles. These are surely the shadows made by the first and second portions of the dilated duodenum. There is a sharp fluid level.

These films are characteristic of duodenal atresia, as was the history. Vomiting began at 4 hours, followed by continuous regurgitation of dark brown fluid containing bile and blood. Meconium was passed several times and there was no distention.

Diagnosis. As one might expect, the symptoms of partial duodenal obstruction appear later, depending on the degree of obstruction, and are more intermittent than are those of complete atresia. In the neonate, vomiting may start at any time, but its onset is usually delayed until at least 4 days after birth. Onset at 10 days or at 1 month or at any time throughout childhood is not at all uncommon. Often, only one or two feedings a day are lost, and there may be weeks or months during which no vomiting whatever occurs. Since most stenoses involve the second and third portions of the duodenum, the vomitus usually contains bile. Stools may be normal in number and nature, or during the periods when vomiting is prominent, constipation may be moderate to severe. Epigastric distention is also variable, as is visible gastric peristalsis.

Flat and upright films of the abdomen should be obtained immediately, but it is important to remember that in partial obstruction they may show nothing abnormal. If so, these should be followed by barium enema films. These may or may not show the cecum to lie in an abnormal position or to be excessively mobile. Only if these procedures have failed to provide diagnostic information is it proper to perform an upper gastrointestinal series. With this, the narrowed segment of bowel may be visualized, with or without dilatation of the loop proximal to it, and the contrast medium may be seen to trickle slowly into the intestine distal to the stenosis.

Treatment. Operative correction is the treatment of choice; if the preoperative studies indicate that malrotation may be present, the operation should be performed immediately. This urgency is dictated by the possibility that symptomatic malrotation is often associated with midgut volvulus.

Jejunal and Ileal Atresia

Atresias of the jejunum and the ileum constitute about 40 per cent of all atresias. The obstruction is in the proximal jejunum in about 31 per cent of the cases, in the distal jejunum in 20 per cent, in the

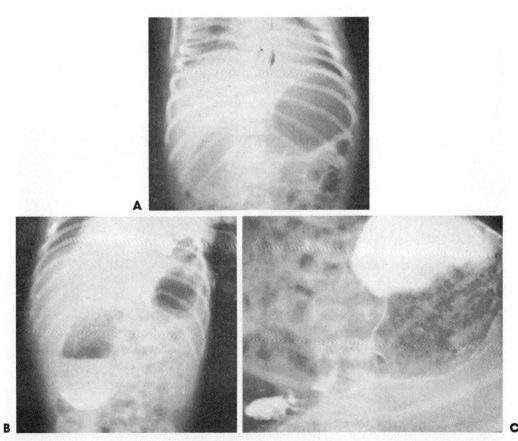

Figure 37–2. *A,* Anteroposterior film in the supine position shows a double-bubble pattern made up of stomach and hugely dilated duodenum. It shows, in addition, some air in the large and small bowels, indicating that obstruction cannot be complete. *B,* Anteroposterior film taken in the erect position after a barium swallow. A fluid level can now be seen in the dilated duodenum. *C,* After 1 hour, a small mass of Lipiodol has passed out of the hugely dilated duodenum visible above it.

proximal ileum in 13 per cent, and in the distal ileum in 36 per cent (DeLorimier et al., 1969).

An unusual condition that is almost always fatal was described by Guttmann and colleagues in 1973. He reported five fatal cases of multiple atresias of the gastrointestinal tract from the stomach to the rectum. They were inherited in an autosomal recessive manner. More recently, Teja and colleagues described a single patient of parents who were second cousins. The infant started vomiting soon after birth and on exploration was found to have the gastric antrum obstructed by a thin diaphragm as well as multiple obstructions of the small and large bowel. At autopsy, the lesions showed evidence of chronic inflammation. The absence of vascular lesions was noted and led to the suggestion that almost all the lesions were postinflammatory.

Classification.   Several classifications have been proposed to assist the clinician. Martin and Zerella suggest the following:

Type I: Single atresia from obstructing membrane as diaphragm.
Type II: Single atresia with discontinuity of bowel wall. The blind ends may be connected by a fibrous strand. Total bowel length may be shortened in this situation.
Type III: Multiple atresias.

Type IV: Discontinuity of bowel wall with distal segment lacking mesentery and receiving blood supply from ileocolic artery.

Associated problems were cystic fibrosis, prematurity, omphalocoele, and cloacal exstrophy.

Diagnosis.   Vomiting may begin a bit later in life, usually at the end of the first day or during the second day, although abdominal distention has been noted in many immediately after birth. Distention becomes considerably more prominent, gradually increasing to involve the entire abdomen symmetrically. Vomitus invariably contains bile and may become fecal. Shrand argues with plausibility that the green staining of the amniotic fluid of his example of multiple jejunal atresia, and presumably of others, must have been due to vomiting in utero, not to meconium staining, for at operation the distal bowel was markedly narrowed and contained white meconium. After the lower bowel has emptied itself of its meconium, no other stools are passed, but passage of five or six meconium stools is not unusual. The stools never become transitional or fecal. Percussion reveals tympany over the entire abdomen, including the flanks, but liver dullness, although elevated, is not obscured. With the stethoscope, the sounds of hyperactive peristalsis are heard, although in a neglected late case they may be absent.

Many dilated loops of bowel are evident on the radiographs. In the erect position, one usually sees fluid levels in many of these dilated loops, at times in the characteristic "stepladder" pattern. Unless per-

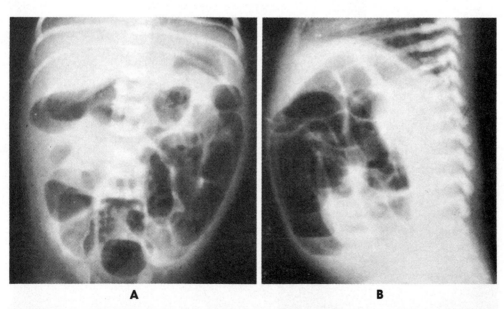

A   **B**

Figure 37–3.   *A,* Supine anteroposterior flat film showing an irregular distribution of grossly dilated loops of bowel of varying sizes throughout the abdomen. The loop in the left lateral abdomen was misinterpreted as large bowel but turned out at operation to be small bowel like all the others. *B,* Lateral erect film. Visible in this position are the fluid levels in all the dilated loops of small bowel that produce the typical "stepladder" design of lower intestinal obstruction. Atresia was discovered in the ileum.

The history was equally typical, with vomiting and distention beginning at 17 hours, passage of a meconium plug but no further stools, and vomiting of bile-stained material.

foration has taken place, no air can be discerned outside the intestinal loops, and no bubble will be seen above the liver. If a barium enema is performed, microcolon is ordinarily seen. The column of barium may not reach the obstruction, but serves to define pathology in the colon.

In differential diagnosis midgut volvulus, meconium ileus, aganglionosis, and paralytic ileus must be considered. It has become clear that jejuno ileal atresias coexist with both volvulus and meconium ileus with surprising frequency. It is probable that prenatal volvulus leads to intestinal atresia by compromising mesenteric blood supply and that prenatal obstruction by the thick, inspissated intestinal contents of cystic fibrosis may have the same effect.

Treatment and Prognosis. The outcome of surgical intervention has improved dramatically in recent years with the advent of neonatal intensive care. Touloukian reports 96 per cent operative survival from resection of atresias of jejunum and ileum. Late morbidity may be the result of other problems, such as prematurity, cardiac malformations, and, in the event of multiple atresias, the too little remaining intestine (short-gut syndrome).

Martin and Zerella report that the rate of mortality before 1968 was 50 per cent, but no deaths were recorded subsequently. They attribute the dramatic improvement to availability of intravenous alimentation.

Atresia of the Colon

Atresia of the colon accounts for less than 10 per cent of intestinal atresias, and stenoses of the colon are even rarer. Boles and coworkers described their experiences with 11 infants seen between 1958 and 1975. The atresia was in the ascending colon in 7 infants, the transverse colon in 1, and the descending colon in 3. In some instances, significant amounts of colon were missing. Other anomalies were found in these infants: gastroschisis in 4 and hydronephrosis in 1.

Diagnosis. The salient clinical features were abdominal distention, vomiting, and failure to pass meconium. On plain radiographs, dilated proximal colon may be present. A barium enema is essential to definitive diagnosis.

Treatment and Prognosis. Ten of Boles's 11 patients survived operation, which was a staged procedure. He advocates initial exteriorization of the proximal end of the atresia to permit decompression and oral feeding; then, after a few weeks or months, intestinal continuity can be re-established with an appropriate anastomosis.

Meconium Ileus

Incidence. Meconium ileus is a relatively frequent cause of intestinal obstruction among the white pop-

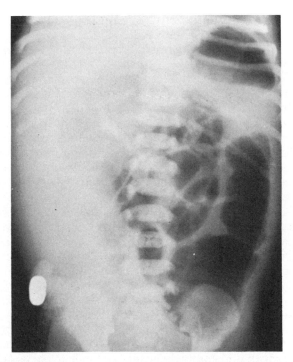

Figure 37–4. X-ray view of abdomen taken in the erect posture. The gas pattern is bizarre. Fewer loops can be seen than is usual, and these are almost confined to the left half of the abdomen; some are hugely dilated. No air is seen in the right half. There are no fluid levels, except in the stomach. The exact point of obstruction cannot be determined. At operation, meconium ileus was found.

One of this infant's two siblings had died of intestinal obstruction in the neonatal period.

ulation. It is very rare among non-Caucasian ethnic groups. From 1940 to 1965 at Children's Hospital in Boston, 164 patients were diagnosed as having meconium ileus (Donnison et al., 1966).

Pathophysiology. Abnormal accumulation of intestinal secretory products and deficient pancreatic enzymes are presumed to make the meconium excessively viscid. Necrosis of the intestinal wall may occur in utero to produce peritonitis. Healing can occur so that only flecks of calcium may persist postnatally on radiographs as silent witnesses of the intrauterine peritonitis. One of the only pathologic findings in cystic fibrosis in neonates is hypertrophy of mucous glands in the gut. The pancreas itself is often normal on histologic examination. Excess albumin in the meconium of infants with cystic fibrosis has been the basis of one neonatal screening test (Shwachman and Antonowicz, 1981).

Diagnosis. For the diagnosis of this condition, an awareness of the physical status of previous children is of great importance. A history of congenital intestinal obstruction or cystic fibrosis in a sibling should immediately alert one to the possibility of meconium ileus. If one's suspicions are aroused, the diagnosis can conceivably be made before the signs of intestinal obstruction make their appearance or even in utero with ultrasonography.

If one has not been forewarned by the family history, the first suggestive sign is apt to be distention. This is noticed between 12 and 24 hours in most cases. Vomiting also occurs, but it is not nearly so prominent as it is in the atresia group and does not make its appearance until the second day in most cases. Failure to pass meconium is absolute, but by the time this is noted the other signs have usually made their appearance.

On physical examination, abdominal distention is the outstanding finding. Visible intestinal patterns are often discernible on the abdominal wall. On palpation, these dilated loops can often be felt, but much more diagnostic is the presence of numerous hard masses throughout the abdomen. Some of these are sausage-shaped; most are hard or doughy balls, freely movable in any direction. Bowel sounds can generally be heard until late in the course. Digital examination of the rectum reveals a normal anus and sphincter and complete absence of meconium as far as the finger can penetrate.

Radiographic examination is helpful. The variably dilated loops of small bowel suggest the presence of intestinal obstruction. In the erect position, fluid levels are seldom seen in the uncomplicated cases. Tiny bubbles of gas may be seen mixed with the meconium in the distal small bowel in some cases and a diffuse granular appearance in others. The locus of obstruction can usually be discerned in the distal small bowel. A cross-table lateral film of the abdomen with the baby in the prone position helps determine whether or not there is air in the rectum.

Proteolytic enzymes are absent from the stools of all infants with complete obstruction. This renders this examination useless for differentiating this type from others. But newborn infants may show the characteristic elevation of sodium chloride in their sweat.

Course and Prognosis. It is imperative that diagnosis be made and treatment instituted early, since complications supervene rapidly and frequently. These are perforation of the intestine, with subsequent meconium and bacterial peritonitis, and volvulus. Indeed, both complications may have already occurred by the time of birth.

Treatment. About half the infants with meconium ileus can be treated by hyperosmolar enemas (Gastrografin). Introduced by Noblett in 1969, this method draws water into the intestinal tract and allows the sticky meconium to be dislodged. Great care should be taken to maintain fluid and electrolyte balance in these babies by intravenous infusion sufficient to keep serum osmolarity below 290 mOsm per liter

(Rowe et al., 1971). In other patients, exploration with irrigation of the intestine may be required. Gross pioneered the modern surgical treatment of these infants, which is resection of distal ileum with establishment of Mikulicz-type ileostomy. Many surgeons now use the Bishop-Koop modification of his approach. "After resection of the dilated portion of the ileum an end-to-side anastomosis is performed, and the free end of the distal ileum brought out in the abdominal wall as an ileostomy." One then irrigates the distal segment with N-acetyl-cysteine to clear it of its firm concretions. Anastomosis is carried out approximately 2 weeks later. An alternative method of management is to evacuate the obstructing firm meconium in the ileum and cleanse the colon of any residual meconium. After this, an end-to-end anastomosis can be performed.

Outcome. The outcome is usually successful from the surgical perspective. The hazards to the infant are due to susceptibility to pulmonary infections and to other problems that may coexist with meconium ileus, such as prematurity. Many survivors of the neonatal period have episodes of fecal impaction in later life, even into adulthood. Shwachman is following 7 patients over 30 years of age who had meconium ileus as infants, indicating that this particular manifestation of cystic fibrosis need not be associated with severe pulmonary symptoms.

Duplications of Colon and Rectum

Cystic masses within or adjacent to the colon or rectum are rare, but they do occur and can cause obstruction. The lesions may present as abdominal masses and require ultrasonographic and radiographic evaluation to distinguish them from presacral teratomas or anterior meningoceles. Cystic duplications are often associated with other anomalies such as imperforate anus and abnormalities of the genitourinary tract.

Excision of the duplication should be performed to avoid the possibility of volvulus, intussusception, or future malignant change, such as that described in six patients by Orr and Edwards.

Congenital Deformities of the Anus and Rectum

The pediatrician need not be concerned too deeply with minute details of all the possible combinations and permutations that abnormal embryologic development may lead to in this area of the body. Essentially all that it is necessary to know is contained in the answers to three questions. Is there atresia with complete obstruction? Is there stenosis with partial obstruction? Is there a fistulous connection between lower bowel and urinary tract, genital tract, or perineum? Associated anomalies occur in over half the infants with imperforate anus. Genitourinary anomalies were found in about 28 per cent of patients and other gastrointestinal anomalies in another 13 per cent (Kiesewetter, 1980).

Embryology. The proctodeum comprises the anus and a canal that extends cephalad a short distance to meet the blind end of the hindgut, which simultaneously moves caudad. At the seventh to eighth week of gestation these should make contact, separated only by the anal membrane. At the same time, the lower urinary tract is developing alongside the lower intestinal tract, and the two anlagen are separated by the urorectal membrane. Malformations of the anus arise locally from maldevelopment within the proctodeum itself, while atresias, stenoses, and fistulas arise from imperfect resolution of the anorectal membrane with or without concomitant failure of the urorectal membrane to separate completely the genitourinary and rectal anlagen.

Classification. Browne classifies deformities of the anus into three groups, each containing several subgroups. Group I includes *stenosis of the anus,* in which the finger meets a fibrous ring just inside the junction of skin and mucosa, and the *microscopic anus,* which is exactly what its name implies. Group II consists of the *ectopic anus,* which is shifted well forward of its normal position to form a "shotgun perineum," with the edges of vagina and anus touching; the *vaginal ectopic anus,* in which the anus actually opens into the lower portion of the vagina (this should not be confused with imperforate anus plus rectovaginal fistula); and the *male ectopic anus,* which is a stenotic opening well forward of its normal position. Group III he calls the *covered anus,* with, in the female, no visible anal opening and feces passing freely through the vulva; and, in the male, a blue line running forward from the anal dimple, representing a sinus tract filled with meconium.

The classification of rectal and anal deformities most often utilized is that of Ladd and Gross. They divide them into the following four types:

Type I: Stenosis at lower rectum or anus (incomplete rupture of anal membrane).

Type II: Membranous form of imperforate anus (persistence of anal membrane).

Type III: Imperforate anus, and rectum ends as a blind pouch a variable distance from the perineum.

Type IV: Anal canal and lower rectum form a distal pouch, separated from a blind rectal pouch by a variable distance.

Fistulas are associated in a high percentage of cases (55 to 82 per cent of all reported series). Most of these involve the type III malformation, and, conversely, almost every type III deformity has an associated fistula. In the female these are almost always rectovaginal, rarely rectoperineal, and never rectourinary. In the male, fistulas are almost always rectourinary, terminating in the bladder or urethra, and are only rarely rectoperineal. In Santulli's series of 62 cases, the type III variety accounted for 53, type

I for four, type II for three, and type IV for only two examples.

Diagnosis. Microscopic anus is obvious from the start, resembling an imperforate anus with a tiny dot of meconium or stool visible at times in its center. Only a fine probe can be passed. A low stenosis usually does not cause symptoms within the neonatal period, difficulty in defecation and ribbon-like stools ordinarily delaying their appearance for several months. The reason may be that the stoma is large enough to permit passage of semiliquid and pasty stools characteristic of early life but not passage of formed stools. When symptoms appear, digital rectal examination confirms the diagnosis.

So rare is the type II membranous diaphragm deformity that Potts encountered only one in his entire career. The anus is normal in appearance; hence, diagnosis usually awaits distention and vomiting, which begins at 24 to 48 hours of age. By then, the bulging green or brown membrane may be visible at the anus, but, if not, it is readily palpable by the probing finger a few centimeters above the sphincter. If a radiograph is taken with the infant held upside down, a thermometer held in place within the anus as far as it will penetrate without forcing, the air in the lowermost loop of bowel will be seen to abut the thermometer bulb closely. This is true only provided one has waited at least 24 hours for air to have entered the entire large bowel and has held the infant inverted for at least 5 minutes so that its most distal loop has filled.

In the type III lesion, one can see the anal dimple, but the anus is clearly imperforate. One expects to find a fistula: rectovaginal in the female, rectourinary in the male, rarely rectoperineal in either sex. One is almost never disappointed in this anticipation. X-ray studies with barium injected vaginally or through the urethra will confirm fistula, as will the appearance of meconium or flatus within the vagina of the female or the urethra of the male.

The diagnosis of the type IV lesion, since the anus looks normal, awaits evidence of lower bowel obstruction, after which rectal examination may reveal the atresia. Thereafter, plain radiographs taken in the inverted position with the mentioned precautions should demonstrate the distance by which blind upper and lower pouches are separated.

Treatment. Briefly, all stenotic lesions are treated by repeated and long-continued dilatations; obstructive lesions with or without fistula must be treated surgically. In the case of membranous lesions surgery is simple, consisting merely of perforation of the diaphragm. Operative repair of the type III malformation in the female may be delayed, since the rectovaginal fistula dilates adequately to permit passage of stools; however, it is best to correct this problem during the first year of life to avoid the psychologic trauma associated with later correction. The infant may require help in the form of mineral oil or Colace by mouth to keep the stools soft and of periodic enemas whenever impaction threatens. Those patients with obstruction due to an imperforate anus in which the blind rectal pouch resides above the levator sling (and/or those with a rectourinary fistula) will require a colostomy to relieve them of obstruction. Definitive surgical repair of the imperforate anus and rectourinary fistula should be performed at 1 to 2 years of age.

Prognosis. The outlook for an infant with imperforate anus depends on the nature of the lesion, the skill of the surgeon, and, probably most critically, on the presence of associated anomalies.

Kiesewetter and Hoon reviewed a 25 year experience in Pittsburgh and reported a 19.4 per cent mortality rate for a series of 284 patients. Three fourths of the survivors in this series had good results. The remaining had incontinence, some of which could be corrected by reoperation. The authors noted gradual improvement in many. They do not advocate permanent colostomy before adolescence.

Rupture of Bowel

Perforations of the gastrointestinal tract may be spontaneous in otherwise well infants or associated

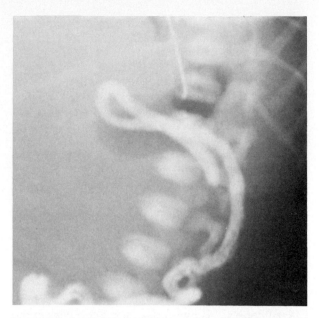

Figure 37–6. This 2-day-old boy had had bile-stained vomitus for 24 hours. This barium enema shows an opaque nasogastric catheter. The barium-filled colon is very narrow and is termed a "microcolon"; this implies nonuse and complete higher obstruction, present for some weeks at least. The course of the left colon is normal, but the right colon is deflected into the left side of the abdomen. The ileocecal valve, the landmark of the lower end of the midgut mesentery, is therefore not in its normal right lower quadrant position, and malrotation must be diagnosed. Operation confirmed midgut malrotation and also showed the suspected volvulus. The volvulus had led to small bowel infarction, necrosis, and cystic dilatation of the infarcted bowel. The child died during surgery. (Courtesy of Dr. N. T. Griscom.)

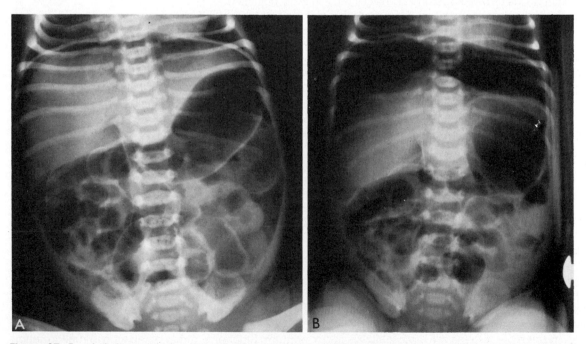

Figure 37–5. *A,* Anteroposterior view of abdomen taken in the erect position at 72 hours of age. There is air in the stomach and intestines, and one gets the distinct impression that some of the air is outside the lumen of the bowel. A layer of air is clearly visible above the liver and below the diaphragm. *B,* Ten hours later. By now, there is a huge accumulation of air between the diaphragm and the liver.

with a history of perinatal asphyxia, prematurity, or diagnostic procedures. Over a 22-year period at Case Western Reserve, Tucker and coworkers described 53 gastrointestinal perforations, 72 per cent of which appeared during the first week of life. The stomach, small intestine, and colon each accounted for 23 to 30 per cent of the total. Forty-nine per cent of the infants survived.

Abdominal distention and failure to pass stools should always alert the physician to the possibility of perforation; diagnosis depends on radiographic evidence of free air. Associated illnesses, such as meconium ileus or necrotizing enterocolitis, may become evident on radiographs as well.

Occasionally, an infant will have free air dissect into the peritoneal cavity from an intrathoracic air leak. In the event of severe respiratory distress syndrome with evidence of pneumothorax and a small amount of intra-abdominal air in the absence of bowel disease, this possibility should be considered.

Treatment consists of immediate laparotomy to repair the site or sites of perforation.

Malrotation with Volvulus

Malrotation may be present alone and may be asymptomatic for life, or it may become symptomatic because volvulus supervenes, owing to excessive mobility of bowel, or because aberrant bands compress a loop of intestine. Volvulus may occur in an apparently normal bowel or in a malrotated one.

This disastrous accident may occur in an infant whose small bowel has failed to re-enter the abdominal cavity in normal fashion and whose mesenteric attachments have not developed properly (see p. 348). The midgut lies free, attached to the posterior abdominal wall at only two points, the duodenum and the proximal colon, and may therefore twist on this narrow axis in either direction. However, when volvulus occurs, it usually does so in a clockwise direction. It may twist only a few degrees or may make as many as three or four complete turns upon itself. Kinking of the entering bowel or of the emergent segment or of both may follow, but the point of obstruction is almost always at the duodenojejunal junction. The circulation to the twisted segment is often obstructed and leads to rapid development of gangrene.

Diagnosis. Diagnosis depends on sudden onset of vomiting and rapid development of distention. Vomiting may not begin at birth, as an infant is rarely born with volvulus, but may be delayed until the third or fourth day in the early cases and until a month or more in the late ones, or it may start at any time in between. Once begun, vomiting usually occurs after every feeding. The vomitus is bile-stained. The degree of distention depends firstly on the tightness of

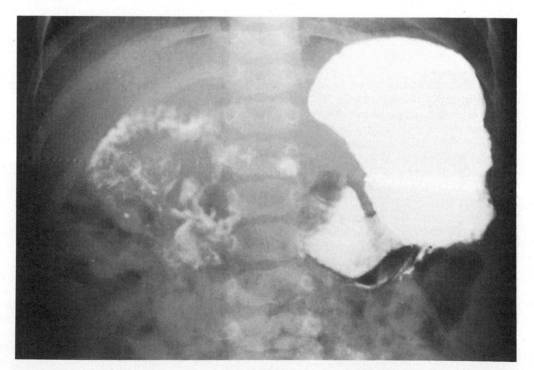

Figure 37–7. Irrefutable evidence for malrotation by upper gastrointestinal series. The body of the stomach is properly placed, but the duodenum wanders far to the right. No ligament of Treitz (duodenojejunal flexure) was seen on films or by fluoroscopy. The upper end of the midgut mesentery is therefore neither properly placed nor properly fixed, and malrotation is present. Shown here is the film of a 6-month-old boy; the findings would be the same in the newborn.

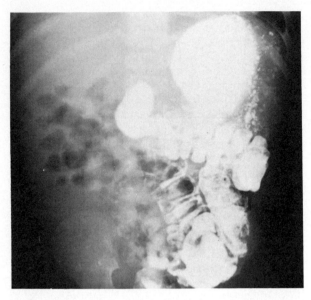

Figure 37–8. Unequivocal malrotation, proved by the presence of the cecum and appendix in the left lower quadrant; the lower end of the midgut mesentery is therefore improperly located. There is also barium in the stomach, but the duodenum and ligament of Treitz are not shown. Same case as that illustrated in Figure 37–7.

the volvulus and the consequent completeness or incompleteness of the obstruction and secondly on how recently vomiting with decompression of the stomach and duodenum has occurred. Since obstruction is often incomplete, all gradations of distention are seen.

Clinically, midgut volvulus must be suspected in any infant with bile-stained vomitus and evidence of incomplete obstruction at the duodenal level. There are even recorded instances of what appears to be complete obstruction at the duodenal level and no air distal to this point, with complete volvulus of the midgut. Compromise of the bowel secondary to the volvulus leads to evidence of peritonitis, sepsis, and shock.

Radiographs of the abdomen are variable. One usually sees not quite complete obstruction in the third or fourth portion of the duodenum with moderate dilatation of the stomach and sparse, scattered accumulations of air in the small bowel. For the rest, the abdomen appears full and homogeneously hazy. Barium introduced by enema may fail to penetrate beyond the transverse colon if the emergent loop is obstructed. If the radiopaque mixture reaches the cecum, it may demonstrate that this structure is displaced from its normal right lower quadrant location.

Treatment. Immediate operation is imperative in any case in which the diagnosis of midgut volvulus cannot be categorically excluded. The danger is not so much that of high intestinal obstruction with its resultant blood chemical dislocations, although this is great, but the rapid development of gangrene of a large segment of bowel due to the vascular constriction caused by the twisted mesentery. It is necessary for the surgeon to decide how much, if any, of the involved intestine is no longer viable and will have to be resected. Extensive resection renders an already serious prognosis more grave.

Inguinal Hernia

Herniated abdominal contents in the newborn may project into the thoracic cavity through the diaphragm, through the abdominal wall at the umbilicus or along the linea alba, through the inguinal ring, or into internal defects of the mesentery. Diaphragmatic hernia has been discussed (see p. 189). This variety seldom incarcerates. Umbilical hernia is also described (see p. 377). We have never seen one of these become incarcerated, although a few have been reported beyond the neonatal period. Internal hernias can be diagnosed only at the time of operation for intestinal obstruction. They too are extremely rare in the neonatal period.

Inguinal hernias, generally of the indirect variety, are not at all an uncommon finding in the nursery or later in the neonate. Boys are affected much more often than girls. The right side is involved more frequently than the left, and bilateral hernias are found not uncommonly. The hernia may be complete or scrotal, abdominal contents descending into a wide-open funicular peritoneal process to fill the scrotum completely. Alternatively, it may be funicular, descending only to some point above the testis where the tunica vaginalis is sealed off. Other varieties, such as direct or femoral, are only rarely encountered.

Diagnosis may rest entirely upon detection of a mass in the inguinal region or within the scrotum. The mass generally appears intermittently, coming out after crying or straining and withdrawing during periods of sleep or inactivity. Later, it may remain visible and palpable constantly. Many of these infants are extraordinarily irritable, crying as though in pain much of the day and night, for as long as 2 or 3 weeks before the hernia becomes apparent. This circumstance undoubtedly has given rise to the lay belief that excessive crying causes hernia. It is probable that the reverse is true.

Anorexia and inordinate crying may be the earliest signs of incarceration; vomiting, distention, blood and mucus in the stools, and an irreducible mass in the inguinal region indicate strangulation.

Differential diagnosis from hydrocele is occasionally difficult. Hydrocele of the testis should not present much trouble, since in this disorder the enlargement clearly encompasses the testis, which can no longer be palpated, and the fluid-filled sac transilluminates brilliantly. In scrotal hernia, the testis can be felt at the bottom of the mass, the whole is generally reducible, and light does not traverse it nearly so brightly. Hydrocele of the cord within the inguinal canal is often harder to differentiate, especially if a funicular hernia here is incarcerated and irreducible. Fortunately for one's conscience, hydrocele and this form of herniation often coexist, so that exploratory operation can be advised without too much hesitation if one remains in doubt after careful examination and after attempted reduction has failed.

The mass in the inguinal canal occasionally proves to be a gonad. A few cases are on record in which the gonad discovered high in the inguinal canal turns out to be one of the sex opposite to that indicated by the conformation of the external genitals. Thus, a number of apparently female infants have been reported in whom the inguinal gonad was discovered to be testis. This situation is discussed in Chapter 56.

Treatment.   The accepted method of dealing with inguinal hernia is to advise operation. This must of course be performed as an emergency if the mass cannot be reduced. If it can, one may wait a few days for a time suitable to the parents, but no longer. The danger of incarceration and strangulation hangs over one always, and the hazard of elective herniorrhaphy is so slim that procrastination is not to be condoned.

When hernias are found in infants in whom general anesthesia poses a risk, such as premature infants with bronchopulmonary dysplasia, it is our practice to temporize. A useful way of reducing an inguinal hernia is to invert the child. Only if it does not reduce during this maneuver do we consider operation urgent.

Because hernia often appears later on the opposite side, more and more surgeons are exploring the other inguinal region after the first one has been repaired and repairing that side too if the vaginal process is open. In 40 per cent of the cases, it will be open, and, without surgical repair, one half of these would go on to develop hernia within months or years (Rowe et al., 1969).

White and his collaborators make a strong case in favor of performing inguinal herniography in children admitted for unilateral hernia in order to outline the opposite peritoneal sac. They believe that if this is also open, the potential hernia should be repaired with the overt one.

Annular Pancreas

Annular pancreas is a thin flat ring of pancreatic tissue that surrounds the second part of the duodenum distal to the ampulla of Vater. The ring of normal pancreatic tissue merges with the head of the pancreas. It usually contains a duct that joins Wirsung's duct or, on occasion, empties by other orifices into the duodenum.

Incidence.   In 1954, Kiesewetter and Koop were able to discover 74 cases of annular pancreas in the literature and added six of their own. They com-

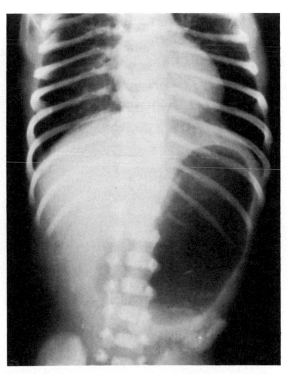

Figure 37–9. The supine plain anteroposterior film shows a hugely dilated stomach and a small bubble lying to its right that is the shadow of dilated first portion of the duodenum. No air is to be seen elsewhere in the abdomen. The diagnosis of complete duodenal obstruction can be made, but its cause, annular pancreas, had to be discovered at operation.

mented that the condition had been described with regularity only in the preceding 10 years and suggested that it may be more common than this small total number suggests. By 1956, Frucht found the number to have increased to 100. Between 1938 and 1977 at Children's Hospital in Boston, 36 cases were seen. It is discovered considerably more often in adults than in newborns, Rickham reporting a ratio of nearly nine older patients to one newborn. Males are affected much more frequently than females. Rarely, it may appear in siblings.

Diagnosis.   It must be remembered that annular pancreas (1) may not constrict the duodenum at all, (2) may constrict the duodenum sufficiently to produce duodenal stenosis, or (3) may completely block the duodenum. Thus, it may cause no symptoms or it may simulate duodenal stenosis or duodenal atresia. Actual stenosis or atresia of duodenum is present in about 40 per cent of infants with annular pancreas. Other congenital defects such as Down syndrome or heart disease may be associated with annular pancreas.

Antenatal ultrasonography in mothers with hydramnios may permit diagnosis of duodenal obstruction. Postnatal radiographs may show the "double

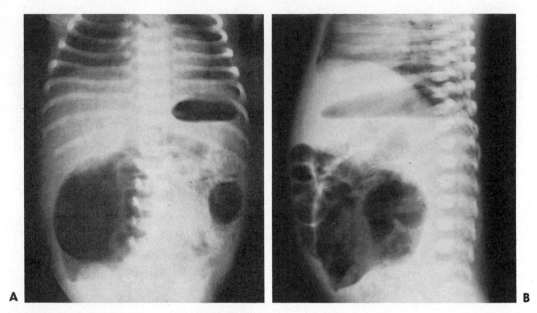

Figure 37–10. *A,* Anteroposterior view of abdomen in the erect position. A bizarre gas pattern is seen in which one can distinguish stomach, with fluid level, and a sparse scattering of gas throughout the small bowel. A large gas bubble filling the right side proved at operation to be a duplicated segment of colon. A smaller one on the left is probably a dilated loop of small bowel. *B,* Lateral view.

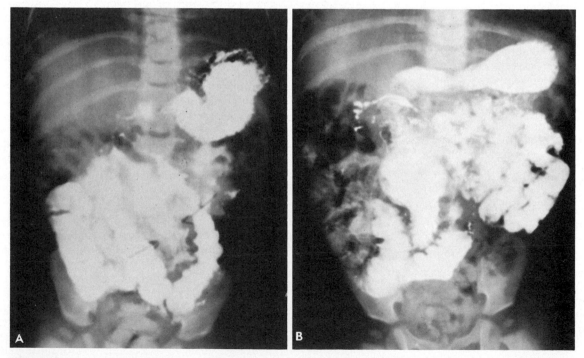

Figure 37–11. Films of barium-filled stomach and bowel show a persistent abnormality of pattern below the stomach. *A,* The pyloric cap is filled, but beyond this the duodenum appears to be almost empty. *B,* This same hiatus is apparent, and at this time the stomach seems to be flattened from below by some ill-defined mass. The duplicated segment of small bowel discovered at operation must have lain immediately caudad to the stomach, displacing it upward and normal small intestine downward.

bubble." Differentiation from duodenal atresia can only be made at operation.

Treatment. Since one of the major pancreatic ducts may be present in the ring, transection of the constricting ring is not advised. The operation of choice is a bypass procedure such as a side-to-side isoperistaltic duodenojejunostomy or a duodeno-duodenostomy. Some infants may have a several-week delay in recovery of normal bowel function and require intravenous alimentation during that interval.

Duplication of Small Intestine

Duplication cysts may be attached to the duodenal wall and are often imbedded in the pancreas. Occasionally, the cyst is lined with gastric mucosa, and peptic ulceration has been described, although the cysts are more commonly lined with intestinal mucosa. They can vary in size and be asymptomatic or obstruct the duodenum.

The majority of duplications are associated with jejunum and ileum. In a report of 246 instances of alimentary tract duplications tabulated by Wrenn, 129 were jejunal and ileal, 43 mediastinal, 35 colonic, 13 rectal, 13 gastric, 8 thoracoabdominal, and 5 cervical.

The diagnosis depends on size and location of the duplication. The ileal-jejunal duplications are within the mesentery and thus, when palpable, are freely movable. Signs of intestinal obstruction may be present, and bleeding can mimic that of Meckel's diverticulum. If pain is prominent, then volvulus or intussusception may be present. Radiographs may help identify displacement of normal structures. Sometimes, vertebral anomalies are present. Septate or double urinary tract structures may also occur as a part of the abortive twinning process that has been evoked to explain these anomalies. Radioisotope scans with technetium are useful ways to identify aberrant gastric mucosa. Ultrasonography and computerized axial tomography may help in preoperative evaluation.

Some tubular duplications communicate with the intestinal lumen at one or more points. All cysts and duplications can become pivotal sites for volvulus, intussusception, or, rarely, malignant change. For these reasons, surgical removal is advised once they are detected. Complete excision of the cyst and attached bowel may be required. If the duplication is very long and resection of that much bowel is contraindicated, the mucosa of the anomalous bowel can be stripped through multiple enterotomies. The remaining muscle coat will not present a problem.

REFERENCES

Agerty, H. A., Ziserman, A. J., and Shollenberger, C. L.: Perforation of the ileum in a newborn. J. Pediatr. *22*:233, 1943.

Aranda, J. V., Stern, L., and Dunbar, J. S.: Pneumothorax with pneumoperitoneum in a newborn infant. Am. J. Dis. Child. *123*:163, 1972.

Beck, W. C., and Chohany, G.: Duodenal atresia. J. Pediatr. *42*:432, 1953.

Boles, E. T., Vassy, L. E., and Ralston, M.: Atresia of the colon. J. Pediatr. Surg. *11*:69, 1976.

Boles, G. T., and Smith, B.: Preduodenal portal vein. Pediatrics *28*:805, 1961.

Boyden, E. A., Cope, J. A., and Bill, A. H., Jr.: Anatomy and embryology of congenital intrinsic obstruction of the duodenum. Am. J. Surg. *114*:190, 1967.

Browne, D.: Congenital deformities of the anus and rectum. Arch. Dis. Child. *30*:42, 1955.

Chamberlain, J. W.: Partial intestinal obstruction in the newborn due to kinking of the proximal small bowel. N. Engl. J. Med. *275*:1241, 1966.

DeLorimier, A. A., Fonkalsrud, E. W., and Hays, D. M.: Congenital atresia and stenosis of the jejunum and ileum. Surgery *65*:819, 1969.

Di Sant' Agnese, P. A., Dische, Z., and Danilczenko, A.: Physicochemical differences of mucoproteins in duodenal fluid of patients with cystic fibrosis of the pancreas and controls. Pediatrics *19*:252, 1957.

Donnison, A. B., Shwachman H., and Gross, R. E.: A review of 164 children with meconium ileus seen at the Children's Hospital Medical Center, Boston. Pediatrics *37*:833, 1966.

Effmann, E. L., Griscom, N. T., Colodny, A. H., and Vawter, G. F. Neonatal gastrointestinal masses arising late in gestation. Am. J. Roentgenol. *135*:681, 1980.

el-Shafie, M., and Rickham, P. P.: Multiple intestinal atresias. J. Pediatr. Surg. *5*:655, 1970.

Favara, B. E., Franciosi, R. A., and Akers, D. R.: Enteric duplications, 37 cases: a vascular theory of pathogenesis. Am. J. Dis. Child. *122*:501, 1971.

Frucht, D. A.: Annular pancreas in infancy. Am. J. Dis. Child. *92*:182, 1956.

Gross, R. E.: An Atlas of Children's Surgery. Philadelphia, W. B. Saunders Co., 1970.

Gross, R. E., Holcomb, G. W., and Farber, S.: Duplications of the alimentary tract. Pediatrics *9*:449, 1952.

Gryboski, J.: Gastrointestinal Problems in the Infant. Philadelphia, W. B. Saunders Co., 1975.

Guttmann, F. M., Braum, P., Garance, P. H., et al.: Multiple atresias and a new syndrome of hereditary multiple atresias involving the gastrointestinal tract from stomach to rectum. J. Pediatr. Surg. *8*:633, 1973.

Holder, T. M., and Leape, L. L.: The acute surgical abdomen in the neonate. N. Engl. J. Med. *278*:605, 1968.

Holsclaw, D. S., Eckstein, H. B., and Nixon, H. H.: Meconium ileus. A 20 year review of 109 cases (1944–1964). Am. J. Dis. Child. *109*:101, 1965.

Hyde, J. S.: Congenital duodenal atresia in four sibs. J. A. M. A. *191*:52, 1965.

Kalayoglu, M., Sieber, W., Rodnan, J. B., and Kiesewetter, W. B.: Meconium ileus: A critical review of treatment and eventual prognosis. J. Pediatr. Surg. *6*:290, 1971.

Kiesewetter, W. B.: Imperforate anus. In Holder, T. M., and Ashcraft, K. W. (Eds): Pediatric Surgery. Philadelphia, W. B. Saunders Co., 1980.

Kiesewetter, W. B., and Hoon, A.: Imperforate anus: an analysis of mortalities during a 25 year period. Progr. Pediatr. Surg. *13*:211, 1979.

Kiesewetter, W. B., and Koop, C. W.: Annular pancreas in infancy. Surgery *36*:146, 1954.

Lee, C. M., Jr., and MacMillan, B. G.: Rupture of the bowel in the newborn infant. Surgery *28*:48, 1950.

Martin, L. W., and Zerella, J. T.: Jejunoileal atresia: a proposed classification. J. Pediatr. Surg. *11*:399, 1976.

McPartlin, J. F., Dickson, J. A. S., and Swain, V. A. J.: Meconium ileus: Immediate and long-term survival. Arch. Dis. Child. *47*:207, 1973.

Mishalany, H. G., Der Kaloustian, I. M., and Ghandour, M.: Familial congenital duodenal atresia. Pediatrics *47*:629, 1970.

Montgomery, R. C., Poindexter, M. H., Hall, G., and Leigh, J. E.: Report of a case of annular pancreas of the newborn in two consecutive siblings. Pediatrics 48:148, 1971.

Neuhauser, E. B. D.: Roentgen changes associated with pancreatic insufficiency in early life. Radiology 46:319, 1946.

Noblett, H. R.: Treatment of uncomplicated meconium ileus by Gastrografin enema: a preliminary report. J. Pediatr. Surg. 4:180, 1969.

Orr, M. M., and Edwards, A. J.: Neoplastic change in duplications of the alimentary tract. Br. J. Surg. 62:269, 1975.

Potts, W. J.: The Surgeon and the Child. Philadelphia, W. B. Saunders Co., 1959.

Prouty, M., and Waskow, W. L.: Duodenal compression by the mesenteric artery. J. Pediatr. 50:734, 1957.

Rickham, P. P.: Annular pancreas in the newborn. Arch. Dis. Child. 29:80, 1954.

Rowe, M. I., Copelson, L. W., and Clatworthy, H. W.: The patent process vaginalis and the inguinal hernia. J. Pediatr. Surg. 4:102, 1969.

Rowe, M. I., Furst, A. J., et al.: The neonatal response to Gastrografin enema. Pediatrics 48:20, 1971.

Santulli, T. V.: The treatment of imperforate anus and associated fistulae. Surg. Gynecol. Obstet. 95:601, 1952.

Scott, J. E. S.: Intestinal obstruction in the newborn associated with peritonitis. Arch. Dis. Child. 38:120, 1963.

Shrand, H.: Vomiting in utero with intestinal atresia: Pediatrics 49:767, 1972.

Shwachman, H., and Antonowicz, I.: Studies on meconium. In Lebenthal, E. (Ed.): Textbook of Gastroenterology and Nutrition in Infancy. New York, Raven Press, 1981.

Shwachman, H., Antonowicz, I., Mahmoodian, A., and Ishida, S.: An approach to screening tests to detect cystic fibrosis. Am. J. Dis. Child. 132:1112, 1978.

Silverman, F. N., and Caffey, J.: Congenital obstructions of the alimentary tract in infants and children: Errors of rotation of the midgut. Radiology 53:780, 1949.

Small, W. T., and Berman, C. Z.: Annular pancreas producing obstruction in infancy. N. Engl. J. Med. 251:191, 1954.

Stewart, D. R., Colodny, A. L., and Daggett, W. C.: Malrotation of the bowel in infants and children. A 15 year review. Surgery 79:716, 1976.

Teja, K., Schnatterly, P., and Shaw, A.: Multiple intestinal atresias: pathology and pathogenesis. J. Pediatr. Surg. 16:194, 1981.

Touloukian, R. J.: Intestinal atresia. Clin. Perinatol. 5:3, 1978.

Touloukian, R. J.: Intestinal atresia and stenosis. In Holder, T. M., and Ashcraft, K. (Eds.): Pediatric Surgery. Philadelphia, W. B. Saunders Co., 1980.

Touloukian, R. J., and Wright, H. F.: Intrauterine villus hypertrophy with jejunal atresia. J. Pediatr. Surg. 8:779, 1973.

Tucker, A. S., Soine, L., and Izant, R. J., Jr.: Gastrointestinal perforations in infancy. Am. J. Roentgenol. 123:755, 1975.

Waggett, J., Bishop, H. C., and Koop, C. E.: Experience with Gastrografin enema in the treatment of meconium ileus. J. Pediatr. Surg. 5:649, 1970.

Waggett, J., Johnson, P. G., et al.: The nonoperative treatment of meconium ileus by Gastrografin enema. J. Pediatr. 77:407, 1970.

White, J. J., Parks, L. C., and Haller, J. A.: The inguinal herniogram: a radiologic aid for accurate diagnosis of inguinal hernia in infants. Surgery 63:991, 1968.

Wrenn, E. L.: Alimentary tract duplications. In Holder, T. M., and Ashcraft, K. (Eds.): Pediatric Surgery. Philadelphia, W. B. Saunders Co., 1980, p. 445.

Young, W. F., Swain, V., and Pringle, E. M.: Long-term prognosis after major resection of the small bowel in early infancy. Arch. Dis. Child. 44:465, 1969.

38

ACQUIRED INTESTINAL OBSTRUCTION

Necrotizing Enterocolitis

Although this problem has been noted for many years, it has come into sharper focus since the publication of the first comprehensive studies of the condition, reported from Babies' Hospital in New York during 1964 and 1965 by Mizrahi and colleagues. A more complete description of a longer experience was summarized by Santulli and coworkers in 1975 and by Kliegman and Fanaroff in 1981. In earlier editions of this book, we discussed pneumatosis intestinalis and *Pseudomonas* enteritis, both of which would probably be presented as necrotizing enterocolitis today.

Incidence. The incidence varies in the same center year by year, giving the impression of being an epidemic disease. It also varies between centers for reasons that are not clear, except that it is much more common among infants whose birth weight is less than 1500 grams. Stoll and colleagues in Atlanta reported necrotizing enterocolitis in 66 per every 1000 livebirths weighing less than 1500 grams between July, 1977 and February, 1979. Males and females are equally affected.

Pathogenesis. No clear sequence of events common to all infants with enterocolitis has been found. Most have been born prematurely, many have had perinatal asphyxia, and some have had sepsis and shock. Many have had umbilical artery or venous catheters. The possibility of bowel ischemia, aggravated by colonization with potential pathogens and subsequent feedings, is viewed as likely. Santulli suggested that the intestinal mucosal cells are injured by ischemia and stop secreting protective mucus. In-

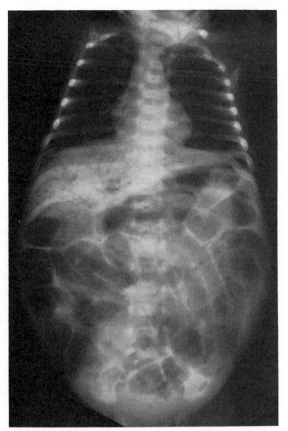

Figure 38–1. This film of the chest and abdomen, obtained because of abdominal distention and bloody stools 5 days after birth, shows extensive gaseous distention of the intestines. The distention clearly involves the small bowel and probably involves the colon as well. Fine linear lucencies projected over the left side of the abdomen represent either intramural gas (pneumatosis intestinalis) or gas in the smaller tributaries of the mesenteric veins. The most striking finding is in the liver; the branching lucent shadows are cast by gas widely distributed in the intrahepatic branches of the portal vein. The radiologic findings strongly support the clinical impression of necrotizing enterocolitis. Born at 1650 grams at a gestational age of 28 weeks.

vacion of the bowel wall by gas-forming microorganisms then allows their proliferation in the production of pneumatosis intestinalis, or hydrogen gas in the wall of the intestinal tract. Much speculation exists about the possible aggravation of the problem by cow's milk formula (in contrast to human milk) or hyperosmolar loads. In some instances formula feeding may upset a delicate balance, but in others we have seen enterocolitis in infants whose only nutrition was human milk.

Bacteria isolated from these infants are the ones commonly found in intensive care nurseries, such as *Escherichia coli, Klebsiella, Aerobacter,* and *Pseudomonas. Clostridium difficile* may produce a pseudomembranous colitis in some of these infants. Attempts to treat the disease with antibiotics have led to equivocal results.

Clinical Aspects. The earliest sign of impending enterocolitis is onset of abdominal distention after the initiation of oral feeding, usually on the third to fifth

day of life but as late as 1 month. The age of onset is inversely related to gestational age, perhaps because very small infants do not start oral feedings as early as larger ones. Sometimes the infants seem less active. Their color may be poor, and, with progression of the disease, sepsis and shock may ensue. The organism most commonly recovered from blood cultures is *E. coli.* Careful monitoring of abdominal events by serial radiographs is necessary to identify bowel perforations. Since the infants have functional intestinal obstruction, they may vomit bile-stained material. Stools are usually few but sometimes blood-streaked.

Laboratory Findings. A low granulocyte count may be present. Thrombocytopenia, probably caused by increased destruction, is the rule. A sudden drop in platelet count is a poor prognostic sign. In severely ill infants, disseminated intravascular coagulation may be present.

Radiologic Diagnosis. The findings are intestinal distention, intramural air, ascites, intrahepatic portal venous gas, and, if rupture has occurred, pneumoperitoneum.

Treatment. We discontinue all oral intake and initiate intravenous alimentation (see Chapter 89). Antibiotics are given on the basis of the sensitivities of organisms cultured from the blood or stool, although there is no evidence that in the absence of sepsis antibiotics alter the course. A nasogastric tube is helpful in preventing gastric distention from swallowed air

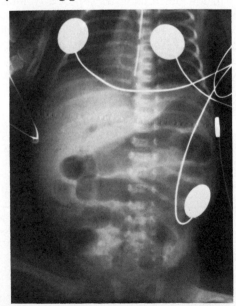

Figure 38–2. This 800-gram infant had massive distention of the abdomen. The thickened bowel walls, some with interstitial air, are characteristic of necrotizing enterocolitis. Air in the biliary tree is a late and ominous finding. This infant died a few hours after this film was taken.

or gastric secretions. Consultation with a surgeon should be undertaken once the diagnosis is suspected, since bowel necrosis with perforations may require immediate intervention. Occasionally, necrotic sections of bowel may require resection, and gastrostomy may be necessary to decompress the bowel. Strictures of the intestine may develop in colon or ileum at a later date and require resection.

Prognosis. Necrotizing enterocolitis is a serious disease. In the first series described, the rate of mortality was about 75 per cent. With wider recognition of the problem, earlier diagnosis, and use of intravenous alimentation, the mortality rate is under 20 per cent. In a given infant, consideration of degree of prematurity and associated problems affects prognosis. Early diagnosis and prompt cessation of oral feedings should further reduce the mortality.

Intussusception

Intussusception is the invagination of one loop of bowel into a loop distal to it. The proximal segment, the intussusceptum, enters the distal portion, the intussuscipiens, as the tip of a glove finger may be inverted and pushed inside out up the length of the finger. The intussusceptum then travels down the bowel for a variable distance, at times reaching and even extruding from the anus. Intussusceptions usually originate in the ileum, although they may arise from the jejunum or the colon. Their danger lies only partially in the obstruction they produce. More important is intestinal gangrene from compression of the blood vessels that are carried along with the intussusceptum.

Incidence. Although intussusception is a common cause of intestinal obstruction in infants, mostly male, 6 to 18 months old, it is extremely rare in the first month of life. Rachelson and coworkers, in 1955, were able to find reports of only 28 cases in newborns in the past 150 years. It has been described in a fetus (Ravitch, 1979).

Table 38–1. Intussusception—Symptoms*

Symptom	Recorded	Not Present	No Mention
Vomiting	20	2	1
As first symptom	14		
Bile staining	9		
Blood in stools	17	2	4
As first symptom	11		
Screaming	5		
As first symptom	4		
As only symptom	1		
Mass felt per rectum	2		
Mass felt abdominally	4		

* Symptoms have not been recorded in three cases.

Table 38–2. Intussusception—Symptoms (Continued)

Age at First Symptom	Number
Up to 48 hours	15
Up to 1 week	5
Up to 1 month	4
Total	24
Died soon after birth	1
Unusual presentation	1

Etiology. An obvious lead point is discovered in 6 to 8 per cent of all cases in most series, much less commonly in infants than in children and adults. These consist of Meckel's diverticula, polyps, intraluminal cysts, duplications, and foci of lymphoid hyperplasia. A number of investigators have found an adenovirus in cultures from infants with intussusception much more often than from controls, and they postulate lymphoid hyperplasia as the trigger lead point. For the remainder, no good reason has been advanced.

Diagnosis. The cardinal symptoms of intussusception in infants are intermittent vomiting, a nondistended abdomen with a mass, usually in the right lower quadrant, and the passage of blood or blood-stained mucus through the rectum.

Talwalker, in 1962, reviewed painstakingly the case histories of 16 newborns with intussusception reported in the British literature and nine more unreported cases from English hospitals, and he added one of his own. Vomiting and blood in the stools were almost always, but by no means always, present, whereas pain and palpable mass were almost always missing. Eight of 26 arose in the jejunum, an unusually high proportion of jejunals to ileocecals (Tables 38–1 to 38–4).

Radiography, in the newborn as in the older infant, reveals a characteristic picture. Flat films show the usual evidences of obstruction in the form of dilated loops of small intestine above and relative airlessness below the level of obstruction. Barium enema shows the column of opaque fluid to end in a meniscus, with a coiled-spring pattern extending just proximal to the meniscus.

Prognosis. Most of the reported patients died. This unfortunate result has often been due to the fact that the classic signs of intussusception have not all been present. The realization that this is the usual state of affairs in the newborn would without doubt lead to a greater awareness of the possibility, hence to more vigorous diagnostic efforts and probably to a higher percentage of cure. *The passage by a newborn of*

Table 38–3. Intussusception—Treatment

	Total	Alive	Dead
Resection	12	6	6
Reduction	10	7	3

blood or blood-stained mucus, without cause in the anus or rectum, calls for proctoscopic inspection and a barium enema study.

Treatment. Rarely, a patient may go on to spontaneous cure by sloughing of the entire intussusception and autoanastomosis. In the case reported by Rachelson and coworkers, sloughing took place, and the gangrenous mass of inverted bowel was passed by rectum after nothing more than a few hours of anorexia! In this instance, autoanastomosis did not follow, and anastomosis had to be accomplished later operatively.

The initial treatment of choice is operation after attempted reduction of the intussusception by hydrostatic pressure of a barium mixture under the fluoroscope. Barium enema reduction alone is successful in a large number of cases occurring in older infants, but in infants less than 6 months old it is often unsuccessful. Zachary compiled some interesting figures pertinent to this problem. The percentage of cure by barium enema was not high in the younger babies. Nevertheless, the partial reduction obtained by hydrostatic pressure is useful in that it renders the subsequent operative procedure less traumatic, since much less "milking" of the bowel is required before reduction is accomplished. Talwalker's results with reduction in newborns were by no means bad. Unfortunately, the authors of some of the largest recent reviews, such as Gierup and associates, who report hydrostatic reduction successful in 81 per cent of 319 attempts—85 per cent if performed within 12 hours of onset—do not separate newborns from other infants and children.

Hayes and Gwinn have recalled to our attention the hazards of delay in arriving at the correct diagnosis, and they remind us that *barium enema under fluoroscopy for diagnosis and possible reduction is not permissible as an office procedure. It should only be undertaken in a setting in which a surgeon is standing by.*

Peritoneal Adhesions

Obstruction may follow the development of adhesions between one hollow viscus and another as a result of healed peritonitis of any kind. Inflammation may have resulted from bacterial infection, chemical irritation, such as bile peritonitis, mechanical irritation, such as talc peritonitis, or previous laparotomy.

This variety of intestinal obstruction requires no further comment.

Mesenteric Thrombosis

Thrombosis of the mesenteric veins has been a well-recognized entity in adults since the 1940s. Pathologists have called our attention to mesenteric arterial thrombosis, most often involving the superior mesenteric artery, for almost as long. In the newborn we encounter both: the venous form almost always secondary to abdominal inflammatory disease, perhaps with dehydration, shock, and increased blood viscosity playing a role; and the arterial form to emboli, either septic or nonseptic, perhaps arising in the contracting ductus arteriosus. In the past decade, this syndrome has surely been initiated by umbilical artery catheterization, a complication found not infrequently by both Kitterman and his associates and Neal and his. Fortunately, only a few of these become symptomatic. Infants of poorly controlled diabetics are susceptible to thromboses in many organs, one of which is the mesentery (Oppenheimer and Avery, 1968).

In 1953, Rothschild and coworkers reported a case of intestinal obstruction due to mesenteric artery occlusion in a newborn in whom no lesion was found that could have initiated the process. The child was born by breech at term. His condition was precarious during the first day, with flaccidity, cyanosis and subnormal temperature, gallop rhythm, and enlarged heart. He improved for a few days but on the fifth day began to vomit, and progressive jaundice and increasing distention developed. Barium meal series was interpreted as showing multiple obstructions, and laparotomy was performed. The peritoneal cavity contained much greenish fluid. Most of the small bowel was gangrenous with scattered areas of plastic exudate. No peristalsis was seen, and no arterial pulsation could be felt in the mesentery. The superior mesenteric artery was found after death to contain a tight thrombus formed before death.

Prevention and Treatment. The condition is so rare that no systematic approach to treatment has been undertaken. It would seem prudent to try to

Table 38–4. Intussusception—Types*

Type of Intussusception	Number	Method of Treatment			Causative Lesion
		Reduction	*Resection*	*None*	
Ileocecal	12	6	3	3	1
Jejunal	8	2	6	—	4
Ileal	3	2	1	—	1
Colic	1	—	1	—	—
Site not mentioned	2				

* Tables 38–1 through 38–4 modified from Talwalker, Y. C.: Arch. Dis. Child. 37:203, 1962.

prevent the problem by appropriate hydration of the infant. (Some instances have been described in association with dehydration and diarrhea.) Better control of diabetes in pregnancy has been associated with fewer complications, including venous thromboses.

Once the lesion is suspected, correction of hemoconcentration is mandatory, and consultation with a pediatric surgeon is appropriate to discuss timing of surgical exploration.

REFERENCES

Barlow, B., Santulli, T. V., et al.: An experimental study of acute neonatal enterocolitis. The importance of breast milk. J. Pediatr. Surg. 9:587, 1974.

Book, L. S., Herbst, J. J., and Jung, A. L.: Carbohydrate malabsorption in necrotizing enterocolitis. Pediatrics 57:201, 1976.

Brown, E. G., and Sweet, A. Y.: Neonatal Necrotizing Enterocolitis. New York, Grune and Stratton, Inc., 1980.

Case Records of the Massachusetts General Hospital. Case 45–1973. N. Engl. J. Med. 289:1027, 1973.

Clark, E. J., Phillips, I. A., and Alexander, E. P.: Adenovirus infection in intussusception in children in Taiwan. J.A.M.A. 208:1671, 1969.

Clatworthy, H. W., Jr., Howard, W. H. R., and Lloyd, J.: The meconium plug syndrome. Surgery 39:131, 1956.

Danis, R. K.: Surgical Hazards with Hydrogen Peroxide. Presented at the Thirty-fifth Annual Meeting of the American Academy of Pediatrics, Surgical Section, Oct. 23, 1966.

Emery, J. L.: Abnormalities in meconium of the foetus and newborn. Arch. Dis. Child. 32:17, 1957.

Frantz, I. D., L'Heureux, P., Engel, R. R., and Hunt C. E.: Necrotizing enterocolitis. J. Pediatr. 86:259, 1975.

Gierup, J., Jorulf, H., and Livaditis, A.: Management of intussusception in infants and children: A survey based on 288 consecutive cases. Pediatrics 50:535, 1972.

Hallum, J. L., and Hatchuel, W. L. F.: Congenital paralytic ileus in a premature baby as a complication of hexamethonium bromide therapy for toxaemia of pregnancy. Arch. Dis. Child. 29:354, 1954.

Hayes, D. M., and Gwinn, J. L.: The changing face of intussusception. J. A.M.A. 195:817, 1966.

Hinden, E.: Meconium ileus with no pancreatic abnormality. Arch. Dis. Child. 25:99, 1950.

Kitterman, J. A., Phibbs, R. H., and Tooley, W. H.: Pediatr. Clin. North Am. 17:895, 1970.

Kliegman, R. M., and Fanaroff, A. A.: Neonatal necrotizing enterocolitis: A nine-year experience. Am. J. Dis. Child. 135:603, 1981.

Mayell, M. J.: Intussusception in infancy and childhood in Southern Africa. Arch. Dis. Child. 47:20, 1972.

Mizrahi, A., Barlow, O., Berdon, W., et al: Necrotizing enterocolitis in premature infants. J. Pediatr. 66:697, 1965.

Neal, W. A., Reynolds, J. W., et al.: Umbilical artery catheterization: Demonstration of arterial thrombosis by aortography. Pediatrics 50:6, 1972.

Necrotizing Enterocolitis in the Newborn Infant. Report of the Sixty-Eighth Ross Conference on Pediatric Research, Moore, T. D., ed. Columbus, Ohio, Ross Laboratories, 1975.

Oppenheimer, E. H., and Avery, M. E.: Clinical-pathological conference. J. Pediatr. 73:143, 1968.

Prouty, M., Bruskewitz, H. W., and Schwei, G. P.: Intussusception in a newborn infant. J. Pediatr. 34:487, 1949.

Rachelson, M. H., Jernigan, J. P., and Jackson, W. F.: Intussusception in the newborn infant with spontaneous expulsion of the intussusceptum. J. Pediatr. 47:87, 1955.

Ravitch, M. M.: Intussusception. In Pediatric Surgery 2. 3rd ed. Chicago, Yearbook Medical Publishers, 1979.

Rothschild, H. B., Storch, A., and Meyers, B.: Mesenteric occlusion in a newborn infant. J. Pediatr. 43:569, 1953.

Rowe, M. I., Copelson, L. W., and Clatworthy, H. W., Jr.: The patent processus vaginalis and the inguinal hernia. J. Pediatr. Surg. 4:102, 1969.

Santulli, T. V., Schullinger, J. N., Heird, W. C., et al.: Acute necrotizing enterocolitis in infancy: a review of 64 cases. Pediatrics 55:376, 1975.

Stoll, B. J., Kanto, W. P., Jr., Glass, R. I., et al.: Epidemiology of necrotizing enterocolitis: a case control study. J. Pediatr. 96:447, 1980.

Talwalker, V. C.: Intussusception in the newborn. Arch. Dis. Child. 37:203, 1962.

Zachary, R. B.: Meconium and faecal plugs in the newborn. Arch. Dis. Child. 32:22, 1957.

39

Hirschsprung's Disease

Revised with the assistance
of Harland S. Winter

Hirschsprung's Disease (Congenital Megacolon, Congenital Aganglionosis)

The etiology of Hirschsprung's disease has been reviewed briefly on page 349. The pathologic criterion, as well as the cause of constipation by virtue of its effect upon orderly peristalsis, is absence of ganglion cells of the plexus of Auerbach in a segment of the large bowel. Passarge's data indicate that in some examples there is a strong familial incidence of aganglionosis, and that in other families other major defects, chiefly Down syndrome, appear in excess, but that in most neither genetic nor chromosomal factors are discoverable.

Incidence. Congenital aganglionosis is one of the less common causes of neonatal intestinal obstruction but is by no means an extreme rarity. Between 1950 and 1960, Kottmeier and Clatworthy found that 41 such patients had been admitted to one hospital, all proved by biopsy, of which 85 per cent had become symptomatic within the first week of life. Forty-five per cent were admitted to the hospital for the first time before the age of 3 months.

Diagnosis. Vomiting, distention, and constipation are the usual presenting signs. Diarrhea is prominent in about one fifth of all cases; it may be intermittent, alternating with periods of constipation, or constant, with no constipation whatever. Diarrhea may also be associated with a form of severe, often lethal enterocolitis.

Vomiting often begins on the first day but may be delayed until the third day or later. Distention may reach an advanced stage, accompanied by intestinal patterning. Meconium stools are usually passed for a variable number of days before constipation appears and becomes obdurate.

A characteristic story is that no meconium is passed in the first 24 hours of life and signs of obstruction that may develop are relieved by enema. Thereafter, the infant may be symptom-free for a period as short as a week or as long as 10 weeks, when vomiting, distention, and constipation recur. This cycle may be repeated a number of times until the clinical and roentgenologic picture becomes typical of Hirschsprung's disease.

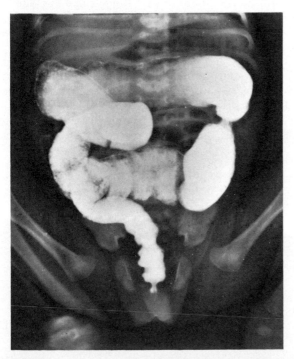

Figure 39–1. Film showing rectosigmoid narrowing and dilatation of colon above. Anorexia and vomiting began in this infant at 1 day of age; he was in hospital 10 days and went home apparently well. He was at home for 5 days, during which time he was anorexic and passed no stool whatever. No stool was found in the rectum, and the barium enema film taken on the thirtieth day of life is shown above. A Swenson procedure was performed. The patient died on the fifty-fourth day of severe ileocolitis, a not uncommon complication of this disease.

Confirmatory Evidence. Early radiographic study shows distended loops throughout the abdomen of both small and large bowel. In the erect posture, numerous fluid levels may be seen. Often, no point of obstruction can be distinguished. Barium enema fluid flows in freely and outlines a normal or slightly dilated rectosigmoid and colon. Only rarely in the first days or weeks of life does one see the characteristic narrowed rectosigmoid segment distal to a slightly dilated sigmoid segment, or the so-called pathognomonic "pigtail" sign. In Ehrenpreis' experience, the typical caliber differential did not become apparent until 3 or 4 weeks of age in most, and until 8 or 9 months in some.

Highly suggestive in the first weeks, however, is the demonstration that barium remains in the lower bowel for 24 hours or more.

Kottmeier and Clatworthy correctly warn us not to accept the radiologic evidence of caliber differential as an absolute indication for operation. In their own experience, several infants were operated upon mistakenly on that indication alone. In all of them, resected bowel showed an abundance of ganglion cells.

Tobon and coworkers have devised a comparatively simple manometric technique that graphically depicts the response of the internal sphincter to transient distention of the rectum by an inserted balloon. Technical advances have altered the apparatus, but the principles remain the same. In the normal situation, this sphincter relaxes after such distention (Fig. 39–2); in Hirschsprung's disease, it paradoxically contracts (Fig. 39–3). In so-called "functional constipation" resulting in "idiopathic megacolon," the sphincteric responses are absolutely normal. Although the manometric evidence may be supportive, some infants will have incomplete relaxation and results will be nondiagnostic.

The only certain method for the diagnosis of Hirschsprung's disease until recently has been the demonstration of absence of ganglion cells in a deep-muscle biopsy specimen of the rectum. Ganglion cells (Fig. 39–4) may be demonstrated by suction biopsy, which does not require anesthesia or an operative procedure. However, if ganglion cells are not found after serial sectioning, a full-thickness biopsy is needed. Some centers use cholinesterase stains to identify biopsies compatible with Hirschsprung's disease. In our experience, this stain is no more sensitive than a careful evaluation by a knowledgeable pathologist. But this technique too is subject to misinterpretation for a variety of reasons. Finding ganglion cells assures one that aganglionosis cannot be the correct diagnosis, but not seeing them may be a matter of too superficial a specimen, poor staining, or some other error.

When aganglionosis involves proximal segments of the colon or the small intestine, the diagnosis is even more difficult. In these instances, it will depend almost

RECTAL MANOMETRY

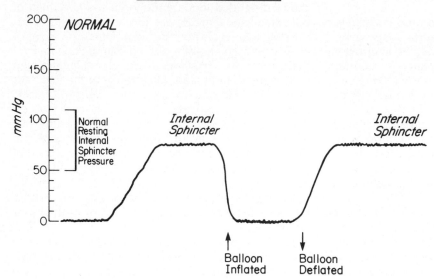

Figure 39–2. Tracing from rectal manometry in a normal infant. (Courtesy of Dr. H. Winter.)

entirely upon the pathologic picture of biopsied or autopsied intestine. Total bowel aganglionosis can occur. Vomitus containing stool or barium from a barium enema makes the diagnosis probable.

Treatment. Definitive treatment of Hirschsprung's disease is operative. For a number of years after Swenson perfected the pull-through operation, this was the only procedure used. Objections were then raised against it in view of persistent fecal incontinence, disturbances in bladder emptying and urinary incontinence in some of the survivors. The State operation, an end-to-end anastomosis of colon from

above the aganglionic segment to the upper portion of the rectum, and the Duhamel operation, which bypasses the rectum but leaves it in situ, were offered as substitutes. Many reports suggest that the latter is superior. The Soave procedure involves excision of the rectal mucosa, with suturing of proximal normal bowel to the denuded rectum.

Most pediatric surgeons are loath to perform definitive repair until the infant has reached the age of 8 months or more, preferring to temporize by performing a colostomy.

An explosive form of enterocolitis may complicate the course of Hirschsprung's disease at any time,

RECTAL MANOMETRY

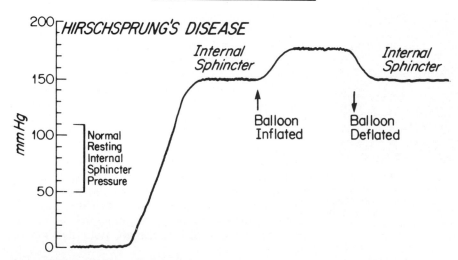

Figure 39–3. Note the elevated rectal pressures in an infant with Hirschsprung's disease. (Courtesy of Dr. H. Winter.)

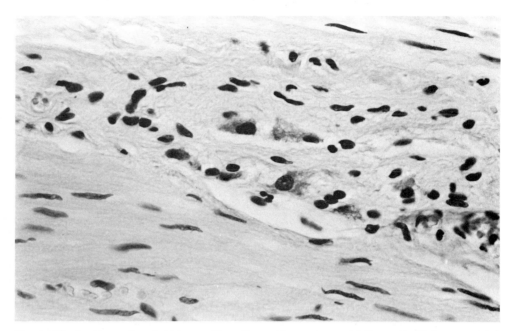

Figure 39–4. Normal rectal biopsy. Ganglion cells are pyramid-shaped with large nuclei. (Courtesy of Dr. H. Winter.)

even after an apparently successful operation. Its exact cause is unknown, but most agree with Swenson that the basic trouble is obstruction, which may contribute to ischemia or sepsis. In addition to rapid intravenous replacement therapy, rectal tubes and colonic irrigations must be used to empty the bowel on an emergency basis. Colostomy is required to relieve obstruction and put an end to the diarrhea.

REFERENCES

Campbell, P. E., and Noblett, H. R.: Experience with rectal suction biopsy in the diagnosis of Hirschsprung's disease. J. Pediatr. Surg. 4:410, 1969.

Duhamel, B.: A new operation for the treatment of Hirschsprung's disease. Arch. Dis. Child. 35:38, 1960.

Ehrenpreis, T.: Hirschsprung's disease in the neonatal period. Arch. Dis. Child. 30:8, 1955.

Hiatt, R. B.: A further description of the pathologic physiology of congenital megacolon and the results of surgical treatment. Pediatrics 21:825, 1958.

Kostia, J.: Results of treatment in Hirschsprung's disease. Arch. Dis. Child. 37:167, 1962.

Kottmeier, R. K., and Clatworthy, H. W., Jr.: Aganglionic and functional megacolon in children: A diagnostic dilemma. Pediatrics 36:572, 1965.

Livaditis, A.: Hirschsprung's disease: long-term results of the original Duhamel operation. J. Pediatr. Surg. 16:484, 1981.

Mahboubi, S., and Schnaufer, L.: The barium enema examination and rectal manometry in Hirschsprung disease. Radiology 130:643, 1979.

Martin, L. W.: Surgical management of total colonic aganglionosis. Ann. Surg. 176:343, 1972.

McDonald, R. G., and Evans, W. A., Jr.: Hirschsprung's disease: Roentgen diagnosis. A.M.A. J. Dis. Child. 87:575, 1954.

Morikawa, Y., Donahoe, P. K., and Hendren, W. H.: Manometry and histochemistry in the diagnosis of Hirschsprung's disease. Pediatrics 63:865, 1979.

Nixon, H. H.: Review article: Hirschsprung's disease. Arch. Dis. Child. 39:109, 1964.

Passarge, E.: The genetics of Hirschsprung's disease. N. Engl. J. Med. 276:138, 1967.

Potts, W. J., Boggs, J. D., and White, H.: Intestinal obstruction in the newborn infant due to agenesis of the myenteric plexus (congenital megacolon). Pediatrics 10:253, 1952.

Rehbein, F., and von Zimmermann, H.: Results with abdominal resection in Hirschsprung's disease. Arch. Dis. Child. 35:29, 1960.

Santulli, T. V.: Intestinal obstruction in the newborn. Bull. N.Y. Acad. Med. 33:175, 1957.

Soave, F.: Surgery of rectal anomalies with preservation of the relationship between the colonic muscular sleeve and the puborectalis muscle. J. Pediatr. Surg. 4:705, 1969.

Soper, R. T., and Figueroa, P.: Surgical treatment of Hirschsprung's disease: Comparison of modifications of the Duhamel and Soave operations. J. Pediatr. Surg. 6:761, 1971.

State, D.: Segmental colon resection in the treatment of congenital megacolon (Hirschsprung's disease). Au. J. Surg. 105:93, 1963.

Stockdale, E. M., and Miller, C. A.: Persistent diarrhea as the predominant symptom of Hirschsprung's disease (congenital dilatation of the colon); report of two cases. Pediatrics 19:91, 1957.

Swenson, O.: Congenital megacolon (Hirschsprung's disease); follow-up on eighty-two patients treated surgically. Pediatrics 8:542, 1951.

Tobon, F., Reid, N. C. R. W., Talbert, J. L., and Schuster, M. M.: Non-surgical test for the diagnosis of Hirschsprung's disease. N. Engl. J. Med. 278:188, 1968.

Tobon, F., and Shuster, M. M.: Megacolon: Special diagnostic and therapeutic features. Johns Hopkins Med. J. 135:91, 1974.

40

Disorders of the Umbilicus

General Considerations

The umbilical cord is a structure of the utmost importance to the fetus, serving as the sole channel bringing oxygen and nutriment to it and carrying from it carbon dioxide and waste products. Any accident that diminishes blood flow through this channel constitutes a grave hazard to the life or health of the fetus or newborn infant.

The prime danger in this regard is compression of the cord. This may take place when the cord, instead of floating freely within the amniotic fluid, becomes wrapped around the body, an extremity or the neck of the fetus. It may also follow when the cord is delivered before the baby, that is, in cases of prolapse of the cord. We must hastily point out the fact that looping about some portion of the fetus or being prolapsed does not necessarily mean that blood flow is impeded. In only a minority of these instances is looping so tight or is the prolapsed cord wedged so firmly between a fetal part and a bony prominence that true compression results. When it does, the obstetrician may note that the prolapsed portion, or the cord distal

to a tight loop, is pulseless. The effects of such asphyxia upon the brain and respiratory system of the newborn infant have been discussed in other sections. One might add here that a tight loop about the neck jeopardizes the fetus no more than one about the wrist if blood flow is completely obstructed. If less tight, it is conceivable that a loop about the neck might obstruct venous return, while arterial flow is not diminished. Venous congestion, petechial hemorrhages, and edema of the brain might be expected to follow, and this would have greater significance than similar congestive alterations in an extremity.

The second dangerous accident to the newborn is that the cord may tear during delivery. This catastrophy may result from a velamentous insertion of cord to placenta.

Although we do not understand what determines the length of the umbilical cord, great variations have been the cause of speculation for many years. Cord length in normal newborns was found by Purola to be 59 ± 12 cm, with a range of 22 to 130 cm. It has been thought that a cord of 35.5 cm is needed for normal progression of vaginal delivery without undue traction.

Miller and coworkers categorized events associated with cords under that length as follows: (a) intrauterine constraint before 6 weeks' gestation in association with amnion rupture, (b) limitation of movement in second trimester as in Potter's syndrome, and (c) structural limb dysfunction as in arthrogryposis.

Since it appears that cord length depends on in-

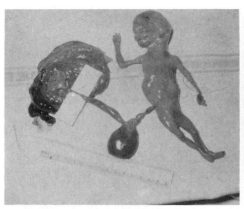

Fig. 40–1

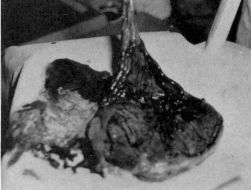

Fig. 40–2

Figure 40–1. Stillborn infant with umbilical cord and placenta attached. The cord is looped and is obstructed at the point of closure of the loop. The fetus is maldeveloped and macerated as a result.

Figure 40–2. Umbilical cord and placenta, showing the former's insertion into the latter after having divided into a number of fine branches. These branches in such a velamentous insertion are liable to be torn during delivery.

trauterine space and fetal movement, Miller and co-workers postulate that umbilical cord growth depends on tensile forces operating on it. Perhaps this fact is useful in the event of random cord entanglements, since linear growth could alleviate pressure.

The obvious clinical significance of a short cord noted in the delivery room is that it alerts the pediatrician to some condition that could have inhibited intrauterine movements before 30 weeks' gestation.

The umbilical region is an extremely busy locale during embryonic life. Originally the widely open communication between the yolk sac and primitive gut, it ends up as a narrow aperture through which course the umbilical artery and vein, the vitelline duct, and the urachus. In the interim the entire midgut has passed through it into a large physiologic umbilical hernia, has remained there some weeks, and has ultimately returned to take up its proper position within the abdominal cavity.

After birth, the umbilical arteries contract strongly, blood flow ceases, and their lumens become narrow. Persistent pulsations, when they occur, are usually associated with hypoxia. Their intimal and medial layers undergo aseptic necrosis, the stump separates, and granulation tissue develops and is quickly covered with epithelium.

It is our practice to ask the obstetricians to note the number of umbilical arteries on the page of information that accompanies each infant to the nursery, since the cord may dry quickly and make later identification uncertain. Single umbilical artery occurs in about 1 per cent of single births and 7 per cent of twin births. Associated abnormalities occur in about one third of the infants and include all systems, but gastrointestinal obstructive lesions are among the most common. The question remains as to what the pediatrician does once a single artery is noted. A meticulous search for all possible congenital defects is indicated, with particular care to palpate the kidneys at a time when the infant is relaxed and the stomach not distended. At least one urinalysis is mandatory. In recent years we have depended on ultrasonographic studies to identify genitourinary abnormali-ties. We also follow the infants with monthly urinalyses. Further radiographic evaluation depends on results of these studies.

Classification. A large number of developmental errors may lead to imperfections in the umbilical region at the time of birth, and the umbilicus is liable to other postnatal disorders. These will be discussed in the following order: (1) infection of the umbilicus, (2) septic umbilical arteritis, (3) granuloma of the umbilicus, (4) umbilical stomach, (5) omphalocele, (6) umbilical hernia, (7) congenital malformations of the vitelline (omphalomesenteric) duct, (8) congenital malformations of the urachus, and (9) single umbilical artery.

Infection of the Umbilicus

We have become accustomed in this aseptic age to consider umbilical infection one of the archaic diseases that have virtually disappeared. Any practicing pediatrician can vouch for the fact that this is not true. Serous, purulent, or sanguineous drainage from the umbilicus for a number of days after the cord has separated is still a common complaint. Furthermore, clinically silent omphalitis and umbilical phlebitis and, more rarely, septic umbilical arteritis may be found after death to have served as portals of entry for sepsis of the newborn.

Tetanus neonatorum, having its origin in contamination of the cord stump, is still a great problem in primitive societies, but it is encountered more and more rarely in medically sophisticated communities. This is discussed in Part 12.

Diagnosis. Omphalitis manifests itself by drainage from the umbilical stump or from its base at its point of attachment to the abdominal wall or from the navel after the cord has separated. Secretions may be thin

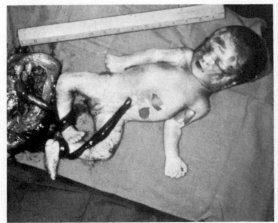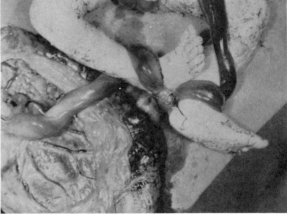

Figure 40–3. All-over and close-up view of a lethal cord entanglement about the extremities of a stillborn fetus.

and serous, sanguineous, or frankly purulent. They must be differentiated carefully from the serous secretions of vitelline duct remnants or the urinous discharge of urachal remnants and from the serous or serosanguineous discharge from umbilical papilloma. At times, they are foul-smelling. Infection may remain restricted to the cord or may spread to involve the surrounding skin. Periumbilical redness and induration result, but true erysipelas, common a generation ago, is a rare sequel today.

Treatment. Simple omphalitis, without evidences of periumbilical spread, responds readily to local application of antibiotic compresses or ointments. Bacitracin or neomycin or a combination of these is the local antibiotic treatment of choice. Oral or parenteral antibiotic medication is indicated if the discharge is frankly purulent or if any evidence of periumbilical spread appears. The hazards of generalized sepsis and metastatic infection of bone or lung, inter alia, must not be overlooked. Final choice of antibiotic will depend upon culture and sensitivity tests.

Septic Umbilical Arteritis

Forshall recalled to our attention this disorder, which was common at the turn of the century but which is now comparatively rare. She pointed out that several clinical pictures may ensue from infection of the umbilical artery. Bacteria may invade, lie latent in, or spread along the lumen, the inner necrosing coats, or the mantle of loose connective tissue of the artery. Thereafter, one of several courses may be followed. If both the iliac and abdominal ends are sealed, the infection remains localized and carries with it the implications of any septic focus. If the artery remains patent externally, the umbilicus drains purulent material. If the mantle zone becomes involved, spread from this region leads to peritonitis. Alternatively, infection may track along the course of the artery to point as an abscess in the scrotum or thigh. If the iliac end of the umbilical artery remains patent, swarms of bacteria may be discharged into the blood stream to lead to rapidly fatal septicemia.

Granuloma of the Umbilicus

Usually, the umbilical cord separates from the abdominal wall 5 to 8 days after birth, and the base epithelializes. Occasionally, delayed separation or infection can stimulate production of granulation tissue.

Serous or serosanguineous discharge from the umbilicus noted after the cord has separated suggests granuloma. If small, this can be seen only as a red button in the depths of the navel after it has been spread open. Large ones project far out of the socket.

Granuloma must be differentiated from everted gastric or intestinal mucosa. The appearances may be remarkably similar. It has been pointed out that they have a different feel. When the tip of the finger is rubbed over a granuloma, the sensation is that of dry velvet, whereas mucous membrane feels velvety but moist, and a thin film of mucus comes away on the examining finger tip. More conclusive evidence is afforded by gentle probing. A granuloma is solid, but everted mucosa should permit the entrance of a fine probe at some point.

The *treatment* usually recommended is desiccation by silver nitrate. Performed with caution, this is satisfactory, but, since silver nitrate can burn normal skin, great care must be taken to touch only the granuloma with the point of the stick and to wash away the excess with toothpick swabs, moistened with saline after the application has been made.

Delay in Separation of the Cord

Delay in separation of the umbilical cord for more than 10 days is abnormal and requires investigation. The causes could include absence of bacteria, as in the case of animals raised in a germ-free environment. Of most concern is the possibility of a defect in neutrophil mobility. Hayward and colleagues in 1979 described six infants (from two families) with multiple infections from which four died. The umbilical cords separated between 3 and 6 weeks. Two additional patients with intervals of 17 and 30 days before cord separation were found to lack killer-cell activity and gamma-interferon production. Both subsequently died of septicemia (Davies et al., 1982).

Aberrant Umbilical Stomach

In Cullen's monumental work on the normal and diseased umbilicus, he comments that "several observers have reported mucosa at the umbilicus that more or less resembles gastric mucosa." He quotes Pillmans, who in 1882 observed "a 13 year old boy who exhibited a tumor the size of a walnut, bright red in color and covered with mucosa, present since birth. After he had eaten, the tumor would sometimes swell perceptibly, become redder, the mucosa thicker. A tenacious mucus was secreted, as much as 2 or 3 cc in 15 minutes. It was acid in reaction and digested fibrin at 39°C."

Wachter and Elman reported two cases of aberrant gastric mucosa at the umbilicus, present since birth, in white female infants 5 and 10 months old respectively. The first patient presented an area of moist induration, 7 mm in diameter, surrounded by a partly cystic, partly solid mass measuring about 5 by 5 cm. It drained clear fluid that was acid to blue litmus and congo red paper and digested coagulated egg albumin. Removed completely, the umbilical structure contained gastric mucosa. The findings in their second case consisted simply of an indurated, reddened umbilicus that constantly drained an acid secretion. The authors point out that the diagnosis can be made at the bedside by a simple test proving that the discharge is acid.

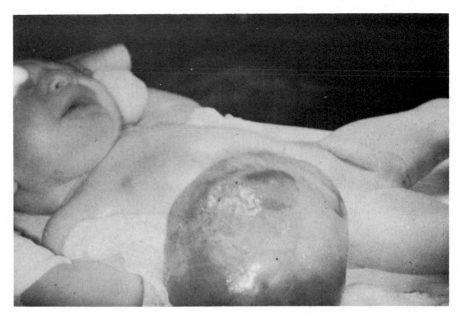

Figure 40–4. A mass is seen protruding from the umbilical region. No specific structures can be identified. It is covered by whitish, glistening membrane and is obviously an omphalocele.

It might be worthwhile to mention in passing that ectopic tissue of other varieties can be discovered in the umbilicus. For example, Harris and Wenzel have reported finding a small, spherical, firm red mass projecting from the surface of the cord 4 cm from the skin margin. This proved to be heterotopic pancreatic tissue plus intestinal mucosa.

Omphalocele (Amniocele, Exomphalos)

After the return of the midgut from the umbilical cord into the abdominal cavity by about the tenth week of gestation, the rectus muscles approach one another from above downward and close the larger circular defect originally present. At times, this closure does not take place. Whether this is due to the circumstance that the abdominal cavity does not enlarge sufficiently to accept the returning bowel or whether for some reason the bowel does not re-enter, hence the muscular defect cannot close, is unknown.

Two types of exomphalos are now recognized, depending on the time at which this failure of closure develops. If early, at about the third week of gestation, the defect is large and involves the midline from umbilicus cephalad, part or all of the way to the xiphoid process. This results in *omphalocele* or *amniocele* (Fig. 40–4). If later, at about the tenth week, the defect is smaller and is located at the umbilicus itself. This has been called *umbilical cord hernia* (Fig. 40–5). In both, the protruding mass is covered by a thin transparent membrane composed of peritoneum and amnion. At times the membrane ruptures prior

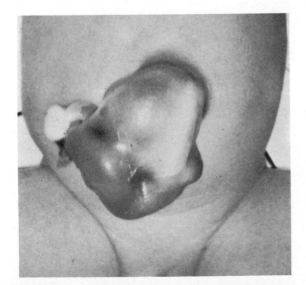

Figure 40–5. Showing a comparatively small mass protruding from the umbilical region. A loop of bowel can readily be recognized running around its lower margin. The mass is completely covered by shiny transparent membrane. This is clearly an "umbilical cord hernia."

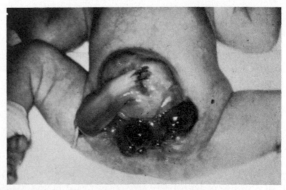

Figure 40–6. A combination of omphalocele and ectopia vesicae. The bright structure below the omphalocele is everted, exstrophic bladder.

to and at other times during the delivery. In the latter case eviscerated intestine lies freely about the gaping hole in the abdominal wall (Fig. 40–7).

An important exception must be added to this statement as we originally wrote it. *A few hernias lie entirely within the base of the umbilical cord and are not obvious herniated masses covered by thin membrane but are manifest only as swellings of the cord for a short distance from the skin margin.* Landor and coworkers have reported two cases in which such swellings were ignored and clamped, whereupon intestinal obstruction immediately ensued.

One third to one half of all infants with exomphalos are born with other congenital defects. Many of these are local, examples being malrotation, Meckel's diverticulum, and patent vitelline duct, but a good number involve the cardiovascular and other systems.

During the years from 1947 through 1973 at Children's Hospital in Boston, 159 infants with omphalocele were evaluated for other malformations. Of these babies, 31 (20 per cent) had congenital heart disease. One of the trisomy syndromes was present in 17 infants (11 per cent), diaphragmatic hernia and other upper midline defects were found in 10 (6 per cent), and multiple anomalies appeared in 8 (5 per cent).

Diagnosis. There is nothing that so closely resembles exomphalos that its diagnosis should be in doubt. The closest approximation to it would be patent omphalomesenteric duct with evagination of ileum. Here the protruding bowel is not covered by membrane. It consists only of one readily identifiable segment of small intestine, turned inside out, not of a mass of intestinal loops.

Small swellings of the umbilical cord near its attachment must be viewed with suspicion. They may be cysts of Wharton's jelly or hematomas or true hernias into the cord.

Treatment. Operative repair of small omphaloceles should be undertaken as soon as feasible. For larger lesions, usually over 6 cm in diameter, a plastic sheet is sewed around the edge of the defect. Steady pressure is applied over a matter of days to reduce the protrusion until surgical closure is possible. If surgery is contraindicated because of other lesions such as congenital heart disease, the sac may be painted with 0.5 per cent Mercurochrome to permit formation of a crust and protection from infection. Epithelialization will progress from the periphery inward and will be complete in 6 to 8 weeks. Surgery can then be deferred until the patient is several years of age.

Prognosis. The prognosis for small omphaloceles is good. When they are large and when they contain liver as well as intestine, the outlook is less good. Even when these infants survive the primary closure, their general condition is precarious. The abdomen, protected by skin and a thin layer of subcutaneous tissue only, protrudes grotesquely, and their weight gain is slow. Many succumb to intercurrent infection or some other disorder before secondary closure can be attempted.

The outlook has improved with conservative and staged repairs to an overall survival rate of 70 per cent.

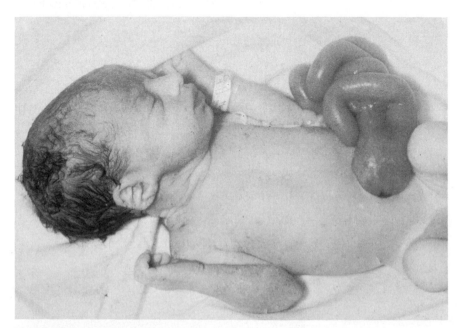

Figure 40–7. Omphalocele in which the containing amniotic-peritoneal membrane must have been torn away during delivery. Loops of bowel lie free upon the abdominal wall. (Case of Dr. Arnold Tramer of Baltimore, reprinted with his kind permission.)

Gastroschisis

In this condition, the abdominal contents are found floating in the amniotic liquid, in association with a defect in the abdominal wall lateral to the umbilicus. Occasionally, they are edematous and matted; sometimes, they are glistening as if only recently eviscerated.

The cord is normally attached to the abdominal wall, most commonly to the left of the defect. No remnant of sac is present. Most infants have some degree of malrotation; gut atresias may also be present.

Pathogenesis. An important insight into pathogenesis of gastroschisis was suggested in 1981 by Hoyme and colleagues. In a review of 26 cases, they identified 10 with an associated structural defect, including intestinal atresia, hydronephrosis, and porencephaly. They postulate that with the exception of hydronephrosis, the other lesions could follow interruption of the vascular supply in utero. The specific defect in gastroschisis could result from occlusion of an omphalomesenteric artery in utero. This would explain why the lesion lies to the right of the umbilicus and why the rectus muscles are intact. The etiology of the vascular deficiency is unknown.

Treatment. In about half the infants, all the viscera can be returned to the abdomen. Intravenous alimentation may be required for some weeks before normal bowel function returns.

Umbilical Hernia

Umbilical hernia differs from omphalocele in that skin and subcutaneous tissue have covered the original defect, while separation of the rectus muscles has persisted.

Incidence. Umbilical hernias are found in about 30 per cent of black infants and 4 per cent of white infants under 6 weeks old. By one year, the incidence is 12.6 per cent in black and 1.9 per cent in white children. The condition is much more common in infants under 1500 gm, 75 per cent of whom have a small hernia in the first months of life, which closes by 1 year of age. Among other conditions associated with large or persisting umbilical hernias are Down syndrome, hypothyroidism, and Beckwith's syndrome.

Diagnosis. Hernia is usually noted immediately after the cord has separated, although it may not attain its maximum size until the end of the first month or later. Umbilical hernias range in size from tiny ones as small as a marble to some as large as a grapefruit. The hernial aperture, located at or just above the umbilicus, may barely admit the tip of a finger or may measure 4 or 5 cm in diameter. The sac contains omentum alone or a loop of bowel from which a quantity of air can be squeezed back into the abdomen.

The diagnosis of umbilical hernias presents no difficulties. They should not be confused with ventral hernias, which appear in the midline at some point between the xiphoid and symphysis. These are protrusions, usually of omentum, through small defects in the linea alba, which seldom exceed the size of a pea.

Treatment. Small umbilical hernias may be left untreated, since their natural course is to close spontaneously within a few months to 3 years. Reducing the hernia by taping does not accelerate healing. We no longer advocate it. Incarceration is possible but very rare. The supine position and cessation of crying promote spontaneous reduction.

Some umbilical hernias should be closed surgically, but it is not easy to lay down arbitrary rules to designate exactly which ones. Large ones whose apertures measure 5 cm or more in diameter probably should be repaired early. Somewhat smaller ones with apertures 2 to 5 cm across should be taped repeatedly and observed. If at the end of 6 to 8 months there has been no or little diminution in size, these too should be closed. Hernias smaller than 2 cm should never be operated on unless they have not

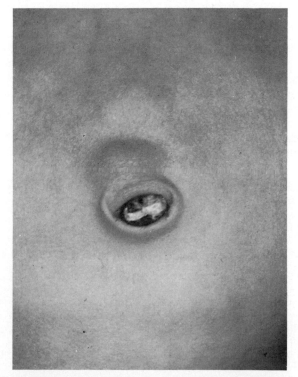

Figure 40–8. Two definite bulges are seen cephalad to the umbilicus, one above the other. Two distinct apertures could be felt in the midline. This represents a minor defect of the abdominal wall.

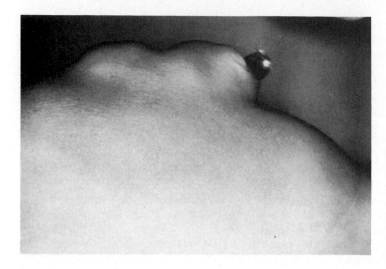

Figure 40–9. Large triangular herniation of and above the umbilicus. The bulge contained easily reducible bowel. A large aperture could be felt just above the umbilicus, and a second, smaller one several centimeters above it. Between them the rectus muscles were diastatic. This is a large defect of the abdominal wall demanding surgical closure.

closed by the age of 4 years. There is room for wide difference of opinion in this matter.

Defect of Abdominal Wall

Some herniations appear to be double or multiple, permitting omentum or bowel to protrude through more than one defect in the region of the umbilicus and above. These are not simple umbilical hernias, nor, since they are covered by skin, can they be termed omphaloceles. We call them, for want of a better name, "defects of the abdominal wall." Figures 40–8 and 40–9 depict two infants with this defect. Treatment is surgical.

Urachus

The urachus is that remnant of the allantois that extends from the bladder portion of the cloaca to the umbilicus. The urachus, like the omphalomesenteric duct, may remain completely patent throughout its length, or its proximal or distal end or its midportion may fail to obliterate.

Embryology. The allantois at first is an outpouching of the yolk sac from its caudal end and is in free communication with it (Fig. 40–10). Its internal end becomes attached to the primitive hindgut, and when the cloaca separates into the lower bowel and urinary system, this segment develops into a portion of the bladder. Its duct becomes incorporated into the umbilical cord, where it courses alongside the vitelline duct. The urachus normally persists as a musculotendinous structure situated between the transversalis fascia and peritoneum, but ordinarily its inner epithelial lining disappears.

Four types of anomalous development of the ur-

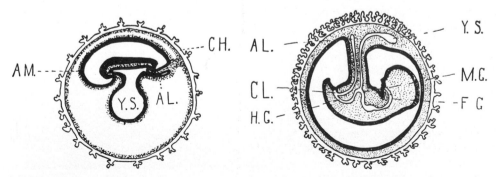

Figure 40–10. Diagrams illustrating formation of the allantois. The proximal portion of the allantois that extends from the cloaca to the umbilicus above the bladder is called the urachus. Abbreviations: *AL.,* allantois; *AM.,* amnion; *CH.,* chorion; *CL.,* cloaca; *FG.,* foregut; *H.G.,* hindgut; *M.G.,* midgut; *Y.S.,* yolk sac. (From Sibley, W. L.: Arch. Surg. *49:*156, 1944.)

achus have been described: (1) completely patent urachus, (2) patency of umbilical end (blind external type), (3) patency of vesical end (blind internal type), and (4) patency of midportion (urachal cyst).

Incidence. All varieties are encountered rarely. By 1937, Herbst was able to find 140 cases in the literature. Three examples were met in 200,000 admissions to the Children's Hospital of Boston.

Completely Patent Urachus

The appearance of the umbilicus at birth is often normal. In some instances, overgrowths of urachal remnants may present as protruding masses. In Nichols and Lowman's case, for example, there was a defect of the umbilicus with a protruding, elongated mass covered with overhanging skin, the center of which contained mucosa grossly resembling that of intestine. The mass was 6.5 cm long and 3.2 cm in diameter. Discharge from the normal or abnormal navel may appear at birth, within the first few days, or may be delayed several months. The fluid has all the characteristics of urine.

Diodrast or other radiopaque fluid injected into the orifice outlines the urachal tract and enters the bladder. Similarly, cystograms demonstrate the tract from below.

The only possible *diagnosis* with which patent urachus might be confused is patency of the vitelline duct. Careful observation of the nature of discharged material resolves doubt. Radiographic visualization supplies the final assurance.

Treatment consists of surgical excision of the umbilicus with the entire urachus and a small portion of the bladder. Results are usually good.

Blind External Type

When only the distal end of the urachus has failed to become obliterated, a draining sinus results. Drainage may become manifest immediately or, as is more usual, after the cord has separated, or only after several months. The discharge is watery, clear, and yellow, and it both looks and smells like urine. A nodule of aberrant mucous membrane may or may not be visible within the umbilicus, or projecting from it. At times a firm cord can be felt coursing beneath the skin and subcutaneous tissue in the direction of the symphysis pubis.

Differential diagnosis must be made between urachal sinus and omphalomesenteric sinus. The urinous discharge of the former is quite different from the serous, seromucous, or serosanguineous secretion of the latter. Biopsy shows bladder-like mucosa in the former, intestinal mucosa in the latter. The sinus tract visualized by radiographic examination courses directly inward if it is vitelline duct, diagonally caudad and inward if it is urachus.

Treatment consists of surgical excision of the sinus tract.

Blind Internal Type

Failure of obliteration of the proximal end of the urachus results in a diverticulum of the bladder near its fundus. This produces no symptoms and no disease and hence has no clinical significance. It can be demonstrated only by cystogram. Nothing need be done about this condition.

Urachal Cyst

Incomplete obliteration of the midportion of the urachus leads to the development of urachal cyst. At times, this is a solitary defect, but not infrequently it is associated with persistent external or internal patency. Cysts may be present at birth, may grow slowly and become obvious at any time during infancy or

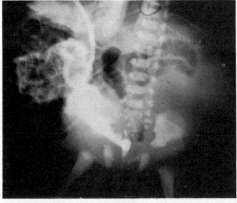 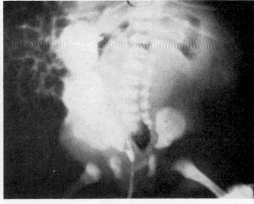

Figure 40–11. *A,* Urachogram showing a catheter traversing the patent urachus to a cyst adjacent to the bladder. The bladder is irregular in shape. *B,* Cystogram showing a catheter entering the bladder from the urethra, the contrast medium filling it, and the urachal cyst above it.

childhood, or may suddenly manifest themselves because of infection. Urachal cysts are highly susceptible to infection and, if not removed after the first episode, to repeated reinfection.

They present as spherical masses of variable size at some point between the umbilicus and the symphysis pubis. They feel and are superficial, since they lie extraperitoneally between the fascia of the transversalis muscle and the peritoneum. When they are infected, the surrounding skin and subcutaneous tissue are thickened, red and edematous, and often purulent material drains from the navel.

Plain radiographs show the round soft tissue mass within or just beneath the abdominal wall. If radiopaque material can be injected through an umbilical sinus, the entire cyst may be filled and visualized. Injection of contrast material into the bladder may or may not fill the cyst from below.

Operation should be performed, preferably before the cyst becomes infected or, if this has already taken place, after infection has been controlled by compresses and antibiotics. The danger of surgical manipulation during active infection is that the peritoneum may be entered and general peritonitis ensue.

Caput Medusae

Failure of fusion or obliteration of the abdominal portion of the umbilical vein early in fetal life demands enlargement of collateral umbilical vessels to carry oxygenated blood to the fetus. Prominent veins over the anterior abdominal wall, arranged spoke-like about the umbilicus, are striking at birth, and regress over the first weeks of life. White and colleagues published the only known instance of such an event in 1969. Their infant was only 2100 gm at term but in all other respects was normal (Fig. 40–12).

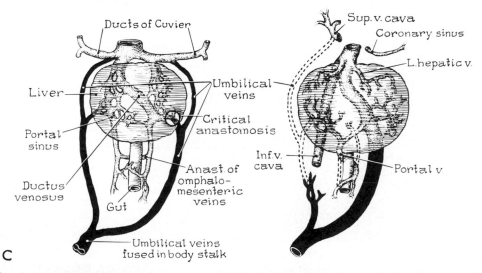

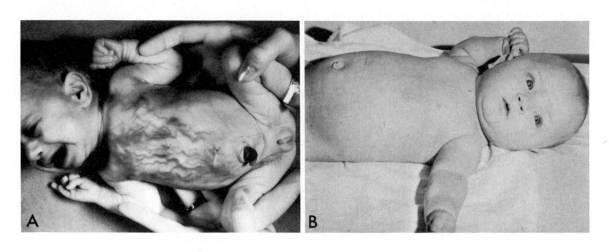

Figure 40–12. *A,* appearance of caput medusae at birth. *B,* At 5 weeks of age. *C,* Diagrammatic sketch of circulation through liver at time of birth.

Aitken, J.: Exomphalos: Analysis of a 10-year series of 32 cases. Arch. Dis. Child. *38*:126, 1963.

Benirschke, K., and Bourne, G. L.: The incidence and diagnostic implication of congenital absence of one umbilical artery. Am. J. Obstet. Gynecol. *79*:251, 1960.

Blichert-Toft, M., and Nielson, O. V.: Congenital patent urachus and acquired variants. Acta. Chir. Scand. *137*:807, 1971.

Crump, E. P.: Umbilical hernia. Occurrence of the infantile type in Negro infants and children. J. Pediatr. *40*:214, 1952.

Cullen, T. S.: Embryology, Anatomy and Diseases of the Umbilicus, Together with Diseases of the Urachus. Philadelphia, W. B. Saunders Company, 1916.

Cunningham, A. A.: Exomphalos. Arch. Dis. Child. *31*:144, 1956.

Davies, E. G., Isaacs, D., and Levinsky, R. J.: A lethal syndrome of delayed umbilical cord separation, defective neutrophil mobility and absent natural killer cell activity. Abstr. Br. Paediatr. Assoc., 1982, p. 46.

Forshall, I.: Septic umbilical arteritis. Arch. Dis. Child. *32*:25, 1957.

Greenwood, R. D., Rosenthal, A., and Nadas, A. S.: Cardiovascular malformations associated with omphalocoele. J. Pediatr. *85*:818, 1974.

Grob, M.: Conservative treatment of exomphalos. Arch. Dis. Child. *38*:148, 1963.

Gryboski, J.: Gastrointestinal Problems in the Infant. Philadelphia, W. B. Saunders Company, 1975.

Harris, L. E., and Wenzel, J. E.: Heterotopic pancreatic tissue and intestinal mucosa in the umbilical cord. N. Engl. J. Med. *268*:721, 1963.

Hayward, A. R., Leonard, J., Wood, C. B. S., et al.: Delayed separation of the umbilical cord, widespread infections and defective neutrophil mobility. Lancet *1*:1099, 1979.

Herbst, cited by R. W. Nichols and R. M. Lowman: Patent urachus. Am. J. Roentgenol. *52*:615, 1944.

Hoyme, H. E., Higginbottom, M. C., and Jones, K. L.: The vascular pathogenesis of gastroschisis: intrauterine interruption of the omphalomesenteric artery. J. Pediatr. *98*:228, 1981.

Landor, J. H., Armstrong, J. H., Dickerson, O. B., and Westerfeld, R. A.: Neonatal obstruction of bowel caused by accidental clamping of small omphalocele: Report of 2 cases. South. Med. J. *56*:1236, 1963.

Lassaletta, L., Fonkalsrud, E. W., Tovar, J. A., Dudgeon, D., and Asch, M. J.: Management of umbilical hernias in infancy and childhood. J. Pediatr. Surg. *10*:405, 1975.

MacMillan, R., Schullinger, J., and Santulli, T. V.: Pyourachus: An unusual surgical problem. J. Pediatr. Surg. *8*:387, 1973.

Miller, M. E., Higginbottom, M., and Smith, D. W.: Short umbilical cord: its origin and relevance. Pediatrics *67*:618, 1981.

Moore, T. C.: Gastroschisis and omphalocele: clinical differences. Surgery *82*:561, 1977.

Ney, C., and Friedenberg, R. M.: Radiographic findings in anomalies of the urachus. J. Urol. *99*:288, 1968.

Nichols, R. W., and Lowman, R. M.: Patent urachus. Am. J. Roentgenol. *52*:615, 1944.

Purola, E.: The length and insertion of the umbilical cord. Ann. Chir. Gynaecol. *27*:621, 1968.

Schuster, S. R.: A new method for the staged repair of large omphalocoeles. Surg. Gynecol. Obstet. *125*:837, 1967.

Schuster, S. R.: Omphalocoele, Hernia of the Umbilical Cord and Gastroschisis. In Ravitch, M. M., et al. (Eds.) Pediatric Surgery. Vol. 2. Chicago, Year Book Medical Publishers, 1979.

Sibley, W. L.: Cyst of the urachus. Am. J. Surg. *79*:465, 1950.

Vohr, B. R., Rosenfield, A. G., and Oh, W.: Umbilical hernia in the low–birth–weight infant (less than 1,500 gm). J. Pediatr. *90*:807, 1977.

Wachter, H. E., and Elman, R.: Aberrant umbilical stomach: Report of two cases. A.M.A. J. Dis. Child. *87*:204, 1954.

Walker, S. H.: The natural history of umbilical hernias. Clin. Pediatr. *6*:29, 1967.

Wesselhoeft, C. W. Jr., and Randolph, J. G.: Treatment of omphalocoele based on individual characteristics of the defect. Pediatrics *44*:101, 1969.

White, J. J., Brenner, H., and Avery, M. E.: Umbilical vein collateral circulation: The caput medusae in a newborn infant. Pediatrics *43*:391, 1969.

41

Congenital Malformations of the Omphalomesenteric (Vitelline) Duct

Embryology. The yolk sac in the very small human embryo is a relatively large structure attached to its ventral surface, its cavity communicating directly with the primitive coelom. It soon shrinks and develops a long narrow stalk that becomes enclosed within the umbilical cord (Fig. 41–1). Its proximal end becomes connected with the primitive midgut, and for a time these two structures communicate freely. In the normal course of ontogeny, the vitelline duct becomes obliterated and disappears.

Under adverse circumstances, the duct or portions of it do not disappear. All the theoretical possibilities of imperfect obliteration are encountered in newborns. The entire duct may remain patent, leading to enteroumbilical fistula. A remnant of mucous membrane may persist at the umbilicus, producing a polyp. The proximal segment may fail to close entirely, leaving a Meckel's diverticulum behind. If the distal segment fails to obliterate, a draining sinus tract remains. When obliteration is complete at both ends, but imperfect somewhere in its midportion, an om-

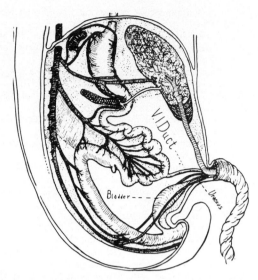

Figure 41–1. Diagram showing the vitelline duct extending from the midgut to the umbilicus. At this stage, the bladder is directly connected with the hindgut at the cloaca; on each side of the bladder, the hypogastric arteries are visible. (From Sibley, W. L.: Arch. Surg. *49*:156, 1944.)

phalomesenteric cyst forms. Finally, the duct may obliterate but not be resolved, leaving behind a fibrous cord that courses from the umbilicus toward the ileum.

Patent Omphalomesenteric Duct (Enteroumbilical Fistula)

This condition manifests itself by drainage from the umbilical stump or from the umbilicus after the cord has separated. Discharge may be noted as early as the first day or as late as the second week of life. Since the connection between the umbilicus and ileum is complete, gas and meconium, later fecal matter, will be seen to be extruded from the navel at irregular intervals. Careful inspection of the well-cleaned area discloses a small orifice through which a fine probe can be passed with ease. There may be a bud or outpouching of the sinus tract, resembling a granuloma, in the center of which the orifice is situated. Injection of a few milliliters of radiopaque fluid permits visualization of the fistulous tract and confirms its communication with the small bowel. Simple fistulous connection between the ileum and umbilicus is not in itself too hazardous. It is true that constant contact with contaminated discharge often leads to omphalitis and periomphalitis, but with care this can be prevented. The great danger of this condition is that *evagination of small bowel* may take place, the attached segment of ileum literally turning itself inside out in the process of protruding through the umbilical

orifice. The result is a T-shaped mass, whose external surface is intestinal mucosa, lying upon the abdominal wall.

Approximately 150 cases of enteroumbilical fistula had been reported by 1952, and 30 of these were complicated by prolapse of the ileum. The prognosis becomes approximately five times as grave when this complication occurs. Scaletter and Mazursky found that 20 of 113 (17 per cent) patients with simple fistula had died after operation, while 26 of 30 (87 per cent) died if evagination had already taken place. These figures indicate clearly that simple enteroumbilical fistula should be repaired surgically at once. Waiting until the infant grows larger in order to make the procedure easier cannot be condoned.

CASE 41–1

A male white infant was born after normal pregnancy and labor, weighing 9 pounds 10 ounces (4365 gm). He was treated repeatedly in the outpatient department for persistent bleeding of an "umbilical granuloma" by silver nitrate applications. At 10 days the cord had fallen away, but it had never healed. With straining, blood was discharged, estimated to amount to one teaspoonful. At times, a white watery fluid was seen to drain from it. From birth, appetite had been poor, vomiting frequent, and weight gain slow.

At 4 months of age he was hospitalized. Weight was at that time 13 pounds 5 ounces (6040 gm). At the umbilicus was a red exuberant mass resembling granulation tissue, measuring 1 by 1 cm. At its apex a dimple could be seen through which it was possible to pass a fine probe measuring several inches (Fig. 41–2A). The whole tract was resected on the ninth hospital day. Its distal end terminated in a Meckel's diverticulum arising from the ileum about 18 inches from the ileocecal valve (Fig. 41–2B). Postoperative course was uneventful.

Comment. This, unfortunately, is an often-encountered story in cases of this sort. The supposed granuloma is treated by cauterizing agents. Failure to heal after months finally brings the realization that granuloma may not be the correct diagnosis. Those infants are fortunate who do not develop evagination and herniation of the ileum through the fistulous tract.

Umbilical Polyp

In this disorder, mucosal remnants of the omphalomesenteric duct persist at the umbilicus. The mucosa secretes mucus, but there is no discoverable orifice and no sinus tract.

After the cord has fallen away, a bright red nodule is seen in the navel. This differs from granuloma in that it is moister. When the nodule is stroked, sticky mucus clings to the finger tip. The skin about the polyp is more likely to be excoriated than that about a granuloma. Biopsy should be performed if any doubt exists. The demonstration of mucous membrane characteristic of small intestine is pathognomonic.

Treatment of choice is cauterization when one is absolutely certain that no sinus tract is present.

Omphalomesenteric Sinus

In this variety of patency of the vitelline duct, only the distal end remains lined with mucosa and in communication with the outside. The proximal segment may or may not have persisted as an obliterated fibrous cord connecting the umbilicus with ileum.

The first sign is persistent discharge after the cord has separated. Discharged material is usually watery but may be slightly bloody. At times, there is bleeding of small amounts from the navel. Examination almost always discloses a red nodule projecting from the base of the umbilical well that at first glance resembles granuloma but that is actually a pouting mucous membrane. One differential point between the two has already been mentioned, that is, that mucus clings to the examiner's finger tip in the latter case but not in the former. Morgan noted another interesting phenomenon. As one watched, the polyp changed its shape intermittently. At times it would

stand, become tense, and protrude for a distance of 1 cm, while at others it would slowly draw inward and almost disappear from view. Careful inspection and exploration with a blunt probe disclose an orifice near the apex of the polyp. Injection of radiopaque material outlines the sinus tract.

Treatment consists of excision of the umbilicus and the sinus tract. The operator should explore the entire region between the umbilicus and small bowel for evidences of other anomalies along the course of the vitelline duct and deal as indicated with any that might be found.

Omphalomesenteric Duct Cyst (Vitelline Cyst)

When both the proximal and distal ends of the vitelline duct become obliterated, but a segment in the middle remains patent, an omphalomesenteric cyst forms from accumulation of its secretions. This variety of cyst must be distinguished from the many

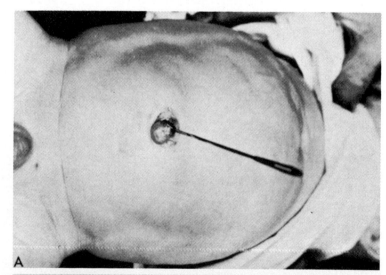

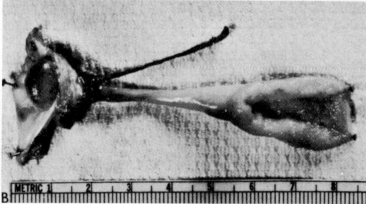

Figure 41–2. *A*, Probe lying within a fistulous tract extending inward from the umbilicus. It has been passed a distance of about 2 inches. *B*, The excised omphalomesenteric fistula in toto. At the umbilical end it presents as a granulomatous-looking bulge. At the ileal end it resembles a cone-shaped Meckel's diverticulum. The film showing barium outlining the entire tract has been lost.

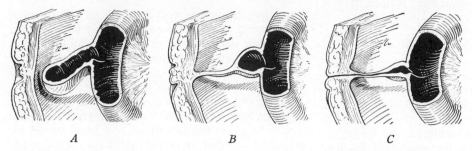

Figure 41–3. Meckel's diverticulum of the ileum. *A*, Ordinary, blind sac. *B*, Diverticulum continued to umbilicus as a cord. *C*, Diverticulum, with fistulous opening at umbilicus. (From Arey, L. B.: Developmental Anatomy. Revised 7th ed., 1974.)

other kinds that are discussed elsewhere. Generally, they present as visible and palpable masses buried shallowly within the abdomen just beneath the umbilicus. They are intimately tied to the navel. When grasped and moved from side to side or pressed inward, the umbilicus can be seen to pucker in conformity with their movement. They are spherical or ovoid, and their feel is distinctly cystic. Patency of the proximal end (i.e., Meckel's diverticulum) or of the distal end, as described in the previous paragraphs, or both, are not infrequently associated defects.

Treatment consists of surgical excision.

Meckel's Diverticulum

When the proximal, or intestinal, end of the omphalomesenteric duct fails to become obliterated completely, an outpouching of the ileum persists. The diverticulum may be as short as 2 cm or as long as 90 cm. It is usually tent-shaped, but it may be tubular. It may arise from any point of the small intestine as close as 3 cm proximal to the cecum or as far as 100 cm distant from it. The junction usually lies at some point in the ileum, rarely in the jejunum, and exceptionally in the duodenum. It must arise from the antimesenteric side of the bowel, a fact that distinguishes Meckel's diverticulum from duplications. Its distal end usually lies free in the peritoneal cavity, but some are attached to the umbilicus by a fibrous cord, and a small minority remain patent to the umbilicus (omphalomesenteric fistula) (Fig. 41–3). Its structure simulates that of small bowel, with well-defined mucosa, submucosa, muscularis, and serosa. Unfortunately, in about one fifth of the cases it is the site of ectopic pancreatic or gastric tissue. Aberrant pan-

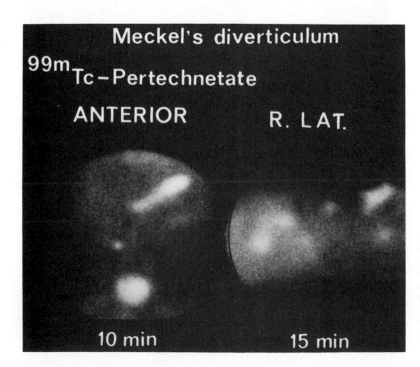

Figure 41–4. Anterior gamma camera view of abdomen of a 2-year-old infant. Note the small well-defined area of increased uptake located in right lower quadrant. The stomach and bladder are also visualized. On the lateral view, some radioactivity is evident on the diaper as well. (Courtesy of Dr. S. Treves, Children's Hospital Medical Center, Boston, Mass.)

creatic tissue is usually present as a small mass in the wall, while gastric mucosa replaces or overlies the usual intestinal mucosa at some point or points. A pancreatic mass may act as a leader to produce intussusception. Gastric mucosa may cause peptic ulceration and bleeding; the latter is the sign that is almost always the presenting one if Meckel's diverticulum becomes symptomatic. The fibrous cord, if present, may produce intestinal obstruction. Rarely, inflammation of the diverticulum may lead to peritonitis.

Incidence. A Meckel's diverticulum can be discovered in 1.5 to 2 per cent of all persons. Only a small proportion of these ever become symptomatic, and, when they do, this usually happens beyond the age of 4 months. The youngest infant to become symptomatic in our experience presented with intestinal obstruction from a volvulus around the diverticulum at 10 days of age (Meguid et al., 1974). Only exceptionally do they cause illness in the neonatal period. Males outnumber females by 3 to 5:1.

Diagnosis. Hemorrhage from the bowel is the definitive sign of Meckel's diverticulum. A few cases in older children and adults may produce the signs and symptoms of diverticulitis, but this condition has never been described in young infants. Hemorrhage is often sudden and catastrophic, causing a precipitous fall in the hematocrit level and a shocklike state within a few hours. The first few stools passed may be composed almost entirely of unchanged blood; later, they become burgundy-colored, then tarry. In other instances, bleeding is constant and occult. About 25 per cent of individuals with Meckel's diverticulum present with intussusception.

Meckel's diverticulum must be differentiated from the other disorders that produce gross bleeding from the bowel. These are peptic ulcer, duplication, and intestinal polyp for the most part. Intussusception, intestinal hemangioma, and a few other even rarer entities may be responsible for an occasional case. Blood dyscrasias usually cause bleeding into the skin and from other sites simultaneously. Fissure in ano, proctitis, and ulcerative colitis ordinarily do not lead to gross hemorrhage, blood loss being confined to the passage of bloody mucus or of stools containing a surface accumulation of blood. Polyps, too, are seldom responsible for massive hemorrhage, so that bleeding peptic ulcer and duplication are the only conditions left that are difficult to distinguish from bleeding Meckel's diverticulum. The most useful differential point is that hematemesis usually coexists with rectal bleeding in the case of peptic ulcer, whereas hematemesis is extremely rare in Meckel's diverticulum. The mass of duplication is sometimes palpable.

We no longer advocate barium studies, since they rarely demonstrate the lesion and may interfere with a technetium scan.

Scans after intravenous injection of ^{99m}technetium pertechnetate are often, but not always, diagnostic of Meckel's diverticulum, since the technetium is concentrated in gastric mucosa. Pentagastrin or cimetidine is useful in enhancing the image of gastric mucosa on subsequent technetium scans.

Treatment. Blood replacement therapy is the prime indication in massive hemorrhage regardless of its cause. If bleeding ceases and the diagnosis has not been ascertained, it is permissible to keep the infant under observation and do nothing more. In the newborn a peptic ulcer, once healed, is not likely to cause further trouble. A second episode of bleeding at some future date strongly suggests some other diagnostic possibility, and Meckel's diverticulum takes first place in this list. Laparotomy is therefore indicated after a recurrent bout of hemorrhage. If a diverticulum is discovered, it must be excised. After its resection, no additional trouble is to be anticipated.

REFERENCES

Brown, A. G., and Cain, F. G.: Evagination of ileum through patent omphalomesenteric duct. Am. J. Surg. *79*:339, 1950.

Christie, A.: Meckel's diverticulum: A pathologic study of 63 cases. Am. J. Dis. Child. *42*:544, 1931.

Craft, A. W., Watson, A. J., and Scott, J. E. S.: "Giant Meckel's diverticulum" causing intestinal obstruction in the newborn. J. Pediatr. Surg. *11*:1037, 1976.

Fox, P. F.: Uncommon umbilical anomalies in children. Surg. Gynecol. Obstet. *92*:95, 1951.

Kittle, C. F., Jenkins, H. P., and Dragstedt, L. B.: Patent omphalomesenteric duct and its relation to the diverticulum of Meckel. Arch. Surg. *54*:10, 1947.

Leonidas, J. C., and Germann, D. R.: 99m-Technetium pertechnetate imaging in diagnosis of Meckel's diverticulum. Arch. Dis. Child. *49*:21, 1974.

Meguid, M., Canty, T., and Eraklis, A. J.: Complications of Meckel's diverticulum in infants. Surg. Gynecol. Obstet. *139*:541, 1974.

Meguid, M. M., Wilkinson, R. H., Canty, T., Eraklis, A. J., and Treves, S.: Futility of barium sulfate in diagnosis of Meckel's diverticulum. Arch. Surg. *108*:361, 1974.

Morgan, J. E.: Patent omphalomesenteric duct: Review of the literature and case report. Am. J. Surg. *58*:267, 1942.

Petrokubi, R. J., Baum, S., and Rohrer, G. V.: Cimetidine administration resulting in improved pertechnetate imaging of Meckel's diverticulum. Clin. Nucl. Med. *3*:385, 1978.

Scaletter, H. E., and Mazursky, M. M.: Congenital entero-umbilical fistula due to a patent vitelline duct. J. Pediatr. *40*:310, 1952.

Soltero, M. J., and Bill, A. H.: The natural history of Meckel's diverticulum and its relation to incidental removal. Am. J. Surg. *132*:168, 1976.

Treves, S., Grand, R. J., and Eraklis, A. J.: Pentagastrin stimulation of technetium-99m uptake by ectopic gastric mucosa in a Meckel's diverticulum. Radiology *128*:711, 1978.

42

Fetal Ascites, Neonatal Ascites, Peritonitis, and Lymphedema

Accumulation of liquid in the abdominal cavity of the fetus is most often found in association with generalized edema. Heart failure from either fetal tachycardia or, as in hydrops fetalis, in association with anemia is the most common underlying cause. Sometimes, the abdominal distention is so great that delivery by cesarean section is necessary. After birth, paracentesis may be indicated to ascertain the nature of the liquid or to relieve respiratory distress from upward displacement of the diaphragm. If there is a question of an associated mass, as in congenital Wilms' tumor or neuroblastoma, ultrasonography is indicated. Obstructive uropathies may present with abdominal distention, and here, too, ultrasonographic studies should delineate the problem. Rupture of the overdistended urinary tract can occur and produce urinary ascites (Griscom et al., 1977).

Peritonitis

Two main categories of peritonitis are encountered in the neonatal period: chemical and bacterial. Together they compose a considerable segment of the urgent surgical disorders of the first week of life. Rickham had to deal with 17 cases of peritonitis in the Newborn Surgical Service of the Alder Hey Hospital of Liverpool in the course of a 3½-year period in which 250 patients were admitted for surgery (7 per cent). He suggests the following classification, somewhat modified:

Peritonitis in the Neonatal Period
I. Meconium peritonitis
  A. Group I (with intestinal obstruction)
    1. In lumen of gut (meconium ileus)
    2. In wall of gut
    3. Outside the gut (volvulus, hernia, bands, etc.)
  B. Group II (without intestinal obstruction)
    1. Defect in muscularis
    2. Vascular accident
II. Acute bacterial peritonitis
  A. Acute appendicitis
  B. Perforation of a hollow viscus
  C. Gangrenous bowel
  D. Trauma
  E. Septicemia
  F. Transmural infection from gastroenteritis
III. Bile peritonitis

Meconium Peritonitis

This is a "sterile, chemical and foreign body reaction resulting from leakage of bowel content into peritoneal cavity during late intrauterine or early neonatal period. Within 24 hours after birth the meconium may become contaminated . . . and the meconium peritonitis converted to a bacterial one" (White, 1956).

Incidence. Although the disorder is not common, it is far from being an extraordinary rarity. Santulli reported 77 cases, 70 of which were associated with intestinal obstruction. Twenty-six of these patients had meconium ileus.

Etiology. As indicated in the classification, meconium may leak as a result of rupture of the intestine

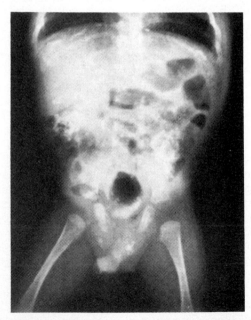

Figure 42–1. Flat film of the abdomen, made on the fourth day of life. One can see many areas of calcium deposition extending from the diaphragm to and including the inguinal canals. Clearly, some of these are situated outside intestinal lumen. There is no evidence of intestinal obstruction. The diagnosis is meconium peritonitis.

at some point proximal to obstruction, either intrinsic or extrinsic. The tear may be obvious or may have healed over so perfectly that it cannot be distinguished at operation or autopsy. To explain bowel rupture without obstruction, various hypotheses have been advanced. The bowel wall may have been congenitally weak from localized defect or may have become weakened by a localized vascular accident or for some other reason. Trauma is not an important factor.

The most frequent predisposing lesions are atresia and meconium ileus. Stenosis does not lead to rupture. Cases have also been reported to follow intussusception, volvulus, incarcerated internal hernia, imperforate anus, and meconium plugs, among others.

The fetus begins to swallow amniotic fluid by about the third month of gestation. Within the next month, meconium begins to form, reaching the ileocecal valve at 4 months, the rectum at 5 months. Theoretically, meconium peritonitis could occur at any time in the last 4 or 5 months of gestation.

Diagnosis. If the bowel has ruptured before birth, abdominal distention at the time of delivery is the outstanding sign. The infant is sick and cyanotic and breathes rapidly and with grunting. The abdominal wall may be covered with dilated veins and may be bluish and edematous. Edema may extend to the flanks, scrotum, or vulva. Anorexia, vomiting, and constipation are prominent, although one or two meconium stools or masses of mucus tinged with blood may be passed.

The aforementioned description fits the great majority of infants born with meconium peritonitis. A minority are born in good or reasonably good condition, manifesting only a moderate degree of abdominal distention. A few of these will also show "hydroceles" at birth, "only to return at 4 weeks of age with hard scrotal . . . masses" (Berdon et al., 1967). Radiograms of these show calcifications that may lead to the incorrect diagnosis of testicular teratoma. Only the additional finding of scattered abdominal calcifications indicates the proper explanation, namely, that the scrotal fluid at birth was ascitic fluid that traversed the normally patent processus vaginalis and induced calcification. Calcified plaques here, as in the peritoneal cavity, can be expected to disappear within a few months.

If rupture occurs after delivery, the infant suddenly becomes obviously sick, and the signs enumerated previously appear rapidly. In prenatal rupture with meconium peritonitis, the physical examination reveals only fluid within the abdominal cavity, whereas if rupture takes place after birth, both fluid and air can be demonstrated within the peritoneum.

Radiographs of rupture occurring before delivery show dilated loops of bowel in an almost completely opaque field; in postnatal rupture, the picture is characteristic of pneumoperitoneum. In the first, scattered plaques of calcified material may be discerned throughout the abdomen.

Treatment. A nasogastric or orogastric tube should be inserted as soon as possible to decompress the stomach. Unless the perforation has obviously healed spontaneously and no obstructive signs are present, immediate operation is indicated. If a tear is discovered, it must be repaired. Obstructive lesions must be searched for and bypassed where found.

Bacterial Peritonitis

Invasion of the peritoneal cavity by bacteria may follow a long list of primary disorders. These include acute appendicitis, sepsis, omphalitis with spread inward via umbilical arteritis or periarteritis, and gastroenteritis. Peritonitis inevitably follows postnatal rupture of the stomach or intestine, which results from peptic ulceration, necrotizing enterocolitis, gangrene of the bowel due to volvulus, intussusception, or mesenteric thrombosis, or which occurs spontaneously, for no known reason.

Scott has reported six cases of peritonitis in infants 3 to 13 days of age, in whom the clinical histories consisted of vomiting but no diarrhea, distention, obvious intestinal obstruction without discoverable structural reason and, in five of the six, rupture and pneumoperitoneum. In all, there was necrotizing inflammation of ileum, jejunum, or colon. *Escherichia coli* was grown from peritoneal swabs of four, and *E. coli* metastatic abscesses complicated one case. *Candida albicans* was seen in the intestinal sections of two. Two of the infants recovered, one after simple colostomy, and one after two resections of segments of gangrenous bowel and subsequent aspirations of osteomyelitis of the head of a femur. The author believes that overwhelming infection is the cause of this necrotizing enteritis but cannot decide whether bacteria—or fungi—invaded from the bowel lumen or from the blood stream (see also Necrotizing Enterocolitis, p. 364).

Diagnosis. The signs of peritonitis are often overshadowed by those of the preceding disorder. Peritonitis adds little to the symptomatology of pneumoperitoneum or of gangrenous bowel subsequent to midgut volvulus. In the purer form, such as that which complicates gangrenous appendicitis or sepsis of the newborn, the onset is marked by anorexia, vomiting, and progressive abdominal distention. On examination, one may or may not be able to demonstrate free fluid within the peritoneal cavity by discovering dullness in the flanks that shifts with change of position. One does not expect to find in the newborn localized muscle spasm or general abdominal rigidity. Fever and leukocytosis are the rule in full-term infants but not in those prematurely born.

Radiographs can be helpful by demonstrating generalized distention of bowel loops with no obvious point of obstruction—unless obstruction is indeed the basis of the peritonitis—and a homogeneous opacity in the flanks and between bowel loops indicating free fluid.

Treatment. Any abdomen showing these signs will have to be laparotomized. If a primary disorder can be attacked surgically, this will be done. If not, drainage and vigorous antibiotic therapy will be the only recourse.

Prognosis. In Rickham's series of 17 patients, seven infants died. This mortality rate of 40 per cent is probably better than that achieved in many other clinics.

Acute Appendicitis

Incidence. Appendicitis can occur in newborn infants, and it accounts for about 2 per cent of childhood appendicitis.

Diagnosis. The diagnosis was made easy for Reed. In his case, reported in 1913, an infant was born with an omphalocele through the transparent membrane of which cecum, small bowel, and appendix could be seen. The appendix was visibly acutely inflamed! It was removed, the intestines were replaced, and cure was effected.

In Hill and Mason's report, an infant was born distended, all fluids offered were vomited, but meconium was passed freely. Distention became extreme, temperature rose to 102°F, and he died on the third day. Autopsy showed a ruptured, inflamed appendix. Cultures from the peritoneal exudate after death were sterile. Other infants have been well for 3 to 4 days or longer and have then begun to vomit and become distended, death occurring a few days after the onset. Polymorphonuclear leukocytosis has been found in several.

We encountered an example of *Pseudomonas* sepsis in a newborn in whom death occurred after 5 days. At postmortem examination, acute appendicitis was found among the multiple foci of infection.

Treatment. A high index of suspicion is required in the presence of signs of abdominal tenderness or distention. The diagnosis is usually made at operation. Cultures and intravenous antibiotics are essential.

Bile Peritonitis

Davies and Elliott-Smith object to the term "bile peritonitis" to describe the disorder that arises from the escape of bile into the peritoneal cavity. They prefer the designation "bile ascites," since, they say, no acute peritonitis, only an outpouring of fluid, results, owing to the higher osmotic pressure of bile.

Incidence. This condition is an extreme rarity. We have been able to discover only five cases involving neonates.

Etiology. Adequate reasons for escape of bile were found in three cases. In one, the common duct had ruptured just above a stenotic point in the common duct; in another, one of a group of tiny cysts at the junction of the cystic and common ducts had ruptured; in the third, the common duct had ruptured just proximal to the point at which a gallstone lay. No cause was found in the other two infants.

Diagnosis. The classic picture of bile peritonitis in the adult—sudden severe illness with abdominal distention, tenderness, fever, and shock—was seen in only one of the aforementioned cases. The others developed abdominal distention rapidly, the stools had been or became white, and mild jaundice appeared. Distention was accompanied in three of them by bilateral inguinal herniation, which was the reason that the infants were brought to the pediatrician. Free fluid was demonstrated in the peritoneal cavity by the usual physical signs. Why one infant became acutely ill at the onset while others were brought for consultation because of hernia alone is not understood.

Most of the infants were slightly jaundiced from birth, and stools had been noted to be without color. Hernias and abdominal distention appeared at 3 to 6 weeks of age. There was obvious discrepancy between the lack of color in the stools and the minor degrees of bilirubinemia and bilirubinuria found. Davies's comment about this point is that "the combination of white stools with only mild jaundice suggests that bilirubin is escaping elsewhere. Abdominal distention and shifting dullness suggest where it has gone."

Treatment. Three of the infants recovered quickly after laparotomy and drainage alone. Anastomosis of the common duct to the duodenum was successfully accomplished in the fourth. The fifth infant died without benefit of operation, although after death a stenotic common duct was found that could have been bypassed surgically. Clearly, one should not rely upon drainage alone when bile peritonitis has been diagnosed, but careful exploration should be performed and any basic defect treated definitively.

Chylous Ascites

Incidence. Although accumulation of chyle within the peritoneal cavity is not too uncommon in adult life, it is a rarity in infancy. Nevertheless, Kessel was able to find 31 cases reported up to 1952, when he added another to the collection. In many of these, the onset was noted at birth or within the first few weeks of life. The disease is twice as common in males as in females.

Pathology and Etiology. Pathologic alterations are limited to the abdomen in most cases. One case is on record in which chylous ascites was associated with chylothorax and lymphedema of one leg and the contralateral hand and forearm. Trauma, commonly a causative factor in adults, seems to play little etiologic part in the newborn. McKendry and co-workers, who found great lymphatic channel dilatation and hypertrophy distally and little or none proximally, concluded that the factor responsible is failure of peripheral channels to communicate with the major ones. This congenital defect, if it indeed is this, appears to be irreversible in many, self-limited in others.

Diagnosis. The abdomen has been noted to be swollen at birth in some cases, whereas in others swelling has begun a few days or weeks later. Kessel's infant was born "swollen all over," but by the age of 3 weeks all the edema had disappeared, while the abdomen remained full. In four examples, scrotal swelling accompanied that of the abdomen, and in two of these tapping was accomplished via the scrotum. Lymphedema preceded the onset of abdominal distention by several weeks in one case.

Physical examination showed little more than abdominal fullness and the presence of fluid within the peritoneal cavity. Veins may become dilated over the surface of the abdomen. Appetite remains good, and vomiting does not occur unless a great excess of ascites causes tight distention.

Paracentesis results in a free flow of milky fluid with a high fat content and 3 to 5 gm of protein per 100 ml. The first few taps before the ingestion of milk may yield straw-colored fluid,

Course. The natural history of this disorder closely resembles that of chylothorax, to which it must be closely related. Some infants become well after one or two tappings. Others require multiple taps, and, in the era before intravenous alimentation, such infants died of inanition and infection.

Treatment. Paracentesis may be required periodically to relieve distention. As much fluid should be withdrawn as comes out freely. Drainage should not be accomplished too rapidly. The interval between tappings depends entirely on the speed with which the abdominal cavity refills. Little is gained by exploratory laparotomy. A low fat diet with medium chain triglycerides is often helpful in lessening the formation of chyle. If chyle formation persists, intravenous alimentation is appropriate to provide nutrition while the bowel is allowed to rest. Cautious reintroduction of elemental formulas can then occur. Most patients undergo an eventual remission.

HEREDITARY LYMPHEDEMA

In this country, hereditary lymphedema is commonly known as Milroy's disease. Nonne described it in 1891, under the title "elephantiasis congenita hereditaria," one year earlier than Milroy. It is marked by firm edema of one or more extremities.

Incidence. The disorder is rare. In 17 years, eight examples were observed in the Toronto Hospital for Sick Children.

Etiology and Pathogenesis. A familial pattern indicating that it is transmitted as a non—sex-linked recessive can be discovered in most instances.

McKendry and associates injected Patent Blue V dye into the first interdigital web of limbs with lymphedema and of the opposite limbs as normal controls. On the normal side, blue-green streaks soon appeared over the dorsum of the foot and ankle and spread upward in the line of the long saphenous vein, reaching the groin in about 20 minutes. Dissection showed lymph channels and glands stained blue-green. Dye then spread upward until the skin of the entire body was discolored. Dye similarly injected on the affected side remained in situ, never ascending even as far as the foot. Tissue examined histologically revealed a mass of dilated lymph channels indistinguishable from lymphangioma. The disorder appears to result from failure of communication between peripheral lymph channels and more centrally placed ones.

Rarely, lymphedema of one or more extremities coexists with manifestations of lymphatic channel blockage in other areas, such as chylothorax and chylous ascites.

Abnormalities in the lymph vessels of the lower extremities, with persistent pedal edema, were associated with obstructive jaundice in two female siblings described by Sharp and Krivit. The jaundice was managed by administration of cholestyramine to reduce the serum bile acids and medium chain triglycerides to improve nutrition, and the outlook was thought to be favorable.

Diagnosis. Edema of one or several extremities is often noted at birth, although later onset at any time during infancy or childhood is not uncommon. The leg is involved much more often than the arm. Originally, only the foot may be affected, but swelling may then extend gradually to the knee or hip. The affected limb may reach a large size, fully justifying the descriptive term "elephantiasis." The tissues feel firmer than those of truly edematous extremities, and deep pressure produces little or no pitting.

There is no pain or tenderness or loss of motility except for some awkwardness that is directly associated with excessive size. The limbs are subject to repeated bouts of an erysipeloid-like infection, with fever, local redness, heat, and increased swelling. These are self-limited, lasting 2 to 7 days.

In the newborn, Milroy's disease must be differentiated from generalized edema of all kinds. This is simple enough, since the swelling in Milroy's disease is never universal and symmetric, even though both feet or both hands may be involved, and because the edema does not pit so deeply. The same differences are found in Turner's disease, and other characteristic anomalies are encountered in this syndrome. Localized lymphangiomas or hemangiomas should cause no confusion.

Treatment. Several operative procedures have been devised with the object of diverting lymph drainage to deeper channels. The most widely used has been the Kondoleon operation, in which long strips of skin and subcutaneous tissue are excised from the entire length of the lymphedematous extremity. This approach to the problem not only is deforming but also is seldom effective.

In a few well-documented cases, cortisone or prednisone has successfully reduced the swelling, and small running doses have maintained the improvement. Panos reports an example of such a cure with prednisone. In this case, 30 mg a day were administered for one week, 25 mg a day for another week, and so on; the dosage was gradually decreased to a maintenance dose of 5 mg a day.

Nonimmune Hydrops

Occasionally, an infant is born with generalized edema. The causes are multiple. In a review of 61 cases, Hutchison and coworkers found an incidence of 1 per every 3748 livebirths. Ultrasonographic examination confirmed the diagnosis when performed

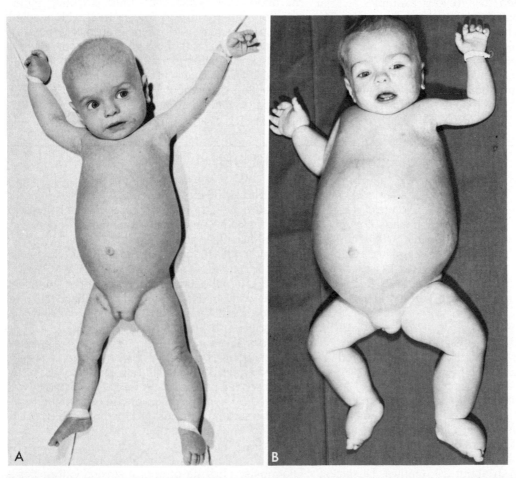

Figure 42–2. *A,* Infant 12 months of age with swelling of the right arm and left leg and some abdominal protuberance. *B,* At 15 months of age. In addition to swelling of the right arm and left leg, there is extreme abdominal enlargement and some generalized edema. (Reprinted from Pediatrics *19:*21, 1957, with the kind permission of Dr. J. B. J. McKendry.)

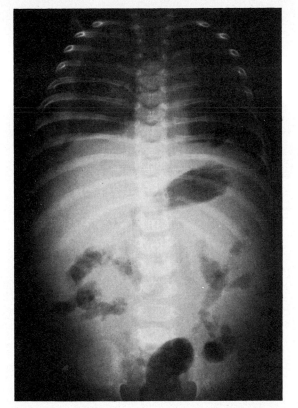

Figure 42–3. X-ray photograph of patient shown in Figure 42–2 made at the age of 4½ months, showing pleural and abdominal effusions.

for detection of preeclampsia or polyhydramnios. No fetal sex predilection was found. Only one of the 61 infants survived. Forty-four per cent of the patients were judged cardiopathic; in 41 per cent, hydrops was associated with a major congenital anomaly (Hutchison, 1982).

REFERENCES

Bartlett, R. H., Eraklis, A. J., and Wilkinson, R. H.: Appenditicis in infants. Surg. Gynecol. Obstet. *130*:99, 1970.

Bendel, W. L., and Michel, M. L.: Meconium peritonitis: review of the literature and report of a case with survival after surgery. Surgery *34*:321, 1953.

Berdon, W. E., Baker, D. H., Becker, J., and De Sanctis, P.: Scrotal masses in healed meconium peritonitis. N. Engl. J. Med. *277*:585, 1967.

Byrne, J. J., and Bottomley, G. T.: Bile peritonitis in infancy. A.M.A. J. Dis. Child. *85*:694, 1953.

Connell, T. H., Jr., and Bogin, M.: Gangrene of the intestine occurring in utero: report of a successful resection. A.M.A. J. Dis Child. *87*:621, 1954.

Davies, P. A., and Elliott-Smith, A.: Bile peritonitis in infancy. Arch. Dis. Child. *30*:174, 1955.

Fonkalsrud, E. W., Ellis, D. G., and Clatworthy, H. W., Jr.: Neonatal peritonitis. J. Pediatr. Surg, *1*:227, 1966.

France, N. E., and Back, E. H.: Neonatal ascites associated with urethral obstruction. Arch. Dis. Child. *29*:565, 1954.

Friedman, A. B., Abellara, R. M., Lidsky, I., and Lubert, M.: Perforation of the colon after exchange transfusion in the newborn. N. Engl. J. Med. *282*:796, 1970.

Griscom, N. T., Colodny, A. H., Rosenberg, H. K., et al.: Diagnostic aspects of neonatal ascites: report of 27 cases. Am. J. Roentgenol. *128*:961, 1977.

Grosfeld, J. L., Weinberger, M., and Clatworthy, H. W., Jr.: Acute appendicitis in the first two years of life. J. Pediatr. Surg. *8*:285, 1973.

Hill, W. B., and Mason, C. C.: Prenatal appendicitis with rupture and death. Am. J. Dis. Child. *29*:86, 1925.

Hutchison, A., Drew, J., Yu, V., Williams, M., et al.: Nonimmunologic hydrops fetalis: a review of 61 cases. Obstet. Gynecol. *59*:347. 1982.

Kessel, I.: Chylous ascites in infancy. Arch. Dis. Child. *27*:79, 1952.

MacRae, C., and Helang, E. B.: Clinicopathological Conference, Alexandria Hospital, Mar. 11, 1966. Personal Communication.

Marx, K., and Dale, W. A.: Neonatal ascites and obstructive uropathy. Pediatrics *27*:29, 1961.

McKendry, J. B. J., Lindsay, W. K., and Gerstein, M. C.: Congenital defects of the lymphatics in infancy. Pediatrics *19*:21, 1957.

Meyer, J. F.: Acute gangrenous appendicitis in a premature infant. J. Pediatr. *41*:343, 1952.

Milroy, W. A.: Chronic hereditary edema: Milroy's disease. J.A.M.A. *91*:1172, 1928.

Morphis, L. G., Arcinus, E. L., and Krause, J. R.: Generalized lymphangioma in infancy with chylothorax. Pediatrics *46*:566, 1970.

Nonne, U.: Vier Fälle von Elephantiasis congenita hereditaria. Arch. Pathol. Anat. *125*:189, 1891.

Panos, T. C.: Prednisone in the management of idiopathic hereditary lymphedema (Milroy's disease). J.A.M.A. *161*:1475, 1956.

Reed, E. M.: Infant disembowelled at birth—appendectomy successful. J.A.M.A. *41*:199, 1913.

Rickham, P. P.: Peritonitis in the neonatal period. Arch. Dis. Child. *30*:23, 1955.

Rosen, F. S., Smith, D., Earle, R., Janeway, C. A., and Gitlin, D.: The etiology of hypoproteinemia in a patient with congenital chylous ascites. Pediatrics *30*:696, 1962.

Sanchez, R. E., Mahour, G. H., Brennan, L. P., and Woolley, W. M.; Chylous ascites in children. Surgery *69*:183, 1971.

Santulli, T. V.: Meconium ileus. *In* Holder, T. M., and Ashcraft, K. W.: Pediatric Surgery. Philadelphia, W. B. Saunders Co., 1980, p. 367.

Scott, J. E. S.: Intestinal obstruction in the newborn associated with peritonitis. Arch. Dis. Child. *38*:120, 1963.

Sharp, H. L., and Krivit, W.: Hereditary lymphedema and obstructive jaundice. J. Pediatr. *78*:491, 1971.

Sinclair, W., Jr., and Driver, M. M.: Meconium ileus, meconium peritonitis and volvulus of ileum with cystic fibrosis of pancreas. A.M.A. J. Dis. Child. *87*:337, 1954.

White, R. B.: Meconium peritonitis. A surgical emergency. J. Pediat. *48*:793, 1956.

PART 6 DISORDERS OF THE GENITOURINARY TRACT

43

General Considerations

By Warren E. Grupe

Embryology. It is not possible to review the ontogeny of the urinary tract in detail in this discussion. Only a few facts will be recalled that have immediate bearing on clinical disorders in the neonatal period.

Morphologic Development. The human kidney develops from the primitive nephrogenic ridge in three successive stages. The earliest structure, the pronephros, consists of a set of tubules in the 1.7-mm embryo. They join distally to form a duct that is the anlage of the mesonephric, or wolffian, duct. The pronephros degenerates, and, more caudally, differentiation of the mesonephros occurs. The importance of the two primitive kidneys is not clear, although it is thought that the mesonephros is capable of urine formation. It is the ureteric bud, arising from the caudal portion of the mesonephric duct and migrating cephalad, that makes contact with the metanephros and then, through a series of dichotomous branchings, induces the mass of metanephric cells to differentiate into the definitive kidney. The ureteral bud, in turn, forms the calyces, renal pelves, and ureters. Defects in nephrogenesis have direct expression in congenital anomalies. For example, the absence of a kidney can reflect any one of several developmental arrests. Absence of the ureteric bud leads to an absence of both kidney and ureter. If the ureteric bud fails to make contact with the metanephros, a short blind ureter with a normal bladder insertion results. If the ureteric bud enters the mass of primitive tissue but failure of induction or differentiation occurs, then one finds a nubbin of aplastic, nonfunctioning tissue at the end of an otherwise normal ureter. Failure of maturation of the primitive kidney may be associated with absence or anomalous development of gonads, sex ducts, adrenals, and lung.

The development of the major and minor calyces is complete by about 10 weeks of gestation, the terminal collecting ducts appear in the subsequent weeks, and by 20 to 22 weeks nephrons are first seen with their collecting ducts near the medulla. Nephrogenesis starts at 7 to 8 weeks, and continues to about 35 weeks. Examination of the glomerular zones of the kidney provides one useful measure of the stage of gestation, at least to distinguish infants born before and after 35 weeks.

Electron microscopic studies by Vernier and colleagues show that glomerular capillaries form in situ in the endothelial cell mass. Foot processes arise by infolding of epithelial cell membranes and are present in 30 per cent of the glomeruli in fetuses 5 months of age.

The secretory and collecting tubules may not effect perfect juncture, and polycystic kidneys are the result. We cannot be sure that this is the proper explanation for this anomaly, but it seems probable. One or both kidneys may not complete normal ascent and may wind up in an ectopic location. If the ureteric buds fuse early in gestation, horseshoe kidney results, which is not only a single conjoint kidney but also generally one that sits lower than normal and in which the pelves face ventrally instead of medially. This is due to the fact that early fusion prevents proper ascent with its concomitant rotation. Not too rarely, collecting systems (i.e., calyces, pelves, and ureters) are duplicated; at times, the entire kidney is a double structure, the ureters of which may join at some point in their course or may empty into the bladder or some abnormal site separately. Stenoses and strictures of the tubular structures are encountered with some frequency, most often at points of junction, but not always. Most of the difficulties that these embryologic deviations produce are associated not with inability to function properly, although this statement is not true for polycystic or hypoplastic organs, but with their propensity for producing obstruction to outflow of urine. This in turn increases the possibility of infection and renders infection, once acquired, difficult to eradicate.

Functional Development. Little is known about renal function in utero, since only recently has it been possible to keep catheters chronically implanted in fetal animal vessels and bladder to allow studies under physiologic conditions. From studies made on abortuses, it is evident that by the third month of fetal life urine is formed; the urine is usually very dilute, with an osmolality of approximately 270 and much lower urea and electrolyte concentrations than are found in postnatal life.

The loop of Henle functions by the fourteenth gestational week, leading to a decrease in the volume and an increase in the quality of the urine produced; this change is accompanied by a continuing increase in glomerular filtration rate. In the early days after birth, urine of premature infants is rarely over 650 milliosmols, or approximately twice the osmolality of serum. When stressed, infants can concentrate more, but even full-term ones do not approach the ability of the adult in concentration. After birth also, urine osmolality will depend on feeding practices. With breast feeding, urine tends to concentrate somewhat on the second and third days of life, and then to achieve a steady range with an average specific gravity of 1.008. When the newborn is fed milk with a content of phosphorus considerably higher than that contained in breast milk, his relatively incompetent kidney cannot prevent its piling up in the blood, and tetany may result. Similarly, excesses of protein may lead to elevation of urea nitrogen in the serum.

The volume of urine produced by the normal fetus at term is not known, but it clearly is an essential source of amniotic liquid. Renal agenesis is regularly associated with oligohydramnios.

The average amount of urine in the bladder of a term infant at birth is said to be about 6 ml, with a wide range up to 44 ml. In the studies by Sherry and Kramer and by Clark, 14 to 17 per cent of infants void in the delivery room, and 92 to 100 per cent void by 24 hours. All normal infants should have voided by 48 hours. Preterm infants tend to void earlier than either term or post-term neonates. Infants of diabetic mothers void early and frequently. Infants born by cesarean section or whose mothers have been sedated behave no differently than other newborns. Urinary retention has been associated with the use of ephedrine.

The role of the kidneys in the regulation of acid-base balance of the fetus is not known, but it must be inconsequential, since infants can be well developed and in normal acid-base balance at birth with agenesis of the kidneys. After birth, however, the kidney assumes the task of excretion of fixed acids. The pH of fetal urine is about 6; after birth, the pH depends on acid production by the fetus and the fluid intake. Acid-loading can increase the hydrogen-ion excretion; however, small premature infants are less able to excrete the hydrogen ions because of a reduced ability to excrete ammonium ions and phosphates. Infants fed human milk excrete about one tenth the amount of titratable acid excreted by infants fed cow's milk, presumably because of the greater amount of phosphate in cow's milk. The renal threshold for bicarbonate has been shown by Edelman and coworkers to be lower in infants than in adults, consistent with the observation that plasma bicarbonate levels in neonatal life are lower than those in subsequent months.

In summary, no sudden renal morphologic events herald or accompany birth. Improvement of functional capability is also a constant that seems to be related more to the time from conception than to the extent of extrauterine life. There is a rapid increase in function in the first few days of life, possibly related to stabilization and distribution of renal blood flow. Thereafter, the pattern and rate of postnatal maturation is similar to that of a fetus of the same conceptual age. The improvement in functional capability is nonlinear, however, with a sudden increase at 34 weeks gestation, which coincides with the completion of nephrogenesis. Prior to 34 weeks, the glomerular filtration rate is low, glycosuria more common, and the urinary excretion of amino nitrogen the

highest. Beyond 34 weeks, the change can be dramatic. For example, the absolute glomerular filtration rate averages 0.45 ml/min prior to 34 conceptual weeks. Between 34 and 37 weeks, it doubles to 1.01 ml/min, only to double again to 2.24 ml/min after 37 weeks. All infants require many months of extrauterine life to reach levels of function comparable to those of the adult when comparisons are made per unit of surface area. Although the exact mechanism is not clear, it is reasonable to presume that functional demand is a very important stimulus to this change in function.

Despite its limitations, the immature kidney is capable of altering function appropriately under stress. The homeostatic controls respond qualitatively but often require greater stimuli to initiate a response that is quantitatively more limited. A comparatively decreased glomerular filtration rate quantitatively hampers the neonate's ability to excrete excessive loads of a variety of substances, including drugs. This is a particularly important consideration for those infants between 25 and 34 conceptual weeks. Glomerulotubular imbalance with glomerular preponderance defines tubular function at an even more reduced level, which is reflected in the infant's limited ability to conserve glucose, phosphates, bicarbonate, and amino acids. Recent evidence would suggest that the extent of glomerulotubular imbalance may not be as great as previously described and that with optimal distribution of intrarenal blood flow, glomerulotubular balance may exist. Arant's reports, for example, noted glomerulotubular balance for glucose in every infant studied, regardless of gestational age or duration of extrauterine life. Aptly suited for growth, the neonatal kidneys are functioning near their maximum capacity with little reserve for the stresses of disease, injudicious management, or unrealistic expectations.

General remarks about the development of the genital tract will be discussed in Chapter 56.

Urinalysis

Examination of a freshly voided specimen of urine provides the most immediate information about the urinary tract and should be part of the physical examination of infants. The normal newborn urine is quite pale in color. Clouds of urates may be present in the first few voidings and may sometimes give the urine a pinkish tinge or stain the diaper a faint red. The benzidine test on the urine or diaper distinguishes between hemoglobin and urate stain. Specific gravity of the newborn's urine is ordinarily quite low. It may be factitiously elevated by high molecular weight solutes such as radiographic contrast material, sugars, and protein. It may also be increased in children with cardiac failure, dehydration, respiratory distress, and inappropriate ADH secretion. In the absence of exogenously administered solute, there is ordinarily a good correlation between urine osmolarity and specific gravity. Using small clinical refractometers, one can measure the specific gravity with as little as two drops of urine. The maximum concentrating ability of the premature is approximately 750 milliosmoles per liter (specific gravity, 1.018) (Table 43–1). Occasionally, concentrations in a full-term infant may reach as high as 1000 milliosmoles per liter (specific gravity, 1.025). The inability of the newborn to concentrate the urine further is due to the fact that growing infants normally excrete such a small solute load. Newborn infants attain the full capacity to concentrate urine by about 3 months of age. In the interim, their limited ability to concentrate influences their ability to tolerate either restricted intake or excessive insensible fluid losses. In older children, the specific gravity increases markedly with water deprivation, whereas in young infants it may not. Therefore, urine volume may become a more useful parameter of hydration than specific gravity or urinary osmolality in the newborn.

Proteinuria

Protein is normally found in small amounts in the urine of the newborn, varying between 30 and 75 mg in a 24 hour period, in a concentration not exceeding 10 mg per 100 ml. Proteinuria may be seen with asphyxia, cardiac failure, massive doses of penicillin, and dehydration and in the presence of x-ray contrast media. Persistent proteinuria must be considered pathologic until proved otherwise and may be the first manifestation of renal disease. Massive proteinuria usually indicates glomerular injury. Persistent massive proteinuria in the newborn should alert one to consider congenital nephrotic syndrome. Renal biopsy may be necessary to establish the diagnosis. Tubular injury without glomerular disease usually results in a modest increase in protein excretion as well. Arant measured the total protein excretion during the first 48 hours of life by sulfosalicylic

acid precipitation in infants of various gestational ages. Protein excretion increased from a mean of 0.9 mg/hr/M^2 (range, 0.2 to 1.3) at 28 weeks to a peak mean of 2.5 mg/hr/M^2 (0 to 13.1) at 34 weeks, only to fall again to 1.3 mg/hr/M^2 (0 to 6.1) at 40 gestational weeks. Only 12 per cent of the infants excreted protein at a rate exceeding 96 mg/M^2/day. With qualitative reagent strips, 24 per cent had no protein detected in the urine, while 73 per cent had a trace or 1 + reaction and 3 per cent had a 2 + reaction. The incidence of positive results falls to less than 1 per cent after removal of urates from the urine.

Albumin is the most abundant of the plasma proteins in the urine. Karlsson and Hellsinc found that immunoelectrophoretically measured albumin in the urine of neonates averaged 1.1 mg/100 ml (range, 0.1 to 9.8). Tamm-Horsfall protein is a high–molecular-weight mucoprotein produced by the kidney; it may account for as much as 25 to 40 per cent of normal urinary protein and seems to be a major constituent of urinary casts. Proteins do penetrate the normal glomerular basement membrane and have been shown by immunofluorescent technique to be reabsorbed in the proximal tubule. Administration of large amounts of plasma proteins or albumin to neonates can be associated with transient proteinuria, which may represent a saturation of the tubular reabsorptive mechanism.

A syndrome in young hypovolemic infants has been described in which transient renal obstruction seems to result from the precipitation of Tamm-Horsfall protein in the renal tubules; rarely, acute renal failure may appear. This is detected on intravenous pyelograms by a prolonged nephrogram that may last for hours or days, as the radiopaque material is detained. Proteinuria has also been reported in children with cyanotic congenital heart disease in the absence of congestive heart failure. This proteinuria is thought to be related to increased venous pressure.

Hematuria

Hematuria is not frequently seen in the newborn, with excretion rates usually less than 100,000 red cells per 12 hours. When hematuria is detected, its origin must be determined. Red blood cells can enter

Table 43–1. Evaluation of Renal Function in the Newborn

Function	Clinical Test	Premature	Full-term Neonate	Two Months	Adult	Age of Maturity
Glomerular filtration rate	Inulin clearance ml/min/ 1.73 M^2	40–60	30–50	70	120	12–18 months
	Creat. clearance ml/min/ 1.73 M^2	13–58	15–60	63–80	120–140	12–18 months
Renal plasma flow	PAH clearance ml/min/ 1.73 M^2	120–150	140–200	300	630	3–6 months
Proximal tubular reabsorption	Tm glucose mg/min/1.73 M^2		60	170	300	12–24 months
Proximal tubule excretion	Tm PAH mg/min/1.73 M^2		16	50	75	12–18 months
Distal tubule transport	Urine concentration (mOsm/kg)	400–700	600–1100	700–1200	1400	3 months
	Maximum U/P Osm ratio		2.5:1	3.4:1	4:1	3 months

the urinary tract anywhere from the renal parenchyma to the urethra. The presence of red blood cell
casts indicates glomerular disease. Other causes of
hematuria include blood dyscrasias, infections, neoplasia, stones, trauma, congenital malformations, disseminated intravascular coagulation, and anoxia. Hematuria can also be associated with nephrotoxic
drugs. In the female, extraurinary sources such as the
vagina must be excluded. Other causes in the newborn include renal vein thrombosis, renal arterial
thrombosis, cortical and medullary necrosis, and obstructive uropathy.

In lower urinary tract bleeding with gross hematuria, it is not uncommon that following centrifugation
the reddish discoloration sediments to the bottom of
the tube, leaving a clear supernate. In glomerular disease, however, hemoglobinuria may also be present,
producing a smoky or brownish color that does not
sediment on centrifugation.

Radiologic examination, cystoscopy, and renal arteriography may be necessary to establish the diagnosis in the newborn. If a urologic evaluation seems
appropriate, it is generally more fruitful if the investigation is performed at that time during which hematuria is present. It is rarely necessary to perform
a renal biopsy to establish a diagnosis in the newborn.

Pyuria

Pyuria, like hematuria, can appear from anywhere
in the genitourinary tract. It can be present in glomerular disease, tubular disease, acidosis, interstitial
nephritis, fever, and dehydration and following instrumentation. White blood cell casts are always an
indication of renal parenchymal disease.

Although commonly associated with urinary tract
infections, pyuria can be associated with any type of
inflammatory process within the genitourinary tract.
In spontaneously voided specimens, pyuria occurs in
only 2 per cent of normal newborn males and in 6
per cent of normal newborn females.

Casts

Casts are the only definitive evidence of upper urinary tract involvement. Cast formation can take place
only in the lumen of the nephron. Red blood cell
casts are most commonly seen in glomerular injury.
White blood cell casts may be seen with infection,
interstitial injury, tubular damage, or renal inflammation. Epithelial cell casts, which may be difficult to
distinguish from white blood cell casts, are seen with
tubular or interstitial injury. Broad casts, which develop in atrophied and dilated nephrons, are indicative of nephron death. Granular casts usually represent partially decomposed cellular casts. They can
be seen in dehydration, interstitial injury, or tubular
injury. When cells are trapped within the substance
of the casts, it indicates that these cells originated in
the parenchyma of the kidney. Hyaline casts may
occasionally be found normally or in states of de-

hydration; they are very common in massive proteinuria.

Radiographic Studies

Evaluation of the anatomy of the neonatal urinary
tract by intravenous urography can be difficult. Given
the infant's relatively low glomerular filtration rate
and poor ability to concentrate urine, visualization
may be inadequate when standard intravenous contrast doses are used, and it may not be entirely satisfactory even when the larger doses of radiopaque
material that are the rule in pediatric radiologic settings are used. Since the radiopaque contrast agents
commonly used have an osmolality approximately
five times that of serum and a sodium concentration
approximately one third of serum, excessive doses
must be avoided, particularly in ill infants. However,
3 ml per kg of diatrizoate can be used safely unless
the infant is markedly dehydrated. Contrast material
is always injected intravenously; the intramuscular
route is to be avoided. Urography can usually be
successful in any infant with a urine creatinine concentration in excess of 15 times the plasma concentration, with the anatomy shown to better advantage
5 to 7 days after delivery. The time sequence of the
normal infant I.V.P. is elongated; the nephrogram
persists longer than in the older child, with pyelogram
phase beginning later and lasting longer as well.

The voiding cystourethrogram is important in outlining the bladder and urethra and in determining the
presence and degree of vesicoureteral reflux. A 15
per cent solution of diatrizoate, instilled at no more
than 100 mm of water pressure by gravity drip infusion under fluoroscopic control in the unanesthe-
tized child using a straight catheter (not a Foley), provides proper and safe filling and yields the most useful
information.

Renal scans and renograms provide both anatomic
and functional information about the kidneys. Their
size, shape, and location can be determined when
conventional urography is contraindicated or unsuccessful. With the renogram, information about renal
blood flow or parenchymal function and obstruction
can also be determined. Ultrasonography is noninvasive, does not use radioactive materials, and requires neither blood flow nor function. It is being increasingly used in localizing kidneys and measuring
renal size, in identifying solid and cystic masses, and
as an aid in renal biopsy.

Clinical Evaluation of Renal Function

GLOMERULAR FILTRATION RATE

It is particularly difficult, and often impossible, to
estimate accurately glomerular filtration rate in the

neonate by standard means, owing to incomplete or inaccurate urine collections. Yet, creatinine clearance remains the most widely available assessment of glomerular filtration. When properly performed, with accurately timed urine specimens, it can be quite reliable. The plasma creatinine concentration in healthy neonates is normally lower than in healthy children. The creatinine clearance in the premature averages 25 to 30 ml/min/1.73 M^2, and in the term neonate 35 to 40 ml/min/1.73 M^2; this gradually rises to 65 to 75 ml/min/1.73 M^2 by 2 months of age. The serum creatinine in cord blood is usually in the range of 0.7 mg/100 ml, falling over the first few weeks of life to 0.3 to 0.4 mg/100 ml. In this light, a serum creatinine of 0.6 to 0.8 mg/100 ml, although below the upper limits of normal for a given laboratory, can reflect a glomerular filtration rate that is half the normal value for that infant. Diatrizoate may interfere with the laboratory determination of creatinine and give a falsely elevated result; therefore, adequate time for clearing diatrizoate from the plasma after intravenous urography should be allowed.

Although most standards for creatinine clearance have been devised on the basis of 24 hour collections, the production of creatinine depends on muscle mass and varies little throughout the day. Providing the time of voiding can be accurately determined and the collections are complete, collection periods as short as 2 hours may be more practical in the nursery. A collection for creatinine clearance in which the infant's urinary excretion rate is less than 15 mg/kg/24 hours should be considered incomplete and the result erroneous.

Inulin clearance has been a standard measure of glomerular filtration rate. It has only recently been applied to neonates in situations in which gestational age rather than weight is used as the measure of prematurity. Oh and coworkers found that the inulin clearance in term infants averaged 20 ml/min/1.73 M^2 at 1 to 12 hours of age, then rose to 33 ml/min/1.73 M^2 at 2 to 5 days of age. Guignard's study of a group of newborns of gestational age of predominantly 35 to 39 weeks and postnatal age of 12 hours to 25 days was very similar. Inulin clearance averaged 19.2 ml/min/1.73 M^2 at 2 to 5 days and 33 ml/min/1.73 M^2 at 6 to 14 days. Clearances ranged from 10 to 55 ml/min/1.73 M^2. Leake and colleagues evaluated a group of immature infants of gestational ages 25 to 42 weeks. When measured at 1 to 9 weeks of age, the inulin clearance in this group averaged 55 ml/min/1.73 M^2. The range was even broader, however, varying from 12 to 117 ml/min/1.73 M^2. Those infants whose gestational age was $\leq$ 34 weeks averaged 33 ml/min/1.73 M^2 when studied at 1 to 2 weeks of age.

An important concept has emerged from the several recent studies of glomerular filtration rate by both inulin and creatinine techniques. All studies have shown that clearance function improves linearly with

postnatal age. Recent studies of immature infants have shown the same relation with gestational age. Studying infants over a broader range has shown in most series that glomerular filtration varies directly with the time since conception, a pattern that continues during extrauterine life. Thus, a premature infant 1 or 2 days after delivery will follow a pattern of renal development that is quantitatively similar to that of a fetus in utero of the same conceptual age. Arant showed that this pattern was not a constant relationship; the glomerular filtration rate was uniformly very low prior to 34 weeks, then abruptly increased at a rapid pace that continued after term status was achieved, whether in utero or in extrauterine life.

A persistent difficulty in the routine measurement of glomerular function has been the requirement for accurate urine collection, which is difficult in the neonate without bladder catheterization. Several available techniques obviate the need for urine collection. The plasma disappearance of ^{131}I sodium iodothalamate and ^{51}Cr–EDTA, when calculated according to a multicompartmental analysis, appears quite accurate at very low doses of radiation. Because of unequal distribution in the small, immature infant, this method tends to overestimate the glomerular filtration rate when compared with the inulin clearance. The individual contribution of each kidney as well as a delineation of the anatomic status of the kidney and collecting system can be ascertained in addition to the glomerular filtration rate when ^{99m}Tc–DTPA is used with nuclear scan techniques. The method is highly reproducible, and a comparison with standard creatinine clearance shows a disparity of about 5 per cent. The radiation dosage is less than that received through standard intravenous pyelography. Leake and collaborators have adapted the constant infusion inulin technique of Cole and colleagues to neonates as small as 25 gestational weeks with ease and accuracy. Like the plasma disappearance methods, the constant infusion technique tends to overestimate the inulin clearance. That these methods require no urine collections is a distinct advantage in the nursery that more than offsets their minor disadvantages when compared with standard inulin clearance techniques.

RENAL PLASMA FLOW

The measurement of renal plasma flow has little clinical diagnostic value in the nursery. It is ordinarily measured by the clearance of para-amino hippurate (PAH), which is virtually completely extracted by the kidney. The extraction in infants is less complete than in the older child, which causes underestimation of the true effective renal plasma flow. When corrected for body surface area, the renal plasma flow is still low at birth, doubles in the first 2 weeks, and reaches mature levels by 6 months of age. Guignard and colleagues measured PAH clearances in newborns of 32 to 39 weeks gestation. Between 12 hours and 25 days of extrauterine life, PAH clearance averaged 43.2 ml/min/1.73 M^2. PAH clearance progressively increased and was directly related to postnatal age, averaging 53 ml/min/1.73 M^2 in the first week of life and doubling to 110 ml/min/1.73 M^2 by the second week. It is felt that much of the improvement in glomerular filtration rate in the newborn is related to a decrease in renal vascular resistance and an increase in renal plasma flow.

GLUCOSE

Normally, glucose is present in the urine in only trace amounts, below the detection levels of glucose oxidase-impregnated paper laboratory strips. Abnormal amounts of glucose in the urine are not interpretable without a simultaneous blood glucose. With the blood glucose below 100 mg/dl, Arant found that 13 per cent of infants below the gestational age of 34 weeks had urinary glucose detected by reagent strips, while none of the neonates above 34 weeks had glycosuria.

Glucose is both filtered and reabsorbed. The renal defect associated with glycosuria is a defect in tubular reabsorption, in which abnormal amounts of glucose appear in the urine at normal or only slightly elevated blood levels. In infants whose gestational age is less than 34 weeks, only 93 per cent of the filtered glucose is reabsorbed. In those above 34 weeks, the fraction reabsorbed increases to 99.2 per cent. Glycosuria may occur as an isolated proximal tubular defect or in combination with aminoaciduria and phosphaturia. Renal glycosuria is not to be confused with diabetes mellitus. The tubular maximum for glucose (TmG) is lower in the newborn than in the adult. Determination of the TmG in the neonate is rarely necessary to establish the diagnosis. Glycosuria may also appear during intravenous infusions of glucose at normal rates because of the infant's relatively lower TmG.

PHOSPHATE

Over 85 per cent of filtered phosphorus is reabsorbed in infants at birth. The absolute level is related to gestational age. The tubular reabsorption of phosphate falls once formula feedings are instituted and serum phosphorus levels rise.

An abnormal loss of phosphate in the urine may be the result of an intrinsic defect of the tubular reabsorption of phosphate or of increased parathormone activity. Hypophosphatemia is the rule in defects of phosphate reabsorption. If hyperparathyroidism is the result of hypocalcemia, elevation of the serum calcium by infusion will reduce parathormone secretion and thus increase the tubular reabsorption of phosphate.

AMINO ACIDS

Amino acids are also reabsorbed by the proximal tubule. Characteristically, plasma amino acid levels are normal when there is a renal defect of amino acid reabsorption. They are elevated in the metabolic de-

fects leading to overproduction, which results in a filtered level that exceeds the normal reabsorption capacity. Both the pattern and the amount of amino acids excreted varies with the age of the child. Infants normally have a higher excretion of amino acids, particularly threonine, serine, proline, glycine, and alanine. Excretion is highest before 34 weeks gestational age, approaching 2 mg of alpha-aminonitrogen per minute per 100 ml of glomerular filtrate. After 34 weeks, the excretion of alpha-aminonitrogen falls to 0.8 mg/min/dl of glomerular filtrate. Formula feedings may increase amino acid excretion.

HYDROGEN ION

The renal tubule excretes hydrogen ion in two phases. In the proximal tubule, hydrogen ion is produced by the dissociation of carbonic acid under the influence of carbonic anhydrase and is excreted into the lumen to neutralize filtered bicarbonate. The system can handle a large quantity of bicarbonate against a low gradient. Defects in this system are manifested in a low threshold for bicarbonate. In the distal nephron, hydrogen ion is excreted in exchange for sodium or potassium. This system can handle a smaller quantity of hydrogen ion but at a much greater gradient. Defects in this system are manifested in an inability to produce adequate amounts of titratable acid.

Proximal renal tubular acidosis can either be an isolated defect or be combined with other proximal tubular defects such as aminoaciduria, glycosuria, and phosphaturia. The isolated defect occurs predominantly in males and is characterized by a bicarbonate resistant, hyperchloremic acidosis. Should the blood bicarbonate fall below the renal threshold, an acid urine may be noted.

The normal newborn, in the first few days of life, may not be able to lower the urinary pH below 6.0. However, by the first week of life, urinary pH below 6.0 should be possible in the face of a systemic acidosis. Also, the threshold for bicarbonate in the normal infant may be as low as 20 mEq/l, while the older child's threshold is usually 24 to 26 mEq/l. Occasionally, a transient form of proximal tubular acidosis can be seen in severely ill infants that resolves as the infant's condition improves.

The diagnosis of proximal renal tubular acidosis is made by demonstrating both a low renal threshold for bicarbonate and the infant's capability to acidify the urine at bicarbonate levels below the threshold. Therapy consists of administering large amounts of either Shohl's solution or bicarbonate; amounts equivalent to 4 to 5 mEq/kg/day of bicarbonate may be necessary, given in divided doses throughout the 24 hours. Some infants may require amounts as high as 20 to 25 mEq/kg/day before adequate control and normal growth can be attained. The state is self-limiting, and the infants do not develop rickets, renal stones, or nephrocalcinosis. Growth can approach normal if vigorous treatment corrects the acidosis, although this level of control is difficult in the proximal form.

Distal renal tubular acidosis is usually an isolated defect occurring predominantly in females. Although it can be inherited as an autosomal dominant trait, it usually presents as an isolated circumstance in the absence of a family history. Most children are diagnosed after the neonatal period because of failure to thrive or polyuria or during an episode of dehydration. These infants fail to produce an acid urine even in the face of profound systemic acidosis. Their ability to handle an administered ammonium chloride load is impaired. Therapy consisting of Shohl's solution or a bicarbonate equivalent to 1 to 2 mEq/kg/day has been standard, although many children require as much as 5 to 14 mEq/kg/day to attain normal growth and avoid nephrocalcinosis. Most children require supplemental potassium as well. The defect is permanent, and the infants may develop renal stones, nephrocalcinosis, or rickets. Growth can be normal with sufficient control of the systemic acidosis, which is more easily attained in this form than in the proximal form.

Normal values for the clinically useful tests of several renal functions in the immature and mature newborn are listed in Table 43–1, compared with the normal adult and the age at which the function matures.

REFERENCES

Arant, B. S.: Developmental pattern of renal functional maturation compared in the human neonate. J. Pediatr. 92:705, 1978.

Arey, L. B.: Developmental Anatomy. Revised 7th ed. Philadelphia, W. B. Saunders Company, 1974.

Bashour, B. N., and Balfe, J. W.: Urinary tract anomalies in neonates with spontaneous pneumothorax and/or pneumomediastinum. Pediatrics 59(s):1048, 1977.

Brodehl, J., Franken, A., and Gellissen, K.: Maximum tubular reabsorption of glucose in infants and children. Acta Pediatr. 61:413, 1972.

Brodehl, J., and Gellissen, K.: Endogenous renal transport of free amino acids in infancy and childhood. Pediatrics 42:395, 1968.

Chantler, C., and Barratt, T. M.: Estimation of glomerular filtration rate from the plasma clearance of 51-chromium edetic acid. Arch. Dis. Child. 47:613, 1972.

Clark, D. A.: Times of first void and stool in 500 newborns. Pediatrics 60:457, 1977.

Cohen, M. L., Smith, F. G., Mindell, R. S., and Vernier, R. L.: A simple, reliable method of measuring glomerular filtration rate, using single, low dose sodium iothalamate I-131. Pediatrics 43:407, 1969.

Cole, B. R., Giangiacomo, J., Ingelfinger, J., and Robson, A.: Measurement of renal function without urine collection. N. Engl. J. Med. 287:1109, 1972.

Dodge, W. F., Travis, L. B., and Daeschner, C. W.: Comparison of endogenous creatinine clearance with insulin clearance. Am. J. Dis. Child. 113:683, 1967.

Edelmann, C. M.: Pediatric Nephrology. E. Mead Johnson Award Address, 1972. Pediatrics 51:854, 1973.

Edelmann, C. M., and Spitzer, A.: The maturing kidney. J. Pediatr. 75:509, 1969.

Edelmann, C. M., Barnett, H. L., Stark, H., Boichis, H., and Rodriguez-Soriano, J.: A standardized test of renal concentrating capacity in children. Am. J. Dis. Child. 114:639, 1967.

Edelmann, C. M., Barnett, H. L., and Troupkou, V.: Renal concentrating mechanisms in newborn infants. Effect of dietary protein and water content, role of urea, and responsiveness to antidiuretic hormone. J. Clin. Invest. 39:1062, 1960.

Edelmann, C. M., Boichis, H., Rodriguez-Soriano, J., and Stark, H.: The renal response of children to acute ammonium chloride acidosis. Pediatr. Res. 1:452, 1967.

Edelmann, C. M., Rodriguez-Soriano, J., Boichis, H., Gruskin, A. B., and Acosta, M. I.: Renal bicarbonate reabsorption and hydrogen ion excretion in normal infants. J. Clin. Invest. 64:1309, 1967.

Gatewood, O. M. B., Glasser, R. J., and Van Houtte, J. J.: Roentgen evaluation of renal size in pediatric age groups. Am. J. Dis. Child. 110:162, 1965.

Glidden, R. S., and DiBona, F. J.: Urinary retention associated with ephedrine. J. Pediatr. 90:1013, 1977.

Greenberg, B. G., Winters, R. W., and Graham, J. B.: The normal range of serum inorganic phosphorus and its utility as a discriminant in the diagnosis of congenital hypophosphataemia. J. Clin. Endocrinol. 20:364, 1960.

Greene, L. F., Feinzaig, W., and Dahlin, D. C.: Multicystic dysplasia of the kidney with special reference to the contralateral kidney. J. Urol. 105:482, 1971.

Guignard, J. P., Torrado, A., DaCunha, O., and Gautier, E.: Glomerular filtration rate in the first three weeks of life. J. Pediatr. 87:268, 1975.

Hansen, J. D. L., and Smith, C. A.: Effects of withholding fluid in the immediate postnatal period. Pediatrics 12:99, 1953.

Hurt, A. S., Jr.: Anomalies of the urinary tract in infants. Am. J. Dis. Child. 38:1202, 1929.

Kainer, G., McIlveen, B., Höschl, R., and Rosenberg, A. R.: Assessment of individual renal function in children using ^{99m}Tc-DTPA. Arch. Dis. Child. 54:931, 1979.

Karlsson, F. A., and Hellsinc, K.: Urinary protein excretion in early infancy. J. Pediatr. 89:89, 1976.

Kathel, B. L.: Radioisotope renography as a renal function test in the newborn. Arch. Dis. Child. 46:314, 1971.

Kuhns, L. R.: Bladder transillumination to facilitate bladder puncture. J. Pediatr. 91:850, 1977.

Leake, R. D., Trygstad, C. W., and Oh, W.: Insulin clearance in the newborn infant; relationship to gestational age and postnatal age. Pediatr. Res. 10:759, 1976.

Lyons, E. A., Murphy, A. V., and Arneil, G. C.: Sonar and its use in kidney disease in children. Arch. Dis. Child. 47:777, 1972.

Mascatello, V., and Lebowitz, R. L.: Malposition of the colon in left renal agenesis and ectopia. Radiology 120:371, 1976.

McCance, R. A., and Widdowson, E. M.: Normal renal function in the first 2 days of life. Arch. Dis. Child. 29:488, 1954.

McCrory, W. W., Forman, C. W., McNamara, H., and Barnett, H. L.: Renal excretion of inorganic phosphate in newborn infants. J. Clin. Invest. 31:357, 1952.

Moore, E. S., and Galvez, M. D.: Delayed micturition in the newborn period. J. Pediatr. 80:867, 1972.

Nash, M. A., and Edelmann, C. M., Jr.: The developing kidney. Immature function or inappropriate standard? Nephron 11:71, 1973.

Oh, W., Oh, M. A., and Lind, J.: Renal function and blood volume in newborn infants related to placental transfusion. Acta Pediatr. Scand. 56:197, 1966.

Parkkulainen, K. V., Hjelt, L., and Sirola, K.: Congenital multicystic dysplasia of the kidney: Report of 19 cases with discussion on the etiology, nomenclature and classification of cystic dysplasia of the kidney. Acta Chir. Scand. 244:1, 1959.

Piepiz, A., Denis, R., Ham, H. R., Dobbeleir, A., Schulman, C., and Erbsmann, F.: A simple method for measuring separate glomerular filtration rate using a simple injection of ^{99m}Tc-DTPA and the scintillation camera. J. Pediatr. 93:769, 1978.

Pratt, E. L., and Snyderman, S. E.: Renal water requirement of infants fed evaporated milk with and without added carbohydrate. Pediatrics 11:65, 1953.

Rodriguez-Soriano, J., and Edelmann, C. M.: Renal tubular acidosis. Ann. Rev. Med. 20:363, 1969.

Royer, P.: Explorations biologiques du métabolism calcique chez l'enfant. Helv. Paediatr. Acta 16:320, 1961.

Saigal, S., and Sinclair, J. C.: Urine solute excretion in growing low birth weight infants. J. Pediatr. 90:934, 1977.

Sakai, T., Leumann, E. P., and Holliday, M. A.: Single injection clearance in children. Pediatrics 44:905, 1969.

Schwartz, G. J., Haycock, G. B., Edelmann, C. M., and Spitzer, A.: Late metabolic acidosis: a reassessment of the definition. J. Pediatr. 95:102, 1979.

Scriver, C. R.: Amino acid transport in the mammalian kidney. In Nyhan, W. L. (Ed.): Amino Acid Metabolism and Genetic Variation. New York, McGraw-Hill, 1967, pp. 327–340.

Sherry, S. N., and Kramer, I.: The time of passage of the first stool and the first urine by the newborn infant. J. Pediatr. 46:158, 1955.

Siegel, S. R., and Oh, W.: Renal function as a marker of human fetal maturation. Acta Pediatr. Scand. 65:481, 1976.

Spence, H. M.: Congenital unilateral multicystic kidney: an entity to be distinguished from polycystic kidney disease and other cystic disorders. J. Urol. 74:693, 1955.

Tausch, M.: Der Fetalharn. Arch. Gynaekol. 162:27, 1936.

Teele, R. L.: Ultrasonography of the genitourinary tract in children. Radiol. Clin. North Am. 15:109, 1977.

Thalassinos, N. C., Leese, B., Latham, S. C., and Joplin, G. F.: Urinary excretion of phosphate in children. Arch. Dis. Child. 45:269, 1970.

Vernier, R. L., and Birch-Anderson, A.: Studies of the human fetal kidney. J. Pediatr. 60:754, 1962.

Vernier, R. L., and Smith, F. G.: Fetal and neonatal kidney. In Assali, N. (Ed.): Biology of Gestation. Vol. II. New York, Academic Press, 1968.

Woolf, L. I., and Nomen, A. P.: The urinary excretion of amino acids and sugars in early infancy. J. Pediatr. 50:271, 1957.

44

Phimosis

The foreskin of the newborn is ordinarily of sufficient length to cover the glans penis completely. It extends beyond the tip and tapers down to a narrow point that, when spread apart, reveals an adequate orifice. At this age and for 2 or 3 months more, the foreskin is fairly tight and rigid and cannot be retracted without tearing. No attempt should be made to retract the foreskin at this time. Phimosis appears to be the normal condition in the neonatal period.

Surgical Circumcision

The practice of circumcision has become almost universal in the United States. It is performed on the eighth day of life by orthodox Jews as a religious rite. On other infants it is usually done the day before discharge from the nursery; that is, on the third or fourth day of life. Early circumcision is a fetish for some obstetricians, reaching its reductio ad absurdum in one instance with which we are familiar in which the operation was performed when the hips had been delivered and before expulsion of the upper half of the body.

The medical value of universal circumcision is still a moot question. No one will quarrel with its performance as a religious rite. The alleged advantages are prevention of permanent phimosis, paraphimosis, condyloma, and balanoposthitis, the greater cleanliness afforded by elimination of the blind space in which smegma may collect and infection develop,

Abnormalities of the Genital Tract

By Warren E. Grupe

a lower incidence of penile carcinoma later in life, and the virtual absence of carcinoma of the cervix in wives of circumcised men. But contraindications of some validity come to mind. Occasionally, surgical trauma results in a penis that is deformed, buried, amputated, denuded, or burned. The penile meatus, deprived of its protective cover, becomes liable to ulceration by ammoniacal urine, and ulceration not infrequently leads to meatal stenosis. A few instances of penile gangrene and more of near gangrene have followed the use of patented bell clamps. Of even greater moment is the suspicion that some cases of sepsis of the newborn originate at the site of surgical circumcision. The data purporting to show lowered incidence of subsequent carcinoma in both circumcised men and their wives are suspect but fairly generally believed. Bolande, in a thoughtful review entitled "Ritualistic Surgery—Circumcision and Tonsillectomy," concludes that arguments in favor of circumcision are not very convincing but that "little serious objection can be raised . . . since its adverse effects seem minimal." Complications, in fact, are probably fewer with circumcision than with almost any other surgical procedure.

The pediatrician is seldom consulted as to the advisability of circumcision. When our advice has been sought, we have in latter years recommended that the operation not be done for other than ritual reasons. When it is not, we carefully attempt to retract the foreskin at subsequent monthly examinations, waiting to complete the retraction until it can be accomplished without trauma, and we then instruct the mother to perform the same procedure two or three times a week until the danger of adhesion is past.

Ulcerative Meatitis and Meatal Stenosis

As far back as 1921, Brenneman taught that meatal ulceration occurred only in the circumcised baby. MacKenzie observed an incidence of such ulceration following circumcision in more than 20 per cent of 140 infants. Ulceration itself is of little consequence, although it does cause some discharge, bleeding, crusting, and dysuria, since it clears promptly after the application of almost any bland ointment.

Allen measured 100 newborn male urethras, finding 40 per cent calibrated to 8 French. However, meatal openings, even as small as 4 French, rarely produce significant obstruction. Therefore, obstruction is best defined by an objective measure, such as obtained with pressure-flow techniques, rather than by observation of a narrowed meatus. Most of these cases cause no trouble, but some seem to be responsible for frequency, dysuria, and, perhaps, enuresis, and a few, which have gone on to the stage of pinpoint meatus, may lead to obstructive symptoms and, perhaps, to an increased incidence of urethritis or even acute pyelonephritis.

Preputial Adhesions

Surgical circumcisions are often incomplete and leave a fringe of foreskin behind. Mothers are ordinarily poorly instructed in the care of this region, with the result that preputial adhesions are permitted to form that become more and more fibrous and firm. One of the duties of the pediatrician at his monthly examinations is to tear these adhesions until glans and foreskin are thoroughly separated, to anoint the raw areas with petroleum jelly, and to instruct the mother to perform this procedure regularly until it is no longer necessary.

Microphallus

The penis of the full-term newborn may appear to be very large or very small. Great care must be exercised in order to avoid error in judgment as to its actual size as contrasted with its apparent size. Commonly, it projects 2 to 3 cm beyond the pubis. In some males it projects not at all, the glans alone being visible, flush with the pubic contour. These infants are usually very well nourished, and a penis of normal length and breadth can be palpated buried within the thick pad of subcutaneous fat. Rarely, the phallus is indeed tiny, measuring less than 2 cm in total palpable length. These infants deserve careful consideration with respect to the other important indices of genital development. Special attention must be given to their chromosomal sex, to the presence or absence and position of gonads, to size and skin characteristics of the scrotum, and to the structure of the urinary and genital excretory ducts. It is an easy matter to confuse an underdeveloped penis with an overgrown clitoris. If the testes are descended and if the urethra is completely penile and without hypospadias, small size of the penis need cause no alarm. The combination of hypogenitalism with polydactyly and obesity might suggest Laurence-Moon-Biedl syndrome.

Guthrie and coworkers demonstrated that considerable penile growth can be induced in boys under 3 years of age by no more than four thrice-weekly injections of Depo-Testosterone (25 mg each). After verification of this observation, it is probable that we should adopt this method in order to spare the child and his parents the problems of psychosexual adjustment that often follow persistent microphallus.

Absence of the Penis

This is a rare abnormality, with under 40 cases reported by 1973. Although ambiguous genitalia can be of concern, the pattern of abnormality in these infants is sufficiently uniform to allow the distinction to be made. The scrotum is usually normally formed and located. Associated hydroceles, hernias, or cryptorchidism is common. The urethral meatus is usually just inside or anterior to the anus, often marked by a small skin tag. Various associated abnormalities are present, including imperforate anus, anal stricture, and rectovesical fistula. However, the infants are generally continent for urine. The lesion can be associated with renal dysplasia or agenesis or both. Endocrine and chromosomal abnormalities are not present.

Megalopenis

When congenital adrenal cortical hyperplasia affects a male infant, penile overgrowth ordinarily does not commence until a year or more after birth. Rarely, the penis has been noted to be larger than usual in the neonatal period. The observation that the penis is unusually large at birth calls for careful study of 17-ketosteroid excretion.

Duplication of the Penis

This is another rare abnormality in which the penis can be bifid, frankly duplicated, or ectopic (accessory). The findings are quite variable in the cases reported, and classification is difficult. All seem to represent a defective development of the gonadal bud. The bifid penis has a vertical longitudinal cleft that can involve the glans alone or extend a variable distance down the shaft of the penis. Each half of the penis contains one corporal body. The urethra is hypospadic in the depth of the cleft.

Diphalia involves two fully formed penises, each with its own urethra and neither joined. The scrotum may be bifid, each sac containing a testicle, or duplicated. The bladder is usually bilobed or duplicated, and each urethra has its own opening into the bladder. Associated abnormalities include diastasis of the symphysis pubis, deformities of the lower spine, duplication of the bowel, and, occasionally, abnormalities of the upper urinary tract. Surprisingly, urinary continence is the rule. Reconstructive surgery is difficult and requires careful planning and thought.

Ectopic or accessory penis is usually nonfunctional, contains no urethra, and behaves like an organized skin tag. Simple excision, once one is assured there is no connection with the bladder, is usually performed.

Scrotal skin can be attached to the ventral surface of the penis, forming a web. The webbed penis is a deformity of the skin that is not associated with other abnormalities of the genitourinary tract. The redundant web can be resected.

Torsion of the Penis

Congenital torsion of the penis is discovered extremely rarely as an isolated defect, somewhat more commonly when associated with other defects of the external genitalia. Hypospadias or epispadias is its usual concomitant. We have encountered one infant who had torsion of the penis, a slit-like balanitic hypospadias, hypoplasia of abdominal musculature, bladder neck obstruction, megacystis, and megaureter. Stenosis of the meatus may coexist and may produce symptoms, but the torsion itself causes no difficulties.

The penis is twisted on its long axis, either clockwise or counterclockwise, so that the frenum of the glans faces upward. In uncomplicated cases, the meatus lies in the exact center of the tip of the glans,

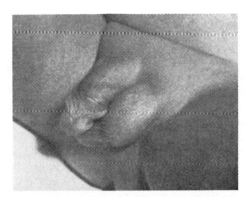

Figure 44–1. Counterclockwise torsion of penis with meatus at 2 o'clock. (Broussard, E. R.: J. Pediat. *46*:456, 1955.)

and urine is expelled forcefully and directly ahead (Fig. 44–1).

No treatment is indicated.

Hypospadias

The penile urethra develops during the tenth to fourteenth weeks of gestation by progressive folding together of the edges of the urogenital groove from behind forward. The progression may stop short to leave the urethral orifice at some point between the scrotal raphe and the base of the glans penis. Figure 44–2 shows the usual locations of abnormal hypospadiac orifices.

Hypospadias is a very common condition, with an incidence of 1 in 700 newborn males. Although on theoretical grounds it implies a deficiency in fetal androgen synthesis or action, the large majority of affected infants have a normal potential for adult sexual function. The familial occurrence in 38 per cent of cases and the concordance rate of 50 per cent in twins found by Sorenson, together with the frequent occurrence in syndromes of multiple phenotypic abnormalities, suggest that many nonendocrine factors contribute to production of hypospadias. However, Aarskog, in 1970, reported that congenital adrenal

Figure 44–2. Anomalies of the male genitalia. *A*, Hypospadias, showing in one drawing a composite of the common locations. *B*, Hypospadias, of a severe degree, in a false hermaphrodite. *C*, Epispadias. (Arey, L. B.: Developmental Anatomy. 7th ed., 1965.)

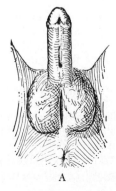

A

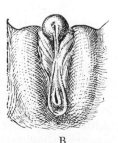

B

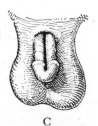

C

hyperplasia, chromosomal abnormalities, and maternal progestin ingestion accounted for 15 of 100 consecutive cases referred for evaluation. Other investigators have cited much lower rates. Application of specific radioimmunoassays of steroid metabolites and recognition that the first 3 months of life are normally an active time for testosterone synthesis may lead to a higher incidence of specific biochemical diagnoses in future series. Noting the type and prevalence of associated lower urinary tract abnormalities in 625 patients led Svensson to postulate an androgen insufficiency or a defective action of müllerian-inhibiting hormone or both in the 60-day fetus as etiologic in at least some infants.

Hypospadias is subdivided into several types, depending upon the location of the meatus. The simplest form is the *balanitic*, or *glandular*, in which the meatus is situated at the base of the glans penis. Usually, this is asymptomatic and requires no treatment. Narrowing of the opening may occasionally require dilatation or meatotomy. In the *penile* form, the opening lies at some point between the glans and scrotum. Associated deformities usually found are absent ventral foreskin (hooded foreskin), ventral angulation of the shaft of the penis (chordee), and flattened glans. This type of deformity should be corrected surgically, but the first stage is not ordinarily performed until the age of 1 to 4 years. The remnant of foreskin should not be circumcised, since it may be useful in later plastic procedures. The *penoscrotal* and *perineal* forms demonstrate these deformities in greater degree. The penis may be underdeveloped, the scrotum bifid, the urinary meatus widely open, and the testes undescended. In these forms, the possibility of pseudohermaphroditism must be carefully explored. Staged operative reconstruction will be attempted some time after the first year of life.

Whether more extensive urographic evaluation is valid in infants with hypospadias is not completely resolved. McArdle and Lebowitz present evidence that anomalies of the upper tract are not frequent enough to warrant screening urography in children with coronal or penile hypospadias. Lutzker and coworkers reviewed 121 of their own patients and studied 1014 reported in the literature. Although the incidence of associated abnormalities varied between 9 and 28 per cent, patients with severe abnormalities such as obstruction, dilatation, renal dysplasia, hypoplasia, aplasia, and cystic disease represented an incidence of 4 per cent, which is at least twice that of the normal population. Abnormalities that require surgical correction (e.g., hydronephrosis and ureteral ectasia and reflux) accounted for 30 per cent of the anomalies found in association with hypospadias. Thus, screening seems valuable on the basis of this information. Contrary to McArdle and Lebowitz, neither Lutzker and colleagues nor Neyman and Schermer found any relationship between the degree

of hypospadias and the prevalence of an associated urinary tract abnormality.

Lower urinary tract abnormalities were also noted in a group of 625 patients with hypospadias evaluated by Svensson in 1979. Cryptorchidism was noted in 6 per cent, bifid scrotum in 4 per cent, penile hypoplasia in 8 per cent, and abnormalities of the prostatic urethra in 44 of 87 examined by voiding cystourethrography. A compromise offered by Lutzker and associates to lower radiation exposure yet assuage concerns about urinary tract abnormalities associated with hypospadias was to use ultrasonography to detect hydronephrosis and abnormalities of renal size and position and to reserve urography for those with urinary tract symptomatology, documented urinary tract infection, or abnormal ultrasonography.

Epispadias

When the urethra is displaced toward the dorsal aspect of the penis and opens at some point proximal to the glans, epispadias is present. The opening may consist of a small meatal orifice or of a long furrow that bisects the upper penile surface for some or all of its length. Epispadias is considerably less common than hypospadias and is generally only one small part of a massive defect that includes exstrophy of the bladder. Plastic repair of epispadias should be attempted at a later date, especially when incontinence of urine coexists.

Diverticulum of the Male Urethra

Congenital diverticula of the urethra are rare. Meiraz and coworkers recently described two examples. The diverticula arise at the penoscrotal junction and present at birth as swellings of variable size from which urine can be expressed. Diagnosis can be readily verified by injection of a radiopaque dye through the meatus. They endanger life because they produce obstruction that may eventuate in hydroureter and hydronephrosis, often with pyelonephritis. For this reason, plastic repair must not be delayed.

Meatal Atresia

Failure to void during the first 24 hours of life should call first for careful examination of the penis. Obstruction to urinary outflow may be discovered in the form of absence of a meatal orifice. Fortunately, the obstructing element in many instances consists of a membranous velum covering and sealing the opening. This can easily be punctured with a fine hemostat and the meatus can be spread apart. Once opened, the orifice remains patent.

Other, more deeply seated obstructions may be responsible for failure to void. Urethral atresia, with or without urachal patency, is a serious malformation that will have to be managed by the urologist. Vesical neck obstruction will be discussed later.

Undescended Testis (Cryptorchidism)

It is customary to separate cryptorchid testes into (1) those whose descent has become halted at some point in their normal route from their original high paralumbar position to the bottom of the scrotum (arrested descent), and (2) those that arrive at an abnormal locus (maldescent). This condition is to be distinguished from absent testes. Descent may be arrested early, the testis remaining within the abdomen, or, later, the gonad ceasing its progression at any point from the internal inguinal ring downward. In maldescent, the testis may come to lie at the lower part of the abdominal wall, the medial aspect of the upper thigh, the femoral area, the base of the penis, the opposite scrotal sac, or within the perineum.

Incidence. Figures reported by various observers for nondescent range from 1 to 14 per cent (Robinson and Engle, 1955). Scorer examined 2700 newborn males and discovered 108 (4 per cent) examples of all stages of arrested descent. A later survey demonstrated an incidence that varied from 0.7 per cent in the full-term infant to 100 per cent in infants whose birth weight was under 1000 gm.

Pathogenesis. The testis arises early in gestation as an outgrowth of the urogenital ridge that bulges into the celomic cavity not far below the diaphragm. By the tenth week, it has migrated caudad to lie at the boundary between the abdomen and the pelvis. There it remains until some time between the seventh and ninth months of gestation, when it passes through the internal inguinal ring and makes its way slowly down the processus vaginalis into the scrotum. The undescended testicle is often abnormal, usually smaller and generally more oblong. It is more susceptible to torsion, and there is often maldevelopment of the testicular appendages. Failure to descend has no singularly satisfactory explanation. Primary testicular failure, abnormal testicular chromosomes, dysgenesis or adhesions, inadequate gonadotropins, shortness of the spermatic cord, persistent abnormal gubernacular slips, and premature tightening of the inguinal ring with mechanical obstruction have all been proposed as causes. Generally, the higher the testis, the more evident the abnormality. Disadvantages of high testes include delayed maturation of germinal elements, fibrosis of tubules, possible trauma, increased susceptibility to malignancy (although this is not great), and psychologic trauma.

Descent is complete in most full-term newborns, but in a few it does not occur until after birth. Over half the arrested testes in Scorer and Farrington's survey finished descent by the first month, and an additional one fourth finished some time between the second month and the end of the first year. The rest remained cryptorchid, so that the incidence of nondescent was only 0.8 per cent at 1 year of age.

Diagnosis. The diagnosis can be made only on the basis of inability to see or palpate both testes in the scrotum. In older children, involvement is usually unilateral, with the right testis involved more often than the left. In the premature, however, it is usually bilateral. If both testes are undescended in a full-term newborn, one should give more than passing thought to the possibility of intersexuality. The size and conformation of the phallus and scrotum and the position and structure of the urethra and its meatus supply invaluable information as to this possibility. Yet Weldon and coworkers have seen five examples of cryptorchidism resulting from adrenal hyperplasia in whom there was *complete* masculinization of the external genitalia, with perfectly placed penile urethras (*see* Pseudohermaphroditism and Hermaphroditism, Chapter 56). Retraction of the testicle due to an active cremasteric reflex is less important in neonates than in older boys. Scorer and Farrington, however, have emphasized the importance of recording testicular descent in the routine neonatal examination when the cremasteric reflex is poor and the scrotum lax. Cryptorchidism is regularly associated with several syndromes, including Noonan's triad (prune belly), Prader-Willi, Smith-Lemli-Opitz, and Lowe's syndromes. Otherwise, urinary tract anomalies are no more frequent than in the general population, suggesting that further radiologic examination is required only if warranted by history or symptoms.

Treatment. No treatment is indicated in the neonatal period for cryptorchidism per se. Suspicion of pseudohermaphroditism demands further studies, namely 24-hour urinary ketosteroid and pregnanetriol excretion, serum electrolytes, and buccal smears, and confirmation calls for appropriate therapy. Surgery is indicated if inguinal hernia, present in 75 to 90 per cent, becomes obvious. During the course of operation for hernia, the undescended testis will be brought down into the scrotum, if possible, and fixed in its normal position. It should be remembered, however, that the testis in the canal or an otherwise ectopic position is more vulnerable to trauma and torsion and is more prone to seminoma or other malignancies. Malignancy, reportedly as high as 40 times greater than that in the normally positioned testis, may be related to the length of time the testis remains in an abnormal location. It is not clear that orchiopexy completely restores spermatogenic potential.

Although the optimal age for corrective surgical therapy is not firmly established, Lattimer and coworkers make the statement, in agreement with many if not all pediatric urologists, that "on the basis of histological, cellular kinetic and clinical studies, but most importantly the psychologic considerations, it appears best to initiate and complete the treatment both for true cryptorchid and for migratory testes between the fourth and fifth birthdays." The treatment for cryptorchidism is operative. Injections of gonadotropins have been used, usually in patients over 2 years of age with incomplete descent, when it is clear that the testis is not ectopic and mechanical obstruction is absent. Some believe that the hormone is effective only in instances of active cremasteric retraction. Others, after great care to exclude retractile testes, have produced descent in as many as 38 per cent of undescended testes. Nevertheless, if it is impossible to assure retractile testes by any other means, a course of gonadotropins may be more practical than surgery.

Anorchia

Three per cent of "cryptorchid" males do not have maldescent but congenital absence of one or both testes. These babies will develop eunuchoidism. They can be identified by low plasma testosterone levels and by a failure of this level to rise after chorionic gonadotropin stimulation. The vas is usually present, and they usually have no stigmata of intersexuality. Urinary gonadotropins are elevated.

It is probable that testes had formed in utero, then regressed for reasons that are not clear. The diagnosis rests on completely adequate exploration for a gonadal remnant. Confirmed monorchia requires no therapy except a cosmetic prosthesis in the scrotal sac. In true anorchia, there is hormonal inadequacy as well as the cosmetic problem. One treats this condition with testosterone therapy at puberty and intrascrotal placement of artificial testes, often using gel-filled silastic implants of appropriate size.

Hydrocele

An accumulation of fluid about the testis constitutes a hydrocele. The processus vaginalis closes late in fetal development. If the processus remains patent throughout its length, fluid will tend to migrate toward the testicle, producing a communicating hydrocele. Reports indicate a patent processus vaginalis in 94 per cent of premature infants and in 57 per cent of 1-year-old children, so hydroceles are not a surprising finding in the nursery. The processus may be patent for only a short distance below the inguinal ring, or patency may include the tunica vaginalis. In the former instance the cord appears thickened for some or all of its length below the ring, while in the latter instance there is also apparent enlargement of the testis. It is difficult to determine the size of the inguinal ring in the presence of communicating hydroceles,

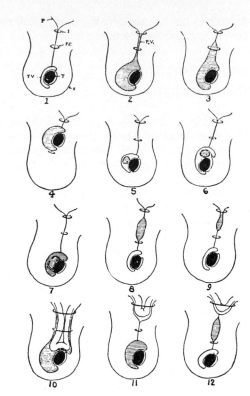

Figure 44–3. Schematic representation of types of hydrocele. *1*, Normal relationship. *2*, Congenital hydrocele. *3*, Infantile. *4*, Hydrocele of undescended testis. *5*, Hydrocele of testis. *6*, Hydrocele of epididymis. *7*, Bilocular. *8*, Hydrocele of cord. *9*, Hydrocele of hernial sac. *10*, With hernia (congenital type). *11*, Hydrocele of tunica vaginalis with hernia. *12*, Hydrocele of cord with hernia. (From Campbell, M. F.: Pediatric Urology.)

but hernia often coexists, and the conditions for herniation are by definition present. Campbell's schematic representation of the various types of hydrocele is still informative (Fig. 44–3).

If the processus vaginalis is sealed but a variable quantity of fluid occupies the space between the tunica vaginalis and the tunica albuginea, a noncommunicating hydrocele is present. If the amount is small, the testis appears to be moderately enlarged and may be relatively soft, but large collections may enlarge it tremendously and render it tense. The mass transilluminates brightly, but the dark round or oval shadow of the testis stands out sharply within it. The cord feels normal unless the processus is open for a distance proximal to the testis (infantile hydrocele), when this portion may be felt to be distended. The external inguinal ring is not dilated.

If the processus is closed at either end, a small cystic hydrocele of the cord can result within the inguinal canal just below the ring. These are much less common than hydroceles involving the testes. If one can feel a normally sized cord above it and an undilated inguinal ring, he can be sure that no hernia is present. If one cannot, and this seems to be the more common situation, differential diagnosis may be impossible without exploration or ultrasonography.

There is usually no difficulty in diagnosing hydroceles and differentiating them from inguinal hernias. They have a fluctuant cystic feel and transilluminate with ease. When palpable, the external inguinal ring is narrow. The size of hydroceles, even communicating ones, is relatively constant, while hernias vary in size or frankly disappear. The hernia often feels crepitant and usually transilluminates poorly, if at all. When the hernia is incarcerated, one must rely on nontranslucency and on the fact that the testis lies free from the mass and below it, while the swelling can be followed as a firm tube from the scrotum all the way into the inguinal canal. Communicating hydroceles that include the testis and the entire cord present a bit more difficulty, but their translucency and the relative absence of fluctuations in size (they may be slightly larger at night than in the morning) and visualization of the testicular shadow within the mass should make the distinction clear. Rarely, a hydrocele may become acutely distended and mimic an incarcerated hernia. Ultrasonography may be quite useful in those few situations in which transillumination is equivocal or absent.

The noncommunicating hydrocele seldom requires treatment. Huge ones that remain large and tense for many months are at times tapped. If fluid reaccumulates promptly, operative intervention may have to be considered. Communicating hydroceles are ordinarily watched closely and repaired only if herniation becomes apparent. The acute hydrocele of the cord may be repaired after exploration has ruled out the presence of strangulated hernia.

Torsion of the Spermatic Cord

Torsion of the testicle produces damage when rotation of the organ compromises circulation. It appears in two forms. Intravaginal torsion is by far the most common in boys beyond the newborn period, usually occurring around the time of puberty. The testis turns on its pedicle within the tunica vaginalis because of a congenital abnormality of its suspension. This produces venous congestion of the organ with pain, fever, erythema, and, eventually, arterial compromise and testicular necrosis. Extravaginal torsion results in rotation of both the testis and the tunica at the external inguinal ring, that is, torsion of the spermatic cord. Although this accounts for only 6 per cent of all instances of testicular torsion in the pediatric population, it is the most common form in the newborn infant. It is not caused by a predisposing congenital anomaly; normally, the tunica vaginalis is not attached to the scrotum at birth, sliding freely within the scrotal sac and subject to twisting by the cremasteric muscle. Since adhesions form quickly on the scrotal wall, spermatic cord torsion becomes rapidly less likely after the newborn period.

Incidence. Peterson reviewed 56 cases of torsion of the testicle in the newborn period that had been reported during the years up to 1961. Twenty-two of these were noted immediately after delivery and hence were classified as torsions in utero. Testicular infarction is often spoken of as being of two types: (1) that resulting from torsion, and (2) the idiopathic form in which no torsion is found at operation. Rhyne and coworkers argue convincingly that these also have resulted from torsion but that spontaneous detorsion had taken place prior to operation.

Diagnosis. Spermatic cord torsion, unlike intravaginal testicular torsion, is usually free of intense symptoms such as fever, nausea, vomiting, and intense pain. It usually becomes evident at or soon after birth as a smooth, painless, firm or stony hard mass in the scrotum accompanied by a thickening of the skin over the mass and a reddish or bluish discoloration of the overlying skin.

The right testis is involved much more often than the left, and bilateral involvement is not too uncommon. To our knowledge, torsion of the testicular appendages (appendix testis and appendix epididymis) has not been reported in a newborn.

Differential diagnosis is comparatively simple. The only other disorders worthy of consideration are traumatic hematoma, strangulated hernia, hydrocele of the testis, orchitis, and testicular neoplasm. The first two should present no difficulty in differential diagnosis. In hydrocele, the mass is usually soft and fluctuant, although it may be tense; it transilluminates, and there is no discoloration of the overlying skin. Orchitis is an extremely rare localization of infection in sepsis of the newborn, and some of the other manifestations of neonatal septicemia should be found in association with it. Epididymitis is even rarer. Testicular tumors, usually dermoids, are rare in the neonatal period, and in them also discoloration and induration of the scrotum are not encountered. When doubt exists, a sodium pertechnetate radionuclide scan to determine blood flow may be helpful.

Treatment. Salvage of the testicle is usually unlikely. Leape was unable to save any of seven examples that he saw in the newborn period, one of which was bilateral. Thus, it may be questioned whether exploration is valid, since diagnosis is rarely in doubt. Nevertheless, most infants are explored with the hope of saving the organ. Under such circumstances, it is prudent to wait at least a few minutes to observe how well circulation returns to the testis after manual detorsion before one takes the irreversible step of excision. A rare instance of bilateral disease has been reported, which has led some to recommend orchiopexy on the uninvolved side. However, a congenital abnormality of suspension is not involved, and bilateral disease occurring on separate occasions has not been reported, suggesting that there is little indication for exploration of the opposite side.

Labial Fusion

True labial fusion is discussed fully under Pseudohermaphroditism (see Chapter 56). It is a developmental defect that at times depends on masculinization of the female external genitalia and excretory ducts by excessive androgen production in early embryonic life.

This should not be confused with another form of fusion not infrequently encountered in which the vaginal orifice is partially or completely obliterated by more or less tight adherence of the labia minora. This false fusion is effected by connective tissue adhesions, at first delicate but later fibrous in consistency, that tie one labium to the other. Ordinarily, this condition produces no symptoms, but in some patients it is the cause of perineal irritation with frequency and dysuria.

The labia should be separated widely as part of the original neonatal examination and every few months thereafter. If this is done, adhesions can be torn painlessly while they are still delicate and friable. After months or years, they may become so tough that the procedure will have to be carried out under anesthesia.

Hypertrophy of the Clitoris

See Pseudohermaphroditism and Hermaphroditism (see Chapter 56).

Hydrometrocolpos

Hydrocolpos signifies an abnormal collection of fluid in the vagina, and *hydrometra* denotes distension of the uterus. Both conditions are due to a combination of excessive cervical and/or vaginal secretions and obstruction to the outflow of this material. The two abnormalities often coexist as hydrometrocolpos. It is encountered more commonly during the neonatal period than during any other time of life. It assumes great importance because misdiagnosis leads to totally unnecessary abdominal operative procedures. Diagnosis is usually simple and treatment often simpler.

Incidence. Antell was able to find 21 cases reported in the literature up to 1952 and added one of his own. Radman and coworkers reported that among 25,000 admissions to the gynecologic service of the Sinai Hospital of Baltimore, there were two cases of hydrometrocolpos, both neonatal, one diagnosed at birth, the other at 9 weeks of age. Reviews of neonatal abdominal masses indicate that about 6 per cent are hydrometrocolpos.

Pathogenesis. Excessive vaginal secretion is noted in many female newborns in the first few weeks of life. Its cause is believed to be transplacental transfer of estrogen from mother to fetus late in gestation. Commonly, this secretion is discharged from the vagina; when bloody, it is called *pseudomenstruation.* If the vaginal introitus is obstructed, such secretions are dammed up and accumulate within the vagina and the uterus. Blockage may be effected by an imperforate hymen or by incomplete involution of the central portion of the vaginal plate, producing stenosis of the uterine cervix, vaginal stenosis, or a persistent urogenital sinus with a transverse vaginal septum at its apex.

Diagnosis. Most girls will present within the first 2 days of life, some with merely a bulging at the vaginal orifice. When larger quantities of fluid accumulate, a fixed, anterior, midline suprapubic mass of considerable size may develop within the pelvis and abdomen. If sufficiently large, the mass may produce respiratory distress, and signs of obstructed venous return may then appear, such as edema and bluish discoloration of the legs and lower part of the abdomen and visible dilatation of the veins and capillary network. Rarely, the tumor may produce hydronephrosis or intestinal obstruction by pressure upon contiguous structures.

A bulging hymen makes the diagnosis obvious (Fig. 44–4). However, 15 per cent of the infants have uterine cervical stenosis, vaginal stenosis, or a persistent urogenital sinus with no perineal signs and an abdominal mass that can be easily confused with a distended bladder. In these instances, it becomes important to locate exactly the urethral orifice as clearly separate from the vaginal opening. A mass that persists after bladder catheterization and yet remains anterior by rectal examination is likely to be of genital tract origin. Ultrasonography or simultaneous opacification of the bladder and rectum can delineate the anatomy more clearly. The external genitalia are usually normal. However, hydrometrocolpos can be associated with anorectal abnormalities. In the review by Reed and Griscom, six of the nine patients had complex abnormalities and five infants had imperforate ani. In four patients, rectovaginal or rectouterine fistulas were present and air from the rectum was visible on a flat plate within the abdominal mass. Sex of the child was in doubt in three cases because of abnormalities of the external genitalia; one child was apparently a true hermaphrodite.

Plain films of the abdomen will show displacement of the bowel. Intravenous pyelograms are usually normal but may demonstrate hydronephrosis, lateral displacement of the ureters, indentation of the bladder, or any combination of these conditions.

Treatment. An imperforate hymen should simply be incised at the apex of the bulge. Nothing further is required. Other serious congenital abnormalities of cloacal or urogenital partition require more specific and complex surgical reconstruction.

Cysts of the ovary usually become evident within the first 2 days of life. They represent 3 to 6 per cent of neonatal abdominal masses. Costin and Kennedy discovered 200 cases reported to 1948 and added but 23 more from the wide experience of the Mayo Clinic. Reis and Koop found 25 ovarian tumors of all kinds in the records of the Children's Hospital of Philadelphia from 1947 to 1961. Ten of these were in babies less than 1 week old, and 10 more were found in those aged 1 week to 6 months. The great majority of these were cystic. Bower and coworkers were able to find 65 cases reported up to 1974. Their own example was the first in which ovarian cysts were bilateral.

Pathology.   Most are cystic teratomas, some are follicular, and a few are cystadenomas. Several students of the problem have stressed the important point that malignant ovarian tumors are extremely rare in the newborn period. Torsion of the pedicle occurs in 70 per cent of all ovarian cysts and produces the presenting signs and symptoms in many older children but not often in the newborn. Cysts may rupture and lead to a picture simulating ascites, and peritonitis may follow rupture.

Diagnosis.   In most patients, a soft to firm, cystic, movable mass is palpated in the midline at the level of the umbilicus. It often extends beyond the midline and may be felt surprisingly high in the abdomen because of a long pedicle. On at least two occasions, the cyst was of sufficient size to interfere with delivery. A plain film often shows the mass clearly, which usually appears more abdominal than pelvic. There is usually no calcification and little if any disturbance of the intestinal gas pattern. Associated congenital ab-

normalities are unusual. Intravenous pyelograms are normal, although occasionally a slight obstruction to the lower ureter can be seen. All, however, demonstrate total body opacification, and some can be shown to transilluminate. One must attempt to distinguish this from other cystic masses. A mobile, anterior, midline mass is most likely to be an ovarian cyst or an intestinal duplication. Catheterization should rule out distended bladder due to bladder neck or urethral obstruction. Careful examination of the vulva and perineum should rule out the possibility of hydrocolpos (see p. 408). Pyelography must be performed in order to exclude hydronephrosis of an ectopic kidney and hydroureter. Cyst of the urachus may or may not be suggested by the appearance of the umbilicus, and its more superficial position may be appreciated by careful palpation. Differentiation from this condition, as well as from mesenteric and pancreatic cyst, may have to await laparotomy.

If torsion complicates the picture, nausea and vomiting, fever, tenderness, and guarding upon palpation of the lower abdomen may be added to the clinical picture.

Treatment.   Immediate surgical removal is indicated. The dangers of malignancy, twisted pedicle, and rupture render this decision mandatory.

Vaginal Agenesis

A total absence of the vagina should be apparent at birth, although many cases are not diagnosed until later in life. The perineal surface between the urethra

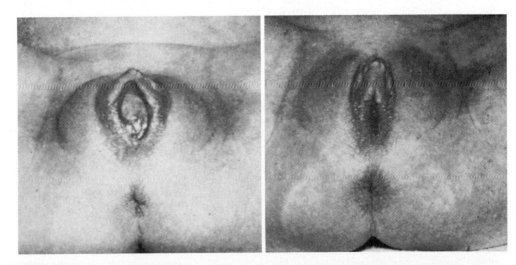

Figure 44–4.   Hydrometrocolpos. *A,* Appearance of external genitalia on admission. Note the bulge of the perineum, the widely spread labia, and the bulging hymen between. *B,* After spontaneous rupture of the hymen. The labia majora are still prominent from edema, but the perineal and hymeneal bulging has disappeared, and the labia minora have assumed a more normal approximation.

and anus is either completely flat or slightly dimpled at the usual vaginal site. The labia and clitoris are usually normal, although vaginal atresia occasionally accompanies ambiguous genitalia and problems of sex determination. Associated renal abnormalities, including unilateral renal agenesis or ectopia, are relatively common. With uncomplicated developmental failure of müllerian duct formation as the common cause, the ovaries are usually present. The uterus is often but not always absent. Any ambiguity over the infant's sex, however, requires a complete evaluation (see p. 511). Vaginal reconstruction is ideally left for a later age unless a lower abdominal mass or another problem with uterine secretions develops.

External Genital Cysts

Merlob and colleagues discovered solitary cysts of the external genitalia in 19 of 3026 phenotypically female newborns (0.6 per cent). Twelve had vaginal cysts attached to the hymen, six had paraurethral cysts located just inferior to the urethral meatus, and one had a clitoral cyst. All the cysts drained spontaneously, and none caused long-term difficulty or required subsequent surgery. The cysts did not interfere with voiding and produced no symptoms.

REFERENCES

Aarskog, P.: Clinical and cytogenetic studies in hypospadias. Acta Paediatr. Scand. 59 (suppl. 203): 1, 1970.

Ahmed, S.: A case of transverse testicular ectopia. J. Urol. 106:308, 1971.

Albin, R., Reyes, H. M., and Replogle, R. L.: A penile testis. J. Pediatr. Surg. 7:308, 1972.

Allen, J. S., Summers, J. L., and Wilkerson, J. E.: Meatal calibration of newborn boys. J. Urol. 107:498, 1972.

Altman, B. L., and Malament, M.: Carcinoma of the testis following orchiopexy. J. Urol. 97:498, 1967.

Andrews, J.: Large penis. Clinical case no. 899. Case Rep. Child. Mem. Hosp., Chicago 14:3824, 1956.

Antell, L.: Hydrocolpos in infancy and childhood. Pediatrics 10:306, 1952.

Bolande, R. P.: Ritualistic surgery—circumcision and tonsillectomy. N. Engl. J. Med. 280:591, 1969.

Bongiovanni, A. M.: Diagnosis and treatment: the undescended testicle. Pediatrics 36:786, 1965.

Bower, R., Dehner, L. P., and Ternberg, J. L.: Bilateral ovarian cysts in the newborn. Am. J. Dis. Child. 128:731, 1974.

Brenneman, J.: The ulcerated meatus in the circumcised child. Am. J. Dis. Child. 21:38, 1921.

Broussard, E. R.: Uncomplicated congenital torsion of the penis. J. Pediatr. 46:456, 1955.

Campbell, M. F.: Stenosis of the external urethral meatus. J. Urol. 50:740, 1943.

Castleman, B. (Ed.): Case records of the Massachusetts General Hospital. Torsion with infarction of normal fallopian tube and ovary. N. Engl. J. Med. 284:491, 1971.

Cecil, A. B.: Hypospadias and epispadias. Pediatr. Clin. North Am. 2:711, 1955.

Charnock, D. A., and Riddle, H. I.: Genital tract diseases in infants and children. Pediatr. Clin. North Am. 2:827, 1955.

Charny, C. W., and Wolgin, W.: Cryptorchism. New York, Paul B. Hoeber, 1957.

Chiles, D. W., and Foster, R. S.: Torsion of the appendix testis in the newborn. Am. J. Dis. Child. 118:652, 1969.

Costin, M. E., Jr., and Kennedy, R. L. J.: Ovarian tumors in infants and children. Am. J. Dis. Child. 76:127, 1948.

Davis, C. B., Jr., and Fell, E. H.: Double hydrometrocolpos and imperforate anus in the newborn infant. Am. J. Dis. Child. 80:79, 1950.

Dickinson, S. J.: Structural abnormalities in the undescended testis. J. Pediatr. Surg. 8:523, 1973.

Donohue, R. E., Utley, W. L. F., and Maling, T. M.: Excretory urography in asymptomatic boys with cryptorchidism. J. Urol. 109:912, 1963.

Dooley, R. T.: Hydrometrocolpos: report of a case in a newborn infant. Am. J. Dis. Child. 103:692, 1962.

Ehrlich, R. M., Dougherty, L. J., Tomashefsky, P., et al.: Effect of gonadotropin in cryptorchism. J. Urol. 102:793, 1969.

Ein, S. H., Darte, J. M., and Stephens, C. A.: Cystic and solid ovarian tumors in children. A 44-year review. J. Pediatr. Surg. 5:143, 1970.

Engel, R. M., and Scott, W. W.: Hypospadias: experience with a one-stage repair. Md. State Med. J. 20:45, 1971.

Farah, R., and Reno, G.: Congenital absence of the penis. J. Urol. 107:154, 1972.

Franzblau, A. H.: Torsion of the spermatic cord in the newborn. A.M.A. J. Dis. Child. 92:179, 1956.

Gillenwater, J. M., and Burros, H. H.: Torsion of the spermatic cord in utero. J.A.M.A. 198:1123, 1966.

Glenn, J. F., and McPherson, H. T.: Anorchism; definition of a clinical entity. Trans. Am. Assoc. Genitourin. Surg. 62:147, 1970.

Graves, G. Y., McIlvoy, D. B., Jr., and Hudson, G. W.: Ovarian cyst in a premature infant. A.M.A. J. Dis. Child. 81:256, 1951.

Gross, R. E., and Jewett, R. C., Jr.: Surgical experience from 1222 operations for undescended testis. J.A.M.A. 160:634, 1956.

Guthrie, R. D., Smith, D. W., and Graham, C. B.: Testosterone treatment for micropenis during early childhood. Pediatrics 83:247, 1973.

Hodgson, N. B.: A one-stage hypospadias repair. J. Urol. 104:281, 1970.

James, T.: Torsion of the spermatic cord in the first year of life. Br. J. Urol. 25:56, 1953.

Kiesewetter, W. B.: Hernias and hydroceles. Pediatr. Clin. North Am. 6:1129, 1959.

Klingerman, J. J., and Nourse, M. H.: Torsion of the spermatic cord. J.A.M.A. 200:97, 1967.

Kolodny, H. D., Kim, S., et al.: Anorchia: a variety of empty scrotum. J.A.M.A. 216:497, 1971.

Kunstadter, R. H., Schultz, A., and Strauss, A. A.: Large ovarian cyst in a newborn infant. Am. J. Dis. Child. 80:993, 1950.

Lattimer, J. K., Smith, A. M., et al.: The optimum time to operate for cryptorchidism. Pediatrics 53:96, 1974.

Leape, L. L.: Torsion of the testis: invitation to error. J.A.M.A. 200:669, 1967.

Leduc, B., Van Campenhout, J., and Simard, R.: Congenital absence of the vagina: observations on 25 cases. Am. J. Obstet. Gynecol. 100:512, 1968.

Lutzker, L. G., Kogan, S. J., and Levitt, S. B.: Is routine intravenous urography indicated in patients with hypospadias? Pediatrics 59:630, 1977.

MacKenzie, A. R.: Meatal ulceration following neonatal circumcision. Obstet. Gynecol. 28:221, 1966.

Maxted, W., Baker, R., McCrystal, H., et al.: Complete masculinization of the external genitalia in congenital adrenocortical hyperplasia: presentation of two cases. J. Urol. 94:266, 1965.

McArdle, R., and Lebowitz, R.: Uncomplicated hypospadias and anomalies of the upper urinary tract. Need for screening? Urology 5:712, 1975.

McKusick, V. A., Bauer, R. L., Koop, C. E., et al.: Hydrometrocolpos as a simply inherited malformation. J.A.M.A. 189:812, 1964.

Meiraz, D., Dolberg, L., et al.: Diverticulum of the urethra in two boys. Am. J. Dis. Child. 122:271, 1971.

Merlob, P., Bahari, C., Liban, E., and Reisner, S. H.: Cysts of the female external genitalia in the newborn infant. Am. J. Obstet. Gynecol. *132*:607, 1978.

Mininberg, D. T., and Bingol, N.: Chromosomal abnormalities in undescended testes. Urology *1*:98, 1973.

Nadel, N. S., Gitter, M. H., Han, L. C., et al.: Preoperative diagnosis of testicular torsion. Urology *1*:478, 1973.

Neyman, M. A., and Schermer, H. K. A.: Urinary tract evaluation in hypospadias. J. Urol. *94*:439, 1965.

Noe, H. N., and Patterson, T. H.: Screening urography in asymptomatic cryptorchid patients. J. Urol. *119*:669, 1978.

Parker, R. M., and Robinson, J. R.: Anatomy and diagnosis of torsion of the testicle. J. Urol. *106*:243, 1971.

Pearman, R. O.: Congenital absence of the testicle: monorchism. J. Urol. *85*:599, 1961.

Peterson, C. G.: Testicular torsion and infarction in the newborn. J. Urol. *85*:65, 1961.

Preston, E. N.: Whither the foreskin? A consideration of routine neonatal circumcision. J.A.M.A. *213*:1853, 1971.

Radman, H. M., Askin, J. A., and Kolodner, L. J.: Hydrometrocolpos and hematometrocolpos. Obstet. Gynecol. *27*:2, 1966.

Redman, J. F.: Noonan's syndrome and cryptorchidism. J. Urol. *109*:909, 1973.

Reed, M. H., and Griscom, N. T.: Hydrometrocolpos in infancy. Am. J. Roentgenol. *118*:1, 1973.

Reis, R. L., and Koop, C. E.: Ovarian tumors in infants and children. J. Pediatr. *60*:96, 1962.

Rhyne, J. L., Mantz, E. A., Jr., and Patton, J. F.: Hemorrhagic infarction of testis in the newborn: relationship to testicular torsion. A.M.A. J. Dis. Child. *89*:240, 1955.

Robinson, J. N., and Engle, E. T.: Cryptorchidism. Pediatr. Clin. North Am. *2*:729, 1955.

Rubinstein, M. M., and Bason, W. M.: Complications of circumcision done with a plastic bell clamp. Am. J. Dis. Child. *116*:381, 1968.

Scorer, C. G.: A treatment of undescended testicle in infancy. Arch. Dis. Child. *32*:520, 1957.

Scorer, C. G., and Farrington, C. M.: Congenital deformities of the testis and epididymis. New York, Appleton-Century-Crofts, 1971.

Scott, L. S.: Fertility in cryptorchidism. Proc. Roy. Soc. Med. *55*:1047, 1962.

Shulman, J., Ben-Hur, N., and Neuman, Z.: Surgical complications of circumcision. Am. J. Dis. Child. *107*:149, 1964.

Smith, R. C.: Simple ovarian cyst in a newborn infant. Pediatrics *14*:232, 1954.

Snyder, W. H., Jr.: Some unusual forms of imperforate anus in female infants. Am. J. Surg. *111*:319, 1966.

Sorensen, M. R.: Hypospadias with special reference to aetiology. Copenhagen, Munksgaard, 1953.

Svensson, J.: Male hypospadias, 625 cases, associated malformations and possible etiologic factors. Acta Pediatr. Scand. *65*:587, 1979.

Tietz, K. G., and Davis, J. B.: Ruptured ovarian cyst in a newborn infant. J. Pediatr. *51*:564, 1957.

Watson, R. A., Lennox, K. W., and Gangai, M. P.: Simple cryptorchidism: the value of excretory urogram as a screening method. J. Urol. *111*:789, 1974.

Weldon, V. V., Blizzard, R. M., and Migeon, C. J.: Newborn girls misdiagnosed as bilateral cryptorchid males. N. Engl. J. Med. *274*:829, 1966.

Whitesel, J. A.: Intrauterine and newborn torsion of spermatic cord. J. Urol. *106*:786, 1971.

45

Congenital Malformations of the Genitourinary Tract

By Warren E. Grupe

Synchronous with the induction of the final kidney from the metanephros, a series of events take place in several separate embryonic tissues that are incorporated in and about the cloaca and allantois. This chapter reviews several developmental anomalies of the genitourinary tract in which the inciting events produce maldevelopment of the urogenital sinus, the mesonephric ducts, or the metanephric ducts.

Exstrophy of the Bladder

This anomaly occurs once in every 30,000 to 40,000 livebirths. It is more common in males but can occur in females, and it does not appear to be familial. It is a defect of midline fusion with a localized deficiency in the abdominal wall, pubis, bladder, and urethra. The result is immediately obvious at birth, with an eversion of bright red bladder mucosa between widely separated rectus muscles that insert into the disconnected pubic bones. The umbilicus is at the top edge of the defect. The trigone and the ure-teral orifices are exposed, and urine dribbles intermittently onto the mucosal surface. The perineum is flattened, the anus more anterior, and the femoral heads externally rotated. Correct diagnosis is usually not difficult.

In males, the penis is flattened, broad, and short. An opened fissure along the dorsal surface represents the epispadiac urethra. Occasionally, the paired rudimentary halves of the phallus remain separated. The testes are usually undescended. In the female,

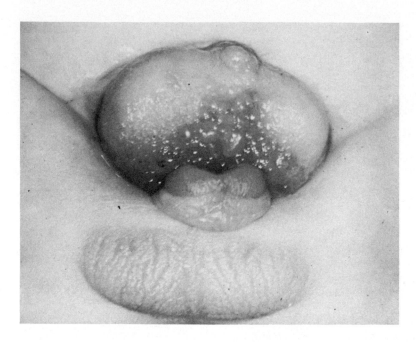

Figure 45–1. Bulging everted bladder lying below the umbilicus. Beneath this, a completely epispadiac penis is seen, and below that is a shallow, poorly developed scrotum devoid of testes.

the clitoris fails to fuse or is deeply fissured, and the labia are widely separated. The vagina may be absent, anteriorly dislocated, or replaced by a rectovaginal cloaca. Inguinal hernias are common.

The exposed bladder should be immediately protected to prevent damage, irritation, tenesmus, and rectal prolapse. Definitive therapy is surgical and is often carried out within a few days or weeks of birth. Such surgery involves repair of the pubic rami, closure of the abdominal defect, and establishment of an anterior wall for the bladder. The goal is to establish a functioning bladder with reasonable capacity and urinary continence. This may take several stages and may not be completely successful. If continuity

of a functional lower tract cannot be established, primary urinary diversion is in order. When the bladder can be reconstructed, subsequent surgery will be required to repair the epispadias, reimplant the ureters, create a bladder sphincter, lengthen the penis in boys, and approximate the labia in girls. Usually, the upper urinary tracts are normal until after closure of the bladder.

About 40 per cent of children with exstrophy of the bladder achieve good bladder control, and another 40 per cent acquire some control. In the remaining 20 per cent, results are not satisfactory, and a urinary diversion must be created, usually by ureterosigmoidostomy. Carcinoma of the recon-

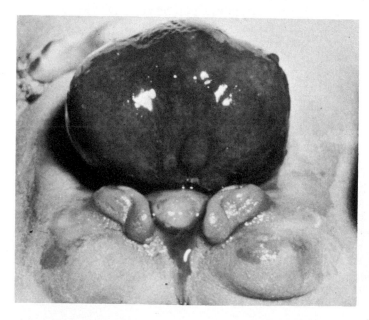

Figure 45–2. Bulging everted bladder lies on the lower part of the abdomen. Below it, the three structures seen are a small, flattened phallus in the midline and widely separated labia to either side. Below and lateral to these are the bulges of indirect inguinal hernias. (Photograph of a case of Dr. Martin A. Robbins of Baltimore, reproduced with his kind permission.)

structed bladder has been reported in 4 to 7.5 per cent of cases.

Cloacal Exstrophy

This anomaly is a more extensive defect that involves a vesicointestinal fissure and imperforate anus. The anomaly is rare, occurring once in every 200,000 to 250,000 births. The infant presents at birth with a large anterior abdominal defect, an omphalocele, and a plate-like structure whose lateral surfaces are covered with bladder mucosa flanking midline colonic mucosa, representing ectopic cecum. The pelvis is widely disjointed, separating the bifid genitalia. Frequently, both internal and external genitalia are absent. When kidneys are present, their ureters are found inserted at the caudal aspect of the bladder mucosa. Ileum may be prolapsed into the defect. Musculoskeletal abnormalities, including meningomyelocele, are common. Many children fail to survive the newborn period; those who do require extensive surgical reconstruction.

Imperforate Anus and Urogenital Abnormalities

The association of imperforate anus with a wide variety of abnormalities in the lower and upper urinary tract is relatively frequent. Embryologically, the cloacal septum is separating the urogenital sinus from the gastrointestinal tract at about the same time that metanephric development is initiated and the lumbosacral spine is formed. Thus, a localized developmental error near the fourth week of gestation can produce a multisystem abnormality.

When formation of the urorectal septum is incomplete, a persistent communication remains between the anterior and posterior portions of the cloaca. When this defect is high (supralevator), a fistulous tract is retained between the blind rectal pouch and urogenital tract. In males, this fistula enters the pros-

tatic urethra, although on rare occasions it may communicate with the bladder. In the female, a rectovaginal fistula results. In those in whom the urorectal defect is low (infralevator), the fistulas communicate with the perineum, emerging at the base of the scrotum in the male and at the posterior fourchette in the female.

Half the infants with high defects have associated genitourinary abnormalities. In 60 per cent of these, the lesions are limited to the upper tract and include renal agenesis, hypoplasia, and dysplasia. Other abnormalities consistent with defective ureteral bud development include vesicoureteral reflux, aberrant insertion of the vas deferens, ureteral obstruction, and duplication of the collecting system.

Only 14 to 20 per cent of infants with infralevator imperforate anus have genitourinary lesions. In this group, renal agenesis is infrequent, although renal malrotation, renal ectopia, and duplicated collecting systems occur.

A neurogenic bladder is present in about 10 per cent of infants and is related either to the presence of sacral lesions or to vigorous surgery to correct the imperforate anus.

The rectourethral and rectovesical fistulas offer no relief of the intestinal obstruction. Air in the bladder may be present with both lesions. A diverting colostomy relieves the situation in those infants with supralevator defects and allows a more studied evaluation of the upper urinary tracts before surgical reconstruction is performed.

VATER, VACTERL, and MURCS Anomalies

Other associations have been noted, often with a variety of mnemonics, linking multiple system abnormalities with the genitourinary tract. The VATER

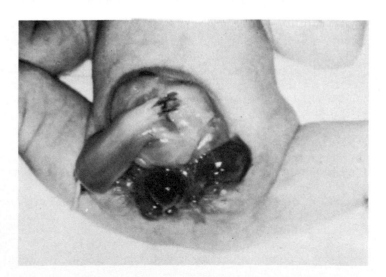

Figure 45–3. The umbilicus, with cord still attached, is herniated so as to form a large omphalocele. Beneath it lies the deep, dark red mucosa of everted bladder. The genitalia cannot be seen in this photograph.

anomaly links *V*ertebra defects, *A*nal atresia, and *T-E* fistula with *E*sophageal atresia and *R*adial and *R*enal dysplasia. The VATER association has been noted in a patient with a deletion of the long arm of chromosome 6. The VACTERL acronym expands the VATER associations to include congenital *C*ardiac disease with the *L*imb abnormalities. One report notes a familial association of the anal, ear, renal, and radial malformations, suggesting an autosomal dominant transmission. The MURCS association includes *MÜ*llerian duct aplasia, *R*enal aplasia, and *C*ervico-thoracic *S*omite dysplasia. These associations, either singly or in groups, suggest that the fetus is most susceptible to the development of genitourinary abnormalities at or about 33 days gestation. This may be of some importance when one considers the defects noted in association with exposure to such external agents as diethylstilbestrol or in the fetal alcohol syndrome. Such associated defects in other organ systems can also alert the physician to consider radiologic evaluation of the infant's genitourinary tract.

Absence of the Abdominal Musculature (Triad Syndrome)

Deficiency of all or nearly all of the abdominal musculature, associated with abnormalities of the urinary tract, has been the central feature of this anomalad, first described in 1839. The term "prune belly," which was first used by Osler to describe the appearance of the abdominal wall, has become the popular idiom and is used interchangeably with the terms Eagle-Barrett syndrome, mesenchymal dysplasia syndrome, and urethral obstruction malformation complex. The incidence of this complex abnormality is not completely known, but it is probably present in one of every 30,000 to 40,000 livebirths.

Etiology and Pathogenesis. The formation of the abdominal wall begins by the fifth gestational week and is completed by the twelfth week, coincident with the beginnings of urine formation. Failure to develop musculature, therefore, must be explained by events in the first trimester. Three possible associations exist: (1) The muscular defect is primary, with laxity of the abdominal wall and decreased intra-abdominal pressure encouraging the dilatation of the developing urinary tract; (2) both the muscular defect and the genitourinary anomalies are separately the result of a primary mesodermal defect; and (3) the genitourinary abnormalities are primary and timed such that secondary abdominal wall changes result.

Recent evidence favors the last possibility for the moment. Pagon and coworkers have presented a compelling argument that attempts to relate all the defects to fetal urethral obstruction. Their first point is that abdominal muscle deficiency can be seen in association with other conditions that produce fetal abdominal distention, including XO Turner's syndrome, fetal ascites, Beckwith-Wiedemann syndrome, primary polycystic kidneys, cystic adenomatoid malformation of the lung, and urethral obstruction. They present evidence that the bladder distention resulting from urethral obstruction presents a secondary mechanical blockade to the descent of the testes, the rotation of the colon, the vascular supply to the lower limbs, and the production of amniotic fluid. By vesicoureteral reflux, the bladder induces dilatation of the urinary tract and inhibits continued nephrogenesis. The severity of the defects may relate either to the completeness of the outlet obstruction or to the relief of entrapped urine through rupture of the bladder or through the urachus. Their postulate is that the anomalies result from the combination of urethral obstruction *plus* urine production coupled with the lack of an early decompression of the urinary tract through an alternative outlet. Resolution of the fetal urethral obstruction in utero, with subsequent decompression and collapse of the severely stretched abdominal wall (hence the wrinkled appearance of a dried prune), accounts for the postnatal absence of demonstrable obstructive lesions in many of these infants. Also, since the morphogenesis of the male urethra is more complex than that of the female urethra, the large excess of males with the triad syndrome is understandable. Since the causes of urethral obstruction are multiple, the recurrence risk for this syndrome is unknown.

Thus, what may distinguish the child with triad syndrome from some infants with Potter's syndrome may be the ability of the former to excrete urine. With severe early urethral obstruction, fetal survival may depend on the ability to decompress the distended bladder followed by regression of the abdominal distention. The escape of urine allows formation of sufficient amniotic fluid, which prevents the external uterine compression that produces the characteristic abnormalities of Potter's syndrome, including pulmonary hypoplasia. Those without prenatal urine extravasation either fail to survive to term or suffer early neonatal death associated with the clinical features of Potter's syndrome.

Diagnosis. The finding of a lax, wrinkled abdominal wall associated with cryptorchidism and urinary tract anomalies completes the classic triad. Additional defects include malrotation of the colon, lower limb defects, rib cage anomalies, imperforate anus, and cardiovascular abnormalities. Although the infant is nearly always male, the syndrome has occasionally been described in females.

There can be a wide spectrum of clinical severity and clinical presentation. Some infants are sufficiently damaged to be stillborn or to die in the early neonatal period from pulmonary hypoplasia. Others are so mildly affected that the diagnosis may become evident only when radiologic investigation demonstrates

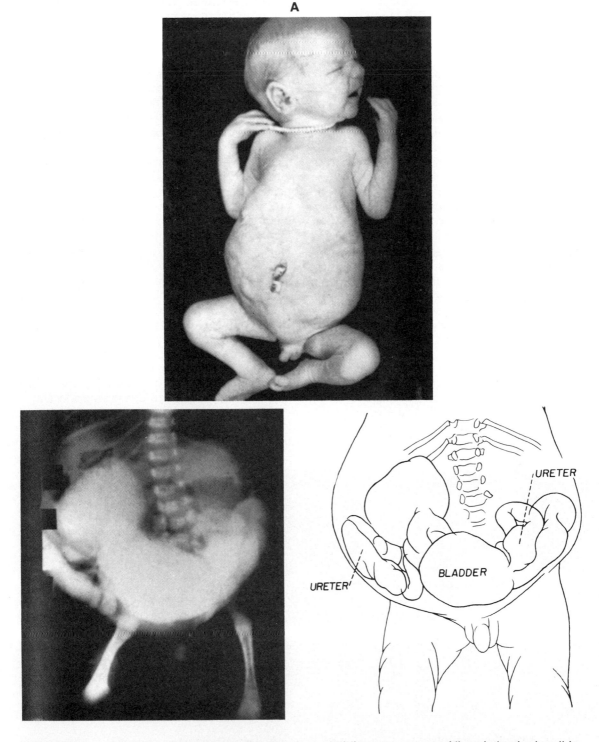

Figure 45—4. *A*, Photograph at birth exhibits the characteristic appearance of the abdominal wall in an infant with the triad syndrome. *B*, Cystogram performed via urethral catheter demonstrating bilateral urethral reflux, bilateral hydronephrosis, and hydroureter. (From McGovern, J. M., and Marshall, V. F.: Surg. Gynecol. Obstet. *108*:289, 1959.)

the urinary tract abnormalities. Still others may have a persistently patent urachus as the initial visible manifestation. In these milder forms, careful examination may be required for discernment of the abdominal wall defect. What can initially appear to be ascites may prove to be a markedly distended bladder on further examination.

Usually, the abdomen has a decided bulge, and the flanks sag limply. The skin is characteristically wrinkled and creased. Intestinal loops may be floridly visible. The palpating hand meets no resistance, so one can feel all the organs and the vertebral column with surprising ease. Often, many discrete masses are palpable, including the large bladder, the dilated ureters, and the prominent kidneys. The testes are invariably undescended and often intra-abdominal.

Radiographically, long, dilated, and tortuous ureters with poor peristalsis and varying calibre are seen to empty into a huge bladder that often has a urachal diverticulum and bizarre contour. The posterior urethra is usually dilated and associated with abnormalities of the prostate. Reflux may be noted into the utricle, the vas deferens, or the seminal vesicles. There will be varying degrees of renal dysplasia. Although urethral stenosis or atresia may be rarely demonstrated, it is more common that no obstructive lesion is detected in these survivors; dilatation does not equate with obstruction. Deficiencies in the corpus spongiosum and in the anterior urethra can also be found.

Treatment. Since there is so little to work with, reconstructive operations to re-establish abdominal tone are not possible. Some continue to use a tight abdominal binder, with some evidence that abdominal tone improves over the years. There is no evidence, however, that such binders improve renal function or facilitate urine drainage, and at least one death from respiratory insufficiency from the zealous use of an elastic binder has beed recorded.

Opinions about the value of surgical intervention have been polarized. Over 20 years ago, the feeling was that "masterful inactivity" should give way to prompt enhancement of urinary egress either by nephrostomy or vesicostomy (McGovern and Marshall, 1959). It was claimed that dilated and tortuous ureters must be shortened, straightened, and reimplanted early. If the bladder remained large and its pressure increased, revision of the bladder neck or urinary diversion was contemplated.

More recently, data have been presented to show that those subjected to vigorous or early surgery in the absence of a demonstrable obstructing site have fared no better and, in some cases, worse than those patients treated with "close medical and urologic examination, with efforts to control bacteremia" (Burke et al., 1969). Current practice would have surgery dictated by problems of incomplete urine drainage or problems with recurrent infections rather than by the degree of radiologic abnormality. Cutaneous vesicostomy, when needed, will usually drain the entire system adequately and avoid the introduction of foreign material. The need for ureteral reimplantation is not clear, and some feel that extensive reconstruction of the ureter worsens the urodynamics of an al-

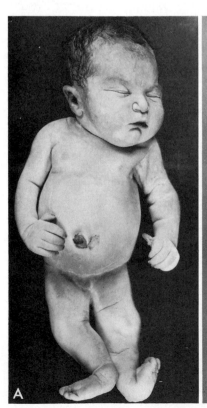 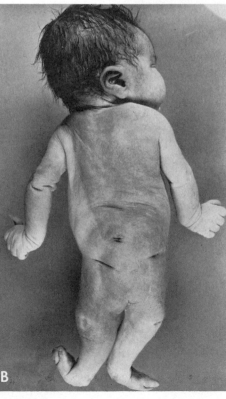

Figure 45–5. Absence of external genitals, together with imperforate anus and facial characteristics suggestive of renal agenesis. (Case of J. D. Kirshbaum. Photographs reprinted with his kind permission from J. Pediatr. *37:*102, 1950.)

ready tenuous system. The efforts of this group are directed toward the prevention of infection with the judicious use of antibiotics, and surgery is performed only when obstruction is carefully demonstrated by adequate pressure-flow measurements. With this itinerary, the triad syndrome does not become a neonatal surgical emergency.

Prognosis.   The ultimate outcome for the infant is, in the final analysis, related to the amount of functioning renal tissue remaining. If the degree of dysplasia is marked, the infant may be faced with months to years of difficulty that eventually leads to the need for mechanical dialysis and renal transplantation. Those with milder degrees of dysgenesis, who constitute a significant proportion of this group of children, may still be alive with reasonable or normal renal function 14 to 25 years later, providing infection is properly controlled.

Bilateral Renal Agenesis (Potter's Syndrome)

Although congenital absence of one kidney may go undetected during a normal lifetime, complete absence of nephrogenesis is incompatible with life. Certain clinical traits were initially described by Potter in association with bilateral renal agenesis that allowed this fatal condition to be recognized during life. Potter found 20 examples in 5000 consecutive autopsies of fetuses and newborns, defining an inci-

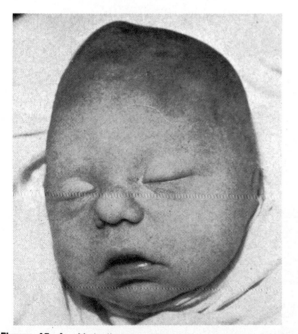

Figure 45–6.   Note the prominent eyes, the fold sweeping in an arc from the inner canthus downward and outward, the depressed nasal bridge and retroussé nose, and the low-set ears. In this case, there was complete absence of the right kidney and hypoplasia of the left kidney. (Case of J. D. Kirshbaum. Photograph reprinted with the author's permission from California Med. *71:*148, 1949.)

dence of 4 per every 1000 neonatal deaths and 1 per every 3000 births.

Diagnosis.   The characteristics that constitute Potter's syndrome have come to be associated with severe impairment of nephrogenesis. The physical appearance is that of an infant, almost always a male, who is small for gestational age with widely spaced eyes flanking a depressed nasal bridge and a retroussé nose. A very prominent skin fold arises from the epicanthus and progresses inferiorly, then extends laterally beneath the eyes. The chin is receded, and the face is prematurely senile. The ears are posteriorly rotated, asymmetrical, floppy, and low-set. Oligohydramnios is inevitably present, and the placenta is abnormal. Those infants with bilateral renal agenesis or aplasia are completely anuric. However, Potter's facies may also be seen in other conditions associated with a severely reduced urine output in utero, including severe renal dysplasia, renal hypoplasia, and bilateral multicystic dysplasia. In a review of 85 children with Potter's syndrome, Roodhooft and Holmes noted that 44 had bilateral agenesis, 30 had bilateral severe dysgenesis, and 11 had agenesis of one kidney with severe dysgenesis of the other. Other associated but inconstant abnormalities include imperforate anus, hydrocephalus, meningomyelocele, arthrogryposis, skeletal anomalies (including hypoplasia of the pelvis), abnormalities of the lower limbs (including equinovarus), and hypoplasia of the lungs. Owing to the lung abnormality, many of these infants surface in the nursery because of spontaneous pneumothorax occurring at or soon after birth or difficult and ineffective resuscitation. Recognition of this composite at birth discourages the multiple investigative, therapeutic, and surgical procedures that might otherwise result in an unsuccessful attempt to diagnose a salvageable condition.

Two reports have noted the association of bilateral and unilateral aplasia in the same families. Roodhooft and Holmes, using ultrasonography, found that 10.8 per cent of parents and first degree relatives of infants with Potter's syndrome had nonlethal malformations of either metanephric or müllerian duct derivatives. These anomalies included renal cysts, double collecting systems, unilateral renal agenesis, absent ovary, and bicornate uterus. Siblings with Potter's syndrome were also noted on two occasions in this survey.

In one reported case of twins, one infant had bilateral agenesis, while the other had unilateral renal dysplasia and an ectopic kidney. Neither twin had the facial, limb, pulmonary, or skin abnormalities of Potter's syndrome. The authors argued that the twins were protected because the one functioning kidney of the four forestalled oligohydramnios. Most now believe that oligohydramnios is responsible for the pulmonary hypoplasia, while the external compression resulting from uterine constraint causes the other associated defects.

Prognosis. Usually, the clinical course declines rapidly. Of Potter's original 20 cases, six died during labor, and the remainder died within 11 hours after delivery. Although almost all patients with this abnormality are anuric, uremia is not the cause of death. Most die from pulmonary complications before uremia can supervene. Generally, dialysis is not instituted.

Some infants with hypoplasia or dysplasia do produce urine, even though the other features of the syndrome are present. They may have varying degrees of remaining renal function and may survive the neonatal period, depending on the degree of pulmonary hypoplasia.

Duplication of the Collecting System

Both incomplete and complete duplication of the ureters, pelvis, and collecting system results from developmental changes in the ureteric bud. The lesions are more common in girls and are more often unilateral.

Partial duplication is commonly asymptomatic and produces no physiologic changes. It results from early division of the advancing ureteric bud. Radiographically, the ureters are Y-shaped. There may be to-and-fro movement of urine from one limb of the Y to the other (ureteroureteral reflux), which has the same effect as urinary stasis and which may become important when associated with urinary tract infection.

Complete duplication results from more than one ureteric bud developing from the mesonephric duct.

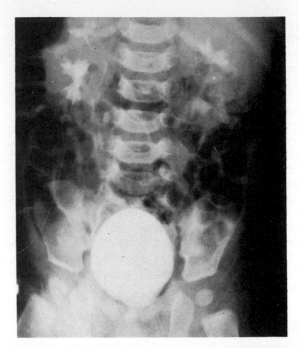

Figure 45–8. Film taken during the course of an intravenous pyelographic study. The left collecting system is definitely duplicated, and two ureters can be seen on that side. The same situation is almost surely present on the right. In spite of this, the pelves are not enlarged, and all the calyces are delicate, sharply outlined, and concave. There is clearly no obstruction to urinary outflow at any point.

This series of films was made in the course of a survey to determine the cause of vomiting. This was clearly an incidental finding that had no bearing on the chief complaint.

The ureter to the upper pole more commonly has an ectopic bladder insertion that is medial and inferior to the insertion of the lower segment ureter or involves an ureterocele. Occasionally, the ureter bypasses the bladder to discharge into the vagina or onto the perineum. Dysplasia and variable degrees

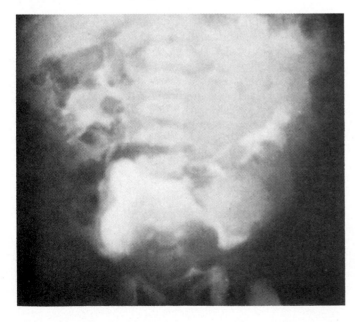

Figure 45–7. Intravenous pyelogram made on the fifth day of life. Two collecting systems can be seen on the right. The collecting system visible on the left is displaced far downward and appears to be flattened by an opaque mass above it.

of obstruction often involve and can totally destroy the superior duplicated segment with or without infection. Vesicoureteral reflux into the lower pole ureter is common.

Diagnosis. This anomaly can never be diagnosed without complete and careful urologic evaluation. Both ureters must be followed in their entirety, and the functional status of both renal segments drained by the system must be established. Occasionally, an enlarged kidney is felt, or the infant develops unexplained fever, pyuria, or sepsis. At times, the obstructed and dilated upper pole will displace the functioning lower pole downward and thus mimic a suprarenal tumor, especially if the upper segment is nonfunctioning.

Treatment. The incomplete duplications rarely require any surgical manipulation. Complete duplications with obstruction and dysplasia can seldom be repaired satisfactorily and generally require eventual heminephrectomy and ureterectomy. If the other half is likewise beyond repair, a total nephrectomy is performed. When the lower pole shows satisfactory function and no obstruction, ureteral reimplantation is performed to correct the vesicoureteral reflux.

REFERENCES

Amolsch, A. L.: Bilateral metanephric agenesia with a report of 4 cases. J. Urol. *38*:360, 1937.

Bain, A. D., and Scott, J. S.: Renal agenesis and severe urinary tract dysplasia: review of 50 cases with particular reference to associated anomalies. Br. Med. J. *5176*:841, 1960.

Bashour, B. N., and Balfe, W.: Urinary tract anomalies in neonates with spontaneous pneumothorax and/or pneumomediastinum. Pediatrics *59*:S1048, 1977.

Belman, A. B., and King, L. R.: Urinary tract abnormalities associated with imperforate anus. J. Urol. *108*:823, 1972.

Berdon, W. E., Baker, D. H., Wigger, H. J., and Blanc, W. A.: The radiologic and pathologic spectrum of the prune belly syndrome: the importance of urethral obstruction in prognosis. Radiol. Clin. North Am. *15*:83, 1977.

Burke, E. C., Shin, M. H., and Kelalis, P. P.: Prune-belly syndrome: clinical findings and survival. Am. J. Dis. Child. *117*:668, 1969.

Cain, D. R., Griggs, D., et al.: Familial renal agenesis and total dysplasia. Am. J. Dis. Child. *128*:377, 1974.

DeBeukelaer, M. M., Randall, C. L., and Stroud, D. R.: Renal anomalies in the fetal alcohol syndrome. J. Pediatr. *91*:759, 1977.

Duncan, P. A., Shapiro, L. R., Stangel, J. J., Klein, R. M., and Addonizio, J. C.: The MURCS association: Mülleran duct aplasia, renal aplasia and cervicothoracic somite dysplasia. J. Pediatr. *95*:399, 1979.

Garrett, R., and Franken, E.: Neonatal ascites: perirenal urinary extravasation with bladder outlet obstruction. J. Urol. *102*:627, 1969.

Gellis, S. S., and Feingold, M.: Picture of the month: congenital absence of abdominal musculature (prune belly). Am. J. Dis. Child. *109*:571, 1965.

Goldstein, G., and Arulanathan, K.: Neural tube defect and renal anomalies in a child with fetal alcohol syndrome. J. Pediatr. *93*:636, 1978.

Henderson, B. E., Benton, B., Cosgrove, M., Baptista, M. A., Aldrich, J., Townsend, D., Hart, W., and Mack, T.: Urogenital tract abnormalities in sons of women treated with diethylstilbestrol. Pediatrics *58*:505, 1976.

Jeffs, R. D.: Exstrophy and cloacal exstrophy. Urol. Clin. North Am. *5*:127, 1978.

Johnson, J. H.: The genital aspects of exstrophy. J. Urol. *113*:701, 1975.

Johnston, J. H., and Kogan, S. J.: The exstrophic anomalies and their surgical reconstruction. *In* Ravitch, M. M. (Ed.): Current Problems in Surgery. Chicago, Year Book Medical Publishers, 1974.

Kelley, J. H., and Eraklis, A. J.: A procedure for lengthening of the phallus in boys with exstrophy of the bladder. J. Pediatr. Surg. *6*:645, 1971.

King, C. R., and Prescott, G.: Pathogenesis of the prune-belly anomalad. J. Pediatr. *93*:273, 1978.

Kirshbaum, J. D.: Facial characteristics of an infant without renal function. California Med. *71*:148, 1949.

Kohn, G., and Borns, P. F.: The association of bilateral and unilateral renal aplasia in the same family. J. Pediatr. *83*:95, 1973.

Kurnit, D. M., Steele, M. W., Pinsky, L., and Dibbins, A.: Autosomal dominant transmission of a syndrome of anal, ear, renal and radial congenital malformations. J. Pediatr. *93*:270, 1978.

Ladd, W. E., and Gross, R. E.: Congenital malformations of anus and rectum: report of 162 cases. Am. J. Surg. *23*:167, 1934.

Lee, M. J.: Prune belly syndrome in a 54 year old man. J.A.M.A. *237*:2216, 1977.

Markland, C., and Fraley, E. E.: Management of infants with cloacal exstrophy. J. Urol. *109*:740, 1973.

Mauer, S. M., Dobrin, R. S., and Vernier, R. L.: Unilateral and bilateral renal agenesis in monoamniotic twins. J. Pediatr. *84*:236, 1974.

McGovern, J. M., and Marshall, V. F.: Congenital deficiency of the abdominal musculature and obstructive uropathy. Surg. Gynecol. Obstet. *108*:289, 1959.

McNeal, R. M., Skoglund, R. R., and Francke, U.: Congenital anomalies including the VATER association in a patient with a del(6)q deletion. J. Pediatr. *91*:957, 1977.

Nunn, I. N., and Stephens, F. D.: The triad syndrome: a composite anomaly of the abdominal wall, urinary system and testes. J. Urol. *86*:782, 1961.

Osler, W.: Congenital absence of the abdominal muscles with distended and hypertrophied bladder. Bull. Johns Hopkins Hosp. *12*:331, 1901.

Pagon, R. A., Smith, D. W., and Shepard, T. H.: Urethral obstruction malformation complex: a cause of abdominal muscle deficiency and the "prune belly." J. Pediatr. *94*:900, 1979.

Passarge, E., and Sutherland, J. H.: Potter's syndrome with chromosome analysis of three cases with Potter's syndrome or related syndromes. Am. J. Dis. Child. *109*:80, 1965.

Potter, E. L.: Bilateral renal agenesis. J. Pediatr. *29*:68, 1946.

Potter, E., and Craig, J.: Pathology of the Fetus and the Infant. 3rd ed. Chicago, Year Book Medical Publishers, 1975.

Pramanik, A. K., Alschuler, G., Light, I. J., and Sutherland, J. M.: Prune belly syndrome associated with Potter's (renal non-function) syndrome. Am. J. Dis. Child. *131*:672, 1977.

Quan, L., and Smith, D. W.: The VATER association. J. Pediatr. *82*:104, 1973.

Raffensperger, J. G.: Anomalies of the female genitalia: *In* Kelalis, P. P., and King, L. R. (Eds.): Clinical Pediatric Urology. Philadelphia, W. B. Saunders Co., 1976, p. 669.

Roberts, P.: Congenital absence of the abdominal muscles with associated abnormalities of the genito-urinary tract. Arch. Dis. Child. *31*:236, 1956.

Rogers, L. W., and Ostrow, P. T.: The prune belly syndrome: report of 20 cases and description of a lethal variant. J. Pediatr. *83*:786, 1973.

Roodhooft, A. M., and Holmes, L. B.: Family studies: Potter's syndrome of renal agenesis and dysgenesis. Am. J. Hum. Genet. *33*:91A, 1981.

Santulli, T. V., Kiesewetter, W. B., and Bill, A. H., Jr.: Anorectal anomalies: a suggested international classification. J. Pediatr. Surg. *5*:281, 1970.

Silverman, F. N., and Huang, N.: Congenital absence of the abdominal muscles associated with malformations of the genitourinary tracts: report of cases and a review of literature. Am. J. Dis. Child. *80*:91, 1950.

Smith, D. W.: Redundant skin folds in the infant—their origin and relevance. J. Pediatr. *94*:1021, 1979.

Smith, M. J. V., and Lattimer, J. R.: The management of bladder exstrophy. Surg. Gynecol. Obstet. *123*:1015, 1966.

Stephens, F. D., and Smith, E. D.: Ano-rectal malformations in children. Chicago, Year Book Medical Publishers, 1971, p. 334.

Tankx, E. S., and Watts, H.: Hyperchloremic acidosis from urethrorectal fistula and imperforate anus. Surgery *63*:837, 1968.

Temtamy, S. A., and Miller, J. D.: Extending the scope of the VATER association: definition of the VATER syndrome. J. Pediatr. *85*:345, 1974.

Texter, J. H., and Murphy, G. P.: The right-sided syndrome: congenital absence of the right testis, kidney and rectum. Urologic diagnosis and treatment. Johns Hopkins Med. Bull. *122*:224, 1968.

Thomas, I. T., and Smith, D. W.: Oligohydramnios, cause of the nonrenal features of Potter's syndrome, including pulmonary hypoplasia. J. Pediatr. *84*:811, 1974.

Timothy, R. P., Decter, A., and Perlmutter, A. D.: Ureteral duplication: clinical findings and therapy in 46 children. J. Urol. *105*:445, 1971.

Ulson, A. C., Lattimer, J. K., and Melicow, M. M.: Types of exstrophy of urinary bladder and concomitant malformations. Report based on 82 cases. Pediatrics *23*:927, 1959.

Welch, K. K., and Kearney, G. P.: Abdominal musculature deficiency syndrome: prune belly. J. Urol. *111*:693, 1974.

Whitaker, R. H.: Investigating wide ureters with ureteral pressure flow studies. J. Urol. *116*:81, 1976.

White, P., and Lebowitz, R. L.: Exstrophy of the bladder. Radiol. Clin. North Am. *15*:93, 1977.

Wiener, E. S., and Kiesewetter, W. B.: Urologic abnormalities associated with imperforate anus. J. Pediatr. Surg. *8*:151, 1973.

Williams, D. I.: Urological complications of imperforate anus. Br. J. Urol. *41*:660, 1969.

Williams, D. I., and Burkholder, G. V.: The prune belly syndrome. J. Urol. *98*:244, 1967.

Williams, D. I., and Keeton, J. E.: Further progress with reconstruction of the exstrophied bladder. Br. J. Surg. *60*:203, 1973.

46

Congenital Malformations of the Kidney

By Warren E. Grupe

The explanation of many developmental anomalies of the kidneys lies in abnormalities of nephrogenesis. Once the ureteric bud has made contact with the metanephros, defects in either the degree of branching or the induction of nephrons can result in dysgenesis of the final kidney. This chapter reviews several renal parenchymal lesions that have their origin in defective nephron development.

Hypoplastic Kidneys

Hypoplasia of the kidneys has been defined as a congenitally decreased amount of normal renal tissue. Unilateral hypoplasia denotes a kidney that is less than 50 per cent of its expected weight. Bilateral hypoplasia is severe if the combined renal mass is less than half the expected weight and moderate if it is one half to two thirds the average weight in proportion to total body weight and length. Although the true incidence is not known, it may be as high as 2 per cent of autopsied cases. There is no clear familial tendency and no predilection for either sex.

These infants are commonly of low birth weight and often have abnormalities of organ systems other than the genitourinary tract. Lateral displacement of the nipples has been said to be an aid to diagnosis in the nursery. Hypertension is not common. Intravenous pyelography and ultrasonography show small kidneys without cysts. In true hypoplasia, the number of reniculi and calyces are reduced, but they appear normal.

Morphologically, the kidneys are well differentiated with a clear cortical medullary junction, and the nephrons are normally arranged. They appear normal microscopically, with no histologic features of dysplasia, although areas of tubular atrophy and interstitial scar are occasionally seen. The degree of dysfunction is determined by the total functioning mass of the kidney. Tubular dysfunction is prominent in hypoplasia, with high volumes of dilute urine, acidosis, and salt wasting. If the amount of renal tissue is totally inadequate, the infant may have severe respiratory problems in the nursery.

Often, the term "hypoplastic dysplasia" is used to describe kidneys that are small and that manifest other evidences of embryonic maldevelopment. However, it is improper to call "dysplastic" any small kidney with bizarre calyces on pyelography.

An interesting subgroup of the renal dysplasias was described in 1962 by Royer and his collaborators. Because there was the simultaneous presence of hypoplasia and hypertrophy of the sparse nephrons, they called the syndrome "oligoméganéphronie."

The infants are often of low birth weight and born to mothers over 35 years of age. Affected males outnumber females 3 to 1. Abnormalities in other organ systems are unusual. Pyelography and ultrasonography reveal small kidneys with normal calyces. Hypertension is unusual, even as renal failure progresses. There is no clear familial tendency. Of the hypoplastic diseases, oligomeganephronia is the most likely to be associated with proteinuria. Tubular dysfunction is prominent, with polyuria, polydipsia, and a decreased concentrating ability. Characteristic of pediatric patients is an early onset of renal insufficiency, which may then remain stable for many years. It may be accompanied by vomiting, failure to thrive, and acidosis. Renal sodium wasting is almost universal, and many develop rickets. Treatment is supportive and symptomatic.

Griffel and coworkers and Van Aker and colleagues have each reported a case of unilateral oligomeganephronia with contralateral aplasia or agenesis associated with a small renal artery. Morphologically, the kidney shows glomerular volume that is seven to ten times the normal value, while the proximal tubular length is four times the normal measurement. No dysplastic elements are found microscopically.

Hypertrophy of the remaining nephrons is the usual renal response to a loss of functional parenchyma by whatever means. Thus, oligomeganephronia may be considered the expected response to insufficient nephron induction. Considered in this light, true hypoplasia could represent a dual developmental defect: first, an insufficient induction of nephrons by the advancing ureteric bud, and second, an inability of the normal hypertrophy response.

Dysplasia

Dysplasia is more common and represents hypoplasia with disordered development of the metanephros. The majority of infants have associated abnormalities in the urinary tract, and it has been postulated on the basis of both experimental grounds and clinical observation that obstruction while nephrons are immature is a major component of the abnormality, even though obstruction may no longer be demonstrable at birth. Animal experiments have shown that the timing of the obstruction is crucial in the production of dysplasia. Others have felt that a primary defect in the ampullae of the ureteric bud causes decreased branching and, therefore, decreased nephron induction and maturation. A third proposal by Mackie and coworkers suggests that the budding of the ureter from the wolffian duct is out of phase and thereby misses the moment at which

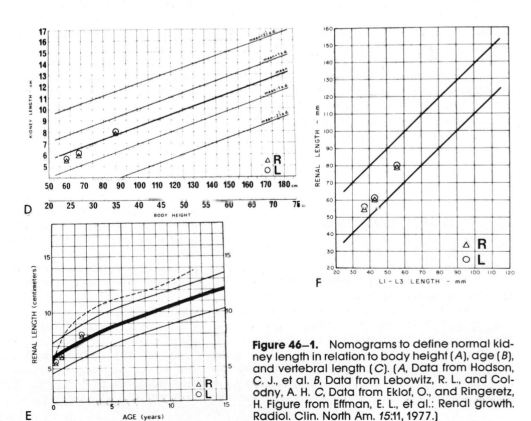

Figure 46–1. Nomograms to define normal kidney length in relation to body height (*A*), age (*B*), and vertebral length (*C*). (*A*, Data from Hodson, C. J., et al. *B*, Data from Lebowitz, R. L., and Colodny, A. H. *C*, Data from Eklof, O., and Ringeretz, H. Figure from Effman, E. L., et al.: Renal growth. Radiol. Clin. North Am. *15*:11, 1977.)

the metanephric tissue has the best potential for nephrogenesis. Ectopic placement of the ureter's bladder insertion in some children with renal dysplasia has been cited in support of this proposal.

Dysplasia is a microscopic diagnosis characterized by primitive ducts, metaplastic cartilage, fetal glomeruli and tubules, and microcysts. The primitive tubules are lined by tall columnar cells with hyperchromic nuclei. These tubules are usually surrounded by a mesenchymal cell mass. Dysplasia can involve one kidney or both. Within the kidney, it can be focal or diffuse, medullary or cortical, solid or cystic.

Familial occurrences of dysplasia have been described occasionally. Dysplasia has also been associated with abnormal development in other organs, notably the central nervous system and lungs. It can be so severe as to mimic agenesis, with oligohydramnios, Potter's facies, renal failure, and death. Patients with dysplasia usually produce urine, whereas those with bilateral agenesis are anuric. Dysplasia has been seen in association with urethral valves, ureteral reflux, ureterocele, ectopic ureters, triad syndrome, Potter's syndrome, imperforate anus, and coarctation of the aorta.

Dysplasia may occur with macrocysts and is not to be confused with the polycystic diseases. These cysts may or may not be associated with any other urinary tract abnormalities or obstruction. Differentiation of multicystic dysplasia, hypoplasia, dysplasia, and aplasia is not always possible because the degree of overlap is so great in the clinical setting. Multicystic dysplastic and aplastic kidneys are nonfunctional, whereas the degree of functional derangement in dysplasia is proportional to the amount of normally differentiated tissue. Multicystic dysplasia is the most common of these conditions. When multicystic dysplasia is unilateral, the prognosis for complete recovery following nephrectomy is excellent. However, since obstructive abnormalities and noncystic dysplasia can exist on the contralateral side in as many as 30 per cent of children, full investigation is warranted.

Segmental Hypoplasia

Segmental hypoplasia (Ask-Upmark kidney) is characterized by hypertension and localized areas of renal hypoplasia. It is the only one of the hypoplastic diseases regularly accompanied by hypertension. The segment of hypoplasia is seen radiologically as a sharp cleft indenting the capsule during the nephrogram phase and appears as a "swallow-tail" deformity of the adjacent calyceal system. There is still a disagreement between those who feel it is a primary disorder of nephrogenesis and those who feel it is the secondary result of infectious or vascular diseases.

The condition has been reported in a 13-month-old infant but to our knowledge has not been reported in the newborn; this could be the result of failure to recognize the disease in newborns rather than clear support for the theory that the lesion is acquired. Most reported patients are older than 10 years of age. Females are affected twice as often as males. Proteinuria is present in half the patients. The lesion is usually unilateral but can occasionally be bilateral. When it is unilateral and detected prior to secondary development of more diffuse vascular disease, removal of the affected segment, or nephrectomy, is associated with disappearance of hypertension and complete recovery. Renal arteriogram is usually normal, while pyelography demonstrates the classic swallow-tail deformity of the calyx with associated loss of overlying parenchyma. Morphologically, the lesion is noted to involve the loss of both cortical and medullary elements. Histologically, the affected segment is sharply demarcated from normal tissue, as in pyelonephritis, but no interstitial infiltrate is detected. The glomeruli are obliterated, and the vessels are numerous and tortuous. Part of the evidence that this is not an acquired disease has come from the studies of the microvasculature.

Horseshoe Kidney

This condition is the result of fusion of the ureteric buds in embryonic life. Partial obstruction to urinary outflow may develop at the point at which the ureters cross the isthmus. Infection may follow. Pathologically, the fused mass lies closer to the midline and a bit lower than the site of the normal kidneys. Fusion has taken place at the lower pole in most cases and at the upper pole in less than 10 per cent. In the process, the kidneys have not been able to complete their normal rotation, so the pelves face anteriorly instead of toward the midline. The pelves are often extrarenal. The two collecting systems commonly develop normally, the ureters descend and enter the bladder in their proper positions, and vesicoureteral reflux is not common.

At times, the midline mass can be felt deep in the hypogastrium. More often, suspicion is directed towards a renal abnormality by the discovery of proteinuria or pyuria or by vomiting for which no other obvious explanation can be found. Diagnosis can be made by intravenous pyelography, ultrasonography, or radionuclide scanning. The characteristic malposition of the pelves and demonstration of the bridge producing one kidney mass rather than two widely separated ones confirm the diagnosis.

Nothing need be done unless infection of the urinary tract supervenes and cannot be controlled. When this complication exists, the urologist may attempt surgical correction. The single kidney should be divided into two halves and fixed in such positions that urinary stagnation is avoided. It may be necessary to resect a portion of the kidney mass that has been irretrievably damaged.

The ascent of the kidney from its low position in early fetal life to its permanent postnatal site has been described. At any point in this migration, ascent may cease. The kidney may then lie within the pelvis or in the lower part of the abdomen, and, since rotation does not take place, the position of the renal pelvis and the course of the short ureter are abnormal.

Diagnosis depends on palpation of a firm fleshy mass in the lower part of the abdomen in a few instances but in the majority rests on visualization of the malpositioned kidney by urography performed because of pyuria or abdominal symptoms. Symptoms are not caused by the ectopia itself but by obstruction to urinary outflow or urinary infection that at times supervenes. Treatment should be as conservative as possible. Removal of the kidney is necessary if pyelonephritis becomes chronic and incurable.

An even rarer positional defect is the unilateral fused kidney, or cross renal ectopia. In this situation, as in the horseshoe kidney, the ureteric buds fuse early in gestation. The one kidney ascends towards its normal position, carrying the other one across the midline and upward with it. This large mass can be readily felt deep in the lower part of the abdomen. Its particular hazard lies in the possibility that it may not be recognized at operation for what it is. Its removal would be a catastrophic error. Hypertension has been described due to constriction of the contralateral renal artery as it passes over the vertebral column.

Cysts of the Kidney

The kidney is the site of a large variety of cystic disorders. These can be classified in ascending order of gravity as solitary cysts, multiloculated cysts, multicystic dysplasia, and polycystic kidneys. Renal cysts have also been noted in association with such hereditary diseases as Meckel's syndrome, Jeune's asphyxiating dystrophy, Zellweger's cerebrohepatorenal syndrome, and trisomy D and E. Not included in this section is the congenital microcystic defect that characterizes congenital nephrosis.

SOLITARY CYSTS

Solitary serous cysts are found in 3 to 5 per cent of all autopsied patients. They are rarely observed by the clinician and become manifest only when they attain very large size. Uncomplicated ones in the newborn are extremely unusual. The cysts usually appear in males and are commonly unilateral, with the left kidney more frequently involved. Diagnostic studies include pyelography, ultrasonography, and, occasionally, percutaneous cyst puncture and aspiration. Some feel that surgical exploration is indicated to rule out malignancy, since solitary cysts are so uncommon.

MULTILOCULATED CYSTS

This term describes an encapsulated mass of multiple distinct cysts and daughter cysts of varying size entrapped within the kidney. The parenchyma surrounding the mass is intact, and there is left a considerable mass of functioning renal tissue. Most often, the lesion must be differentiated from multicystic dysplasia or Wilms' tumor. The diagnosis is made by discovery of an enlarged kidney and demonstration of a mass lesion, often polar, producing irregular distortion of the calyceal system that is revealed by intravenous pyelography. Ultrasonography shows multiple cysts. Arteriography shows a well-circumscribed mass with prominent capsular vessels. Exploration is often necessary to make the diagnosis with certainty.

There can be some difficulty in distinguishing these kidneys from those containing Wilms' tumor. Some authors have characterized locular cysts as a "differentiated" nephroblastoma. Clear cell carcinoma has been seen in two cases reported by Uson and Melicow. Differentiation of multiloculated cysts from multicystic dysplasia is made on the basis of recognition of the following characteristics of the former condition: the contralateral kidney is usually normal, the ureter is entirely patent, there is function on intravenous pyelography, no dysplastic tissue is seen microscopically, and the mass usually involves a pole rather than the entire kidney. Treatment consists of resection of the mass.

MULTICYSTIC KIDNEYS

This category differs from the preceding ones in that cysts compromise all or almost all of the mass of the kidney, there being practically no functional renal parenchyma between them. This disease needs to be differentiated from all other cystic diseases of the kidney. It is the most common cystic mass of the newborn and, depending on the series, either the first or second most common abdominal mass in infants.

The infants are often of low birth weight and usually born to mothers less than 30 years of age, of whom 60 per cent are primigravidas. There does not appear to be a familial tendency. The number of affected males is equal to that of affected females.

It is usually noted as an abdominal mass that feels irregularly nodular. It is more common on the left than on the right and is usually unilateral. Intravenous pyelography usually shows a nonfunctioning kidney with a negative imprint by total body opacification. However, there is a spectrum of function, and some visualization may be present at 24 to 48 hours, or one may see on the nephrogram a thin rim representing cords of functioning tissue between the cysts. Ultrasonography can distinguish this lesion from hydronephrosis and infantile polycystic kidneys. Radionuclide scanning shows poor or no perfusion of the mass. There may be compensatory hypertrophy of the contralateral kidney. Abnormalities in the contralateral kidney (usually ureteropelvic junction obstruction) have been noted with an incidence as high as 30 per cent.

The cysts are usually superficial and of varying size. The ureter is usually atretic, and the renal pelvis is often absent. Histologically, the tissue between the cysts is quite dysplastic with primitive ducts, cartilage, and mesenchymal stroma and immature glomeruli and tubular structures. The cysts themselves are lined with epithelium and are thought to represent dilated ampullae of the ureteric buds.

De Klerk and coworkers found that the status of the ureter is predictive of the status of the contralateral kidney and the ultimate prognosis. In those patients in whom ureteric atresia was limited at the level of the pelvis, contralateral renal abnormalities were unusual, and 93 per cent of the infants survived the first year of life. However, in 40 per cent of those in whom there was atresia in either the lower ureter or the entire ureter, contralateral abnormality was noted, and over half the infants failed to survive the first year.

Treatment consists of removal of the affected kidney. When the disease is unilateral, complete recovery occurs. Nephrectomy need not be done as an emergency. There really is no good study of what happens to these infants if the kidney is left in place. Hypertension has been reported in some, however. There have also been several instances in which the lesion has been diagnosed incidentally in adult life.

JUVENILE NEPHRONOPHTHISIS

This lesion is characterized by microscopic cysts, occasionally reaching 1 centimeter in diameter, lo-

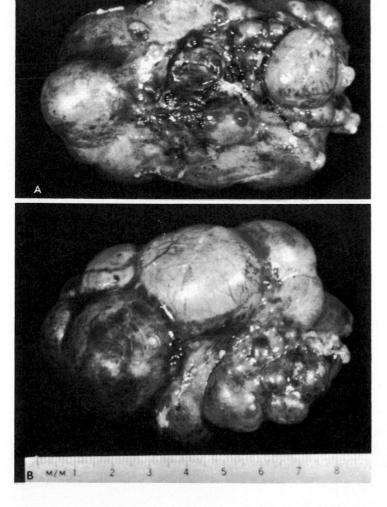

Figure 46–2. *A,* Anterior view of multicystic kidney. *B,* Medial view. The atretic ureter and blood vessels cannot be seen. (Case of Lipton, E. L., and Scordamaglia, L. J.: J. Pediatr. *50:*730, 1957.)

cated at the corticomedullary junction. These cysts represent diverticula of the distal nephron and collecting ducts. The major clinical manifestation is disordered tubular function with polyuria, polydipsia, defective urinary concentration, impaired urinary acidification, growth retardation, and, occasionally, salt wasting. There may also be the insidious onset of a normochromic, normocytic anemia. The juvenile form has an autosomal recessive inheritance, whereas the adult onset medullary cystic disease, which is morphologically and clinically similar, is an autosomal dominant trait. Family history for renal disease is often negative in the juvenile form. There is no sex predilection. The disease has been described in twins. The juvenile form may have a more rapid progression to renal failure. Intravenous urography rarely defines the small cystic lesions and may be limited to showing smaller than normal kidneys with reduced function. Ultrasonography, however, can define the larger of the cysts. Although the lesion is rarely defined in the nursery, the more ubiquitous use of noninvasive ultrasonography may serendipitously define corticomedullary cysts at younger ages. Treatment is supportive until renal insufficiency develops.

POLYCYSTIC KIDNEYS

This group of cystic lesions is entirely distinguishable from those described previously. They are always bilateral, have no dysplastic elements morphologically, and have a defined mode of inheritance. Polycystic disease should also be distinguished from other hereditary diseases that may be associated with cysts in the kidney. There is no therapy. Classification is still uncertain, and morphogenesis is not clear. The disease is often subdivided into neonatal, infantile, juvenile, and adult types, but it is probable that such subdivisions do not define distinct entities, although not all agree. However, on the basis of morphology, associated system involvement, and mode of inheritance, at least two patterns emerge. It is often difficult to differentiate the two clinically in the nursery and thus impossible to provide intelligent genetic counseling.

Infantile Polycystic Disease

This lesion can become clinically apparent at any age through childhood. In all cases, cysts are found in the liver as well as in the kidneys, although the degree of involvement of both organs may vary. Cysts may also be found in the pancreas and lungs, rarely in other organs. The length of survival seems to depend on the amount of functioning renal tissue. The more severely affected kidneys become evident soon after birth. They may be so large as to have interfered with delivery. Some patients may be stillborn, while others have Potter's facies and oligohydramnios. There may be associated abnormalities in the nervous, genitourinary, cardiovascular, and pulmonary systems. Death during the neonatal period may be the result of either uremia or respiratory failure.

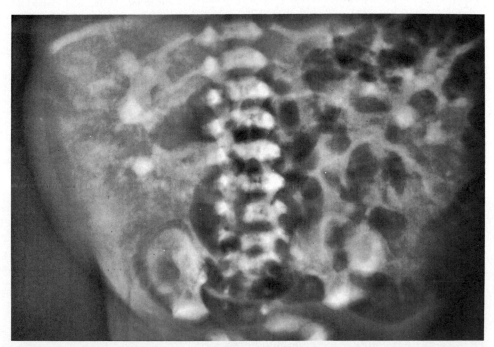

Figure 46–3. Intravenous pyelogram shows a bizarre distribution of calyces that are dilated and rounded. Separating some of the calyces are rounded radiolucent areas suggestive of cystic masses.

Other children may survive the neonatal period or not be diagnosed until later in infancy. Hypertension is common in this group and may be associated with cardiac failure. Progressive renal failure inevitably develops. Portal hypertension, with a palpable liver and esophageal varices, may also develop. Some of these children live several years before uremia becomes evident.

In other children, generally older, hepatic involvement is more prominent. In the past, the conditions of these children have been grouped under "juvenile polycystic disease" or "congenital hepatic fibrosis." They may present with portal hypertension and esophageal varices, with the renal involvement almost incidental. Others will manifest hypertension or uremia, along with the evidence of hepatic dysfunction.

The lesion is inherited as an autosomal recessive trait. Morphologically, the renal cysts are uniformly distributed, fusiform, and arranged radially. There is dilatation of the collecting ducts and distal nephrons with ectatic medullary ducts. There is relatively little early fibrosis. The kidneys are bilaterally enlarged by palpation, with a nodular, irregular feel. Urinalysis may show proteinuria, hematuria, and decreased concentrating ability. The intravenous pyelogram shows delayed appearance of the contrast material, with a mottled, irregular nephrogram and a distorted calyceal system. Retention of contrast material occurs in the radially oriented fusiform cysts, and pyelotubular backflow is occasionally seen on retrograde pyelography. Although the sonographic appearance is similar for adult and infantile polycystic disease, ultrasonography is an ideal mode for screening young patients at risk.

Both neonatal death and prolonged survival may be seen in one sibship, suggesting that the different clinical courses are reflections of the same genetic defect rather than separate entities. In other families, only a single pattern emerges, compatible with the different clinical progressions representing separate genetic abnormalities. Whether these subvarieties are truly distinct or represent variations in the natural history of the same disease is still unclear.

Adult Polycystic Disease

This is an extremely uncommon illness in the nursery, although it may appear in early childhood. It differs from the childhood types by an autosomal dominant pattern of inheritance and a relatively minimal hepatic involvement. The renal cysts are irregularly distributed; both cortical and medullary cysts are present. Intravenous pyelography shows large, lobulated kidneys, with deformity of the pelvocalyceal system by the large cysts. Although progressive renal insufficiency eventually develops, this is unusual in childhood. Hypertension generally does not appear until renal insufficiency is advanced. Ultrasonography, which can detect cystic abnormalities in affected infants before the kidneys become palpable, should be performed in infants with a positive family history.

REFERENCES

Ahey, J. B.: Cystic lesions of the kidney in infants and children. J. Pediatr. 54:429, 1959.

Bacopoulos, C., Karpathios, T., Nicolaidou, P., Thomaidis, T., and Matsaniotis, N.: Acute infantile pyelonephritis simulating polycystic kidney disease. J. Pediatr. 94:437, 1979.

Baxter, T. J.: Polycystic kidney of infants and children: Morphology, distribution and relation of the cysts. Nephron 2:15, 1965.

Bernstein, J.: Heritable cystic disorders of the kidney: The mythology of polycystic disease. Pediatr. Clin. North Am. 18:435, 1971.

Bernstein, J.: Developmental abnormalities of the renal parenchyma; renal hypoplasia and dysplasia. Pathol. Ann. 3:213, 1968.

Bernstein, J.: The classification of renal cysts. Nephron 11:91, 1973.

Blyth, H., and Ockenden, B. G.: Polycystic disease of kidneys and liver presenting in childhood. J. Med. Genet. 8:257, 1971.

Branch, C. F.: Some observations of solitary cysts of the kidney. J. Urol. 21:451, 1929.

Chamberlin, B. C., Hagge, W. W., and Stickler, G. B.: Juvenile nephronophthisis and medullary cystic disease. Mayo Clin. Proc. 52:485, 1977.

Currarino, G.: Roentgenographic estimation of kidney size in normal individuals with emphasis on children. Am. J. Roentgenol. 93:464, 1965.

DeKlerk, D. P., Marshall, F. F., and Jeffs, R. D.: Multicystic dysplastic kidney. J. Urol. 118:306, 1977.

Elkin, M., and Bernstein, J.: Cystic diseases of the kidney—radiological and pathological considerations. Clin. Radiol. 20:65, 1969.

Fetterman, G. H., and Habib, R.: Congenital bilateral oligonephronic renal hypoplasia with hypertrophy of nephrons (oligoméganéphronie). Am. J. Clin. Pathol. 52:199, 1969.

Gatewood, O. M. B., Glasser, R. J., and Van Houtte, J. J.: Roentgen evaluation of renal size in pediatric age groups. Am. J. Dis. Child. 110:162, 1965.

Greenberg, L. W., and Nelsen, C. E.: Crossed fused ectopia of the kidney. Am. J. Dis. Child. 122:175, 1971.

Greene, L. F., Feinzaig, W., and Dahlin, D. C.: Multicystic dysplasia of the kidney: with special reference to the contralateral kidney. J. Urol. 105:482, 1971.

Griffel, B., Pewzner, S., and Berandt, M.: Unilateral "oligoméganéphronie" with agenesis of the contralateral kidney, studied by microdissection. Virchows Arch. Pathol. Anat. 357:179, 1972.

Hodson, C. J., et al.: Renal size in normal children. Arch. Dis. Child. 37:616, 1962.

Johnson, D. E., Ayala, A. G., Medellin, H., et al.: Multilocular renal cystic disease in children. J. Urol. 109:101, 1973.

Kanasawa, M., Moller, J., Good, R. A., and Vernier, R. L.: Dwarfed kidneys in children. Am. J. Dis. Child. 109:130, 1965.

Kaplan, B. S., Rabin, I., Nogrady, M. B., and Drummond, K. N.: Autosomal dominant polycystic renal disease in children. J. Pediatr. 90:782, 1977.

Kaye, C., and Lewy, P. R.: Congenital appearance of adult type (autosomal dominant) polycystic kidney disease. J. Pediatr. 85:807, 1974.

Lieberman, E., et al.: Infantile polycystic diseases of the kidneys and liver. Medicine 50:277, 1971.

Lipton, E. L., and Scordamaglia, L. J.: Congenital unilateral multicystic kidney associated with maternal rubella. J. Pediatr. 50:730, 1957.

Ljungqvist, A., and Lagergren, C.: The Ask-Upmark kidney: a congenital renal anomaly studied by micro-angiography and histology. Acta Pathol. Microbiol. Scand. 56:277, 1962.

Mackie, G. G., Awang, H., and Stephens, F. D.: The ureteric orifice: the embryologic key to radiologic status of duplex kidneys. J. Pediatr. Surg. 10:473, 1975.

Makker, S. P., Grupe, W. E., Perrin, E., and Heymann, W.: Identical progression of juvenile hereditary nephronophthisis in monozygotic twins. J. Pediatr. 82:773, 1973.

Mauseth, R., Lieberman, E., and Heuser, E. T.: Infantile polycystic disease of the kidneys and Ehlers-Danlos syndrome in an 11 year old patient. J. Pediatr. 90:81, 1977.

Melicow, M. M., and Uson, A. C.: Palpable abdominal masses in infants and children: a report based on a review of 653 cases. J. Urol. 81:705, 1959.

Mozziconacci, P., Attal, C., Boisse, J., et al: Hypoplasie segmentaire du rein avec hypertension artérielle. Ann. Pediatr. 15:337, 1968.

Orathanondh, V., and Potter, E. L.: Pathogenesis of polycystic kidneys. Arch. Pathol. 77:459, 1964.

Pathak, I. G., and Williams, D. I.: Multicystic and cystic dysplastic kidneys. Br. J. Urol. 36:318, 1963.

Peterman, M. G., and de la Pena, A.: Horseshoe kidney. Am. J. Dis. Child. 38:799, 1929.

Risdon, R. A.: Renal dysplasia: I. A clinico-pathological study of 76 cases. J. Clin. Pathol. 24:57, 1971.

Rosenfeld, J. B., Cohen, L., Garty, I., et al.: Unilateral renal hypoplasia with hypertension (Ask-Upmark kidney). Br. Med. J. 2:217, 1973.

Royer, P., et al.: Pediatric Nephrology. Philadelphia, W. B. Saunders Co., 1974.

Royer, P., Habib, R., Mathieu, H., et al.: L'hypoplasie rénale bilatérale congénitale avec réduction du nombre et hypertrophie des néphrons chez l'enfant. Ann. Pediatr. (Paris) 38:133, 1962.

Rubenstein, M., Meyer, R., and Bernstein, J.: Congenital abnormalities of the urinary system. J. Pediatr. 58:356, 1961.

Sears, W. G.: Congenital cystic disease of kidneys, liver and pancreas. Guy's Hosp. Rep. 76:31, 1926.

Shapiro, I. J.: Congenital polycystic kidneys. J. Urol. 21:308, 1929.

Uson, A. C., and Melicow, M. M.: Multilocular cysts of kidney with intrapelvic herniation of a "daughter" cyst: report of 4 cases. J. Urol. 89:341, 1963.

Van Acker, K. J., Vincke, H., et al: Congenital oligonephronic renal hypoplasia with hypertrophy of nephrons (oligonephronia). Arch. Dis. Child. 46:321, 1971.

Vlachos, J., and Tsakraklidis, V.: Glomerular cysts: an unusual variety of polycystic kidneys. Am. J. Dis. Child. 114:379, 1967.

Vuthibhadgee, A., and Singleton, E. B.: Infantile polycystic disease of the kidney. Am. J. Dis. Child. 125:167, 1973.

47

Hydronephrosis

By Warren E. Grupe

Hydronephrosis denotes dilatation of the renal pelvis, usually associated with dilatation of the calyces. Strictly speaking, any excess of fluid within the collecting system constitutes hydronephrosis, regardless of whether or not the total kidney volume is increased. In the majority of instances, however, the one accompanies the other.

Hydronephrosis can be subdivided into several categories on the basis of anatomic etiology, as shown in Table 47–1, taken from a retrospective study of 146 newborns by Lebowitz and Griscom. Hydronephrosis, confined to the kidney by an abnormality of the ureteropelvic junction, is usually obstructive, although a few patients will show no definitive intrinsic abnormality. Hydronephrosis accompanied by hydroureter is either a primary ureteral abnormality, such as obstruction or infection, or an abnormality of the vesicoureteral junction leading to reflux. Congenital megaureter is always accompanied by reflux. Lesions of the bladder such as megacystis or of the urinary outlet such as urethral valves can also result in hydronephrosis, as can extrinsic lesions such as hydrometrocolpos, teratoma, or tumors. Identification and prompt diagnosis are of immense value, since the lesion is often treatable with at least some improvement. The infant kidney does not tolerate the destructive effects of obstruction well, especially when infection is added, as is frequently

the case. Since urine is formed and excreted by the fetal kidney from the twelfth week of gestation, the immature kidney has been exposed to abnormal drainage for months. It is not surprising, therefore, that considerable irreversible damage may be manifest at birth. Examples of fetal and neonatal ascites may have their origin in obstructive uropathy, and at least one case of prenatal bladder rupture was related to urethral valves. Although the remarkable capability of the immature kidney to hypertrophy is not realized until after birth, even significant renal insufficiency should not of itself deter precise diagnosis and prompt therapy.

Diagnosis. Over half the infants present with one or more palpable abdominal masses, usually in the flank (Table 47–1). In some series, hydronephrosis or hydroureteronephrosis is the most common reason for a neonatal abdominal mass, with multicystic dysplasia a close second. While no symptoms are evident in most, some infants may come to medical attention because of feeding problems, vomiting, failure to thrive, unexplained fevers, or urinary tract infection. In any newborn with sepsis, the possibility of a congenital urinary tract anomaly must be considered. Instances in which renal enlargement is extraordinarily advanced may manifest visible abdominal enlargement, with a fullness in one or both flanks. The mass, usually situated deep in the flank, is easily caught and rolled between the palpating hands and is firm, round, regular, and smooth. It is rarely tender and moves with respirations. By palpation alone, tumor or polycystic kidney is a frequent erroneous diagnosis. The larger ones transilluminate brightly. The discovery of such a mass in a newborn infant calls for further investigation. The urinalysis may be normal or may contain variable amounts of protein, white cells, and red blood cells. Blood urea nitrogen and serum creatinine may or may not be elevated, depending on the amount of functional renal tissue remaining.

More boys than girls are affected, except in instances of meningomyelocele and ectopic ureterocele (Table 47–1). Structural anomalies of the genitourinary tract other than hydronephrosis occur in approximately one fourth of the patients, often on the contralateral side. This is more common in patients with ureteropelvic junction abnormalities than in those with urethral valves or ureteroceles. The highest rate of associated urinary tract abnormalities

appears with ureteral or ureterovesical obstruction. Hydronephrosis sometimes exists with dysplasia of various types.

Anomalies outside the urinary tract occur in approximately one third of the patients and may be reason alone for one to suspect hydronephrosis (Table 47–1). Lesions such as imperforate anus, congenital vertebral anomalies, malformed ears, facial skeletal anomalies, myelodysplasia, absent or deficient abdominal musculature, unexplained pneumothorax or pneumomediastinum, absence or dysplasia of the radius, hypoplasia of the bony pelvis, severe hypospadias, and unexplained septicemia should alert the physician to the possibility of an associated urinary tract abnormality. Although associated abnormalities of clinical importance can exist in patients with undescended testicle, coronal or penile hypospadias, or a single umbilical artery, they are quite infrequent.

The radiographic signs of hydronephrosis include a mass in the renal area with delayed excretion of the contrast material shown by intravenous pyelography. There may be opacification of the ducts of Bellini appearing as a row of beads. The filled collecting tubules can appear as a dense crescent enclosing the proximal end of the calyces. A rim of relatively dense renal tissue can appear in the early films adjacent to the lucent unfilled pelvis during total body opacification. The calyces, when visualized, are full, and the papillae are flattened or frankly concave "cysts." Ultrasonography is quite helpful in those patients with large kidneys and a nondiagnostic intravenous pyelogram, and it has provided an early alert by defining hydronephrosis in utero as an unsus-

Table 47–1. Hydroureteronephrosis in Newborns

Affected Newborns	Category	Males	With Flank or Suprapubic Mass(es)	With Urinary Infection or Sepsis	With Ipsilateral or Contralateral Dysplasia*	With Other Urinary Structural Abnormalities[†]	With Extraurinary Anomalies
32	Ureteropelvic junction obstruction	18	26	2	7	9[‡]	6
27	Posterior urethral valves	27	12	2	0	2	6
20	Ectopic ureterocele	8	11	2	2	1[§]	3
18	Deficient abdominal musculature	18	4	3	6		6[‖]
11	Lower ureteral and ureterovesical obstruction	8	5	2	1	6	4
8	Infection without reflux or obstruction	6	1	8	1	3	5
7	Reflux without obstruction	4	2	2	2	2	3
7	Neurogenic hydronephrosis	2	1	0	0	0	0[**]
5	Bladder diverticulum or septation	4	3	0	1	2	2
4	Hydronephrosis of unknown cause	4	2	0	0	1	3
3	Obstruction of nonduplicated ectopic ureter	2	2	0	2	0	3
2	Simple ureterocele	1	2	0	1	0	0
2	Other urethral lesions	2	0	0	0	2	0
146							

* Probably an underestimate; does not include agenesis.
[†] Includes agenesis.
[‡] Does not include contralateral ureteropelvic obstruction.
[§] In addition to ipsilateral or bilateral duplication anomalies, which each of these children had.
[‖] In addition to undescended testicles and deficient musculature.
[**] Does not include myelomeningocele, which all these children had.
(From Lebowitz, R. L., and Griscom, N. T.: Radiol. Clin. North Am. 15:49, 1977.)

pected, incidental finding on many occasions. Ultrasonic scans can usually differentiate between hydronephrosis and multicystic dysplasia. The ultrasonographic signs of hydronephrosis include an oval "ring" of pelvicalyceal echoes with a central lucency, a series of uniform "cysts" radiating from the pelvis, or, in advanced degrees, a large sonolucent sac that may cross the midline.

Sometimes, the collecting systems are outlined by reflux with cystography. However, ureteroceles may be obscured by the density of the contrast material or collapsed by the intravesicular pressure. Oblique or lateral films during intravenous pyelography outline ureteroceles best. Radionuclide scans of the kidneys provide information when renal function is poor. Antegrade pyelography, by injection of contrast material through a percutaneous catheter situated in the dilated renal pelvis, may help distinguish ureteropelvic obstruction from lower ureteral disease when delayed pyelography provides equivocal information. In those instances in which an umbilical artery catheter is present, an aortogram can be obtained as part of the intravenous pyelogram. With the techniques currently available, it is rare that retrograde pyelography is required.

Obstruction at the Ureteropelvic Junction

Ureteropelvic junction obstruction is the most common cause of neonatal hydronephrosis. In the study by Lebowitz and Griscom, such obstruction ac-

counted for 20 per cent of cases of hydroureteronephrosis in newborns. Many childhood cases are discovered in the neonatal period. Uson and colleagues reported on 130 infants and children up to 14 years of age. Thirty-nine were diagnosed before 2 years of age, and 16 of these were diagnosed earlier than 6 months. In a similar study by Drake and coworkers, 32 of 88 children were diagnosed within the first 3 years of life. A palpable mass is the reason for study in 80 per cent of these infants. Males predominate, and the disease is bilateral in 15 to 20 per cent of children. There does not appear to be a definite predilection for either side. Anomalies in other parts of the genitourinary tract occur in half the children, with contralateral dysplasia and agenesis the most common. Other abnormalities include horseshoe kidneys, ectopia, malrotation, duplication of the collecting system, multicystic dysplasia, and agenesis.

On some occasions, obstruction may be equivocal. This can often be resolved noninvasively during routine urography with furosemide, administered 1 mg/kg intravenously. With no or minimal obstruction, there is prompt dilution and drainage of the contrast material and no distention of the renal pelvis. With true obstruction, the renal pelvis distends even more, and the contrast material is retained without further dilution. Pressure-flow studies through a percutaneous catheter placed into the renal pelvis are very sensitive in distinguishing spurious from significant obstruction but are invasive.

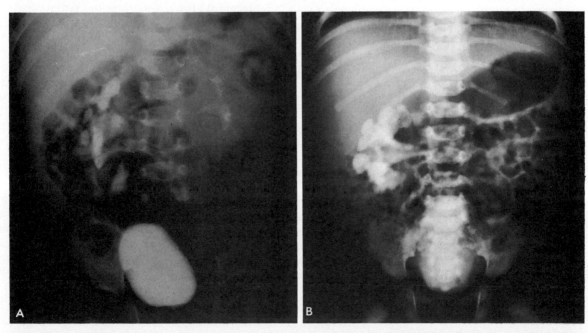

Figure 47–1. *A,* Intravenous pyelogram made on the fifth day of life. The collecting system on the left appears to be perfectly normal. Calyces and pelvis of the right kidney are dilated, the calyces club-shaped. The right ureter cannot be seen. *B,* Later film shows that excretion from the right side is considerably slower than from the left. The enlargement and clubbing of calyces are more striking now, and the absence of right hydroureter strongly suggests obstruction at the ureteropelvic junction.

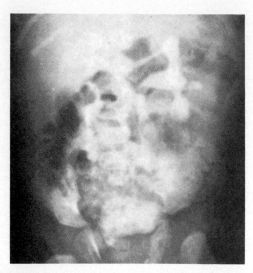

Figure 47–2. Intravenous pyelogram made on the fourth day of life of an infant whose history is not abstracted in the text. The left kidney, palpably enlarged from birth, contains enlarged, pear-shaped calyces. The pelvis and upper portion of the ureter on that side are also dilated. No dye is visible on the right side. The reason for the nonfunctioning of the right kidney was not determined, since studies were delayed by a concomitant and severe congenital cardiac defect.

Pathology. Although much has been made of the extramural obstruction produced by aberrant renal arteries, these can rarely be incriminated as the cause of obstruction. For example, in no case did the vessel appear to be the primary cause in the review by Lebowitz and Griscom. The most frequent cause is intrinsic narrowing of the ureter from atresia, fibrosis, muscle hypertrophy, local adynamic segments, and polyps. Extrinsic fibrous bands narrowing the ureteral lumen are the second most common cause of obstruction.

The reason for the hydronephrotic change is not well understood. Although increased back pressure caused by the continued formation of urine against an obstructed outflow seems logical, direct measurements of intrarenal hydrostatic pressure are not always elevated, and, in a few, no clear evidence of obstruction is defined. Ischemic necrosis of papillae with subsequent re-epithelialization is common. Some feel that the ischemia is predominantly arterial, while others feel that it is the result of venous congestion. In either state, the cause of ischemia is not clear if different from increased intrapelvic pressure. Since urine is produced from the twelfth gestational week, while nephrogenesis is still proceeding in primordial and unsupported mesenchyme, small degrees of intrauterine obstruction could produce distention of the more elastic immature kidney without demonstrable changes in intrarenal pressure.

Treatment. The aim of therapy is to restore the continuity of the tract and establish the unobstructed flow of urine from the renal pelvis. Although many changes in operative technique have occurred in recent years, the current tendency is towards dismemberment pyeloplasty. Dismemberment permits the effective removal of redundant pelvis and the narrowed ureteral segment with the relocation of the pelviureteric junction to the most dependent point. Y-V pyeloplasty of the ureter is rarely performed, and attempted dilatation with bougies has no place.

Immediate nephrectomy is discouraged. In those situations in which the functional capacity of the kidney is in doubt, a temporizing diverting procedure or a nephrostomy permits evaluation of the recuperative capacity of the unobstructed kidney. Subsequently, functionless kidneys can be removed and others repaired.

Ureteropelvic narrowing is not always progressive, even if untreated. Occasional infants with a mild degree of obstruction, in whom there is no lower tract involvement, no infection, and normal renal function, can be observed carefully and re-evaluated radiologically and functionally at regular intervals. Some may resolve, while others with evidence of progressive obstruction or renal parenchymal destruction will eventually require surgical correction.

Ureteral and Ureterovesical Obstruction

Ureteral obstruction is an uncommon cause of hydronephrosis in the newborn, accounting for less than 10 per cent of cases. About 80 per cent of patients are boys, and an abdominal mass is the initial finding in about half the infants. Disease appears to be more common on the left than on the right.

The obstruction is in the extravesicular portion of the ureter in about 50 per cent of patients. Half the infants have other abnormalities of the genitourinary tract, and one third have extraurinary abnormalities.

A demonstration that hydronephrosis exists is usually simple. However, specifically defining the site and cause of the obstruction is more difficult. Since reflux is unusual in this group, cystourethrography is generally normal. It may be difficult to visualize the ureter by intravenous pyelography because of an insufficient delay to allow the dilated ureter to fill. Thus, an erroneous diagnosis of ureteropelvic junction abnormality is common. Percutaneous antegrade pyelography can be diagnostic, but so can ultrasonography by demonstrating a dilated proximal ureter in continuity with a distended renal pelvis. The dilated distal ureter can also be seen as an echolucent ring behind the posterior wall of the bladder.

Ureterocele

Ureteroceles account for approximately 15 per cent of the episodes of hydroureteronephrosis. Ectopic ureteroceles, over half of which occur in girls, are decidedly the most common. Again, an abdominal mass is the most common reason for study, although prolapse of the ureterocele occurs in one third of the infants and is recognized as an intermittent protuberance at the introitus. Even though bilateral ureteroceles are unusual, contralateral obstruction and reflux by a unilateral ureterocele is common. Most of the ureteroceles are of the stenotic type. About half the infants have bilateral complete ureteral duplication or a contralateral bifid ureter. Associated urinary tract or extrarenal abnormalities are unusual. Current therapy involves excision of the obstructed pole (usually the upper pole) of the kidney together with its ureter to within a few centimeters of the bladder. The ureterocele is then left in situ, where it remains collapsed. With this approach, no additional surgery of the bladder is necessary. The previously popular procedure of incising the ureterocele to relieve obstruction invariably transformed an obstructed system into a massively refluxing system often associated with infection. Attempts to remove the ureterocele completely usually require the additional reimplantation of the unobstructed ureter. Recent evidence, however, would suggest that such extensive surgery is no longer necessary.

Urinary Infection Without Reflux

It is now quite clear that acute infection, even without underlying congenital obstructive defects, can give rise to hydroureteronephrosis of considerable magnitude and that one is justified in treating these with appropriate antibiotics while closely monitoring the outcome. Pais and Retik have noted reversible nonobstructive hydronephrosis in the neonate related to urinary tract infection, while Makker and coworkers have seen the same condition associated with generalized peritonitis. Lebowitz and Griscom noted eight newborns, six of them males, who fell into this category; in four, the hydronephrosis was bilateral. Three of the children had imperforate anus with rectourethral or rectovesical fistulas, one had ambiguous genitalia, and two had severe anomalies elsewhere. In only one of these children was a hydronephrotic kidney palpable. It is probable that the hydronephrosis is secondary to atony of the drainage system produced by the infection. If treatment of the infection is not accompanied by prompt resolution of the hydroureteronephrosis, further studies to define obstruction should be undertaken.

Deficient Abdominal Musculature

The prune-belly, or triad, syndrome is discussed in Chapter 45.

Neurogenic Bladder

Neurogenic bladder accounts for approximately 5 per cent of the cases of hydronephrosis in infants. It is usually associated with meningomyelocele in the newborn. Dilatation of the renal pelvis is not always evident on physical examination and may be detected by urography only because of a suspicion generated by the presence of the meningomyelocele. Occasionally, a suprapubic mass will be detected. Other children may be investigated because of abnormalities of micturition. Virtually all newborns with myelodysplasia have normal kidneys, and only one third have reflux, so prompt recognition is important. If adequate therapy is not initiated, vesicoureteral reflux, hydroureter, hydronephrosis, and renal parenchymal damage can ensue, associated with urinary tract infections and pyelonephritis.

Initial therapy is directed towards the preservation of normal kidneys and the assurance of adequate bladder emptying. The Credé maneuver, reducing outlet resistance, drug therapy, and intermittent catheterization should be attempted before surgical diversion of the upper tracts is even comtemplated. Urinary diversion, in fact, is reserved for those in whom upper tract damage develops despite all efforts. Even when hydronephrosis is already present, urethral dilatation, the Credé maneuver, and intermittent bladder catheterization can return the upper tracts to normal.

Bladder diverticula, often near the ureteric orifice, are an unusual cause of hydronephrosis. At times, the ureter can open directly into the diverticulum, an event associated with massive reflux. Diverticulectomy, sometimes accompanied by ureteral reimplantation, can restore normal renal function and markedly improve the urographic appearance.

Bladder Outlet Obstruction

Posterior urethral valves are recognized with increasing frequency and currently represent a cause of hydronephrosis second only to ureteropelvic junction obstruction. Urethral valves are almost exclusively a male disease. They have been grouped into three classic types. In type 1, the valves pass from the verumontanum to the anterolateral urethral wall; in type 2, the valves pass from the verumontanum toward the bladder neck; and in type 3, a diaphragmatic valve is located at the level of the verumontanum. The true incidence of valves is unknown. Tsingoglu and Dickson found them in 91 of 165 examples of lower urinary tract obstruction in infancy. Lebowitz and Griscom found that they represented 90 per cent of urethral obstructions. A mass in one or both flanks or a palpable bladder is what usually prompts investigation in the nursery. In many infants, however, the obstruction is totally asymptomatic and may be diagnosed during an evaluation for such nonspecific symptoms as vomiting, failure to thrive, anorexia, hematuria, edema, fever, or sepsis.

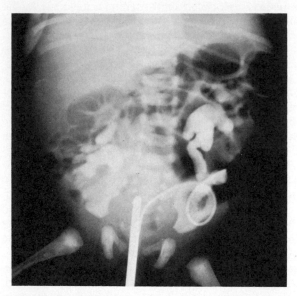

Figure 47–3. Retrograde urogram. The cystoscope can be seen in the bladder, and a catheter is in the left ureter. The right side has already been filled with dye. The bladder is enlarged, and both calyceal systems are greatly dilated and blunted. Both pelves are large. The right ureter cannot be visualized in this film, but the left ureter is dilated and tortuous.

Vesicoureteral reflux, which is a sign, not a diagnosis, is present in 70 per cent of the infants and is bilateral in one third. The infants with severe outlet obstruction and reflux will be diagnosed in the nursery, while those with milder degrees of obstruction may not be diagnosed until later. Dysplasia and poor renal function are common in the immature kidney exposed to reflux; however, dysplasia can be seen with posterior urethral valves in the absence of demonstrable reflux. In 5 per cent of all patients with hydronephrosis and in 15 per cent of newborns with refluxing ureters, obstruction cannot be demonstrated. Many of the obstructing abnormalities that produce reflux require primary surgical repair of the ureterovesical insertion. However, reflux secondary to infection, inflammation, or urethral valves can respond to correction of the primary problem without surgical correction of the ureteral insertion.

Ten per cent of the patients with posterior urethral valves have ascites. France and Back pointed out that ascites in the neonatal period is associated with organic posterior urethral obstruction in practically all the cases. Of 103 patients with neonatal ascites, there were 22 with dilatation of the urinary tract, and 18 of these were born with lesions obstructing urinary outflow at the bladder. In some, the ascites is fully developed at birth. A review by Griscom and coworkers describes 7 of 27 liveborn neonates with massive ascites from urinary causes. Abdominal distention was found at birth in 24 infants, and seven

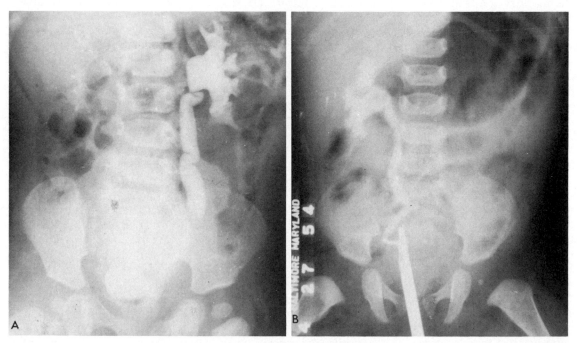

Figure 47–4. *A*, Intravenous pyelogram. The collecting system on the right side cannot be seen well. The left ureter and pelvis are definitely dilated, but the calyces are concave and sharp. *B*, Retrograde pyelogram, right. On this side the reverse is true. The right ureter and pelvis are not at all or are questionably dilated, but the calyces are blunt and convex.

This was a 6-week-old infant whose symptoms of onset were diminution in number of voidings, episodes of stiffening and crying, and puffiness of the eyes. Bladder was not palpable, but there were 30 ml of residual and a B.U.N. of 60. A median bar was found, and after resection the infant did well.

also had edema of the extremities or abdominal wall or both. Cystourethrography and urography, therefore, are extremely useful in determining the etiology of neonatal ascites. The gross appearance of the fluid, the concentration of creatinine or urea, and the presence or absence of white and red blood cells are also useful in differentiating uriniferous ascites from other causes. Protein concentration of the ascitic fluid varies markedly, with no detectable pattern indicative of urinary tract disease. Although posterior urethral valves are a common cause of ascites, it can also be seen in association with ureterocele, bladder neck obstruction, urethral strictures, pelvic neuroblastoma, bladder perforation, congenital nephrosis, ureteric stenosis, and renal vein thrombosis. A urinary leak, as the cause of ascites, can be verified by a cystogram that shows spillage of contrast material from the bladder into the peritoneal cavity. Marx and Dale reported such a case in which tremendous ascites developed by the age of 4 weeks and subsided after catheter decompression of the bladder.

By far, the most reliable means of determining outlet obstruction is the voiding cystourethrogram. Urethral valves can be clearly seen on voiding films, even when they are missed by cystoscopy; vesicoureteral reflux can also be determined best by this radiologic technique. It is important to obtain a voiding cystourethrogram prior to cystoscopy to determine which areas require special attention. Valves can be difficult to visualize by cystoscopy, and it becomes easy to confuse the secondary hypertrophy of the bladder neck as the primary lesion. Since surgical revision of the bladder neck is accompanied by a high incidence of sterility in the male, overdiagnosis and unnecessary surgery for want of a voiding cystourethrogram should be avoided.

The characteristic radiologic finding with urethral valves is dilatation of the posterior urethra just proximal to the valve and poor filling of the urethra distally. The bladder neck is often prominent, giving the posterior urethra the appearance of a "spinning top." Reflux into one or both ureters is common, often accompanied by filling of the entire pelvocalyceal system, and can be associated with blunting and distortion of calyces. The bladder may show evidence of the obstructive process, with thickened walls and diverticula, but at other times may show little change, presumably protected by the relief of vesicoureteral reflux at the expense of the kidneys.

Intravenous pyelograms in the neonatal period do not always adequately define the outflow tract. When they do, dilatation of the bladder will be seen with or without variable degrees of dilatation of ureters, pelves, and calyces. Reflux up one or both ureters need not be seen early, but it almost always follows long-term, increased intravesical tension or infection as a result of loss of competence at the ureterovesical junction. This, together with the voiding urethrogram, precisely defines the functional and anatomic condition of lower ureters, bladder, and urethra.

The passage of a rubber catheter may be difficult when the tip reaches the level of the stenosed bladder neck. In many instances, however, the catheter passes into the bladder with the greatest of ease. This is because mucosal flaps are situated so as to cause obstruction only from above downward; that is, they behave as check valves rather than stop valves.

Estimation of residual urine is not easy in the newborn and offers little diagnostic help in the presence of diagnostic radiographs. The infant must be watched closely until he voids. Either prompt catheterization or ultrasonographic determination of the

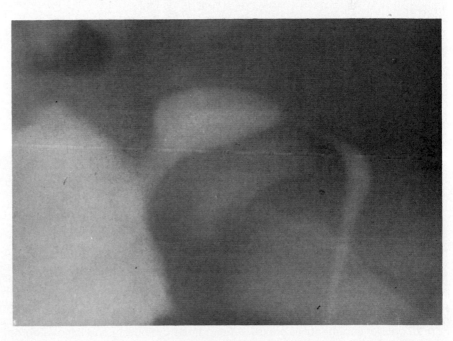

Figure 47–5. One of the films of the cineurographic series shows the greatly dilated posterior urethra, which then tapers to a fine point at the level of the external sphincter. Its caliber remains threadlike for several centimeters and then reverts to normal.

size of the bladder should follow, and the amount of urine remaining in the bladder must be measured. In the normal newborn, there should be no more than 1 or 2 ml of residual urine.

The urine is not abnormal unless infection has supervened. Blood chemical determinations may fall within normal limits, but obstructions of sufficient magnitude rapidly lead to retention of nitrogenous end products, with elevation of creatinine and blood urea nitrogen values.

The final diagnostic step is cystoscopy. The urologist skilled in the use of the infant's cystoscope will not only confirm the presence of posterior urethral obstruction by the appearance of the bladder but also determine its nature by direct inspection.

Treatment. Therapy is directed toward assuring quick and permanent relief from obstruction to urinary outflow. We stress the adjectives "quick" and "permanent" because halfway measures cannot be sanctioned. The kidneys of the newborn do not tolerate prolonged back pressure well, and, when infection is added to pressure, their function may be irretrievably damaged in a short time.

Surgical removal of the urethral valves can be approached by one of several techniques. Most favor resection through the endoscope as the simplest and most effective method associated with the lowest morbidity. It is unusual that any surgical alteration of the bladder neck is necessary, and in the overwhelming majority the abnormal radiologic findings at the outlet resolve after simple excision of the valve. The same is true with the upper tracts, where reflux often disappears with no further surgery.

It may be technically impossible in rare situations to resect the valves through the cystoscope, and a more radical approach may be required, either by suprapubic cystotomy or by a perineal approach.

Repeated dilatation of the stenosis by bougienage from below may be, but often is not, adequate therapy. It cannot be expected to help when the basic defect consists of mucosal valves, nor does it relieve for more than a few hours or days many narrowings due to fibrous or muscular hyperplasia. Obstructions due to membranous diaphragms constitute the favorable exceptions.

Other Forms of Obstructive Uropathy

Obstruction to urinary outflow can be caused by a host of congenital abnormalities other than those discussed already. Other abnormalities of the urinary tract accounting for less than 10 per cent of cases of hydronephrosis in newborns include complete urethral occlusion, urethral diverticula, bladder diverticula, ectopic ureters, bladder septation, reflux without obstruction, agenesis of the bladder, or agenesis of

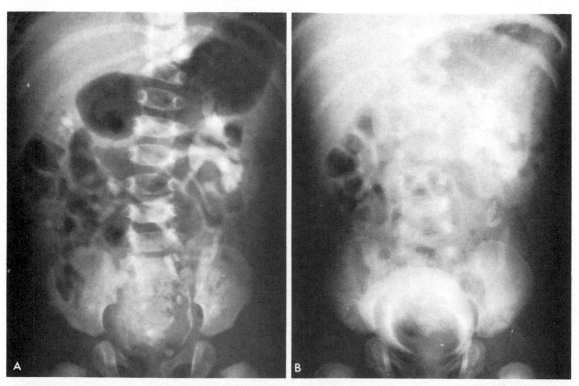

Figure 47-6. *A*, Intravenous pyelogram does not outline the right collecting system. On the left, the calyces are dilated and somewhat blunted, and the pelvis is a bit dilated. The ureter, however, seems to be of normal caliber throughout its course. *B*, Retrograde cystogram and left pyelogram. A large filling defect is seen within the bladder. Again, the left-sided hydronephrosis is visible.

the urethra. Lesions extrinsic to the urinary tract, such as hydrometrocolpos, teratoma, or tumors contiguous with the ureters, bladder, or urethra, can produce urinary obstruction and hydronephrosis. The actual diagnosis of obstructive uropathy will depend on ancillary studies that include testing for residual urine, intravenous pyelography, ultrasonography, cystourethrography, renal nuclide scan, occasionally cystoscopy, and, only rarely, retrograde pyelography. In the course of these studies, the specific abnormality will come to light. The treatment will depend on the outcome of these studies.

Congenital Megaloureter (Megacystis, Megaureter Syndrome)

Megacystis is distinguished as a thin-walled, unobstructed bladder of large capacity that empties completely with no evidence of obstruction. Vesicoureteral reflux through gaping ureteral orifices is inevitably present. The condition is usually associated with dilatation of the renal pelves and blunting of the calyces. The etiology of megacystis syndrome is unexplained. In some examples, gross lesions of the spinal cord have been detected, such as meningomyelocele, lipomyelomeningocele, and dural or cord tears sustained during difficult breech delivery. The ureteral insertions in the bladder appear to be more laterally displaced with a very short or absent intramural or submucosal tunnel. A primary defect in trigonal development has been proposed. A congenital imperfection of the autonomic nervous control has been suspected in some, but no proof has ever been offered for this hypothesis. Cystometrograms in megacystis syndrome usually have a normal configuration. Swenson suggested that megaloureter, like megacolon, with which it is occasionally associated, may be due to a congenital defect in the pelvic parasympathetic system associated with absence or underdevelopment of the intrinsic nerve supply to the ureters and bladder. He believes that he has demonstrated this defect in some cases. This explanation, however, has not been supported by Lebowitz and Bodian. Baker found no alteration from the normal peristaltic pattern other than slightly lower voltage, indicated by electroureterogram. He points out that the intrinsic nerve supply is not indispensable for orderly contraction and that contraction waves seem to originate within muscle fibers independently. Stevens has proposed a congenital disorder of the ureteric bud that produces hyperexpansion of the bladder. Obstruction seems unlikely, since the bladders are not trabeculated and empty completely despite their large size.

Diagnosis. The diagnosis of megacystis depends almost entirely on the discovery of urinary tract infection and the symptoms associated with it. Most of these patients void large quantities of urine infrequently. On rare occasions, a child may present with urinary retention as a result of bladder decompensation in association with severe vesicoureteral reflux.

The bladder may be palpable on examination. Since infection may be delayed months or years, the condition does not often become manifest in the nursery. The diagnosis is established by excluding neurogenic or obstructive disorders of the lower urinary tract. Patients can have the bladder extend as high as the fifth lumbar vertebral space. However, voiding is generally complete, with no residual urine found. Any apparent urinary residue is the result of urine refluxed into the dilated upper tract returning to the bladder. The neurologic examination is normal, and cystometrography demonstrates that the bladder has a large capacity but normal pressure. Flow studies are normal. The characteristic finding at cystoscopy is a smooth, nontrabeculated, thin-walled bladder. The trigone is two or three times normal size with laterally placed, incompetent ureteral orifices. Saculation and diverticula of the bladder are not present. Excretory urography may show varying degrees of hydronephrosis and renal scar, depending on the presence and severity of the vesicoureteral reflux and the presence or absence of infection. Reflux, however, is almost always demonstrated by voiding cystourethrography. Final confirmation is made by intravenous urography and voiding cystourethrography.

Treatment. The treatment of megacystis is correction of the vesicoureteral reflux and prevention of urinary stagnation. Several large series have shown a success rate that exceeds 90 per cent when the insertion of the ureter into the bladder is revised. Since there is no abnormality of the bladder neck or the urethra in this condition, surgery in or dilatation of these areas is not needed even if the bladder is very large. Operations on the autonomic nervous system, based on the assumption that sympathetic-parasympathetic imbalance is the causative defect, have been uniformly unsuccessful.

The prognosis seems to depend on the amount of renal damage present initially. Often, complicating urinary tract infections and pyelonephritis can be controlled by appropriate antibiotics, but infections tend to recur as soon as therapy is stopped. In some, without surgical correction, infection can become chronic and intractable. The prognosis, however, is usually good. With successful reimplantation of the ureters, progressive renal damage is unusual, even if subsequent bladder infections occur. The children generally develop normally, and megacystis by itself is not a disorder incompatible with normal life.

REFERENCES

Allen, R. P., Condon, V. R., and Collins, R. E.: Multilocular cystic hydronephrosis secondary to congenital (ureteropelvic) obstruction. Radiology 80:203, 1963.

Alton, D. J.: Pelviureteric obstruction in childhood. Radiol. Clin. North Am. 15:61, 1977.

Askin, J. A., Reichelderfer, T., Salik, J., and Merritt, J.: Indications for excretory urography in children. Pediatrics 20:1033, 1957.

Baker, R.: Ureteral electromyography in congenital megaloureter. A.M.A. J. Dis. Child. 87:7, 1954.

Bearn, A. R.: Hydronephrosis in infancy. Arch. Dis. Child. 31:110, 1956.

Berman, L. B., Crotty, J. J., and Tina, L. U.: The pediatric implications of bladder neck obstructions. Pediatrics 28:816, 1961.

Colodny, A. H.: Evaluation and management of infants and children with neurogenic bladder. Radiol. Clin. North Am. 15:71, 1977.

Condit, L.: Convulsions. Case Histories Child. Mem. Hosp. Chicago 14:3803, 1956.

DeSanctis, P. N., and Lattimer, J. K.: Management of meningomyelocele: plea for earlier urologic consultation. Urology 3:421, 1974.

Drake, D. P., Stevens, P. S., and Eckstein, H. B.: Hydronephrosis secondary to ureteropelvic obstruction in children. Review of 14 years experience. J. Urol. 119:649, 1978.

Eklöf, O., and Ringertz, H.: Pre- and post-operative urographic findings in posterior urethral valves. Pediatr. Radiol. 4:43, 1975.

Felson, B., and Cussen, L. J.: The hydronephrotic type of unilateral congenital multicystic disease of the kidney. Semin. Roentgenol. 10:113, 1975.

Flocks, R. H.: Lower urinary tract obstructions in infants and children. Pediatr. Clin. North Am. 2:755, 1955.

France, N. E., and Back, E. H.: Neonatal ascites associated with urethral obstruction. Arch. Dis. Child. 29:565, 1954.

Griscom, N. T.: The roentgenology of neonatal abdominal masses. Am. J. Roentgenol. 93:447, 1965.

Griscom, N. T., Colodny, A. H., Rosenberg, M. K., Fliegel, C. P., and Hardy, B. E.: Diagnostic aspects of neonatal ascites: report of 27 cases. Am. J. Roentgenol. 128:961, 1977.

Griscom, N. T., Vawter, G. F., and Fellers, F. X.: Pelvoinfundibular atresia, the usual form of multicystic kidney: 44 unilateral and 2 bilateral cases. Semin. Roentgenol. 10:125, 1975.

Jewett, H. J.: Upper urinary tract obstructions in infants and children. Pediatr. Clin. North Am. 2:737, 1955.

Johnston, J. H.: The pathogenesis of hydronephrosis in children. Br. J. Urol. 41:724, 1969.

Kasper, T. E., Osborne, R. W., Jr., Semerdjian, H. S., and Miller, H. C.: Urologic abdominal masses in infants and children. J. Urol. 116:629, 1976.

Kozakewich, H., and Lebowitz, R. L.: Congenital megacalyces. Pediatr. Radiol. 2:251, 1974.

Kretchmer, H. L., and Pierson, L. E.: Congenital valves of the posterior urethra. Am. J. Dis. Child. 38:804, 1929.

Lapides, J., et al.: Clean, intermittent self-catheterization in the treatment of urinary tract disease. Trans. Am. Assoc. Genitourin. Surg. 63:92, 1971.

Lebowitz, R. L., and Griscom, N. T.: Neonatal hydronephrosis: 146 cases. Radiol. Clin. North Am. 15:49, 1977.

Lebowitz, S., and Bodian, M.: A study of the vesical ganglia in children and the relationship of the megaureter, megacytis syndrome and Hirschsprung's disease. J. Clin. Pathol. 16:342, 1963.

Longino, L. A., and Martin, L. W.: Abdominal masses in newborn infant. Pediatrics 21:596, 1958.

Makker, S. P., Izant, R., Tucker, A., and Heymann, W.: Nonobstructive hydronephrosis associated with generalized peritonitis. N. Engl. J. Med. 287:535, 1972.

Martin, D. J., Gilday, D. L., and Reilly, B. J.: Evaluation of the urinary tract in the neonatal period. Radiol. Clin. North Am. 13:359, 1975.

Marx, K., and Dale, W. A.: Neonatal ascites and obstructive uropathy: a case report with a four-year follow-up. Pediatrics 27:29, 1961.

Mascatello, V., and Lebowitz, R. L.: Malposition of the colon in left renal agenesis and ectopia. Radiology 120:371, 1976.

McDonald, J., and Murphy, A. V.: Neonatal ascites from spontaneous rupture of the bladder. Arch. Dis. Child. 50:956, 1975.

Michaelson, G.: Percutaneous puncture of the renal pelvis, intrapelvic pressure and the concentrating capacity of the kidney in hydronephrosis. Acta Med. Scand. Supp. 559, 1974.

Moncada, R., Wang, J. W., Love, L., and Bush, I.: Neonatal ascites associated with urinary outlet obstruction (urine ascites). Radiology 90:1165, 1968.

Murnagham, G. F.: Experimental aspects of hydronephrosis. Br. J. Urol. 31:370, 1959.

Nogrady, M. B., and Dunbar, J. S.: The technique of roentgen investigation of the urinary tract in infants and children. Progr. Pediatr. Radiol. 3:3, 1969.

Pais, V. M., and Retik, A. B.: Reversible hydronephrosis in the neonate with urinary sepsis. N. Engl. J. Med. 292:465, 1975.

Rickham, P. P.: Advanced lower urinary obstruction in childhood. Arch. Dis. Child. 37:122, 1962.

Ridlon, H. C., et al.: Myelomeningocele: suggested minimal urological evaluation and surveillance. Pediatrics 56:477, 1975.

Robson, W. J., et al.: Pelvic-ureteric obstruction in infancy. J. Pediatr. Surg. 11:57, 1976.

Shopfner, C. E.: Nonobstructive hydronephrosis and hydroureter. Am. J. Roentgenol. 98:172, 1966.

Stern, L., Fletcher, B. D., Dunbar, J. S., Levant, M. N., and Fawcett, J. S.: Pneumothorax and pneumomediastinum associated with renal malformations in the newborn infants. Am. J. Roentgenol. 116:785, 1972.

Stevens, F. D.: Idiopathic dilation of the urinary tract. J. Urol. 112:819, 1974.

Swenson, O.: Congenital defects in the pelvic parasympathetic system. Arch. Dis. Child. 30:1, 1955.

Teele, R. L.: Ultrasonography of the genitourinary tract in children. Radiol. Clin. North Am. 15:109, 1977.

Toulowkian, R. J., and Weiss, R. M.: Obstructed bladder syndrome in the neonate. Surg. Gynecol. Obstet. 143:965, 1976.

Tsingoglu, S., and Dickson, J. A. S.: Lower urinary obstruction in infancy: a review of lesions and symptoms in 165 cases. Arch. Dis. Child. 47:215, 1972.

Uson, A. C., Cox, L. A., and Lattimer, J. K.: Hydronephrosis in infants and children. J.A.M.A. 205:323, 1968.

Whitaker, R. H.: Equivocal pelvi-ureteric obstruction. Br. J. Urol. 47:771, 1976.

Williams, D. I., and Karlaftis, C. M.: Hydronephrosis due to pelvi-ureteric obstruction in the newborn. Br. J. Urol. 38:138, 1966.

Williams, D. I., and Kenawi, M. M.: The prognosis of pelvi-ureteric obstruction in childhood. Eur. Urol. 2:57, 1976.

Williams, D. I.: The natural history of reflux—a review. Urol. Int. 26:350, 1971.

48

Renal vascular occlusions in the neonate share the common pathogenic mechanism of altered parenchymal blood flow, either through vasoconstriction or intravascular coagulation. In the past, renal venous thrombosis has been the most common. Renal arterial thrombosis, however, has become increasingly prevalent in recent years, a trend that is associated with the more frequent use of umbilical catheters. Although extensive parenchymal necrosis can be noted without vascular lesions, most episodes of both cortical and medullary necrosis are accompanied by either venous or arterial thrombosis.

The kidney in the newborn is particularly at risk for vascular thromboses. The vessels are small in caliber, the renal blood flow is relatively low, and the vascular resistance is comparatively high. Hypoxia, particularly if accompanied by hypercapnea, further decreases renal plasma flow. The newborn also has a more active renin-angiotensin system. There is a proportionately higher insensible water loss and fluid turnover, which places the infant at a greater risk for hypovolemia. The neonate is relatively more polycythemic. There may even be immaturity in the fibrinolytic mechanisms. Therefore, small changes in any one or combination of these factors provide ample opportunity for either venous or arterial thrombosis to occur.

Renal Vein Thrombosis

Renal venous thrombosis may occur at any age, but the newborn is particularly prone to this accident. Over two thirds of the patients with this disorder are under 1 month of age.

Incidence. The incidence of this disorder in newborn nurseries is incompletely defined. Oppenheimer and Esterly, in reviewing 4000 consecutive neonatal postmortem examinations, found 14 infants with renal vein thrombosis, five of whom were infants of diabetic mothers. The first diagnosis in vivo was made by Campbell in 1942. Currently, renal venous thrombosis is recognized during life with increasing frequency. Nevertheless, most estimates of frequency are still based on postmortem examinations. Current estimates vary between 1.9 and 2.7 per cent of neonatal deaths.

Etiology. Renal venous thrombosis is usually divided into primary and secondary forms, the latter resulting from extension of the thrombus from the vena cava. The primary form, in which thrombosis originates in the smaller intrarenal veins themselves, is the one encountered in the newborn. The most important predisposing factors are hypovolemia and hyperosmolality. In most instances, the thrombus probably starts in the smaller intrarenal veins, the result of venous stasis, subsequently spreading distally to involve the renal cortex or medulla and simultaneously extending into larger veins. In the secondary form, which is rare in the newborn and more common in adults, a thrombus in a main vein extends distally into the kidney.

Other factors contributing to venous stasis include hypotension, low renal plasma flow, polycythemia, anoxia, septicemia, cyanotic congenital heart disease, congenital renal anomalies, and severe pyelonephritis. Angiocardiography in infants with congenital heart lesions, possibly related to hyperosmolality, has also been implicated as a contributing factor. Thrombosis also has been reported in association with maternal diabetes mellitus or prediabetes. This association, however, has not been as common in recent years, and, in one study of 115 Scottish children, there was no recognized incidence of maternal diabetes. Injury from a severely traumatic or breech delivery has also been implicated. In many cases, however, no predisposing disorder has been discovered. There is clear evidence that the lesion can occur prenatally, which is unusual and accounts for less than 5 per cent of all cases. In this situation, calcification of the kidney can be detected in utero or in the first weeks of life. Prenatal thrombosis of one kidney followed by postnatal thrombosis of the second has been reported occasionally.

Diagnosis. The characteristic presentation of renal venous thrombosis is the sudden enlargement of one kidney in association with a sudden deterioration of the infant's clinical status accompanied by hematuria, metabolic acidosis, tachypnea, pallor, and failure to thrive. This usually occurs during the course of a complex illness or several days after a traumatic delivery. In all series, more males than females are affected, and the ratio of affected males to affected females may be as high as 2:1 in the newborn period. There

437

is no obvious seasonal, socioeconomic, or ethnic pre-dilection. A history of maternal diabetes, trauma, congenital cyanotic heart disease, recent arteriography, dehydration, asphyxia, shock, or sepsis may be obtained. A firm, palpable kidney is present in only 60 per cent. At times, renal enlargement is unaccompanied by symptoms; at other times, vomiting, abdominal distention, shock, and fever may appear along with enlargement. Diarrhea, vomiting, or shock have been noted in 10 to 20 per cent of cases. The blood pressure is usually normal or low, although hypertension can be present at levels generally not as severe as that seen with renal arterial thrombosis. Anuria and oliguria can be present, but edema is usually absent. Hemoperitoneum has been recorded in some cases.

Gross hematuria is frequently present and may be the first sign. Two thirds of the patients, however, have microscopic hematuria, and, in other cases, hematuria may be absent entirely. The urine may contain an excess of protein and white cells, alone or in addition to red blood cells. Azotemia is usual, and metabolic acidosis is present in half the infants. The serum sodium concentrations are variable, while the serum potassium level can be elevated.

Thrombocytopenia, when present, probably is the result rather than the cause of the thrombosis. Over 50 per cent of the infants have microangiopathic hemolytic anemia that is often accompanied by changes in the coagulation factors and thrombocytopenia, suggesting that the renal thrombosis is the manifestation of intravascular coagulation. It is possible that anoxic damage to endothelial cells leading to platelet consumption could promote secondary thrombus formation in at least some of these infants.

Intravenous pyelography and radionuclide scans usually reveal complete absence of excretory function or only a slight opacification after a long delay on the involved side. Renal ultrasonography, however, usually shows a large kidney with a disordered central collection of echoes. If doubt persists, inferior vena cavagrams may help outline the renal vasculature.

Treatment. Immediate nephrectomy or thrombectomy was considered the ideal treatment in the past. Unfortunately, operative intervention is at times contraindicated by concomitant disease such as active diarrhea with dehydration, fever, severe jaundice with sepsis, electrolyte disorders with a disturbed acid base state, shock, and oliguria. In such situations everything possible must be done to correct shock, and supportive care to correct the primary disorder seems more essential than emergency surgery. Besides, the thrombosis usually begins in the small vessels of the kidney, often associated with zones of hemorrhagic infarction, making thrombectomy of little consequence to the kidney. Since the extent of

kidney recovery is not predictable, emergency nephrectomy would also eliminate any chance of renal recuperation.

Belman and his collaborators have demonstrated the effectiveness of medical treatment for unilateral renal vein thrombosis. Six of the seven infants they treated survived, and in only one of the survivors was the kidney found to be atrophic. Ghai and associates reported thrombosis in one kidney in each of a pair of conjoined twins; they too did well with conservative management. Duncan and coworkers, who used supportive therapy alone, avoiding administration of anticoagulants, also reported encouraging results. Thus, nephrectomy and thrombectomy are rarely indicated at present.

Bilateral thrombosis is much more serious, with mortality in half the infants. Many have thrombosis of the vena cava as well. However, recent reports of recovery with conservative management, peritoneal dialysis, or heparin are encouraging even in this serious state. In some series, almost half have been bilateral.

When there is evidence of continuing intravascular coagulation, or if thrombosis of the inferior vena cava is present, anticoagulation with heparin may be indicated. Heparin is usually continued for at least 5 days or until the platelet count returns to normal. The effectiveness of anticoagulation, however, has not been established. Nephrectomy, even in this serious situation, is rarely indicated and is usually reserved for those few patients with malignant hypertension.

Outcome. Mortality has been alarmingly high in some series. In most reports, the outcome depends, to a large extent, on the severity of the underlying, primary medical condition. Those who appear to be at particularly high risk are males with congenital heart defects and those subjected to early nephrectomy. If the infant's general condition and underlying problems can be managed satisfactorily, there is a reasonable possibility of survival.

Recovery of renal function on the affected side is not uncommon, which is compelling reason to avoid nephrectomy during the acute phases. Of some concern have been reports of renal atrophy developing some months later and renal mediated hypertension, which may necessitate subsequent nephrectomy. Tubular dysfunction, including proteinuria, amino aciduria, glycosuria, phosphaturia, metabolic acidosis with growth failure, and rickets, have been reported as late sequelae of renal venous thrombosis. Some degree of renal atrophy can be expected in all patients. Many patients may also show calyceal clubbing and renal calcification. The discovery of a small kidney with calyceal clubbing in a patient who has had previously undiagnosed renal vein thrombosis may lead to the erroneous diagnosis of either chronic pyelonephritis or dysplasia. Under these circumstances, the calcification pattern in the kidney becomes important. A reticular pattern to the renal calcification is highly suggestive, if not pathognomonic, of a previous renal vascular thrombosis.

Until the last decade, thrombosis of the renal artery was much less common than renal venous thrombosis. Now the prevalence of renal arterial occlusions in infants has increased considerably with the more ubiquitous use of umbilical artery catheterization. Woodard and colleagues alerted us to the fact that renal arterial thrombosis, until then only a pathologic finding, could be diagnosed in vivo and treated successfully. Their two patients had failing hearts followed by proteinuria, hematuria, and hypertension. Azotemia was looked for and found in one. The kidneys were not enlarged, and pyelograms revealed no excretion of dye on the affected side. Operation was performed on one in the expectation of finding renal venous thrombosis, but the kidney was dark blue and not enlarged, and a thrombus was found in the main renal artery. Removal of the kidney resulted in a cure. In their other cases, the correct diagnosis was suspected, but the infant died before operation could be attempted.

In an earlier review of arterial occlusion in infants, Gross noted that of 47 patients with lesions at various sites, four had thrombosis of the renal artery. Zuelzer and coworkers found four occurrences of renal artery thrombosis among 2058 postmortem examinations in newborns. Such a high incidence in the Zuelzer series suggests that partial arterial occlusion of the renal artery may occur more frequently than previously diagnosed.

Diagnosis. The symptoms and signs of renal artery thrombosis are secondary to the renal infarction. Although the kidney may be acutely enlarged, it is unusual that a mass is palpable. Anuria, oliguria, and hematuria are common. There may be evidence of thrombosis occurring in other organs, including gangrenous areas of skin. Vomiting and abdominal tenderness may be seen. Blood urea and creatinine may be either elevated or normal. There is usually variable function of the kidney shown by intravenous pyelography or radionuclide scanning. Renal arterial thrombosis has been increasingly associated with umbilical artery catheterization, particularly when hypertonic fluids have been administered or when the level of the catheter tip has been placed too high.

Treatment. Aggressive support of the infant, including dialysis when necessary, constitutes the preferred treatment. The value of anticoagulation therapy has not been adequately determined, although occasional reports support their use. Thrombectomy has little support. Meticulous attention to the fluid and electrolyte status and a vigorous advance on the primary causes of vasoconstriction, hypovolemia, asphyxia, and intravascular coagulation provide the best hope of survival and recovery for these infants. Management of the hypertension can be particularly difficult, requiring aggressive pharmacologic therapy with dosages that, at times, are proportionally higher than those used in older children (see Chapter 49).

Authors who report failure with antihypertensive therapy generally have used doses of medications that are lower than the doses used by those who report success. Early nephrectomy is probably not warranted, since the extent of involvement is variable and the recovery cannot be predicted. Renal atrophy with or without hypertension can be a late sequela.

Renal Cortical and Medullary Necrosis

It is appropriate to consider cortical and medullary necrosis together, since they are virtually indistinguishable clinically, often coexist, and are both the result of renal vascular compromise. Complete data concerning incidence or prevalence are not available. Davies and coworkers found 18 clinically unsuspected cases in 3516 autopsies. Nevertheless, it is probably misleading to give the impression that these conditions are rare. The two factors regularly implicated in the pathogenesis are vasoconstriction and intravascular coagulation, which are commonly associated with neonatal vascular thromboses of every sort.

The disorder commonly follows serious illness at birth, including profound perinatal asphyxia, hyperosmolality, hypovolemia, shock, sepsis, severe anemia, pneumonia, congenital heart disease, hemorrhage, obstructive uropathy with infection, gastroenteritis, and disseminated intravascular coagulation. To the usual signs of respiratory distress may be added later bouts of apnea, flaccidity, and lethargy. Cortical necrosis is the more common lesion associated with sepsis, while medullary necrosis is more commonly seen following hypovolemia or hyperosmolality.

Diagnosis. Characteristically, there is complete anuria, or, if urine is passed, it is scanty and nonconcentrated and contains low levels of protein and red blood cells. Occasionally, grossly bloody urine is present. The kidneys are often palpable, and examination may show evidence of clotting in other organs. Edema is unusual, and hypertension that is resistant to therapy can develop rapidly, particularly with arterial lesions. The BUN is usually mildly elevated, unless renal damage is extensive. With medullary necrosis, there may be a short, 2- to 3-day phase of oliguria that is frequently missed in the complexity of the primary illness. This is followed by a period of polyuria and sodium wasting. In cortical necrosis, serum potassium may be elevated disproportionately to sodium or the degree of renal insufficiency. Thrombocytopenia and microangiopathic hemolytic anemia may be present as evidence of intravascular coagulation, as might other abnormalities of coagulation.

Radiographically, there is usually poor visualization of the kidneys by intravenous pyelography or nuclide scanning. When visualization is achieved, a prolonged nephrogram may be seen after some delay with dense opacification of the pyramids, which is characteristic of medullary necrosis. In about half the cases, this prolonged opacification is limited to the medulla alone, while in the others it involves the entire kidney. This effect may be related to a leakage of contrast material into the interstitium. Prolonged opacification is not unique to medullary necrosis; it can also be seen in acute tubular injury and with intraluminal precipitation of Tamm-Horsfall protein. However, to the trained eye, it is distinctive. With cortical necrosis, the necrotic renal tissue calcifies rapidly. The lesions of cortical necrosis are usually bilateral, while bilaterality is less common in medullary necrosis.

Treatment. The required treatment consists of vigorous supportive care, careful management of fluid and electrolyte balance, and active handling of renal failure, including peritoneal dialysis or hemodialysis when appropriate. This has improved the outlook for these children. The efficacy of anticoagulation has not been demonstrated in these lesions.

Outcome. The ultimate outcome depends on the degree to which the kidneys have been damaged. Severely affected infants commonly die before the fourth day of life. Most survivors have a significant return of excretory function. Permanent impairment of concentrating ability may be present with medullary necrosis because of extensive loss of juxtamedullary nephrons. Functional studies in children who have survived cortical necrosis, however, have shown a relative preservation of tubular function, which has been attributed to a relative sparing of the juxtamedullary nephrons. Growth of the kidney with either insult can be impaired.

Medullary necrosis, because of the location of the injury, will often demonstrate pyelocalyceal deformities, partial atrophy, irregular renal outlines, and clubbing of calyces on follow-up intravenous pyelography. Such deformities may be easily confused with chronic pyelonephritis, segmental renal hypoplasia, or dysplasia, unless previous knowledge of the infant's perinatal course is available. Within a few weeks, cortical necrosis will demonstrate a characteristic granular pattern of cortical calcification with occasional streaks radiating along the columns of Bertin into the medulla.

Reports of relatively longer survivals and recovery are increasing. Some of those who recover will have late sequelae, including hypertension, tubular dysfunction, and, in a few, renal insufficiency that eventually requires dialysis and renal transplantation.

Perirenal Hematoma

Perirenal hematoma may likewise simulate either renal vein or renal artery thrombosis. There may be a flank mass, a history of obstetric trauma, anemia, hematuria, oliguria, and a rising BUN. The importance of distinguishing this lesion is that a perirenal hematoma, unless evacuated, has the potential to organize and contract, leading to renal atrophy and hypertension of the sort seen experimentally after induced renal ischemia.

REFERENCES

Abeshouse, B. S.: Thrombosis and thrombophlebitis of the renal veins. Urol. Cutan. Rev. 49:661, 1945.

Adelman, R. D., Merten, D., Vogel, J., et al.: Non-surgical management of neurovascular hypertension in the newborn. Pediatrics 62:71, 1978.

Anand, S. K., Northway, J. D., and Smith, J. A.: Neonatal renal papillary and cortical necrosis. Am. J. Dis. Child. 13:773, 1977.

Arneil, G. C., MacDonald, A. M., Murphy, A. V., and Sweet, E. M.: Renal venous thrombosis. Clin. Nephrol. 1:119, 1973.

Avery, M. E., Oppenheimer, E. M., and Gordon, H. H.: Renal vein thrombosis in newborn infants of diabetic mothers. N. Engl. J. Med. 256:1134, 1957.

Barenberg, L. H., Greenstein, N. M., Levy, W., and Rosenbluth, S. B.: Renal thrombosis with infarction complicating diarrhea of the newborn. Am. J. Dis. Child. 62:362, 1941.

Belman, A. B., Susmano, D. F., Burden, J. J., and Kaplan, G. W.: Nonoperative treatment of unilateral thrombosis in the newborn. J.A.M.A. 211:1165, 1970.

Berdon, W. E., Schwartz, R. H., Becker, J., and Baker, D. H.: Prolonged nephrogram in oliguric patients due to precipitation of Tamm-Horsfall proteinuria. Its relationship to prolonged nephrogram in infants and children and to renal failure following intravenous urography in adults with multiple myeloma. Radiology 92:714, 1969.

Campbell, M. F., and Matthews, W. F.: Renal thrombosis in infants: report of two cases in male infants urologically examined and cured by nephrectomy at 13 and 33 days of age. J. Pediatr. 20:604, 1942.

Chrispin, A. R.: Medullary necrosis in infancy. Br. Med. Bull. 28:233, 1972.

Chrispin, A. R., Hull, D., Lillie, J. G., and Risdon, R. A.: Renal tubular necrosis after gastroenteritis in infants. Br. Med. J. 1:140, 1970.

Clatworthy, H. W., Jr., Dickens, D. R., and McClave, C. R.: Renal thrombosis complicating epidemic diarrhea in the newborn: nephrectomy with recovery. N. Engl. J. Med. 248:628, 1953.

Davies, D. J., Kennedy, A., and Roberts, C.: Renal medullary necrosis in infancy and childhood. J. Pathol. 99:125, 1969.

Duncan, R. E., Evans, A. T., and Martin, L. W.: Natural history and treatment of renal vein thrombosis in children. J. Pediatr. Surg. 12:639, 1977.

Fallon, M. L.: Renal venous thrombosis in the newborn. Arch. Dis. Child. 24:125, 1949.

Fraley, E. E., Fish, A. J., and Najarian, J. S.: Bilateral renal vein thrombosis in infancy: report of a survivor following surgical intervention. J. Pediatr. 78:509, 1971.

Ghai, O. P., Singh, M., et al.: Acute renal failure following renal vein thrombosis in conjoined twins. Am. J. Dis. Child. 121:57, 1971.

Gilbert, E. F., Khoury, G. H., Hogan, G. R., and Jones, B.: Hemorrhagic renal necrosis in infancy: relationship to radiopaque compounds. J. Pediatr. 76:49, 1970.

Groshong, T. D., Taylor, A. A., Nolph, K. D., Esterly, J., and Maher, J. F.: Renal function following cortical necrosis in childhood. J. Pediatr. 78:269, 1971.

Gross, R. E.: Arterial embolism and thrombosis in infancy. Am. J. Dis. Child. 70:61, 1945.

Gruskin, A. B., Oetliker, O. H., Wolfish, N. M., Gootman, N. I., Bernstein, J., and Edelmann, C. M.: Effects of angiography on renal function and histology in infants and piglets. J. Pediatr. 76:14, 1970.

Husband, P., and Howlett, K. A.: Renal papillary necrosis in infancy. Arch. Dis. Child. 48:116, 1973.

Kaufmann, H. J.: Renal vein thrombosis. Am. J. Dis. Child. 95:377, 1958.

Leonidas, J. C., Berdon, W. E., and Gribetz, D.: Bilateral renal cortical necrosis in the newborn infant: roentgenographic diagnosis. J. Pediatr. 79:623, 1971.

Lowry, M. F., Mann, J. R., Abrams, L. D., and Chance, G. W.: Thrombectomy for renal vein thrombosis in infant of diabetic mother. Br. Med. J. 3:687, 1970.

Mauer, S. M., and Nosgrady, M. B.: Renal papillary and cortical necrosis in a newborn infant: report of a survivor with roentgenologic documentation. J. Pediatr. 74:750, 1969.

Mauer, S. M., Fraley, E. E., Fish, A. J., et al.: Bilateral renal vein thrombosis in infancy: report of a survivor following surgical intervention. J. Pediatr. 78:509, 1971.

McDonald, P., Tarar, R., Gilday, D., and Reilly, B. J.: Some radiologic observations in renal vein thrombosis. Am. J. Roentgenol. Radium Ther. Nucl. Med. 120:368, 1974.

McFarland, J. B.: Renal venous thrombosis in children. Q. J. Med. 34:269, 1965.

Oppenheimer, E. H., and Esterly, J. R.: Thrombosis in the newborn; comparison between infants of diabetic and non-diabetic mothers. J. Pediatr. 67:549, 1965.

Renfield, M. L., and Kraybill, E. N.: Consumptive coagulopathy with renal vein thrombosis. J. Pediatr. 82:1054, 1973.

Stark, H., and Geiger, R.: Renal tubular dysfunction following vascular accidents of the kidneys in the newborn. J. Pediatr. 83:933, 1973.

Sutton, T. J., Leblanc, A., Gauthier, N., and Hassan, M.: Radiologic manifestations of neonatal renal vein thrombosis on follow-up examinations. Radiology 122:435, 1977.

Verhagen, A. D., Hamilton, J. P., and Genel, M.: Renal vein thrombosis in infants. Arch. Dis. Child. 42:214, 1965.

Walters, T. R., and Holder, T. M.: Neonatal hyperbilirubinemia and renal vein thrombosis in infants: occurrence in a newborn infant of a diabetic mother. Am. J. Dis. Child. 111:433, 1966.

Warren, H., Birdsong, M., and Kelley, R. A.: Renal vein thrombosis in infants. J.A.M.A. 152:700, 1953.

Woodard, J. R., Patterson, J. H., and Brinsfield, D.: Renal artery thrombosis in newborn infants. Am. J. Dis. Child. 114:191, 1967.

Zuelzer, W. W., Charles, S., Kurnetz, R., Newton, W. A., Jr., and Fallon, R.: Circulatory diseases of the kidneys in infancy and childhood. I. Am. J. Dis. Child. 81:1, 1951.

Zuelzer, W. W., Kurnetz, R., and Newton, W. A., Jr.: Circulatory diseases of the kidneys in infancy and childhood. IV. Occlusion of the renal artery. Am. J. Dis. Child. 81:21, 1951.

49

Hypertension

By Warren E. Grupe

Hypertension is very uncommon in children under 1 year of age and a rare occurrence in the nursery. Although the exact incidence is unknown, Ingelfinger noted hypertension recorded in 0.2 per cent of 10,000 deliveries. Reports from intensive care nurseries indicate an incidence of at least 1 to 2.5 per cent. The recent increase in reported cases since 1976 may reflect either better infant observation or the increased use of indwelling umbilical artery catheters in high-risk neonates. Often its existence is first detected by the appearance of congestive heart failure. When discovered, a cause must be sought and established even if the blood pressure can be controlled by antihypertensive medication; essential hypertension in the neonate is so unusual as to be a virtual nonentity in this already uncommon clinical state.

Until recently, the accurate determination of the blood pressure in the newborn was difficult. This probably has accounted as much for the absence of good surveys in normal infants as for the proliferation of techniques. The use of the Doppler ultrasound method has greatly enhanced the accuracy and simplicity of obtaining blood pressures in the small infant and appears, at the moment, to be the method of choice. A cuff approximating two thirds of the length of the upper extremity should be used (in small infants, a 4 by 9 cm cuff works well), with the transducer placed over the brachial artery. In this fashion, the blood pressure can be taken in the infant at rest. A cuff too small will overestimate the blood pressure, and a cuff too large will underestimate it. In general, the mean systolic blood pressure is slightly lower and the mean diastolic blood pressure is slightly higher with the Doppler technique than with the intra-aortic pressures, but the accuracy and reliability are excellent in the clinical situation.

Hypertension is defined as pressure levels above the ninety-fifth percentile for size and age. Normal pressures for neonates, obtained by umbilical artery catheter, are listed in Appendix III.

Etiology. Renal vascular disease has replaced coarctation of the aorta in recent years as the most common cause of hypertension in the newborn. Published reports since 1976 implicate renal arterial occlusion in approximately 75 per cent of cases. This is primarily due to an increase in thromboembolic occlusion of renal vessels accompanying the widespread use of indwelling umbilical artery catheters. The association between umbilical catheters and vascular thrombosis has been well documented, with an incidence of at least 3 to 10 per cent. The renal vessels are particularly at risk when the catheter tip is in the aorta above the origin of the renal arteries. Often, thrombotic or embolic blockage of other vessels, especially in the legs, is also demonstrable. There is no clearly demonstrated relationship between the development of hypertension and the interval for which the catheter has been in place.

Congenital renal artery stenosis is a less common but still significant etiology, accounting for perhaps 20 per cent of the cases of hypertension in neonates. This may accompany aortic stenosis or atresia. Cardiac failure without valvular disease has led, in some reports, to the initial diagnoses of myocarditis, endocardial fibroelastosis, and cardiomyopathies, including glycogen storage disease, before renal artery stenosis has been detected.

An association also exists between patent ductus arteriosus and renal artery occlusion leading to severe hypertension. Since an increasing number of immature infants with a persistent patency of the ductus are surviving, this might be anticipated to become an increasing cause of neonatal hypertension. In three of 17 hypertensive neonates evaluated by Adelman, hypertension developed shortly after closure of the ductus, suggesting the possibility of renal embolism. Another patient reported by Dimmick and coworkers had occlusion of the right renal artery associated with aneurysmal dilatation and thrombosis of the ductus arteriosus. Of the eight infants reported by Durante and associates, six had thrombosis of the ductus arteriosus. Zuelzer and colleagues, Dimmick and coworkers, and Gross (who provided the original description) reported infants who also had a major cerebral vascular infarct as part of this phenomenon. Coarctation of the aorta (see p. 267) still remains a prevalent cause of hypertension. For this reason, the blood pressure measurement should be obtained in both the upper and lower extremities; pressure normally should be higher in the leg than in the arm. Synchronism of brachial and femoral pulses is probably of more value in coarctation than attempts to judge the relative force of the femoral pulse.

Raised intracranial pressure, from any cause, including tumor, subdural hematoma, and meningitis, may cause an acute increase in blood pressure in the neonate. Pheochromocytoma and fibromuscular dysplasia have not been diagnosed in the newborn.

Hypertension has been reported in association with obstructive uropathy. Crossed renal ectopia with hypertension has been reported in a male infant with a left to right ectopia and one renal mass on the right.

Table 49–1. Causes of Hypertension in Infancy

Vascular
  Coarctation of the thoracic aorta
  Coarctation of the abdominal aorta
  Anomalies of the renal pedicle, including arterial stenosis and
    hypoplasia
  Hypoplasia of the aorta
  Renal artery thrombosis

Renal
  Infantile polycystic kidney
  Hypoplastic kidney
  Obstructive uropathy with hydronephrosis
  Crossed renal ectopia
  Acute and chronic renal insufficiency
  Renal tumors
  Medullary cystic diseases
  Multicystic kidney

Other
  Increased intracranial pressure
  Neural crest tumors
  Adrenogenital syndrome
  Cushing's disease
  Primary hyperaldosteronism
  Fluid and electrolyte overload
  Ocular phenylephrine

This was associated with an imperforate anus and rectourethral fistula. Hypertension was corrected by removal of the ectopic kidney. There was hydronephrosis of the crossed left kidney, and arteriography showed a small narrow renal artery. Another case was reported by Palmer and coworkers in a young patient with a solitary kidney and ureteropelvic obstruction. Peripheral and renal vein renin activity was normal. Removal of the obstruction resulted in a massive postoperative diuresis and cure of the hypertension. It was proposed that sodium and water retention, on the basis of renal insufficiency, suppressed the release of the expected increased amounts of renin.

Hypertension is not usual in patients with congenital anomalies of the urinary tract, however. Only infantile polycystic kidneys and segmental hypoplasia are commonly associated with elevated blood pressures. It is interesting that most patients with developmental anomalies such as hypoplasia or dysplasia seem quite resistant to the development of hypertension, even after the development of renal insufficiency. The reason for this is not evident.

Other causes of hypertension in the neonate include adrenal hyperplasia, fluid and electrolyte overload, neuroblastoma, Cushing's disease, and primary hyperaldosteronism. These other causes are quite rare in the nursery. Systemic hypertension has also been reported following the ocular administration of 10 per cent phenylephrine in the neonate. Causes of hypertension reported in infancy are listed in Table 49–1.

Renin-Angiotensin System

The renin-angiotensin system is undoubtedly involved in renovascular hypertension and has been implicated as a final common pathway in several other hypertensive states. Renin is released from the juxtaglomerular cells of the renal cortex in response to decreased renal plasma flow, decreased plasma volume, or sodium depletion. An enzyme, renin acts on a liver-produced glycoprotein substrate to release a decapeptide, angiotensin I. Another enzyme from lung converts angiotensin I to an octapeptide, angiotensin II, which both causes vasoconstriction and stimulates the adrenal cortex to produce aldosterone. Although the regulating mechanisms are not clearly defined, the advantage of this system in the maintenance of plasma volume, sodium regulation, and intravascular pressure is obvious. The role of renin-angiotensin in the fetus and newborn is not clear. However, increased renal vascular resistance seems to be a major factor in the relatively decreased glomerular filtration rate and renal plasma flow in the neonate. Its role may also include maintaining functionally significant levels of aldosterone in a relatively refractory adrenal cortex.

Information about the renin-angiotensin system in the neonate is just becoming available. Based on morphology, it appears that the human fetus produces renin as early as the seventeenth week of gestation; sustained hypertension has been produced in the fetal lamb by renal artery constriction in utero, presumably related to the renin-angiotensin system. Using immunoassays, the level of plasma renin activity (PRA) 1 to 12 hours after birth is significantly elevated compared with normal adult standards and is similar to that found in adults following the combined stimulus of salt deprivation and upright position. Kotchen and coworkers, using immunoassay, found that the mean PRA for the neonate is 8.8 ng/ml/hr ± 2.8 S.E.M. By 3 to 6 days, the PRA rises still higher to 11.6 ng/ml/hr. Three to 6 weeks later, activity falls slightly to 2.3 ng/ml/hr, but it is still higher than in the average adult. Although some reports in prematures and term neonates do not find plasma renin levels different from those of older children, other groups measuring PRA in children between the ages of 2 months and 19 years have shown that PRA is higher in the younger children and gradually declines during the first 6 years to approximately adult levels. This decline with age does not seem to be related to an increase in sodium intake, since sodium excretion, corrected for body surface area, does not vary with age in normal children on normal diets.

Plasma renin substrate in the newborn is also significantly elevated over normal adult controls and seems to stay relatively stable between birth and 6 weeks of age. Plasma renin activity depends on both enzyme and substrate concentrations. However, it is probable that the increased PRA in the neonate is primarily a reflection of elevations of the enzymes rather than the level of substrate. The substrate concentration is only modestly elevated, while PRA is over 10 times that of the adult. Also, in 3- to 6-week-old infants, PRA is significantly lower than in the younger infant, while the elevated substrate concentration persists at roughly the same level.

PRA levels vary with both gestational and postnatal age. Therefore, diagnostic and therapeutic decisions must allow for the higher normal levels of both PRA and substrate in the neonate. Like creatinine, the normal values for the laboratory are not always the normal values for the infant.

Peripheral PRA is elevated in most, but not all, infants with renal vascular hypertension. However, levels may also be elevated in nonhypertensive infants with respiratory distress syndrome, renal failure, hypovolemia, and severe lung disease. Plasma levels may also be altered by drugs that stimulate renin release, such as hydralazine, or by agents that inhibit renin production, such as propranolol. Although the level in renal vascular disease usually exceeds that seen in these conditions, an elevated PRA in a hypertensive, ill infant is not absolute evidence of renal artery disease.

It is not clear whether one can implicate the renin-angiotensin system in all cases of hypertension of the newborn. For example, elevations of PRA are not universal in coarctation of the aorta, and the role of the kidney or renal plasma flow in this hypertensive state is controversial. The same is true for hypertension associated with either increased intracranial pressure or fluid and electrolyte overload.

Diagnosis. The signs and symptoms of hypertension in the newborn are often nonspecific until congestive heart failure develops. The infants can show irritability, lethargy, anorexia, failure to thrive, vomiting, diarrhea, fever, tachypnea, apnea, cyanosis, seizures, opisthotonus, hemiparesis, coma, polyuria, hypokalemia, alkalosis, and hypotonia. Physical findings may include cardiomegaly, hepatomegaly, asymmetric reflexes, and hypertonicity. Since the initial findings are so protean, it becomes evident that accurate blood pressure determinations should be a part of the evaluation of the ill newborn, regardless of the initial impression.

Each of the causes listed in Table 49–1 must be considered and evaluated by appropriate radiologic and chemical techniques. The routine measurement in every infant of 17-hydroxysteroids, 17-ketosteroids, VMA, catecholamines, and aldosterone secretion, without some other indication, most often increases the expense and postpones definitive therapy with little diagnostic return. Radiologic and electrocardiographic evaluations of heart size are important, as is every effort to diagnose coarctation of the aorta. Urinalysis, tests of renal function, renal ultrasonography, radionuclide renal scan, and intravenous pyelography should also be performed to determine the presence of renal parenchymal disease and congenital abnormalities of the urinary tract. Peripheral plasma renin activity is helpful if significantly elevated, but it may be deceiving if normal. Since most reports of hypertension in the neonate in the absence of coarctation of the aorta are related to renovascular disease, a major effort to define this entity should be made.

The diagnosis of renal vascular hypertension is made best by arteriography, often performed through the indwelling umbilical catheter, with which information about abnormal size, caliber, and contours of the renal vessels becomes readily available. Accessory vessels become apparent as do areas of stenosis or poststenotic dilatation or both. The nephrogram also provides the size and shape of the kidney and the homogeneity of its vascular supply. Renal vein samples for plasma renin activity should be obtained at the same time that the arteriography is performed.

When the levels in both renal veins are compared, a ratio of greater than 2½ to 1 is highly suggestive of unilateral disease and implies a good prognosis following nephrectomy. Normal renal vein PRA does not clearly exclude unilateral disease, since blood from a small ischemic area may not be detected because of dilution of the blood from the remainder of the kidneys. However, selective sampling from branches of the renal vein is almost impossible in the infant. It is often difficult enough just to get a sampling catheter into the major renal vessels.

Reports of infants with renal vascular hypertension in whom rapid sequence pyelography has been used are insufficient to assess the value of this test. Reports in older children indicate that most, but by no means all, children with renal vascular hypertension will have some abnormality of either size or function or in the appearance of contrast material in the affected kidney. Localized areas of poor or delayed visualization, as well as those of nonvisualization, provide valuable information. It has been noted that delayed appearance of contrast material on one side, when coupled with increased density on the same side, is consistent with an abnormality of the renal pedicle. Since intravenous pyelography is difficult to assess in the newborn, it is unlikely that the rapid sequence pyelogram would negate the use of arteriography in an infant with hypertension. It would seem wise to proceed to aortography in a hypertensive newborn whether or not the pyelogram is suggestive of a renal lesion. Differential renal function studies are technically difficult in the child and practically impossible in the neonate. Radionuclide studies, however, can measure blood flow and excretory function in each kidney. Likewise, in the infant who no longer has an indwelling arterial catheter, nuclide studies can demonstrate renal vascular disease and thus possibly obviate the need for an invasive femoral catheter for arteriography. It would appear that tests such as the urea washout pyelogram and renal biopsy are of less value than the arteriogram in neonates with renal vascular hypertension. However, information on this is virtually nonexistent.

Significant alteration of renal function indicates bilateral renal disease, either primary parenchymal involvement or secondary to hypertension. With any significant hypertension, secondary damage to cerebral, retinal, and renal vessels can be expected. The renal lesion is a nephrosclerosis primarily affecting the afferent arteriole but can progress to hyalinization of the glomeruli. The glomerular lesion is irreversible. Early control of hypertension seems to prevent progression of this secondary lesion, and the reversibility of the arteriolar damage appears more common in children than in adults. Therefore, the clinical evaluation must be prompt and complete and must include consideration of bilateral or irreversible renal involvement.

Treatment. The major reason for pursuing the clinical evaluation to completion and to a precise diagnosis is to provide the opportunity for a surgical cure or sensible pharmacologic control. When the result is unilateral artery stenosis, and if diagnosed early enough, nephrectomy is curative. Most feel that nephrectomy is better than attempts to reconstruct a renal artery, since most attempts to revascularize in the infant result in thrombosis of the repaired vessels. Bilateral stenotic disease is a more difficult problem. Some will attempt surgical repair on one side at a time with some reported success. There has been some success using autotransplantation in the treatment of bilateral disease. This has not been reported in an infant but has been performed successfully in an 8-year-old. Successful medical management may be a more prudent approach in bilateral disease, the surgical approach being reserved for those in whom control of the blood pressure cannot be maintained.

Treatment for renal vascular occlusion has traditionally been immediate nephrectomy. However, severe concomitant disease may increase the risk of surgery, and recent results with aggressive pharmacologic management may render surgery obsolete as primary therapy. The fact that mortality is higher in patients subjected to early nephrectomy is not easily interpreted, but it certainly does not support nephrectomy as first line treatment. Since the extent of irreversible damage is not easily determined or predicted, early nephrectomy would clearly thwart the significant renal recovery that can occur.

For those infants in whom surgery is not possible or appropriate, pharmacologic agents become the mainstay of medical management. Treatment must be individualized not only in terms of the type, amount, or combinations of antihypertensive agents but also in terms of the goal of the specific therapy. For example, an infant with inoperable renal artery stenosis and renin-angiotensin–mediated hypertension should be considered in a different manner than one with chronic renal insufficiency whose major difficulty may be fluid and electrolyte excess.

Information about the long-term effects of antihypertensive drugs begun in infancy or about the effects of these agents on development in the immature is virtually nonexistent. The controversy over whether reserpine is related to breast cancer is a typical example of the lack of information. Whether the drugs themselves have an influence on growth or development is not known. Children with hypertension and normal renal function do not grow normally until the hypertension is brought under control. The mechanism by which hypertension might alter growth is unknown, and the long-term effect of the treatment is also not certain.

When considering an approach to therapy, one should keep in mind the pharmacologic effects and sites of action of the agents employed. Drugs that alter peripheral vascular resistance include thiazides, reserpine, hydralazine, methyldopa, guanethidine, diazoxide, and nitroprusside. Drugs that interfere with the renin-angiotensin system include propranolol and methyldopa. Drugs that alter cardiac output include propranolol, hydralazine, and reserpine. Drugs that decrease plasma volume include the thiazides, furosemide, ethacrynic acid, and spironolactone.

Mild hypertension may respond to diuretics alone. The majority of infants requiring further medication can be managed with a single antihypertensive agent. Hydralazine and propranolol, either alone or in combination, are effective for most infants, providing sufficient medication is given. Newborns seem to tolerate the higher dosages usually required to control hypertension from renal vascular disease. Those authors recommending surgery for medical failure have usually used doses that are substantially lower for periods that are shorter than those of authors reporting medical success. One must provide aggressive treatment, occasionally even using larger doses than recommended for older children.

Hypertensive emergencies should be treated with parenteral medication. The drugs available include reserpine, hydralazine, methyldopa, diazoxide, and nitroprusside. Many infants will respond promptly to intramuscular reserpine and hydralazine, with the other medications being held in reserve; these two agents should have discernible effects within 1 hour of administration. Tachycardia from the hydralazine and flushing, somnolence, or irritability from the reserpine are the usual side effects.

In resistant patients, diazoxide, given rapidly intravenously, is the next step. To be effective, the drug must be administered by bolus within 30 seconds. The effect is almost immediate and may persist for hours after a single administration with no other antihypertensive drug. Few side effects have been reported. Transient tachycardia is usual. A report of nonfatal arrhythmia in an infant, related to diazoxide injected through a central venous line, is cause for concern. Thus, it is probably more prudent to use a peripheral vessel for diazoxide, even if a central catheter is available. Hyperglycemia and hyperuricemia have also been reported with diazoxide.

Parenteral nitroprusside has yet to fail to reduce blood pressure. Its effect is immediate (within seconds), the desired level of blood pressure can be virtually titrated by control of the intravenous rate, and hypotension from overdose can be reversed almost

instantaneously by discontinuing the infusion. Its major drawback is also its main virtue; since changes in its effect are directly related to the rate of parenteral administration, it requires intense monitoring under constant observation by professional personnel familiar with its use. Experience with the drug is very limited in the neonate, and side effects, other than hypotension, have not been well documented.

Dialysis or plasmapheresis may be the most effective treatment for severe hypertension from fluid and electrolyte overload that does not respond to diuretics and restriction of intake.

In the medical management of persistent or chronic hypertension, one should also keep in mind the etiology of the hypertension. Patients with fluid and electrolyte overload, either iatrogenic or related to renal insufficiency, should have their intake appropriately decreased and their output increased with diuretics. At the same time, consideration must be given to the potential of increasing the stimulus for renin release by producing a low plasma volume; therefore, in an infant with renin-angiotensin–mediated hypertension, vigorous treatment with diuretics has at least the theoretical possibility of enhancing rather than controlling hypertension. It would seem more profitable in such a circumstance to consider those drugs known to suppress plasma renin activity, such as methyldopa or propranolol.

The starting oral doses for antihypertensive agents in common use are given in Table 49–2. These are a guideline; there is no routine dose, no routine order of increasing effectiveness, no fixed combination of agents. The best dose is one that attains the goal of a normal blood pressure with absent or clinically tolerable side effects and that is within the capability of the family to administer. The timing and frequency of medication depend on the diurnal variability of the infant's pressures and the duration of action of the medications. The aim should be to maintain as normal a blood pressure as possible throughout the day.

Table 49–2. Antihypertensive Medications in Neonates

Medication	Parenteral Dose	Oral Dose
Reserpine	0.001–0.02 mg/kg I.M.	0.02 mg/kg/day divided into 2 doses
Hydralazine	0.15 mg/kg I.M.	0.25 mg/kg/day divided into 3–6 doses
Methyldopa	2–4 mg/kg I.M. or I.V.	10 mg/kg/day divided into 3–4 equally spaced doses
Guanethidine		0.2 mg/kg/day single dose
Propranolol		1.5 mg/kg/day divided into 2–3 doses
Diazoxide	3–5 mg/kg I.V.	
Nitroprusside	0.004 µg/kg/min. I.V.	

Outcome. For the newborn, hypertension remains a serious disease accompanied by a significant rate of mortality. Death, sometimes the result of uncontrolled blood pressure, occurs in about 30 per cent of infants with hypertension. However, these neonates who die are often seriously ill and in a poor clinical state from catastrophic underlying primary disease to which surgery may have added an unbearable stress. The results with medical management in the infants presented by Adelman are encouraging. All 17 neonates, including nine with angiographically proved renal arterial occlusion, responded to pharmacologic treatment; none required nephrectomy. Three required less than 2 weeks of therapy, while in 13 others medications were discontinued 3 to 6 months later. In all, blood pressure remained normal over a mean of 15.2 months, as did renal function, urinalysis, and growth, even though renal atrophy was present in many and renal nuclide scan was completely normal in only one. Adelman's experience is not unique. Nevertheless, long-term follow-up of such infants is required, since the ultimate outcome of the survivors of neonatal hypertension remains unclear.

REFERENCES

Adelman, R. D.: Neonatal Hypertension. Pediatr. Clin. North Am. 25:99, 1978.

Adelman, R. D., Merten, D., Vogel, J., et al.: Non-surgical management of renovascular hypertension in the newborn. Pediatrics 62:71, 1978.

Adelman, R. D., and Sherman, M. P.: Hypertension in the neonate following closure of abdominal wall defects. J. Pediatr. 97:642, 1980.

Anand, S. K., Northway, J. D., and Smith, J. A.: Neonatal renal papillary and cortical necrosis. Am. J. Dis. Child. 131:773, 1977.

Belman, A. B., Kropp, K. A., and Simon, N. M.: Renal pressor hypertension secondary to unilateral hydronephrosis. N. Engl. J. Med. 278:1133, 1968.

Berens, S. C., Linde, L. M., and Goodwin, W. E.: Transitory hypertension following urologic surgery. Pediatrics 38:194, 1966.

Black, I. F. S., Kotrapu, N., and Massie, H.: Application of Doppler ultrasound to blood pressure measurement in small infants. J. Pediatr. 81:932, 1972.

Bonomeo-Megrail, V., Bordiuk, J. M., and Keitel, H.: Systemic hypertension following ocular administration of 10% phenylephrine in the neonate. Pediatrics 51:1032, 1973.

Carella, J. A., and Silber, I.: Hyperreninemic hypertension in an infant secondary to pelviureteric obstruction treated successfully by surgery. J. Pediatr. 88:987, 1976.

Chen, J. J., Anand, S. K., and Porter, P. J.: Neonatal hypertension associated with renal artery hypoplasia. Pediatrics 41:524, 1968.

Cook, G. T., Marshall, V. F., and Todd, J. E.: Malignant renovascular hypertension in a newborn. J. Urol. 96:863, 1966.

Coran, A. G., and Schuster, S. R.: Renovascular hypertension in childhood. Surgery 64:572, 1968.

deSwiet, M., Fayers, P., and Shinebourne, E. A.: Systolic blood pressure in a population of infants in the first year of life: The Brompton Study. Pediatrics 65:1028, 1980.

Dimmick, J. E., Patterson, M. W. H., and Andrew-Wu, H. W.: Systemic hypertension in a newborn infant. J. Pediatr. 95:321, 1979.

Durante, D., Jones, D., and Spitzer, R.: Neonatal renal artery embolism syndrome. J. Pediatr. 89:978, 1976.

Ford, K. T., Teplick, S. K., and Clark, R. E.: Renal artery embolism causing neonatal hypertension. Radiology 113:169, 1974.

Foster, J. H., Pittinger, W. A., Oates, J. A., et al.: Malignant hypertension secondary to renal artery stenosis in children. Ann. Surg. 164:700, 1966.

Goddard, C., Riondel, A. M., Veyrat, R., Megevand, A., and Muller, A. F.: Plasma renin activity and aldosterone secretion in congenital adrenal hyperplasia. Pediatrics 41:883, 1968.

Gross, R. E.: Arterial embolism and thrombosis in infancy. A.M.A. J. Dis. Child. 70:61, 1945.

Gupta, J. M., and Scopes, J. W.: Observations on blood pressure in newborn infants. Arch. Dis. Child. 40:637, 1965.

Hernandez, A., Goldring, D., Hartmann, A. F., Crawford, C., and Reed, G. N.: Measurement of blood pressure in infants and children by the Doppler ultrasound technique. Pediatrics 48:788, 1971.

Hiner, L. B., Gruskin, A. B., Bacuarte, H. J., and Cote, M. L.: Plasma renin activity in normal children. J. Pediatr. 89:258, 1976.

Imai, M., Igarashi, Y., and Sokabe, H.: Plasma renin activity in congenital virilizing adrenal hyperplasia. Pediatrics 41:879, 1968.

Ingelfinger, J. R.: Hypertension in the first year of life. In Ingelfinger, J. R. (Ed.): Pediatric Hypertension. Philadelphia, W. B. Saunders Co., 1982.

Kirkendall, W. M., Culbertson, J. W., and Eckstein, J. W.: Renal hemodynamics in patients with coarctation of the aorta. J. Lab. Clin. Med. 53:6, 1959.

Kirkland, R. T., and Kirkland, J. L.: Systolic blood pressure measurement in the newborn infant with the transcutaneous Doppler method. J. Pediatr. 80:52, 1972.

Kitterman, J. A., and Phibbs, R. H.: Aortic blood pressure in the normal newborn: hazards of the umbilical artery catheter. Pediatrics 45:893, 1970.

Kotchen, T. A., Strickland, A. L., Rice, T. W., and Walters, D. R.: A study of the renin-angiotensin system in newborn infants. J. Pediatr. 80:938, 1972.

Lindesmith, G. G., Stanton, R. E., Stiles, Q. R., et al.: Coarctation of the thoracic aorta. Ann. Thorac. Surg. 11:482, 1971.

Ljungquist, A., and Wallgren, G.: Unilateral renal artery stenosis and fatal arterial hypertension in a newborn infant. Acta Paediatr. Scand. 51:575, 1962.

Loggie, J. M. H., New, M. I., and Robson, A. M.: Hypertension in the pediatric patient: a reappraisal. J. Pediatr. 94:685, 1979.

Londie, S., and Gollub, S. W.: Arm position and blood pressure. J. Pediatr. 94:617, 1979.

Lum, L. G., and Jones, M. D.: The effect of cuff width on systolic blood pressure measurements in neonates. J. Pediatr. 91:963, 1977.

Makker, S. P., and Lubahn, J. D.: Clinical features of renovascular hypertension in infancy: report of a 9 month old infant. Pediatrics 56:108, 1975.

Marie, J., Royer, P., Gabilan, J. C., and Vandevoorde, J.: Le traitement médical de l'hypertension artérielle permanente chez l'enfant. Ann. Pediatr. (Paris) 4:251, 1965.

Mininberg, D. T., Roze, S., Yoon, H. J., and Pearl, M.: Hypertension associated with crossed renal ectopia in an infant. Pediatrics 48:454, 1971.

Monin, P., Gerbaux, A., and Vert, P.: Arterial dysplasia and neonatal hypertension. Arch. Fr. Pediatr. 31:517, 1974.

Morse, R. O., Brownell, G. L., and Currens, J. H.: The blood pressure of newborn infants. Indirect determination by an automated recorder. Pediatrics 25:50, 1960.

Munoz, A. I., Baralt, J. F., and Melandez, M. T.: Arterial hypertension in infants with hydronephrosis. Am. J. Dis. Child. 131:38, 1977.

Neal, W. A., Reynolds, J. W., Jarvis, C. W., et al.: Umbilical artery catheterization: demonstration of arterial thrombosis by aortography. Pediatrics 50:6, 1972.

Olinger, G. N., and Mulder, D. G.: Direct monitoring of arterial pressure in the newborn and infant: a difficult procedure made easy. Ann. Thorac. Surg. 21:557, 1976.

Palmer, J. M., Zweiman, F. G., and Assaykeen, T. A.: Renal hypertension secondary to hydronephrosis with normal plasma renin activity. N. Engl. J. Med. 283:1032, 1970.

Plumer, L. B., Mendoza, S. A., and Kaplan, G. W.: Hypertension in infancy: the case for aggressive management. J. Urol. *113*:555, 1975.

Plumer, L. B., Kaplan, G. W., and Mendoza, S. A.: Hypertension in infants—a complication of umbilical artery catheterization. J. Pediatr. *89*:802, 1976.

Reder, R. F., Dimich, I., Cohen, M. L., and Steinfeld, L.: Evaluating indirect blood pressure measurement techniques: a comparison of three systems in infants and children. Pediatrics *62*:326, 1978.

Schmidt, D. M., and Rambo, O. N.: Segmental intimal hyperplasia of the abdominal aorta and renal arteries producing hypertension in an infant. Am. J. Clin. Pathol. *44*:546, 1965.

Siegler, R. L., Crouch, R. H., Hackett, T. N., et al.: Potassium-renin-aldosterone relationships during the first year of life. J. Pediatr. *91*:52, 1977.

Skinner, S. L., Lumbers, E. R., and Symonds, E. M.: Renin concentration in human fetal and maternal tissues. Am. J. Obstet. Gynecol. *101*:529, 1968.

Snyder, C. H., Bast, R. B., and Platau, R. V.: Hypertension in infancy with anomalous renal artery. Pediatrics *15*:88, 1955.

Stalker, H. P., Holland, N. H., Kotchen, J. M., and Kotchen, T. A.: Plasma renin activity in healthy children. J. Pediatr. *89*:256, 1976.

Timmis, G. C., and Gordon, S.: A renal factor in hypertension due to coarctation. N. Engl. J. Med. *270*:814, 1964.

Uhari, M., Remes, M., Lanning, P., and Seppanen, J.: Severe hypertension in a patient with unilateral obstructive hydronephrosis and renal artery stenosis. J. Pediatr. *93*:458, 1978.

Walker, C. H. M., West, P. J., Simons, S. L., and Whytock, A. R.: Indirect estimation of systolic and diastolic blood pressure in the newborn. Pediatrics *50*:387, 1972.

Wernig, C., Schonbeck, M., Weidmann, P., et al.: Plasma renin activity in patients with coarctation of the aorta. Circulation *40*:731, 1969.

Zuelzer, W. W., Kurnetz, R., and Newton, W. A., Jr.: Circulatory diseases of the kidneys in infancy and childhood. IV. Occlusion of the renal artery. Am. J. Dis. Child. *81*:121, 1951.

50

Differential Diagnosis of the Enlarged Kidney

By Warren E. Grupe

The surprising discovery of an abdominal mass, often asymptomatic, during the routine examination of a newborn should be worrisome to the physician and often initiates a series of invasive investigations that eventually lead to surgery. If tragedy is to be averted, the approach to the patient must be thoughtful, meticulous, and organized. A rush to surgery is often not the best way to solve the unknown, since few of these masses are malignant. Nevertheless, surgery either cures or significantly helps most infants, and thus it is imperative that an early and complete diagnosis be efficiently made. Waiting for the mass to disappear or for the infant to grow larger may add to the complications and thwart the infant's rehabilitation.

In most instances, the discovery of the abdominal mass is the crucial manifestation of disease and often the only physical finding. Since a mass unfelt is a mass ignored, there is no diagnostic substitute for a good physical examination. The best time to feel a mass is within the first few days of life, when intestinal contents are few and abdominal musculature hypotonic. Not surprisingly, most studies indicate that the masses have been discovered within the first 48 hours. In the study by Wedge and coworkers, 30 of 63 masses became apparent in the first 24 hours of life, whereas in Griscom's series, 62 per cent of all abdominal masses, over half the renal masses, and all the genital tract masses were evident within the first 48 hours.

Abdominal masses are unusual in the newborn nursery. Sherwood and colleagues surveyed 12,160 newborns, finding abdominal masses in 24 (0.2 per cent). Museles and coworkers found 71 newborns with suspected abdominal masses by deep palpation on their initial examination, of which 55 (0.6 per cent of the 10,000 total) were confirmed by radiologic examination. In a recent survey, Perlman and Williams, who examined the abdomens of about 11,000 infants within the first 3 days of life, found suspected renal anomalies by palpation in 82 otherwise normal infants. The diagnosis of a renal anomaly was confirmed in 51 of the 71 infants fully investigated (0.4 per cent of the total).

There seems to be wide agreement that the genitourinary tract is the most common source of palpable abdominal masses in the newborn. Melicow and Uson reviewed 653 infants and older children with masses who were admitted to a pediatric urologic service. Of these, 139 had masses of genitourinary tract origin. A review of 10 series involving 529 newborn infants shows that over two thirds of abdominal masses were of renal origin. In some series, the percentage has been as high as 85 per cent and 93 per cent. When more infants have been included in the study, the percentage associated with renal anomalies is higher.

Etiology. The etiology of the various renal masses, defined by several studies, is outlined in Table 50–1, which provides some sense of the prevailing di-

Table 50–1.   Distribution of Renal Masses in 191
Neonates*

Lesion	Number	Percentage
Hydronephrosis	74	39
Multicystic dysplasia	59	31
Polycystic kidneys	16	8
Ectopia	12	6
Tumor	10	5
Renal vein thrombosis	5	3
Horseshoe kidney	4	2
Other†	11	6

* Data extracted from Sherwood et al. (1956); Griscom (1965); Emanuel and White (1968); Raffensperger and Abousleiman (1968); and Wedge et al. (1971).

† "Other" includes multilocular cysts, multiple cysts, solitary cysts, leiomyoma, cystic hamartoma, rupture of renal pelvis, abscess, agenesis, malrotation, and duplication.

agnostic probabilities. Although slight variances exist, most studies show either hydronephrosis or multicystic dysplastic kidneys as the most common. In both Griscom's series and the review by Emanuel and White, multicystic disease occurred more often than hydronephrosis during the first few days of life, after which hydronephrosis was the more common. In any event, hydronephrosis and multicystic kidneys together account for 70 per cent of neonatal urinary tract masses and for at least 40 per cent of all abdominal masses found in the first month of life. Polycystic kidneys and ectopia are the next most common lesions. No other condition accounts for more than 10 per cent of the total. Not all authors agree. Museles and colleagues and Perlman and Williams, for example, found horseshoe kidney the most prominent, accounting for 26 per cent of masses. Ectopia was more common than either hydronephrosis or multicystic dysplasia in the three series reported by Museles and coworkers, Perlman and Williams, and Sherwood and colleagues. In some reviews, multicystic kidneys and hydronephrosis each accounts for less than 10 per cent of masses. In no series limited to neonates has malignancy exceeded 15 per cent of the total. In the two studies by Melicow and Uson and by Kaspar and associates, which included older children, malignant tumors were the most frequent cause and hydronephrosis second.

Physical Examination.   Since normal kidneys are palpable to the experienced examiner during the first or second day of life in almost all newborns, even a small deviation in size or position should prompt investigation. It is difficult at times to be sure whether or not a kidney is enlarged. However, palpability is not synonymous with enlargement. A method of palpation proposed by Sherwood and colleagues and modified by Museles and coworkers takes only 30 seconds in the well-relaxed infant. Palpating in both upper quadrants, the examiner supports the flank with one hand while palpating with the other. Moving the palpating hand medially, the first encounter is with the anterolateral aspect of the lower pole. The normal kidney is located above the level of the umbilicus. When the lower pole projects well below this level, the organ is either enlarged or dislocated downward. Since the long axis of the kidney usually parallels the long axis of the body, medial displacement of the lower pole should suggest a horseshoe kidney. By palpating directly over the lumbar vertebrae, moving the palpating hand medially, one can detect the isthmus. Both lower quadrants are then examined for the presence of a pelvic kidney. Finally, the examiner places a hand in each flank, compressing medially and raising the hand slightly to allow the abdominal contents to pass between the fingers of the opposing hands. This helps in detecting a freely movable mass, such as an intestinal duplication or a cyst.

An equally efficient technique has been proposed by Perlman and Williams. In this procedure, the infant is held in a semireclining position, facing the examiner, whose hand is behind the infant's shoulders and neck supporting the occiput. Flexing the legs of the supine infant is another way to relax the abdomen. The fingers of the opposite hand are placed behind the flank to allow the thumb to explore all portions of that side of the abdomen systematically. The thumb and fingers are gently opposed subcostally for deep palpation, entrapping the upper pole of the kidney between them. As the thumb is moved caudally, while maintaining gentle pressure, the size, shape, axis, and consistency of the contents of the renal fossa are determined. The thumb is then moved through the lower quadrant toward the midline, continuing up the lumbar vertebrae to the xyphoid. Reversing the hands allows examination of the opposite side. The authors feel that the technique was mastered after examining 20 infants, and it took only 30 seconds to perform. The major difference from previous techniques is the use of the thumb, which is not ordinarily considered sufficiently sensitive. Nevertheless, it works well and offers the examining physician yet another option.

The size of the mass is of little diagnostic significance. However, the location can be helpful. Renal masses tend to be more superficial than one expects, and competent examiners have been surprised to find that a mass felt quite anterior or inferior was actually kidney. It is not unusual for left renal vein thrombosis, for example, to be mistaken for an enlarged spleen. A flank mass is usually renal or adrenal, whereas bilateral flank masses are likely to be polycystic or hydronephrotic kidneys. Bilateral multicystic renal dysplasia is rare. Unilateral flank masses are typically multicystic dysplasia, tumor, or hydronephrosis. Lower abdominal masses generally indicate bladder, ovaries, hydrocolpos, or hydrometra. A midline mass arising from or fixed to the pelvis is more frequently bladder, hydrometra, or hydrometrocolpos, whereas a more mobile and more anterior mass is probably an ovarian cyst or intestinal duplication.

Renal masses tend to be smooth and move with respirations. A perfectly smooth, rounded mass is likely to be hydronephrotic kidney, but the infarcted and displaced kidney may feel the same. Grossly irregular masses presenting one or more rounded knobs may be multicystic, whereas the surface of polycystic kidneys is apt to feel homogeneously and finely nodular. Tumors tend to be firm, but so do hydronephrosis and renal vein thrombosis. Neuroblastoma seldom presents as unilateral kidney displacement alone in the newborn, although this may constitute part of the picture. A usual presenting sign is the huge, smooth liver of metastatic involvement. The primary tumor may not be felt, although a normal, displaced kidney might be.

Examination of the perineum can expose a bulging hydrocolpos, a ureterocele protruding through the urethra, or an imperforate anus. Clues to the renal origin of an abdominal mass can be obtained from associated abnormalities such as meningomyelocele, abnormal ears, microcephaly, aniridia, hypertension, hemihypertrophy, pneumomediastinum, and absent abdominal musculature.

Diagnostic Procedures.   Urine examination may be helpful, but results are often within normal limits. Excess albumin is often found in polycystic kidneys and renal vein thrombosis, although it may occur in some cases of hydronephrosis and mesoblastic nephroma. Microscopic hematuria is often viewed as evidence of tumor but, in fact, can occur in any of the diagnoses under consideration. Pyuria and cylindruria are also found in infarcted kidneys and are present in the others only if infection has supervened.

The urea nitrogen level rises rapidly when the renal vein becomes thrombosed. It may be elevated early in hydronephrosis and in polycystic disease, but elevation commonly awaits a later date. If there is no superimposed pyelonephritis, the urea nitrogen level should not be high in any of the other conditions being contemplated.

The definitive differentiation of renal masses relies heavily on the resources of radiology, ultrasonography, and nuclear medicine. Even when the mass does not seem to be renal by location or palpation, intravenous urography is still indicated. The great majority of masses and practically all the large masses will be readily detected on a plain abdominal scout film through displacement of gas-containing viscera, although small posterior masses may be seen better on a lateral film. Masses involving the kidney are usually of uniform water density. Large masses sometime balloon the flanks. Lesions of the upper right kidney may displace the colon inferiorly and anteriorly and may even displace the second portion of the duodenum, whereas lesions of the left kidney may deviate the spleen upward and laterally. Absence or ectopia of the left kidney is suggested by malpositioned colon in the renal fossa, best seen on a lateral film. Adrenal enlargement will depress the kidney and rotate its upper pole laterally. Calcifications in

renal masses at birth are virtually nonexistent and should, therefore, direct attention toward tumor, meconium peritonitis, intestinal atresia, or, later, vascular accidents and abnormal adrenals.

The intravenous urogram provides information through both excretion urography and total body opacification. Total body opacification is the uniform slight opacification produced by contrast material in the vascular compartment. The effect allows avascular or cystic lesions not seen on the preliminary film to appear as a negative shadow a few minutes after the intravenous injection of contrast material. The effect will then slowly disappear as the kidneys extract the contrast material from the blood. Since over 75 per cent of neonatal masses are cystic or otherwise avascular, total body opacification can be quite useful in the differential diagnosis. The neonatal masses most commonly delineated are multicystic kidneys, ovarian cysts, hydronephrotic kidneys, polycystic kidneys, and renal vein thrombosis.

The nephrogram and subsequent films will define the position and structure of the kidneys. If there is nonvisualization on the early films, films delayed up to 24 hours later are essential. For example, a unilaterally nonfunctioning kidney generally implies multicystic dysplasia or renal vein thrombosis. However, later opacification of the collecting system and pelvis could define hydronephrosis. In the review by Emanuel and White, eight of ten patients with proven hydronephrosis had delay in the visualization of contrast material. A still later film might outline the ureter and distinguish ureteropelvic junction stenosis from ureterovesical obstruction. A late film may also outline the septa of cysts in multicystic dysplasia.

If malignancy is of concern, the inferior vena cava can be visualized during injection of the contrast material through a leg vein. A prolonged nephrogram, lasting several days and occasionally associated with an elevated serum creatinine, can be obtained from neonates who are dehydrated or oliguric prior to intravenous pyelography. The main functions of cystourethrography are to determine the presence or absence of reflux and to outline obstructing urethral valves.

Ultrasonography can be quite helpful in the delineation of the nonvisualized and poorly visualized kidney. It is particularly helpful in differentiating solid from cystic structures and can show renal size, the status of the collecting systems, and the position of the kidneys, even when no excretory function exists. A large kidney suggests hydronephrosis, multicystic dysplasia, or renal vein thrombosis. Ultrasonography can usually differentiate between these lesions. In fact, when a diagnosis of multicystic dysplasia can be made with certainty, invasive diagnostic procedures are often unnecessary. Radioactive nuclide scanning is a most accurate procedure for defining renal blood flow and function in nonvisualized kidneys. One can also use appropriate isotopes to determine differentially the percentage of filtration function contributed by each kidney. Scans also distinguish renal pseudotumors from the space-taking lesions.

Although still important in their place, arteriography and retrograde pyelography are becoming less useful. Antegrade pyelography can be used occasionally to define the poorly functioning hydronephrotic kidney further. Percutaneous insertion of the needle into the renal pelvis with ultrasonic guidance has enhanced the success and safety of this procedure. It can also define retroperitoneal cystic lesions. Transillumination enhanced by the use of a fiberoptic light source may detect the cystic nature of a palpable mass. Although the majority of hydronephrotic and multicystic kidneys transilluminate, it is not clear that transillumination has any advantage over ultrasonography.

Multicystic Renal Dysplasia

The vast majority of cases of multicystic kidney are found during the first few days of life. The disease is almost always unilateral, and the left is involved more commonly than the right. It often produces considerable abdominal distention. The palpating hand is met by a soft, lobular, and often palpably cystic mass. Veins over the stretched abdominal wall can be prominent. It is seldom symptomatic, and results of urinalysis are generally within normal limits. Other congenital abnormalities are unusual. However, in the series reported by Wedge and coworkers, 6 of 15 infants with multicystic renal disease had other urinary tract abnormalities that in several cases affected the contralateral kidney. Careful evaluation of the contralateral side, therefore, is imperative. Nevertheless, when the opposite kidney is normal at the time of the initial evaluation, it is extremely unusual for subsequent abnormalities to appear. A nonfunctioning kidney in a neonate usually represents multicystic kidney or renal vein thrombosis. However, function in a dilated hydronephrotic kidney may be delayed several hours. Most multicystic kidneys will transilluminate, and many are definitively diagnosed by ultrasonography as an echolucent mass with multiple septa. Nuclide scanning confirms the lack of both function and flow. Occasionally, individual cysts are faintly seen by intravenous pyelography or nuclide scanning as round lucent areas separated by slightly opacified septa. This appearance in a flank mass is diagnostic of multicystic dysplasia. The mass is usually radiolucent by total body opacification. The treatment of choice is nephrectomy.

Hydronephrosis

This lesion is usually unilateral and commonly related to ureteropelvic obstruction. Although often found within the first few days of life, it is clearly the most common cause of a renal abdominal mass thereafter. In cases found later in the neonatal period, infection has often intervened, causing fever, anorexia, vomiting, somnolence, and failure to thrive. Results of the urinalysis are generally negative unless infection is present. Hydronephrotic kidneys commonly feel smooth and vary in consistency from boggy to hard and tense. Voiding abnormalities are not always present, even when urethral obstruction can be demonstrated, although an enlarged bladder is occasionally palpable. With urography, a thin rim of functioning renal parenchyma will be visible as a crescent about the dilated collecting system. Early films will show a nonopacified, globular, noncompartmented mass. Ureteroceles, often obstructing and producing hydronephrosis in the upper pole, are visualized as filling defects within the bladder more clearly by intravenous urography than by cystourethrography. The degree of function determined by urography or nuclide scanning depends on the amount of functioning tissue and thus can vary from poor to almost normal. The ultrasonic feature of hydronephrosis is an ovoid pelvis surrounded by a series of uniform cysts.

Ectopic Kidney

A malpositioned but otherwise normal kidney can present as an abdominal mass. Crossed renal ectopia is not uncommon, however. Although these masses often feel like kidneys, intravenous pyelography makes the diagnosis obvious.

Renal Vein Thrombosis

Renal vein thrombosis usually presents as a unilaterally enlarged, tense, nonfunctioning kidney in the infant of a diabetic mother. The mass is rarely present at birth but often appears within the first 24 hours. Ultrasonography defines a large renal mass with centrally disordered echoes. It is occasionally accompanied by proteinuria and often by hematuria. The condition of the infant may provide the first clue to differential diagnosis. Only renal vein thrombosis and adrenal hemorrhage would be likely to make the child severely ill. A long-standing tumor might also have adverse effects, as would other congenital malformations if they were complicated by urinary infection.

Polycystic Renal Disease

Often, these infants are primarily investigated because of hypertension and failure to thrive rather than because of a palpable mass. A family history of polycystic disease is diagnostically quite helpful but not always present with the usual recessive inheritance of the infantile form. Renal enlargement varies from moderate to extreme but is always bilateral. Function evaluated by urography and nuclide scanning varies from poor to almost normal. Occasionally, cystic defects pressing upon the calyces and pelvis will suggest the cause. A radial arrangement of non-opacified shadows are seen in the early phases of urography, filling later as dilated and distorted tubules. Ultrasonography is similar in both infant and adult polycystic disease. Both kidneys are large with distortion of the renal contour and with multiple interfaces representing cyst walls in the renal cortex. The cysts are more variable in size than the dilated calyces of hydronephrosis, and a dilated renal pelvis is less common. In contrast to multicystic dysplasia, polycystic renal disease demonstrates a pelvocalyceal outline on the ultrasonogram.

Summary

The multiplicity of minimally invasive techniques available to the physician allow a rapid and accurate differential diagnosis of enlarged kidneys to be made in the nursery. Proper surgical correction or medical therapy can then be knowledgeably planned rather than hastily contrived. In Griscom's experience with 117 newborns, 60 per cent of the abdominal masses were surgically cured, and an additional 20 per cent of infants were significantly helped by either surgery or an appropriate medical program. These encouraging results are not unique.

REFERENCES

Boles, E. T., Jr.: Diagnosis of abdominal masses. Postgrad. Med. 42:237, 333, 1967.
Emanuel, B., and White, H.: Intravenous pyelography in the differential diagnosis of renal masses in the neonatal period. Clin. Pediatr. 7:529, 1968.
Goldberg, B. B., Pollack, H. M., Capitanio, M. A., et al.: Ultrasonography: an aid in the diagnosis of masses in pediatric patients. Pediatrics 56:421, 1975.

Griscom, N. T.: The roentgenology of neonatal abdominal masses. Am. J. Roentgenol. 93:447, 1965.
Grossman, M.: The evaluation of abdominal masses in childhood with emphasis on non-invasive methods: a roentgenographic approach. Cancer 35:885, 1975.
Henderson, K. C., and Torch, E. M.: Differential diagnosis of abdominal masses in the neonate. Pediatr. Clin. North Am. 24:557, 1977.
Hendren, W. H.: Abdominal masses in newborn infants. Am. J. Surg. 107:502, 1964.
Holder, T. M., Stuber, J. L., and Templeton, A. W.: Sonography as a diagnostic aid in the evaluation of abdominal masses in infants and children. J. Pediatr. Surg. 7:532, 1972.
Kasper, T. E., Osborne, R. W., Jr., Semerojian, M. S., and Miller, H. C.: Urologic abdominal masses in infants and children. J. Urol. 116:629, 1976.
Lebowitz, R. L., and Griscom, N. T.: Neonatal hydronephrosis; 146 cases. Radiol. Clin. North Am. 15:49, 1977.
Longino, L. A., and Martin, L. W.: Abdominal masses in the newborn infant. Pediatrics 21:596, 1958.
Melicow, M. M., and Uson, A. C.: Palpable abdominal masses in infants and children: a report based on a review of 653 cases. J. Urol. 81:705, 1959.
Museles, M., Gaudry, C. L., and Bason, M. W.: Renal anomalies in the newborn found by deep palpation. Pediatrics 47:97, 1971.
Perlman, M., and Williams, J.: Detection of renal anomalies by abdominal palpation in newborn infants. Br. Med. J. 2:347, 1976.
Raffensperger, J., and Abousleiman, A.: Abdominal masses in children under one year of age. Surgery 63:514, 1968.
Richmond, H., and Dougall, A. J.: Neonatal renal tumors. J. Pediatr. Surg. 5:413, 1970.
Sherwood, D. W., Smith, R. C., Lemmon, R. H., and Vrabel, I.: Abnormalities of the genitourinary tract discovered by palpation of the abdomen of the newborn. Pediatrics 18:782, 1956.
Tank, S., Poznanski, A. K., and Holt, J. F.: The radiologic discrimination of abdominal masses in infants. J. Urol. 109:128, 1973.
Teele, R. L.: Ultrasonography of the genitourinary tract in children. Radiol. Clin. North Am. 15:109, 1977.
Wedge, J. J., Grosfeld, J. L., and Smith, J. P.: Abdominal masses in the newborn: 63 cases. J. Urol. 106:770, 1971.

51

Nephropathies

By Warren E. Grupe

Glomerulonephritis

Glomerulonephritis in the neonate is an infrequent occurrence and is not as clearly understood as nephritis in the older child. The acute and the persistent glomerulonephritides common in childhood have not been established in the neonate by currently accepted techniques. Most reports of glomerular injury in the neonate are associated with the nephrotic syndrome (see p. 453). In this circumstance minimal lesion glomerulonephropathy, focal segmental sclerosis, membranous glomerulonephropathy, and diffuse mesangial sclerosis have been described. Other forms of renal injury that may also involve the glomerulus include bacterial and nonbacterial pyelonephritis and hereditary nephritis.

One difficulty in evaluating glomerulonephritis in the neonate involves the characteristics of the immature renal glomeruli. In both humans and experimental animals, these include a small diameter of the glomerular tuft with a narrow Bowman's space, splitting of the lamina densa, a nonfenestrated broad rim of the endothelial cytoplasm around the periphery of the glomerular tuft, and a relatively narrow capillary lumen. Palisading of adjacent visceral epithelial cells over the capillary loop and broad extension of epithelial cytoplasm covering the basement membrane contrast with the discrete foot processes noted in the older child or adult. In addition, glomerular senescence and hyalinization are common in the newborn, appearing to be normal processes of glomerular involution. Sclerotic glomeruli account for approximately 10 per cent of the glomerular population in newborns dying of other diseases, although sclerosis has been reported in as many as 20 per cent of glomeruli. One may see the other hallmarks of nephron involution, including focal tubular atrophy and slight interstitial reaction. It is presumed that the mechanism of this normal glomerular involution is ischemia, but the hyalinized and sclerotic glomeruli can appear similar to those seen in chronic glomerulonephritis in the older child. Many of the clinical and pathologic descriptions of neonatal nephritis are difficult to evaluate in light of the current recognition of this normal involutional process. It is also quite possible that some examples of neonatal nephritis have been confused with renal cortical and medullary necrosis.

Occasionally, acute and chronic pyelonephritis may also be associated with proliferative changes. This has raised questions about the relationship between infectious processes and neonatal glomerulonephritis.

Porter and Giles make a strong argument that identifies the basic defect in their five cases as pyelonephritis rather than glomerulonephritis. In their first case, the pyelonephritis was acute and unmistakable. In their other four cases the alterations were of longer duration, death having occurred between 14 and 20 weeks of age, and were therefore more difficult to evaluate. In all five cases, the urine culture was positive for *Escherichia coli*, and in two the blood grew out the same organism. All met the pathologic criteria established by Weiss and Parker for the diagnosis of chronic pyelonephritis. They include (1) infiltration of interstitium with lymphocytes, plasma cells and eosinophils, (2) pericapsular fibrosis, with or without intracapsular crescent formation, and (3) colloid casts in dilated tubules lined by atrophic epithelium. They point out that their cases differ from chronic glomerulonephritis in that many glomeruli are unaffected, the glomerular tufts are often uninvolved where pericapsular fibrosis is evident, involved glomeruli are apt to be found in wedge-shaped clusters, and interstitial inflammation is notable. Absence of much fibrosis they attribute to the relatively short course, and the presence of numerous crescents they discount with the statement that crescents seem to form more readily in infants than in adults and are found in many conditions other than glomerulonephritis.

These same authors wondered why all five of their patients were males when chronic pyelonephritis beyond the neonatal period is predominantly a disorder of females. They investigated the possibility of a congenital defect of the kidney being responsible for persistent infection and were gratified to find that in four of the five cases microdissection revealed the proximal tubules shorter than normal and almost devoid of convolutions. The fact that two of their patients were brothers strengthened their conviction that a congenital anomaly was at the root of the disorder.

Pyelonephritis that involves a hypoplastic or dysplastic kidney seems more likely to become chronic and progressive than the same infection that becomes lodged in a normal kidney.

Collins and others maintain, and the descriptions of the kidneys in their cases suggest, that chronic glomerulonephritis, whose pathogenesis is unclear, may be in some examples the correct pathologic diagnosis. Claireaux and Pearson disagree with Collins' conclusion, maintaining that the histologic alterations he described in the kidneys of his case, as in theirs, are compatible with chronic pyelonephritis.

Congenital syphilis can cause both an acute proliferative and chronic membranous glomerulonephropathy. The acute lesion is characterized by hematuria, proteinuria, cylinduria, and moderate azotemia. The clinical diagnosis can be suspected when other stigmata of congenital syphilis are evident and positive serologic tests are noted. Renal biopsy reveals a proliferative glomerulonephritis with interstitial infiltrates of plasma cells and lymphocytes. The lesion usually responds completely to antibiotic therapy, with complete resolution of the glomerular lesion. Other infants with congenital syphilis may present with an infantile nephrotic syndrome including massive proteinuria, edema, hypoproteinemia, and hypercholesterolemia. This also responds completely to antibiotic therapy.

An instance of nonluetic membranous glomerulonephropathy has been reported secondary to infantile systemic lupus erythematosus. The lesion was reportedly responsive to steroids.

Nephritis has also been implicated in other congenital infections, including cytomegalic inclusion disease, herpesvirus, rubella virus and toxoplasmosis. These are usually mild both clinically and morphologically. The association of cytomegalovirus and toxoplasmosis with congenital nephrotic syndrome is not clear and is considered by some to be a coincidental or incidental finding.

Chronic glomerulonephritis has been described in newborns and in some cases has had a rapidly progressive course. Glomeruli are described as sclerotic and hyalinized, with severe epithelial proliferation and crescent formation. Tubular atrophy, casts, interstitial infiltrate, fibrosis, and vascular sclerosis have also been described. The incidence of this disorder in the nursery has not been established.

Infantile Nephrotic Syndrome

The infantile nephrotic syndrome is a heterologous group of diseases that may have in common only the fact that onset occurs in the first year of life (Table 51–1). Although with current knowledge an exact classification is not entirely possible, several distinct subgroups and several recurrent associations have been noted. It is clear that infantile microcystic disease (Finnish type) is not the only morphologic type and that the outcome of infantile nephrosis need not always be progressive loss of renal function leading inevitably to uremia and death. Because of the complexity of this group of diseases, renal biopsy is virtually mandatory to diagnose the condition correctly and to provide adequate guidance for therapy and prognosis. The presentation in these children differs little from that of the nephrotic syndrome in the older child. Massive proteinuria, often detected in the first specimen voided at birth, and hypoproteinemia, hypoalbuminemia, and, eventually, anasarca are the hallmarks. Although hypercholesterolemia and hyperlipemia are also present, the serum lipids may not be as significantly elevated in the young infant as might be expected for the degree of hypoalbuminemia. The forms of infantile nephrotic syndrome have been subdivided on the basis of morphology, mode of inheritance, clinical course, and response to appropriate therapy.

Infantile Microcystic Disease. This has been the most widely recognized form of infantile nephrotic syndrome, is probably still the most common lesion noted, and has contributed most to the idea that infants with nephrotic syndrome will inevitably die of renal failure. It is a familial disease with an autosomal recessive mode of inheritance. It has been commonly reported in children of Finnish extraction but is by no means restricted to that lineage. Outside Finland, it is still the most common cause of infantile nephrosis. Prematurity with a large edematous placenta is common, as is a high incidence of toxemia during the pregnancy. The placenta may account for 40 per cent of the birth weight and be the most important early clue to the disease. Signs of fetal asphyxia are common, and many patients have a family history of

high perinatal mortality. Males and females are equally affected. The pathogenesis is unknown.

Proteinuria is present at birth in all and is usually highly selective. Anasarca develops in 50 per cent of the infants by the end of the first postnatal week and in all by 3 months of age. The protein concentration in the ascitic fluid varies but can be as high as 1 gm/dl. Microhematuria is common but not universal. Glycosuria and aminoaciduria are frequently present. Renal insufficiency is not a feature in the newborn period. Diarrhea, malnutrition, infections, and severe electrolyte disorders are the rule.

The characteristic lesion is microcystic dilatation of the proximal tubule, more so in the cortex than in the medulla; the dilated tubules have flattened epithelial cells and intact basement membranes. Microdissection studies have demonstrated the cystlike dilatations in the proximal tubule.

Confirming this diagnosis by biopsy is essential. Steroids and cytotoxic drugs are ineffective in the treatment of this lesion, and, since infection is such a problem with these children, it is probably in the child's best interest that this form of therapy not be tried. Genetic counseling of the parents is very important, since there is one chance in four that subsequent children will be affected by the same lesion.

Practically all patients fail to thrive and remain in poor general condition throughout the course of their disease. Growth is meager, bone age is severely retarded, and motor development is poor. In the experience of most physicians, death is inevitable within the first 2 years, with only 25 per cent surviving to their first birthday. The immediate cause of death is usually infection, not uremia. However, an approach by Broyer, using constant-rate, low-flow, nasogastric feedings of a high protein formula with intramuscular gamma globulin and careful treatment of each infection, has prolonged life to 1.5 to 5.8 years in four of five children and has resulted in good growth, improved general condition, and normal psychomotor development as well. Uremia eventually ensues, but at a size and age favorable to successful dialysis and transplantation. Successful renal transplantation without recurrence of the original disease has been reported in several infants.

Prenatal diagnosis as early as 15 weeks gestation

Table 51–1. Types of Infantile Nephrotic Syndrome

Primary	
Infantile microcystic disease	Congenital glomerulosclerosis
Diffuse mesangial sclerosis	Nail-patella syndrome
Idiopathic membranous glomerulonephropathy	Interstitial nephritis
Minimal lesion nephrotic syndrome	Focal glomerulosclerosis

Secondary	
Syphilis	Mercury toxicity
Toxoplasmosis	Renal vein thrombosis
Cytomegalovirus	Nephroblastoma

is possible by the detection of elevated levels of alpha-fetoprotein in both the amniotic fluid and maternal plasma. Even though other fetal and obstetric problems can cause an elevated maternal level in the third trimester, the results to date have been quite accurate. Although this has led some to recommend therapeutic abortion on the basis of the fact that the disease is universally fatal, recent improvements in survival with supportive therapy, infantile dialysis, and renal transplantation of the very young may warrant some modification of this recommendation.

Minimal Lesion Nephrotic Syndrome. This lesion is clinically and morphologically similar to the lipoid nephrosis more common in the older child. The nephrotic syndrome is not accompanied by persistent azotemia, hematuria, hypertension, or evidence of systemic disease. The renal histology by light microscopy appears entirely normal; immunofluorescence microscopy shows no evidence of antibody deposition, and only fusion of the epithelial cell foot processes is seen by electron microscopy. Recovery from this disease, either spontaneously or following treatment with steroids, is not uncommon. Although some infants progress to chronic renal insufficiency, their course is longer than with the microcystic form of the disease. Clear definition by renal biopsy is important in planning treatment. No etiology is known, and no hereditary pattern has been established.

Focal Glomerulosclerosis. The nephrotic syndrome associated with this lesion is usually accompanied by microscopic hematuria. No etiology is known, and there is no evidence of a pattern of inheritance. This is the third most common morphologic finding by biopsy of nephrotic infants. The lesion is usually steroid resistant, and there is no clear evidence that steroids with cytotoxic agents alter the course or the prognosis of this lesion. A recurrence of this lesion has been seen in older children following renal transplantation.

Diffuse Mesangial Sclerosis. In many cases, the onset of this disease occurs beyond the neonatal period, although it can present in the first week of life. The clinical course is that of a steroid-resistant nephrotic syndrome with progressive loss of renal function. Renal insufficiency may not occur until the second year of life, although the age of death has varied from 10 to 36 months. Many of the reported infants have abnormal or ambiguous genitalia with penoscrotal hypospadias. Familial involvement may be present, although not clearly in all patients; the mode of inheritance has not been established. The renal pathologic features include diffuse mesangial sclerosis involving all glomeruli, with retraction of the glomerular tuft, which is surrounded by a crescent of epithelial cells. There is also interstitial inflammation

and fibrosis. There are few reports of this lesion, and results with renal transplantation are not clear.

Congenital Glomerulosclerosis. Completely hyalinized glomeruli are an expected finding in infant kidneys but normally do not exceed 20 per cent of glomeruli. However, two infants have been reported with the nephrotic syndrome, ophthalmologic changes, and progressive renal failure leading to death before 1 month of age in whom glomerulosclerosis was extensive and involved virtually every glomerulus. One infant may have had intrauterine rubella exposure, while in the other patient congenital toxoplasmosis was diagnosed. Neither child responded to intravenous albumin or diuretic therapy.

Extramembranous Glomerulonephritis (Membranous Glomerulonephropathy). This form has been described in a few infants, most often in association with congenital syphilis. A proliferative glomerulonephritis can also be seen in congenital syphilis (see Chapter 88). In one patient, immunofluorescent microscopy showed granular deposition of IgG, IgA, IgM, and β-1-C, suggesting that the renal lesion in congenital syphilis is immunologically mediated. Other reports have shown nodular deposition of IgG and fibrin without β-1-C. Light microscopy shows thickening of the glomerular basement membrane with minimal proliferation or infiltration. The tubules and interstitium are normal. The lesions respond well to penicillin, with complete recovery. Again, morphologic diagnosis becomes important so that the use of steroids or cytotoxic drugs can be avoided.

Epimembranous glomerulonephropathy has also been seen in association with toxoplasmosis and cytomegalic inclusion disease. In others, no cause can be identified.

Interstitial Nephritis. One case, with onset at birth, has been described in which the primary renal abnormality was a chronic interstitial nephritis with widespread interstitial fibrosis. There were collections of lymphocytes in the interstitium but no plasma cells and no polymorphonuclear leukocytes, with no indication of an infectious etiology. The child had abnormal external genitalia and progressed to chronic renal failure and death at 9 months of age.

Nail-Patella Syndrome (Hereditary Onycho-Osteodysplasia). This is a rare disease that usually presents after 3 months of age, but it has been reported in the neonate. Renal disease is present in 30 to 40 per cent of patients with this syndrome. Inheritance is autosomal dominant and apparently linked to the gene locus of ABO blood groups. The clinical characteristics are malformed nails, absent or hypoplastic patella, abnormal radial head, and iliac horns. The radiographic demonstration of the iliac horns can be the presenting clue in the neonate. Proteinuria is the characteristric presentation of renal disease. Approximately 25 per cent of those with the renal lesion will eventually suffer renal insufficiency.

Other Forms of Infantile Nephrotic Syndrome.

Nephrotic syndrome has been reported in association with nephroblastoma and pseudohermaphroditism. Mercury intoxication, which may also be a cause, usually responds to withdrawal of the toxic agent. Although cytomegalovirus infection and toxoplasmosis have been described in association with the nephrotic syndrome, many believe that such findings are merely coincidental.

With such morphologic heterogeneity, the differences in response to therapy, and the need for intelligent genetic counseling, clear diagnosis becomes important. Genetic counseling is clear only in the case of infantile microcystic disease, which has an autosomal recessive mode of inheritance. Some cases of diffuse mesangial sclerosis appear to be familial. Some authors feel that even the minimal lesion form that appears in the first year of life may be familial. Habib reports that four of seven children with minimal lesion disease and a family history of nephrosis experienced onset of their disease in the first year of life.

In those instances in which renal failure is developing or will inevitably occur, preparation for dialysis must be planned prospectively. Arteriovenous fistulas for hemodialysis vascular access take as long as 4 months to mature in infants to the point of usability. If one waits until uremia is present, dialysis must be instituted either by the peritoneal route or by a femoral shunt until a fistula can be constructed.

REFERENCES

Anand, S. K., Northway, J. D., and Vernier, R. L.: Congenital nephrotic syndrome: report of a patient with cystic tubular changes who recovered. J. Pediatr. 95:265, 1979.

Aula, P., Rapola, J., Karjalainen, O., et al.: Prenatal diagnosis of congenital nephrosis in 23 high-risk families. Am. J. Dis. Child. 132:984, 1978.

Beale, M. G., Strayer, D. S., Kissane, J. M., and Robson, A. M.: Congenital glomerulosclerosis and nephrotic syndrome in two infants. Am. J. Dis. Child. 133:842, 1979.

Bouton, J. M., and Coulter, J. B. S.: The nephrotic syndrome of infancy. Acta. Paediatr. Scand. 63:769, 1974.

Braunstein, G. D., Lewis, E. J., Galvanek, E. G., Hamilton, A., and Bell, W. R.: The nephrotic syndrome associated with secondary syphilis. An immune deposit disease. Am. J. Med. 48:643, 1970.

Broyer, M. Cathelineau, L., Loirat, C., et al.: Congenital nephrotic syndrome, Finnish type: A new therapeutic approach. Proc. VII Internatl. Congr. Nephrol. 0–5, 1975.

Claireaux, A. E., and Pearson, M. G.: Chronic nephritis in a newborn infant. Arch. Dis. Child. 30:366, 1955.

Cocuzza, S., and Perfetto, V.: Su due casi di glomerulonefrite neonatale. Min. Pediatr. 20:559, 1968.

Collins, R. D.: Chronic glomerulonephritis in a newborn child. A.M.A. J. Dis. Child. 87:478, 1954.

Giles, H. M., Pugh, R. C., Darmady, E. M., Stranack, F., and Woolf, L. I.: The nephrotic syndrome in early infancy: a report of three cases. Arch. Dis. Child. 32:167, 1957.

Grupe, W. E., Cuppage, F. E., and Heymann, W.: Congenital nephrotic syndrome and interstitial nephritis. Am. J. Dis. Child. 111:482, 1966.

Habib, R., and Bois, E.: Hétérogénéité des syndromes néphrotiques à début précoce du nourrisson (syndrome néphrotique "infantile"). Helv. Paediatr. Acta 28:91, 1973.

Hallman, N., Hjelt, L., and Ahvenainen, K.: Nephrotic syndrome in newborn and young infants. Ann. Paediatr. Fenn. 2:227, 1956.

Hallman, N., and Hjelt, L.: Congenital nephrosis syndrome. J. Pediatr. 55:152, 1959.

Hallman, N., Norio, R., and Kouvalainen, K.: Main features of the congenital nephrotic syndrome. Acta Paediatr. Scand. (suppl.) 172:75, 1967.

Hallman, N., Norio, R., and Rapola, J.: Congenital nephrotic syndrome. Nephron 11:101, 1973.

Hill, L. L., Singer, D. B., Falletta, J., and Stasney, R.: The nephrotic syndrome in congenital syphilis: an immunopathy. Pediatrics 49:260, 1972.

Hoyer, J. R., Michael, A. F., Jr., Good, R. A., and Vernier, R. L.: The nephrotic syndrome of infancy: clinical morphologic and immunologic studies of four infants. Pediatrics 40:233, 1967.

Hoyer, J. R., Raig, L., Vernier, R. L., Simmons, R. L., Najarian, J. S., and Michael, A. F.: Recurrence of idiopathic nephrotic syndrome after renal transplantation. Lancet 2:343, 1972.

Hoyer, J. R., Kjellstrand, C. M., Simmons, R. L., et al.: Successful renal transplantation in 3 children with congenital nephrotic syndrome. Lancet 1:1410, 1973.

Hoyer, J. R., Mauer, S. M., Kjellstrand, C. M., Buselmeier, T. J., Simmons, R. L., Michael, A. F., Najarian, J. S., and Vernier, R. L.: Successful treatment of the congenital nephrotic syndrome by renal transplantation. Pediatr. Res. 7:292, 1973.

Hoyer, J. R., and Anderson, C. E.: Congenital nephrotic syndrome. Clin. Perinatol. 8:333, 1981.

Hoyer, J. R., Michael, A. F., and Vernier, R. L.: Renal disease in nail-patella syndrome: clinical and morphologic studies. Kidney Int. 2:231, 1972.

Huttunen, N. P.: Congenital nephrotic syndrome of Finnish type: study of 75 patients. Arch. Dis. Child. 51:344, 1976.

Huttunen, N. P., Savilahti, E., and Rapola, J.: Selectivity of proteinuria in congenital nephrotic syndrome of Finnish type. Kidney Int. 8:255, 1976.

Kaplan, B. S., Bureau, M. A., and Drummond, K. N.: The nephrotic syndrome in the first year of life: Is a pathologic classification possible? J. Pediatr. 85:255, 1975.

Kjessler, B., Johansson, S. G. D., Sherman, M., Gustavsson, K. H., and Jultquist, G.: Antenatal diagnosis of congenital nephrosis. Lancet 2:553, 1975.

Kohaut, E. C., and Hill, L. L.: Atypical nephrotic syndrome in the first year of life. J. Pediatr. 90:415, 1977.

Kunstadter, R. H., and Rosenblum, L.: Neonatal glomerulonephritis and nephrotic syndrome in a 1320 gm prematurely born infant. A.M.A. J. Dis. Child. 88:611, 1954.

McDonald, R., Wiggelinkhuizen, J., and Kaschula, R. O. C.: The nephrotic syndrome in very young infants. Am. J. Dis. Child. 122:507, 1981.

Milunsky, A., Alpert, E., Frigoletto, F. D., et al.: Prenatal diagnosis of the congenital nephrotic syndrome. Pediatrics 59:770, 1977.

Norio, R.: Heredity in the congenital nephrotic syndrome. Ann. Paediatr. Fenn. 12(suppl. 27):1, 1966.

Papaioannou, A. C., Asrow, G. G., and Schuckmell, N. H.: Nephrotic syndrome in early infancy as a manifestation of congenital syphilis. Pediatrics 27:636, 1961.

Porter, K. A., and Giles, H. M.: A pathological study of five cases of pyelonephritis in the newborn. Arch. Dis. Child. 31:303, 1956.

Simila, S., Vesa, L., and Wasz-Hockert, O.: Hereditary onycho-osteodysplasia (nail-patella syndrome) with nephrosis-like renal disease in a newborn boy. Pediatrics 46:61, 1970.

Ty, A., and Fine, B.: Membranous nephritis in infantile systemic lupus erythematosus associated with chromosomal abnormalities. Clin. Nephrol. 12:137, 1979.

Weiss, S., and Parker, F., Jr.: Pyelonephritis: its relation to vascular lesions and arterial hypertension. Medicine 18:221, 1939.

Wiggelinkhuizen, J., Nelson, M. M., Berger, G. M. B., and Kaschula, R. O. C.: Alpha-fetoprotein in the antenatal diagnosis of the congenital nephrotic syndrome. J. Pediatr. 89:452, 1976.

Worthen, H. G., Vernier, R. L., and Good, R. A.: The syndrome of infantile nephrosis. A.M.A. J. Dis. Child. 96:585, 1958.

52

Acute Renal Failure

By Warren E. Grupe

Acute renal failure implies a potentially reversible reduction in filtration function, with or without a concomitant reduction in tubular function, that produces a significant metabolic or physiologic derangement. Although oliguria is a common symptom in these infants, the volume of urine bears no relation to the degree of functional impairment. Renal function can be severely curtailed during polyuria, whereas severe oliguria is compatible with only mild changes in function. Maneuvers that improve urine flow, such as diuretics, may have no demonstrable effect on solute excretion and thus not alter renal function. Azotemia is also an unreliable indicator, since the blood level of urea can be as influenced by increased production as by defective excretion. Conversely, a noncatabolic infant with virtually no protein intake may have a normal or near normal BUN with severely compromised renal function. Therefore, changes in serum creatinine remain the most reliable indicator of the degree of altered renal functional capacity.

Acute renal failure is a clinical syndrome with multiple causes, not a diagnosis. Acute renal insufficiency is usually perceived as a rapid change in previously normal kidneys with the potential, at least, for complete reversal. Nevertheless, the diagnostic and therapeutic approach is the same for an infant with a known renal abnormality whose function becomes suddenly worse. Even though management is dictated by the degree, not the etiology, of the renal insufficiency, precise diagnosis of the commonly

present precipitating event allows correction of the causative factor(s) when possible. The newborn infant differs from the older child, having a higher prevalence of congenital and structural abnormalities, a constrained response to renal injury, a delay in compensatory renal hypertrophy until after delivery, and metabolic demands that are high in relation to body mass.

Problems that require urgent attention, regardless of etiology, are hyperkalemia, circulatory collapse, sepsis, metabolic acidosis, hypertension, severe hypervolemia, hypocalcemia, and osmolar disequilibrium. Vigorous and attentive management can thwart mortality. Nevertheless, acute renal failure is still a serious condition from which one third to one half of the infants will die and from which one third to one half of the survivors will have continued impairment of renal function.

Incidence. Few reports define the incidence of acute renal insufficiency during the neonatal period. Norman and Asadi found 72 instances of altered renal function among 314 consecutive admissions (23 per cent) to a children's hospital infant intensive care unit. Their selected population consisted of infants who were born elsewhere and transferred to the nursery for medical or surgical problems. Most of these neonates had perinatal hypoxia and shock associated with complicated labor. Of the 72 infants, 52 responded immediately to plasma volume expansion, leaving 20 (6 per cent) with apparent intrinsic renal failure.

Etiology

Hypoperfusion. Most instances of acute renal failure in the nursery occur within the first 48 hours of life in association with major perinatal complications, of which hypoxia and hypovolemia are prom-

Table 52–1. Etiologies of Neonatal Acute Renal Insufficiency

I. Inadequate perfusion	II. Renal parenchymal damage	III. Obstructive uropathy
A. Hypovolemia	A. Acquired	A. Hydronephrosis
1. Hemorrhage	1. Vascular occlusion	B. Urethral valves
2. Dehydration	2. Cortical or medullary necrosis	C. Ureterocele
a. gastrointestinal	3. Acute tubular injury	D. Genital agenesis
b. excessive insensible water loss	4. Nephrotoxins	E. Urate nephropathy
B. Hypoxia	5. Intravascular coagulation	F. Tumor
1. Respiratory distress syndrome	6. Acute pyelonephritis	
2. Pneumonia	7. Rhabdomyolysis	
3. Perinatal asphyxia	8. Hemolysis	
C. Cardiac failure	9. Congenital nephrosis	
D. Hypotension	B. Structural	
1. Sepsis	1. Agenesis, aplasia	
2. Hemorrhage	2. Dysplasia	
3. Hypothermia	3. Polycystic kidney disease	

inent. In series published since 1976, practically all reported infants have had renal insufficiency develop in concert with the respiratory distress syndrome, perinatal anoxia, pneumonia, meconium aspiration, hemorrhage (maternal or infant), sepsis, or shock. Many infants have more than one contributing factor.

The newborn kidney appears precariously susceptible to alterations in blood flow. The fetal kidney receives a smaller proportion of cardiac output than does the kidney in the more mature individual. Renal vascular resistance is normally high in the newborn period and is the major factor in the neonate's low glomerular filtration rate and renal plasma flow. Plasma renin activity is regularly high. Hypoxia is known to increase renal vascular resistance further. In studies of neonates without overt renal failure, hypoxia lowers glomerular filtration rate, renal plasma flow, and urinary acidification. Intrarenal blood flow is also diverted to juxtamedullary areas in the kidney, further depriving the superficial nephrons. Acidosis per se does not seem to be a cause.

However, hypoxia alone may not be the sole factor. Guignard and coworkers showed that the degree of renal functional change correlated with the radiologic severity of respiratory distress. However, patients with only moderate alteration of inulin or PAH clearances could have the same Pa_{O_2} as those with severe renal impairment. Intermittent positive pressure ventilation increases already high vascular resistance, lowers cardiac output, and diminishes renal plasma flow still further. Daniel and James have noticed that hypoxia with hypocapnia in the immature of some species promotes diuresis and increased free water and electrolyte excretion, whereas hypercapnia decreases renal plasma flow, urine output, and electrolyte loss. Hypoxia and hypercapnia also influence the vasopressin and the renin-angiotensin system. These mechanisms adequately explain the development of renal insufficiency in the hypoxic infant and provide ample reason to focus as much therapeutic attention toward the reversal or prevention of asphyxia as on the flow of urine or the reduction of urea. The rapid resolution of renal failure in many infants following improved ventilation not only emphasizes this therapeutic focus but also supports the functional nature of the renal abnormality in many of these infants. Congenital heart disease with hypoperfusion or congestive heart failure or following cardiac surgery is increasing as rapidly as the quality of cardiac care expands the number of survivors.

Parenchymal Injury. Many types of insults can lead to direct damage of the renal parenchyma. Acquired lesions contributing to acute parenchymal damage generally appear after the third day of life, whereas those related to perinatal hypoperfusion usually become manifest within the first 24 to 72 hours.

Vascular accidents, often accompanying indwelling arterial catheters, have recently assumed increasing significance, producing renal arterial emboli, renal venous thrombosis, renal cortical and medullary necrosis, and intravascular coagulation. Nephrotoxic

Table 52–2. Urinary Indices of Parenchymal Damage

Index	Parenchymal Failure	Hypoperfusion
U_{Na}	63.4 ± 34.7	31.4 ± 19.5
U/S_{Na}	0.45 ± 0.22	0.23 ± 0.14
U/S urea	5.8 ± 2.9	29.6 ± 17.9
U/S creatinine	9.7 ± 3.6	29.2 ± 15.6
RFI	11.6 ± 9.6	1.3 ± 0.8
FE_{Na}	4.3 ± 2.2	0.9 ± 0.6

(Modified from Mathew, O. P., et al.: Pediatrics 65:57, 1980.)

drugs, usually aminoglycoside antibiotics, are becoming more important. The effect is dose-related and generally reversible upon discontinuation of the antibiotic. Common antibiotics often implicated are gentamicin, kanamycin, cephaloridine and colistin. Large doses can induce frank tubular necrosis.

Disseminated intravascular coagulation, often secondary to sepsis or other systemic disease, is another important cause. Prematurity, maternal diabetes, and acute gastroenteritis have been reported as predisposing factors. Severe DIC can lead to renal vein thrombosis or acute cortical necrosis.

Other acquired causes of parenchymal injury include rhabdomyolysis, myoglobinuria, systemic candidiasis, acute pyelonephritis, congenital nephrosis, and hemoglobinuria.

Congenital Structural Abnormalities of the Kidneys. These anomalies, with or without obstructive uropathy, still play a major etiologic role. However, although several authors have published inclusive medical reviews since 1976, only Reimold and colleagues have reported that congenital structural abnormalities have primary importance in the nursery.

Clinical Presentation and Diagnosis. Acute renal failure usually occurs within the first week of life. In the series by Anand and coworkers, 79 per cent appeared within the first 3 days of life. In the review by Reimold and associates, 21 of their 52 children had renal failure detectable on the first day of life, 18 of whom had congenital or structural abnormalities.

In most infants, the clinical findings reflect the primary medical or surgical condition. There is no sex predilection. Most but not all infants have oliguria or anuria. Oliguria is generally defined as less than 10 to 15 ml of urine/kg/24 hours. In some series, it has been the cardinal feature of the renal failure. Oliguria, however, can be hidden and therefore may be recognized only in retrospect. In contrast, complete anuria is ominous, indicating bilateral agenesis, severe dysgenesis, urinary tract obstruction, vascular accidents, or ischemic necrosis (cortical or medullary).

Ninety-two per cent of normal infants void in the first 24 hours of life, with 98 per cent voiding by 48 hours. Delayed micturition may be mistaken for anuria or oliguria. The most common cause of delay is hypovolemia with inadequate perfusion of the kidney. Other causes have been carefully reviewed by Moore and Galvez. The low incidence of serious problems in their series when delayed micturition was the only sign indicates that a cautious and thoughtfully expectant approach may be very appropriate in this group of infants, particularly in the absence of azotemia or elevated serum creatinine. Urinary frequency may not increase normally until after the first 72 hours of life. Some have suggested urethral catheterization as the quickest way to determine whether there has been urine formation. Although the exact risk to the infant of introducing infection with catheterization has not been established, it must be considered in the decision, since ultrasonography may provide the same information and is considerably less invasive.

A delay in micturition following a period of asphyxia and associated with adequate urine formation has been attributed to asphyxiation of the bladder. These infants had distended bladders from which urine was readily expressed, normal external genitalia, and no other evidence of renal abnormality. Although the behavior of the infants was similar to that of the patients with posterior urethral valves, no anatomic abnormalities were detected, and no other cause for urine retention was defined. This again emphasizes that urine flow rate in no way reflects the degree of renal insufficiency.

Measurement of the electrolyte composition of the urine appears to be the most sensitive means of differentiating between hypoperfusion and intrinsic renal damage (Table 52–2). Measurements of urinary sodium concentration, urine/plasma sodium, urine/plasma urea, urine/plasma creatinine, renal failure index, and fractional excretion of sodium show statistically significant differences between patients with hypoperfusion and those with renal parenchymal damage. However, the overlap is broad, and the ability to diagnose differentially for any particular infant is incomplete. The best discrimination appears to result from evaluation of either the fractional excretion of sodium or the renal failure index. Any infant with a fractional excretion of sodium in excess of 2.5 to 3 per cent probably has acute renal parenchymal damage, whereas the infant whose excretion is less than 1 per cent almost always has hypoperfusion. Urinary indices suggestive of parenchymal disease are often present in obstructive uropathy, whereas the indications of hypoperfusion are common with glomerular disease. Falsely high fractional excretions of sodium can be produced, however, by a large sodium load, vigorous volume expansion, diuretics (particularly loop diuretics), and mannitol.

Urinalysis alone may not distinguish the etiology of renal insufficiency. Specific gravity is normally low, and the urine pH is often greater than 6. Hematuria is common in all forms of acute renal failure, although it may be more pronounced in vascular accidents or with cortical and medullary necrosis. Proteinuria is variable. Numerous granular casts may be present, especially with hypoperfusion injury. In fact, the presence of casts in the urine should raise concern about renal injury in the infant with respiratory distress syndrome.

Other aspects of the physical examination may provide clues to the etiology of renal failure. Potter's facies, unexplained pneumothorax, high ventilation pressures, and anuria are consistent with agenesis, aplasia, and severe bilateral dysgenesis. Irritability, pallor, emesis, poor feeding, and lethargy, although nonspecific, are suggestive of uremia, particularly when accompanied by oliguria. Enlarged kidneys connote acute tubular injury, renal vein thrombosis, polycystic kidneys, obstructive uropathy, multicystic dysplasia, or neoplasm. Seizures are usually due to hyponatremia or hypocalcemia. Ascites in the newborn may indicate obstructive uropathy or may be part of the congenital nephrotic syndrome.

Radiologic investigation is important in almost all these infants. Intravenous pyelography generally cannot distinguish the etiology of parenchymal renal damage but can be helpful in diagnosing obstructive diseases, tumors, or hydronephrosis. Its value can become limited in the face of rising urea and creatinine levels. A nonvisualized kidney may connote agenesis, aplasia, multicystic dysplasia, or vascular occlusion. Chrispin noted heavy medullary opacification as a sign of acute medullary damage. Transient intrarenal obstruction, apparently the result of tubular obstruction from precipitated Tamm-Horsfall protein, produces a persistent and prolonged nephrogram with IVP. Acute renal failure may rarely occur in this condition. A prolonged dense nephrogram may also indicate tubular injury or uric acid obstruction. The contrast medium, diatrizoate, has been reported to interfere with the laboratory measurement of creatinine by producing the false appearance of elevated levels of the substance. This must be taken into consideration in the clinical evaluation of a child with acute renal insufficiency whose creatinine has suddenly increased after intravenous pyelography. Voiding cystourethrography will rapidly outline the bladder and lower tract, define outlet obstruction, and reveal reflux. It is often an important procedure in the neonate. Ultrasonography can often define obstructive disease noninvasively. Likewise, renal vein thrombosis may be identifiable by increased and disordered central echogenicity. Polycystic kidney disease, aplasia, and multicystic dysplasia are also recognized by ultrasonography. Radionuclide techniques may define the size and position of the kidneys when other standard radiographic measures have failed. A renogram may be prolonged in tubular injury and the excretion phase prolonged in obstructive uropathy.

Infants in whom renal failure is the first sign of congenital or structural abnormality often demonstrate major congenital malformations in other organ systems. An abnormal urinary stream, a palpable bladder, a palpably enlarged kidney, or evidence of a urinary tract infection (with or without septicemia) is certainly suggestive of a structural abnormality requiring further investigation. The symptoms of lower urinary tract obstruction in infants, as reported by Tsingoglou and Dickson, were of a nonspecific nature, with failure to thrive, vomiting, and fever of unknown origin the most frequent. Acute retention or dribbling micturition were the most frequent signs related to the urinary tract. In this series, the peak incidence of urinary obstruction occurred in the first 2 weeks of life, with a rapid decline thereafter. Accrued mortality was, at 32.5 per cent, highest in infants whose first symptoms appeared before 1 month of age. It was 18 per cent in all cases in which there was a follow-up of at least 1 year. Radiologic and urologic investigations are usually necessary before a diagnosis of obstructive uropathy can be made or excluded. Posterior urethral valves are the most common cause in males, whereas an ectopic ureterocele accounts for approximately 75 per cent in girls.

Treatment

Initial Assessment and Support. The extent of renal function cannot be fully evaluated until the plasma volume is adequate. If the infant is clearly well hydrated, further attempts to increase plasma volume can be damaging. However, the presence of hypovolemia should be corrected carefully over a 1- to 3-hour period with administration of 15 to 25 ml/kg of either isotonic fluids or 5 per cent dextrose containing 75 mEq/l sodium, 50 mEq/l chloride, and 25 mEq/l bicarbonate. If urine output fails to increase yet weight does, a trial of intravenous mannitol (0.2 to 0.5 gm/kg I.V.) or a loop diuretic such as furosemide or ethacrynic acid (1 to 3 mg/kg) can be initiated. Preservation of renal blood flow and GFR is more important than merely producing adequate urine flow. In the series reported by Norman and Asadi, 52 of 72 infants with oliguria responded with an immediate and sustained increase in urine output and a fall in blood urea with proper fluid and electrolyte replacement.

A lack of a response to fluid replacement or diuretics or both is forceful evidence of intrinsic renal dysfunction, regardless of urinary biochemical values. Any further attempts to increase urine output by overhydrating the infant or increasing doses of diuretics may be disastrous for the patient. Hyponatremia with seizures is often the result of sustained and inappropriate fluid replacement. Carried to the extreme, overzealous replacement of both fluids and electrolytes may precipitate hyperosmolarity, pulmonary edema, cerebral edema, convulsions, coma, or cardiac failure. Loop diuretics have aggravated renal failure or caused deafness when administered to hypovolemic patients. Finally, the production of increased urine flow rates may give the physician a false assurance rather than improve renal function.

Fluid Maintenance. Fluid intake should equalize urine output, insensible losses, gastrointestinal losses, losses through surgical drains, endogenous water of oxydation, and preformed water. Changes in weight are still the most accurate and easily obtained indicators of the patient's overall fluid status. Urine output can be measured over a timed period and used in conjunction with accurate weights to determine the fluid requirement for the subsequent time period. Usually, insensible losses from skin, stool, and lungs approximate 20 to 25 ml/kg/day during the first 3 days of life. Premature infants may require more than double this amount. There is additional need to increase insensible losses by 15 to 20 ml/kg/day if phototherapy and radiant warmers are used. Fluid requirements are further increased by fever, hyperventilation, and hypercatabolism, and they are decreased by a humidified environment and hypothermia. These insensible losses should be replaced as electrolyte-free water. Weight should remain constant when caloric intake is adequate. However, for most infants, a loss of 0.5 to 1 per cent of body weight per day should be allowed as body solids are reduced to extracellular fluids. A stable weight in a starving infant indicates progressive overhydration.

None of the calculations commonly used to define fluid balance is a substitute for frequent and accurate weighing of the patient. In fact, accurate recording of fluid input and measured output combined with weighing of the patient at least twice daily allows more precise planning of fluid therapy than does any biochemical measurement. With the scales currently available, it is possible to weigh even the most critically ill infant.

Sodium Balance. The proper sodium balance is usually maintained with less than 1 mEq/kg/day. When fluid balance is accurately controlled, sodium requirements can be derived from changes in serum levels and urinary losses. Hypernatremia, often the result of vigorous sodium replacement, occurs in approximately 10 per cent of patients, whereas hyponatremia occurs in about 13 per cent of patients, usually representing iatrogenic overhydration. Urine sodium concentration is generally high in patients with acute parenchymal injury and does not itself reflect sodium balance. Therefore, accurate measurement of the total urinary sodium lost is more important for the calculation of daily requirements. Sodium bicarbonate may be used instead of sodium chloride for fulfillment of sodium requirements in order to correct metabolic acidosis.

Hyperkalemia. During anuria, serum potassium concentrations generally rise from 0.4 to 0.8 mEq/l/day. This rate is accelerated by hemolysis, acidosis, bleeding, tissue necrosis, infection, catabolism, or malnutrition. Administered fluids should be potassium-free until the patient's ability to avoid hyperkalemia is firmly established. If concerted efforts cannot maintain the serum potassium concentration below 6 mEq/l, potassium can be removed with enteral sodium polystyrene sulfonate, an ion exchange resin. One gm/kg of the exchange resin will decrease serum potassium levels by 1 mEq/l. It should be understood, however, that 1 mEq of sodium is absorbed for each mEq of potassium removed. Therefore, the amount of sodium retained should enter into the calculations of sodium balance. If the serum potassium concentration rises abruptly, immediate therapy includes sodium bicarbonate (2 to 3 mEq/kg I.V.), glucose and insulin (0.25 units of insulin and 0.5 gm of glucose/kg I.V.), and calcium gluconate (0.5 ml/kg I.V. of a 10 per cent calcium gluconate solution). Such treatment either shifts potassium temporarily from one fluid compartment to the other or counteracts its cardiotoxicity. Only ion resin effects a net removal of potassium from the infant.

Metabolic Acidosis. This condition can often be managed by the administration of the patient's sodium requirement as a bicarbonate source to maintain the serum bicarbonate level between 15 and 20 mEq/l. Attempts to correct completely the serum values complicate the infant's management. Since the therapy for acidosis usually involves sodium-containing agents, the amount of sodium should be included in the calculations of total sodium balance to avoid fluid overload, hypernatremia, pulmonary congestion, or cardiac failure. The need for dialysis can be indicated by the patient's inability to tolerate the therapeutic sodium load rather than by specific problems with either potassium, hydrogen ion, or urea.

Hypertension. Although renal hypertension exists occasionally in acute renal failure, the cause is usually fluid and sodium overload. Reduction of the fluid intake or the use of diuretics or both may suffice, occasionally supplemented with a partial exchange transfusion. Blood transfusion or infusion of colloid may also provoke sudden hypertension, central venous congestion, and decreased peripheral perfusion. The drugs commonly used for the treatment of hypertension are quite effective in the newborn infant (see Chapter 49). Diazoxide is extremely reliable when a rapid response is necessary.

Calcium and Phosphorus. Reduction of hyperphosphatemia must precede attempts to correct hypocalcemia so that metastatic calcifications are avoided. Also, any attempts to elevate serum calcium intravenously with calcium infusions is at best transitory while phosphorus remains high. Limiting phosphorus intake through low phosphorus formulas and preventing intestinal absorption with aluminum hydroxide (50 to 100 mg/kg/day, taken with feedings) will diminish serum phosphorus concentrations. Hypocalcemia is usually asymptomatic but may become clinically manifest as tetany or convulsions. Intravenous calcium gluconate (0.5 ml/kg of a 10 per cent solution) administered immediately and 20 to 30 mg/kg/day of oral elemental calcium supplementation will usually control these symptoms.

Nutrition. Starvation increases endogenous protein catabolism and thus results in endogenous water production, hyperkalemia, acidosis, and hyperphosphatemia. This is thwarted only by the provision of adequate calories in the form of carbohydrates and fats. Oral feedings provide more calories with less fluid than do parenteral formulas. The intake should

Table 52–3. Drugs and Renal Failure

Drug	Elimination		Half-Life (hr)		Dose Change for Renal Failure	Loss with Dialysis
	Hepatic	*Renal (%)*	*Normal*	*Anephric*		
Penicillin	Slight	75–90	1	7–20	Interval q 12 hr	Slight
Ampicillin	Slight	50–90	1	6	Dose 20 mg/kg/day	Moderate
Isoxazolyl penicillin	Moderate	40–70	0.5	1	None	Slight
Carbenicillin	Moderate	50	1	16	¼ dose q 12 hr	Moderate
Cephalothin	30%	70	0.5	15	Interval q 12–24 hr	Considerable
Cephalexin	Slight	90	1	20	Interval q 24–60 hr	Considerable
Cefamandole	—	90	0.5	9	q 12 hr	Slight
Cefazolin	—	60–90	2	40	Interval q 48 hr	Considerable
Cephradine	—	80	1.3	15	25% dose	Considerable
Chloramphenicol	Major	—	3	3–7	None	Considerable
Aminoglycosides	—	100	2–4	4–100	Follow levels	Considerable
Erythromycin	Major	<15	1–2	4–6	None	Slight
Tetracycline	Slight	45	6–12	35–75	Avoid	Slight
Aspirin	Variable	—	2–5	2–5	Avoid	Considerable
Acetaminophen	Major	—	2	2	None	Considerable
Opiates	Major	<15	3	?	None	Unknown
Digitalis	Moderate	60	36	120	25% dose; follow levels	Slight
Diazepam	Major	<20	30	?	None	Slight
Phenobarbital	Major	<10	50	120	Interval q 12 hr	Considerable
Phenytoin	Major	<15	15	8	None	Slight
Hydralazine	Major	10–50	2	8	Interval q 8–24 hr	Slight
Methyldopa	Moderate	>50	2–8	3–16	Interval q 12–24 hr	Moderate

(From Grupe, W. E., and Harmon, W. E.: Acute renal insufficiency. *In* Welch, K. J. [Ed.]: Complications of Pediatric Surgery. Philadelphia, W. B. Saunders Co., 1982.)

include 1 to 1.5 grams of protein/kg/day and a minimum of 40 to 60 cal/kg in the form of carbohydrates and fats. This should all be provided in accord with the infant's ability to manage fluid, sodium, potassium, and phosphorus. To this end, human breast milk offers several advantages to the newborn infant.

For infants with inadequate oral intake, intravenous supplementation must be provided. The solutions must be modified from the usual neonatal formulas so that fluid overload, hypercalcemia, and hyperphosphatemia are avoided. The use of essential amino acids has been advocated in adults with acute renal failure for promotion of protein synthesis and prevention of rapid rises in BUN. However, such therapy has not been sufficiently evaluated in the neonate and has been associated with hyperammonemia and metabolic acidosis in the older child.

Drug Therapy. Pharmaceuticals that are metabolized or excreted by the kidney should be administered in dosages modified in proportion to the degree of renal dysfunction. Table 52–3 provides some guidelines with data obtained from older children and adults.

Dialysis Therapy. The indications for dialysis are (1) severe hyperkalemia not correctable by ion exchange resin, (2) intractable fluid overload, especially if accompanied by pulmonary edema or hypertension, (3) uncontrollable severe acidosis, (4) uncontrollable hypernatremia or hyponatremia, and (5) signs of encephalopathy. Absolute levels of urea or creatinine are not in themselves reliable indications for dialysis. The choice between peritoneal dialysis and hemodialysis usually depends on experience with small hemodialyzers and the presence of a vascular access.

Peritoneal dialysis has been more commonly used in the neonate because it requires less highly trained personnel, needs less complex equipment, is technically easier, and demands less preparation. The technique for the neonate differs little from that described for the older child. After the urinary bladder is emptied by a catheter, a peritoneal cannula is inserted percutaneously in the midline just below the umbilicus or by direct surgical placement if the infant is severely ill with ileus, bowel distention, or coagulation defect. Warm dialysate, 20 to 40 ml/kg, is instilled then drained as rapidly and as completely as possible by gravity flow after 15 to 30 minutes. In some infants, the acetate solution is poorly metabolized, a problem that leads to an organic metabolic acidosis. Careful measurement of the fluid balance and frequent recording of weights are mandatory for accurate maintenance of fluid equilibrium. Complications are unusual with careful attention to detail.

Experience with hemodialysis in neonates is limited. Success, even in premature infants, is possible, however, when one uses umbilical vessels and small dialyzers with priming volume and filtration characteristics appropriate to the infant. Complications can include hypovolemia from excessive ultrafiltration, dysequilibrium syndrome from vigorous solute removal, bleeding from heparinization, clotting of the dialyzer from inadequate blood flow, acid-base disturbance from excessive acetate absorption, and infection of the vascular access. Most complications can be avoided, however, by meticulous care.

Outcome. Acute renal failure in the neonatal period still has a very poor prognosis. Modern therapeutic techniques have had little impact on the ultimate outcome. In most cases, acute renal failure in the neonate accompanies catastrophic underlying medical diseases or multiple congenital anomalies. Thus, almost all infants have more than one life-threatening clinical problem, with the renal insufficiency a contributing factor. When the primary disease dominates the clinical picture, the management of such infants is more effectively directed toward the primary condition, with treatment of the renal failure not the most pressing priority. In some cases, the many abnormalities are not compatible with life.

Death occurs in approximately 50 per cent of the infants. The residua of hypovolemia and shock, infection, multiple congenital anomalies, and disseminated intravascular coagulation are the most common reasons for death. Acute renal damage is the cause of death in only 9 per cent of instances. There is no discernible difference between survivors and nonsurvivors defined by initial blood pressure, Pa_{O_2}, Pa_{CO_2}, BUN, or urine flow rates. In one series, initial creatinine clearance correlated with ultimate outcome.

In those who survive the acute episode, approximately one half have chronically impaired renal function. Only 23 per cent of infants with neonatal acute renal failure recover completely. It seems unlikely, therefore, that improvements in dialysis or transplantation techniques alone will alter the outcome in any of these children. Early institution of therapy directed toward the primary clinical problem of preventing the development of renal failure appears to have more lifesaving potential.

REFERENCES

Ahmadian, Y., and Lewy, P. R.: Possible urate nephropathy of the newborn infant as a cause of transient renal insufficiency. J. Pediatr. 91:96, 1977.

Anand, S. K., Northway, J. D., and Crussi, F. G.: Acute renal failure in newborn infants. J. Pediatr. 92:985, 1978.

Aschinberg, L. C., Petros, M. Z., Hageman, J. R., and Vidyasagar, D.: Acute renal failure in the newborn. Crit. Care. Med. 5:36, 1977.

Barratt, T. M.: Renal failure in the first year of life. Br. Med. Bull. 27:115, 1971.

Barratt, T. M.: Post-operative complications of children with congenital heart disease. Bull. Assoc. Eur. Pediatr. Cardiol. 9:54, 1973.

Bashour, B. N., and Balfe, J. W.: Urinary tract anomalies in neonates with spontaneous pneumothorax and/or pneumomediastinum. Pediatrics 59 (suppl.): 1048, 1977.

Basso, A., and Marshall, V. F.: Postoperative fatalities in pediatric urology. J. Urol. *108*:177, 1972.

Bock, G. H., Campos, A., Thompson, T., Maher, S. M., and Kjellstrand, C. M.: Hemodialysis in the premature infant. Am. J. Dis. Child. *135*:178, 1981.

Boichis, H., and Winterborn, M. H.: Acute renal failure in childhood. Pediatr. Ann. *3*:58, 1974.

Chesney, R. W., Kaplan, B. S., Freedon, R. M., Haller, J. A., and Drummond, K. N.: Acute renal failure: an important complication of cardiac surgery in infants. J. Pediatr. *87*:381, 1975.

Chrispin, A. R.: Medullary necrosis in infancy. Br. Med. J. *28*:233, 1972.

Daniel, S. S., and James, L. S.: Abnormal renal function in the newborn infant. J. Pediatr. *88*:856, 1976.

Dauber, T. M., Krauss, A. N., Symchych, P. S., and Auld, P. A. M.: Renal failure following perinatal anoxia. J. Pediatr. *88*:851, 1976.

Day, R. E., and White, R. H. R.: Peritoneal dialysis in children. Arch. Dis. Child. *52*:56, 1977.

Dobrin, R. S., Larsen, C. D., and Holliday, M. A.: The critically ill child: acute renal failure. Pediatrics *48*:286, 1971.

Falco, F. G., Smith, H. M., and Arcieri, G. M.: The nephrotoxicity of aminoglycosides and gentamycin. J. Infect. Dis. *119*:406, 1969.

Fleisher, D. S.: Cation exchange resin therapy for hyperkalemia in infants and children. J. Pediatr. *58*:436, 1961.

Grupe, W. E.: The kidney. *In* Klaus, M. H., and Fanaroff, A. A. (Eds.): Care of the High-Risk Neonate. 2nd ed. Philadelphia, W. B. Saunders Co., 1979, pp. 324–340.

Guignard, J. P., Torrado, A., Mazouni, S. M., and Gautier, E.: Renal function in respiratory distress syndrome. J. Pediatr. *88*:845, 1976.

Haftel, A. J., Eichner, J., Haling, J., and Wilson, M. L.: Myoglobinuric renal failure in a newborn infant. J. Pediatr. *93*:1015, 1978.

Harmon, W. E., Spinozzi, N., Meyer, A., and Grupe, W. E.: The use of protein catabolic rate to monitor pediatric hemodialysis. Dial. Transpl. *10*:324, 1981.

Heckmatt, J. Z., Meadow, S. R., and Anderson, C. K.: Acute anuric renal failure in an infant with systemic candidiasis. Arch. Dis. Child. *54*:70, 1979.

Hodson, E. M., Kjellstrand, C. M., and Mauer, S. M.: Acute renal failure in infants and children: outcome of 53 patients requiring hemodialysis treatment. J. Pediatr. *93*:756, 1978.

Ivey, H. H.: Asphyxiated bladder as a cause of delayed micturition in the newborn. J. Urol. *120*:498, 1978.

Jain, R.: Acute renal failure in the neonate. Pediatr. Clin. North Am. *24*:605, 1977.

Kjellstrand, C. M., Mauer, S. M., Buselmeier, T. J., et al.: Haemodialysis of premature and newborn babies. Proc. Eur. Dial. Transplant Assoc. *10*:349, 1973.

Kjellstrand, C. M., Campbell, D. C., von Hartitzsch, B., et al.: Hyperuricemic acute renal failure. Arch. Intern. Med. *133*:349, 1974.

Lay, K. S., Bancalari, E., Malkus, H., Baker, R., and Strauss, J.: Acute effects of albumin infusion on blood volume and renal failure in premature infants with respiratory distress syndrome. J. Pediatr. *97*:619, 1980.

Lieberman, E.: Management of acute renal failure in infants and children. Nephron *11*:193, 1973.

Makela, P., Ahola, T., Bjorkman, H., et al.: Infant dialysis. Proc. Eur. Dial. Transplant Assoc. *9*:187, 1972.

Manley, G. L., and Gollipp, J. J.: Renal failure in the newborn: treatment with peritoneal dialysis. Am. J. Dis. Child. *115*:127, 1968.

Mathew, O. P., Jones, A. S., James, E., Bland, M., and Groshong, T.: Neonatal renal failure: usefulness of diagnostic indices. Pediatrics *65*:57, 1980.

Mofenson, H. C., and Greensher, J.: Peritoneal dialysis, an outline of the procedure. Clin. Pediatr. *11*:534, 1972.

Moore, E. S., and Galvez, M. B.: Delayed micturition in the newborn period. J. Pediatr. *80*:867, 1972.

Nash, M. A., and Russo, J. C.: Neonatal lactic acidosis and renal failure: the role of peritoneal dialysis. J. Pediatr. *91*:101, 1977.

Norman, M. E., and Asadi, F. K.: A prospective study of acute renal failure in the newborn infant. Pediatrics *63*:475, 1979.

Reimold, E. W., Don, T. D., and Worthen, H. G.: Renal failure during the first year of life. Pediatrics *59* (suppl.):987, 1977.

Segar, W. E., Gibson, R. K., and Rhamy, R.: Peritoneal dialysis in infants and small children. Pediatrics *27*:603, 1961.

Thomas, G. I.: A large-vessel applique arteriovenous shunt for hemodialysis. Trans. Am. Soc. Artif. Intern. Organs *15*:288, 1969.

Torrado, A., and Guignard, J. P.: Renal failure in respiratory distress syndrome (RDS). J. Pediatr. *85*:443, 1974.

Tsingoglou, S., and Dickson, J. A. S.: Lower urinary obstruction in infancy: review of lesions and symptoms in 165 cases. Arch. Dis. Child. *47*:215, 1972.

Wiggelinkhuizen, J., and Pokroy, M. V.: Acute renal failure in infancy and childhood. S. Afr. Med. J. *48*:2129, 1974.

PART 7 DISORDERS OF MINERAL METABOLISM AND THE ENDOCRINE SYSTEM

53

Disorders of Mineral and Bone Metabolism

By Constantine S. Anast

Endocrine Control of Calcium and Phosphate Metabolism

The normal serum total calcium concentration varies only slightly with age and ranges between 8.8 and 10.6 mg/dl, with an average of 10 mg/dl. A normal serum calcium level of 10 mg/dl consists of approximately 5.5 mg/dl of diffusible calcium and 4.5 mg/dl of protein-bound calcium. Of the diffusible fraction, approximately 4.5 mg/dl is ionized, while the remainder is complexed to anions. The physiologically important fraction of extracellular calcium, which is the concentration that is closely controlled, is the ionized calcium. The serum inorganic phosphate concentration varies with age and sex and is highest during infancy, with a gradual decline to adulthood. Approximately 10 per cent of inorganic phosphate in serum is noncovalently bound to protein, while 90 per cent circulates as ions or complexes of HPO_4^{-2} and $H_2PO_4^{-1}$. The majority of total body calcium and phosphate is in the skeleton, in which the hydroxyapatite $Ca_5(OH)(PO_4)_3$ provides mechanical support as well as a reservoir of these important minerals. The principal hormones that control calcium and phosphate metabolism are parathyroid hormone, calcitonin, and vitamin D.

Parathyroid hormone (PTH) is a single chain polypeptide consisting of 84 amino acids with a molecular weight of 9500. The hormone is synthesized in the cell as a larger molecule, proPTH, which is converted intracellularly into PTH by splitting off a hexapeptide at the aminoterminal end of the peptide chain. Following secretion, PTH is further cleaved into fragments. The aminoterminal portion (1-34) of the PTH molecule possesses full biological activity, whereas the carboxyterminus is devoid of activity. Gel-filtration studies indicate that most of the circulating immunoassayable PTH consists of a carboxyterminal fragment(s) and intact PTH with a relatively small amount of the biologically active aminoterminal fragment(s). The reason for this is that the carboxyterminal fragment(s) persists for a longer period of time in the circulation than the aminoterminal frag-

ment(s). Immunocytologic studies indicate the presence of immunoreactive PTH-containing cells in the parathyroid gland of the fetus at 10 weeks gestation (Leroyer-Alizon et al., 1981).

A fall in circulating ionized calcium level is the primary stimulus for secretion of PTH. The action of PTH at end organs is mediated through the adenylate cyclase–cyclic AMP system. PTH promotes the resorption of calcium and phosphate from bone, increases the tubular renal reabsorption of calcium, and decreases the tubular renal reabsorption of phosphate. PTH stimulates the synthesis of 1,25-dihydroxyvitamin D in the kidney, which, in turn, increases the intestinal absorption of calcium and phosphate. The net effect of the action of PTH at the end organs is an increase in circulating calcium and a decrease in circulating phosphate.

Calcitonin is produced by the parafollicular "C" cells of the thyroid gland. Immunocytologic studies indicate the presence of immunoreactive calcitonin in the C cells of the human fetal thyroid gland as early as 14 weeks gestation (Leroyer-Alizon et al., 1980). The C cell population and the concentration of immunoreactive calcitonin in the thyroid gland of newborn infants are much greater than in older subjects (Wolfe et al., 1975). Calcitonin is a single chain polypeptide consisting of 32 amino acids with an aminoterminal seven-membered disulfide ring and a carboxyterminus of prolinamide. The primary stimulus for calcitonin secretion is a rise in the circulating calcium concentration. Calcitonin lowers the serum calcium and phosphate levels primarily by inhibiting bone resorption.

Vitamin D produced in the skin or absorbed by the gastrointestinal tract is transported to the liver, where it is converted to 25-hydroxyvitamin D (25-OH-D). 25-OH-D is transported to the kidney, where it is converted to 1,25-dihydroxyvitamin D (1,25-$(OH)_2$-D) by renal tubular mitochondria. 1,25-$(OH)_2$-D is considered the most biologically active metabolite of vitamin D. The synthesis of 1,25-$(OH)_2$-D is increased by PTH and by phosphate depletion. Vitamin D, 25-OH-D, and 1,25-$(OH)_2$-D all circulate bound to an alpha globulin (D-Binding Protein, or DBP) with a molecular weight of 55,000. Protein-binding assays are available for measurement of circulating 25-OH-D and 1,25-$(OH)_2$-D. The normal circulating level of 25-OH-D is 10 to 50 ng/ml. The normal circulating concentration of 1,25-$(OH)_2$-D is approximately 1/1000 of 25-OH-D and ranges from 30 to 75 pg/ml. Circulating 25-OH-D levels are increased by sunshine exposure and by the ingestion of vitamin D and are decreased in vitamin D deficiency and in hepatocellular disorders. Circulating

1,25-$(OH)_2$-D levels are increased in hyperparathyroidism and in phosphate depletion and are reduced in hypoparathyroidism. Interestingly, circulating 1,25-$(OH)_2$-D levels may be either depressed or normal in vitamin-D–deficient states (Mawer, 1980; Chesney et al., 1981). The normal levels are in all probability secondary to increased conversion of low substrate concentrations of 25-OH-D to 1,25-$(OH)_2$-D by increased circulating PTH levels and depressed circulating inorganic phosphate levels that occur in vitamin D deficiency. 1,25-$(OH)_2$-D acts on the intestine to increase the absorption of calcium and phosphate and acts on bone to enhance the skeletal resorption of calcium and phosphate.

Perinatal Calcium Metabolism

PARATHYROID HORMONE AND CALCITONIN

During pregnancy, the maternal total serum calcium concentration declines progressively, reaching a nadir at the midthird trimester and then increases slightly over the last month or two of gestation (Pitkin and Gebhardt, 1977). In general, the serum calcium level during pregnancy parallels that of serum albumin, which declines in association with the well-known increase in extracellular fluid volume. Whether or not there is a significant change in maternal serum ionized calcium during pregnancy remains controversial. The maternal serum inorganic phosphate and magnesium levels exhibit patterns similar to that of total calcium during pregnancy. Although there is not complete agreement, most studies have demonstrated a gestational increase in maternal PTH levels, with some discrepancies in the pattern and extent of augmentation. Several reports suggest that maternal serum calcitonin increases during pregnancy. However, in one longitudinal study during pregnancy, 25 per cent of mothers exhibited relatively constant levels of calcitonin, 25 per cent a progressive decline, and 50 per cent a progressive increase to a maximum in the second trimester, followed by a decrement (Pitkin et al., 1979).

The total, ultrafilterable, ionized calcium and inorganic phosphate levels are higher in cord than in maternal plasma (Delivoria-Papadopoulis, 1967; Pitkin et al., 1979). This indicates that calcium and phosphate are transferred from mother to fetus against concentration gradients. There is no evidence that PTH and calcitonin cross the placenta. In normal newborns, the plasma calcium decreases progressively after birth so that by the second or third day of life the level is often lower than that found in older infants and children. The plasma calcium usually returns to normal by 5 to 10 days of age in normal full-term infants. The serum PTH levels tend to be low in cord blood, whereas the calcitonin levels are normal or somewhat elevated (Samaan et al., 1975; Hillman et al., 1977; Anast and Dirksen, 1978; Wieland et al., 1980). As the serum calcium normally decreases during the first 48 hours of life, the serum

PTH increases to the normal range, and the serum calcitonin increases sharply to a peak at 13 to 24 hours of age. After 36 hours of age, there is a progressive decrease in serum calcitonin, but the level remains relatively high and above normal at the end of the first week of life (Hillman et al., 1977). The high serum calcitonin in the neonatal period is consistent with the high C cell population and calcitonin concentration in the thyroid gland of the newborn infant. It is possible that the elevated levels of calcitonin in the neonatal period contribute to the early fall in serum calcium and that the serum PTH increases as an appropriate physiologic response to the fall in serum calcium.

PERINATAL VITAMIN D METABOLISM

Maternal serum 1,25-$(OH)_2$-D increases during pregnancy, whereas the serum 25-OH-D varies with the season and vitamin D intake (Hillman and Haddad, 1974; Kumar et al., 1979; Bouillon et al., 1981). The transport protein (DBP) for vitamin D and its metabolites increases in maternal serum during pregnancy and can be correlated with the rise in maternal serum 1,25-$(OH)_2$-D concentration (Haddad et al., 1976; Bouillon et al., 1981). The calculated free concentration of 1,25-$(OH)_2$-D in maternal serum remains normal up to 35 weeks of gestation but increases significantly during the last 5 weeks of pregnancy (Bouillon et al., 1981). The human placenta can synthesize 1,25-$(OH)_2$-D, but the destination(s) of this placenta-produced vitamin D metabolite is uncertain (Weissman et al., 1979; Tanaka et al., 1979; Whitsett and Tsang, 1980).

There is a close correlation between maternal and cord serum 25-OH-D levels consistent with a passive or facilitative transfer of this metabolite by the placenta. Within the normal range, infant values are 70 to 80 per cent of maternal values, at high values the infant levels are considerably lower, and at very low levels the infant values may exceed maternal values. Low levels may be found in infants born of mothers with low circulating levels of 25-OH-D resulting from poor dietary intake of vitamin D and lack of exposure to sunlight (Rosen et al., 1974; Heckmatt et al., 1979). The serum 25-OH-D concentrations remain relatively stable during the first week of life in term infants who will begin to correct low levels of this metabolite, if present. Although controversial, one study suggest that premature infants may have impaired ability to correct low levels or maintain normal serum levels of 25-OH-D (Hillman and Haddad, 1975).

The cord serum total 1,25-$(OH)_2$-D at term has variously been reported to be less than (Steichen et al., 1980; Fleischman et al., 1980), equal to (Wieland et al., 1980), and greater than (Gertner et al., 1980; Seino et al., 1980) the level in normal nonpregnant older subjects. Similarly, there is no unanimity regarding the correlation between maternal and cord serum total 1,25-$(OH)_2$-D levels, as there are some reports of a direct linear correlation and others of no correlation. The reason for these divergent results is unknown. However, all studies agree that cord serum total levels of 1,25-$(OH)_2$-D at term are lower than the elevated maternal levels. In a report of relatively low cord serum total 1,25-$(OH)_2$-D, the level increased to normal by 24 hours of age. By contrast, in a report of relatively high cord serum total 1,25-$(OH)_2$-D, the level remained constant during the first week of life. The finding of higher levels of 1,25-$(OH)_2$-D in arterial than in venous cord blood suggests that the fetus synthesizes this metabolite (Wieland et al., 1980).

The concentration of cord serum vitamin D transport protein (DBP) is lower than that of the elevated level in maternal serum as well as that of normal nonpregnant females. Although the total 1,25-$(OH)_2$-D is higher in maternal than cord serum, the calculated free 1,25-$(OH)_2$-D is higher in cord serum at term with a positive correlation in paired samples of maternal and cord blood (Bouillon et al., 1981).

Neonatal Hypocalcemia

Neonatal hypocalcemia may be divided into the following clinical categories: (1) hypocalcemia that occurs during the first 24 to 48 hours of life (early neonatal hypocalcemia), which is observed primarily in premature infants, sick infants, and infants born of abnormal labor and pregnancy; (2) hypocalcemia found at the end of the first week of life (late neonatal hypocalcemia), which frequently appears in babies who have been fed cow's milk formulas with their inherent high phosphorus load; (3) neonatal hypocalcemia associated with maternal hyperparathyroidism; (4) neonatal hypocalcemia associated with hypomagnesemia; (5) other clinical entities including primary hypoparathyroidism and renal abnormalities. This classification is chosen for convenience, recognizing that in some cases the clinical separation may not be distinct (Anast, 1975).

Authors have variously defined neonatal hypocalcemia as a plasma calcium less than 8 mg/100 ml, less than 7.5 mg/100 ml, or less than 7 mg/100 ml. The total circulating calcium concentration and the distribution between bound and ionized fractions are influenced by the protein concentration and pH of plasma. As indicated previously, approximately 45 to 50 per cent of plasma calcium is bound to protein, but it is the ionized fraction that is biologically important. In cases of hypoproteinemia, the depressed plasma calcium concentration is not accompanied by

a parallel depression in ionized calcium, which can be demonstrated if the ionized fraction is measured directly. If this is not possible, a simple "correction" for the effect of hypoproteinemia on total serum calcium is to adjust total serum calcium +1 mg/dl for each 1 gm/dl reduction of serum albumin. Acidosis results in a decrease in binding of calcium to protein resulting in a higher ionized fraction. A precise definition of hypocalcemia in premature infants is particularly difficult and will probably be best defined by the level of ionized calcium. However, there is limited information regarding ionized calcium levels in premature infants, and a distinction between hypocalcemia and normocalcemia based on ionized calcium awaits further studies.

EARLY NEONATAL HYPOCALCEMIA

Early neonatal hypocalcemia is most frequently seen in premature infants. Premature infants demonstrate an exaggeration of the fall in serum calcium seen in term infants, with a nadir occurring earlier (24 hours) and lower, and the decrease being inversely proportional to the gestation. The total serum calcium levels not uncommonly fall below 7.0 mg/dl in premature infants. However, the fall in ionized calcium is not comparable to the fall in total calcium and the ratio of ionized to total calcium is higher in these infants (Scott et al., 1979). The reason for the lesser fall in ionized calcium is uncertain but, in part, is probably related to the low serum protein concentration and the frequent acidosis found in premature infants. The sparing effect of the ionized calcium may, in part, explain the frequent lack of signs of hypocalcemia in premature infants.

The pathogenesis of early neonatal hypocalcemia in premature infants is uncertain. The finding of elevated circulating levels of parathyroid hormone in several studies is consistent with an appropriate physiologic response of the parathyroid glands to hypocalcemia in prematures (Anast and Dirksen, 1977, 1978; David et al., 1977, 1981; Hillman et al., 1977). Moreover, these studies indicate that factors other than parathyroid insufficiency act to lower the serum calcium in most premature infants.

The possibility that an abnormality in vitamin D metabolism plays a pathogenic role in the hypocalcemia of premature infants has been considered, but there is only limited information regarding this point. Studies have been performed on premature infants greater than 31 weeks gestation, and there is little or no information in infants of lower gestational age. In one study, serum 25-OH-D levels remained low in premature infants who received 400 IU of vitamin D per day orally or intravenously, suggesting impaired ability to convert vitamin D to 25-OH-D in the liver (Hillman and Haddad, 1975). However, in a more recent study, the oral administration of 2100 IU of vitamin D per day during the first 5 days of life in premature infants resulted in a significant increase in both 25-OH-D and 1,25-$(OH)_2$-D, indicating that the infants had the ability to synthesize both these metabolites (Glorieux et al., 1981). Moreover, the presence of hypocalcemia in premature infants with normal circulating 25-OH-D and 1,25-$(OH)_2$-D levels suggests that impaired vitamin D metabolism is not a pathogenic factor in early hypocalcemia of prematurity (Glorieux et al., 1981).

Available evidence indicates that hypercalcitonemia may be an etiologic factor in the hypocalcemia of prematurity (David et al., 1977, 1981; Anast and Dirksen, 1977, 1978; Salle et al., 1977; Schedewie et al., 1978). An inverse correlation between gestational age and serum calcitonin levels as well as between serum calcitonin and serum calcium levels has been reported.

The finding of reduced phosphaturic and renal cyclic AMP responses to parathyroid extract in premature infants during the first few days of life suggests that refractoriness to parathyroid hormone is a pathogenic factor (Linarelli et al., 1973). However, in contrast to the impaired renal response to parathyroid extract, a significant calcemic response to the parathyroid hormone in premature infants has been reported (Tsang et al., 1973b). The role that refractoriness to parathyroid hormone plays in the pathogenesis of neonatal hypocalcemia has not been clearly established.

Early neonatal hypocalcemia is frequently observed in asphyxiated infants. Elevated circulating calcitonin and parathyroid hormone have been reported in these infants, but there is little information concerning vitamin D metabolites (Schedewie et al., 1978). Thus, the pathogenesis of hypocalcemia in these infants remains uncertain, although hypercalcitonemia may play a role.

Early neonatal hypocalcemia is also frequent in infants of diabetic mothers. No consistent abnormality in vitamin D metabolism has been observed (Fleischman et al., 1978; Steichen et al., 1981), and serum calcitonin is not unusually increased (Schedewie et al., 1979). A tendency to higher serum phosphorus concentration and to a delay in the neonatal increase in circulating parathyroid hormone has been reported in infants of diabetic mothers (Tsang et al., 1975; Schedewie et al., 1979).

An increase in circulating phosphate leads to a reciprocal fall in calcium. An increase in phosphate release secondary to tissue hypoxia has been postulated to play a role in the hypocalcemia of asphyxiated infants. However, in general, the relative frequency and etiologic significance of hyperphosphatemia in early neonatal hypocalcemia is uncertain.

LATE NEONATAL HYPOCALCEMIA

Late neonatal hypocalcemia most often occurs in full-term infants but may occur in premature infants. Usually, the delivery has been uneventful, and there is no correlation with birth trauma or anoxia. The incidence is higher in males than in females. The signs and symptoms of hypocalcemia usually occur at the end of the first week of life, most often in infants fed cow's milk formulas but occasionally in breast-fed infants. Human milk contains 150 mg/l of phosphorus as compared to 1000 mg/l in cow's milk and 500 mg/l in infant feedings prepared from cow's milk whey or isolated soy bean protein. Although hyperphosphatemia is of uncertain significance in early neonatal hypocalcemia, it is a prominent feature of late neonatal hypocalcemia. The ingestion of a relatively high phosphate load coupled with a low glomerular filtration rate in the neonatal period leads to an increase in serum inorganic phosphate and a reciprocal decrease in serum calcium. The normal physiologic response to hypocalcemia is an increase in parathyroid secretion, which would lead to an increase in both urinary excretion of phosphate and tubular resorption of calcium. However, we and others (Fakraee et al., 1980) have observed low circulating parathyroid hormone levels in infants with late neonatal hypocalcemia, which reflect a state of functional hypoparathyroidism. An increase in serum calcium is frequently observed in these infants when they are placed on a milk feeding with a low phosphate concentration and calcium supplements. After several days to weeks, the serum parathyroid hormone level increases, and the infants are able to tolerate higher phosphate loads. The pathogenesis of this "transient hypoparathyroidism" in infants with late neonatal hypocalcemia is unknown.

Some studies suggest that the incidence of late neonatal hypocalcemia is higher in infants of mothers who have received low or marginal vitamin D intakes during pregnancy (Purvis et al., 1973; Cockburn et al., 1980). In addition, a high incidence of enamel hypoplasia of incisor teeth is reported in these infants, reflecting a defect in mineralization in the last trimester of pregnancy. However, it is not clear how the relative vitamin D deficiency would lead to impaired parathyroid secretion in the neonate. It is possible that impaired parathyroid secretion and relative maternal vitamin D deficiency are independent but additive factors in the pathogenesis of late neonatal hypocalcemia. Further studies are needed to either confirm or refute this possibility.

NEONATAL HYPOCALCEMIA ASSOCIATED WITH MATERNAL HYPERPARATHYROIDISM

Hypocalcemia is commonly observed in infants born of hyperparathyroid mothers (Hartenstein and Gardner, 1966; Anast, 1976). These infants frequently manifest symptoms of increased neuromuscular irritability during the first 3 weeks of life. The serum calcium levels range from 5.0 to 7.5 mg/dl, and the serum inorganic phosphate levels are usually

8.0 mg/dl or higher. The hypocalcemia and increased neuromuscular irritability appear to be more prominent in infants who receive cow's milk formulas with their inherent high phosphate loads. Indeed, there are reports of two infants born of hyperparathyroid mothers who exhibited symptoms of hypocalcemia for the first time at ages 5 months (Friderichsen, 1938) and 1 year (Bruce and Strong, 1955), respectively, shortly after addition of cow's milk to the infant's diet. In some instances, symptoms are severe in the infants born of hyperparathyroid mothers, and resistance to antitetany therapy may be observed. As a rule, however, there is eventual improvement with calcium therapy, which in some cases must be continued for several weeks.

It is postulated that in maternal hyperparathyroidism, the increase in serum calcium and circulating maternal parathyroid hormone facilitates calcium transport across the placenta to the fetus. As a result, fetal hypercalcemia develops and fetal parathyroid gland suppression may be even greater than in normal pregnancy, with an increase in tendency of the development of neonatal hypocalcemia. One study conducted by us on an infant born of a hyperparathyroid mother is consistent with this hypothesis (Anast and Burns, 1978). The mother had hypercalcemia and elevated circulating levels of parathyroid hormone, whereas the hypocalcemic infant had inappropriately low levels of circulating parathyroid hormone. In contrast to our findings, there is a report of elevated circulating parathyroid hormone in a hypocalcemic, hypomagnesemic infant born to a hyperparathyroid mother (Monteleone et al., 1975). It was speculated that impaired end-organ responsiveness to parathyroid hormone, secondary to hypomagnesemia, was the cause of the hypocalcemia in this infant. The reason for the hypomagnesemia observed in some infants born of hyperparathyroid mothers is uncertain but conceivably could be (1) secondary to maternal magnesium depletion, which could be a complication of hyperparathyroidism; (2) secondary to transient neonatal hypoparathyroidism; and (3) secondary to hyperphosphatemia, which may result from transient hypoparathyroidism or the high phosphate level of cow's milk formulas or both.

The mothers of affected infants are hypercalcemic and hypophosphatemic. They may be asymptomatic, or hyperparathyroidism may be indicated clinically or radiologically or both. In many recorded cases, hypocalcemic tetany occurring in the infant led to the diagnosis of hyperparathyroidism in an asymptomatic mother. Because there is an increased incidence of complications and of fetal morbidity and mortality in pregnancy complicated by primary hyperparathyroidism, it has been advocated that an exploration for parathyroid adenoma should be performed when hyperparathyroidism is diagnosed during pregnancy.

NEONATAL HYPOCALCEMIA ASSOCIATED WITH HYPOMAGNESEMIA

Hypomagnesemia may impair parathyroid function by at least two mechanisms and thereby produce hypocalcemia. The accumulated evidence indicates that hypomagnesemia impairs parathyroid hormone secretion (Anast et al., 1972, 1976; Suh et al., 1973; Rude et al., 1978) and in some instances also blunts the end-organ response to parathyroid hormone (Muldowney et al., 1970; Rude et al., 1976). Newborn infants with depressed serum magnesium levels may be divided into two groups (Salet and Fournet, 1970; Anast, 1975): (1) chronic congenital low serum magnesium or primary hypomagnesemia with secondary hypocalcemia, and (2) transient low serum magnesium. Chronic congenital hypomagnesemia with secondary hypocalcemia is a relatively rare disease that is due to an isolated defect in the intestinal transport of magnesium. The serum magnesium level is frequently less than 0.8 mg/dl (normal 1.6 to 2.8 mg/dl), and circulating levels of parathyroid hormone are low in the presence of hypocalcemia. The administration of magnesium to these patients leads to spontaneous parallel increases in serum parathyroid hormone, serum calcium, and renal phosphate clearance. Relapses occur in the absence of continuous magnesium therapy.

Transient low serum magnesium levels in the newborn period may occur in association with hypocalcemia, or, less commonly, the plasma calcium may be normal. The serum magnesium level in infants with transient hypomagnesemia is usually higher than in infants with chronic hypomagnesemia, frequently ranging from 0.8 to 1.4 mg/dl. Depressed serum magnesium levels have been observed in some infants with early as well as late neonatal hypocalcemia.

In many infants with transient hypomagnesemia, the plasma magnesium level increases spontaneously as the plasma calcium level returns to normal following the administration of calcium supplements. However, in other cases the hypocalcemia responds poorly to calcium therapy, but when magnesium salts are given, the plasma calcium as well as the plasma magnesium rises. In contrast to infants with primary hypomagnesemia, infants with transient hypomagnesemia require only a short course of magnesium therapy to avoid relapses.

The reason for the depressed serum magnesium levels in infants with transient hypomagnesemia is unknown. It is possible that extracellular magnesium may be subjected to the same physiologic or pathologic influences as calcium during the neonatal period. Thus, it has been established that depressed serum magnesium levels may result from phosphate loads and may occur in parathyroid insufficiency. Conversely, hypomagnesemia may impair parathyroid secretion. Whether or not transient neonatal hypomagnesemia contributes to the hypocalcemia by impairing parathyroid function, as has been described in infants with chronic primary hypomagnesemia, is uncertain. It is possible that this factor plays a contributory role in neonates with hypocalcemia associated with transient hypomagnesemia that is resistant to calcium therapy but responsive to magnesium therapy.

CONGENITAL HYPOPARATHYROIDISM

On a rare occasion neonatal hypocalcemia is secondary to congenital hypoparathyroidism. The hypocalcemia is associated with hyperphosphatemia and low circulating parathyroid hormone levels. The hypoparathyroidism in these infants is permanent. Congenital hypoparathyroidism may be due to the isolated absence of parathyroid glands. Most cases are sporadic, but both X-linked recessive and autosomal recessive inheritance occur. Congenital absence of the parathyroid glands may be associated with congenital absence of the thymus and a variety of congenital aortic arch or conotruncal anomalies (DiGeorge's syndrome). This syndrome occurs as a sporadic disorder in both males and females. Infants with congenital hypoparathyroidism require lifelong treatment with vitamin D preparations.

CLINICAL FINDINGS IN NEONATAL HYPOCALCEMIA

Signs and symptoms are variable and are not necessarily related to the degree of hypocalcemia. While some infants are severely affected, others may be asymptomatic with equally depressed serum calcium levels.

The major manifestation of hypocalcemia is tetany, which is hyperexcitability of the central and peripheral nervous system. Increased neuromuscular irritability and convulsions are characteristic symptoms of neonatal tetany. The factors that lead to the development of tetany are not clearly understood, and they do not appear to be a direct function of the absolute concentrations of serum calcium or magnesium or their sum or ratio.

Infants with tetany tend to be jittery and hyperactive, and they frequently exhibit muscle jerking and twitching. There may be a heightened response to sensory stimuli such as loud sounds or jarring of the bed. Laryngospasm with inspiratory stridor, at times severe enough to cause anoxia, is occasionally observed. Carpopedal spasm and ankle clonus may be present. The peroneal sign is frequently present, whereas Chvostek's sign may or may not be elicited; however, these signs may be present in newborn infants without any relation to the level of serum calcium.

Frank convulsions of a clonic type, which are not distinctive in nature, may occur either early or late in the course of the disorder. The seizures may be unilateral and at times alternate from one side to the other. They may recur at irregular intervals or persist for prolonged periods of time.

Vomiting occurs relatively frequently in neonatal tetany, and in a small number of cases there may be hematemesis or melena. At times, the gastrointestinal symptoms are severe enough to dominate the clinical picture and to suggest intestinal obstruction. It is possible that the vomiting results from spasms of the smooth muscles of the gastrointestinal tract that may be induced by hypocalcemia.

In 1929, Shannon reported the frequent finding of edema in neonatal tetany and attributed it to increased capillary permeability. Although the mechanism has not been clearly elucidated, the occurrence of edema in association with neonatal tetany has since been reported in several infants. Sixteen of 33 patients reported by Dodd and Rapoport in 1949 manifested edema, and in nine it was of a severe degree. In 1971, Chiswick reported an association between edema and hypomagnesemia in term infants with hypocalcemic tetany. The edema in these infants was attributed to the high solute load in the cow's milk formula fed to the infants. It was postulated that fluid retention led to secondary aldosteronism, which, in turn, increased the urinary excretion of magnesium and thereby contributed to the production of hypomagnesemia.

Other signs that have been described in neonatal tetany include apnea, tachycardia, tachypnea, and cyanosis. It has not been established that the nonspecific manifestations of tetany are causally related to the concentration of calcium in the serum (Silverman, 1961).

TREATMENT OF NEONATAL HYPOCALCEMIA

The treatment of neonatal hypocalcemia consists primarily of the administration of calcium salts. The commonly used compounds are calcium gluconate, calcium lactate, and calcium chloride. In evaluating these therapeutic agents, one should remember that the calcium content of calcium chloride is 30 per cent, as compared with 17 per cent in calcium lactate and 9 per cent in calcium gluconate.

For emergency treatment of acute tetany, a 10 per cent solution of calcium gluconate may be given intravenously at a rate not to exceed 1 ml per minute. The calcium solution should be administered slowly to avoid reactions such as circulatory collapse or vomiting. Careful observation of the infant is essential, and the injection should be discontinued at the first sign of bradycardia or as soon as the desired clinical result is obtained. The intravenous dose of calcium gluconate necessary to stop convulsions usually is 1 to 3 ml. Toxic reactions may be avoided if the maximum intravenous dose of calcium gluconate administered at any one time does not exceed 2.0 ml/kg; doses above 3.0 ml/kg should be administered with caution. If necessary, intravenous calcium therapy may be repeated three or four times in 24 hours to help control acute symptoms. Leakage of calcium gluconate into the tissues surrounding the vein should be avoided, since it is a tissue irritant and may cause necrosis. For this same reason, none of the calcium salts should be administered intramuscularly. Because of its acid properties, calcium chloride should not be given intravenously or by gavage.

After acute symptoms have been controlled, calcium therapy should be continued as needed to maintain the serum calcium between 8.0 and 9.0 mg/100 ml. In part, the level of serum calcium to be achieved will depend on the level of serum protein. In hypoproteinemic infants, lower levels of total serum calcium are normally present. In premature and other infants in whom the oral intake is limited, 5.0 ml/kg of 10 per cent calcium gluconate may be infused with intravenous fluids over a 24-hour period. If oral feedings are tolerated, Neo-Calglucon (calcium glubionate), which contains approximately 24 mg of Ca/ml, may be given in a dose of 2 ml/kg/day divided into four to six doses. Intravenous or oral calcium supplements may be continued until the serum calcium stabilizes above 8.0 mg/dl.

There is no unanimity regarding indications for treatment of hypocalcemic infants who are completely asymptomatic. Decisions may be particularly difficult in premature infants with early neonatal hypocalcemia who are frequently asymptomatic. Although there are no known long-term consequences of transient neonatal early hypocalcemia in prematures, this point remains uncertain. In making a decision regarding treatment of asymptomatic hypocalcemic infants, the serum protein concentration and pH should be taken into consideration, and, if possible, the ionized calcium level should be determined. Values of total serum calcium less than 7.5, 7.0, 6.5, and 6.0 mg/dl and serum ionized calcium less than 2.5 and 3.0 mg/dl are variously and arbitrarily used as indications for treatment of asymptomatic hypocalcemia in premature infants with early neonatal hypocalcemia. The method of treatment outlined in the previous paragraph can be applied to these infants.

In late neonatal tetany, dietary factors are of importance, and measures should be taken to reduce the phosphate load and to increase the Ca:P ratio of milk feedings to 4:1. This can be accomplished by the use of low phosphorus feedings such as Similac PM 60/40 or human milk in conjunction with calcium supplements. The serum calcium and phosphorus levels should be monitored weekly and the calcium supplements discontinued in a stepwise fashion after 2 to 6 weeks.

Although there are reports of the use of vitamin D metabolites in the treatment and prevention of early neonatal hypocalcemia in premature infants, this approach cannot be recommended at this time, especially in view of evidence that the prematures greater than 31 weeks gestation have the capacity to synthesize 25-OH-D and 1,25-$(OH)_2$-D. It is recommended that premature infants routinely receive 400 to 600 IU of vitamin D daily.

The administration of magnesium salts may be indicated in infants with neonatal tetany who have depressed serum magnesium levels. Magnesium may be administered intramuscularly as a 50 per cent solution of magnesium sulfate (there are 4 mEq of magnesium in 1.0 ml of 50 per cent USP $MgSO_4 \cdot 7H_2O$). The suggested intramuscular or intravenous dose of 50 per cent magnesium sulfate is 0.1 to 0.2 ml/kg. If given intravenously, the infusion should be introduced slowly and cautiously, with electrocardiographic monitoring to detect acute disturbances, which may include prolongation of atrioventricular conduction time and sinoatrial or atrioventricular block. The magnesium dose may be repeated every 12 to 24 hours, depending on clinical response and monitoring of serum magnesium levels. In many infants with transient hypomagnesemia, one or two injections of magnesium are sufficient, whereas in other infants magnesium therapy may need to be continued for 2 to 4 days. Serum magnesium levels should be carefully monitored to guard against hypermagnesemia. Infants with primary hypomagnesemia will have permanently low serum magnesium levels and require lifelong treatment with oral magnesium supplements.

Neonatal Hypercalcemia

Hypercalcemia may be defined as a total serum calcium concentration greater than 11.0 mg/dl and an ionized calcium concentration greater than 5.0 mg/dl. Neonatal hypercalcemia is found in association with a number of clinical entities and, if severe, presents as a medical emergency. The clinical findings in neonatal hypercalcemia include poor feeding, vomiting, hypotonia, lethargy, polyuria, hypertension, respiratory difficulties, and seizures. Hypercalcemia causes polyuria and polydipsia by interfering with the action of the antidiuretic hormone on the collecting ducts. Dehydration results from the excessive loss of water in the urine and poor feeding. The central nervous system manifestations result from a direct effect of calcium on nerve cells as well as from hypertensive encephalopathy and cerebral ischemia. The hypertension is probably secondary to a direct vasoconstriction effect of calcium and, possibly, to increased activity of the renin angiotensin system resulting from renal arteriolar constriction. Persistent hypercalcemia may result in metastatic calcification in the kidney, skin, subcutaneous tissue, falx cerebri, arteries, myocardium, lung, and gastric mucosa.

The first principle in the medical management of hypercalcemia is to increase the urinary excretion of calcium by maximizing glomerular filtration and the urinary excretion of sodium (for review see Neer and Potts, 1979). In the normal kidney, sodium clearance and calcium clearance are very closely linked during water or osmotic diuresis. Infants with severe neonatal hypercalcemia are frequently dehydrated. Two thirds to full strength saline containing 30 mEq of potassium chloride per liter is infused intravenously at a rate (frequently 1½ × maintenance) to correct dehydration and maximize glomerular filtration rate. In addition, Lasix in a dose of 1 mg/kg may be given intravenously at 6- to 8-hour intervals or sooner to inhibit tubular reabsorption of calcium as well as sodium and water. In situations in which severe hypercalcemia is associated with hypophosphatemia, oral or intravenous phosphorus may be given in a dose of 30 to 50 mg/kg/day of phosphorus as a phosphate salt. Unlike sodium, phosphate does not remove calcium from the body but causes a redistribution of calcium in the body. The aim of phosphate therapy is to maintain the serum inorganic phosphate concentration in a range of 3 to 5 mg/dl. The oral route for phosphate therapy is preferable, since serious immediate reactions have been reported with intravenous phosphate treatment, possibly due to the formation of intravascular calcium-phosphate aggregates. The aforementioned mode of therapy usually results in a significant reduction in serum calcium concentration over a 24- to 48-hour period. In more severe and resistant cases, cortisone 10 mg/kg up to 300 mg/day or prednisone 2 mg/kg up to 60 mg/day can be added to the therapeutic regimen. Although effective in several types of hypercalcemic states, glucocorticoids are relatively ineffective in the treatment of hypercalcemia associated with primary hyperparathyroidism. More definitive and specific therapy depends on the underlying cause of the hypercalcemia.

NEONATAL PRIMARY HYPERPARATHYROIDISM

Neonatal primary hyperparathyroidism is an uncommon but life-threatening disorder (Pratt et al., 1947; Hillman et al., 1964; Rhone et al., 1975; Speigel et al., 1977; Proesmans et al., 1977; Thompson et al., 1978; Marx et al., 1982). With few exceptions, the birth weights in the reported cases have been normal. The infants usually appear normal at birth, but there are reported observations of a depressed sternum, elfin facies, thoracic-lumbar kyphosis, and one dysmature infant with a narrow thorax and short femora. Symptoms of hypercalcemia usually develop during the early days of life. Repeated serum calcium levels usually range between 15 and 30 mg/dl, whereas serum inorganic phosphate concentration is frequently less than 3.5 mg/dl. The serum alkaline phosphatase activity may be normal or increased. In addition to these findings, unexplained anemia, splenomegaly, and hepatomegaly have been reported. Skeletal roentgenograms reveal demineralization, subperiosteal resorption, and pathologic fractures. Renal calcinosis is a common radiographic finding. The characteristic pathologic finding in the parathyroid glands is clear cell hyperplasia.

In some cases of neonatal primary hyperparathy-

roidism, there has been no evidence of familial disease, although there have been few details concerning family screening. In other cases, consanguinity in normocalcemic parents or hypercalcemia in siblings or both suggest autosomal recessive transmission. In still others, the presence of hypercalcemia in one parent as well as in one or more siblings suggests autosomal dominant transmission. Of great interest is the recent observation of an association between neonatal severe primary hyperparathyroidism and familial hypocalciuric hypercalcemia (FHH) (Marx et al., 1982). FHH is an autosomal dominant trait in which family members have modest and usually asymptomatic hypercalcemia (Marx et al., 1980, 1981). There is usually significant hypophosphatemia and a modest increase in serum magnesium concentration. In contrast to patients with primary hyperparathyroidism, patients with FHH have hypocalciuria rather than hypercalciuria. The circulating parathyroid hormone levels are either normal or modestly elevated. The pathophysiology of FHH is unknown, although functional parathyroid glands are needed for full expression. Patients with FHH usually require no specific therapy, although parathyroidectomy is occasionally required in a patient who becomes symptomatic. The reason for the occurrence of severe neonatal hyperparathyroidism in kindreds with FHH is unknown. It is apparent, however, that serum calcium determinations should be carried out on all family members of infants with neonatal primary hyperparathyroidism.

Neonatal primary hyperparathyroidism is usually, but not always, considered a surgical emergency. If untreated, most infants die between 2 and 7 months of age. Total parathyroidectomy has been advocated because of the high recurrence rate that occurs following subtotal parathyroidectomy. Infants subjected to total parathyroidectomy require lifelong treatment for hypoparathyroidism. Recent reports indicate that neonatal primary hyperparathyroidism may occasionally present in a milder form and not necessitate surgical intervention (Eftekhari and Yousefzadeh, 1982).

Recently, we treated a neonate with severe primary hyperparathyroidism with total parathyroidectomy and autotransplantation of ⅓ of one parathyroid gland to the muscle in the forearm. Both the mother and grandfather of the infant had asymptomatic hypercalcemia. Hypocalciuria (calcium clearance/creatinine clearance less than 0.0125) was present in the infant and the mother but not in the grandfather. Preoperatively, the bones of the infant were severely demineralized, the serum calcium ranged between 20 and 30 mg/dl, and the serum parathyroid hormone level was ten times greater than normal. Postoperatively, serum calcium fell to a range of 11 to 12 mg/dl, the serum parathyroid hormone level was at the upper limit to somewhat above

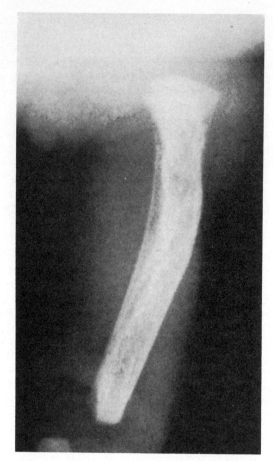

Figure 53—1. Note the bony demineralization, bowing, and subperiosteal resorption, findings quite consistent with the features of hyperparathyroidism. (From Bronsky, D., et al.: Pediatrics *42*:606, 1968.)

normal, and there was marked improvement in bone mineralization. The infant is asymptomatic and at 10 months of age is growing and developing well. Further observations are necessary to determine the long-term effects of the autotransplantation and to determine whether this mode of therapy is superior to total parathyroidectomy.

NEONATAL HYPERPARATHYROIDISM ASSOCIATED WITH MATERNAL HYPOPARATHYROIDISM

Congenital hyperparathyroidism may occur in infants born to mothers with poorly treated idiopathic or surgical hypoparathyroidism (Bronsky et al., 1968; Landing and Kamoshita, 1970; Sann et al., 1976; Anast, 1976). The birth weight of these infants is frequently less than 2500 gm. The infants usually appear normal at birth, although there is one report of a baby with deformity of the skull and chest. Roentgenograms in the neonatal period demonstrate

changes consistent with hyperparathyroidism, including generalized skeletal demineralization and subperiosteal resorption (Fig. 53–1). In the one case in which it was measured, serum parathyroid hormone was elevated (Sann et al., 1976). In contrast to infants with neonatal primary hyperparathyroidism, these infants frequently have low birth weights, serum calcium levels that are frequently depressed or normal rather than elevated, and serum inorganic phosphate levels that are normal to somewhat elevated rather than depressed. The reason for these differences in biochemical findings between the two groups is unknown. In one hyperparathyroid infant born of a hypoparathyroid mother, there was radiographic evidence of rickets as well as hyperparathyroidism, and the serum 25-OH-D level was low (Sann et al., 1976). The authors concluded that hyperparathyroidism in the infant induced a state of vitamin D deficiency, possibly by increasing the requirement for vitamin D, as has been reported in some adults with primary hyperparathyroidism (Woodhouse et al., 1971). The mortality rate in infants born of poorly or untreated hypoparathyroid mothers is high, especially in infants with birth weights less than 2000 gm. In the infants who survive, the osseous abnormalities regress spontaneously, and roentgenograms are normal by 4 to 7 months of age.

The findings in these infants demonstrate the effects of maternal parathyroid deficiency on the offspring. It is postulated that when hypocalcemia secondary to hypoparathyroidism is present in the mother, there is a decrease in calcium transport from mother to fetus. As a result, the fetus is exposed to hypocalcemia in utero, which leads to hyperplasia of the fetal parathyroid glands. The increased secretion of fetal parathyroid hormone mobilizes calcium from the fetal skeleton. Following birth, the infant skeleton avidly takes up calcium, and, over time, the parathyroid hyperplasia subsides and bone lesions heal spontaneously. Correction of hypocalcemia in hypoparathyroid women during pregnancy will prevent the development of hyperparathyroidism in the fetus.

IDIOPATHIC HYPERCALCEMIA

A large number of cases of hypercalcemia were observed in infants in Britain during and shortly after World War II (Harrison and Harrison, 1979). Radiographic findings consistent with hypervitaminosis D were found, including osteoporosis, particularly in the bones of the face and skull, and dense bands of mineralization at the metaphyseal ends of long bones. These infants were receiving 3000 to 4000 units of vitamin D per day as part of a concerted effort to prevent nutritional deficiencies in babies subjected to the disruptions of wartime. The serum inorganic phosphate concentrations were usually not reduced as in hyperparathyroidism. With the reduction of vitamin D intake to 400 units per day, the incidence of "idiopathic hypercalcemia" decreased markedly, indicating that the previously high intake of vitamin

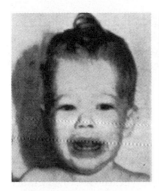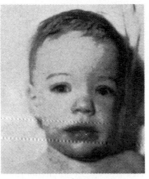

Figure 53–2. Photographs of two unrelated infants with idiopathic hypercalcemia, in order to show their striking facial similarity. The facies is described in the text. (From O'Brien, D., Peppers, T. D., and Silver, H. K.: J.A.M.A. *173*:1106, 1960. Reproduced with the kind permission of the senior author.)

D played a prominent role in the production of the infantile hypercalcemia.

Idiopathic hypercalcemia may be found in association with the Williams elfin facies syndrome (Williams et al., 1961; White et al., 1977). The phenotypic features of this syndrome include depressed nasal bone, receding mandible, prominent maxilla, hypertelorism, short turned up nose, prominent upper lip, and low-set ears (Fig. 53–2). Premature suture fusion leading to craniostenosis may be present. There may be evidence of prenatal growth deficiency, and these infants characteristically manifest failure of weight gain and growth starting in early infancy. Cardiovascular disturbances are common, including supravalvular aortic stenosis, and peripheral pulmonic arterial stenosis. Although it is sometimes difficult to ascertain the date of onset of the various phenotypic features of Williams syndrome, cardiac murmurs may be heard at birth. Many of the infants manifest a late psychomotor development. Roentgenographic studies may demonstrate osteosclerosis at the base of the skull and at the metaphyseal ends of long bones as well as evidence of nephrocalcinosis and other extraskeletal calcification. Submetaphyseal rarefaction similar to that seen in vitamin D intoxication is occasionally observed. The hypercalcemia associated with normal or increased serum inorganic phosphate levels and the radiographic findings differentiate Williams syndrome from primary hyperparathyroidism. Hypercalcemia may be present at the time of diagnosis in some infants. In others the serum calcium level is normal, but the presence of nephrocalcinosis and other soft tissue calcification suggests the previous presence of hypercalcemia. In still other infants with phenotypic features of Williams syndrome, there is neither present nor past evidence of hypercalcemia as reflected in normal serum calcium levels and the absence of soft tissue calcification (Jones and Smith, 1975).

The pathogenesis of hypercalcemia in Williams syndrome is uncertain. Excessive vitamin D intake has been considered a possible etiologic factor. However, hypercalcemia in Williams syndrome has been observed in the absence of excessive vitamin D intake in either the mother or the infant. Hypercalcemia appears to be a variable feature of Williams syndrome. It is possible that some infants with Williams syndrome have an increased sensitivity to vitamin D, which might reflect a lack of adequate control of the production of one or more of the bioactive vitamin D metabolites. Further studies are needed to either confirm or refute this possibility. One treats idiopathic hypercalcemia by feeding a low-calcium, low–vitamin-D diet and by administering glucocorticoids.

NEONATAL HYPERCALCEMIA ASSOCIATED WITH SUBCUTANEOUS FAT NECROSIS

Infantile hypercalcemia occurs in association with subcutaneous fat necrosis (Sharlin and Hollenger, 1970). In the afflicted infants, indurated subcutaneous masses with bluish-red discoloration of the overlying skin develop in the early weeks of life. The masses frequently occur at sites of pressure and contain fatty acid crystals with lymphocytes, giant cells, and histiocytes in the subcutaneous adipose tissue. The serum phosphate level and the alkaline phosphatase activity are normal. Radiographs of the long bones are usually normal, although periosteal elevation has been described in one case, and findings similar to those in Williams syndrome were reported in another. Ectopic calcification may be present. The reason for the hypercalcemia in these infants is unknown. In one study, serum parathyroid hormone levels were low, serum 25-OH-D and 1,25-$(OH)_2$-D levels were normal, and urinary prostaglandin E levels were elevated (Veldhuis et al., 1979). It is known that prostaglandins have potent bone resorptive actions and can thereby induce hypercalcemia. It is uncertain whether fat necrosis may either follow or elicit prostaglandin release. In contrast to the elevated urinary prostaglandin observed in the aforementioned study, normal plasma levels of prostaglandin E_2 and E_3 were reported in another infant with subcutaneous fat necrosis (Metz and Hassal, 1980). The hypercalcemia associated with subcutaneous fat necrosis may persist for several days or weeks and has primarily been treated with glucocorticoids and low calcium diet. If further studies confirm that prostaglandin production is a pathogenic factor in this disorder, inhibitors of prostaglandin synthetase such as aspirin or indomethacin may be effective therapeutic agents.

BLUE DIAPER SYNDROME

This is a rare familial disease in which hypercalcemia and nephrocalcinosis are associated with a defect in the intestinal transport of tryptophan (Drummond et al., 1964). Bacterial degradation of the tryptophan in the intestine leads to excessive indole production, which is converted to indican in the liver. The oxidative conjugation of two molecules of indican following elimination from the body forms the water-insoluble dye indigotin (indigo blue), which results in blue discoloration of the diaper. The clinical course is characterized by failure to thrive, recurrent unexplained fever, infections, marked irritability, and constipation. A bluish discoloration of the diaper is noted in early infancy. Nephrocalcinosis has been observed in the reported cases, and roentgenograms of the long bones have revealed increased density and transverse bands at the metaphysis. The mechanism of the hypercalcemia is uncertain, although oral tryptophan-loading in both humans and experimental animals produces an increase in serum calcium. Treatment consists of glucocorticoid administration and a low-calcium, low–vitamin-D diet.

HYPERCALCEMIA ASSOCIATED WITH ADRENAL INSUFFICIENCY

Modest hypercalcemia may occur in acute adrenal failure. The pathogenesis is uncertain, but there is evidence that the total but not the ionized calcium concentration is increased in adrenal insufficiency. It has been suggested that three alterations combine to produce the hypercalcemia in adrenal failure (Walser et al., 1963): (1) an elevated plasma protein concentration due to hemoconcentration, (2) an increase in the affinity of plasma protein for calcium due to the hyponatremia and low ionic strength of plasma, and (3) an increase in calcium complexes, especially calcium citrate and calcium phosphate. The increased serum calcium concentration does not depend on increased intestinal absorption, since it occurs in the presence of a calcium-free diet. The serum calcium returns to normal with glucocorticoid replacement.

HYPERCALCEMIA ASSOCIATED WITH PHOSPHATE DEPLETION

Hypercalcemia occurs in phosphate depletion, which, in the neonatal period, is seen most commonly in low birth weight infants who are fed human milk (Rowe et al., 1979; Sagy et al., 1980). The low phosphate concentration in human milk leads to hypophosphatemia, which, in turn, leads to an increase in circulating $1,25\text{-}(OH)_2\text{-}D$ with attendant increased intestinal absorption of calcium. In the presence of hypophosphatemia, only limited amounts of calcium can be deposited in bone, and rickets with hypercalcemia and hypercalciuria results. The treatment of this condition is discussed in the following section.

Osteopenia in Premature Infants

Osteopenia in the context of this discussion is defined as radiologic evidence of diminished bone density. Osteopenia is present in rickets, osteomalacia, and osteoporosis.

Rickets is defined as a disturbance in growing bone in which there is a lag in the mineralization of matrix so that uncalcified cartilage matrix and uncalcified bone matrix (osteoid) accumulate to an abnormal extent. Histologically, the ratio of bone mineral to bone matrix is reduced. The delay of crystallization of bone salt in rickets is secondary to a decrease in the concentrations of the essential ions, inorganic phosphate or calcium or both in the extracellular fluid phase of bone. Whether or not the vitamin D metabolites play a direct role in bone formation is uncertain. Roentgenographic findings in rickets include osteopenia (decreased bone density) and characteristic findings at the cartilage-shaft junction of growing bones, including an increase in the width of the growth plate, cupping, and fraying. In rickets, the serum inorganic phosphate or calcium or both are characteristically depressed, and the serum alkaline phosphatase level is elevated.

Osteomalacia is rickets that occurs in the presence of little or no linear skeletal growth such as might occur in some premature infants. The biochemical findings and histologic lesion of reduced ratio of mineral to matrix are the same as in rickets. Radiologically, osteomalacia is characterized by osteopenia but lacks the radiologic features of rickets at the cartilage-shaft junction.

Osteoporosis is defined as a state of reduced bone mass per unit volume with a normal ratio of mineral to matrix. Unlike rickets and osteomalacia, in which the primary abnormality is a defect in mineralization, the primary abnormality in osteoporosis is either a decrease in matrix formation or an increase in matrix and mineral resorption. Osteoporosis may not be distinguishable from osteomalacia radiographically, since both are characterized by an osteopenia without the characteristics of rickets at the cartilage-shaft junction. The two are differentiated histologically by the finding of reduced ratio of mineral to matrix in osteomalacia in contrast to a normal ratio in osteoporosis. In contrast to patients with rickets and osteomalacia, patients with osteoporosis have normal serum concentrations of calcium, inorganic phosphate, and alkaline phosphatase. In some disorders, histologic examination reveals evidence of both osteoporosis and osteomalacia.

Osteopenia with or without radiologic evidence of rickets at the cartilage shaft junction is not uncommonly observed between 3 and 12 weeks of age in premature infants, especially those with birth weights less than 1500 gm. There have been limited pathologic studies of osteopenic bones of premature infants, so that the relative contributions of osteoporosis and rickets or osteomalacia to the pathogenesis of the reduced bone density is uncertain. It is pertinent, however, that histopathologic studies in three preterm infants who died after prolonged intravenous feeding and artificial ventilation revealed pronounced osteoporosis in addition to osteomalacia (Oppenheimer and Snodgrass, 1980). It is possible, therefore, that osteoporosis, secondary to either reduced bone matrix formation or increased bone matrix destruction, is present to a lesser or greater degree in osteopenic bones of premature infants. Nevertheless, the remainder of this discussion will deal primarily with rickets and osteomalacia in the premature infant, since most studies and attention have been addressed to this defect in bone mineralization.

The clinical findings in premature infants with rickets include craniotabes, bony expansion at the wrists, costochondral beading, and fractured ribs (Geigel et al., 1978). Respiratory distress may occur secondary to demineralization and softening of the thoracic cage (Glasgow and Thomas, 1977).

The biochemical findings of rickets in premature infants are similar to those found in older children and adults with rickets and osteomalacia and include a low to low-normal serum calcium, low to low-normal serum inorganic phosphate, elevated alkaline phosphatase activity, and elevated circulating parathyroid hormone, which occurs secondary to the hypocalcemia. In premature infants, there may not be a good correlation between serum alkaline phosphatase activity and the other biochemical or radiologic findings of rickets. Generalized aminoaciduria may be present and is secondary to elevated circulating parathyroid hormone. The aforementioned biochemical abnormalities are found in infants with radiologic evidence of frank rickets and may be found in some infants with osteopenia in which there is no radiographic evidence of rickets (Hillman et al., 1979). The abnormal biochemical findings in the latter suggest a component of osteomalacia. Two factors have received primary consideration in the pathogenesis of a bone mineral defect in premature infants: (1) mineral deficiency, and (2) relative vitamin D deficiency with possible impaired metabolism of vitamin D.

Until recently, the majority of premature infants in the United States were fed commercial formulas that contained from 440 to 550 mg/l calcium, from 330 to 460 mg/l phosphorus, and 400 IU/l vitamin D. It is estimated that 80 per cent of bone mineralization in the fetus occurs during the last trimester, when fetal calcium and phosphorus requirements are 100 to 120 mg/kg/day and 60 to 75 mg/kg/day, respectively (Ziegler et al., 1976). The mineral content of the standard commercial formulas coupled with a relatively low intestinal calcium absorption rate in premature infants does not allow for in utero accretion of calcium and phosphate. As a means of circumventing this problem, milk formulas have been modified to contain approximately 1200 mg/l of calcium and 600 mg/l of phosphorus. Reported studies suggest that feeding of these high–mineral-content formulas increases the retention of calcium and phosphorus to levels that approximate in utero accretion rates and increases bone mineral content as evaluated by photon absorptiometry (Steichen et al., 1980). Moreover, rickets has been observed in low birth weight infants (BW 800 to 1200 gm) receiving standard formulas (Similac 20, Ross Laboratories, or ProSobee, Mead Johnson) and 400 to 800 infant IU, and rapid improvement was observed following the administration of high–mineral-content formulas (Ca 1260 mg/l and P 630 mg/l) and 800 to 1200 IU of vitamin D/day (Steichen et al., 1981). With one exception, there was no evidence of vitamin D deficiency in these infants as reflected in normal serum 25-OH-D levels and elevated serum 1,25-$(OH)_2$-D levels. The elevated serum 1,25-$(OH)_2$-D was thought to be secondary to elevated circulating parathyroid hormone levels. It is of interest that there was a pronounced increase in serum 25-OH-D levels (3–9-fold) following treatment with the high–mineral-content formula, during which time there was only a modest increase in vitamin D intake from a range of 400 to 800 IU/day to a range of 800 to 1200 IU/day. The reason for the dramatic increase in serum 25-OH-D and the role it played in healing the rickets in these cases is uncertain.

Biochemical and radiologic evidence of rickets has been observed in very low birth weight infants (BW 750 to 1160 gm) in whom the serum 25-OH-D levels were extremely low (Hoff et al., 1979). Serum 1,25-$(OH)_2$-D levels were not measured. The infants had received either a low-calcium "human milk–like" (Similac PM 60/40) formula or a soy protein formula. The mean daily intake of vitamin D since birth had been 300 ± 181 IU. The administration of 4000 IU of vitamin D daily without a change in formula resulted in an increase in serum 25-OH-D to normal or above and healing of the rickets. The low-circulating 25-OH-D levels in these infants suggests either reduced intestinal absorption of vitamin D or impaired conversion of vitamin D to 25-OH-D in the liver. Results of limited studies regarding this point are not in agreement with possible impaired intestinal absorption and/or hepatic 25-hydroxylation of vitamin D suggested in one study (Hillman and Haddad, 1975) but not in others (Glorieux et al., 1981; Robinson et al., 1981). Further work is needed to settle this issue more clearly. The available evidence indicates that the premature infant of postconceptual age of greater than 31 weeks can hydroxylate 25 OH-D to 1,25-$(OH)_2$-D in the kidney normally (Glorieux et al., 1981). Whether or not premature infants of younger postconceptual age have this capacity is unknown.

The preceding discussion has focused on the occurrence of rickets and osteopenia in low birth weight infants who received various commercial milk formulas. For a variety of reasons, human milk has recently been prescribed as a food source for premature infants. Because human milk has a low phosphate content, feeding it to rapidly growing premature infants has resulted in rickets associated with phosphate depletion (Rowe et al., 1979; Sagy et al., 1980). Characteristically, these infants have hypophosphatemia, hypercalcemia, hypercalciuria, normal or depressed serum parathyroid hormone levels, normal 25-OH-D levels, and elevated serum 1,25-$(OH)_2$-D levels. The hypophosphatemia is the stimulus for the production of 1,25-$(OH)_2$-D, which, in turn, increases the intestinal absorption of calcium. In the presence of hypophosphatemia, only limited amounts of calcium can be deposited in bone, and hypercalcemia and hypercalciuria result. The hypercalcemia inhibits parathyroid hormone secretion. Rickets in this disorder does not respond to vitamin D therapy but responds promptly to an increase in the ingestion of inorganic phosphate. This can be accomplished either by supplementing human milk with 20 to 25 mg/kg/day of phosphorus as potassium phosphate or by switching from human milk to a proprietary formula with a higher phosphate content. The phosphate supplements may reduce serum calcium levels to subnormal values and require the addition of calcium supplements in a dose of 30 mg/kg/day of calcium.

Human milk contains small quantities of 25-OH-D (0.3 μg/l) and 1,25-$(OH)_2$-D (5 ng/l) (Hollis et al., 1981). The total antirachitic activity is only 25 IU/l, and it is apparent that premature infants fed human milk should receive vitamin D supplements, probably at a dose of 400 to 600 IU daily.

In summary, rickets has been reported in premature infants in whom there is no evidence of vitamin D deficiency (normal serum 25-OH-D and elevated serum 1,25-$(OH)_2$-D). These infants have responded favorably to a milk formula high in mineral content (Ca 1200 mg/l and P 600 mg/l) and to an increase in vitamin D intake from a range of 400 to 800 IU/day to a range of 800 to 1200 IU/day. On the other hand, rickets has also been observed in premature infants with evidence of vitamin D deficiency (low 25-OH-D levels). Some physicians have treated these infants successfully by increasing the vitamin D intake from 300 ± 180 IU/day to 4000 IU/day while continuing a low calcium "human milk–like" formula or a soy protein formula. The possibility that there may be impaired metabolism of vitamin D in some premature infants has been raised, but there is no unanimity concerning this point. The accumulated evidence indicates that premature infants should receive at least 400 to 600 IU of vitamin D daily (Lewin et al., 1971). At least one study suggests that prophylaxis against osteopenia in premature infants may be achieved by providing a high mineral content formula in addition to 1000 IU of vitamin D per day (Steichen et al., 1980). Further observations are needed to determine the adequacy of this prophylaxis as well as to determine whether there is impaired metabolism of vitamin D in premature infants. Finally, premature infants who receive human milk are at high risk for development of rickets associated with phosphate depletion. It would seem advisable to add phosphate supplements routinely to human milk being fed to premature infants.

Copper deficiency is an unusual cause of osteopenia in premature infants. In a case reported by Tanaka and coworkers in 1980, the osteopenia was associated with flaring and cupping of the metaphyses of the long bones and irregular thickening of the provisional zones of calcification. The serum copper and ceruloplasmin concentrations were decreased. The serum alkaline phosphate activity was increased, whereas the serum calcium, phosphate, and 25-OH-D levels were normal. The administration of copper sulfate resulted in marked improvement in the radiographic appearance of the bones. The copper deficiency was attributed to the low copper concentration of the milk formula fed to the infant.

Magnesium Metabolism

Magnesium is the second most common intracellular cation, and it is required for many enzymatic reactions, particularly those that also require ATP. About 50 per cent of total body magnesium is in bone, and most of the rest is intracellular. Normal serum magnesium levels range between 1.6 and 2.8 mg per 100 ml. Roughly 35 per cent of total magnesium is bound to serum protein. Fetal magnesium levels are higher than maternal levels because of active transport across the placenta. However, in experimental magnesium deficiency in rats, the fetus becomes relatively more deficient than the mother (Dancis et al., 1971). Following birth, there is a rise in serum magnesium levels, except in infants receiving cow's milk formulas with an inherent high phosphate load (Anast, 1964; David and Anast, 1974).

HYPOMAGNESEMIA

This condition is discussed in a preceding section entitled "Neonatal Hypocalcemia Associated with Hypomagnesemia."

HYPERMAGNESEMIA

Magnesium sulfate continues to be used in the management of eclampsia. Magnesium given to the mother readily crosses the placenta and causes elevation of fetal magnesium levels and depression of the newborn infant. In 1967, Lipsitz and English studied 16 infants born to toxemic mothers who had received 16 to 60 gm of magnesium by continuous intravenous infusion for from 12 to 24 hours prior to delivery. The mothers' blood levels of magnesium ranged from 3.6 to 17 mg/dl, and the babies' levels were between 4.9 and 14.0 mg/dl. A majority of the babies were cyanotic, flaccid, and unresponsive. Others had less severe signs, including delayed passage of meconium. Nine infants required tracheal intubation and respiratory support. The medication may or may not have played a part in the deaths of three of the 10 premature infants. There was no absolute correlation between cord blood levels and depth of depression, but symptoms disappeared within 24 to 48 hours pari passu with the steady fall in magnesium levels. Exchange transfusion has been advocated as a means of lowering magnesium more rapidly, and infusion of calcium salts has been used to antagonize some of the adverse effects of excess magnesium (Lipsitz, 1971).

In 1973, Outerbridge and colleagues reported the tragic case of a full-term newborn who was treated with an enema of 100 ml of 50 per cent magnesium sulfate solution for presumed hyaline membrane disease. Ninety minutes later respiratory arrest occurred, and the serum magnesium was 5.6 mg/dl. In spite of calcium and exchange transfusion, the baby died at 46 hours of age.

There seems no room for doubt that magnesium enemas should no longer be used for the treatment of respiratory distress, and that it is dangerous for the obstetrician to continue the intravenous infusion of magnesium salts into toxemic mothers for more than 24 hours. Intramuscular injections and infusion for shorter periods may not be hazardous (Lipsitz, 1971).

REFERENCES

Anast, C. S.: Serum magnesium levels in the newborn. Pediatrics 33:969, 1964.
Anast, C. S.: Tetany of the newborn. In Gardner, L. I. (Ed.): Endocrine and Genetic Diseases of Childhood and Adolescence. W. B. Saunders Co., Philadelphia, 1975, pp. 377–399.
Anast, C. S.: Parathyroid hormone during pregnancy and effect on offspring. In New, M. I., and Fiser, R. H. (Eds.): Diabetes and Other Endocrine Disorders during Pregnancy in the Newborn. New York, Alan R. Liss, Inc., 1976, pp. 235–248.
Anast, C. S., and Burns, T. W.: Impaired neonatal parathyroid function and maternal hyperparathyroidism. Pediatr. Res. 12:276, 1978.
Anast, C., and Dirksen, H.: Neonatal hypocalcemia. In Norman, A. W., Schaefer, K., Coburn, J. W., DeLuca, H. F., Fraser, D., Grigoleit, H. G., and Herrath, D. B. (Eds.): Vitamin D Biochemical, Chemical and Clinical Aspects Related to Calcium Metabolism. New York, Walter De Gruyter and Co., 1977, p. 727.
Anast, C. S., and Dirksen, H.: Studies related to the pathogenesis of neonatal hypocalcemia. In Copp, D. H., and Talmadge, R. V. (Eds.): Endocrinology of Calcium Metabolism. Amsterdam, Excerpta Medica Foundation 421:12, 1978.
Anast, C. S., Mohs, J. M., Kaplan, S. L., and Burns, T. W.: Evidence for parathyroid failure in magnesium deficiency. Science 177:606, 1972.
Bouillon, R., Van Assche, F. A., Van Baelen, H., Heyns, W., and De Moor, P.: Influence of the vitamin D–binding protein on the serum concentration of 1,25-dihydroxyvitamin D_3: significance of the free 1,25-dihydroxyvitamin D_3 concentration. J. Clin. Invest. 67:589, 1981.
Bronsky, D., Kiamko, R. T., Moncada, R., and Rosenthal, I. M.: Intrauterine hyperparathyroidism secondary to maternal hypoparathyroidism. Pediatrics 42:606, 1968.
Brown, J. K., Cockburn, F., and Forfar, J. O.: Clinical and chemical correlates in convulsions of the newborn. Lancet 1:135, 1972.
Bruce, J., and Strong, J. A.: Maternal hyperparathyroidism and parathyroid deficiency in child, with account of effect of para-

thyroidectomy on renal function and of attempt to transplant part of tumor. Q. J. Med. 24:307, 1955.
Chesney, R. W., Zimmerman, J., Hamstra, A., De Luca, H. F., and Mazess, R. B.: Vitamin D metabolite concentrations in vitamin D deficiency. Am. J. Dis. Child. 135:1025, 1981.
Chiswick, M. L.: Association of oedema and hypomagnesaemia with hypocalcaemic tetany of the newborn. Br. Med. J. 3:15, 1971.
Cockburn, F., Belton, N. R., Purvis, R. J., Giles, M. M., Brown, J. K., Turner, T. L., Wilkinson, E. M., Forfar, J. O., Barrie, W. J. M., McKay, F. S., and Pocock, S. J.: Maternal vitamin D intake and mineral metabolism in mothers and their newborn infants. Br. Med. J. 288:11, 1980.
Dancis, J., Springer, D., and Cohlan, S. Q.: Fetal homeostasis in maternal malnutrition. II. Magnesium deprivation. Pediatr. Res. 5:131, 1971.
David, L., and Anast, C.: Calcium metabolism in newborn infants: the interrelationship of parathyroid function and calcium, magnesium, and phosphorus metabolism in normal, "sick," and hypocalcemic newborns. J. Clin. Invest. 54:287, 1974.
David, L., Salle, B., Chopard, P., and Grafmeyer, D.: Studies on circulating immunoreactive calcitonin in low birth weight infants during the first 48 hours of life. Helv. Paediatr. Acta 32:39, 1977.
David, L., Salle, B. L., Putet, G., and Grafmeyer, D.: Serum immunoreactive calcitonin in low birth weight infants. Description of early changes; effect of intravenous calcium infusion; relationships with early changes in serum calcium, phosphorus, magnesium, parathyroid hormone, and gastrin levels. Pediatr. Res. 15:803, 1981.
Delivoria-Papadopoulis, M., Battaglia, F. C., Bruns, P. D., and Meschia, G.: Total, protein-bound, and ultrafilterable calcium in maternal and fetal plasma. Am. J. Physiol. 213:363, 1967.
Dodd, K., and Rapoport, S.: Hypocalcemia in neonatal period. Am. J. Dis. Child. 78:537, 1949.
Drummond, K. N., Michael, A. F., Ulstrom, R. A., and Good, R. A.: The blue diaper syndrome: familial hypercalcemia with nephrocalcinosis and indicanuria. Am. J. Med. 37:928, 1964.
Eftekhari, F., and Yousefzadeh, D. K.: Primary infantile hyperparathyroidism: clinical, laboratory, and radiographic features in 21 cases. Skeletal Radiol. 8:201, 1982.
Fakraee, S., Bell, M., and Hillman, L. S.: Hypomagnesemia and parathyroid hormone (PTH) deficiency in classical late neonatal hypocalcemia (CLNH) and surgically related late neonatal hypocalcemia (SLNH). Pediatr. Res. 14:571, 1980.
Fleischman, A. R., Rosen, J. F., Cole, J., Smith, C. M., and DeLuca, H. F.: Maternal and fetal serum 1,25-dihydroxyvitamin D levels at term. J. Pediatr. 97:640, 1980.
Fleischman, A. R., Rosen, J. F., and Nathenson, G.: 25-hydroxyvitamin D: serum levels and oral administration of calcifediol in neonates. Arch. Intern. Med. 138:869, 1978.
Friderichsen, C.: Hypocalcemie bei einem Brustkind und Hypercalcemie bei der Mutter. Mschr. Kinderheilk. 75:146, 1938.
Geggel, R. L., Pereira, G. R., and Spackman, T. J.: Fractured ribs: unusual presentation of rickets in premature infants. J. Pediatr. 93:680, 1978.
Gertner, J. M., Glassman, M. S., Coustan, D. R., and Goodman, D. B. P.: Fetomaternal vitamin D relationships at term. J. Pediatr. 97:637, 1980.
Glasgow, J. F. T., and Thomas, P. S.: Rachitic respiratory distress in small preterm infants. Arch. Dis. Child. 52:268, 1977.
Glorieux, F. H., Salle, B. L., Delvin, E. E., and David, L.: Vitamin D metabolism in preterm infants: serum calcitriol values during the first five days of life. J. Pediatr. 99:640, 1981.
Haddad, J. G., Hillman, L., and Rojanasathit, S.: Human serum binding capacity and affinity for 25-hydroxyergocalciferol and 25-hydroxycholecalciferol. J. Clin. Endocrinol. Metab. 43:86, 1976.
Harrison, H. E., and Harrison, H. C.: Hypercalcemic states. In Harrison, H. E., and Harrison, H. C. (Eds.): Disorders of Calcium and Phosphate Metabolism in Childhood and Adolescence. Philadelphia, W. B. Saunders Company, 1979.

Hartenstein, H., and Gardner, L. I.: Tetany of the newborn associated with maternal parathyroid adenoma: report of the seventh affected family. N. Engl. J. Med. 274:266, 1966.

Hillman, D. A., Scriver, C. R., Pedvis, S., and Shragovitch, I.: Neonatal familial primary hyperparathyroidism. N. Engl. J. Med. 270:483, 1964.

Hillman, L. S., and Haddad J. G.: Human perinatal vitamin D metabolism. I: hydroxyvitamin D in maternal and cord blood. J. Pediatr. 84:742, 1974.

Hillman, L. S., and Haddad, J. G.: Perinatal vitamin D metabolism. II: Serial concentrations in sera of term and premature infant. J. Pediatr. 86:928, 1975.

Hillman, L., Hoff, N., Martin, L., and Haddad, J.: Osteopenia, hypocalcemia, and low 25-hydroxyvitamin D (25-OHD) serum concentrations with use of soy formula. Pediatr. Res. 13:400, 1979.

Hillman, L., Rojanasathit, S., Slatopolsky, E., and Haddad, J.: Serial measurements of serum calcium, magnesium, parathyroid hormone, calcitonin, and 25-hydroxyvitamin D in premature and term infants during the first week of life. Pediatr. Res. 11:739, 1977.

Hoff, N., Haddad, J., Teitelbaum, S., McAlister, W., and Hillman, L: Serum concentrations of 25-hydroxyvitamin D in rickets of extremely premature infants. J. Pediatr. 94:460, 1979.

Hollis, B. W., Roos, B. A., Draper, H. H., and Lambert, P. W.: Vitamin D and its metabolites in human and bovine milk. J. Nutr. 111:1240, 1981.

Landing, B. H., and Kamoshita, S.: Congenital hyperparathyroidism secondary to maternal hypoparathyroidism. J. Pediatr. 77:842, 1970.

Leroyer-Alizon, E., David, L., Anast, C. S., and Dubois, P. M.: Immunocytological evidence for parathyroid hormone in human parathyroid glands. J. Clin. Endocrinol. Metab. 52:513, 1981.

Leroyer-Alizon, E., David, L., and Dubois, P. M.: Evidence for calcitonin in the thyroid gland of normal and anencephalic human fetuses: immunocytological localization, radioimmunoassay, and gel filtration of thyroid extracts. J. Clin. Endocrinol. Metab. 50:316, 1980.

Lewin, P., Reid, M., Reilly, B. J., Swyer, P., and Fraser, D.: Iatrogenic rickets in low-birthweight infants. J. Pediatr. 78:207, 1971.

Linarelli, L. G., Bobik, C., and Bobik, J.: Urinary cAMP and renal responsiveness to parathormone in premature hypocalcemic infants. Pediatr. Res. 7:329, 1973.

Lipsitz, P. J.: The clinical and biochemical effects of excess magnesium in the newborn. Pediatrics 47:501, 1971.

Lipsitz, P. J., and English, J. C.: Hypermagnesemia in the newborn infant. Pediatrics 40:856, 1967.

Marx, S. J., Attie, M. F., Levine, M. A., Spiegel, A. M., Downs, R. W., Jr., and Lasker, R. D.: The hypocalciuric or benign variant of familial hypercalcemia: clinical and biochemical features in fifteen kindreds. Medicine 60:397, 1981.

Marx, S. J., Attie, M. F., Spiegel, A. M., Levine, M. A. Lasker, R. D., and Fox, M.: An association between severe primary hyperparathyroidism and familial hypocalciuric hypercalcemia in three kindreds. N. Engl. J. Med. 306:257, 1982.

Marx, S. J., Spiegel, A. M., Brown, E. M., et al.: Familial hypocalciuric hypercalcemia. In DeLuca, H. F., and Anast, C. S. (Eds.): Pediatric Diseases Related to Calcium. New York, Elsevier North-Holland, 1980, pp. 413–431.

Mawer, B. E.: Clinical implications of measurements of circulating vitamin D metabolites. Clin. Endocrinol. Metab. 9:63, 1980.

Metz, S. A., and Hassal, E.: PGE, hypercalcemia and subcutaneous fat necrosis. J. Pediatr. 97:336, 1980.

Monteleone, J. A., Lee, J. B., Tashjian, A. H., Jr., and Cantor, H. E.: Transient neonatal hypocalcemia, hypomagnesemia, and high serum parathyroid hormone with maternal hyperparathyroidism. Ann. Intern. Med. 82:670, 1975.

Muldowney, F. P., McKenna, T. J., Kyle, L. H., Fresney, R., and Suan, M.: Parathormone-like effect of magnesium replenishment in β-steatorrhea. N. Engl. J. Med. 282:61, 1970.

Oppenheimer, S. J., and Snodgrass, G. J. A. I.: Neonatal rickets. Arch. Dis. Child. 55:945, 1980.

Outerbridge, E. W., Papageorgiu, A., and Stern, L.: Magnesium sulfate enema in a newborn, J.A.M.A. 224:1392, 1973.

Paunier, L., Lacourt, G., Pilloud, P., Schlaeppi, P., and Sizonenko, P.: 25-hydroxyvitamin D and calcium levels in maternal, cord and infant serum in relation to maternal vitamin D intake. Helv. Paediatr. Acta 33:95, 1978.

Pitkin, R. M., and Gebhardt, M. P.: Serum calcium concentrations in human pregnancy. Am. J. Obstet. Gynecol. 127:775, 1977.

Pitkin, R. M., Reynolds, W. A., Williams, G. A., and Hargis, G. K.: Calcium metabolism in pregnancy: a longitudinal study. Am. J. Obstet. Gynecol. 133:781, 1979.

Pratt, E. L., Geren, B. B., and Neuhauser, E. B. D.: Hypercalcemia and idiopathic hyperplasia of the parathyroid glands in an infant. J. Pediatr. 30:388, 1947.

Purvis, R., MacKay, G., Cockburn, F., Barrie, W., Wilkinson, E., Belton, N., and Forfar, J.: Enamel hypoplasia of the teeth associated with neonatal tetany: a manifestation of maternal vitamin D deficiency. Lancet 2:811, 1973.

Robinson, M. J., Merrett, A. L., Tetlow, V. A., and Compston, J. E.: Plasma 25-hydroxyvitamin D concentrations in preterm infants receiving oral vitamin D supplements. Arch. Dis. Child. 56:144, 1981.

Rosen, J. F., Roginsky, M., Nathenson, G., and Finberg, L.: 25-hydroxyvitamin D: Plasma levels in mothers and their premature infants with neonatal hypocalcemia. Am. J. Dis. Child. 127:220, 1974.

Rowe, J. C., Wood, D. H., Rowe, D. W., and Raisz, L. G.: Nutritional hypophosphatemic rickets in a premature infant fed breast milk. N. Engl. J. Med. 300:293, 1979.

Rude, R. K., Oldham, S. B., and Singer, F. R.: Functional hypoparathyroidism and parathyroid hormone end-organ resistance in human magnesium deficiency. Clin. Endocrinol. 5:209, 1976.

Saan, L., David, L., Thomas, A., Frederich, A., Chapuy, M. D., and Francois, R.: Congenital hyperparathyroidism and vitamin D deficiency secondary to maternal hypoparathyroidism. Acta Paediatr. Scand. 65:381, 1976.

Sagy, M., Birenbaum, E., Balin, A., Orda, S., Barzilay, Z., and Brish, M.: Phosphate depletion syndrome in a premature infant fed human milk. J. Pediatr. 96:683, 1980.

Salet, J., and Fournet, J. P.: Les hypomagnésémies néo-natales. Ann. Pediatr. 17:837, 1970.

Salle, B. L., David, L., Chopard, J. P., Grafmeyer, D. C., and Renaud, H.: Prevention of early neonatal hypocalcemia in low birth weight infants with continuous calcium infusion: effect on serum calcium, phosphorus, magnesium, and circulating immunoreactive parathyroid hormone and calcitonin. Pediatr. Res. 11:1180, 1977.

Schauberger, C. W., and Pitkin, R. M.: Maternal-perinatal calcium relationships. Obstet. Gynecol. 53:74, 1979.

Schedewie, H., Fisher, D., Odell, W., Deftos, L. J., Elders, M. J., Cantor, T. L., and Dodge, M.: Etiology of first day hypocalcemia (FDH) role of PTH and calcitonin? Pediatr. Res. 12:512, 1978.

Schedewie, H. K., Odell, W. D., Fisher, D. A., Drutzik, S. R., Dodge, M., Cousins, L., and Fiser, W. P.: Parathormone and perinatal calcium homeostasis. Pediatr. Res. 13:1, 1979.

Scott, S. M., Ladenson, J. H., Aguanno, J. J., and Hillman, L. S.: Ionized calcium in the sick neonate. Pediatr. Res. 13:505, 1979.

Seino, Y., Shimotsuji, T., Yamaoka, K., Ishida, M., Ishu, T., Matsuda, S., Ikehara, C., Yabuuchi, H., and Ookoh, S.: Plasma 1,25-dihydroxyvitamin D concentrations in cords, newborns, infants and children. Calcif. Tissue Int. 30:1, 1980.

Shannon, W. B.: Generalized edema in association with tetany in the newborn. Arch. Pediatr. 46:5, 1929.

Sharlin, D. N., and Koblenzer, P.: Necrosis of subcutaneous fat with hypercalcemia. A puzzling and multifaceted disease. Clin. Pediatr. 9:290, 1970.

Steichen, J. J., Gratton, T. L., and Tsang, R. C.: Osteopenia of prematurity: the cause and possible treatment. J. Pediatr. 96:528, 1980.

Steichen, J., Tsang, R., Gratton, T., Hamstra, A., and DeLuca, H.: Vitamin D homeostasis in the perinatal period. N. Engl. J. Med. 302:315, 1980.

Steichen, J. J., Tsang, R. C., Greer, F. R., Ho, M., and Hug, G.:

Elevated serum 1,25-dihydroxyvitamin D concentrations in rickets of very low birth weight infants. J. Pediatr. *99*:293, 1981.

Steichen, J. J., Tsang, R. C., Ho, M., Knowles, H., Lavin, J., and Miodovnik, M.: 1,25(OH)$_2$ vitamin D (1,25(OH)$_2$D) and incidence of hypocalcemia in infants of diabetic mothers (IDM) in relation to prospective randomized treatment during pregnancy. Pediatr. Res. *15*:683, 1981.

Tanaka, Y., Hatano, S., Nishi, Y., and Usui, T.: Nutritional copper deficiency in a Japanese infant on formula. J. Pediatr. *96*:255, 1980.

Thompson, N. W., Carpenter, L. C., Kessler, D. L., and Nishiyama, R. H.: Hereditary neonatal hyperparathyroidism. Arch. Surg. *113*:100, 1978.

Tsang, R., Chen, I. W., Friedman, M., and Chen, I.: Neonatal parathyroid function: role of gestational age and postnatal age. J. Pediatr. *83*:728, 1973a.

Tsang, R. C., Chen, I. W., Friedman, M. A., Gigger, M., Steichen, J., Koffler, H., Fenton, L., Brown, D., Pramanik, A., Keenan, W., Strub, R., and Joyce, T.: Parathyroid function in infants of diabetic mothers. J. Pediatr. *86*:399, 1975.

Tsang, R. C., Light, I. J., Sutherland, J. M., and Kleinman, L. I.: Possible pathogenetic factors in neonatal hypocalcemia of prematurity. J. Pediatr. *82*:423, 1973b.

Veldhuis, J. D., Kulin, H. E., Demers, C. M., and Lambert, P. W.: Infantile hypercalcemia with subcutaneous fat necrosis: endocrine studies. J. Pediatr. *95*:460, 1979.

Walser, M., Robinson, B. H. B., and Duckett, J. W., Jr.: The hypercalcemia of adrenal insufficiency. J. Clin. Invest. *42*:456, 1963.

Weissman, Y., Harrell, A., Edelstein, S., David, M., Spirer, Z., and Golander, A.: 25-dihydroxy vitamin D$_3$ and 24,25-dihydroxy vitamin D$_3$ in vitro synthesis by human decidua and placenta. Nature *281*:317, 1979.

White, R. A., Preus, M., Watters, G. V., and Fraser, F. C.: Familial occurrence of the Williams syndrome. J. Pediatr. *91*:614, 1977.

Wieland, P., Fischer, J., Trechsel, U., Roth, H. R., Vetter, K., Schneider, H., and Huch, A.: Perinatal parathyroid hormone, vitamin D metabolites, and calcitonin in man. Am. J. Physiol. *239*:E385, 1980.

Williams, J. C. P., Barratt-Boyes, B. G., and Lowe, J. B.: Supravalvular aortic stenosis. Circulation *24*:1311, 1961.

Wolfe, H., DeLellis, R., Voelkel, E., and Tashjian, A.: Distribution of calcitonin-containing cells in the normal neonatal human thyroid gland: a correlation of morphology with peptide content. J. Clin. Endocrinol. Metab. *41*:1076, 1975.

Ziegler, E. E., O'Donnell, A. M., Nelson, S. E., and Forman, S. J.: Body composition of the reference fetus. Growth *40*:329, 1976.

54

General Considerations

The mammalian adrenal gland is a dual endocrine organ, consisting of cortex and medulla within a common capsule. The two glands have distinct embryologic origins and different functions. In the fifth week of fetal life, the primitive adrenal cortex is formed from cells of the coelomic mesoderm. A thin layer of more compact cells gradually surrounds the fetal cortex. This structure will eventually constitute the permanent, or definitive, adrenal cortex. During the seventh week, the cortex is invaded by ectodermal neural crest cells that aggregate to form a central cell mass, the adrenal medulla.

Adrenal cortical cells produce a variety of steroid hormones, and the medulla produces the catecholamines norepinephrine and epinephrine. As a consequence of its special anatomic relationship to the adrenal cortex, the medulla is exposed to very high steroid levels in venous blood draining the cortex. Wurtman and Axelrod have shown that the enzymatic conversion of norepinephrine to epinephrine is enhanced by a high local concentration of cortisol. In all other respects, the adrenal cortex and medulla appear to function independently. Adrenal catecholamine deficiency in the neonatal period may contribute to hypoglycemia. The consequences of cat-

Disorders of the Adrenal Glands and Sodium Metabolism

Revised by Constantine S. Anast*

echolamine excess are discussed in the section on neuroblastoma. This chapter will focus on development and function of the adrenal cortex.

Adrenal steroid production can be detected by the ninth week of gestation, and by the twelfth week the adrenal glands are fully as large as the kidneys. The primitive, or fetal, zone of the adrenal cortex accounts for most of its bulk. This zone involutes slowly during the third trimester and more rapidly after birth. There is no intrinsic difference between male and female adrenal function in utero, and the adrenal does not contribute to normal genital differentiation. The fetal adrenal cortex is relatively deficient in 3β-hydroxysteroid dehydrogenase, an enzyme required for the

* This chapter includes some contributions from previous authors, Drs. John S. Parks and Alexander Schaffer.

synthesis of C-21 glucocorticoids and mineralocorticoids. The primary role of the fetal adrenal appears to be production of inactive metabolites such as dehydroepiandrosterone sulfate, which the placenta can convert to estrogens. These estrogens may in turn help maintain the pregnancy. Monitoring of maternal urinary estriol excretion has been used to provide insight into fetal and placental well-being in high risk pregnancies.

During the second half of pregnancy, the permanent adrenal cortex emerges as a distinct anatomic structure and begins to synthesize the glucocorticoids and mineralocorticoids that will be required for successful adaptation to extrauterine life (Fig. 54–1). Glucocorticoids, of which cortisol is the most important in man, play a major role in carbohydrate metabolism. They promote gluconeogenesis and synthesis of liver glycogen and act to elevate blood glucose levels. Levels of glucocorticoids in amniotic fluid show a marked increase between the thirty-sixth and fortieth weeks of pregnancy. Cortisol has enzyme-inducing capabilities that doubtless affect many organs and thus prepare the infant for postnatal life. This aspect of glucocorticoid action has been most completely delineated in the discussion of fetal lung maturation (see Chapter 11).

Available evidence suggests that HCG is adreno-corticotropic in the fetus during the first half of pregnancy, when the maternal plasma concentration of HCG is high and appreciable amounts are delivered to the fetus (Kaplan and Grumbach, 1976). HCG stimulates steroidogenesis in the fetal adrenal and produces ultrastructural changes similar to those induced by ACTH (Johannisson, 1968). Moreover, normal adrenal development is observed in the ACTH-deficient anencephalic fetus until midgestation, and thereafter the adrenals become atrophic. In the second half of pregnancy, the growth and secretory activity of the adrenal depend on ACTH.

The ACTH concentration is relatively high in fetal-neonatal and maternal plasma (Winters, 1974; Similia et al., 1977). Winters and coworkers reported mean afternoon ACTH values of 43 ± 4 pg/ml in normal adults, values of 194 ± 29 in maternal plasma during labor, 241 ± 33 pg/ml in cord blood prior to 34 weeks gestation, $143 \pm 7\mu$/ml in cord blood at term, and $120 \pm 8\mu$g/ml during the first week of life. Although the ACTH values during the first 3 to 5 days of life are higher than those of prepubertal children, the values are equivalent to those of prepubertal children by 1 week of age. Measurement of fetal and neonatal plasma ACTH reflects secretion of this hormone by the fetal pituitary, since ACTH does not cross the placenta. The ACTH levels of infants born to diabetic mothers are not significantly different from those of normal infants, despite the presence of hypoglycemia in the former (Cacciari et al., 1975).

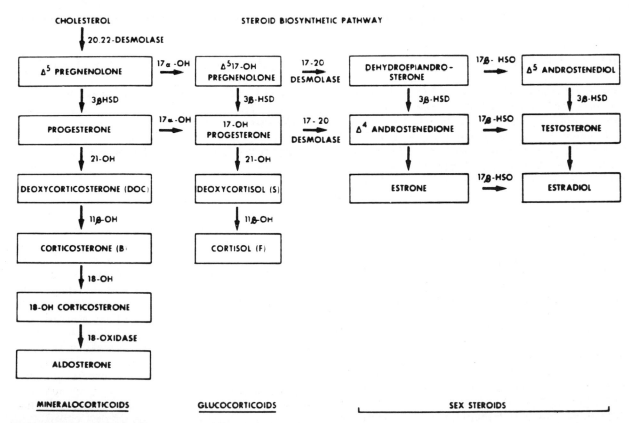

Figure 54–1. Steroid biosynthetic pathway. OH = hydroxylase; 3β-HSD = 3β-hydroxysteroid dehydrogenase Δ^5 isomerase, and 17-β-HSO = 17-β-hydroxysteroid oxidoreductase. (Adapted from Grumbach and Conte, 1981.)

There is limited information regarding plasma cortisol concentrations during fetal life. In 1973, Beitins and coworkers reported a mean value of 2.1 ± 1.2 µg/dl in fetuses of 3 to 6 months gestation as compared with a mean value of 6.3 ± 2.9 µg/dl in the cord blood of infants born at term by cesarean section. Although the fetal plasma cortisol concentration may increase between midpregnancy and term, there is not the abrupt increase in late pregnancy that has been observed in some nonprimate animals (Simmer et al., 1974; Ohrlander et al., 1976). Cortisol crosses the placenta, but approximately 80 per cent of maternal cortisol is converted to cortisone when it traverses the placenta (Murphy et al., 1974; Murphy, 1975, 1977; Campbell and Murphy, 1977). Cord arterial levels are higher than cord venous levels, indicating that a significant amount of circulating cord cortisol is of fetal origin. It has been estimated that near term, 50 to 75 per cent of fetal plasma cortisol is derived from the fetal adrenal, and 25 to 50 per cent originates from maternal cortisol that traverses the placenta (Beitins et al., 1973). The concentrations of corticosteroid binding globulin (CBG), total cortisol, and unbound cortisol are lower in fetal than in maternal plasma (Simmer et al., 1974; Ohrlander et al., 1976).

Although fetal plasma cortisol rises in association with a stress-induced increase in maternal plasma cortisol during labor (Ohrlander et al., 1976), there is no evidence to indicate that fetal plasma ACTH or cortisol is altered in response to fetal stress. Fetal ACTH is similar after labor and vaginal delivery and after elective cesarean section (Winters et al., 1974). Maternal ACTH and cortisol increase during labor, and the increase in fetal plasma cortisol that occurs during this period is thought to be of maternal origin (Kauppila et al., 1974; Ohrlander et al., 1976; Tuimala et al., 1976). There is no evidence to support the concept that the human fetal adrenal cortex plays the role in the initiation of labor that it seems to have in the case of several other mammalian species.

The plasma cortisol concentrations fall after birth, reaching a nadir at 24 to 36 hours of age, and then rapidly increase to levels that are equal to or greater than later in infancy (Sperling, 1980). Perinatal stress results in a rise in plasma cortisol levels. The response to exogenous ACTH is normal immediately after birth, but there is a smaller response in the initial days of life corresponding to the period of low plasma cortisol levels. After 5 days of life, there is a pronounced increase in serum cortisol in response to exogenous ACTH (Gutai et al., 1972; Sperling, 1980). The age at which the circadian rhythm of ACTH and cortisol secretion become established is not known. The adult pattern of high morning and low nocturnal plasma 17-hydroxycorticosteroids does not appear to be present before 1 to 3 years of age (Franks, 1967). However, a decrease in urinary free cortisol during daytime sleep and increases before and after the sleep have been reported in 1-year-old infants (Tennes and Vernadakis, 1977).

Cortisol production is regulated by a hypothalamic-pituitary-adrenal homeostatic system. The hypothalamus produces a peptide corticotropin releasing factor that provokes release of ACTH from the pituitary. This system is activated by low circulating cortisol levels and by stressful stimuli. ACTH stimulates adrenal steroid production. High cortisol levels directly inhibit the secretion of ACTH by the pituitary as well as corticotropin releasing factor by the hypothalamus, thus closing a negative feedback loop. The fetal plasma ACTH declines during the last trimester of pregnancy (Winters et al., 1974), which may reflect an increasing sensitivity of the pituitary hypothalamic axis to circulating cortisol.

Mineralocorticoids differ from glucocorticoids in structure, activity, site of synthesis, and regulation. Aldosterone is the most important natural mineralocorticoid in man. In contrast to cortisol, aldosterone lacks a 17-hydroxyl group and contains an aldehyde group at carbon 19. It acts to promote conservation of sodium and loss of potassium by renal tubules and sweat glands. Aldosterone deficiency results in hyponatremia and hyperkalemia. The hormone is produced by the zona glomerulosa, the outermost zone of the permanent adrenal cortex.

ACTH contributes relatively little to the regulation of aldosterone synthesis. The main homeostatic mechanism involves release of renin from renal juxtaglomerular cells in response to diminished renal arteriolar pressure. Renin acts to increase angiotensin II, which, in turn, increases aldosterone secretion and has a direct effect on vascular contractility. Increased pressure and volume act to diminish renin production, thus closing the feedback loop. Low sodium intake and high potassium intake also enhance aldosterone secretion, the latter by a mechanism that does not depend on the renin-angiotensin system.

The newborn is able to regulate aldosterone secretion in an appropriate manner. Kowarski and colleagues found that aldosterone levels in umbilical and newborn venous plasma were comparable to adult values. The levels rose to values above the adult range between 11 days and 1 year of age.

The fetus does not depend on endogenous glucocorticoid or mineralocorticoid production. Its needs can be met by transplacental passage of maternal hormones, and deficiencies, per se, are not evident at delivery. However, the catastrophic consequences of defective organogenesis or of enzymatic errors soon become apparent. Glucocorticoid deficiency can result in hypoglycemia within hours of birth, and mineralocorticoid deficiency manifests as salt loss and adrenal crisis within days or weeks.

Adrenal Hemorrhage

The large adrenal glands of the newborn infant are vulnerable to mechanical trauma during labor and delivery. Focal hemorrhage at the junction of the fetal zone and the permanent cortex is a common finding in infants dying of other causes (Boyd, 1967). Minor bleeding into the adrenal cortex may not produce symptoms but is often responsible for adrenal calcifications noted incidentally later in life. Massive adrenal hemorrhage is an uncommon but lifethreatening event. Predisposing factors include high birth weight, prolonged or difficult labor, placental bleeding, and perinatal anoxia. Adrenal hemorrhage may occur in premature infants without obvious trauma. The adrenal may be the site of hemorrhage in infants with sepsis or with primary coagulopathies. In most published series, male infants outnumber females by three to one.

The affected infant shows signs of hypovolemic shock within the first few days of life. Pallor, apnea, hypothermia, listlessness and failure to suck are accompanied by a falling hematocrit and jaundice. A large flank mass may be palpated, more commonly on the right side, and may require differentiation from a neuroblastoma. In 5 to 10 per cent of cases the hemorrhage is bilateral. The condition must be differentiated from renal vein thrombosis. In both conditions, there may be azotemia, proteinuria, and hematuria, but in adrenal hemorrhage the hematuria is of a lesser degree. Intravenous pyelograms reveal no function on the affected side when a renal vein or artery has been thrombosed. As shown in Figure 54–2, adrenal hemorrhage typically displaces the kidney downward and rotates it laterally, with flattening of the upper calyces.

Signs of adrenal insufficiency may be subtle and delayed. Hypoglycemia is a more common finding than is salt loss. Even with massive bilateral hemorrhage, functioning islands of zona glomerulosa cells are generally preserved. Destruction of greater than 90 per cent of the adrenal cortex is required to produce adrenal insufficiency.

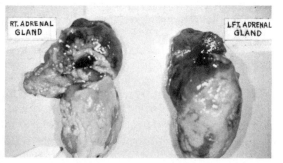

Figure 54–2. Kidneys and adrenal glands, with an enlarged hemorrhagic adrenal capping each kidney. The kidneys were also the sites of hemorrhagic necrosis, plus left-sided renal vein thrombosis.

This was an 11 pound 7 ounce boy born after excessive manipulation and traction and 22½ hours of labor. Asphyxia neonatorum was followed by facial twitchings, fever, and hematuria, and then convulsions. On the fourth day, a large mass was palpable in the left flank.

Immediate management is directed at blood and volume replacement. Indications for steroid replacement include bilateral hemorrhage, failure to respond to volume expansion, hypoglycemia, polyuria, hyponatremia, hyperkalemia, or an anticipated need from general anesthesia.

Within 1 to 3 weeks after the hemorrhage, a thin zone of calcification appears at the periphery of the gland. As blood and necrotic adrenal tissue are resorbed, the area of calcification shrinks and assumes the shape and size of the original gland. Such calcification may persist for life. Adrenal function generally improves with resolution of the hemorrhage. ACTH stimulation with measurement of plasma or urinary corticoid responses is indicated after the acute phase of the illness. Late adrenal insufficiency has been reported, and one of Black and Williams' eight patients developed renal vascular hypertension.

Transient Adrenal Insufficiency

In 1946, Jaudon described a series of 14 infants with dehydration, salt loss, and failure to gain weight. All responded to steroid replacement, and in each case it was eventually possible to discontinue treatment without a recurrence of symptoms. Others have reported additional infants with an apparent delay in maturation of adrenal cortical function. Bongiovanni described a premature infant with marked hyponatremia and hyperkalemia and no detectable serum cortisol or urinary corticoids. The infant did well on cortisol replacement, and, at age 6 months, following discontinuation of steroid treatment, he showed normal cortisol and aldosterone responses to ACTH. He has not developed adrenal calcifications. Kreines and De Vaux described a similar course in an infant born to a mother with Cushing's syndrome due to an adrenal adenoma.

Rarely, transient adrenal insufficiency is observed in a neonate whose mother received glucocorticoids during pregnancy (Yackel et al., 1966). The type of glucocorticoid administered to the mother may be important in this regard. Substantial amounts of cortisol and prednisolone are converted to cortisone and prednisone, respectively, during their traversal across the placenta as well as in the fetal circulation by both the placenta and other fetal tissues. Thus, when the mother is treated with cortisol or prednisolone, the fetal plasma concentration of these active steroids is only a small fraction of that in the mother. However, following administration of dexamethasone to the mother, the concentrations in fetal and maternal plasma are similar (Osathanondh et al., 1977).

The combination of hyponatremia, hyperkalemia, and polyuria may occur in acutely ill infants under a variety of other circumstances that do not involve adrenal insufficiency. Infants recovering from hypovolemic shock and acute tubular necrosis demonstrate these features, as do infants treated with furosemide without replacement of sodium. In doubtful cases, one may collect serum and urine specimens during a therapeutic trial of desoxycorticosterone acetate. This agent, given intramuscularly in a dosage of 0.5 mg per kg per day, provides a potent mineralocorticoid effect and does not inhibit pituitary ACTH or interfere with serum cortisol or urinary corticoid estimation. If steroid measurements do not support a diagnosis of adrenal insufficiency, and if serum sodium does not rise and serum potassium decline in response to desoxycorticosterone acetate, then the medication may safely be discontinued.

Adrenal Hypoplasia

In the absence of pituitary gland function, the adrenal glands fail to develop normally. The adrenal glands of anencephalic infants weigh less than 0.5 gm at birth, as opposed to normal combined weights greater than 6 gm. Arrested development of the adrenals has been attributed to a lack of trophic stimulation by ACTH. Interestingly, the adrenal glands of anencephalic fetuses at midgestation are histologically normal, suggesting the involvement of nonpituitary factors such as HCG in early adrenal morphogenesis.

Pituitary hypoplasia can also occur in infants without major central nervous system malformations. In these infants, severe hypoglycemia can result in death within the first 48 hours of life. Blizzard and Alberts described a male infant who had, in addition, microphallus and cryptorchidism. The association has been noted in several other cases and probably reflects a lack of trophic hormone stimulation of both adrenal and testis. Prompt glucocorticoid replacement is required.

Adrenal hypoplasia occurs as well in infants with anatomically and functionally intact pituitary glands (Roselli and Barbosa, 1965; Sperling et al., 1973; Pakravan et al., 1974). Isolated and familial forms, with either X-linked or autosomal recessive transmission, have been described. In the autosomal recessive form, the adrenal histology is similar to that observed in neonates with pituitary insufficiency in that the fetal zone is primarily affected, while the cortex is well differentiated but small. In contrast, the adrenal cortex in the X-linked form is disorganized and contains large cells resembling those of the fetal cortex.

Early recognition, cortisol replacement, and prolonged survival have permitted studies of the mechanisms that underlie familial adrenal hypoplasia. The disease is manifested in infancy or early childhood by hyperpigmentation as a consequence of elevated ACTH levels and by hypoglycemia as a consequence of glucocorticoid deficiency. In contrast to congenital adrenal hyperplasia, familial adrenal hypoplasia has no associated excess of abnormal steroid metabolites. Mineralocorticoid production is generally unimpaired. Migeon and colleagues provided evidence that the disorder may result from an end-organ unresponsiveness to ACTH. A possible defect might involve the adrenal membrane receptor for this polypeptide hormone. The family reported by Moshang and coworkers had features that suggested an inherited degenerative disease of the zona fasciculata and zona reticularis. Five of seven siblings were affected by the disease. Of these, two developed glucocorticoid deficiency some months after testing had shown normal adrenal function. Aldosterone excretion was normal in the basal state and rose after ACTH, indicating a normal response of the zona glomerulosa to the trophic hormone.

Congenital Adrenal Hyperplasia

Adrenal steroid biosynthesis requires a sequence of enzymatic reactions that are illustrated in Figure 54–1. Genetically determined deficiency in the activity of any of the required enzymes results in a serious disease. The disease states in this category have several features in common. Each condition is inherited in an autosomal recessive manner. Thus, multiple sibling involvement is common, and recurrence risk in subsequent pregnancies is 25 per cent. Each, with the exception of 18-hydroxysteroid dehydrogenase deficiency, involves hyperplasia of the adrenal cortex under the stimulus of elevated ACTH levels. Combined adrenal weights of 30 gm are not uncommon. In each case, the disorder may be managed quite well with appropriate steroid replacement.

Clinical manifestations of adrenal hyperplasia depend on the site and severity of the enzymatic block. With a block, precursors accumulate and are diverted into alternative metabolic pathways. Laboratory confirmation of a suspected defect involves measurement of these metabolites. The metabolites may have major physiologic effects, particularly on the differentiation of the external genitalia. For example, defects in both 21-hydroxylase and 11-hydroxylase lead to overproduction of androgens that produce virilization of female external genitalia. In other instances, the enzymatic defect impairs testicular testosterone synthesis and leads to undervirilization of the male fetus. Deficiencies of both 17α-hydroxylase and of 20,22 desmolase have such an effect. The 3β-hydroxysteroid dehydrogenase defect demonstrates both features of congenital adrenal hyperplasia in that females tend to be virilized and males tend to be undervirilized at birth. The defects listed in Table 54–1 will be discussed individually.

Deficiency of 21-Hydroxylase

The 21-hydroxylase deficiency is the most common form of congenital adrenal hyperplasia as well as the most common cause of ambiguous genitalia in general. The incidence of 21-hydroxylase deficiency is estimated to be between 1 in 4000 to 1 in

15,000 in Caucasians in the United States and Europe. However, the gene frequency varies in different ethnic groups, and an unusually high prevalence of the disorder (1 in 490) has been reported in the Yupik Eskimos of Alaska (Hirschfeld and Fleshman, 1969). The gene that codes for 21-hydroxylation is located on the short arm of chromosome 6 in proximity to the locus of the histocompatibility gene HLA-B (Levine et al., 1978; New et al., 1981). Knowledge of this genetic linkage has led to the use of HLA typing in families with affected individuals for detection of heterozygotes and cryptic homozygotes as well as for the prenatal diagnosis of affected fetuses (Levine et al., 1980; Pollack et al., 1981; New et al., 1981).

Hydroxylation at the C-21 position is required for synthesis of glucocorticoids and mineralocorticoids, but this enzymatic reaction is not involved in the synthesis of androgens or estrogens. Hydroxylation at the C-21 position has been demonstrated in both the zona fasciculata and zona glomerulosa of the adrenal cortex. Recent studies have been presented in support of the concept that the zona fasciculata and the zona glomerulosa function as two separate glands under separate regulation and, possibly, under different genetic control (Kuhnle et al., 1981). According to this concept, ACTH stimulates steroidogenesis in the zona fasciculata, the site of cortisol synthesis, while renin-angiotensin stimulates steroidogenesis in the zona glomerulosa, the site of aldosterone synthesis.

There are two basic clinical syndromes of congenital adrenal hyperplasia due to a 21-hydroxylation defect: simple virilization and virilization with salt wasting. In both forms, defective cortisol synthesis leads to increased secretion of ACTH, which, in turn, stimulates the adrenal to produce increased amounts of cortisol precursors, including androgens and androgen precursors, proximal to the block in the biosynthetic pathway. The plasma concentrations of 17-hydroxyprogesterone, androstenedione, and testosterone are elevated in affected patients, and the metabolites of these steroids result in increased urinary excretion of 17-ketosteroids and pregnanetriol. As a result of high circulating fetal androgen levels, female neonates demonstrate varying degrees of virilization, ranging from mild clitoral enlargement to severe clitoral enlargement with complete labial fusion and a phallic urethra. Affected males are formed normally at birth. If untreated, both females and males show progressive virilization during infancy and early childhood with rapid linear growth and skeletal and somatic maturation. In addition to virilization, some infants show signs of salt wasting and aldosterone deficiency with failure to thrive, hyponatremia, hyperkalemia, and, ultimately, vascular collapse. Salt-losing crisis is uncommon before 6 days of age but occurs in about 50 per cent of affected infants between 6 and 14 days of age. Patients with virilization and salt wasting are aldosterone-deficient, as reflected by reduced circulating aldosterone levels and increased plasma renin activity. By contrast, patients with simple virilization have normal or elevated serum aldosterone levels and plasma renin activity in the baseline state that increase further in response to sodium restriction. The reason for the increased circulating aldosterone in patients with simple virilization is uncertain, but it has been postulated that the increased secretion of aldosterone is a compensatory response to natriuretic hormones secreted by the adrenals in these patients. However, the existence of such hormones has not been proved.

Recent studies indicate that in the simple virilizing form of 21-hydroxylation deficiency there is a defect in 21-hydroxylation in the zona fasciculata that results in impaired cortisol secretion, whereas the zona glomerulosa is spared this defect (Kuhnle et al., 1981). In individuals affected with both virilization and salt wasting, the defect in 21-hydroxylation involves both the zona fasciculata and zona glomerulosa and leads to both impaired cortisol (fasciculata) and aldosterone (glomerulosa) secretion. Additional observations have demonstrated even greater heterogeneity of 21-hydroxylase deficiency. In eight of 124 families, a total of 16 siblings and parents of affected patients have been shown by HLA typing and steroid analyses to have asymptomatic 21-hydroxylase deficiency (Levine et al., 1980). These

Table 54–1. Enzymatic Defects in Adrenal Steroid Biosynthesis

Enzyme	Virilization	Incomplete Masculinization	Salt Loss	Hypertension	Urinary 17-Ketosteroids	Plasma 17-OHP	Predominant Abnormal Urinary Steroid
20,22-Desmolase	−	+	+	−	↓	↓	Virtually absent
3β-Hydroxysteroid dehydrogenase	+	+	+	−	↑	N or ↑ *	Pregnenetriol
17-Hydroxylase	−	+	−	+	↓	↓	Tetrahydro DOC
21-Hydroxylase	+	−	±	−	↑	↑↑	Pregnanetriol
11-Hydroxylase	+	−	−	+	↑	↑	Tetrahydro DOC, S
18-Hydroxysteroid dehydrogenase	−	−	+	−	N	N	Tetrahydro corticosterone

* Possibly reflects an increase in 3β-hydroxysteroid dehydrogenase activity of hepatic or testicular origin under separate genetic control.

family members have been designated as individuals with cryptic 21-hydroxylase deficiency. Accumulated evidence suggests that classic congenital adrenal hyperplasia, "acquired or late onset" adrenal hyperplasia, and "cryptic" adrenal hyperplasia are all forms of 21-hydroxylase deficiency with a wide range of clinical and biochemical abnormalities (Levine et al., 1980; Lorenzen et al., 1980; Pollack et al., 1981; New et al., 1981).

Congenital adrenal hyperplasia should be suspected in all infants with ambiguous genitalia or a family history of either this condition or unexplained infant death and in all infants with vomiting, sluggish feeding, dehydration, or failure to thrive.

The initial step of evaluation of an infant with ambiguous genitalia is to obtain a buccal smear for sex chromatin analysis. A karyotype is performed to confirm the sex chromatin analysis. The steroidal biochemical findings include elevated urinary excretion of 17-ketosteroids and pregnanetriol and elevated plasma levels of 17-hydroxyprogesterone and Δ^4 androstenedione. The most useful test is the determination of plasma 17-hydroxyprogesterone (17-OHP). The concentration of 17-OHP is normally elevated in umbilical cord blood with a mean value of 1700 ng/dl but rapidly decreases to 100 to 200 ng/dl after 24 hours of age (Grumbach and Conte, 1981). Although cord blood levels of 17-OHP may not be diagnostic of 21-hydroxylase deficiency, after 24 hours of age both 17-OHP and Δ^4 androstenedione levels usually distinguish infants with 21-hydroxylase deficiency from normal infants. It is well to be aware, however, that sick unaffected infants may have elevated 17-OHP and Δ^4 androstenedione levels that confuse the diagnosis of 21-hydroxylase deficiency. In affected patients, the plasma 17-OHP levels usually range from 3000 to 40,000 ng/dl, depending on the age and severity of 21-hydroxylase deficiency (Grumbach and Conte, 1981). Borderline levels of plasma 17-OHP may be found in patients with mild 21-hydroxylase deficiency or in heterozygotes. In these instances, the effect of ACTH administration on the rise of plasma 17-OHP and ratio of 17-OHP/cortisol will usually identify affected infants (Levine et al., 1981). In families with an affected member, HLA genotyping will distinguish between heterozygosity and a mild form of the disorder in a homozygous infant.

The urinary excretion of 17-ketosteroids and pregnanetriol is also useful in the diagnosis of 21-hydroxylase deficiency. It is necessary to be aware that during the first few days of life, the urinary 17-ketosteroids may be as high as 2 to 4 mg per 24 hours in normal infants, while urinary pregnanetriol may be normal in affected infants. After the early days of life, urinary 17-ketosteroid excretion values of greater than 2.5 mg per 24 hours and pregnanetriol values greater than 0.5 mg per 24 hours are of diagnostic value.

The combined use of HLA typing of amniotic fluid cells and the determination of 17-OHP and Δ^4 androstenedione in amniotic fluid permits the definitive prenatal diagnosis of 21-hydroxylase deficiency. Amniotic fluid concentrations of 17-OHP and Δ^4 androstenedione are elevated in affected fetuses between 14 and 20 weeks gestation (Milunsky and Tulchinsky, 1977; Nagamani et al., 1978; Pang et al., 1980). HLA typing of amniotic fluid cells obtained from mothers who had a previously affected offspring permits identification of fetuses who are homozygous or heterozygous for 21-hydroxylase deficiency (Pollack et al., 1979).

In the infant with severe salt loss, initial treatment requires volume expansion with isotonic saline in 5 or 10 per cent dextrose administered intravenously at a rate of 100 to 120 ml per kg per day with 25 per cent of this amount given in the first 2 hours. Fifty mg per M^2 of hydrocortisone sodium succinate should be given as a bolus intravenously and another 50 to 100 mg per M^2 added to the infusion fluid over the first 24 hours. When hyponatremia and hyperkalemia are present, desoxycorticosterone acetate (DOCA) may be given intramuscularly in a dosage of 1 mg every 24 hours.

Chronic medical treatment of congenital adrenal hyperplasia requires provision of sufficient cortisol to suppress adrenal androgen production and protect against stress. The required dosage is generally in the range of 15 to 20 mg per M^2 of hydrocortisone per day, given in three divided oral doses. Cortisone acetate may be given intramuscularly every 3 days for long-term replacement. The dosage should be doubled or tripled during acute illnesses, and intramuscular cortisone acetate should be substituted in a dosage of 25 to 50 mg per M^2 per day during protracted vomiting or surgical stress. Inadequate dosage permits excessive production of androgens and excessively rapid growth and skeletal maturation. Overdosage produces slowing of growth and other features of Cushing syndrome.

Infants with proved or suspected salt loss should also receive mineralocorticoid replacement and salt supplements (1 to 3 gm per day orally). Florinef (9-flurohydrocortisone) in an oral dose of 0.025 to 0.1 mg per day is commonly used for mineralocorticoid replacement. During the first 2 years of life, some prefer to implant one or two 125 mg DOCA pellets rather than prescribe Florinef. The pellets are absorbed slowly and last for 6 to 9 months. Suboptimal growth occurs with inadequate replacement, and excessive doses produce failure to thrive as well as hypertension.

In addition to the evaluation of growth, skeletal maturation, and signs of virilization, adequacy of glucocorticoid therapy is assessed by monitoring urinary excretion of 17-ketosteroids and pregnanetriol and plasma levels of 17-OHP (Hughes and Winter, 1976). In this regard, plasma levels of 17-OHP have not been found more useful than urinary 17-ketosteroids (Grumbach and Conte, 1981). Indeed, there is uncertainty regarding the value of plasma 17-OHP measurements in assessing the quality of treatment (Frisch et al., 1981). Plasma levels of sodium and potassium and plasma renin activity are useful in evaluating the adequacy of mineralocorticoid therapy.

Surgical correction of mild to moderate clitoral enlargement is generally not required. Clitoral size tends to remain stable or even decrease as the child grows. When indicated, surgery may be performed at 4 to 12 months of age. The best age for correction of labial fusion is probably about 2 years. Some girls may require more complicated vaginoplasty at a later age. The prognosis for normal psychosexual development and reproductive function is excellent in boys and girls with 21-hydroxylase deficiency.

Deficiency of 20,22-Desmolase

Conversion of cholesterol to pregnenolone is an essential step in the synthesis of mineralocorticoids, glucocorticoids, androgens, and estrogens. This conversion requires a complex mitochondrial mixed function oxidase system including cytochrome P-450. The adrenal mitochondrial content of cytochrome P-450 has been reported to be decreased in patients with 20,22-desmolase deficiency (Kazumi et al., 1977). Defects in this early set of reactions lead to severe salt and water loss and hypoglycemia. Female infants have normal genitalia at birth but will be incapable of producing estrogens at the time of puberty. Male infants with this defect usually have female external genitalia with a blind vaginal pouch but absent Müllerian duct derivatives. No distinctive steroid precursors are present in serum or urine. Little or no C_{21} or C_{19} steroids are detectable in plasma or urine. The adrenal glands and gonads are enlarged and filled with cholesterol and other lipids, hence the name "lipoid adrenal hyperplasia." In the cases of Prader and Gurtner and of Comacho and coworkers, the defect was confirmed at autopsy. Most patients have died in infancy, but, in a few (who, perhaps, have less severe defects), steroid treatment has permitted prolonged survival.

Deficiency of 3β-Hydroxysteroid Dehydrogenase

Conversion of pregnenolone to progesterone requires oxidation at the 3 position and isomerization of a double bond from the Δ^5 to the Δ^4 position. The defect results in defective synthesis of cortisol, aldosterone, and potent androgens and estrogens. Bongiovanni originally described several infants with defects in this crucial enzyme complex. Such infants have severe salt and water loss and, despite adequate

steroid replacement, may not survive infancy. Urinary and plasma steroid metabolites are predominantly of the $\Delta^5,3\beta$-hydroxy configuration and include pregnenetriol and dehydroepiandrosterone. However, during the first few weeks of life, the $\Delta^5,3\beta$-hydroxysteroids may be elevated in normal premature and full-term infants. It is, therefore, necessary to interpret the levels of these steroids in early infancy in relation to normal values for age. As a result of accumulation of dehydroepiandrosterone, a weak androgen, and defective conversion to the more potent androgens, androstenedione and testosterone, both males and females have "partial" virilization. Males have hypospadias and may have a bifid scrotum with or without cryptorchidism. Females have slight to moderate clitoral enlargement, which may be associated with labial fusion. Affected males have developed gynecomastia at puberty. Mild forms of 3β-hydroxysteroid dehydrogenase deficiency may not become clinically evident until adolescence (Rosenfield et al., 1980). Schneider and coworkers reported an elevated ratio of Δ^5-androstenediol to testosterone, which provides evidence of persistent deficiency of testicular 3β-hydroxysteroid dehydrogenase activity and supports the hypothesis that the adrenal and testicular enzymes are under common genetic control. With increasing age in XY males, the presence of low normal concentrations of plasma testosterone, increased estrogen levels, and a diminishing ratio of urinary pregnenetriol to pregnanetriol has been attributed to the maturation of hepatic 3 β-hydroxysteroid dehydrogenase activity under different genetic control (Bongiovanni et al., 1971). In infancy, urinary 17-ketosteroids and pregnanetriol are elevated. The latter finding differentiates the defect from the more common deficiency of 21-hydroxylase. Both glucocorticoid and mineralocorticoid replacement are required throughout life. Male fertility and female puberty have yet to be described in this syndrome.

Deficiency of 11-Hydroxylase

Hydroxylation at the C-11 position is required for cortisol and aldosterone synthesis. As originally reported by Eberlein and Bongiovanni, deficiency of 11β-hydroxylase results in virilization of the female infant together with a variable degree of hypertension. There is accumulation of the immediate precursors, 11-deoxycortisol (compound S) and desoxycorticosterone (DOC) in the plasma and increased urinary excretion of their tetrahydro metabolites. Recent studies suggest that the adrenal 11β- and 18-hydroxylating activities are related and may involve the same enzyme protein and catalytic step (Levine et al., 1980). Whereas compound S is biologically inert, DOC has mineralocorticoid effects and contributes to the hypertensive state. Neither compound is recognized by the hypothalamic-pituitary regulatory system, and an increase in ACTH secretion occurs. Although 11β- and 18-hydroxylations are reduced in the zona fasciculata, the 11β- and 18-hydroxylase pathway in the zona glomerulosa is functional, and normal amounts of aldosterone can be secreted under the influence of the renin-angiotensin system (New et al., 1981). In the untreated state the excessive circulating DOC reduces plasma renin and, hence, aldosterone secretion. Hydrocortisone replacement suppresses ACTH production and thereby prevents further virilization and relieves hypertension. Transient hyponatremia and hyperkalemia may occur soon after the initiation of glucocorticoid therapy as a result of inhibition of ACTH-stimulated DOC secretion before the inhibited renin-angiotensin-aldosterone system has had time to recover (Holcomb et al., 1980). Monitoring of treatment requires management of urinary 17-ketosteroid or tetrahydro-S excretion.

The 11β-hydroxylase gene is not linked to the HLA loci. The frequency of 11β-hydroxylase deficiency is from 10 to 20 per cent of that of 21-hydroxylase deficiency, except in certain Middle Eastern populations in which the two defects occur with equal frequency. The defect may be partial, and hypertension either may be absent or may not appear until late childhood or adulthood. Similarly, signs of virilization in the female may not appear until adolescence (Cathelineau et al., 1980).

Deficiency of 17α-Hydroxylase

Hydroxylation at the C-17 position is required for cortisol, androgen, and estrogen synthesis, but it is not involved in the synthesis of mineralocorticoids. Biglieri described four adult females with lack of secondary sexual development, hyperkalemic alkalosis, and hypertension who proved to have deficiency of this enzyme. They demonstrated excessive plasma levels of DOC and corticosterone and excessive excretion of their urinary metabolites. Aldosterone levels tended to be low, presumably owing to inhibition of the renin-angiotensin system. In affected XX females, both internal and external genitalia are normal female. In males, impaired testosterone synthesis by the fetal testes results in either phenotypic female external genitalia or ambiguous genitalia, but the female duct derivatives are absent. Failure of pubertal development in females and defective virilization in males, as described by New, provide evidence that adrenal and gonadal 17α-hydroxylase activities are under common genetic control. Cortisol replacement inhibits ACTH production and relieves hypertension. Exogenous androgens or estrogens are required at the age of puberty.

Deficiency of 18-Hydroxysteroid Dehydrogenase

The final steps in aldosterone synthesis involve hydroxylation and dehydrogenation at C-18. Deficiency at this level results in aldosterone deficiency

and salt loss without any alteration in the synthesis of cortisol or the sex steroids. Ulick and coworkers described a patient with these features in 1964. Several authors have postulated that the transient salt wasting of infancy described by Jaudon might be due to delayed maturation of this enzyme. Appropriate therapy consists of a mineralocorticoid and supplemental sodium chloride. Glucocorticoid replacement is not required.

Adrenal Overactivity

Glucocorticoid excess results in hyperphagia, obesity, and impairment of linear growth, together with hypertension, osteoporosis, and polycythemia. The Cushing syndrome is extremely rare in infancy except as a result of administration of glucocorticoids or ACTH. The cases that have been reported show a preponderance of adrenal tumors, both adenomas and carcinomas. There may be overproduction of androgens as well as glucocorticoids. There is no suppression with administration of dexamethasone. Surgical treatment involves unilateral or bilateral adrenalectomy, with attendant glucocorticoid replacement to prevent acute adrenal insufficiency.

Other Abnormalities of Sodium Metabolism

Both hypernatremia and hyponatremia may affect newborn infants. In both conditions, convulsions and severe alterations in the sensorial state may result either from obtunding of the sensorium, with effects ranging from unresponsiveness to coma, or from overstimulation of it leading to irritability, irrational behavior, and convulsions. Brain cells should become dehydrated as a result of hyperosmolality of the extracellular fluids in which they bathed or swell from overhydration because of hypotonicity of these same fluids.

HYPERNATREMIA

Serum sodium concentrations in excess of 160 mEq per liter, usually associated with chloride levels greater than 110 mEq per liter, are encountered in the newborn period as well as in later infancy and childhood. The most common causes of hypernatremia are as follows:

1. *Severe diarrhea,* with loss of proportionally more water than sodium chloride in the intestinal discharges.

2. *Excessive intake of sodium salts.* This occurs fairly frequently when babies are treated for diarrhea with electrolyte solutions prepared improperly or of-

fered in excess. In 1972, Taitz and Byers reminded us that the use of heaping rather than level scoops of milk powder in the preparation of formula is often sufficient to produce dangerous hypernatremia. Insufficiently diluted liquid products can have the same effect. Serious epidemics of hypernatremia have reportedly followed the inadvertent substitution of salt for sugar in the preparation of infant formulas in hospital milk rooms.

That the use of large quantities of sodium bicarbonate increases the risk of intracranial hemorrhage is strongly suggested by the 1972 study by Simmons and coworkers. "Intakes of more than 5 mg per kg per 24 hours should be regarded as excessive."

3. *Nephrogenic diabetes insipidus.* In this condition, excessive quantities of water are lost via polyuria.

Treatment consists of withholding sodium salts and *slow* rehydration for the hypernatremia, plus whatever other therapy seems indicated for the underlying condition.

HYPONATREMIA

Serum levels of sodium below 135, usually but not always accompanied by levels of chloride below 95 mEq per liter, are discovered in a variety of conditions in the newborn infant. The presenting symptom of hyponatremia is, in the majority of cases, convulsions, but irritability, mental confusion, and coma characterize some examples. Hyponatremia may be encountered under the following conditions:

1. *Severe burns.* Salt is lost in the profuse serous exudate from the denuded areas. It is our impression that this loss may be accentuated by treatment with silver nitrate, which exerts a specific leeching action upon the body store of sodium.

2. *Cerebrospinal fluid-to-ureter shunting* in the attempt to control advancing hydrocephalus.

3. *Inappropriate antidiuretic hormone secretion.* This is uncommon in the newborn but does occur in this age period. Mor and colleagues, with convincing documentation, ascribed the convulsions of their 6-week-old male patient with severe pneumonia to inappropriate ADH secretion. The last example we saw was in an infant with a subdural hematoma. In this situation there is oliguria, high urine specific gravity, low sodium and chloride serum concentrations but normal potassium and nonprotein nitrogen, and falling hematocrit and total serum solids.

4. *Water intoxication.* An example of this was observed in a 2-month-old infant who had been fed a formula consisting of 390 ml of evaporated milk, 2 liters of water, and some sugar. Since he always seemed hungry, he drank four or five 240-ml bottles of water a day in addition. His calculated intake was 400 ml per kilogram per 24 hours!

Water intoxication has also been observed in a newborn infant whose mother had received large quantities of 5 per cent dextrose without added salt for 24 hours or longer prior to delivery.

5. *Pseudohypoaldosteronism (end-organ unresponsiveness to aldosterone).* This is a salt-wasting disorder that results from renal tubular unresponsiveness to aldosterone (Proesmans et al., 1973). Characteristically, there is urinary sodium wasting, hyponatremia, hyperkalemia, vomiting, and dehydration in early infancy. Urinary 17-ketosteroids and plasma androgens are normal, whereas plasma aldosterone and renin concentrations are elevated. The infants do not respond to mineralocorticoid therapy, and treatment with supplemental sodium chloride is necessary.

REFERENCES

Baden, M., Bauer, C. R., Colle, E., Klein, G., Papageorgiou, A., and Stern, L.: Plasma corticoids in infants with the respiratory distress syndrome. Pediatrics 52:782, 1973.

Beitins, I. Z., Bayard, F., Ances, I. G., Kowarski, A., and Migeon, C. J.: The metabolic clearance rate, blood production, interconversion and transplacental passage of cortisol and cortisone in pregnancy near term. Pediatr. Res. 7:509, 1973.

Biglieri, E. G., Herron, M. A., and Brust, N.: 17-Hydroxylation deficiency in man. J. Clin. Invest. 45:1946, 1966.

Black, J., and Williams, D. I.: Natural history of adrenal haemorrhage in the newborn. Arch. Dis. Child. 48:183, 1973.

Blizzard, R. M., and Alberts, M.: Hypopituitarism, hypoadrenalism and hypogonadism in the newborn infant. J. Pediatr. 48:782, 1956.

Bongiovanni, A. M.: Disorders of adrenal steroid biogenesis. In Stanbury, J. B., Wyngaarden, J. B., and Fredrickson, D. S. (Eds.): The Metabolic Basis of Inherited Disease. New York, McGraw-Hill Book Co., 1972, p. 857.

Bongiovanni, A. M.: Adrenogenital syndrome with deficiency of 3β-hydroxysteroid dehydrogenase. J. Clin. Invest. 41:2086, 1962.

Bongiovanni, A. M., Eberlein, W. R., and Moshang, T. M.: Urinary excretion of pregnanetriol and Δ5-pregnenetriol in two forms of congenital adrenal hyperplasia. J. Clin. Invest. 50:2751, 1971.

Boyd, J. F.: Disseminated fibrin thromboembolism among neonates dying within 48 hours of birth. Arch. Dis. Child. 42:401, 1967.

Cacciari, E., Cicognani, A., Pirazzoli, P., Dallacasa, P., Mazzaracchio, M. A., Tassoni, P., Bernardi, F., Salardi, S., and Zappula, F.: Plasma ACTH values during the first seven days of life in infants of diabetic mothers. J. Pediatr. 87:943, 1975.

Camacho, A. M., Kowarski, A., Migeon, C. J., and Brough, A. J.: Congenital adrenal hyperplasia due to a deficiency of one of the enzymes involved in the biosynthesis of pregneneolone. J. Clin. Endocrinol. Metab. 28:153, 1968.

Campbell, A. L., and Murphy, B. E. P.: The maternal-fetal cortisol gradient during pregnancy and delivery. J. Clin. Endocrinol. Metab. 45:435, 1977.

Cathelineau, G., Brerault, J., Fiet, J., Julien, R., Dreux, C., and Canivet, J.: Adrenocortical 11-β-hydroxylation defect in adult women with post menarcheal onset of symptoms. J. Clin. Endocrinol. Metab. 51:287, 1980.

Eberlein, W. R.: Steroids and sterols in umbilical cord blood. J. Clin. Endocrinol. Metab. 25:1101, 1965.

Eberlein, W. R., and Bongiovanni, A. M.: Plasma and urinary corticosteroids in hypertensive form of congenital adrenal hyperplasia. J. Biol. Chem. 223:85, 1956.

Finberg, L., Kravath, R. E. and Fleischman, A. R.: Water and Electrolytes in Pediatrics. Philadelphia, W. B. Saunders Co., 1982.

Franks, R. D.: Diurnal variation of plasma 17-hydroxycorticosteroids in children. J. Clin. Endocrinol. Metab. 27:75, 1967.

Frisch, H., Parth, K., Schober, E., and Swoboda, W.: Circadian patterns of plasma cortisol, 17-hydroxyprogesterone, and testosterone in congenital adrenal hyperplasia. Arch. Dis. Child. 56:208, 1981.

Grumbach, M. M., and Conte, F. A.: Disorders of sex differentiation. In Williams, R. H. (Ed.): Textbook of Endocrinology. Philadelphia, W. B. Saunders Company, 1981, p. 423.

Gutai, J., George, R., Koeff, S., and Bacon, G. E.: Adrenal response to stress and the effect of adrenocorticotropic hormone in newborn infants. J. Pediatr. 81:719, 1972.

Hirschfeld, A. J., and Fleshman, J. K.: An unusually high incidence of salt-losing congenital adrenal hyperplasia in the Alaskan Eskimo. J. Pediatr. 75:492, 1969.

Holcombe, J. A., Keenan, B., Nichols, B., Kirkland, R., and Clayton, G.: Neonatal salt loss in the hypertensive form of congenital adrenal hyperplasia. Pediatrics 65:777, 1980.

Hughes, I. A., and Winter, J. S. D.: The application of a serum 17-OH-progesterone radioimmunoassay to the diagnosis and management of congenital adrenal hyperplasia. J. Pediatr. 88:766, 1976.

Jaudon, J. C.: Addison's disease in an infant. J. Clin. Endocrinol. Metab. 6:558, 1946.

Johannisson, E.: The foetal adrenal cortex in the human. Acta Endocrinol. (Suppl.) 130:7, 1968.

Kaplan, S. L., and Grumbach, M. M.: The ontogenesis of human foetal hormones. II. Luteinizing hormone (LH) and follicle-stimulating hormone (FSH). Acta Endocrinol. 81:808, 1976.

Kauppila, A., Tuimala, R., and Haapalahti, J.: Maternal adrenocorticotrophic hormone and cortisol during labour and vaginal delivery. J. Obstet. Gynaecol. Br. Comm. 81:691, 1974.

Koizumi, S., Kyoya, S., Miyawaki, K. H., Funabashi, T., Nakashima, H., Ohta, G., and Katajiri, M.: Cholesterol side-chain cleavage enzyme activity and cytochrome P-450 content in adrenal mitochondria of a patient with congenital lipoid adrenal hyperplasia (Prader disease). Clin. Chem. Acta 77:301, 1977.

Kowarski, A., Katz, H., and Migeon, C. J.: Plasma aldosterone concentration in normal subjects from infancy to adulthood. J. Clin. Endocrinol. Metab. 38:489, 1974.

Kreines, K., and De Vaux, W. D.: Neonatal adrenal insufficiency associated with maternal Cushing's syndrome. Pediatrics 47:516, 1971.

Kuhnle, U., Chow, D., Rapaport, R., Pang, S., Levine, L. S., and New, M. I.: The 21-hydroxylase activity in the glomerulosa and fasciculata of the adrenal cortex in congenital adrenal hyperplasia. J. Clin. Endocrinol. Metab. 52:534, 1981.

Levine, L. S., Dupont, B., Lorenzen, F., Pang, S., Pollack, M., Oberfield, S. E., Kohn, B., Lerner, A., Cacciari, E., Mantero, F., Cassio, A., Scaroni, C., Chiumello, G., Rondanini, G. F., Gargantini, L., Giovannelli, G., Virdis, R., Bartolotta, E., Migliori, C., Pintor, C., Tato, L., Barboni, F., and New, M. I.: Genetic and hormonal characterization of cryptic 21-hydroxylase deficiency. J. Clin. Endocrinol. Metab. 53:1193, 1981.

Levine, L. S., Dupont, B., Lorenzen, F., Pang, S., Pollack, M., Oberfield, S., Kohn, B., Lerner, A., Cacciari, E., Mantero, F., Cassio, A., Scaroni, C., Chiumello, G., Rondanini, G. F., Gargantini, L., Giovannelli, G., Virdis, R., Bartolotta, E., Migliori, C., Pintor, C., Tato, L., Barboni, F., and New, M. I.: Cryptic 21-hydroxylase deficiency in families of patients with classical congenital adrenal hyperplasia. J. Clin. Endocrinol. Metab. 51:1316, 1980.

Levine, L. S., Rauh, W., Gottesdiener, K., Chow, D., Gunczler, P., Rapaport, R., Pang, S., Schneider, B., and New, M. I.: New studies of the 11β-hydroxylase and 18-hydroxylase enzymes in the hypertensive form of congenital adrenal hyperplasia. J. Clin. Endocrinol. Metab. 50:258, 1980.

Levine, L. S., Zachmann, M., New, M. I., Prader, A., Pollack, M. S., O'Neill, G. J., Yang, S. Y., Oberfield, S. E., and Dupont, B.: Genetic mapping of the 21-hydroxylase–deficiency gene within the HLA linkage group. N. Engl. J. Med. 299:911, 1978.

Lorenzen, F., Pang, S., New, M., Pollack, M., Oberfield, S., Dupont, B., Chow, D., Schneider, B., and Levine, L.: Studies of the C-21 and C-19 steroids and HLA genotyping in siblings and parents of patients with congenital adrenal hyperplasia due to 21-hydroxylase deficiency. J. Clin. Endocrinol. Metab. 50:572, 1980.

Migeon, C. J., Kenny, F. M., and Kowarski, A.: The syndrome of congenital unresponsiveness to ACTH. Pediatr. Res. 2:501, 1968.

Milunsky, A., and Tulchinsky, D.: Prenatal diagnosis of congenital adrenal hyperplasia due to 21 hydroxylase deficiency. Pediatrics 59:768, 1977.

Mor, J., Ben-Galim, E., and Abrahamov, A.: Inappropriate antidiuretic hormone secretion in an infant with severe pneumonia. Am. J. Dis. Child. 129:133, 1975.

Moshang, T. M., Jr., Rosenfield, R. L., Bongiovanni, A. M., Parks, J. S., and Amrhein, J. A.: Familial glucocorticoid insufficiency. J. Pediatr. 82:821, 1973.

Murphy, B. E.: Chorionic membrane as an extra-adrenal source of foetal cortisol in human amniotic fluid. Nature 266:179, 1977.

Murphy, B. E. P.: Non-chromatographic radio transinassay for cortisol: application to human adult serum, umbilical cord serum and amniotic fluid. J. Clin. Endocrinol. Metab. 41:1050, 1975.

Murphy, B. E. P., Clark, S. J., Donald, I. R., Pinsky, M., and Vedady, D.: Conversion of maternal cortisol to cortisone during placental transfer to the human fetus. Am. J. Obstet. Gynecol. 118:538, 1974.

Nagamani, M., McDonough, P., Ellegood, J., and Mahesh, V.: Maternal and amniotic fluid 17α hydroxyprogesterone levels during pregnancy. Diagnosis of congenital adrenal hyperplasia in utero. Am. J. Obstet. Gynecol. 130:791, 1978.

New, M. I., Dupont, B., Pang, S., Pollack, M., and Levine, L. S.: An update of congenital adrenal hyperplasia. Recent Prog. Horm. Res. 37:105, 1981.

New, M. I., and Suvannakul, L.: Male pseudohermaphroditism due to 17α-hydroxylase deficiency. J. Clin. Invest. 49:1930, 1970.

Ohrlander, S., Gennser, G., and Encroth, P.: Plasma cortisol levels in human fetus during parturition. Obstet. Gynecol. 48:381, 1976.

Osathanondh, R., Tulchinsky, D., Kamali, H., Fenel, M., and Taeusch, H. W.: Dexamethasone levels in treated pregnant women and newborn infants. J. Pediatr. 90:617, 1977.

Pakravan, P., Kenny, F. M., Depp, R., and Allen, A. C.: Familial congenital absence of adrenal glands: evaluation of glucocorticoid, mineralocorticoid, and estrogen metabolism in the perinatal period. J. Pediatr. 84:74, 1974.

Pang, S., Levine, L., Cederquist, M., Fuentes, M., Riccardi, V., Holcomb, H., Nitowsky, G., and New, M.: Amniotic fluid concentrations of Δ^5 and Δ^4 steroids in fetuses with congenital adrenal hyperplasia due to 21 hydroxylase deficiency and in anencephalic fetuses. J. Clin. Endocrinol. Metab. 51:223, 1980.

Parks, G. A., New, M. I., Bermudez, J. A., Anast, C. S., and Bongiovanni, A. M.: A pubertal boy with the 3β-hydroxysteroid dehydrogenase defect. J. Clin. Invest. 33:269, 1971.

Pollack, M. S., Levine, L. S., O'Neill, G. J., Pang, S., Lorenzen, F., Kohn, B., Rondanini, G. F., Chiumello, G., New, M. I., and Dupont, B.: HLA linkage and B14, DR1, BfS haplotype association with the genes for late onset and cryptic 21-hydroxylase deficiency. Am. J. Hum. Genet. 33:540, 1981.

Prader, A., and Gurtner, H. P.: Das Syndrom des Pseudohermaphroditismus masculinus bei kongenitaler Nebennierenrinden hyperplasie ohne Androgenüberproduktion (adrenaler Pseudohermaphroditismus masculinus). Helvet. Paediatr. Acta 10:397, 1955.

Proesmans, W., Geussens, H., Corbeel, L., and Eeckels, R.: Pseudohypoaldosteronism. Am. J. Dis. Child. 126:510, 1973.

Roselli, A., and Barbosa, L. T.: Congenital hypoplasia of the adrenal glands: Report of 2 cases in sisters, with necropsy. Pediatrics 35:70, 1965.

Rosenfield, R. L., Rich, B., Wolfsdorf, J., Cassorala, F., Parks, J., Bongiovanni, A., Wu, C., and Shackelton, H.: Pubertal presentation of congenital Δ^5-3β-hydroxysteroid dehydrogenase deficiency. J. Clin. Endocrinol. Metab. 51:345, 1980.

Schneider, G., Genel, M., Bongiovanni, A. M., Goldman, A. S., and Rosenfield, R. L.: Persistent testicular Δ5-isomerase-3β-hydroxysteroid dehydrogenase deficiency in the Δ5-3β-HSD form of congenital adrenal hyperplasia. J. Clin. Invest. 55:681, 1974.

Similä, S., Kauppila, A., Ylikorkala, O., Koivisto, M., Mäkelä, P., and Haapalahti, J.: Adrenocorticotrophic hormone during the first day of life. Eur. J. Pediatr. *124*:173, 1977.

Simmer, H. H., Frankland, M. V., and Greipel, M.: Unbound unconjugated cortisol in umbilical cord and corresponding maternal plasma. Gynecol. Invest. *5*:199, 1974.

Simmons, M. A., Adcock, E. W., et al.: Hypernatremia and intracranial hemorrhage in neonates. Arch. Dis. Child. *47*:257, 1972.

Sperling, M. A.: Newborn adaptation: Adrenocortical hormones and ACTH. *In* Tulchinsky, D., and Ryan, K. J. (Eds.): Maternal-Fetal Endocrinology. Philadelphia, W. B. Saunders Co., 1980, p. 387.

Sperling, M. A., Wolfsen, A. R., and Fisher, D. A.: Congenital adrenal hypoplasia: an isolated defect of organogenesis. J. Pediatr. *82*:44, 1973.

Taitz, L. S., and Byers, H. D.: High calorie/osmolar feeding and hypertonic dehydration. Arch. Dis. Child. *47*:257, 1972.

Tennes, K., and Vernadakis, A.: Cortisol excretion levels and daytime sleep in one-year-old infants. J. Clin. Endocrinol. Metab. *44*:175, 1977.

Tuimala, R., Kauppila, A., Ronnberg, L., Jouppila, R., and Haapalahti, J.: The effects of labour on ACTH and cortisol levels in amniotic fluid and maternal blood. Br. J. Obstet. Gynecol. *83*:707, 1976.

Ulick, S., Gautier, E., Vetter, K. K., Markello, J. R., Yaffe, S., and Lowe, C. U.: An aldosterone biosynthetic defect in a salt-losing disorder. J. Clin. Endocrinol. Metab. *24*:669, 1964.

Wilkins, L., Fleishman, W., and Howard, J. E.: Macrogenitosomia precox associated with hyperplasia of the androgenic tissue of the adrenal and death from corticoadrenal insufficiency. Endocrinology *25*:385, 1940.

Winters, A. J., Oliver, C., Colston, C., MacDonald, P. C., and Porter, J. C.: Plasma ACTH levels in the human fetus and neonate as related to age and parturition. J. Clin. Endocrinol. Metab. *39*:269, 1974.

Wurtman, R. J., and Axelrod, J.: Adrenaline synthesis. Control by the pituitary gland and adrenal glucocorticoids. Science *150*:1464, 1956.

Yackel, D. B., Kempers, R. D., and McConahey, W. M.: Adrenocorticosteroid therapy in pregnancy. Am. J. Obstet. Gynecol. *96*:985, 1966.

55

Disorders of the Thyroid Gland

By Constantine S. Anast

The Hypothalamic-Pituitary-Thyroid System

The secretion of thyroid hormones is under the control of a negative feedback system that involves the hypothalamus and the pituitary gland. Thyrotropin-releasing hormone (TRH), a small tripeptide molecule (pyroglutamyl-histidyl-proline amide), is secreted by the hypothalamic neuroendocrine cells into the pituitary portal system, where it is transported to the anterior pituitary gland. TRH stimulates the pituitary thyrotrope cells to synthesize and secrete thyroid-stimulating hormone (TSH), a glycoprotein with an estimated molecular weight of 28,300 daltons. TSH is a tropic hormone that stimulates the thyroid gland to synthesize and secrete the iodothyronines. The metabolic steps involved in the synthesis of the iodothyronines include (1) active transport of iodide into the thyroid gland, (2) iodination at carbon 3 and/or 5 of tyrosine residues within thyroglobulin to form monoiodotyrosine (MIT) and diiodotyrosine

(DIT), and (3) the coupling of MIT and DIT residues within thyroglobulin to form the following iodothyronines: T_4 (thyroxine), or 3,5,3'5' tetraiodothyronine, T_3, or 3,5,3' triiodothyronine, rT_3 (reverse T_3), or 3,3'5' triiodothyronine. In a fourth metabolic step, thyroglobulin is enzymatically hydrolyzed, and the free iodothyronines are released into the blood stream; in a fifth step, intrathyroidal iodine is recycled by dehalogenation of hormonally inactive iodotyrosines and iodothyronines.

In the blood, 99.98 per cent of T_4 and 99.7 per cent of T_3 and of rT_3 are bound to the serum proteins, thyroxine-binding globulin (TBG), thyroxine-binding prealbumin (TBA), and albumin. In general, it is thought that the circulating T_4 and T_3 not bound to plasma proteins (i.e., the "free T_4" and "free T_3") are the biologically important fractions that are available to the tissues, while the protein-bound hormones serve as a reservoir. However, recent evidence indicates that much of protein-bound T_3 can enter cells during a single passage of blood through the liver or brain, while a small fraction of protein-bound T_4 may also be available to cells (Pardridge, 1979; Pardridge and Mietus, 1980). Additional work is needed to determine the physiologic significance of this observation.

The thyroid gland is the sole source of T_4, but thyroidal secretion is only one of two sources of T_3. Most of circulating T_3 is derived from nonglandular sources by monodeiodination of T_4 in peripheral tissues. In experimental animals, the conversion of T_4 to T_3 has been identified in the liver, kidney, anterior pituitary, brain, and skeletal muscle (Larsen et al., 1981; Kaplan, 1982), whereas T_4 conversion to rT_3 has been identified in liver, kidney, and brain but not in anterior pituitary (Gavin et al., 1980; Kaplan and Yaskoski, 1980; Kaplan, 1982).

Accumulated evidence indicates that T_3 is the predominant active intracellular thyroid hormone and that T_4 does not have a major intracellular hormonal role. According to this thesis, T_4 has little intrinsic biological activity and serves primarily as a precursor for T_3. In thyroidectomized animals, the conversion of T_4 to T_3 is significantly increased in the cerebral cortex, which serves to defend the intracellular T_3 against reductions in plasma T_4 (Kaplan and Yaskoski, 1980; Leonard et al., 1981). T_3 binds to nuclear receptors in target organs and stimulates synthesis of messenger RNA for several thyroid hormone–dependent proteins and subsequent synthesis of the proteins themselves (Oppenheimer et al., 1976; Baxter et al., 1979). This leads to a variety of physiologic actions, including effects upon growth and development, oxygen consumption, heat production, nerve function, the action of other hormones, and the metabolism of carbohydrates, lipids, proteins, nucleic acids, and inorganic ions. In contrast to T_3, which has important biological actions, rT_3, according to current evidence, is metabolically inactive. In normal older children and adults, the serum concentration of T_4 ranges from 5 to 13 µg/dl and is 50 to 100 times greater than the serum concentration of T_3, which ranges from 80 to 200 ng/dl. The serum concentration of rT_3 in normal nonfasted older children and adults is approximately one third that of T_3. Of particular relevance to this discussion is the observation that elevated serum levels of rT_3 are present during pregnancy and the early days of life (Chopra et al., 1975).

In the feedback control of thyroid secretion, TSH increases the synthesis and secretion of T_3 and T_4, and, in turn, circulating free T_3 and T_4 inhibit TSH secretion. The inhibition of TSH secretion by T_3 and T_4 occurs at the level of the pituitary. (For extensive reviews and discussions, see Florsheim, 1974; Reichlin, 1978; Ingbar and Woeber, 1981.) Current evidence indicates that T_3, derived from the circulation and from T_4 conversion in the pituitary itself, plays the major role in suppression of TSH secretion. TRH initially stimulates the release and later the synthesis of TSH. Although the subject of many studies, there is no convincing evidence that T_3 and T_4 suppress TSH secretion by directly inhibiting the release of TRH by the hypothalamus. Moreover, the inhibitory effects of T_3 and T_4 on TSH secretion are not merely a direct antagonism of the effects of TRH, since they are observed when the hypothalamic source of TRH is destroyed. The accumulated evidence suggests that T_3 and T_4 mediate the feedback regulation of TSH secretion, whereas TRH determines its set point.

In addition to the control of thyroid activity by the hypothalamic-pituitary axis, intrinsic mechanisms in the thyroid gland regulate thyroid function independent of the influence of TSH and TRH (Ingbar, 1978; Ingbar and Woeber, 1981). These autoregulatory responses are demonstrated under conditions in which circulating TSH is totally lacking or kept constant by infusion. This is exemplified by the fact that in the absence of TSH in hypophysectomized animals, the rate of iodide transport by the thyroid gland is inversely related to the iodine intake. Moreover, it is the organic iodine (iodinated tyrosine) rather than the inorganic iodine content of the thyroid gland that exerts an autoregulatory influence on iodide transport. The organic iodine content of the thyroid also exerts an intrinsic effect on glandular morphology. Thus, iodine deficiency results in an increase in thyroid size in the absence of TSH in hypophysectomized animals. In general, it is thought that the feedback control of thyroid function mediated by TSH attempts to maintain normal circulating and tissue levels of thyroid hormones, whereas the autoregulatory mechanism serves to maintain constancy of hormone stores in the thyroid gland.

ONTOGENESIS OF HYPOTHALAMIC-PITUITARY-THYROID FUNCTION

Under normal conditions, the human fetal hypothalamic-pituitary-thyroid system appears to develop free of maternal influence, since the placenta is impermeable to T_4, T_3, rT_3, and TSH. Although TRH crosses the placenta, there is no evidence that it influences fetal pituitary-thyroid development under normal circumstances. Fisher and Klein suggest that the fetal-thyroid system ontogenesis can be separated into three phases. Phase I, or embryogenesis, occurs during the first 10 to 12 weeks of gestation, when the fetal thyroid gland develops characteristic histology and the capacity to concentrate iodine and to synthesize iodothyronines. During this period, the fetal pituitary also differentiates histologically and contains TSH. Moreover, TSH as well as T_4 are measurable in fetal serum.

Phase II, or hypothalamic maturation, proceeds from the fourth or fifth week through the thirtieth to thirty-fifth weeks of gestation. During this period, maturation of the hypothalamus and the pituitary-portal vascular system takes place. TRH is detectable in hypothalamic tissue at 10 to 12 weeks gestation.

Phase III involves the functional maturation of the thyroid system. Although the capacities for syntheses of TRH, TSH, and iodothyronines are present in the first trimester, thyroid function is relatively dormant until midgestation (18 to 22 weeks), when serum TSH and T_4 begin to increase. Fetal serum TSH levels peak at a mean value of about 15 µU/ml (normal children and adults <5 µU/ml) at 20 to 24 weeks and then gradually decrease to a mean value of 10 µU/ml at term. Fetal serum T_4 progressively increases from midgestation to term, reaching a mean peak value of 11.5 µg/dl (normal children and adults 5 to 13 µg/dl). The progressive increase in fetal serum T_4 after 24 weeks gestation in the presence of a modest decline in serum TSH suggests an apparent increase in thyroid responsiveness to T_3 during Phase III. This is not due to increasing thyroid mass, since thyroid weight per unit of body weight remains constant during this time.

The TSH response to TRH is present early in the third trimester, and the human infant born after 26 to 28 weeks gestation responds to exogenous TRH with an increase in serum TSH levels comparable to those observed in adults (Jacobsen et al., 1975, 1977). Less is known regarding the iodothyronine control of TSH secretion during human fetal life, although it has been demonstrated that TSH secretion can be inhibited by T_4 administration at term (Fisher et al., 1977; Klein et al., 1978). The intrinsic autoregulation of the thyroid gland that allows it to modify iodide transport relative to iodine intake, independent of the influence of TSH, is lacking until after 36 to 40 weeks gestation (Theodoropoulos et al., 1979; Castaign et al., 1979).

The conversion of T_4 to T_3 by peripheral tissues is relatively low during fetal life (Abuid et al., 1973; Fisher et al., 1977). Fetal serum T_3 levels are unmeasurable before 30 weeks gestation and then progressively increase to 50 ng/dl at term. During this period, there is a decrease in fetal serum rT_3 from about 250 ng/dl at 30 weeks to 150 ng/dl at term (Chopra et al., 1975; Oddie et al., 1979). At term, the serum level of T_3 is relatively low and that of rT_3 relatively high when compared with levels in normal older children and adults. Iodothyronine beta-ring monodeiodination is necessary for both T_4 conversion to T_3 and rT_3 conversion to $3,3'-T_2$. Therefore, reduced iodothyronine beta-ring monodeiodination could account for the reduced serum T_3 and elevated serum rT_3 concentrations that characterize Phase III of thyroid ontogeny (Fisher and Klein, 1981).

Little is known concerning the maturation of iodothyronine receptors and responses to thyroid hormones in the human fetus and newborn. However, it is pertinent that brain-cell T_3 binding in the rat fetus is comparable to that in the adult, whereas hepatic T_3 receptors do not mature until the first few weeks after birth (Schwartz et al., 1978; Naidoo et al., 1979). Moreover, neonatal thyroidectomy in the rat increases the number of T_3-binding sites in the brain. However, the relation between T_3 nuclear-receptor binding and brain-tissue responsiveness is unclear, since neither the adult nor the neonatal brain appears to respond to exogenous T_3 administration with an increase in oxygen consumption.

Neonatal Thyroid Function

FULL-TERM INFANT

The exposure of the fetus to the extrauterine environment results in a pronounced increase in the activity of the pituitary-thyroid system (Fisher et al., 1977; Klein et al., 1979; Jacobsen and Hummer, 1979; Fisher and Klein, 1981). At birth, there is an acute increase in circulating TSH that reaches a peak level of 70 µU/ml at 30 minutes followed by a rapid decrease during the first 24 hours, with a slower decrease over the next four days to levels less than 5 µU/ml (Fig. 55–1). The initial rise in TSH is thought to be due to cooling in the extrauterine environment.

Serum T_4 and free T_4 increase rapidly after birth, with the mean cord serum T_4 concentration increasing from 11 to 12 µg/dl to a mean peak value of 16 µg/dl at 24 to 36 hours of life. Thereafter, the serum T_4 slowly decreases to a mean value of 11 to 12 µg/dl at 6 weeks of age (Fig. 55–1). The serum T_3 and

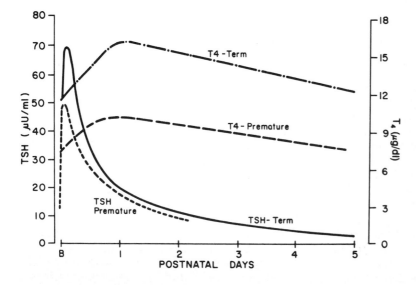

Figure 55–1. Changes in serum TSH and T_4 concentrations in full-term and premature infants during the first 5 days of life. The neonatal TSH surge peaks at 30 minutes at a level approximating 70µU per milliliter in term infants. Mean serum T_4 increases from the cord-blood value of 11 to 12µg per deciliter to a mean level of about 16µg per deciliter at 24 to 36 hours, falling gradually thereafter. In premature infants, the TSH surge and the subsequent T_4 response are both blunted. The degree of blunting is greater in small premature infants. (Data of Fisher, D. A., and Klein, A. H. Reprinted, by permission, from the New England Journal of Medicine *304*:702, 1981.) The serum T_4 in prematures may remain 20 to 40 per cent below those of full-term infants during the first 4 to 6 weeks of life (Cuestas, 1978; Jacobsen and Hummer, 1979).

free T_3, which are relatively low at birth, increase by 3- to 6-fold during the first 4 hours of life. Studies in sheep suggest this initial increase in T_3 is in large part due to an abrupt increase in peripheral conversion of T_4 to T_3 (Fisher et al., 1977; Wu et al., 1978). The stimulus for the increased conversion is unknown. Between 4 and 24 to 36 hours of life, there is a further increase in serum T_3 and free T_3 (Fig. 55–2). The second delayed T_3 peak coincides with the postnatal peak in T_4 and is thought to be due both to an increase in T_3 secretion by the thyroid and to an increase of T_4 substrate for conversion to T_3 in peripheral tissues. After 24 to 36 hours of life, the serum T_3 decreases over a 5- to 6-day period and then plateaus at a level that is within the upper normal level of older children and adults. The serum rT_3, which is relatively high at birth, remains relatively constant during the first 2 weeks of life and then gradually decreases over the next 2 to 3 weeks to levels that are equal to those found in normal older children and adults (Fig. 55–2).

PRETERM INFANT

The response of the hypothalamic-pituitary-thyroid system to birth in the preterm infant qualitatively resembles but is quantitatively less than that of the term infant (Cuestas, 1978; Uhrmann et al., 1978; Klein et al., 1979; Fisher and Klein, 1981). Circulating TSH and T_4 increase in the preterm infant in response to parturition but to a lesser degree than in the term infant (Fig. 55–1). Moreover, the serum T_4 concentration in prematures may remain 20 to 40 per cent below those of full-term infants during the first 4 to 6 weeks of life, with the lowest levels in infants under 34 weeks estimated gestational age (EGA) (Cuestas, 1978; Jacobsen and Hummer, 1979). As in full-term infants, the serum TSH decreases to less than 5 µU/ml by 1 week of age. As in term infants, there is an abrupt, albeit lesser, increase in serum T_3 levels in preterm infants during the first 2 to 4 hours of life. However, in contrast to

the further increase in term infants during the next 24 to 36 hours, there is a decrease in the serum T_3 in preterm infants. After a few days, the serum T_3 gradually increases, eventually reaching levels comparable to those of term infants at 2 to 3 weeks of age (Fig. 55–2). At birth, the serum rT_3 is higher in preterm than in term infants, but after a few days it declines to levels similar to those of term infants (Fig. 55–2).

Serum T_4 and T_3, but not rT_3, levels have reportedly been lower in small for gestational age (SGA) infants of 1 to 3 weeks of age than in appropriate for gestational age (AGA) preterm infants of comparable gestational age (Uhrmann et al., 1978).

Congenital Hypothyroidism

THYROID DYSGENESIS

Thyroid dysgenesis refers to a disorder in which there is ectopic, hypoplastic, or total agenesis of thyroid tissue. It accounts for most cases of decreased thyroid function detected by newborn screening programs. Some thyroid tissue, as detected by thyroid scanning and uptake studies, is present in 40 to 60 per cent of the infants, which accounts for the varying degree of thyroid deficiency observed in these infants. In some instances, neither thyroid scanning nor uptake testing is sensitive enough to detect small amounts of functioning tissue. Normal or near normal serum T_3 levels with low T_4 levels indicate the presence of residual thyroid tissue, even in the absence of detectable uptake on thyroid scanning (Fisher and Klein, 1981).

The etiology of thyroid dysgenesis is unknown. The disorder is most prevalent in females, with a female to male ratio of $2:1$. Although usually sporadic, familial cases have been reported and the risk is suf-

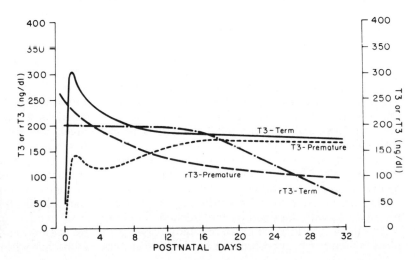

Figure 55–2. Changes in serum T_3 and rT_3 concentrations in term and premature infants during the first month of life. Values in premature infants vary with gestational age and with postnatal morbidity. (Reprinted, by permission, from the New England Journal of Medicine *304*:702, 1981.)

ficiently high to justify early thyroid hormone testing in subsequent siblings. There may be a positive family history of chronic lymphocytic thyroiditis or hyperthyroidism, particularly on the maternal side. Blizzard reported a strikingly high incidence (29 per cent) of positive antithyroid antibodies in the mothers of hypothyroid infants. However, the great majority of mothers with antibodies give birth to infants with normal thyroid function. In some infants with thyroid dysgenesis, there are other somatic abnormalities that indicate a more generalized disturbance of embryologic development. Prenatal infection has not been proved a major etiologic factor, but several reported infants have had both congenital toxoplasmosis and hypothyroidism (Andersen, 1961).

Clinical Findings. Most infants with hypothyroidism associated with thyroid dysgenesis are asymptomatic, and few have signs (except, possibly, retarded bone maturation) during the early weeks of life. Thyroid hormone is not required for fetal growth. Hypothyroid infants tend to be longer and heavier than average at birth. Lack of thyroid hormone is, however, reflected in slow skeletal maturation. Sixty to 70 per cent of infants with congenital hypothyroidism have retarded bone maturation at birth, in spite of the fact that clinical signs of hypothyroidism are absent in the great majority (Wolter et al., 1980; Klein et al., 1981). Palpation of abnormally large anterior and posterior fontanels provides an early indication of delayed skeletal development. Subtle signs of hypothyroidism in the neonatal period include lethargy, a weak suck, and poor feeding. Hypothermia and prolonged jaundice may raise suspicion of sepsis. Respiratory distress and cyanosis may also be noted. Contis and coworkers observed that the latter two findings together with heart murmurs and low-voltage P, R, and T waves led to a suspicion of congenital heart disease in one fourth of their series of hypothyroid infants. These symptoms were readily reversed by treatment.

Deviations from normal development become more apparent with age. Linear growth and weight gain are severely impaired. Feeding is listless, and the quantity of formula consumed is small. Constipation may be a very prominent complaint. Delay in motor and social development is particularly noticeable to experienced mothers. New parents may misinterpret these signs and report that theirs is an exceptionally good baby.

The complete picture of congenital hypothyroidism is unmistakable (Fig. 55–3) and includes the following criteria: The facies is grotesque, owing to widely separated eyes with puffy lids, a short retrousse nose with flattened bridge, thickened tongue protruding from the mouth held constantly open, and a low hairline over a corrugated forehead. The skin

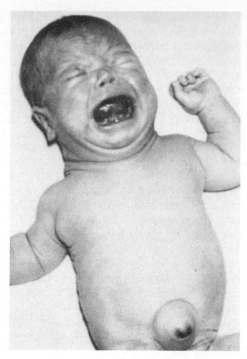

Figure 55–3. Athyrotic cretin at the age of 4 weeks. Only a few of his unusual characteristics can be distinguished from the picture. Noteworthy are the flattened bridge and uptilted tip of his shortened nose, widely separated eyes, puffiness about the eyes, large tongue, and a large umbilical hernia.

is remarkable for its pallor and coldness and is often mottled. Varying degrees of myxedema are found, chiefly involving the periorbital regions, the dorsa of the hands, and the back of the neck. Excessive fat deposition may be apparent as a "buffalo hump" or as "fatty tumors" of the anterior neck. An umbilical hernia usually crowns a protuberant abdomen. The legs are short, the hands square and spade-shaped, the fingers stubby and broad. The pulse rate is slow, even in the presence of anemia. Behavior is as characteristic as appearance. Sluggish and unresponsive, the baby moves infrequently and cries little and hoarsely. The baby is slow to cry following an unpleasant stimulus, and the crying is not sustained.

Infants with complete thyroid agenesis may attain this extreme state of clinical hypothyroidism as early as 2 months after birth. Others, with definite but ultimately inadequate remnants of thyroid tissue, may have a much milder and slower course.

Laboratory Findings. The implementation of neonatal thyroid screening programs has played an invaluable role in the early diagnosis of congenital hypothyroidism before the appearance of clinical signs or symptoms. The serum T_4 concentration is usually less than 6.5 μg/dl, and the serum TSH is greater than 60 to 70 μU in cord blood and greater than 20 μU after the second day of life. More detailed information regarding the circulating T_4 and TSH levels is found in the section on Neonatal Screening for Hypothyroidism that follows.

Although the serum T_3 may be depressed (<100 µg/ml), many infants with congenital hypothyroidism have a normal serum T_3 concentration in the presence of a low serum T_4 and elevated serum TSH (Klein et al., 1976; Larsen et al., 1981). The severity of symptoms of congenital hypothyroidism has been correlated with the concentration of T_3 in the serum. Moreover, it has been suggested that the normal serum T_3 concentration accounts for the euthyroid appearance during the early weeks of life of many neonates with congenital hypothyroidism. An elevated serum TSH in the presence of a normal serum T_3 is seemingly a paradox, since, as discussed earlier, it is the intracellular T_3 concentration in anterior pituitary cells that is of primary importance in the negative feedback regulation of TSH secretion. A possible explanation of this finding is obtained from studies that indicate that tissues such as the liver, kidney, and cardiac and skeletal muscle derive most of the intracellular T_3 from plasma, whereas in the pituitary and cerebral cortex, a substantial portion of intracellular T_3 is derived from intracellular conversion of T_4 to T_3 (Kaplan and Yaskoski, 1980; Larsen et al., 1981). Based in part on this observation, Larsen et al. have postulated the following: As the plasma T_4 declines in hypothyroidism, there is less T_4 available for conversion to T_3 in the pituitary cells, which leads to an increased secretion of TSH. In turn, the high circulating level of TSH stimulates the synthesis and release of hormone by the thyroid, with an increase in the ratio of T_3 to T_4. As a result of the shift toward direct secretion of T_3 by the thyroid, the plasma T_3 concentration is maintained at or near normal, despite a reduction in plasma T_4. The result of this compensatory change is that tissues such as kidney, liver, and cardiac and skeletal muscle, which depend on plasma T_3 for intracellular T_3, can remain metabolically euthyroid despite physiologically significant increases in TSH. Since a normal plasma T_3 in the presence of reduced plasma T_4 is not sufficient to provide normal quantities of intracellular T_3 in the pituitary and cerebral cortex, the elevated TSH secretion required to maintain this compensated state persists.

The anemia of congenital hypothyroidism may be macrocytic or normocytic and is associated with a low reticulocyte count that does not improve until thyroid replacement is begun. Unconjugated hyperbilirubinemia, secondary to delayed development of the bilirubin conjugating system, is a common associated finding.

Additional tests are helpful in assessing the severity, duration, and classification of hypothyroid states. Radiographs showing a lack of distal femoral and proximal tibial ossification centers suggest that the process begins before birth. Some epiphyseal centers may be irregularly formed, fragmented, or stippled. Uptake of radioiodine at 24 hours is zero in athyreotics and generally less than 10 per cent in infants with thyroid hypoplasia. Iodine or technetium scanning discloses a feeble uptake in the normal infant or an ectopic location of the thyroid in a substantial number of infants, conditions that would otherwise be classified as athyreosis.

Treatment. Synthetic L-thyroxine is the drug of choice for treatment of hypothyroidism. The cost is low and the potency is more uniform than desiccated thyroid. Combinations of thyroxine and T_3 produce unphysiologic and probably undesirable peaks of T_3 shortly after ingestion. By contrast, a single daily oral dose of thyroxine produces steady physiologic levels of both hormones. The initial starting dose of L-thyroxine is 10 µg/kg rounded off to the nearest 12.5, 25.0, and 37.5 µg to coincide with the potency of available thyroxine tablets (Klein, 1979). After 3 to 4 months, when the initially high normal values of circulating T_4 and T_3 have returned close to the normal values of older children and adults, the dose is 7 µg/kg/day up to 10 kg, plus 3.0 to 3.5 µg for each kg between 11 and 20 kg, plus 1.5 µg for each kg over 20 kg. These are average values and are adjusted according to the clinical response of the child and circulating T_4 and TSH concentrations. The therapeutic aim in early infancy is to maintain the circulating T_4 level between 10 and 14 µg/dl and the circulating TSH at less than 20 µU/ml. Early in infancy, the TSH response to adequate thyroxine replacement may be sluggish. In some patients with adequate replacement therapy, the TSH concentrations are normal 2 to 6 weeks after beginning treatment. In others, however, the TSH falls to about 40 µU/ml and remains around this level for 6 months to 1 year. The reason for this is unknown but reflects resistance of TSH suppression by normal circulating levels of T_4 and T_3 levels in the early months of treatment of congenital hypothyroidism.

Prognosis. The initiation of thyroid hormone replacement brings rapid improvement in appearance, appetite, activity, skin color, myxedema, and constipation. It is useful to warn the parents that their child will experience hair loss as a new crop of growing hairs displaces the resting hairs. With lifelong thyroid hormone replacement, the prospects for normal health and physical growth are excellent. However, the prospects for mental development are less certain. In general, it is believed that the prognosis for mental development depends on the severity of hypothyroidism and the duration of the disorder prior to treatment. Thyroid hormone deficiency during the proliferative phase of brain growth may result in permanent impairment of brain function. Human brain DNA content and, therefore, cell number undergo a rapid increase in the third trimester and approach adult levels by 5 years of age (Winick, 1968). Several studies of the outcome of hypothyroid infants emphasize the importance of early recognition and treatment (Collipp et al., 1965; Raiti and Newns, 1971; Klein et al., 1972; Mäenpää, 1972). Both Mäenpää and Klein and coworkers reported that 80 per cent of hypothyroid infants treated before 3 months of age had I.Q. scores above 85 as opposed to about 45 per cent of those treated after that age.

The goals of neonatal thyroid screening programs are to prevent mental retardation and more subtle neuropsychologic handicaps by early diagnosis and treatment of congenital hypothyroidism. Careful follow-up studies are required to assess the results of the screening programs fully and accurately. However, encouraging early results were recently reported by the New England Regional Screening Program (Klein et al., 1981). In this study, psychometric testing was carried out at 1 and 2 years with the Bayley developmental scales and at 3 and 4 years with the revised Stanford-Binet scales in the following groups of children: (1) those with congenital hypothyroidism treated at age of 25 ± 10 days—before the appearance of clinical manifestation, (2) those with congenital hypothyroidism who were diagnosed at birth because of gross clinical findings and treated at 5 to 15 days, and (3) those constituting the control group—normal siblings and euthyroid children. The mean I.Q. scores of the infants treated before the appearance of clinical signs were similar to those of the control group (106 ± 16) and showed a normal distribution. By contrast, low I.Q. scores were observed in three of four children in whom hypothyroidism was diagnosed at birth. This study suggests that children with congenital hypothyroidism treated adequately before clinically diagnostic signs and symptoms appear are protected against mental retardation seen in hypothyroid infants treated only after a clinical diagnosis can be made. Whether or not the children with apparently normal I.Q. scores will manifest specific learning disabilities or other neuropsychologic handicaps at an older age remains to be seen.

INBORN ERRORS OF THYROID HORMONE SYNTHESIS

The second most frequent cause of permanent congenital hypothyroidism is an inborn error of thyroid synthesis, which accounts for 10 to 15 per cent of cases of congenital hypothyroidism. The estimated incidence is one in 30,000 to 50,000 livebirths in North America and Europe (Fisher and Klein, 1981). Hereditary defects may occur during any one of the five enzymatic steps required for thyroid hormone synthesis and release. A detailed discussion of the various enzymatic abnormalities is beyond the scope of this discussion but may be found in an excellent recent review (Stanbury et al., 1979). In each case,

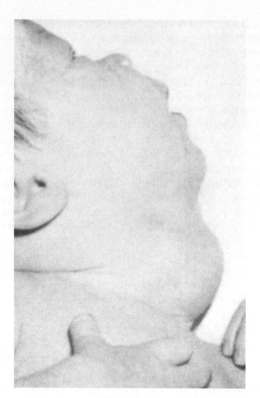

Figure 55–4. Note the large mass bulging forward in the midline of the neck. No details of the cretinoid facies can be detected in this lateral view.

the disease has an autosomal recessive mode of inheritance. Female infants with an inborn error of thyroid synthesis only slightly outnumber similarly affected males. Goiter may occur at birth in association with this disorder, but in most instances it develops in the early months or years of life (Fig. 55–4). Except in infants with a defect in iodine-concentrating ability, there is normal or increased thyroid radioiodine uptake in infants with an inborn error of thyroid synthesis in contrast to the reduced uptake in infants with thyroid dysgenesis. As in infants with thyroid dysgenesis, the serum T_4 is depressed, and the serum TSH is elevated. Some may be partly compensated with low serum T_4, normal T_3, and elevated TSH (Delange et al., 1980), and others may be totally compensated with normal T_4 and T_3 but elevated TSH levels.

Treatment of hypothyroidism due to an inborn error of thyroid synthesis is identical with treatment of hypothyroidism associated with thyroid dysgenesis. The goiters regress with adequate treatment. The prognosis for mental development depends on both the severity of the defect and the duration of hypothyroidism prior to treatment.

DEFICIENT TSH SECRETION OR EFFECT

Congenital hypothyroidism results from TSH deficiency, which may occur as a primary disorder of pituitary secretion of TSH or secondary to TRH deficiency or insensitivity. Affected infants may have anomalous hypothalamic or pituitary development or a sporadic or familial deficiency in TRH or TSH secretion with or without other pituitary hormone deficiencies. Several syndromes have been reported, including hypothalamic hypothyroidism with TRH deficiency or insensitivity, isolated TSH deficiency, congenital absence of the pituitary, and familial panhypopituitarism with absence of the sella turcica (Miyai et al., 1976; Stanbury et al., 1979; Dussault et al., 1980). TSH deficiency that occurs in association with growth hormone deficiency may present with hypoglycemia as well as micropenis in male infants. Infants with hypothalamic (tertiary) hypothyroidism due to TRH deficiency have low serum T_4, T_3, and free T_4 levels, whereas the serum TSH may be either in a low range or slightly elevated. The administration of TRH to these infants produces a normal or prolonged TSH response. Infants with pituitary TSH deficiency (secondary hypothyroidism) have low serum T_4, T_3, and free T_4 levels with low or unmeasurable levels of TSH and do not manifest a TSH response to TRH. Hypothyroidism that occurs secondary to hypothalamic-pituitary disorders is usually less severe than that observed in infants with primary hypothyroidism.

Thyroid gland unresponsiveness to TSH is a rare cause of congenital hypothyroidism (Stanbury et al., 1968, 1979; Codaccioni et al., 1980). The affected patients have depressed serum T_4 and T_3 concentrations and elevated serum TSH levels. Thyroid uptake of radiolabeled iodine and thyroid scan are normal. An inborn error of thyroid hormone synthesis is ruled out by appropriate biologic investigations. The stimulatory effect of TSH is mediated through the adenylate cyclase system. In vivo and in vitro evidence indicates that the thyroid gland unresponsiveness to TSH in these patients is due to a defect in the coupling mechanism between the TSH receptor and adenylate cyclase. Treatment of hypothyroidism associated with these disorders is identical with treatment of primary hypothyroidism, described previously.

TRANSIENT HYPOTHYROIDISM

Transient hypothyroidism, characterized by low serum T_4 and elevated serum TSH, is usually due to the ingestion of goitrogenic substances by the mother. The goitrogenic substances that have been implicated include iodides, thioureas, sulfonamides, and hematinic preparations containing cobalt. In the affected neonates, hypothyroidism is usually associated with goiter. It is of interest that transient hypothyroidism has been reported in infants bathed with iodine-containing antiseptic agents or exposed to iodine or iodine-containing agents during gestation (Castaign et al., 1979; Rodesch et al., 1976). Hypothyroidism and goiter may occur in infants of mothers receiving more than 300 mg of propylthiouracil per day. Doses of 300 mg or less of propylthiouracil are thought to afford satisfactory control

of maternal hyperthyroidism and are not ordinarily regarded as causes of clinically evident thyroid dysfunction in the neonate. However, a recent report indicates that infants born to hyperthyroid mothers treated with low dose propylthiouracil (100 to 200 mg/day) are clinically euthyroid but have biochemical evidence (low T_4 and elevated TSH) of mild, transient hypothyroidism (Cheron et al., 1981). Neonatal goiter and hypothyroidism secondary to maternal ingestion of goitrogens are usually of short duration and disappear spontaneously. If the goiter is sufficiently large to cause dyspnea or if hypothyroidism is present, it is advisable to treat with full substitution with thyroid hormone. It may be necessary to interrupt breast feeding, since thiourea drugs and iodides are secreted in breast milk. If tracheal compression by the goiter is severe, tracheal decompression by surgical resection of the thyroid isthmus is indicated.

Transient neonatal hypothyroidism and endemic cretinism have been related to iodine deficiency in certain parts of the world (Delange et al., 1980). Endemic cretinism is usually, but not always, associated with goiter at birth.

Neonatal thyroid screening programs have turned up a small number of infants with transient hypothyroidism in whom there is no history of either maternal ingestion of goitrogen or iodine deficiency (LaFranchi et al., 1977; Delange et al., 1978; Mitchell and Larsen, 1980; Dussault et al., 1980). These infants have low serum T_4, low or normal serum T_3, and elevated serum TSH levels during the early days and weeks of life. In one study most, but not all, cases occurred in premature infants, whereas in other studies the relative prevalence in premature and full-term infants was not reported. In six infants with transient hypothyroidism reported by Delante and coworkers in 1978, the bone ages were normal and the thyroid gland was in a normal position, as indicated by scintigram; the physical and psychomotor development of these infants appeared normal in the follow-up period. The infants did not appear hypothyroid, and the abnormal thyroid function tests reverted to normal by 2 to 4 months of age. The prevalence of this abnormality ranged from one in 46,000 to one in 150,000 in the different screening programs. These infants were recognized in one of two ways. First, after initial screening values indicated hypothyroidism, some infants were lost to recall temporarily so that treatment was not started. Serum for confirmation was not obtained until 4 to 8 weeks of age, at which time the hormonal values were normal. Second, in some children normal hormonal values and clinical conditions were maintained when replacement therapy was discontinued after several years. Infants with transient neonatal hypothyroidism are usually diagnosed as having primary hypothyroidism, which is considered permanent, and are treated accordingly. Therefore, in many cases the definitive diagnosis will be delayed until thyroid medication is withheld at some later date in childhood. It is possible that future studies will demonstrate that the prevalence of transient neonatal hypothyroidism is greater than that currently reported by neonatal screening programs. The cause of transient neonatal hypothyroidism, in which there is no history of maternal ingestion of goitrogen or iodine deficiency, is unknown. It has been speculated that the disorder is secondary to transient decreased thyroid gland responsiveness to TSH or to a transient block in thyroid hormone synthesis (Fisher and Klein, 1981).

TRANSIENT LOW T_4 LEVELS IN PRETERM INFANTS

Serum T_4 levels increase with gestational age, so it is not surprising that relatively low serum levels are observed in premature infants. In a recent study of 215 consecutive premature births, 53 per cent of infants born after 28 to 30 weeks gestation and 25 per cent of all premature infants under 37 weeks gestation had cord serum T_4 levels below 6.5 µg/dl (Hadeed et al., 1981; Fisher and Klein, 1981). These low levels persisted during the first week in association with low free T_4 values, normal serum TSH levels, and normal responses of TSH and T_4 to TRH. Serum T_4 levels increased gradually to normal over a period of 4 to 20 weeks. Growth and development of these infants were reportedly normal, as were the Gesell developmental scores at 12 months of age. In another study, serum T_4 levels below 3 µg/dl with normal TSH levels were common among preterm infants during the early days of life, especially among infants with hyaline membrane disease and SGA infants (Uhrmann, 1981). The T_3-charcoal uptake, an indirect measurement of serum T_4–binding capacity, was normal. By 3 weeks of age, the serum T_4 had risen to at least 4 µg/dl in most of the infants.

The transient low serum T_4 levels in these infants is most probably due to hypothalamic immaturity (Fisher and Klein, 1981). The low serum free T_4 levels and normal serum TSH associated with a normal TSH response to TRH are characteristic of hypothalamic hypothyroidism. Moreover, the pattern and course of maturation of serum T_4 levels and, presumably, hypothalamic-pituitary function appear similar in the intrauterine fetus and premature infant.

NEONATAL SCREENING FOR HYPOTHYROIDISM

The incidence of apparent permanent congenital hypothyroidism detected by screening programs is one in every 3500 to 5000 livebirths. Screening for hypothyroidism in the newborn period can be per-formed by measuring T_4 or TSH concentrations in cord blood or in the infant's capillary blood in the first week of life. Screening with TSH gives fewer false-positive results but will miss the unusual case of hypothyroidism that is due to circulating TSH deficiency. T_4 concentrations less than 6.5 µg/dl and TSH concentrations greater than 60 to 70 µU/ml are found in the cord blood of infants with congenital primary hypothyroidism (Klein et al., 1974; Walfish, 1976). The relatively high level of TSH (up to 60 or 70 µU/ml) that may be found in the cord blood of normal infants reflects the neonatal surge in circulating TSH that occurs on exposure to the extrauterine environment and peaks at 30 minutes.

In North America, screening is usually accomplished by measuring T_4 concentrations on filter paper specimens of capillary blood that are drawn concomitantly with blood specimens for PKU testing at 2 to 5 days of life. In the New England Screening Program (Klein, 1979), other filter paper specimens are analyzed for TSH if the T_4 concentration is less than 6.0 µg/dl. An infant with a T_4 concentration less than 6.0 µg/dl and a TSH level of greater than 20 µU/ml is considered to have primary hypothyroidism, and the physician is advised to draw blood and to begin treatment while awaiting results of confirmatory tests unless there are known factors suggesting transient hypothyroidism, such as maternal ingestion of iodine or antithyroid drugs. In the experience of the New England Screening Program, only one third of the infants have permanent hypothyroidism when the TSH concentration is between 20 and 40 µU/ml. The other two thirds have either transient hypothyroidism or a low T_4 concentration for other reasons and a slightly elevated TSH because the blood specimen was drawn before the TSH had reverted to below 20 µU/ml after the initial postnatal TSH rise.

In 2.5 per cent of newborns in the New England Screening Program, the T_4 concentrations are less than 6 µg/dl, and the circulating TSH concentrations are normal. Most of these instances are associated with prematurity, obstetric or neonatal stress, or illness, but some are unrelated to any known factors. In 98 per cent of the infants who have screening values of T_4 less than 6 µg/dl and normal TSH the T_4 will return to normal by 1 month of age. From a practical standpoint, it has been observed that no infant with a T_4 concentration between 4 and 6 µg/dl and normal TSH has turned out to have hypothyroidism, hypopituitarism, or TBG deficiency; such infants are no longer followed by the New England Screening Program.

In this program, a screening serum T_4 value below 4 µg/dl and a concomitant normal TSH occur in 0.9 per cent of all births and in 8 to 16 per cent of premature infants. In these instances, repeat testing is performed at 6 to 8 weeks. If the T_4 value remains unchanged in the presence of normal TSH, it suggests either TBG deficiency or hypothalamic-pituitary deficiency. The incidence of TBG deficiency is one per 9000 to one per 14,000 births, and the diagnosis of this disorder is made by measuring TBG in serum (see later section). If TBG is normal, then provocative testing with TRH is advised for testing for hypothyroidism secondary to hypothalamic-pituitary deficiency (approximate incidence, one per 110,000 births). As discussed earlier, the circulating TSH response to TRH serves to differentiate hypothalamic (tertiary) from pituitary (secondary) hypothyroidism. Other tests of pituitary function such as growth hormone and ACTH secretion may be indicated.

In an occasional infant with a screening T_4 less than 4.0 μg/dl and a normal TSH, the serum T_4 will remain low and the TSH will increase to abnormally high values over the first few weeks of life. This evolution of biochemical findings of primary hypothyroidism may be associated with the gradual appearance of subtle clinical manifestations of hypothyroidism (Mitchell and Larsen, 1980). It is apparent that these infants should be treated with L-thyroxine.

As noted earlier, in most premature infants with low screening T_4 values and normal TSH, the serum T_4 levels gradually rise to normal over a 4- to 20-week period, and the infants grow and develop normally. It would appear, therefore, that only selected premature infants with low screening serum T_4 and normal serum TSH levels will require additional studies, although follow-up determinations of serum T_4 and TSH levels should be performed routinely.

In one neonatal screening program, falsely elevated serum TSH values were found in infants with normal serum T_3 and T_4 levels (Gendrel et al., 1981). The falsely elevated TSH levels were due to the placental transfer of an antirabbit factor from mothers who recently received injections of a microbial vaccine cultured on a rabbit lung–containing medium. The antirabbit factor interfered with the immunoassay procedure for TSH, producing artificially elevated values of this hormone.

Euthyroid Sick (Low T_3) Syndrome

The euthyroid sick (low T_3) syndrome is observed in acutely or chronically ill premature infants, including those with the respiratory distress syndrome. The increases in both serum TSH and T_4 that normally occur after delivery may be blunted, and T_4 levels may remain lower than those of well premature infants. Although an abrupt increase in serum T_3 occurs after delivery in affected infants, the levels usually decrease by 12 hours, probably as a result of secondary inhibition of T_4 to T_3 conversion. Serum rT_3 levels resemble those of otherwise well premature infants or may be increased. Free T_4 levels are normal for fetal age and size in most infants. Low total serum T_4 levels are occasionally observed, possibly as a result of an inhibitor of T_4 binding to TBG. In summary, the characteristic biochemical features of the low T_3 syndrome are (1) low serum T_3, (2) normal or elevated serum rT_3, (3) variable serum T_4 with normal or possibly elevated free T_4, and (4) normal serum TSH.

The low T_3 syndrome is not strictly a functional maturational defect but appears to be the effect of nonthyroidal illnesses on various aspects of thyroid metabolism resembling what is observed in acutely or chronically ill older children and adults (Cavalieri and Rapoport, 1977; Chopra et al., 1978; Fisher and Klein, 1981). In small premature infants, the low T_3 syndrome may, in part, be related to a state of malnutrition that is sometimes present in these infants. Weight loss or malnutrition is known to be associated with low T_3 levels. It has been suggested that a decrease in serum T_3 level and an increase in inactive rT_3 may protect the body by reducing the metabolic rate and protein catabolism during illness. This could serve to protect the premature infant if tissue oxygenation is marginal. The abnormal thyroid functions return to normal as the sick premature infants improve.

Some studies have suggested that thyroid function, as reflected in low T_4 and T_3 and elevated TSH in cord blood, is decreased in infants who develop RDS (Redding et al., 1974; Cuestas et al., 1976; Abbassi et al., 1977). However, other authors have not been able to substantiate this observation (Uhrmann et al., 1978; Klein et al., 1979, 1981), suggesting that the maturation of the hypothalamic-pituitary-thyroid axis and the pathways of peripheral metabolism of thyroid hormone are not delayed in infants who subsequently develop RDS. This is consistent with the thesis that the abnormal thyroid hormone values found during the early days of life in infants with RDS are secondary to illness (euthyroid sick syndrome) rather than to a defect in thyroid system maturation.

Alterations in Serum T_4 and T_3 Secondary to Alterations in TBG

As previously discussed, 99.98 per cent of total serum T_4 and 99.7 per cent of total serum T_3 are bound to protein. The major transport protein for both is TBG. TBG appears at about the twelfth week of intrauterine life and doubles between 24 and 30 weeks gestation with no further change up to birth (Greenberg et al., 1970; Fisher et al., 1977). In the newborn infant, serum TBG is about 1.5 times higher than the normal adult level, probably as a result of transplacental passage of maternal estrogens. The serum TBG concentrations are not significantly different in term, AGA preterm and SGA infants (Jacobsen and Hummer, 1979).

Familial TBG deficiency is transmitted as an X-linked trait. TBG-binding capacity is low or undetectable in affected males and approximately half-normal in affected females (Stanbury et al., 1979). The total serum T_4 and T_3 levels vary similarly and are reduced, whereas the serum free T_4 and T_3 levels are normal. Occasionally, there is an artificially low free T_4 level with very low or absent TBG levels that is presumably due to technical difficulties in measuring the dialyzable T_4 fraction. The serum TSH levels are normal, as is the TSH response to TRH. The infants are clinically euthyroid.

Familial TBG excess also appears to be transmitted as an X-linked trait (Stanbury et al., 1979). Affected males have markedly elevated TBG-binding capacity, whereas females have an intermediate elevation. In TBG excess, serum T_4, T_3, and free T_4 levels are high-normal or elevated, whereas free T_3 is usually normal.

Like those infants with TBG deficiency, infants with TBG excess are clinically euthyroid and have normal serum TSH levels and a normal TSH response to TRH.

Neonatal Hyperthyroidism

Thyrotoxicosis is a rare condition in the newborn and usually occurs in infants born to mothers known to have Graves' disease either prior to or during pregnancy. Most, but not all, of the infants have a brief self-limited disorder that disappears spontaneously in approximately 3 months. It is thought that neonatal thyrotoxicosis results from transplacental passage of thyroid-stimulating immunoglobulins of the IgG class from the mother. The association of neonatal thyrotoxicosis with maternal Graves' disease and the self-limited course of the disorder are consistent with this thesis. One such immunoglobulin that has been found in both mother and neonate with Graves' disease is long-acting thyroid stimulator, or LATS. LATS is determined by a bioassay procedure in the mouse. However, there has been doubt concerning the pathogenic role of LATS because (1) neonatal thyrotoxicosis may occur in infants without detectable LATS in their serum, (2) mothers with detectable serum LATS may give birth to normal infants, and (3) the course of neonatal thyrotoxicosis does not necessarily correspond with the disappearance rate of LATS (Hollingsworth et al., 1975). Moreover, more recent evidence indicates that LATS, which is present in the serum of about 50 per cent of adults with Graves' disease, happens to have the ability to stimulate the mouse thyroid gland but may not be able to stimulate the human thyroid. More recent attention has focused on other Graves'-related IgG's that interact with human thyroid tissue. The Graves' IgG's are polyclonal and of various specificities, especially for

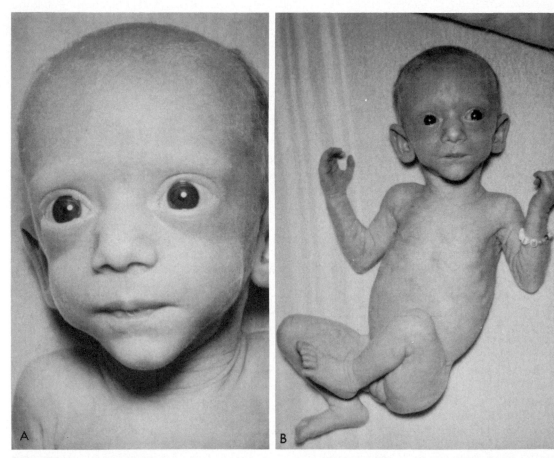

Figure 55–5. This transiently hyperthyroid infant of a hyperthyroid mother had a persistent stare and tachycardia, and she failed to gain weight despite a ravenous appetite. Her thyroid gland was not palpable. (Photograph of a case of Drs. R. T. and J. Kirkland, reproduced with their kind permission.)

nonhuman TSH receptors. Almost all the patients negative in the LATS assay have IgG's that block the ability of LATS$^+$ serum to stimulate the mouse thyroid (i.e., that block receptors but do not stimulate). However, almost all these patients' IgG's (LATS$^+$ and LATS$^-$ alike) stimulate human thyroid tissue and appear to be the probable cause of the hyperthyroidism. This has not been looked at specifically in neonatal Graves' disease but is probably true in that situation as well.

In addition to goiter, prematurity, exophthalmos, hyperirritability, enormous appetite, failure to gain weight, tachycardia, congestive failure, jaundice, hepatosplenomegaly, and thrombocytopenia are among the clinical features of hyperthyroidism in the newborn (Fig. 55–5). Tracheal obstruction due to a large goiter may occur. Premature synostosis of cranial sutures in some of the infants is attributable to high levels of thyroid hormone, since a similar association has been observed in hypothyroid infants treated with extremely high doses of thyroid hormone. Although neonatal hyperthyroidism is usually transient, it may persist for years. It is possible that the pathogenesis of the transient and persistent forms of the disorder are different. Neonatal thyrotoxicosis is not innocuous, and mortality rates of 15 to 20 per cent have been reported. Thyroid storm may produce a rapidly downhill course.

Treatment is based on severity of the symptoms. Close observation with no specific therapy is appropriate for mildly affected infants with a self-limited course. In moderately affected infants, 10 mg of propylthiouracil may be given every 8 hours orally. In more severe cases, propranolol in a dosage of 2 mg/kg/day may be used. Although iodides, 1 drop every 8 hours, may be used in conjunction with propylthiouracil, it is suggested that iodides be used only in the most severe cases (i.e., those requiring rapid metabolic control) because the thyroid-blocking effect is of limited duration and high thyroidal iodine opposes the action of propylthiouracil (Van Wyk and Fisher, 1977). Supportive measures include oxygen, digitalis when needed, provision of adequate nutrition (calories/glucose), and precautions to prevent tracheal obstruction by a large goiter. Rarely surgery may be necessary to relieve tracheal obstruction.

REFERENCES

Abbassi, V., Merchant, K., and Abramson, D.: Postnatal triiodothyronine concentrations in healthy preterm infants and in infants with respiratory distress syndrome. Pediatr. Res. 11:802, 1977.

Abuid, J., Stinson, D. A., and Larsen, P. R.: Serum triiodothyronine and thyronine in the neonate and acute increases in these hormones following delivery. J. Clin. Invest. 52:1195, 1973.

Andersen, H. J.: Studies in hypothyroidism in children. Acta Paediatr. 125:(Suppl.)1, 1961.

Baxter, J. D., Eberhardt, N. L., Apriletti, J. W., Johnson, L. K., Ivarie, R. D., Schachter, B. S., Morris, J. A., Seeburg, P. H., Goodman, H. M., Latham, K. R., Polansky, J. R., and Martial, J. A.: Thyroid hormone receptors and responses. Recent Prog. Hormone Res. 35:97, 1979.

Blizzard, R. M., Chandler, R. W., Landing, B. H., Petit, M. D., and West, D. C.: Maternal autoimmunization as a probable cause of athyreotic cretinism. N. Engl. J. Med. 263:327, 1960.

Castaign, H., Fournet, J. P., Leger, F. A., et al.: Thyroid of the newborn and postnatal iodine overload. Arch. Fr. Pediatr. 36:356, 1979.

Cavalieri, R. R., and Rapoport, B.: Impaired peripheral conversion of thyroxine to triiodothyronine. Annu. Rev. Med. 28:57, 1977.

Cheron, R. G., Kaplan, M. M., Larsen, R. P., Selenkow, H. A., and Crigler, J. F., Jr.: Neonatal thyroid function after propylthiouracil therapy for maternal Graves' Disease. N. Engl. J. Med. 304:525, 1981.

Chopra, I. J., Sack, J., and Fisher, D. A.: Circulating 3,3',5'-triiodothyronine (reverse T$_3$) in the human newborn. J. Clin. Invest. 55:1137, 1975.

Chopra, I. J., Solomon, D. H., Chopra, U., Wu, S. Y., Fisher, D. A., and Nakamura, Y.: Pathways of metabolism of thyroid hormones. Recent Prog. Hormone Res. 34:521, 1978.

Codaccioni, J. L., Carayon, P., Michael-Bechet, M., Foucault, F., Lefort, G., and Pierron, H.: Congenital hypothyroidism associated with thyrotropin unresponsiveness and thyroid cell membrane alterations. J. Clin. Endocrinol. Metab. 50:932, 1980.

Collipp, P. J., Kaplan, S. A., Kogut, M. D., et al.: Mental retardation in congenital hypothyroidism: improvement with thyroid replacement therapy. Am. J. Ment. Defic. 40:432, 1965.

Contis, G., Nadas, A. S., and Crigler, J. F., Jr.: Cardiac manifestations of congenital hypothyroidism in infants. Pediatrics 38:452, 1966.

Cuestas, R. A.: Thyroid function in healthy premature infants. J. Pediatr. 92:963, 1978.

Cuestas, R. A., Lindall, A., and Engel, R. R.: Low thyroid hormones and respiratory distress syndrome of the newborn. N. Engl. J. Med. 295:297, 1976.

Delange, F., Dodion, J. Wolter, R., et al.: Transient hypothyroidism in the newborn infant. J. Pediatr. 92:974, 1978.

Delange, F., Beckers, C., Höfer, R. König, M. P., Monaco, F., and Varrone, S.: Progress report on neonatal screening for congenital hypothyroidism in Europe. In Burrow, G. N., and Dussault, J. H. (Eds.): Neonatal Thyroid Screening. New York, Raven Press, 1980, pp. 107–131.

Dussault, J. H., Mitchell, M. L., LaFranchi, S., and Murphey, W. H.: Regional screening for congenital hypothyroidism: results of screening one million North American infants with filter paper spot T4-TSH. In Burrow, G. N., and Dussault, J. H. (Eds.): Neonatal Thyroid Screening. New York, Raven Press, 1980, pp. 155–165.

Fisher, D. A., Dussault, J. H., Sack, J., and Chopra, I. J.: Ontogenesis of hypothalamic-pituitary-thyroid function and metabolism in man, sheep, and rat. Recent Prog. Hormone Res. 33:59, 1977.

Fisher, D. A., and Klein, A. H.: Thyroid development and disorders of the thyroid in the newborn. N. Engl. J. Med. 304:702, 1981.

Florsheim, W. H.: Control of thyrotropin secretion. In Knobil, E., and Sawyer, W. H. (Eds.): Handbook of Physiology, Section 7: Endocrinology. Vol. IV, The Pituitary Gland and Its Neuroendocrine Control. Baltimore, Williams and Wilkins, 1974.

Gavin, L. A., Bui, F., McMahon, F., and Cavalieri, R. R.: Sequential deiodination of thyroxine to 3,3'-diiodothyronine via 3,5,3'-triiodothyronine and 3,3',5'-triiodothyronine in rat liver homogenate. The effects of fasting versus glucose feeding. J. Biol. Chem. 254:49, 1980.

Gendrel, D., Feinstein, M. C., Grenier, J., et al.: Falsely elevated serum TSH in newborn infants: transfer from mothers to infants of a factor interfering in the TSH radioimmunoassay. J. Clin. Endocrinol. Metab. 52:62, 1981.

Greenberg, A. H., Czernichow, P., Reba, R. D., Tyson, J., and Blizzard, R. M.: Observations on the maturation of thyroid function in early fetal life. J. Clin. Invest. 49:1790, 1970.

Hadeed, A., Asay, L., Klein, A. H., and Fisher, D. A.: The significance of transient hypothyroxinemia in premature infants with and without respiratory distress syndrome. Pediatrics 68:494, 1981.

Hollingsworth, D. R., and Marby, C. C.: Congenital Graves' disease. In Fisher, D. A., and Burrow, G. N. (Eds.): Perinatal Thyroid Physiology and Disease. New York, Raven Press, 1975, pp. 163–183.

Ingbar, S. H.: Effects of iodine: autoregulation of the thyroid. In Werner, S. C., and Ingbar, S. H. (Eds.): The Thyroid. Hagerstown, Harper and Row, 1978.

Ingbar, S. H., and Woeber, K. A.: The thyroid gland. In Williams, R. H. (Ed.): Textbook of Endocrinology. Philadelphia, W. B. Saunders Co., 1981, pp. 117–247.

Jacobsen, B. B., Andersen, H., Dige-Petersen, H., and Hummer, L.: Thyroid response to thyrotropin-releasing hormone in full-term, euthyroid, and hypothyroid newborns. Acta Paediatr. Scand. 65:433, 1975.

Jacobsen, B. B., Andersen, H., Dige-Petersen, H., and Hummer, L.: Pituitary-thyroid responsiveness to thyrotropin-releasing hormone in preterm and small-for-gestational age newborns. Acta Paediatr. Scand. 66:541, 1977.

Jacobsen, B. B., and Hummer, L.: Changes in serum concentrations of thyroid hormones and thyroid hormone–binding proteins during early infancy. Acta Paediatr. Scand. 68:411, 1979.

Kaplan, M. M.: Thyroid metabolism in adult, fetal, and neonatal life. In Dussault, J. H. (Ed.): Congenital Hypothyroidism. New York, Marcel Dekker (In press.)

Kaplan, M. M., and Yaskoski, K. A.: Phenolic and tyrosyl ring iodothyronine deiodination in rat brain homogenates. J. Clin. Invest. 66:551, 1980.

Klein, A. H., Agustin, A. V., and Foley, T. P.: Successful laboratory screening for congenital hypothyroidism. Lancet 2:77, 1974.

Klein, A. H., Foley, B., Foley, T. P., MacDonald, M. M., and Fisher, M. D.: Thyroid function studies in cord blood from premature infants with and without RDS. J. Pediatr. 98:818, 1981.

Klein, A. H., Foley, B., Kenny, F. M., and Fisher, D. A.: Thyroid hormone and thyrotropin responses to parturition in premature infants with and without the respiratory distress syndrome. Pediatrics 63:380, 1979.

Klein, A. H., Foley, T. P., Jr., Larsen, P. R., Agustin, A. V., and Hopwood, N. J.: Neonatal thyroid function in congenital hypothyroidism. J. Pediatr. 89:545, 1976.

Klein, A. H., Hobel, C. J., Sack, J., and Fisher, D. A.: Effect of intraamniotic thyroxine injection on fetal serum and amniotic fluid iodothyronine concentrations. J. Clin. Endocrinol. Metab. 47:1034, 1978.

Klein, A. H., Meltzer, S., and Kenny, F. M.: Improved prognosis in congenital hypothyroidism treated before 3 months. J. Pediatr. 81:912, 1972.

Klein, R. Z.: Neonatal screening for hypothyroidism. In Barness, L. A. (Ed.): Advances in Pediatrics. Chicago, Year Book Publishers, 1979, pp. 417–440.

Klein, R. Z.: Effects of screening for hypothyroidism: prevention of mental retardation by treatment before clinical manifestations. New England Congenital Hypothyroid Collaborative. Lancet 2:1095, 1981.

LaFranchi, S. H., Buist, N. R. M., Murphey, W. H., Larsen, P. R., and Foley, T. P., Jr.: Transient neonatal hypothyroidism detected by newborn screening program. Pediatrics 60:538, 1977.

Larsen, P. R., Silva, J. E., and Kaplan, M. M.: Relationships between circulating and intracellular thyroid hormones: physiological and clinical implications. Endocrine Rev. 2:87, 1981.

Leonard, J. G., Kaplan, M. M., Visser, T. J., Silva, J. E., and Larsen,

R. P.: Cerebral cortex responds rapidly to thyroid hormones. Science 214:571, 1981.

Mäenpää, J.: Congenital hypothyroidism: aetiological and clinical aspects. Arch. Dis. Child. 47:914, 1972.

Mitchell, M. L., and Larsen, P. R.: Screening for congenital hypothyroidism in New England using the T4-TSH strategy. In Burrow, G. N., and Dussault, J. H. (Eds.): Neonatal Thyroid Screening. New York, Raven Press, 1980, pp. 95–105.

Miyai, K., Azukizawa, M., Onishi, T., et al.: Familial isolated thyrotropin deficiency. In James, V. H. T. (Ed.): Endocrinology. Amsterdam, Excerpta Medica, 1976, pp. 345–349. (International Congress Series no. 403.)

Naidoo, S., Valcana, T., and Timiras, P. S.: Thyroid hormone receptors in the developing rat brain. Am. Zool. 18:545, 1979.

Oddie, T. H., Bernard, B., Klein, A. H., and Fisher, D. A.: Comparison of T4, T3, rT3, and TSH concentrations in cord blood and serum of infants up to 3 months of age. Early Hum. Dev. 3:239, 1979.

Oppenheimer, J. H., Schwartz, H. L., Surks, M. I., Koerner, D., and Dillman, W. H.: Nuclear receptors and the initiation of thyroid hormone action. Recent Prog. Hormone Res. 32:529, 1976.

Pardridge, W. M.: Carrier-mediated transport of thyroid hormones through the rat blood-brain barrier: primary role of albumin-bound hormone. Endocrinology 105:605, 1979.

Pardridge, W. M., and Mietus, L. J.: Influx of thyroid hormones into rat liver in vivo. J. Clin. Invest. 66:367, 1980.

Raiti, S., and Newns, G. H.: Cretinism: early diagnosis and its relation to mental prognosis. Arch. Dis. Child. 46:692, 1971.

Redding, R. A., and Pereria, C.: Thyroid function in respiratory distress syndrome (RDS) of the newborn. Pediatrics 54:423, 1974.

Reichlin, S.: Neuroendocrine control. In Werner, S. C., and Ingbar, S. H., (Eds.): The Thyroid. Hagerstown, Harper and Row, 1978.

Rodesch, F., Camus, M., Ermans, A. M., Dodion, J., and Delange, F.: Adverse effect of amniofetography on fetal thyroid function. Am. J. Obstet. Gynecol. 126:723, 1976.

Schwartz, H. L., and Oppenheimer, J. H.: Ontogenesis of 3,5,3′-triiodothyronine. Endocrinology 103:943, 1978.

Stanbury, J. B., Aiginger, P., and Harbison, M. D.: Familial goiter and related disorders. In DeGroot, L. J., Cahill, J. F., Jr., Odell, W. D., et al. (Eds.): Endocrinology. New York, Grune & Stratton, 1979, pp. 523–539.

Stanbury, J. B., Rocmans, P., Buhler, U. K., and Ochi, Y.: Congenital hypothyroidism with impaired thyroid response to thyrotropin. N. Engl. J. Med. 279:1132, 1968.

Theodoropoulos, T., Braverman, L. E., and Vagenakis, A. G.: Iodide-induced hypothyroidism: a potential hazard during perinatal life. Science 205:502, 1979.

Uhrmann, S., Marks, K. H., Maisels, M. J., et al.: Thyroid function in the preterm infant: a longitudinal assessment. J. Pediatr. 92:968, 1978.

Uhrmann, S., Marks, K. H., Maisels, M. J., Kuhn, H. E., Kaplan, M., and Utiger, R.: Frequency of transient hypothyroxemia in low birth weight infants. Potential pitfalls for neonatal screening programs. Arch. Dis. Child. 56:214, 1981.

Van Wyk, J. J., and Fisher, D. A.: Thyroid. In Rudolph, A. M. (Ed.): Pediatrics. New York, Appleton-Century-Crofts, 1977.

Walfish, P. G.: Evaluation of three thyroid-function screening tests for detecting neonatal hypothyroidism. Lancet 1:1208, 1976.

Winick, M.: Changes in nucleic acid and protein content of the human brain during growth. Pediatr. Res. 2:353, 1968.

Wolter, R., Noel, P., and DeCock, P.: Neuropsychological study in treated thyroid dysgenesis. Acta Paediatr. Scand. 277:(Suppl.)41, 1980.

Wu, S. Y., Klein, A. H., Chopra, I. J., and Fisher, D. A.: Alterations in tissue thyroxine-5′-monodeiodinating activity in the perinatal period. Endocrinology 103:235, 1978.

56

General Considerations

Anatomic differentiation of the external genitalia is usually complete in the human infant by birth. This fortunate circumstance enables the obstetrician and proud parents to proclaim, "It's a girl" or, "It's a boy." Permanent gender assignment is made instantaneously. Occasionally, genital differentiation is incomplete or ambiguous. The physician's reactions to these medical emergencies will have an immense impact on the children and their families. It is important to have a sound understanding of normal sexual differentiation, to understand what can go wrong in development, and to be able to initiate steps that will lead to appropriate gender assignment, diagnosis, and management.

Two principles emerge in the consideration of embryologic sexual differentiation. The first is that sexual organs at all three levels—gonads, internal duct structures, and external genitalia—develop from identical undifferentiated structures in the male and female fetus. The second principle is that the female form predominates unless opposed by active male determinants.

Male and female gonads develop from anlagen located on the urogenital ridge, next to the kidney and primitive adrenal. Primordial germ cells migrate into the gonads from the endoderm of the yolk sac. These cells later form either oogonia or spermatogonia. Prior to 6 weeks of gestational age, testis and ovary are indistinguishable. In the fetus with a 46,XY chromosome constitution, definite testicular differentiation occurs rapidly over the ensuing weeks. By 12 weeks, both testicular testosterone concentration (Reyes et al., 1973) and the ability to convert pregnenolone to testosterone enzymatically (Siiteri and Wilson, 1974) are maximal. Peak concentrations of testosterone in the fetal circulation, comparable to those of the adult male, are reached at 16 weeks. Thereafter, the testosterone concentration falls, and, after 24 weeks, the concentration is in the early pubertal range (Kaplan and Grumbach, 1978). Proliferation and activity of fetal Leydig cells are stimulated by chorionic gonadotropin, which reaches peak levels in the fetal circulation at about 12 weeks and then decreases to low levels at 24 weeks. The pattern of testosterone secretion early in gestation follows that of chorionic gonadotropin. The low level of circulating testosterone after 15 to 18 weeks is maintained by both chorionic gonadotropin and LH (luteinizing hormone). As circulating chorionic gonadotropin decreases, circulating LH and FSH (follicle stimulating hormone) increase, reaching peak levels at 22 to 24 weeks and then decreasing to low or undetectable

Abnormalities of Sexual Differentiation

Revised by Constantine S. Anast*

levels later in gestation. Early development and function of the testis have important effects on genital development.

In contrast, ovarian differentiation occurs later and is not required for normal female genital development. In the fetus with a 46,XX chromosome complement, oocytes appear at about the twelfth week. Primordial follicles, containing oocytes surrounded by a layer of granulosa cells, are recognizable by the twentieth week. Despite the discordance between the respective times at which histologically recognizable primordial testis and ovary appear, there is a report of the simultaneous development at 8 weeks of gestation of the capacity of the fetal testis to synthesize testosterone and of the exclusive synthesis of estradiol by the fetal "ovary" (George and Wilson, 1979). Testosterone is synthesized by fetal Leydig cells, but the site of synthesis of estradiol in the primitive ovary is unknown. The circulating estrogens in the fetus are primarily of placental origin, with little contribution from the fetal ovary. The ovary has no apparent role in sex differentiation of the female genital tract.

The mechanisms involved in the translation of genetic sex into a testis or ovary are poorly understood. Recent studies of the H-Y (histocompatibility Y) antigen provide some insight into genes and testicular organogenesis (Ohno, 1979; Ohno et al., 1979; Watchel and Ohno, 1979). The H-Y antigen, a protein with a molecular weight of 16,500 to 18,000, is a male-specific component that has been detected in the membranes of all cells from normal XY males except immature germ cells. The locus of the structural gene for H-Y antigen is not known. It is postulated that the pericentromeric region of the Y chromosome contains a locus or loci that either codes for the plasma membrane H-Y antigen or regulates its expression. The H-Y antigen is disseminated by cells in the gonadal blastema, binds to gonad-specific H-Y receptors, and induces differentiation of the primitive gonad as a testis. The critical factor in testis organogenesis is not the presence or absence of a de-

---

* This chapter includes contributions from previous authors, Drs. John S. Parks and Alexander Schaffer.

503

tectable Y chromosome but the expression of the H-Y antigen. The embryonic gonad has an inherent tendency to form an ovary in the absence of H-Y antigen or its specific gonad receptor.

Genes for normal ovarian differentiation are located on both the long and the short arms of the human X chromosome. Accumulated evidence supports the view that two X chromosomes are required for differentiation of the indifferent gonad. It is unknown whether a counterpart to the H-Y antigen exists in the female and is involved in ovarian differentiation.

A schematic representation of fetal genital development is shown in Figure 56-1. At 7 weeks of gestation, the fetus has precursors of both male and female genital ducts. The müllerian ducts are anlagen of the fallopian tubes, uterus, and proximal vagina. Wolffian ducts are anlagen for the epididymis, vas deferens, seminal vesicles, and ejaculatory duct of the male. The brilliant experiments of Josso have shown that the fetal testis produces a locally active macromolecular hormone that induces regression of the müllerian ducts. This action cannot be mimicked by

androgens. However, high local concentrations of testosterone, produced by the fetal testis, are required for further development of the wolffian ducts. Genital duct development is nearly complete by 12 weeks of gestation.

Male and female external genitalia are also identical during the second month of pregnancy. Three structures are easily recognizable, as shown in Figure 56-1. These structures are the genital tubercle, the genital folds, and the genital swellings. Testosterone, and, more specifically, its active intracellular metabolite dihydrotestosterone, is required for male differentiation. Without testosterone, the genital tubercle remains small and forms the clitoris, the genital folds remain separate and form the labia minora, and the genital swellings form the labia majora. Virilization causes the genital tubercle to enlarge and form the penis. The genital folds fuse to form a phallic urethra, and the genital swellings fuse to form the scrotum. Fusion is complete by the twelfth week of gestation, but phallic enlargement continues to term.

Following birth, the pituitary gonadotropins LH and FSH rise to reach a peak at 1 to 3 months. In the male infant, there is an accompanying rise in testicular testosterone synthesis that has been shown by Forest and coworkers to produce plasma testosterone levels equivalent to those achieved in midpuberty.

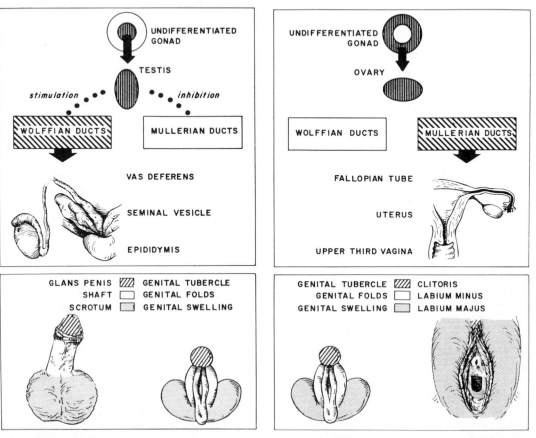

Figure 56-1. Outline of genital development. Note that gonadal development occurs from a common indifferent gonad, the internal genitalia develop from separate primordia present in both sexes, and the external genitalia develop in a continuous transformation of anlage common to both sexes. (From Federman, D. D.: N. Engl. J. Med. 277:351, 1967.)

Table 56–1. Classification of Abnormalities of Sexual Differences

I. Disorders of gonadal differentiation
   A. Klinefelter syndrome. 47,XXY and variants
   B. Turner syndrome (gonadal dysgenesis). 45,X and variants
   C. "Pure" gonadal dysgenesis. 46,XX and 46,XY
   D. True hermaphroditism
II. Virilization of the female fetus. 46,XX
   A. Due to maternal ingestion of drugs
   B. Due to virilizing maternal tumor
   C. Due to congenital adrenal hyperplasia
      1. 21-Hydroxylase deficiency
      2. 3β-Hydroxysteroid dehydrogenase deficiency
      3. 11β-Hydroxylase deficiency
III. Undervirilization of the male fetus. 46,XY
   A. Anorchia or vanishing testis
   B. Genetic defects in testosterone biosynthesis
      1. Defects common to cortisol and testosterone pathways
         a. 3β-Hydroxysteroid dehydrogenase deficiency
         b. 17α-Hydroxylase deficiency
      2. Defects unique to androgen and estrogen synthesis
         a. 17,20 Desmolase deficiency
         b. 17β-Hydroxysteroid oxidoreductase deficiency
   C. End-organ insensitivity to testosterone
      1. 5α-Reductase deficiency
      2. Testicular feminization
      3. Partial testicular feminization
   D. Testicular unresponsiveness to HCG and LH
   E. Maternal ingestion of progestins and estrogens
IV. Anatomic Abnormalities
   A. As isolated findings
      1. Hypospadias
      2. Cryptorchidism
      3. Persistence of müllerian structures
   B. Associated with other birth defects

This burst of activity is not accompanied by clinical signs of further virilization and is succeeded by a decline of testosterone to barely detectable levels by the end of the first year.

Most of the known errors of human sexual differentiation can be provisionally explained by genetic or biochemical alterations in the aforementioned sequence of events. Federman as well as Grumbach and Conte have written excellent detailed reviews of this area. This discussion will follow the classification scheme shown in Table 56–1. The first category entails disorders of gonadal differentiation, usually in association with abnormal number or structure of the X or Y chromosomes. The second category involves virilization of the female fetus, and the third undervirilization of the male fetus. A fourth category involves anatomical defects that, in most cases, do not have a definite chromosomal or hormonal etiology.

Disorders of Gonadal Differentiation

KLINEFELTER SYNDROME

Klinefelter syndrome is one of the most common sex chromosome anomalies, occurring once in every 1000 male births. The 47,XXY chromosome constitution arises during meiotic division in either parent or, less commonly, from mitotic nondisjunction in the zygote at the time of or following fertilization and is associated with advanced maternal age. Infants with 47,XXY karyotype as a group have lower birth weights than controls and have an increased incidence of major and minor congenital anomalies, especially clinodactyly. Although the testes may be noticeably small during infancy, there are seldom any genital abnormalities, and the diagnosis is seldom made during early childhood. Presenting features in older children and adolescents include low verbal I.Q., behavioral disorders, poor gross motor control, eunuchoid habitus, gynecomastia, and variable virilization.

Infertility is accompanied by the histologic finding of hyalinization of the seminiferous tubules. Patients with the variant karyotypes 48,XXYY, 48,XXXY, and 49,XXXXY generally have severe mental retardation and may be recognized earlier in childhood. De la Chapelle has reviewed 45 cases in which phenotypic males were found to have 46,XX karyotypes. Most had testicular morphology resembling that of 47,XXY males. However, Kasdan and coworkers have reported a family in which this karyotype was compatible with fertility.

TURNER SYNDROME AND VARIANTS

Turner syndrome is defined as gonadal dysgenesis due to a missing or structurally defective X chromosome. The 45,X karyotype is associated with a high intrauterine mortality. Its frequency is one per every 20 spontaneous abortuses but only one per every 2700 live newborn females. An increased incidence of the 45,X karyotype has been reported in the conceptuses of teen-aged mothers (Warburton, 1980). Infants with this condition often have distinctive physical features that have nothing to do with their gonadal abnormalities. The condition should be suspected and appropriate diagnostic tests should be done in female infants with webbing of the neck, edema of the extremities, or coarctation of the aorta. Such an infant is shown in Figure 56–2. In this infant, as in the great majority with gonadal dysgenesis, the external genitalia and internal duct structures were unequivocally female. More subtle findings include low birth weight for gestational age, ptosis, hypertelorism, micrognathia, hypertension, low-set and/or deformed ears, renal abnormalities, cubitus valgus, and dysplasia of finger and toe nails. In the neonate, pleural effusions and ascites that clear spontaneously are not uncommon (Gordon and O'Neill, 1969), and, rarely, pericardial effusion has been reported. In other children, somatic abnormalities are minimal and the condition is suspected because of short stature, failure of breast development, and primary amenorrhea at the age of puberty. A lack of feedback inhibition of hypothalamic-pituitary axis by the dysgenic ovary is reflected in elevated serum FSH and LH levels in affected infants as early as 5 days of age (Conte et al., 1980).

Roughly 85 per cent of girls with gonadal dysgenesis have a 45,X karyotype, and the diagnosis can be made by finding a chromatin-negative buccal smear. The remainder have either mosaicism, for example, 46,XX/45,X, or a structural abnormality of the X chromosome. Structural abnormalities include isochromosomes of either the short (XXpi) or long arm (XXqi), deletion of the short (XXp⁻) or long arm (XXq⁻), and ring chromosomes. Mosaicism and structural abnormalities can be detected only by karyotyping.

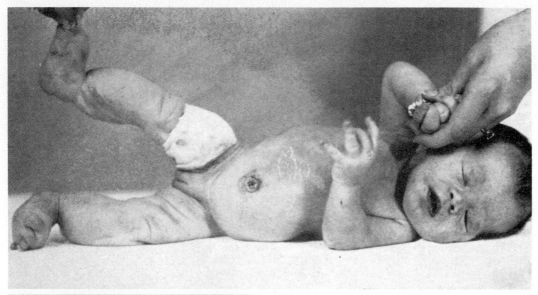

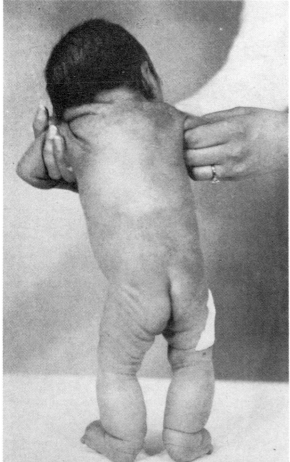

Figure 56–2. Edema of the feet extending to the midthigh and of the hands. The neck is short, and the scalp hair extends to a low level. There are loose folds of skin over the neck.

In this infant an oral mucosal smear showed the chromatin-negative pattern. This is a typical instance of gonadal dysgenesis. (Reproduced from Pediatrics, 20:743, 1957, with the kind permission of Dr. Melvin M. Grumbach, the author.)

Suspicion and confirmation of gonadal dysgenesis in a newborn infant confers an unusual responsibility upon the physician. There is seldom any doubt about gender assignment, for these infants are females. However, their ovaries have in most instances regressed to vestigial streaks by the time of birth. The great majority of these girls will be short and infertile as adults. Chromosomal findings are confusing to most parents and probably should not be mentioned during early discussions. The parents should be told that their child will be shorter than average and probably infertile and will require hormone replacement at the age of puberty to foster a growth spurt, breast development, and menstrual cycles. However, it is well to be aware that although streak gonads are the rule in 45,X gonadal dysgenesis, exceptions have been documented. Primary follicles have been observed in the ridges of some 45,X individuals in adolescence, and this correlates with the rare occurrence of menarche and a variable but attenuated period of regular menses (Kohn et al., 1980). Moreover, conceptions have been documented in some women in whom extensive karyotypic studies revealed only 45,X cell line in multiple tissues (King et al., 1978; Kohn et al., 1980). It is possible that some fertile 45,X women may be unrecognized sex chromosome mosaics. Alternatively, it is possible that the presence of oogonia in 45,X individuals results from mitotic nondisjunction in a certain number of 45,X germ cells with the formation of 46,XX oogonia.

Mosaicism involving the Y chromosome is less common than classic Turner syndrome and produces a wider variety of phenotypes. Infants with 45,X/46,XY karyotypes commonly have ambiguous genitalia. Gender assignment should be in accordance with the expected potential for adult sexual function. Gonads generally consist of bilateral dysgenetic testes or a dysgenetic testis and a contralateral gonadal streak. Either or both gonads may have failed to produce müllerian-inhibiting substance, and there may be a uterus and unilateral or bilateral fallopian tubes. Depending on the extent and timing of intrauterine testosterone production, there may also be well-developed wolffian structures. Short stature and the somatic abnormalities of Turner syndrome are inconstant findings. Dysgenetic gonads are predisposed to neoplasia and should be removed at an early age. Hormone replacement at the age of puberty must be concordant with the sex of rearing. It is useful to consider the syndrome of gonadal dysgenesis and its variants as a continuum of clinical features ranging from those of the typical 45,X phenotype to a normal female or male. Any of the features of the 45,X phenotype may be modified by the presence of lesser degrees of sex chromosome deficiency. The functional importance of chromosomal additions to the basic 45,X karyotype is reflected in the extent to which they modify toward normal the dwarfism, sexual infantilism and somatic anomalies characteristic of the complete sex chromosome monosomy (Grumbach and Conte, 1981).

PURE GONADAL DYSGENESIS

Pure gonadal dysgenesis is a term applied to phenotypic females with bilateral streak gonads who lack the somatic stigmata of Turner syndrome and who are of normal or tall stature. Karyotype may be either 46,XX or 46,XY. The internal and external genitalia of the 46,XX individuals with gonadal dysgenesis are normal female. The 46,XX patients seldom show clitoral enlargement, may show some ovarian function at puberty, and are not prone to gonadal neoplasms. Familial cases are not uncommon in 46,XX gonadal dysgenesis, and transmission is consistent with an autosomal recessive trait. Sensorial deafness is an associated finding in some families with 46,XX gonadal dysgenesis (Simpson, 1976).

Familial aggregates as well as sporadic cases of 46,XY gonadal dysgenesis have been described (Simpson, 1976; German et al., 1978). Inheritance consistent with an X-linked or male-limited dominant trait has been observed. Usually, the external and internal genital tract is completely female, and the patient is sexually infantile (complete form). However, clitoral enlargement is not uncommon, and affected siblings may have ambiguous external genitalia and development of the genital ducts and urogenital sinus (incomplete or variant form). The spectrum of genital ambiguity suggests that the mutant gene exhibits variable expressivity. Both H-Y antigen—positive and H-Y antigen—negative forms have been described, findings that further reflect the genetic heterogeneity of this syndrome (Dorus et al., 1977; Ghosh et al., 1978; Wolf, 1979).

TRUE HERMAPHRODITISM

True hermaphroditism requires the presence of both ovarian and testicular tissue in the same individual. The tissue may be present in the same or opposite gonads. In almost one half there is an ovotestis on one side and an ovary or testis on the other, in one fifth there are bilateral ovotestes, and in one third there is an ovary on one side and a testis on the other. The external genitalia are extremely variable, but roughly three fourths of patients have had phallic enlargement, generally with hypospadias, and have been raised as males. Cryptorchidism is common, and an inguinal hernia that may contain a gonad or uterus is present in about one half of the cases. A uterus is usually present and often is asymmetric. Genital ducts develop in accordance with the function of the ipsilateral gonad. Most patients with an ovotestis have predominantly female development of the genital ducts. Chromosomal findings are varied and do not correlate with gonadal histology or external genital appearance. Approximately 70 percent of true hermaphrodites are X chromatin—

positive. Von Niekerk reported that of 148 patients, 89 were 46,XX, 18 were 46,XY, 21 were XX/XY chimeras, and the remainder were sex chromosome mosaics. All true hermaphrodites are H-Y antigen–positive. The presence of H-Y antigen in 46,XX true hermaphrodites supports the postulate that the structural gene for H-Y antigen is on an autosome and not the Y, and therefore an autosomal mutation affecting the structural gene for H-Y antigen results in the differentiation of a testis or ovotestis in an XX individual (Fraccaro et al., 1979). However, until the sites of the putative regulatory genes that may affect the expression of H-Y are determined, the pathogenesis of true hermaphroditism in relationship to H-Y antigen remains uncertain.

At puberty, breast development is common, menses occurs in over half the patients, and a large number virilize. Although spermatogenesis is rare, ovulation is not uncommon, and pregnancy and childbirth have been observed in several patients with an XX karyotype (Kim et al., 1979).

True hermaphroditism should be considered in any infant or child with ambiguous genitalia in whom an alternative explanation cannot be established from chromosomal, hormonal, and radiologic contrast studies. Diagnosis requires laparotomy and biopsy of gonads. Management involves surgical removal of gonads, internal duct structures, and features of the external genitalia that are incongruous with gender assignment.

VIRILIZATION OF THE FEMALE FETUS

Virilization of the female fetus is the most common category of disorders producing ambiguity of the external genitalia. Its mechanisms and consequences are also the most easy to understand. Androgens may enter the maternal and fetal circulation following ingestion or as a result of a virilizing tumor. The female fetus may produce excessive androgens as a result of congenital adrenal hyperplasia. In these instances, the fetal ovaries and genital ducts are normal. Fusion of the genital folds or the genital swellings or both is a result of androgen exposure prior to the twelfth gestational week. Clitoral enlargement can occur with exposure at any time. Buccal smears are chromatin positive, and karyotypes are 46,XX. Medical management of congenital adrenal hyperplasia and surgical correction of anatomic abnormalities are followed by normal pubertal development and normal adult sexual and reproductive function.

VIRILIZATION BY MATERNAL DRUGS

Virilization of the female fetus has been attributed to testosterone, the 19-nortestosterone progestins,

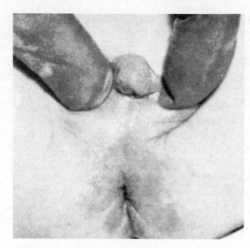

Figure 56–3. External genitals of an infant whose mother received large quantities of dehydroxyprogesterone in order to forestall abortion. One can see an enlarged clitoris, with no urethral meatus at its tip, a fused labioscrotum containing no gonads. The single urogenital orifice can be seen to open at the base of the phallus only when this is lifted away.

progesterone, and even, paradoxically, diethylstilbestrol. In each case, a fairly small proportion of exposed infants had clinically evident virilization. There was seldom evidence of virilization in the mother. It is not known which of these compounds act directly on the external genitalia and which act indirectly through altering androgen synthesis by the mother or fetus. It seems reasonable to speculate that differences in maternal, placental, or fetal metabolism of the synthetic steroids may determine which infants are affected.

The incidence of this condition has diminished as the use of synthetic estrogens and progestins for management of threatened abortion has waned. However, the condition is still seen in offspring of women who unknowingly continue to take birth control pills following conception. Severity of virilization is quite variable, ranging from mild clitoral enlargement to complete labial fusion with a phallic urethra. The infant will not show progressive virilization or accelerated growth and skeletal maturation after birth. Even in the presence of a positive history of maternal hormone ingestion, it is mandatory to obtain a buccal smear and a 24-hour urine for 17-ketosteroids to exclude other possible diagnoses.

VIRILIZATION BY MATERNAL OVERPRODUCTION OF ANDROGENS

Severe disorders of maternal androgen production generally preclude pregnancy. However, artificial induction of ovulation in a virilized woman or development of a virilizing neoplasm during pregnancy can set the stage for virilization of a female infant. In their review of 12 cases, Haymond and Weldon found only one case of adrenal tumor. The remaining 11 mothers had ovarian lesions. In most cases, the mother had clinical signs of virilization such as hirsutism, acne, clitoromegaly and deepening of the voice. In other cases, the fetus had a lower threshold for showing virilization than the mother. Virilization has been observed in a female infant born to a mother with a virilizing form of congenital adrenal hyperplasia (Kai et al., 1979). The clinical features of the offspring of virilized mothers are identical with those described previously for girls whose mothers received sex hormones. Diagnosis requires demonstration of elevated urinary 17-ketosteroids or plasma testosterone in the mother, as well as exclusion of alternative diagnoses in the infant.

CONGENITAL ADRENAL HYPERPLASIA

This category of diseases is discussed more fully in Chapter 54. Inherited enzymatic blocks in the synthesis of cortisol lead to overproduction of androgens and virilization of the female fetus. Defects in 21-hydroxylase, 3β-hydroxysteroid dehydrogenase, and 11-hydroxylase can each produce this result. Buccal smear is chromatin positive, and urinary excretion of 17-ketosteroids remains above 2.5 mg per 24 hours. In infants with a defect in 21-hydroxylase, the plasma 17-hydroxyprogesterone level is elevated. Treatment with cortisol suppresses adrenal androgen production and prevents further virilization and excessively rapid growth and skeletal maturation. In infants with salt-losing forms of congenital adrenal hyperplasia, cortisol and mineralocorticoid replacement are lifesaving.

UNDERVIRILIZATION OF THE MALE FETUS

Complete male genital differentiation requires the presence of testes, the ability of testes to produce testosterone, and the ability of the genital anlagen to recognize and respond to testosterone. Defects can occur at each of these levels and result in genitalia that are either ambiguous or unambiguously female and discordant with a normal 46,XY male karyotype.

ANORCHIA (Vanishing Testes Syndrome)

A spectrum of genital anomalies is observed in patients with a 46,XY karyotype resulting from cessation of testicular function during the critical stages of male sexual differentiation between 8 and 14 weeks gestation. Deficiency of testicular function before 8 weeks gestation results in female external and internal genitalia, whereas lack of testicular function beginning between 8 and 10 weeks gestation results in ambiguous genitalia (Cleary et al., 1977). The latter has been referred to as the "XY gonadal dysgenesis syndrome" (Coulam, 1979). Loss of testicular function after 14 weeks gestation results in "anorchia," in which there is normal male differentiation both internally and externally but no gonadal tissue. The diagnosis of anorchia is made in male infants with apparent cryptorchidism, elevated circulating gonadotropins, and failure of testosterone response

to human chorionic gonadotropin administration. Kirschner and coworkers have demonstrated by selective venous catheterization and testosterone measurements that some androgen production may persist despite the absence of morphologically distinct testicular tissue.

DEFECTS IN THE SYNTHESIS OF TESTOSTERONE

In several varieties of congenital adrenal hyperplasia, the enzymatic defect is shared by adrenal and gonadal tissue. The result is undervirilization of the affected male due to impairment of fetal testosterone production. Specific defects include 3β-hydroxysteroid dehydrogenase and 17α-hydroxylase deficiencies, discussed in Chapter 54. In these conditions, the enzyme deficiency impairs synthesis of cortisol as well as testosterone.

Defects may also occur in metabolic pathways unique to the synthesis of sex steroids. The 17,20-desmolase enzyme converts 17α-hydroxypregnenolone to dehydroepiandrosterone and 17α-hydroxyprogesterone to androstenedione. Deficiency, as in the family reported by Zachmann and coworkers, leads to severe hypospadias, with or without cryptorchidism, and an elevated urinary excretion of pregnenetriol and 11-ketopregnanetriol, suggesting elevated plasma levels of 17α-hydroxyprogesterone and 17α-hydroxypregnenolone. Occurrence in siblings and an "aunt" indicated X-linked recessive or male-limited autosomal dominant inheritance. In 1976, Goebelsman subsequently reported a 46,XY phenotypic female with normal external genitalia, no müllerian structures, atrophic wolffian derivative, abdominal testes, and biochemical findings suggestive of a defect in 17,20-desmolase.

The next step in testosterone synthesis involves 17β-hydroxysteroid oxidoreductase, which converts dehydroepiandrosterone to Δ5-androstenediol, androstenedione to testosterone, and estrone to estradiol. Deficiency results in ambiguous genitalia and elevated plasma androstenedione and estrone levels in postpubertal patients (Grumbach and Conte, 1981). Puberty in the patients reported by Saez and colleagues was characterized by virilization and gynecomastia. The latter finding was attributed to elevated concentrations of the estrogen estrone.

End-Organ Insensitivity to Testosterone

DEFICIENCY OF 5α-REDUCTASE

The external genital anlagen of the fetus normally possess 5α-reductase activity and are able to convert testosterone to the active metabolite dihydrotestosterone. This transaction seems to be required for complete male genital development, and a defect at this level may explain an autosomal recessive condition known as "pseudovaginal perineoscrotal hypospadias." An interesting aspect of this condition, also known as the "penis at twelve" syndrome, is marked virilization and phallic growth at puberty. In the adult, the ratio of circulating testosterone to dihydrotestosterone is increased.

TESTICULAR FEMINIZATION

Recognition of testosterone or dihydrotestosterone by target tissues requires the participation of a cytoplasmic receptor protein that binds the steroid, enters the nucleus, and interacts with nuclear chromatin to alter gene expression. Genetic disorders in the rat and mouse have been shown to involve receptor defects and closely parallel the human condition of testicular feminization.

In the complete form of the disorder, 46,XY infants have unambiguously female external genitalia. Unless there are inguinal hernias containing testes, recognition may be delayed until puberty, when these girls show normal breast development but lack sexual hair and fail to menstruate. The vagina ends blindly, and the uterus and fallopian tubes are absent, reflecting the intrauterine production of and response to müllerian inhibiting substance. The disorder is familial, with multiple sibling involvement and occurrence in maternal aunts suggesting X-linked recessive or male-limited autosomal dominant inheritance. The gender assignment is unquestionably female. Gonads should be removed because of a high incidence of malignant degeneration. Estrogen replacement at puberty enhances breast development but does not induce menses because there is no uterus.

Partial testicular feminization implies a partial defect in recognition of testosterone with an attendant partial inhibition of male genital differentiation. Wilson and coworkers have suggested that many familial cases of microphallus, hypospadias, and gynecomastia with normal testosterone production at puberty fall in this category. They propose the term "familial, incomplete male pseudohermaphroditism, type I" to encompass conditions described separately by Reifenstein, Lubs, Gilbert-Dreyfus and Rosewater.

Studies of dihydrotestosterone binding by cultured fibroblasts from genital skin have shown two patterns in both the complete and partial forms of testicular feminization (Kaufman et al., 1979; Griffen and Wilson, 1980). In one, there are quantitatively reduced or absent (complete form) cytosol receptors for dihydrotestosterone and testosterone; in the other, cytosol binding and nuclear binding of dihydrotestosterone are normal. The latter, in receptor-positive patients, presumably represents an as yet undefined postreceptor defect or subtle qualitative abnormality in the androgen receptor itself.

TESTICULAR UNRESPONSIVENESS TO HCG AND LH

A new form of male pseudohermaphroditism has been described in which there is Leydig cell hypoplasia or agenesis apparently secondary to a deficiency or abnormality of the HCG-LH receptor on the plasma membrane of the fetal and postnatal Leydig cell (Berthezene et al., 1976; Brown et al., 1978; Grumbach and Conte, 1981). The external genitalia in these 46,XY patients were female except for slight posterior labial fusion and clitoromegaly in one patient. Separate vaginal and urethral openings were present, but uterus and fallopian tubes were absent. Plasma LH was elevated, and plasma FSH was normal or elevated. Plasma testosterone was low and did not increase in response to HCG. It is thought that the resistance of undifferentiated embryonic and fetal Leydig cells to HCG results in fetal testicular deficiency with female or predominantly female differentiation of the external genitalia.

MATERNAL INGESTION OF PROGESTINS AND ESTROGENS

Animal studies have suggested an antiandrogen effect of progestins on the male fetus. Maternal ingestion of progestins and estrogens has been implicated but not proved as a rare cause of male pseudohermaphroditism in humans. Some studies have suggested an association between progestins and hypospadias (Sweet et al., 1974; Lorber et al., 1979; Aarskag, 1979); another report describes male pseudohermaphroditism in a boy whose mother received large doses of diethylstilbestrol during early pregnancy (Kaplan, 1959). In vitro studies have demonstrated that progestins can inhibit 5α-reductase activity (Voight et al., 1973), which, as discussed earlier, converts testosterone to dihydrotestosterone, the active metabolite that is required for complete male development.

Isolated Anatomical Abnormalities

CRYPTORCHIDISM

For a discussion of cryptorchidism, see Chapter 44.

PERSISTENCE OF MÜLLERIAN DUCTS

A fully developed uterus and fallopian tubes may be discovered incidental to surgery in phenotypic males with normal 46,XY karyotypes. The theoretical explanation of this finding is a failure of production or recognition of müllerian inhibiting substance. The condition may be transmitted as an autosomal recessive trait, although X-linked recessive inheritance and genetic heterogeneity have not been excluded (Summit, 1979). Treatment consists of removal of organs that are discordant with the patient's gender.

Anatomic Abnormalities in Association with Other Defects

Malformations of the external genitalia may be a part of a more complicated embryopathy. In females, genital abnormalities may be associated with imperforate anus, renal agenesis, or congenital nephritis and other congenital malformations of the lower intestine and genitourinary tract. Drash and associates have reported an association between degenerative renal disease, Wilms' tumor, and ambiguity of the external genitalia in males. Rimoin and Schimke's monograph has an excellent discussion of associations between genital abnormalities and largely nonendocrine syndromes. In many instances, such infants have severe defects incompatible with life, but there is still the problem of assigning gender.

Evaluation of Infants with Ambiguous Genitalia

It is extremely important that the evaluation of a newborn with ambiguous genitalia be carried out immediately after birth. A flow chart in Figure 56–4 indicates studies that can be carried out to provide a provisional diagnosis and a firm gender assignment in the first 72 hours. The parents should be advised that their infant's genital development had not been completed by birth, that the baby is all girl or all boy and not a little bit of both, that tests will be done to determine the correct sex, and that announcement of the birth to friends and relatives should be delayed until the tests are returned.

Inspection of the external genitalia will reveal a phallic structure that is small for a male or large for a girl. There is likely to be chordee with hypospadias. The genital swellings may be fused or open. A urologic surgeon should be involved quite early in the examination of the infant. If the phallus shows little potential for penile function, a female gender assignment will be made regardless of further findings. However, the converse is not true. The degree of phallic enlargement should not preclude a female gender assignment. Palpation for gonads is extremely important, for these gonads are usually testes.

The buccal smear for determination of sex chromatin should be done on the first day of life. Although the number of positive chromatin bodies may be diminished in comparison to adult values, there should be no overlap of results between 46,XX females and 46,XY males. The chromatin-positive infant should be considered to have virilizing congenital adrenal hyperplasia until proved otherwise. Lymphocyte karyotyping should be done on the same indications as the buccal smear, but analysis takes weeks rather than hours.

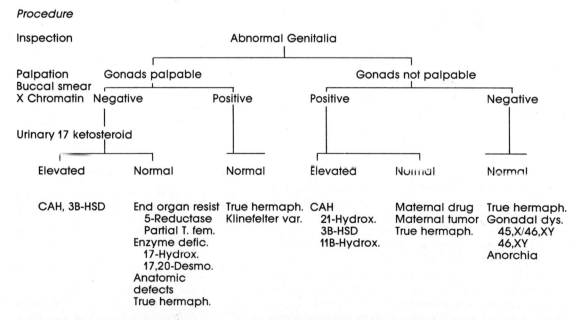

Figure 56–4. Investigation of the infant with ambiguous genitalia. Palpation of gonads is useful in that it usually is associated with an X chromatin negative buccal smear and a 46,XY karyotype. However, testicular non-descent can occur in virtually all of the enzymatic deficiency syndromes. Infants with 21-hydroxylase deficiency have elevated plasma levels of 17-hydroxyprogesterone.

Determination of 17-ketosteroid and pregnanetriol excretion can be accomplished in the first 72 hours. Infants with congenital adrenal hyperplasia due to a deficiency of 21-hydroxylase or 3β-hydroxysteroid dehydrogenase will show an increase rather than a decrease in 17-ketosteroid excretion during the first week, with levels remaining above 2.5 mg per 24 hours. A striking increase in plasma 17-hydroxyprogesterone is found in infants with defective 21-hydroxylation. Vomiting, dehydration, hyperkalemia, and hyponatremia are observed in salt-losing forms of 21-hydroxylase and 3β-hydroxysteroid dehydrogenase deficiencies.

Obtaining the history is extremely important. There should be a complete inquiry about all medications taken during pregnancy. Family history may reveal unexplained infant deaths among siblings of infants with salt-losing congenital adrenal hyperplasia. Infants with defects in testosterone synthesis or with partial testicular feminization commonly have hypogonadal maternal uncles, or maternal "aunts" with primary amenorrhea.

By 72 hours, a definite gender assignment will have been made in most cases. Chromatin-positive infants will almost always be female. Those who do not have congenital adrenal hyperplasia, virilization due to maternal drugs or tumor, or associated birth defects will probably require laparotomy and gonadal biopsy in later infancy. Chromatin-negative infants may have a male or female gender assignment, depending on phallic structure. They will require karyotyping to exclude 45,X/46,XY mosaicism, further serum and urinary steroid measurement to define rare abnormalities of adrenal or gonadal steroid synthesis, and contrast studies of the genitourinary tract to search for müllerian duct structures. Laparotomy and gonadal biopsy can safely be deferred to a later age.

The pioneering studies of Money and colleagues have shown that karyotype, gonads, internal ducts, and hormones have very little to do with behavior and psychosexual inclinations. These features are chiefly influenced by gender assignment and home environment. If the parents are secure about their boy or girl, the gender role is firmly established in early infancy and can rarely be reversed. The physician's role is to be sure that the physical and hormonal state of the growing child is not seriously at odds with the gender assignment. In the girl with congenital adrenal hyperplasia, this involves glucocorticoid replacement, consideration of clitorectomy and vaginoplasty if needed in infancy, and continued follow-up after maturity. In the male with hypospadias and deficient testosterone production, it means surgical repair of hypospadias and evaluation of the need for testosterone replacement at the age of puberty. The genetic male with a female gender assignment needs protection from confusing information about chromosomes and may require gonadectomy before puberty to prevent virilization.

Prenatal Diagnosis of Abnormalities of Sexual Differentiation

Amniocentesis, ultrasonography, and studies of maternal blood and urine provide tools for the prenatal diagnosis of abnormalities of sexual differentiation. Abnormalities of sex chromosome number and structure can be determined by karyotypic analysis of chromosomes from amniotic fluid obtained as early as 14 to 16 weeks gestation (Milunsky, 1979). HLA typing of amniotic fluid cells may aid in the prenatal diagnosis of 21-hydroxylase deficiency, since the gene for 21-hydroxylase has been shown to be closely linked to the HLA locus on the short arm of chromosome 6. Moreover, elevated amniotic fluid levels of 17-hydroxyprogesterone and androstenedione are present in male and female fetuses with 21-hydroxylase deficiency (Pang et al., 1980). Similarly, a fetus affected with 11β-hydroxylase deficiency can be detected by measurement of 11-deoxycortisol in amniotic fluid or in maternal plasma and urine (Rösler et al., 1979; Schumert et al., 1980). Estriol concentrations in maternal plasma and urine reflect the functional integrity of the fetal adrenal and placenta; low levels are observed in disorders of fetal hypothalamic-pituitary adrenal function (Davies, 1980).

Fetal sexing is now possible with ultrasonography after 28 weeks gestation (LeLann, 1979).

REFERENCES

Aarskog, D.: Clinical and cytogenetic studies in hypospadias. Acta Paediatr. Scand. 203(suppl.):1, 1970.

Aarskog, D.: Maternal progestins as a possible cause of hypospadias. N. Engl. J. Med. 300:75, 1979.

Berthezene, F., Forest, M. G., Grimaud, J. A., Claustrat, B., and Mornex, R.: Leydig cell agenesis: a cause of male pseudohermaphroditism. N. Engl. J. Med. 295:969, 1976.

Brown, D. M., Markland, C., and Dehner, L. P.: Leydig cell hypoplasia: a cause of male pseudohermaphrodism. J. Clin. Endocrinol. Metab. 46:1, 1978.

Cleary, R. E., Caras, J., Rosenfeld, R. L., and Young, P. C. M.: Endocrine and metabolic studies in a patient with male pseudohermaphrodism and true agonadism. Am. J. Obstet. Gynecol. 128:862, 1977.

Conte, F. A., Grumbach, M. M., Kaplan, S. C., and Reiter, E. O.: Correlation of luteinizing hormone–releasing factor, induced luteinizing hormone, and follicle-stimulating hormone release from infancy to 19 years with the changing pattern of gonadotropin secretion in agonadal patients: relation to restraint of puberty. J. Clin. Endocrinol. Metab. 50:163, 1980.

Coulam, C. B.: Testicular regression syndrome. Obstet. Gynecol. 53:44, 1979.

Davies, J.: The fetal adrenal. In Tulchinsky, D., and Ryan, K. (Eds.): Maternal-Fetal Endocrinology. Philadelphia, W. B. Saunders Co., 1980.

de la Chappelle, A.: Nature and origin of males with XX sex chromosomes. Am. J. Hum. Genet. 24:71, 1972.

Dorus, E., Amarose, A. P., Koo, G., and Wachtel, S. S.: Clinical, pathologic and genetic findings in a case of 46,XY pure gonadal dysgenesis (Swyer's syndrome). II. Presence of H-Y antigen. Am. J. Obstet. Gynecol. *127*:829, 1977.

Drash, A., Sherman, F., Hartmann, W. H., and Blizzard, R. M.: A syndrome of pseudohermaphroditism, Wilm's tumor, hypertension, and degenerative renal disease. J. Pediatr. *76*:585, 1970.

Federman, D. D.: Abnormal Sexual Development. Philadelphia, W. B. Saunders Co., 1967.

Forest, M. G., Sizonenko, P. C., Cathiard, A. M., and Bertrand, J.: Hypophyso-gonadal function in humans during the first year of life. I. Evidence for testicular activity in early infancy. J. Clin. Invest. *53*:819, 1974.

Fraccaro, M., Tiepolo, L., Zuffardi, D., Chiumello, G., DiNatale, B., Gargantini, L., and Wolf, U.: Familial XX true hermaphrodism and the H-Y antigen. Hum. Genet. *48*:45, 1979.

George, F. W., and Wilson, J. D.: The regulation of androgen and estrogen formation in fetal gonads. Ann. Biol. Anim. Biochem. Biophys. *19*:1297, 1979.

German, J., Simpson, J. L., Chaganti, R. S. K., Summit, R., Reid, B. C., and Merkatz, I. R.: Genetically determined sex reversal in 46,XY humans. Science *202*:53, 1978.

Ghosh, S. N., Shah, P. N., and Gharpure, H. M.: Absence of H-Y antigen in XY females with dysgenetic gonads. Nature *276*:180, 1978.

Goebelsmann, U., Zachmann, M., Darajan, R., Israel, R., Mestman, J., and Mishell, D. R.: Male pseudohermaphrodism consistent with 17,20-desmolase deficiency. Gynecol. Invest. 7:138, 1976.

Gordon, R. R., and O'Neill, E. M.: Turner's infantile phenotype. Br. Med. J. 1:483, 1969.

Griffen, J. E., and Wilson, J. D.: The syndrome of androgen resistance. N. Engl. J. Med. *302*:198, 1980.

Grumbach, M. M., and Conte, F. A.: Disorders of sex differentiation. *In* Williams, R. H. (Ed.): Textbook of Endocrinology. Philadelphia, W. B. Saunders Co., 1981.

Haymond, M. W., and Weldon, V. V.: Female pseudohermaphroditism secondary to a maternal virilizing tumor. J. Pediatr. *82*:682, 1973.

Imperato-McGinley, J., Guerrero, L., Gautier, T., and Peterson, R. E.: An unusual form of male pseudohermaphroditism: a model of 5α-reductase deficiency in man. Science *186*:1214, 1974.

Josso, N.: Permeability of membranes to the mullerian-inhibiting substance synthesized by the human fetal testis in vitro: a clue to its biochemical nature. J. Clin. Endocrinol. Metab., *34*:265, 1972.

Kai, H., Nose, O., Iida, Y., Ono, J., Harada, T., and Yabuuchi, H.: Female pseudohermaphrodism caused by maternal congenital adrenal hyperplasia. J. Pediatr. *95*:418, 1979.

Kaplan, N. M.: Male pseudohermaphrodism: report of a case, with observations on pathogenesis. N. Engl. J. Med. *261*:641, 1959.

Kaplan, S. L., and Grumbach, M. M.: Pituitary and placental gonadotropins and sex steroids in the human and sub-human primate fetus. Clin. Endocrinol. Metab. 7:487, 1978.

Kasdan, R., Nankin, H. R., Troen, P., Wald, N., Pan, S., and Yanaihara, T.: Paternal transmission of maleness in XX human beings. N. Engl. J. Med. *288*:539, 1973.

Kaufman, M., Pinsky, L., Baird, P. A., and McGillivany, B. C.: Complete androgen insensitivity with a normal amount of 5α-dihydrotestosterone–binding activity in labium majus skin fibroblasts. Am. J. Med. Genet. 1:101, 1979.

Kim, M. H., Gumpel, J. A., and Graff, P.: Pregnancy in a true hermaphrodite("es"). Obstet. Gynecol. *53*(3 suppl.):40S, 1979.

King, C. R., Magenis, E., and Bennett, S.: Pregnancy and the Turner syndrome. Obstet. Gynecol. *52*:617, 1978.

Kirschner, M. A., Jacobs, J. B., and Fraley, E. E.: Bilateral anorchia with persistent testosterone production. N. Engl. J. Med. *282*:240, 1970.

Kohn, G., Yarkoni, S., and Cohen, M. M.: Two conceptions in a 45,X woman. Am. J. Med. Genet. 5:339, 1980.

LeLann, D.: Diagnostic echographique antinatal du sexe masculin et feminin. Nouv. Presse Med. 8:2760, 1979.

Lorber, C. A., Cassidy, Z. B., and Engel, E.: Is there an embryo-fetal exogenous sex steroid exposure syndrome (EFESSES)? Fertil. Steril. *31*:21, 1979.

Milunsky, A.: Genetic Disorders and the Fetus. New York, Plenum Press, 1979.

Money, J., Hampson, J. G., and Hampson, J. L.: Hermaphroditism: recommendations concerning assignment of sex, change of sex and psychologic management. Bull. Johns Hopkins Hosp. *96*:253, 1955.

Ohno, S.: Major Sex Determining Genes. Berlin, Springer-Verlag, 1979.

Ohno, S., Nagai, Y., Ciccarese, S., and Iwata, H.: Testis-organizing H-Y antigen and the primary sex-determining mechanism of mammals. Recent Prog. Horm. Res. *35*:449, 1979.

Pang, S., Levine, L. S., Cederquist, L. C., Fuentes, M., and New, M. I.: Amniotic fluid concentrations of Δ^5 and Δ^4 steroids in fetuses with congenital adrenal hyperplasia due to 21-hydroxylase deficiency and in anencephalic fetuses. J. Clin. Endocrinol. Metab. *51*:223, 1980.

Reyes, F. I., Winter, J. S. D., and Faiman, C.: Studies on human sexual development. I. Fetal gonadal and adrenal sex steroids. J. Clin. Endocrinol. Metab. *37*:74, 1973.

Rimoin, D. L., and Schimke, R. N.: Genetic Disorders of the Endocrine Glands. Saint Louis, The C. V. Mosby Company, 1971.

Rösler, A., Leiberman, E., Rosenmann, A., Ben-Uzilio, R., and Weedenfeld, J.: Prenatal diagnosis of 11-β-hydroxylase deficiency congenital adrenal hyperplasia. J. Clin. Endocrinol. Metab. *49*:546, 1979.

Saez, J. M., Morera, A. M., dePeretti, E., and Bertrand, J.: Further in vivo studies in male pseudohermaphroditism with gynecomastia due to a testicular 17-ketosteroid reductase defect (compared to a case of testicular feminization). J. Clin. Endocrinol. Metab. *34*:598, 1972.

Schumert, Z., Rosenmann, A., Landau, H., and Rösler, A.: 11-deoxycortisol in amniotic fluid: prenatal diagnosis of congenital adrenal hyperplasia due to 11-β-hydroxylase deficiency. Clin. Endocrinol. *12*:257, 1980.

Siiteri, P. K., and Wilson, J. D.: Testosterone formation and metabolism during male sexual differentiation in the human embryo. J. Clin. Endocrinol. Metab. *38*:113, 1974.

Simpson, J. L.: Disorders of Sexual Differentiation: Etiology and Clinical Delineation. New York, Academic Press, 1976.

Sorenson, H. R.: Hypospadias, with Special Reference to Aetiology. Copenhagen, Munksgaard, 1953.

Summitt, R. L.: Genetic forms of hypogonadism in the male. *In* Steinberg, A. G., Bearn, A. G., Motulsky, A. G., and Childs, B. (Eds.): Progress in Medical Genetics. Vol. III. Philadelphia, W. B. Saunders Co., 1979.

Sweet, R. A., Schrott, H. G., Kurland, R., and Culp, O. S.: Study of the incidence of hypospadias in Rochester, Minnesota, 1940–1970, and a case control comparison of possible etiologic factors. Mayo Clinic Proc. *49*:52, 1974.

van Niekerk, W. A.: True Hermaphrodism. Hagerstown, Harper and Row, 1974.

van Niekerk, W. A.: True hermaphroditism. An analytic review with a report of 3 new cases. Am. J. Obstet. Gynecol. *126*:890, 1976.

Voight, W., and Hsia, S. L.: Further studies on testosterone 5α-reductase of human skin: structural features of steroid inhibitors. J. Biol. Chem. *248*:4280, 1973.

Wachtel, S. S., and Ohno, S.: The immunogenetics of sexual development. *In* Steinberg, A. G., Bearn, A. G., Motulsky, A. G., and Childs, B. (Eds.): Progress in Medical Genetics. Vol. III. Philadelphia, W. B. Saunders Co., 1979.

Warburton, D.: Monosomy X: a chromosomal anomaly associated with young maternal age. Lancet 1:167, 1980.

Wilson, J. D., Harrod, M. J., Goldstein, J. L., Hemsell, D. L., and MacDonald, P. C.: Familial incomplete male pseudohermaphroditism, type I. Evidence for androgen resistance and variable clinical manifestations in a family with the Reifenstein syndrome. N. Engl. J. Med. *290*:1097, 1974.

Wolf, U.: XY gonadal dysgenesis and the H-Y antigen. Hum. Genet. *47*:269, 1979.

Zachmann, M., Völlmin, J. A., Hamilton, W., et al.: Steroid 17,20-desmolase deficiency: a new cause of male pseudohermaphroditism. Clin. Endocrinol. 1:369, 1972.

57

Disorders of Carbohydrate Metabolism

By Kenneth H. Gabbay*

This chapter is included in the section on disorders caused by endocrine dysfunction even though abnormalities in carbohydrate homeostasis may result from deficiencies in specific enzymes (e.g., galactosemia, hereditary fructose intolerance), availability or utilization of a variety of substrates (e.g., ketones, lactate, glycerol, alanine), and relative or absolute hyperinsulinism or hypoinsulinism (transient diabetes mellitus, pituitary "aplasia," adenomatous dysplasia, hyperplasia). A variety of organs, such as the endocrine pancreas, pituitary, thyroid, adrenal cortex, and medulla, as well as the liver, all play important roles in carbohydrate metabolism. One or several of these regulatory factors may operate to interfere with proper blood sugar homeostasis. Sufficient clinical experience and laboratory data are now available to provide useful clinical and pathologic classifications.

Development of the Endocrine Pancreas

The islets of Langerhans contain at least four endocrine cell types: the beta or (B) cell, which secretes insulin, the alpha (A) cell, which secretes glucagon, the delta (D) cell, which produces somatostatin, and a pancreatic polypeptide (PP) cell, which is the source of the compound for which it is named. In the human, the A cell is evident by 9 weeks, and the others appear shortly thereafter. Although the A cells are more prominent initially, the B cells become more numerous during the latter stages of gestation and early life until the adult ratio of at least 1:3 is reached.

Insulin is present in the pancreas from at least the eleventh week of fetal life, earlier than the B cells can be seen; glucagon has been identified as early as 50 days and increases throughout fetal life. The B-cell response to glucose is influenced by both gestational and postnatal age, with rapid maturation occurring postnatally. Amino acids stimulate insulin secretion earlier than does glucose and act synergistically with glucose as insulin secretagogues (Grasso et al., 1968) in the fetus at term. Glucagon release is stimulated by arginine and epinephrine but is not affected by glucose or acetylcholine. Insulin increases glycogen accumulation in fetal liver explants after 7 weeks gestation, whereas glucagon depletes hepatic glycogen.

Indirect evidence supports a central role for insulin as a growth factor during fetal life. In the rare instances of congenital absence of the pancreas, the fetus has been severely growth retarded. Infants born with transient diabetes mellitus, thought to be from a delay in maturation of the B cells, are small for gestational age. Indeed, decreased insulin levels are found in other growth-retarded infants as well. By contrast, excess insulin during fetal life is in part responsible for the macrosomia of the infant of the diabetic mother, and hyperinsulinemia is an important associated feature in the Beckwith-Wiedemann syndrome.

In addition to hormonal excess or deficiencies, abnormalities in insulin receptors or function or both may also play a role in growth and carbohydrate homeostasis. In normal infants, the number of insulin receptors on monocytes from cord blood is six times higher than in adults, and the affinity for insulin is twice that of adults, according to the data of Thorsson and Hintz. Leprechaunism was recently shown to be caused by a postreceptor defect that interferes with the insulin signal transduction, resulting in insulin resistance. In this syndrome, hyperglycemia and poor growth are the major features. It is inevitable that many more syndromes caused by defects at the receptor and postreceptor levels will be recognized in the near future.

General Considerations of Carbohydrate Metabolism

It is necessary to understand the blood sugar pattern of the normal newborn before one can evaluate the deviations from normal. In order to understand the state of carbohydrate metabolism properly, it is essential to measure the true glucose levels in blood rather than total reducing substances. We shall not here go into details of the methodology involved because this has been covered thoroughly by Cornblath and Schwartz and by others.

---

*This chapter was revised from the contribution of Dr. Marvin Cornblath, which appeared in the 4th edition of this book.

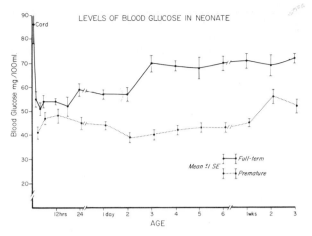

Figure 57–1. A total of 206 determinations of blood glucose levels was obtained in 179 full-sized infants (>2.5 kg), and a total of 442 determinations was made in 104 low birth weight infants (<2.5 kg) throughout the neonatal period. (From Cornblath and Reisner, N. Engl. J. Med. *273*:378, 1965.)

The blood glucose level in umbilical cord blood is proportional to, but lower than, maternal blood. At birth, the scatter is great, depending on a like scatter in the mother's blood glucose levels (i.e., whether or not she has eaten recently, whether or not she has been receiving intravenous fluids, etc.). In presumably normal full-term babies, the blood glucose level drops to 55 to 60 mg/dl at 2 to 4 hours. Cornblath and Reisner found a range of 30 to 120 mg/dl in 95 per cent of these babies. Subsequently, the mean blood glucose rises until it reaches the 70- to 80-mg/dl level from 72 hours onward. After this time, a level of whole blood glucose below 40 or exceeding 125 mg/dl would be considered abnormal (Fig. 57–1).

Most series include blood glucose values in the 40s and 30s, a few in the 20s, and an occasional one below 20 mg/dl some time within the first 24 hours of life. Cornblath and coworkers, in their 1961 study, found 14 per cent of their full-term infants born of normal mothers to have at least one true blood sugar level of less than 30 mg/dl some time within the first 24 hours of life. More recently, Lubchenco and Bard found 11.4 per cent of a general nursery population with blood glucose levels lower than 30 mg/dl before 6 hours of age and prior to the first feed. In none of these normal infants with blood sugar levels in the range considered hypoglycemic for older persons were these low concentrations a problem.

There is general agreement with respect to the glucose levels in the blood of low birth weight infants. Gittleman and Pincus found the mean level to be 39, with a range of 20 to 73 mg/dl, whereas in an earlier study utilizing exactly the same methods, they had reported a mean of 55 mg/dl in full-term normal infants. Lubchenco and Bard found a greater incidence of blood glucose levels below 30 mg/dl in preterm than in term infants, and Beard and colleagues reported an increased frequency with delayed feedings. Baens and coworkers carried on their study for a

longer period and found that after the rise from 3 to 12 hours of age, the true blood sugar of their small infants fell to its lowest level on the third and fourth days, when the mean was as low as 39. They noted that a single hypoglycemic value was not accompanied by signs or symptoms but that repeatedly low values often were. Pildes and her coworkers found hypoglycemia (levels less than 20 mg/dl) in at least two successive readings in 5 to 6 per cent of all infants weighing less than 2500 gm at birth. All these infants fell below the fiftieth percentile for weight in relation to gestational age, and half of them fell below the tenth percentile. Of four sets of twins who were 25 per cent or more discordant in birth weight and of whom the smaller weighed less than 2000 gm, hypoglycemia was found in the smaller twin. Thus, intrauterine growth retardation is an important causal factor in the production of neonatal hypoglycemia. It is likely that hypoglycemia in the infant of low birth weight can not always but often be forestalled by early feeding. The condition should be treated vigorously like all other neonatal hypoglycemias.

The Hypoglycemias

Virtually everyone now accepts the definition of neonatal hypoglycemia as a whole-blood glucose level of less than 30 mg/dl (less than 35 mg/dl in serum or plasma) in the first 72 hours of life or of less than 40 mg/dl (less than 45 mg/dl in serum or plasma) after the third day in full-term, full-size infants. In infants of low birth weight, the lower limit of normal is set at 20 mg/dl in whole blood or 25 mg/dl in plasma or serum. A single low value accompanied by hypoglycemic symptoms is adequate indication for initiating therapy, although a second blood analysis should be obtained. However, in asymptomatic infants, repeatedly low values must be obtained to establish a definitive diagnosis.

Pathogenesis. There are many pathogenic mechanisms involved in the production of hypoglycemia. The majority are listed in Table 57–1.

We propose to discuss these various disorders in the sequence in which the attending physician would normally consider them.

Blood glucose determinations should be performed on certain newborns routinely. They are mandatory for all infants of diabetic mothers and for all low birth weight babies who fall below the tenth percentile for gestational age. Such studies might well be done on all who fall below the fiftieth percentile, especially if an elevation of the hematocrit coexists. It is important that glucose values be obtained on all infants with severe hemolytic disease of the newborn, before and often after exchange transfusion.

It would seem wise to monitor the glucose level in

Table 57–1. Pathogenic Factors in Hypoglycemia

I. Inadequate substrate availability
   A. Malnutrition
      1. Small for gestational age infants
      2. Starvation
      3. Transient diabetes mellitus
   B. Block in gluconeogenesis and substrate availability
      1. Enzymatic immaturity or deficiencies (e.g., fructose-diphosphatase deficiency)
II. Excess substrate utilization
   A. Organic
      1. Hyperinsulinemia
         a. Transient (e.g., IDM, erythroblastosis)
         b. Persistent (e.g., nesidioblastosis, adenomatoid dysplasia, hyperplasia, Beckwith-Wiedemann syndrome)
      2. Isolated or multiple endocrine deficiencies (e.g., hypothalamic deficiency or congenital hypopituitarism, adrenal deficiency)
   B. Functional
      1. Hypersensitivity to amino acids (e.g., leucine)
      2. Hypersensitivity to glucose (e.g., IDM, iatrogenic I.V. glucose administration)
      3. Stress
         a. Sepsis
         b. Hypothermia
         c. Perinatal asphyxia (term, appropriate or large for gestational age)
         d. Anoxia, polycythemia

all undergrown preterm infants regularly, perhaps all those weighing 1500 gm or less, through the first 4 days of life. We would recommend a few determinations on all hypothermic newborns as well as on all macrosomic ones, especially if exomphalos is present (e.g., in the Beckwith-Wiedemann syndrome) or if there is associated micropenis or midline defects such as cleft lip or palate.

The attending physician will do this in order not to miss hypoglycemia, even if it is totally asymptomatic. There is no established schedule for the performance of these tests. Since hypoglycemia occurs as late as the third or even fourth day in small, preterm, or small for gestational age infants, clearly several tests should be made on them in the first 4 days. Infants of diabetic mothers, however, are usually in jeopardy for only the first 24 hours; therefore, determinations should be made at perhaps 2- to 4-hour intervals until it is evident that the initial drop is not too low or until the initial fall has been followed by a substantial compensatory rise. In erythroblastosis fetalis, frequent tests are particularly desirable after the beginning of exchange transfusions with acid-citrate and dextrose (ACD) blood.

Classification.   Recent data permit the differentiation of at least four clinical categories of neonatal hypoglycemia. As modified from Cornblath and Schwartz, these include the following categories:
  I. Early transitional
  II. Secondary

III. Classic, or transient symptomatic
IV. Severe, recurrent, or persistent

Category I occurs during the first 6 to 12 hours of life, is associated with perinatal distress, increased frequency of diabetes mellitus in the mother, and moderately severe erythroblastosis but with a normal frequency of toxemia and twins. There is no sex predilection. Delayed feedings may be important. Over 80 per cent of the infants are asymptomatic. The hypoglycemia is usually of short duration (12 hours) and recurs infrequently. The hypoglycemia usually responds to relatively small quantities of glucose (6 mg/kg/min).

Category II can be characterized as hypoglycemia associated with or secondary to a specific event, usually in a symptomatic infant. Thus, hypoglycemia has been reported with the following: (1) congenital and acquired defects in the central nervous system, (2) sepsis (Yeung, 1970), (3) congenital heart disease, (4) asphyxia, anoxia, and preterminal states, (5) hypothermia, (6) drugs administered to the mother, (7) abrupt cessation of hypertonic glucose, (8) endocrine deficiency (hypothyroidism and adrenal hemorrhage), (9) multiple congenital anomalies, and (10) hypocalcemia. These combinations are important because a low blood glucose should not eliminate the consideration of other pathology and because some of the symptomatology and residual damage in the multiple entities enumerated may be secondary to hypoglycemia.

Category III, classic transient hypoglycemia, is associated with a high incidence of toxemia (hypertensive disease of pregnancy) in the mother and of twinning. The infants are usually small for gestational age; males predominate (2.5:1), and close to 80 per cent have clinical manifestations of hypoglycemia ranging from episodes of tremor, cyanosis, apnea, and irritability to convulsions. Often associated with this type of hypoglycemia are (1) polycythemia (15 per cent), (2) hypocalcemia (12 per cent), (3) central nervous system pathology (10 to 15 per cent), and (4) cardiac enlargement with or without pulmonary edema (15 per cent). Treatment must be vigorous (8 to 10 mg glucose/kg/min) and sustained for 48 to 72 hours or more. As many as 10 per cent of the infants will have recurrent hypoglycemia later in infancy.

Category IV represents severe, recurrent, or persistent hypoglycemia and includes specific syndromes associated with relative or absolute hyperinsulinism or specific enzymatic or metabolic abnormalities. A useful classification is outlined in Table 57–2.

Thus, hypoglycemia in the neonate may have multiple etiologies, pathogeneses, and degrees of significance.

EARLY TRANSITIONAL HYPOGLYCEMIA (CATEGORY I)

Infants with this type of hypoglycemia include those with perinatal distress, delayed feeding, and

Table 57–2. Conditions Associated with Category IV Hypoglycemia

I. Hormone deficiencies
   A. Glucagon deficiency
   B. Multiple (pituitary aplasia or hypoplasia)
   C. Primary (pituitary, thyroid, adrenal cortex or medulla)
II. Hormone excess (hyperinsulinism)
   A. Exomphalos-macroglossia-gigantism syndrome of Beckwith-Wiedemann
   B. Islet cell pathology including:
      1. Adenomatoid dysplasia
      2. Nesidioblastosis
III. Hereditary defects in carbohydrate metabolism
   A. Glycogen storage disease, Type I
   B. Fructose intolerance
   C. Galactosemia
   D. Glycogen synthetase deficiency
   E. Fructose, 1-6 diphosphatase deficiency
IV. Hereditary defects in amino acid metabolism
   A. Maple syrup urine disease
   B. Propionic acidemia
   C. Methylmalonic acidemia
   D. Tyrosinosis

moderately severe erythroblastosis and those of mothers with gestational (IGDM) or insulin dependent diabetes mellitus (IDM).

Infants of Diabetic Mothers

Although as many as 50 per cent of infants of diabetic mothers (IDM) and 25 per cent of infants of gestational diabetic mothers (IGDM) have blood glucose levels of less than 30 mg/dl during the first 2 to 6 hours of life, the majority of these infants show no untoward effects from their hypoglycemia. Many will recover spontaneously, others will respond dramatically to glucagon (300 μg or 0.3 mg per kg intramuscularly or intravenously, not to exceed 1.0 mg total), whereas a few have persistently low values that may be associated with clinical manifestations and require parenteral glucose to maintain normoglycemia. However, there appears to be little if any correlation between low glucose levels and either mortality or morbidity. Many infants with low levels have been alert and lively when their blood glucose was at its lowest. Early oral feeds frequently are adequate to prevent very low blood glucose levels.

Since C-peptide, a byproduct of the conversion of proinsulin to insulin, is secreted by B cells in equimolar amounts with insulin, it can provide a good indication of endogenous fetal insulin secretion, particularly in infants of insulin-dependent diabetic mothers who have insulin antibodies. Sosenko and colleagues found elevated levels of C-peptide in cord sera of infants of diabetic mothers compared with infants of nondiabetic mothers. The levels were directly related to the severity of maternal diabetes.

The hyperglycemia of poorly controlled maternal diabetes stimulates fetal pancreatic islet cell hypertrophy and leads to hypersecretion of insulin. In fact, it was shown by Sosenko and coworkers (Fig. 57–2) that IDMs at an early gestational age already had significantly higher C-peptide levels than did infants of nondiabetic mothers. Indeed, the low tolerance of premature infants of nondiabetic mothers to glucose infusions can be explained by the low C-peptide levels in these infants.

The multiple problems of the IGDM and IDM, including frequency of respiratory distress (see p. 135), hyperbilirubinemia, polycythemia, hypocalcemia, and, perhaps, hypomagnesemia as well as congenital malformations render hypoglycemia in these patients only one aspect of concern in management. Again, if the blood sugar remains low with or without symptoms, parenteral glucose support in addition to oral feedings is indicated. The objective is to support the maintenance of a blood glucose level of approximately 50 mg/dl while allowing the B cell response to decline.

Erythroblastosis Fetalis

Islet hyperplasia has long been recognized in erythroblastosis. In general, the more severe the hemolytic process, the more profound the hypoglycemia. Raivio and Osterlund found it present before, during, or after exchange transfusion in 18 per cent of infants with cord hemoglobin of less than 10 gm/dl. Exchange transfusion with ACD blood produces a temporary hyperglycemia that leads to hypersecretion of insulin and a postexchange reactive hypoglycemia. The problem is less severe in premature infants who are less apt to oversecrete insulin in response to the I.V. glucose. Hyperinsulinism is probably not a problem in erythroblastotic infants before birth, since they are not macrosomic.

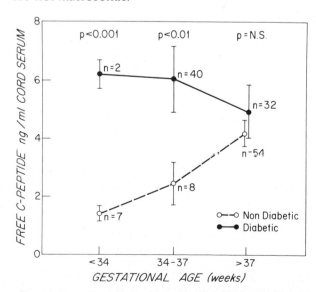

Figure 57–2. Relation of cord serum C-peptide levels to gestational age in infants of nondiabetic and diabetic mothers (mean ± S.E.M.). (From Sosenko, I., et al. Reprinted, by permission, from the New England Journal of Medicine *301*:859, 1979.)

SECONDARY HYPOGLYCEMIA (CATEGORY II)

Hypoglycemia has been reported closely associated with or precipitated by a number of events, ranging from the abrupt cessation of hypertonic glucose infusion to infections and central nervous system abnormalities, including congenital defects, birth injury, microcephaly, hemorrhage, and kernicterus. Thus, it is important that a hypoglycemic glucose level not preclude the possibility of other pathology. Furthermore, some of the manifestations and damage in a number of neonatal pathologic states may be due to associated hypoglycemia.

An unusual iatrogenic hypoglycemia was described by Nagel and coworkers in an infant in whom an umbilical artery catheter must have permitted infusions to the pancreatic vessels. The patient was profoundly hypoglycemic; repositioning of the catheter led to an immediate and sustained rise in blood glucose. The authors postulated that the tip of the catheter was positioned in such a way that dextrose infusions were delivered directly to pancreatic vessels and stimulated insulin secretion.

In two reported series (Koivisto et al. 1972; Fluge, 1974) of a total of 447 infants with hypoglycemic blood levels, 238, or 53.2 per cent, were considered to have "secondary hypoglycemia."

CLASSIC TRANSIENT HYPOGLYCEMIA (CATEGORY III)

It was not until 1959 that the occurrence of hypoglycemia in groups of newborn infants other than infants of diabetic mothers was noted by Cornblath and associates. They described eight infants, born of mothers with toxemia, who had tremors, cyanosis, and, occasionally, convulsions in association with hypoglycemia. The time of recognition of symptoms was between $2\frac{1}{2}$ hours and 7 days, with the peak between 24 and 48 hours. Since then, many clinics have described similar hypoglycemia in groups of infants, the majority of whom are of low birth weight for gestational age.

This syndrome is associated with an increased frequency of maternal toxemia and twinning as well as with central nervous system abnormalities (10 to 15 per cent), polycythemia (15 per cent), hypocalcemia (12 per cent), and cardiomegaly (15 per cent).

The symptoms of hypoglycemia include tremors, convulsions, bouts of apnea, apathy, refusal to feed, cyanosis, irritability, and limpness, all of which are nonspecific and may exist for a variety of other reasons. Their nonspecific nature has led some to challenge their relationship to hypoglycemia. However, when two or more successive blood glucose values are low, and these symptoms disappear with the ad-

ministration of parenteral glucose, it is hard to avoid the conclusion that they are related.

The frequency of hypoglycemia is two to three per 1000 livebirths. Of infants less than 2500 gm birth weight, who have blood glucose levels determined daily, 5 to 6 per cent will show blood glucose levels of less than 20 mg/dl on at least two occasions, according to Wybregt and associates.

Once one finds a blood glucose level of either less than 30 mg/dl in a full-term infant or less than 20 mg in one weighing less than 2500 gm, the determination is repeated if the baby is asymptomatic, as is the case with approximately 20 per cent of such patients. If the result of this second evaluation is also low or if the original low figure was accompanied by any of the aforementioned symptoms, treatment is begun promptly. Symptomatic infants are given 0.5 to 1.0 gm per kg of 25 per cent glucose in water intravenously at the rate of 8 to 10 mg/kg/min. Thus, for a daily fluid requirement of 65 to 85 ml/kg/day, use 20 per cent glucose solution. After 12 to 24 hours, add 40 mEq/l of NaCl, and after 24 to 48 hours of intravenous therapy, add 1 to 2 mEq/kg/day of KCl. Oral feedings should be started as soon as the child's condition permits. Some infants remain hypoglycemic even after this amount of supplementary glucose is administered. Glucagon is of no help to these babies because their stores of glycogen appear to be exhausted. Diazoxide is not recommended because of its unfavorable side effects. Cortisone, however, may be very effective in raising the blood sugar level. If this is truly transient symptomatic hypoglycemia, both the added glucose and the cortisone will be able to be withdrawn after a few days.

Initial studies to be performed when hypoglycemia is discovered and verified include a lumbar puncture to rule out intracranial bleeding, a hematocrit determination, a urinalysis for galactose or other reducing sugars and for acetone (with glycogen storage disease in mind), and a blood calcium. A roentgenogram of the chest for heart size is also indicated.

The blood glucose levels should be followed by determinations every 4 to 6 hours, and further studies are indicated if the symptoms persist or recur. If the serum calcium is found to be below 7.0 mg per 100 ml (as it not infrequently is in these babies), calcium should be given as described for the hypocalcemias (see p. 466).

All agree that symptomatic infants must be treated vigorously. Whether or not low blood glucose values are physiologic and without hazard in asymptomatic infants remains to be determined. Newborns may not respond to unusually low blood glucose levels with tremors or convulsions because of availability of other substrates (e.g., ketones and lactate) to support cerebral function or because of some cerebral refractoriness comparable to their ability to withstand prolonged hypoxia. Indeed, the study of Anderson and coworkers revealed "extensive degeneration of nerve cells in the central nervous system" in three infants who died with untreated hypoglycemia, whereas in three others who had hypoglycemia that was corrected but who later died from other causes, only slight abnormalities were found in the brain. For this reason, it is advised that all hypoglycemic infants, symptomatic or not, be treated.

Follow-up of babies with transient hypoglycemia reveals that the great majority recover completely, although a few may have recurrences at some later date. In a prospective controlled 5- to 7-year follow-up of 39 hypoglycemic and 41 normoglycemic matched controls, Pildes and coworkers found no differences in mean height or weight or EEG records. However, the hypoglycemic group had smaller head circumferences, a higher incidence of neurologic abnormalities, and a larger number of children with I.Q. scores below 86 than did the control group. Asymptomatic infants had a better prognosis than did those with convulsions.

SEVERE RECURRENT OR PERSISTENT HYPOGLYCEMIA (CATEGORY IV)

If hypoglycemia proves recalcitrant to the aforementioned management or if it disappears only to recur promptly, one must begin a search for other causes, as outlined in Table 57–2. Only a few of the syndromes in this category will be discussed here.

Multiple Endocrine Deficiencies

At least 22 cases of multiple endocrine deficiencies associated with anterior pituitary "aplasia" or hypoplasia or, in some patients, a hypothalamic abnormality have been reviewed by Sadeghi-Nejad and Senior and by Cornblath and Schwartz. The infants tend to have an increased birth weight (mean 3.81 kg for 14), males predominate 2:1, and, in 20 per cent, a sibling was affected to a varying degree. In addition to an 85 per cent frequency of severe symptomatic hypoglycemia in the first hours and days of life, jaundice, hypocalcemia, hepatomegaly, and edema were relatively common. Another noteworthy abnormality in the males was a small phallus, or micropenis, reported in nine of 11 patients. A few infants had midline deformities, including clefts of the palate and lip. To date, the prognosis is guarded. A high index of suspicion must be maintained, and critical laboratory studies such as a blood sample for glucose, HGH, ACTH, cortisol, T$_4$, TSH, and insulin must be performed prior to initiating therapy. Therapy requires immediate parenteral glucose plus steroids. Further replacement therapy may be introduced as specific endocrine deficiencies are documented. Recognizing its familial occurrence, Sadeghi-Nejad and Senior reported a patient who survived normally as a result of prompt therapy initiated on the basis of the history of the death of a previous sibling. They suggest all future pregnancies be monitored with maternal plasma or urinary estriol levels to anticipate affected fetuses.

Hypoglycemia from Glucagon Deficiency

The first patient in whom glucagon deficiency was postulated as the cause of persistent neonatal hypoglycemia was reported by Vidnes and Oyasaeter in Norway in 1977. The disorder is apparently inherited as an autosomal recessive, since two siblings of this Pakistani child died at 4 months of age with symptoms of hypoglycemia. The patient described had convulsions, hypotonia, and a weak cry on the third day of life, with a blood glucose level of 15 mg/dl. He responded to intravenous glucose. He was shown to be glucagon-deficient, with barely measurable plasma glucagon levels and no elevation in blood glucose after alanine infusions. The patient responded to glucagon injections. Normal insulin secretion was present.

Hyperinsulinemia

Hypoglycemia of Infancy with Nesidioblastosis. Nesidioblastosis is a pathologic diagnosis made by microscopic examination of the pancreas. The findings include the presence of beta and other islet cells in the interstitial spaces of the pancreas as well as endocrine cells apparently arising from the pancreatic ducts. The associated clinical syndrome has recently been more frequently recognized, owing to the earlier and more aggressive surgical approach to hypoglycemia in infancy, coupled with advances in understanding pancreatic histology by special staining, electron microscopy, and specific immunofluorescent techniques (Orci and Zuppinger, 1976; Hirsch et al., 1977). Since 1971, the number of infants in whom this diagnosis has been made by biopsy or pancreatectomy has increased (Yakovac et al., 1971; Harken et al., 1971; Grampa et al., 1974; Zuppinger, 1975; Hirsch et al., 1977; Gabbay, 1978).

The clinical syndrome is characterized by the occurrence of persistent hypoglycemia at birth or shortly thereafter. A family history of similar hypoglycemia of infancy states has been described in an appreciable number of cases. There are at least five known families with more than one affected sibling. The infant is frequently symptomatic with severe signs of hypoglycemia, including seizures. In its milder form, the infant may have only mildly low blood glucose levels (40 to 50 mg/dl), remaining asymptomatic because of the frequency of feedings. In such cases, the infant may not be recognized as having significant hypoglycemia until the nightly feedings are withdrawn at 6 weeks or later. In all cases, the insulin levels are inappropriately elevated with respect to the blood glucose levels. The serum insulin levels are usually low, under 20 μU/ml (range, 6 to 30 μU/ml), which is nevertheless quite high in the face of a blood glucose of 20 to 30 mg/dl. The fasting serum proinsulin fraction, which is often elevated in adult cases of insulinoma, is usually low (below 10 per cent) and is of no help in making the diagnosis. The finding of inappropriately elevated insulin levels and the frequent need to maintain a high parenteral glucose infusion rate of 10 to 20 mg/kg min to attain normoglycemia make the diagnosis almost certain.

The patients with severe hypoglycemia are equally refractory to medical therapy with diazoxide or steroids. While glucagon can be given to elevate the blood glucose acutely, the majority of patients have normal or slightly elevated glucagon levels. Hirsch and coworkers reported elevated plasma glucagon values in two patients who responded normally to exogenous glucagon and who had normal intravenous glucagon tolerance tests. That the inappropriate secretion of insulin and the consequent relative hyperglycemia is in large part responsible for the severe persistent hypoglycemia was evident in a few reported cases of euglycemia after a combination of somatostatin and glucagon was given by continuous infusion.

A variety of measures are useful for emergency treatment pending operation. The infant's blood glucose should be monitored every 4 hours, and he should be fed frequently. Continuous glucose infusions, via a central venous line if necessary, are necessary to maintain normoglycemia until surgery. Maintenance of normoglycemia prior to surgery has been credited with virtually complete prevention of neurologic damage in these infants (Gabbay, 1978). It is probably sufficient to maintain blood glucose levels of 50 to 60 mg/dl, and the glucose infusion rate should be adjusted accordingly.

Since no laboratory tests are specific or diagnostic, early surgical intervention for biopsy and a partial (75 to 85 per cent) pancreatectomy are indicated. If the hypoglycemia recurs, a repeat pancreatectomy, with removal of up to 95 per cent of the pancreas, may be necessary. At the time of surgery, special handling of the biopsy or surgical specimen is essential to preparing the tissue for electron microscopy and immunofluorescent studies. In addition to demonstrating the wide scattering of islet cells among ductular and acinar tissue (Yakovac et al., 1971; Hirsch et al., 1977; Gabbay, 1978), various authors have shown that the diffuse islets include beta cells containing insulin, alpha cells containing glucagon, and D cells containing somatostatin. Thus, nesidioblastosis may provide important leads in understanding the interactions of these three hormones as well as the importance of organized surface contact between these cell types in regulating glucose homeostasis.

Instances of normal basal plasma insulin levels and increased insulin *binding* sites have been described in infants with nesidioblastosis, leucine sensitivity, and Type I glycogen storage disease. Chrousos and coworkers speculate that chronic hypoglycemia may stimulate the increase in insulin receptors, which in turn would increase the bioeffect of insulin and reduce glucose secretion from the liver. However, this mechanism is presumably secondary and remains speculative.

Adenomatoid Dysplasia and/or Islet Cell Adenoma. Before 1959, only one neonate with questionable islet cell adenoma had been reported (Sherman, 1947). Since then, several infants with islet cell adenoma have been reported.

There is no way at the present time to distinguish an islet cell adenoma from the much more frequent hypoglycemia of infancy with nesidioblastosis just described. The only clinical and laboratory finding is a relatively high insulin to glucose ratio (i.e., the plasma insulin values exceeded 10 µU/ml when the blood glucose was less than 15 to 20 mg/dl); thus, a relative hyperinsulinemia was apparent. Another usual feature is that glucose infusion rates of 15 to 20 mg/kg/min may be needed to attain normoglycemia. In most patients, diazoxide is ineffective in normalizing the blood glucose, as is every other type of medical therapy.

At operation, discrete areas resembling isolated tumors are found in the majority of infants, but frequently two or more "adenomata" are found. In most cases, these areas are not well-delineated, encapsulated adenomas but rather areas that show dysplastic changes with diffuse involvement and spread. These adenomatoid dysplasias are distinctly different from what one sees in the adult form of an insulinoma (Gabbay, 1978). In one case, the "adenoma" showed evidence of ductules and nesidioblastosis within the lesion. Since the majority of infants had a partial to almost complete pancreatectomy, one is hard put to determine whether these "adenomas" are the sole cause of the hypoglycemia or part of a more diffuse dysplastic process similar to that seen in nesidioblastosis. It is probable that both nesidioblastosis and adenomatoid dysplasia represent a continuum in islet dysmorphogenesis.

Lesions are found in the tail, the head, and the body as well as at the junction of the head and the body of the pancreas. The majority of infants have immediate hyperglycemia of significant magnitude following surgery. The pre- and postoperative management of these infants is identical with that of the infants with nesidioblastosis. In both conditions, diagnoses have been made earlier, and a number of infants are alive and well at follow-up. Others have moderate to severe neurologic or mental defects or both. Early diagnosis and therapy are critical and depend on rigorous maintenance of normoglycemia in these infants until surgery as well as reliable blood glucose and plasma insulin assays of blood obtained when the infant is hypoglycemic.

The Exomphalos-Macroglossia-Gigantism (EMG) Syndrome of Beckwith-Wiedemann (see p. 320). Although not a constant finding, hypoglycemias of varying severity and duration have been reported in many of these infants during the first days of life. Much of the neonatal mortality and subsequent morbidity have been attributed to untreated hypoglycemia, but the evidence is far from conclusive. Carbohydrate tolerance tests, hormonal measurements (insulin levels are frequently higher than 50 μU/ml in contrast to much lower values in nesidioblastosis), and microscopic examination of the pancreas support the idea that hyperinsulinemia is responsible for the hypoglycemia.

This syndrome is characterized by omphalocele, muscular macroglossia, gigantism, visceromegaly, and mild microcephaly as well as by diffuse cytomegaly of the adrenal fetal cortex and hyperplasia of the kidneys, endocrine pancreas, and gonadal interstitial cells. Advanced bone age, abnormal insertion of the diaphragm, flame nevus of the face, earlobe fissures, and hemihypertrophy also occur. Over 50 patients have been reported, and extensive reviews of the syndrome have been published.

Leucine Sensitivity. This functional aberration is not considered a specific cause of hypoglycemia and may be present with multiple types of beta-cell abnormalities, either functional or structural. If present, a low leucine diet is both diagnostic and therapeutic. Roth and Segal as well as Snyder and Robinson have reported the details of patients who received successful dietary management.

The hypoglycemia in some of these patients has responded to zinc glucagon, in some to diazoxide, and in others to cortisone. In almost all, medication has been discontinued without further trouble after 2 to 7 months.

It is well known that hypoglycemia plays a role in the symptomatology of congenital galactosemia, hereditary fructose intolerance, and the glycogen storage diseases. These disorders are discussed elsewhere. Hypoglycemia can also occur in certain hereditary defects in amino acid metabolism, including maple syrup urine disease, propionic acidemia, methylmalonic acidemia, and tyrosinosis.

In 1963, Lewis and coworkers reported hypoglycemia caused by an inability to synthesize glycogen because of congenital and familial deficiency of the enzyme glycogen synthetase. In 1965, Parr and coworkers recorded another example. Their babies did not become symptomatic in the neonatal period, probably because they were receiving feedings throughout the night. Trouble appeared when night feedings were discontinued.

Transient Diabetes Mellitus (Temporary Idiopathic Neonatal Hyperglycemia)

Reversible diabetes mellitus is an almost unheard of phenomenon in any period of life except the neonatal. Gentz and Cornblath were able to find 50 reports of hyperglycemia in the first 6 weeks of life in the literature up to 1969. Of these cases, 11 appeared to be permanent diabetes, nine were uncertain, and 20 were transient. Subsequently, additional patients have been reported by Milner and colleagues, including three siblings born over a 7-year interval.

Hyperglycemia occurs in small for gestational age infants, presenting with marked dehydration and wasting but with a history of adequate food intake and absence of vomiting or diarrhea. Both sexes are affected equally, and a positive family history for diabetes is present in about one third of cases. Ketosis is mild and may appear after hydration. The diagnosis is based on glycosuria and hyperglycemia with blood sugars in excess of 250 mg/dl. Where measured, acid-base derangements are not uncommon. Of 10 infants in whom electrolytes were measured, six had normal serum sodiums, one had hypernatremia, and three were hyponatremic. Thus, the observations of Jung and Done of two infants with transient hyperglycemia secondary to hyperosmolarity and profound hypernatremia resulting from the ingestion of a concentrated formula are the exception and not the rule.

Although the exact etiology of this syndrome is unknown, several infants have had relative hypoinsulinemia; that is, inappropriately low plasma immunoreactive insulin values in relation to the degree of hyperglycemia. Thus, the data support the hypothesis that a temporary aberration in beta-cell function in the islet of Langerhans may be responsible. In a few of the reported cases, hyperglycemia was preceded by a period of symptomatic hypoglycemia.

These infants differ from true diabetics in the reversibility of their disease without recurrence in follow-ups of 3 to 25 years. For this reason, insulin treatment is optional. Certainly, insulin is indicated when hyperosmolality is great because of glucose levels of 500 to 1000 mg/dl, which they often can reach. This may represent a real hazard to the cells of the central nervous system and possibly to the kidney, since renal cortical necrosis and hyperglycemia have been found associated a number of times. The infants are usually insulin-sensitive, and clinical improvement occurs with blood sugar values between 130 and 200 mg/dl. Hypoglycemia must be avoided.

True fetal onset diabetes is even rarer than the transient form. Liggins reported such an infant, whose birth weight at term was only 1800 grams. That infant was permanently diabetic.

REFERENCES

Anderson, J. M., Milner, R. D. G., and Strich, S. J.: Effects of neonatal hypoglycemia on the nervous system: a pathological study. J. Neurol. Neurosurg. Psychiatry 30:295, 1967.

Baens, G., Lundeen, E., and Cornblath, M.: Studies of carbohydrate metabolism in the newborn infant. VI. Levels of glucose in blood in premature infants. Pediatrics 31:580, 1963.

Beard, A. G., Panos, T. C., Marasigan, B. V., Eminians, J., Kennedy, H. F., and Lamb, J.: Perinatal stress and the premature neonate: II. Effect of fluid and calorie deprivation on blood glucose. J. Pediatr. 68:329, 1966.

Beard, A., Cornblath, M., Gentz, J., Kellum, M., Person, B., Zetterstrom, R., and Haworth, J. C.: Neonatal hypoglycemia: a discussion. J. Pediatr. 79:314, 1971.

Benzing, F. III, Schubert, W., Hug, G., and Kaplan, S.: Simultaneous hypoglycemia and acute congestive heart failure. Circulation 40:209, 1969.

Bloomgarden, Z. T., Sundell, H., Rogers, L. W., et al.: Treatment of intractable neonatal hypoglycemia with somatostatin plus glucagon. J. Pediatr. 96:148, 1980.

Chrousos, G. P., Rodbard, H. W., and Adams, A. J.: Increased ^{125}I-insulin receptor binding to erythrocytes of hypoglycemic infants and children. Pediatr. Res. 15:1345, 1981.

Cochrane, W. A.: Idiopathic infantile hypoglycemia and leucine sensitivity. Metabolism 9:386, 1960.

Combs, J. T., Grunt, J. A., and Brandt, I. K.: New syndrome of neonatal hypoglycemia: association with visceromegaly, macroglossia, microcephaly and abnormal umbilicus. N. Engl. J. Med. 275:236, 1966.

Cornblath, M., Ganzon, A. F., Nicolopoulos, D., Baens, G. S., Hollander, R. J., Gordon, M. H., and Gordon, H. H.: Studies of carbohydrate metabolism in the newborn infant. III. Some factors influencing the capillary blood sugar and the response to glucagon during the first hours of life. Pediatrics 27:378, 1961.

Cornblath, M., Levin, E. Y., and Marquetti, E.: Studies of carbohydrate metabolism in the newborn. II. The effect of glucagon on the concentration of sugar in capillary blood of the newborn infant. Pediatrics 21:885, 1958.

Cornblath, M., Odell, G. B., and Levin, E. Y.: Symptomatic neonatal hypoglycemia associated with toxemia of pregnancy. J. Pediatr. 55:545, 1959.

Cornblath, M., and Reisner, S. H.: Blood glucose in the neonate and its clinical significance. N. Engl. J. Med. 273:378, 1965.

Cornblath, M., and Schwartz, R.: Disorders of Carbohydrate Metabolism in Infancy. 2nd ed. Philadelphia, W. B. Saunders Co., 1976.

Cornblath, M., Wybregt, S. H., Baens, G. S., and Klein, R. I.: Studies of carbohydrate metabolism in the newborn infant. VIII. Symptomatic neonatal hypoglycemia. Pediatrics 33:388, 1964.

Cser, A., and Milner, R. D. G.: Glucose tolerance and insulin secretion in very small babies. Acta Paediatr. Scand. 64:457, 1975.

Dubois, P. M., Paulin, C., Assan, R., et al.: Evidence for immunoreactive somatostatin in the endocrine cells of the human fetal pancreas. Nature 256:731, 1975.

Dweck, H. S., and Cassady, G.: Glucose intolerance in infants of very low birth weight. I. Incidence of hypoglycemia in infants of birth weights 1100 gms. or less. Pediatrics 53:189, 1974.

Ehrlich, R. M., and Martin, J. M.: Diazoxide in the management of hypoglycemia in infancy and childhood. Am. J. Dis. Child. 117:411, 1969.

Filippi, G., and McKusick, V.: The Beckwith-Wiedemann syndrome. Medicine 49:279, 1970.

Fluge, G.: Clinical aspects of neonatal hypoglycaemia. Acta Paediatr. Scand. 63:826, 1974.

Gabbay, K. H.: Hypoglycemia in a three-month-old infant (CPC). N. Engl. J. Med. 299:241, 1978.

Garces, L. Y., Drash, A., and Kenny, F. M.: Islet cell tumor in the neonate. Pediatrics 41:789, 1968.

Gentz, J. C. H., and Cornblath, M.: Transient diabetes of the newborn. Adv. Pediatr. 16:345, 1969.

Gittleman, I. F., and Pincus, J. B.: Blood sugar and citric acid levels in newborn infants. Pediatrics 9:38, 1952.

Grampa, G., Gargantini, L., Grigolato, P. G., and Ghiumello, G.: Hypoglycemia in infancy caused by beta cell nesidioblastosis. Am. J. Dis. Child. 128:226, 1974.

Grasso, S., Palumbo, G., Rugolo, S., et al.: Human fetal insulin secretion in response to maternal glucose and leucine administration. Pediatr. Res. 14:782, 1980.

Grasso, S., Saporito, N., Messina, A., and Reitano, G.: Plasma

insulin, glucose and free fatty acid (FFA) response to various stimuli in the premature infant. Diabetes 17:306, 1968.

Guest, G. M.: Infantile diabetes mellitus: three cases in successive siblings, two with onset at three months of age and one at nine days of age. Am. J. Dis. Child. 75:461, 1948.

Hamilton, J. P., Baker, L., Kaye, R., and Koop, C. E.: Subtotal pancreatectomy in the management of severe persistent idiopathic hypoglycemia. Pediatrics 39:49, 1967.

Hansson, S., and Redin, B.: Familial neonatal hypoglycemia: syndrome resembling foetopathic diabetica. Acta Paediatr. 52:145, 1963.

Harken, A. H., Filler, R. M., Av Ruskin, J. W., and Crigler, J. F., Jr.: The role of "total" pancreatectomy in the treatment of unremitting hypoglycemia of infancy. J. Pediatr. Surg., 6:284, 1971.

Hazeltine, F. G.: Hypoglycemia and Rh erythroblastosis fetalis. Pediatrics 39:696, 1967.

Heitz, P. U., Kloppel, G., Hack, W. H., et al.: Nesidioblastosis: the pathologic basis of persistent hyperinsulinemic hypoglycemia in infants. Diabetes 26:632, 1977.

Hirsh, H. J., Loo, S. W., and Gabbay, K. H.: The development and regulation of the endocrine pancreas. J. Pediatr. 3:518, 1977.

Hirsch, H. J., Loo, S., Evans, N., Crigler, J. F., Jr., Filler, R. M., and Gabbay, K. H.: Hypoglycemia of infancy and nesidioblastosis: studies with somatostatin. N. Engl. J. Med. 296:1323, 1977.

Jung, A. L., and Done, A. K.: Extreme hyperosmolality and "transient diabetes." Am. J. Dis. Child. 118:859, 1969.

Keidan, S. E.: Transient diabetes in infancy. Arch. Dis. Child. 39:291, 1955.

King, A. C., and Cuatrecasas, P.: Peptide hormone-induced receptor mobility, aggregation and internalization. N. Engl. J. Med. 305:77, 1981.

Kitzmiller, J. L., Cloherty, J. P., Younger, M. D., et al.: Diabetic pregnancy and perinatal morbidity. Am. J. Obstet. Gynecol. 131:560, 1978.

Koivisto, M., Blanco-Sequeiros, M., and Krause, U.: Neonatal symptomatic and asymptomatic hypoglycaemia: a follow-up study of 151 children. Develop. Med. Child Neurol. 14:603, 1972.

Lewis, G. M., Spencer-Peet, J., and Stewart, K. M.: Infantile hypoglycemia due to inherited deficiency of glycogen synthetase in the liver. Arch. Dis. Child. 38:40, 1963.

Liggins, G. C.: The influence of the fetal hypothalamus and pituitary on growth. In Size at Birth, Ciba Foundation Symposium 27 (new series), Elsevier North-Holland, 1974.

Lubchenco, L. O., and Bard, H.: Incidence of hypoglycemia in newborn infants classified by birth weight and gestational age. Pediatrics 47:831, 1971.

McQuarrie, I.: Idiopathic spontaneously occurring hypoglycemia in infants. A.M.A. J. Dis. Child. 87:399, 1954.

Milner, R. D. G., Ferguson, A. W., and Naidu, S. H.: Aetiology of transient neonatal diabetes. Arch. Dis. Child. 46:724, 1971.

Milner, R. D. G.: Neonatal hypoglycemia. J. Perinat. Med. 7:185, 1979.

Milner, R. D. G.: Growth and development of the endocrine pancreas. In Davis, J., and Dobbing, J. (eds.): Scientific Foundation of Pediatrics. London, William Heineman Medical Books, 1981.

Nagel, J. W., Sims, J. S., and Alpin, C. E.: Refractory hypoglycemia associated with a malpositioned umbilical artery catheter. Pediatrics 64:315, 1979.

Orci, L., and Zuppinger, K. A.: Nesidioblastosis. Chapter V Appendix. In Cornblath, M., and Schwartz, R., (Eds.): Disorders of Carbohydrate Metabolism in Infancy. 2nd ed. Philadelphia, W. B. Saunders Co., 1976.

Parr, J., Teree, T. M., and Larner, J.: Symptomatic hypoglycemia, visceral fatty metamorphosis and aglycogenosis in an infant lacking glycogen synthetase and phosphorylase. Pediatrics 35:770, 1965.

Pildes, R. S., Cornblath, M., Warren, I., Page-El, E., diMenza, S., Merritt, D. M., and Peeva, A.: A prospective controlled study of neonatal hypoglycemia. Pediatrics 54:5, 1974.

Raivio, K. O., and Hallman, N.: Neonatal hypoglycemia. I. Occurrence of hypoglycemia in patients with various neonatal disorders. Acta Paediatr. Scand. 57:517, 1968.

Raivio, K. O., and Osterlund, K.: Hypoglycemia and hyperinsulinemia associated with erythroblastosis fetalis. Pediatrics 43:217, 1969.

Roe, T. F., Kershnar, A. K., Weitzman, J. J., and Madrigal, L. S.: Beckwith's syndrome with extreme organ hyperplasia. Pediatrics 52:372, 1973.

Roth, H., and Segal, S.: The dietary management of leucine-sensitive hypoglycemia, with report of a case. Pediatrics 34:831, 1964.

Sadeghi-Nejad, A., and Senior, B.: A familial syndrome of isolated aplasia of the anterior pituitary. J. Pediatr. 84:79, 1974.

Sadeghi-Nejad, A., Loridan, L., and Senior, B.: Studies of factors affecting gluconeogenesis and glycolysis in glycogenosis of the liver. J. Pediatr. 76:561, 1970.

Sherman, H.: Islet cell tumor of pancreas in a newborn infant (nesidioblastoma). Am. J. Dis. Child., 74:58, 1947.

Snyder, R. D., and Robinson, A.: Leucine-induced hypoglycemia. Am. J. Dis. Child. 113:566, 1967.

Sosenko, I., Kitzmiller, J., Loo, S., et al.: The infant of the diabetic mother: correlation of increased cord C-peptide levels with macrosomia and hypoglycemia. N. Engl. J. Med. 301:859, 1979.

Thorsson, A. V., and Hintz, R. L.: Insulin receptors in the newborn: an increase in affinity and number. N. Engl. J. Med. 297:908, 1977.

Vidnes, J., and Oyasaeter, S.: Glucagon deficiency causing severe neonatal hypoglycemia in a patient with normal insulin secretion. Pediatr. Res. 11:943, 1977.

Wybregt, S. H., Reisner, S. H., Patel, R. K., Nelhaus, G., and Cornblath, M.: The incidence of neonatal hypoglycemia in a nursery for premature infants. J. Pediatr. 64:796, 1964.

Yakovac, W. C., Baker, L., and Hummeler, K.: Beta cell nesidioblastosis in idiopathic hypoglycemia in infancy. J. Pediatr. 79:226, 1971.

Yeung, C. Y.: Hypoglycemia in neonatal sepsis. J. Pediatr. 77:812, 1970.

Zuppinger, K. A.: Hypoglycemia in childhood: Evaluation of diagnostic procedures. In Falkner, F., Kretchmer, N., and Rossi, E. (Eds.): Monographs in Paediatrics. Basel, S. Karger, 1975.

PART 8 INBORN ERRORS OF METABOLISM

58

General Considerations

By Harvey L. Levy

The inborn errors of metabolism are among the most exciting and challenging disorders in medicine. This is particularly true for those that cause clinical disease in the newborn infant or that are identified by routine newborn screening. As newly recognized inborn errors are added to an already long list, it becomes increasingly obvious that they represent not only a substantial percentage of known genetic disorders but also a growing percentage of newborn disease.

Three factors account for the increased recognition that inborn errors of metabolism are an important part of neonatal medicine: (1) the greater awareness of clinical signs of these disorders in the newborn, (2) the increased availability of reliable methods for detecting and measuring biochemical substances in physiologic fluids, (3) the emergence of newborn screening for metabolic disorders as a routine procedure that identifies biochemical disorders in infants who may be *clinically normal* and in whom timely treatment will *prevent* clinical manifestations from ever occurring (see Newborn Screening, Part 2).

The inborn error of metabolism is genetic in origin. As in other genetic disorders, the basic abnormality is a mutant gene. The gene, acting as a template, directs the synthesis of a complementary mRNA (messenger RNA) that travels from the nucleus, where it was synthesized, to the cytoplasm, where it attaches to ribosomes and directs the arrangement of amino acids into a polypeptide chain (Fig. 58–1). If the gene is abnormal as a result of a mutation, the resulting polypeptide chain is abnormal.

In an inborn error, the protein that contains this polypeptide is functionally as well as structurally abnormal. If this protein is an enzyme, which it usually is in an inborn error of metabolism, the result is deficient activity. The cause of this deficiency may be inadequate binding of substrate or, less commonly, insufficient binding of coenzyme (Fig. 58–2). In either instance, the result is accumulation of substrate and reduced synthesis of product (Fig. 58–3). Metabolic byproducts of the substrate (secondary metabolites) may also accumulate as a result of the increased substrate concentration.

An example of this is phenylketonuria (PKU), as illustrated in Fig. 58–1 (see Chapter 60). Deficient activity of phenylalanine hydroxylase in the liver results in increased concentrations of phenylalanine and related metabolites in body fluids and tissues and a concomitant decrease in the concentration of tyrosine, the product of phenylalanine hydroxylation. In PKU, the basic phenylalanine hydroxylase enzyme (apoenzyme) is abnormal. Phenylalanine hydroxylation may also be impaired if the necessary cofactor, tetrahydrobiopterin (BH_4), is deficient. This may result from a defect in dihydropteridine reductase, which is essential for the regeneration of BH_4 from quinonoid dihydropteridine ($_qBH_2$), or a defect in the synthesis of biopterin, a precursor of BH_4.

The basis of the clinical abnormalities in the inborn errors of metabolism is presumed to be the accumulation of substrate and/or related metabolites, which in increased concentrations may be toxic to certain body tissues. The precise mechanism by which this toxicity occurs, however, is not known.

The excitement surrounding the inborn errors of metabolism is based on the recognition that a number of them can be treated so that the irreversible clinical

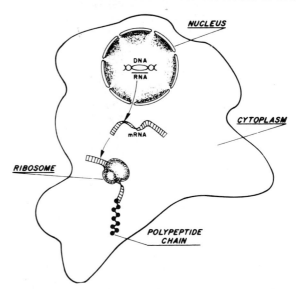

Figure 58–1. The gene, or DNA, serves as a template for the synthesis of RNA that has a nucleic acid sequence complementary to the nucleic acid sequence of the DNA. This RNA, which becomes processed to mRNA (messenger RNA), enters the cytoplasm and attaches to the ribosomes. Here it directs the formation of a polypeptide chain that has an amino acid sequence in the precise order determined by the mRNA. If the nucleic acid sequence of the DNA is altered as the result of a mutation (inherited or spontaneous), the altered sequence is reflected through altered mRNA in an altered amino acid sequence in the polypeptide chain. Thus, the protein that contains this altered polypeptide chain is abnormal.

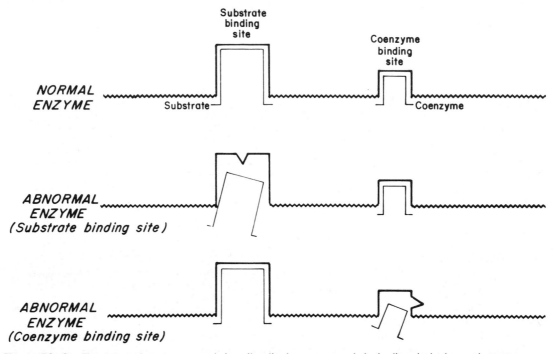

Figure 58–2. The normal enzyme contains sites that accommodate both substrate and coenzyme. A genetic mutation results in structural abnormality at either the substrate or the coenzyme binding site. When this occurs, the substrate or the coenzyme cannot bind properly to the enzyme, and enzyme activity is reduced.

complications are prevented. Thus, mental retardation, liver disease, and eye disease that, once present, cannot be treated can be prevented with early diagnosis and treatment. Furthermore, the potential for prevention of certain types of heart and kidney disease, which may be at least partly due to metabolic disorders, renders the field that much more exciting.

At present, there are two forms of specific therapy. The most important is a dietary change that results in lowered concentrations of the presumed toxic biochemicals and normalization of the deficient product. The second type of therapy is the administration of a large amount of a specific vitamin that is utilized as a cofactor by the deficient enzyme system. This latter therapy, which results in activation of the enzyme, is possible only when the defect is in binding of the coenzyme (Fig. 58–2) or in deficient production of the cofactor. Optimal effectiveness from either of these therapeutic modes, however, is often possible only when the metabolic disorder is identified in the neonate by routine screening or through prompt recognition of the clinical signs and appropriate biochemical testing.

Antenatal diagnosis of an inborn error of metabolism (see Prenatal Genetic Diagnosis, Part I) has potential therapeutic value. For this diagnosis, the presence of an inborn error is suspected in the fetus, perhaps on the basis of occurrence of the disorder in the family. Through amniocentesis and examination of the cultured amniotic cells or the fluid, the diagnosis is made. "Therapy" in most instances is usually induced abortion, which, although not actually treatment, may be extremely important to the family. A significant alternative to abortion is intrauterine therapy for the fetus. Vitamin B_{12} treatment was administered to a mother who was carrying a fetus with B_{12}-responsive methylmalonic acidemia.

NORMAL METABOLISM

SUBSTRATE —ENZYME→ PRODUCT

INBORN ERROR OF METABOLISM

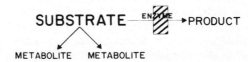

Figure 58–3. In the presence of a normal enzyme, the substrate interacts with the enzyme so that it is converted to its product. In an inborn error of metabolism, the abnormal enzyme cannot interact with the substrate (or with the coenzyme). The result is an increased substrate concentration, the formation of secondary metabolites of the substrate, and reduced concentration of the product.

The infant was normal at birth and had very low levels of biochemical abnormalities. This principle of antenatal therapy may be applicable to other metabolic disorders.

Other forms of therapy, such as direct administration of enzymes and organ transplantation, are under investigation for certain disorders. As yet, there is no evidence that these methods can be effectively used. However, this is one of the most active and important areas under study, and we can anticipate substantial advances in the years ahead. The technique of recombinant DNA is particularly promising for the production of enzymes in sufficiently large amounts and, perhaps, for engineering human genes.

Specific Diagnosis

Whenever the possibility of an inborn error of metabolism is suspected in a newborn because of either clinical signs in the infant or a family history of a particular disorder, it is important to contact a screening facility or other appropriate laboratory to determine whether it performs tests that can detect metabolic disorders in the newborn. If the tests are available at the laboratory, it is then important to be certain that the proper blood and/or urine specimens are submitted. Since some of these tests are quite complicated, they may not be available in certain states or even regions. This is particularly true for organic acid analyses. In this case, the physician should check with a medical center laboratory or a screening facility to determine where they can be performed. Certain large laboratories perform comprehensive screening for inborn errors and will accept specimens from throughout the United States as well as from other countries. The American Academy of Pediatrics has published a list of regional facilities with the names and addresses of individuals who can be contacted about this matter.

The type of specimen that is most desirable depends on the inborn error of metabolism suspected. For instance, one is much more likely to detect phenylketonuria (PKU) by examining a blood specimen than by evaluating a urine specimen. Conversely, one may detect argininosuccinic acidemia far more readily by testing urine than by examining blood. For other diseases, such as galactosemia, both blood and urine tests are desirable for a definite diagnosis. In general, however, whenever there is any reason to suspect an inborn error of metabolism, both blood and urine should be submitted for examination. Often, the filter-paper blood specimen sent for routine neonatal screening is sufficient for a specific diagnosis, although in other instances it may be desirable to test a specimen of plasma, serum, or liquid whole blood. Similarly, a urine specimen impreg-

Table 58–1. Major Clinical Signs in the Neonatal Period That Suggest the Presence of an Inborn Error of Metabolism

Signs	Possible Disorder(s)
Jaundice Hepatomegaly Lethargy Weight loss Poor feeding	Galactosemia
Lethargy Hypotonicity or spasticity Vomiting Poor feeding Metabolic acidosis	Maple syrup urine disease Methylmalonic acidemia Isovaleric acidemia Propionic acidemia (Other) organic acidemias
Lethargy Poor feeding Hypotonicity Hyperammonemia	Urea cycle disorder
Lethargy Poor feeding Hypotonicity Poor respirations	Nonketotic hyperglycinemia
Obstipation Abdominal distention Vomiting	Cystic fibrosis

nated into filter paper may be sufficient for the detection of certain disorders, but a liquid urine specimen is often desirable. The determination of the type of specimen to be sent can be accurately made only after consultation with the staff of the laboratory at which the testing will be performed.

Certain clinical signs in the neonate should alert one to the possibility of the presence of an inborn error of metabolism. These signs, which are listed in Table 58–1, include prolonged and unexplained jaundice, lethargy, weight loss or failure of weight gain, vomiting, poor feeding, and neurologic signs such as convulsions or spasticity. At times, a distinctive odor can be appreciated. Two general biochemical findings can be associated with any one or a number of these signs and may be part of several different inborn errors of metabolism. These findings are hyperammonemia and metabolic acidosis. Thus, among the first tests that should be obtained when one or more of these clinical signs appear are the determination of blood ammonia and of the state of acid-base balance. If the former is increased, there would be reason to suspect one of the urea cycle disorders. In the event of metabolic acidosis, maple syrup urine disease or one of the inborn errors of organic acid metabolism may be present. These disorders will be discussed in more detail later. Interestingly, a neonate with an organic acid metabolic disorder may have hyperammonemia as well as metabolic acidosis, although the hyperammonemia in this instance is usually less severe than that noted in association with the urea cycle disorders. Conversely, metabolic acidosis is usually not present with a urea cycle disorder.

It is important to remember that routine newborn screening for metabolic disorders, even when multiple testing is performed, does not cover most inborn errors of metabolism (see Newborn Screening, Part 2). Thus, any neonate with acute clinical signs or, later on, with signs of chronic illness (e.g., developmental delay, hepatomegaly) should be tested for an inborn error by the comprehensive examination of blood *and* urine. Delays in the diagnosis and treatment of these disorders are often due to the mistaken notion that an infant who has received newborn screening with presumed negative results cannot have a metabolic disorder. This is a severe tragedy to the families of these patients, one that need not occur.

REFERENCES

American Academy of Pediatrics, Committee on Nutrition: Special diets for infants with inborn errors of amino acid metabolism. Pediatrics 57:783, 1976.

Ampola, M. G., Mahoney, M. J., et al.: Prenatal therapy of a patient with vitamin B$_{12}$-responsive methylmalonic acidemia. N. Engl. J. Med. 293:313, 1975.

Miller, W. L.: Recombinant DNA and the pediatrician. J. Pediatr. 99:1, 1981.

59

Inborn Errors of Carbohydrate Metabolism

By Harvey L. Levy

Galactosemia

Galactosemia is an inborn error of metabolism that may produce clinically recognizable illness within the first few days of life. However, the results of routine newborn screening for galactosemia indicate that this disorder is more frequently overlooked in the newborn than it is diagnosed, despite the fact that a simple urine test for reducing substances can quickly lead to the diagnosis. Early diagnosis and the prompt institution of a relatively simple dietary therapy will likely lead to a normal life for an affected infant who otherwise faces the possibilities of neonatal death or the development of cataracts, cirrhosis, and mental retardation. The salient clinical features of galactosemia in the neonate include jaundice, hepatomegaly, lethargy, poor feeding, excessive and continuing weight loss, vomiting, and diarrhea. Many or perhaps most galactosemic infants will become septic, usually with *Escherichia coli*, by the age of 10 to 14 days unless dietary treatment has been given before that time. Sepsis in a galactosemic infant is usually fatal despite antibiotic therapy. If death from sepsis or other causes does not occur, the untreated neonate may spontaneously recover from the clinical illness but develop the chronic complications of cataracts, cirrhosis, and mental retardation. The urine in the untreated galactosemic is strongly positive for reducing substance (galactose) but is negative on specific testing for glucose. Albuminuria and hyperaminoaciduria may also be present. The diagnosis is confirmed by specific testing of blood, which will reveal markedly increased concentrations of galactose and galactose-1-phosphate and the absence of red blood cell galactose-1-phosphate uridyl transferase (transferase) activity. Treatment consists of withdrawal of all foods containing lactose and galactose

from the diet. The prognosis for normal physical and mental development is excellent when treatment is begun early in the neonatal period and continued throughout life.

The presence of increased galactose in blood and urine may be due to defects in two other galactose metabolic enzymes. These two entities, galactokinase deficiency and uridine diphosphate galactose 4-epimerase deficiency, will be discussed in the following section, and the term "galactosemia" will refer only to the deficiency in transferase activity. Even within galactosemia, however, there are a number of variants, each representing a different genetic disorder. These variants, listed in Table 59–1, may or may not result in clinical disease, depending on the degree of residual transferase activity and perhaps on other factors that are as yet undetermined. Since galactose accumulates in blood and urine in "classic" galactosemia and in the much rarer clinically important transferase variants, the initial diagnostic means are identical, as is the therapy.

Incidence.   The average frequency of galactosemia throughout the world is about one case per 50,000 infants, as based on data from routine newborn screening. This frequency varies from one case per

30,000 in some countries (e.g., Switzerland) to less than one case per 100,000 in other countries. These differences in the observed frequency, however, may to some extent be a result of differences in screening methods. It has become quite clear in the past few years that infants with galactosemia may be "missed," even in well-organized and well-conducted screening programs.

Etiology.   Galactosemia is a genetic disorder transmitted as an autosomal recessive. The mutant gene codes for the synthesis of an altered protein that has little or no transferase activity. This protein may also have electrophoretic mobility that is different from that of the normal enzyme (Table 59–1). This indicates that the structure of the protein is abnormal, possibly in the substitution of a single amino acid residue, as in the case of sickle hemoglobin. Heterozygotes (carriers) usually have about 50 per cent of normal red blood cell transferase activity, as expected, and often have abnormalities in the galactose tolerance curve. However, they are clinically normal and do not have detectable galactose and/or galactose-1-phosphate in blood or galactose in urine when on a normal diet.

Pathology.   In the neonate or young infant, the liver is enlarged and there is a striking fatty change with no excess glycogen deposition. This fatty change should lead to the suspicion of galactosemia in an undiagnosed neonate who dies with hepatomegaly, lethargy, and, perhaps, *E. coli* sepsis. Blood obtained from the heart postmortem and impregnated into filter paper (PKU-type specimen) can be sent to a newborn screening program to test for galactosemia. In addition, the original newborn blood specimen that was submitted for routine metabolic screening (see Newborn Screening, Part 2) can be recovered from the screening laboratory and tested (or retested) for galactosemia.

Later in infancy or in childhood, the alterations of portal cirrhosis are seen, including periportal fibrosis and bile-duct regeneration, which may progress to full-blown nodular cirrhosis of the Laennec type. The ocular lenses may show the characteristic opacification of cataract formation.

Pathogenesis.   Galactose enters the body as a result of the ingestion of lactose, the disaccharide of milk. When milk or a milk product is ingested, the lactose is hydrolyzed by intestinal lactase to its monosaccharide constituents, glucose and galactose. These monosaccharides are transported through the intestinal wall into the portal system and thus carried to the liver. In the normal state, the galactose is phosphorylated, exchanged for the glucose moiety of uridine diphosphate (UDP) glucose, epimerized to glucose from the galactose moiety of UDP galactose, and eventually converted to carbon dioxide through the glucose monophosphate shunt. This specific metabolic pathway involves several enzymes (Fig. 59–1) that are normally expressed in erythrocytes, leukocytes, liver, intestinal mucosa, and cultured skin fibroblasts. In galactosemia, activity of the *transferase* enzyme is markedly deficient or undetectable when assayed in these cells or tissues. As a result, galactose-1-phosphate accumulates in body cells. This accumulated galactose-1-phosphate inhibits the activity of galactokinase (product or feedback inhibition), so galactose itself accumulates. Because galactose-1-phosphate cannot leave the cell, it is detectable only in erythrocytes or in other body cells. Galactose, however, freely exchanges between intracellular and extracellular spaces and as a result is detectable either within cells or in extracellular compartments such as plasma or serum and urine. The free galactose in the ocular lens is converted to galactitol, which establishes an osmotic gradient that draws fluid into the lens. This causes swelling of the lens, denaturation and precipitation of lenticular protein, and, eventually, cataract formation. It is believed that the damage to other organs, primarily brain, liver, and kidney, results from intracellular toxicity of galactose-1-phosphate. According to this concept of pathogenesis, galactose-1-phosphate accumulates in neurons, hepatocytes, and renal tubular cells, causing damage that

Table 59–1.   Characteristics Regarding Variants of Galactose-1-Phosphate Uridyl Transferase

Variant	Erythrocyte Transferase Activity (% of Normal)	Starch-gel Electrophoretic Mobility (Related to Normal)	Other Biochemical Characteristics	Clinical Characteristics
"Classic"	0*	—	—	Disease†
Duarte	50*	Faster	—	Benign
"Negro"	0*	—	10% activity in liver and intestine	Disease
Indiana	0–45	Slower	Unstable in heparinized blood and isotonic phosphate buffer	Disease
Rennes	7	Slower	—	Disease
Los Angeles	140	Faster	—	Benign

* This represents the activity in individuals homozygous for the variant.
† Jaundice, other neonatal signs with complications of cataracts, liver disease, and mental retardation.

eventually results, respectively, in mental retardation, cirrhosis, and renal tubular dysfunction characterized by the renal Fanconi syndrome.

There are a number of secondary abnormalities for which there is as yet no clear explanation. Most prominent among these is the marked hypoglycemia that is often present when there is acute neonatal illness from galactosemia. This may be due to reduced gluconeogenesis as a direct result of the enzyme deficiency, but it is perhaps more likely that the hepatocellular disease results in impaired gluconeogenesis and the hypoglycemia, as occurs in liver disease from other causes. The hepatocellular disease does account for the marked aberrations in liver function and, most probably, for the hyperaminoacidemia in which tyrosine and methionine are most notably elevated but that also includes almost all the measurable free amino acids in the blood.

Diagnosis. The clinical picture associated with galactosemia in the neonate varies widely from clinical normality to very severe and often precipitous disease characterized by marked jaundice, hepatosplenomegaly, vomiting, lethargy, and weight loss that, if untreated, will result in death. This clinical spectrum is usually associated with a range of transferase activity that varies from virtually undetectable in the very ill infant to as much as 10 per cent of residual activity in the neonate who is clinically normal. However, some infants with no detectable transferase activity do not develop neonatal illness. Furthermore, the black infant may have the "Negro variant," in which transferase is virtually undetectable in erythrocytes but present in low activity in liver and in which there may be no symptoms in the neonatal period. Thus, routine newborn screening for galactosemia is very valuable in the early identification of infants who would otherwise not be diagnosed until clinical illness occurs.

In the infant who is ill, the greatest immediate danger appears to be sepsis, most often due to *E. coli*. As a result of routine newborn screening it is now known that a number of neonates with galactosemia have died with sepsis, the galactosemia unrecognized until the screening test abnormalities directed attention to this disorder.

The clinically ill neonate usually develops jaundice on the second or third day of life. The jaundice increases, and by the fifth or sixth day of life the infant has hepatomegaly, perhaps splenomegaly, vomiting, excessive weight loss, lethargy, and often diarrhea. Cataracts are not present at this time, although careful ophthalmologic examination will reveal a "water drop" clouding of the optic lenses. If milk is not withdrawn, these clinical signs worsen and sepsis may intervene, at which point death may be unavoidable. In some instances, however, sepsis does not develop and the signs of disease may spontaneously disappear, despite the continuation of milk. In these patients, the chronic abnormalities of galactosemia will develop later in infancy or in childhood.

Laboratory Investigations

Galactosemia and Melituria. Within less than 1 hour after the ingestion of milk, galactose-1-phosphate can be demonstrated in whole blood, and galactose appears in blood and urine. The diagnosis can be readily made by testing a filter-paper blood specimen ("PKU" specimen) for galactose and galactose-1-phosphate, using either a bacterial assay or a chemical test. These procedures may be most efficiently performed in a central state or regional laboratory that conducts routine newborn screening for metabolic disorders (see Newborn Screening, Part 2). The large amount of urinary galactose can be detected as reducing substance by a strongly positive reaction to Benedict's solution. This is most readily shown by testing the urine with a test tablet for reducing substance.

When testing the urine, one should be aware that it is very important to recognize that the commonly used dipstick method utilizes glucose oxidase to obtain the test result and thus is specific for glucose. When this is the only method used in the nursery or

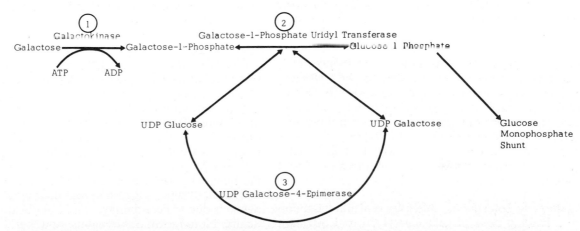

Figure 59–1. Pathway of galactose metabolism. The known human disorders in this pathway are indicated by the numbered enzyme deficient in each disorder.

in the laboratory that tests urine specimens from the nursery, galactosemia will be missed. Thus, whenever a urinalysis is performed in the newborn, the test for urinary sugar should always be one that detects reducing substances rather than the dipstick type. If there is reducing substance in the urine, a dipstick test for glucose should then be performed. In galactosemia, this latter test will be negative or at most only slightly positive, consistent with the fact that most or all of the reducing substance is galactose. The identity of galactose in urine can be verified by a chromatographic method for sugars or by a specific chemical or bacterial assay.

Two facts should be kept in mind when examining urine from an infant suspected of having galactosemia. The first is that some normal neonates excrete detectable amounts of reducing substance, mostly lactose or glucose. Occasionally, the quantity is sufficient to produce a strong reaction with Benedict's solution. These infants will have a negative blood test for galactosemia. The other fact is that the urine remains free of galactose in galactosemic infants unless milk is fed. This obvious fact may be overlooked when a sick infant is brought into the hospital and given only intravenous fluids. This infant, however, will have increased galactose-1-phosphate in erythrocytes, so an appropriate blood test (e.g., bacterial assay that responds to galactose-1-phosphate as well as to galactose) will be positive and will verify suspected galactosemia.

Proteinuria. Albumin is usually present during acute illness due to galactosemia and disappears within 2 to 4 days after milk is withdrawn. The albuminuria varies from a trace to a moderately large amount.

Formed Elements in the Urine. Red blood cells, white blood cells, and casts of various kinds may be present in the urine.

Hyperaminoaciduria. A marked increase in the excretion of virtually all free amino acids in the urine occurs during acute illness. Although this hyperaminoaciduria is accompanied by an increased concentration of blood amino acids, it is far in excess of what is expected in "overflow" from blood and is caused by the renal tubular damage and resulting impaired renal transport of amino acids. The hyperaminoaciduria is not a specific type but is similar to that seen in small premature infants or in those with renal tubular malabsorption due to other causes of the renal Fanconi syndrome. When milk is withdrawn, the hyperaminoaciduria disappears in 2 to 4 days.

Galactose Tolerance. After the oral administration of a loading dose of galactose (1.25 to 1.50 g/kg), the blood galactose and galactose-1-phosphate concentrations increase to an inordinately high level (100

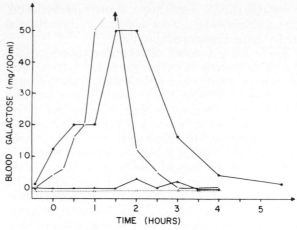

Figure 59–2. Galactose tolerance curves following the ingestion of milk that contains 0.78 gm of galactose (in the form of lactose) per kilogram of body weight for normal control subjects ($\triangle\cdots\triangle$); a Duarte/"classic" galactosemia mixed heterozygous patient ($\blacktriangle$——$\blacktriangle$); a "classic" galactosemic patient on dietary treatment ($\bullet$——$\bullet$); and a patient with Rennes variant on dietary treatment ($\bigcirc$——$\bigcirc$). (From Hammersen, Houghton, and Levy: Rennes-like variant of galactosemia: Clinical and biochemical studies. J. Pediatr. *87*:50–57,1975. Reproduced by permission of the Journal of Pediatrics.)

to 200 mg/100 ml) and remain markedly elevated for 5 or more hours.

Galactose tolerance tests probably should not be performed in infants with proven galactosemia or in those even suspected of having galactosemia. For clinical diagnosis and therapy, galactosemia can be very adequately studied on the basis of response to a milk feeding, which produces a response in blood galactose and galactose-1-phosphate that is less dramatic and shorter lived than that following a galactose load and that can be used to differentiate infants with transferase variants from those with "classic" galactosemia (Fig. 59–2). The much greater accumulations of galactose and galactose-1-phosphate, as well as the hypoglycemia, that follow a loading dose of galactose in galactosemic infants and children could result in irreversible organ damage. Furthermore, enzyme assays using the readily available erythrocytes or cultured skin fibroblasts will almost always determine the specific type and degree of galactosemia, thus rendering a galactose loading test unnecessary.

Liver Function. One of the first signs of galactosemia is neonatal jaundice. By the third to fifth day of life jaundice is often quite substantial, with total serum bilirubin concentrations of approximately 14 to 18 mg/100 ml. If the galactosemia remains untreated, the serum bilirubin level will usually continue to increase, and by 7 to 9 days of life it may be as high as 20 mg/100 ml or higher. It is often stated that the bilirubin is predominantly of the direct-reacting (conjugated) type, suggesting that the hyperbilirubinemia is due to liver damage, perhaps obstructive in nature. More recent observations, however, indicate that the early hyperbilirubinemia of the galactosemic neonate may be predominantly indirect-reacting (unconjugated). This can still be explained by liver damage in that the bilirubin conjugating mechanism may be inhibited by galactose-1-phosphate or other toxic metabolites that accumulate in galactosemia. Other indicators of liver damage, such as elevated levels of SGOT and of serum alkaline phosphatase and increased prothrombin time and partial thromboplastin time, may be present, but often these findings do not appear until the second week of life. Within 2 to 3 days after the withdrawal of milk, the serum bilirubin concentration begins to recede, and the other indicators of liver dysfunction begin to return to normal.

Renal Function. Basic kidney function seems to be retained intact, despite the impaired tubular transport of amino acids. The blood urea nitrogen concentration, the specific gravity of urine, and the excretion of electrolytes remain within normal limits.

Blood Elements. There is usually little or no alteration in the indices of hematologic function. In particular, evidence of hemolysis is almost always absent. Hemoglobin usually remains normal, as does the reticulocyte count. If neonatal sepsis intervenes, however, any of the hematologic signs of this dire complication may be present. These signs include anemia, evidence of hemolysis, alterations in the white blood cell count, and thrombocytopenia.

Treatment. Treatment consists of the complete discontinuance of milk and milk products from the diet at the moment the diagnosis is established. This means that breast-feeding or feeding of any milk-containing formula or of whole milk must cease, and a nonmilk formula must be substituted. Two types of nonmilk formulas are used. One type is soybean-based, and several of these products are readily available. The carbohydrate source in soybean-based formulas is sucrose, a disaccharide consisting of glucose and fructose. The other type of acceptable formula is casein hydrolysate–based, in which the carbohydrate source is usually glucose. If there is substantial hypoglycemia and if the infant is feeding poorly or is dehydrated, it may be wise to institute nonspecific intravenous fluid therapy for replacement and maintenance. A blood culture should be obtained, and antibiotic therapy effective against *E. coli* and other gram-negative organisms should be given *before* the results of the blood culture are available. This is particularly important, since galactosemia is so often associated with sepsis.

The galactosemic individual will probably have to remain on a diet that avoids or at least severely restricts the intake of milk and milk products for the remainder of his life. In contrast to infants with many other inborn errors of metabolism, galactosemic patients may readily ingest protein-rich foods such as meat and fish. Thus, the diet in galactosemia can be relatively easily administered and tolerated. It should be monitored at regular intervals in a specific pediatric metabolic unit.

Prognosis. Unless the diagnosis is made during the first week or two of life, the infant may die with sepsis.

Should the infant survive, the cirrhosis and cataracts may remain or they may regress after having been present for surprisingly long periods. Each day that the infant is exposed to the toxicity of galactose and its metabolites, his chances for an optimal recovery diminish.

The prognosis with respect to mental development is not yet known with certainty; however, there appears to be little doubt that the frank mental deficiency observed in untreated or late-treated galactosemia is to a great extent, if not entirely, a result of the disease. This mental deficiency is largely or completely preventable by early and correct treatment. The diagnosis can and should be made early in the neonatal period; a delay of a week or two may mean the difference between mental normality and mental retardation. The rapidly growing brain of the newborn cannot be insulted for many days with impunity.

CASE 59–1

A male infant was born to a primigravida mother after a normal pregnancy and full-term gestation. Delivery was by breech extraction under spinal anesthesia. Apgar scores were 6 at 1 minute and 9 at 5 minutes. Birth measurements were as follows: weight, 3180 gm (7 pounds), length, 50 cm, and head circumference, 35.5 cm. Breast-feeding was attempted but was abandoned on the third day, and the infant was formula-fed thereafter.

Jaundice was noted on the fourth day with total serum bilirubin level 15.8 mg/100 ml (1.2 mg/100 ml direct-reactive). Phototherapy was instituted. On the sixth day, the total serum bilirubin level was 14.0 mg/100 ml, but the patient was lethargic and had excessive weight loss. Sepsis was suspected, and cultures of blood, CSF, and urine were initiated. Antibiotic therapy was begun. The CSF contained a total sugar concentration of 235 mg/100 ml, and the blood total sugar concentration was 300 mg/100 ml. The sugar was not further characterized, and a form of neonatal diabetes mellitus was initially suspected. On the seventh day, the state newborn screening program reported by telephone that the results of screening tests on the routine blood specimen (obtained on the third day) indicated the presence of galactosemia. Specifically, this specimen contained a very large amount of galactose and galactose-1-phosphate (greater than 50 mg/100 ml) and the enzyme spot screening test for transferase activity revealed no evidence of activity. Blood amino acid analysis at this time revealed a generalized increase with particularly prominent increases in methionine and tyrosine. The infant was immediately switched from regular formula to a casein hydrolysate–based formula.

By the ninth day, the infant began to improve with reduction in the degree of jaundice and initiation of weight gain. The cultures that were obtained on the sixth day were reported as negative, so the antibiotic therapy was discontinued. Ophthalmologic examina-

tion with slit-lamp disclosed a small amount of opacity in both lenses consistent with the early cataract of galactosemia but thought to be reversible.

On the tenth day (three days after milk was withdrawn), the blood galactose and galactose-1-phosphate level was only 4 mg/100 ml, and by the thirteenth day, neither galactose nor galactose-l-phosphate was detectable in blood or urine. Blood and urine amino acid levels were also normal. At this time, the patient was no longer jaundiced, was gaining weight, and was active. He was discharged on the twenty-first day.

At home, the casein hydrolysate–based formula continued. The infant was allowed to have all baby foods and, later, other solid foods that do not contain milk or milk products. When he was weaned from the bottle, he was given fruit juices as a substitute and a daily calcium supplement to supply calcium needs that are ordinarily fulfilled by normal milk intake.

His growth and development have been normal. He has no signs of liver disease, and his ocular lenses are clear with no evidence of cataracts. He did have delayed speech with some minor speech and language difficulties (common in almost all treated galactosemic children), but these were overcome with speech therapy. He is now 6 years old, is physically normal, has intelligence in the superior range, and has performed well in the first grade.

Confirmatory enzyme studies of erythrocytes revealed no detectable transferase activity in this boy and approximately 50 per cent of normal transferase activity in each parent. These findings are consistent with the autosomal recessive mode of inheritance known to be present in galactosemia.

Comment. This patient developed many of the characteristic findings of galactosemia in the newborn nursery, including unexplained jaundice, lethargy, and excessive weight loss. Galactosemia was not initially recognized because the elevated sugar in blood and CSF was mistakenly reported from the laboratory as "glucose." Simple urine tests for reducing substance and for glucose (the latter would have been negative) would have established the diagnosis of galactosemia, but, unfortunately, these were not performed. However, routine newborn screening in the state does include testing for galactosemia, so a potential tragedy was avoided.

Galactokinase and UDPG-4-Epimerase Deficiencies

Galactose may appear in blood and urine as a result of deficient activity of galactokinase or UDPG-4-epimerase (Fig. 59–1). Galactokinase deficiency has been identified in the newborn as well as in older children. In contrast to galactosemia, this condition is not associated with an accumulation of galactose-1-phosphate. In the untreated state, cataracts will develop during infancy or early childhood, but, unlike galactosemia, galactokinase deficiency manifests no neonatal symptoms, and other complications such as liver disease and mental retardation do not occur. The diagnosis is suspected upon discovery of large amounts of galactose in the blood and urine and confirmed by demonstration of markedly reduced or absent galactokinase activity in erythrocytes. The treatment is identical with that for galactosemia in that milk and milk products are excluded from the diet. Neonatal screening in which an assay for galactose is performed (see Newborn Screening, Part 2) should detect galactokinase deficiency as well as galactosemia. It is important to identify and treat this disorder in the neonatal period in order to prevent the formation of cataracts.

UDPGalactose-4-epimerase (epimerase) deficiency has been described in only a few families. The affected infants or older individuals accumulate a small amount of galactose in blood and a much larger amount of galactose-1-phosphate in erythrocytes. No signs of disease have been noted, suggesting that this may be a benign disorder. The diagnosis is confirmed by the demonstration of reduced epimerase activity in erythrocytes.

Glycogen Storage Diseases

At least eight different inherited abnormalities of glycogen metabolism can lead to the same effect, an excessive accumulation of glycogen in tissues. Some of these may produce clinical abnormalities in the neonatal period, whereas others do not become symptomatic until later in life. The three types that can produce neonatal findings are discussed in the subsequent paragraphs.

TYPE I (VON GIERKE'S DISEASE)

In this rare disorder, there is a striking accumulation of glycogen in liver and kidneys. It is due to a deficiency in glucose-6-phosphatase activity and is inherited as an autosomal recessive trait.

Clinical Findings. The affected newborn has hepatomegaly but is otherwise asymptomatic. By several months of age, however, abdominal enlargement due to massive hepatomegaly, loss of appetite, and vomiting appear. In some instances, "sinking spells" and even convulsions due to hypoglycemia are noted.

Diagnosis. Type I glycogen storage disease is suspected because of hepatomegaly. Withdrawal of food for a few hours leads to hypoglycemia, lactic acidemia, and pyruvic acidemia. The hypoglycemia is unresponsive to epinephrine and glucagon. Other laboratory findings include elevated serum triglycerides, phospholipids, cholesterol, and uric acid. Liver biopsy reveals liver cells that contain vacuoles filled with glycogen. Reduced or absent glucose-6-phosphatase activity is demonstrated by enzyme assay of liver tissue.

Prognosis. Many infants fail to grow adequately, and some die within the first years of life. Those who are less severely afflicted survive but have stunted growth, persistent hypoglycemia, and a bleeding diathesis. If the affected individuals live beyond age 4 years, the abdomen becomes less prominent, and the prognosis progressively improves.

Treatment. Affected infants are given frequent feedings to counteract the hypoglycemia. These feedings may need to be given every 3 or 4 hours, day and night, for many months. Hypoglycemic crises must be treated vigorously with glucose infusions. Portacaval shunts have recently been shown to produce dramatic improvement in a number of patients.

TYPE II (GENERALIZED GLYCOGENOSIS; POMPE'S DISEASE)

This type of glycogen storage disease usually comes to attention because of its effects on the heart. There is massive cardiomegaly, accompanied by an extremely abnormal electrocardiogram. There is also marked hypotonia, although the muscles are firm and of normal mass. The tongue may be enlarged, and there is a failure to thrive. Diagnosis is confirmed by muscle biopsy demonstrating increased concentration of glycogen with normal structure. Enzyme confirmation is obtained by demonstration of virtual absence of alpha-glucosidase in leukocytes. There is no known effective treatment.

TYPE III ("DEBRANCHER" DISEASE)

These patients may have a clinical appearance that is similar to that of those babies with Type I glycogen storage disease. Hepatomegaly develops early in infancy, and growth retardation may be striking. There is also hypoglycemia and hyperlipidemia. Unlike those with Type I disease, however, these patients may have splenomegaly but no renal involvement.

The enzyme deficiency is in amylo-1,6-glucosidase (debrancher) activity. The diagnosis is confirmed by complicated enzyme studies of muscle and liver. The disorder is inherited as an autosomal recessive trait. Treatment includes frequent feedings with a high protein diet to offset the hypoglycemic tendency. The prognosis may be good, since Type III disease is milder than Type I and the hepatomegaly may disappear at puberty.

Essential Benign Fructosuria

Fructosuria appears in infants who have an inherited deficiency of fructokinase, an enzyme that phosphorylates fructose to fructose-1-phosphate. The disorder is transmitted as an autosomal recessive trait. The diagnosis is made through discovery of urinary reducing substance that is identified as fructose and through demonstration of prolonged and high curves of blood fructose concentration after the oral or intravenous administration of fructose. The disorder is asymptomatic, and no treatment is required.

Hereditary Fructose Intolerance

This inborn error of fructose metabolism is inherited as an autosomal recessive trait and produces clinical abnormalities when fruit or sucrose, a disaccharide consisting of fructose and glucose, is ingested. Following fructose ingestion, fructose and fructose-1-phosphate accumulate in the body, a result of deficient fructose-1-phosphate aldolase activity. Virtually coincidental with the first ingestion of fructose in these infants are poor feeding, vomiting, failure to thrive, and hepatomegaly. Symptoms such as lethargy and clinical findings such as pallor, hemorrhages, and jaundice may also be present.

The diagnosis is suspected when an infant with these findings has a history of fructose ingestion. Formerly, this did not occur until about the second month of life or later, when fruit is first added to the infant's diet. Fructose ingestion may now occur much earlier in life, however, since a number of formulas (particularly those that are soybean-based) contain sucrose as the source of carbohydrate. Thus, clinical illness from hereditary fructose intolerance can occur early in the neonatal period.

Laboratory. The laboratory findings include the presence of reducing substance in the urine (which consists of both fructose and glucose), hyperaminoaciduria, abnormal liver function test results such as elevations in SGOT, serum alkaline phosphatase, and prothrombin time, hypolkalemia, and hypophosphatemia. Blood amino acid analysis may reveal increased tyrosine and methionine and may be confused with hereditary tyrosinemia (see Hereditary Tyrosinemia, Chapter 60).

Diagnosis. The differential diagnosis in an infant with this clinical picture who has ingested fructose includes galactosemia, hereditary tyrosinemia, sepsis, neonatal hepatitis, and liver dysfunction of unknown origin. Galactosemia and sepsis are respectively excluded on the basis of negative tests for galactose and galactose-1-phosphate in blood (see Galactosemia) and negative cultures. The other possibilities are more difficult to exclude and the diagnosis of hereditary fructose intolerance may be confirmed by an intravenous fructose tolerance test. For this, a fructose dose of 0.2 to 0.3 gm/kg is given in a single injection. Within 20 to 40 minutes, blood glucose and serum phosphate decrease markedly. A fructose tolerance test should be performed *only* in a hospital under carefully controlled conditions with intravenous fluid administered, since marked hypoglycemia and, perhaps, hypokalemia can occur precipitously in an affected infant. The finding of decreased liver fructose-1-phosphate aldolase activity by direct enzyme assay provides definitive evidence for the diagnosis.

Treatment. When the diagnosis is established, treatment must begin immediately by withdrawal of sources of fructose from the diet. This includes the elimination of all fruits, sugar, and formulas that contain sucrose.

Prognosis. Following treatment the symptoms and signs, except hepatomegaly, usually clear almost immediately. Fatty changes in the liver may persist for many months, but this symptom also eventually clears.

REFERENCES

Baerlocher, K., Gitzelmann, R., et al.: Hereditary fructose intolerance in early childhood: a major diagnostic challenge. Helv. Paediatr. Acta 33:465, 1978.

Beutler, E., Matsumoto, F., et al.: Galactokinase deficiency as a cause of cataracts. N. Engl. J. Med. 288:1203, 1973.

Donnell, G. N., Koch, R., et al.: Clinical aspects of galactosaemia. In Burman, D., Holton, J. B., and Pennock, C. A. (Eds.): Inherited disorders of carbohydrate metabolism. Lancaster, MTP Press, 1980, pp. 103–115.

Donnell, G. N., Ng, W. G., et al.: Galactose metabolism in the newborn infant. Pediatrics 39:829, 1967.

Fernandes, J.: Hepatic glycogen storage diseases. In Raine, D. N. (Ed.): The treatment of inherited metabolic disease. Lancaster, MTP Press, 1975, pp. 115–149.

Fishler, K., Donnell, G. N., et al.: Intellectual and personality development in children with galactosemia. Pediatrics 50:412, 1972.

Gitzelmann, R., Steinmann, B., et al.: Uridine diphosphate galactose 4'-epimerase deficiency. IV. Report of eight cases in three families. Helv. Paediatr. Acta 31:441, 1976.

Greene, H. L., Slonim, A. E., et al.: Continuous nocturnal intragastric feeding for management of type I glycogen-storage disease. N. Engl. J. Med. 294:423, 1976.

Hammersen, G., Houghton, S., and Levy, H. L.: Rennes-like variant of galactosemia: clinical and biochemical studies. J. Pediatr. 87:50, 1975.

Ichiba, Y., Namba, N., and Misumi, H.: Uridine diphosphate galactose 4-epimerase deficiency. Am. J. Dis. Child. 134:995, 1980.

Komrower, G. M., and Lee, D. H.: Long-term follow-up of galactosaemia. Arch. Dis. Child. 45:367, 1970.

Levy, H. L., and Hammersen, G.: Newborn screening for galactosemia and other galactose metabolic defects. J. Pediatr. 92:871, 1978.

Levy, H. L., Pueschel, S. M., and Hubbell, J. P., Jr.: Unconjugated hyperbilirubinemia. N. Engl. J. Med. 292:923, 1975.

Levy, H. L., Sepe, S. J., et al.: Galactose-1-phosphate uridyl transferase deficiency due to Duarte/galactosemia combined variation: clinical and biochemical studies. J. Pediatr. 92:390, 1978.

Levy, H. L., Sepe, S. J., et al.: Sepsis due to Escherichia coli in neonates with galactosemia. N. Engl. J. Med. 297:825, 1977.

Nadler, H. L., Inouye, T., and Hsia, D. Y.-Y.: Classical galactosemia: a study of fifty-five cases. In Hsia, D. Y.-Y. (Ed.): Galactosemia. Springfield, Ill., Charles C Thomas, 1969, pp. 127–139.

Reuser, A. J. J., Koster, J. F., et al.: Biochemical, immunological, and cell genetic studies in glycogenosis type II. Am. J. Hum. Genet. 30:132, 1978.

Sadeghi-Nejad, A., Presente, E., et al.: Studies in type I glycogenosis of the liver. J. Pediatr. 85:49, 1974.

Segal, S.: The Negro variant of congenital galactosemia. In Hsia, D. Y.-Y. (Ed.): Galactosemia. Springfield, Ill., Charles C Thomas, 1969, pp. 176–185.

Segal, S., Rutman, J. Y., and Frimpter, G. W.: Galactokinase deficiency and mental retardation. J. Pediatr. 95:750, 1979.

Thalhammer, O., Gitzelmann, R., and Pantlitschko, M.: Hypergalactosemia and galactosuria due to galactokinase deficiency in a newborn. Pediatrics 42:441, 1968.

Van den Berghe, G.: Biochemical aspects of hereditary fructose intolerance. In Hommes, F. A., and van den Berg, C. J. (Eds.): Normal and Pathological Development of Energy Metabolism. New York, Academic Press, 1975.

60

Inborn Errors of Amino Acid Metabolism

By Harvey L. Levy

Metabolic testing for the evaluation of clinical illness and for routine newborn screening usually includes the measurement of blood or urine amino acids or both. Consequently, amino acid disorders are among the most frequently identified metabolic derangements. It is neither necessary nor desirable to discuss all the 40 or more inborn errors in this category. Many of these are very rare and therefore are not likely to be encountered. Others, however, are more likely to be seen because of their clinical presentation in the newborn period or as a result of routine newborn screening (see Newborn Screening, Part 2). It is important to note that in many of these disorders, therapy may prevent irreversible damage, but for optimal benefit the treatment must begin during the first days or weeks of life. It is also important to emphasize that identification of the specific disorder may be difficult and requires confirmation by an experienced laboratory directed by a physician or other professional. A laboratory of this type is probably available in only one or two places within each state or region. This laboratory should be contacted before specific therapy is given and whenever a question concerning one of these disorders arises.

Phenylketonuria (PKU)

PKU is an inborn error of metabolism involving the amino acid phenylalanine. It should always come to attention as a result of routine newborn screening. Treatment must begin in the neonatal period or at least during early infancy if brain damage with mental retardation is to be prevented. The early institution of appropriate dietary therapy, well before clinical signs appear, will prevent mental retardation and other neurologic sequelae.

Incidence. Based on the results of routine newborn screening for PKU in the United States and in many other countries, the general frequency is about one in 15,000 individuals. Among different countries and even among different states within the United States, the frequency varies between one per 6000 to less than one per 25,000. These differences presumably relate to genetic variations among different ethnic groups. The highest frequencies are reported in Ireland and among Americans of Irish descent. Relatively high frequencies are also reported in Poland. PKU is rarely found among blacks and Ashkenazi Jews. Approximately 1 to 2 per cent of individuals institutionalized for mental retardation are found to have PKU.

Etiology and Pathogenesis. PKU is inherited as an autosomal recessive trait. Approximately 1 per cent of the population are carriers of the gene. In affected individuals, the genetic abnormality results in an almost total lack of phenylalanine hydroxylase activity, which in turn results in an inability to convert phenylalanine to tyrosine (Fig. 60–1). This causes a marked accumulation of phenylalanine in the blood, urine, and tissues when the diet is normal. The urine may also contain excessive amounts of phenylalanine metabolites, including phenylpyruvic acid, phenyllactic acid, phenylacetic acid, phenylacetylglutamine, and o-hydroxyphenylacetic acid. In the neonate, however, there may be little or no urinary excretion of these metabolites, since their formation depends on activity of phenylalanine transaminase, an enzyme that may have very low activity until the infant is several months of age.

It seems that the brain damage in untreated PKU is a direct or indirect result of the accumulation of phenylalanine or its metabolites or both. Thus, when these concentrations have been controlled by the use of a special diet, mental retardation and other signs of brain damage do not appear. However, the precise cause of the brain toxicity is not known. The theories

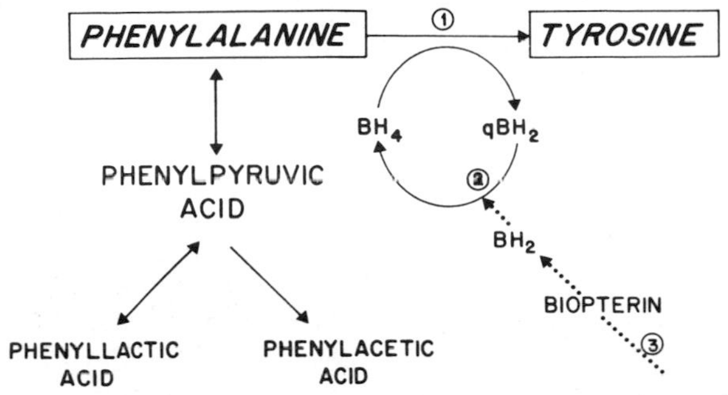

Figure 60–1. Pathway of phenylalanine hydroxylation. The hydroxylating enzyme, phenylalanine hydroxylase (1), requires tetrahydrobiopterin (BH_4) for activity. The reduced pterin is oxidized to quininoid dihydrobiopterin (qBH_4) in this reaction. The qBH_4 is reduced back to BH_4 via activity of dihydropteridine reductase (2). Dihydrobiopterin (BH_2) also enters this cycle as a reduced product of biopterin.

The most frequent cause of increased phenylalanine concentration and the accumulation of phenylpyruvic acid and other metabolites is a defect in apoenzyme phenylalanine hydroxylase. This produces PKU, atypical PKU, and mild hyperphenylalaninemia. In rare cases, phenylalanine and metabolite accumulations are caused by a defect in dihydropteridine reductase or a defect in the synthesis of biopterin, both of which result in BH_4 deficiency. This produces a marked reduction in phenylalanine hydroxylase activation and must be differentiated from PKU.

regarding pathogenesis include (1) direct toxic effect of phenylalanine or one of its metabolites, (2) toxicity secondary to a reduction in the intracellular concentrations of amino acids other than phenylalanine produced by an inhibition of cellular uptake by the increased phenylalanine, (3) reduction in synthesis of neurotransmitters, (4) reduced protein synthesis in brain caused by phenylalanine-induced disaggregation of polyribosomes, and (5) inhibition by phenylalanine or phenylpyruvate of key glucose metabolic enzymes in brain. Regardless of the immediate pathogenic mechanism, reduction in the accumulation of phenylalanine and its metabolites by the low phenylalanine diet currently in use is the most effective available therapy.

Diagnosis. PKU should always be identified in the neonate by the process of newborn screening. PKU cannot otherwise be suspected in the neonate or young infant, since the clinical signs of brain damage do not appear until later in infancy or childhood. By this time, the brain damage is to some extent irreversible. The frequency of prenatal, perinatal, and neonatal complications is no greater among phenylketonuric infants than in the general newborn population. Affected infants usually appear to be normal.

Identification in the neonate is based on an increased concentration of phenylalanine in the blood. If PKU is already known to be present in the family, particularly in a sibling, the suspicion of PKU must be high, since the disorder is inherited. For example, if a sibling has PKU, each parent is presumed to carry the gene, and thus the chance that any additional child will have PKU is one in four. Regardless of family history, however, a PKU test should be performed on every newborn infant (see Newborn Screening, Part 2). In most infants with PKU, the blood phenylalanine concentration, which is normally 2 mg/100 ml or less, will be at least 6 mg/100 ml or greater by the third day of life. An occasional infant with PKU, however, will have only a slightly increased phenylalanine level in the screened blood specimen. In order not to overlook this occasional infant, one must obtain another blood specimen from any newborn infant whose blood phenylalanine concentration is at least 4 mg/100 ml or greater.

It is important to remember that urine from a newborn with PKU rarely has a detectable increase in phenylalanine metabolites. Thus, the urine ferric chloride test that responds to phenylpyruvic acid is almost always negative and therefore ineffective in detecting PKU in the newborn period, although it may be effective in identifying PKU in older infants and children. Consequently, a urine test is *not* reliable in the detection of PKU in the newborn infant.

Upon identification by newborn screening, the infant with an increased blood phenylalanine level should be referred to a pediatric metabolic center that is experienced in the diagnosis and treatment of PKU. If a referral such as this is impossible, at least direct contact with this type of center should be established so that the proper confirmatory and treatment procedures are initiated as soon as possible. For confirmation, all amino acids should be measured in blood by an accurate quantitative technique (e.g., amino acid analyzer). A specific elevation of the phenylalanine concentration that is as least 20 mg/100 ml or greater when the infant is on a normal diet indicates that PKU is present. When the confirmatory blood phenylalanine concentration is less than 20 mg/100 ml but is still increased, another type of biochemical defect may be present (Table 60–1). Since the biochemical defect in PKU results in failure of phenylalanine to convert to tyrosine (Fig. 60–1), the blood tyrosine concentration in the phenylketonuric infant is usually at the lower end of the normal range.

Treatment. When the diagnosis of PKU has been confirmed, the infant should be given a low-phenylalanine diet. For optimal effects, this should begin within the first 3 weeks of life. This treatment regimen must be planned and carefully monitored under the guidance of physicians, nutritionists, and others who are experienced and knowledgeable in the treatment of PKU. The regular infant formula or breast-feeding is discontinued, and a special low-phenylalanine formula is substituted. This special formula must not be given alone, however, but must be mixed with a certain amount of milk in order to supply the infant with his minimum requirements of phenylalanine. If this is not supplied, the body will be quickly depleted of phenylalanine, and a low or undetectable blood phenylalanine concentration and severe complications such as growth retardation, brain damage, and even death will result. The amount of milk necessary as a dietary supplement varies from one infant to another and is added to the low-phenylalanine formula on the basis of the blood phenylalanine concentration. For optimal therapeutic effects, this concentration should be maintained within the range of 4 to 10 mg/100 ml. Foods added to the diet later in infancy should be low in protein, generally fruits and vegetables.

It is possible to continue breast-feeding on a low-phenylalanine diet. Only two or three breast-feedings per day are allowable, however, and the other feedings must consist of the special low-phenylalanine formula. The infant must be carefully weighed on an accurate scale before and after each breast-feeding so that the amount of phenylalanine ingested at each feeding can be calculated from the quantity of ingested breast milk.

The policy in most centers is to recommend continuation of a low-phenylalanine diet indefinitely. Formerly, many centers recommended discontinuation of the diet when the child reached 5 or 6 years of age, but recent information indicates that the I.Q. scores may decrease in some children who have discontinued the diet. Whether the diet should be continued into adult years or perhaps can be safely dis-

Table 60–1. Metabolic Disorders Associated with an Increased Blood Phenylalanine Concentration

Disorder	Blood Phe (mg/dl)	Enzyme Defect	Treatment
PKU	>20	Phe hydroxylase (<1%)	Diet
"Atypical" PKU	12–20	Phe hydroxylase (2–3%)	Diet
Mild hyphe*	>2–<12	Phe hydroxylase (2–5%)	None
Transient hyphe*	>2–20	?	None
DHPR deficiency†	12–20	DHPR (<1%) Neurotransmitter precursors	
Biopterin synthetase deficiency	12–20	Unknown	

* Hyperphenylalaninemia.
† Dihydropteridine reductase deficiency.

Hyperphenylalaninemias

There are inborn errors of metabolism other than phenylketonuria that are associated with reduced activity of phenylalanine hydroxylase. These defects result in mild to moderate degrees of increase in the blood phenylalanine level, rather than the more severe increase associated with PKU (Table 60–1). These entities are sometimes included under the rubric of phenylketonuria, but they are clearly distinct entities.

"ATYPICAL PHENYLKETONURIA"

An infant whose blood phenylalanine concentrations in the untreated state are consistently greater than 12 mg/100 ml but less than 20 mg/100 ml is usually considered to have "atypical PKU." The result in the newborn screening test often is a lower phenylalanine level than that in the truly phenylketonuric infant. The frequency of "atypical PKU" is less than that of phenylketonuria, approximating 1:40,000. It is not known to what extent clinical complications may occur in this disorder, although it is believed that if it is left untreated, lowered intellectual performance or a mild degree of mental retardation may result. In most centers, a low-phenylalanine diet is administered to these infants just as in PKU. However, these infants have a greater tolerance for phenylalanine than do infants with PKU, so the diet in these infants must be monitored with particular care.

MILD PERSISTENT HYPERPHENYLALANINEMIA

As is "atypical PKU," this entity is usually genetically distinct from PKU. The untreated infant with mild persistent hyperphenylalaninemia has a blood phenylalanine concentration that is consistently higher than the normal 2 mg/100 ml but that is no greater than 12 mg/100 ml. The frequency of this entity is similar to that of "atypical PKU," about 1:40,000. It seems to be clinically benign and thus probably should not be treated (Table 60–1). For this reason, it is important to differentiate mild persistent hyperphenylalaninemia from both "atypical PKU" and true PKU.

TETRAHYDROBIOPTERIN DEFICIENCY

About 1 per cent of infants with hyperphenylalaninemia have a defect in synthesis of tetrahydrobiopterin (BH_4), the necessary cofactor for phenylalanine hydroxylase (Fig. 60–1). When BH_4 is not available in sufficient amounts, hydroxylations of tyrosine and tryptophan, as well as that of phenylalanine, are reduced. Thus, neurotransmitters such as dopamine and norepinephrine (products of tyrosine hydroxylation) and serotonin (product of tryptophan hydroxylation) are deficient.

These infants have usually been incorrectly diagnosed initially as having PKU or "atypical PKU." They come to attention when, unlike infants with PKU, they show signs of severe brain damage despite treatment with the low-phenylalanine diet. These signs include lethargy, delayed development, and seizures, usually myoclonic in type. The brain damage probably results from the deficiencies in neurotransmitters.

At least two genetically distinct metabolic defects result in lack of sufficient BH_4. Each is inherited as an autosomal recessive trait. The first described, *dihydropteridine reductase deficiency*, results in lack of BH_4 regeneration from qBH_2 (Fig. 60–1). The second, termed *biopterin synthetase deficiency*, is a defect in the synthesis of biopterin (Fig. 60–1). The precise location of this block is unknown. The diagnosis of each is established by enzyme assay in biopsied liver. Dihydropteridine reductase deficiency can also be confirmed by assay for this enzyme activity in cultured skin fibroblasts.

All newborn infants with any degree of hyperphenylalaninemia should be tested for a defect in tetrahydrobiopterin synthesis. Two methods are now available for this testing. One is a challenge with BH_4, in which BH_4 is administered orally in a dose of 10 mg/kg or intravenously in a dose of 2 mg/kg when the infant is on a normal diet. The blood phenylalanine level is measured before the BH_4 load and at 6 hours after this administration. Infants with biopterin synthetase deficiency will respond by lowering their blood phenylalanine concentration to less than 50 per cent of the pre-BH_4 level. Infants with dihydropteridine reductase deficiency may not show this response. Infants with PKU, "atypical PKU," or mild persistent hyperphenylalaninemia will show little or no change in the blood phenylalanine level under these conditions. The second method of testing newborns for tetrahydrobiopterin deficiency is to measure neopterin and biopterin in urine. In biopterin synthesis deficiency, urinary biopterin is very low, so the neopterin:biopterin ratio is high. Conversely, in dihydropteridine reductase deficiency, urinary biopterin is increased, so the neopterin:biopterin ratio is low. In PKU, this ratio is essentially unchanged from that seen in normal infants. These tests are difficult to perform and should be conducted only at a pediatric metabolic center.

The current treatment of tetrahydrobiopterin deficiency consists of supplying the immediate precursors of the deficient neurotransmitters. Thus, L-dopa (and carbidopa) are given to provide the infant with dopamine and norepinephrine, and hydroxytryptophan is given to provide the infant with serotonin.

This therapy has not reversed the severe neurologic signs in affected children, although it has increased the activity and muscle tone in some patients. It is possible that this therapy would be beneficial in preventing the neurologic sequelae if it began in the newborn period. Other modes of therapy, such as treatment with BH_4 or BH_4 analogues, are currently under investigation.

Maternal Phenylketonuria

Women with PKU may have nonphenylketonuric children who are mentally retarded. These offspring may also have microcephaly, low birth weight, and congenital heart disease. The microcephaly may be quite striking in the neonate and has often led to an extensive evaluation for neonatal microcephaly prior to nursery discharge. An evaluation for neonatal microcephaly should always include a maternal blood phenylalanine measurement ("PKU test" of the mother). This should be performed regardless of whether the mother is mentally retarded, since an occasional phenylketonuric individual will be mentally normal despite not receiving treatment for PKU.

These offspring abnormalities are presumed to be a consequence of fetal damage resulting from the maternal biochemical derangements that cross the placenta. The damage to offspring in maternal PKU, therefore, is due to the aberrant intrauterine environment and not to a genetic defect in the offspring. Those few offspring who are phenylketonuric are shown to have PKU by newborn screening and are treated, but they are nevertheless adversely affected by the maternal PKU.

Maternal PKU is important, since, as a result of newborn screening programs and the early treatment of PKU, there will be in the coming decades many women who have PKU but who are mentally normal and will want to bear children. Will these women have offspring who are mentally retarded?

Those women with true PKU who have blood phenylalanine concentrations of 20 mg/100 ml or greater and perhaps some women with "atypical PKU" seem to be at greatest risk of bearing damaged offspring. Women with mild hyperphenylalaninemia may be at less risk or may be at no greater than normal risk of having retarded children.

Treatment during pregnancy with a low-phenylalanine diet that controls the maternal biochemical abnormalities may prevent fetal damage in maternal PKU. Several such cases with normal offspring have been reported. Treatment during pregnancy has not always resulted in normal offspring, however, and one determinant may be how soon in pregnancy the treatment begins. For optimal results, treatment may have to begin preconceptually so that it is in effect throughout pregnancy.

Maple Syrup Urine Disease (Branched-Chain Ketoaciduria)

This is an inborn error of metabolism involving the branched-chain amino acids (leucine, isoleucine, and valine) and their ketoacid analogues. It is inherited as an autosomal recessive trait and is rare, occurring in approximately one per 200,000 infants. The basic defect is in the mechanism that controls the activity of the three branched-chain α-ketoacid decarboxylases. As a result of this defect, the affected infant develops increased concentrations of the branched-chain amino acids and their corresponding ketoacids.

Clinical Characteristics. There are at least three different disorders within the "maple syrup urine disease" category. The first described and the most dramatic is that termed *maple syrup urine disease* itself. In this disorder, the defect in branched-chain decarboxylation is virtually complete. The infant usually has a normal prenatal and perinatal history. On about the third day of life he may become lethargic, and by the fourth or fifth day of life he develops vomiting, increasing lethargy, poor feeding, and weight loss. Neurologic signs such as hypotonia or hypertonia, seizures, and loss of basic reflexes may appear. Metabolic acidosis due to the accumulation of ketoacids is clearly evident by this time. If vigorous treatment is not begun, the clinical course rapidly declines, and death ensues within the first month of life in almost all such infants.

The second disorder is known as the *intermediate variant of maple syrup urine disease*. The branched-chain decarboxylation defect is not complete in this disorder, with about 2 to 5 per cent of residual enzyme activity remaining. Affected infants are usually asymptomatic during the neonatal period. They may continue to be clinically normal until they are several months old, when developmental delay is noted. Subsequently, mental retardation is evident and episodes of metabolic acidosis, often mild and associated with acute febrile illnesses, develop.

The third disorder, *intermittent variant of maple syrup urine disease*, is associated with about 5 to 15 per cent of residual branched-chain decarboxylase activity. As patients with the intermediate variant, these infants are clinically normal during the neonatal period. They usually remain asymptomatic through infancy and childhood, except when there is an acute febrile episode or trauma, such as that due to surgery or an accident. At these times the branched-chain ketoacids accumulate to an extraordinary extent, and severe metabolic acidosis with all the acute signs of maple syrup urine disease may occur. Several affected children have died during these acute episodes.

Diagnosis. As in virtually all other inborn errors of metabolism, the most effective means of diagnosing maple syrup urine disease is by routine newborn screening (see Newborn Screening, Part 2). In an infant with the severe or intermediate form of maple syrup urine disease, this may be the only effective means of instituting therapy before death or irreversible brain damage has occurred. For infants with the intermittent variant of maple syrup urine disease, this may be the only means by which the disease is suspected, and the clinical complications can be anticipated.

If maple syrup urine disease is suspected on the basis of clinical signs or family history, blood and urine specimens should be obtained and sent to a laboratory in which tests for amino acids and organic acids can be performed. During acute episodes in any of the maple syrup urine disease disorders, the branched-chain amino acid concentrations in blood, particularly leucine, will be many times greater than the normal 2 mg/100 ml, perhaps as high as 50 or 60 mg/100 ml. The urine may have an odor reminiscent of maple syrup. The branched-chain ketoacid concentrations in the urine will be very high and may be detected by a screening test using the dinitrophenylhydrazine reagent. When this reagent is acidified and added to urine containing a large concentration of ketoacids, dinitrophenylhydrazones will form, resulting in a cloudy reaction and a precipitate, whereas there is no change in a normal urine. Amino acid analysis of urine will reveal increased branched-chain amino acid concentrations.

In the intermediate variant of maple syrup urine disease, the only finding may be a mildly increased blood leucine concentration (4 to 10 mg/100 ml), except during acute episodes, when all the other findings appear. In the intermittent variant, blood amino acid levels as well as those of urine amino acids and ketoacids may be normal except, again, during an acute episode. The intermittent variant, therefore, may be particularly difficult to diagnose and usually is suspected only when an acute episode has occurred. In the neonate, the blood leucine concentration should be increased after the first or second day of life in severe maple syrup disease as well as in the intermediate variant, but this concentration may be normal in the intermittent variant.

Treatment. The treatment of maple syrup urine disease is dietary. The diet must be reduced in branched-chain amino acid content, especially that of leucine, and is very difficult to prepare and administer. The dietary therapy should be attempted only at a pediatric metabolic unit staffed by physicians, nutritionists, and others who have the expertise and experience to deal properly with this difficult disorder. The basic diet consists of a mixture composed of the necessary free amino acids excluding the branched-chain amino acids and including minerals, carbohydrate, and fat. This diet must be prepared so that it will be reasonably palatable. It is supplemented with a small amount of milk or other food containing the branched-chain amino acids. Allowable foods include fruits and vegetables.

Thiamine (vitamin B_1) might be helpful in the treatment of certain infants and children with maple syrup urine disease. A coenzymatically active derivative of thiamine is necessary for branched-chain decarboxylase activity. Large amounts of thiamine might stimulate this activity in some individuals with maple syrup urine disease or the variants, although thiamine therapy is at best adjunctive and cannot replace dietary restriction.

Sulfur Amino Acid Abnormalities

There are several disorders within this group, each due to a specific metabolic block in the methionine pathway. Some are associated with severe clinical disease and others appear to be benign. Each is inherited as an autosomal recessive trait. All are potentially identifiable by routine newborn screening if particular methods are used for this screening (see Newborn Screening, Part 2).

HYPERMETHIONINEMIA

Several infants with methionine adenosyltransferase deficiency (Fig. 60–2) have been described. They have markedly elevated concentrations of methionine in blood. These infants have reduced enzyme activity in liver but normal activity in cultured skin fibroblasts. They are clinically normal, possibly because the enzyme deficiency is not generalized throughout the body. Thus, this may be a benign disorder.

Increased concentrations of methionine in blood may be induced in a normal neonate by feeding a high protein diet. This is a transient state that will disappear in 2 or 3 days when a lower protein diet is given. If the increased protein ingestion continues, the hypermethioninemia will spontaneously disap-

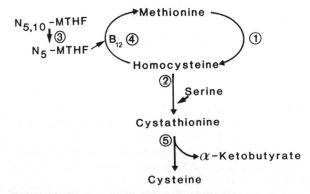

Figure 60–2. Transsulfuration in methionine metabolic pathway. The inborn errors in this diagram include (1) *hypermethioninemia* due to methionine adenosyltransferase deficiency; (2) *homocystinuria* due to cystathionine β-synthase deficiency; (3) *methionine remethylation defect* due to N5,10-methylenetetrahydrofolate reductase deficiency and to (4) B_{12} metabolic defect; and (5) cystathioninemia due to cystathionase deficiency.

pear by the time the infant is about 3 months old. No clinical abnormality is known to result from transient hypermethioninemia. With the recent trend back to breast-feeding and, consequently, a lower protein intake in the neonate, transient hypermethioninemia is much less frequent than it formerly was.

Increased blood methionine concentrations may also occur in association with neonatal liver disease. This is most commonly noted in neonatal hepatitis but is also seen in hereditary tyrosinemia, galactosemia, and fructosemia. It is presumed that the hypermethioninemia (and tyrosinemia) of liver disease are secondary to hepatocellular damage. The amino acid abnormalities are important only in that they may serve as indicators of liver disease and perhaps also as measures of the severity of damage.

HOMOCYSTINURIA

This disorder results from a deficiency in cystathionine β-synthase activity. This is an enzyme that is responsible for the conversion of homocysteine to cystathionine (Fig. 60–2). In the neonates with homocystinuria, the most striking biochemical abnormality is an increase in the blood methionine level. There is also a small accumulation of homocystine in blood and urine. Later in infancy and in childhood, the homocystine accumulation becomes more prominent and the hypermethioninemia is less striking. The concentration of cystine in blood is low. The frequency of homocystinuria is approximately one per 200,000 infants.

Clinical Characteristics. Homocystinuria does not usually produce clinical signs in the neonate. Detection of the disease at this early age, therefore, depends on routine newborn screening (see Newborn Screening, Part 2) or suspicion due to family history. If undetected and untreated, homocystinuria leads to brain damage with mental retardation, dislocation of the ocular lenses (ectopia lentis), skeletal abnormalities including osteoporosis and elongated limbs, and thromboembolic phenomena. The clinical complications are highly variable, however, and some individuals may not have brain or skeletal involvement.

The propensity for thromboembolic complications in this disease may result in cerebral occlusion, even in infancy. Thus, infants with a stroke should always be tested for homocystinuria.

Diagnosis. The diagnosis of homocystinuria is based on the presence of homocystine in blood and urine and an increased blood methionine level. The demonstration of homocystine in particular may require a careful and quantitative analysis for amino acids, preferably with an amino acid analyzer. Less sensitive methods of amino acid analysis such as thin-layer or paper chromatography or screening methods such as the urine cyanide-nitroprusside test, may be insufficient to detect the small amount of homocystine present in the affected neonate or young infant.

Treatment. Treatment consists of a special low-methionine diet supplemented with cystine. This diet is difficult to administer and should be given only at pediatric metabolic centers. Perhaps as many as 50 per cent of homocystinuric individuals respond to pharmacologic doses of pyridoxine (vitamin B_6). In these individuals, large amounts of pyridoxine (25 to 200 mg/day), perhaps in association with a modified low-methionine diet, may be all that is necessary to control the biochemical manifestations. Treatment begun early in infancy may prevent most if not all the clinical complications. Even when begun after the clinical complications have appeared, treatment has sometimes been beneficial.

METHIONINE REMETHYLATION DEFECTS

Methionine must be remethylated from homocysteine for adequate methionine conservation (Fig. 60–2). Otherwise, methionine is depleted in the body. The major pathway for methionine remethylation is via $N5$-methyltetrahydrofolate-homocysteine methyltransferase, an enzyme that requires $N5$-methyltetrahydrofolate and homocysteine as substrates. This enzyme also requires methyl-B_{12}, a vitamin B_{12} product, as a cofactor.

Two metabolic blocks result in a reduction in methionine remethylation. One of these is a primary defect in $N5,10$-methylenetetrahydrofolate reductase, an enzyme that is responsible for the synthesis of $N5$-methyltetrahydrofolate. $N5,10$-methylenetetrahydrofolate reductase deficiency results in an accumulation of homocystine in blood and urine and in a reduced blood methionine level. Failure to thrive and mental retardation have been described as consequences of this disease. Treatment is with folinic acid and, possibly, methionine supplementation.

The other block is due to reduced activity of $N5$-methyltetrahydrofolate-homocysteine methyltransferase secondary to lack of sufficient methyl-B_{12}. Vitamin B_{12} deficiency as a result of breast-feeding from a vegetarian mother may produce this. These infants have failure to thrive and present with megaloblastic anemia at 3 to 5 months of age. Vitamin B_{12} treatment is curative. More often reported as a cause of this block is an inborn error in B_{12} metabolism. These infants have normal serum total B_{12} levels, but they cannot synthesize sufficient amounts of methyl-B_{12}. They generally have evidence of intrauterine growth retardation with low birth weight and microcephaly. They continue to grow poorly after birth and usually present at 2 to 4 months of age with failure to thrive, microcephaly, developmental delay, and megaloblastic anemia. They as well as infants with vitamin B_{12} deficiency have accumulations of homocystine and cystathionine in blood and urine, a low blood methionine level, and accumulations of methylmalonic acid (see Methylmalonic Acidemia, Chapter 61). The biochemical abnormalities and the megaloblastosis may respond partially or completely to pharmacologic doses of B_{12} (hydroxocobalamin). Whether there is clinical benefit from treatment has not been determined.

CYSTATHIONINEMIA

This inborn error is caused by deficient activity of the enzyme cystathionase, which results in increased cystathionine in blood and urine (Fig. 60–2). As in homocystinuria, there are two forms of this disorder: One is biochemically responsive to pyridoxine (vitamin B_6), but the other shows no such response, even to massive amounts of pyridoxine. Most affected individuals (perhaps 90 per cent or more) respond to pyridoxine. The diagnosis of either form depends on the demonstration of persistently increased amounts of cystathionine in urine and of the presence of cystathionine in blood. Present evidence indicates that cystathioninemia (cystathionase deficiency) is benign and that there are no clinical consequences in either the early infantile or later periods of life. Should one wish to treat this disorder, therapy consists of pyridoxine hydrochloride supplementation in oral doses of 25 to 200 mg/day for the B_6-responsive form. The B_6-nonresponsive form might respond to a low methionine diet.

Tyrosinemia

An increase in the concentration of tyrosine may occur either transiently or as a persistent condition in the newborn.

TRANSIENT NEONATAL TYROSINEMIA

This finding formerly occurred in as many as 5 to 10 per cent of all newborns. As with transient hypermethioninemia, however, the recent reduction in neonatal protein intake through greater use of breastfeeding has substantially decreased the frequency of transient tyrosinemia. It is initiated by delayed maturation of parahydroxyphenylpyruvic acid oxidase, an enzyme that metabolizes parahydroxyphenylpyruvic acid, a product of tyrosine oxidation. Reduced activity of this enzyme results in the accumulation of tyrosine and parahydroxyphenylpyruvate as well as secondary metabolites such as parahydroxyphenyllactate and parahydroxyphenylacetate. The blood tyrosine level is often markedly increased, sometimes in excess of 20 mg/100 ml (the normal blood tyrosine concentration is less than 4 mg/100 ml). Tyrosine and the aforementioned metabolites are present in greatly excessive quantities in the urine.

There are several interesting characteristics of this common entity. First, transient tyrosinemia is much more frequent among premature than among fullterm infants. This is presumably related to the tendency toward immaturity of many enzyme systems in premature infants. Second, a high protein intake either causes the findings to appear or increases the degree of tyrosinemia. Third, ascorbic acid (vitamin C) therapy activates the enzyme in most infants and thus remedies the biochemical abnormalities.

Transient tyrosinemia usually appears after the first week of life and reaches its peak during the second or third month, especially when the protein intake has been substantially increased. There is debate as to whether this finding causes clinical problems. Some centers have reported slightly reduced intellectual performance among children who had transient neonatal tyrosinemia, whereas other centers have found no such reduction. No physical problems have been reported. It is probably advisable to limit the protein intake of infants to less than 4 gm/kg/day and to maintain a daily ascorbic acid intake of 25 to 50 mg/day so as to lessen the chances that significant tyrosinemia will occur.

Tyrosinemia can occasionally confuse the results of newborn screening for phenylketonuria. A markedly elevated blood tyrosine level may be associated with an increased concentration of phenylalanine, since phenylalanine is the immediate precursor of tyrosine (Fig. 60–1). When this occurs, an increased phenylalanine concentration in the newborn blood specimen may be incorrectly interpreted as an indication of phenylketonuria. If a complete blood amino acid analysis is performed, however, the differentiation between phenylketonuria and tyrosinemia is unmistakable, since phenylketonuria is associated with a normal or reduced tyrosine concentration and tyrosinemia causes a markedly increased tyrosine concentration. This type of analysis should be performed on all infants whose newborn screening results suggest the presence of phenylketonuria.

HEREDITARY TYROSINEMIA

This genetic disorder is inherited as an autosomal recessive trait. It is very rare except among those of French-Canadian ancestry, in whom a relatively high frequency has been found. The precise metabolic defect has not been identified. Deficient enzyme activities of both parahydroxyphenylpyruvic acid oxidase and tyrosine transaminase have been reported in the liver of patients. The most prominent amino acid findings are increased tyrosine and methionine in blood and increased tyrosine and tyrosine metabolites in urine. These derangements in tyrosine metabolism may be a secondary feature of this disease. The serum alpha-fetoprotein concentration is markedly elevated.

Clinical Characteristics. The disease presents in two ways. The most dramatic is severe liver disease that is apparent within the first week or two of life. Hepatomegaly and jaundice appear. Liver-function test results are abnormal, particularly the prothrombin and partial thromboplastin times. This presentation is usually associated with a rapidly progressive course characterized by deteriorating liver function, recurrent gram-negative sepsis, bleeding, and death by 2 to 3 months of age.

More often, however, there is a less dramatic presentation. These affected infants are usually clinically normal until the end of the first or second month of life, when jaundice and hepatomegaly are noted. At this time, liver function test results are abnormal, and there may be a urinary pattern of the renal Fanconi syndrome with glycosuria, generalized hyperaminoaciduria, and proteinuria. During the next few months, the hepatic disease progresses to cirrhosis, and rickets may appear. If untreated, death due to liver disease occurs later, usually during the first few years of life. Notably, mentality remains normal, and there are no signs of CNS involvement.

Diagnosis. The diagnosis of hereditary tyrosinemia is often controversial. Liver disease from several causes, including hepatitis, galactosemia, and hereditary fructosemia, may be associated with increased tyrosine and tyrosine metabolites as well as increased methionine. Consequently, these biochemical abnormalities are not specific for hereditary tyrosinemia, and in this disorder as in other disorders they may be secondary to the type of hepatocellular disease that is present. The cause of the liver disease in hereditary tyrosinemia, therefore, may be an agent that is as yet unidentified. Thus, there are no particular confirmatory findings in hereditary tyrosinemia. The diagnosis usually depends on the presence of typical clinical and biochemical findings, family history and ethnic characteristics, and the elimination of other disorders that may produce similar findings.

Treatment. Treatment includes therapy for the complications of liver disease and control of the amino acid abnormalities through the use of a special diet. This diet, which is low in both tyrosine and phenylalanine, results in reversal of the renal abnormalities and of the rickets, but, except in a few isolated instances, it has not been effective in arresting the progression of the liver disease.

TYROSINOSIS

This inborn error, unlike hereditary tyrosinemia, appears to be an authentic primary disorder of tyrosine metabolism. Only a few cases have been de-

scribed. In these families, the disorder seems to have been transmitted as an autosomal recessive trait. The metabolic defect may be a deficiency of cytosolic tyrosine transaminase with normal mitochondrial tyrosine transaminase. The transaminase deficiency results in primary accumulations of tyrosine in blood and urine and, secondarily, in accumulations of tyrosine metabolites in urine. Despite these accumulations, which are identical with and in greater quantity than those noted in hereditary tyrosinemia, there are no abnormalities of liver, kidney, or bone. However, all the reported patients have been mentally retarded. The mental retardation appears to be similar to that seen in phenylketonuria, with developmental delay during the first year of life and obvious intellectual retardation noted by the second or third year. In addition, affected individuals have painful hyperkeratotic lesions on the hands and feet. The third feature of this disease is a keratitis with corneal ulcerations that causes photophobia and increased lacrimation. The skin and eye lesions can be controlled by a low-tyrosine, low-phenylalanine diet that reduces the levels of tyrosine and tyrosine metabolites. If tyrosinosis is analogous to phenylketonuria, the diet would have to be initiated during the first weeks of life in order to prevent the mental retardation.

Urea Cycle Disorders

Each of the disorders in this important group of inborn errors may present with dramatic clinical symptoms and signs during the neonatal period. The underlying cause of the clinical state appears to be ammonia toxicity due to ammonia accumulation that results from a block in the urea cycle, that cycle which allows the human to convert ammonia to urea (Fig.

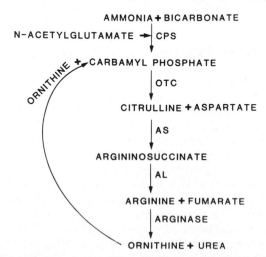

Figure 60–3. Urea cycle. Ammonia is metabolized to urea through a series of five major enzymatic reactions. There is an inborn error of metabolism for each of the enzymes. The abbreviations refer to enzymes as follows: CPS (carbamylphosphate synthetase); OTC (ornithine transcarbamylase); AS (argininosuccinate synthetase); and AL (argininosuccinate lyase).

60–3). In the severe form of any of these disorders, there is a characteristic clinical presentation of hyperammonemia in the neonate that includes lethargy, hypotonia, poor feeding, and even collapse and unresponsiveness if the blood ammonia concentration rises to levels of greater than 10 times normal. In less severe forms, clinical disease appears later in infancy with signs such as lethargy, failure to thrive, and developmental delay.

The sick neonate may require immediate lifesaving measures. These include exchange transfusion, peritoneal dialysis, or hemodialysis as well as supportive parenteral therapy. Chronic treatment for the recovered neonate and the infant who presents with a less severe form of the disorder consists of a low-protein diet. Other measures relate to the specific disorder and are discussed subsequently.

CARBAMYL PHOSPHATE SYNTHETASE (CPS) DEFICIENCY

This autosomal recessive disorder is caused by a deficiency in activity of the first enzyme within the urea cycle. Severe clinical illness may occur in the neonatal period. Otherwise, the disorder becomes evident later in infancy. The signs of illness include failure to thrive, developmental delay, and periodic hyperammonemic coma during acute febrile periods. The blood ammonia level is usually 3 to 5 times normal but may be higher. Blood amino acid analysis reveals reduced levels of citrulline and arginine. The diagnosis is confirmed by enzyme analysis of liver obtained by biopsy. Treatment consists of low-protein diet, but this has had limited effectiveness in the few reported cases. Sodium benzoate may be an effective adjunct in acute and chronic therapy.

ORNITHINE TRANSCARBAMYLASE (OTC) DEFICIENCY

This disorder is caused by deficient activity of the second enzyme within the urea cycle. It is probably the second most frequent of the urea cycle disorders. It is inherited as an X-linked trait, unlike most inborn errors, which are autosomal recessive. Thus, affected male infants, who are hemizygotes (since they have only one X chromosome), have virtually no activity of this enzyme, and they become profoundly hyperammonemic during the first days of life. Characteristically, these infants are normal at birth, but by the second or third day of life they develop marked lethargy and hypotonia. This may rapidly progress to unresponsiveness. The blood ammonia level at this time is usually at least 10 times greater than normal. Amino acid analysis of blood reveals reduced levels of citrulline and arginine, as in CPS deficiency. Despite the fact that ornithine is a cosubstrate of OTC, the blood ornithine level remains normal. A key finding is increased orotic acid in urine, which distin-

guishes this disorder from CPS deficiency, in which there is a normal or reduced level of urinary orotic acid. Despite dramatic treatment, only one or two male infants with OTC deficiency have lived beyond the neonatal period. The diagnosis is confirmed by enzyme assay in biopsied or postmortem liver.

The female with OTC deficiency is a heterozygote (since she has a second X chromosome that has a normal gene for OTC). She has approximately 50 per cent of normal enzyme activity in the liver. She may remain clinically normal, or she may develop signs of mild to moderate hyperammonemia in infancy or childhood. These signs, which include vomiting, lethargy, and ataxia, usually appear when the protein intake is increased. Treatment consists of a reduction in dietary protein.

CITRULLINEMIA

This autosomal recessive disorder is caused by a deficiency in argininosuccinate synthetase, the third enzyme within the urea cycle. It may present as acute neonatal disease or as chronic disease later in infancy or childhood. There may also be a benign variant of citrullinemia. There is marked hyperammonemia in the sick neonate but a less severe degree of hyperammonemia in the older infant. The major amino acid abnormality is an increased level of citrulline in blood and urine. The urine also contains an increased orotic acid concentration. The diagnosis is confirmed by enzyme assay in cultured skin fibroblasts or liver. Treatment consists of a low-protein diet. Supplementation with arginine may also be helpful in the treatment of this disorder.

ARGININOSUCCINIC ACIDEMIA (ASA)

This is the most frequent urea cycle disorder. It is an autosomal recessive trait caused by deficient activity of argininosuccinate lyase (argininosuccinase), the fourth enzyme within the urea cycle. There are at least three forms of this disorder. The most severe form presents in the neonate with marked hyperammonemia and huge accumulations of argininosuccinate in blood and urine. These neonates may rapidly progress from lethargy and hypotonia to unresponsiveness. Few have survived despite dramatic therapeutic measures. A less severe form presents during the third or fourth month of life with developmental lag and hepatomegaly after a clinically normal neonatal period. Signs of brain damage progress and convulsions usually appear. These infants have moderate hyperammonemia and high concentrations of argininosuccinate in blood, urine, CSF, and tissues. Treatment consists of a low-protein diet and supplementation with arginine. The third form appears to be benign. These infants are discovered by routine newborn screening on the basis of increased urinary argininosuccinate. They have normal or only slightly increased concentrations of blood ammonia, and most have remained clinically normal despite receiving little or no treatment.

The diagnosis of argininosuccinic acidemia can be readily confirmed by enzyme studies of erythrocytes. Enzyme studies can also be performed in cultured skin fibroblasts, liver, kidney, and brain. The precise enzymatic differences among infants with these different clinical pictures have not been clearly defined.

ARGININEMIA

This is an autosomal recessive disorder due to deficient activity of arginase, the fifth and final enzyme within the urea cycle. Only a few cases have been reported. The clinical picture has been progressive neurologic degeneration, usually appearing in late infancy or early childhood, characterized by developmental delay, ataxia, and spasticity. A mild hyperammonemia has been present in most cases. Arginine is increased in blood and urine. The diagnosis is confirmed by enzyme assay in erythrocytes. Liver arginase is also deficient in this disorder. Attempted treatment has included a low-protein diet.

Hyperglycinemia

This term should not imply a specific disorder but a biochemical abnormality noted in a number of disorders that may produce neonatal disease. When increased glycine is associated with ketosis and metabolic acidosis, the general term "ketotic hyperglycinemia" has been applied. This includes several inborn errors of organic acid metabolism in which the hyperglycinemia is a secondary feature (see Chapter 61). Hyperglycinemia may also be present as an isolated but striking finding in the absence of ketosis or acidosis and, when so, is termed nonketotic hyperglycinemia.

"KETOTIC HYPERGLYCINEMIA"

Any of the organic acidemias (propionic acidemia, methylmalonic acidemia, etc.) may be associated with secondary hyperglycinemia (see Chapter 61). Signs of metabolic acidosis may appear during the first 2 or 3 days of life. These signs include lethargy, tachypnea, vomiting, and poor feeding. Amino acid analysis of blood reveals a glycine concentration that is two to four times normal. Urinary glycine is markedly increased, but there is no other amino acid ab-

normality. CSF glycine is increased but less so than the blood glycine. Tests for urinary ketones, such as with the Acetest* tablet or the Ketostix,* will be positive. The basic disorder involves a defect in the metabolism of an organic acid, and the disease should be named accordingly. Thus, "ketotic hyperglycinemia" is an obsolete term.

NONKETOTIC HYPERGLYCINEMIA

Hyperglycinemia as a specific finding in the absence of ketosis and acidosis is seen with several clinical pictures. These are sufficiently distinct to suggest that nonketotic hyperglycinemia, as the ketotic hyperglycinemias, may also be a secondary finding in many of the disorders with which it is associated.

Acute Neonatal Type

The clinical presentation in this autosomal recessive disorder is one of the most striking in neonatal medicine. The infant, who is usually born after a normal pregnancy and delivery, appears to be normal for the first 24 to 36 hours of life. At this time, he becomes noticeably lethargic, and by the end of the second day of life he is so inactive and hypotonic as to be characterized by "acute neonatal collapse." Mechanical ventilation and other supportive therapy may be necessary at this point. There are no other clinical findings. Routine laboratory data are surprisingly normal for such a serious clinical state. In particular, there is no acidosis or hyperammonemia. Amino acid studies, however, reveal a markedly increased glycine concentration in blood, sometimes as high as 10 times normal, and a huge urinary excretion of glycine. Even more striking is the CSF glycine concentration, which often is 30 to 50 times normal. This greater increase in the CSF glycine level as compared with the blood glycine level results in a reduced plasma–to–CSF-glycine ratio. Organic acids, including short-chain fatty acids, are normal. Glycine cleavage enzyme activity is reduced to about 20 per cent of normal in the liver but to about 5 per cent or less of normal in the brain. Therefore, this form of nonketotic hyperglycinemia may be due to a primary defect in glycine metabolism.

There is no effective therapy for this disorder. Exchange transfusion and peritoneal dialysis have not produced clinical improvement. Strychnine therapy in the form of strychnine sulfate 100 μg/kg/day may improve muscle tone and responsiveness but does not prevent the progressive and profound brain damage. Sodium benzoate in large doses (500 mg to 1 gm/day orally) may reduce the peripheral accumulation of free glycine by conjugating with glycine to form hippurate (benzoylglycine), but it has no effect on glycine in the central nervous system, since it does

---

*Ames Company, Elkhart, IN 46514

not cross the blood-brain barrier. Infants with this disorder either die within the first few weeks of life or live to develop progressive neurologic deterioration, severe myoclonic seizures with a hypsarrhythmic electroencephalographic pattern, and a virtual vegetative state.

Infantile Type

These infants are clinically normal until 1 to 2 months of age, when poor head control and other signs of developmental lag become evident. There are no abnormal physical findings. Myoclonic seizures develop by 3 to 4 months of age. As in the acute neonatal disease, amino acid analysis reveals specifically increased concentrations of glycine in blood, urine, and CSF with a reduced plasma–to–CSF-glycine ratio. The glycine concentrations, however, are usually less markedly increased than in the acute neonatal disease. Several of these children have had a peculiar transient comatose reaction to the administration of valine, but the pathogenesis of this response is unknown. There is no known treatment for this form of nonketotic hyperglycinemia. The disease is not progressive, and the children develop a stable mental retardation.

Other Forms

Several children with nonketotic hyperglycinemia have had only mild to moderate mental retardation without seizures. An unusual type of spinal motor neuron disease involving the legs and beginning in childhood or adolescence has been described in association with nonketotic hyperglycinemia. There might also be a benign form, although this has not been clearly documented.

Histidinemia

This autosomal recessive disorder results from a defect in the conversion of histidine to urocanic acid. It does not produce neonatal disease and is probably benign, but it is included in this chapter because it is identified in some newborn screening programs. The major biochemical finding is a 3- to 7-fold increase in the blood histidine level and an even greater increase in urinary histidine. A low-histidine diet is available for treatment, but there is no clear evidence that treatment is necessary.

academic achievement of children treated early for phenylketonuria. Dev. Med. Child. Neurol. 21:311, 1979.

Bickel, H.: Phenylketonuria: past, present, future. J. Inher. Metab. Dis. 3:123, 1980.

Butler, I. J., O'Flynn, M. E., et al.: Neurotransmitter defects and treatment of disorders of hyperphenylalaninemia. J. Pediatr. 98:729, 1981.

Kang, E. S., Solle, N. D., and Gerald, P. S.: Results of treatment and termination of diet in phenylketonuria (PKU). Pediatrics 46:881, 1970.

Kaufman, S.: Phenylketonuria: biochemical mechanisms. In Agranoff, B. W., and Aprison, M. H. (Eds.): Advances in Neurochemistry. Vol. 2. New York, Plenum Press, 1976, pp. 1–132.

Levy, H. L.: Treatment of phenylketonuria. In Papadatos, C. J., and Bartsocas, C. S. (Eds.): The Management of Genetic Disorders. New York, Alan R. Liss, 1979, pp. 171–182.

O'Flynn, M. E., Holtzman, N. A., et al.: The diagnosis of phenylketonuria. A report from the Collaborative Study of Children Treated for Phenylketonuria. Am. J. Dis. Child. 134:769, 1980.

Scriver, C. R., and Clow, C. L.: Phenylketonuria: epitome of human biochemical genetics. N. Engl. J. Med. 303:1336 and 1394, 1980.

Waisbren, S. E., Schnell, R. R., and Levy, H. L.: Diet termination in children with phenylketonuria: a review of psychological assessments used to determine outcome. J. Inher. Metab. Dis. 3:149, 1980.

Williamson, M. L., Koch, R., et al.: Correlates of intelligence test results in treated phenylketonuric children. Pediatrics 68:161, 1981.

Hyperphenylalaninemia

Berlow, S.: Progress in phenylketonuria: defects in the metabolism of biopterin. Pediatrics 65:837, 1980.

Berman, J. L., and Ford, R.: Intelligence quotients and intelligence loss in patients with phenylketonuria and some variant states. J. Pediatr. 77:764, 1970.

Brewster, T. G., Moskowitz, M. A., et al.: Dihydropteridine reductase deficiency associated with severe neurologic disease and mild hyperphenylalaninemia. Pediatrics 63:94, 1979.

Güttler, F.: Hyperphenylalaninemia. Diagnosis and classification of the various types of phenylalanine hydroxylase deficiency in childhood. Acta Paediatr. Scand. Suppl. 280:7, 1980.

Kang, E. S., Kaufman, S., and Gerald P. S.: Clinical and biochemical observations of patients with atypical phenylketonuria. Pediatrics 45:83, 1970.

Kaufman, S.: Differential diagnosis of variant forms of hyperphenylalaninemia. Pediatrics 65:840, 1980.

Kaufman, S., Berlow, S., et al.: Hyperphenylalaninemia due to a deficiency of biopterin. A variant form of phenylketonuria. N. Engl. J. Med. 299:673, 1978.

Levy, H. L., Shih, V. F., et al.: Persistent mild hyperphenylalaninemia in the untreated state: a prospective study. N. Engl. J. Med. 285:424, 1971.

Task Force on Biopterin: New developments in hyperphenylalaninemia. Pediatrics 65:844, 1980.

Maternal Phenylketonuria

Lenke, R. R., and Levy, H. L.: Maternal phenylketonuria and hyperphenylalaninemia. An international survey of the outcome of untreated and treated pregnancies. N. Engl. J. Med. 303:1202, 1980.

Levy, H. L., Lenke, R. R., and Crocker, A. C. (Eds.): Maternal PKU. DHHS Pub. No. (HSA) 81:5299. Washington, U.S. Government Printing Office, 1981.

Levy, H. L., and Shih, V. E.: Maternal phenylketonuria and hyperphenylalaninemia. A prospective study. Pediatr. Res. 8:391, 1974.

REFERENCES

Phenylketonuria

Berry, H. K.: The diagnosis of phenylketonuria. A commentary. Am. J. Dis. Child. 135:211, 1981.

Berry, H. K., O'Grady, D. J., et al.: Intellectual development and

MacCready, R. A., and Levy, H. L.: The problem of maternal phenylketonuria. Am. J. Obstet. Gynecol. 113:121, 1972.

Maple Syrup Urine Disease

Committee for Improvement of Hereditary Disease Management: Management of maple syrup urine disease in Canada. Can. Med. Assoc. J. 115:1005, 1976.

Danner, D. J., Wheeler, F. B., et al.: In vivo and in vitro response of human branched chain α-ketoacid dehydrogenase to thiamine and thiamine pyrophosphate. Pediatr. Res. 12:235, 1978.

Hammersen, G., Wille, L., et al.: Maple syrup urine disease: treatment of the acutely ill newborn. Eur. J. Pediatr. 129:157, 1978.

Naylor, E. W., and Guthrie, R.: Newborn screening for maple syrup urine disease. Pediatrics 61:262, 1978.

Pueschel, S. M., Bresnan, M. J., et al.: Thiamine-responsive intermittent branched-chain ketoaciduria. J. Pediatr. 94:628, 1979.

Sulfur Amino Acid Abnormalities

Carmel, R., Bedros, A. A., et al.: Congenital methylmalonic aciduria-homocystinuria with megaloblastic anemia: observations on response to hydroxocobalamin and on the effect of homocysteine and methionine on the deoxyuridine suppression test. Blood 55:570, 1980.

Gaull, G. E., and Tallan, H. H.: Methionine adenosyltransferase deficiency: new enzymatic defect associated with hypermethioninemia. Science 186:59, 1974.

Gaull, G. E., Tallan, H. H., et al.: Hypermethioninemia associated with methionine adenosyltransferase deficiency: clinical, morphologic, and biochemical observations on four patients. J. Pediatr. 98:734, 1981.

Harpey, J.-P., Rosenblatt, D. S., et al.: Homocystinuria caused by 5,10-methylenetetrahydrofolate reductase deficiency: a case in an infant responding to methionine, folinic acid, pyridoxine, and vitamin B_{12} therapy. J. Pediatr. 98:275, 1981.

Levy, H. L., and Mudd, S. H.: Cystathioninuria and homocystinuria. Clin. Chim. Acta 58:51, 1975.

Levy, H. L., Mudd, S. H., et al.: A derangement in B_{12} metabolism associated with homocystinemia, cystathioninemia, hypomethioninemia and methylmalonic aciduria. Am. J. Med. 48:390, 1970.

Mudd, S. H., and Levy, H. L.: Disorders of transsulfuration. In Stanbury, J. B., Wyngaarden, J. B., Fredrickson, D. S., Goldstein, J. L., and Brown, M. S. (Eds.): The Metabolic Basis of Inherited Disease. 5th Ed. New York, McGraw-Hill, 1982, pp. 522–559.

Narisawa, K., Wada, Y., et al.: Infantile type of homocystinuria with $N^{5,10}$-methylenetetrahydrofolate reductase defect. Tohoku J. Exp. Med. 121:185, 1977.

Pascal, T. A., Gaull, G. E., et al.: Cystathionase deficiency: evidence for genetic heterogeneity in primary cystathioninuria. Pediatr. Res. 12:125, 1978.

Pullon, D. H. H.: Homocystinuria and other methioninemias. In Bickel, H., Guthrie, R., and Hammersen, G. (Eds.): Neonatal Screening for Inborn Errors of Metabolism. Berlin, Springer Verlag, 1980, pp. 29–44.

Scott, C. R., Dassell, S. W., et al.: Cystathioninemia: a benign genetic condition. J. Pediatr. 76:571, 1970.

Valle, D., Pai, G. S., et al.: Homocystinuria due to cystathionine β-synthase deficiency: clinical manifestations and therapy. Johns Hopkins Med. J. 146:110, 1980.

Whitehead, P. D., Clayton, B. E., et al.: Changing incidence of neonatal hypermethioninemia: implications for the detection of homocystinuria. Arch. Dis. Child. 54:593, 1979.

Wilcken, B., and Turner, G.: Homocystinuria in New South Wales. Arch. Dis. Child. 53:242, 1978.

Tyrosinemia

Bienfang, D. C., Kuwabara, T., and Pueschel, S. M.: The Richner-Hanhart Syndrome. Report of a case with associated tyrosinemia. Arch. Ophthalmol. 94:1133, 1976.

Carson, N. A. J., Biggart, J. D., et al.: Hereditary tyrosinaemia. Clinical, enzymatic, and pathological study of an infant with the acute form of the disease. Arch. Dis. Child. 51:106, 1976.

Gray, G. F., Patrick, A. D., et al.: Acute hereditary tyrosinaemia Type I: Clinical, biochemical and haematological studies in twins. J. Inher. Metab. Dis. 4:37, 1981.

Holston, J. L., Levy, H. L., et al.: Tyrosinosis: a patient without liver or renal disease. Pediatrics 48:393, 1971.

Mamunes, P., Prince, P. E., et al.: Intellectual deficits after transient tyrosinemia in the term neonate. Pediatrics 57:675, 1976.

Martin, H. P., Fischer, H. L., et al.: The development of children with transient neonatal tyrosinemia. J. Pediatr. 84:212, 1974.

Nutrition Committee of the Canadian Paediatric Society: Vitamin C prophylaxis of tyrosinemia in the newborn. Can. Med. Assoc. J. 114:447, 1976.

Pelet, B., Antener, I., et al.: Tyrosinemia without liver or renal damage with plantar and palmar keratosis and keratitis (Hypertyrosinemia type II). Helv. Paediatr. Acta 34:177, 1979.

Strife, C. F., Zuroweste, E. L., et al.: Tyrosinemia with acute intermittent porphyria: aminolevulinic acid dehydratase deficiency related to elevated aminolevulinic acid levels. J. Pediatr. 90:400, 1977.

Urea Cycle Disorders

Batshaw, M. L., and Brusilow, S. W.: Treatment of hyperammonemic coma caused by inborn errors of urea synthesis. J. Pediatr. 97:893, 1980.

Batshaw, M. L., Thomas, G. H., and Brusilow, S. W.: New approaches to the diagnosis and treatment of inborn errors of urea synthesis. Pediatrics 68:290, 1981.

Burgess, E. A., Oberholzer, V. G., et al.: Acute neonatal and benign citrullinaemia in one sibship. Arch. Dis. Child. 53:179, 1978.

Campbell, A. G. M., Rosenberg, L. E., et al.: Ornithine transcarbamylase deficiency. A cause of lethal neonatal hyperammonemia in males. N. Engl. J. Med. 288:1, 1973.

John, E. G., Bhat, R., and Vidyasagar, D.: Neonatal survival after early diagnosis and treatment of argininosuccinic aciduria. J. Pediatr. 97:867, 1980.

Mantagos, S., Tsagaraki, S., et al.: Neonatal hyperammonemia with complete absence of liver carbamyl phosphate synthetase activity. Arch. Dis. Child. 53:230, 1978.

Shih, V. E.: Congenital hyperammonemic syndromes. Clin. Perinatol. 3:3, 1979.

Hyperglycinemia

Kølvraa, S., Brandt, N. J., and Christensen, E.: Nonketotic hyperglycinemia. Clinical, biochemical and therapeutic aspects. Acta Paediatr. Scand. 68:629, 1979.

Perry, T. L., Urquhart, N., et al.: Nonketotic hyperglycinemia. Glycine accumulation due to absence of glycine cleavage in brain. N. Engl. J. Med. 292:1269, 1975.

van Wendt, L., Similä, S., et al.: Failure of strychnine treatment during the neonatal period in three Finnish children with nonketotic hyperglycinemia. Pediatrics 65:1166, 1980.

Warburton, D., Boyle, R. J., et al.: Nonketotic hyperglycinemia. Effects of therapy with strychnine. Am. J. Dis. Child. 134:273, 1980.

Histidinemia

Coulombe, J. T., Rosenmann, A., et al.: Histidinemia: Retrospective and prospective studies. Pediatr. Res. 14:521, 1980.

Levy, H. L., Shih, V. E., and Madigan, P. M.: Routine newborn screening for histidinemia. Clinical and biochemical studies. N. Engl. J. Med. 291:1214, 1974.

Popkin, J. S., Scriver, C. R., et al.: Is hereditary histidinaemia harmful? Lancet 1:721, 1974.

61

Inborn Errors of Organic Acids

By Harvey L. Levy

The term "organic acid" applies to biochemical compounds that do not fit into categories such as amino acids, carbohydrates, or lipids. They are intermediary metabolites within amino acid metabolic pathways. The disorders of organic acid metabolism are considered separately from the disorders of amino acid metabolism, however, because of two important distinctions. First, *metabolic acidosis* is a prominent feature of the organic acid disorders, whereas acidosis is rarely seen in a primary aminoacidopathy. Second, in an organic acid disorder it is an *organic acid* rather than an amino acid that is abnormal. Thus, if biochemical analyses are performed only for amino acids, as is often the case, an organic acid disorder will be overlooked.

The most frequently identified organic acid disorders in the neonate are due to defects in the metabolic pathways of the branched-chain amino acids (leucine, isoleucine, and valine). These include isovaleric acidemia, propionic acidemia, and methylmalonic acidemia. They will be specifically discussed in this chapter. Pyruvic acidemia and glutaric acidemia will also be described, since they are prominent among these disorders. A number of other organic acid disorders that can cause disease in the neonate or in early infancy, however, have also been reported. These include multiple holocarboxylase deficiency, α-methylacetoacetyl-CoA thiolase deficiency, succinyl-CoA:3 ketoacid CoA transferase deficiency, and, possibly, pyroglutamic acidemia. Thus, any infant with *metabolic acidosis* should receive an organic acid analysis of urine. This analysis should be performed by appropriate screening procedures, including gas chromatography, that can identify any known organic acid abnormality.

Isovaleric Acidemia

This autosomal recessive disorder has been termed the "sweaty foot syndrome" because of the offensive odor noted on the body and in the blood and urine of affected individuals. It is caused by a defect in the leucine metabolic pathway at the point at which isovaleryl-CoA is converted to β-methylcrotonyl-CoA. Isovaleric acid, a short-chain fatty acid, accumulates and is detectable in blood, urine, and CSF. The free isovaleric acid is presumably responsible for the unique odor reminiscent of dried sweat or rancid cheese.

Clinical Characteristics. Metabolic acidosis and associated odor are the characteristic features of this disease. The acidosis usually presents in the neonatal or early infancy periods with vomiting, lethargy, and weight loss. There are no specific abnormalities on physical examination. With general supportive therapy, these acute symptoms will disappear, and the infant will remain clinically normal until infection, a high protein intake, or some other intercurrent event precipitates another acute episode of metabolic acidosis. Thus, recurrent metabolic acidosis is the usual history, as with other organic acid disorders. Death can occur during one of these acute episodes. The surviving infant usually becomes mentally retarded unless specific therapy is initiated in infancy.

Diagnosis. The diagnosis is made on the basis of demonstrating increased isovaleric acid in blood and the presence of isovalerylglycine in urine. Other laboratory findings during acute episodes include ketonuria and leukopenia or pancytopenia. Amino acids may be normal, or there may be a mild hyperglycinemia.

Treatment. Aside from supportive therapy during acute episodes, isovaleric acidemia may be controlled with a low-leucine diet or glycine supplementation. The mental retardation can be prevented by prompt institution of this diet.

Propionic Acidemia

The prominent feature of this autosomal recessive disorder is recurrent metabolic acidosis, usually beginning in the neonatal period. The metabolic defect is near the end of the isoleucine and valine degradative pathways. As shown in Figure 61–1, both these branched-chain amino acids are degraded to propionyl-CoA which, in propionic acidemia, cannot be converted to methylmalonyl-CoA because of deficient propionyl-CoA carboxylase activity. Propionic acid accumulates in the blood, but even more striking is the markedly increased urinary excretion of metabolites such as hydroxypropionate, hydroxyisovalerate, methylcitrate, and propionyl-glycine.

Clinical and Laboratory Characteristics. The usual history is that of severe metabolic acidosis presenting in the neonate or young infant. The infant is lethargic, feeds poorly, may vomit, and fails to gain weight. Tachypnea is often a presenting sign in the neonate. Blood pH is low, sometimes near or even less than 7.0. Blood total carbon dioxide is usually less than 15. Ketonuria is present, often in large amounts. The blood ammonia level is increased. Blood amino acid analysis sometimes reveals an increased glycine concentration, but other amino acid concentrations are normal. Analysis of serum for short-chain fatty acids may disclose an increased concentration of propionic acid, but, strangely, this seems to be normal in many affected infants. The diagnosis is made on the basis of urine organic acid analysis, which reveals the aforementioned characteristic metabolites. Specific enzyme analysis of cultured skin fibroblasts will confirm the diagnosis.

Treatment. Without prompt treatment of the acute episodes, death often occurs in the neonatal period. If the infant survives but does not receive treatment, the usual sequelae are recurrent acidosis, failure to thrive, recurrent infection, and mental retardation. These chronically ill children usually die within the first few years of life.

Treatment of the acute acidotic episodes consists of supportive intravenous fluids. The infant often recovers rapidly. If the acidosis is particularly severe or prolonged, bicarbonate is added to the therapy. Chronic therapy includes a low-protein diet. The amount of protein in this diet is disputed. Some authorities believe that these infants should receive no more than 1.0 gm of protein/kg/day, whereas others recommend 1.5 to 1.7 gm/kg/day. Adequate calories and other nutrients must be provided. Supplemental biotin (5 to 10 mg/day) is recommended by some, since propionyl-CoA carboxylase is a biotin-dependent enzyme, but this is not of proven therapeutic benefit.

A male infant, one of dizygotic twins, was born to a gravida 3, para 2 mother after an uneventful full-term pregnancy. Labor and delivery were normal. Birth weight was 2820 gm. Apgar scores were 9 at 1 and 5 minutes. On the evening of the second day of life, his very observant mother noted that he was irritable, that he fed poorly from the breast, and that his breathing was rapid. By the third day of life, he had marked tachypnea and was increasingly lethargic. Blood gases at this time revealed pH 7.25 and TCO_2 10. Cultures of blood and CSF were negative. His twin brother remained normal. Family history at this time revealed that a sibling born 6 years before died at 13 days of age after a neonatal course that was characterized by lethargy, tachypnea, poor feeding, and dehydration. There was no specific diagnosis in this sibling, and no metabolic studies were performed.

Physical examination on the third day revealed a tachypneic neonate with poor skin turgor and mild hepatomegaly. Urine was strongly positive for ketones. Complete blood count revealed leukopenia with a white blood count of only 5500. Blood ammonia was 394 μg/dl (normal 40 to 75 μg/dl). All other laboratory data were normal, including serum electrolytes, serum creatinine, liver function indicators, and blood urea nitrogen.

Supportive therapy with intravenous fluids was begun. Within 12 hours, the patient's blood gases became normal, and he was markedly improved with increasing activity and subsiding tachypnea. Specific metabolic studies were initiated at this time. Blood amino acid analysis disclosed slight hyperglycinemia but otherwise normal findings. Thus, maple syrup urine disease was eliminated. Urine organic acid analysis revealed no methylmalonic acid (ruling out methylmalonic acidemia) and no elevation of lactic acid (ruling out pyruvic acidemia). A more elaborate urine organic acid analysis (by gas chromatography) was pending. There was no body odor, so isovaleric acidemia was unlikely. The working diagnosis was propionic acidemia.

Intravenous therapy was maintained, and the infant continued to improve. On the sixth day of life, he began to accept clear fluids orally. Blood ammonia became normal by the ninth day, and 1.0 gm/kg/day protein feedings were begun. He tolerated these well, and by discharge at 18 days of age he was tolerating 2.0 gm of protein/kg/day without difficulty. The diagnosis of

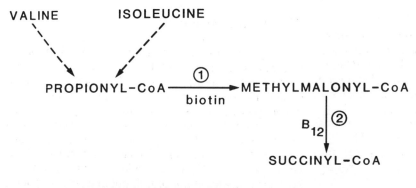

Figure 61–1. Metabolism of propionic acid and methylmalonic acid. This organic acid pathway begins with propionyl-CoA, which derives from the amino acids valine and isoleucine. Normally, propionyl-CoA is carboxylated to methylmalonyl-CoA. In propionic acidemia, propionyl-CoA carboxylase activity is reduced, and propionic acid and its metabolites accumulate. Under normal conditions, methylmalonyl-CoA is converted to succinyl-CoA. In methylmalonic acidemia, however, methylmalonyl-CoA mutase activity is deficient, and methylmalonic acid and its metabolites accumulate.

VALINE   ISOLEUCINE

PROPIONYL-CoA → METHYLMALONYL-CoA
(1) biotin

B_{12} (2)

SUCCINYL-CoA

(1) PROPIONYL-CoA CARBOXYLASE
(2) METHYLMALONYL-CoA MUTASE

propionic acidemia was substantiated by the characteristic urinary findings of increased hydroxypropionate, hydroxyisovalerate, methylcitrate, and propionylglycine as determined by gas chromatographic analysis.

Chronic treatment consists of a low-protein diet and oral biotin supplementation of 10 mg daily. For the first six months of life, the infant's daily protein intake was 1.5 to 2.0 gm/kg. His growth was at the third percentile, and his development was about 1 month delayed. He had numerous episodes of metabolic acidosis, however, usually associated with an acute febrile respiratory illness. Consequently, his daily protein intake was reduced to 1.0 gm/kg. Until the age of 11 months (his present age) he has continued to progress, and he has had fewer episodes of acidosis.

Methylmalonic Acidemia

This autosomal recessive organic acid disorder presents either as severe metabolic acidosis in the neonate or as metabolic acidosis in the young infant who has previously been well. The enzymatic defect is of methylmalonyl-CoA mutase, a B_{12}-dependent enzyme that is responsible for the conversion of methylmalonyl-CoA to succinyl-CoA (Fig. 61–1). The metabolic block results in a marked accumulation of methylmalonic acid in blood, urine, and CSF.

Clinical and Laboratory Characteristics. The most striking presentation is that in the neonate. This usually is a fulminant and rapidly lethal course. The neonate is noted to be lethargic and to feed poorly by the second day of life. There may be hepatomegaly but no other physical findings. Studies reveal severe metabolic acidosis. The blood ammonia level may be markedly increased. There are numerous striking elevations in the blood amino acids. Analysis of urine for organic acids discloses a huge concentration of methylmalonic acid. Methylmalonic acid will also be demonstrable in serum. Urinary organic acid metabolites similar to those seen in propionic acidemia may also be present, but the quantities are much less in methylmalonic acidemia.

In the delayed presentation, the previously well 2- or 3-month-old infant becomes lethargic, vomits, and refuses to feed. This usually coincides with an increase in the amount of dietary protein. Metabolic acidosis, hyperammonemia, and, often, hyperglycinemia are present. Urine and serum analysis for organic acids reveals increased methylmalonic acid as the predominant finding. The diagnosis may be confirmed by the subsequent assay of methylmalonyl-CoA mutase in cultured skin fibroblasts.

Treatment. The fulminant neonatal presentation or the acute phase of the delayed presentation requires aggressive therapeutic measures. Exchange transfusion or peritoneal dialysis may be lifesaving. Hemodialysis may be the most effective measure. Supportive therapy through intravenous fluid with adequate calories must be maintained. Vitamin B_{12} (cyanocobalamin or hydroxocobalamin) 1 mg intramuscularly should be administered.

Chronic therapy consists of a low-protein diet. About 50 per cent of affected infants who have the delayed presentation respond to the administration of B_{12} with marked reduction in the levels of blood and urine methylmalonic acid. These B_{12}-responsive patients have a defect in the synthesis of deoxyadenosylcobalamin (deoxyadenosyl-B_{12}), the specific B_{12} cofactor for methylmalonyl-CoA mutase, rather than a defect in the mutase per se. They should receive weekly or biweekly injections of B_{12} and continue on a modified low-protein diet. Patients who do not respond to B_{12} have a defect in the mutase and must be on a standard low-protein diet.

Other Causes. Methylmalonic acid may be present in urine (and blood) in infants with a B_{12} metabolic defect (see Sulfur Amino Acid Abnormalities, Chapter 60). These infants also have amino acid abnormalities such as homocystinuria(emia), cystathioninuria(emia), and hypomethioninemia. Methylmalonic acid may also appear in the urine as a transient finding in normal breast-fed infants. Finally, there appears to be a benign form of mutase deficiency in which the infant has persistent but mild methylmalonic acidemia. These healthy infants have generally been identified by routine newborn urine screening. No treatment is indicated for this condition.

Pyruvic Acidemia

Pyruvate is an intermediary metabolite in the degradation of glucose. Products of pyruvate oxidation enter the citric acid cycle. Several inherited enzyme deficiencies in pyruvate oxidation have been described. The defects that cause disease in the neonate are in the pyruvate dehydrogenase complex.

These infants develop tachypnea, lethargy, and hypotonia during the first few days of life. Laboratory data reveal metabolic acidosis and increased blood lactate and pyruvate. Urine is positive for ketones and contains large amounts of lactate and β-hydroxybutyrate on organic acid analysis. Blood amino acid analysis reveals an increased concentration of alanine but is otherwise normal. The diagnosis is confirmed by enzyme studies of cultured skin fibroblasts or of postmortem tissue.

Therapy consists of intravenous infusion with maintenance fluids, bicarbonate, and glucose. These infants have usually died in early infancy or have suffered neurologic damage.

Glutaric Aciduria

Glutaric acid is an intermediate in the metabolism of the amino acids lysine, hydroxylysine, and tryptophan. Two inherited disorders of glutaric acid degradation have been described. Glutaric aciduria type

I seems to result from a deficiency in glutaryl-CoA dehydrogenase. This disorder is associated with a progressive neurologic deterioration during infancy, but this is not noticeable until about 3 months of age.

Glutaric aciduria type II, however, causes metabolic acidosis with lethargy and hypotonia in the newborn. Routine laboratory studies may reveal hypoglycemia. Amino acids are usually normal, but organic acid analysis of urine reveals markedly increased concentrations of glutaric acid and lactic acid as well as moderate increases in several other organic acids. The precise metabolic defect in this disease is unknown. Treatment consists of intravenous fluids with glucose during the acute phase. A low-protein diet has been given for long-term treatment after the neonatal period, but these infants nevertheless manifest poor growth and development and usually die during infancy.

REFERENCES

Isovaleric Acidemia

Cohn, R. M., Yudkoff, M., et al.: Isovaleric acidemia: use of glycine therapy in neonates. N. Engl. J. Med. 299:996, 1978.
Levy, H. L., Erickson, A. M., et al.: Isovaleric acidemia: results of family study and dietary treatment. Pediatrics 52:83, 1973.

Propionic Acidemia

Robert, M. F., Schultz, D. J., et al.: Treatment of a neonate with propionic acidaemia and severe hyperammonemia by peritoneal dialysis. Arch. Dis. Child. 54:962, 1979.
Wolf, B.: Reassessment of biotin-responsiveness in "unresponsive" propionyl CoA carboxylase deficiency. J. Pediatr. 97:964, 1980.

Methylmalonic Acidemia

Packman, S., Mahoney, M. J., et al.: Severe hyperammonemia in a newborn infant with methylmalonyl-CoA mutase deficiency. J. Pediatr. 92:769, 1978.
Shapiro, L. J., Bocian, M. E., et al.: Methylmalonyl-CoA mutase deficiency associated with severe neonatal hyperammonemia: activity of urea cycle enzymes. J. Pediatr. 93:986, 1978.

Pyruvic Acidemia

Robinson, B. H., Taylor, J., and Sherwood, W. G.: The genetic heterogeneity of lactic acidosis: occurrence of recognizable inborn errors of metabolism in a pediatric population with lactic Pediatr. 96:1020, 1980.
Strömme, J. H. Borud, O., and Moe, P. J.: Fatal lactic acidosis in a newborn attributable to a congenital defect of pyruvate dehydrogenase. Pediatr. Res, 10:60, 1976.

Glutaric Aciduria

Goodman, S. I., McCabe, E. R. B., et al.: Multiple acyl-CoA dehydrogenase deficiency (glutaric aciduria type II) with transient hypersarcosinemia and sarcosinuria; possible inherited deficiency of an electron transfer flavoprotein. Pediatr. Res. 14:12, 1980.
Sweetman, L., Nyhan, W. L., et al.: Glutaric aciduria type II. J. Pediatr. 96:1020, 1980.

62

Inborn Errors of Lipid Metabolism

By Harvey L. Levy

This chapter includes two general areas of aberrant lipid metabolism. The better known of these is the category of inherited hyperlipidemia, which includes conditions that are associated with increased blood cholesterol and triglyceride concentrations. A great deal of attention has been given to the possible role of these conditions in the production of atherosclerosis leading to coronary artery disease and strokes.

The second of these categories is that of the lysosomal storage diseases. This category includes those inborn errors of metabolism in which there is an abnormal accumulation of lipid in certain cells of the body. Many of these disorders cause severe and progressive neurologic disease, but these manifestations usually do not appear until late infancy or childhood.

Familial Hyperlipidemias

At least six distinct disorders are recognized within this group. These are classified as types I through VI. Each type is characterized by a particular pattern of lipoprotein abnormality. Inheritance is either autosomal dominant or autosomal recessive. All except type II present in childhood or adult years. Although type II rarely presents in the neonatal period, an awareness of this disorder is important, since in some instances it may be desirable to begin dietary therapy in early infancy so that later clinical complications might be prevented. Only type II will be described in this discussion.

Type II hyperlipidemia, known as familial hypercholesterolemia, is the best-known and most frequent hyperlipidemia. The inheritance is autosomal dominant. In the homozygous state it is characterized by extremely high concentrations of cholesterol and low-density lipoprotein (LDL) in plasma and a moderately increased plasma triglyceride concentration. Xanthomas (yellowish fatty modules) are present on the eyelids or over the elbows, extensor tendons of the hands, and the Achilles tendon. These xanthomas may be present at birth. Ischemic heart disease and other complications of severe atherosclerosis develop in childhood or during adolescence.

Type II hyperlipidemia is rare in the homozygous state, but in the heterozygous (carrier) state it may have a frequency as high as 1 per cent of the population. These individuals will have increased plasma cholesterol, triglyceride, and LDL. The degree of increase, however, will be far less than that in the homozygous state. These individuals tend to develop premature atherosclerosis with ischemic heart disease and other complications. These clinical problems usually appear in the middle adult years.

The biochemical defect in type II hyperlipidemia appears to be a deficiency of cellular LDL receptor activity. Thus, LDL cannot enter peripheral cells in the normal manner and is thereby increased in the circulation. This increased LDL with its cholesterol is picked up by reticuloendothelial cells, and in this manner forms the basis for atheromas. The usual therapy is a low-cholesterol diet so that the amount of body cholesterol can be reduced. Other therapeutic measures are sometimes used, but their effectiveness has not been proved.

Lysosomal Storage Diseases

In these inherited disorders, the defective enzymes are located in the lysosomes of the cell, in contrast to other inborn errors of metabolism in which the enzyme in question is in the mitochondria or cytosol of the cell.

There are several categories of these disorders. These categories include (1) the lipidoses, in which lipid material accumulates in cells, often neurons, (2) the mucopolysaccharidoses, in which the cellular accumulation is a mucopolysaccharide, (3) generalized glycogen storage disease (Pompe's disease), and (4) other diseases of complex carbohydrate metabolism (fucosidosis, mannosidosis, aspartylglucosaminuria, and Wolman's disease).

Most of the lysosomal storage diseases present later than the neonatal period. However, several may produce neonatal findings, which will be discussed. In addition, Tay-Sachs disease (GM$_2$ gangliosidosis) will be described, since it is a prominent lipidosis.

TAY-SACHS DISEASE

This is the best known of the lipidoses. It is transmitted as an autosomal recessive trait and is most frequent among Ashkenazi Jews, although it may also occur in other ethnic groups. GM$_2$ ganglioside accumulates in neurons because of a deficiency in hexosaminidase-A activity. This results in severe and progressive mental and motor deterioration, which begins between 3 and 6 months of age. Death is inevitable, usually occurring by 3 years of age, following a tragic clinical course that includes deafness, blindness, convulsions, and spasticity. There is no treatment for this disease. Antenatal diagnosis is available (see Prenatal Genetic Diagnosis, Part I).

GM$_1$ GANGLIOSIDOSIS (TYPE 1)

This is one of the few lipidoses that presents in the neonate. In this autosomal recessive disease, GM$_1$ ganglioside accumulates in neurons. There are foam cells throughout the reticuloendothelial system and in other visceral organs such as the kidney. The enzyme defect is in β-galactosidase activity. Shortly after birth, the infant becomes lethargic, sucks poorly, and loses weight. He is noted to have dysmorphic facial features and hepatosplenomegaly. Growth and development are severely limited, and severe neurologic impairment develops during the first year of life. The symptoms are progressive, and death occurs by 2 years of age.

GAUCHER'S DISEASE (TYPE 2)

Gaucher's disease of the infantile, or type 2, form usually presents at 3 to 4 months of age with hepatosplenomegaly and failure to thrive. Occasionally, the affected infant is abnormal at birth, with lethargy and poor feeding as well as hepatosplenomegaly. Glucocerebroside accumulates in the brain and other organs owing to a deficiency of glucocerebrosidase activity. The infants show progressive deterioration and usually die by 1 or 2 years of age. There is no treatment. Enzyme replacement has been attempted but so far this has not proved clinically beneficial.

NIEMANN-PICK (TYPE A)

In the infantile, or Type A, form of Niemann-Pick disease, the infant may have hepatomegaly within the first days of life. Feeding difficulties ensue, and severe progressive neurologic involvement with hepatosplenomegaly develops during the next few months with death by 3 years of age. The accumulating lipid is sphingomyelin, which is found in increased quantities in the brain and viscera of patients. Sphingomyelinase appears to be the defective enzyme. The disease is inherited as an autosomal recessive trait and is most frequent among Ashkenazi Jews. There is no specific treatment.

WOLMAN'S DISEASE

This disease is characterized by vomiting, failure to thrive, and hepatosplenomegaly during the first week or two of life. An additional and striking finding is calcification of the adrenal glands. Triglycerides and cholesterol ester are the predominant lipids that accumulate in this disease. These accumulations are noted in the liver and spleen; plasma cholesterol and triglyceride levels are normal. The proposed enzyme defect in this autosomal recessive disease is in acid lipase. The disease is progressive, with death usually occurring by 3 to 6 months of age. There is no specific therapy.

I-CELL DISEASE

This autosomal recessive disease, often referred to as mucolipidosis II, is one of the few lipidoses that is expressed at birth. These infants have somewhat low birth weight, coarse facies, and orthopedic abnormalities such as clubfeet, congenital hip dislocation, thoracic deformities, and kyphosis. Affected males have congenital inguinal hernias. Cultured skin fibroblasts from these patients contain very large lysosomes that are filled with mucopolysaccharide material. Levels of lysosomal hydrolases are increased in body fluids and decreased in cultured fibroblasts, suggesting that in this disease the hydrolases are structurally deficient and therefore unable to remain in or re-enter cells. The diagnosis of I-cell disease is made on the basis of the characteristic clinical phenotype and the measurement of increased hydrolase activities in serum and urine. There is no specific treatment, and most of the children die by the age of 6 years.

REFERENCES

Breslow, J. L.: Pediatric aspects of hyperlipidemia. Pediatrics 62:510, 1978.

Cipolloni, C., Boldrini, A., et al.: Neonatal mucolipidosis II (I-cell disease): clinical, radiological and biochemical studies in a case. Helv. Paediatr. Acta 35:85, 1980.

Crocker, A. C.: Inborn errors of lipid metabolism: early identification. Clin. Perinatol. 3:99, 1976.

Goldstein, J. L., and Brown, M. S.: The LDL receptor locus and the genetics of familial hypercholesterolemia. Ann. Rev. Genet. 13:259, 1979.

Kolodny, E. H.: Current concepts in genetics. Lysosomal storage diseases. N. Engl. J. Med. 294:1217, 1976.

Spritz, R. A., Doughty, R. A., et al.: Neonatal presentation of I-cell disease. J. Pediatr. 93:954, 1978.

63

Miscellaneous Inborn Errors of Metabolism

By Harvey L. Levy

Menkes' Steely-Hair Disease

Clinical Characteristics. This disease, also referred to as kinky-hair syndrome, is inherited as an X-linked recessive. Affected males often express the disease at birth. Delivery may be premature at 34 to 36 weeks gestation with appropriate birth weight. The newborn infant may be lethargic and feed poorly. Temperature instability as manifested by hypothermia may also be present in the neonate. These problems continue, and by the age of 2 months the infant has poor weight gain and is flaccid. By the age of 4 to 5 months, he has developmental delay, marked temperature instability, and, often, convulsions. At this time or even before, his hair becomes depigmented and sparse. The hair strands break easily, leaving short stubbles that feel like "steely" hair. Microscopic examination of the hair strand reveals changes of pili torti. The clinical course is one of progressive neurologic deterioration, with death usually occurring during the first year of life.

Etiology. Menkes' disease appears to be a disorder of copper metabolism or transport. Levels of copper in serum and CSF are low. Serum ceruloplasmin levels are also low. Tissue copper, however, varies between low levels in liver and brain to very high levels in kidney and intestinal mucosa. Copper is also increased in cultured skin fibroblasts. Orally administered copper is poorly absorbed, but intravenously or intramuscularly administered copper is handled normally. The mechanism for this disease may be the trapping of copper in certain tissues, particularly intestinal mucosa and kidney, perhaps by metallothionein, a copper-binding protein.

Diagnosis and Treatment. The diagnosis of Menkes' disease is based on the characteristic clinical phenotype and the presence of reduced levels of copper and ceruloplasmin in serum. Liver biopsy with the demonstration of reduced copper concentration provides further evidence of this disease as does the demonstration of increased copper in cultured skin fibroblasts. Treatment with parenterally administered copper raises the serum copper and ceruloplasmin concentrations to normal levels but has neither improved the clinical manifestations nor stemmed the progression of the disease.

Neonatal Hypophosphatasia

This disorder appears to be inherited as an autosomal recessive trait. It occurs as a severe neonatal form, a less severe childhood form, or a relatively mild adult form. The differentiation is largely based on the age of onset of the bone lesions and the clinical course of the disease.

Diagnosis. Neonatal hypophosphatasia may present at birth with respiratory distress and gross skeletal deformities. The affected infant can develop generalized seizures during the first 2 to 4 days of life. He is usually hypotonic and may vomit his feedings. Roentgenograms reveal poorly mineralized bones with rachitic changes at the ends of the long bones. The skull is poorly ossified, and the sutures are widened.

Laboratory data include a markedly reduced serum alkaline phosphatase level. There is also an increased serum calcium level, which presumably results from hyperparathyroidism. In the two cases in which serum parathyroid hormone levels were measured, they were found to be elevated. The urine contains phosphoethanolamine.

The diagnosis is made on the basis of the bone abnormalities (particularly the rachitic changes) that are demonstrated radiographically, the reduced serum alkaline phosphatase level, and the presence of urinary phosphoethanolamine as determined by amino acid analysis.

Treatment and Prognosis. There is no effective therapy for this disease. A low-calcium diet lowers the hypercalcemia but does not result in clinical improvement. Therapy with steroids and vitamin K, designed to increase bone mineralization, has also been ineffective. Most infants with the neonatal form of hypophosphatasia have failed to gain weight, and a number have developed increased intracranial pressure, sometimes associated with craniostenosis. Death due to respiratory insufficiency or recurrent infections usually occurs during the first year of life. Those who survive become dwarfed and grotesquely deformed.

Nephrogenic Diabetes Insipidus

This is an inherited defect in which there is lack of response to antidiuretic hormone (ADH) by the renal tubule. There is excessive loss of water from the kidneys because the renal tubules cannot reabsorb water. Chemical abnormalities in the blood are secondary to this water loss.

Etiology. This is an X-linked genetic disease. Males are hemizygotes and are more frequently and usually much more severely affected than females. The few females who have had clinical evidence of nephrogenic diabetes insipidus are presumably heterozygotes who by Lyon randomization have inherited an unusually large number of cells with the defect.

Diagnosis. Affected infants usually come to attention within the first few months of life. Failure to thrive with unexplained fever are the most frequent clinical signs at presentation. Diarrhea or constipation may also be present. Further history reveals that there is polyuria and that the infant may also be almost continuously thirsty (polydipsia). Recurrent urinary tract infection has been noted in some infants. On examination, the infant is dehydrated and might show signs of developmental delay. In older children, mild mental retardation is frequent, and hydronephrosis as well as hydroureters may be present.

The urine output is voluminous, and the urine specific gravity is usually below 1.010. Except when infection is present, the urine is otherwise normal. There is no glycosuria or proteinuria, and urine amino acids are normal. Serum sodium, chloride, and creatinine and blood urea nitrogen levels are elevated. Plasma ADH levels are normal or elevated. Injections of vasopressin fail to increase the urine specific gravity or decrease urine output.

Treatment. There is no specific therapy. Adequate hydration must be maintained. In acute episodes of dehydration, this may require parenteral therapy that consists of a minimum of glucose (so as not to promote solute diuresis) and a low sodium-chloride content.

Diuretics such as the chlorothiazides may reduce urine flow and increase urine concentration when given chronically to patients with nephrogenic diabetes insipidus. This effect is enhanced when the patient is maintained on a low-sodium diet.

Neonatal Myasthenia Gravis

Approximately 12 per cent of the offspring of women with myasthenia gravis will have transient neonatal myasthenia gravis.

Etiology.   Neonatal myasthenia gravis is caused by the passive transfer of antiacetylcholine receptor antibody across the placenta. The antibody blocks the acetylcholine receptor at the neuromuscular junction, resulting in a lack of response by the muscle to the nerve impulse. For reasons unknown, the fetus generally appears to be protected from the effects of this blocking action, since fetal movements and other characteristics of pregnancy are normal in most cases. At birth or shortly after birth, however, clinical effects become apparent.

Diagnosis.   The infant is usually normal at delivery with good Apgar scores. Within hours of birth, however, weakness is noted. This is most commonly manifested by difficulty in feeding. The infant is hungry and begins to suck vigorously, but sucking weakens so rapidly that adequate nourishment is impossible. Generalized weakness and hypotonia are present, sometimes producing respiratory difficulty. Many infants have a weak cry and flat facial expression. Features of permanent myasthenia gravis, such as oculomotor paresis and ptosis, are usually absent.

The most important feature of family history is maternal myasthenia gravis. An intramuscular or subcutaneous injection of 0.1 mg of edrophonium chloride will confirm the diagnosis. There is a clear improvement in suck and muscle strength within 10 to 15 minutes of this injection. Neostigmine methylsulfate, 0.15 mg intramuscularly, may also be used as a therapeutic test, often with atropine sulfate, 0.03 mg intramuscularly. However, edrophonium is preferred, since neostigmine may give a false-negative response.

Treatment and Prognosis.   In 20 per cent of cases, the symptoms are mild and drug therapy is unnecessary. Adequate nutrition can be maintained with frequent small feedings. In severely affected infants, respirations and feeding should be carefully supported. Neostigmine methylsulfate, 0.1 mg intramuscularly, should be initially administered 20 minutes prior to feeding. More exact dosages should be determined by the response in terms of respirations and feeding. If oral doses are used when adequate swallowing has been established, they should be 10 times the intramuscular doses. The need for medication may persist for several weeks. Periodic attempts to withdraw the drug should be made.

The outlook for the newborn with myasthenia gravis is good, provided one makes the diagnosis promptly and treats properly. The symptoms may persist for as short a time as a few hours or for as long as 7 weeks. Once muscle strength has returned, it never again is lost.

Cystic Fibrosis

Cystic fibrosis is an inherited disorder that affects many different organs of the body, most notably the lungs and the pancreas. It is probably an inborn error of metabolism, although the precise metabolic system(s) involved has yet to be defined.

Incidence.   The disease is inherited in an autosomal recessive manner. In the United States, it is far more common among whites than among blacks, having an incidence of approximately 1 per 1600 in whites to 1 per 30,000 in blacks. In general, it has a similar frequency among most white Europeans. It is very rare in Orientals. The risk of producing a child with cystic fibrosis in the Caucasian population varies with the family history (Table 63–1).

Pathophysiology.   The most prominent biochemical abnormality found is increased concentrations of sodium and chloride in sweat. The viscosity of mucus secreted by many exocrine glands is markedly increased. This leads to inspissated mucus in many organs, including the trachea and bronchial tree, the pancreas, the intestinal tract, the bile ductules and ducts of the liver, and the testis. The viscid mucus in the tracheobronchial system leads to chronic pulmonary infection. In other organs, the outflow tracts

Table 63–1.   Risks of Producing a Child with Cystic Fibrosis (CF)*

One Parent	Other Parent	Risk of Cystic Fibrosis in Each Pregnancy
With no CF history	With no CF history	1:1600
With no CF history	With 1st cousin having CF	1:320
With no CF history	With aunt or uncle having CF	1:240
With no CF history	With sib having CF	1:120
With no CF history	With CF child by previous marriage	1:80
With no CF history	With parent having CF	1:80
With no CF history	Has CF	1:40
With sib having CF	With sib having CF	1:9
With CF child	With CF child	1:4

* Based on prevalence of cystic fibrosis of 1:1600 in the Caucasian population, its mode of inheritance being autosomal recessive with complete penetrance. (From Bowman, B.H., and Mangos, J.A.: N. Engl. J. Med. *294*:937, 1976. Reprinted by permission of the New England Journal of Medicine.)

become chronically obstructed and the secretions collect within the organ, causing tissue damage. In the pancreas, this results in a reduction in the flow of digestive enzymes to the intestine. In the liver, biliary cirrhosis may eventually occur.

The basic defect in cystic fibrosis is unknown. Studies during the past decade have suggested abnormalities in glycoproteins, glycosaminoglycans, polyamines, RNA methylation, cell membranes, and lysosomal enzymes. There has been a focus on the ability of serum or the media of cultured skin fibroblasts from patients with cystic fibrosis to inhibit ciliary activity in oyster gills. This has been designated the "ciliotoxic factor." Fibroblasts from patients with cystic fibrosis are also said to manifest resistance to ouabain toxicity and to accumulate less sodium in the presence of ouabain than normal cells. Attempts to confirm all these findings, however, have produced conflicting results. Thus, these findings may be secondary to the basic process.

Clinical Manifestations.
Most infants with cystic fibrosis appear to be normal during the neonatal period. However, an occasional affected infant will have meconium ileus. When this is present, the diagnosis of cystic fibrosis is almost certain. The meconium plug syndrome has also been described in neonates with cystic fibrosis. Occasionally, excessive sweating is evident in the neonate. The sweat will contain increased electrolyte quantities. This sweat may be noted to have a "salty taste" by the mother when she kisses the infant. Respiratory infections may also present during the first days of life, with the most consistent feature being hyperinflation of the chest. Failure to gain weight and hypoproteinemia may become evident in the weeks after birth. Bulky and fatty stools, usually the first signs of the deficiency of pancreatic enzymes, may be noted during the early months of life. Prolonged obstructive jaundice may also be an early manifestation of the disease.

Diagnosis.
The collection of sweat by iontophoresis for analysis of sodium and chloride, or measurement of electrical conductivity, which depends on the concentrations of these ions, is the definitive diagnostic test. It may be difficult to collect a sufficient amount of sweat from infants in the first weeks of life for these chemical assays, although in expert hands this is usually possible. If an infant has an affected sibling or any signs or symptoms suggesting cystic fibrosis, sweat analysis is essential before making or excluding the diagnosis.

Treatment.
No consensus exists on how vigorous one should be in treating the asymptomatic infant with cystic fibrosis. Most would agree on a normal diet and the addition of water-soluble vitamins. The prompt identification and treatment of pulmonary infections is imperative and probably preferable to chemoprophylaxis. Some hold that the initial staphylococcal pneumonia is so harmful that antibiotics should be given daily in an attempt to prevent it.

Pancreatic supplements are recommended as tolerated.

Prognosis.
Each year the prognosis for this disease improves, in part because of wider recognition and detection of milder cases, and in part, no doubt, in relation to therapy. Many afflicted individuals are now adults, and some of the females are parents. Sterility in the males is very common. The severity of the disease varies greatly among siblings; hence, prognostication about the life span of an affected infant is unwise.

REFERENCES

Antonowicz, I., Ishida, S., and Shwachman, H.: Studies in meconium: disaccharidase activities in meconium from cystic fibrosis patients and controls. Pediatrics 56:782, 1975.

Barlow, C. F.: Neonatal myasthenia gravis. Am. J. Dis. Child. 135:209, 1981.

Blumenthal, I., and Fielding, D. W.: Hypoproteinaemia, oedema, and anaemia: an unusual presentation of cystic fibrosis in dizygotic twins. Arch. Dis. Child. 55:812, 1980.

Bowman, B. H., and Mangos, J. A.: Current concepts in genetics: cystic fibrosis. N. Engl. J. Med. 294:937, 1976.

Breslow, J. L., McPherson, J., and Epstein, J.: Distinguishing homozygous and heterozygous cystic fibrosis fibroblasts from normal cells by differences in sodium transport. N. Engl. J. Med. 304:1, 1981.

Danks, D. M., Campbell, P. E., et al.: Menkes's kinky hair syndrome. An inherited defect in copper absorption with widespread effects. Pediatrics 50:188, 1972.

Davis, P. B., and Di Sant'Agnese, P. A.: A review. Cystic fibrosis at forty—quo vadis? Pediatr. Res. 14:83, 1980.

Di Sant'Agnese, P. A., and Davis, P. B.: Research in cystic fibrosis. N. Engl. J. Med. 295:481, 534, 597, 1976.

Donaldson, J. O., Penn, A. S., et al.: Antiacetylcholine receptor antibody in neonatal myasthenia gravis. Am. J. Dis. Child. 135:222, 1981.

Drachman, D. B.: Myasthenia gravis. N. Engl. J. Med. 298:136, 186, 1978.

Elias, S. B., Butler, I., et al.: Neonatal myasthenia gravis in the infant of a myasthenic mother in remission. Ann. Neurol. 6:72, 1979.

Fenichel, G. M.: Clinical syndromes of myasthenia in infancy and childhood. Arch. Neurol. 35:97, 1978.

Hen, J., Jr., Dolan, T. F., Jr., and Touloukian, R. J.: Meconium plug syndrome associated with cystic fibrosis and Hirschsprung's disease. Pediatrics 66:466, 1980.

Holmes, L. B., Driscoll, S. G., et al.: Contractures in a newborn infant of a mother with myasthenia gravis. J. Pediatr. 96:1067, 1980.

Knox, G. E., Palmer, M. D., and Huddleston, J. F.: Fetal cystic fibrosis presenting as dystocia due to midgut volvulus with lethal perforation. Am. J. Obstet. Gynecol. 131:698, 1978.

Labadie, G. U., Hirschhorn, K., et al.: Increased copper metallothionein in Menkes cultured skin fibroblasts. Pediatr. Res. 15:257, 1981.

Lott, I. T., DiPaolo, R., et al.: Abnormal copper metabolism in Menke's steely-hair syndrome. Pediatr. Res. 13:845, 1979.

Maesaka, H., Niitsu, N., et al.: Neonatal hypophosphatasia with elevated serum parathyroid hormone. Eur. J. Pediatr. 125:71, 1977.

Maldonado, P., Pino, S., et al.: Diabetes insípida nefrogénica: presentación de tres casos. Breve revisión del tema. Rev. Child. Pediatr. 51:61, 1980.

McPartlin, J. F., Dickson, J. A. S., and Swain, V. A. J.: Meconium ileus—immediate and long term survival. Arch. Dis. Child. 47:252, 1972.

Nooijen, J. L., De Groot, C. J., et al.: Trace element studies in three patients and a fetus with Menkes' disease. Effect of copper therapy. Pediatr. Res. 15:284, 1981.

Oppenheimer, E. H., and Esterly, J. R.: Hepatic changes in young infants with cystic fibrosis: possible relation to focal biliary cirrhosis. J. Pediatr. 86:683, 1975.

Rao, G. J. S., and Nadler, J. L.: Arginine esterase in cystic fibrosis of the pancreas. Pediatr. Res. 8:684, 1974.

Rosenstein, B. J.: Cystic fibrosis presenting with the meconium plug syndrome. Am. J. Dis. Child. 132:167, 1978.

Schreiner, R. L., Skafish, P. R., et al.: Congenital nephrogenic diabetes insipidus in a baby girl. Arch. Dis. Child. 53:906, 1978.

Shapiro, B. L., Smith, Q. T., and Warwick, W. J.: Serum glutathione reductase and cystic fibrosis. Pediatr. Res. 9:885, 1975.

Ten Bensel, R. W., and Peters, E. R.: Progressive hydronephrosis, hydroureter, and dilatation of the bladder in siblings with congenital diabetes insipidus. J. Pediatr. 77:439, 1970.

Wolfish, N. M., and Heick, H.: Hyperparathyroidism and infantile hypophosphatasia: effect of prednisone and vitamin K therapy. J. Pediatr. 95:1079, 1979.

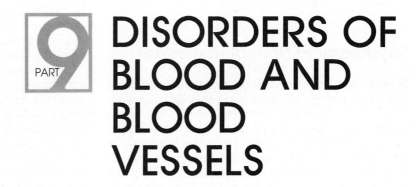

DISORDERS OF BLOOD AND BLOOD VESSELS

64

Bleeding Disorders in the Newborn Infant

By Bertil E. Glader

Physiology of Normal Hemostasis

Normal hemostasis is a complicated process involving vascular integrity, platelets, and coagulation proteins (Fig. 64–1). Bleeding disorders can be due to abnormalities in any one of these parameters. Hemorrhage caused by vascular problems (anatomic or physiologic) may be responsible for some of the serious bleeding episodes (pulmonary and CNS) seen in premature infants. Unfortunately, the pathophysiology of vascular-related bleeding is poorly understood. The major defects discussed in this chapter are directly related to abnormalities in platelets and coagulation proteins.

Platelets are activated following exposure to subendothelial collagen of the severed blood vessel. In the presence of collagen, platelets release several hemostatic factors including serotonin, adenosine diphosphate (ADP), and platelet membrane lipid (platelet factor 3). Serotonin enhances vasoconstriction. Platelet factor 3 is utilized in the clotting scheme (see subsequently). Released ADP causes platelets to aggregate reversibly into clumps, thus forming the primary, or loose, hemostatic plug. In conditions associated with thrombocytopenia or abnormal platelet function (inability to release cellular components),

formation of the primary hemostatic plug will be defective. The production of a firm, definitive hemostatic plug depends on normal plasma coagulation in addition to platelets and vasoconstriction. This process requires the sequential activation of a series of clotting proteins, the end result of which is the formation of a fibrin clot. As seen in Fig. 64–1, there are two different pathways for initiating coagulation. The "intrinsic pathway" is stimulated when factor XII reacts with subendothelial collagen. Following this, sequential interaction with other factors (XI, IX, VIII, and platelet factor 3) results in the activation of factor X. The "extrinsic" pathway is stimulated when injured tissues release a tissue thromboplastin that reacts with factor VII to activate factor X. Thus the intrinsic and extrinsic pathways activate factor X via different reactions, but beyond this step the clotting pathways are identical. Activated factor X, factor V, and platelet factor 3 together convert prothrombin (factor II) into thrombin. Thrombin is a proteolytic enzyme that converts fibrinogen (factor I) into a loose fibrin clot. Factor XIII (fibrin stabilizing factor) then converts the friable clot into tight fibrin polymers. The definitive hemostatic plug consists of irreversible platelet aggregates and tight fibrin polymers. Irreversible platelet clumps are formed when thrombin reacts with reversible platelet aggregates. This brief summary indicates how the vasculature, platelets, and coagulation proteins are separately and interdependently involved in normal hemostasis.

A group of physiologic clot-limiting controls react in parallel with the coagulation process. These regulating reactions are very important because plasma contains sufficient coagulant potential to convert the entire blood volume into one large thrombus once coagulation is activated. Most of these limiting controls are poorly characterized.

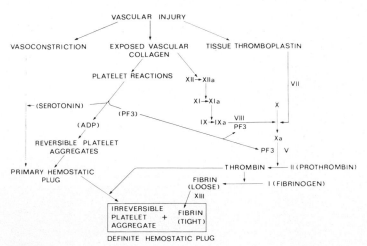

Figure 64–1. Physiology of normal hemostasis.

Table 64–1. Blood Clotting Factors

Number	Synonyms
I	Fibrinogen
II	Prothrombin
III	Thromboplastin
IV	Calcium
V	Proaccelerin (labile factor)
VI	Activated factor V (term not used)
VII	Proconvertin (stable factor)
VIII	Antihemophiliac factor (AHF)
IX	Plasma thromboplastin component (PTC) Christmas factor
X	Stuart-Prower factor
XI	Plasma thromboplastin antecedent (PTA)
XII	Hageman factor, contact factor
XIII	Fibrin stabilizing factor

1. Antithrombins are proteins that neutralize the action of thrombin. When thrombin production is excessive, however, antithrombins may be consumed, thus leading to increased clotting. Neonates are relatively deficient in antithrombin III.

2. Fibrinolysis is characterized by the conversion of plasminogen, an inactive plasma protein, to plasmin, an active protein. The proteolytic activity of plasmin breaks down fibrin deposited at sites of vessel injury. In addition, plasmin degrades factors V, VIII, and fibrinogen. The degradation products of fibrin and fibrinogen are known as fibrin split products (FSPs). Fibrinolysis is stimulated by many of the same factors that activate coagulation. Under normal conditions, this is a beneficial process that limits the extent of fibrin deposition and maintains vascular patency. In certain pathologic conditions, however, persistent activation of clotting and fibrinolysis can deplete factors V, VIII, and fibrinogen and thereby lead to bleeding. In addition, markedly increased fibrin split products enhance the hemorrhagic tendency directly by inhibiting the normal conversion of fibrinogen to fibrin.

General Approach to the Bleeding Infant

Medical History and Physical Examination. Evaluation of any bleeding infant requires historical

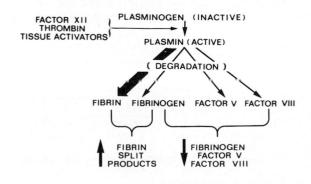

Figure 64–2. Physiology of fibrinolysis.

information regarding outcome of previous pregnancies, family bleeding problems, maternal illnesses (especially infections), drug administration (maternal and neonatal), and documentation that vitamin K was given at birth. Simple observations on physical examination (localized versus diffuse bleeding; healthy or sick infant) have tremendous importance for classifying hemorrhagic disorders. Normal infants frequently have petechiae over presenting parts secondary to venous congestion and the trauma of delivery. These petechiae are seen shortly after birth but gradually disappear and are not associated with bleeding. Infants with isolated platelet disorders generally appear healthy except for progressive petechiae, ecchymoses, and/or mucosal bleeding. Hemorrhages due to vitamin K deficiency or inherited coagulation defects characteristically occur in apparently healthy children with large ecchymoses or localized bleeding (large cephalhematomas, umbilical cord bleeding, or gastrointestinal hemorrhage). Bleeding due to disseminated intravascular coagulation (DIC) or liver injury generally is seen in sick infants with diffuse bleeding from several sites.

Laboratory Evaluation of Bleeding Infant. The etiology of hemorrhage frequently can be identified by simple diagnostic tests. A differential diagnosis based on the platelet count, prothrombin time (PT), and partial thromboplastin time (PTT) is presented in Table 64–2.

1. Platelet Count. In emergency situations or when quantitative platelet counts cannot be obtained, a reliable estimate of the platelet count can be made by examining the peripheral blood smear. The average number of platelets per high-power field is determined after observing several fields under the microscope. This number multiplied by 15,000 is a valid estimate of the platelet count. For example, if one observes 50 platelets after examining 20 high-power fields, there is an average of 2.5 platelets per field, and the approximate platelet count is 37,500 (2.5 multiplied by 15,000). The peripheral blood smear also should include an evaluation of platelet size. Thrombocytopenia associated with normal-sized platelets generally reflects a bone marrow production defect, whereas the presence of large platelets indicates rapid production and destruction of circulating platelets.

The platelet count in term and healthy premature neonates is the same as that in older children. Previously, it was thought that prematures had significantly lower platelet counts than normal term infants. This was partly due to the fact that many laboratories included all premature infants in establishing their normal values. It is now generally agreed, however, that healthy prematures have platelet counts in the same range as term infants and older children. A corollary of this is that sick premature infants frequently have low platelet counts. A platelet count less than 100,000 is definitely abnormal.

2. **Bleeding Time.** This functional test, although seldom used in the newborn period, measures the quality and quantity of platelets and their interaction with the vasculature. This procedure has its major value in bleeding patients with normal platelet counts and coagulation studies. A prolonged bleeding time is seen in von Willebrand's disease and functional platelet disorders. Since abnormal results are seen when the platelet count is less than 100,000, this test should not be done in patients with significant thrombocytopenia. The bleeding time in normal term and premature infants is the same as in older children.

3. **Prothrombin Time and Partial Thromboplastin Time.** These two tests should be used as the initial coagulation screening procedures in any bleeding infant:

PROTHROMBIN TIME (PT). This test measures the extrinsic activation of factor X by factor VII as well as the remainder of the coagulation scheme (factors V, II, and fibrinogen).

PARTIAL THROMBOPLASTIN TIME (PTT). This test measures the intrinsic pathway (activation of factor X by factors XII, XI, IX, and VIII) as well as the final coagulation reactions (V, II and fibrinogen). Most laboratories use an activated partial thromboplastin time (APTT). This test is similar to the PTT except that material is added to hasten the activation of factor XII and thereby speed up the overall reaction.

Two important variables must be considered when collecting venous blood for neonatal coagulation studies. First, the ratio of blood to anticoagulant (3.8 per cent sodium citrate) should be 19:1 (Koepke et al., 1975). The usual ratio (9:1) may give spurious results in neonates with hematocrits over 60 per cent. Second, *blood should not be drawn from heparinized catheters, since even minute amounts of this anticoagulant can prolong the PTT.*

Neonates have decreased levels of certain clotting factors, particularly those dependent on vitamin K (Table 64–3). Consequently, the PT and PTT in healthy term infants are slightly prolonged compared to that seen in older children. These physiologic factor deficiencies are exaggerated in premature infants, and thus the PT and PTT in prematures may be even slightly more prolonged. It is important to emphasize that the differences in clotting parameters between older children and infants are physiologically normal. Any questionable abnormality must be compared to these "normal" neonatal values. Furthermore, each individual hospital must establish its own normal values, since slight modifications in blood collection or assay methods exist between different laboratories.

4. **Fibrinogen Determination.** One measures this factor when attempting to differentiate DIC or liver disease from other clotting abnormalities. Reduced fibrinogen synthesis occurs in liver disease. Increased degradation of fibrinogen is seen in DIC.

5. **Fibrin Split Products (FSPs).** These degradation products of fibrin and fibrinogen are increased in patients with DIC. Increased levels occasionally are seen in liver disease and are possibly due to decreased clearance of FSPs. Since DIC frequently coexists with liver disease, it is often difficult to distinguish these two entities. Fibrin split products are not increased in normal infants when blood samples are properly collected.

6. **Apt Test.** This simple test distinguishes gastrointestinal blood loss due to neonatal hemorrhage from that caused by swallowed maternal blood.

a. Mix 1 volume of stool or vomitus with 5 volumes of water.

b. Centrifuge mixture and separate clear pink supernatant (hemolysate).

c. Add 1 ml of 1 per cent NaOH to 4 ml hemolysate. Mix and observe color change after 2 minutes. Hemoglobin A changes from pink to yellow-brown color (this indicates maternal blood). Hemoglobin F resists denaturation and remains pink (this indicates fetal blood).

Approximately 30 per cent of all episodes of gastrointestinal bleeding are due to swallowed maternal

Table 64–2. Differential Diagnosis of Bleeding in the Neonate

| Clinical Evaluation | Laboratory Studies | | | Likely Diagnosis |
	Platelets	*PT*	*PTT*	
"Sick"	↓	↑	↑	DIC
	↓	N	N	Platelet consumption (infection, necrotizing enterocolitis, renal vein thrombosis)
	N	↑	↑	Liver disease
	N	N	N	Compromised vascular integrity (associated with hypoxia, prematurity, acidosis, hyperosmolality)
"Healthy"	↓	N	N	Immune thrombocytopenia
				Occult infection or thrombosis
				Bone marrow hypoplasia (rare)
	N	↑	↑	Hemorrhagic disease of newborn (vitamin K deficiency)
	N	N	↑	Hereditary clotting factor deficiencies
	N	N	N	Bleeding due to local factors (trauma, anatomic abnormalities)
				Qualitative platelet abnormalities (rare)
				Factor XIII deficiency (rare)

blood (Sherman and Clatworthy, 1967). In those cases in which blood loss is neonatal in origin, less than 25 per cent of infants have detectable platelet or coagulation abnormalities. Underlying abnormalities of the gastrointestinal tract are responsible for some of these bleeding episodes, although in many cases there is no *apparent cause* of hemorrhage.

Blood Components Used in Therapy of Bleeding Infants

Platelet Transfusions. A unit of platelets is defined as that number of platelets obtained from one unit of blood. Platelets are suspended in plasma, approximately 1 unit of platelets in 15 ml of plasma. In order to prevent neonatal red blood cell injury, donor platelets should be type-specific (A, B, O), since the donor plasma may contain antibodies that react with recipient RBCs. Platelets do not contain the Rh antigen, but virtually all platelet concentrates contain some RBCs. Rh-negative infants, therefore, are given platelets from Rh-negative donors. If emergency conditions require that Rh-negative girls be given platelets from an Rh-positive donor, the use of anti-Rh immune serum should be considered in order to protect against red blood cell isoimmunization. In cases of neonatal isoimmune thrombocytopenia, maternal platelets are obtained, washed free of antibody, and resuspended in AB-negative plasma. As a rule of thumb, the administration of 1 unit of fresh platelets per 5 kg of body weight elevates the platelet count over 100,000. Subsequently, the platelet count should decline slowly over 4 to 6 days. Failure to sustain a platelet increase indicates platelet incompatibility due to sensitization or increased platelet destruction (sepsis, DIC, anti-platelet antibody).

Fresh Frozen Plasma. Plasma that is frozen and stored immediately after separation contains adequate concentrations of all clotting factors. Fresh frozen plasma (10 ml/kg) given every 12 hours provides adequate hemostasis for most causes of bleeding due to lack of factors. One unit of clotting factor is defined as that concentration present in 1 ml of normal pooled plasma. Whenever coagulation factors and

platelets are given at the same time, the volume of platelet suspension (largely plasma) must be accounted for in calculating plasma therapy.

Clotting Factor Concentrates. Patients with factor VIII deficiency (classic hemophilia) or factor IX deficiency (Christmas disease) occasionally require very high levels in cases of severe bleeding. In order to avoid problems with fluid volume overload, one should use concentrated factor preparations.

Hemorrhagic Disease of the Newborn

The American Academy of Pediatrics has defined this disorder as any bleeding problem due to vitamin K deficiency and decreased activity of factors II, VII, IX, and X. These clotting proteins are synthesized and stored in the liver until activated by vitamin K. Newborn infants are capable of normal factor synthesis, but because they are relatively deficient in vitamin K, coagulant activity of these factors is decreased. Normally, vitamin K is obtained from the diet and from intestinal bacterial synthesis. Neonates, however, get variable amounts of dietary vitamin K during the first few days of life, and the intestine is not colonized with bacteria at birth. Therefore, as maternally derived vitamin stores are depleted during the first day of life, vitamin K deficiency actually becomes worse, clotting studies become more abnormal, and significant bleeding episodes can occur between 24 and 72 hours of age.

Sanford and coworkers demonstrated that neonatal hemorrhagic disease could be prevented by institution of early feedings with cow's milk. This effect was due to the significantly higher vitamin K content of cow's milk compared with that of breast milk (Dam et al., 1942). Neonatal hemorrhagic disease is extremely unusual today, since vitamin K is given routinely to infants at birth. When bleeding does occur, it is generally because someone has failed to admin-

Table 64–3. Coagulation Profile of Newborn Infants

	Normal Children	Term Infants	Premature Infants
Platelet count	200,000–400,000	200,000–400,000	150,000–350,000
Bleeding time (BT)	2.5–5.5 min	2.5–5.5 min	2.5–5.5 min
Prothrombin time (PT)	12–14 sec	13–20 sec	13–21 sec
Partial thromboplastin time (PTT)	37–50 sec	45–65 sec	45–75 sec
Activated partial thromboplastin time (APTT)	25–35 sec	30–45 sec	35–55 sec
Clotting Factors			
Normal	All factors	Fibrinogen V, VIII, XII, XIII	Fibrinogen V, VIII, XII, XIII
Slightly decreased	—	II, VII, IX, X, XI	XI
Moderately decreased	—	—	II, VII, IX, X

(Data based on normal values published by Hathaway, W. E.: Semin. Hematol. *12*:175, 1975 and on normal values at Children's Hospital Medical Center, Boston, MA.)

ister the vitamin. Rarely, hemorrhagic disease is seen in children born to epileptic mothers under treatment with Dilantin or phenobarbital (Mountain et al., 1970). These drugs can interfere with vitamin K and thereby cause abnormal clotting studies, extremely low factor levels, and bleeding at birth. Infants born to mothers receiving coumarin compounds (vitamin K antagonists) also can bleed because these drugs cross the placenta and cause low levels of factors that depend on vitamin K. Heparin does not cross the placenta. Therefore, in those maternal conditions that require anticoagulation, heparin should be substituted for coumarin a few days prior to delivery (Hirsh et al., 1970). Heparin also should be used instead of coumarin in the first trimester of pregnancy, since coumarin compounds have been associated with teratogenic effects (Fillmore and McDevitt, 1970).

Hemorrhage due to vitamin K deficiency characteristically occurs in otherwise healthy thriving infants. Bleeding may be localized to one area (frequently gastrointestinal) or there may be diffuse ecchymoses. In cases of classic vitamin K deficiency, hemorrhage generally is seen after the first 24 hours of age. In contrast, bleeding secondary to maternal drugs such as phenobarbital, Dilantin, and coumarin derivatives frequently occurs within the first 24 hours of life. The following laboratory test results suggest vitamin K deficiency in a bleeding infant: a normal platelet count, a prolonged PTT, and a prolonged PT. Bleeding infants with these criteria should be given vitamin K (1 mg I.V.). The PT and PTT will begin to normalize after a 4-hour period, and clinical bleeding will cease if the abnormality is due to vitamin K deficiency. Failure to note improvement in bleeding and clotting tests after giving vitamin K suggests another diagnosis, such as liver disease or isolated factor deficiency. Life-threatening hemorrhages due to vitamin K deficiency are unusual, but if they occur fresh frozen plasma (10 ml/kg) should be given in addition to vitamin K.

In most centers, prophylactic vitamin K (0.5 to 1.0 mg) is given intramuscularly at the time of delivery or when the infant enters the nursery. The natural, or fat soluble, form of vitamin K (vitamin K_1 oxide) is safe and nontoxic. High concentrations of some water soluble analogues (menadione), however, may cause hemolysis, hyperbilirubinemia, and kernicterus (Lucey and Dolan, 1959). The minimal dose of vitamin K that prevents the fall in PT and bleeding is 0.025 mg; higher concentrations have no more beneficial effect (Aballi and DeLamerens, 1962). Nevertheless, we continue to give doses that greatly exceed the minimum requirement. Previously, it was thought that premature infants did not respond to vitamin K. Aballi and his coworkers, however, have demonstrated that healthy prematures do respond, although sick prematures may manifest a less than optimal change in clotting studies. It is our policy to administer

vitamin K (0.5 mg) 1 to 2 times each week to ill prematures and infants receiving total parenteral alimentation. Vitamin K given to mothers during labor has proved effective in preventing neonatal bleeding, although one is never quite certain how much actually crosses the placenta. It is more rational to administer vitamin K at the time of birth, since the response to the vitamin is rapid, and bleeding rarely occurs in the first 24 hours of life. Infants of mothers receiving antiseizure medications are an exception to this rule, for these neonates can bleed during the first 24 hours. In these cases, vitamin K should be given during labor in order to prevent any bleeding secondary to the trauma of delivery. Following birth, vitamin K should be given as usual to the neonate.

CASE 64–1

A 3000-gm male infant was born to a healthy gravida 1, para 1 mother after an uneventful 40-week gestation. Apgar score at birth was 9. Physical examination was normal. Breast feedings were started at 18 hours of age. On the second day of life, a bruise appeared over the right buttock. Several bloody stools were noted on the third day. There were no other abnormalities. No petechiae were seen. An Apt test on the stool samples indicated that the source of blood was the infant rather than the mother. The prothrombin time and partial thromboplastin time were markedly prolonged. Examination of the peripheral blood smear indicated that the platelet count was greater than 200,000. The infant was given 1 mg of vitamin K intravenously. After 5 hours no gastrointestinal bleeding was evident, and the PT and PTT had decreased to nearly normal levels. The subsequent clinical course was uneventful.

Comment. This is a classic case of neonatal hemorrhagic disease due to vitamin K deficiency: delayed onset of bleeding, gastrointestinal hemorrhage, normal platelet count, abnormal coagulation studies, and a definite clinical and laboratory response to vitamin K administration. Although there was no apparent cause of bleeding, a check of the medical record indicated that vitamin K had not been given at birth. At the time this child entered the nursery, most of the medical personnel were actively administering to two other critically ill infants. In the midst of this confusion, the infant under discussion failed to receive vitamin K.

Hereditary Clotting Factor Deficiencies

Infants with hereditary clotting factor deficiencies usually are healthy and do not bleed. When hemorrhage does occur, it most commonly is manifested by local blood loss, such as gastrointestinal hemorrhage, bleeding from circumcision or umbilical stump, and large cephalhematomas. The PTT and PT usually are prolonged, but the platelet count is normal. Neither bleeding nor abnormal coagulation studies respond to vitamin K. Diagnosis of most factor deficiencies can be made in the newborn period, since coagulation proteins do not cross the placenta (Cade et al., 1969). In some cases the specific diagnosis is obscured by physiologic factor deficiencies, but virtually all hereditary clotting defects can be detected by 4 months of age.

FACTOR VIII DEFICIENCY (CLASSIC HEMOPHILIA, HEMOPHILIA A)

Classic hemophilia is a sex-linked disorder characterized by decreased activity of factor VIII or antihemophilic factor (AHF). Production of normal factor VIII activity is controlled by two separate genes, one autosomal and the other sex-linked. The autosomal gene regulates production of factor VIII protein, whereas the sex-linked gene regulates coagulant activity of factor VIII protein. Classic hemophilia, a sex-linked disorder, is characterized by normal amounts of factor VIII protein (also known as factor VIII antigen) with markedly diminished factor VIII coagulant activity (Ratnoff, 1972). Von Willebrand's disease (see following discussion) is an autosomal disorder characterized by decreased AHF protein and coagulant activity.

The spectrum of hemorrhagic problems in hemophiliac children is well known to most physicians. For unknown reasons, however, severe neonatal bleeding due to factor VIII deficiency is unusual. Hemorrhage that does occur generally follows traumatic procedures. In a retrospective study, Baehner and Strauss observed that less than 40 per cent of hemophiliacs hemorrhaged following circumcision, and in most cases hemorrhage was very mild. One explanation of this minimal bleeding may be that tissue injury liberates thromboplastin and thereby activates the extrinsic pathway (which bypasses factor VIII). The severe muscle and joint hemorrhages characteristic of hemophilia in older children do not begin until infants start to crawl and walk.

As a sex-linked disorder, hemophilia occurs in male children. There is no problem making this diagnosis in the newborn period, since factor VIII levels in the neonate are the same as those in older children. Although the platelet count and PT are normal, the PTT is prolonged. A specific factor assay should be done if possible because similar values are seen in deficiencies of factors IX, XI, and XII. In the absence of a factor assay, however, most laboratories can make a presumptive diagnosis by modifying the PTT test. Factor VIII is absent from normal serum but is present in plasma. Therefore, if the patient's plasma is mixed with equal amounts of normal serum or plasma, the abnormal PTT will be corrected by plasma but not by serum. This result is very suggestive of factor VIII deficiency. Nevertheless, a specific factor VIII determination is ultimately necessary to confirm the diagnosis. Knowledge of the factor level also can be of prognostic significance. Children with severe hemophilia have less than 1 per cent normal factor VIII

activity, whereas cases of mild to moderate disease are characterized by 1 to 20 per cent factor VIII levels.

In the absence of bleeding, no specific therapy is necessary. Mild bleeding from circumcison or umbilical stump usually can be corrected by local measures such as topical thrombin or Gelfoam. Nonabsorbable substances should not be used because bleeding may start again when the material is removed. In those cases in which bleeding is more severe, factor VIII must be given to raise the plasma concentration to 20 per cent of normal. One factor VIII unit administered per kilogram of body weight elevates the plasma concentration 2 per cent. Thus, to achieve a level that is 20 per cent of normal requires 10 factor VIII units per kilogram of body weight, or 30 factor VIII units for a 3-kg infant. This can be achieved by 30 ml of plasma, since 1 factor VIII unit is by definition equal to that activity in 1 ml of normal plasma. Alternatively, commercial concentrates that provide factor VIII in a much smaller volume can be used to avoid volume overload problems. Factor VIII concentrates should be used whenever possible, especially in conjunction with surgery or with those rare life-threatening hemorrhages in which factor VIII levels of 50 to 100 per cent of normal are required. The in vivo half-life of factor VIII is relatively short, thus infusions need to be repeated every 12 hours until bleeding is under control.

VON WILLEBRAND'S DISEASE

This common autosomal dominant disorder is characterized by abnormal platelet function, decreased factor VIII levels, and, in contrast to classic hemophilia, reductions in both factor VIII coagulant activity and factor VIII protein (i.e., factor VIII antigen) (Ratnoff, 1972). The platelet defect in von Willebrand's disease is due to decreased levels of this protein, since normal platelet function requires interaction with factor VIII. This explanation is supported by the clinical observation that plasma transfusions, even plasma from classic hemophiliacs, can correct the platelet abnormality (i.e., bleeding time) in von Willebrand's disease. In addition, plasma infusions correct the defect in factor VIII coagulant activity. Factor VIII replacement in hemophiliacs results in a transient increase in factor VIII coagulant activity (half-life of 12 hours). In von Willebrand's disease, however, a single factor VIII infusion produces an increase in factor VIII activity that is sustained for several days. Presumably, the patient with von Willebrand's disease can generate the coagulant component of the factor VIII molecule once the protein factor is present.

Little is known about the neonatal course of children with von Willebrand's disease. In older children, bleeding is milder than in classic hemophilia and most often is characterized by severe epistaxis. Occasionally, severe hemorrhage may occur after trauma or surgery. The diagnosis of this disorder can be difficult, since coagulation studies are not always abnormal. In some cases the PTT is prolonged, but this is not an invariable finding. Factor VIII levels of 20 to 50 per cent of normal usually are seen. The concentration of factor VIII antigen also is 20 to 50 per cent of normal. One of the most useful diagnostic tests is that of bleeding time. Mild cases are characterized by a mildly abnormal bleeding time, and these children rarely have significant hemorrhagic manifestations. In severe cases of von Willebrand's disease, however, the bleeding time is prolonged. A more definitive diagnosis can be made by separately measuring factor VIII coagulant activity and factor VIII antigen. Treatment of a bleeding neonate suspected of having von Willebrand's disease (usually on the basis of family history) is similar to that of the infant with classic hemophilia, with the major difference that only one factor VIII infusion is required to provide adequate hemostasis. Platelet transfusions are not needed, since the platelet defect is corrected by administration of factor VIII.

FACTOR IX DEFICIENCY (CHRISTMAS DISEASE, HEMOPHILIA B)

Although it is less common than classic hemophilia, factor IX deficiency accounts for 15 per cent of all cases of hemophilia. This disorder is also sex-linked, and the clinical manifestations are indistinguishable from those of factor VIII deficiency. Coagulation studies are the same as for infants with factor VIII deficiency: normal platelets, normal PT, and prolonged PTT. However, the PTT in factor IX deficiency, unlike that in factor VIII deficiency, is normalized by mixing normal plasma or serum with the patient's plasma (factor IX present in plasma and serum). Definitive diagnosis requires a specific factor assay, preferably done after 2 months of age.

When excess bleeding is present in a child thought to have Christmas disease, fresh frozen plasma should be given. One unit of factor IX increases plasma IX activity by 1 per cent. For minor bleeding, 10 ml per kilogram of body weight every 12 hours provides adequate hemostasis. With severe bleeding or in conjunction with surgery, factor IX activity should be increased to 40 to 50 per cent of normal. Commercial factor IX concentrates are used to achieve these high levels.

FACTOR XI DEFICIENCY (HEMOPHILIA C)

This autosomal recessive factor deficiency occurs primarily in Jewish families. Bleeding is rarely a serious problem because the factor is not completely absent from plasma. It is difficult to make a specific diagnosis in neonates, since factor XI levels remain low for the first several months of life. Factor therapy rarely is required, even for surgical procedures. In a bleeding patient thought to have factor XI deficiency, fresh frozen plasma (10 ml/kg) should be given.

FACTOR XIII DEFICIENCY

Factor XIII (fibrin stabilizing factor) deficiency is characterized by delayed bleeding from the umbilical stump. Deficiency of this factor results in an inability to form stable fibrin polymers, and thus a very friable clot is produced. Between 24 and 48 hours after a period of apparent adequate hemostasis, the clot begins to ooze. The screening coagulation tests (platelet count, PT, PTT) are all normal. Diagnosis requires both a high index of suspicion and definitive laboratory tests. Normal fibrin clots are not dissolved by reagents such as 5M urea or monochloroacetic acid, whereas the friable clot produced in factor XIII deficient plasma is rapidly broken down by these agents. Fibrin stabilizing factor is present in plasma and should be administered if there is significant bleeding.

MISCELLANEOUS FACTOR DEFICIENCIES

Hereditary deficiencies of virtually all other clotting factors have been described. These are extremely rare, and significant neonatal bleeding associated with these deficiencies is even more infrequent. Diagnosis of individual factor deficiencies is suggested by unexplained abnormalities in coagulation tests, but specific factor assays are required for confirmation. As in factor IX deficiency, diagnosis of the other vitamin K–dependent factors cannot be made with certainty until the infant is 2 months of age. Fresh frozen plasma should be given for serious hemorrhage in any bleeding neonate thought to have a factor deficiency.

Intravascular Coagulation Syndromes

The intravascular coagulation syndromes are caused by inappropriate activation of the clotting process. These events are inappropriate in that coagulation is stimulated by factors other than vascular injury. Intravascular coagulation is not a disease; it is a response to local or systemic pathology. Occasionally, however, the effects of accelerated coagulation are more severe than the initiating causes.

DISSEMINATED INTRAVASCULAR COAGULATION (DIC)

Several years ago the term "secondary hemorrhagic disease" was applied to sick infants with severe

Table 64–4. Disseminated Intravascular Coagulation

Clinical Diagnosis
Sick infant
Usually diffuse petechiae/bleeding
Rarely diffuse thrombosis (skin necrosis)

Laboratory Diagnosis
Decreased platelets
Prolonged PT and PTT
Decreased factors V, VIII, and fibrinogen
Increased fibrin split products
Microangiopathic RBC changes

Therapy
1. Vigorous treatment of underlying condition (correction of hypoxia, acidosis and hypovolemia; antibiotics)
2. Plasma and platelet infusions
3. If serious bleeding continues:
   (a) consider exchange transfusion
   (b) continue plasma and platelet infusions as required
4. If clinical presentation is mainly thrombotic:
   (a) administer heparin intravenously
   (b) after heparinization, give plasma and platelets

bleeding not related to vitamin K deficiency. It is now apparent that this syndrome includes many infants with disseminated intravascular coagulation. Disseminated intravascular coagulation is caused by widespread activation of the clotting mechanism, brought about by a variety of systemic problems. The clinical effects of accelerated coagulation are thrombosis and bleeding. Thrombotic manifestations are due to diffuse intravascular fibrin deposition. Bleeding occurs for the two following reasons:

1. During accelerated coagulation, certain clotting factors (II, V, VIII, and fibrinogen) are consumed at a faster rate than they are synthesized.

2. Persistent stimulation of clotting activates fibrinolysis, and fibrin split products are produced. These fibrin degradation products contribute to hemorrhage by inhibiting the normal conversion of fibrinogen to fibrin.

DIC is associated with a variety of conditions in the newborn period: shock, sepsis, acidosis, hypoxia, hypothermia, abruptio placentae, and retention of a dead twin fetus. Unlike bleeding caused by lack of vitamin K or inherited factor deficiencies, DIC occurs in sick infants. Commonly, these neonates are premature and are thus most likely to suffer from the problems known to cause DIC. The severity of DIC is generally related to the duration of the activating stimulus. Subsequent coagulation abnormalities are less severe in cases of acute and self-limited activation, such as transient hypothermia or abruptio placentae, than in those conditions associated with more prolonged disease, such as sepsis or respiratory distress syndrome. Some infants have no clinical manifestations of DIC in spite of marked laboratory abnormalities. In most cases, however, there is diffuse bleeding characterized by petechiae, oozing from venipuncture sites, and gastrointestinal hemorrhages. In a small number of infants the clinical picture is dominated by thrombosis (gangrenous necrosis of skin).

The laboratory diagnosis of DIC is characterized by several distinct abnormalities:

1. Invariably, there is thrombocytopenia due to increased platelet utilization.

2. The PT and PTT are prolonged owing to factor depletion.

3. Fibrinogen usually is decreased. If facilities are available for the measurement of factors V and VIII, their levels will also be found to be decreased.

4. Fibrin split products are increased because of enhanced fibrinolysis.

5. Microangiopathic red blood cell changes (cell fragments, distorted cells) are seen on the peripheral blood smear. Fragment formation is presumably due to RBC interaction with fibrin deposited on the vascular wall.

There is general agreement that successful management of infants with DIC depends on effective removal of conditions activating coagulation. Thus, the most critical therapeutic considerations must be directed at associated infection, hypoxia, acidosis, hypotension, and other physiologic abnormalities. Beyond this observation, there are few data to support the concept that specific therapy for the coagulopathy alters survival (Gross et al., 1982).

Most commonly, DIC is characterized by diffuse cutaneous bleeding. In these infants, our initial approach is to replace platelets and clotting factors with fresh frozen plasma. Occasionally, this is all that is necessary, particularly in neonates who are not very ill and who have minimally abnormal clotting studies. If bleeding persists after plasma and platelet replacement, we proceed with an exchange transfusion using red blood cells (CPD) reconstituted with fresh frozen plasma (hematocrit of 50 to 60). Platelets also are given during and following the exchange. This procedure provides clotting factors and platelets, but it also may remove fibrin split products and some of the toxic factors causing DIC. In addition, adult red blood cells deliver oxygen more readily than do neonatal red blood cells (see Chapter 66), and this may reduce tissue damage from hypoxia. Gross and Melhorn have reported the beneficial effects of exchange transfusion in several infants with DIC. In some of these neonates, exchange transfusion corrected bleeding and coagulation problems before the associated conditions (sepsis, respiratory distress) were under control.

We occasionally see infants with DIC manifested by gangrenous necrosis of the skin (purpura fulminans). Rarely, DIC produces kidney necrosis caused by the thrombosis of large renal vessels. Teleologically, these conditions are due to a relative increase in fibrin deposition compared with factor depletion (i.e., clotting greater than fibrinolysis). Therefore, anticoagulation is a logical therapeutic modality in children with thrombotic problems. Intravenous heparin (15 mg/kg/hr) is given continuously for a total duration of 2 to 3 days. Once heparin has been started, platelet and plasma transfusions can be given. From a theoretical perspective, it seems important that platelets and plasma be replaced after heparin, otherwise one merely provides substrate for more thrombus formation.

It should be pointed out that a few centers employ heparin in cases of DIC in which there is bleeding without thrombotic manifestations. This therapeutic approach is based on the assumption that hemorrhage is due in part to depletion of clotting factors. Thus, heparin transiently interferes with normal coagulation and allows these factors to regenerate. There are several reports that heparin has corrected the laboratory abnormalities in DIC. The studies of Corrigan and Jordan, however, clearly demonstrate that heparin has no effect on the overall mortality from DIC.

CASE 64–2

A 1090-gm female infant was born by spontaneous delivery after 31 weeks' gestation. At birth the child was well, but by 5 hours of age respiratory distress developed, with frequent apneic episodes. At 15 hours of age, bleeding from the umbilical catheter and skin was noted. Vitamin K had been given at birth. Laboratory studies revealed a markedly prolonged PT and PTT. The platelet count was 32,000. Fibrinogen was less than 100 mg per 100 ml. Fibrin split products were markedly elevated. The infant was transfused with fresh frozen plasma and platelets, but bleeding continued unabated. Intravenous heparin (15 mg/kg/hr) was started, and more platelets and factors were given. At 26 hours of age, the infant died. Autopsy revealed hemorrhage into the cerebral ventricles and lungs.

Comment.   This child was born at a time when we believed in early heparinization for DIC. Nowadays we rarely anticoagulate bleeding infants, mainly because there is no proof that it is efficacious. Furthermore, we are never certain whether fatal hemorrhages are due to DIC or to heparin therapy. Our current approach to cases like this would be to perform an exchange transfusion after the initial failure. In view of the child's gestational age and respiratory disease, one could argue that exchange transfusion should be the initial therapy once DIC is diagnosed.

LOCALIZED INTRAVASCULAR COAGULATION

Specific organ pathology can lead to deposition of fibrin and platelets. Generally, these effects are limited to localized thrombosis in the area of activation, although depletion of platelets and coagulation factors occasionally is seen. The hemolytic-uremic syndrome (HUS) is an example of localized intravascular coagulation. This disorder generally occurs in children less than 2 years of age and rarely may be seen in neonates. HUS is characterized by local deposition of fibrin and platelets within the renal vasculature. In most cases there is thrombocytopenia, but consumption of clotting factors occurs infrequently. Bleeding usually is due to decreased platelets. Intravascular fibrin interacts with red blood cells, forming distorted red blood cells or schistocytes (fragments, helmet cells). These cells are fragile and are rapidly destroyed, thus producing hemolytic anemia. Renal failure is the major clinical problem in HUS, and most therapeutic efforts are directed toward the management of this process (early peritoneal dialysis). If systemic bleeding occurs, platelets and fresh frozen plasma should be given as needed. Heparinization has not been demonstrated to be beneficial.

Localized intravascular coagulation is seen in a variety of other conditions: renal vein thrombosis, portal vein thrombosis, necrotizing enterocolitis, and large hemangiomas (see section on thrombocytopenia).

Bleeding Associated With Liver Disease

Since the liver produces all clotting factors with the exception of factor VIII, it is not surprising that bleeding is a main clinical manifestation of serious liver disease. Neonatal bleeding due to liver injury generally occurs in sick infants following hypoxia or hypotension. The characteristics of this type of bleeding are very similar to those of DIC, and DIC is frequently associated with liver disease. The PT and PTT are both prolonged, and there is no significant change following vitamin K administration. The platelet count may be normal or decreased, depending on whether there is associated DIC or significant portal hypertension. Fibrin split products may be increased, owing to decreased hepatic clearance, even in the absence of DIC. A normal factor VIII level is the only feature of liver disease that distinguishes this syndrome from DIC.

Therapy for bleeding due to liver disease is largely factor replacement (10 ml plasma/kg/12 hr). Platelets are given if there is significant thrombocytopenia.

CASE 64–3

A female infant weighing 1810 gm was born to a healthy mother after 33 weeks' gestation. Shortly after birth, respirations became labored, with grunting and cyanosis. The chest radiograph was characteristic of hyaline membrane disease. Blood gases revealed the following: pH 7.26, P_{CO_2} 39.6 mm Hg, and P_{O_2} 30 mm Hg. The child was given assisted ventilation with a Bennett respirator and oxygen. Over the next 4 days, her clinical status improved somewhat. On the fourth day, however, there was bleeding from the umbilical catheter, and a large ecchymosis was noted on the right leg. There were no petechiae or other physical abnor-

malities. The platelet count was 165,000, but the PT and PTT were both markedly prolonged. Vitamin K (1.0 mg) given intravenously had no effect on the bleeding or clotting studies. The fibrinogen level was less than 100 mg per 100 ml. Fibrin split products were slightly increased. There was no alteration in RBC morphology. The child was given plasma infusions over the next 3 days. Clotting studies improved, and there was no further bleeding. At the same time the infant's respiratory status improved considerably.

Comment. In view of the relatively normal platelet count, this child's bleeding was probably due to liver disease rather than DIC. Presumably, liver injury was due to hypoxia during the course of respiratory disease. Fresh frozen plasma and improvement in respiratory status resulted in cessation of all bleeding. It should be pointed out, however, that this is an atypical case of bleeding associated with liver disease. In most cases, the patients are refractory to therapy and the prognosis is grave.

Bleeding Due to Platelet Abnormalities

Platelet-related bleeding usually is due to thrombocytopenia, although hereditary and acquired platelet dysfunction are seen rarely. Bleeding due to platelet disturbances generally is petechial and superficial (skin and mucosa) in contrast to the large ecchymoses and muscle hemorrhages seen in coagulation disturbances. The major causes of neonatal thrombocytopenia include (1) DIC (dicussed previously), (2) immune reactions, and (3) infection. In the absence of DIC, the PTT and PT usually are normal.

ISOIMMUNE THROMBOCYTOPENIA

This condition is analogous to erythroblastosis due to ABO and Rh incompatibility. The infant's platelets contain an antigen that is lacking on maternal platelets. During pregnancy, fetal platelets enter the maternal circulation and stimulate antibody production against fetal platelet antigens (Harrington et al., 1953). Maternal platelets are not affected. Although the antibody is specific for one of several platelet antigens, 50 per cent of cases are due to Pl^{A1} antigens (mother is Pl^{A1}-negative, infant is Pl^{A1}-positive) (Shulman, 1964).

Children with isoimmune thrombocytopenia manifest increasing petechiae and mucosal bleeding during the first 48 hours of life (Pearson et al., 1964). Generally, this is the only symptom in an otherwise healthy neonate. The platelet count is decreased and may be as low as 2000. Platelets appear very large on the peripheral blood smear. Coagulation studies are normal. This disorder is suspected when isolated thrombocytopenia is seen in a thriving infant whose

mother is healthy and has a normal platelet count. Definitive diagnosis requires demonstration of a neonatal platelet antigen that is lacking on maternal platelets. This can only be done in a specialized platelet laboratory.

Studies reported several years ago suggested a 10 to 15 per cent mortality with this disorder, with death usually due to CNS hemorrhage. (Undoubtedly, many of these cases were in fact due to DIC.) In most cases, infants with neonatal isoimmune thrombocytopenia do not have serious bleeding, particularly if the platelet count is greater than 20,000. The platelet count remains low until the neonate clears maternal antibody, generally within a period of 4 to 8 weeks. In spite of this persistent thrombocytopenia, significant bleeding is seen only in the first few days of life.

It should be recognized that the appropriate therapy for this disorder is controversial. Our policy is to treat all children who have platelet counts of less than 30,000, even in the absence of overt bleeding. The mainstay of therapy is transfusion of maternal platelets that have been washed and resuspended in AB-negative plasma. Random donor platelets are of little value in cases due to Pl^{A1} sensitivity, since 97 per cent of donors will be Pl^{A1}-positive. In the absence of facilities to separate platelets, a unit of maternal whole blood can be removed and transported to the closest institution that can fractionate blood. In this way platelets are provided for the infant, and red blood cells can be reinfused into the mother. In most cases, a single transfusion of maternal platelets produces a sustained elevation in the neonatal platelet count. Recently, however, we observed a clearly documented case of isoimmune thrombocytopenia (mother Pl^{A1}-negative, infant Pl^{A1}-positive) that required three separate platelet transfusions in order to elevate the peripheral platelet count. This delayed response most probably was due to the fact that this infant also was infected.

Neonates with significant bleeding or with very low platelet counts also are given hydrocortisone (10 mg every 12 hours, intravenously) until the response to maternal platelets can be assessed. The efficacy of steroid therapy in thrombocytopenias has never been clearly established, but there is a general impression that these drugs increase the platelet count. In any event, it is our belief that a short course of steroids to bleeding but otherwise healthy infants is not significantly deleterious. When maternal platelets are not immediately available to treat severe hemorrhage, steroids and random donor platelets should be given. The survival time of these platelets is short, although they may be transiently functional before being coated with antibody and removed from the circulation. Exchange transfusion prior to giving random donor platelets has been advocated in order to remove circulating antibody partially.

Isoimmune thrombocytopenia differs from Rh disease in that 50 per cent of all cases occur in the first pregnancy (Shulman, 1964). Furthermore, once this entity has occurred, there is a 70 to 85 per cent probability of recurrence in subsequent pregnancies. There is at present no satisfactory assay that can detect whether an infant will be born with thrombocytopenia. Maternal antiplatelet antibody titers have been followed but have been of little prognostic value. The approach to high-risk pregnancies (i.e., previous history of isoimmune thrombocytopenia) also is controversial. We currently advocate the following:

1. Maternal platelets are removed the day before delivery.

2. Delivery is by elective cesarean section in order to prevent serious neonatal bleeding during passage through the birth canal.

3. Maternal platelets are transfused immediately after birth if the infant is thrombocytopenic. With this rather aggressive approach we have successfully avoided any major complications in thrombocytopenic infants.

CASE 64–4

A 3200-gm male infant was born to a gravida 1, para 1 mother after an uneventful pregnancy. At the time of birth, the infant's physical examination was entirely normal except for a few petechiae over his chest. The infant did well until 16 hours of age, at which time he passed a grossly bloody stool. (Apt test revealed blood to be of neonatal origin.) At this time more petechiae were noted over his abdomen and shoulders. A CBC revealed the following: Hgb 16 gm/100 ml, WBC 16,000, platelet count 4500. The PT and PTT were normal. Skin, nose, throat, and blood cultures were obtained, although there was no obvious infection. The mother's platelet count was 290,000, and further study of her past medical history revealed nothing to explain her infant's thrombocytopenia. The child was given 1 unit of random donor platelets from the blood bank. By 1 hour after the transfusion, his platelet count increased to 28,000 and 6 hours later was down to 6000. During this interval, the infant had several bloody stools, but otherwise he appeared to be thriving. A unit of blood was obtained from the infant's mother, and platelets were separated. One hour after the neonate was transfused with maternal platelets, the platelet count was 120,000, and 6 hours later it was 102,000. During the remainder of the neonatal course, there was no more bleeding. All previous cultures were negative. At 7 days of age, the child's platelet count was 14,000. He was given another unit of maternal platelets and sent home.

Comment. Although platelet typing was not done on this particular child and his parents, the clinical history is classic for isoimmune thrombocytopenia. The two following features of this management deserve further comment:

1. Steroids were not given with the initial platelet transfusion, although it was apparent the child probably had some form of immune thrombocytopenia. Currently, we add steroids early in the therapy until we can assess the bleeding response to platelet transfusions. This is certainly a controversial area, and obviously this child did well without steroids.

2. At the time of discharge, the infant was given another unit of maternal platelets. Bleeding beyond the first week of life, regardless of the platelet count, is extremely rare in isoimmune thrombocytopenia. However, since maternal platelet transfusions are relatively innocuous and potentially protective, we currently continue this practice.

IMMUNE THROMBOCYTOPENIA SECONDARY TO MATERNAL DISEASE

In contrast to isoimmune thrombocytopenia, this disease involves an antiplatelet antibody that is directed against maternal platelets. The neonate is affected to the extent that the antibody crosses the placenta and injures fetal platelets. The reasons for decreased platelets in the mother are as varied as the causes of adult immune thrombocytopenia (idiopathic, systemic lupus erythematosus, etc.). The likelihood that thrombocytopenia will develop in a child will be determined in large part by the state of the maternal disease (Goodhue and Evans, 1963). If the mother had ITP in the past but now has a normal platelet count, the probability that her infant will develop thrombocytopenia is low. On the other hand, if the mother has evidence of active disease, or a low platelet count, it is likely (50 to 85 per cent) that the neonate will have thrombocytopenia. It should be noted that some splenectomized women with a history of ITP have normal platelet counts but continue to have high titers of antiplatelet antibodies. These individuals also have a high risk of bearing infants with thrombocytopenia. In the future, direct measurement of maternal antiplatelet antibody titers may prove to have prognostic importance.

The major risk to the fetus who may be thrombocytopenic is bleeding in the central nervous system during vaginal delivery. McMillan recommends cesarean section if the mother has been splenectomized, regardless of her platelet count, or if the platelet count is less than 100,000 per cubic millimeter. Since section may be hazardous to the mother, another approach was advocated by Ayromlooi. He measured platelet counts on fetal scalp blood early in labor. If the count was over 50,000 per cubic millimeter, vaginal delivery was undertaken. If less than that, section was performed.

Steroid administration to the mother during pregnancy (or at least during the last days of pregnancy) is associated with higher platelet counts in the infant. Karpatkin and coworkers reviewed their experience among mothers who had received 10 to 20 mg of prednisone daily for 10 to 14 days before delivery compared with others who did not receive steroids, and they demonstrated significantly higher platelet counts in the infants of steroid-treated mothers.

These neonates are clinically identical with those with isoimmune thrombocytopenia. Rarely, an infant of a mother with lupus erythematosus will transiently develop the total symptoms of SLE, including thrombocytopenia, malar rash, and L-E cells in the peripheral blood (Nathan and Snapper, 1958). Generally, however, these thrombocytopenic infants are healthy and thriving. The clinical course also is similar to the isoimmune disorder, although the platelet count may remain low for a longer period of time (up to 12 weeks). The prognosis usually is good, and significant bleeding beyond the first few days of life is most unusual.

Appropriate treatment of this disorder also is controversial. We give steroids to infants who have platelet counts less than 20,000 or any evidence of bleeding. Initial therapy is with hydrocortisone (10 mg I.V. every 12 hours). If for any reason steroids are required beyond 2 or 3 days (evidence of bleeding or platelets persistently less than 10,000) oral prednisone (1 mg/kg/day) is used for a maximum period of 3 weeks. In contrast to treatment of isoimmune thrombocytopenia, management of this disease does not greatly involve platelet transfusions. The maternal antiplatelet antibody usually is directed against a "public antigen" that is shared by maternal and neonatal platelets. Thus, random donor platelets are removed rapidly by the reticuloendothelial system. Nevertheless, in the presence of life-threatening hemorrhage, platelet transfusions should be given. Occasionally, incompatible platelets may be utilized for hemostasis before they are destroyed by antibody (i.e., delayed antigen-antibody reaction). Rarely, platelet responsiveness to random donor platelet transfusions may appear after previous failures to achieve an increased platelet count. Presumably, this is due to "soaking up" of antibodies by previous platelet transfusions. In severely bleeding infants refractory to steroids and random donor platelets, exchange transfusion followed by administration of platelets is indicated.

IMMUNE THROMBOCYTOPENIA DUE TO DRUG-INDUCED MATERNAL THROMBOCYTOPENIA

Certain drugs (quinine, quinidine, sulfonamides, digitoxin) given to mothers can cause both maternal and neonatal thrombocytopenia on an immune basis (Mauer et al., 1957). An antibody to the drug is produced by the mother. This antibody reacts with the drug, and the drug-antibody complex then attaches to the platelets ("innocent bystanders"), resulting in the removal of coated platelets from the circulation. The neonate is affected to the extent that drug and antibody cross the placenta into the fetal circulation. These children are clinically indistinguishable from other neonates with thrombocytopenia due to maternal disease. Significant bleeding is rare, but if it

occurs platelet transfusions are indicated. This form of neonatal thrombocytopenia clears rapidly, the rate-limiting factor being the neonatal clearance of drug. Once drug is removed from the neonate, platelet counts will increase even though the antibody may persist for several weeks.

THROMBOCYTOPENIA ASSOCIATED WITH INFECTION

Thrombocytopenia frequently accompanies infection. The most commonly implicated infections are bacterial sepsis, cytomegalic inclusion disease, toxoplasmosis, syphilis, rubella, and generalized herpes simplex. These infants may be relatively asymptomic or severely ill. Rarely is thrombocytopenia the only abnormality, and in most cases it is not the major problem. Occasionally, however, significant bleeding may occur. Hepatosplenomegaly is a common clinical finding not seen in the other neonatal thrombocytopenias.

The mechanism of thrombocytopenia is multifactorial:

1. Many infections are associated with DIC, a common cause of decreased platelets.

2. Megakaryocyte platelet production may be inhibited directly by causative agents or their metabolites.

3. Reticuloendothelial hyperplasia associated with infection may lead to platelet sequestration.

4. Infectious agents may react with circulating platelets (similar to platelet plus antibody) and thereby lead to their sequestration and removal.

In the absence of DIC, thrombocytopenia rarely is severe enough to cause serious bleeding. The major therapeutic effort must be directed to the underlying infection. Steroids are of no value. If serious bleeding does occur, platelet transfusions are indicated.

THROMBOCYTOPENIA ASSOCIATED WITH GIANT HEMANGIOMAS

Hemangiomas commonly appear in the neonatal period, grow during the first few months of life, and then begin to recede in size. Rarely, large superficial hemangiomas are associated with thrombocytopenia and bleeding (Kasabach and Merritt, 1940). Studies with [51]chromium-labeled platelets have demonstrated that thrombocytopenia is due to sequestration and destruction of platelets within the vascular tumor (Kontras et al., 1963). In addition, recent reports have indicated decreased levels of factors V, VIII, and fibrinogen in many patients, thus suggesting that localized intravascular coagulation also occurs in these lesions.

Hemorrhage most commonly occurs after several

weeks of age when the tumors are largest. Occasionally, however, bleeding is seen earlier, and at least 50 per cent of hemorrhagic angiomas initially bleed during the first month of life. Angiomas of the placenta (chorioangiomas) also can cause neonatal thrombocytopenia. Bleeding hemangiomas characteristically darken in color, enlarge, and become firm to palpation. Petechiae may appear around the periphery of the hemangioma as well as at distant sites. Systemic bleeding secondary to thrombocytopenia or depletion of clotting factors or both may occur. In some cases, however, the major clinical problems are not due to blood loss but rather are secondary to compression of vital structures (i.e., airway obstruction) as bleeding occurs into the hemangioma.

In the absence of symptoms, the best therapy for large hemangiomas is benign neglect, since almost all lesions regress spontaneously with time. Furthermore, most modes of therapeutic intervention produce serious side effects (scarring after surgery, bone growth retardation following radiation). No treatment is indicated for isolated thrombocytopenia in the absence of bleeding. If symptomatic hemorrhage occurs, platelets and fresh frozen plasma should be given as needed. In addition, attempts should be made to eradicate the angioma. The initial and most conservative approach is to attempt shrinkage of the tumor, using steroids (prednisone, 20 mg/day for 2 weeks) (Fost and Esterly, 1968). In those angiomas refractory to steroids, radiotherapy may be useful. Radiation occasionally produces a rapid reduction in tumor size, and therefore this modality is most useful when enlarging hemangiomas cause compression of vital structures (Duncan and Halnan, 1968). Rarely, it is necessary to resort to surgical excision in situations that do not respond to steroids or radiation. Surgery should be done under cover of platelets and fresh frozen plasma, but even with these precautions, blood loss is usually excessive. It is difficult to remove the entire hemangioma surgically, but frequently the immediate threat to life can be decreased. The major complication in surviving patients is disfigurement brought about by the extensive surgery involved in tumor removal.

THROMBOCYTOPENIA DUE TO BONE MARROW HYPOPLASIA

Thrombocytopenia due to decreased platelet production is usually associated with other congenital abnormalities or evidence of systemic disease. The diagnosis of a production defect is suggested by a decreased quantity of normal-sized platelets on peripheral blood smear. Examination of the bone marrow is mandatory in cases of suspected marrow failure in order to rule out aplasia, leukemia, and other neoplasms. Bleeding episodes are treated with platelet transfusions.

Thrombocytopenia and Bilateral Absence of Radii. Several cases of these two isolated congenital abnormalities have been reported (Hall et al., 1969). These infants frequently manifest a leukemoid reaction (markedly elevated leukocyte count with many immature forms) in the peripheral blood. Bleeding should be treated with platelet transfusions. Beyond the neonatal period, the platelet count frequently increases over the next several years.

Fanconi's Hypoplastic Anemia. This syndrome usually becomes apparent later in childhood, at which time there is pancytopenia (anemia, neutropenia, thrombocytopenia). In rare instances thrombocytopenia during infancy may be the initial manifestation of this disorder. Invariably, most patients have one or more congenital abnormalities, such as short stature, renal deformities, skeletal defects, hyperpigmentation, and microphthalmia.

Congenital Leukemia. Bleeding due to thrombocytopenia may be the presenting sign of congenital leukemia (see Chapter 107).

Thrombocytopenia Secondary to Maternal Drug Ingestion. Although the maternal ingestion of thiazides was previously considered to be a relatively common cause of neonatal thrombocytopenia, the general consensus now is that this is an extremely rare cause, if it exists at all (Merenstein et al., 1970). It is difficult to document maternal drug ingestion as a cause of neonatal megakaryocyte failure when maternal platelets are not affected. In this category of thrombocytopenia the physician must rely upon a diagnosis of exclusion, since it is much more important not to overlook other, more subtle, causes of decreased platelet production.

Decreased Platelet Production Associated with Infection. This group (considered in the previous discussion) is mentioned here only to emphasize that the thrombocytopenia of infection can be caused by suppression of normal megakaryocyte production. Presumably, this is the mechanism of thrombocytopenia that occurs in some cases of rubella.

HEREDITARY THROMBOCYTOPENIAS

Wiskott-Aldrich Syndrome. Thrombocytopenia, eczema, and frequent infections due to immunologic defects characterize this disorder (Baldini, 1966). In rare instances, bleeding in the neonatal period may be the initial manifestation. Thrombocytopenia is due to an intrinsic platelet defect leading to decreased platelet survival. Unlike the large platelets seen in other thrombocytopenias characterized by a decreased life span, those in the Wiskott-Aldrich syndrome are much smaller than normal (microplatelets). This is a sex-linked disorder affecting male children. The prognosis is poor, and children die of severe infections during the first years of life. Bone marrow transplantation has been successful in curing some of these infants.

Miscellaneous Hereditary Thrombocytopenias. This group includes several poorly understood thrombocytopenias caused by either decreased platelet life span or decreased platelet production. Family members frequently manifest thrombocytopenia. Serious neonatal bleeding problems are unusual.

Hemorrhage Due to Platelet Dysfunction. Platelet function can be assessed in vivo by the bleeding time or in vitro by observing platelet aggregation in response to known stimulants (ADP, thrombin, collagen). Neonatal platelet aggregation reportedly is abnormal, but this must not be of major significance, since the bleeding time of infants and older children is the same. Nevertheless, abnormal platelet function is suspected in any bleeding infant whose platelets are adequate and in whom coagulation studies are normal. In rare instances, hereditary disorders of platelet function (Glanzmann's thrombasthenia) may present with bleeding in the newborn period. A more important fact, however, is that neonates frequently acquire platelet dysfunction secondary to drug exposure.

Aspirin is known to cause abnormal platelet function. (Acetylation of platelet membrane by ASA inhibits release of platelet ADP and thereby prevents platelet aggregation.) In some individuals, this results in bleeding. Several studies have demonstrated that aspirin taken by mothers within 2 or 3 days of delivery produces both maternal and neonatal platelet dysfunction (Corby and Schulman, 1971; Bleyer and Breckenridge, 1970). Furthermore, some infants with aspirin-induced platelet dysfunction have had suspicious hemorrhages (large cephalhematomas). Other drugs also have been implicated in neonatal platelet abnormalities. Corby and Schulman observed decreased platelet aggregation in neonates born to mothers given Demerol and Phenergan prior to delivery. No effect on maternal platelet function was noted.

A bleeding time should be done on any infant with a suspected platelet functional defect. Patients with von Willebrand's disease may present in a similar way, although the PTT usually is abnormal. Transfusion of random donor platelets is the treatment of choice for bleeding due to platelet dysfunction. Circulating drugs will not affect the function of transfused platelets over a short period of time.

Hemostatic Abnormalities Associated With Serious Local Hemorrhage

We have become relatively sophisticated in our understanding of normal hemostasis, and many major bleeding problems are currently being studied at the molecular level. The pathophysiology of the most serious neonatal bleeding problems, however, remains to be defined. These major pulmonary and central nervous system hemorrhages are discussed elsewhere in this text. The point to be emphasized here is that fatal bleeding episodes in neonates are not necessarily due to coagulation or platelet abnormalities. Massive pulmonary hemorrhage is occasionally associated with laboratory evidence of DIC or liver injury, but usually no hemostatic abnormality is detected. Similarly, coagulation abnormalities (liver injury, DIC) often are seen with the respiratory distress syndrome, and children with RDS frequently have intraventricular hemorrhages. Clotting defects, however, are seen in only a small number of these infants with CNS hemorrhages. In most cases of intraventricular hemorrhage, local vascular factors must be important, since there often is no bleeding outside the CNS.

REFERENCES

General and Neonatal Hemostasis

Bleyer, W. A., Hakami, N., and Shepard, T. H.: The development of hemostasis in the human fetus and newborn infant. J. Pediatr. 79:838, 1971.

Chessells, J. M., and Hardisty, R. M.: Bleeding problems in the newborn infant. Progress in hemostasis and thrombosis. 2:333, 1974.

Craig, W. S.: On real and apparent external bleeding in the newborn. Arch. Dis. Child. 36:575, 1961.

Fogel, B. J., Arias, D., and Kung, F.: Platelet counts in healthy premature infants. J. Pediatr. 73:108, 1968.

Hathaway, W. E.: The bleeding newborn. Semin. Hematol. 12:175, 1975.

Jensen, A. H., Josso, F., Zamet, P., Monset-Couchard, M., and Minkowski, A.: Evolution of blood clotting factor levels in premature infants during the first 10 days of life: a study of 96 cases with comparison between clinical status and blood clotting factor levels. Pediatr. Res. 7:638, 1973.

Koepke, J. A., Rodgers, J. L., and Ollivier, M. J.: Preinstrumental variables in coagulation testing. Am. J. Clin. Pathol. 64:591, 1975.

Oski, F. A., and Naiman, J. L.: Hematologic Problems in the Newborn. 3rd ed. Philadelphia, W. B. Saunders Co., 1982.

Sell, E. J., and Corrigan, J. J., Jr.: Platelet counts, fibrinogen concentrations, and factor V and factor VIII levels in healthy infants according to gestational age. J. Pediatr. 82:1028, 1973.

Sherman, N. J., and Clatworthy, H. W., Jr.: Gastro-intestinal bleeding in neonates: a study of 94 cases. Surgery 62:614, 1967.

Hemorrhagic Disease of the Newborn

Aballi, A. J., and DeLamerens, S.: Coagulation changes in neonatal period and early infancy. Pediatr. Clin. North Am. 9:785, 1962.

Aballi, A. J., Lopez Banus, V., DeLamerens, S., and Rozengvaig, S.: Coagulation studies in the newborn period. I. Alterations of thromboplastin generation and effects of vitamin K on full-term and premature infants. Am. J. Dis. Child. 94:594, 1957.

Committee on Nutrition, American Academy of Pediatrics: Vitamin K compounds and the water-soluble analogues: use in therapy and prophylaxis in pediatrics. Pediatrics 28:501, 1961.

Dam, H., Glavind, J., Larsen, H., and Plum, P.: Investigations into the cause of physiological hypoprothrombinemia in newborn children. IV. The vitamin K content of woman's milk and cow's milk. Acta Med. Scand. *112*:210, 1942.

Fillmore, S. J., and McDevitt, E.: Effects of coumarin compounds on the fetus. Ann. Intern. Med. *73*:731, 1970.

Gellis, S. S., and Lyon, R. A.: The influence of diet of the newborn infant on the prothrombin index. J. Pediatr. *19*:495, 1941.

Hilgartner, M. W., Solomon, G. E., and Kutt, H.: Diphenylhydantoin induced coagulation abnormalities. Pediatr. Res. *5*:408, 1971.

Hirsh, J., Cade, J. F., and O'Sullivan, E. F.: Clinical experience with anticoagulant therapy during pregnancy. Br. Med. J. *1*:270, 1970.

Lucey, J. F., and Dolan, R. G.: Hyperbilirubinemia of newborn infants associated with the parenteral administration of a vitamin K analogue to the mothers. Pediatrics *23*:553, 1959.

Mountain, K. R., Hirsh, J., and Gallus, A. S.: Neonatal coagulation defect due to anticonvulsant drug treatment in pregnancy. Lancet *1*:265, 1970.

Nammacher, M. A., Willemin, M., Hartmann, R. R., and Gaston, L. W.: Vitamin K deficiency in infants beyond the neonatal period. J. Pediatr. *76*:547, 1970.

Sanford, H. M., Gesteyer, T. H., and Wyat, L.: The substances involved in the coagulation of blood of the newborn. Am. J. Dis. Child. *43*:58, 1932.

Townsend, C. W.: The hemorrhagic disease of the newborn. Arch. Pediatr. *11*:559, 1894.

Hereditary Clotting Factor Deficiencies

Abildgaard, C. F.: Current concepts in the management of hemophilia. Semin. Hematol. *12*:223, 1975.

Baehner, R. L., and Strauss, H. S.: Hemophilia in the first year of life. N. Engl. J. Med. *275*:524, 1966.

Britten, A. F. H.: Congenital deficiency of factor XIII (fibrin-stabilizing factor). Am. J. Med. *43*:751, 1967.

Cade, J. F., Hirsh, J., and Martin, M.: Placental barrier to coagulation factors: its relevance to the coagulation defect at birth and to haemorrhage in the newborn. Br. Med. J., *1*:281, 1969.

Donaldson, V. H., and Kisker, C. T.: Blood coagulation in hemostasis. *In* Nathan, D. G. and Oski, F. A. (Eds.): Hematology of Infancy and Childhood. Philadelphia, W. B. Saunders Co., 1974, pp. 561–610.

Hartmann, J. R., Howell, D. A., and Diamond, L. K.: Disorders of blood coagulation during the first weeks of life. A.M.A.J. Dis. Child. *90*:594, 1955.

Ratnoff, O. D.: The molecular basis of hereditary clotting disorders. *In* Spaet, T. (Ed.): Progress in Hemostasis and Thrombosis. Vol. 1. New York, Grune & Stratton, 1972, pp. 39–74.

Weiss, H. J.: Von Willebrand's disease. *In* Williams, W. J., et al. (Eds.): Hematology. New York, McGraw-Hill Book Co., 1972.

Intravascular Coagulation Syndromes

Abildgaard, C. F.: Recognition and treatment of intravascular coagulation. J. Pediatr. *74*:163, 1969.

Alstatt, L. B., Dennis, L. H., Sundell, H., Malan, A., Harrison, V., Hedvall, G., Eichelberger, J., Fogel, B., and Stahlman, M.: Disseminated intravascular coagulation and hyaline membrane disease. Biol. Neonate *19*:227, 1971.

Chessells, J. M., and Wigglesworth, J. S.: Secondary haemorrhagic disease of the newborn. Arch. Dis. Child. *45*:539, 1970.

Chessells, J. M., and Wigglesworth, J. S.: Haemostatic failure in babies with rhesus isoimmunization. Arch. Dis. Child. *46*:38, 1971.

Chessells, J. M., and Wigglesworth, J. S.: Coagulation studies in preterm infants with respiratory distress and intracranial haemorrhage. Arch. Dis. Child. *47*:564, 1972.

Corrigan, J. J., and Jordan, C. M.: Heparin therapy in septicemia with disseminated intravascular coagulation. N. Engl. J. Med. *283*:778, 1970.

Deykin, D.: The clinical challenge of disseminated intravascular coagulation. N. Engl. J. Med. *283*:636, 1970.

Du, J. N. H., Briggs, J. N., and Young, G.: Disseminated intravascular coagulopathy in hyaline membrane disease: massive thrombosis following umbilical artery catheterization. Pediatrics *45*:287, 1970.

Glaun, B. P., Weinberg, E. G., and Malan, A. F.: Peripheral gangrene in a newborn. Arch. Dis. Child. *46*:105, 1971.

Gross, S. J., Filston, H. C., and Anderson, J. C.: Controlled study of treatment for disseminated intravascular coagulation in the neonate. J. Pediatr. *100*:445, 1982.

Gross, S., and Melhorn, D. K.: Exchange transfusion with citrated whole blood for disseminated intravascular coagulation. J. Pediatr. *78*:415, 1971.

Hathaway, W. E., Mull, M. M., and Pechet, G. S.: Disseminated intravascular coagulation in the newborn. Pediatrics *43*:233, 1969.

Karpatkin, M., Sacker, I., and Ackerman, N.: Respiratory distress syndrome and disseminated intravascular coagulation in two siblings. Lancet *1*:102, 1972.

Lowry, M. F., Mann, J. R., Abrams, L. D., and Chance, G. W.: Thrombectomy for renal venous thrombosis in infant of diabetic mother. Br. Med. J. *3*:687, 1970.

Markarian, M., Cohen, R. J., and Milbauer, B.: Disseminated intravascular coagulation in a neonate treated with heparin. J. Pediatr. *78*:74, 1971.

Roberts, J. T., Davies, A. J., and Bloom, A. L.: Coagulation studies in massive pulmonary hemorrhage of the newborn. J. Clin. Pathol. *19*:334, 1966.

Rowe, S., and Avery, M. E.: Massive pulmonary hemorrhage in the newborn. II. Clinical considerations. J. Pediatr. *69*:12, 1966.

Platelet Disorders

Adner, M. M., Fisch, G. R., Starobin, S. G., and Aster, R. H.: Use of "compatible" platelet transfusions in treatment of congenital isoimmune thrombocytopenic purpura. N. Engl. J. Med. *280*:244, 1969.

Anthony, B., and Krivit, W.: Neonatal thrombocytopenic purpura. Pediatrics *30*:776, 1962.

Ayromlooi, J.: A new approach to the management of immunologic thrombocytopenic purpura in pregnancy. Am. J. Obstet. Gynecol. *130*:235, 1978.

Baldini, M.: Idiopathic thrombocytopenic purpura. N. Engl. J. Med. *274*:1245, 1302, 1360, 1966.

Bleyer, W. A., and Breckenridge, R. T.: Studies in the detection of adverse drug reactions in the newborn. II. The effects of prenatal aspirin on newborn hemostasis. J.A.M.A. *213*:2049, 1970.

Chessells, J. M., and Wigglesworth, J.S.: Haemostatic failure in babies with rhesus isoimmunization. Arch. Dis. Child. *46*:38, 1971.

Corby, D. G., and Schulman, I.: The effects of antenatal drug administration on aggregation of platelets of newborn infants. J. Pediatr. *79*:307, 1971.

Corrigan, J. J.: Thrombocytopenia: a laboratory sign of septicemia in infants and children. J. Pediatr. *85*:219, 1974.

Duncan, W., and Halnan, K. E.: Giant hemangioma with thrombocytopenia. Clin. Radiol. *15*:224, 1964.

Fost, N. C., and Esterly, N. B.: Successful treatment of juvenile hemangiomas with prednisone. J. Pediatr. *72*:351, 1968.

Goodhue, P. A., and Evans, T. S.: Idiopathic thrombocytopenic purpura in pregnancy. Obstet. Gynecol. Surg. *18*:671, 1963.

Hall, J. G., Levin, J., Kuhn, J. P., Ottenheimer, E. J., Van Berkum, K. A. P., and McKusick, V. A.: Thrombocytopenia with absent radius. Medicine *48*:411, 1969.

Harrington, W. J., Sprague, C. C., Minnich, V., Moore, C. V., Aulvin, R. C., and Dubach, R.: Immunologic mechanisms in idiopathic and neonatal thrombocytopenic purpura. Ann. Intern. Med. *38*:433, 1953.

Karpatkin, M., Porges, R. F., and Karpatkin, S.: Platelet counts in infants of women with autoimmune thrombocytopenia. N. Engl. J. Med. *305*:936, 1981.

Kasabach, H. H., and Merritt, K. K.: Capillary hemangioma with extensive purpura. Report of a case. Am. J. Dis. Child. *59*:1063, 1940.

Kontras, S. B., Green, O. C., King, L., and Duran, R. J.: Giant hemangioma with thrombocytopenia; case report with survival and sequestration studies of platelets labeled with chromium 51. Am. J. Dis. Child. *105*:188, 1963.

Mauer, A. M., DeVaux, L. O., and Lahey, M. E.: Neonatal and maternal thrombocytopenic purpura due to quinine. Pediatrics *19*:84, 1957.

McIntosh, S., O'Brien, R. T., Schwartz, A. D., and Pearson, H. A.: Neonatal isoimmune purpura: response to platelet infusions J. Pediatr. *82*:1020, 1973.

McMillan, R.: Chronic idiopathic thrombocytopenic purpura. New Engl. J. Med. *304*:1145, 1981.

Merenstein, G. B., O'Loughlin, E. P., and Plunket, D. C.: Effects of maternal thiazides on platelet counts of newborn infants. J. Pediatr. *76*:766, 1970.

Nathan, D. J., and Snapper, I.: Simultaneous placental transfer of factors responsible for L.E. cell formation and thrombocytopenia. Am. J. Med. *25*:647, 1958.

Pearson, H. A., Shulman, N. R., Marder, V. J., and Cone, T. E.,
Jr.: Isoimmune neonatal thrombocytopenic purpura. Clinical and therapeutic considerations. Blood *23*:154, 1964.

Schulman, I.: Clinical Disorders of the Platelets. *In* Nathan, D. G., and Oski, F. A. (Eds.): Hematology of Infancy and Childhood. Philadelphia, W. B. Saunders Co., 1974, pp. 639–654.

Seip, M.: Systemic lupus erythematosus in pregnancy with haemolytic anaemia, leucopenia and thrombocytopenia in the mother and her newborn infant. Arch. Dis. Child. *35*:364, 1960.

Shulman, N. R., Marder, V. J., Hiller, M. C., and Collier, E. M.: Platelet and leukocyte isoantigens and their antibodies: Serologic, physiologic and clinical studies. Progr. Hematol. *4*:222, 1964.

Stuart, M. J.: Inherited defects of platelet function. Semin. Hematol. *12*:233, 1975.

65

Neonatal Leukocyte Disorders

By Bertil E. Glader

Leukocytes have a central role in host defense against infection. The pathophysiology of lymphocyte disorders is discussed in the section on Immunology (see Chapter 82). This chapter is mainly concerned with disorders of blood neutrophils. Many infants with granulocyte abnormalities have clinical problems in the newborn period. In most cases, however, the diagnosis of specific neutrophil disorders occurs after repeated infectious episodes, generally a few weeks to months after birth.

Normal Granulocyte Physiology

Development of myeloid cells into circulating neutrophils takes 6 to 10 days (Fig. 65–1). Approximately one third of bone marrow myeloid cells are in some phase of cell division (blasts, promyelocytes, myelocytes), while the remaining, more differentiated cells (metamyelocytes, bands, mature granulocytes) are maintained in a storage pool. Myeloid cells continue to mature in this storage pool, although they can be released if needed in the periphery. After release from the bone marrow, neutrophils are equally distributed between circulating cells and granulocytes marginated on the vascular wall. The peripheral blood count measures only circulating cells. Granulocytes remain in the circulation for less than 24 hours before being mobilized into peripheral tissues. It is here that neutrophils begin their major function, phagocytosis of bacteria.

The term phagocytosis includes several independent but related processes: chemotaxis, opsonization, ingestion, and intracellular killing (Fig. 65–2). *Chemotaxis* is the directed movement of neutrophils to areas of injury or bacterial infection. This is a metabolically dependent response of granulocytes to chemoattractants in peripheral tissues. Factors known to

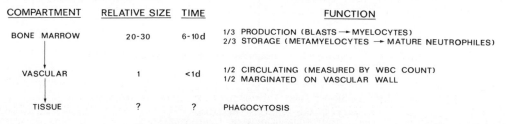

Figure 65–1. Neutrophil life cycle.

stimulate leukocyte migration include soluble bacterial products, complement components, and antigen-antibody complexes. In vivo, chemotaxis is assessed by sequential observation of cell migration into an abraded area of skin pretreated with chemoattractants such as DPT or typhoid vaccine (Rebuck skin window). Under these conditions, granulocytes initially appear within 3 to 6 hours, but by 12 hours monocytes predominate. In vitro, chemotaxis is evaluated by measuring the rate at which granulocytes traverse a filter that separates cells and chemotactically active material (Boyden chamber). This method is useful in determining what substances have chemotactic activity, but it is of questionable validity when used to compare chemotactic function of different granulocytes. Leukocyte migration through filters is a measure of several cell properties in addition to chemotactic responsiveness.

Opsonization is the process whereby bacteria are made more "edible" for phagocytes. The granulocyte ingestion of bacteria normally is a very slow process unless the bacterial membrane surface is first modified by various serum proteins. There are three fundamental modes of opsonization:

1. Rarely, increased concentrations of specific antibody alone can prepare bacteria for ingestion.

2. More commonly, opsonization follows the reaction of small amounts of antibody with complement proteins.

3. Opsonization can also occur by bacterial complement fixation in the presence of properdin proteins. This properdin-dependent, or "alternate," pathway is important, since it does not require antibody.

Ingestion is an active metabolic process in which the neutrophil membrane surrounds opsonized bacteria and forms an internalized vacuole, or phagosome. This ingestion-related movement (as well as chemotaxis itself) probably depends on contractile proteins. It has been suggested that reversible polymerization and depolymerization of neutrophil "actin" is responsible for this active motion.

Intracellular killing is the last stage of phagocytosis.

One of the essential reactions in this process is the generation of superoxide and hydrogen peroxide in the area of the phagosome. The specificity and intracellular location of the enzyme responsible for this reaction are not definitely known. An equally important process is the fusion of neutrophilic granules with the phagosome, following which digestive enzymes are thrust upon the enclosed bacteria. Neutrophils contain two types of granules. Primary granules are first noted in young myeloid cells (promyelocytes) and contain several hydrolytic enzymes, including myeloperoxidase. This enzyme potentiates the bactericidal effect of hydrogen peroxide. The secondary, or specific, granules develop in older cells (late myelocytes). These secondary lysosomal structures contain alkaline phosphatase in addition to other hydrolytic enzymes.

Granulocyte Physiology and Neonatal Infection

In older infants and children, the total and differential leukocyte count can be used to diagnose infection and frequently can help distinguish between bacterial and viral processes. During the neonatal period, wide variations in the quantity and distribution of leukocytes limit the utility of these simple laboratory measurements. The total white blood cell (WBC) count shortly after birth ranges from 10,000 to 30,000 per μl, owing mainly to an increase in neutrophils, bands, and metamyelocytes (Table 65–1). Occasionally, younger myeloid forms are seen also, particularly in premature infants. During the first week of life, the WBC count decreases (6000 to 15,000 per μl), immature myeloid cells disappear, and neutrophils decrease to a level that equals the number of lymphocytes. In view of these marked changes, physicians frequently ignore neonatal WBC counts in the diagnosis of infection, although this is a controversial topic currently under investigation in many centers. Xanthou has noted that the absolute neutrophil count (4000 to 7000 per μl) actually is quite stable in healthy infants after 72 hours of age. Furthermore, she observed that neonates with suspected or proved infection (after 3 days of age) manifested significant qualitative or quantitative neutro-

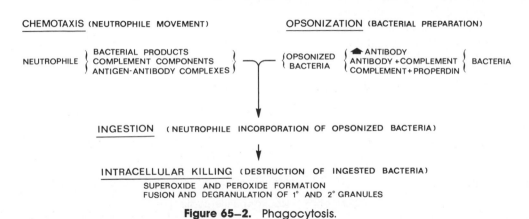

CHEMOTAXIS (NEUTROPHILE MOVEMENT)   OPSONIZATION (BACTERIAL PREPARATION)

NEUTROPHILE { BACTERIAL PRODUCTS / COMPLEMENT COMPONENTS / ANTIGEN-ANTIBODY COMPLEXES } { OPSONIZED BACTERIA } { ANTIBODY / ANTIBODY + COMPLEMENT / COMPLEMENT + PROPERDIN } BACTERIA

INGESTION (NEUTROPHILE INCORPORATION OF OPSONIZED BACTERIA)

INTRACELLULAR KILLING (DESTRUCTION OF INGESTED BACTERIA)
SUPEROXIDE AND PEROXIDE FORMATION
FUSION AND DEGRANULATION OF 1° AND 2° GRANULES

Figure 65–2. Phagocytosis.

Table 65–1. Leukocyte Values in Term and Premature Infants (10^3 Cells/μl)

Age (hrs)	Total WBC	Neutrophils	Bands/Metas	Lymphocytes	Monocytes	Eosinophils
Term infants						
0	10.0–26.0	5.0–13.0	0.4–1.8	3.5–8.5	0.7–1.5	0.2–2.0
12	13.5–31.0	9.0–18.0	0.4–2.0	3.0–7.0	1.0–2.0	0.2–2.0
72	5.0–14.5	2.0–7.0	0.2–0.4	2.0–5.0	0.5–1.0	0.2–1.0
144	6.0–14.5	2.0–6.0	0.2–0.5	3.0–6.0	0.7–1.2	0.2–0.8
Premature infants						
0	5.0–19.0	2.0–9.0	0.2–2.4	2.5–6.0	0.3–1.0	0.1–0.7
12	5.0–21.0	3.0–11.0	0.2–2.4	1.5–5.0	0.3–1.3	0.1–1.1
72	5.0–14.0	3.0–7.0	0.2–0.6	1.5–4.0	0.3–1.2	0.2–1.1
144	5.5–17.5	2.0–7.0	0.2–0.5	2.5–7.5	0.5–1.5	0.3–1.2

(Data modified from Xanthou, M.: Arch. Dis. Child. *45:*242, 1970.)

phil changes or both. Either the absolute granulocyte count was elevated above 7000/μl or there was an increased number of circulating immature myeloid cells. More recent studies suggest that serious neonatal sepsis most commonly is associated with neutropenia (Manroe et al. 1979; Christensen et al., 1981). Under these conditions, the absolute band count is not elevated, although the *ratio* of immature granulocytes to mature segmented cells is increased (Christensen et al., 1981). It also has been found that the sedimentation rate often increases with neonatal infection (Adler, 1975), and the activity of leukocyte alkaline phosphatase activity may be elevated in neonatal bacterial infections (Donato et al., 1979). Much also has been written about the histochemical nitroblue tetrazolium dye reduction test as an indicator of bacterial infection in older children and infants. It is now clear that this test is nonspecific and probably has little clinical significance in detecting the presence or absence of infection. *In summary, the best criteria for the diagnosis of infection remain appropriate cultures and good clinical judgment, with a high index of suspicion.* Other studies assessing the importance of qualitative granulocyte changes, however, may prove clinically useful.

Each stage of phagocytosis has been examined in neonatal granulocytes. The in vivo movement of neutrophils to an area of inflammation is normal, although there is a delay in the subsequent appearance of mononuclear cells. The clinical significance of this is not known. In vitro studies (Boyden chamber) suggest that chemotaxis is decreased in neonatal granulocytes. For the aforementioned reasons, however, it is not clear whether this reflects abnormal chemotaxis or merely some other physical property regulating neonatal neutrophil movement. Decreased opsonic activity of neonatal serum is one phagocytic abnormality on which there is general agreement. This may be due to decreased IgM, low complement levels (C3), or defects in the properdin pathway. Approximately 15 per cent of neonates are severely deficient in certain properdin proteins (see Chapter 82). Once bacteria are opsonized, neonatal granulocytes are capable of normal ingestion and intracellular killing.

Neutropenic Disorders

Neutropenia is defined as an absolute granulocyte count less than 1500 cells per μl. This may occur as a transient phenomenon associated with infection (discussed previously) or as a chronic process. The general mechanisms of neutropenia are the same as those that produce anemia and thrombocytopenia: decreased production and increased destruction or utilization. Viral infections are the most common cause of transient neutropenia, presumably due to suppression of normal myeloid production. This form of neutropenia is of little consequence. Bone marrow aplasia or neoplasia also can present as neutropenia, and for this reason bone marrow examinations are mandatory in all noninfected children with unexplained persistent neutropenia. Formerly we thought that a paucity of bone marrow myeloid precursors characterized production defects, whereas myeloid hyperplasia was seen in granulocytopenias due to increased peripheral destruction. Unfortunately, there are too many exceptions to this generalization, and we now consider the bone marrow as diagnostically useful only in those neutropenias due to aplasia or neoplastic invasion.

Table 65–2. Diagnostic Evaluation of Infants with Persistent Neutropenia

1. *Bone marrow examination*
   To rule out leukemia, neoplasm, and aplastic anemia
2. *Maternal neutrophil counts*
   To rule out maternal disease or drugs
3. *Neutrophil counts on family members*
   To rule out hereditary neutropenia
4. *Antineutrophil antibody determination*
   To rule out immune neutropenia
5. *Repeat neutrophil counts on baby (2 times per week for 1 month)*
   To rule out cyclic neutropenia

The spectrum of clinical severity in neutropenic children is extremely variable. Most children have no clinical problems, some manifest frequent infections of moderate severity, and a few develop serious life-threatening infections. The difference between children with mild disease and those with severe disease is related to the capacity for neutrophils to be mobilized at sites of infection, and this probably is a function of the absolute neutrophil count. Severe infections are unusual with consistent mean granulocyte levels greater than 500 cells per μl. At lower neutrophil levels, however, the frequency and severity of infections increase dramatically. The degree of monocytosis may be important also, since these macrophages can partially compensate for the loss of neutrophil phagocytic function.

In the absence of infection, no treatment for neutropenic children is indicated. Steroids have no role in the management of these disorders. If infection is present, however, vigorous antibiotic therapy with bactericidal drugs is indicated. In some children with severe neutropenia and frequent life-threatening infections with one particular organism, prophylactic antibiotic therapy may be indicated. There are many inherent difficulties with this approach, but unfortunately there are few therapeutic alternatives for some of these children. Granulocyte transfusions are effective in sepsis associated with leukemia and aplastic anemia but have not yet been systematically used in neonatal sepsis. One report of leukocyte transfusions used to treat neonatal sepsis suggests that this therapeutic modality may be efficacious (Laurenti et al., 1981). The remainder of this section summarizes the more common neonatal neutropenic syndromes.

ISOIMMUNE NEUTROPENIA

This disorder is the neutrophil equivalent of isoimmune thrombocytopenia and isoimmune anemia (ABO and Rh incompatibility). Fetal granulocytes possess an antigen not present on maternal neutrophils, and maternal sensitization results in antibody production against fetal granulocytes. Maternal neutrophils are not affected. The measurement of neutrophil antibodies is more difficult than the detection of antibodies in other isoimmune disorders. Consequently, these assays are done only in specialized laboratories. The clinical significance of antigranulocyte antibodies is not completely understood, since 20 to 25 per cent of all multiparous women have antineutrophil antibodies, yet neutropenia rarely is seen in these infants. The prognosis for infants with isoimmune neutropenia is very good, and severe infections are unusual. The granulocytopenia resolves as soon as the infant clears maternal antibody (6 to 12 weeks). An increase in the neutrophil count after this period of time also helps differentiate this isoimmune disorder from other nonimmune causes of neutropenia.

NEUTROPENIA ASSOCIATED WITH MATERNAL DISEASE

Antibodies that cause maternal neutropenia may passively cross the placenta and secondarily injure fetal granulocytes. Rare cases of maternal idiopathic neutropenia have been associated with neonatal granulocytopenia. Similarly, maternal lupus erythematosus has been implicated as a cause of immune neonatal neutropenia. In association with maternal systemic disease, however, anemia and thrombocytopenia frequently are present and usually are more important than any coexistent neutropenia.

IDIOPATHIC CONGENITAL NEUTROPENIA

This diverse group includes a number of poorly understood granulocytopenias that can occur as isolated entities or associated with other abnormalities. The most severe syndrome in this group is *congenital agranulocytosis*. Clinically this profound neutropenia is characterized by the neonatal onset of fulminant infections and early death. The bone marrow manifests marked myeloid hypoplasia, although rarely there are adequate early myeloid precursors. Some cases are familial. A rare and unusual variant of this disorder is known as *reticular dysgenesis*. Infants with this syndrome have no circulating neutrophils or lymphocytes. Similarly, the bone marrow contains no myeloid or lymphoid elements. All children reported with reticular dysgenesis have died within the first few weeks of life. Thymic atrophy and lymphocyte depletion of lymph nodes have been noted on autopsy.

In contrast to these severe idiopathic neutropenias, there is a group of disorders known as benign granulocytopenias. These disorders are benign in that infections are not life-threatening and some children may be completely asymptomatic. Rarely do these children have serious neonatal infections. In most cases, the bone marrow contains myeloid precursors, and the granulocytopenia is not as low as in the severe syndromes. Chronic granulocytopenia may be the only abnormality, or there may be additional clinical features: pancreatic insufficiency, inborn errors of metabolism, or immunoglobulin abnormalities. *Cyclic neutropenia* is another variant, characterized by a fluctuating granulocyte count that cycles every 21 days. At the nadir of this neutropenia, there frequently is an increased incidence of fevers and mild infections (stomatitis, gingivitis).

NEUTROPENIA SECONDARY TO DRUGS

Many drugs have been implicated in the etiology of neutropenia. Phenothiazines, antithyroid medications, and certain antibiotics (chloramphenicol, sulfonamides) have gained the most notoriety. A current list of drugs associated with neutropenia can be obtained from the Registry on Blood Dyscrasias of the Council on Drugs of the American Medical Association. Drugs should be considered in the etiology of any obscure neutropenia.

NEUTROPENIA DUE TO LEUKEMIA AND OTHER NEOPLASMS

Neutropenia in these conditions is secondary to invasion and destruction of normal bone marrow elements. In contrast to that in adults, chronic neutropenia in children rarely converts to leukemia.

Disorders of Leukocyte Function

Recurrent bacterial infections can occur in the presence of adequate numbers of circulating and bone marrow neutrophils. Most commonly, these infections are due to decreased serum opsonic activity caused by a lack of specific antibody (i.e., hypogammaglobulinemic states). Occasionally, abnormal granulocyte function itself is responsible. The diagnosis of neutrophil dysfunction syndromes rarely is made in the newborn period, although these infants frequently are infected. Some of these functional disorders are outlined subsequently.

LAZY LEUKOCYTE SYNDROME

This rare condition is characterized by recurrent fevers, frequent mild infections, and neutropenia. In contrast to most other neutropenias, however, the bone marrow contains normal numbers of all myeloid cells. The main functional defect in this disorder thus may be due to abnormal membrane deformability, which limits granulocyte release from the bone marrow. This is supported by the observation that neutrophils released into the circulation do not migrate normally in response to chemotactic stimulants in vitro (Boyden chamber). Serum opsonic activity, neutrophil ingestion, and intracellular killing are normal. The prognosis for children with this disorder is good.

NEUTROPHIL MUSCULAR DYSTROPHY

Another neutrophil mobility defect has been described (Boxer et al., 1974).

CASE 65–1

A 5-month-old male infant was admitted with recurrent infections of the skin, abdominal wall, and gastrointestinal tract. The infant's total leukocyte count was elevated (17,000 to 133,000), and most of the cells

were mature granulocytes. In spite of marked neutrophilia, pus never formed at sites of infection. Biopsies of infected areas contained necrotic tissue, histiocytes, and lymphocytes, but no granulocytes. It was of particular interest that pus was formed following therapeutic granulocyte transfusions. Neutrophil chemotaxis was abnormal in vitro (Boyden chamber) and in vivo (Rebuck skin window). Granulocyte ingestion also was abnormal. The other stages of phagocytosis were intact. The child's clinical condition deteriorated in spite of vigorous antibiotic therapy and granulocyte transfusions. A bone marrow transplant was attempted but was unsuccessful, and the patient died.

Comment. The unique motility defect in these granulocytes was attributed to an abnormality of neutrophil actin. The cell content of actin was normal, but the protein was qualitatively abnormal in that it manifested poor polymerization in vitro. As stated in the section on neutrophil physiology, reversible polymerization of actin is probably responsible for granulocyte movement associated with chemotaxis and ingestion.

CHRONIC GRANULOMATOUS DISEASE (CGD)

This rare hereditary disorder is characterized by recurrent granulomatous infections involving lymph nodes, skin, viscera, and bones. After the first few months of age hepatosplenomegaly is present. The peripheral blood neutrophil count and bone marrow are entirely normal. Chemotaxis is normal, ingestion is intact, and there are no opsonic defects. The fundamental abnormality in this condition is an inability of neutrophils to kill certain ingested bacteria (Holmes et al., 1967). Pathologically, the persistence of viable intracellular bacteria stimulates granulomata formation in tissues to which neutrophils are transported. The molecular basis for decreased intracellular killing is not completely understood, although it is related to reduced hydrogen peroxide production in the phagosome. When CGD granulocytes ingest latex particles coated with an enzyme that generates peroxide, the intracellular killing defect is corrected. This finding partially explains the spectrum of clinical infections in children with CGD. Severe problems commonly are due to *Staphylococcus aureus*, although infections also occur with *Klebsiella*, *Escherichia coli*, *Serratia marcescens*, and *Candida albicans*. Each of these microorganisms contains catalase, an enzyme potentially capable of destroying whatever small amounts of peroxide are formed in the phagosome. Infections with organisms lacking catalase are not a clinical problem; presumably, the trivial amount of peroxide present in CGD neutrophils is bactericidal for these agents. CGD is diagnosed by observing granulocyte inability to kill catalase-positive organisms or by failure of NBT reduction in circulating neutrophils. NBT dye reduction correlates with intracellular peroxide formation, and thus the diagnosis of CGD is one situation in which this screening test is useful. The clinical course of children with CGD is quite variable. No specific therapy is available to correct the intracellular lesion. In view of the predominance of staphylococcal infections, however, our patients currently are maintained on prophylactic dicloxacillin. There is no controlled datum to evaluate the efficacy of this therapy, but it is our impression that the frequency and intensity of infections are less. Chronic granulomatous disease is classically a sex-linked disorder affecting male children, although some cases may be autosomal recessive. In accord with the Lyon hypothesis, female carriers have both normal and abnormal neutrophils, and this is seen most clearly when the NBT slide test is performed. Clinically, female CGD carriers manifest no increased evidence of infection.

CHEDIAK-HIGASHI SYNDROME

This autosomal recessive disorder is characterized by oculocutaneous albinism, photophobia, and recurrent infections. During the course of disease, hepatosplenomegaly also develops. Most patients ultimately die from infection, although death is occasionally due to a lymphoma-like illness. Thrombocytopenia is frequently present. Anemia is rare. The total white blood cell count can be normal, but neutropenia is common in severe cases. The pathognomonic laboratory finding is the presence of large granules in granulocytes and lymphocytes. Within neutrophils, these giant lysosomal structures contain peroxidase activity, and thus represent abnormal primary granules. It has been observed that these giant lysosomes fail to degranulate their contents into phagocytic vacuoles at a normal rate, and intracellular killing of certain bacteria also is abnormal. In spite of these interesting findings, however, increased susceptibility to infections is correlated best with the degree of neutropenia. The relationship of granule abnormalities to rare malignant transformation is unknown.

Eosinophilia in Premature Infants

Eosinophilia (>500 eosinophils/μl blood) in older children is associated with allergy, drug reactions, parasitic infestations, immunodeficiency syndromes, collagen-vascular diseases, and adrenal insufficiency. Eosinophila also frequently is observed in premature infants, although the significance of this finding is unknown. Usually, there are no obvious explanations for this eosinophilia. A recent report suggests eosinophilia in premature infants may reflect a normal growth process, the onset of positive nitrogen balance (Gibson et al., 1979).

REFERENCES

Normal Granulocyte Physiology

Boggs, D. R.: The kinetics of neutrophilic leukocytes in health and disease. Semin. Hematol. 4:359, 1967.

Harris, M. C., Strovbant, J., Cody, C. S., Douglas, S. D., and Polin, R. A.: Phagocytosis of group B streptococcus by neutrophils from newborn infants. Pediatr. Res. 17:358, 1983.

Keller, H. U., Hess, M. W., and Cotlier, H.: Physiology of chemotaxis and random motility. Semin. Hematol. 12:47, 1975.

Klebanoff, S. J.: Antimicrobial mechanisms in neutrophilic polymorphonuclear leukocytes. Semin. Hematol. 12:117, 1975.

Rebuck, J. W., and Crowley, J. H.: A method of studying leukocyte function in vivo. Ann. N.Y. Acad. Sci. 59:757, 1951.

Stossel, T. P.: Phagocytosis. N. Engl. J. Med. 290:717, 1974.

Granulocyte Physiology and Neonatal Infection

Adler, S. M., and Denton, R. L.: Erythrocyte sedimentation rate in the newborn period. J. Pediatr. 86:942, 1975.

Christensen, R. D., Bradley, P. B., and Rothstein, G.: The leukocyte shift in clinical and experimental sepsis. J. Pediatr. 98:101, 1981.

Donato, H., Gebara, E., deCosen, R. H., and Gioseffi, O.: Leukocyte alkaline phosphatase activity in the diagnosis of neonatal bacterial infections. J. Pediatr. 94:242, 1979.

Gregory, J., and Hey, E.: Blood neutrophil response to bacterial infection in the first month of life. Arch. Dis. Child. 47:747, 1972.

Manroe, B. L., Weinberg, A. G., Rosenfeld, C. R., and Browne, R.: The neonatal blood count in health and disease. I. Reference values for neutrophilic cells. J. Pediatr. 95:89, 1979.

Miller, M. E.: Chemotactic function in the human neonate: humoral and cellular aspects. Pediatr. Res. 5:492, 1971.

Miller, M. E.: Phagocytosis in the newborn infant: humoral and cellular factors. J. Pediatr. 74:255, 1969.

Nathan, D. G.: NBT reduction by human phagocytes. N. Engl. J. Med. 290:280, 1974.

Steigbigel, R. T., Johnson, P. K., and Remmington, J. S.: The nitroblue tetrazolium reduction test versus conventional hematology in the diagnosis of bacterial infection. N. Engl. J. Med. 290:235, 1974.

Xanthou, M.: Leukocyte blood picture in healthy full-term and premature babies during neonatal period. Arch. Dis. Child. 45:242, 1970.

Xanthou, M., Tsomides, K., Nicolopoulos, D., and Matsaniotis, N.: Leukocyte blood picture in newborn babies during and after exchange transfusion. Pediatr. Res. 6:59, 1972.

Neutropenic Disorders

Ackerman, B. D.: Dysgammaglobulinemia: Report of a case with a family history of a congenital gamma globulin disorder. Pediatrics 34:211, 1964.

de Vaal, O. M., and Seynhaseve, V.: Reticular dysgenesis. Lancet 2:1123, 1959.

Gitlin, D., Vawter, G., and Craig, J. M.: Thymic alymphoplasia and congenital aleukocytosis. Pediatrics 33:184, 1964.

Good, R. A., and Zak, S. J.: Disturbances in gamma globulin synthesis as "experiments of nature." Pediatrics 18:109, 1956.

Hanson, J. W., and Smith, D. W.: The fetal hydantoin syndrome. J. Pediatr. 87:285, 1975.

Huguley, C. M., Jr.: Drug-induced blood dyscrasias. II. Agranulocytosis. J.A.M.A. 188:817, 1964.

Kauder, E., and Mauer, A. M.: Neutropenias of childhood. J. Pediatr. 69:147, 1966.

Kostmann, R.: Infantile genetic agranulocytosis (agranulocytosis infantilis hereditaria). A new recessive lethal disease in man. Acta Paediatr. (suppl. 105) 45:1, 1956.

Lalezari, P., Nussbaum, M., Gelman, S., and Spaet, T. H.: Neonatal neutropenia due to maternal isoimmunization. Blood 15:236, 1960.

Laurenti, F., Ferro, R., Isacchi, G., Panero, A., Savignoni, P. G., Malagnino, F., Palermo, D., Mandelli, F., and Bucci, G.: Polymorphonuclear leukocyte transfusion for the treatment of sepsis in the newborn infant. J. Pediatr. 98:118, 1981.

Page, A. R., and Good, R. A.: Studies on cyclic neutropenia. A clinical and experimental investigation. A.M.A. J. Dis. Child. 94:623, 1957.

Payne, R.: Neonatal neutropenia and leukoagglutinins. Pediatrics 33:194, 1964.

Shwachman, H., Diamond, L. K., Oski, F. A., and Khaw, K-T.: The syndrome of pancreatic insufficiency and bone marrow dysfunction. J. Pediatr. 65:645, 1964.

Disorders of Leukocyte Function

Baehner, R. L., and Johnston, R. B., Jr.: Chronic granulomatous disease: correlation between pathogenesis and clinical findings. Pediatrics 48:730, 1971.

Baehner, R. L., Nathan, D. G., and Karnovsky, M. L.: Correction of the metabolic deficiencies in the leukocytes of patients with chronic granulomatous disease. J. Clin. Invest. 49:860, 1970.

Blume, R. S., and Wolff, S. M.: The Chediak-Higashi syndrome: studies in four patients and a review of the literature. Medicine 51:247, 1972.

Boxer, L. A., Hedley-Whyte, E. T., and Stossel, T. P.: Neutrophil actin dysfunction and abnormal neutrophil behavior. N. Engl. J. Med. 291:1093, 1974.

Holmes, B., Page, A. R., and Good, R. A.: Studies of the metabolic activity of leukocytes from patients with a genetic abnormality of phagocyte function. J. Clin. Invest. 46:1422, 1967.

Johnston, R. B., Jr., and Baehner, R. L.: Improvement of leukocyte bactericidal activity in chronic granulomatous disease. J. Clin. Invest. 49:860, 1970.

Klebanoff, S. J.: Intraleukocytic microbicidal defects. Ann. Rev. Med. 22:39, 1971.

Miller, M. E.: Pathology of chemotaxis and random mobility. Semin. Hematol. 12:59, 1975.

Miller, M. E., Oski, F. A., and Harris, H. B.: Lazy-leukocyte syndrome. A new disorder of neutrophil function. Lancet 1:665, 1971.

Quie, P. G.: Pathology of bactericidal power of neutrophils. Semin. Hematol. 12:143, 1975.

Eosinophilia in Premature Infants

Gibson, E. L., Vaucher, Y., and Corrigan, J. J.: Eosinophilia in premature infants: relationship to weight gain. J. Pediatr. 95:99, 1979.

66

Erythrocyte Disorders in Infancy

By Bertil E. Glader

Normal Erythrocyte Physiology in the Fetus and Neonate

FETAL ERYTHROPOIESIS

Fetal erythropoiesis occurs in three different sites: yolk sac, liver, and bone marrow. Yolk sac formation of RBCs is maximal between the second and tenth weeks of gestation. The liver is a major site of erythropoiesis between the tenth and twenty-sixth weeks of gestation. Myeloid, or bone marrow, production of red blood cells begins around the eighteenth week, and by the thirtieth week of fetal life bone marrow is the major erythropoietic organ. At birth, almost all RBCs are produced in the bone marrow, although a low level of hepatic erythropoiesis persists through the first few days of life. Sites of fetal erythropoiesis are occasionally reactivated in older patients with hematologic disorders such as myelofibrosis, aplastic anemia, and severe hemolytic anemia.

Red blood cell production in extrauterine life is controlled in part by erythropoietin, a humoral erythropoietic stimulating factor (ESF) produced by the kidney. The role of erythropoietin in the developing fetus has not been completely defined. Current thoughts are that ESF does not influence yolk sac or hepatic erythropoiesis, but it may partially regulate myeloid RBC production (Finne and Halvorsen, 1972). Erythropoietic stimulating factor is detected in fetal blood and amniotic fluid during the last trimester of pregnancy. The concentration of this hormone increases directly with the period of gestation, and thus, erythropoietin levels in term neonates are significantly higher than in premature infants. This difference may reflect some degree of fetal hypoxia during late intrauterine life. Increased ESF titers also are seen in placental dysfunction, fetal anemia, and maternal hypoxia (Finne, 1966). Fetal RBC formation is not influenced by maternal erythropoietin, since transfusion-induced maternal polycythemia (decreased maternal ESF levels) has no effect on fetal erythropoiesis (Jacobson et al., 1959). Maternal nutritional status also is not a significant factor in the regulation of fetal erythropoiesis, since iron, folate, and vitamin B_{12} are trapped by the fetus irrespective of maternal stores. Most studies have demonstrated that women with severe iron deficiency bear children with normal total body hemoglobin content (Lanzkowsky, 1961).

Hemoglobin, hematocrit, and RBC count increase throughout fetal life (Table 66–1). Extremely large RBCs (MCV 180) with an increased hemoglobin content (MCH 60) are produced early in fetal life. The size and hemoglobin content of these cells decrease throughout gestation, but the concentration of hemoglobin (MCHC) does not change significantly. Even at birth, the MCV and MCH are larger than those seen in older children and adults. Many nucleated RBCs and reticulocytes are present early in gestation, and the percentage of these cells also decreases as the fetus ages.

Hemoglobin production increases markedly during the last trimester of pregnancy. The actual hemoglobin concentration increases, but, more importantly, body weight, blood volume, and total body hemoglobin triple in size during this period. Fetal iron accumulation parallels the increase in total body hemoglobin content. The neonatal iron endowment at birth, therefore, is directly related to total body hemoglobin content and length of gestation. Term infants have more iron than prematures.

RBC PHYSIOLOGY AT BIRTH

In utero, fetal blood (umbilical vein) is approximately 50 per cent saturated with oxygen. This relative hypoxia may be responsible for the increased content of erythropoietin and signs of active erythropoiesis (nucleated RBCs, increased reticulocytes) seen in neonates at birth. When lungs become the source of oxygen, hemoglobin-O_2 saturation increases to 95 per cent, and erythropoiesis decreases. Within 72 hours of age, erythropoietin is undetectable, nucleated RBCs disappear, and reticulocytes decrease to less than 1 per cent.

The concentration of hemoglobin during the first few hours of life increases to values greater than those seen in cord blood. This is a relative increase due to a reduction in plasma volume (Gairdner et al., 1958) and an absolute increase due to placental blood transfusion (Usher et al., 1963). The umbilical vein remains patent long after umbilical arteries have constricted, and thus transfusion of placental blood occurs when neonates are held at a level below the placenta. The placenta contains approximately 100 ml of fetal blood (30 per cent of the infant's blood volume). Approximately 25 per cent of placental blood enters the neonate within 15 seconds of birth, and by 1 minute, 50 per cent is transfused. The time of cord clamping is thus a direct determinant of neonatal blood volume. The blood volume of term infants (mean of 85 ml per kg) varies considerably (50 to 100 ml per kg) because of different degrees of placental transfusion (Usher et al., 1963). These differences are readily apparent when the effects of early versus delayed cord clamping are compared at 72 hours of age: 82.3 ml per kg (early clamping) versus 92.6 ml per kg (delayed clamping). These changes are largely due to differences in RBC mass (early clamping 31 ml per kg, delayed clamping 49 ml per kg). The blood volume of premature infants (89 to 105 ml per kg) is slightly greater than that of term infants, but in large part this is due to an increased plasma volume (Usher and Lind, 1965). The RBC mass of premature infants is the same as in term neonates.

FETAL AND NEONATAL HEMOGLOBIN FUNCTION

A variety of hemoglobins are present during fetal and neonatal life (see discussion under Hemoglobinopathies). Fetal hemoglobin (Hgb F) is the major hemoglobin in utero, whereas hemoglobin A is the normal hemoglobin of extrauterine life. Both are present in the same cell, but the relative proportion of each varies with gestational and postnatal age. One major difference between hemoglobins A and F is related to oxygen transport.

The transport of oxygen to peripheral tissues is regulated by several factors, including blood oxygen ca-

Table 66–1. Mean Red Cell Values During Gestation

Age (Weeks)	Hb (gm/dl)	Hematocrit (%)	RBC (10^6/mm³)	Mean Corpusc. Vol. (fl)	Mean Corpusc. Hb (pg)	Mean Corpusc. Hb Conc. (gm/dl)	Nuc. RBC (% of RBCs)	Retic. (%)	Diam. (μ)
12	8.0–10.0	33	1.5	180	60	34	5.0–8.0	40	10.5
16	10.0	35	2.0	140	45	33	2.0–4.0	10–25	9.5
20	11.0	37	2.5	135	44	33	1.0	10–20	9.0
24	14.0	40	3.5	123	38	31	1.0	5–10	8.8
28	14.5	45	4.0	120	40	31	0.5	5–10	8.7
34	15.0	47	4.4	118	38	32	0.2	3–10	8.5

(From Oski, F. A., and Naiman, J. L.: Hematologic Problems in the Newborn. 3rd ed. Philadelphia, W. B. Saunders Co., 1982.)

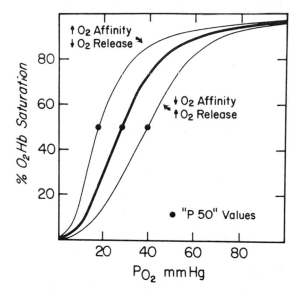

Figure 66–1. The oxygen dissociation curve of normal adult hemoglobin (dark line). The per cent oxygen saturation (ordinate) is plotted for arterial oxygen tensions between 0 and 100 mm Hg (abscissa). As the curve shifts to the right, more oxygen is released at any given P_{O_2}. Conversely, as the curve shifts to the left, more oxygen is retained on hemoglobin at any given P_{O_2}. The "P 50" refers to that P_{O_2} where hemoglobin is 50 per cent saturated with oxygen. This term is useful in comparing the oxygen affinity of different hemoglobins. (Oski, F. A., and Delivoria-Papadopoulos, M.: J. Pediatr. *77*:941, 1970.)

DPG to any significant extent (Bauer et al., 1968); consequently, cells containing hemoglobin F have a higher oxygen affinity than those containing hemoglobin A.

The increased oxygen affinity of fetal RBCs is obviously advantageous for extracting oxygen from maternal blood within the placenta. A few months after birth, however, infant blood acquires the same oxygen affinity as that of older children (Fig. 66–2). The postnatal decrease in O_2 affinity is due to a reduction in hemoglobin F and an increase in hemoglobin A (which interacts with 2,3-DPG). It is an interesting fact that oxygen delivery (the difference in arterial and venous O_2 content) actually increases while oxygen capacity (hemoglobin concentration) decreases during the first week of life (Fig. 66–3). This enhanced delivery is largely a reflection of the decreased oxygen affinity of infant blood (Delivoria-Papadopoulos et al., 1971). The oxygen affinity of blood from premature infants is higher than that of term infants, and the normal postnatal changes (decrease in oxygen affinity, increase in oxygen delivery) occur much more gradually in prematures (Fig. 66–3).

pacity, cardiac output, and hemoglobin-oxygen affinity. (1) Oxygen capacity is a direct function of hemoglobin concentration (1 gm hemoglobin combines with 1.34 ml oxygen). (2) Compensatory changes in cardiac output can maintain normal O_2 delivery under conditions in which oxygen capacity is significantly reduced. (3) The oxygen affinity of hemoglobin also influences oxygen delivery to tissues. Hemoglobin A is 95 per cent saturated at arterial oxygen tensions (100 mm Hg), but this decreases to 70 to 75 per cent saturation at a venous P_{O_2} of 40 mm Hg. The difference in O_2 content at arterial and venous oxygen tensions reflects the amount of oxygen that can be released. Changes in hemoglobin affinity for oxygen can influence O_2 delivery (Fig. 66–1). At any given P_{O_2}, more oxygen is bound to hemoglobin when oxygen affinity is increased. Stated in physiologic terms, increased hemoglobin-oxygen affinity reduces oxygen delivery, whereas decreased hemoglobin-oxygen affinity increases oxygen release to peripheral tissues.

The oxygen affinity of hemoglobin A in solution is greater than that for hemoglobin F. Paradoxically, however, whole blood from normal children (Hgb A) has a lower oxygen affinity than neonatal blood (Hgb F) (Allen et al., 1953). This difference is related to an intermediate of RBC metabolism known as 2,3-diphosphoglycerate (2,3-DPG). This organic phosphate compound interacts with hemoglobin A to decrease its affinity for oxygen and thereby enhance O_2 release. Fetal hemoglobin does not interact with 2,3-

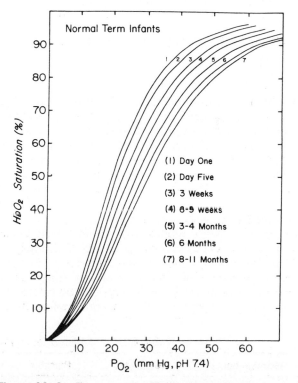

Figure 66–2. The oxygen affinity of blood from term infants at birth and at different postnatal ages. The gradual rightward shift of the oxygen saturation curve indicates increased oxygen release from hemoglobin as infants get older. This decreased oxygen affinity is due to a decrease in hemoglobin F and an increase in hemoglobin A. (Oski, F. A., and Delivoria-Papadopoulos, M.: J. Pediatr. *77*:941, 1970.)

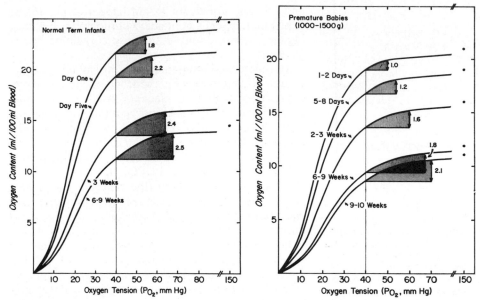

Figure 66–3. Oxygen delivery in normal term and premature infants. Oxygen content (a function of total hemoglobin) is on the ordinate. Oxygen tension is on the abscissa. Oxygen delivery is measured by the difference in oxygen content at arterial (100 mm Hg) and venous (40 mm Hg) oxygen tensions. For both term and premature infants, oxygen delivery (shaded areas) increases with age. This occurs in spite of a decrease in oxygen content. (Delivoria-Papadopoulos, M., Roncevic, N. P., and Oski, F. A.: Pediatr. Res. 5:235, 1971.)

General Approach to Anemic Infants

Medical History and Physical Examination. The etiology of anemia frequently can be ascertained by medical history and physical examination. Particular importance is given to family history (anemia, cholelithiasis, unexplained jaundice, splenomegaly), maternal medical history (especially infections), and obstetric history (previous pregnancies, length of gestation, method and difficulty of delivery). The age at which anemia becomes manifest also is of diagnostic importance. Significant anemia at birth invariably is due to blood loss or isoimmune hemolysis. After 24 hours, internal hemorrhages and other causes of hemolysis become manifest. Anemia that appears several weeks after birth can be caused by a variety of conditions, including abnormalities in the synthesis of hemoglobin-beta chains, hypoplastic RBC disorders, and the physiologic anemia of infancy or prematurity.

Infants with chronic blood loss anemia may appear pale, without other evidence of clinical distress. Acute blood loss can produce hypovolemic shock and a clinical state similar to severe neonatal asphyxia. Neonates with hemolytic anemia frequently show a greater than expected degree of icterus. In addition, hemolysis often is associated with hepatosplenomegaly, and in cases due to congenital infection other stigmata may be present.

Laboratory Evaluation of Anemia. A simple classification of neonatal anemia based on physical examination and simple laboratory tests is presented in Table 66–2.

RBC Count, Hemoglobin, Hematocrit, and RBC Indices. Red blood cell values during the

Table 66–2. Differential Approach to Anemia in Newborn Period

Hemoglobin	Reticulocytes	Bilirubin	Coombs' Test	Clinical Considerations
Decreased	Normal/decreased	Normal	Negative	Physiologic anemia of infancy/prematurity Hypoplastic anemia
Decreased	Normal/increased	Normal	Negative	Hemorrhagic anemia
Decreased	Normal increased	Increased	Positive	Immune-mediated hemolysis
Decreased	Normal/increased	Increased	Negative	Acquired or hereditary RBC defects Enclosed hemorrhage with resorption of blood Coombs'-negative ABO incompatibility

neonatal period are more variable than at any other time of life. The diagnosis of anemia must therefore be made in terms of "normal" values appropriate for an infant's gestational and postnatal age. The mean cord blood hemoglobin of healthy term infants ranges between 14 and 20 gm per 100 ml (Table 66–3). Shortly after birth, however, hemoglobin concentration increases. This increase is both relative (owing to a reduction of plasma volume) and absolute (owing to placental RBC transfusion). Failure of hemoglobin to increase during the first few hours of life may be the initial sign of hemorrhagic anemia. RBC values at the end of the first week are virtually identical with those seen at birth. Anemia during the first week of life is thus defined as any hemoglobin less than 14 gm per 100 ml. A significant hemoglobin decrease during this time, although within the normal range, is suggestive of hemorrhage or hemolysis. For example, 14.5 gm hemoglobin at 7 days of age is abnormal for a term infant whose hemoglobin was 18.5 gm at birth. A slight hemoglobin reduction normally occurs in premature infants during the first week. Beyond the first week, however, the hemoglobin concentration decreases in both term and premature infants (see Physiologic Anemia of Infancy and Prematurity).

The electronic equipment currently used for blood counts also gives statistical information regarding erythrocyte size (mean corpuscular volume [MCV] and hemoglobin content (mean corpuscular hemoglobin [MCH]). The normal MCV ($\mu\mu$) in older children ranges from 75 to 90. Mean corpuscular volumes less than 75 are considered microcytic, whereas those over 100 indicate macrocytosis. Normal infant RBCs are large (MCV 105 to 125), and not until 8 to 10 weeks of age does cell size approach that of older children. Neonatal microcytosis is defined as an MCV less than 95 at birth. The RBC hemoglobin content of neonatal cells (MCH 35 to 38) is greater than that seen in older children (MCH 30 to 33). Neonatal hypochromia is defined as an MCH less than 34. Hypochromia and microcytosis generally occur together, and invariably these abnormalities are due to hemoglobin production defects. Neonatal hypochromic microcytosis is seen with iron deficiency (chronic blood loss, late anemia of prematurity) and

thalassemia disorders (alpha and gamma thalassemias).

The site at which blood is obtained is important, since peripheral stasis leads to higher hemoglobin concentrations in capillary blood compared with simultaneously obtained central venous samples. This difference can be minimized by warming an extremity to obtain "arteriolized capillary blood" (Oh and Lind, 1966). In the face of acute hemorrhage, however, central venous samples must be obtained because of marked peripheral vasoconstriction.

Reticulocyte Count. The normal reticulocyte count of children and older infants is 1 to 2 per cent. The reticulocyte count in term infants ranges between 3 to 7 per cent at birth, but this decreases to 1 to 3 per cent by 4 days and to less than 1 per cent by 7 days of age (Table 66–3). In prematures, reticulocyte values at birth are higher (6 to 10 per cent) and may remain elevated for a longer period of time. Nucleated red blood cells are seen in newborn infants, but they generally disappear by the third day of life in term infants and in 7 to 10 days in premature infants. The persistence of reticulocytosis or nucleated RBCs suggests the possibility of hemorrhage or hemolysis. Hypoxia, in the absence of anemia, also can be associated with increased release of reticulocytes and nucleated RBCs.

Peripheral Blood Smear. Examination of the peripheral blood smear is an invaluable aid in the diagnosis of anemia. In particular, the smear is evaluated for alterations in the size and shape of RBCs as well as abnormalities in leukocytes and platelets. Erythrocytes of older children are approximately the size of a small lymphocyte nucleus, whereas those of neonates are slightly larger. Red blood cell hemoglobinization (e.g., hypochromia) is estimated by observing the area of central pallor, which is one third the diameter of normal RBCs and over one half the diameter of hypochromic cells. Spherocytes are detected by the complete absence of central pallor. The degree of reticulocytosis can be estimated, since these cells are larger and have a bluish coloration

Table 66–3. RBC Values in Term and Premature Infants During First Week of Life

	Hgb (gm/100 ml)	Hct (%)	Reticulocytes (%)	Nucleated RBCs (cells/1000 RBCs)
Term				
Cord blood	17.0 (14–20)	53.0 (45–61)	<7	<1.00
Day 1	18.4	58.0	<7	<0.40
Day 3	17.8	55.0	<3	<0.01
Day 7	17.0	54.0	<1	0
Premature (less than 1500 gm)				
Cord blood	16.0 (13.0–18.5)	49	<10	<3.00
Day 7	14.8	45	<3	<0.01

(due to RNA) when viewed in the blood smear. In order to obtain good peripheral smears in neonates, one should dilute high hematocrit blood (1:1) in saline.

Serum Bilirubin. Bilirubin is a normal breakdown product of hemoglobin (see Chapter 68). In cases of hemolytic anemia (increased RBC destruction), bilirubin levels are increased to above normal neonatal levels. Hyperbilirubinemia is not seen with anemia caused by external hemorrhage, although resorption of blood from large enclosed hemorrhages can produce icterus.

Haptoglobin. This glycoprotein binds free hemoglobin, and the hemoglobin-haptoglobin complex is cleared from the circulation. Decreased serum haptoglobin is a sign of hemolysis in older children, but it is not a useful measurement in neonates, since haptoglobin is normally decreased at this time of life. Normal haptoglobin levels generally are present by 1 month of age.

Coombs' Test. The vast majority of neonatal hemolytic anemias are due to isoimmunization. The Coombs' test detects the presence of antibody on RBCs (direct Coombs') or in the plasma (indirect Coombs'). One must search diligently to rule out an isoimmune disorder before embarking on a more esoteric workup of hemolysis.

Blood Transfusions in the Treatment of Anemia. A hemoglobin of 15 gm per 100 ml corresponds to an RBC mass of 30 ml per kg. This implies that a transfusion of 2 ml RBC per kg will increase the hemoglobin concentration 1 gm per 100 ml. Packed RBCs (hematocrit approximately 67 per cent) contain 2 ml of RBC per 3 ml packed RBC. Whole blood (hematocrit approximately 33 per cent) contains 2 ml RBC per 6 ml whole blood. Thus, the transfusion of 3 ml packed RBC per kg or 6 ml whole blood per kg will increase hemoglobin concentration 1 gm per 100 ml.

EXAMPLE. *A 3.5-kg infant with a hemoglobin of 6.5 gm per 100 ml is to be transfused to a hemoglobin of 12.0 gm per 100 ml. The difference between the desired and present hemoglobin is 5.5 gm per 100 ml. The volume of packed RBCs to be administered is 58 ml (3.5 kg × 5.5 gm per 100 ml hemoglobin difference × 3 ml packed RBC per kg). Alternatively, 116 ml whole blood will produce the same hemoglobin increase.*

Whenever possible, packed RBCs should be used in order to avoid fluid volume overload. Whole blood (or packed RBCs reconstituted with fresh-frozen plasma), however, is the therapy of choice for large acute hemorrhages, since this blood loss usually is associated with hypovolemia (see discussion under Hemorrhagic Anemia). Infants with hemolytic disorders occasionally need RBC replacement therapy, although exchange transfusions are usually required if there is significant hyperbilirubinemia. Fresh whole blood can be used for exchange transfusions, although packed RBCs reconstituted with fresh frozen plasma are more commonly utilized.

Blood currently available in most blood banks is anticoagulated with acid-citrate-dextrose (ACD) or citrate-phosphate-dextrose (CPD). The use of CPD blood is now more common and is preferred for several reasons: (1) The pH of CPD blood is less acidic than ACD blood. (2) The level of 2,3-DPG is maintained better in CPD, and therefore oxygen delivery of these RBCs presumably is greater. (3) Red blood cell potassium loss is less in CPD stored blood, and this decreases the risk of hyperkalemia when older bank blood is transfused.

It is well known that in utero infection with cytomegalovirus can cause damage to the fetus. It now also is apparent that blood transfusions can produce serious CMV infections in premature infants. In a recent study, it was observed that 24 per cent of infants born to CMV seronegative mothers (hemagglutinin titers less than 1:8) developed CMV infection when the neonates were transfused with red blood cells from donors who were CMV seropositive (hemagglutinin titer greater than 1:8) (Yeager et al., 1981). These investigators also observed that 50 per cent of these CMV infections were either "serious or fatal." Most importantly, however, no CMV infection was detected in neonates born to CMV seronegative mothers when the infants were transfused with CMV seronegative red blood cells. The use of RBCs from CMV seronegative donors did not reduce the incidence of CMV infection in neonates born to mothers who were CMV seropositive; however, the overall-nursery excretion of cytomegalovirus decreased significantly when CMV seronegative blood products were utilized. This important study, which suggests that neonates should receive CMV seronegative blood products, has major implications related to the future of neonatal transfusion therapy. In all likelihood, a policy statement regarding this matter will be considered by the American Association of Blood Banks in the near future.

Graft-versus-host (GVH) disease rarely follows intrauterine blood transfusions for severe erythroblastosis (Naiman et al, 1969; Parkman, et al., 1974). This is presumably due to transfusion of viable lymphocytes into immunologically incompetent fetuses. There is no current evidence that direct or exchange transfusion of neonates leads to GVH disease. Theoretically, however, some small premature infants (30 to 32 weeks' gestation) may be unable to reject foreign lymphocytes in transfused blood. Whether blood given to small premature infants should be irradiated prior to administration, however, remains to be determined.

Hemorrhagic Anemia

Anemia frequently follows fetal blood loss, bleeding from obstetric complications, and internal hemorrhages associated with birth trauma. The clinical

Fetal hemorrhage
  Spontaneous fetomaternal hemorrhage
  Hemorrhage following amniocentesis
  Twin-twin transfusion

Placental hemorrhage
  Placenta previa
  Abruptio placentae
  Multilobed placenta (vasa previa)
  Velamentous insertion of cord
  Placental incision during cesarean section

Umbilical cord bleeding
  Rupture of umbilical cord with precipitous delivery
  Rupture of short or entangled cord

Postpartum hemorrhage
  Bleeding from umbilicus
  Cephalhematomas, scalp hemorrhages
  Hepatic rupture, splenic rupture
  Retroperitoneal hemorrhages

presentation of anemia depends on the magnitude and acuteness of blood loss.

Infants with anemia subsequent to moderate hemorrhage or chronic blood loss are generally asymptomatic. The only physical findings are pallor of the skin and mucous membranes. Laboratory studies can range from a mild normochromic-normocytic anemia (hemoglobin 9 to 12 gm per 100 ml) to a more severe hypochromic-microcytic anemia (hemoglobin 5 to 7 gm per 100 ml). The only therapy required for asymptomatic children is iron (2 mg elemental iron per kg, t.i.d. for 3 months). RBC replacement is indicated only if there is evidence of clinical distress (tachycardia, tachypnea, irritability, feeding difficulties). In most cases, raising the hemoglobin to 10 to 12 gm per 100 ml will remove all signs and symptoms due to anemia. Since severely anemic infants are frequently in incipient heart failure, however, these children should be transfused very slowly (2 ml per kg per hr). If signs of congestive heart failure appear, a rapid-acting diuretic (furosemide, 1 mg per kg intravenously) should be given before proceeding with the transfusion. An alternative approach is to exchange transfuse severely anemic infants with packed RBCs for anemic whole blood. This increases the hemoglobin concentration without the danger of increasing blood volume and precipitating congestive heart failure.

Infants who rapidly lose large volumes of blood appear in acute distress (pallor, tachycardia, tachypnea, weak pulses, hypotension, and shock). This presentation is distinct from that seen in neonatal respiratory asphyxia (slow respirations with intercostal retractions, bradycardia, and pallor with cyanosis). The clinical response to assisted ventilation and oxygen is also different: Infants with respiratory problems manifest a marked improvement, whereas there is little change in anemic neonates. Cyanosis is not a feature of severe anemia because the hemoglobin concentration is too low (clinical cyanosis indicates at least 5 gm per 100 ml of deoxygenated hemoglobin). The hemoglobin concentration immediately after an acute hemorrhage may be normal, since the initial response to acute volume depletion is vasoconstriction. A decreased hemoglobin may not be seen until the plasma volume has re-expanded several hours later. In view of these hemodynamic considerations, it is apparent that the diagnosis of acute hemorrhagic anemia is based largely on physical findings and evidence of blood loss. It is important to recognize these clinical features, for immediate therapy is required. Treatment is directed at rapid expansion of the vascular space (20 ml fluid per kg). The ideal fluid is cross-matched and type-specific packed RBCs reconstituted with fresh-frozen plasma, although this is usually not available in most emergency situations. Group O, Rh-negative blood that is not cross-matched can be given as an alternative. If no blood is available, other plasma expanders (plasma, saline with albumin, dextran) should be given. An additional 10 ml per kg of packed RBCs should be administered as soon as it is available. This procedure usually improves the clinical status of infants with hypovolemia due to fetal blood loss. Neonates with serious internal hemorrhages, however, generally show a poor response.

FETAL HEMORRHAGE

Fetomaternal Hemorrhage. Significant bleeding into the maternal circulation occurs in approximately 8 per cent of all pregnancies and thus represents one of the most common forms of fetal bleeding. Small amounts of fetal blood are lost in most cases, but in 1 per cent of pregnancies fetal blood loss may be as great as 40 ml (Cohen et al., 1964). Fetomaternal hemorrhage occasionally follows amniocentesis and placental injury (Zipursky et al., 1963), although anemia is seen only after unsuccessful amniocentesis or when there is evidence of a bloody tap (Woo Wang et al., 1967). For this reason, infants born to mothers who have had amniocentesis should be observed closely for signs of anemia. The effects of anemia due to fetomaternal hemorrhages are quite variable. Large acute hemorrhages can produce hypovolemic shock (Raye et al., 1970), whereas slower, more chronic blood loss results in hypochromic microcytic anemia due to iron deficiency (Pearson and Diamond, 1959). Some infants with severe chronic anemia (hemoglobin as low as 4 to 6 gm per 100 ml) may have minimal symptoms. An examination of the maternal blood smear for the presence of fetal cells (Kleihauer-Betke preparation) is necessary in any infant with suspected fetomaternal hemorrhage. (For details of this procedure see Oski and Naiman, Hematologic Disorders of the Newborn, W. B. Saunders Co., 1982, page 63.) This test is based on the principle that hemoglobin A is eluted from RBCs at an acid pH, whereas hemoglobin F is not affected by these conditions. Consequently, when alcohol-fixed and acid-treated RBCs are stained with eosin, those containing hemoglobin A are colorless, whereas those containing hemoglobin F (fetal RBCs) appear normally colored (Table 66–5). Approximately 50 ml of fetal blood must be lost to produce significant neonatal anemia. This volume is greater than 1 per cent of the maternal blood volume, and therefore fetal cells within the maternal circulation may be detected quite readily. This test is not valid when there is coexistence of maternal hemoglobinopathies with increased hemoglobin F levels. In addition, fetal-maternal ABO incompatibility may cause rapid removal of fetal RBCs and thus obscure any significant hemorrhage. For this reason, it is important to examine maternal blood as soon as anemia due to fetal hemorrhage is suspected.

Twin–Twin Transfusion. Transfusion of blood from one homozygous twin to another can result in anemia in the donor twin and polycythemia in the recipient. Significant hemorrhage is seen only in monochorionic monozygous twins (approximately 70 per cent of all monozygous twins). In approximately 15 per cent of these pregnancies, there is a twin-to-twin transfusion (Rausen et al., 1965). Bleeding occurs because of vascular anastomosis in monochorionic placentas. The anemic donor twin is usually smaller than the polycythemic recipient. Polyhydramnios is frequently seen in the recipient twin and oligohydramnios is seen in the donor. Twin-to-twin transfusions should be suspected when the hemoglobin concentration of identical twins differs by more than 5 gm per 100 ml.

PLACENTAL BLOOD LOSS

Placental bleeding during pregnancy is quite common, but in most cases hemorrhage is from the maternal aspect of the placenta. In placenta previa, however, the thin placenta overlying the cervical os frequently results in fetal blood loss. The vascular communications between multilobular placental lobes are also very fragile and are easily subjected to trauma during delivery. Vasa previa is the condition in which one of these connecting vessels overlies the cervical os and thus is prone to rupture during delivery. The perinatal death rate in vasa previa may be

greater than 50 per cent. Abruptio placentae generally causes fetal anoxia and death, although surviving infants can be severely anemic. Bleeding also follows inadvertent placental incision during cesarean sections (Montague and Krevans, 1966), and thus the placenta should be inspected for injury following all cesarean sections.

UMBILICAL CORD BLEEDING

The normal umbilical cord is resistant to minor trauma and does not bleed. The umbilical cord of dysmature infants, however, is weak and liable to rupture and hemorrhage (Raye et al., 1970). In cases of precipitous delivery, a rapid increase in cord tension can rupture the fetal aspect of the cord and cause serious acute blood loss. Short or entangled umbilical cords and abnormalities of umbilical blood vessels (velamentous insertions into the placenta) are also liable to rupture and hemorrhage. Bleeding from injured umbilical cords is rapid but generally ceases after a short period of time, owing to arterial constriction. The umbilical cord should always be inspected for abnormalities or signs of injury, particularly after unattended, precipitous deliveries.

CASE 66–1

A 2950-gm white male infant was born by vaginal delivery to a gravida 1, para 0, white female at 38 weeks' gestation. Vaginal bleeding was excessive at the time of delivery, and inspection of the cord and placenta revealed a velamentous insertion of umbilical vessels into the placenta. The infant's Apgar score was 7, although he was pale and manifested moderate tachycardia and tachypnea. There were no intercostal retractions or cyanosis. Spleen and liver were not palpable. The hemoglobin concentration of blood from the umbilical vein was 13.4 gm per 100 ml. Bilirubin was 2.3. The infant was transfused with 60 ml of type-specific whole blood, following which his color improved and cardiac and respiratory status returned to normal. Eight hours after the blood transfusion, the infant's hemogloblin was 14.4 gm per 100 ml. The subsequent clinical course was unremarkable, and no further transfusions were required.

Comment. Physical findings and a history of excessive bleeding at birth suggested some degree of blood loss. The nearly normal hemoglobin concentration at birth probably was due to immediate va-

Table 66–5. Comparative Clinical Findings in Neonatal Respiratory Distress and Acute Hemorrhage

	Neonatal Asphyxia	Acute Blood Loss
Heart rate	Decreased	Increased
Respiratory rate	Decreased	Increased
Intercostal retractions	Present	Absent
Skin color	Pallor with cyanosis	Pallor without cyanosis
Response to oxygen and assisted ventilation	Marked improvement	No significant change

soconstriction associated with loss of blood volume. Transfusion with whole blood certainly improved the infant's clinical state, although the increase in hemoglobin was less than expected. A 60-ml transfusion of whole blood (20 ml per kg) should increase hemoglobin concentration around 3 gm per 100 ml. Failure to see this increase presumably was due to the initial vasoconstriction and subsequent vascular expansion following whole-blood transfusion. This case clearly demonstrates the dramatic response to blood transfusion given to neonates with moderate but self-limited blood loss.

POSTPARTUM HEMORRHAGE

Hemorrhagic anemia due to internal bleeding is occasionally associated with birth trauma. Characteristically, internal hemorrhages are asymptomatic during the first 24 to 48 hours of life, with signs and symptoms of anemia developing after this time. Cephalhematomas can be sufficiently large to cause anemia and hyperbilirubinemia, owing to the resorption of blood (Leonard and Anthony, 1961). Scalp hemorrhages ("hemorrhagic caput") also can produce severe anemia (Pachman, 1962). These hemorrhages are frequently more extensive than cephalhematomas, since bleeding is not limited by periosteum. Adrenal and kidney hemorrhages occasionally follow difficult breech deliveries. Splenic rupture and hemorrhage occur most commonly in association with splenomegaly, as in erythroblastosis fetalis (Philipsborn et al., 1955). Hepatic hemorrhages are generally subcapsular and many be asymptomatic. Rupture of the hepatic capsule results in hemoperitoneum and hypovolemic shock. Hepatic hemorrhages are suspected when a previously healthy infant goes into shock with clinical manifestations of an increasing right upper quadrant abdominal mass, shifting dullness on percussion, and evidence of free fluid on abdominal radiographs. In contrast to neonates with acute blood loss due to fetomaternal or umbilical vessel bleeding, infants with hepatic hemorrhage generally demonstrate a poor clinical response to blood replacement. Exploratory laparotomy is usually required for confirmation of diagnosis and possible repair of the hemorrhagic site.

HEMOLYTIC ANEMIA

Red blood cells from children and adults normally circulate for 100 to 120 days. Erythrocyte survival in neonates is somewhat shorter: 70 to 90 days in term infants, 50 to 80 days in prematures (Pearson, 1967). Hemolytic anemia is the clinical consequence of RBC abnormalities leading to shorter than normal erythrocyte survival. The precise mechanism of cell destruction is not known, although membrane deformability is thought to be an important determinant (LaCelle, 1970). Erythrocytes are 7 to 8 micrometers wide, whereas the vascular diameter in some areas

Table 66–6. Hemolytic Anemia During the Newborn Period

Immune
  Isoimmune: Rh and ABO incompatibility
  Maternal immune disease: autoimmune hemolytic anemia, systemic lupus erythematosus
  Drug induced: penicillin

Acquired RBC disorders
  Infection: CID, toxoplasmosis, syphilis, bacterial sepsis
  Disseminated and localized intravascular coagulation, respiratory distress syndrome

Hereditary RBC disorders
  Membrane defects: hereditary spherocytosis, hereditary elliptocytosis
  Enzyme abnormalities: G6PD, pyruvate kinase
  Hemoglobinopathies: alpha-thalassemia syndromes, gamma/beta–thalassemia

of the microcirculation may be less than 3. Consequently, RBCs must deform their membranes and intracellular contents in order to pass through these narrow channels. This is no problem for normal RBCs. Abnormalities in RBC metabolism, hemoglobin, or cell shape, however, all lead to decreased RBC membrane deformability. The consequence of this decreased membrane flexibility is RBC sequestration and removal by reticuloendothelial cells of the spleen and liver.

In older infants and children, the usual response to increased RBC destruction is enhanced erythropoiesis, and there may be little or no anemia if the rate of production matches the accelerated rate of destruction. In these cases of well-compensated hemolysis, the major manifestations are due to increased erythrocyte destruction (hyperbilirubinemia) and augmented erythropoiesis (reticulocytosis). During the early neonatal period, however, increased oxygen-carrying capacity of blood (see Physiologic Anemia of Infancy) may obviate any compensatory erythropoietic activity in cases of mild hemolysis. Consequently, hyperbilirubinemia in excess of normal neonatal levels may be the only apparent manifestation of hemolysis. In most cases of significant hemolysis, however, some degree of reticulocytosis is usually present. The degree of hyperbilirubinemia and reticulocytosis obviously must be interpreted in terms of values appropriate for gestational and postgestational age.

Therapeutic Considerations for Infants With Hemolytic Disease

As for older children and adults, the general therapeutic principles for neonates with hemolytic disease include maintenance of normal oxygen delivery (adequate levels of circulating hemoglobin) and rectification of causative hemolytic factors (treatment of infection, removal of hemolytic drugs, etc.). An additional important therapeutic consideration is prevention of kernicterus. This condition is a clinical consequence of increased unconjugated bilirubin levels, transport of "free" bilirubin (not bound to albumin) across the blood-brain barrier, and bilirubin-staining of the cerebellum and basal ganglia. The molecular explanation for bilirubin toxicity in neural tissue is not understood. Kernicterus generally does not occur at bilirubin levels less than 20 mg/dl, although numerous factors modify this (acidosis, low serum albumin, prematurity, etc.), and serious problems can occur at lower bilirubin concentrations. It should be noted, however, that hyperbilirubinemia is not a problem for erythroblastotic fetuses, since bilirubin is effectively cleared by the placenta and maternal liver. Since normal infant bilirubin levels may reach 12 to 15 mg/dl, the increased bilirubin load due to hemoglobin degradation (1 gm hemoglobin = 34 mg bilirubin) may further aggravate the "physiologic" hyperbilirubinemia. Clinical features of kernicterus include lethargy, poor feeding, loss of Moro reflex, high-pitched crying, and spasms leading to opisthotonos. Once these clinical signs of kernicterus appear, over 75 per cent of affected infants die. Surviving infants have problems ranging from moderate hearing loss to spastic diplegia, choreoathetosis, and mental retardation. Thus, to prevent kernicterus, one should attempt to keep bilirubin levels reduced. This is accomplished by two different procedures: exchange transfusion and phototherapy.

Exchange transfusion is an effective means of reducing serum bilirubin concentration and removing potential sources of bilirubin (i.e., red blood cells). The usual two-volume exchange transfusion effectively removes 85 per cent of circulating RBCs, although the resultant serum bilirubin decrease is less than expected from the removed blood volume. This discrepancy reflects that bilirubin is distributed in both extracellular fluid and intracellular compartments. During exchange transfusion, bilirubin rapidly equilibrates between blood and interstitial fluids, but there is a much slower bilirubin redistribution between tissues and extracellular fluid. Consequently, there commonly is a "rebound" increase in bilirubin within 30 to 60 minutes after an exchange transfusion. Exchange transfusion is much more effective for removing "potential bilirubin" than for lowering the actual serum bilirubin concentration, and, thus, it is important to consider early exchange transfusion for those neonatal conditions in which persistent RBC destruction is likely (i.e., hemolysis due to Rh incompatibility).

Phototherapy is the second means available for reducing serum bilirubin concentration. This therapy is based on the principle that light (450 to 460 nm) and oxygen convert bilirubin to water-soluble degradation products that are excreted in bile and urine.

These photodegradation products are relatively nontoxic and do not cause or influence the development of kernicterus. Occasional mild complications of phototherapy include transient bronze skin discoloration, skin rashes, and frequent loose stools. The rate of light-induced bilirubin oxidation is relatively slow, and thus the value of this procedure is limited to conditions associated with mild hyperbilirubinemia. It has proved particularly effective in the hyperbilirubinemia of prematurity and, in mild cases of ABO incompatibility, and as an adjuvant procedure following exchange transfusions. It should not be used as the initial treatment for marked hyperbilirubinemia or when significant RBC destruction is likely. Also, once phototherapy is instituted, it is necessary to monitor the serum bilirubin concentration closely, since photo-oxidation nullifies the use of "jaundice" as a clinical sign of hyperbilirubinemia.

IMMUNE HEMOLYSIS

The most common cause of neonatal hemolysis is transplacental passage of maternal antibodies that injure fetal erythrocytes. Maternal antibodies generally are directed against specific antigens on fetal RBCs, and thus hemolysis occurs only in the fetus. Occasionally, autoimmune maternal antibodies produce hemolysis in both mother and neonate.

Rh Hemolytic Disease ("Erythroblastosis Fetalis"). The role of the Rh antibody in classic erythroblastosis fetalis was first elucidated in 1941 by Levine and Katzin. It is now recognized that the Rh antigen is a large protein molecule with several antigenic sites and that each of these antigens reflects a specific chemical or structural protein characteristic. There are several recognized Rh antigens (C, c, D, E, e), each of which is detected by specific antibodies. The most important of these is the D antigen, and RBCs possessing this antigen are Rh-positive. The symbol "d" (used to denote the absence of D, or Rh-negative) is not a specific antigen, since no anti-d serum has been identified. Proteins are produced under the direction of paired chromosomes, and thus red blood cell Rh proteins have two determinants of each antigen (CC, cc, or Ce; DD, dd, or Dd; and EE, ee, or Ee). Individuals with DD or dD are considered Rh-positive, whereas those with dd are Rh-negative. The frequency of the Rh-negative genotype varies in different racial groups. It is high in whites (15 per cent), lower in American blacks (5 per cent), and virtually nonexistent in Orientals. The frequency of Rh-incompatible matings in Caucasians is relatively high (85 per cent Rh-positive × 15 per cent Rh-negative = 12.5 per cent, or one of every eight matings).

The pathophysiology of isoimmune hemolysis due to Rh incompatibility includes the following: (1) an Rh-negative mother, (2) an Rh-positive fetus, (3) leakage of fetal RBCs into maternal circulation, (4) maternal sensitization to D antigen on fetal RBCs, (5) produc-lion and transplacental passage of maternal anti-D antibodies into fetal circulation, (6) attachment of maternal antibodies to Rh-positive fetal RBCs, and (7) destruction of antibody-coated fetal RBCs. Rh hemolytic disease is rare (1 per cent) during the first pregnancy involving an Rh-positive fetus, but the likelihood of having an affected infant increases with each subsequent pregnancy. The first pregnancy generally is characterized by maternal sensitization to fetal RBCs. Small volumes of fetal RBCs enter the maternal circulation throughout gestation, although the major fetal-maternal bleeding responsible for sensitization occurs during delivery (Zipursky et al., 1963) (see disucssion of prevention of Rh sensitization further on). In those cases in which significant hemolysis occurs during the first pregnancy, it is thought that earlier isoimmunization may have occurred with previous abortions (Lee et al., 1969), ruptured tubal pregnancies (Katz and Marcus, 1972), amniocentesis (Misenheimer, 1966), or transfusion with Rh-positive blood. Also, it recently has been suggested that Rh-negative girls born to Rh-positive mothers may be sensitized at birth as a result of maternal-fetal hemorrhage (i.e., penetration of maternal RBCs into fetal circulation (Bowen and Renfield, 1976). Regardless of the mechanism of initial sensitization, small amounts of fetal blood that enter the maternal circulation during subsequent pregnancies are sufficient to elicit an anamnestic response. The initial maternal response is production of IgM anti-D, and this subsequently is followed by the formation of IgG anti-D. The titer of IgM anti-D (detected by RBC agglutination in saline) and IgG anti-D (detected by agglutination with Coombs' serum) can be followed in maternal serum. Since IgM antibodies do not cross the placenta, however, only the concentration of IgG anti-D is important. With elevated IgG antibody titers, there is an increased likelihood of neonatal hemolytic disease.

The clinical severity of Rh erythroblastosis is variable (Table 66–7) but ultimately depends on the

quantity of maternal antibody that binds to fetal RBCs. In general, the clinical course is mild, moderate, or severe (Bowman, 1975).

Mild Hemolytic Disease. Approximately 50 per cent of affected infants with a positive direct Coombs' test have a minimal hemolysis manifested by no anemia (cord blood hemoglobin greater than 14 gm/dl) and minimal hyperbilirubinemia (cord blood bilirubin less than 4 mg/dl). These neonates generally do not require specific therapy unless the postnatal bilirubin rise is greater than expected (Fig. 66–4). In some of these infants, however, the persistence of maternal antibody may result in an exaggerated "physiologic anemia" at 2 to 3 months of age.

Moderate Hemolytic Disease. In approximately 25 per cent of affected infants there is significant hemolysis, as manifested by mild to moderate anemia (cord blood hemoglobin less than 14 gm/dl) and increased cord blood bilirubin levels (greater than 4 mg/dl). The peripheral blood of moderately affected neonates may contain numerous nucleated RBCs, decreased numbers of platelets, and, occasionally, a leukemoid reaction with marked numbers of immature granulocytes. The etiology of thrombocytopenia is not understood, but it is unlikely that it is due to an immune reaction, since platelets lack the Rh antigen. Similarly, the cause of leukemoid reactions is not defined, although these rarely may be of such a magnitude as to be confused with congenital leukemia. Infants with leukemoid reactions also may manifest marked hepatosplenomegaly, a consequence of several factors: extramedullary hematopoiesis, sequestration of antibody-coated RBCs, and reticuloendothelial hyperplasia. This group of neonates will develop kernicterus if not treated, and thus early exchange transfusion with type-specific Rh-negative fresh RBCs is mandatory. There is minimal morbidity and mortality from this procedure, and clearly it has been responsible for the favorable outcome of this group of infants with moderate isoimmune hemolysis. It is not uncommon for neonates treated with exchange transfusion to manifest a lower than normal hemoglobin at the nadir of their physiologic anemia. This may reflect the decreased P 50 and enhanced oxygen delivery of adult RBCs utilized for the exchange process.

Severe Hemolytic Disease. A significant fraction of remaining affected infants (25 per cent) have more severe disease and are either stillborn or hydropic at birth. The etiology of fetal death and hydrops is related to anemia-induced cardiac failure. In addition, there usually is some degree of hypoproteinemia (Driscoll, 1966). Therapy for these seriously affected fetuses is directed at prevention of severe anemia and death. In order to accomplish this, it is first necessary to identify the "severely" affected fetus and then institute appropriate therapy.

Table 66–7. Clinical and Laboratory Features of Isoimmune Hemolysis Due to Rh Disease and ABO Incompatibility

	Rh Disease	ABO Incompatibility
Clinical Features		
Frequency	Unusual	Common
Pallor	Marked	Minimal
Jaundice	Marked	Minimal to moderate
Hydrops	Common	Rare
Hepatosplenomegaly	Marked	Minimal
Laboratory Features		
Blood type		
Mother	Rh($-$)	O
Infant	Rh($+$)	A or B
Anemia	Marked	Minimal
Direct Coombs' test	Positive	Frequently negative
Indirect Coombs' test	Positive	Usually positive
Hyperbilirubinemia	Marked	Variable
RBC morphology	Nucleated RBCs	Spherocytes

As discussed previously, elevated maternal titers of IgG anti-D will detect those pregnancies associated with isoimmune disease. Unfortunately, however, elevated maternal antibody titers do not clearly distinguish between mild and severe fetal hemolytic disease. A better indicator of fetal jeopardy has been the measurement of amniotic fluid bilirubin. The bilirubin concentration in amniotic fluid normally is very low (0.1 mg/dl), and this decreases further as gestation progresses. Even in cases of severe erythroblastosis, the bilirubin concentration rarely exceeds 0.8 mg/dl, and this also may decrease as pregnancy proceeds. In view of these difficulties in accurately measuring low bilirubin levels, a more sensitive technique has been employed in which the absorption of amniotic fluid is measured spectrophotometrically at different wavelengths (from 350 nm to 700 nm) (Liley, 1963). Normally, the optical density of amniotic fluid increases linearly as the wavelength decreases. In the presence of increased bilirubin levels, however, there is increased absorption (deviation from linearity) at a wavelength of 450 nm (Fig. 66–4). Furthermore, it has been established that the magnitude of increased absorption at 450 nm can reliably predict the probability of severe fetal erythroblastosis (Liley, 1963). This is true in spite of the fact that the absolute change in amniotic fluid optical density decreases throughout gestation. The current indications for amniocentesis include a previous history of neonatal hemolytic disease and an increased maternal anti-D antibody titer determined by the indirect Coombs' test. In the absence of these criteria, amniocentesis should not be performed, since small fetal-maternal hemorrhages frequently occur, and these can lead to sensitization or increased antibody production or both. It is important to identify "high-risk" fetuses early in pregnancy, since over 50 per cent of stillborns occur before 32 weeks' gestation. Currently, it is recommended that initial amniocentesis be performed at 22 weeks' gestation. If the fetus is found to be in the "minimal-risk" category, amniocentesis should be repeated in 2 weeks. Once a "high-risk" fetus is identified, therapeutic intervention is required (Bowman, 1975).

Two therapeutic approaches are possible: early induction of labor or intrauterine RBC transfusions. After 30 to 32 weeks' gestation, induction of early labor can salvage 60 per cent of erythroblastoic fetuses destined to be stillborn if pregnancy were continued to term (Bowman, 1975). Depending on the stage of gestation, however, premature infants may be subject to other serious consequences, the major problem being the respiratory distress syndrome (hyaline membrane disease). In order to determine the probability of this complication, one can assess fetal lung maturation by measuring the lecithin:sphingomyelin ratio in amniotic fluid (Gluck et al., 1971). If this ratio indicates that fetal lung ma-

turation is adequate, premature delivery should be induced. For those severely affected fetuses who cannot be delivered early because of low gestational age (less than 32 weeks) or a low lecithin:sphingomyelin ratio or both, the only possible therapy is intrauterine RBC transfusions. This procedure has proved effective in salvaging many fetuses with all the indications of severe hemolytic anemia in utero (Liley, 1963). The principle of this technique is based on the observation that RBCs injected into the peritoneal cavity are absorbed by the lymphatic system and effectively enter the circulating blood volume. Details of the specific procedures and complications of intrauterine transfusions are found in several review articles (Bowman, 1975). One general protocol is as follows: 50 ml packed RBCs (80 per cent hematocrit, Rh-negative cells) are administered at 24 weeks' gestation, 110 ml RBCs are given at 30 weeks, and subsequent transfusions are given every 2 weeks until delivery. Since Rh-negative RBCs replace fetal erythrocytes, affected infants often are born with a negative Coombs' test and little, if any, fetal hemoglobin. In spite of this, severe hyperbilirubinemia commonly

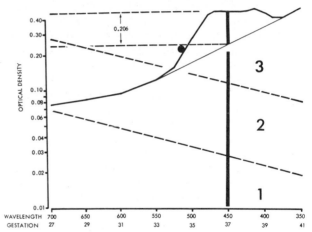

Figure 66–4. This composite graph depicts how spectrophotometric estimation of amniotic fluid bilirubin levels can be utilized as an indicator of fetal jeopardy from hemolytic disease. (1) The optical density of amniotic fluid (ordinate) is measured from 700 to 350 nm (abscissa—top). This absorption curve is depicted as the heavy solid line. (2) The contribution of bilirubin to this absorption is then calculated by subtracting the optical density of the projected baseline (fine solid line) from the measured optical density at 450 nm. In this case, the calculated value is 0.206. (3) This calculated contribution of bilirubin is then plotted as a function of gestational age (abscissa—bottom). In this particular patient, the gestational age of 34.5 weeks and the bilirubin absorption of 0.206 determine the point indicated by the solid dot. (4) The dashed lines demarcate three zones (1, 2, and 3): Zone 1 indicates an Rh negative infant or very mild hemolytic disease. Zone 2 indicates mild to moderate hemolytic disease. Zone 3 represents severe hemolytic disease with impending fetal death. Since the bilirubin concentration of amniotic fluid decreases with gestational age, the absolute optical density that places a fetus in zone 3 decreases as the length of gestation increases. In the case depicted here, an absorption of 0.206 at 34.5 weeks' gestation indicated this fetus was in zone 3 and thus seriously at risk. (From Bowman, J. M., and Pollock, J. M.: Pediatrics 35:815, 1965.)

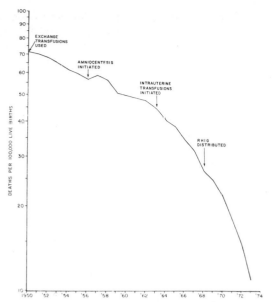

Figure 66–5. Infant death rates from hemolytic disease of the newborn, United States, 1950 to 1973. (From Center for Disease Control: Rh Hemolytic Disease Surveillance Annual Report, June 1975, with kind permission.)

occurs (owing to destruction of newly formed RBCs), and exchange transfusions generally are required.

As seen in Figure 66–5, neonatal exchange transfusion, amniocentesis, selective-early induction of delivery, and intrauterine fetal blood transfusions all have reduced the neonatal death rate from Rh incompatibility. Without question, however, the major factor responsible for reduced death rate has been the advent of immune therapy to prevent maternal sensitization. Approaches toward this goal initially were based on two separate observations: (1) The bulk of fetal-maternal RBC transfer (and presumably sensitization) occurs during delivery. (2) The frequency of Rh immune hemolytic disease is much lower in ABO incompatible pregnancies (maternal RBC type O, fetal RBC type A or B). The beneficial effect of ABO incompatibility presumably is mediated by maternal isoantibodies that cause the destruction of fetal RBCs before sensitization occurs. On the basis of these observations, attempts were made to prevent maternal sensitization by injection of immune-globulin–containing antibodies to the "Rh-positive antigen (anti-D)." Several years later, it is now well established that the administration of such an immune globulin within 74 hours of delivery effectively reduces maternal sensitization to less than 1 per cent of all pregnancies at risk (Freda et al., 1975). Failure to achieve 100 per cent effectiveness is due to sensitization earlier in gestation or to the occurrence of large fetal-maternal bleeds not adequately treated with the standard (300 μg anti-D) dose of gamma globulin. In addition to administering anti-Rh globulin to all Rh-negative mothers shortly after delivery, one should, according to current recommendations, give immune globulin to females at risk following abortions (Freda et al., 1975). The beneficial effects of immune globulin therapy earlier in gestation also are under evaluation (Bowman, 1975).

ABO Incompatibility. Hemolysis associated with ABO incompatibility is similar to Rh hemolytic disease in that maternal antibodies enter the fetal circulation and react with A or B antigens on the erythrocyte surface (Table 66–7). In type A and B individuals, naturally occurring anti-B and anti-A isoantibodies largely are IgM molecules that do not cross the placenta. In contrast, the isoantibodies present in type O individuals are predominantly IgG molecules (Abelson and Rawson, 1961). For this significant reason, ABO incompatibility is largely limited to type O mothers with type A or B fetus. The presence of IgG anti-A or anti-B antibodies in type O mothers also explains why hemolysis due to ABO incompatibility frequently occurs during the first pregnancy without prior "sensitization." A set-up for ABO incompatibility is present in approximately 12 per cent of pregnancies, although red blood cell–antibody reactions (i.e., positive direct Coombs' test) are found in only 3 per cent of births, and less than 1 per cent of live-births are associated with significant hemolysis (Zipursky et al., 1963; Kaplan et al., 1976).

The relative mildness of neonatal ABO hemolytic disease contrasts sharply with the findings in Rh incompatibility. In large part, this is because A and B antigens are present in many tissues besides RBC; consequently, only a small fraction of anti-A or anti-B antibody that crosses the placenta actually binds to erythrocytes, the remainder being absorbed by other tissues.

Although ABO incompatibility is clinically milder than Rh disease, severe hemolysis occasionally occurs, and hydrops fetalis has been reported. In most cases, infants are minimally pale and jaundiced (Table 66–7). Hepatosplenomegaly is uncommon. Laboratory features include minimal to moderate hyperbilirubinemia and, occasionally, some degree of anemia. The direct Coombs' test frequently is negative, although the indirect Coombs' test (neonatal serum plus type-specific adult RBCs) more commonly is positive. This paradox is related to the fact that adult RBCs, compared with neonatal erythrocytes, have more type-specific antigen on their surface (Voak and Williams, 1971). The peripheral blood smear is characterized by marked spherocytosis, which is thought to be due to the reduced RBC surface area that results as antibody and membrane are removed by splenic macrophages. Autoimmune hemolytic anemia in older children is associated with antibodies directed against the Rh locus, and these cases also are characterized by spherocytosis. For unknown reasons, however, spherocytes are not a prominent feature of neonatal hemolysis due to Rh incompatibility.

Mild cases of ABO incompatibility generally require phototherapy, whereas exchange transfusion is indicated with more severe hemolysis (Fig. 66–4). In some cases of ABO incompatibility not treated with exchange transfusion, the persistence of maternal antibody may be responsible for prolonged low-grade hemolysis and an exaggerated physiologic anemia of infants at 8 to 12 weeks of age. In view of the generally mild clinical course of ABO incompatibility, amniocentesis is not indicated.

Minor Blood Group Incompatibility. Approximately 1 per cent of all cases of isoimmune hemolysis are due to other RBC antigens (Kell, Duffy and Luthern, etc.). The pathophysiology of these disorders is similar to that of Rh and ABO incompatibility. The infrequency of minor group incompatibility is primarily a reflection of the relatively reduced antigenicity of these RBC antigens. Diagnosis of minor group incompatibility is suggested by Coombs'-positive hemolytic anemia in the absence of ABO or Rh incompatibility and a negative maternal direct Coombs' test. Definitive diagnosis requires identification of the specific antibody in neonatal serum or an eluate from neonatal RBCs. This is readily accomplished by testing serum against a variety of known RBC antigens. Maternal serum should contain elevated titers of the antibody in question.

Immune Hemolytic Anemia Due to Maternal Disease. Maternal autoimmune hemolytic anemia (AIHA) during pregnancy may be associated with passive transfer of IgG antibody to the fetus. The degree of hemolysis in the fetus depends largely on amount and the specificity of transferred antibody. In one review of 19 cases of maternal AIHA, four infants were stillborn, three infants had severe postnatal hemolysis, and the remaining 12 were normal (Chaplin et al., 1973). Autoimmune hemolytic anemia also occurs with connective tissue disorders such as lupus erythematosus and rheumatoid arthritis. In these cases, maternal antibody may not be specific for red cells, and immune neutropenia or thrombocytopenia or both also occur (Seip, 1960). The diagnosis of neonatal hemolysis is suggested by the presence of Coombs'-positive neonatal hemolytic disease, lack of set-up for Rh or ABO incompatibility, and Coombs'-positive hemolysis in the mother. Treatment with prednisone (2 mg/kg/day) may reduce both maternal hemolysis and neonatal morbidity. As in other cases of neonatal hemolysis, attempts are made to prevent hyperbilirubinemia and kernicterus.

Drug-Induced Immune Hemolysis. The classic example of drug-induced immune hemolysis is seen with penicillin and appears when an antibody is directed to a complex of penicillin bound to the red blood cell membrane. No hemolysis occurs in the absence of penicillin, even though antibody persists in the circulation. This type of drug-mediated immune hemolysis has been reported in newborn infants. In a mother who had a penicillin antibody but who was not on penicillin, neonatal hemolysis occurred when the infant was given penicillin (Clayton et al.). The Coombs' test in these cases may be positive only when the test is done in the presence of penicillin. Hemolysis ceases once the drug is withdrawn.

NONIMMUNE ACQUIRED HEMOLYTIC DISEASE

Infection. Cytomegalic inclusion disease, toxoplasmosis, syphilis, and bacterial sepsis all can be associated with hemolytic anemia. In most of these conditions, some degree of thrombocytopenia also exists. Generally, there is hepatosplenomegaly. In cases of bacterial sepsis, both the direct and indirect bilirubin may be elevated. The mechanism of hemolysis is not clearly defined, but it may be related to RBC sequestration in the presence of marked reticuloendothelial hyperplasia associated with infection. Documentation of infection as the cause of hemolysis is made by the presence of other clinical and laboratory stigmata of neonatal infections. Hemolysis due to infections may present early in the neonatal period, or it can be delayed for several weeks.

Disseminated Intravascular Coagulation. This coagulation abnormality is discussed in detail elsewhere (see p. 566). The hemolytic component of this disorder is secondary to the deposition of fibrin within the vascular walls. When erythrocytes interact with fibrin, fragments of RBCs are broken off, producing fragile, deformed red blood cells, or schistocytes. These cells are relatively rigid and thus incapable of normal deformation within the microcirculation. The hemolytic-uremic syndrome represents a localized form of intravascular coagulation that is characterized by thrombocytopenia, renal disease, and hemolytic anemia. Hemolysis is characterized by RBC fragmentation, presumably for the aforementioned reasons.

HEREDITARY RBC DISORDERS

Membrane Defects. Several RBC membrane abnormalities are associated with hemolytic anemia, but aside from hereditary spherocytosis (HS) these disorders are relatively uncommon.

Hereditary Spherocytosis

This is an autosomal dominant disorder manifested by the presence of spherocytic RBCs. Spherocytes are characterized by a decreased membrane surface area to volume ratio. The volume (MCV) of HS red blood cells is relatively normal, and thus it is thought that spherocytes result from a decrease in membrane surface area. In fact, it has been established that HS erythrocytes lose membrane lipid during their life span. Spherocytes in vitro are susceptible to osmotic lysis (i.e., the release of hemoglobin when RBCs swell in hypotonic salt solutions). It is unlikely that this is an important hemolytic mechanism in vivo (Crosby and Conrad, 1960). More likely, the rigid membrane properties of spherocytes lead to splenic sequestration and hemolysis.

The clinical manifestations of hereditary spherocytosis include mild to moderate hemolysis with reticulocytosis, hyperbilirubinemia, and splenomegaly. This is usually a well-compensated process with little or no anemia. There is a neonatal history of hemolysis and hyperbilirubinemia in approximately 50 per cent of all cases (Stamey and Diamond, 1957).

The diagnosis of HS is suspected when there is laboratory evidence of hemolysis and presence of spherocytes on the peripheral blood smear. The incubated osmotic fragility test (24 hours, 37°C) indicates that the RBCs are osmotically more fragile. This incubated osmotic fragility is most useful in bringing out the membrane defect in severe cases of HS in which few if any circulating spherocytes may be present. This paradox is due to the fact that severely affected spherocytes are rapidly removed by the spleen and do not circulate. A Coombs' test and blood typing are essential in any case of spherocytosis, since the clinical and laboratory presentation of HS is sim-

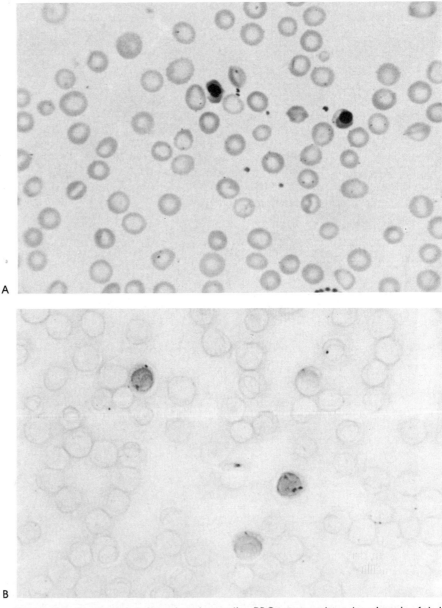

Figure 66–6. *A*, Hypochromic-microcytic RBCs secondary to chronic fetal blood loss. *B*, Fetal RBCs in the maternal blood after a fetomaternal hemorrhage (acid-elution technique).

Illustration continued on following page

ilar to that seen in ABO incompatibility. Unfortunately, however, the Coombs' test in ABO incompatibility is occasionally negative, thus obscuring the correct diagnosis. Examination of family members for spherocytes may be useful in these cases, although no family history of hereditary spherocytosis is found in 25 per cent of patients. Alternatively, definitive diagnosis can be deferred until maternal antibody is cleared by the neonate (after 4 months). Persistence of spherocytes at this time indicates hereditary spherocytosis.

The important hemolytic role of the spleen in HS is manifested by the rapid decrease in bilirubin and reticulocytes following splenectomy. Spherocytes persist following surgery, but the survival of these cells is normal once the spleen is removed. There is no question regarding the efficacy of splenectomy in reducing hemolysis in cases of HS. Nevertheless, surgery is usually deferred until 5 years of age, since young splenectomized children have an increased susceptibility to overwhelming pneumococcal and *H. influenzae* sepsis (Diamond, 1969). The risk of these serious infections is somewhat decreased after 5 years of age. The most important aspect of therapy in the neonatal period is prevention of kernicterus (phototherapy, exchange transfusion). Packed RBCs should be given if there is significant anemia without hyperbilirubinemia. Survival of transfused cells is normal unless there is significant hypersplenism. Folic acid (50 μg per day) should be administered pro-

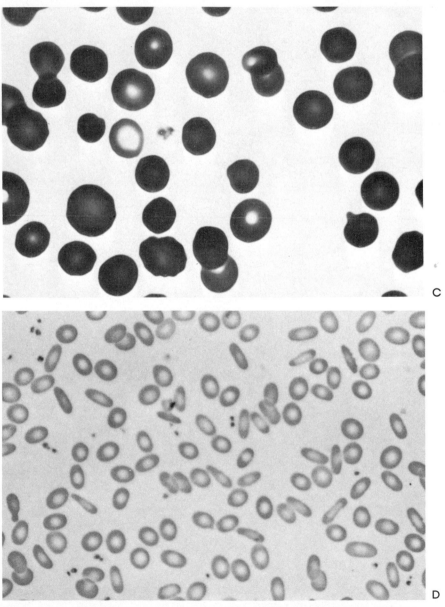

C

D

Figure 66–6. *Continued* C, Hereditary spherocytosis. D, Hereditary elliptocytosis.

Illustration continued on opposite page

phylactically to prevent folate-induced erythroid hypoplasia.

CASE 66–2

A 15-month-old female infant was evaluated for severe chronic hemolytic anemia. This was the first child born to a gravida 1, para 0, white female after an uneventful pregnancy and delivery. Shortly after birth, the infant was noted to be icteric, and a spleen tip was easily palpable 1 to 2 cm below the left costal margin. The remainder of the physical examination was normal. At 36 hours of age, the bilirubin concentration was 16 mg per 100 ml, hemoglobin was 12 gm per 100 ml, and reticulocytes were 15 per cent. Maternal blood type was O-positive, and that of the infant was A-positive. Direct and indirect Coombs tests were negative. The peripheral blood smear revealed marked variation in RBC size and shapes, but there was no predominant cell shape. An osmotic fragility test on a fresh blood sample was within normal limits. There was no evidence of G6PD or PK deficiency. RBC indices were normal. Hemoglobin F was 70 per cent, and no abnormal hemoglobins were seen on hemoglobin electrophoresis. The infant's parents were both hematologically normal. The infant was exchange transfused with O-positive blood.

At 5 weeks of age, she again was noted to be anemic (hemoglobin 6 gm per 100 ml, reticulocytes 9 per cent, total bilirubin 2.3). Physical examination was remarkable for a palpable spleen 3 to 4 cm below the left costal margin. The child was transfused with packed RBCs.

The infant's hemolytic anemia persisted during the next 14 months, and RBC transfusions were required

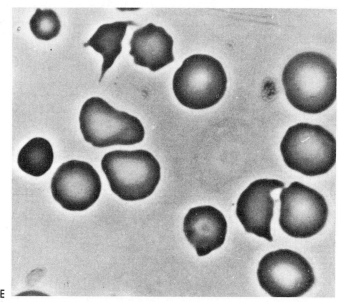

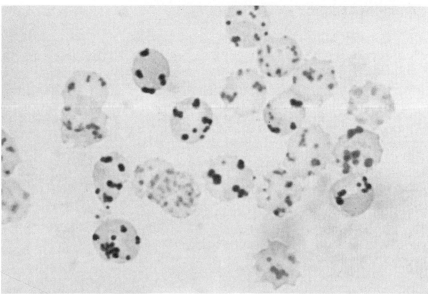

Figure 66–6. *Continued E,* G6PD deficient RBCs during acute hemolytic episode. *F,* Heinz bodies in patient with G6PD deficient hemolysis (stained with supravital dye).

at 6- to 8-week intervals. Repeat laboratory evaluation at 15 months was unchanged from previous studies with one exception: The incubated osmotic fragility was abnormal, with a large population of osmotically fragile RBCs. Rare spherocytes were seen on the peripheral blood smear. The patient subsequently underwent splenectomy, and 6 weeks after surgery hemolysis had markedly diminished: Hemoglobin increased to 12 gm per 100 ml, reticulocytes decreased to 1.2 per cent, and numerous spherocytes were present in the peripheral blood. The child was placed on prophylactic penicillin in view of her risk for developing sepsis.

Comment. This is a case of severe hereditary spherocytosis with several unusual features: (1) Spherocytosis was not a characteristic feature of the peripheral blood until after splenectomy. Prior to surgery, these cells were rapidly removed from the circulation. (2) The initial negative osmotic fragility test points out the fallibility of testing fresh blood rather than blood that has been incubated (37°C for 24 hours) in order to bring out the membrane defect. (3) Transfusion-dependent HS is very unusual, but it does occur. The decision to remove her spleen was based on splenomegaly with transfusion-dependent hemolytic anemia. The rapid cessation of hemolysis following surgery indicates that splenectomy was beneficial for this infant. Nevertheless, it must be emphasized that splenectomy before 5 years of age is quite risky because of the possibility of overwhelming sepsis due to *H. influenzae* or *Pneumococcus* or both. Whenever possible, surgical removal of the spleen should be deferred until age 5 years.

Hereditary Elliptocytosis

Normal individuals may have up to 15 per cent elliptical cells, but patients with this autosomal dominant disorder have 25 to 75 per cent elliptical RBCs in the peripheral blood. Approximately 0.04 per cent of people in the United States are affected by this abnormality, but only a small fraction (12 per cent) of individuals with elliptocytosis ever have significant hemolytic anemia (Penfold and Lipscomb, 1943). The mechanism of hemolysis is not known, and no biochemical abnormality has been demonstrated. In those rare cases in which both parents manifest elliptocytosis, significant hemolytic anemia may occur in the newborn period (Nielson and Strunk, 1968). The clinical features of this disorder are extremely variable. Elliptocytosis is usually an incidental finding in an otherwise healthy child. In other cases, the disorder may be characterized by splenomegaly, anemia, and jaundice, all of which can occur in neonates. Elliptocytosis associated with hemolysis has a clinical course very similar to that of hereditary spherocytosis.

RBC ENZYME ABNORMALITIES

Hemolysis has been reported in association with several erythrocyte enzyme deficiencies, but only two of these are of major clinical significance: glucose-6-phosphate dehydrogenase (G6PD) deficiency and pyruvate kinase (PK) deficiency (Sullivan and Glader, 1980).

Glucose-6-Phosphate Dehydrogenase Deficiency

This RBC enzyme deficiency affects millions of people throughout the world, with the highest frequency occurring in Mediterranean countries, Africa, and China (Beutler, 1971). Approximately 10 per cent of blacks in the United States are G6PD-deficient. Generally, this is a mild hemolytic disorder, although it can cause life-threatening anemia in certain individuals. Hemolysis occurs because enzyme-deficient RBCs are unable to defend against the external oxidant stresses associated with infection and the administration of certain drugs (Fig. 66–7). Generation of hydrogen peroxide near or within RBCs is the common denominator of all oxidants, and the intracellular accumulation of peroxide leads to an oxidative assault on the RBC membrane, enzymes, and hemoglobin. The oxidant attack on hemoglobin results in globin degradation (Heinz bodies), and this in turn produces membrane injury leading to decreased deformability and hemolysis. Normal RBCs contain reduced glutathione (GSH), a sulfhydryl-containing tripeptide that functions as an intracellular buffer that degrades peroxide and protects other cell proteins from oxidant injury. In order to sustain this protection one must maintain intracellular levels of GSH. G6PD is one of the vital enzymes required for GSH regeneration. In G6PD-deficient RBCs, there is a limited capacity to sustain GSH, and thus these cells are vulnerable to oxidant injury and hemolysis.

The severity of hemolysis in G6PD deficiency is obviously related to the magnitude of the oxidant

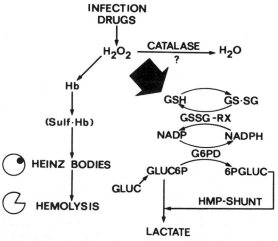

Figure 66–7. G6PD hemolysis—pathophysiology.

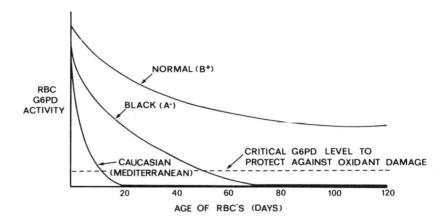

Figure 66–8. Decay of RBC-G6PD activity.

stress, but two other variables also are important: racial origin and sex. As erythrocytes age, G6PD activity decreases, but in normal individuals the lowest activity in older RBCs is more than sufficient to protect against oxidant injury (Fig. 66–8). The defect in black G6PD-deficients is due to instability of the enzyme: G6PD activity in young cells is normal, but that in older cells is severely deficient. This is in accord with the clinical observation that hemolysis in black G6PD-deficients is self-limited, affecting only older cells in which the enzyme has decayed below a critical threshold. The abnormality in G6PD-deficient whites is due to even greater enzyme instability, and RBCs of all ages are affected. Consequently, hemolysis in white deficients can be severe and result in the destruction of the entire circulating RBC mass. Rare cases of death due to G6PD deficiency have been reported in these patients. Manifestations of the Oriental G6PD variant are similar to those seen in whites. Favism is an idiopathic reaction resulting in massive and rapid hemolysis of G6PD deficient RBCs after eating or inhaling pollen of the fava bean. The mechanism of this reaction is unknown, although it is seen only in whites and Orientals.

Glucose-6-phosphate dehydrogenase deficiency is a sex-linked disorder that causes hemolysis primarily in males. Females are variably affected, since they possess one normal X chromosome in addition to the X chromosome bearing the G6PD-deficient gene (Fig. 66–9). In accord with the Lyon hypothesis, however, only one X chromosome is active in a given cell line, since the other chromosome is randomly inactivated early in embryonic life (Lyon, 1961). As a consequence of this, G6PD-deficient females are affected to the extent that they have lyonized to the abnormal chromosome. A female with 50 per cent of normal G6PD activity has 50 per cent normal RBCs and 50 per cent G6PD-deficient cells. The deficient cells are as vulnerable to hemolysis as are deficient male RBCs.

A few variants of G6PD deficiency seen in whites are associated with chronic nonspherocytic hemolytic

anemia in the absence of obvious oxidant stresses. In most cases, however, G6PD-deficient individuals are not anemic, and hemolysis is seen only with infection and drugs. It should be emphasized that infection (bacterial and viral) is the most common cause of hemolysis. Hepatosplenomegaly is unusual.

The diagnosis of G6PD deficiency is suggested by Coombs'-negative hemolytic anemia associated with drugs or infection. Special stains of the peripheral blood (brilliant cresyl blue) may reveal Heinz bodies during hemolytic episodes. Cells that look as if a "bite" had been removed (due to splenic removal of Heinz bodies) occasionally are seen on the routine peripheral blood smear. Specific diagnosis of G6PD deficiency can be made with commercially available screening kits. Unfortunately, most of these tests are relatively insensitive, and false-negative results frequently are obtained if abnormal RBCs have been removed by hemolysis. This is not a problem in white males, but it certainly is a factor in diagnosing some white females and most blacks. In these cases, more sensitive tests can be employed (Fairbanks and Fer-

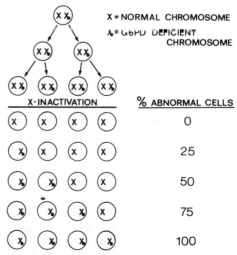

Figure 66–9. Lyon hypothesis of G6PD deficiency.

Disorders of Blood and Blood Vessels

nandez, 1969), or family members can be studied. If the propositus is male, his mother should also be affected, whereas an affected female can have a mother or father with G6PD deficiency. Alternatively, one can wait until the hemolytic crisis is over and reevaluate the patient when his RBC mass has been repopulated with cells of all ages (approximately 8 to 12 weeks).

Hemolysis due to G6PD deficiency is well documented in the newborn period. The usual causal factors (drugs and infection) can be responsible, although in many cases there is no obvious oxidant threat. It is generally agreed that term black infants with G6PD deficiency manifest no increased incidence or severity of hemolysis and hyperbilirubinemia (O'Flynn and Hsia, 1963). In premature black infants with G6PD deficiency, however, hyperbilirubinemia has been reported, but significant hemolysis is rare (Eshaghpour et al., 1967). Severe hemolysis and hyperbilirubinemia are seen only in whites and Orientals with G6PD deficiency. In one study from Greece (Doxiadis and Valaes, 1964), approximately 30 per cent of all exchange transfusions for hyperbilirubinemia were done in G6PD-deficient infants with no evidence of isoimmune hemolytic anemia.

Therapy for hemolysis due to G6PD deficiency is as follows: (1) Prevent kernicterus by managing hyperbilirubinemia with phototherapy or exchange transfusion or both. (2) Replace RBCs if there is significant anemia. Transfused cells will survive normally. (3) Attempt to remove all potential oxidants. Treat infections and avoid all possible offending drugs. (4) Folic acid (50 µg per day) should be given to those rare individuals with chronic nonspherocytic hemolysis. No specific therapy is required in the absence of hemolysis.

CASE 66–3 (MENTZER AND COLLIER, 1975)

A male infant weighing 2722 gm was born at 38 weeks gestation to a 30-year-old Chinese, gravida 3, para 1, aborta 1, mother. Apgar score at birth was 1. Despite intensive resuscitative measures, the infant died after 2 hours, never having established spontaneous respirations. Hemoglobin was 9.8 gm per 100 ml, and the WBC count was 7200. There was marked polychromatophilia (reticulocytosis), and numerous nucleated RBCs were seen in the peripheral smear. The infant's blood type was AB-positive, mother's blood type was B-positive, and the Coombs' test (direct and indirect) was negative. Hemoglobin electrophoresis revealed 52 per cent hemoglobin F, 45 per cent hemoglobin A, and no evidence of Bart's hemoglobin or hemoglobin H. Erythrocyte G6PD activity was decreased. The infant's mother also was G6PD-deficient (heterozygote). During her pregnancy, the mother had an upper respiratory infection 4 weeks prior to delivery. Ascorbic acid (250 to 500 mg per day) was adminis-

Comment. Severe hemolysis and hyperbilirubinemia are not uncommon in G6PD-deficient whites and Orientals. As a result of this case, however, G6PD deficiency can also be considered a cause of hydrops fetalis. The reason for the disastrous course in this neonate is not known. Infection, ascorbic acid (an intracellular oxidant), or fava-bean exposure could have been responsible.

Pyruvate Kinase Deficiency

This autosomal recessive disorder occurs throughout the world and in all ethnic groups. Although its frequency is much less than that of G6PD deficiency, several hundred cases of hemolytic anemia due to this enzyme defect have been identified (Tanaka and Paglia, 1971). Pyruvate kinase is one of two key enzymatic steps during which adenosine triphosphate (ATP) can be generated in RBCs. This high-energy compound has a variety of functions, including the maintenance of normal RBC deformability. It is no surprise that impaired ATP production of PK-deficient cells leads to a short survival in the circulation.

Pyruvate kinase deficiency is characterized by a variable degree of anemia and hemolysis. Some children manifest a moderate chronic hemolytic anemia (hemoglobin 8 to 10 gm per 100 ml, hyperbilirubinemia, reticulocytosis, and splenomegaly). In other children hemolysis is much more severe, often requiring frequent blood transfusions to maintain an adequate circulating hemoglobin. Severely affected children often benefit from splenectomy, since the spleen adds a further insult to metabolically inferior RBCs. Most children with PK deficiency have neonatal jaundice, and many require exchange transfusion. Kernicterus has been reported in PK-deficient neonates.

The diagnosis of PK deficiency is considered in the presence of unexplained jaundice and a Coombs'-negative hemolytic anemia not related to infection or drugs. The anemia is normochromic-normocytic, hemoglobin electrophoresis is normal for age, and the maternal medical history usually is negative. The peripheral blood smear is nonspecific, although irregularly contracted and densely staining erythrocytes may be seen. Specific diagnosis requires a definitive enzyme assay for pyruvate kinase. Parents manifest biochemical heterozygosity (decreased enzyme activity), but they are not anemic and there is no hemolysis.

Treatment of PK deficiency during the newborn period is symptomatic and directed at the prevention of kernicterus (phototherapy, exchange transfusion). In the presence of severe anemia, RBC transfusions should be given. Transfused cells will survive normally. Folic acid (50 µg per day) should be given to

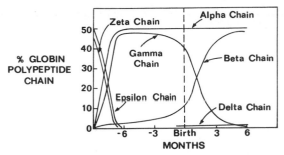

Figure 66–10. Fetal and neonatal hemoglobin production.

meet the requirements of increased RBC production. Children who require frequent RBC transfusions may benefit from splenectomy, although this decision should be deferred for several months if possible.

HEMOLYSIS DUE TO HEMOGLOBIN DISORDERS

In order to appreciate the unique hemoglobinopathies that occur in neonates, one must have an understanding of in utero hemoglobin production. Hemoglobin is a tetrameric protein consisting of 4 hemes (iron-protoporphyrins), each of which is associated with a specific globin polypeptide chain. The heme groups in all known hemoglobins are identical, although there are major differences in the various globin chains (alpha, beta, gamma, delta, epsilon, and zeta). Most functional hemoglobins produced beyond early embryonic life consist of two alpha chains and two non-alpha globin chains.

Gower 1 (zeta 2, epsilon 2) is the earliest detectable embryonic hemoglobin. Currently, it is thought that zeta chains are the embryonic equivalent of alpha chains.

Gower 2 (alpha 2, epsilon 2) is another embryonic hemogloblin present in early fetal life.

Hemoglobin Portland (zeta 2, gamma 2) is the embryonic equivalent of fetal hemoglobin.

Fetal hemoglobin (alpha 2, gamma 2) accounts for 90 to 95 per cent of all hemoglobin production, and thus it is the major hemoglobin of fetal life. This maximal synthetic rate decreases after 35 weeks gestation, and at birth fetal hemoglobin accounts for 50 to 60 per cent of hemoglobin production. This rate continues to decrease, and at 3 months of age only 5 per cent of synthesis is due to fetal hemoglobin.

Hemoglobin A is the major extrauterine hemoglobin. At 20 weeks gestation, Hgb A accounts for 5 to 10 per cent of hemoglobin synthesis, and this increases to 35 to 50 per cent of new hemoglobin production at birth.

The hemoglobin composition of cord blood is a reflection of past and present synthesis (Fig. 66–11). The concentration of hemoglobin F is 60 to 85 per cent, and the remaining 15 to 40 per cent is due to hemoglobin A. Trace amounts of other hemoglobins are also present in cord blood. Hemoglobin A_2 is a minor hemoglobin (less than 3 per cent of total hemoglobin in children and adults), and it may be present in small concentrations in cord blood. Bart's hemoglobin is a tetramer of gamma chains (gamma 4) which is increased in alpha thalassemic disorders (see following discussion). Normal cord blood contains less than 1 per cent Bart's hemoglobin.

Hemolysis is associated with quantitative and qualitative hemoglobin defects. Qualitative disorders are due to the production of abnormal globin chains (sickle cell disease). Quantitative disorders are due to decreased synthesis of normal globin chains (thalassemia syndromes). Hemoglobinopathies related to beta-chain abnormalities are usually not clinically apparent in the neonatal period. On the other hand, gamma-chain abnormalities may be clinically manifest in neonates and then disappear as infants get older and beta-chain synthesis increases. Alpha-chain disorders are seen in both infants and children.

Thalassemia Syndromes

This group of autosomal recessive disorders is a result of decreased synthesis of normal hemoglobin polypeptides. Decreased hemoglobin production leads to anemia characterized by small RBCs (microcytes) containing less hemoglobin per cell (hypochromia). An associated hemolytic component aggravates the magnitude of anemia. Hemolysis is a consequence of continued synthesis of the remaining globin chains (e.g., decreased beta-chain production in beta thalassemia is associated with alpha-chain accumulation in developing RBCs). The excess of unbalanced globin chains interact to form tetramers (α_4, β_4, or hemoglobin H, and γ_4, or Bart's hemoglobin). Globin tetramers are unstable and tend to precipitate and produce cell membrane injury. The severity of injury is directly related to the instability of globin chain tetramers ($\alpha_4 > \gamma_4 > \beta_4$).

	HEMOGLOBIN	GLOBIN POLYPEPTIDES	% IN CORD BLOOD
EMBRYONIC	GOWER-1	Zeta-2, Epsilon-2 ($\zeta_2\epsilon_2$)	0
	GOWER-2	Alpha-2, Epsilon-2 ($\alpha_2\epsilon_2$)	0
	PORTLAND	Zeta-2, Gamma-2 ($\zeta_2\gamma_2$)	0
FETAL	BARTS	Gamma-4 (γ_4)	<1%
	Hgb F	Alpha-2, Gamma-2 ($\alpha_2\gamma_2$)	60-85%
ADULT	Hgb A	Alpha-2, Beta-2 ($\alpha_2\beta_2$)	15-40%
	Hgb A_2	Alpha-2, Delta-2 ($\alpha_2\delta_2$)	<1%

Figure 66–11. Hemoglobin composition of cord blood.

Alpha Thalassemia. This form of thalassemia is seen worldwide with a particularly high incidence in Asia and Africa, although its manifestation is milder in blacks than in Orientals. Defects in alpha-chain production are apparent at birth, since alpha chains constitute half the globin moiety of fetal hemoglobin. In the absence of alpha chains, gamma-chain tetramers (Bart's hemoglobin) are formed. Severity of the alpha-chain defect is proportional to the cord blood content of Bart's hemoglobin. The clinical and laboratory signs of alpha thalassemia are best understood if one accepts the theory that four genes (two from each parent) regulate the normal production of alpha polypeptide chains (Table 66–8).

Silent Carrier State. These individuals lack one of the four genetic loci regulating alpha-chain production. There are no clinical or hematologic abnormalities. Cord blood contains a slightly increased level of Bart's hemoglobin (1 to 2 per cent).

Alpha Thalassemia Trait. Deficiency of two determinants of alpha-chain production results in a mild hypochromic microcytic anemia. There is no significant hemolysis or reticulocytosis. No therapy is required. In older children, the diagnosis is made by excluding iron deficiency, beta-thalassemia trait, and other causes of hypochromic microcytic anemia. In affected neonates, alpha-thalassemia trait is manifested by an MCV (less than 95) that is decreased compared with that of normal infants (100 to 120) (Schmaier et al.). The content of Bart's hemoglobin in cord blood is increased (5 to 6 per cent).

Hemoglobin H Disease. This disorder results from a deficiency of three determinants of alpha-chain production. One parent has alpha-thalassemia trait, whereas the other is a silent carrier. Anemia is more severe than in alpha-thalassemia trait, globin chain imbalance is greater, and hemolysis may be

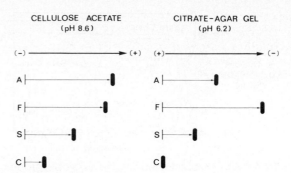

Figure 66–13. Migration of various hemoglobins at pH 8.6 and at pH 6.2.

more intense. Bart's hemoglobin accounts for 20 to 40 per cent of cord blood hemoglobin. Small amounts of hemoglobin H (β_4) also may be present. Both these tetrameric hemoglobins are readily detected on hemoglobin electrophoresis.

Homozygous Alpha Thalassemia ("Hydrops"). This disorder is caused by the absence of all four genetic loci for alpha-chain synthesis. Both parents have alpha-thalassemia trait. In the absence of alpha chains, cord blood contains Bart's hemoglobin and hemoglobin H. In addition, small amounts of hemoglobin Portland, the embryonic form of fetal hemoglobin, can be present. (In the absence of alpha-chain production, zeta synthesis persists during fetal life.) Most affected infants are stillborn, although some may live for a few hours after birth. Death is due to severe anemia. The gamma- and beta-chain tetramers have a high oxygen affinity, which also contributes to the degree of asphyxia. These infants are hydropic at birth and thus are similar in appearance to neonates with severe erythroblastosis due to Rh incompatibility. Invariably, there is hepatosplenomegaly. The mother has a hypochromic microcytic anemia. There is no Rh or ABO incompatibility, and the Coombs' test on cord blood is negative. This homozygous form of alpha thalassemia is seen only in Orientals.

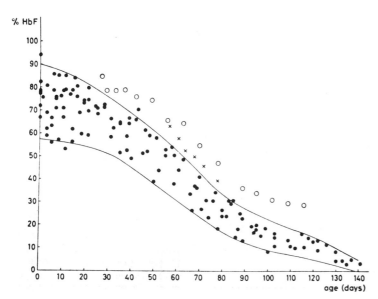

Figure 66–12. Decreasing concentration of fetal hemoglobin after birth. (Garby, L., Sjölin, S., and Vuille, J. C.: Acta Paediatr. *51*:245, 1962.)

Beta Thalassemia. This hemolytic anemia occurs throughout the world, but the incidence is increased in countries surrounding the Mediterranean Sea. In the United States, it is the most common form of thalassemia seen in older children and adults. This is not specifically a neonatal problem, since this disorder is due to decreased beta-chain production. Infants with beta thalassemia are not anemic at birth. Symptoms and signs first appear after 2 or 3 months age, when the bulk of hemoglobin synthesis is due to beta chain production. The heterozygous state (thalassemia minor) is characterized by a mild hypochromic-microcytic anemia. This is a benign disorder that requires no specific therapy. Affected individuals have a normal life span. Conversely, homozygous beta thalassemia (thalassemia major, or Cooley's anemia) is a severe hypochromic-microcytic anemia associated with marked hemolysis (due to accumulation of alpha chains). Most children with this disorder have a lifelong RBC transfusion requirement. Death commonly occurs before 20 years of age, usually from complications of iron overload (iron from RBC transfusions and increased intestinal absorption). Most cases of thalassemia major are diagnosed after 3 months of age but before 1 year. A severe hemolytic anemia associated with marked hepatosplenomegaly occurs in late infancy. Hemoglobin electrophoresis indicates that almost all hemoglobin is of the fetal type, with a small amount of hemoglobin A_2. There is virtually no hemoglobin A.

Gamma Thalassemia. The production of gamma polypeptides is regulated by four genes. The complete absence of gamma chains is incompatible with fetal life. Intermediate reduction of gamma-polypeptide synthesis may produce a mild to moderate neonatal anemia characterized by a reduced percentage of fetal hemoglobin (Stamatoyannopoulos, 1971). This type of anemia resolves when significant beta-chain synthesis begins.

CASE 66–4 (KAN ET AL., 1972)

A full-term 2300-gm girl was noted to be jaundiced at 24 hours of age (bilirubin 13.7 mg). Hemoglobin was 10.4 gm per 100 ml, hematocrit 32 per cent, RBC count 3.8 × 10⁶ μl, WCV 84 μ³, and MCH 27 pg. The reticulocyte count was 26 per cent, and there were 400 nucleated RBCs per 100 white cells. There was no Rh or ABO incompatibility, Coombs' test was negative, iron and iron-binding capacity were normal, and there was no detectable RBC-enzyme deficiency. Hemoglobin F content was 52 per cent (normal 60 to 85 per cent), and no Bart's hemoglobin was detected. The infant was transfused with packed RBCs, and over the next few days nucleated RBCs disappeared, reticulocytes decreased, and the hematocrit remained stable. The infant's mother was hematologically normal, but her father had a hypochromic microcytic anemia that was diagnosed as beta-thalassemia trait. At several months of age, this infant was doing well, although she had a mild hypochromic microcytic anemia that clearly was due to beta-thalassemia trait.

Comment. We frequently see neonates with severe hemolytic anemia that spontaneously disappears by several months of age, thus suggesting that some unique feature of the fetal RBC is responsible for hemolysis. This case is such an example. The presence of a hypochromic-microcytic anemia not related to iron deficiency (which occurs with chronic fetal blood loss) suggested one of the thalassemia disorders. Either alpha or gamma thalassemia could produce this degree of anemia. Alpha thalassemia was ruled out by the absence of Bart's hemoglobin in cord blood. With very sophisticated techniques to measure the synthesis of separate globin chains, it was found

Table 66–8. **Alpha-Thalassemia Syndromes**

		Anemia	Hemolysis	α:β Chain Synthesis	Abnormal Hemoglobins Cord Blood		Adult Blood
Normal	α/α $\overline{\alpha/\alpha}$	None	None	0.95–1.10	0–1%	γ4	—
Silent carrier	$\alpha/-$ $\overline{\alpha/\alpha}$	None	None	0.85–0.95	1–2%	γ4	—
α-thalassemia trait	$-/-$ $\overline{\alpha/\alpha}$	Mild Hypochromic Microcytic	None	0.72–0.82	5–6%	γ4	—
Hemoglobin "H" disease	$-/-$ $\overline{\alpha/-}$	Moderate Hypochromic Microcytic	Moderate	0.30–0.52	20–40% 0–5%	γ4 β4	20–40% β4
Homozygous α-thalassemia ("hydrops")	$-/-$ $\overline{-/-}$	Severe Hypochromic Microcytic	Severe	0	70–80% 15–20% 0–10%	γ4 β4 ζ2γ2	

that this child produced decreased amounts of gamma chains (i.e., gamma-thalassemia trait). In addition, she manifested a lower than anticipated rate of beta-chain synthesis (beta-thalassemia trait), and thus her defect is best described as beta-gamma thalassemia. Neonatal hemolytic anemia was presumably a result of increased alpha-chain accumulation in the absence of normal beta and gamma polypeptides. Hemolysis diminished as the infant got older and began to synthesize more beta chains. Her father had beta-thalassemia trait, and as the patient became older she also developed the classic laboratory evidence of heterozygous beta thalassemia.

Sickle Cell Anemia

Sickle cell anemia is caused by the production of abnormal beta globin chains. The resultant hemoglobin (alpha 2, beta-S 2) gels at low oxygen tension and thereby distorts the cell membrane forming sickled cells. Approximately 10 per cent of all blacks in the United States are carriers of the sickle gene, and since this is an autosomal recessive disorder, one in 400 black infants has sickle cell anemia. Individuals heterozygous for this abnormality (sickle cell trait) are asymptomatic and are not anemic. Homozygotes have sickle cell anemia and suffer from all the known vaso-occlusive and infectious problems associated with this disease. There is no anemia or sickling problem in the newborn period, since this is a beta-chain abnormality. The small number of sickle cells present, however, may explain the hyperbilirubinemia occasionally seen in these neonates. The presence of sickle hemoglobin can be detected by the metabisulfite screening test ("sickle prep"). This screening procedure does not distinguish between sickle trait and sickle cell anemia, and therefore hemoglobin electrophoresis is required for definitive diagnosis. Both A and S hemoglobins are present in sickle trait, but only S hemoglobin (and some fetal hemoglobin) is found in homozygous sickle cell anemia. With conventional hemoglobin electrophoretic methods (pH 8.6, cellulose acetate), it is difficult to demonstrate the presence of small amounts of hemoglobin A when fetal hemoglobin is increased, as it is in the newborn period. It is difficult, therefore, to determine whether a newborn infant is heterozygous or homozygous for the sickle gene. By altering the conditions of electrophoresis (pH 6.3), one can distinguish hemoglobins A and F and thus diagnose sickle cell disease in the newborn period (Schroeder et al., 1973).

Individuals heterozygous for the sickle gene and an additional hemoglobin abnormality may also have problems beyond the newborn period (Figure 66–14). Heterozygosity for the sickle gene and beta thalassemia (each parent must have one defect) produces sickle cell thalassemia. If one parent has he-

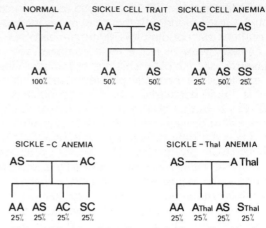

Figure 66–14. Genetics of sickle cell variants.

moglobin C (another beta-chain variant) while the other carries the sickle gene, there is a 25 per cent chance that offspring will develop hemoglobin S-C disease. Both these conditions (S-thalassemia, and S-C disease) manifest many of the same problems seen in sickle cell anemia, although the overall course generally is milder. These infants have no problems in the first 3 months of life.

Our approach to infants of mothers with sickle trait is as follows:

1. Whenever possible, the father is evaluated for thalassemia trait (hypochromic-microcytic anemia) and hemoglobin S or C (hemoglobin electrophoresis). In the absence of these abnormalities, it is unlikely that a child will have one of the sickle syndromes.

2. Hemoglobin electrophoresis (pH 8.6) is done in the newborn period. This will reveal whether sickle hemoglobin is present. S-C disease can be detected at this time, since hemoglobin F has an electrophoretic migration distinct from both S and C.

3. If hemoglobin S is detected on routine electrophoresis at birth, the procedure is repeated (at pH 6.3) when there is a clear resolution of hemoglobins A and F. This allows one to differentiate sickle trait from sickle cell anemia.

4. A practical alternative to (3) is to repeat the routine electrophoresis at 3 months of age. Hemoglobin F is decreased at this time, and the presence of hemoglobin A can be easily detected. Waiting 3 months for a definitive diagnosis is justified medically, since the severe vaso-occlusive and infectious problems associated with sickle cell anemia usually are not seen before this time.

Infants born to mothers with sickle cell disease present more of a neonatal problem than those destined to develop sickle cell anemia after several months of age. It is well established that maternal morbidity and mortality are increased in pregnant women with sickle cell disease, although recent studies suggest that good obstetric management can minimize these problems (Pritchard et al., 1973). Nevertheless, fetal wastage and prematurity remain serious problems in these pregnancies. Approximately 35 per cent of all pregnancies end in early abortion, 17 per cent are associated with stillborns or neonatal deaths, and only 48 per cent result in surviving children. Furthermore, 40 per cent of all viable infants are born premature, and 15 per cent are small for gestational age. These statistics reflect the inordinate vulnerability of the placenta to sickling. Current attempts to maintain normal placental function and decrease fetal wastage include exchange transfusion of maternal (sickle) blood for normal (hemoglobin A) blood early in the third trimester of pregnancy. It is known that this type of procedure is beneficial in other clinical conditions such as severe pulmonary sickling and central nervous system sickling. The clinical problems of neonates born to mothers with sickle cell disease (SS, S-C, S-thalassemia) are directly related to their degree of prematurity. These infants have no hematologic disease, although they will be carriers of the S, C, or thalassemia gene as they begin to produce beta chains. In those cases in which the father also carries a gene for one of these hemoglobinopathies, the infant may develop hemolytic anemia at a later age. (For prenatal diagnosis, see Chapter 2 and Boehm et al., 1983).

Hypoplastic Anemia

Anemia due to an isolated defect in erythropoiesis is known as congenital hypoplastic anemia, or the Blackfan-Diamond syndrome. Clinical manifestations of this rare idiopathic disorder generally become manifest during the first 6 months of life, although some degree of anemia is usually present at birth. Characteristically, there is a moderate-to-severe normochromic-normocytic anemia associated with reticulocytopenia. Bilirubin is not increased. No platelet or leukocyte abnormalities are present. Bone marrow cellularity is normal to slightly decreased, but there is a striking paucity of erythroid precursors. Physical abnormalities (usually of the upper extremities) frequently are present (Alter, 1980).

Corticosteroids are the backbone of therapy for children with Blackfan-Diamond anemia. In most cases, prednisone (4 mg per kg per day) produces a reticulocytosis after 1 to 2 weeks of therapy, and subsequently the steroid dose can be reduced to much lower levels. Alternate-day therapy should be used for children requiring long-term steroid administration. In most cases, this will sustain a clinical remission while preventing many of the known side effects of prolonged steroid therapy. In some cases, clinical remission can be maintained on steroid doses that are actually within the normal physiologic range of hormone production by the adrenal gland. The reason for this inordinate erythropoietic sensitivity to steroids is unknown. Packed RBC transfusions are given to symptomatic children who fail to respond to prednisone. Iron, folate, and other hematinics have no specific role in the therapy of this disorder.

The prognosis for children who respond to steroids is very good. Nonresponders, however, generally de-

velop hemosiderosis secondary to their lifelong RBC transfusion requirement. These children usually succumb to complications of iron storage during the second to third decade of life. Rare cases of acute leukemia also have been reported after the third decade of life (Wasser et al., 1979).

CASE 66–5

A 2650-gm girl born after 38 weeks of gestation was noted to be pale at birth. Physical examination revealed no tachycardia, tachypnea, hepatosplenomegaly, or other abnormality. Bleeding was not excessive at the time of delivery, and there was no abnormality of the placenta or umbilical cord. The following laboratory data were obtained: hemoglobin 11.4 gm per 100 ml, MCV 102, MCH 34, reticulocytes 2.4 per cent, WBC count 17,400, platelet count 230,000, bilirubin 2.8 mg per 100 ml. The mother's blood type was O-positive; the infant's was B-positive. Coombs' test was negative. A Kleihauer-Betke preparation of the maternal blood smear did not reveal RBCs with fetal hemoglobin.

At this time, it was thought that anemia was due to a fetomaternal bleed, and iron therapy (2 mg Fe per kg, tid) was started. At 7 weeks, her hemoglobin had fallen to 6.8 gm per 100 ml, and she was transfused with packed RBCs up to a hemoglobin of 11.5 gm per 100 ml. By 3 months of age, her hemoglobin again decreased to 7.5 gm per 100 ml and the reticulocyte count was only 0.1 per cent. Bone marrow examination was normal except that erythroid precursors were virtually nonexistent. The infant was started on prednisone (4 mg per kg), and within 9 days reticulocytosis was noted. Prednisone was decreased to 0.2 mg per kg over the next 6 weeks, after which the hemoglobin was 9.2 mg per 100 ml. The steroid dose was further reduced to 0.2 mg every other day, and, at 7 months of age (when her hemoglobin was 11.9 gm per 100 ml), prednisone was discontinued altogether. Approximately 3 months later, hemoglobin again had decreased (7.8 gm per 100 ml), and the reticulocyte count was only 0.2 per cent. Steroids were restarted and erythropoiesis again was stimulated. Subsequently, the child has been able to maintain a normal hemoglobin while on a small maintenance dose of prednisone (0.2 mg per kg, qod).

Comment. The initial diagnosis was thought to be anemia due to a fetomaternal blood loss. The absence of fetal cells in the maternal circulation could have been caused by ABO incompatibility between mother and child. The diagnosis of congenital hypoplastic anemia was suspected because of the lower than expected hemoglobin and also because of a failure to respond to iron therapy. This suspicion was confirmed by the absence of erythroid precursors in the marrow and the dramatic response to corticosteroids. Newborn infants normally manifest erythroid hypoplasia during the first few weeks of life, and it is frequently difficult to distinguish this from the marrow picture of congenital hypoplastic anemia. The obvious difference is that erythropoiesis resumes spontaneously in normal infants (see Physiologic Anemia of Infancy and Prematurity).

Physiologic Anemia of Infancy and Prematurity

At birth the mean hemoglobin of term infants (17.0 gm per 100 ml) is slightly greater than in prematures (16.0 gm per 100 ml). The hemoglobin concentration in term infants subsequently decreases to a plateau at which it remains throughout the first year of life (Table 66–9). This is known as the *physiologic anemia of infancy*. A similar process occurs in premature infants except that hemoglobin falls more rapidly and reaches a lower concentration. This is known as the *anemia of prematurity*. After 1 year of age, there is little difference between the hemoglobin values of term and premature infants.

PHYSIOLOGIC ANEMIA OF INFANCY

The hemoglobin-oxygen saturation at birth increases from 50 per cent to 95 per cent, thus producing an increase in blood oxygen content and a cessation of erythropoiesis. Subsequently, the hemoglobin concentration begins to decrease, since there is no replacement of aged RBCs as they are normally removed from the circulation. Iron from degraded RBCs is stored in tissue for future hemoglobin synthesis. The hemoglobin concentration continues to fall until a point is reached at which tissue oxygen needs are greater than oxygen delivery. This occurs sometime between 6 and 12 weeks of age, when hemoglobin has reached a level of 9.5 to 11.0 gm per 100 ml. Erythropoiesis resumes at this time, and iron previously stored in reticuloendothelial tissues is utilized for hemoglobin synthesis. These stores provide normal term infants with sufficient iron for hemoglobin synthesis until 20 weeks of age. It is unnecessary to administer iron during this period, since it will not prevent the physiologic decrease in hemoglobin. Any iron that is given will be added to stores for future use. It must be emphasized that this physiologic hemoglobin decrease does not represent "anemia" in the true sense of the term. Rather, it is a reflection of the excess oxygen delivery relative to tissue O_2 needs. There is no hematologic problem, and no therapy is required.

ANEMIA OF PREMATURITY

The magnitude of anemia in prematures is directly related to birth weight, and in large measure it is an exaggeration of the physiologic anemia of infancy. The anemia of prematurity, however, differs in several respects from that seen in term infants:

1. The hemoglobin nadir is reached at an earlier age (4 to 8 weeks). Presumably, this is due to the relatively decreased RBC survival of premature infants compared with that of term neonates (Pearson, 1967).

2. The hemoglobin nadir is lower in prematures (6.5 to 9.0 gm per 100 ml) compared with that of term infants (9.5 to 11.0 gm per 100 ml). This difference may be a function of decreased tissue oxygen requirements, because premature infants consume less oxygen (ml O_2 per kg per min) than do term neonates (Mestyan et al., 1964). In accord with this concept, erythropoietin is produced by term infants at hemoglobins of 10 to 11 gm per 100 ml, whereas no erythropoietin is detected in prematures at significantly lower hemoglobin concentrations (Buchanan and Schwartz, 1974; McIntosh, 1975). It is unlikely that this merely represents blunted erythropoietin responsiveness, for hypoxic prematures with respiratory or cardiac disease readily generate increased erythropoietin levels. The lower hemoglobin concentrations seen in premature infants may thus represent a physiologic state of balanced oxygen delivery and oxygen needs. This is supported by the clinical observation that many premature infants with hemoglobin levels of 6 to 7 gm per 100 ml are quite

Table 66–9. Hemoglobin Changes During First Year of Life

Week	Term	Premature (1.2–2.5 kg)	Premature (<1.2 kg)
0	17.0 (14.0–20.0)	16.4 (13.5–19.0)	16.0 (13.0–18.0)
1	18.8	16.0	14.8
3	15.9	13.5	13.4
6	12.7	10.7	9.7
10	11.4	9.8	8.5
20	12.0	10.4	9.0
50	12.0	11.5	11.0
Lowest hemoglobin (mean)	10.3 (9.5–11.0)	9.0 (8.0–10.0)	7.1 (6.5–9.0)
Time of nadir	6–12 weeks	5–10 weeks	4–8 weeks

healthy, with no evidence of cardiac or respiratory distress.

3. Although the hemoglobin concentration of premature and term infants is similar at birth, the total body hemoglobin (an iron) content is significantly less in prematures. Consequently, iron depletion occurs earlier in prematures than in term infants. Most prematures are endowed with sufficient iron to maintain hemoglobin synthesis for 10 to 14 weeks. Iron administered before this time is stored for later use, but it does not influence the rate or level of the physiologic decrease in hemoglobin (Schulman, 1959). In fact, iron given to prematures during the first weeks of life may actually aggravate the anemia of prematurity (see following discussion of vitamin E). After 2 months of age, however, iron supplements must be given in order to maintain hemoglobin synthesis and to prevent iron deficiency (the late anemia of prematurity). Iron is given as ferrous sulfate (2 mg of elemental iron per kg per day for a period of 6 months). This iron requirement is met by currently available iron-fortified formulas.

4. *Role of vitamin E deficiency.* Vitamin E is an antiperoxidant compound vital to the integrity of erythrocytes. Red blood cells are susceptible to membrane injury and hemolysis in the absence of this vitamin (Fig. 66–15). Three factors are integrally related to the pathophysiology of this hemolysis: lipid composition of RBC membrane, catalysts of lipid peroxidation, and vitamin E: (1) Lipid composition of erythrocytes is influenced by the quality of lipids in plasma and diet. An increase in dietary polyunsaturated fatty acids (PUFA) increases RBC membrane PUFA content. (2) Unsaturated bonds in PUFA undergo oxidation with the formation of free radicals and lipid peroxides. High concentrations of oxygen and certain heavy metals (iron) catalyze this reaction. Once free radicals and lipid peroxides are formed, these compounds further catalyze the peroxidation

Table 66–10.   Vitamin E Responsive Hemolytic Anemia in Premature Infants*

	Pretreatment	Post-treatment
Vitamin E (mg/dl)	0.25 ± 0.15	0.95 ± 0.23
H_2O_2 Hemolysis (%)	80 ± 14	8 ± 10
Hgb (gm/100 ml)	7.6 ± 1.1	9.8 ± 0.8
Reticulocytes (%)	8.2 ± 2.9	3.0 ± 1.5

* Vitamin E dependent hemolytic anemia in premature infants (1480 ± 205 gm) diagnosed at 6 to 11 weeks of age. Infants were treated with 270 to 1094 international units (IU) of vitamin E. The mean response to treatment was seen in 10 days. (Data from Oski, F. A., and Barness, L. A.: J. Pediatr. 70:211, 1967.)

of PUFA (a chain reaction). (3) Vitamin E inactivates lipid peroxides and thereby inhibits further lipid peroxidation. The requirement for vitamin E is increased when dietary PUFA are increased or in the presence of excessive catalytic activity from O_2 or metals. Lipid peroxides produce RBC membrane injury and hemolysis in the absence of adequate vitamin E.

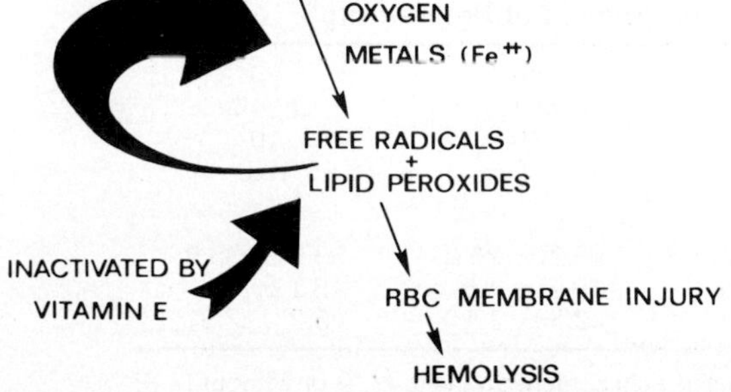

Premature infants are endowed with significantly less vitamin E than are term neonates. This deficiency state persists for 2 to 3 months, at which time their intestinal absorption of vitamin E becomes similar to that of term infants. Hemolytic anemia occurring in premature infants (less than 1500 gm) at 6 to 10 weeks of age is one known consequence of vitamin E deficiency (Oski and Barness 1967; Ritchie et al., 1968). This anemia is characterized by decreased hemoglobin, reticulocytosis, reduced vitamin E levels, and increased RBC peroxide hemolysis (a measure of RBC vitamin E content). Signs of hemolytic anemia rapidly disappear following vitamin E administration (Table 66–10).

This observation suggests that the anemia of prematurity may in part be due to vitamin E deficiency. Oski and Barness demonstrated that premature infants given daily vitamin E (15 IU per day) had higher hemoglobins and lower reticulocytes than a control group not given the vitamin (Table 66–11). Similar results have been reported in several outstanding studies by Melhorn and Gross. Thus it appears that vitamin E deficiency may contribute to the *magnitude* of anemia in prematurity. In a more recent study, it has been demonstrated that vitamin E given to infants weighing less than 1500 gm resulted in a bilirubin level that was significantly reduced compared with that of control infants (Gross, 1979). Moreover, the duration of phototherapy was significantly less in the vitamin E–supplemented group.

Since iron catalyzes the peroxidation of PUFA in vitro, Melhorn and Gross questioned whether iron therapy aggravated the anemia of prematurity. After 6 weeks of age, they observed lower hemoglobins and higher reticulocytes in neonates given iron (8 mg per kg per day) compared with those in infants given no additional supplements. Because this study was

DIETARY UNSATURATED FATTY ACIDS

↓

PLASMA UNSATURATED FATTY ACIDS

↕

RBC UNSATURATED FATTY ACIDS
(MOSTLY IN PHOSPHATIDYLETHANOLAMINE)

OXYGEN
METALS (Fe^{++})

FREE RADICALS
+
LIPID PEROXIDES

INACTIVATED BY
VITAMIN E

RBC MEMBRANE INJURY

HEMOLYSIS

Figure 66–15. Hemolysis of vitamin E deficient erythrocytes.

Disorders of Blood and Blood Vessels

Table 66–11.   Effect of Supplemental Vitamin E on Anemia of Prematurity*

	Control	Vitamin E (15 IU/day)
Birth weight	1176 ± 182 gm	1278 ± 180 gm
6–8 weeks of age		
Vitamin E (mg/100 ml)	0.22 ± 0.10	1.00 ± 0.25
H_2O_2 hemolysis (%)	66 ± 21	9 ± 9
Lowest Hgb (gm/100 ml)	7.7 ± 1.5	9.2 ± 1.3
Highest reticulocytes (%)	6.7 ± 2.5	3.1 ± 0.7

* Premature infants were given prophylactic vitamin E (15 international units per day) and the vitamin E level, peroxide hemolysis, hemoglobin concentration and reticulocyte count were measured after 6 to 8 weeks. These values were compared to a group of control infants not given vitamin E supplements. (Data from Oski, F. A., and Barness, L. A.: J. Pediatr. *79:*211, 1967.)

done in prematures receiving therapeutic, rather than prophylactic, iron dosages, Williams and her co-workers re-examined this problem in neonates given artificial formulas fortified with iron (approximately 10 to 15 mg iron per liter formula or 3 to 4 mg iron per day). The results of this limited but provocative study emphasize the importance of dietary fatty acid composition in addition to iron content (Table 66–12). Infants fed formulas low in linoleic acid (similar to breast milk) manifested the same hemoglobin and reticulocyte count, with or without added iron. Neonates fed with formulas containing an increased content of linoleic acid (with or without iron) demonstrated a positive peroxide hemolysis test, thus indicating a state of relative vitamin E deficiency. Reticulocytosis and decreased hemoglobins, however, were seen only in neonates fed formulas with both increased linoleic acid and iron.

In summary, the anemia of prematurity can be separated into early and late phases. The two components of the early anemia are due to (1) an aggravation of the normal physiologic anemia of infancy (not preventable), and (2) a low grade of hemolysis due to vitamin E deficiency (preventable). The late phase of anemia occurs at 3 to 4 months after erythropoiesis resumes and iron stores are depleted (preventable).

On the basis of our current concepts of anemia in prematures, an ideal physiologic approach to the nutritional management of these infants can be devised:

1. Vitamin E (25 IU or 0.5 ml of Aquason E) should be given daily until 8 to 10 weeks of age. There is no known toxic effect of vitamin E given in these dosages to premature infants.

2. Formulas similar to mother's milk (low in linoleic acid) should be used in order to maintain a low content of RBC polyunsaturated fatty acids. Currently, this is satisfied by all commercially available formula preparations.

3. During the first 2 months, iron supplements are not needed.

4. After 2 months of age, iron supplements (2 mg per kg per day) must be given in order to prevent the late anemia of prematurity.

Polycythemia

An increased hematocrit may reflect a relatively decreased plasma volume or an absolute increase in RBC mass. True polycythemia is due to an increased RBC mass.

Polycythemia in older children is seen with arterial hypoxemia (cyanotic heart disease, pulmonary disorders), tumors (renal, hepatic, cerebellar) and abnormal hemoglobins (increased oxygen affinity). Polycythemia vera or primary erythrocytosis is rare. Neonatal polycythemia is generally due to fetal hypertransfusion or to one of the placental dysfunction syndromes. Hypertransfusion occurs with delayed umbilical cord clamping (see RBC Physiology at

Table 66–12.   Influence of Iron Supplementation on Anemia of Prematurity*

Formula	(1)	(2)	(3)	(4)
Linoleic acid content	12.8%	12.8%	32.4%	32.4%
Vitamin E (IU/liter)	10	10	10	10
Iron (mg/liter)	0	13.3	0	12.0
5 Weeks				
Peroxide hemolysis (%)	1.8 ± 4.7	3.2 ± 2.2	62.2 ± 26.0	53.0 ± 35.5
Hemoglobin (gm/100 ml)	10.4 ± 1.8	9.6 ± 0.6	10.6 ± 1.5	8.1 ± 1.3
Reticulocytes (%)	2.7 ± 1.3	1.8 ± 1.5	2.3 ± 1.1	5.2 ± 2.5

* Premature infants were fed formulas with low (1,2) or high (3,4) linoleic acid content and with (2,4) or without (1,3) added iron. All formulas contained low supplements of vitamin E. The peroxide hemolysis, hemoglobin, and reticulocyte count were measured after 5 weeks. (Data obtained from Williams, M. L., et al.: N. Engl. J. Med. *292:*887, 1975.)

Table 66–13. Etiology of Neonatal Polycythemia

Placental hypertransfusion
  Delayed cord clamping
  Twin-twin transfusion
  Maternal-fetal transfusion

Placental insufficiency syndromes
  Small for gestational age infants
  Toxemia
  Postmaturity
  Placenta previa

Birth) or maternal blood loss into the fetal circulation (Michael and Mauer, 1961). In addition, twin-to-twin transfusions can produce polycythemia in one infant (usually the larger) and anemia in the other twin (Sacks, 1959). Neonatal polycythemia occasionally is associated with toxemia, placenta previa, postmaturity, and small for gestational age infants (Humbert et al., 1969). It is thought that the increased RBC mass associated with these placental insufficiency syndromes reflects fetal hypoxia and increased erythropoietin production. Oh and his coworkers, however, have suggested an additional mechanism to explain hypoxia-induced polycythemia. They observed that acute maternal (and fetal) hypoxia increased the fetal RBC mass by augmenting the fraction of placental blood transfused into the fetus.

Blood viscosity increases at hematocrits greater than 60 per cent, and this in turn leads to a reduction of blood flow (Fig. 66–16). Oxygen transport, which is determined by hemoglobin (oxygen content) and blood flow, is maximal in the normal hematocrit range. At low hematocrits, oxygen transport is decreased because of limited oxygen capacity, whereas at higher hematocrits, decreased oxygen transport is due to reduced blood flow. These changes are further modified when the effects of normovolemia and hypervolemia are compared. Hypervolemia is advantageous, since this distends the vasculature, decreases peripheral resistance, and thereby increases blood flow and oxygen transport at any given hematocrit. These physiologic concepts are of therapeutic importance, since most cases of polycythemia are associated with an increased blood volume (i.e., hypervolemia).

Most polycythemic infants are asymptomatic. The physical examination is normal except for a plethoric appearance and occasionally cyanosis. Cyanosis is due to relative stasis of high hematocrit blood. Symptoms of hyperviscosity may occasionally be present: respiratory distress, convulsions, congestive heart failure, priapism, and renal vein thrombosis. Hyperbilirubinemia is common, because an elevated RBC mass increases the bilirubin load to the liver (1 gm hemoglobin produces 34 mg bilirubin). Hypoglycemia and hypocalcemia are also associated with neonatal polycythemia.

The diagnosis of neonatal polycythemia is not as clear-cut as that of anemia. Certainly, most infants are polycythemic if adult or childhood criteria of polycythemia are applied. In neonates, however, polycythemia is defined as a hemoglobin greater than 22 gm per 100 ml, or a hematocrit greater than 65 per cent. The etiology of polycythemia can often be ascertained by history (twin pregnancy, delayed cord clamping) or physical examination (small for gestational age infant). In many cases, however, there is no apparent cause.

It is our policy to decrease the RBC mass of all infants with symptomatic polycythemia: respiratory difficulties, CNS symptomatology, congestive heart failure. Whenever possible, partial exchange transfusion with fresh plasma is preferred over simple phlebotomy, since oxygen transport is better in the face of hypervolemia. If signs of congestive heart failure persist following hematocrit reduction, diuretics and digitalization are indicated. The general principles for the partial exchange have been outlined by Oski and Naiman:

Volume of blood exchanged for plasma = Blood volume
$$\times \frac{Observed\ Hct\ -\ Desired\ Hct}{Observed\ Hct}$$

Assume blood volume of 100 ml per kg. Desired Hct is 55 per cent, since viscosity is relatively normal at this level. Exchange should be done in volumes of 3 ml blood/kg body weight.

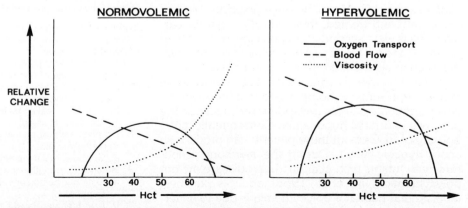

Figure 66–16. Effect of hematocrit on viscosity, blood flow, and oxygen transport.

Methemoglobinemia

Example: A 3 kg dyspneic infant with an 80 per cent hematocrit requires a partial exchange.

$$Blood\ volume = 3\ kg \times 100\ ml/kg = 300\ ml$$

$$\frac{Observed\ Hct\ -\ Desired\ Hct}{Observed\ Hct} = \frac{80\ -\ 55}{80} = 0.31$$

Therefore, volume of exchange = 300 ml × 0.31 = 93 ml.

The treatment of asymptomatic neonates with polycythemia is not as clearly defined. In view of the frequency of hyperbilirubinemia and in order to prevent the emergence of problems related to hyperviscosity, our current approach is to do a "prophylactic" partial exchange in neonates with hematocrits greater than 65 to 70 percent. Close monitoring for signs of hypoglycemia and hypocalcemia is necessary in all polycythemic infants.

CASE 66–6

A gravida 2, para 1, white female delivered a 2950-gm male infant following a normal pregnancy, labor, and delivery. At birth, the child had an Apgar score of 6. Physical examination revealed a cyanotic infant with a grade III/VI systolic heart murmur. The liver edge was palpable 2 cm below the right costal margin, and the spleen tip was palpable. Chest radiograph revealed a markedly enlarged heart with increased pulmonary vascular markings. The hemoglobin was 26 gm per 100 ml, and the hematocrit was 79 per cent. There were no other hematologic abnormalities. The child was partially exchanged with plasma and the post-exchange hematocrit was 62 per cent. Subsequently, the child's color improved, heart murmur disappeared, and there were no remaining signs of congestive heart failure.

Comment. The clinical findings in this infant were initially very suggestive of organic heart disease. All cardiac signs cleared rapidly once polycythemia was recognized and treated, thus indicating that the cardiac effects were secondary to polycythemia-induced hyperviscosity. This series of events is distinct from that seen in older children with cyanotic heart disease and polycythemia. The increased RBC mass in these infants represents a compensatory adjustment by which adequate oxygen transport is maintained in the presence of arterial hypoxemia. Consequently, phlebotomy of RBCs from these patients can produce an acute hypoxic insult. During the newborn period, however, infants with cyanotic heart disease are not polycythemic (Gatti et al., 1966), and it is extremely unlikely that neonatal polycythemia is due to underlying organic heart disease.

Hemoglobin iron is normally in the reduced or ferrous (Fe^{++}) state. Methemoglobin is an oxidized derivative of hemoglobin in which iron is in the ferric (Fe^{+++}) state. In contrast to ferrohemoglobin, ferrihemoglobin (methemoglobin) does not complex with oxygen. Significant methemoglobinemia, therefore, reduces blood oxygen capacity and transport.

In vivo, small amounts of hemoglobin are continually being oxidized by endogenous agents including oxygen itself (auto-oxidation). Normally, however, less than 1 per cent of hemoglobin is methemoglobin, because RBCs can reduce the relatively low levels of ferrihemoglobin that are formed:

1. *NADH-methemoglobin reductase* is the enzyme that catalyzes the reduction of methemoglobin under physiologic conditions. Hereditary deficiency of this enzyme produces methemoglobinemia. NADH (dihydronicotinamide adenine dinucleotide) is a required cofactor produced by metabolic reactions.

2. *NADPH-methemoglobin reductase* by itself is unable to reduce methemoglobin to any significant extent. Individuals lacking this enzyme do not have methemoglobinemia. In the presence of certain redox compounds (e.g., methylene blue), however, this enzyme rapidly reduces methemoglobin to ferrohemoglobin. Thus, this enzyme is important in the treatment of methemoglobinemia with methylene blue. NADPH (dihydronicotinamide adenine dinucleotide phosphate) is a required cofactor that is generated by cell metabolism. G6PD is one of the main sites of NADPH production in RBCs.

Table 66–14. Approach to Infants with Cyanosis and Methemoglobinemia

Cyanosis associated with respiratory and cardiac findings
  Blood turns red when mixed with air
  Decreased arterial P_{O_2}
  Consider pulmonary, cardiac, or CNS disease

Cyanosis with or without respiratory and cardiac findings
  Blood turns red when mixed with air
  Normal arterial P_{O_2}
  Consider polycythemia syndromes (αOCBC)

Cyanosis without respiratory or cardiac findings
  Blood remains dark after mixing with air
  Arterial P_{O_2} normal
  Consider methemoglobinemia syndromes:
  1. Rapid clearing of methemoglobin following methylene blue
    a. Consider toxic methemoglobinemia (look for environmental oxidants)
    b. Consider NADH-methemoglobin reductase deficiency (do enzyme assay)
  2. Reappearance of methemoglobinemia after initial response to methylene blue
    a. Consider NADH-methemoglobin reductase deficiency
  3. No change in methemoglobin following methylene blue
    a. Consider hemoglobin M disorders (do hemoglobin electrophoresis)
    b. Consider associated G6PD deficiency (do enzyme assay)

3. *Reduced glutathione (GSH)* can directly and nonenzymatically reduce ferrihemoglobin. Quantitatively, this reaction is less important than NADH-methemoglobin reductase.

An increased methemoglobin concentration is caused by disruption of the delicate balance between oxidation and reduction of hemoglobin iron. Two forms of methemoglobinemia are seen: acquired or toxic methemoglobinemia (common) and congenital methemoglobinemia (rare).

Acquired methemoglobinemia occurs in normal individuals exposed to increased concentrations of chemicals that oxidize hemoglobin iron. During the first weeks of life, neonates are particularly susceptible to this form of methemoglobinemia for the following reasons: (1) Fetal hemoglobin is more readily oxidized to the ferric state than is hemoglobin A (Martin and Huisman, 1963). (2) Neonates are transiently deficient in NADH-methemoglobin reductase activity (Ross, 1963), a deficiency that persists for the first 3 or 4 months of life (Bartos and Desforges, 1966). One class of chemicals that will readily oxidize hemoglobin iron includes nitrite and nitrate compounds. Nitrite is the active agent. Nitrates are converted to nitrites by intestinal bacteria. Neonates given ''well water'' with an increased nitrate content occasionally develop methemoglobinemia (Comly, 1945). Also, the feeding of vegetable preparations with high levels of nitrate (cabbage, spinach, beets, and, occasionally, carrots) can produce methemoglobinemia in infants. Aniline derivatives constitute another class of chemicals that will oxidize hemoglobin, and methemoglobinemia has been caused in neonates by marking nursery diapers with aniline dyes. Drugs administered prior to delivery can also produce methemoglobinemia in mothers and newborn infants. Prilocaine, a local anesthetic used for obstetric purposes, is such an agent (Climie et al., 1967). It should be noted that most agents capable of oxidizing hemoglobin will, in fact, produce methemoglobin in normal individuals if the concentration of oxidant chemical is sufficiently high. Increased infant susceptibility to these chemicals during the first weeks of life is relative to fetal hemoglobin content and the degree of NADH-methemoglobin reductase deficiency.

Congenital methemoglobinemia can be due to inherited hemoglobin or enzyme abnormalities:

1. *Hemoglobin M disorders* are rare autosomal dominant defects brought about by amino acid substitutions in the normal globin chain. As a result of these substitutions, heme iron is more stable in the ferric than in the ferrous state. The normal methemoglobin reductive capacity cannot compensate for this instability of ferrous heme. M hemoglobins can be caused by alpha- or beta-chain defects, but only alpha-chain abnormalities are present in the newborn period. Heterozygotes have increased methemoglobin levels and some degree of cyanosis but otherwise are asymptomatic. No therapy is indicated (and none is possible). The homozygous state is obviously incompatible with life.

2. *NADH-methemoglobin reductase deficiency* is a rare autosomal recessive disorder in which the rate of ferrihemoglobin reduction is markedly reduced. Heterozygotes are asymptomatic and do not have methemoglobinemia unless challenged by toxic agents. Homozygote deficients generally have 15 to 40 per cent methemoglobin levels. These patients are cyanotic but otherwise asymptomatic.

The cardinal clinical manifestation of methemoglobinemia is cyanosis without evidence of cardiac or respiratory disease (normal physical examination, chest radiograph, EKG, and arterial Po_2). Cyanosis may be present at birth (suggesting hereditary methemoglobinemia) or may suddenly appear in an otherwise asymptomatic infant (suggesting toxic or acquired methemoglobinemia). Blood appears dark in color, but, in contrast to deoxygenated blood, does not change in color to bright red when it is mixed with air. This is the basis of the following simple screening test for detection of methemoglobin (Harley and Celermajer, 1970):

A drop of blood is placed on filter paper and then allowed to dry while the filter paper is waved in air. Blood that is not saturated with oxygen turns red, whereas methemoglobin remains brown. This test detects levels of ferrihemoglobin greater than 10 per cent of total hemoglobin. Methemoglobin concentrations can be measured with spectrophotometric techniques in most laboratories (Evelyn and Malloy, 1938). Cyanosis is apparent at methemoglobin levels of 1.5 gm per 100 ml (10 per cent of total hemoglobin). Symptoms due to decreased oxygen transport are generally not apparent until 30 to 40 per cent of hemoglobin is oxidized to methemoglobin. Levels greater than 70 per cent are incompatible with life. Methemoglobinemia is not associated with anemia, hemolysis, or other hematologic abnormalities.

Neonates with greater than 15 to 20 per cent methemoglobin are treated with methylene blue (1 mg per kg as a 1 per cent solution in normal saline). The response to methylene blue is both therapeutic and diagnostic. A rapid decrease in methemoglobin occurs within 1 to 2 hours if the cause of methemoglobin is an acquired toxic agent or a deficiency of NADH-methemoglobin reductase. Failure to note improvement following methylene blue suggests one of the M hemoglobins, and this can be confirmed by hemoglobin electrophoresis. Decreased NADPH generation (i.e., G6PD deficiency) also produces a less than optimal response to methylene blue. (It should be pointed out that G6PD deficiency per se is not a *cause* of methemoglobinemia but rather a possible cause of poor response to methylene blue.) A reappearance of methemoglobinemia after an initial response to methylene blue suggests a deficiency of NADH-methemoglobin reductase, although the persistence of an occult oxidant must be kept in mind. The diagnosis of NADH-methemoglobin reductase deficiency requires an enzyme assay, which is done in specialized hematology laboratories. Most infants with hereditary methemoglobinemia are asymptomatic and require no therapy. In older children, therapy is occasionally given for cosmetic reasons to decrease cyanosis. This is readily accomplished with daily oral administration of ascorbic acid or methylene blue. Methylene blue will produce blue urine, but this is harmless.

REFERENCES

Normal Erythrocyte Physiology in the Fetus and Neonate

Allen, D. W., Wyman, J., and Smith, G. A.: The oxygen equilibrium of fetal and adult hemoglobin. J. Biol. Chem. 203:81, 1953.

Bauer, C., Ludwig, I., and Ludwig, M.: Different effects of 2,3-diphosphoglycerate and adenosine triphosphate on oxygen affinity of adult and fetal hemoglobin. Life Sci. 7:1339, 1968.

Delivoria-Papadopoulos, M., Roncevic, N. P., and Oski, F. A.: Postnatal changes in oxygen transport of term, premature, and sick infants: the role of red cell 2,3-diphosphoglycerate and adult hemoglobin. Pediatr. Res. 5:235, 1971.

Finne, P. H.: Erythropoietin levels in cord blood as an indicator of intrauterine hypoxia. Acta Paediatr. Scand. 55:478, 1966.

Finne, P. H., and Halvorsen, S.: Regulation of erythropoiesis in the fetus and newborn. Arch. Dis. Child. 47:683, 1972.

Gairdner, D., Marks, J., Roscoe, J. D., and Brettell, R. O.: The fluid shift from the vascular compartment immediately after birth. Arch. Dis. Child. 33:489, 1958.

Jacobson, L. O., Marks, E. K., and Gaston, E. O.: Studies on erythropoiesis. XII. The effect of transfusion-induced polycythemia in the mother on the fetus. Blood 14:644, 1959.

Lanzkowsky, P.: The influence of maternal iron deficiency on the haemoglobin of the infant. Arch. Dis. Child. 36:205, 1961.

Oski, F. A., and Delivoria-Papadopoulos, M.: The red cell, 2,3-diphosphoglycerate, and tissue oxygen release. J. Pediatr. 77:941, 1970.

Usher, R., and Lind, J.: Blood volume of the newborn premature infant. Acta Paediatr. Scand. 54:419, 1965.

Usher, R., Shepard, M., and Lind, J.: The blood volume of the newborn infant and placental transfusion. Acta Paediatr. Scand. 52:497, 1963.

General Approach to Anemic Infants

Gill, F. M., and Schwartz, E.: Anemia in early infancy. Pediatr. Clin. North Am. 19:841, 1972.

Matoth, Y., Zaizor, R., and Varsano, I.: Postnatal changes in some red cell parameters. Acta Paediatr. Scand. 60:317, 1971.

Naiman, J. L., Punett, H. H., Lischner, H. W., Destine, M. L., and Arey, J. B.: Possible graft-versus-host reaction after intrauterine transfusion for Rh erythroblastosis fetalis. N. Engl. J. Med. 281:697, 1969.

Oh, W., and Lind, J.: Venous and capillary hematocrit in newborn infants and placental transfusion. Acta Paediatr. Scand. 55:38, 1966.

Parkman, R., Mosier, D., Umansky, I., Cochran, W., Carpenter, C. B., and Rosen, F. S.: Graft-versus-host disease after intrauterine and exchange transfusions for hemolytic disease of the newborn. N. Engl. J. Med. 209:359, 1974.

Schwartz, A. D.: Differential diagnosis of neonatal anemia. Paediatrician 3:107, 1974.

Seip, M.: The reticulocyte level and erythrocyte production judged from reticulocyte studies in newborn infants during the first week of life. Acta Paediatr. Scand. 44:355, 1955.

Yeager, A. S., Grumet, F. C., Hafleigh, E. B., Arvin, A. M., Bradley, J. S., and Prober, C. G.: Prevention of transfusion-acquired cytomegalovirus infections in newborn infants. J. Pediatr. 98:281, 1981.

Hemorrhagic Anemia

Cohen, F., Zuelzer, W. W., Gustafson, D. C., and Evans, M. M.: Mechanisms of isoimmunization. I. The transplacental passage of fetal erythrocytes in homo-specific pregnancies. Blood 23:621, 1964.

Grobbelaar, B. G., and Dunning, E. K.: A method of calculating the volume of transplacental foetomaternal haemorrhage. Br. J. Haematol. 17:231, 1969.

Kirkman, H. N., and Riley, H. D.: Posthemorrhagic anemia and shock in the newborn due to hemorrhage during delivery: a report of 8 cases. Pediatrics 24:92, 1959.

Kirkman, H. N., and Riley, H. D.: Posthemorrhage anemia and shock in the newborn. A review. Pediatrics 24:97, 1959.

Leape, L. L., and Bordy, M. D.: Neonatal rupture of the spleen. Report of a case successfully treated after spontaneous cessation of hemorrhage. Pediatrics 47:101, 1971.

Leonard, S., and Anthony, B.: Giant cephalohematoma of newborn. Am. J. Dis. Child. 101:170, 1961.

Montague, A. C. W., and Krevans, J. R.: Transplacental hemorrhage in cesarean section. Am. J. Obstet. Gynecol. 95:1115, 1966.

Oski, F. A., and Naiman, J. L.: Hematologic Problems in the Newborn. 3rd. ed. Philadelphia, W. B. Saunders Co., 1982.

Pachman, D. J.: Massive hemorrhage in the scalp of the newborn infant. Hemorrhagic caput succedaneum. Pediatrics 29:907, 1962.

Pearson, H. A., and Diamond, L. K.: Fetomaternal transfusion. Am. J. Dis. Child. 97:267, 1959.

Phillipsborn, H. F., Traisman, H. S., and Greer, D.: Rupture of the spleen: a complication of erythroblastosis fetalis. N. Engl. J. Med. 252:159, 1955.

Ratten, G. J.: Spontaneous haematoma of the umbilical cord. Aust. N. Z. J. Obstet. Gynaecol. 9:125, 1969.

Rausen, A. R., Seki, M., and Strauss, L.: Twin transfusion syndrome. A review of 19 cases studied at one institution. J. Pediatr. 66:613, 1965.

Raye, J. R., Gutberlet, R. L., and Stahlman, M.: Symptomatic posthemorrhagic anemia in the newborn. Pediatr. Clin. North Am. 17:401, 1970.

Sacks, M. O.: Occurrence of anemia and polycythemia in phenotypically dissimilar single ovum human twins. Pediatrics 24:604, 1959.

Schwartz, J., Surchin, H., Lupu, H., and Cooperberg, A. A.: Severe hypochromic anemia in a newborn due to fetal-maternal transfusion. Can. Med. Assoc. J. 95:369, 1966.

Siddall, R. S., and West, R. H.: Incision of placenta at cesarean section: a cause of fetal anemia. Am. J. Obstet. Gynecol. 63:425, 1952.

Woo Wang, M. Y. F., McCutcheon, E., and Desforges, J. F.: Fetomaternal hemorrhage from diagnostic transabdominal amniocentesis. Am. J. Obstet. Gynecol. 97:1123, 1967.

Zipursky, A., Pollock, J., Chown, B., and Israels, L. G.: Transplacental fetal maternal hemorrhage after placental injury during delivery or amniocentesis. Lancet 2:493, 1963.

Hemolytic Anemia

Abelson, N. M., and Rawson, A. J.: Studies of blood group antibodies. V. Fractionation of examples of anti-B, anti-A,B, anti-M, anti-P, anti-JKa, anti-Lea, anti-D, anti-CD, anti-K, anti-Fya, anti-S, and anti-Good. Transfusion 1:116, 1961.

Austin, R. F., and Desforges, J. F.: Hereditary elliptocytosis: an unusual presentation of hemolysis in the newborn associated with transient morphologic abnormalities. Pediatrics 44:196, 1969.

Bard, H.: The postnatal decline of hemoglobin F synthesis in normal full-term infants. J. Clin. Invest. 55:395, 1975.

Baumann, R., and Rubin, H.: Autoimmune hemolytic anemia during pregnancy with hemolytic disease in the newborn. Blood 41:293, 1973.

Beutler, E.: Abnormalities of the hexosemonophosphate shunt. Semin. Hematol. 8:311, 1971

Boehm, C. D., Antonarakis, S. E., Phillips, J. A., et al.: Prenatal diagnosis using DNA polymorphisms. N. Engl. J. Med. 308:1054, 1983.

Bowen, F. W., and Renfield, M.: The detection of anti-D in Rho(D)-negative infants born of Rho(D)-positive mothers. Pediatr. Res. 10:213, 1976

Bowen, J. M.: Rh erythroblastosis fetalis. Semin. Hematol. 12:110, 1975.

Clayton, E. M., Hyun, B. H., Palumbo, V. N., and Dean, V. M.: Penicillin induced positive Coombs' test in a newborn. Am. J. Clin. Pathol. 52:370, 1969.

Crosby, W. H., and Conrad, M. E.: Hereditary spherocytosis: observations on hemolytic mechanisms and iron metabolism. Blood 15:662, 1960.

Diamond, L. K.: Splenectomy in childhood and the hazard of overwhelming infection. Pediatrics 43:886, 1969.

Doxiadis, S. A., and Valaes, T.: The clinical picture of glucose-6-phosphate dehydrogenase deficiency in early infancy. Arch. Dis. Child 39:545, 1964.

Driscoll, S. G.: Hydrops fetalis. N. Engl. J. Med. 275:1432, 1966.

Eshaghpour, E., Oski, F. A., and Williams, M.: The relationship of erythrocyte glucose-6-phosphate dehydrogenase deficiency to hyperbilirubinemia in Negro premature infants. J. Pediatr. 70:595, 1967.

Fairbanks, V. F., and Fernandez, M. N.: The identification of metabolic errors associated with hemolytic anemia. J.A.M.A. 208:316, 1969.

Forget, B. G., and Kan, Y. W.: Thalassemia and the genetics of hemoglobin. In Nathan, D. G., and Oski, F. A. (Eds.): Hematology of Infancy and Childhood. Philadelphia, W. B. Saunders Co., 1974, p. 450.

Freda, V. J., Gorman, J. G., Pollack, W., and Bowe, E.: Prevention of Rh hemolytic disease—10 years' clinical experience with Rh immune globulin. N. Engl. J. Med. 292:1014, 1975.

Friedman, S., Atwater, J., Gill, F. M., and Schwartz, E.: α-Thalassemia in Negro infants. Pediatr. Res. 8:955, 1974.

Glader, B. E., Fortier, N., Albala, M. M., and Nathan, D. G.: Congenital hemolytic anemia associated with dehydrated erythrocytes and increased potassium loss. N. Engl. J. Med. 291:491, 1974.

Glader, B. E., and Nathan, D. G.: Haemolysis due to pyruvate kinase deficiency and other glycolytic enzymopathies. Clin. Haematol. 4:123, 1975.

Gluck, L., Kulovich, M. V., Borer, R. C., Brenner, P. H., Anderson, G. G., and Spellacy, W. N.: Diagnosis of the respiratory distress syndrome by amniocentesis. Am. J. Obstet. Gynecol. 109:440, 1971.

Gross, G. P., and Hathaway, W. E.: Fetal erythrocyte deformability. Pediatr. Res. 6:593, 1972.

Kan, Y. W., Allen, A., and Lowenstein, L.: Hydrops fetalis with alpha thalassemia. N. Engl. J. Med. 276:18, 1967.

Kan, Y. W., Forget, B. G., and Nathan, D. G.: Gamma-beta thalassemia: A cause of hemolytic disease of the newborn. N. Engl. J. Med. 286:129, 1972.

Kan, Y. W., Schwartz, E., and Nathan, D. G.: Globin chain synthesis in the alpha thalassemia syndromes. J. Clin. Invest. 47:2515, 1969.

Kaplan, E., Herz, F., and Scheye, E.: ABO hemolytic disease of the newborn, without hyperbilirubinemia. Am. J. Hematol. 1:279, 1976.

Katz, J., and Marcus, R. G.: Risk of Rh isoimmunization in ruptured tubal pregnancy. Br. Med. J. 3:667, 1972.

Krueger, H. C., and Burgert, E. O., Jr.: Hereditary spherocytosis in 100 children. Mayo Clin. Proc. 41:821, 1966.

LaCelle, P. L.: Alteration of membrane deformability in hemolytic anemias. Semin. Hematol. 7:355, 1970.

Lee, D., Nnatu, S. N. N., and Houston, J. K.: Incidence of fetomaternal transfusion in spontaneous abortion. J. Obstet. Gynaecol. Br. Comm. 76:1120, 1969.

Levine, P., Katzin, E. M., et al.: Isoimmunization in pregnancy, its possible bearing on the etiology of erythroblastosis fetalis. J.A.M.A. 116:825, 1941.

Liley, A. W.: Liquor amnii analysis in the management of pregnancy complicated by rhesus sensitization. Am. J. Obstet. Gynecol. 82:1359, 1961.

Liley, A. W.: Errors in the assessment of hemolytic disease from amniotic fluid. Am. J. Obstet. Gynecol. 86:485, 1963.

Liley, A. W.: Intrauterine transfusion of foetus in hemolytic disease. Br. Med. J. 2:1107, 1963.

Lyon, M. F.: Gene action in the X-chromosome of the mouse. Nature 190:372, 1961.

Mentzer, W. C., Jr. and Collier, E.: Hydrops fetalis associated with erythrocyte G-6-PD deficiency and maternal ingestion of fava beans and ascorbic acid. J. Pediatr. 86:565, 1975.

Miller, D. R., Rickles, F. R., Lichtman, M. A., LaCelle, P. L., Bates, J., and Weed, R. I.: A new variant of hereditary hemolytic anemia with stomatocytosis and erythrocyte cation abnormality. Blood 38:184, 1971.

Milner, P. F.: The sickling disorders. Clin. Haematol. 3:289, 1974.

Misenheimer, H. R.: Fetal hemorrhage associated with amniocentesis. Am. J. Obstet. Gynecol. 94:1133, 1966.

Nielson, J. A., and Strunk, K. W.: Homozygous hereditary elliptocytosis as a cause of hemolytic anemia in infancy. Scand. J. Haematol. 5:486, 1968.

Nienhaus, A. W., and Propper, R. D.: The thalassemias: disorders of hemoglobin synthesis. In Nathan, D. G., and Oski, F. A., (Eds.): Hematology of Infancy and Childhood. Vol II. 2nd ed. Philadelphia, W. B. Saunders Co., 1981.

O'Flynn, M. E. D., and Hsia, D. Y.: Serum bilirubin levels and glucose-6-phosphate dehydrogenase deficiency in newborn American Negroes. J. Pediatr. 63:160, 1963.

Orkin, S. H., and Goff, S. C.: The duplicated human α-globin genes: their relative expression as measured by RNA analysis. Cell 24:345, 1981.

Oski, F. A., and Diamond, L. K.: Erythrocyte pyruvate kinase deficiency resulting in congenital nonspherocytic hemolytic anemia. N. Engl. J. Med. 269:763, 1963.

Pearson, H. A.: Life-span of the fetal red blood cell. J. Pediatr. 70:166, 1967.

Pearson, H. A., Shanklin, D. R., and Brodine, C. R.: Alpha-thalassemia as a cause of nonimmunologic hydrops. Am. J. Dis. Child. 109:168, 1965.

Penfold, J. B., and Lipscomb, J. M.: Elliptocytosis in man, associated with hereditary hemorrhagic telangiectasia. Quart. J. Med. 12:157, 1943.

Platt, O., and Nathan, D. G.: Sickle cell disease. In Nathan, D. G., and Oski, F. A. (Eds.): Hematology of Infancy and Childhood. Philadelphia, W. B. Saunders Co., 1981, p. 687.

Pritchard, J. A., Scott, D. E., Whalley, P. J., Cunningham, F. G., and Mason, R. A.: The effects of maternal sickle cell hemoglobinopathies and sickle cell trait on reproductive performance. Am. J. Obstet. Gynecol. 117:662, 1973.

Schmaier, A. H., Maurer, H. M., Johnston, C. L., and Scott, R. B.: Alpha thalassemia screening in neonates by mean corpuscular volume and mean corpuscular hemoglobin determination. J. Pediatr. 83:794, 1973.

Schroeder, W. A., Jakway, J., and Powers, D.: Detection of hemoglobins S and C at birth: a rapid screening procedure by column chromatography. J. Lab. Clin. Med. 82:303, 1973.

Seip, M.: Systemic lupus erythematosus in pregnancy with hemolytic anemia, leucopenia and thrombocytopenia in the mother and her newborn infant. Arch. Dis. Child. 35:365, 1960.

Stamatoyannopoulos, G.: Gamma-thalassemia. Lancet 2:192, 1971.

Stamey, C. C., and Diamond, L. K.: Congenital hemolytic anemia in the newborn. Am. J. Dis. Child. 94:616, 1957.

Sullivan, D. W., and Glader, B. E.: Erythrocyte enzyme disorders in children. Pediatr. Clin. North Am. 27:449, 1980.

Tanaka, P. R., and Paglia, D. E.: Pyruvate kinase deficiency. Semin. Hematol. 8:367, 1971.

Trucco, J. T., and Brown, A. K.: Neonatal manifestations of hereditary spherocytosis. Am. J. Dis. Child. 113:263, 1967.

Valaes, T., Karaklis, A., Stravrakakis, D., Bavela-Stravrakakis, K., Perakis, A., and Doxiadis, S. A.: Incidence and mechanism of neonatal jaundice related to glucose-6-phosphate dehydrogenase deficiency. Pediatr. Res. 3:448, 1969.

Voak, D., and Williams, M. A.: An explanation of the failure of the direct antiglobulin test to detect erythrocyte sensitization in ABO hemolytic disease of the newborn and observations on pinocytosis of IgG anti-A antibodies by infant (cord) red cells. Br. J. Haematol. 20:9, 1971.

Wasi, P., Na-Nakorn, S., and Pootrakul, S.: The α-thalassaemias. Clin. Haematol. 3:383, 1974.

Zarkowsky, H. S., Oski, F. A., Sha'afi, R., Shohet, S. B., and Nathan, D. G.: Congenital hemolytic anemia with high sodium, low potassium red cells. I. Studies of membrane permeability. N. Engl. J. Med. 278:573, 1968.

Zipursky, A., Pollock, J., Chown, B., and Israels, L. G.: Transplacental foetal hemorrhage after placental injury during delivery or amniocentesis. Lancet 2:493, 1963.

Hypoplastic Anemia

Alter, B. P.: Childhood red cell aplasia. Am. J. Pediatr. Hematol./Oncol. 2:121, 1980.

Diamond, L. K., Allen, D. M., and Magill, F. B.: Congenital (erythroid) hypoplastic anemia. Am. J. Dis. Child. 102:149, 1961.

Diamond, L. K., and Blackfan, K. D.: Hypoplastic anemia. Am. J. Dis. Child. 56:464, 1938.

Hughes, D. W. O.: Hypoplastic anemia in infancy and childhood. Arch. Dis. Child. 36:349, 1961.

Pearson, H. A., and Cone, T. E.: Congenital hypoplastic anemia. Pediatrics 19:192, 1957.

Wasser, J. S., Yolken, R., Miller, D. R., and Diamond, L. K.: Congenital hypoplastic anemia (Diamond-Blackfan syndrome) terminating in acute myelogenous leukemia. Blood 53:504, 1979.

Physiologic Anemia of Infancy and Prematurity

Buchanan, G. R., and Schwartz, A. D.: Impaired erythropoietin response in anemic premature infants. Blood 44:347, 1974.

Dallman, P. R.: Iron, vitamin E, and folate in preterm infant. J. Pediatr. 85:742, 1974.

Delivoria-Papadopoulos, M., Roncevic, N. P., and Oski, F. A.: Postnatal changes in oxygen transport of term, premature, and sick infants: the role of red cell 2,3-diphosphoglycerate and adult hemoglobin. Pediatr. Res. 5:235, 1971.

Gross, S., and Milhorn, D. K.: Vitamin E dependent anemia in the premature infant. III. Comparative hemoglobin, vitamin E, and erythrocyte phospholipid responses following absorption of either water-soluble or fat-soluble d-alpha tocopherol. J. Pediatr. 85:753, 1974.

Gross, S. J.: Vitamin E and neonatal bilirubinemia Pediatrics 64:321, 1979.

Halvorsen, S., and Finne, P. H.: Erythropoietin production in the human fetus and newborn. Ann. N.Y. Acad. Sci. 149:576, 1968.

McIntosh, S.: Erythropoietin excretion in the premature infant. J. Pediatr. 86:202, 1975.

Melhorn, D. K., and Gross, S.: Vitamin E–dependent anemia in the premature infant I. Effects of large doses of medicinal iron. J. Pediatr. 79:569, 1971.

Melhorn, D. K., and Gross, S.: Vitamin E–dependent anemia in the premature infant II. Relationships between gestational age and absorption of vitamin E. J. Pediatr. 79:581, 1971.

Mestyan, J., Fekete, M., Bata, G., and Jarai, I.: The basal metabolic rate of premature infants. Biol. Neonatol. 7:11, 1964.

O'Brien, R. T., and Pearson, H. A.: Physiologic anemia of the newborn infant. J. Pediatr. 79:132, 1971.

Oski, F. A., and Barness, L. A.: Vitamin E deficiency: a previously unrecognized cause of hemolytic anemia in the premature infant. J. Pediatr. 70:211, 1967.

Pearson, H. A.: Life-span of the fetal red blood cell. J. Pediatr. 70:166, 1967.

Ritchie, J. H., Fish, M. B., McMasters, V., and Grossman, M.: Edema and hemolytic anemia in premature infants. N. Engl. J. Med. 279:1185, 1968.

Schulman, I.: The anemia of prematurity. J. Pediatr. 54:663, 1959.

Shojania, A. M., and Gross, S.: Folic acid deficiency and prematurity. J. Pediatr. 64:323, 1964.

Stockman, J. A., III: Anemia of prematurity. Semin. Hematol. 12:163, 1975.

Stoutenborough, K. A., Sutherland, J. M., Meineke, H. A., and Light, I. J.: Erythropoietin levels in cord blood of control infants and infants with respiratory distress syndrome. Acta Paediatr. Scand. 58:121, 1969.

Williams, M. L., Shott, R. J., O'Neal, P. L., and Oski, F. A.: Role of dietary iron and fat in vitamin E deficiency anemia of infancy. N. Engl. J. Med. 292:887, 1975.

Polycythemia

Baum, R.: Viscous forces in neonatal polycythemia. J. Pediatr. 69:975, 1966.

Danks, D. M., and Stevens, L. H.: Neonatal respiratory distress associated with a high hematocrit reading. Lancet 2:499, 1964.

Gatti, R. A., Muster, A. J., Cole, R. B., and Paul, M. H.: Neonatal polycythemia with transient cyanosis and cardiorespiratory abnormalities. J. Pediatr. 69:1063, 1966.

Gross, G. P., Hathaway, W. E., and McGaughey, H. R.: Hyperviscosity in the neonate. J. Pediatr. 82:1004, 1973.

Humbert, J. R., Abelson, H., Hathaway, W. E., and Battaglia, F. C.: Polycythemia in small for gestational age infants. J. Pediatr. 75:812, 1969.

Kontras, S. B.: Polycythemia and hyperviscosity syndromes in infants and children. Pediatr. Clin. North Am. 19:919, 1972.

Michael, A. F., Jr., and Mauer, A. M.: Maternal-fetal transfusion as a cause of plethora in the neonatal period. Pediatrics 28:458, 1961.

Minkowski, A.: Acute cardiac failure in connection with neonatal polycythemia (in monovular and single newborn infants). Biol. Neonatol. 4:61, 1962.

Oh, W., Omori, K., Emmanouilides, G. C., and Phelps, D. L.: Placenta to lamb fetus transfusion in utero during acute hypoxia. Am. J. Obstet. Gynecol. 122:316, 1975.

Sacks, M. O.: Occurrence of anemia and polycythemia in phenotypically dissimilar single-ovum human twins. Pediatrics 24:604, 1959.

Stone, H. O., Thompson, H. K., Jr., and Schmidt-Nielsen, K.: Influence of erythrocytes on blood viscosity. Am. J. Physiol. 214:913, 1968.

Wood, J. L.: Plethora in the newborn infant associated with cyanosis and convulsions. J. Pediatr. 54:143, 1959.

Methemoglobinemia

Bartos, H. R., and Desforges, J. F.: Erythrocyte DPNH dependent diaphorase levels in infants. Pediatrics 37:991, 1966.

Climie, C. R., McLean, S., Starmer, G. A., and Thomas, J.: Methaemoglobinaemia in mother and foetus following continuous epidermal analgesia with prilocaine. Br. J. Anaesthesiol. 39:155, 1967.

Comly, H. R.: Cyanosis in infants caused by nitrates in well water. J.A.M.A. 129:112, 1945.

Evelyn, K. A., and Malloy, H. T.: Microdetermination of oxyhemoglobin, methemoglobin, and sulfhemoglobin in a single sample of blood. J. Biol. Chem. 126:655, 1938.

Farmer, M. B., Lehmann, H., and Raine, D. N.: Two unrelated patients with congenital cyanosis due to haemoglobinopathy M. Lancet 2:786, 1964.

Fisch, R. O., Berglund, E. B., Bridge, A. G., Finley, P. R., and Raile, R.: Methemoglobinemia in a hospital nursery. A search for causative factors. J.A.M.A. 185:124, 1963.

Gerald, P. S.: The electrophoretic and spectroscopic characterization of hemoglobin M. Blood 12:936, 1958.

Harley, J. D., and Celermajer, J. M.: Neonatal methaemoglobinaemia and the "red-brown" screening test. Lancet 2:1223, 1970.

Jaffe, E. R., and Hsieh, H-S.: DPNH-methemoglobin reductase deficiency and hereditary methemoglobinemia. Semin. Hematol. 8:417, 1971.

Keating, J. P., Lell, M. E., Strauss, A. W., Zarkowsky, H., and Smith, G. E.: Infantile methemoglobinemia caused by carrot juice. N. Engl. J. Med. 288:24, 1973.

Lees, M. H., and Jolly, J.: Severe congenital methaemoglobinaemia in an infant. Lancet 2:1147, 1957.

Lo, S. S., Hitzig, W. H., and Martin, H. R.: Hereditary methemoglobinemia due to diaphorase deficiency. Acta Haematol. 43:177, 1970.

Martin, H., and Huisman, T. H. J.: Formation of ferrihaemoglobin of isolated human haemoglobin types by sodium nitrite. Nature 200:898, 1963.

Nurse, D. S.: Congenital methaemoglobinaemia. Med. J. Austr. 47:692, 1960.

Quie, P. G., Fisch, R. O., and Raile, R.: Methemoglobinemia and hemolytic anemia in normal newborns and normal prematures. Lancet 82:428, 1962.

Ross, J. D.: Deficient activity of DPNH-dependent methemoglobin diaphorase in cord blood erythrocytes. Blood 21:51, 1963.

Shearer, L. A., Goldsmith, J. R., Young, C., Kearns, O. A., and Tamplin, B. R.: Methemoglobin levels in infants in an area with high nitrate water supply. Am. J. Pub. Health 62:1174, 1972.

Smith, R. P., and Olson, M. V.: Drug-induced methemoglobinemia. Semin. Hematol. 10:253, 1973.

Vigil, J., Warburton, S., Haynes, W. S., and Kaiser, L. R.: Nitrates in municipal water supply cause methemoglobinemia in infants. Pub. Health Rep. 80:1119, 1965.

67

Rheumatic Disorders

By Mandel R. Sher

Infantile Polyarteritis Nodosa

Infantile polyarteritis nodosa (IPN) is an uncommon disease of early childhood and rarely occurs in neonates. The clinical presentation and pathologic findings of IPN differ from those of other forms of polyarteritis nodosa; however, IPN and the more recently described mucocutaneous lymph node syndrome (MLNS, or Kawasaki's disease) are very similar. The clinical presentations of IPN and MLNS have common features, and the pathologic vasculitic lesions of both entities are indistinguishable. IPN is usually fatal, whereas MLNS is associated with a low mortality rate. Therefore, IPN and MLNS may represent different expressions of the same disease process.

IPN usually presents with prolonged or intermittent fever, upper respiratory tract symptoms, and rash. The rash is typically erythematous and macular but can be urticarial or similar to erythema multiforme. Conjunctivitis, lymphadenopathy, hepatosplenomegaly, diarrhea, and peripheral edema are frequent clinical manifestations. Less frequent but significant clinical characteristics include nuchal rigidity, limb paresis, congestive heart failure, hypertension, and digital and extremity infarcts.

Leukocytosis and either pyuria or albuminuria are frequent findings. Cardiomegaly and pulmonic infiltrates can be seen on the chest roentgenogram. The EKG in 20 per cent of cases reveals evidence of left ventricular hypertrophy or myocardial ischemia. Cerebrospinal pleocytosis with increased protein occurs in 20 per cent.

The course of IPN averages 27 days and usually terminates in sudden death from coronary thrombosis or rupture. The pathologic hallmark of IPN is the presence of coronary artery vasculitis, with thromboses and aneurysms seen in over 90 per cent of cases. Vasculitis and thrombosis of other medium-sized vessels are common. These include, in order of decreasing frequency, renal, periadrenal, intestinal, pancreatic, splenic, and iliac arteries. Myocardial and renal infarcts are frequently seen.

Pathology. The histologic appearance of IPN is primarily characterized by a segmental panarteritis of medium-sized vessels. Different stages of inflamma-

Table 67–1. Common Features of Infantile Polyarteritis Nodosa

Symptom	Frequency (Per Cent)
Fever	95
Upper respiratory symptoms	90
Rash	80
Conjunctivitis	50
Lymphadenopathy	40
Cardiomegaly	20
Digital desquamation	15
Hypertension	10
Extremity infarcts	10
Leukocytosis	95
Pyuria	45
CSF pleocytosis	20
EKG changes	20

tion and repair can be seen in the same artery. The exudative phase is marked by intimal proliferation with destruction of the internal elastic lamina and media. Thrombi, when present, merge with the intima. Fibrinoid changes are not seen, as the rate of the disease process allows time for repair. However, aneurysms may develop during the reparative phase.

Diagnosis. Rarely has the diagnosis of IPN been made during life. Chamberlain and Perry as well as Glanz and colleagues diagnosed IPN in infants after documentation of coronary aneurysms by coronary angiography. The diagnosis of IPN should be suspected when the typical clinical characteristics are present. Documentation of coronary thromboses and aneurysms by two-dimensional echocardiography will help establish the diagnosis. Coronary angiography may be performed when a diagnosis cannot be confirmed by other means. Since this procedure has a significant risk in the presence of active coronary vasculitis, it should be performed only in the healing stages of disease. Differentiating IPN from MLNS may be difficult. Diagnostic criteria are estab-

Table 67–2. Diagnostic Criteria for Mucocutaneous Lymph Node Syndrome

1. Fever, persisting for more than 5 days
2. Bilateral conjunctival injection
3. Erythematous rash
4. Mucous membrane changes (at least one)
   a. Injected or fissured lips
   b. Injected pharynx
   c. Strawberry tongue
5. Extremity changes (at least one)
   a. Erythema of palms or soles
   b. Edema of the hands and feet
   c. Generalized or periungual desquamation
6. Cervical lymphadenopathy (at least one node 1.5 cm in diameter)

(From Report from MCLS Research Committee of the Ministry of Health and Welfare 1971–1972. Japanese Government, 1972, pp. 9–10.)

lished in MLNS (Table 67–2). Although the pathology of MLNS and IPN are indistinguishable, very few cases of IPN fulfill the clinical criteria for a firm diagnosis of MLNS.

The diagnosis of IPN is even more difficult to make in the neonatal period. Of the 50 cases of documented IPN, four cases involved neonates presenting between 10 days and 5 weeks of age. Only one of these four infants had the typical clinical course of

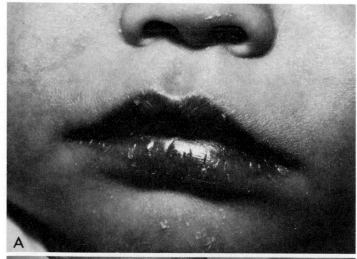

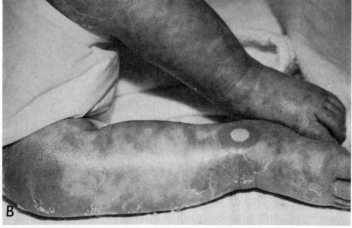

Figure 67–1. 11-week-old male infant with diagnosis of MLNS. Erythematous macular rash, injected lips, and edema of extremities are also typical of IPN.

IPN. Roberts and Fetterman reported a 5-week-old child with fever, upper respiratory infection, and macular rash who went on to develop congestive heart failure and arterial thrombosis of an arm and leg. Pathologic findings were typical of IPN.

Wilmer reported two cases of neonates with IPN. The first child began to vomit on the eighth day and developed dyspnea on the tenth day. There was a purulent omphalitis, and the child died that day in shock. Necropsy revealed an umbilical arteritis and umbilical venous thrombosis in addition to vasculitis of many arteries. Wilmer's second patient presented with a rash and puffy eyelids during the third week and went on to have fever, diarrhea, hematemesis, and petechiae. He developed thrombocytopenia and died after a right-sided convulsion. Necropsy revealed a large adrenal hemorrhage in addition to polyarteritis nodosa. In 1954, Liban and coworkers reported a child who failed to thrive and had intermittent episodes of fever from birth. The child died at 9 months after developing progressive congestive heart failure. Necropsy revealed extensive vasculitic involvement of pulmonary and coronary arteries. Although Wilmer's cases are atypical, Liban's case could have been diagnosed today by echocardiography.

The pathogenesis of IPN is unknown. Studies by Rich and Gregory implicate a hypersensitivity mechanism in these forms of systemic vasculitis. This is supported by a report of increased serum concentrations of IgE in two patients with IPN.

Treatment. Treatment for this very rare condition remains controversial. Chamberlain and Perry as well as Glanz and coworkers treated their two patients with steroids and cytotoxic agents with satisfactory results. Older children and adults with polyarteritis nodosa respond well to this regimen. In contrast, steroids may be harmful to patients with the coronary aneurysms of MLNS, whereas treatment with antiplatelet drugs such as aspirin may be efficacious (Kato et al., 1979). Owing to the great similarities of IPN and MLNS, antiplatelet drug therapy alone may be appropriate in the treatment of IPN.

Systemic Lupus Erythematosus

Primary systemic lupus erythematosus (SLE) in the newborn is extremely rare. Transient SLE phenomena have been well documented in infants of mothers with SLE. These phenomena are presumably caused by the transplacental passage of maternal autoantibodies. These antibodies in similar titers may also occur in asymptomatic offspring of mothers with SLE.

Congenital complete heart block (CCHB) is increasingly recognized in infants of mothers with SLE, rheumatoid arthritis, and other connective tissue diseases (CTD). CCHB in these infants is often permanent and results in significant morbidity. Transient SLE phenomena infrequently occur in these infants.

PRIMARY NEONATAL SLE

There exist only a few reports that may be consistent with the diagnosis of primary neonatal SLE. Nice reported a child born of a normal mother who had persistent Coombs'-positive hemolytic anemia, thrombocytopenia, and positive LE cell tests. The child developed recurrent bronchopneumonias and chronic anemia and died at 4 years of age of congestive heart failure. Necropsy was not performed. Ty and Fine reported a 3-month-old infant who had positive antinuclear antibodies (ANA) and membranous nephritis. Hogg and Hull each described a case of an infant whose mother had SLE who died shortly after birth with extensive myocardial fibrosis.

TRANSIENT NEONATAL SLE

Although more than 25 cases of transient neonatal SLE have been reported, the incidence is not known. The female-to-male ratio in adult SLE is $9:1$; it is $2:1$ in neonatal SLE.

Transient neonatal SLE is usually characterized by the scaly and erythematous rash of discoid lupus. The distribution of the skin lesions includes the face, particularly the periorbital area, the trunk, and the upper extremities. The rash may be present at birth or appear anytime during the first several months of life. It commonly resolves by 6 months of age but may leave residual skin atrophy and telangiectasis (Vonderheid et al., 1976).

Hematologic abnormalities, including hemolytic anemia, leucopenia, and thrombocytopenia, are seen in 10 per cent of cases. These abnormalities may occur in association with other clinical manifestations or as isolated findings and tend to resolve within a few weeks. Although the pathogenesis of these hematologic abnormalities is presumed to be based on autoimmunity, antibodies directed at blood cell elements have rarely been documented (Nathan and Snapper, 1958).

Other less frequent transient neonatal SLE manifestations include hepatosplenomegaly and pericarditis (Nolan et al., 1979).

The clinical manifestations of transient neonatal SLE will frequently be associated with positive tests for antinuclear antibodies (ANA) and LE cells. The presence of these antibodies is believed to occur from the transplacental passage of maternal antibodies. They typically disappear within 3 to 4 weeks, a course that parallels that of the disappearance of transplacentally transferred maternal immunoglobulins. Positive tests for ANA and LE cells also occur in asymptomatic infants.

Although the pathogenesis of transient neonatal SLE is unknown, the transplacental passage of maternal immunoglobulins is probably involved. Deposition of immunoglobulin and complement in skin lesions of infants with transient neonatal SLE has been documented.

Of particular interest are the infants of normal mothers who develop transient neonatal SLE. Some of these mothers have subsequently developed connective tissue disorders. This phenomenon suggests that unidentified maternal serum factors may be involved in the pathogenesis of transient neonatal SLE and other connective tissue disorders.

Transient neonatal SLE is usually benign and self-limited. No specific treatment is required except for severe hemolytic anemia or thrombocytopenia, which may benefit from corticosteroid therapy. The discoid skin lesions may rarely persist (Brustein et al., 1977). There have been two case reports of infants with transient neonatal SLE who subsequently developed systemic lupus erythematosus in adolescence (Fox et al., 1979; Jackson and Gulliver, 1979).

CONGENITAL COMPLETE HEART BLOCK

Over 70 cases of congenital complete heart block (CCHB) in infants of mothers with SLE or connective tissue disorders have been reported. The estimated incidence of CCHB in all infants is 1 in 20,000 births, and it is possible that as many as 30 to 60 per cent of these patients may be offspring of mothers with SLE and other CTD (Esscher and Scott, 1979; McCue et al., 1977).

Congenital complete heart block in these infants commonly presents antenatally or at birth with bradycardia. The diagnosis is frequently confused with bradycardia secondary to fetal distress, which may result in premature delivery of the infant. The infants with CCHB can be asymptomatic or present with congestive heart failure. A cardiomyopathy present in some of these infants contributes to the development of failure. Other congenital heart defects seen in about 20 per cent of these cases include corrected transposition, patent ductus arteriosus, and partial anomalous venous return. Transient neonatal SLE phenomenon is observed in less than 10 per cent of infants with CCHB.

The mortality rate of CCHB in infants of mothers with SLE and CTD is between 20 and 30 per cent. The contributing factors are the frequency of congestive heart failure and the increased incidence of low birth weight and prematurity seen in infants of mothers with systemic lupus erythematosus. The development of heart block has been postulated to result from inflammation of myocardial tissue that occurs during organogenesis and causes conduction system malformation and scarring. Supporting evidence may be found in the pathologic findings of focal degeneration and fibrosis of the conduction system, failure to identify the atrioventricular node, and the presence of subendocardial fibroelastosis. Myocardial injury may be secondary to maternal antibodies directed against phase-specific antigens at the time of fetal conduction system development (Esscher and Scott, 1979).

Asymptomatic infants with CCHB require only observation, whereas those infants with CCHB and congestive failure need meticulous medical management as well as cardiac pacing when indicated.

REFERENCES

Beck, J. S., and Rowell, N. R.: Transplacental passage of antinuclear antibody. Lancet 1:134, 1963.

Berlyne, G. M., Short, I. A., and Vickers, C. F. H.: Placental transmission of the LE factor. Lancet 2:15, 1957.

Brustein, D., Rodriguez, J. M. Minkin, W., and Rabhan, N. B.: Familial lupus erythematosus. J.A.M.A. 238:2294, 1977.

Chamberlain, J. L., and Perry, L. W.: Infantile periarteritis nodosa with coronary and brachial aneurysms—a case diagnosed during life. J. Pediatr. 78:1039, 1971.

Esscher, E., and Scott, J. S.: Congenital heart block and maternal systemic lupus erythematosus. Br. Med. J. 1:1235, 1979.

Fox, R. J., McCuistion, C. H., and Schoch, E. P.: Systemic lupus erythematosus. Arch. Dermatol. 115:340, 1979.

Fraga, A., Mintz, G., Drozas, J., et al.: Sterility rates, fetal wastage and maternal morbidity in systemic lupus erythematosus. J. Rheumatol. 1:293, 1974.

Glanz, S., Bittner, S. J., Berman, M. A., Dolan, T. F., and Talner, N. S.: Regression of coronary-artery aneurysms in infantile polyarteritis nodosa. N. Engl. J. Med. 294:939, 1976.

Hess, E. V., and Spencer-Green, G.: Congenital heart block and connective tissue disease. Ann. Intern. Med. 91:645, 1979.

Hogg, G. R.: Congenital acute lupus erythematosus associated with subendocardial fibroelastosis. Report of a case. Am. J. Clin. Pathol. 28:648, 1957.

Hull, D., Binns, B. A. O., and Joyce, D.: Congenital heart block and widespread fibrosis due to maternal lupus erythematosus. Arch. Dis. Child. 41:688, 1966.

Jackson, R., and Gulliver, M.: Neonatal lupus erythematosus progressing into systemic lupus erythematosus. Br. J. Dermatol. 101:81, 1979.

Kato, H., Koike, S., and Yokoyama, T.: Kawasaki disease: effect of treatment on coronary artery involvement. Pediatrics 63:175, 1979.

Kawasaki, T., Kosaki, F., Okawa, S., Shrigematsu, I., and Yanagawa, H.: A new infantile acute febrile mucocutaneous lymph node syndrome (MLNS) prevailing in Japan. Pediatrics 54:271, 1974.

Krous, H. F., Clausen, C. R., and Ray, C. G.: Elevated immunoglobin E in infantile polyarteritis nodosa. J. Pediatr. 84:841, 1974.

Landing, B. H., and Larson, E. J.: Are infantile periarteritis nodosa with coronary artery involvement and fatal mucocutaneous lymph node syndrome the same? Comparison of 20 patients from North America with patients from Hawaii and Japan. Pediatrics 59:651, 1977.

Liban, E., Shamir, Z., and Schorr, S.: Periarteritis nodosa in a nine month old infant. Am. J. Dis. Child. 88:210, 1954.

McCue, C. M., Mantakas, M. E., Tingelstad, J. B., and Ruddy, S.: Congenital heart block in newborns of mothers with connective tissue disease. Circulation 56:82, 1977.

Mund, A., Simson, J., Rothfield, N.: Effect of pregnancy on course of systemic lupus erythematosus. J.A.M.A. 183:917, 1963.

Nathan, D. J., and Snapper, I.: Simultaneous placental transfer of factors responsible for LE cell formation and thrombocytopenia. Am. J. Med. 25:647, 1958.

Nice, C. M., Jr.: Congenital disseminated lupus erythematosus. Am. J. Roentgenol. Radium Ther. Nucl. Med. 88:585, 1962.

Nolan, R. J., Shulman, S. T., and Victorica, B. E.: Congenital complete heart block associated with maternal mixed connective tissue disease. J. Pediatr. 95:420, 1979.

Rich, A. R.: The role of hypersensitivity in periarteritis nodosa as indicated by 7 cases developing during serum sickness and sulfonamide therapy. Bull. Johns Hopkins Hosp. *71*:123, 1942.

Rich, A. R., and Gregory, J. E.: Experimental demonstration that periarteritis nodosa is a manifestation of hypersensitivity. Bull. Johns Hopkins Hosp. *72*:65, 1943.

Roberts, F. B., and Fetterman, G. H.: Polyarteritis nodosa in infancy. J. Pediatr. *63*:519, 1963.

Schaller, J. G.: Lupus phenomena in the newborn. Proceedings of the first conference on childhood rheumatic diseases. Arthritis Rheum. (suppl. 2) *20*:312, 1977.

Seip, M.: Systemic lupus erythematosus in pregnancy with haemolytic anaemia, leucopenia and thrombocytopenia in the mother and her newborn infant. Arch. Dis. Child. *35*:364, 1960.

Tanaka, N., Sekimoto, K., and Naoe, S.: Kawasaki disease. Relationship with infantile polyarteritis nodosa. Arch. Pathol. Lab. Med. *100*:81, 1976.

Ty, A., and Fine, B.: Membranous nephritis in infantile systemic lupus erythematosus associated with chromosomal abnormalities. Clin. Nephrol. *12*:137, 1979.

Vonderheid, E. C., Koblenzer, P. J., Ming, P. M. L., and Burgoon, C. F.: Neonatal lupus erythematosus. Arch. Dermatol. *112*:698, 1976.

Wilmer, H. A.: Two cases of periarteritis nodosa occurring in the first month of life. Bull. Johns Hopkins Hosp. *77*:275, 1945.

PART 10 JAUNDICE

68

General Considerations

By Frank A. Oski

Jaundice is the visible manifestation of chemical hyperbilirubinemia. Most adults are visibly jaundiced when serum bilirubin concentrations exceed 2.0 mg per 100 ml, whereas neonatal icterus is rarely perceptible until the serum bilirubin concentration exceeds 7.0 mg per 100 ml.

Chemical hyperbilirubinemia, a serum bilirubin of 2.0 mg per 100 ml or more, is virtually universal in newborn infants during the first week of life. Although some degree of jaundice may be considered a normal physical finding in both term and preterm infants, the findings from the National Collaborative Perinatal Project indicate that only 6.2 per cent of white infants and 4.5 per cent of black infants weighing more than 2500 gm at birth will have bilirubin values in excess of 12.9 mg per 100 ml (221 µmol/l). In contrast, 10 to 20 per cent of infants weighing less than 2500 gm at birth will have bilirubin values that exceed 15 mg per 100 ml during the first week of life.

Bilirubin Formation and Excretion

Bilirubin is derived from the catabolism of heme proteins. Heme-containing proteins include hemoglobin, myoglobin, and heme-containing enzymes such as the cytochromes, catalase, and tryptophan pyrrolase. Virtually all cells of the body are a potential source of bilirubin, although, under usual circumstances, this pigment is primarily due to the destruction of hemoglobin contained within erythrocytes. The catabolism of 1 gm of hemoglobin results in the production of 34 mg of bilirubin.

Bilirubin IXα, the naturally occurring isomer in humans, is ultimately derived from the enzymatic opening of the protoporphyrin IX ring of heme at the alpha carbon bridge (Fig. 68–1) with the initial formation of carbon monoxide and biliverdin. This oxidation is catalyzed by the enzyme microsomal heme oxygenase. Biliverdin, the initial tetrapyrrolic product of the ring-opening reaction, is then rapidly reduced to bilirubin by the enzyme, biliverdin reductase.

One molecule of carbon monoxide is produced for

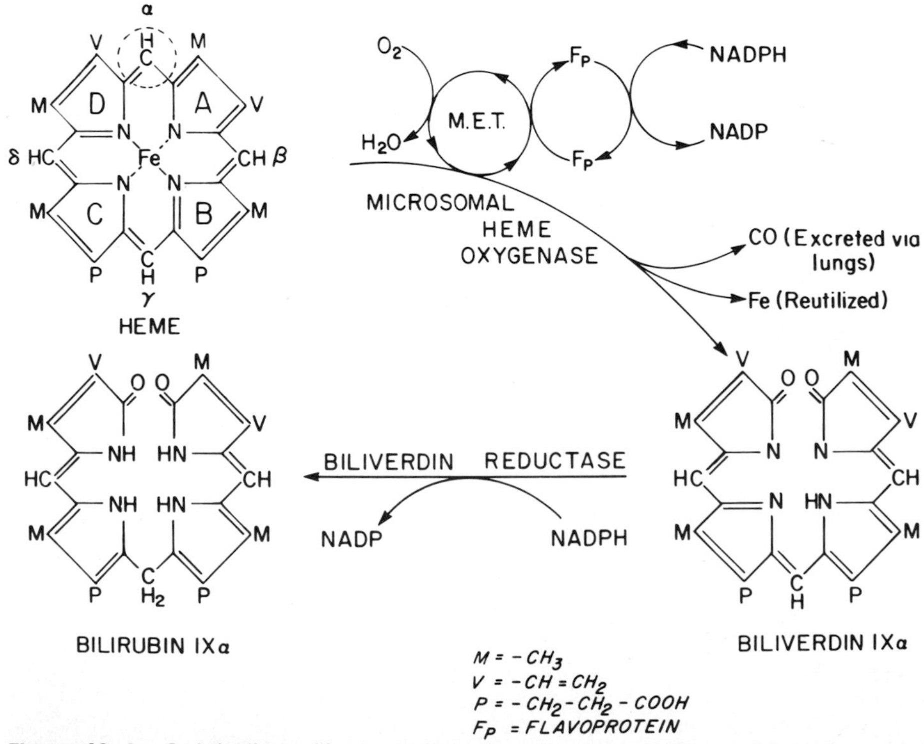

$M = -CH_3$
$V = -CH = CH_2$
$P = -CH_2 - CH_2 - COOH$
$F_P = FLAVOPROTEIN$

Figure 68–1. Catabolism of heme to bilirubin IXα by microsomal heme oxygenase and biliverdin reductase. M.E.T. = microsomal electron transport system. (Modified from Tenhunen et al. by Berlin, N. I., and Berk, P. D.: Blood 57:983, 1981.)

every molecule of bilirubin produced. This pathway represents the only known source of both bilirubin and carbon monoxide in humans. The measurement of either carbon monoxide production rates or carboxyhemoglobin levels has proved useful in documenting the magnitude of heme catabolism and in providing insights into the mechanism of hyperbilirubinemia in both infants and adults.

The destruction of circulating erythrocytes accounts for approximately 75 per cent of the daily bilirubin production in the normal newborn infant. In the normal adult, the death of senescent red cells is the source of 85 to 90 per cent of the bilirubin produced each day. About 25 per cent of the daily bilirubin production in the neonate comes from sources other than the circulating red blood cell. These alternate sources include a nonerythrocytic component resulting from the catabolism of heme proteins and free heme, primarily in the liver, and an erythropoietic component that results from the destruction of red cell precursors in the bone marrow or soon after their release into circulation. This destruction of nonsenescent red blood cells is termed "ineffective erythropoiesis."

The normal newborn produces 8.5 ± 2.3 mg bilirubin per kg per day, which is more than double the bilirubin production of 3.6 mg per kg per day observed in the adult. This difference is a result of the fact that the newborn has a larger red cell mass per kilogram of body weight, red cells with a life span that is only two thirds that of red cells produced by normal adults, and a larger production of bilirubin from nonerythrocytic sources. This increase in bilirubin production is reflected in the higher carbon monoxide production rates observed in normal term infants. Endogenous carbon monoxide production

averages 14 to 15 µl/kg/hr in term infants as compared with an average value of 6.1 µl/kg/hr in normal adults. Carbon monoxide production rates in preterm infants display wide variability but average about 20 per cent more than those observed in term infants.

Bilirubin produced in the peripheral regions of the body and the reticuloendothelial system is transported, tightly bound to albumin, to the liver. Binding to albumin is essential for transport because the solubility of unbound bilirubin at pH 7.4 is extremely low, averaging 0.4 µg per 100 ml. Uptake of the bilirubin from this bilirubin-albumin complex occurs on the surface of the liver parenchymal cells. Bilirubin, but not albumin, is transferred across the cell membrane into the hepatocyte, where it is bound to soluble intracellular proteins. The uptake from the circulation into the liver cell displays the kinetic properties of carrier-mediated transport and may be facilitated by a distinct bilirubin-binding protein located on the membrane surface of the hepatocyte.

Bilirubin within the hepatocyte is bound primarily to ligandin (Y protein, glutathione S-transferase B) but also to other glutathione S-transferases and to Z protein. This binding within the cell prevents backflow of bilirubin into the circulation. Phenobarbital increases the concentration of ligandin, thus providing more intracellular binding sites for bilirubin.

The bound intracellular bilirubin is next transported to the smooth endoplasmic reticulum for conjugation. The unconjugated (or indirect-reacting) bilirubin, which is poorly soluble in aqueous solutions at a pH of 7.4, is converted to its water-soluble con-

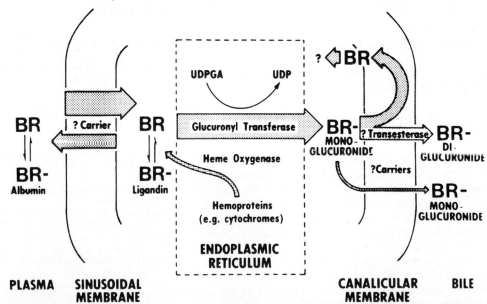

Figure 68–2. Bilirubin transport and conjugation in the hepatocyte. Bilirubin (BR) that has been transferred across the sinusoidal membrane is converted to bilirubin monoglucuronide by glucuronyl transferase located in the endoplasmic reticulum. The monoglucuronide is then either excreted into the bile or converted to bilirubin diglucuronide by a glucuronyl transferase believed to be located in the canalicular membrane. (From Schmid, R.: Gastroenterology 74:1307, 1978.)

jugate, direct-reacting bilirubin, prior to excretion. In adults, the major product of conjugation is bilirubin diglucuronide. In newborns during the first 48 hours of life, only monoglucoronides are formed. After 48 hours of life, bilirubin diglucuronide is the major excretory product. It appears that two separate enzymes participate in the conjugation process. The first is bilirubin uridine diphosphate glucuronyl transferase (UDPG-T), an enzyme associated with the smooth endoplasmic reticulum and inducible by phenobarbital. UDPG-T catalyzes the formation of bilirubin monoglucuronide. This monoglucuronide may be excreted, stored, or converted to the diglucuronide. The formation of the bilirubin diglucuronide appears to be catalyzed by a transferase enzyme located in the plasma membrane of the hepatocyte. This complex series of steps is diagramatically illustrated in Figure 68–2.

After conjugation, bilirubin is excreted into the bile. This is an active, energy-dependent process because the conjugated bilirubin is excreted against a large concentration gradient. Conjugated bilirubin is not reabsorbed once it enters the intestinal tract. In the normal adult, most of the conjugated bilirubin is reduced to stercobilin by bacteria and only a very small fraction is hydrolyzed to unconjugated bilirubin and reabsorbed via the enterohepatic circulation. In the sterile intestine of the newborn infant, the reduction of bilirubin to stercobilin does not occur. In addition, the newborn gut is rich in β-glucuronidase, an enzyme that hydrolyzes the ester linkage of bilirubin glucuronide yielding unconjugated bilirubin. This unconjugated bilirubin is now capable of being reabsorbed and returned to the circulation, where it must again be transported to the liver for conjugation and excretion. This enterohepatic phase of bilirubin metabolism appears to play a major role in the hyperbilirubinemia of some newborn infants.

Fetal Bilirubin Metabolism

Bilirubin formed from heme catabolism during fetal life must also be eliminated. Disposal in utero appears to occur by two mechanisms. Bilirubin that enters the placental circulation is cleared across the placenta into the maternal circulation. The concentration of bilirubin in the venous blood returning from the placenta has been found to be lower than the concentration in the umbilical arteries that transport blood to the placenta. Only unconjugated bilirubin is cleared via the placental circulation. Conjugated bilirubin, when formed in utero, remains in the fetus and may accumulate in fetal plasma and other tissues. Infants with severe hemolytic disease may be born with increased concentrations of conjugated bilirubin in their blood.

The second route for bilirubin clearance in the fetus is by way of the fetal liver. This excretory pathway is limited in the fetus as a consequence of reduced hepatic blood flow, low levels of hepatocyte ligandin, and limited UDP glucuronyl transferase activity. Conjugated bilirubin that is excreted into the fetal gut is largely hydrolyzed and reabsorbed into the fetal circulation.

Bilirubin can be found in normal amniotic fluid about the twelfth week of gestation. It usually disappears from the amniotic fluid by the thirty-sixth to thirty-seventh week of pregnancy. Increased levels of bilirubin are found in the amniotic fluid of infants with severe hemolytic disease and in association with fetal intestinal obstruction.

The mechanism by which bilirubin gets into the amniotic fluid is still a matter of speculation. It has been suggested that bilirubin reaches the amniotic fluid from tracheobronchial secretions, fetal urine, meconium, diffusion across the umbilical vessels, diffusion from the skin, or direct transfer from the maternal circulation. In rabbits, there is a close relationship between the concentration of unconjugated bilirubin in the plasma and that found in tracheal fluid.

In the chapters to follow the various causes of neonatal hyperbilirubinemia will be discussed. Jaundice is usually the result of one or more of the following mechanisms:

1. Overproduction of bilirubin.
2. Defective uptake and transport of bilirubin within the hepatocyte.
3. Impaired conjugation within the hepatic microsomes.
4. Defects in bilirubin excretion.
5. Increased reabsorption of bilirubin from the intestinal tract.

REFERENCES

Berlin, N. I., and Berk, P. D.: Quantitative aspects of bilirubin metabolism for hematologists. Blood 57:983, 1981.

Bernstein, L. H., Ezzer, J. B., Gartner, L., and Arias, I. M.: Hepatic intracellular distribution of tritium-labelled unconjugated and conjugated bilirubin in normal and Gunn rats. J. Clin. Invest. 45:1194, 1966.

Hardy, J. B., Drage, J. S., and Jackson, E. C.: The first year of life. The Collaborative Perinatal Project of the National Institutes of Neurological and Communicative Disorders and Stroke. Baltimore, The Johns Hopkins University Press, 1979, p. 104.

Maisels, M. J.: Bilirubin. On understanding and influencing its metabolism in the newborn infant. Pediatr. Clin. North Am. 19:447, 1972.

Odell, G. B.: Neonatal Hyperbilirubinemia. New York, Grune & Stratton, 1980.

Paumgartner, G., and Reichen, J.: Kinetics of hepatic uptake of unconjugated bilirubin. Clin. Sci. Mol. Med. 51:169, 1976.

Schenker, S., Dawlser, N., and Schmid, R.: Bilirubin metabolism in the fetus. J. Clin. Invest. 43:32, 1964.

Schmid, R.: Bilirubin metabolism: State of the art. Gastroenterology 74:1307, 1978.

Stevenson, D. K., Ostrander, C. R., Cohen, R. S., and Johnson, J. D.: Relationship of heme catabolism to jaundice. Bilirubin production in infancy. Perinatol. Neonatol. 5:35, 1981.

Tenhunen, R., and Marver, H. S.: The enzymatic conversion of heme to bilirubin by microsomal heme oxygenase. Proc. Natl. Acad. Sci. U.S.A. 61:748, 1968.

Wolkoff, A. W., Goresky, C. A., Sellin, J., Gatmaitan, Z., and Arias, I. M.: Role of ligandin in transfer of bilirubin from plasma into liver. Am. J. Physiol. 236:638, 1979.

69

Physiologic Jaundice

By Frank A. Oski

An understanding of bilirubin production and catabolism, as described in the preceding chapter, provides a basis for an understanding of what has long been called "physiologic" jaundice of the newborn. The normal newborn has one or more defects in bilirubin metabolism and transport that regularly result in the occurrence of increased concentrations of serum unconjugated bilirubin during the first week of life.

The general limits of hyperbilirubinemia vary as a function of the gestational age and the race of the infant. In Tables 69–1 and 69–2, the results of the National Collaborative Perinatal Project are presented. In this project, serum bilirubin concentrations were obtained on more than 35,000 infants. Bilirubin concentration was measured at 48 hours of age and then repeated daily if the initial value exceeded 10 mg per 100 ml. Sampling was continued until the serum bilirubin concentration decreased to less than 10 mg per 100 ml. Although this project included all infants, both well ones and those with known hemolytic disease, in 97 per cent the maximum serum bilirubin concentration did not exceed 12.9 mg per 100 ml.

This survey, as well as many other studies of serum bilirubin values in seemingly normal term and preterm infants, has provided guidelines for what is and is not physiologic jaundice. Maisels has proposed five criteria that can be used to exclude the diagnosis of physiologic jaundice (Table 69–3). It must be remembered, however, that the absence of these criteria does not guarantee that the jaundice is physiologic and that the infant has no underlying pathologic process.

This pattern of hyperbilirubinemia, physiologic jaundice, results from an interaction of several developmental abnormalities and has been classified by Gartner and coworkers into two functionally distinct periods. The first period, designated as Phase I, includes the first 5 days of life in the term infant and is characterized by a relatively rapid rise in serum unconjugated bilirubin concentrations from an average cord blood value of 1.5 mg per 100 ml to a peak value of 6 to 7 mg per 100 ml on the third day of life. In the preterm infant, the peak value averages 10 to 12 mg per 100 ml and does not occur until the fifth to seventh day of life. In the term infant, after the third day of life, the bilirubin begins to decline quickly until the fifth day of life, at which point Phase II begins. Phase II is characterized by a relatively stable serum unconjugated bilirubin concentration of about 2 mg per 100 ml that persists until the end of the second week of life. After this time, the serum bilirubin concentration declines again to values observed in normal adults. Normal adults' serum bilirubin concentrations are usually less than 1.0 mg per 100 ml. Phase II may persist in the preterm infant for a month or more, depending on the gestational age of the infant at birth.

Studies in newborn rhesus monkeys by Gartner have disclosed a similar pattern, although the overall course of the disease is shorter. This animal model has provided insight into the biochemical basis for human neonatal physiologic jaundice. Phase I hyperbilirubinemia is caused by excessive bilirubin production coupled with deficient hepatic conjugation. The impaired hepatic conjugation appears to be primarily a result of deficient glucuronyl transferase activity. The excessive bilirubin load presented to the

Table 69–1. Highest Total Serum Bilirubin by Birth Weight in White Newborns

mg/dl	Under 2500 gm			Over 2500 gm			Total		
	Live Births	Per cent	Cumulative Per cent	Live Births	Per cent	Cumulative Per cent	Live Births	Per cent	Cumulative Per cent
0–7	488	42.73	100.00	11908	73.73	100.00	12396	71.69	100.00
8–12	336	29.42	57.27	3243	20.08	26.27	3579	20.70	28.31
13–15	128	11.21	27.85	531	3.29	6.19	659	3.81	7.62
16–19	114	9.98	16.64	315	1.95	2.90	429	2.48	3.81
20+	76	6.65	6.65	153	0.95	0.95	229	1.32	1.32
Subtotal	1142	100.00		16150	100.00		17292	100.00	
Unknown	177	13.42		1012	5.90		1189	6.43	
TOTAL	1319	100.00		17162	100.00		18481	100.00	

(From Hardy, J. B., et al.: The Collaborative Perinatal Project of the National Institutes of Neurological and Communicative Disorders and Stroke. Baltimore, The Johns Hopkins University Press, 1979.)

liver is due to the accelerated destruction of red cells and the increased enterohepatic circulation of bilirubin. The exaggerated physiologic jaundice of the premature infant is the result of a delay in maturation of glucuronyl transferase activity coupled with an even greater rate of red cell destruction than is observed in the normal term infant.

Phase II physiologic jaundice is less well understood. Evidence derived from the study of rhesus monkeys suggests that this phase of hyperbilirubinemia results from the simultaneous occurrence of delayed hepatic uptake of bilirubin and a continued increased bilirubin load that is largely due to excessive enteric bilirubin absorption. This delay in maturation of hepatic bilirubin uptake may be a result of inadequate production of ligandin, the hepatic cytoplasmic bilirubin-binding protein that was discussed in Chapter 68.

Both term and premature newborn infants are in an ever-changing situation with respect to the various steps in bilirubin metabolism. Slight perturbations in any of the developmental processes may result in excessive hyperbilirubinemia. Some of these possibilities are listed in Table 69–4 and are discussed again in Chapter 75. It should be emphasized that although unconjugated hyperbilirubinemia may be a manifestation of either a pathologic process or an exaggerated developmental process, the presence of conjugated hyperbilirubinemia is always an indication of the presence of a pathologic process.

Factors Influencing Serum Bilirubin Levels

It is now recognized that genetic and ethnic factors, perinatal events, maternal diseases, drugs administered to the mother, and infant feeding practices may all influence the degree and course of neonatal hyperbilirubinemia.

Serum bilirubin values appear to be significantly

Table 69–3. Criteria That Rule Out the Diagnosis of Physiologic Jaundice

1. Clinical jaundice in the first 24 hours of life.
2. Total serum bilirubin concentration increasing by more than 5 mg/dl (85 μmol/l) per day.
3. Total serum bilirubin concentration exceeding 12.9 mg/dl (221 μmol/l) in a full-term infant or 15 mg/dl (257 μmol/l) in a premature infant.
4. Direct serum bilirubin concentration exceeding 1.5 to 2 mg/dl (26–34 μmol/l).
5. Clinical jaundice persisting for more than 1 week in a full-term infant or 2 weeks in a premature infant.

(From Maisels, M. J.: In Avery, G. B. (Ed.): Neonatology. 2nd ed. Philadelphia, J. B. Lippincott, 1981, p. 484.)

higher in apparently normal Chinese, Japanese, Korean, and American Indian infants. In certain areas of Greece, there is a very high incidence of hyperbilirubinemia of unexplained origin. It has not as yet been established whether this exaggerated hyperbilirubinemia is a consequence of increased bilirubin production or a maturational delay in bilirubin conjugation and excretion.

Perinatal events that have been reported to be associated with an increased incidence of hyperbilirubinemia include delayed cord clamping, delivery by vacuum extraction, the use of forceps, breech delivery, the use of oxytocin, and the administration of epidural (bupivacaine) analgesia to the mother. Delayed cord clamping is believed to result in higher peak bilirubin concentrations as a result of the fact that the infant has a larger red cell mass and thus a greater capacity to produce bilirubin. Vacuum extraction, the use of forceps, and breech delivery may all produce bruising in an infant, and the resorption of red cells from such entrapped hemorrhages will result in hyperbilirubinemia. Although not all surveys have demonstrated an association between the use of oxytocin and hyperbilirubinemia, Buchan has found that infants delivered following oxytocin induction had evidence of hemolysis. In addition, the oxytocin group had decreased erythrocyte deformability that was ascribed to osmotic swelling of the red cells produced by the action of oxytocin on the red cell membrane resulting in increased water uptake. The mechanism by which bupivacaine pro-

Table 69–2. Highest Total Serum Bilirubin by Birth Weight in Black Newborns

mg/dl	Under 2500 gm			Over 2500 gm			Total		
	Live Births	Per cent	Cumulative Per cent	Live Births	Per cent	Cumulative Per cent	Live Births	Per cent	Cumulative Per cent
0–7	1137	50.29	100.00	11734	74.48	100.00	12871	71.45	100.00
8–12	719	31.80	49.71	3309	21.00	25.52	4028	22.36	28.55
13–15	225	9.95	17.91	412	2.62	4.51	637	3.54	6.19
16–19	113	5.00	7.96	202	1.28	1.90	315	1.75	2.66
20+	67	2.96	2.96	97	0.62	0.62	164	0.91	0.91
Subtotal	2261	100.00		15754	100.00		18015	100.00	
Unknown	356	13.60		1133	6.71		1489	7.63	
TOTAL	2617	100.00		16887	100.00		19504	100.00	

(From Hardy, J. B., et al.: The Collaborative Perinatal Project of the National Institutes of Neurological and Communicative Disorders and Stroke. Baltimore, The Johns Hopkins University Press, 1979.)

duces hyperbilirubinemia is presently unknown, but this agent is soluble in the membrane of the erythrocyte and may produce changes in red cell deformability that could result in accelerated destruction of the cell.

Infants of diabetic mothers are more likely to develop hyperbilirubinemia. This may be a consequence of hypoxia, plethora in the infant, or delay in the maturation of hepatic uptake of bilirubin. It has been observed that hyperbilirubinemia only occurs in macrosomic infants of diabetic mothers.

The introduction of early feeding, now a common practice, as opposed to a 48-hour fast after birth, results in a lower peak serum bilirubin concentration. The feeding may stimulate gut motility and reduce the enterohepatic circulation of bilirubin. Delay in passage of the first stool is known to be associated with increased peak serum bilirubin concentrations.

BREAST-FEEDING AND HYPERBILIRUBINEMIA

Surveys have indicated that somewhere between one in 50 and one in 200 breast-fed infants will develop significant delayed onset and protracted hyperbilirubinemia. The recurrence rate in future siblings may approximate 70 per cent.

This form of late-onset neonatal jaundice was initially ascribed to the inhibition of hepatic glucuronyl transferase activity by an abnormal hormonal component in the human milk. More recent studies have not confirmed this hypothesis.

The typical late-onset breast-milk jaundice usually occurs after the third day of life. Bilirubin concentration, rather than falling as is the usual course in the normal term infant, continues to rise and may achieve peak concentrations of 20 to 25 mg per 100 ml by the end of the second week of life. These infants do well with good appetites, good weight gain, and no evidence of hemolytic disease or other recognized causes of jaundice. If nursing continues, serum bilirubin concentrations gradually decline to normal over a period of 1 to 4 months. An interruption in nursing will produce a fall in serum bilirubin concentration in 24 to 72 hours. Failure of bilirubin concentration to decline significantly within 3 days of cessation of breast-feeding eliminates human milk as the cause of the jaundice. Resumption of breast-feeding is associated with either a cessation of the previously observed decline in serum bilirubin concentration or a rise of only 2 to 3 mg per 100 ml. Kernicterus has never been reported with breast-milk jaundice, but long-term prospective studies have never been conducted. The mechanism for the association of breast-feeding with jaundice is still unsettled. It has been proposed that the milk of such mothers may contain large quantities of unsaturated fatty acids that may inhibit hepatic bilirubin conjugation. Preliminary evidence also suggests that this milk may not inhibit the enterohepatic circulation of bilirubin, whereas normal milk does. Perhaps more than one mechanism is responsible.

Temporary cessation of breast-feeding in a jaundiced infant should be performed only when bilirubin values have approached presumably toxic levels of approximately 20 mg per 100 ml or when such interruption is crucial in establishing the etiology of the protracted jaundice.

It is commonly believed that early-onset hyperbilirubinemia is more common among breast-fed infants. Two prospective studies have failed to demonstrate any significant difference between bottle-fed and breast-fed infants with respect to serum bilirubin concentrations during the first 3 days of life. It is possible that infants who are not being breast-fed at sufficiently frequent intervals (every 2 to 3 hours during the first days of life) may become extremely jaundiced as a result of caloric deprivation.

Table 69–4.   Possible Factors Involved in Producing "Physiologic Jaundice"

Factor	Clinical Correlate
1. Increased bilirubin load to liver cell. Newborns have increased blood volume, erythrocytes with a reduced lifespan, increased ineffective erythropoiesis, and increased bilirubin reabsorption from gut.	Bilirubin levels tend to be higher in infants with polycythemia or delayed cord clamping. Infants with reduced bowel motility tend to have higher bilirubin levels.
2. Defective uptake of bilirubin from the plasma. Decreased Y protein.	Caloric deprivation may reduce formation of hepatic binding proteins. Decreased caloric intake results in higher bilirubin levels.
3. Defective bilirubin conjugation. Decreased UDP glucuronyl transferase activity.	UDP glucuronyl transferase activity decreased with inadequate caloric intake. Enzyme may be inhibited by factors in some mothers' breast milk. Hypothyroidism reduces enzyme activity.
4. Defective bilirubin excretion.	Congenital infections.
5. Inadequate hepatic perfusion.	May occur with hypoxia or in patients with congenital heart disease. Both situations associated with increased incidence of hyperbilirubinemia.
6. Increased enterohepatic circulation of bilirubin.	Increased bilirubin values in babies with delayed passage of meconium or with intestinal obstruction.

Table 69–5. Guidelines for Use of Phototherapy in Newborn Period

Birth Weight (gm)	Indication for Phototherapy
<1500	Start phototherapy during first 24 hours of life regardless of serum bilirubin concentration.
1500–1999	Without hemolysis start phototherapy at 10 mg/dl. With hemolysis start phototherapy at 8 mg/dl.
2000–2499	Without hemolysis start phototherapy at 12 mg/dl. With hemolysis start phototherapy at 10 mg/dl.
>2500	Without hemolysis in healthy infant withhold use of phototherapy. With hemolysis or in presence of factors that contraindicate use of exchange transfusion start phototherapy at 15 mg/dl.

Phototherapy to be continued until serum bilirubin concentration has stabilized at or fallen to less than one half of exchange transfusion indication level listed in Table 69–6.

(From Gartner, L. M.: *In* Nathan, D. G., and Oski, F. A. (Eds.): Hematology of Infancy and Childhood. 2nd ed. Philadelphia, W. B. Saunders Co., 1981, p. 107.)

Diagnosis and Management

The diagnosis of physiologic jaundice remains largely a diagnosis of exclusion (Table 69–3). The steps in the differential diagnosis of jaundice are described in Chapter 75. In brief, any infant in whom the serum bilirubin concentration exceeds the usual limits of normal for weight or gestational age should be studied. Initial evaluation consists of a review of the maternal and perinatal history, a repeat physical examination, and laboratory studies that consist of a hemoglobin or hematocrit, a reticulocyte count, a white cell count with differential, an examination of a peripheral blood film, blood typing of mother and infant, and the performance of direct and indirect Coombs' test on the infant's erythrocytes and serum. It has been estimated that these simple procedures will provide clues to the correct diagnosis in one half of all infants studied.

Blood tests as well as liver function studies will be normal in infants with physiologic jaundice.

Treatment is obviously directed to the prevention of bilirubin encephalopathy. Guidelines for the use of phototherapy and exchange transfusion are described in Tables 69–5 and 69–6, respectively. Nomograms designed to reduce the need for unnecessary phototherapy have been prepared by Cockington and may provide helpful guidance.

PHOTOTHERAPY

Cremer and coworkers reported in 1958 that the exposure of premature infants to sunlight or blue fluorescent light produced a decline in serum bilirubin concentration. Since that initial report, visible light has been used extensively for the prevention and treatment of hyperbilirubinemia. Brown and McDonagh have reviewed the efficacy, toxicity, and current concepts of the mechanism of action of phototherapy.

In a number of well-controlled studies, the effectiveness of phototherapy as a method of preventing or treating moderate degrees of hyperbilirubinemia has been documented. Prophylactic phototherapy in infants at 24 hours of age can reduce serum bilirubin levels by 30 to 50 per cent during the first week of life. Continuous phototherapy in preterm infants will result in bilirubin levels in excess of 12 mg per 100 ml in only 8 per cent of the group; in a control group not receiving phototherapy, the incidence will be 44 per cent.

Data from the collaborative study on phototherapy sponsored by the National Institute of Child Health and Human Development indicate that when phototherapy is used prophylactically in preterm infants between 24 and 120 hours of age, the decrement in bilirubin is greatest in the first 24 hours of exposure. The decreases in serum bilirubin concentration attributable to phototherapy averaged 2.4 and 1.6 mg/100 ml per day for infants with birth weights below 1500 gm and between 1500 and 1999 gm, respectively. The use of phototherapy reduced the rate of exchange transfusion for infants less than 2000 gm from 24.4 per cent in the control group to 4.1 per cent in the treated group.

Table 69–6. Serum Bilirubin Concentrations (mg/dl) at Which Exchange Transfusions Are Indicated During the Neonatal Period

	Birth Weight (gm)					
Infants	<1000	1000–1249	1250–1499	1500–1999	2000–2499	>2500
Healthy infants	10	13	15	17	18	20
High-risk infants*	10	10	13	15	17	18

* High-risk infants include those with perinatal asphyxia, hypoxia, acidosis, hypoalbuminemia, hemolysis, hypothermia, and septicemia (all septicemic infants with proven or highly suspected bacterial infection should be treated as <1000 gm birth weight infants, regardless of birth weight).

(From Gartner, L. M.: *In* Nathan, D. G., and Oski, F. A. [Eds.]: Hematology of Infancy and Childhood. 2nd ed. Philadelphia, W. B. Saunders Co., 1981, p. 105.)

Despite its widespread use, it is still unclear as to how phototherapy works. Phototherapy is thought to reduce serum bilirubin by two possible mechanisms. It was initially believed that light resulted in the photo-oxidation of bilirubin. Bilirubin absorbs light maximally in the blue wavelengths between 420 and 480 nm. Light reaching the bilirubin raises the pigment to a higher energy state. This energy is then transferred to oxygen with the production of singlet oxygen molecules. The singlet oxygen reacts with the bilirubin to produce a variety of oxidation products. The products of photo-oxidation include biliverdin, dipyrroles, and monopyrroles. Many of these products are colorless and, in the van den Bergh test, nonreactive, and they are presumably excreted by the liver and kidneys without requiring conjugation. Animal studies have suggested that these photo-oxidation products are nontoxic. Unfortunately, there is very little evidence to support the hypothesis that the photo-oxidation of bilirubin plays a major role in the lowering of serum bilirubin concentration by phototherapy.

Despite the widespread use of phototherapy, the mechanism by which it reduces serum bilirubin concentration has only recently been elucidated. Phototherapy reduces serum bilirubin primarily by facilitating biliary excretion of unconjugated bilirubin. The work of McDonagh and associates suggests that the major reacton to phototherapy is the rapid conversion of unconjugated bilirubin to two configurational isomers termed "photobilirubin." A small percentage of bilirubin is also converted to the structural isomer "lumirubin."

The first step in the process occurs when light shines on the skin. Part of this light is absorbed by the tissues, and bilirubin IX_a is instantly isomerized into photobilirubin, a more polar compound. Next, the photobilirubin moves from the tissues to the blood by a passive, diffusion-controlled reaction. In the blood, the photobilirubin is bound to albumin and transported to the liver, where the photobilirubin is removed from the circulation. Finally, the photobilirubin is secreted by the hepatocyte into the biliary canaliculus and excreted with normal bile into the duodenum. The excretion of photobilirubin is independent of the bilirubin concentration and does not require hepatic conjugation. Upon entry into the bile, the photobilirubin may be reisomerized to the original bilirubin IX_a.

Various oxidation products of bilirubin are also formed when it is exposed to light in the presence of oxygen. These photodegradation products are excreted in the urine. Photoisomerization rather than photodegradation is believed to be the primary and major mechanism by which phototherapy serves to reduce the concentration on bilirubin in the plasma.

The efficiency of phototherapy depends on the irradiance at the level of the infant's skin. (Irradiance is expressed as microwatts per square centimeter per nanometer.) It has been reported that most standard phototherapy units, fitted with eight 20-w daylight fluorescent lamps, will provide an irradiance of 5 to 6 $\mu w/cm^2/nm$ at a distance of 42 to 45 cm below the lamp, inside the incubator. For most infants with nonhemolytic hyperbilirubinemia, this should produce an average fall in bilirubin of about 2.4 mg/100 ml in 24 hours. Raising the irradiance to 8.6 $\mu w/cm^2/nm$ may produce a decrease in bilirubin of 3.5 mg/100 ml in 24 hours, but an increase above 8.6 $\mu w/cm^2/nm$ confers no additional benefit and may, in fact, increase the incidence of undesirable side effects. A minimum irradiance of 4 $\mu w/cm^2/nm$ appears to be necessary for effective phototherapy.

In 1981, Wu published the following recommendations regarding the indications and technique of phototherapy:

1. Individual centers should establish limits for serum bilirubin concentration that are acceptable for infants of various gestational ages and with various clinical conditions.

2. Phototherapy should be initiated in the presence of values 2.5 to 3 mg below this acceptable limit.

3. The light source should generally not be greater than 45 to 50 cm above the infant to provide an irradiance of 5 to 6 $\mu w/cm^2/nm$.

4. The irradiance should not be less than 4 $\mu w/cm^2/nm$ at the effective spectral bandpass of 400 to 500 nm (maximum bilirubin reduction can be achieved with irradiances between 8 and 9 $\mu w/cm^2/nm$ with a combination of 4 daylight and 4 blue 20-w lamps).

5. The phototherapy unit must have a thermoplastic cover (0.25 in. thick).

6. Infants, naked except for eye patches, can best be treated inside a servo-controlled incubator. Lights may be briefly discontinued and patches removed during feeding or visiting time of parents or relatives.

7. There should be a space of about 2 in. between the thermoplastic incubator hood and the cover of the lamp. This minimizes overheating of the incubator by allowing free flow of air between the two sections of thermoplastic.

8. The hospital line voltage should be no less than 100 v (preferably between 115 and 120 v).

9. Infants receiving phototherapy should be given extra fluid (10 to 15 ml per kg of body weight) to compensate for increased insensible water loss. When possible, caloric intake should be at least 60 calories per kg of body weight every 24 hours (preferably more), since oral caloric intake improves efficiency of phototherapy.

10. In infants weighing 1500 gm with nonhemolytic jaundice, a rebound of 1 to 2 mg of bilirubin should be anticipated when phototherapy is discontinued after serum bilirubin concentration has decreased to <10 mg/100 ml and after the infant is 72 to 144 hours of age. For larger infants, overt rebound may not be present.

Phototherapy may produce a transient rash, transient loose green stools, lethargy, and abdominal distention. Phototherapy may result in the "bronze baby" syndrome, which occurs almost exclusively in infants with an increased concentration of direct-reacting bilirubin in their sera, usually as a result of associated liver disease.

Other metabolic effects of phototherapy include a mild reduction in the platelet count, a reduction in the serum calcium concentration, and an increase in water loss via the skin and respiratory tract. In view of this increased insensible water loss and the increase in stool water content, infants receiving phototherapy require an increase in fluid intake of approximately 15 to 25 ml/kg/24 hours.

During phototherapy, the infant's eyes should be shielded. If the eye shields remain in place and are opaque, damage to vision will not occur. It has been suggested that the phototherapy be intermittently discontinued and the eyeshields removed so that the infant and mother may enjoy visual contact.

REFERENCES

Brown, A. K., and McDonagh, A. F.: Phototherapy for neonatal hyperbilirubinemia: efficacy, mechanism and toxicity. Adv. Pediatr. 27:341, 1980.

Brown, A. K., and Wu, P. Y. K.: Efficacy of phototherapy in prevention of hyperbilirubinemia. Pediatr. Res. 13:277, 1979.

Brown, W. R., and Boon, W. H.: Ethnic group differences in plasma bilirubin levels of full-term healthy Singapore newborns. Pediatrics 36:745, 1965.

Buchan, P. C.: Pathogenesis of neonatal hyperbilirubinemia after induction of labor with oxytocin. Br. Med. J. 2:1255, 1959.

Chalmers, I., Campbell, H., and Turnbull, A. C.: Use of oxytocin and incidence of neonatal jaundice. Br. Med. J. 2:116, 1975.

Cockington, R. A.: A guide to phototherapy in the management of neonatal hyperbilirubinemia. J. Pediatr. 95:281, 1979.

Cohen, A. N., and Ostrow, J. D.: New concepts in phototherapy: photoisomerization of bilirubin IX alpha and potential toxic effects of light. Pediatrics 65:740, 1980.

Cremer, R. J., Perryman, P. W., and Richards, D. H.: Influence of light on the hyperbilirubinemia of infants. Lancet 1:1094, 1958.

Dahm, B. B., Krauss, A. N., Gartner, L. M., Klain, D. B., Soodalter, B. A., and Auld, P. A. M.: Breast feeding and serum bilirubin values during the first 4 days of life. J. Pediatr. 83:1049, 1973.

Davis, D. R., Yeary, R. A., and Lee, K.: The failure of phototherapy to reduce plasma bilirubin levels in the bile-ligated rat. J. Pediatr. 99:956, 1981.

Gartner, L. M., Lee, K. S., et al.: Development of bilirubin transport and metabolism in the newborn rhesus monkey. J. Pediatr. 90:513, 1977.

Hardy, J. B., Drage, J. S., and Jackson, E. C.: The first year of life. The Collaborative Perinatal Project of the National Institutes of Neurological and Communicative Disorders and Stroke. Baltimore, The Johns Hopkins University Press, 1979, p. 104.

Kaplan, E., Herz, F., Scheye, E., and Robinson, L. D., Jr.: Phototherapy in ABO hemolytic disease of the newborn infant. J. Pediatr. 79:911, 1971.

Kopelman, A. E., Brown, R. S., and Odell, G. B.: The bronze baby syndrome: a complication of phototherapy. J. Pediatr. 81:466, 1972.

Kramer, L. I.: Advancement of dermal icterus in the jaundiced newborn. Am. J. Dis. Child. 118:454, 1969.

Lucey, J., Ferreiro, M., and Hewitt, J.: Prevention of hyperbilirubinemia of prematurity by phototherapy. Pediatrics 41:1047, 1968.

Maisels, J. M.: Bilirubin. Pediatr. Clin. North Am. 19:447, 1972.

McDonagh, A. F.: Phototherapy: A new twist to bilirubin. J. Pediatr. 99:909, 1981.

McDonagh, A. F., Palma, L. A., and Lightner, D. A.: Blue light and bilirubin excretion. Science 208:145, 1980.

Romagnoli, G., Polidore, L., Cataldi, G., et al.: Phototherapy-induced hypocalcemia. J. Pediatr. 94:815, 1979.

Shennon, A. T.: The effect of phototherapy on the hyperbilirubinemia of Rh incompatibility. Pediatrics 54:417, 1974.

Winfield, C. R., and MacFaul, R.: Clinical study of prolonged jaundice in breast- and bottle-fed babies. Arch. Dis. Child. 53:506, 1978.

Wu, P. Y. K.: Phototherapy update. Factors affecting efficiency of phototherapy. Perinatol. Neonatol. 5:49, 1981.

70

Unconjugated Hyperbilirubinemia

By Frank A. Oski

A variety of pathologic conditions may result in severe or prolonged jaundice in which the predominant or exclusive pigment that accumulates in the serum is unconjugated (indirect) bilirubin. The conditions in which unconjugated hyperbilirubinemia is primarily responsible for the jaundice are listed in Table 70–1. The most common cause of hyperbilirubinemia is hemolytic disease. The red cell disorders resulting in excessive bilirubin production are discussed in Chapter 66.

The role of swallowed blood and entrapped hemorrhage in the genesis of hyperbilirubinemia have been discussed in Chapter 69.

Intestinal obstruction is frequently associated with hyperbilirubinemia. Jaundice in such circumstances is believed to be the consequence of enhanced enterohepatic circulation of bilirubin and the impairment of hepatic bilirubin conjugation that results from inadequate caloric intake. When the passage of meconium is delayed, the bilirubin that has been excreted into the gut during fetal life may be reabsorbed. Bilirubin cleared from the circulation in the early neonatal period is also reabsorbed and results in presentation of an increased bilirubin load to the liver for repeated conjugation. Martin and Siebenthal

Table 70–1. Pathologic Causes of Unconjugated Hyperbilirubinemia

1. Hemolytic disorders:
   Isoimmunization
   Inherited defects of red cell metabolism
   Acquired hemolytic disorders secondary to infections, drugs, and microangiopathies
2. Extravasation of blood; petechiae, hematomas, pulmonary, cerebral, or retroperitoneal hemorrhages; cephalhematomas
3. Swallowed blood
4. Increased enterohepatic circulation of bilirubin:
   Intestinal obstruction
   Pyloric stenosis
   Meconium ileus
   Paralytic ileus, drug-induced ileus
   Hirschsprung's disease
5. Hypothyroidism
6. Hypopituitarism
7. Familial nonhemolytic jaundice:
   Types 1 and 2
   Gilbert's disease
8. Lucey-Driscoll syndrome
9. Mixed disturbances in which both unconjugated and conjugated hyperbilirubinemia may be present:
   Galactosemia
   Tyrosinosis
   Hypermethionemia
   Cystic fibrosis

were the first to describe the association of jaundice with hypertrophic pyloric stenosis. It has been estimated to occur with a frequency ranging from 2.6 to 17 per cent. No satisfactory explanation for this particular association has yet been demonstrated, although liver biopsies obtained at operation in some infants with prolonged undernutrition have been found to have profoundly decreased glucuronyl transferase activity.

The association of congenital hypothyroidism with hyperbilirubinemia was first documented by Akerrén in 1954. Subsequent studies have found that approximately 10 per cent of all neonates with hypothyroidism will have hyperbilirubinemia or protracted jaundice. When hyperbilirubinemia occurs in association with a gestation of 42 weeks, a birth weight of more than 4.0 kg, a large posterior fontanel, respiratory distress, hypothermia, peripheral cyanosis, hypoactivity, lethargy, lag in stooling beyond 20 hours of life, abdominal distention, or edema, a diagnosis of hypothyroidism should be strongly considered. It is unclear as to whether the protracted jaundice is a consequence of delayed maturation of hepatic conjugating capacity, but a similar picture of protracted jaundice, often in association with refractory hypoglycemia, is seen in infants with congenital hypopituitarism. The presence of a cleft palate or a small penis in association with hypoglycemia and jaundice should alert the physician to the possible presence of hypopituitarism.

The inherited disorders of bilirubin metabolism (the nonhemolytic unconjugated hyperbilirubinemias) can be conveniently, but perhaps oversimplis-

tically, divided into three major types according to the degree of bilirubin–UDPG T activity and their response to enzyme-inducing agents such as phenobarbital. The principal features of these three forms of the disorder are described in Table 70–2.

The Type I disorder was first described by Crigler and Najjar and often is referred to by this eponym. These authors described seven patients in whom the diagnosis was certain and eight others in whom the diagnosis seemed highly probable in retrospect. All fifteen patients could be traced to two common ancestors of a consanguineous marriage. This extremely rare disorder in the past often produced kernicterus, but now patients who are treated with phototherapy and agents that reduce the enterohepatic circulation of bilirubin may lead normal lives.

The Type II disorder is more frequently encountered but is difficult to recognize during the first week of life. The inheritance of the Type II disorder differs from Type I in that it is autosomal dominant. A conjugating defect can generally be demonstrated in one of the parents. Siblings or parents may have bilirubin concentrations in the 2.0 to 4.0 mg per 100 ml range. The administration of phenobarbital will control the hyperbilirubinemia during the neonatal period and may be used in later life if the hyperbilirubinemia proves to be cosmetically unacceptable to the patient.

Gilbert's disease is probably the most common cause of mild, chronic, or intermittent unconjugated hyperbilirubinemia that occurs in the absence of a hemolytic disorder or intrinsic liver disease. The diagnosis is rarely made in infancy, the mean age of recognition being approximately 18 years, although about half the patients with confirmed Gilbert's disease will have a history of significant neonatal hyperbilirubinemia. It is estimated that 2 to 6 per cent of the population have Gilbert's disease. In view of the fact that caloric deprivation results in hyperbilirubinemia in the child or adult with this disease, it seems highly probable that many infants with unexplained hyperbilirubinemia are actually demonstrating the earliest manifestations of this disease. Unfortunately, no follow-up studies have been performed on infants with unexplained hyperbilirubinemia to determine whether they do, in fact, have Gilbert's disease. The hyperbilirubinemia of this disease is also corrected with phenobarbital therapy.

The Lucey-Driscoll syndrome was originally described in 24 infants born of eight mothers. Four of the infants in the original report developed kernicterus as a result of their intense hyperbilirubinemia. The sera from the mothers of these infants contained a substance that markedly inhibited the conjugation, in vitro, of aglycones such as O-aminophenol. This inhibitory material was also detected in the sera of the infants and was postulated to have been transplacentally acquired. The substance eventually dis-

Table 70–2. Congenital Nonhemolytic Unconjugated Hyperbilirubinemia: Clinical Syndromes

Characteristics	Marked (Crigler-Najjar Syndrome) (Arias Type I)	Moderate (Arias Type II)	Mild (Gilbert's Disease)
Steady state serum bilirubin:	>20 mg/dl	<20 mg/dl	<5 mg/dl
Range of bilirubin values	14–50 mg/dl	5.3–37.6 mg/dl	0.8–10 mg/dl
Bilirubin in bile:			
Total	<10 mg/dl (increased with phototherapy)	50–100 mg/dl	Normal
Conjugated	Absent	Present (only monoglucuronide)	Present (50% monoglucuronide)
Bilirubin–UDPG-T activity in vitro	None detected	None detected	20–30% of normal
Bilirubin clearance	Extremely decreased	Markedly decreased	20–30% of normal
Hepatic bilirubin uptake	Normal	Normal	Reduced
Glucuronide formation with other substrates	Decreased	Decreased	Decreased?
Response to phenobarbital:			
Plasma bilirubin	Unchanged	Decreased but remains above normal range	Within normal range
Bilirubin–UDPG-T activity	None detected	None detected	Within normal range
Glucuronidation of other substrates	Increased from previous subnormal levels	Increased from previous subnormal levels	Increased
Smooth endoplasmic reticulum	Hypertrophy	Hypertrophy	Hypertrophy
Bilirubin encephalopathy	Usually present	Uncommon. May occur only in the neonatal period	Not present
Genetics	Autosomal recessive. Parents often related, both demonstrate impairment of glucuronidation but have normal bilirubin levels.	Heterogeneity of defect distinctly possible. Autosomal dominant? Double heterozygotes? No parental consanguinity. Abnormal glucuronidation or Gilbert's defect in one of the parents.	Autosomal dominant (heterozygotes). Usually one of the parents demonstrates similar abnormality

(From Valaes, T.: Clin. Perinatol. *3*:177, 1976.)

appears from the circulation of both the mother and the infant and is believed to be a gestational hormone. This syndrome should be considered in those circumstances in which siblings experience intense, transient hyperbilirubinemia of unexplained cause.

REFERENCES

Akerrén, Y.: Prolonged jaundice in the newborn associated with congenital myxedema, a syndrome of practical importance. Acta Paediatr. *43*:411, 1954.

Arias, I. M.: Inheritable and congenital hyperbilirubinemia. N. Engl. J. Med. *285*:1416, 1971.

Bleicher, M. A., Reiner, M. A., Rapaport, S. A., and Track, N. S.: Extraordinary hyperbilirubinemia in a neonate with idiopathic hypertrophic pyloric stenosis. J. Pediatr. Surg. *14*:527, 1979.

Copland, K. C., Franks, R. C., and Ramamurthy, R.: Neonatal hyperbilirubinemia and hypoglycemia in congenital hypopituitarism. Clin. Pediatr. *20*:523, 1981.

Crigler, J. F., Jr., and Najjar, V. A.: Congenital familial nonhemolytic jaundice with kernicterus. Pediatrics *10*:169, 1952.

Eden, A. N., and Weinstein, V.: Neonatal jaundice and cretinism. N. Y. State J. Med. *64*:2914, 1964.

Lucey, J. F., Arias, I., and McKay, R.: Transient familial neonatal hyperbilirubinemia. Am. J. Dis. Child. *100*:787, 1960.

Martin, J. W., and Siebenthal, B. J.: Jaundice due to hypertrophic pyloric stenosis. J. Pediatr. *47*:95, 1955.

McGillivray, M. H., Crawford, J. D., and Robey, J. S.: Congenital hypothyroidism and prolonged neonatal hyperbilirubinemia. Pediatrics *40*:283, 1967.

Porto, S. O.: Jaundice in congenital malrotation of the intestine. Am. J. Dis. Child. *117*:684, 1969.

Powell, L. W., Hemingway, E., Billing, B. H., and Sherlock, S.: Idiopathic unconjugated hyperbilirubinemia (Gilbert's syndrome): a study of 42 families. N. Engl. J. Med. *227*:1108, 1967.

Schärli, A., Sieber, W. K., and Kiesewetter, W. B.: Hypertrophic pyloric stenosis at the Children's Hospital of Pittsburgh from 1912 to 1967. J. Pediatr. Surg. *4*:108, 1969.

Talamo, R. C., and Hendren, W. H.: Prolonged obstructive jaundice: report of a case with meconium ileus and jejunal atresia. Am. J. Dis. Child. *115*:74, 1968.

Valaes, T.: Bilirubin metabolism. Review and discussion of inborn errors. Clin. Perinatol. *3*:177, 1976.

Woolley, M. M., Felsher, B. F., Asch, M. J., et al.: Jaundice, hypertrophic pyloric stenosis, and glucuronyl transferase. J. Pediatr. Surg. *9*:359, 1974.

71

In 1904, Schmorl coined the term "kernicterus" to describe the characteristic yellow staining of the nuclear centers of the brain that was commonly observed in jaundiced infants who died from severe erythroblastosis fetalis. In kernicterus, the basal ganglia, globus pallidus, putamen, and caudate nuclei are most intensely affected, but cerebellar and bulbar nuclei as well as white and gray matter of the cerebral hemispheres may also be involved. If the affected infant survives the neonatal period and subsequently dies, the yellow staining may no longer be present, but the basal ganglia will display microscopic evidence of cell injury, neuronal loss, and glial replacement.

The "Classic" Disease

The classic form of the disease, which was generally observed in term infants with hemolytic disease, is virtually unknown today. In these infants, the earliest physical findings are a blunted Moro reflex with incomplete flexion of the extremities and opisthotonic posturing (Fig. 71–1). The suck becomes weak, and nursing is difficult. As the disease progresses, the Moro reflex disappears, and vomiting and a high-pitched cry are observed. Hyperpyrexia and seizures are frequently present. Muscle rigidity, paralysis of upward gaze, periodic oculogyric crises, and irregular respirations are often present in the terminal phases of the disease, and infants may die with oozing of bloody froth from the nose and pharynx as a result of pulmonary hemorrhage. Approximately 50 per cent of infants demonstrating these symptoms will die. Surviving infants display the postkernicteric syndrome consisting of high-frequency nerve deafness, choreoathetoid cerebral palsy, dental enamel dysplasia, and, less commonly, mental retardation. In such surviving infants, lessening of spasticity usually occurs at about the end of the first week of life and may incorrectly suggest that the infant has recovered from his neurologic insult. The late sequelae generally reappear by about 6 weeks of age, with neurologic evidence of spasticity progressing to choreoathetosis. Even among infants with no apparent neurologic abnormalities during the newborn period, subsequent follow-up may reveal subtle motor, cognitive, and behavioral disorders.

Zuelzer and Kaplan diagnosed kernicterus in four of 38 ABO-incompatible infants with deep jaundice. Two died promptly, the third died at 6 months, and the fourth was grossly retarded at 8 months. One more of the group, undiagnosed in the neonatal period, demonstrated ataxia, athetosis, and mental retardation later in life. Crosse and her collaborators

Kernicterus

By Frank A. Oski

followed the 16 survivors of their 60 kernicteric prematures. At the age of 1 year, the 13 who could be examined were all retarded. Hearing was impaired in seven, speech delayed in all. Three were already rigid, six were having "stiffening spells," and four had oculogyric crises. Retrospective studies done in schools for cerebral spastics have been revealing. Asher and Schonell found among 368 such children 55 athetotics; 19 of these had had hemolytic disease of the newborn, and 12 more had had severe jaundice in the neonatal period for other reasons. Among the 313 nonathetoid spastics, only seven gave such a history. The association of athetosis with deafness makes the retrospective diagnosis of neonatal kernicterus likely, although this combination is also frequent among children who survived fetal rubella.

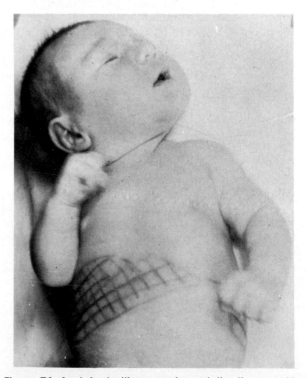

Figure 71–1. Infant with severe hemolytic disease of the newborn in whom kernicterus has developed. Note the enlarged liver and spleen. The posture is typical of athetosis, the head turned sharply to one side, one arm rigidly extended, the other just as rigidly flexed. Movements were characteristically writhing.

Mental retardation without motor defect may follow untreated or incompletely treated hyperbilirubinemia of the newborn, according to Day and his collaborators. They found highly significant differences between the I.Q.'s of untreated newborns with hemolytic disease of the newborn, who recovered without motor defect, and those of their "normal" siblings.

Kernicterus Today

In recent years, improved and aggressive therapy directed at controlling hyperbilirubinemia with phototherapy and exchange transfusions has virtually eliminated clear-cut clinical signs of kernicterus in infants. Unfortunately, kernicterus is still being observed at autopsy. At present, the population at greatest risk for the development of kernicterus appears to be sick, small premature infants. In these infants, kernicterus has been found even when bilirubin levels have remained in a range formerly regarded as "safe."

It has been postulated that kernicterus develops in such infants as a consequence of potentiating factors that act by affecting serum albumin binding of bilirubin or by enhancing the tissue uptake of bilirubin. Potentiating factors that have been proposed include birth weight of less than 1500 gm, hypothermia, asphyxia, acidosis, hypoalbuminemia, sepsis, meningitis, and a variety of pharmacologic agents. Critical analysis of low birth weight infants who died and who were found at autopsy to have kernicterus has failed to reveal any relationship between these potentiating factors and the presence or absence of kernicterus. It may not be possible with presently available criteria to distinguish those infants who are at risk for kernicterus from other premature infants who appear to be as critically ill.

Despite this problem, it has been claimed that the incidence of kernicterus can be reduced by the use of phototherapy and exchange transfusion based on the use of critical bilirubin concentrations adjusted according to birth weight or gestational age and clinical status. Guidelines for the use of exchange transfusions that have apparently produced a reduction in the incidence of kernicterus are outlined in Table 69–6.

Pathogenesis. Although there is a substantial body of evidence to implicate bilirubin in the pathogenesis of kernicterus, its precise role and the relevant modifying factors have not been thoroughly defined.

The direct association between severe unconjugated hyperbilirubinemia and neurologic damage was first convincingly demonstrated in 1952 by Hsia and coworkers and by Mollison and Cutbush. Table 71–1 illustrates the data from which such conclusions were drawn. It should be noted that not all infants

Table 71–1.   Relation Between Maximum Bilirubin Concentration in the Plasma and Kernicterus in Hemolytic Disease of Newborn

Maximum Bilirubin Concentration (mg/dl)	Total Number of Cases	Number with Kernicterus
30–40	11	8
25–29	12	4
19–24	13	1
10–18	24	0

(From the data of Mollison, P. L., and Cutbush, M.: *In* Gairdner, D. (Ed.): Recent Advances in Pediatrics. New York, Blakiston, 1954.)

developed kernicterus, even when bilirubin concentrations reached values of 30 to 40 mg per 100 ml.

It has been repeatedly demonstrated that exchange transfusions in term infants with hemolytic disease, designed to prevent the serum bilirubin level from exceeding 20 mg per 100 ml, virtually eliminates the risk of fatal kernicterus. Other studies have provided evidence that the risk of kernicterus is extremely low in infants weighing more than 1500 gm with nonhemolytic hyperbilirubinemia if serum bilirubin concentrations are kept below 24 mg per 100 ml.

The mechanism by which bilirubin produces neuronal injury once it gains entry into the cell is still a matter of speculation. It has been postulated that bilirubin may interfere with oxidative phosphorylation, cell respiration, protein synthesis, and glucose metabolism. Attempts to demonstrate mitochondrial poisoning in vivo through the perfusion of bilirubin into animals have been largely unsuccessful. In many animal models of kernicterus, asphyxiation in conjunction with bilirubin infusion is necessary to produce the characteristic lesion. Premature infants without apparent hypoxia, however, have been found to have kernicterus at postmortem examination.

The fact that kernicterus may be observed both in the Gunn rat and in patients with the Crigler-Najjar syndrome, in which the cause of the hyperbilirubinemia is an absence of hepatic glucuronyl transferase activity, is persuasive evidence that unconjugated bilirubin, when present in high concentrations, can be neurotoxic.

REFERENCES

Arnold, D. P., Witebsky, E., Selkirk, G. H., and Alford, K. M.: Clinical and serological experience in treating hemolytic disease of the newborn. J. Pediatr. 46:520, 1955.

Asher, P., and Schonell, F. E.: Survey of 400 cases of cerebral palsy in childhood. Arch. Dis. Child. 25:360, 1950.

Crosse, V. M., Meyer, T. C., and Gerrard, J. W.: Kernicterus and prematurity. Arch. Dis. Child. 25:360, 1950.

Day, R.: Kernicterus: further observations on the toxicity of heme pigments. Pediatrics 17:925, 1956.

Gartner, L. M.: Disorders of bilirubin metabolism. *In* Nathan, D. G., and Oski, F. A. (Eds.): Hematology of Infancy and Childhood. 2nd ed. Philadelphia, W. B. Saunders Co., 1981, pp. 86–118.

Gartner, L. M., Snyder, R. N., Chabon, R. S., and Bernstein, J.: Kernicterus: high incidence in premature infants with low serum bilirubin concentrations. Pediatrics 45:906, 1970.

Harris, R. C., Lucey, J. F., and Maclean, J. R.: Kernicterus in premature infants associated with low concentrations of bilirubin in the plasma. Pediatrics 21:875, 1958.

Hsia, D. Y.-Y., Allen, F. H., Gellis, S. S., and Diamond, L. K.: Erythroblastosis fetalis. VIII. Studies of serum bilirubin in relation to kernicterus. N. Engl. J. Med. 247:668, 1952.

Johnson, L., Garcia, M. L., Figueroa, E., and Sarmiento, F.: Kernicterus in rats lacking glucuronyl transferase. A.M.A. J. Dis. Child. 101:322, 1961.

Meyer, T. C.: A study of serum bilirubin levels in relation to kernicterus and prematurity. Arch. Dis. Child. 31:75, 1956.

Mollison, P. L., and Cutbush, M.: Haemolytic disease of the newborn. In Gairdner, D. (Ed.): Recent Advances in Pediatrics. New York, Blakiston, 1954.

Mollison, P. L., and Walker, W.: Controlled trials of the treatment of hemolytic disease of the newborn. Lancet 1:429, 1952.

Pearlman, M. A., Gartner, L. M., Lee, K.-S., Morecki, R., and Horoupian, D. S.: Absence of kernicterus in low birth weight infants from 1971 through 1976: comparison with findings in 1966 and 1967. Pediatrics 62:460, 1978.

Schmorl, G.: Zur Kenntnis des Ikterus neonatorum, insbesondere der Dabei auftretenden Gehirnveranderungen. Verhand d. Deutsch Path. Ges. 6:109, 1903.

Stern, L., and Denton, R. L.: Kernicterus in small premature infants. Pediatrics 35:483, 1965.

Turkel, S. B., Guttenberg, M. E., Moynes, D. R., and Hodgman, J. E.: Lack of identifiable risk factors for kernicterus. Pediatrics 66:502, 1980.

Wishingrad, L., Cornblath, M., Takakuwa, P., Rosenfeld, I. M., Elegant, L. D., Kauffman, A., Lassers, E., and Klein, R. I.: Studies of non-hemolytic hyperbilirubinemia in premature infants. Prospective randomized selection for exchange transfusion with observations on the levels of serum bilirubin with and without exchange transfusion and neurologic evaluations one year after birth. Pediatrics 36:162, 1965.

Zuelzer, W. W., and Kaplan, E.: ABO heterospecific pregnancy and hemolytic disease: a study of normal and pathological variants. IV. Pathological variants. A.M.A. J. Dis. Child. 88:319, 1954.

72

Hydrops Fetalis

By Frank A. Oski

The term *hydrops fetalis* is used to describe generalized edema in the neonate. There is no precise standard concerning the degree of edema that is sufficient to be described accurately as hydrops fetalis, although the condition is usually indicated by obvious widespread subcutaneous edema that is often associated with ascites.

The topic of hydrops fetalis has usually been included in discussions of jaundice because for many years severe Rh isoimmunization was the major cause of profound fetal edema. With the gratifying decline in the incidence of Rh sensitization, other hemolytic anemias as well as a variety of nonhematologic conditions are now assuming more prominent roles in the etiology of hydrops fetalis.

Listed in Table 72–1 are the recognized causes of fetal edema. In general, the causes of hydrops fetalis can be broadly classified into three major categories: chronic intrauterine anemia, intrauterine heart failure, and hypoproteinemia. A single etiologic agent may produce edema by more than one pathophysiologic mechanism.

Although severe intrauterine anemia, usually secondary to Rh isoimmunization, has long been considered the classic mechanism for the production of hydrops fetalis, there is a body of both clinical and laboratory evidence to suggest that anemia alone may not be responsible. Infants with Rh isoimmunization and cord blood hemoglobin concentrations as low as 4 gm per 100 ml may be born without obvious edema. Conversely, intrauterine transfusions for severe Rh disease have resulted in infants born with hydrops despite sustained levels of hemoglobin in utero and with cord blood hemoglobin values of 10.0 gm per 100 ml. There is no consistent relationship between venous hematocrit and the presence or absence of hydrops fetalis in infants with Rh disease. The experimental production of chronic anemia in sheep fetuses has failed to produce a hydropic state. Infants with homozygous alpha thalassemia are born grossly hydropic with hemoglobin values in the range of 9 to 12 gm per 100 ml. In these infants, the primary hemoglobin, Bart's hemoglobin, has a very high affinity for oxygen (a left-shifted oxygen-hemoglobin equilibrium curve), and the release of oxygen to the tissues is severely compromised despite the seeming adequacy of the hemoglobin concentration. It seems that anemia alone is unlikely to be the primary cause of hydrops fetalis.

Congestive heart failure in utero, perhaps precipitated by profound chronic anemia, may play a major role in the etiology of hydrops fetalis. Other pathologic processes leading to myocardial failure, such as paroxysmal atrial tachycardia and arteriovenous fistula, are recognized causes of fetal edema.

A decrease in colloid osmotic pressure, often as a result of hypoalbuminemia, may play a central role

Table 72–1. Causes of Hydrops Fetalis

Infections
  Toxoplasmosis
  Cytomegalic inclusion virus disease
  Leptospirosis
  Chagas' disease
  Syphilis
  Congenital hepatitis
Chronic anemia
  Blood group incompatibility
  Alpha thalassemia
  G6PD deficiency
  Gaucher's disease
  Parabiotic syndrome
  Chronic fetomaternal transfusion
Cardiac disease or failure
  Bradyarrhythmias: heart block
  Calcific myocarditis (Coxsackie virus)
  Tachyarrhythmias: paroxysmal auricular tachycardia, atrial
    flutter
  Truncus arteriosus
  Right or left ventricular endocardial fibroelastosis and mitral
    insufficiency
  Congenital insufficiency of the pulmonary valve
  Premature closure of the foramen ovale
  Arteriovenus fistulas
  UHLs anomaly, pulmonary atresia
  Cardiac neoplasm
  Twin pregnancy with "parasitic fetus"
Renal disease
  Congenital nephrosis
  Renal vein thrombosis
Malformations and congenital tumors
  Pulmonary hypoplasia
  Hemangioendothelioma
  Chorioangioma of the placenta
  Aneurysm of the umbilical artery
  Angiomyxoma of the umbilical cord
  Congenital neuroblastoma
  Cystic hygroma
  Cervical teratoma
  Pulmonary lymphangiectasia
  Cystic adenomatoid malformation of the lung
  Down's syndrome
  Trisomy E
  Turner's syndrome
  Sacrococcygeal teratoma
Miscellaneous
  Idiopathic arterial calcification
  Fetal retroperitoneal fibrosis
  Umbilical vein thrombosis
  Intrauterine intracranial hemorrhage
  Storage disease
  Small bowel volvulus
  Tuberous sclerosis
Maternal disorders
  Diabetes mellitus
  Toxemia of pregnancy
  Polyhydramnios
Idiopathic

(Modified from Giacoia, G. P.: Clin. Pediatr. *19*:334, 1980).

in the genesis of hydrops fetalis. Although infants with severe hemolytic disease frequently have hypoproteinemia, there is no consistent relationship between the degree of edema and the cord blood protein concentration. In analbuminemia, a rare hereditary disorder characterized by the virtual absence of albumin from the plasma, hydrops fetalis is not observed. Colloid osmotic pressure is reduced in such patients but may not be as low as that observed in neonates with congenital nephrosis, despite the fact that infants with nephrosis may have serum albumin concentrations of 1 to 2 gm per 100 ml.

The role of the placenta in the pathogenesis of hydrops fetalis has not been carefully studied, although edema of the placenta is a consistent finding in association with hydrops fetalis.

In summary, it would appear that fetal hydrops fetalis may require the presence of more than one physiologic disturbance. Anemia, impaired cardiac function, decreased colloid oncotic pressure, altered capillary permeability, hypoxemia, and placental perfusion abnormalities may act in concert to produce fetal edema.

Therapy for infants with hydrops fetalis must be directed at the pathologic alterations. Prompt resuscitation and stabilization of the infant are frequently required in the delivery suite. When marked ascites impairs attempts at ventilation, abdominal paracentesis should be performed immediately. Hydrothorax may require thoracentesis. The presence of pulmonary edema should indicate the institution of constant airway pressure. Central arterial and venous pressure should be monitored and used as guidelines in treatment. Infants who are adequately oxygenated but who exhibit poor tissue perfusion may require volume expanders. In anemic hydropic infants, partial exchange transfusion with packed red blood cells is indicated. When a decrease in colloid osmotic pressure is primarily responsible for the generalized edema, the administration of fresh-frozen plasma may prove effective. Tachyarrhythmias may require digitalis or cardioversion. After stabilization of the infant, attention must be given to fluid therapy. Fluid restriction and the use of diuretics may be required in infants with significant pulmonary edema.

Hydrops fetalis should not be regarded as a uniformly fatal process. The prognosis in such infants largely depends on the skill of the physician in instituting prompt effective therapy and the basic underlying pathologic process.

REFERENCES

Baum, J. D., and Harris, D.: Colloid osmotic pressure in erythroblastosis fetalis. Br. Med. J. *1*:601, 1972.

Becker, M. J.: Hydrops fetalis. Arch. Dis. Child. *50*:665, 1975.

Etches, P. C., and Lemons, J. A.: Nonimmune hydrops fetalis: report of 22 cases including three siblings. Pediatrics *64*:326, 1979.

Giacoia, G. P.: Hydrops fetalis (fetal edema). Clin. Pediatr. *19*:334, 1980.

McFadyen, I. R., Boonyaprakob, U., and Hutchinson, D. C.: Experimental production of anemia in fetal lambs. Am. J. Obstet. Gynecol. *100*:686, 1968.

Phibbs, R. H., Johnson, P., Kitterman, J. A., et al.: Cardiorespiratory status of erythroblastotic infants. I. Relationship of gestational age, severity of hemolytic disease, and birth asphyxia to idiopathic respiratory distress syndrome and survival. Pediatrics *49*:5, 1972.

Phibbs, R. H., Johnson, P., and Tooley, W. H.: Cardiorespiratory status of erythroblastotic infants. II. Blood volume, hematocrit and serum albumin concentration in relation to hydrops fetalis. Pediatrics *53*:12, 1973.

73

Obstructive Jaundice Due to Biliary Atresia and Neonatal Hepatitis

By Frank A. Oski

In the last decade we have witnessed a major reorientation in our thinking with respect to the entity termed *congenital atresia of the bile ducts*. In the past, clinicians attempted to distinguish hepatitis from atresia by a variety of diagnostic procedures and deferred operative intervention for several months in hopes that patients with hepatitis would get better, while assuming that little or nothing could be done for infants with anatomic abnormalities.

There is now a growing consensus that neonatal hepatitis and biliary atresia may be opposite ends of a single spectrum of disease and that the pathologic process observed is dynamic. The pathologic picture observed depends on the time and nature of intrauterine insult and the age at which the infant is examined.

Loose and ambiguous use of the term *biliary atresia* has led to confusion concerning the approach to therapy. Only surgical exploration, an operative cholangiogram if a gallbladder is present, a careful dissection of the porta hepatis, and microscopic examination of liver tissue can enable one to classify the patient's disease as intrahepatic or extrahepatic biliary obstruction with or without atresia.

With this information, one can make the following diagnostic classification:

1. Complete intrahepatic biliary atresia
   a. Normal extrahepatic biliary system
   b. Hypoplastic extrahepatic biliary system
   c. Complete extrahepatic biliary atresia
2. Complete extrahepatic biliary atresia
   a. Normal number of intrahepatic ducts
   b. Decreased number of intrahepatic ducts
3. Hypoplasia of the extrahepatic biliary trees
   a. Normal number of intrahepatic ducts
   b. Decreased number of intrahepatic ducts

Such classification is essential now that it has become apparent (owing to the pioneering work of Kasai and the later success of Lilly) that infants with functioning intrahepatic ducts may benefit from surgical procedures that employ a variety of anastomotic techniques that result in adequate biliary drainage. Patients without intrahepatic ducts cannot be saved. Intrahepatic ducts may disappear over a period of several months in the presence of complete extrahepatic obstruction; thus, early surgical intervention is necessary in order to be beneficial.

Pathology. Almost every conceivable pattern of absence or atresia of one or more of the components of the biliary outflow tract has been encountered. All the extrahepatic ducts or, rarely, all the intrahepatic ducts may be absent. The hepatic, cystic, or common duct may be atretic. The gallbladder may be absent or hypoplastic, or it may have no connection with the liver or the duodenum. Stenosis rather than complete atresia may be found.

The liver shows all gradations of damage ranging from biliary stasis to advanced biliary cirrhosis, depending on the length of time the particular infant survives. This is discussed in greater detail in the discussion entitled Liver Biopsy. The spleen enlarges as portal hypertension advances. The bones may become rachitic or osteoporotic because of defective absorption of both vitamin D and calcium. In advanced cases, foci of destruction of skeletal muscle may be discovered after careful search. Weinberg and coworkers correlate this lesion with prolonged deprivation of vitamin E.

Etiology. There is little evidence that congenital biliary atresia is familial or hereditary. One must presume that it results from some noxious process that adversely affects the development of the bile duct system early in gestation. Congenital rubella and cytomegalovirus infections have been associated with biliary atresia, as have prenatal infection by *Listeria monocytogenes*. The final pattern evolves from two distinct portions of the liver anlage: the larger cranial part forming parenchyma as well as hepatic and common ducts and the small caudal part eventuating in gallbladder and cystic duct. These two portions must accomplish juncture secondarily. Congenital defects of many kinds are the end results of imperfections in this complex evolution.

Diagnosis. The prime sign of congenital biliary atresia is persistent jaundice. Many times, the icterus appears to be a continuation of physiologic icterus of the newborn, and one begins to suspect serious trouble only when the color fails to fade at the expected time. In other cases, jaundice is not noted until 1, 2, or even 3 or more weeks have passed, after which it persists and deepens. A history dating the onset of jaundice after 6 weeks of age is good evidence (after 4 weeks, fair evidence) that the disorder is something other than atresia. Surprisingly enough, jaundice often appears variable in intensity, alternately deepening and lightening. Because one would expect complete atresia to give rise to jaundice that steadily increases in intensity, such variability tends to be misleading. The second diagnostic sign is absence of bile in the stools. In some cases, infants pass the typical clay-colored stools from the fourth or fifth day on. In other instances, confusion arises because stools fail to become absolutely white for several weeks or months or because some are clay-colored while others contain a tinge of brown or green. The usual phenomenon is that heavily jaundiced intestinal epithelial cells may be sloughed off and incorporated in the bulk of the stool. These two factors, variability in intensity of jaundice and delay and variability in absoluteness of acholia in stools, cause uncertainty regarding the congenital origin and completeness of the obstruction. One can only warn that not too much weight be assigned to these "red herrings." Within these limitations, jaundice and acholic stools constitute the pathognomonic signs. Jaundice steadily increases to its maximum degree, ultimately imparting to the infant a deep yellow color, due to bilirubin, that is mixed with a greenish discoloration, due to biliverdin. The liver soon becomes large and extremely firm. In the first few months, the baby does not appear or act as though he is ill. Venous dilatation appears over the surface of the protuberant abdomen, greatest over its upper half, and ascites develops. The spleen enlarges.

Fat-soluble vitamins are poorly absorbed in the absence of bile salts from the intestine, but deficiencies in vitamins A, D, and K do not become manifest until after the neonatal period. Vitamin E deficiency may be demonstrated by laboratory tests, and the absorption of an orally administered dose of Aquasol E has been proposed as a simple test for distinguishing hepatitis from biliary atresia.

Blood is normal in the neonatal period. Hemoglobin content and red and white blood cell counts fall within the usual range, and there is no excess of nucleated erythrocytes or reticulocytes. The urine contains bile in large quantities but no urobilinogen. By 4 to 6 weeks of age, most patients are anemic with elevations in their reticulocyte counts.

Serum bilirubin becomes elevated by the end of the first week and gradually rises to a maximum, where it remains throughout life, with minor fluctuations. Much of the bilirubin is of the direct type.

Liver function tests may indicate liver damage but not until considerably later in life, after cirrhotic alterations have begun to develop.

Blood cholesterol level tends to rise gradually pari passu with increasing liver damage. This never happens as early as the neonatal period.

Several transaminating enzymes have been measured in the sera of infants with persistent jaundice. Values for serum glutamic-oxaloacetic transaminase (SGOT) in normal adults range from 8 to 40 units (in normal newborns, from 13 to 120 units) per milliliter of serum per minute. From 5 to 35 units of glutamic-pyruvic transaminase (SGPT) are present in adult serum, and in newborn serum there are 12 to 90 units (Kove et al., 1958). In bile duct atresia, the activities of these enzymes may increase to levels ranging from 500 to 700 units, whereas in hepatitis this figure may rise to as high as more than 1000 units. Unfortunately, there is a good deal of overlapping in these two conditions. The ratio of serum gamma-glutamyl transpeptidase to SGOT is elevated in infants with obstructive cholangiopathy. Platt and coworkers have proposed that the measurement of this ratio may be a sensitive means of distinguishing

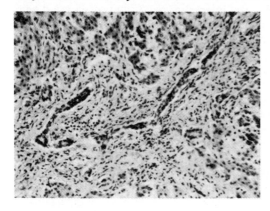

A

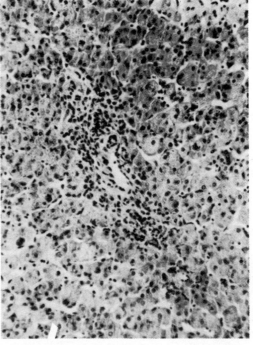

B

Figure 73–1. *A,* Bile duct proliferation and portal fibrosis in an infant with obstruction of the common duct by a plug of inspissated secretions. (Original magnification, 200×.) *B,* Hepatitis with moderate portal inflammation; hepatocellular changes are mild, and multinucleated cells are few. (Original magnification, 200×.) (Brough, A. J., and Bernstein, J.: Pediatrics *43:*519, 1969.)

infants with extrahepatic biliary atresia from those with neonatal hepatitis. This distinction may be evident as early as 5 to 14 days of life. The ratio may also be elevated in neonates with alpha₁-antitrypsin deficiency who demonstrate bile duct proliferation.

A promising diagnostic aid is the measurement of serum alpha-fetoprotein. Zeltzer and coworkers found this to be elevated in 10 of 11 patients with neonatal hepatitis and in only 1 of 6 infants with biliary atresia.

Thaler and Gellis made a strong case for the rose bengal ^{131}I excretion test as the most reliable, although still not perfect, diagnostic test of biliary atresia. Excretion of less than 10 per cent of the dye in the stool was found in all their patients with extrahepatic obstructions, whereas in their patients with hepatitis, the average was 32 per cent. Nevertheless, 20 per cent of those infants in the latter group were obstructed also, with less than 10 per cent of the dye excreted. Most centers now employ rose bengal ^{131}I scintigraphy in the initial evaluation of infants with obstructive jaundice.

In an infant with persistent jaundice and apparent biliary obstruction, efforts should be made by 6 to 8 weeks of age to determine the precise etiology. In addition to conventional measurements of liver enzymes, diagnostic procedures should include one or more of the following in an attempt to determine whether obstruction is present: rose bengal ^{131}I excretion, duodenal intubation and analysis for bile acids, and laparoscopy with biopsy and cholangiogram. If the tests are equivocal or indicate the presence of obstruction, surgery should be performed in an attempt to establish a precise diagnosis and possibly correct or ameliorate the problem. Surgery should be performed by a surgeon who is familiar with the problem and capable of performing an anastomosis if indicated. At the time of exploratory laparotomy, a cholangiogram as well as a liver biopsy should be obtained.

Liver Biopsy. There has been some alteration in the thinking of neonatal pathologists about the pictures that characterize biliary atresia versus those of the other causes of persistent neonatal jaundice with a high percentage of direct-reacting bilirubin. Brough and Bernstein believe, as did several others before

Table 73–1. Anatomic Distribution of the Atretic Areas in 189 Patients with Biliary Atresia Studied Between 1953 and 1979

Level of Atresia	Total	Operated On	Whose Jaundice Disappeared
Common bile duct	29	29	15 (52)
Common hepatic duct	34	34	6 (18)
Total extrahepatic biliary system	126	124*	38 (31)
Total	189	187	59 (32)

* Nine underwent surgical exploration only.
(From Kling, S.: CMA Journal 123:1218, 1980.)

Table 73–2. Correlation Between Postoperative Bile Flow and Age of Patients at the Time of Surgical Correction of Biliary Atresia Between 1971 and 1979

Age (days) at Time of Operation	Number (and per cent) of Patients			
	Total	Good Flow	Poor Flow	No Flow
≤60	13	12 (92)	1	0
61–70	21	13 (62)	7	1
71–90	16	8 (50)	7	1
≥91	7	2 (29)	2	3
Total	57	35 (61)	17	5

(From Kling, S.: CMA Journal 123:1218, 1980.)

them, that bile duct and ductular proliferation is the most reliable sign of biliary atresia. The second most accurate sign consists of hypertrophic changes in hepatic artery branches. Bile plugs in dilated ducts, fibrosis (largely portal), inflammatory changes, and giant-cell transformation are seen, but in less than one half of the cases. These findings contrast with those of neonatal hepatitis, in which hepatocellular damage and inflammation, mostly portal infiltration with mononuclear cells, are the outstanding signs. Giant-cell transformation is far from universal in them, and duct proliferation is only rarely seen (Fig. 73–1).

Kasai has recently reported the long-term follow-up results in his series of 189 proven cases of biliary atresia studied between 1953 and 1979. In one third of the cases, the common bile duct or the common hepatic duct was involved; the atresia was therefore of the "correctable type." In general, the operative results have markedly improved in the last 10 years, with jaundice disappearing in 61 per cent of the patients who have been operated on since 1971. There was a close correlation between the postoperative bile flow and the age of the patient at operation: The younger the patient, the better the result. When the operation was performed before 60 days of age, 90 per cent of the infants achieved satisfactory bile drainage. In contrast, when operation was performed after 120 days of life, no patient displayed active postoperative bile flow. The results of the Kasai experience are depicted in Tables 73–1, 73–2, and 73–3.

Table 73–3. Outcome for 187 Patients with Biliary Atresia Treated Surgically Between 1953 and 1979

Outcome	Number of Patients	
Death	129	
In hospital		44
After discharge		
Within 1 year		36
After 1 year		49
Survival	58	
With jaundice		4
Without jaundice		54

(From Kling, S.: CMA Journal 123:1218, 1980.)

Results in North America do not, as yet, approximate the results obtained in Japan. Fewer patients may have the correctable type of lesion. The major complications of portoenterostomy are recurrent cholangitis, increased intrahepatic fibrosis, and eventual portal hypertension. These complications appear more common in North America than in Japan. Even with these limitations, the chances for long-term survival have clearly improved. Prior to attempts at corrective surgery of the Kasai type, only 1.1 per cent of infants experienced apparent cures, and the average age of death was 12 months.

If anastomosis proves impossible, one is left with the tasks of keeping the infant comfortable, as well-nourished as possible, and free of vitamin deficiencies. Fat-soluble vitamins should be given in the water-miscible form. Drisdol with vitamin A is superior to oily preparations. Vitamin K_1 may be indicated later in the course. It is possible that added tocopherol may avert some muscle damage due to vitamin E deficiency. The distressing itching that is a feature in some infants may prove unresponsive to all forms of sedative and antihistaminic therapy. Treatment with cholestyramine is worthy of trial, although Lottsfeldt and coworkers believe that this anion-exchange resin will be ineffective in cases of complete biliary obstruction.

Prognosis. Death will supervene in all cases of biliary atresia that cannot be surgically corrected. An occasional infant on whom this diagnosis has been made may suddenly and spontaneously be relieved of jaundice after many months. This does not mean that atresia is reversible but indicates that the diagnosis has been incorrect. Errors of this sort have been made even after careful exploration in reputable clinics. One must therefore qualify the grave prognosis when communicating it to the parents by pointing out that this slim possibility exists. Most deaths will be caused by either hepatic failure or the bleeding of portal hypertension and will occur between 6 months and 2 years of age. A few children live years longer. Kernicterus does not complicate biliary atresia because much of the accumulated bilirubin is of the direct kind, and dangerous levels of indirect hyperbilirubinemia are not reached.

Atresia of the Intrahepatic Bile Ducts

This extraordinary variant of the biliary atresia group has been studied most carefully and described most completely by Ahrens and colleagues. Its clinical course differs in some particulars from that of atresia of extrahepatic ducts.

Incidence. Only 10 cases had been reported until 1951, when 264 cases of extrahepatic atresia appeared in the literature. Among 110 cases of neonatal obstructive jaundice, Danks and Bodian found seven of intrahepatic atresia versus 58 of the extrahepatic variety and 45 of neonatal hepatitis. It is therefore extremely infrequent.

Pathology. The absence of bile ducts of any size within the liver substance is characteristic. Bile capillaries are present within each lobule, and these often are dilated and contain plugs of inspissated bile. Extrahepatic ducts are usually absent also, but in three of the 10 early reported cases the extrahepatic duct system seemed perfectly normal. No remnants of compressed, chronically inflamed, or fibrosed ducts are found, and there is no apparent pericholangiolitis. Fibrosis is minimal, and cirrhosis develops extremely slowly and seldom reaches the degree it does when atresia is extrahepatic. Ahrens and coworkers believe that this slow development of cirrhosis stems from the absence of intrahepatic ducts, a condition in which there cannot, of course, be liver injury by distention, backflow of bile, and periductal inflammation.

Diagnosis. The chief difference between intrahepatic and extrahepatic atresia regarding clinical course is that the former disease progresses more slowly than the latter. Jaundice appears at the same time and is equally persistent, but the liver enlarges much more slowly in intrahepatic atresia and does not become so hard and nodular. The nutritional state remains fairly good, and the life span is long. Infants with intrahepatic atresia show a great tendency to develop cutaneous xanthomatosis. This sign is not seen before 18 months of age, usually later, and it may be more apparent in this group because of the increased life expectancy of the infants. Xanthomas appear and disappear with fluctuations in the serum lipid content.

Laboratory Investigations. The blood, stool, and urine findings are exactly the same as those in extrahepatic atresia. Blood lipid content gradually increases over the course of months or years of biliary obstruction of any type.

Treatment. No specific treatment is available. Cholestyramine is more likely to produce lowering of the bilirubin level and subsidence of itching in this form of jaundice than in the extrahepatic obstructive variety.

Prognosis. As has been indicated, the life span of patients with this variety of biliary atresia appears to be considerably longer than that of those in the extrahepatic group. Patients living 10 years or more have been observed. The ultimate prognosis is grave.

Choledochal Cyst

Cystic dilatation of the common duct results from congenital defect of the duct wall, a mucosal valve, or abnormal course of the duct through the duodenal wall. The dilatation is confined to the common duct itself and does not involve the hepatic or cystic ducts or the gallbladder. It may reach the size of an orange or grow even larger.

Incidence. Over 200 cases have been reported in all age groups, but it is extremely rare for choledochal cyst to become symptomatic and to be diagnosed within the neonatal period. In Brough and Bernstein's experience with 39 proven cases of obstructive lesions causing persistent neonatal jaundice, 36 were extrahepatic atresias, one was an obstructive bile plug, and two were choledochal cysts.

Diagnosis. In older persons, a triad consisting of jaundice, abdominal pain, and an upper abdominal tumor strongly suggests the diagnosis. In the neonatal period, the mass is not necessarily large enough to palpate, but it may be huge, filling the entire abdomen. This was true in the last example we saw. Pain is not prominent or easy to localize. When a cystic mass is felt within the abdomen in the presence of jaundice, the possibility must be considered seriously. Wide fluctuations in the depth of the jaundice are highly suggestive. In the final analysis, differential diagnosis can be made only by cholecystography or by direct observation after laparotomy.

Laboratory Investigations. Since jaundice results from blockage by the expanding cyst of entry of bile into the duodenum, the findings will be those of obstructive jaundice. Stools become acholic, the urine contains bile but no urobilin, and the serum bilirubin level rises, with a large percentage of the total bilirubin being direct. Biopsy of the liver will reveal a picture indistinguishable from that of extrahepatic atresia.

Treatment. After the cyst has been visualized by cholecystography or by exploratory laparotomy, its walls should be anastomosed to that of the duodenum.

Prognosis. Cholecystoduodenostomy should result in cure. Again, if operative intervention is delayed, irreversible liver damage may occur.

Pseudocholedochal Cyst

Whereas choledochal cyst results from a congenital defect of the common duct, pseudocholedochal cyst is an iatrogenic disorder that follows injury to the common duct at operation.

Only one case has been observed originating in the neonatal period. This case, reported by Smith and Seeley, is of sufficient interest to be abstracted briefly.

CASE 73–1

A previously normal male infant began to vomit at 3 weeks and was operated on for pyloric stenosis shortly

thereafter. Ten days after the Fredet-Ramstedt operation was performed, vomiting, diarrhea, anorexia, and low-grade fever appeared. Thirty-six hours later jaundice was noted, and the stools became white, the urine dark. After 3 weeks, the abdomen was greatly distended. Paracentesis yielded 1000 ml of amber fluid. The fluid promptly reappeared, and two additional taps were done. On admission at 14 weeks, the presumed diagnosis was cirrhosis of the liver with ascites. The infant was pale and emaciated, and the abdomen was distended and covered with dilated veins. Icterus had disappeared. The liver was not enlarged, but the spleen was palpable. The radiograph showed a large soft tissue density almost filling the right side of the abdomen. At operation, a cyst was seen whose friable wall was inadvertently ruptured, releasing 550 ml of dark green fluid. The fibrous wall was adherent to the small and large bowel, peritoneum, and liver. A transected common duct was found. This was ligated, and cholecystogastrostomy was performed. Convalescence was uneventful.

Neonatal Hepatitis

Between one third and one half of infants with persistent obstructive jaundice do not have primary biliary atresia. Although, as previously indicated, biliary atresia and neonatal hepatitis may be different behaviors of the same disease process, in many instances an entity defined as neonatal hepatitis can be recognized as distinct in its pathologic picture and clinical course. The distinctive pathologic picture is the presence of a cholestatic inflammatory process. Giant-cell transformation occurs, but significant bile duct proliferation is absent. Biopsy specimens may demonstrate disorganized lobular architecture, fibrosis, round cell infiltration, and extramedullary hematopoiesis.

Incidence. This disorder cannot be considered rare, since it is observed in two or three patients every year in most large children's hospitals. Milder forms of this entity are much more common and may occur in great numbers during certain viral epidemics such as rubella.

Etiology. Neonatal hepatitis has multiple etiologies. Viral agents recognized to produce the disease include rubella, cytomegalovirus, herpes simplex, Epstein-Barr virus, coxsackievirus and the hepatitis B virus. Hepatitis may also be observed in infants born with congenital infections due to toxoplasmosis and syphilis. In addition, a clinical picture indistinguishable from that observed with infectious agents may be seen in some infants with severe hemolytic disease or galactosemia. In many instances, an etiologic agent is not determined. Familial cases do occur, and in such patients the disease appears to carry a much worse prognosis.

Mothers who are carriers of the hepatitis B antigen,

formerly known as the virus of serum hepatitis, may transmit this virus transplacentally. Stevens and associates were able to demonstrate such an occurrence in approximately 20 per cent of pregnancies in which mothers were known carriers. Such infants rarely demonstrate any neonatal evidence of hepatic disease. Many infants born of mothers carrying the hepatitis B antigen will themselves become antigen-positive postnatally, either as a result of virus acquisition during the birth process or because of close maternal-infant contact during the first few weeks of life. Kattamis and coworkers were able to demonstrate the presence of hepatitis B antigen in the sera of 10 of 23 infants with hepatitis in whom clinical manifestations of disease appeared between 2 and 4 months of age. Kohler and colleagues were able to prevent the acquisition of hepatitis B antigen by infants of carrier mothers by administering gamma globulin high in hepatitis B antibody to babies during the first week of life.

Hsia and coworkers have presented statistical data that suggest that some cases of this disease might be hereditary, dependent upon a single autosomal gene defect. Danks and Bodian's examination of this question yielded equivocal results. Scott reported a fascinating family in whom an apparently healthy mother gave birth to three infants who became jaundiced at 1 month, 7 days, and 4 months, respectively, and to two other infants who never became ill. Since homologous serum hepatitis has an incubation period of 60 to 150 days, this situation might be explained by virus crossing the placenta of the carrier mother at different times during gestation or not crossing at all in the course of two of her pregnancies or by Hsia's hypothesis.

Lawson and Boggs reviewed 23 patients with neonatal hepatitis and found two classes of patients: familial (five patients) and sporadic (18 patients). The patients with the familial form of the disease had significantly more serious morbidity and higher mortality rates than did those with the sporadic form, independent of any form of surgical procedures.

Pathology. The microscopic pictures of the livers of these children have been compared with those of children suffering from congenital extrahepatic duct atresias (see p. 638). In most but not all patients, the distinction can be made by the histologic pattern.

Diagnosis. Jaundice is the primary sign of neonatal hepatitis. It has been observed at birth, but usually it becomes apparent days or weeks after birth. Onset more than 4 weeks after birth probably, after 6 weeks surely, makes this diagnosis more likely than that of biliary atresia. Abdominal distention and hepatic enlargement appear with or soon after the jaundice. Later, with advancing cirrhosis, the liver may shrink in size and become hard. At this stage, splenomegaly

becomes prominent, and ascites may develop. Fever is usually absent. These infants, in contrast to those with biliary atresia, may appear ill, eat poorly, and vomit. Stools become acholic within the first few weeks, but this sign may be intermittent. Striking intermittence may strongly, but not absolutely, indicate the absence of congenital atresia. The urine darkens at the same time that color disappears from the stool.

Fletcher and coworkers reported an extraordinary case of an infant with neonatal hepatitis who was born with massive ascites. He was greatly improved by exchange transfusion and, thanks to excellent supportive care, made a complete recovery after 7 weeks of being very ill indeed.

In many instances, the clinical differentiation of hepatitis from biliary atresia is not possible with absolute certainty.

Laboratory Investigations. The differentiation between obstructive jaundice on the basis of hepatocellular disease due to neonatal hepatitis and that due to obstruction of the extrahepatic biliary tree is very difficult in many instances. This is because hepatitis often produces prolonged and essentially complete obstruction of the passage of bile from the liver into the gastrointestinal tract. Certain diagnostic procedures, however, may aid in making a distinction.

A gradually rising serum bilirubin level suggests atresia, whereas an irregularly declining serum bilirubin suggests hepatitis.

The presence of a serum that is positive for alpha-fetoprotein suggests the diagnosis of neonatal hepatitis.

The rose bengal radioactive test may also aid in diagnosis. Patients with obstructive jaundice who have patent bile ducts excrete 5 to 20 per cent of the injected dye in their stools, whereas those with biliary atresia excrete 8 per cent or less (in 72 hours). Newer radiopharmaceuticals such as technetium 99m derivatives of iminodiacetic acid are promising agents for visualization of the biliary tree.

The fat-soluble vitamin E is poorly absorbed when bile salts do not reach the small intestine. Measurement of vitamin E absorption as described by Lubin and coworkers or by Melhorn and associates is a simple procedure that correlates well with the results of rose bengal testing and the pathologic picture found at laparotomy.

Administration of phenobarbital or cholestyramine increases the rose bengal excretion and lowers the serum bilirubin and bile salts in many patients with intrahepatic obstruction.

Recovery of a viral agent or serologic demonstration of an infection with rubella, hepatitis B virus, cytomegalovirus, or toxoplasmosis strongly suggests the presence of neonatal hepatitis, although some of these agents may be observed in the presence of a pathologic picture of biliary atresia.

Many infants will ultimately require surgical exploration, cholangiography, and liver biopsy so that the etiology of the persistent jaundice may be determined. Before such procedures are performed, other diseases that may produce liver diseases must also be excluded. These include alpha₁-antitrypsin deficiency, galactosemia, tyrosinemia, and cystic fibrosis.

It is now the consensus that operative diagnosis should not be postponed beyond 2 months of age so that those patients with correctable forms of biliary atresia can be cured.

Prognosis. The prognosis for infants presenting with evidence of hepatitis is largely a function of the etiology of the disease. In general, the majority of infants with viral and bacterial causes of hepatitis recover without residual evidence of chronic liver disease of cirrhosis. Rapid resolution of hepatic dysfunction will occur in neonates with galactosemia if diagnosis is promptly established and galactose-containing feeds are removed from the diet. In contrast, hepatitis as a result of cystic fibrosis, alpha₁-antitrypsin deficiency, cystic fibrosis, or tyrosinemia often progresses to chronic liver disease. The prognosis for infants with idiopathic forms of neonatal giant cell hepatitis is extremely variable. Approximately 20 to 40 per cent of such patients will die within the first year of life, another 20 to 40 per cent will develop chronic liver disease, and the remainder will recover entirely.

Treatment. No uniformly effective treatment is currently available for the management of patients with hepatitis. Steroids produce erratic results.

REFERENCES

Ahrens, E. H., Harris, R. C., and MacMahon, H. E.: Atresia of the intrahepatic bile ducts. Pediatrics 8:628, 1951.

Becroft, D. M. O.: Biliary atresia associated with prenatal infection by Listeria monocytogenes. Arch. Dis. Child. 47:656, 1972.

Brough, A. J., and Bernstein, J.: Liver biopsy in the diagnosis of infantile obstructive jaundice. Pediatrics 43:519, 1969.

Danks, D., and Bodian, M.: A genetic study of neonatal obstructive jaundice. Arch. Dis. Child. 38:378, 1963.

Danks, D., Campbell, P. E., Clarke, A. M., Jones, P. G., and Solomon, J. R.: Extrahepatic biliary atresia. The frequency of potentially operable cases. Am. J. Dis. Child. 128:684, 1974.

Dickinson, E. H., and Spencer, F. C.: Choledochal cyst: report of a case with unusual features. J. Pediatr. 41:462, 1952.

Fletcher, C. B., Eakin, E. L., and Rothman, P. E.: Fetal ascites—liver giant-cell transformation. Am. J. Dis. Child. 108:554, 1964.

Gellis, S. S.: Biliary atresia. Pediatrics 55:8, 1975.

Gellis, S. S., Craig, J. M., and Hsia, D.Y.-Y.: Prolonged obstructive jaundice in infancy. IV. Neonatal hepatitis. A.M.A. J. Dis. Child. 88:285, 1954.

Henriksen, N. T.: Cholestatic jaundice in infancy. The importance of familial and genetic factors in aetiology and prognosis. Arch. Dis. Child. 56:622, 1981.

Hsia, D.Y.-Y., Boggs, J. D., Driscoll, S. G., and Gellis, S. S.: Prolonged obstructive jaundice in infancy. V. The genetic component in neonatal hepatitis. A.M.A. J. Dis. Child. 95:485, 1958.

Hsia, D.Y.-Y., Patterson, P., Allen, F. H., Jr., Diamond, L. K., and

Gellis, S. S.: Prolonged obstructive jaundice in infancy. Pediatrics 10:243, 1952.

Kasai, M., Kimura, S., Asakura, Y., Suzuki, H., Taira, Y., and Onashi, E.: Surgical treatment of biliary atresia. J. Pediatr. Surg. 3:665, 1968.

Kasai, M., Watanabe, I., and Ohi, R.: Follow-up studies of long-term survivors after hepatic portoenterostomy for "noncorrectable" biliary atresia. J. Pediatr. Surg. 10:173, 1975.

Kasai, M.: Long term follow-up after surgery for biliary atresia. In Long-term Follow-up in Congenital Anomalies. Paper and discussion presented at a Pediatric Surgical Symposium, Sept. 14 and 15, 1980, Children's Hospital of Pittsburgh; Kiesewetter, W. B., Coordinator and Editor. Cited by Kling, S.: Neonatal jaundice: the surgical viewpoint. CMA Journal 123:1218, 1980.

Kattamis, C. A., Demetrios, D., and Matsaniotis, M.: Australia antigen and neonatal hepatitis syndrome. Pediatrics 54:175, 1974.

Kohler, P. F., Dubois, R. S., Merrill, D. A., and Bowes, W. A.: Prevention of chronic neonatal hepatitis B virus infection with antibody to the hepatitis B surface antigen. N. Engl. J. Med. 291:1378, 1974.

Kove, S., Goldstein, S., and Wróbleski, F.: Serum transaminase activity in neonatal period: valuable aid in differential diagnosis of jaundice in the newborn infant. J.A.M.A. 168:860, 1958.

Landing, B. H.: Considerations of the pathogenesis of neonatal hepatitis, biliary atresia and choledochal cyst—the concept of infantile obstructive cholangiopathy. In Bill, A. H., and Kasai, M. (Eds.): Progress in Pediatric Surgery. Vol. 2. Baltimore, University Park Press. 1974, pp. 113–139.

Lawson, E. E., and Boggs, J. D.: Long-term follow-up of neonatal hepatitis: safety and value of surgical exploration. Pediatrics 53:650, 1974.

Lilly, J. R.: The Japanese operation for biliary atresia: remedy or mischief? Pediatrics 55:12, 1975.

Lottsfeldt, F. I., Krivit, W., Aust, J. B., and Carey, J. B., Jr.: Cholestyramine therapy in intrahepatic biliary cirrhosis. N. Engl. J. Med. 269:186, 1963.

Lubin, B. H., Baehner, R. L., Schwartz, E., Shohet, S., and Nathan, D. G.: Red cell peroxide hemolysis test in differential diagnosis of obstructive jaundice in the newborn period. Pediatrics 48:562, 1971.

Melhorn, D. K., Gross, S., and Izant, R. J., Jr.: The red cell hydrogen peroxide hemolysis test and vitamin E absorption in the differential diagnosis of jaundice in infancy. J. Pediatr. 81:1082, 1972.

Mowat, A. P., Psacharopoulos, H. T., and Williams, R.: Extrahepatic biliary atresia versus neonatal hepatitis. Review of 137 prospectively investigated infants. Arch. Dis. Child. 51:763, 1976.

Platt, M. S., Potter, J. L., Boeckman, C. R., and Jaberg, C.: Elevated GGTP/SGOT ratio. An early indicator of infantile obstructive cholangiopathy. Am. J. Dis. Child. 135:834, 1981.

Scott, R. B., Wilkens, W., and Kessler, A.: Viral hepatitis in early infancy. Pediatrics 13:442, 1954.

Stevens, C. E., Beasley, R. P., Tseu, J., and Lee, W. C.: Vertical transmission of hepatitis B antigen in Taiwan. N. Engl. J. Med. 292:771, 1975.

Thaler, M. M., and Gellis, S. S.: Studies in neonatal hepatitis. Am. J. Dis. Child. 116:257, 262, 271, 280, 1968.

Weinberg, T., Gordon, H. H., Oppenheimer, E. H., and Nitowsky, H. M.: Myopathy in association with tocopherol deficiency in cases of congenital biliary atresia and cystic fibrosis of the pancreas. Am. J. Pathol. 34:565, 1958.

Zeltzer, P. M., Neerhout, R. C., Fonkalsrud, E. W., and Stiehm, E. R.: Differentiation between neonatal hepatitis and biliary atresia by measuring serum-alpha-protein. Lancet 1:373, 1974.

74

Conjugated Hyperbilirubinemia Other Than That Due to Hepatitis and Biliary Atresia

By Frank A. Oski

Although the clinician commonly associates the accumulation of conjugated bilirubin in the serum of the newborn infant with the possible presence of either neonatal hepatitis or biliary atresia, it must be appreciated that a large number of heterogeneous disorders are associated with laboratory evidence of conjugated hyperbilirubinemia (see Table 74–1).

Metabolic Defects

Conjugated bilirubin may be retained as a result of an isolated specific defect in hepatic bilirubin transport, as occurs in the Dubin-Johnson and Rotor syndromes, or as a result of a more generalized disturbance in hepatic biliary secretion. This more generalized defect is termed *cholestasis*. Obstruction of a mechanical nature may produce cholestasis, but not all cases of cholestasis result from obstructive jaundice.

Dubin-Johnson syndrome and Rotor syndrome are rarely diagnosed in the neonatal period, although both may initially manifest themselves during this period by the elevation in conjugated ("direct"-reacting) bilirubin. The Dubin-Johnson syndrome is caused by a deficiency in the canalicular secretion of conjugated bilirubin and other anions. Bile salt secretion occurs normally and affected patients are not pruritic. The most characteristic laboratory feature of this disease is the markedly increased urinary excretion of the Type I isomer of coproporphyrin. This metabolic error is inherited as an autosomal recessive trait. Liver biopsy is normal except for the presence of brownish-black granules that have many of the characteristics of melanin. Jaundice in patients with

Table 74–1.   Disorders of the Newborn Infant Associated with Conjugated (Direct-Reacting) Hyperbilirubinemia

I. *Obstruction to biliary flow*:
1. Extrahepatic biliary atresia
2. Paucity of intrahepatic ductules (intrahepatic biliary atresia)
3. Choledochal cyst (bile duct stenosis)
4. Bile-plug syndrome (inspissated bile syndrome)
5. Cystic fibrosis
6. Choledocholithiasis
7. Tumors
8. Hepatic hemangioendotheliomas
9. Lymphadenopathy

II. *Hepatic cell injury*:
1. Infection:
   Bacterial:
      Syphilis
      Listeriosis
      Tuberculosis
   Viral:
      Rubella
      Cytomegalovirus
      Herpes
      Coxsackie B
      (?) Hepatitis B
      (?) Hepatitis A
   Parasitic:
      Toxoplasmosis
   Idiopathic:
      Neonatal hepatitis (giant cell hepatitis)
2. Toxic:
   Bacterial sepsis (*E. coli, Proteus, Pneumococcus*)
   Intravenous alimentation
   Drugs
3. Metabolic errors:
   Galactosemia
   Fructosemia
   Tyrosinemia
   α_1-Antitrypsin deficiency
   Cystic fibrosis
   Infantile Gaucher's disease
   Glycogenosis Type IV
   Wolman's disease
   Idiopathic neonatal hemochromatosis
   Niemann-Pick disease
   Cerebro-hepato-renal syndrome (Zellweger's disease)
   Byler's disease
   Trihydroxycoprostanic acidemia
   Indian childhood cirrhosis (?)
   Rotor syndrome
   Dubin-Johnson syndrome

III. *Chronic bilirubin overload*:
1. Erythroblastosis fetalis
2. Glucose-6-phosphate dehydrogenase deficiency and other erythrocyte enzyme deficiencies
3. Spherocytosis, elliptocytosis, pyknocytosis
4. Congenital erythropoietic porphyria

(From Gartner, L. M.: Disorders of bilirubin metabolism. *In* Nathan, D. G., and Oski, F. A. (Eds.): Hematology of Infancy and Childhood. 2nd ed. Philadelphia, W. B. Saunders Co., 1981, p. 108.)

the Dubin-Johnson syndrome becomes more intense during the last trimester of pregnancy and when estrogen-containing oral contraceptives have been used prior to pregnancy.

Rotor syndrome is also inherited as an autosomal recessive trait and is characterized by the presence of life-long mild conjugated hyperbilirubinemia. No pigment accumulates in the liver of affected patients, in contrast to the biopsy findings in patients with the Dubin-Johnson syndrome. The defect in this disorder is believed to be the result of a disturbance in the hepatic storage of anions.

Other rare metabolic defects may produce injury to the hepatocytes and often, but not always, result in the retention of conjugated bilirubin. Alpha$_1$-antitrypsin deficiency may be the most common of the inherited metabolic defects associated with liver disease in the newborn period. Presentation in the neonatal period may mimic that of neonatal hepatitis with jaundice, abnormal liver function tests, and bilirubinuria. The homozygous form of the severe deficiency, designated as the PiZZ genotype by protein electrophoresis, is the only mutant form of the disease associated with liver disease in childhood. This same genotype is associated with emphysema in adults. It is estimated that between 10 and 20 per cent of individuals with the PiZZ genotype will present with conjugated hyperbilirubinemia or cirrhosis or both during infancy or early childhood. When the disease is symptomatic in the neonatal period, it usually leads to fatal cirrhosis. The finding of little or no alpha$_1$-globulin on routine protein electrophoresis suggests that the disease is present. The diagnosis can be made by demonstration that serum is deficient in trypsin-inhibitory activity and that the patient possesses a PiZZ type on electrophoresis. Liver biopsy in affected patients will demonstrate hepatocytes containing amorphous clumps of pink-staining material in the cytoplasm of the cell. These granules are PAS-positive and resistant to diastase digestion. Unfortunately, no effective therapy is presently available to halt the progress of the disease.

Galactosemia, tyrosinemia, fructosemia, Niemann-Pick disease, Gaucher's disease, glycogenosis Type IV, and cystic fibrosis are other metabolic disorders in which conjugated hyperbilirubinemia may be observed in the newborn period. In general, other features of the disease dominate the clinical picture, and the patients rarely present as a simple problem in the differential diagnosis of conjugated hyperbilirubinemia.

Gatzimos and Jowitt first called attention to the association between jaundice and cystic fibrosis. Many of these infants may have a history of delayed passage of the first meconium stool. These infants can be demonstrated to have thick tenacious bile plugging their biliary tree. Needle biopsy of the liver may demonstrate the characteristic eosinophilic plugs in the portal bile ducts, which may be accompanied by hyperplasia. The jaundice usually resolves spontaneously. One can establish a diagnosis of cystic fibrosis in the newborn period by demonstrating the increased concentration of sweat chloride.

Sepsis

Both generalized sepsis and severe urinary tract infections during the first month of life may be accompanied by an increase in the serum concentration of conjugated bilirubin. Bacterial products are believed to produce a toxic injury to the hepatocellular excretory system. Liver biopsy of infected and jaundiced neonates reveals cholestasis, focal liver cell necrosis, and other nonspecific changes. Direct infection of the liver is not evident. Despite the marked increases in the concentration of bilirubin that may accompany infection, the serum values for alkaline phosphatase and the transaminases are either normal or only slightly elevated. Treatment of the infection produces a decline in the bilirubin concentrations without evidence of residual liver damage.

"Toxic" Hepatitis

Although bacterial infections may produce a toxic hepatitis, this term is more commonly applied to circumstances in which exposure to exogenous substances produces cholestasis with variable degrees of hepatocellular injury, inflammation, or fibrosis.

The most common cause of toxic hepatitis or cholestatic jaundice observed in neonatal intensive care nurseries at the present time is the prolonged use of total parenteral nutrition.

Cholestatic jaundice induced by parenteral nutrition is seen with greatest frequency in the most immature infants. It is estimated that at least 10 per cent of infants with a gestational age of less than 32 weeks will develop this complication if they receive parenteral nutrition for periods of 3 to 4 weeks. In contrast, only about 1 per cent of infants with gestational ages of more than 36 weeks will develop cholestatic jaundice under similar circumstances.

Bacterial infections appear to contribute to the development of cholestasis.

Liver biopsies in infants who develop cholestatic jaundice in association with parenteral nutrition demonstrate both hepatocellular damage and cholestasis. Giant-cell transformation may also be observed. The etiology of the cholestasis is unclear but may relate to the fact that amino acids inhibit bile flow. Evidence of hepatic dysfunction, but not clinical jaundice, can be demonstrated within 1 week of the initiation of total parenteral nutrition. This effect appears to be independent of the neonate's underlying condition and unrelated to the concomitant use of intravenous lipid. The initial effect of the amino acid infusion appears to be on the canalicular membrane and is reflected by increases in the serum concentrations of gamma glutamyl transpeptidase and 5'-nucleotidase.

Discontinuation of the parenteral nutrition usually produces a prompt disappearance of the hepatic abnormalities, although evidence of hepatocellular damage and fibrosis occasionally may persist. Neonates receiving total parenteral nutrition should be monitored, at least weekly, with conjugated bilirubin values and serum bile acids.

The Bile-Plug Syndrome

It had been suspected for many years that obstructive jaundice could be caused by plugs in the extrahepatic bile ducts. Bernstein and coworkers proved this theory by demonstrating such plugs in two infants, one of whom became jaundiced as early as 6 days, and the other as late as 7 weeks of age. The second baby was saved after demonstration by cholangiogram of obstruction in the distal end of the common duct and following the removal of an impacted mass of dark, granular, bile-colored material.

REFERENCES

Bernstein, J., Braylan, R., and Brough, A. J.: Bile-plug syndrome. A correctible cause of obstructive jaundice in infants. Pediatrics 43:273, 1969.

Bernstein, J., Chang, C.-H., Brough, A. J., et al.: Conjugated hyperbilirubinemia in infants associated with parenteral alimentation. J. Pediatr. 90:361, 1977.

Black, D. D., Suttle, A., Whitington, P. F., et al.: The effect of short-term total parenteral nutrition on hepatic function in the human neonate: a prospective randomized study demonstrating alteration of hepatic canalicular function. J. Pediatr. 99:445, 1981.

Colon, A. R., and Sandberg, D. H.: Presently recognized forms of inherited jaundice in infancy. A summary and review. Clin. Pediatr. 12:326, 1973.

Escobedo, M. B., and Barton, L. L.: The frequency of jaundice in neonatal bacterial infections. Clin. Pediatr. 13:656, 1974.

Gatzimos, C. D., and Jowitt, R. H.: Jaundice in mucoviscidosis (fibrocystic disease of the pancreas). A.M.A. J. Dis. Child. 80:182, 1955.

Heathcote, J., Deodhar, K. P., Scheuer, P. J., et al.: Intrahepatic cholestasis in childhood. N. Engl. J. Med. 295:801, 1975.

Mowat, A. P.: Liver Disorders in Childhood. London, Butterworth and Co., 1979.

Odievre, M., Martin, J. P., et al.: Alpha-1-antitrypsin deficiency in liver disease in children, phenotypes, manifestations, and prognosis. Pediatrics 57:226, 1976.

Pereira, G. R., Sherman, M. S., DiGiacomo, J., et al.: Hyperalimentation-induced cholestasis. Increased incidence and severity in premature infants. Am. J. Dis. Child. 135:842, 1981.

Taylor, W. F., and Qaqundah, B. Y.: Neonatal jaundice associated with cystic fibrosis. Am. J. Dis. Child. 123:161, 1972.

Touloukian, R. J., and Downing, S. E.: Cholestasis associated with long-term parenteral hyperalimentation. Arch. Surg. 106:58, 1973.

75

Differential Diagnosis of Jaundice

By Frank A. Oski

A thoughtful attempt should be made to establish the etiology of jaundice in all infants who meet one of the following criteria:

1. Clinical jaundice in the first 24 hours of life.

2. Total bilirubin concentration increasing at a rate in excess of 5 mg per 100 ml per day.

3. Term infants in whom the total serum bilirubin concentration exceeds 12.9 mg per 100 ml.

4. Preterm infants in whom the total serum bilirubin concentration exceeds 15.0 mg per 100 ml.

5. All infants in whom the conjugated bilirubin (direct) concentration exceeds 2.0 mg per 100 ml or more than 15 per cent of the total bilirubin value.

6. The persistence of clinical jaundice beyond the first week of life in a term infant or the persistence of clinical jaundice beyond the second week of life in a preterm infant.

The initial diagnostic procedures should be directed at determining whether the jaundice is a result of increased production of bilirubin, impaired bilirubin conjugation, impaired bilirubin excretion, increased reabsorption of bilirubin from the intestinal tract, or a combination of these factors.

Guidelines for the collection and interpretation of historical data, the pertinent physical findings, and laboratory tests are listed in Table 75–1. Maisels and Gifford have reported that the measurement of direct and total bilirubin and hemoglobin or hematocrit, performed with the determination of the blood type of mother and infant, direct Coombs' test on the infant's erythrocytes, the measurement of the infant's reticulocyte count, and examination of the peripheral

Table 75–1. Data Collection in the Diagnosis of Neonatal Jaundice

Information	Significance
Family History	
Parent or sibling with history of jaundice or anemia	Suggests hereditary hemolytic anemia such as hereditary spherocytosis
Previous sibling with neonatal jaundice	Suggests hemolytic disease due to ABO or Rh isoimmunization
History of liver disease in siblings or disorders such as cystic fibrosis, galactosemia, tyrosinemia, hypermethioninemia, Crigler-Najjar syndrome or alpha$_1$-antitrypsin deficiency	All associated with neonatal hyperbilirubinemia
Maternal History	
Unexplained illness during pregnancy	Consider congenital infections such as rubella, cytomegalovirus, toxoplasmosis, herpes, syphilis, hepatitis A or B, Epstein-Barr virus
Diabetes mellitus	Increased incidence of jaundice among infants of diabetic mothers
Drug ingestion during pregnancy	Ingestion of sulfonamides, nitrofurantoins, anti-malarials may initiate hemolysis in G6PD deficient infant
History of Labor and Delivery	
Vacuum extraction	Increased incidence of cephalhematoma and jaundice
Oxytocin induced labor	Increased incidence of hyperbilirubinemia
Delayed cord clamping	Increased incidence of hyperbilirubinemia among polycythemic infants
Apgar score	Increased incidence of jaundice in asphyxiated infants
Infant's History	
Delayed passage of meconium or infrequent stools	Increased enterohepatic circulation of bilirubin. Consider intestinal atresia, annular pancreas, Hirschsprung's disease, meconium plug, drug-induced ileus (hexamethonium)
Caloric intake	Inadequate caloric intake results in delay in bilirubin conjugation
Vomiting	Suspect sepsis, galactosemia, or pyloric stenosis; all associated with hyperbilirubinemia.
Infant's Physical Exam	
Small for gestational age	Infants frequently polycythemic and jaundiced
Head size	Microcephaly seen with intrauterine infections associated with jaundice
Cephalhematoma	Entrapped hemorrhage associated with hyperbilirubinemia
Plethora	Polycythemia
Pallor	Suspect hemolytic anemia
Petechiae	Suspect congenital infection, overwhelming sepsis, or severe hemolytic disease as cause of jaundice
Appearance of umbilical stump	Omphalitis and sepsis may produce jaundice
Hepatosplenomegaly	Suspect hemolytic anemia or congenital infection
Optic fundi	Chorioretinitis suggests congenital infection as cause of jaundice
Umbilical hernia	Consider hypothyroidism
Congenital anomalies	Jaundice occurs with increased frequency among infants with trisomic conditions
Laboratory Data	
Maternal	
Blood group and indirect Coomb's test	Necessary for evaluation of possible ABO or Rh incompatibility
Serology	Rule out congenital syphilis
Infant	
Hemoglobin	Anemia suggests hemolytic disease or large entrapped hemorrhage. Hemoglobin above 22 gm/100 ml associated with increased incidence of jaundice
Reticulocyte count	Elevation suggests hemolytic disease
Red cell morphology	Spherocytes suggest ABO incompatibility or hereditary spherocytosis. Red cell fragmentation seen in disseminated intravascular coagulation
Platelet count	Thrombocytopenia suggests infection
White cell count	Total white cell count less than 5000/mm^3 or band/neutrophil ratio >0.2 suggests infection
Sedimentation rate	Values in excess of 5 during the first 48 hours indicate infection or ABO incompatibility
Direct bilirubin	Elevation suggests infection or severe Rh incompatibility
Immunoglobulin M	Elevation indicates infection
Blood group and direct and indirect Coombs' test	Required to rule out hemolytic disease as a result of isoimmunization
Carboxyhemoglobin level	Elevated in infants with hemolytic disease or entrapped hemorrhage
Urinalysis	Presence of reducing substance suggests diagnosis of galactosemia

smear, will define or suggest the cause of jaundice in approximately 50 per cent of all infants with hyperbilirubinemia.

Jaundice that appears within the first 24 hours of life is usually due to increased production of bilirubin as a result of a hemolytic process. In general, the more severe hemolytic anemias will be manifested by early jaundice rather than by late appearance of pallor. Rh incompatibility and ABO incompatibility are the most common causes of hemolytic disease associated with jaundice during the first day of life. Other congenital defects of red cell metabolism may also be associated with jaundice during this period and must be considered in the differential diagnosis of an infant with unexplained hemolytic anemia. In some instances, jaundice associated with severe infection may appear during the first day. Some features that are useful in distinguishing ABO, Rh, and infectious origins of jaundice are described in Table 75–2.

Physical examination supplies a few valuable differentiating points. If the newborn is jaundiced but is neither sick nor pale, is not covered with petechiae and ecchymoses, and has little or no enlargement of the spleen or liver, ABO or mild Rh hemolytic disease is most likely the correct diagnosis. If he looks very sick, he may have either severe hemolytic disease or nonbacterial infection. Skin hemorrhages and a large liver and spleen strongly suggest the latter.

Further diagnostic studies may have to be postponed and transfusion started at this point if the infant is in shock or is obviously very anemic. The first blood withdrawn will then be subjected to a number of tests. The mother's and father's blood may also have to be investigated.

One should act according to the following guidelines:

1. Evaluate the infant's hemoglobin, serum bilirubin and its partition, red blood cell count, number of spherocytes, nucleated red blood cell number, reticulocyte percentage, white cell count and differential platelet count, direct and indirect Coombs' test results, and the infant's and parents' isoimmunologic and Rh grouping.

2. If Rh is negative and if direct Coombs' test result is strongly positive, search for rare antigens (e.g., Kell, Duffy).

3. If Rh is positive and if direct Coombs' test result is strongly positive, search for circulating Rh antibodies.

4. If Rh is negative and if direct Coombs' test result is negative or weakly positive, and if infant belongs to group A or B and mother to group O, perform an indirect Coombs' test and search for circulating anti-A or anti-B antibodies. Presence and number of spherocytes should be noted.

5. If no blood group incompatibility exists and if this observation is confirmed by negativity of both Coombs' test results, perform blood culture, urine culture for viruses, and serologic studies ("STORCH"). These latter tests should be performed on the mother's serum as well. The infant's IgM concentration and the presence or absence of IgM's against specific diseases will be extremely helpful.

One may interpret these results using the data in Table 75–2. The qualifications are pointed out in footnotes.

Jaundice beginning during the second or third day is probably physiologic. If, however, the infant appears ill, if the liver or spleen is enlarged, if urobilin or bile appears in excess in the urine, or if conjugated bilirubin is found in the blood, other explanations should be sought.

Jaundice first appearing at 4 days or later is usually not due to hemolytic disease of the newborn. Intranatally or postnatally acquired virus infection (cytomegalic disease, generalized herpes simplex) must be thought of as well as the bacterial infections. Neonatal hepatitis cannot be ignored, since its onset may take place at any time from birth to 4 months.

Icterus that persists beyond the usual duration of physiologic jaundice may be hemolytic, functional, or obstructive. If hemolytic, it may be the result of persistent sepsis, pyelonephritis, hereditary erythrocyte malformation, or, very rarely indeed, congenital

Table 75–2. Laboratory Tests in Jaundice That Begins Within the First 24 Hours

Disease Process	Blood Smear			Infant's Erythrocytes			Infant's Bilirubin			Antibodies			Special Tests for Infection
	Sphero-cytes	Erythro-blasts	Reduced Platelets	Group O	Rh-Positive	Direct Coombs'	Direct	In-direct	Indirect Coombs'	A or B	Rh	
ABO hemolytic disease	+	+	Rarely and later	Never*	0 or +	Weak	No > 2.0 mg.%	+	+	+	0	0
Rh hemolytic disease	0	+	Rarely and later	±	+†	+ and strong	Rarely > 2.0 mg.%	+	+	0	+	0
Infection	0	+	+ often	±	0	0	+	+	0	0	0	+†‡

* The infant's blood group is usually A.

† In hR (little c, d, or e) sensitization and those caused by other rare antigens, the Rh will be negative.

‡ In toxoplasmosis, Sabin's dye test becomes positive early, whereas complement fixation becomes positive later. At this stage, dye tests should be positive in the mother and infant, complement fixation only in the mother. If cytomegalic inclusion disease is the cause, the urinary sediment should show inclusion bodies and should yield the virus upon culture. Specific IgM tests are highly desirable.

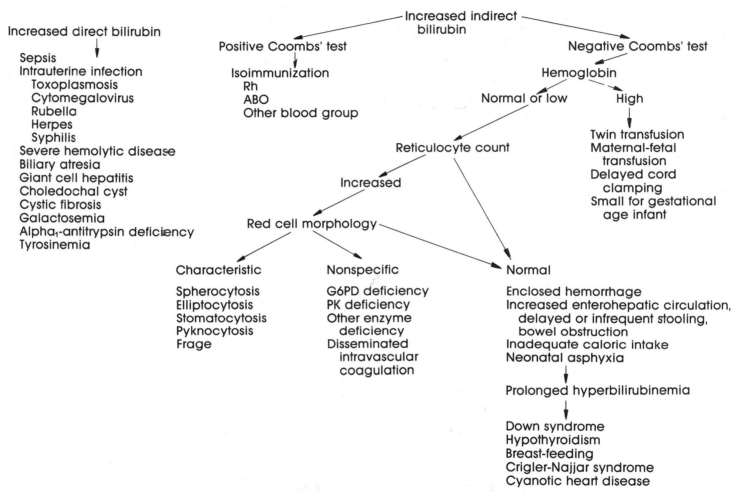

Increased direct bilirubin

Sepsis
Intrauterine infection
 Toxoplasmosis
 Cytomegalovirus
 Rubella
 Herpes
 Syphilis
Severe hemolytic disease
Biliary atresia
Giant cell hepatitis
Choledochal cyst
Cystic fibrosis
Galactosemia
Alpha$_1$-antitrypsin deficiency
Tyrosinemia

Increased indirect bilirubin

Positive Coombs' test

Isoimmunization
 Rh
 ABO
 Other blood group

Negative Coombs' test

Hemoglobin

Normal or low   High

Reticulocyte count

Twin transfusion
Maternal-fetal
 transfusion
Delayed cord
 clamping
Small for gestational
 age infant

Increased

Red cell morphology

Characteristic   Nonspecific   Normal

Spherocytosis   G6PD deficiency
Elliptocytosis   PK deficiency
Stomatocytosis   Other enzyme
Pyknocytosis   deficiency
Frage   Disseminated
                         intravascular
                         coagulation

Enclosed hemorrhage
Increased enterohepatic circulation,
 delayed or infrequent stooling,
 bowel obstruction
Inadequate caloric intake
Neonatal asphyxia

Prolonged hyperbilirubinemia

Down syndrome
Hypothyroidism
Breast-feeding
Crigler-Najjar syndrome
Cyanotic heart disease

Figure 75–1. Schematic approach to the diagnosis of neonatal jaundice.

hemoglobin disorders or erythrocyte enzyme defects. The morphology of the red cells, their osmotic fragility, as well as electrophoretic studies, enzyme studies, and repeated blood cultures should differentiate this group.

If bilirubinemia is pronounced and if the serum bilirubin is almost entirely of the indirect type when there is no evidence of increased hemolysis (reticulocytosis, normoblastosis, and erythroblastosis in the blood; increased urobilin in the stool or urine), one should think first of events that can predispose the patient to hepatic recirculation of bilirubin absorbed from the intestine, and, if this is not the cause, should next consider hypothyroidism. If the latter diagnosis is also incorrect, one can then justifiably think seriously of congenital familial nonhemolytic jaundice.

Persistent obstructive jaundice is a sign that causes much diagnostic perplexity. Its characteristics include a high proportion of direct-reacting bilirubin in the serum (usually 35 per cent or more of the total), diminished or absent bilirubin and urobilin in stools, and increased bile in the urine. Diagnostic possibilities include (1) anatomic obstructions (atresia of bile ducts, bile duct plug, choledochus or pseudocholedochus cyst, or, rarely, cystic fibrosis, hypertrophic pyloric stenosis, intestinal atresia, or malrotation of the intestine); (2) neonatal hepatitis (following erythroblastosis fetalis or congenital or acquired hemolytic anemia or appearing independent of any known underlying disease); and (3) neonatal cirrhosis of the liver. Clinically, there are few features that allow one to differentiate among these possibilities. A fairly reliable one is that infants with bile duct atresia do not appear ill during the neonatal period. They eat well and gain fairly well at first. Likewise, those infants who have obstructive jaundice that follows hemolytic disease do not initially appear ill. Infants with hepatitis and especially those with cirrhosis look and act sick, eat poorly, and may have fever and may vomit often. Infants with hemolytic disease of the newborn will usually have gone through a stage of nonobstructive jaundice within the first week of life, and the obstructive condition either will have followed the first stage directly or will have appeared a few days or weeks after subsidence of the nonobstructive episode. The knowledge that hemolytic disease had been manifest earlier makes the diagnosis of inspissated bile syndrome secondary to this disorder simple. If one does not have this knowledge, retrospective tests as described previously will still be diagnostic.

Liver function tests are of little differentiating value. The rose bengal excretion test may be of greater use, since the dye is well excreted in a large number of patients in the hepatitis group, but poorly in infants with atresia. Serum transaminase activities have some differential diagnostic value.

Promising new approaches to the evaluation of hepatobiliary disease have followed the development of pharmaceutical agents derived from ^{99m}technetium iminodiacetic acid. Acceptable visualization of the biliary tree is achievable with modest hyperbilirubinemia. Many preparations now being evaluated will probably increase our ability to use the most appropriate radiopharmaceutical in given circumstances. Rose bengal (^{131}I) remains the most widely used compound.

An approach to all the potential clinical possibilities discussed in the previous chapters is illustrated in Figure 75–1. It is designed to serve as a reminder of some of the less common clinical entities that often lead to diagnostic confusion.

REFERENCES

Adler, S. M., and Denton, R. L.: The erythrocyte sedimentation rate. J. Pediatr. 86:942, 1975.

Alden, E. R., et al.: Carboxyhemoglobin determination in evaluating neonatal jaundice. Am. J. Dis. Child. 127:214, 1974.

Freeman, L. M., and Weissmann, H. S. (Eds.): Nuclear Medicine Annual. New York, Raven Press, 1981.

Gartner, L. M.: Disorders of bilirubin metabolism. In Nathan, D. G., and Oski, F. A. (Eds.). Hematology of Infancy and Childhood. 2nd ed. Philadelphia, W.B. Saunders Co., 1981, pp. 86–118.

Maisels, M. J., and Gifford, K.: Neonatal jaundice and breast-feeding. Pediatr. Res. 9:308, 1975.

Thaler, M. M.: Algorithmic diagnosis of conjugated and unconjugated hyperbilirubinemia. J.A.M.A. 237:58, 1977.

PART 11

DISORDERS OF THE NERVOUS SYSTEM

76

Neurologic Evaluation of the Newborn Infant

By John H. Menkes*

Introduction

The ontogenesis of the human nervous system can be divided into four stages. The initial stage is one of embryogenesis and induction and occurs during the first 30 days of development. During this period, the neural plate and groove and, subsequently, the neural tube are formed, the vascular primordia are elaborated, and the anlagen for the facial structures are laid down, the latter process being activated by the rostral neural tube. Interference with ontogenesis during this period results in such dysraphic or facial-forebrain anomalies as anencephaly, myelomeningocele, and the holoprosencephalies (Friede, 1975).

The second ontogenetic stage begins at the end of the first month of development. It is one of neuronal proliferation and outward migration from the area surrounding the neural tube. As a rule, earlier cells form the deeper layers, and later arrivals pass through these to form the more superficial regions of the cerebral and cerebellar cortex. The peak period for neuronal proliferation is 2 to 4 months' gestation; for neuronal migration it is 3 to 5 months. In the cerebral cortex, the process continues for as long as the sixth month of postnatal life. In the cerebellum, cellular proliferation begins later and lasts longer, with migration continuing well into the second postnatal year.

By 25 weeks' gestation, the cerebral cortex has reached its full neuronal complement, neuronal proliferation has probably ceased, and electrical activity has become recognizable. Insults to morphogenesis during this period give rise to the various disorders of cellular proliferation and migration, such as the microcephalies, schizencephaly, and polymicrogyria.

At the beginning of the last trimester of gestation, a rapid multiplication of glial cells commences. This event is accompanied by an elaboration of neural processes, the formation of synapses, and the ultimate alignment and orientation of the cortical neurons. These events continue throughout the neonatal period into the first few years of postnatal life. A number of disorders, including perinatal insults, may affect this developmental stage.

Myelination occurs over a long time span. It commences during the second trimester of gestation, is maximal during the first year of postnatal life, and may continue into the third decade.

The brain of the term newborn infant weighs 325 to 435 gm, only one fourth the weight of the average adult brain, but accounts for approximately 10 per cent of the total body weight at birth. All primary and secondary fissures and sulci are present, but the tertiary sulci are only partly developed. The four major lobes are clearly distinguishable, although the frontal and temporal poles are relatively shorter than those of the older child, and the demarcation between cortical gray matter and underlying white matter is not yet distinct. On microscopic examination, the cerebral cortex of the term newborn exhibits lamination similar to that of the adult brain. Nissl bodies are not yet present in cortical neurons, except in certain Betz cells in the motor cortex. The cerebellum in the newborn is notable for its prominent external granular cell layer, composed of 8 to 12 rows of densely packed cells, which gradually disappear during the first postnatal year. Myelin, elaborated from proliferating oligodendrocytes, appears, generally speaking, in a caudocranial order. At birth, all cranial nerves except the optic are myelinated, as are the spinal roots, the olivary and cerebellar connections, and the tracts of the spinal cord posterior columns. Myelination of the corticospinal tract, the corticocerebellar fibers, and the optic nerve commences just prior to birth.

The rapid brain growth that occurs during the first postnatal year is largely the result of continued myelination and tremendous elaboration of dendritic processes, events that establish the neuronal connections necessary for the complex behavior that is characteristic of the older infant and child.

Neurologic Examination

Neurologic examination of the newborn infant is an observational art that requires a certain degree of knowledge of the variations of neonatal behavior, a considerable degree of patience, and a conservative attitude regarding the significance and the predictive value of certain deviations of performance that can be influenced by many systemic and environmental factors. A single examination may suffice to document the presence of neurologic integrity in a newborn and may be adequate when signs of disease are obvious and definite. When signs are marginal or only suggestively abnormal, however, a second exami-

---

* This chapter includes some contributions from a previous author, Dr. William E. Bell.

nation or even daily evaluations will yield more reliable information regarding the nature of the problem. Many of our present concepts of neurologic and behavioral function of the newborn infant are derived from the detailed and astute observations of André-Thomas, Saint-Anne Dargassies, and Illingworth.

Neurologic examination of the newborn child should begin with an adequate period of observation, first before removal of the clothing and then in more detail with the infant completely undressed. Ideally, the baby should be awake, not crying, and not cool or exposed to a cold environment, and approximately 2 hours should have elapsed since his last feeding. General aspects to be noted because of their possible association with neurologic function include the respiratory rate and rhythm, cutaneous abnormalities such as plethora, jaundice, or evidence of sepsis, and the presence of external minor anomalies, especially of the hands, feet, external ears, eyes, or genitalia.

Important components of the infant's behavior to be observed include the state of alertness, the resting posture the child assumes in the supine and prone positions, the capability of the child to perform similar but not necessarily symmetric movements of the limbs on the two sides, and the character of the cry.

Several factors influence the normal infant's state of alertness. These include time of last feeding, environmental stimuli, and gestational age. By 28 weeks' gestation, an infant may be aroused by persistent stimulation or may alert spontaneously. Sleep-wake cycles are clearly apparent by 32 weeks.

The posture of the normal term infant in the prone position is one of partial flexion of the arms and legs, with legs adducted so that the thighs are maintained under the abdomen. When awake, the baby on his abdomen is able to rotate the head from side to side and temporarily elevate it from the surface of the crib. The awake neonate lying on his back will exhibit purposeless, poorly coordinated limb movements, usually consisting of alternating flexion and extension in reciprocal fashion on the two sides. Minimal or absent motor activity, or strikingly asymmetric motor activity in which one arm or one side of the body is little moved, is clearly suggestive of neurologic dysfunction. The cry of an intact newborn is a vigorous and reasonably sustained one, easily elicited by flicking the bottom of the foot or sometimes by eliciting the Moro response. A high-pitched shrill cry, a cry that on repeated observations on different examinations is weak and unsustained, or an inability to provoke a cry are indicators of probable neurologic abnormalities.

Muscle tone is evaluated by passive movement of various parts of the body, ideally with the infant awake and not crying. Since limb tone, like various reflexes, is influenced or altered by tonic neck reflexes, it is important to have the child's head in a neutral position when these assessments are made. In the infant of 28 weeks' gestation, there is minimal resistance to passive movements of the limbs. By 32 weeks, flexor tone appears in the lower extremities

and is prominent by 36 weeks. The normal term infant assumes a flexed posture of both upper and lower extremities with a certain degree of resistance being present at the elbows and knees. Muscle tone should be symmetrical when one side is compared with the other. A reduction in muscle tone is an important diagnostic sign but by itself is without localizing value. Flaccidity is most often encountered in the comatose infant but can also result from traumatic insults to the upper portion of the spinal cord, disease of the spinal anterior horn cells, and abnormalities of the muscles or neuromuscular junction.

Certain deep tendon reflexes can be elicited in the neonate but have limited value except when definitely asymmetric reactions are elicited. The triceps jerk and brachioradialis jerk cannot usually be obtained during the period of flexor tone predominance. The knee jerk is moderately brisk and is often associated with adduction of the opposite thigh. Unsustained ankle clonus of up to 10 beats is common in the days immediately after birth and does not represent an abnormal finding. The plantar response to stimulation of the lateral surface of the sole of the foot is a much discussed phenomenon but of limited usefulness in the clinical assessment of the newborn. The claim that all newborn and young infants have Babinski signs is an overstatement in need of qualification. Although it is true that extension of the great toe is often part of the response to plantar stimulation in early infancy, this normal response is usually quite different from the slow, tonic extension associated with fanning of the other toes seen in the 3- or 4-month-old with spastic lower limbs. The normal response to plantar stimulation is frequently a quick withdrawal with flexion of the knee and prompt but unsustained extension of the great toe. Hogan and Milligan have shown that the first, and most important, response to stroking of the sole of the newborn's foot is a flexor reaction of the great toe, which may then be followed by other movements.

Of the several tests designed to assess cranial nerve function, we have found those discussed subsequently to be the most useful in the neurologic evaluation of the newborn.

Visual responses can first be demonstrated at 28 weeks' gestation. At that time, the infant will blink consistently when confronted by a bright light. By 32 weeks, light induces persistent closure of the lids. The pupillary light reflex appears at 29 weeks and is consistently present at 32 weeks. An optokinetic nystagmus is elicitable at term. Although more complex visual behavior is demonstrable with special techniques, these tests have little value in the routine neurologic examination. In contrast, the funduscopic examination is of considerable importance. The examiner must keep in mind the fact that the newborn's optic disc has a grayish-white appearance and that the macular light reflex is normally absent.

Eye movements are difficult to assess during the first few weeks of life. Discrete following movements are not expected at that time, but an alert infant often appears to fixate on the examiner's face, and some degree of conjugate ocular activity is usually seen. Abrupt, transient horizontal nystagmus is commonly present in the newborn, especially on movement of the child, and should not be judged to be abnormal. The response to the doll's head maneuver is first noted at 30 weeks' gestation and usually is elicitable in the full-term infant. Oculovestibular responses can best be elicited by spinning the infant while he is held in the upright position, facing the examiner.

The amplitude and symmetry of facial movements are noted with the infant at rest and when he is crying or sucking.

After 28 weeks' gestation, an infant will blink or startle to sudden loud noises. In the full-term infant, the sound of a bell may elicit more complex responses, such as cessation of sucking and opening of eyes.

Examination of the head of a newborn infant should include observation and description of its shape, measurement in centimeters of the occipitofrontal circumference, palpation and estimation of degree of separation of sutures, and palpation and measurement of the size of the anterior fontanel. Care must be used in determining the head circumference, and the same landmarks should be used with each estimate. A disposable paper tape is preferred to a metal one and should extend around the head from a point approximately 1 cm above the supraorbital margin anteriorly to the farthest point on the occiput posteriorly. In some instances, auscultation and transillumination of the head are useful additional procedures. The status of the cranial sutures and anterior fontanel, especially on serial examinations over the course of weeks or months, is one of the most reliable indicators of conditions that induce increased intracranial pressure or those that have interfered with continued normal brain growth. The anterior fontanel is best evaluated with the infant quiet and held in the sitting position. The range of normal fontanel size and the conditions that retard fontanel closure have been reviewed by Popich and Smith. In addition to indicating primary neurologic conditions in which increased intracranial pressure is present, a tense fontanel in infancy occurs in some cases with cardiac failure. An unusual finding on examination of the head is a parietal bony defect along the sagittal suture, located approximately 2 cm anterior to the posterior fontanel. This is referred to as a third fontanel but is in fact not a fontanel in that it is not located at the junction of the parietal and adjacent bones. This bony defect results from failure of completion of ossification in the parasagittal parietal region and has been identified especially in infants with Down syndrome and the congenital rubella syndrome (Tan 1971; Chemke and Robinson, 1969).

An important aspect of the neurologic assessment of the newborn pertains to the evaluation of a group of responses termed *neonatal reflexes*. These aspects of newborn function are generally attributed to mechanisms at the brain-stem level that can be provoked by the appropriate stimulus because of the relative lack of cerebral inhibition (Paine and Oppe, 1966).

From a clinical standpoint, we have found those reflexes discussed subsequently to be the most useful.

The Moro response is the best known of the var-

Table 76–1. Percentage of Normal Babies Showing Various Infantile Reflexes with Increasing Age

	Signs That Disappear with Age			Signs That Appear with Age				
	Moro	*Tonic Neck Reflex*	*Crossed Adduction to KJ*	*Neck Righting Reflex*	*Supporting Reaction*	*Landau*	*Parachute*	*Hand Grasp*
	Extension even without flexor phase	Imposable even for 30 degrees or inconstant	Strong or slight	Imposable but transient	Fair or good	Head above horizontal and back arched	Complete	Thumb to forefinger alone
Age (months)								
1	93	67	?*	13	50	0	0	0
2	89	90	?*	23	43	0	0	0
3	70	50	41	25	52	0	0	0
4	59	34	41	26	40	0	0	0
5	22	31	41	38	61	29	0	0
6	0	11	21	40	66	42	3	0
7	0	0	12	43	74	42	29	16
8	0	0	15	54	81	44	40	53
9	0	0	6	67	96	97	76	63
10	0	0	3	100	100	100	79	84
11	0	0	3	100	100	100	90	95
12	0	0	2	100	100	100	100	100

* Divergence of experience and opinion between different examiners.
(From Paine, R. S., and Oppe, T. E.: Clin. Dev. Med. *20*:1, 1966.)

ious neonatal reflexes. It can be elicited in a number of ways, such as abrupt but gentle hyperextension of the neck by allowing the head to fall backward or by abruptly releasing both hands, after pulling the child up slightly from the supine position. The response consists of sudden abduction of the proximal portions of the arms, extension at the elbows, and opening of the fists with abduction of the fingers (Parmelee, 1963). Normal infants frequently cry immediately after the response is provoked. The Moro response gradually diminishes, disappearing by 3 to 4 months of age, or even later in prematurely born infants. Its persistence significantly beyond its expected date of disappearance or its absence or diminished intensity in the first few weeks of life represents abnormalities indicative of neurologic dysfunction (Table 76–1). Marked and persistent asymmetry of the response occurs with brachial plexus injuries or conditions associated with hemiparesis.

The palmar grasp response appears at 28 weeks' gestation, is well established by 32 weeks, and normally disappears by 2 to 4 months of age.

The tonic neck response is elicited by rotation of the head while the chest is maintained in a flat position. It consists of extension of the upper extremity to which the face has been rotated and flexion of the contralateral upper extremity. The lower extremities respond similarly. Asymmetric tonic neck responses are abnormal, as is an obligatory and sustained tonic neck pattern (i.e., one that can be imposed on the infant for prolonged periods and from which he is unable to escape). Inconstant tonic neck responses can be elicited for as long as 6 months (Table 76–1) and may even be momentarily present, particularly during sleep, in the normal 2- or 3-year-old.

Reflex placing and stepping responses are of lesser value. The former is elicited by stimulating the dorsum of the foot against the edge of the examining table. Reflex stepping, which is at least partly a function of the flexion response to noxious stimuli, is present in the normal newborn when he is supported in the standing position. The response disappears by the fourth to fifth month of life.

The neurologic examination, when performed in the aforementioned manner, can be interpreted as normal, abnormal, or suspect. The predictive value of the examination in terms of subsequent neurologic deficits is considerable. In the Collaborative Perinatal Project of the National Institutes of Health, 16 per cent of neonates who had an abnormal neurologic examination were subsequently found to have cerebral palsy. Conversely, a suspect or abnormal examination was seen in only 11 per cent and 0.5 per cent, respectively, of subsequently normal children but in 34 per cent and 23 per cent, respectively, of cerebral palsied children (Nelson and Ellenberg, 1979).

Every physician examining infants suspected of having sustained a cerebral birth injury has encountered a group of patients who appear to have clear-cut neurologic deficits during the neonatal period but who on subsequent examinations have lost all signs of motor dysfunction. Some of these infants may show delayed milestones and ultimately are found to be grossly retarded, whereas others may only demonstrate visual perceptual handicaps, speech defects, nonfebrile seizures, or hyperkinetic behavior (Paine, 1964; Nelson and Ellenberg, 1982).

Assessment of Gestational Age

When it was recognized that infants of low birth weight could be small because of short gestation (premature infant) or because of retardation of intrauterine growth (small for dates infant), methods of distinguishing the two on the basis of clinical assessment became important. External characteristics, including skin texture and color, lanugo, nipple formation, breast size, external ear form and firmness, and external genitalia, correlate with gestational age but are less than precise (Farr et al., 1966; Dubowitz et al., 1970; Volper, 1981) (Table 76–2). They can be used in conjunction with a system of assessing

Table 76–2. External Characteristics Useful for Estimation of Gestational Age

External Characteristics	Gestational Age			
	28 Weeks	*32 Weeks*	*36 Weeks*	*40 Weeks*
Ear cartilage	Pinna soft, remains folded.	Pinna slightly harder, but remains folded.	Pinna harder, springs back.	Pinna firm, stands erect from head.
Breast tissue	None	None	1–2 mm nodule	6–7 mm nodule
External genitalia: male	Testes undescended, smooth scrotum.	Testes in inguinal canal, few scrotal rugae.	Testes high in scrotum, more scrotal rugae.	Testes descended, pendulous scrotum covered with rugae.
External genitalia: female	Prominent clitoris, small, widely separated labia.	Prominent clitoris, larger separated labia.	Clitoris less prominent, labia majora cover labia minora.	Clitoris covered by labia majora.
Plantar surface	Smooth	1–2 anterior creases.	2–3 anterior creases.	Creases cover sole.

(From Volpe, J. J.: Neurology of the Newborn. Philadelphia, W. B. Saunders, Co., 1981. Modified from Usher, R.: Pediatr. Clin. North Am. *13*:835, 1966.)

neurologic maturity as devised by Robinson (Table 76–3). This scheme utilizes five reflex responses, including pupillary reaction, traction response, glabellar tap, neck-righting, and head-turning to diffuse light. Gestational age can be roughly estimated by these observations, since pupillary reaction to light develops from 29 to 31 weeks of gestation, glabellar tap reflex from 32 to 34 weeks, traction response from 33 to 36 weeks, neck-righting reflex from 34 to 37 weeks, and head-turning to diffuse light from 32 to 36 weeks. The method developed by Amiel-Tison is largely dependent on the gradual increase of muscle tone that occurs progressively with increasing gestational age (Fig. 76–1). This scheme is sensitive to a variety of exogenous factors, notably maternal sedation, method of delivery, and the position of the fetus in utero.

Additional methods of differentiating the low birth weight infant due to short gestation from the small for dates infant include measurements of the ulnar nerve conduction velocity (Schulte et al., 1968; Moosa and Dubowitz, 1972; Dubowitz et al., 1968). The mean conduction velocity for the ulnar nerve of the term newborn infant is approximately 30 meters per second and is progressively slower with progressively shorter gestational ages. Electroencephalographic methods have also been used to judge gestational age by determination of the latency of photoevoked responses from the occipital cortex (Engel and Butler, 1963). Infants of a conceptual age of 40 weeks were found to have a mean latency of the response to photic stimulation of approximately 153 milliseconds. At 38 weeks the latency was 169 milliseconds, at 36 weeks 203 milliseconds, at 32 weeks 221 milliseconds, and at 29 weeks 230 milliseconds.

Neurodiagnostic Procedures

TRANSILLUMINATION

Transillumination of the head is a valuable technique that is inexpensive and entirely safe, but it requires the examiner to recognize and to be familiar with normal variations, especially in the low birth weight infant. The examiner should use the same flashlight powered with two D batteries for all examinations so that the intensity of illumination remains constant. The room must be entirely darkened, and one should wait briefly before making the evaluation to permit adaptation to the dark. The light, with a soft rubber adapter, must be placed flush with the head of the child. The glow of light extends 2 to 2.5 cm from the rim of the light source in the frontal region of the term infant and about 1 cm farther in the premature child. Transillumination in the occipital region is significantly less and changes little with gestational age.

Abnormally increased transillumination can result from various extracranial factors such as the infiltration of intravenous solutions into the scalp. Reduced transillumination is normally encountered in black children or in the presence of a subgaleal hematoma. Enhanced transillumination is seen in a variety of conditions that cause increased fluid collection in the subdural space, the subarachnoid space, and the ventricular system. In the Dandy-Walker syndrome, increased transillumination may be localized to the region over the posterior fossa.

LUMBAR PUNCTURE

The method of performing a lumbar puncture and examining the cerebrospinal fluid in the newborn infant is similar to that used in the older child. The procedure is quite safe, because the spinal cord in the term neonate terminates at approximately the level of the second lumbar vertebral body and because the patent cranial sutures and open fontanels diminish the possibility of internal herniations in conditions with increased intracranial pressure. The procedure is preferably done with the infant in the sitting position. A short, 22-gauge needle, with or without a stylet, is preferred by most. Concern has been raised that a penetrating needle without a stylet might possibly introduce epithelial fragments into the subarachnoid space that later might give rise to intraspinal epidermoid tumors (Shaywitz, 1972). This remains speculative and is more applicable to the child who requires multiple spinal taps and the injection of intrathecal medication. Points to remember in the performance of the procedure are the short distance from the skin surface to the subarachnoid space, especially in the premature child, and the absolute re-

Table 76–3. Reflexes of Value in Assessing Gestational Age

Reflex	Stimulus	Positive Response	Gestation (wk.) if Reflex is:	
			Absent	Present
Pupil reaction	Light	Pupil contraction	<31	29 or more
Traction	Pull up by wrists from supine	Flexion of neck or arms	<36	33 or more
Glabellar tap	Tap on glabella	Blink	<34	32 or more
Neck-righting	Rotation of head	Trunk follows	<37	34 or more
Head-turning	Diffuse light from one side	Head-turning to light	Doubtful	32 or more

Note: Twenty-nine weeks means 203 days after the first day of the last menstrual period. If there is a conflict between two results, the reflex placed higher in the table is more likely to give the true gestational age.
(From Robinson, R. J.: Arch. Dis. Child. 41:437, 1966.)

quirement to maintain the tip of the needle in the midline as it is directed through the soft tissues towards the subarachnoid space. The slightest deviation of the plane of the needle is likely to result in an unsuccessful tap.

Measurement of the pressure of cerebrospinal fluid is entirely unreliable in the crying, struggling infant and is best not attempted when these circumstances prevail. The time required and the manipulation of the needle incurred by attaching the manometer increase the risk of dislodging the tip from the subarachnoid space, thus eliminating the opportunity to obtain a CSF specimen uncontaminated by blood. When coma or lack of response to needle penetration prevails, an opening pressure may be obtained, but only after a small quantity of fluid has been secured for cell count and culture.

In the normal term infant, the cerebrospinal fluid is usually crystal clear, whereas variable degrees of xanthochromia are more often seen in the premature baby. Xanthochromia can be due to the presence of approximately 400 to 500 red blood cells per cubic millimeter or may be secondary to hyperbilirubinemia. Studies have shown that there is no direct relationship between the levels of serum and spinal fluid bilirubin in the newborn child, probably reflecting the individual variations in the blood-CSF and blood-brain barriers (Stempfel and Zetterström,

1955). A number of red blood cells and up to 10 white blood cells per mm^3 can be accepted as insignificant in the first few days after birth. White cells are largely mononuclear, although two or three neutrophils per mm^3 can be present in the absence of infection. The range of values for cerebrospinal fluid protein is far greater in the intact newborn infant than in the older child. In the full-term infant, levels between 45 and 100 mg per 100 ml can be considered normal, whereas in the premature baby, a protein content of up to 180 mg per 100 ml can occur without evident neurologic disease (Otila, 1948; Bauer et al., 1965). The CSF protein concentration bears a roughly inverse relationship to weight of the premature child and thus either is a function of degree of maturity of vascular permeability and the blood-CSF barrier (Arnhold and Zetterström, 1958) or reflects the frequency of intracranial hemorrhages in the smaller preterm infant.

Up to the last few years, a carefully performed lumbar puncture was one of the principal diagnostic procedures for establishing the presence of an intracranial hemorrhage in the newborn, and judicious evaluation of whether or not the tap was traumatic

POSTURE AND PASSIVE TONE FROM 28 TO 40 WEEKS GESTATIONAL AGE

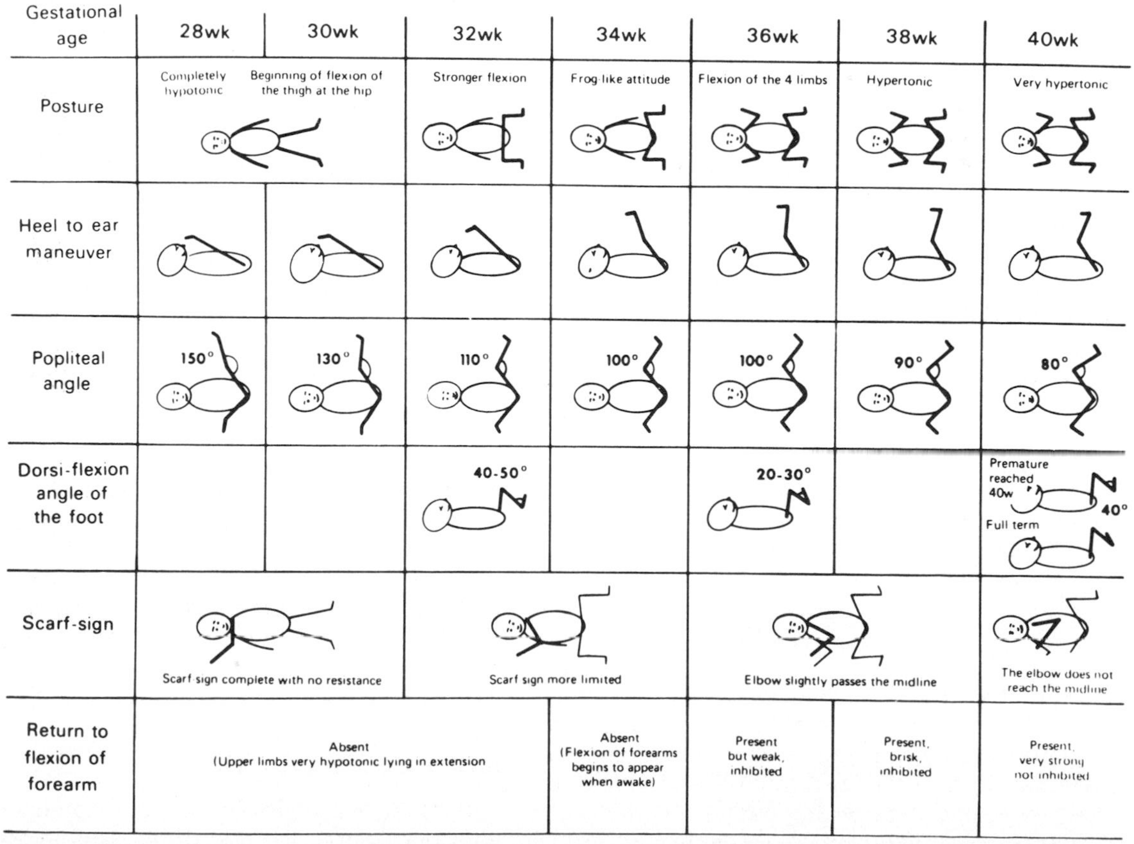

Gestational age	28wk	30wk	32wk	34wk	36wk	38wk	40wk
Posture	Completely hypotonic	Beginning of flexion of the thigh at the hip	Stronger flexion	Frog like attitude	Flexion of the 4 limbs	Hypertonic	Very hypertonic
Heel to ear maneuver							
Popliteal angle	150°	130°	110°	100°	100°	90°	80°
Dorsi-flexion angle of the foot			40-50°		20-30°		Premature reached 40w 40° Full term
Scarf-sign	Scarf sign complete with no resistance		Scarf sign more limited		Elbow slightly passes the midline		The elbow does not reach the midline
Return to flexion of forearm	Absent (Upper limbs very hypotonic lying in extension)			Absent (Flexion of forearms begins to appear when awake)	Present but weak, inhibited	Present, brisk, inhibited	Present, very strong, not inhibited

Figure 76–1. Posture and passive tone from 28 to 40 weeks of gestation, indicating increasing muscle tone in upper and lower extremities, which develops with increasing gestational age. (From Amiel-Tison, C.: In Rudolph, A. M., Barnett, H. L., and Einhorn, A. H. [Eds.]: Pediatrics. 16th ed. New York, Appleton-Century-Crofts, 1977. Reprinted with permission.)

was usually required. For that purpose, the physician had to pay particular attention to the red cell count in the first and last specimen of fluid. It is now clear that traumatic lumbar punctures are less common than had been appreciated, and, conversely, the studies of Silverboard and coworkers have made it evident that in some 30 per cent of infants the presence of clear CSF is compatible with an intracranial hemorrhage of considerable proportions.

By far, the most important reason for cerebrospinal fluid examination in the newborn is to ascertain the presence or absence of an infection.

The cerebrospinal fluid alterations associated with bacterial meningitis in the newborn period are generally similar to those at any other age. The protein value is commonly much higher than the usual value in the older child with meningitis, probably indicative of the greater necrotizing effect of bacterial infection on the immature brain. It is important to recognize that it is possible, although unusual, for a child to have meningitis even though the cerebrospinal fluid is clear to gross observation, contains few cells, and has a normal glucose content (Sarff et al., 1976). For this reason, gram stain and appropriate cultures should be made on every spinal fluid specimen obtained from the neonate, regardless of the other findings

SUBDURAL TAPS

In the past, a transfontanel subdural tap was used primarily for the diagnosis of a convexity subdural hematoma. For this procedure, the hair should be shaved well beyond the site of the needle penetration, and the scalp should be properly cleansed with the appropriate substances. After application of a sterilizing agent to the skin, it should be allowed to dry, or it can be wiped dry before insertion of the needle. The site chosen for the tap should be as close as possible to the junction of the fontanel with the coronal suture in order to avoid injury to the midline superior sagittal sinus.

For ascertaining the presence of blood in the subdural space, a CT scan is a preferable procedure, and in most·instances subdural taps have been relegated to a therapeutic role in the treatment of effusions complicating bacterial meningitis.

ELECTROENCEPHALOGRAPHY

In the older infant or child, the electroencephalogram, when interpreted by a competent individual, is a valuable diagnostic tool. It is useful in confirming a convulsive disorder, in localizing a supratentorial mass lesion, and in providing additional evidence of the absence of structural brain disease in the presence of certain symptoms or signs. Even in the patient with a mature nervous system, however, one must rec-

ognize the limitations of electroencephalography, namely, that minor deviations from normal need not be of clinical significance and that the results of an electroencephalogram must be used in conjunction with the historical data, the physical findings, and the information accumulated from other studies.

In the newborn period, the electroencephalogram has even greater restrictions on its clinical applicability, in part because of the limited ability of the immature cerebral cortex to produce recordable electrical potentials. The electroencephalogram of the premature infant is characterized by discontinuous and disorganized activity that gradually becomes synergistic over the two hemispheres with increasing gestational age (Dreyfus-Brisac, 1962). Before the twenty-sixth week of gestational age, the recording is irregular, with bursts of up to 1-per-second waves alternating with periods of near electrical silence lasting several seconds. Beyond 28 weeks, bursts become more regular, and some intermittent fast activity begins to emerge (Engel, 1965). By about 37 weeks, the tracing becomes continuous. In the full-term infant, the electroencephalogram reveals low-voltage activity, generally less than 50 microvolts, with occasional 3- to 5-per-second waves of slightly higher voltage than the general background (Anderson and Gibbs, 1970; Engel, 1975).

The value of the electroencephalogram in assessing the neonate lies in its prognostic rather than its diagnostic applications. This is because the tracing reflects the state of functional impairment of the brain, and, consequently, identical abnormalities can be seen regardless of the nature of the infant's encephalopathy. The prognostic value of the electroencephalogram is considerable, however, and has been placed on firm footing by the longitudinal studies of Rose and Lombroso and of Sarnat and Sarnat. In the former study, a normal interictal tracing in a neonate with seizures was followed by normal development in 86 per cent of the cases, whereas 88 per cent of infants whose electroencephalogram demonstrated multifocal abnormalities either died or were left with major neurologic deficits. Unifocal electroencephalographic abnormalities were associated with a good prognosis, whereas a flat electroencephalogram, or one that showed bursts of high-voltage discharges, was almost invariably indicative of a poor clinical outcome.

The interpretation of the electroencephalogram in the premature infant is difficult because electrical bursts are a normal phenomenon prior to 37 weeks' gestation, and, consequently, a paroxysmal electroencephalogram in an early premature does not carry the certainty of a poor prognosis, as it would in a term infant.

SKULL RADIOGRAPHS

With the availability of computed tomography and ultrasonography, the role of the skull radiograph in the evaluation of the newborn has become of relatively small importance. As a rule, this study is obtained when there are abnormalities in the shape of the head not explained by molding secondary to the delivery process or when the possibility of a fracture exists on the basis of a cephalhematoma or a traumatic delivery.

COMPUTED TOMOGRAPHY

Computed tomography (CT scan) has a wide spectrum of application to the diagnostic evaluation of the newborn with neurologic disease. The procedure is useful not only in the evaluation of infants suspected of harboring an intracranial hemorrhage but also in the diagnosis of a wide variety of congenital malformations of the nervous system.

Whereas certain pathologic appearances (e.g., those of hemorrhage) are readily interpreted, difficulties are encountered in the CT analysis of parenchymal changes. This occurs because of the frequent presence of alternating areas of high and low densities within the cerebral substance that do not have adult equivalents. However, both gray and white matter have lower attenuation coefficients in neonates than in older children, and the difference in density between gray and white matter is greater than that in adults. Sulci and subarachnoid spaces are often quite prominent and should not be interpreted as cerebral atrophy.

In the preterm infant, interpretation of the CT scan is even further complicated by the poor visualization of the ventricular system. This is due to its small volume in relationship to brain parenchyma and to the similarity of its density to that of the parenchyma. Localized areas of low density in the periventricular region have little significance, as do hypodense parenchymal areas. In most instances, these changes are transient and may reflect a developmental stage.

ULTRASONOGRAPHY

The advantage of ultrasonographic scanning of the neonate is that examinations can be performed at the bedside and serially without harmful effects to the infant. Generally, the brain is examined in two planes: coronal and sagittal. This technique provides excellent visualization of the ventricular system, the basal ganglia, choroid plexus, and corpus callosum. Studies can be completed in a few minutes without sedating or disturbing the infant (Shields and Manger, 1983; Babcock and Han, 1981) (Fig. 76–2).

Intraventricular hemorrhages produce strong echoes in the normally echo-free ventricles. Subependymal and intracerebral hemorrhages are also readily identified, particularly when fresh during the first few days of life. Studies by Bejar and coworkers and by Levene and colleagues suggest that the sensitivity of this technique in detecting small intraventricular and subependymal hemorrhages and organized clots may be superior to that of the CT scan. However, in many instances artefacts may simulate the appearance of small hemorrhages.

Ultrasonography is also useful in visualizing porencephalic cysts and in diagnosing changes in ventricular size produced by hydrocephalus.

BRAIN-STEM-EVOKED–RESPONSE AUDIOMETRY

No physiologic test available can yield the equivalent of a pure-tone audiogram or indicate exactly what a subject hears. The brain-stem–evoked re-

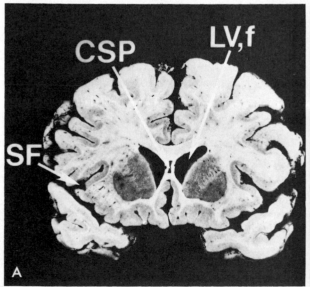
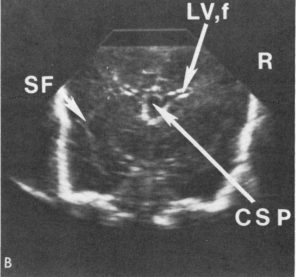

Figure 76–2. Coronal ultrasonographic scan of normal brain with corresponding anatomic sections. LV,f = frontal horns of lateral ventricles; CSP = cavum septum pellucidum; SF = sylvian fissure. (From Babcock, D. S., and Bokyung, K. H.: Radiology *139*:665, 1981.)

sponse (BSER) is a new diagnostic test that is gaining acceptance among pediatricians, audiologists, otolaryngologists, neurologists, and others. Briefly stated, the BSER is a computerized test that averages and records electrical changes that occur at the eighth cranial nerve and brain stem in response to auditory stimuli. These electrical events consist of six waves in the first 10 milliseconds after the acoustic stimulus and can be recorded from scalp electrodes of the infant. It is generally agreed that wave I with a latency of 1.5 milliseconds is generated by the auditory nerve activity, wave II by the cochlear nucleus, wave III by the superior olive, wave IV by the lateral lemniscus, and wave V by the inferior colliculus. The shape of the BSER and the latencies of its various peaks depend on several factors: the stimulus intensity, the repetition rate of the stimulus, and the maturity of the infant. The latency of these waves systematically shorten as the baby develops during the first year of life. The latencies systematically increase as the intensity of the stimulus decreases. Neonates with hearing deficits deviate from the normal latency in ways characteristic of the type of deafness, either conductive or sensorineural (Despland and Galambos, 1980; Hecox and Cone, 1981; Starr et al., 1977).

The BSER is recordable from neonates as young as 25 weeks' gestation. However, the BSER has some limitations. First, the BSER is difficult to elicit with auditory stimuli of a frequency less than 1000 Hz. Thus, an infant who is found to have no positive response to auditory stimuli may have undetected residual hearing in the speech frequency range below 1000 Hz. Second, BSER represents electrical activity only, which is different from the psychoacoustic phenomenon of hearing. Thus, the BSER can only estimate a hearing threshold, and it may differ with thresholds derived by behavioral audiometry. Finally, the BSER depends on detection of minute changes in brain stem electrical activity, and therefore background noise, muscular activity, and particularly electrical interference can have an effect on the observed BSER pattern. Undoubtedly, with technical improvements and further experience, the BSER will become a more precise clinical test of children with hearing problems.

Those neonates who deserve close attention and follow-up are those who are at risk for sensorineural hearing loss. These include (1) those with a family history of sensorineural hearing loss, (2) those exposed in utero to maternal rubella or other viral illness, (3) those with congenital anomalies of the head and neck, including cleft palate, microtia, and so forth, (4) those who weigh less than 1500 gm at birth, (5) those with bilirubin levels greater than 20 mg, and (6) those with neonatal meningitis.

Patients identified as having a negative response to these basic acoustic stimuli should be seen by an otolaryngologist and speech and hearing pathologist who can perform behavioral audiometry under soundproof environmental conditions.

OTHER PROCEDURES

Abnormalities of the visually evoked responses have been described in hypoxic infants and in those with posthemorrhagic hydrocephalus. The clinical value of this procedure is, however, not of the magnitude of the auditory-evoked responses.

Although positron emission tomography (PET) scans have proved useful in delineating focal abnormalities in cerebral blood flow and metabolism, their applicability to neonatal neurology remains to be demonstrated. Similarly, nuclear magnetic resonance (NMR) imaging, a procedure that offers a striking differentiation between gray and white matter and that provides valuable information in disorders of myelination, has not yet been found applicable to neurologic problems in the neonate.

REFERENCES

Ahmann, P. A., Lazzara, A., Dykes, F. D., Brann, H. W., and Schwartz, J. F.: Intraventricular hemorrhage in the high-risk preterm infant: incidence and outcome. Ann. Neurol. 7:118, 1980.

Amiel-Tison, C.: Neurological evaluation of the maturity of newborn infants. Arch. Dis. Child. 43:89, 1968.

Anderson, E., and Gibbs, E.: The normal and abnormal electroencephalogram of the neonate. Clin. Electroencephalogr. 1:30, 1970.

André-Thomas, Chesni, Y., and Saint-Anne Dargassies, S.: The neurological examination of the infant. Little Club Clinics in Developmental Medicine No. 1, 1960.

Arnhold, R. G., and Zetterström, R.: Proteins in the cerebrospinal fluid in the newborn. Pediatrics 21:279, 1958.

Babcock, D. S., and Han, B. K.: The accuracy of high-resolution, real-time ultrasonography of the head in infancy. Radiology 139:665, 1981.

Bauer, C. H., New, M. I., and Miller, J. H.: Cerebrospinal fluid protein values of premature infants. J. Pediatr. 66:1017, 1965.

Bejar, R., Curbelo, V., Coen, R. W., Leopold, G., James, H., and Gluck, L.: Diagnosis and follow-up of intraventricular and intracerebral hemorrhages by ultrasound studies of infants' brain through the fontanelles and sutures. Pediatrics 66:661, 1980.

Chemke, J., and Robinson, A.: The third fontanelle. J. Pediatr. 75:617, 1969.

Despland, P. A., and Galambos, R.: The auditory brainstem response (ABR) is a useful diagnostic tool in the intensive care nursery. Pediatr. Res. 14:154, 1980.

Dreyfus-Brisac, C.: The electroencephalogram of the premature infant. World Neurol. 3:5, 1962.

Dreyfus-Brisac, C.: Neonatal electroencephalography. Rev. Perinatal Pediatr. 3:397, 1979.

Dubowitz, L. M. S., Dubowitz, V., and Goldberg, C.: Clinical assessment of gestational age in the newborn infant. J. Pediatr. 77:1, 1970.

Dubowitz, V., Whittaker, G. F., Brown, B. H., and Robinson, A.: Nerve conduction velocity—an index of neurological maturity of the newborn infant. Dev. Med. Child Neurol. 10:741, 1968.

Engel, R.: Maturational changes and abnormalities in the newborn electroencephalogram. Dev. Med. Child Neurol. 7:498, 1965.

Engel, R.: Abnormal Electroencephalograms in the Neonatal Period. Springfield, Charles C Thomas, 1975.

Engel, R., and Butler, B. V.: Appraisal of conceptual age of newborn infants by electroencephalographic methods. J. Pediatr. 63:386, 1963.

Farr, V., Mitchell, R. G., Neligan, G. A., and Parkin, J. M.: The definition of some external characteristics used in the assessment of gestational age in the newborn infant. Dev. Med. Child Neurol. 8:507, 1966.

Friede, R. L.: Developmental Neuropathology. New York, Springer Verlag, 1975.

Hecox, K. E., and Cone, B.: Prognostic importance of brainstem auditory evoked responses after asphyxia. Neurology 31:1429, 1981.

Hogan, G. R., and Milligan, J. E.: The plantar reflex of the newborn. N. Engl. J. Med. 285:502, 1971.

Illingworth, R. S.: An introduction to developmental assessment in the first year. Little Club Clinics in Developmental Medicine No. 3, 1962.

Levene, M., Wigglesworth, J. S., and Dubowitz, V.: Cerebral structure and intraventricular haemorrhage in the neonate: a real-time ultrasound study. Arch. Dis. Child. 56:416, 1981.

Menkes, J. H.: Perinatal trauma. In Textbook of Child Neurology. 2nd ed. Philadelphia, Lea and Febiger, 1980.

Moosa, A., and Dubowitz, V.: Assessment of gestational age in newborn infants: nerve conduction velocity versus maturity score. Dev. Med. Child Neurol. 14:290, 1972.

Nelson, K. B., and Ellenberg, J. H.: Neonatal signs as predictors of cerebral palsy. Pediatrics 64:225, 1979.

Nelson, K. B., and Ellenberg, J. H.: Children who "outgrew" cerebral palsy. Pediatrics 69:529, 1982.

Otila, E.: Studies on the cerebrospinal fluid in premature infants. Acta Paediatr. (suppl. 35)8:1, 1948.

Paine, R. S.: The evolution of infantile postural reflexes in the presence of chronic brain syndromes. Dev. Med. Child Neurol. 6:345, 1964.

Paine, R. S., and Oppe, T. E.: Neurological examination of children. Clin. Dev. Med. 20:1, 1966.

Parmelee, A. H., Jr.: A critical evaluation of the Moro reflex. Pediatrics 33:773, 1964.

Picard, L., et al.: Cerebral computed tomography in premature infants, with an attempt at staging developmental features. J. Comput. Assist. Tomogr. 4:435, 1980.

Popich, G. A., and Smith, D. W.: Fontanels: range of normal size. J. Pediatr. 80:749, 1972.

Robinson, R.: Cerebral function in the newborn. Dev. Med. Child Neurol. 8:561, 1966.

Robinson, R. J.: Assessment of gestational age by neurological examination. Arch. Dis. Child. 41:437, 1966.

Rose, A. L., and Lombroso, C. T.: Neonatal seizure states. A study of clinical, pathological, and electroencephalographic features in 137 full-term babies with a long-term follow-up. Pediatrics 45:404, 1970.

Saint-Anne Dargassies, S.: La maturation neurologique du prématuré. Etud. Néonatal. 4:71, 1955.

Saint-Anne Dargassies, S.: Neurodevelopmental symptoms during the first year of life. Dev. Med. Child Neurol. 14:235, 1972.

Sarff, L. D., Platt, L. H., and McCracken, G. H., Jr.: Cerebrospinal fluid evaluation in neonates. Comparison of high risk infants with and without meningitis. J. Pediatr. 88:473, 1976.

Sarnat, H. B., and Sarnat, M. S.: Neonatal encephalopathy following fetal distress. Arch. Neurol. 33:696, 1976.

Schulte, F. J., Michaelis, R., Linke, I., and Nolte, R.: Motor nerve conduction velocity in term, preterm, and small-for-dates newborn infants. Pediatrics 42:17, 1968.

Shaywitz, B. A.: Epidermoid spinal cord tumors and previous lumbar punctures. J. Pediatr. 80:638, 1972.

Shields, D., and Manger, M.: Ultrasound evaluation of neonatal intraventricular hemorrhage. Perinat. Neonatol. (In press.)

Silverboard, G., Lazzara, A., Ahmann, P. A., and Schwartz, J. A.: Comparison of lumbar puncture with computed tomography scan as an indicator of intracerebral hemorrhage in the preterm infant. Pediatrics 66:432, 1980.

Starr, A., Amlie, R. N., Martin, W. H., and Sanders, S.: Development of auditory function in newborn infants revealed by auditory brainstem potentials. Pediatrics 60:831, 1977.

Stempfel, R., and Zetterström, R.: Concentration of bilirubin in cerebrospinal fluid in hemolytic disease of the newborn. Pediatrics 16:184, 1955.

Tan, K. L.: The third fontanelle. Acta Paediatr. Scand. 60:329, 1971.

Volpe, J. J.: Neurology of the Newborn. Philadelphia, W.B. Saunders Co., 1981.

77

Introduction

The immediate and delayed consequences of perinatal trauma constitute the most important neurologic problems of the neonatal period. Several factors, acting solely or in concert, may traumatize the infant brain in utero, in the course of the birth process, or in the immediate postnatal period. Mechanical trauma to the central or peripheral nervous system is probably the insult that is understood best. A focal or generalized disorder of cerebral circulation occurring during the prenatal or early postnatal period and acting in isolation is probably an uncommon cause of brain damage. When present, the occlusion usually is in the distribution of the middle cerebral artery and is presumed to result from embolization due to placental infarcts or from thrombosis caused by vascular

Perinatal Trauma and Asphyxia

By John H. Menkes*

maldevelopment, sepsis, or (in the case of a twin to a macerated fetus) the exchange of thromboplastic material from the dead infant (Friede, 1975).

Most often, neurologic symptoms are the result of perinatal asphyxia. This state induces hypoxemia plus a variety of metabolic alterations within the brain

---

* This chapter includes some contributions from a previous author, Dr. William E. Bell.

that, in turn, may lead to cerebral edema and circulatory disturbances (Volpe, 1981) (Fig. 77–1).

Mechanical Trauma and Its Consequences

Mechanical trauma to the fetal head may produce extracranial lesions, notably molding of the head, caput succedaneum, and cephalhematoma.

MOLDING OF THE HEAD AND CAPUT SUCCEDANEUM

The fetal head is frequently asymmetrically shaped as a consequence of pressure while it is still within the uterus or in the birth canal. The sutures override one another, the fontanelles are small or obliterated, and the soft tissues overlying the skull may be soft and boggy because of caput succedaneum. When molding of the fetal head is extreme, tears of the tentorium or cerebral falx may ensue. These can be accompanied by lacerations of the venous structures and thus give rise to a subdural hematoma or other varieties of intracranial hemorrhage.

A caput usually appears at the vertex, and it is commonly accompanied by marked molding of the head. The hemorrhage and edema are situated beneath the skin and may extend under the aponeurosis (subgaleal hemorrhage) but are still external to the periosteum (Fig. 77–2A). In rare instances, sufficient blood is sequestered to produce a significant anemia. Kozinn and coworkers have pointed out that massive scalp hemorrhages may indicate an underlying coagulation defect such as hemophilia or hemorrhagic disease of the newborn (Robinson and Rossiter, 1968).

CEPHALHEMATOMA

Cephalhematoma refers to a usually benign traumatic subperiosteal hemorrhage in the parietal region of the newborn skull (Fig. 77–2B). Bleeding is characteristically restricted in its location by the suture lines, across which it cannot extend. The incidence of neonatal cephalhematoma has been found to range from 1.5 to 2.5 per cent of deliveries. It is twice as common in males, and approximately 15 per cent occur bilaterally. Vaginal delivery is not necessarily a prerequisite for occurrence of this lesion, since it has been encountered in infants born by cesarean section. Linear skull fractures are found in the underlying parietal bones in about 18 per cent of infants with bilateral cephalhematomas. When the cephalhematoma is unilateral, the current incidence of linear frac-

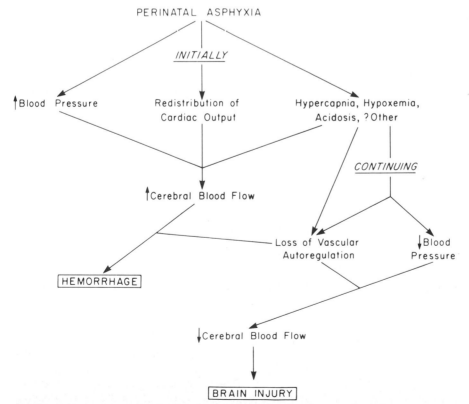

Figure 77–1. Interrelationships between perinatal asphyxia, alterations in cerebral blood flow, and brain damage. In addition to the mechanisms depicted, acidosis may induce focal or generalized cerebral edema, which reduces cerebral blood flow. (From Volpe, J. J.: Neurology of the Newborn. Philadelphia, W. B. Saunders Co., 1981.)

tures is much less, probably about 5 per cent (Zelson et al., 1974). Rarely, a cephalhematoma is found in the occipital region, where its midline location may cause it to be confused with an encephalocele.

The cephalhematoma in the newborn appears in the form of a firm, localized mass that does not transilluminate. Within a few days after birth, change in the consistency of the clotted blood gives rise to a sharp, palpable ridge, or "crater edge," near the periphery that can be confused with a fracture by the inexperienced examiner. Depending on the size of the lesion, a cephalhematoma is usually gradually absorbed by 2 to 8 weeks.

In many patients, roentgenographic examination will reveal hyperostosis of the outer table of the skull that persists for several months after clinical evidence of the lesion has disappeared. Much less often there is persistent thickening of the parietal calvarium at the site of the original lesion, at times with widening

of the diploic space, or cystic defects in the region. In some cases, calcium deposition within the clot occurs in a surprisingly short period of time and can be visualized roentgenographically.

Cephalhematomas of large volume can be associated with anemia or, more often, hyperbilirubinemia, as a consequence of absorption of the blood products (Kozinn et al., 1964). An infrequent but dangerous complication is abscess formation within a cephalhematoma in a septic newborn infant or secondary to contamination during attempted needle aspiration of the lesion (Burry and Hellerstein, 1966; Lee and Berg, 1971). Suppuration within a cephalhematoma may be associated with obvious signs of localized infection or can remain surprisingly silent

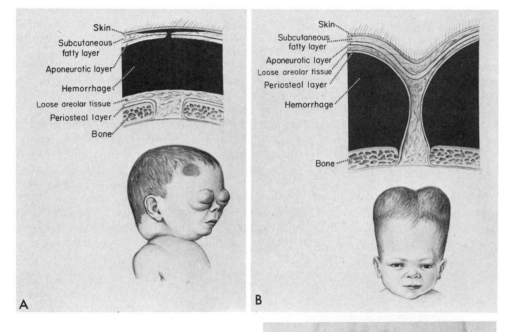

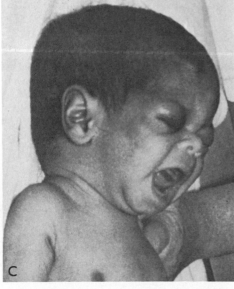

Figure 77–2. *A,* Location of edema and hemorrhage in caput succedaneum. *B,* Location of hemorrhage in cephalhematoma. *C,* Patient with massive hemorrhagic caput succedaneum, whose hemoglobin level fell to 2.2 gm per 100 ml by the age of 48 hours. (Reprinted with the permission of Daniel J. Pachman, M.D., of the University of Illinois Pediatric Department. The photograph, but not the diagrammatic sketches, appeared in Pediatrics 29:907, 1962.)

during progression of the lesion. It should be suspected whenever there is rapid enlargement of the mass several days after birth, the development of cutaneous erythema over the lesion, or otherwise unexplained fever and leukocytosis. An infected cephalhematoma may be complicated by osteomyelitis of the underlying skull or by meningitis, either associated with sepsis or secondary to intracranial extension through an adjacent skull fracture or a cranial suture (Levy et al., 1967; Ellis et al., 1974). Diagnosis is established by needle aspiration whenever an infected cephalhematoma is suspected.

Management of a cephalhematoma in the newborn infant is fundamentally conservative but should include the obtaining of skull films to determine the presence or absence of an underlying fracture as well as periodic checks of the hemoglobin and serum bilirubin, especially the latter if the child becomes jaundiced. Needle aspiration of the uncomplicated cephalhematoma is not indicated, since spontaneous resolution is expected and because of the hazard of bacterial contamination by needle penetration. Underlying skull fractures do not create a management problem and need no specific therapy unless there is significant depression of bone fragments.

SKULL FRACTURES IN THE NEWBORN INFANT

The skull of the infant at birth is less mineralized than it is later in childhood and also is more pliable because of the patency of the cranial sutures. For these reasons, there can be considerable distortion of the infant's head shape in utero and during the birth process without injury to the skull itself. Fractures can occur, however, and may be acquired in utero, during labor or secondary to the application of forceps. Intrauterine fracture of the infant's skull is usually the result of compression of the skull against the promontory of the sacrum (Alexander and Davis, 1969) and can complicate a traumatic event to the mother's abdomen or pelvis or can occur secondary to the forces of uterine contraction.

Most skull fractures identified in the neonate are parietal or frontal in location and linear in type (Chasler, 1967). Some are associated with an overlying cephalhematoma. Simple linear fractures are radiographically visible as lines of decreased density and may be seen only in one view. Such nondisplaced fractures are considered to be benign lesions that are expected to heal spontaneously and that need no therapeutic measures. A depressed skull fracture may result from pressure of the head against the pelvis or may be induced by incorrect application of the obstetric forceps. It is associated with inward buckling of the parietal bone, much like the indentation in a ping-pong ball (Fig. 77–3). A break in the continuity of the bone may not be present or may be evident over only a short length at the margin of the depression. This form of depressed skull injury is best seen in the anteroposterior or posteroanterior views of the skull and sometimes is not apparent at all on the lateral skull views. Depressed skull fractures acquired before or during the birth process should usually be corrected. Nonsurgical methods of elevation of depressed fractures have been successful in some cases (Raynor and Parsa, 1968; Schrager, 1970), and several instances of spontaneous elevation have also been recorded (Natelson and Sayers, 1973). However, in view of the simplicity of the surgical proce-

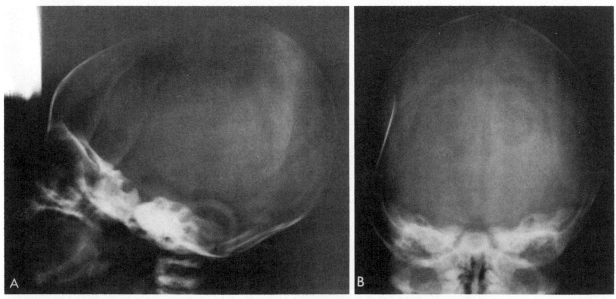

Figure 77–3. *A* and *B*, Lateral and AP skull x-ray films of 1-day-old infant. Depressed skull injury is visualized clearly on the AP view as a linear streak of increased density. Such injuries are the result of inward buckling of the poorly mineralized skull of the newborn infant. The actual break in the continuity of the bone is present over a short distance only.

dure and the possibility that an uncorrected fracture may act as a seizure focus, this author opts for early operative intervention.

SUBDURAL HEMORRHAGE

Mechanical trauma to the infant's brain during delivery may induce lacerations in the tentorium or falx with subsequent subdural hemorrhage. With improved obstetric techniques, these injuries have become relatively uncommon, and they are now generally restricted to large full-term infants delivered through a birth canal that is too small (cephalopelvic disproportion) or to premature infants whose skulls are unusually compliant (Wigglesworth and Husemeyer, 1977). Compression of the head along its occipitofrontal diameter, resulting in vertical molding, may occur with vertex presentations, whereas compression of the skull between the vault and the base, resulting in an anterior-posterior elongation, is likely to be the outcome of face and brow presentations. Tears of the falx and of the tentorium can be caused by both forms of overstretch. The damage is usually located in the region in which the falx joins the anterior edge of the tentorium. Tears and thromboses of the dural sinuses and of the larger cerebral veins, including the vein of Galen, are commonly accompanied by subdural hemorrhages. These may be either major and potentially fatal or minor and clinically unrecognizable. The hemorrhages are mainly localized to the base of the brain, but when the tears extend to involve the straight sinus and the vein of Galen, they can expand into the posterior fossa.

Overriding of the parietal bones occasionally produces a laceration of the superior sagittal sinus and a major fatal hemorrhage. Another uncommon traumatic lesion is a laceration of the occipital sinus associated with occipital osteodiastasis, a separation of the cartilaginous joint between the squamous and lateral portions of the occipital bone (Wigglesworth and Husemeyer, 1977). This injury is most often seen in infants delivered in the breech position.

Tearing of the superficial cerebral veins is probably a relatively common phenomenon. The subsequent hemorrhage results in a thin layer of blood over the cerebral convexity. Bleeding is often unilateral and is usually accompanied by a subarachnoid hemorrhage. Because the superficial cerebral veins of the premature infant are still underdeveloped, this type of a hemorrhage is limited to full-term infants (Gröntoft, 1954).

Subdural hemorrhage over the cerebral convexities usually results in minimal or no clinical signs. When these do occur, they are variable and nonspecific. Volpe has stressed the presence of focal cerebral signs, including hemiparesis, deviation of the eyes, and a nonreactive or poorly reactive pupil. In addition, nonspecific signs indicative of acute subdural collections of blood include pallor, lethargy, irritability, vomiting, a poor Moro response, and bulg-

ing of the anterior fontanel. (Deonna and Oberson, 1974). In some instances, a clinically inapparent subdural hematoma of the neonatal period may not be identified until a few months after birth, when it presents with progressive heart enlargement, seizures, developmental delay, and anemia (McLaurin et al., 1971; Matson, 1969).

Subdural hemorrhage within the posterior fossa is being increasingly recognized by CT scanning. Typically, symptoms appear following a lag period of 12 hours to 4 days (Blank et al., 1978). They include decreased responsiveness, apnea, bradycardia, opisthotonus, and seizures (Fishman et al., 1981). As the subdural hematoma enlarges, the fourth ventricle is displaced forward and soon becomes obstructed, producing signs of increased intracranial pressure, including a bulging fontanel and progressive enlargement of the head circumference. Posterior fossa hemorrhage may be accompanied by intraventricular hemorrhage or an intracerebellar hematoma (Ravenel, 1979).

The diagnosis of neonatal subdural hemorrhage rests mainly on demonstration of the lesion by CT scan. This procedure is indicated in infants who have had a traumatic delivery and who develop nonspecific neurologic signs.

Treatment is usually inadequate for the neonate who has sustained major subdural hemorrhage, although rapid surgical evacuation of the clot has saved some infants with extensive posterior fossa bleeding. Subdural taps are indicated solely to reduce increased intracranial pressure and should not be performed when the infant is asymptomatic. A subdural hematoma that produces a persistent increase in intracranial pressure may require a subdural-peritoneal or other shunting procedure (Moyes et al., 1965). As in the other forms of intracranial hemorrhage, hydrocephalus may ensue and may require neurosurgical intervention.

In some instances, mechanical trauma may induce a hemorrhage that is primarily within the subarachnoid space, with the bleeding presumed to be of venous or subpial origin (Friede, 1975). Rarely, the hemorrhage is localized to the epidural space (Takagi et al., 1978).

PERINATAL TRAUMA TO THE SPINAL CORD

Although spinal birth injuries were first described during the nineteenth century, much of our understanding of perinatal spinal trauma can be attributed to the classic papers of Crothers, Ford, and Crothers and Putnam. Relatively common several decades ago, this type of birth injury has become less frequent with improved obstetric practice, and it accounted for only 0.6 per cent of the series of patients with cerebral palsy encountered by Crothers and Paine. The apparent rarity of this lesion may in part reflect the fact that few infants with major spinal cord damage survive the neonatal period, and in those who do survive, mild injuries to the lower cervical and upper thoracic spinal cord with attendant spastic paraparesis can easily be confused with the similar constellation of findings characteristic of the cerebral diplegic form of cerebral palsy occurring in the premature infant.

Perinatal traumatic lesions of the spinal cord result more commonly from stretching of the cord than from compression or transection (Towbin, 1969). Longitudinal or lateral traction to the infant's neck or excessive torsion, particularly during a difficult breech delivery, stretches the cord, its covering meninges, the surface vessels, and the nerve roots. Lesions are most frequent in the lower cervical and upper thoracic regions. The most common gross pathologic findings are epidural hemorrhage, dural laceration with subdural hemorrhage, tears of the nerve roots, laceration and distortion of the cord, and focal hemorrhage and malacia within the cord (Towbin, 1969). Ischemic lesions of the cord are less common. Gross or petechial hemorrhages may also be seen within the substance of the cord, and myelination of the tracts may be impaired above the transection (Hedley-Whyte and Gilles, 1974).

A difficult breech delivery can be recorded in 75 per cent of infants who have suffered a spinal birth injury (Stern and Rand, 1959). When damage to the cord is severe, death of the neonate occurs during labor or soon after. With a less extensive injury, infants show respiratory depression and generalized hypotonia, or flaccid paraplegia (Bucher et al., 1979). An associated urinary retention and abdominal distention with paradoxical respirations occur. In addition to impaired motor function, there is absence of sensation and perspiration below the level of injury. The deep tendon reflexes are usually unelicitable during the neonatal period, and mass reflex movements do not become apparent until later.

In about 20 per cent of cases, damage to the brachial plexus can also be documented. In others, the lower brain stem is involved as well, with consequent bulbar signs.

The clinical picture following complete transection of the cord evolves from the stage of spinal shock seen during the neonatal period to the appearance of reflex flexion withdrawal movements and a final picture of pure reflex activity of the isolated cord. A great number of survivors have normal intelligence.

The presence of poor muscle tone and flaccid weakness involving all extremities or only the legs following a breech delivery should suggest a cord injury. One should always look for loss of sensory function, even though demonstration of this problem is difficult. Sensory evaluation is usually best performed by demonstration of impaired autonomic response. Shortly after the injury, the dermatomes below the lesion are dry and often have a defective vasomotor response.

Neuromuscular disorders, notably spinal muscular atrophy, are not associated with loss of either sensory function or sphincter control. Of the other neuromuscular disorders, congenital myasthenia gravis is diagnosed by reversibility of symptoms following injection of anticholinesterase drugs (see Chapter 80). Occasionally, an infant with a congenital tumor of the cervical or lumbar cord may present a clinical picture similar to that of a spinal cord injury. Abnormalities of the skin along the posterior lumbosacral midline, including dimpling, hemangiomata, or tufts of hair are commonly seen in the latter (see Chapter 81).

In some cases, the immediate problem is respiratory support. Fractures or fracture dislocations of the spine are generally absent, and there is no specific treatment for the injured spinal cord. Although the majority of clinically apparent spinal birth injuries are severe and irreversible, milder degrees of injury are potentially reversible.

BIRTH INJURIES TO THE CRANIAL NERVES

Facial Nerve

The most common cranial nerve to be injured during birth is the facial nerve. The incidence of such a lesion has been reported to be between 0.25 per cent and 6.4 per cent (McHugh et al., 1969; Hepner, 1951) of live births.

It is generally believed that unilateral facial weakness noted at birth is the result of compression of the facial nerve, although the precise site of injury and time of occurrence have been a subject of debate. Trauma to the nerve distal to its emergence from the stylomastoid foramen by forceps application has been regarded as one important cause, but Hepner found the incidence of facial palsy to be the same in infants born with and without the use of forceps. He assumed that pressure on the maternal sacrum during labor was responsible for most cases of unilateral facial paralysis in the newborn infant. Parmelee proposed that some cases were the result of intrauterine posture of the fetal head in which marked flexion and rotation of the head resulted in compression of the mandible and lateral neck against the shoulder with associated compression of the peripheral portion of the facial nerve. Involvement of the seventh nerve as it traverses the facial canal within the mastoid is probably unusual but has been reported (McHugh, 1963).

The degree of facial paresis ranges from complete loss of function in all three main branches to weakness limited to a small group of muscles. Unilateral facial weakness is most obvious when the infant cries, at which time there is lack of complete eyelid closure along with lack of normal lower facial muscle contraction on the paretic side. Experience with electrodiagnostic tests is limited in infants with congenital facial paresis as compared to older children and adults with acquired facial nerve deficits. The facial nerve excitability test in some instances can, however, distinguish complete from partial denervation, thus providing information concerning the extent of nerve damage (McHugh et al., 1969). The ability to produce contraction of the muscle by stimulating the nerve implies that the conductivity of the nerve is only partially interrupted and suggests a favorable prognosis. However, good recovery is possible even when electric reactions are completely absent (Douglas and Kessler, 1971). It is important to wait at least 3 to 4 days before undertaking these studies to allow any injured fibers to degenerate.

The prognosis for recovery is good. In most instances, the facial nerve palsy is mild, and some improvement becomes evident within a week. In the more severe cases, the start of recovery may be delayed for several months.

Treatment of facial nerve palsy is limited to protection of the eye by application of methylcellulose drops and taping of the paralytic lid. Electric stimulation of the nerve does not hasten recovery. Neurosurgical repair of the nerve should be considered only when there is evidence that the nerve is severed.

Congenital Hypoplasia of the Depressor Anguli Oris Muscle. In recent years, there has been recognition of a syndrome with localized facial weakness in which the lower lip on one side fails to be depressed on crying, resulting in an "asymmetric crying facies" (Nelson and Eng, 1972; Papadatos et al., 1974). It is now believed that this localized muscle deficit is the result of congenital hypoplasia of the depressor anguli oris muscle, whose normal function is to draw the lower corner of the lip downward and evert it. The resulting facial symmetry when the child cries is often misinterpreted by the parents, who may assume the normal side of the face is the abnormal one because they observe the lower lip on the intact side to be pulled down. The abnormal side is, in fact, the side on which the lower lip remains unaltered in position when crying occurs. The cosmetic significance of this minor anomaly lessens as the child gets older, probably largely because the older child is engaged in crying far less than in infancy.

Localized facial paresis causing an asymmetric crying facies can occur in isolated fashion; however, observations have revealed a variable association with other anomalies. Of 44 infants with this syndrome, Pape and Pickering found 27 to have major anomalies of the skeletal, genitourinary, respiratory, or cardiovascular systems. A much lower incidence of associated defects was reported by Perlman and Reisner, who found two patients with significant anomalies among 41 with the localized facial defect. The disorder most strongly associated with this facial defect is congenital cardiac disease, an observation made by Cayler in 1967. The most commonly associated cardiac defect has been ventricular septal defect, but other cardiac lesions have also been described.

Other Cranial Nerves

Conjunctival and retinal hemorrhages are common in the newborn infant, but birth injury involving the optic nerve exclusively is relatively rare. Unilateral and bilateral optic atrophy have been reported, the result of direct injury to the nerve through fracture of the orbit or, less often, of the base of the skull.

A transient postnatal paralysis of the abducens and oculomotor nerves is occasionally encountered. Paralysis of the latter may take the form of a transient postnatal ptosis. Congenital weakness of the musculature of the face, tongue, and palate unassociated with atrophy has been termed "congenital suprabulbar paresis." This condition may appear in isolation or may be accompanied by bilateral cerebral lesions, as in spastic quadriplegia, or extrapyramidal cerebral palsy. Although Worster-Drought in 1974 postulated a developmental defect of the corticobulbar tract, pathologic studies supporting this suggestion are lacking.

Although impaired hearing is seen in about one fourth of children, its association with intraventricular hemorrhage prompts discussion in the section on perinatal asphyxia (Spector et al., 1978).

BIRTH INJURIES TO THE PERIPHERAL NERVES

Brachial Plexus Palsy

Traction, stretch, or avulsion injuries during birth to part or all of the brachial plexus are potentially serious from the functional standpoint. In most instances, the injury and resulting limb weakness are unilateral, with the right arm being affected approximately twice as often as the left. Rarely, the disorder is bilateral, giving rise to serious disabilities if recovery does not occur. The incidence of this type of birth injury has not been well documented, but it is generally agreed that it has decreased considerably in recent decades with improved obstetric techniques. In one series extending from 1932 to 1962, brachial plexus palsy was found in 0.38 per 1000 live births (Adler and Patterson, 1967).

Etiology. The two factors most consistently associated with birth injury to the brachial plexus are excessive weight of the child and complications of the labor and delivery process. Prolonged and difficult labor accompanied by heavy sedation of the mother resulting in a relaxed, large infant represent a combination of factors that increase the vulnerability of the child to this lesion. Breech delivery occurred in 9 per cent of the series of 123 patients described by Adler and Patterson, thus being a less important factor than the size of the infant.

The most common form of brachial plexus injury is one involving the fifth and sixth cervical roots. In most instances, this is the consequence of stretching of the plexus resulting from traction of the shoulder in the course of delivering the aftercoming head in a breech presentation or of turning the head away from the shoulder in a difficult cephalic presentation. In most instances, the brachial plexus is compressed by hemorrhage and edema within the nerve sheath. Less often, there is an actual tear of the nerves or avulsion of the roots from the spinal cord with segmental damage to the gray matter of the spinal cord. With traction, the fifth cervical root gives way first, then the sixth, and so on down the plexus. Thus, the mildest plexus injuries only involve C_5 and C_6, and the more severe involve the entire plexus.

Clinical Features. In about 80 per cent of infants, the paralysis is confined to the upper brachial plexus (Erb-Duchenne paralysis). In about 90 per cent, involvement is unilateral, more often on the right. The weakness is recognized soon after delivery. It affects the deltoid, serratus anterior, biceps, teres major, brachioradialis, and supinator muscles. Weakness of these muscles, which are innervated by the fifth and sixth cervical roots, results in the characteristic clinical picture in which the affected arm is in a position of tight adduction and internal rotation at the shoulder, in addition to extension and pronation at the elbow. Added involvement of the seventh cervical root causes weakness of the extensors of the wrist and fingers leading to a flexion deformity of the hand due to sustained contraction of the flexor muscles supplied by the median nerve. Denervation of the serratus anterior, rhomboids, and other periscapular muscles adds to the motor disability around the shoulder and produces winging of the scapula.

In addition to the characteristic posture of the affected arm, there is an absent or diminished Moro reflex on the denervated side but an intact grasp reflex. The biceps reflex is absent or less active than the triceps reflex, a picture that is the converse of normal. In most instances, one is unable to demonstrate a sensory loss, although occasionally the examiner can convince himself of a loss of cutaneous sensation over the deltoid region and the adjacent radial surface of the upper arm. Fractures of the clavicle or of the humerus, slippage of the capital head of the radius, and subluxation of the shoulder and the cervical spine often accompany an Erb-Duchenne injury (Babbitt and Cassidy, 1968). When a significant degree of injury to the fourth cervical root is present, phrenic nerve paralysis may accompany injury to the upper brachial plexus. Such an infant may show signs of respiratory distress, including tachypnea, cyanosis, and decreased movement of the affected hemithorax. When phrenic nerve palsy is unaccompanied by injury to the brachial plexus, as occurs occasionally, the condition may mimic congenital pulmonary or heart disease (Smith, 1972).

Klumpke's paralysis, or birth injury to the lower brachial plexus, is relatively uncommon (2.5 per cent of brachial plexus birth palsies). In this lesion, the paralysis involves the intrinsic muscles of the hand, with weakness of the flexors of the wrist and fingers. The grasp reflex is absent, and there is often a unilateral Horner's syndrome caused by involvement of the cervical sympathetic nerves. Loss of sensation and sudomotor function over the hand may also be found. Interference with the sympathetic innervation of the eye results in a delay or failure in pigmentation of the iris.

More commonly, the entire brachial plexus is damaged, resulting in a complete paralysis of the arm (Fig. 77–4).

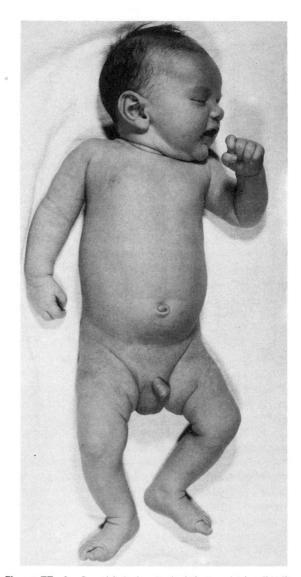

Figure 77–4. Brachial plexus stretch paralysis affecting the right arm. Child was the result of a difficult vertex delivery, birth weight was 4350 grams. In addition to the paresis of the right arm, Horner's syndrome occurred on the infant's right side. The right arm is virtually immobile and is held in a position of adduction and partial internal rotation.

Diagnosis. The diagnosis of brachial plexus injuries is usually readily apparent from the posture of the affected arm and from the absence of voluntary and reflex movements. Congenital Horner's syndrome may occur in the absence of trauma and may be associated with anomalies of the cervical vertebrae, enterogenous cysts, or congenital nerve deafness. Radiographic examinations to detect associated fractures and fluoroscopy to ascertain any limitation of diaphragmatic movement are indicated. In severe injuries causing avulsion of the spinal roots and bleeding into the subarachnoid space, the cerebrospinal fluid may be bloody. Myelography can be used to demonstrate root avulsion. Electromyography performed 2 to 3 weeks after the injury may confirm the extent of denervation.

Management. Treatment is directed primarily toward prevention of contractures. Gentle passive exercises of the affected arm should be begun about 1 week after birth. The infant's sleeve should be pinned in a natural position, rather than in abduction and external rotation as was recommended in the past. Follow-up studies indicate that overimmobilization of the affected arm is conducive to contractures and deformities that can persist despite spontaneous recovery of nerve function.

Reconstructive orthopedic surgery is indicated in certain instances to improve function of the permanently affected arm and hand, but it is not usually performed until 4 years of age or later.

Prognosis. Probability of recovery is difficult to predict in the immediate newborn period, although the child with a partial plexus lesion who shows definite improvement of motor function by 1 to 2 weeks after birth will probably recover completely or with only minor deficits. For some children with Erb-Duchenne palsy, recovery may be complete within a few weeks; for others, the maximum recovery is achieved within 1 to 18 months. In complete brachial plexus injury and in Klumpke's paralysis, the outlook is less good and the majority of children are left with serious difficulties (Eng, 1971). Permanent lesions are accompanied by muscle atrophy, contractures, and impaired limb growth. Some infants have an apparently good return of neuromuscular function and sensation yet are unable to use the affected arm (Eng, 1971). It is likely that transitory sensory motor deprivation in early life impairs the development of normal movement patterns and the organization of cortical body image.

Sciatic Nerve Palsy

The sciatic nerve is ordinarily not susceptible to birth injury; however, it can be damaged in the infant by injection of materials or drugs into the umbilical artery or by misplaced gluteal injections. Injuries to the sciatic nerve can result in either temporary or permanent deficits and may be of variable degrees

of severity. In some cases, weakness of dorsiflexion of the foot along with sensory loss on the dorsal surface of the foot are the only obvious deficits. More severe injuries are associated with extensive weakness and eventual atrophy of all muscle groups below the knee, in addition to weakness of the hamstring muscles on the affected side.

Ischemic sciatic neuropathy in the infant has been described following injections into the umbilical artery (Mills, 1949; San Agustin et al., 1962) and secondary to accidental intra-arterial injection of drugs administered to the region of the buttocks (Knowles, 1966). Sciatic nerve involvement in such cases has been attributed to spasm or occlusion of the inferior gluteal artery. Motor and sensory deficits corresponding to the innervation supplied by the sciatic nerve are accompanied by signs of vascular insufficiency in the region of the buttocks and throughout the affected lower limb. Improvement usually follows the insult, but permanent sequelae, including weakness and atrophy, are not uncommon.

Direct trauma to the sciatic nerve can result from misplaced gluteal injections of antibiotics or other substances (Gilles and Matson, 1970; Scheinberg and Allensworth, 1957; Combes et al., 1960). The young infant, and especially the premature one, is particularly susceptible to this type of nerve injury, mainly because of the much smaller size of the gluteal musculature. Early recognition of this complication of intramuscular injection is important to allow one to institute physical therapy and other measures promptly to minimize joint contractures. Gilles and Matson advise surgical resection of the damaged nerve segment if clinical improvement does not occur within 6 months following the injury.

Birth injuries to the other peripheral nerves are relatively uncommon. Injury to the lumbosacral plexus may occur after a frank breech delivery. Palsies of the radial nerve, laryngeal nerve, and obturator nerve have also been recorded.

Perinatal Asphyxia and its Consequences

Mechanical damage to the brain, while contributing significantly to mortality during the neonatal period, is a rare cause of persistent neurologic deficits. More commonly, these are the consequence of asphyxia, a condition in which the brain is subjected not only to hypoxia but also to ischemia and hypercarbia.

Pathogenesis and Pathology. The biochemical and physiologic changes attending acute asphyxia have been studied extensively. Within seconds after its induction, NAD converts to NADH, and the ion permeability of neuronal membranes increases. This results in depolarization of neurons and loss of spontaneous electrical activity. Accompanying these alterations is an increased rate of glycolysis, which causes an increased production of lactate. Within 3 minutes of induction of asphyxia, there is a rapid increase in brain lactate (Vanucci and Duffy, 1977). At the same time, the concentration of tricarboxylic acid cycle intermediates falls, and the production of high-energy phosphates diminishes. This results in a rapid fall in phosphocreatine and a slower reduction in brain ATP concentrations. Brain glucose and glycogen also decrease rapidly. The water content of brain increases, and within 15 minutes after induction of asphyxia, some brain swelling may already be evident.

Alterations in cerebral blood flow induced by asphyxia are equally important in understanding the genesis of birth injuries (Volpe, 1981). (Fig. 77–1). Initially, there is a redistribution of cardiac output so that a large proportion enters the brain. This results in a 30 to 175 per cent increase in cerebral blood flow. At the same time, there is a loss of cerebral vascular autoregulation (Lou et al., 1979). As a consequence, cerebral arterioles fail to respond to changes in perfusion pressure and carbon dioxide concentrations, resulting in a pressure-passive cerebral blood flow. As asphyxia persists, cardiac output drops and hypotension follows. Since cerebral autoregulation is no longer functional, the arteriolar system is unable to respond to the decreased perfusion pressure with vasodilation, and the result is a striking reduction of cerebral blood flow (Lou et al., 1979). Cerebral blood flow may be further compromised by the development of localized or generalized brain edema.

After an undetermined period, a point of irreversibility is reached. The exact mechanism of tissue damage is still unclear. The studies of Brann and Myers have stressed the role of intracellular and generalized brain edema induced by the combination of hypoxia, acidosis, hypocarbia, and hypotension. Volpe, on the other hand, believes that the loss of vascular autoregulation coupled with hypotension reduces cerebral blood flow to a degree sufficient to produce tissue necrosis and subsequent cerebral edema. The role of postischemic impairment of microvascular perfusion ("No-reflow phenomenon") in the genesis of tissue damage in the asphyxiated human neonate is still unclear.

Three other factors—neonatal hypoglycemia, which hastens the depletion of energy stores under anoxic conditions (Vanucci and Vanucci, 1978), maternal hyperglycemia, which enhances lactic acid production (Myers, 1977), and the ability of the newborn brain to utilize ketone bodies as a source of energy through induction of beta-hydroxybutyric acid dehydrogenase—have not been studied sufficiently to be assessed in terms of their contribution to the production of anoxic brain damage.

Whatever the biochemical and physiologic mechanisms for brain damage, the relative resistance of newborn brain to oxygen lack has been known for some time. It is likely that this phenomenon reflects a reduction in overall cerebral metabolism and decreased energy demands by the newborn brain in comparison with the adult organ. Total metabolism of the newborn mouse brain is about one tenth that of the adult, and glycolysis also proceeds at a much slower rate (Thurston and McDougal, 1969). A relative resistance of the cardiovascular system to hypoxic injury may also be operative.

By themselves, the aforementioned biochemical and physiologic alterations fail to explain the remarkable regional variations in the pathology of the brain of asphyxiated infants. For many years, several distinct pathologic lesions have been known to occur singly or jointly.

When the primate fetus is subjected to acute total asphyxia, a reproducible pattern of brain pathology ensues. This includes bilaterally symmetric lesions in the thalamus and in a number of brain stem nuclei, notably those of the inferior colliculi, the superior olive, and the lateral lemniscus. The neurons of the cerebral cortex, particularly the hippocampus, are especially vulnerable, as are the Purkinje cells of the cerebellum (Norman, 1978). On electron microscopy, the first changes are observed in the neuronal mitochondria, whose internal structure becomes swollen and disrupted (Brown and Brierley, 1973). These pathologic changes, seen soon after the initial insult, are followed by the gradual appearance of widespread transneuronal degeneration. With progressively longer periods of total asphyxia, the destructive changes in the thalamus become more extensive, and damage appears in the putamen and in the deeper layers of the cortex. In its extreme form, the brain of asphyxiated animals shows an extensive cystic degeneration of both cortex and white matter with connective tissue replacement of the damaged areas in the forebrain but a relative lack of cellular reaction in the central nuclear areas (Myers, 1977).

This experimentally produced picture resembles cystic degeneration of the infant brain, a condition characterized by the formation of cystic cavities in white matter (Fig. 77–5). When small, the cysts are trabeculated and do not communicate with the ventricular system. In their most extensive form, they may involve both hemispheres, leaving only small remains of cortical tissue. The cavities are generally believed to be the products of insufficient glial reaction, perhaps the result of cerebral immaturity, or reflections of the sudden and massive tissue damage from circulatory or anoxic events. In 1981, Lyen and coworkers suggested that in some instances fetal viral encephalitis may induce a similar pathologic picture. Infants surviving this type of insult generally go on to develop a severe form of spastic quadriparesis.

One form of brain damage that occurs with par-

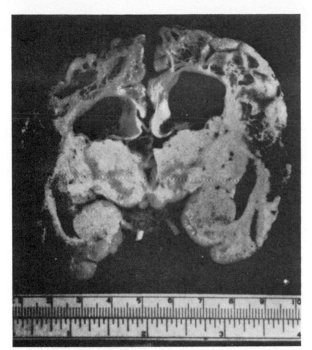

Figure 77–5. Cystic degeneration of dorsal parts of the hemispheres. Coronal section of brain. (From Malamud, N.: Neuropathol. Exp. Neurol. *18*:146, 1959.)

branches of the middle cerebral and posterior cerebral arteries (deReuck et al., 1972). Episodes of serious cardiorespiratory embarrassment and hypotension can be documented in most of the infants and could account, in part, for the lesions. (Young et al., 1982). Gilles found that exposure to *Escherichia coli* endotoxin produces white matter destruction in neonatal experimental animals and suggested that transient bacteremia may at least contribute to this pathologic picture. The condition in the older child that is commensurate with this cerebral lesion is spastic diplegia.

In the full-term infant, the most common site of brain damage is the cortex. Infarctions in this area are secondary to arterial or venous stasis and thromboses. One common pattern for the distribution of lesions (arterial "border zone," or "watershed") is usually the direct result of a sudden fall in systolic blood pressure. The lesions characteristically involve the territory supplied by the most peripheral branches of the three large cerebral arteries (Fig. 77–7) (Freytag and Lindenberg, 1967). Damage is maximal in the posterior parietal-occipital region, becoming less marked in the more anterior portions of the cortex (Volpe and Pasternak, 1977). When gray matter is affected, the brunt of the damage involves the portions around the depths of the sulci. In part, this distribution may reflect the effect of cerebral edema on the drainage of the cortical veins, and in part, it may

ticular frequency in the premature infant is periventricular leukomalacia (Fig. 77–6) (Banker and Larroche, 1962). Essentially, this condition consists of a bilateral (but not necessarily symmetric) necrosis having a periventricular distribution. Tissue destruction is accompanied by proliferation of astrocytes and microglia, a loss of ependyma, and areas of subcortical degeneration. In about 25 per cent of infants, there is hemorrhage into the lesion (Armstrong and Norman, 1974). The distribution of these lesions suggests inadequate circulatory perfusion with subsequent infarction of the vascular border zones between the

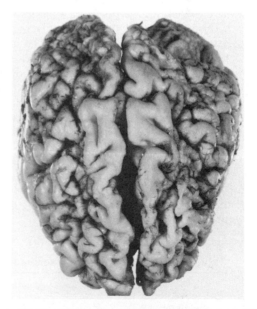

Figure 77–7. Watershed pattern in a 10-year-old patient with history of prolonged labor, subsequent spastic quadriparesis. Symmetric atrophy in border zones of anterior, middle, and posterior cerebral arteries. (Courtesy of Dr. Richard Lindenberg, Towson, Md.)

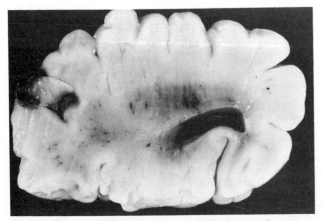

Figure 77–6. Periventricular leukomalacia. Prematurely born child with perinatal asphyxia. There is hemorrhagic softening of the cerebral white matter adjacent to the lateral ventricle.

be the consequence of the impoverished vascular supply of this area in the normal human newborn (Takashima et al., 1978).

This type of lesion has been termed *ulegyria* (mantle sclerosis) (Friede, 1975). It is a common abnormality, accounting for about one third of clinical defects caused by circulatory disorders during the neonatal period (Freytag and Lindenberg, 1967). Ulegyria may be extensive or so restricted that the appearance of the brain is grossly normal. When ulegyria is widespread, an associated cystic defect in the subcortical white matter (porencephalic cyst) and dilation of the lateral ventricles often occur. Less often, ulegyria involves the cerebellum. This neuropathologic picture accounts for many cases of both spastic quadriparesis and congenital spastic hemiparesis.

Abnormalities within the basal ganglia are seen in the majority of infants subjected to perinatal asphyxia (84 per cent in the series of Christensen and Melchior, 1967). One common lesion seen in this area has been termed *status marmoratus*. This picture is characterized by gross shrinkage of the striatum, particularly the globus pallidus, associated with defects in myelination. In some cases myelinated nerve fibers may be found in coarse networks resembling the veining of marble, hence the name of the condition (Fig. 77–8); in other cases, the principal pattern is one of a symmetric demyelination. It is clear that both hypermyelination and demyelination represent different responses to the same insult. Nerve cells in the affected areas are usually conspicuously reduced in number, with the smaller neurons in the putamen and caudate appearing to be more vulnerable. Although the abnormalities within the basal ganglia are the most striking, a variety of associated cortical lesions can be demonstrated in most instances.

The cause of this condition is still under dispute. Fundamentally, the pathologic picture is one of glial scarring corresponding to the areas of tissue destruction (Malamud, 1959).

In the opinion of Friede, damage to the basal ganglia incurred before the onset of myelination deranges the subsequent deposition of myelin and the course, density, and caliber of fibers passing through the affected area. These pathologic alterations are seen in the vast majority of children suffering from extrapyramidal cerebral palsy.

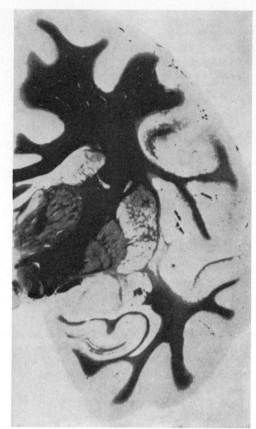

Figure 77–8. Status marmoratus. This coronal section is stained for myelin fibers and demonstrates aggregations of myelinated fibers throughout the basal ganglia. (Courtesy of Dr. E. P. Richardson, Harvard Medical School, Boston. From Cooke, R. E.: The Biologic Basis of Pediatric Practice, 1968. Courtesy of McGraw-Hill Book Co., New York.)

Rarely, the major structural alterations resulting from perinatal asphyxia are localized to the cerebellum. In the majority of instances, the involvement is diffuse with widespread disappearance of the cellular elements of the cerebellar cortex and dentate nucleus (Friede, 1975).

Circulatory lesions of the brain stem secondary to perinatal asphyxia have received relatively little attention. Neuronal necrosis of the ventral portion of the pons has been observed in premature and term infants, particularly those having a history of respiratory distress. This picture may occur as a selective brain stem lesion or may be accompanied by widespread cerebral damage (Friede, 1972). In addition, transient compression of the vertebral arteries in the

Table 77–1. Major Types of Neonatal Intracranial Hemorrhage and Usual Clinical Setting

Type of Hemorrhage	Usual Clinical Setting
Subdural	Full-term > premature; trauma
Primary subarachnoid	Premature > full-term; trauma or "hypoxic" event(s)
Intracerebellar	Premature; "hypoxic" event(s); trauma(?)
Periventricular-intraventricular	Premature > full-term; "hypoxic" event(s)

(From Volpe, J. J.: Neurology of the Newborn. Philadelphia, W. B. Saunders Co., 1981.)

course of rotation or hyperextension of the infant's head during delivery may also be a cause for circulatory lesions of the brain stem (Yates, 1959).

Intracranial hemorrhage can result from factors other than mechanical trauma to the brain. Whereas subdural hemorrhage and, to a lesser extent, primary subarachnoid hemorrhage are related to mechanical trauma, the relationship of periventricular-intraventricular hemorrhage, the most common form of neonatal intracranial hemorrhage, to prematurity and, most likely, to complications of superimposed asphyxia appears well substantiated (Hill and Volpe, 1981; Dykes et al., 1980; Pape and Wigglesworth, 1979) (Table 77–1).

Bleeding originates in the capillaries of the germinal matrix (usually over the body of the caudate nucleus) and, less commonly (as when an intraventricular hemorrhage occurs in term infants), in the choroid plexus (Hambleton and Wigglesworth, 1976; Pape and Wigglesworth, 1979). The hemorrhage does not occur at the time of delivery, but rather commences during the second or third day of life (Tsiantos et al., 1974). The extent of the hemorrhage ranges from slight oozing to a massive intraventricular bleed with extension into the subarachnoid space of the posterior fossa (Babcock and Han, 1981) (Figs. 77–9 and 77–10).

The pathogenesis of this lesion is not completely understood. Although it has been seen in full-term neonates (Lacey and Terplan, 1982), it is clear that its incidence rises with increasing immaturity, so that when CT scanning or ultrasonography is performed on infants with birth weights under 1800 gm, a hemorrhage can be documented in as many as 50 per cent (Shinnar et al., 1982). The predisposition of the premature to periventricular-intraventricular hemorrhages relates to the presence of a highly vascularized subependymal germinal matrix to which a major portion of the blood supply of the immature cerebrum is directed. Furthermore, the capillaries of the premature have less basement membrane than those of the mature brain. Finally, abnormalities in the au-

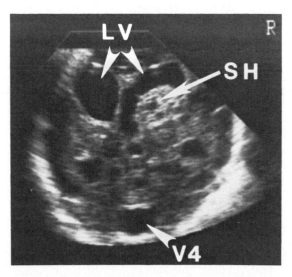

Figure 77–10. Intraventricular hemorrhage in a 1400 gm infant of 30 weeks gestation who suffered birth asphyxia. Coronal ultrasonographic scan. There is moderate hydrocephalus and a large subependymal hemorrhage (SH) in the wall of the right lateral ventricle. (LV = lateral ventricles; V4 = fourth ventricle). (From Babcock, D. S., and Bokyung, K. H.: Radiology *139*:665, 1981.)

toregulation of arterioles in premature and distressed term infants impair their response to hypoxia and hypercarbia and thus permit the transmission of increased arterial pressure to the fragile periventricular capillary bed. Other contributing factors may include alveolar rupture secondary to positive pressure ventilation (Milligan, 1981; Dykes et al., 1980; Hill et al., 1982), increased venous pressure secondary to myocardial failure, severe hyaline membrane disease, hypothermia, and hyperosmolarity induced by excess administration of sodium bicarbonate.

Blood usually clears rapidly from the intraventricular and subarachnoid spaces. Nevertheless, brain injury is a relatively common result of intraventricular hemorrhage. In part, this relates to the antecedent asphyxial injury that predisposes the infant to the bleed. Other factors are also operative. Intracerebral extension of the hemorrhage is not unusual, and a major intracerebral hematoma is seen in one third of the severe hemorrhages (Volpe, 1981; Sauerbrei et al., 1981) (Fig. 77–11). This lesion results in tissue destruction and formation of cystic cavities. In addition, arterial vasospasm may accompany the hemorrhage (Bada et al., 1979).

A progressive ventricular dilation is a common sequel to intraventricular hemorrhage (Fig. 77–12). It evolves 1 to 3 weeks after the hemorrhage and is due to a fibrotic reaction that obliterates the subarachnoid spaces and induces ventricular dilation

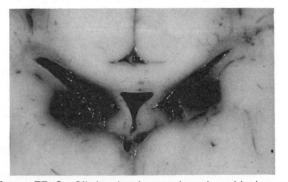

Figure 77–9. Bilateral subependymal matrix hemorrhage in a premature newborn infant. There is extensive intraventricular spread of bleeding in addition to periventricular leukomalacia in the form of hemorrhagic softening extending out from the angles of the lateral ventricles.

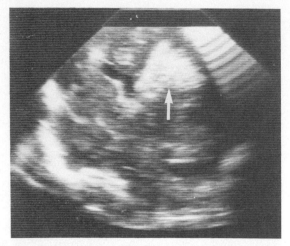

Figure 77–11. Intracerebral hemorrhage in neonate. The arrow indicates the presence of the hematoma. There is displacement of the ventricular system. Coronal ultrasonographic scan. (Courtesy of Dr. Eric E. Sauerbrei, Kingston General Hospital, Kingston, Ontario.)

with or without increased intracranial pressure (Hill and Volpe, 1981).

In addition to mechanical trauma and asphyxia, malformations of the central nervous system play an important role in the genesis of the lesions of perinatal trauma. There is little doubt that, particularly in the premature infant, both faulty maturation of the nervous system and a greater vulnerability to mechanical trauma and asphyxia are responsible for the high incidence of neurologic deficits (Drillien, 1972).

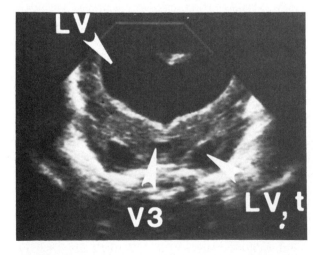

Figure 77–12. Hydrocephalus in a 2-day-old infant with lumbosacral meningomyelocele. Coronal ultrasonographic scan. There is marked dilatation of the bodies of the lateral ventricles (LV) and their temporal horns (LV,t). The third ventricle (V3) is also enlarged but to a lesser degree. (From Babcock, D. S., and Bokyung, K. H.: Radiology 139:665, 1981.)

Clinical Aspects. The degree of functional abnormality of the newborn secondary to asphyxia incurred during labor and delivery depends on the severity, timing, and duration of the insult. In the large series of asphyxiated infants studied by Brown and coworkers in 1974, hypoxia occurred primarily antepartum in 51 per cent, intrapartum in 40 per cent, and postpartum in 9 per cent.

Intrauterine asphyxia can be ascertained by alterations in fetal heart rate (see Chapter 10) and by the in utero passage of meconium. In particular, passage of large amounts of meconium upon rupture of the fetal membranes prior to or during the early stages of labor correlates highly with the presence of neurologic deficits.

After birth, the infant subjected to perinatal asphyxia can be expected to show certain alterations of alertness, muscle tone, and respirations whose severity depends on the extent of oxygen deprivation (Brown et al., 1974; Volpe, 1981). The mildly affected infant may have essentially normal muscle tone but may be jittery with tactile stimulation and exhibit irritability as well as some degree of feeding difficulty. A greater hypoxic insult gives rise to more definite signs, including irritability, vomiting, increased muscle tone, excessive clonus, and a high-pitched, poorly sustained cry. Tremulousness, especially when provoked by abrupt changes of limb position or tactile stimulation, can closely resemble clonic seizures. The severely asphyxiated newborn is either deeply stuporous or in coma. He has marked hypotonia or flaccidity and exhibits little spontaneous limb movements. Periodic breathing or other respiratory irregularities are prominent, and they are often complicated by episodes of apnea with bradycardia. These episodes can sometimes be triggered by handling the infant. The severely asphyxiated infant does not cry on painful stimulation and has minimal, if any, Moro or grasp reactions and absent sucking and swallowing responses. The pupils tend to be the size of a pinpoint, and the blink response to light is absent. Seizures occur in approximately 50 per cent of the infants by 6 to 12 hours following birth.

The Apgar score has been used to quantitate the severity of the initial intrauterine insult. Although a depressed score at 1 and 5 minutes implies the possibility of a hypoxic insult, the value of the score becomes significant in terms of measuring neurologic deficits only when it is obtained at 10 minutes or even later (Nelson and Ellenberg, 1979), and it is evident that 1- and 5-minute scores do not usually reflect the degree of the infant's acidosis (Sykes et al., 1982).

After 12 to 48 hours of age, there may be a change in the clinical picture of the previously hypotonic infant. He becomes jittery, his cry is shrill and monotonous, the Moro reflex becomes exaggerated, there is an increased startle response to sound, and the face assumes a staring or "worried" appearance. The deep tendon reflexes become hyperactive, and an increased extensor tone develops. Seizures may make their first appearance at this time. These signs of cerebral irritation are particularly common in the infant who has experienced a major intracranial hemorrhage. In the series of Brown and coworkers, 24 per cent of infants who were subjected to perinatal hypoxia demonstrated hypotonia progressing to extensor hypertonus. In the experience of De Souza and Richards, this clinical course has an ominous prognosis, and none of the infants following it were ultimately free of neurologic deficits.

In other instances (24 per cent in the series of Brown and colleagues), an infant who has sustained perinatal hypoxia exhibits hypertonia and rigidity during the neonatal period. The clinical picture of spasticity in the neonate is modified by the immaturity of some of the higher centers. In the spastic infant, the deep tendon reflexes are not exaggerated and in fact may even be depressed as a result of muscular rigidity. Hyperreflexia becomes evident only during the second half of the first year of life. More reliable physical signs indicating spasticity include the presence of a sustained tonic neck response. The presence of a spastic hemiparesis is manifest during the neonatal period in only 10 per cent of infants, usually by a unilateral reduction of spontaneous movements or excessive fisting in one extremity. Obvious paralyses during the neonatal period are rarely caused by cerebral damage; rather, they should suggest a peripheral nerve or spinal cord lesion.

The evolution of a periventricular-intraventricular hemorrhage may go clinically unnoted in more than one half of infants (Lazzara et al., 1980; Dubowitz et al., 1981). In others, there may be a sudden, sometimes catastrophic deterioration, highlighted by alterations in consciousness, abnormalities of eye movements, and respiratory irregularities. Deterioration may continue over several hours, then stop, only to resume hours or days later (Volpe, 1981). The presence of a full fontanel is noted in about one third of asphyxiated infants (Brown et al., 1974). It may be the consequence of a massive intracranial hemorrhage, cerebral edema, or (less often) an acute subdural hemorrhage.

Infants surviving a major asphyxial insult begin to improve toward the end of the first week of life. Seizures usually come under control, and there is a gradual change from the generalized hypotonia of the newborn period to the spasticity of later life. As a rule, the longer the duration of hypotonia, the more severely handicapped the child will be. Feeding disturbances are frequent, and the infant may require tube feeding.

CT scans performed in asphyxiated infants 1 to 2 weeks after birth demonstrate local areas of hyperperfusion, with a dense network of proliferating capillaries that almost completely replace the parenchyma. This alteration is most commonly observed in the basal ganglia but may also occur in the brain stem and cerebellum, the periventricular area, the depth of the cortical sulci, and the hippocampus. Shewmon and coworkers consider this hypervascu-

larity a response to the antecedent hypoxia and reduced cerebral blood flow.

The ultimate manifestations of neonatal asphyxia and mechanical birth trauma to the brain are so varied that their full description and the relationship between the clinical and neuropathologic pictures are outside the scope of this chapter. The interested reader is referred to several texts of child neurology (e.g., Menkes, 1980) for a full discussion of the concept of "cerebral palsy."

Diagnosis. The diagnosis of a neurologic disorder that has resulted from neonatal asphyxia depends on the following:

1. A history of intrauterine distress. This may include evidence in alteration of fetal heart rate, the passage of meconium, and a second stage of labor lasting more than 30 minutes, often accompanied by sufficient maternal or fetal distress to require blood transfusion or administration of oxygen. Breech presentation and the application of midforceps are both significantly associated with both mechanical and asphyxial birth injury.

2. A history of an abnormal neonatal course. This includes delayed or impaired respiration requiring such resuscitative measures as endotracheal intubation and assisted ventilation, Apgar scores of less than 3 at 1 minute and less than 5 at 5 minutes, and abnormal neurologic signs during the neonatal period. These may be as obvious as seizures, hypotonia, and a bulging fontanel, or they may be confined to feeding difficulties, irritability, excessive jitteriness, and an abnormal cry.

3. Laboratory studies that reveal findings suggestive of neonatal asphyxia. Examination of the cerebrospinal fluid can provide evidence of a recent intracranial hemorrhage. In the presence of perinatal asphyxia, the concentration of cerebrospinal fluid protein may be above the normal range. It must be remembered, however, that the presence of blood from any source raises the total protein by 1.5 mg/dl of fluid for every 1000 fresh red cells per mm^3. An elevation in the ratio of CSF lactate to pyruvate has been found to persist in asphyxiated infants for several hours after normal oxygenation has been re-established, as does a striking elevation of the blood creatine kinase-BB isoenzyme (Walsh et al., 1982). It should be stressed, however, that a normal cerebrospinal fluid does not exclude the possibility of perinatal asphyxia. CT scanning or, preferably, ultrasonography is invaluable in diagnosing the presence and the extent of an intracranial hemorrhage (Figs. 77–10 and 77–11).

Rarely, an intraventricular hemorrhage may result from a congenital arteriovenous malformation or a ruptured aneurysm (Schum et al., 1979). Intraventricular hemorrhage can also arise from small hemangiomata of the choroid plexus (Doe et al., 1972). Clinical signs of aneurysms of the vein of Galen in the neonate sometimes include bleeding but usually consist of those caused by obstructive hydrocephalus and high-output cardiac failure. Intraventricular bleeding in early infancy can arise from a papilloma of the choroid plexus, but the customary syndrome produced by this unusual tumor is rapid and progressive head enlargement.

Despite the frequency of recurrent apneic spells, their pathogenesis and their relationship to neurologic dysfunction are poorly understood. The occurrence of apneic episodes in an infant with a markedly irregular respiratory pattern usually suggests structural brain disease. Recurrent apnea in the premature newborn with tachypnea secondary to hyaline membrane disease is more frequent. In this situation, apnea can be related to medullary "immaturity," or it may be associated with other factors, such as abnormalities of blood gases, increase in the environmental temperature, electrolyte disturbance, and sepsis. Apneic episodes in infants beyond the immediate newborn period can represent seizure manifestations. Fenichel and coworkers have attempted to distinguish convulsive and nonconvulsive apnea on the basis of the infant's heart rate during the episode. They found the heart rate unchanged in convulsive apnea but discovered a drop in heart rate in nonconvulsive apnea, particularly in spells lasting more than 20 seconds.

Convulsions in the newborn infant are commonly observed in association with other signs of intracranial injury (see Chapter 79). Other causes of neonatal seizures must always be considered, however. These include hypoglycemia, hypocalcemia, hypomagnesemia, sepsis, and meningitis. Convulsions in the newborn can also occur with congenital cerebral anomalies, intrauterine acquired infections, aminoacidurias, and disturbances of pyridoxine metabolism. They can also be secondary to a maternal intake of narcotics, barbiturates, or other drugs.

Hypotonia in the neonatal period is seen in many conditions other than those caused by perinatal insults to the brain and spinal cord. Such conditions as Down syndrome and other trisomic states, glycogen storage disease, and cyanotic congenital heart diseases are readily recognized by the associated physical and biochemical abnormalities (see Chapter 81). Familial dysautonomia, although rare, is another disorder characterized by decreased muscle tone, sucking and swallowing dysfunction, and respiratory difficulty in the newborn period.

Other causes of neonatal hypotonia that may be confused with cerebral insults acquired during the birth process include a variety of disorders of the motor unit (see Chapter 80). Spinal muscular atrophy (Werdnig-Hoffmann disease) is usually identified a few months after birth but can result in abnormalities in the immediate newborn period. Neonatal myasthenia gravis is a rare disease that can be suspected by the presence of the condition in the mother. Myotonic dystrophy can manifest itself during the newborn period, particularly when the disease is transmitted from an affected mother. Congenital myopathies, notably nemaline myopathy, are rare causes of hypotonia in neonates.

Treatment.   The prevention of perinatal asphyxia is largely the task of the obstetrician and therefore is outside the scope of this text.

The immediate and long-term supportive care of the asphyxiated infant is discussed in Chapter 10.

There is no unanimity with respect to the importance of cerebral edema in producing the sequelae of neonatal asphyxia. Accordingly, the value of treating this complication with the accepted methods—avoiding fluid overload and using hypertonic solutions (e.g., mannitol), glucocorticoids, and high doses of barbiturates—is still a matter of considerable controversy.

The control of neonatal seizures is discussed in Chapter 79. The management of neonatal periventricular-intraventricular hemorrhage consists of its prevention in highly susceptible immature infants. For this purpose, treatment with phenobarbital has been advocated. Donn and coworkers suggest a loading dose of 10 mg/kg, administered intravenously at or before 6 hours of age, with subsequent 12 hourly maintenance doses of 2.5 mg/kg for the first 7 days of life. It appears likely, however, that this treatment, as well as the use of ethamsylate, a capillary stabilizing agent, only reduces the incidence of small and thus relatively benign hemorrhages (Morgan et al., 1981).

Little can be done to alleviate the immediate effects of an intraventricular hemorrhage. Serial ultrasonographic scans will provide information as to its extent and, inferentially, ultimate prognosis. Serial lumbar punctures are ineffectual in preventing death or subsequent hydrocephalus. When progressive ventricular dilation ensues after intraventricular hemorrhage, surgical decompression is indicated. Generally, this takes the form of a ventriculoperitoneal shunt (Bada et al., 1979). However, the decision as to when to temporize and when to proceed with surgical intervention and risk the associated high morbidity is difficult, especially in the small premature infant who also has suffered significant asphyxia. Therapy with drugs expected to reduce the production of cerebrospinal fluid (acetazolamide, digoxin) or with osmotic agents such as isosorbide or glycerol has not been consistently effective in patients with posthemorrhagic hydrocephalus (Lorber, 1975).

Occasionally, porencephaly resulting from focal brain necrosis or a periventricular-intracerebral hemorrhage (Pasternak et al., 1980), may expand, producing increased intracranial pressure or increasing head size. Under these circumstances, surgical drainage of the cyst is indicated (Tardieu et al., 1981).

Prognosis. The prognosis of the asphyxiated infant depends on the severity and duration of the asphyxia and is modified by the maturity of the fetus and any pre-existing cerebral anomalies. Since most of the asphyxial insults occur in utero, electronic monitoring of the fetal heart rate should prove invaluable. Preliminary prospective studies have already indicated that one fourth of high-risk infants whose fetal heart rate pattern showed severe variable decelerations, defined as two or more periods of bradycardia (70 to 80 beats/min for more than 60 seconds or less than 70 beats/min for 30 to 60 seconds), and/or late decelerations were neurologically abnormal at 1 year of age (Painter et al., 1978).

Fetal blood sampling may also provide prognostic information, but it must be stressed that there are no absolute values of blood P_{O_2}, P_{CO_2}, or pH beyond which irreparable brain damage is certain to ensue.

The predictability of the 1- and 5-minute Apgar scores is somewhat limited. Nevertheless, term infants with 5-minute Apgar scores of 6 or less are three times more likely to be neurologically abnormal at 1 year of age than are those with scores of 6 to 10 (Drage et al., 1966). The likelihood of permanent brain damage increases even more significantly when depressed Apgar scores persist. Sixty-eight per cent of infants with scores of 3 or less at 10 minutes die during the first year of life, and 12.5 per cent of survivors are neurologically damaged. The prognosis is even worse when an Apgar score of 3 or less persists for 20 minutes. Of those infants, 87 per cent die, and 36 per cent of survivors develop cerebral palsy (Nelson and Ellenberg, 1979).

Conversely, if an asphyxiated infant fails to show neurologic or behavioral abnormalities during his neonatal period on repeated careful examinations, he is unlikely to develop neurologic or intellectual sequelae. In this respect, it is important to note that Nelson and Ellenberg failed to find a statistically significant increase in mental retardation in children with low Apgar scores who did not also have cerebral palsy. They concluded that when mental retardation is a consequence of perinatal asphyxia it is usually severe and is accompanied by evidence of neurologic damage, notably spastic quadriparesis or athetosis or both.

Survivors of perinatal asphyxia demonstrate reduced cerebral blood flow for the first week of life (Sankaran et al., 1981). In preliminary studies, Lou and coworkers have suggested that a reduction of cerebral blood flow to 20 ml/min/100 gm or less (normal, 50 to 56 ml/min/100 gm) during the first few hours after birth is accompanied by cerebral atrophy on CT scan and neurologic deficits at 9 to 12 months of age.

Recovery of an asphyxiated infant is more likely to occur (1) if the infant shows hypertonia rather than hypotonia, (2) if an intracranial bleed is in the form of a subarachnoid hemorrhage rather than an intraventricular hemorrhage, and (3) if the EEG is normal or demonstrates a single focus rather than a periodic or multiple one (De Souza and Richards, 1978). The hearing, speech, and language deficits of survivors of severe perinatal asphyxia have been described by De Souza and Richards.

REFERENCES

Adler, J. B., and Patterson, R. L., Jr.: Erb's palsy. Long-term results of treatment in eighty-eight cases. J. Bone Joint Surg. 49A:1052, 1967.

Alexander, E., Jr., and Davis, C. H., Jr.: Intra-uterine fracture of the infant's skull. J. Neurosurg. 30:446, 1969.

Armstrong, D., and Norman, M. G.: Periventricular leukomalacia in neonates: Complications and sequelae. Arch. Dis. Child. 49:367, 1974.

Babbitt, D. P., and Cassidy, R. H.: Obstetrical paralysis and dislocation of the shoulder in infancy. J. Bone Joint Surg. 50A:1447, 1968.

Babcock, D. S., and Han, B. K.: The accuracy of high-resolution, real-time ultrasonography of the head in infancy. Radiology 139:665, 1981.

Bada, H. S., Salmon, J. H., and Pearson, D. H.: Early surgical intervention in post-hemorrhagic hydrocephalus. Childs Brain 5:109, 1979.

Bada, H. S., et al.: Noninvasive diagnosis of neonatal asphyxia and intraventricular hemorrhage by Doppler ultrasound. J. Pediatr. 95:775, 1979.

Banker, B. Q., and Larroche, J. C.: Periventricular leukomalacia of infancy. Arch. Neurol. 7:386, 1962.

Bejar, R., et al.: Diagnosis and follow-up of intraventricular and intracerebral hemorrhages by ultrasound studies of infant's brain through the fontanelles and sutures. Pediatrics 66:661, 1980.

Blank, N. K., Strand, R., and Gilles, F. H.: Posterior fossa subdural hematomas in neonates. Arch. Neurol. 35:108, 1978.

Brann, A. W., and Dykes, F. D.: The effects of intrauterine asphyxia on the full-term neonate. Clin. Perinatol. 4:149, 1977.

Brann, A. W., and Myers, R. E.: Central nervous system findings in the newborn monkey following severe in utero partial asphyxia. Neurology 25:327, 1975.

Brown, A. W., and Brierley, J. B.: The earliest alterations in rat neurones and astrocytes after anoxia-ischaemia. Acta Neuropathol. 23:9, 1973.

Brown, J. K., Purvis, R. J., Forfar, J. O., and Cockburn, F.: Neurologic aspects of perinatal asphyxia. Dev. Med. Child Neurol. 16:567, 1974.

Bucher, H. U., Boltshauser, E., Friderich, J., and Isler, W.: Birth injury to the spinal cord. Helv. Paediatr. Acta 34:517, 1979.

Burry, V. F., and Hellerstein, S.: Septicemia and subperiosteal cephalhematomas. J. Pediatr. 69:1133, 1966.

Cayler, G. G.: An "epidemic" of congenital facial paresis and heart disease. Pediatrics 40:666, 1967.

Cayler, G. G.: Cardiofacial syndrome. Congenital heart disease and facial weakness, a hitherto unrecognized association. Arch. Dis. Child. 44:69, 1969.

Chasler, C. N.: The newborn skull. The diagnosis of fracture. Am. J. Roentgenol. 100:92, 1967.

Christensen, E., and Melchior, J.: Cerebral palsy—a clinical and neuropathological study. Clin. Dev. Med. 25:1, 1967.

Combes, M. A., Clark, W. K., Gregory, C. F., and James, J. A.: Sciatic nerve injury in infants. Recognition and prevention of impairment resulting from intragluteal injections. J.A.M.A. 173:1336, 1960.

Crothers, B.: Injuries of the spinal cord in breech extraction as an important cause of fetal death and paraplegia in childhood. Am. J. Med. Sci. 165:94, 1923.

Crothers, B., and Paine, R. S.: The Natural History of Cerebral Palsy. Cambridge, Harvard University Press, 1959.

Crothers, B., and Putnam, M. C.: Obstetrical injuries of the spinal cord. Medicine (Baltimore) 6:41, 1927.

Deonna, T., and Oberson, R.: Acute subdural hematoma in the newborn, Neuropaediatrie 5:181, 1974.

deReuck, J., Chattha, A. S., and Richardson, E. P.: Pathogenesis and evolution of periventricular leukomalacia in infancy. Arch. Neurol. 27:229, 1972.

De Souza, S. W., and Richards, B.: Neurological sequelae in newborn babies after perinatal asphyxia. Arch. Dis. Child. 53:564, 1978.

Doe, F. D., Shuangshoti, S., and Netsky, M. G.: Cryptic hemangioma of the choroid plexus. Neurology 22:1232, 1972.

Donn, S. M., Roloff, D. W., and Goldstein, G. W.: Prevention of intraventricular haemorrhage in preterm infants by phenobarbitone. Lancet 2:215, 1981.

Douglas, D. B., and Kessler, R. E.: Significance of electrical reactions in facial palsy of newborn. Behav. Neuropsychiatry 2:6, 1971.

Drage, J. S., et al.: The Apgar score as an index of infant morbidity. Dev. Med. Child Neurol. 8:141, 1966.

Drillien, C. M.: Aetiology and outcome in low-birthweight infants. Dev. Med. Child Neurol. 14:563, 1972.

Dubowitz, L. M. S., et al.: Neurologic signs in neonatal intraventricular hemorrhage: a correlation with real-time ultrasound. J. Pediatr. 99:127, 1981.

Dykes, F. D., et al.: Intraventricular hemorrhage—a prospective evaluation of etiopathogenesis. Pediatrics 66:42, 1980.

Ellis, S. S., Montgomery, J. R., Wagner, M., and Hill, R. M.: Osteomyelitis complicating neonatal cephalhematoma. Am. J. Dis. Child. 127:100, 1974.

Eng, G. D.: Brachial plexus palsy in newborn infants. Pediatrics 48:18, 1971.

Fenichel, G. M., Olson, B. J., and Fitzpatrick, J. E.: Heart rate changes in convulsive and non-convulsive neonatal apnea. Ann. Neurol. 7:577, 1980.

Fishman, M. A., et al.: Successful conservative management of cerebellar hematomas in term neonates. J. Pediatr. 98:466, 1981.

Ford, F. R.: Breech delivery in its possible relation to injury of the spinal cord, with special reference to infantile paraplegia. Arch. Neurol. Psychiatry 14:742, 1925.

Freytag, E., and Lindenberg, R.: Neuropathological findings in patients of a hospital for the mentally deficient: a survey of 359 cases. Johns Hopkins Med. J. 121:379, 1967.

Friede, R. L.: Ponto-subicular lesions in perinatal anoxia. Arch. Pathol. 94:343, 1972.

Friede, R. L.: Developmental Neuropathology. New York, Springer Verlag, 1975.

Gilles, F. H., Averill, D. R., and Kerr, C. S.: Neonatal endotoxin encephalopathy. Ann. Neurol. 2:49, 1977.

Gilles, F. H., and Matson, D. D.: Sciatic nerve injury following misplaced gluteal injection. J. Pediatr. 76:247, 1970.

Goldstein, G. W.: Pathogenesis of brain edema and hemorrhage: Role of the brain capillary. Pediatrics 64:357, 1979.

Gröntoft, O.: Intracranial hemorrhage and blood-brain barrier problems in the newborn. Acta Pathol. Microbiol. Scand. 100(suppl.):1, 1954.

Hambleton, G., and Wigglesworth, J. S.: Origin of intraventricular haemorrhage in the preterm infant. Arch. Dis. Child. 51:651, 1976.

Hedley-Whyte, E. T., and Gilles, F. H.: Observations on myelination of human spinal cord and some effects of parturitional transection. J. Neuropathol. Exp. Neurol. 33:436, 1974.

Hepner, W. R., Jr.: Some observations on facial paresis in the newborn infant: etiology and incidence. Pediatrics 8:494, 1951.

Hill, A., Perlman, J. M., and Volpe, J. J.: Relationship of pneumothorax to occurrence of intraventricular hemorrhage in the premature newborn. Pediatrics 69:144, 1982.

Hill, A., and Volpe, J. J.: Normal pressure hydrocephalus in the newborn, Pediatrics 68:623, 1981.

Hill, A., and Volpe, J. J.: Seizures, hypoxic-ischemic brain injury, and intraventricular hemorrhage in the newborn, Ann. Neurol. 10:109, 1981.

Jones, R., Cummins, M., and Davies, P.: Infants of very low birthweight. Lancet 1:1335, 1979.

Knowles, J. A.: Accidental intra-arterial injection of penicillin. Am. J. Dis. Child. 111:552, 1966.

Kozinn, P. J., Ritz, N. D., Moss, A. H., and Kaufman, A.: Massive hemorrhage—scalps of newborn infants. Am. J. Dis. Child. 108:413, 1964.

Lacey, D. J., and Terplan, K.: Intraventricular hemorrhage in full-term neonates. Dev. Med. Child Neurol. 24:332, 1982.

Lazzara, A., et al.: Clinical predictability of intraventricular hemorrhage in preterm infants. Pediatrics 65:30, 1980.

Lee, Y., and Berg, R. B.: Cephalhematoma infected with Bacteroides. Am. J. Dis. Child. 121:77, 1971.

Levy, H. L., O'Connor, J. F., and Ingall, D.: Bacteremia, infected cephalhematoma, and osteomyelitis of the skull in a newborn. Am. J. Dis. Child. 114:649, 1967.

Lipscomb, A. P., et al.: Pneumothorax and cerebral haemorrhage in preterm infants. Lancet 1:414, 1981.

Lorber, J.: Isosorbide in treatment of infantile hydrocephalus. Arch. Dis. Child. 50:431, 1975.

Lou, H. C., Skov, H., and Pedersen, H.: Low cerebral blood flow as a risk factor in the neonate. J. Pediatr. 95:606, 1979.

Lou, H. C., et al.: Pressure passive cerebral blood flow and breakdown of the blood-brain barrier in experimental fetal asphyxia. Acta Paediatr. Scand. 68:57, 1979.

Lyen, K. R., et al.: Multicystic encephalomalacia due to fetal viral encephalitis. Eur. J. Pediatr. 137:11, 1981.

Malamud, N.: Sequelae of perinatal trauma. J. Neuropathol. Exp. Neurol. 18:141, 1959.

Matson, D.: Neurosurgery of Infancy and Childhood. Springfield, Ill., Charles C Thomas, 1969.

McHugh, H. E.: Facial paralysis in birth injury and skull fractures. Arch. Otolaryngol. 78:443, 1963.

McHugh, H. E., Sowden, K. A., and Levitt, M. N.: Facial paralysis and muscle agenesis in the newborn. Arch. Otolaryngol. 89:131, 1969.

McLaurin, R. L., Isaacs, E., and Lewis, H. P.: Results in nonoperative treatment in 15 cases of infantile subdural hematoma. J. Neurosurg. 34:753, 1971.

Menkes, J. H.: Textbook of Child Neurology. 2nd ed., Philadelphia, Lea and Febiger, 1980, Chapter V.

Milligan, D. W. A.: Positive pressure ventilation and cranial volume in newborn infants. Arch. Dis. Child. 56:331, 1981.

Mills, W. G.: A new neonatal syndrome. Br. Med. J. 2:464, 1949.

Morgan, M. E. I., Benson, J. W. T., and Cooke, R. W. I.: Ethamsylate reduces the incidence of periventricular haemorrhage in very low birth-weight babies. Lancet 2:830, 1981.

Moyes, P. D., Thompson, G. B., and Cluff, J. W.: Subdural peritoneal shunts in the treatment of subdural effusions in infants. J. Neurosurg. 23:584, 1965.

Myers, R. E.: Experimental models of perinatal brain damage: relevance to human pathology. In Gluck, L. (Ed.): Intrauterine Asphyxia and Developing Fetal Brain. Chicago, Year Book Medical Publishers, 1977, pp. 37–97.

Natelson, S. E., and Sayers, M. P.: The fate of children sustaining severe head trauma during birth. Pediatrics 51:169, 1973.

Nelson, K. B., and Ellenberg, J. H.: Neonatal signs as predictors of cerebral palsy. Pediatrics 64:225, 1979.

Nelson, K. B., and Ellenberg, J. H.: Apgar Scores as predictors of chronic neurologic disability. Pediatrics 68:36, 1981.

Nelson, K. B., and Eng, G. C.: Congenital hypoplasia of the depressor anguli oris muscle: differentiation from congenital facial palsy. J. Pediatr. 81:16, 1972.

Norman, M. G.: Perinatal brain damage. Perspect. Pediatr. Pathol. 4:41, 1978.

Painter, M. J., Depp, R., and O'Donoghue, M. N.: Fetal heart rate patterns and development in the first year of life. Am. J. Obstet. Gynecol. 132:271, 1978.

Papadatos, C., Alexiou, D., Nicolopoulos, H., Mikropoulos, H., and Hadzigeorgiou, E.: Congenital hypoplasia of depressor anguli oris muscle. Arch. Dis. Child. 49:927, 1974.

Pape, K. E., and Pickering, D.: Asymmetric crying facies: an index of other congenital anomalies. J. Pediatr. 81:21, 1972.

Pape, K. E., and Wigglesworth, J. S.: Haemorrhage, Ischaemia, and the Perinatal Brain. Philadelphia, J. B. Lippincott, 1979.

Papile, L. A., et al.: Cerebral intraventricular hemorrhage (CVH) in infants < 1500 grams: developmental follow-up at one year. Pediatr. Res. 13:528, 1979.

Parmelee, A. H.: Molding due to intra-uterine posture. Facial paralysis probably due to such molding. Am. J. Dis. Child. 42:1155, 1931.

Pasternak, J. F., Mantovani, J. F., and Volpe, J. J.: Porencephaly from periventricular intracerebral hemorrhage in a premature infant. Am. J. Dis. Child. 134:673, 1980.

Perlman, M., and Reisner, S. H.: Asymmetric crying facies and congenital anomalies. Arch. Dis. Child. 48:627, 1973.

Ravenel, S. D.: Posterior fossa hemorrhage in the newborn. Pediatrics 64:39, 1979.

Raynor, R., and Parsa, M.: Nonsurgical elevation of depressed skull fracture in an infant. J. Pediatr. 72:262, 1968.

Robinson, R. J., and Rossiter, M. A.: Massive subaponeurotic hemorrhage in babies of African origin. Arch. Dis. Child. 43:684, 1968.

Ruiz, M. P. D., et al.: Early development of infants of birth weight less than 1000 gm with reference to mechanical ventilation in newborn period. Pediatrics 68:330, 1981.

San Agustin, M., Nitowsky, H. M., and Borden, J. N.: Neonatal sciatic palsy after umbilical vessel injection. J. Pediatr. 60:408, 1962.

Sankaran, K., Peters, K., and Finer, N.: Estimated cerebral blood flow in term infants with hypoxic-ischemic encephalopathy. Pediatr. Res. 15:1415, 1981.

Sauerbrei, E. E., et al.: Ultrasonic evaluation of neonatal intracranial hemorrhage and its complications. Radiology 139:677, 685, 1981.

Scheinberg, L., and Allensworth, M.: Sciatic neuropathy in infants related to antibiotic injections. Pediatrics 19:261, 1957.

Schrager, G. O.: Elevation of depressed skull fracture with a breast pump. J. Pediatr. 77:300, 1970.

Schum, T. R., et al.: Neonatal intraventricular hemorrhage due to an intracranial arteriovenous malformation: a case report. Pediatrics 64:242, 1979.

Shewmon, D. A., et al.: Postischemic hypervascularity of infancy: a stage in the evolution of ischemic brain damage with characteristic CT scan. Ann. Neurol. 9:358, 1981.

Shinnar, S. et al.: Intraventricular hemorrhage in the premature infant. New Engl. J. Med. 306:1464, 1982.

Smith, B. T.: Isolated phrenic nerve palsy in the newborn. Pediatrics 49:449, 1972.

Spector, G. J., et al.: Fetal respiratory distress causing CNS and inner ear hemorrhage. Laryngoscope 88:764, 1978.

Stern, W. E., and Rand, R. W.: Birth injuries to the spinal cord. Am. J. Obstet. Gynecol. 78:498, 1959.

Sykes, G. S., et al.: Do Apgar scores indicate asphyxia? Lancet 1:494, 1982.

Takagi, T., et al.: Extradural hemorrhage in the newborn as a result of birth trauma. Childs Brain 4:306, 1978.

Takashima, S., Armstrong, D. L., and Becker, L. E.: Subcortical leukomalacia, relationship to development of the cerebral sulcus and its vascular supply. Arch. Neurol. 35:470, 1978.

Tardieu, M., Evrard, P., and Lyon, G.: Progressive expanding congenital porencephalies: a treatable cause of progressive encephalopathy. Pediatrics 68:198, 1981.

Thurston, J. H., and McDougal, D. B.: Effect of ischemia on metabolism of the brain of the newborn mouse. Am. J. Physiol. 216:348, 1969.

Towbin, A.: Latent spinal cord and brainstem injury in newborn infants. Dev. Med. Child Neurol. 11:54, 1969.

Tsiantos, A., et al.: Intracranial hemorrhage in the prematurely born infant: timing of clots and evaluation of clinical signs and symptoms. J. Pediatr. 85:854, 1974.

Vanucci, R. C., and Duffy, T. E.: Cerebral metabolism in newborn dogs during reversible asphyxia. Ann. Neurol. 1:528, 1977.

Vanucci, R. C., and Vanucci, S. J.: Cerebral carbohydrate metabolism during hypoglycemia and anoxia in newborn rats. Ann. Neurol. 4:73, 1978.

Volpe, J. J.: Perinatal hypoxic-ischemic brain injury. Pediatr. Clin. North Am. 28:383, 1976.

Volpe, J. J.: Neonatal intraventricular hemorrhage. N. Engl. J. Med. 304:886, 1981.

Volpe, J. J.: Neurology of the Newborn. Philadelphia, W.B. Saunders Co., 1981, pp. 243–248.

Volpe, J. J., and Pasternak, J. F.: Parasagittal cerebral injury in neonatal hypoxic-ischemic encephalopathy: clinical and neuroradiologic features. J. Pediatr. 91:472, 1977.

Walsh P., et al.: Assessment of neurologic outcome in asphyxiated infants by use of several CK-BB isoenzyme measurements. J. Pediatr. 101:988, 1982.

Wigglesworth, J. S., and Husemeyer, R. P.: Intracranial birth trauma in vaginal breech delivery: the continued importance of injury to the occipital bone. Br. J. Obstet. Gynaecol. 84:684, 1977.

Worcester-Drought, C.: Spinabulbar paresis. Dev. Med. Child Neurol. 16:1 (suppl. 30), 1974.

Yates, P. O.: Birth trauma to vertebral arteries. Arch. Dis. Child. 34:436, 1959.

Young, R. S. K., Hernandez, M. J., and Yagel, S. K.: Selective reduction of blood flow to white matter during hypotension in newborn dogs: a possible mechanism of periventricular leukomalacia. Ann. Neurol. 12:445, 1982.

Zelson, C., Lee, S. J., and Pearl, M.: The incidence of skull fractures underlying cephalhematomas in newborn infants. J. Pediatr. 85:371, 1974.

78

Malformations of the Central Nervous System

By John H. Menkes*

Only those congenital malformations of the nervous system that are apparent in the neonate will be discussed in this chapter. They will be subdivided into disorders of induction and of cellular migration and proliferation.

Embryrogenic Induction Disorders

These disorders represent a failure in the mutual induction of mesoderm and neuroectoderm. The primary defect is a failure of the neural folds to fuse and form the neural tube, with secondary maldevelopment of skeletal structures enclosing the CNS. The defects range from anencephaly to sacral meningomyelocele in the cephalic to caudal direction of the neural tube and from holoprosencephaly to craniospinal rachischisis (midline posterior splitting of skull and vertebral column) in the anterior to posterior direction.

ANENCEPHALY

Anencephaly is a lethal malformation in which the vault of the skull is absent and the exposed brain is amorphous. The insult responsible for this defect is believed to occur after the onset of neural fold development (16 days) but before closure of the anterior neuropore (24 to 26 days). Between 75 and 80 per cent of infants are stillborn, and the remainder succumb within hours or a few weeks after birth. The etiology of this grotesque anomaly is unknown, although epidemiologic studies suggest a familial predisposition. The malformation is stimulus nonspecific because a variety of genetic, infectious, and chemical insults have been implicated in its formation. In the United States, anencephaly has been found in 0.5 to 2 per 1000 births, whereas in Ireland the prevalence rate has been as high as 5.9 per 1000 births (Alter,

1962; Nakano, 1973; Coffey and Jessop, 1957). For unknown reasons, the incidence of this anomaly has fallen over the past few years, not only in Ireland but also in other parts of the world (Windham and Edmonds, 1982). Most investigators have favored nonclosure of the neural tube in early embryonic life as the cause of this defect.

Anencephaly occurs two to four times more often in girls than in boys. A high percentage of these babies are premature, and associated polyhydramnios is not uncommon. The cranial defect is associated with open spinal cord anomalies in as many as half the cases (Friede, 1975). In addition to the grossly anomalous character of the cerebral hemispheres, the hypothalamus is quite malformed, and the cerebellum is usually rudimentary or absent. Brain stem tissue is identifiable. The internal carotid arteries are hypoplastic, a condition probably secondary to the lack of normal brain formation (Vogel, 1961). The anterior lobe of the pituitary gland is present in the anencephalic infant, but the adrenal glands are abnormally small.

Diagnosis of anencephaly is obvious at the moment of birth. Liveborn subjects do not survive infancy. During their few weeks of life they exhibit slow, stereotyped movements and frequent decerebrate posturing. Head, facial, and limb movements may be spontaneous or pain-induced. Some brain stem functions and automatisms, such as sucking, rooting, and righting responses and the Moro reflex, are present and are more readily and more reproducibly elicited than in normal infants. The "bowing reflex," which occasionally can be demonstrated in normal premature infants of 7 months' gestation, is invariably present in anencephalics. It can be elicited by placing the infant into the supine position and extending the thighs at the hip joints. The head then lifts itself slowly, followed by the trunk, so that the infant ultimately achieves the sitting position. The presence of reflexes such as these reflect the absence of cortical inhibitory influences on subcortical and brain stem function.

The presence of anencephaly and other open neural tube defects may be predicted by measuring alpha-fetoprotein (AFP) in amniotic fluid or maternal serum. AFP is the major serum protein in early embryonic life, representing 90 per cent of total serum globulins. It is a fetus-specific alpha-1-globulin probably involved in preventing fetal immune rejection, and it is produced first by the yolk sac and later by fetal liver and gastrointestinal tract. Normally, it passes from fetal serum into fetal urine and then into amniotic fluid. Because of a substantial leak of fetal blood components directly into amniotic fluid, AFP

* This chapter includes portions written by Dr. William E. Bell that appeared in previous editions.

concentrations and maternal serum AFP levels are elevated in anencephaly and open spina bifida or cranium bifidum.

Mothers who have borne one or more children with neural tube defects, spinal dysraphism, or multiple vertebral anomalies, or who have a pedigree history of any of these disorders, or who have themselves survived with spina bifida are at risk to bear children with neural tube defects. Measurements of maternal AFP levels at 14 weeks' gestation serve as a preliminary screen. Normal AFP in adult serum is less than 10 nanograms (ng) per ml, and in normal maternal serum and amniotic fluid it ranges from 15 to 500 ng/ml. During 15 to 20 weeks' gestation, an AFP concentration of 1000 ng/ml or greater strongly suggests an open neural tube defect. A positive test on maternal serum is followed-up by measurement of amniotic fluid AFP or sonography for anatomic configuration of the fetus or both (Milunsky, 1980). Measurement of amniotic fluid acetylcholinesterase activity has been suggested as another secondary test to confirm the elevated AFP (Hullin et al., 1981).

With all diagnostic techniques now available, the detection efficiency approaches 100 per cent for anencephaly. Of the neural tube defects, 4.9 per cent are closed and will go undetected. False-positive results are obtained in a variety of unrelated conditions, including omphalocele, duodenal atresia, Turner's syndrome, and several other fetal defects (Milunsky, 1980).

CRANIUM BIFIDUM AND SPINA BIFIDA

These defects are caused by a failure in fusion of the posterior midline of the skull (cranium bifidum) or the vertebral column (spina bifida). The result is a bony cleft through which varying quantities of brain or spinal cord tissue protrude.

Like anencephaly, these defects are time-specific and stimulus-nonspecific. The insult must occur before 26 to 28 days gestation—the time of closure of the posterior neuropore. Several genetic and envi-

ronmental factors are believed to act in conjunction, with the former accounting for about 20 per cent of cases. In the majority of instances (65 to 70 per cent) the cause is unknown and may be multifactorial (Matson, 1960).

Cranium Bifidum with Encephalocele

In cranium bifidum, the neural herniation is termed *encephalocele* and may consist of brain parenchyma and meninges or only meninges. These cranial defects were classified by Emery and Kalhan in 1970. A practical and simple way of classifying these defects is to consider those lesions containing only meningeal tissue or meningeal tissue and glial elements to be cranial meningoceles and those harboring components of brain to be cranial encephaloceles. The incidence of the latter significantly exceeds that of the former. Approximately 75 to 80 per cent occur in the occipital region, and the remainder are in the parietal, frontonasal, intranasal, or nasopharyngeal region.

Clinical Aspects. Cranium bifidum with occipital encephalocele affects girls more than boys (Guthkelch, 1970). Although the cranial lesion may be the only abnormality, a significant number of cases will be associated with other defects, such as meningomyelocele, midline facial clefts, deformities of the extremities, or congenital heart disease. Unless the encephalocele is small and covered by hair, it is readily apparent at birth in the form of a soft, round, midline mass that is usually partially or totally covered by skin and that varies in size from a centimeter in diameter up to two or three times the circumference of the infant's head (Fig. 78–1). The head size of the neonate with occipital encephalocele is normal in some cases; in others, microcephaly is present initially, and hydrocephalus subsequently develops.

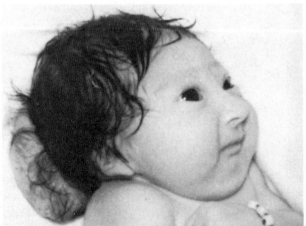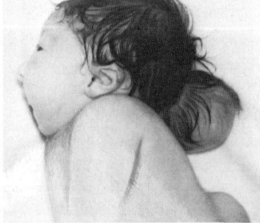

Figure 78–1. Occipital meningoencephalocele. The sloping forehead and small head circumference are evident, although progressive ventricular enlargement often subsequently occurs in such children.

A frontonasal encephalocele presents as a rounded mass at the base of the nose, usually associated with widening of the nasal root and separation of the eyes. Basal encephaloceles, including the intranasal and nasopharyngeal types, differ from the aforementioned, more common, types in that there is no visible external mass, and thus diagnosis is not usually established until later in childhood or even until adulthood (Pollock et al., 1968). The intranasal (transethmoidal) encephalocele is accompanied by a widened nasal root and increased intraocular distance but does not ordinarily become symptomatic until the occurrence of nasal obstruction, epistaxis, or recurrent episodes of bacterial meningitis (Blumenfeld and Skolnik, 1965). Less common types of basal encephaloceles are located in the nasopharynx, sphenoid sinus, or posterior orbit, and they likewise are not usually identified in the infant age group (Pollock et al., 1968).

Diagnosis. Occipital and parietal encephaloceles are quickly identified in the newborn infant by the character of the lesion and the common but not invariable roentgenographic demonstration of the associated skull defect (Fig. 78–2). Transillumination of the lesion is of some diagnostic value in certain cases, and CT scans or ultrasonographic studies before and after surgical repair provide information about associated cerebral anomalies and the presence and degree of hydrocephalus (Byrd et al., 1978).

Frontonasal encephalocele must be differentiated from the so-called nasal "glioma" and dermoids or teratomas in the same region. Pulsation of the mass or bulging with brief bilateral jugular vein compression suggests that it communicates with the suba-

rachnoid space and therefore indicates it to be an encephalocele. In many instances, a precise diagnosis is not available until histologic examination following surgical removal. Intranasal encephalocele should be suspected when an intranasal mass is identified in the child or adult who has a broad nasal bridge and wide-set eyes. It should also be considered in any child who has unexplained recurrent meningitis. This lesion is occasionally biopsied, the preoperative assumption being that it represents a polyp. Specimens obtained from the nasal cavity by biopsy should be submitted for histologic examination because, if not diagnosed, a biopsied encephalocele is likely to lead to cerebrospinal fluid rhinorrhea and subsequent meningitis. Appropriate radiographs and especially CT scans are of great importance in the diagnosis of basal encephaloceles, regardless of their location (Pollock et al., 1968).

Treatment. Whenever possible, an encephalocele should be surgically removed early in life. Hydrocephalus complicates surgical repair in a significant number of cases and is handled by some form of shunt procedure when it occurs. Certain cases must be managed conservatively when the head is distinctly small and the sac contains large amounts of brain tissue, especially if the contained brain includes brain stem or cervical spinal cord elements. Prognosis in terms of survival and intellectual development is far better for infants with meningoceles and considerably worse for those whose lesions contain brain tissue (Lorber, 1967; Mealey et al., 1970).

Spina Bifida Cystica (Meningocele, Meningomyelocele, and Lipomeningocele)

The newborn infant with a meningomyelocele complicated by the usual motor and sensory defects of the lower extremities, the associated intracranial abnormalities, and neurogenic sphincter dysfunction represents a great tragedy for the family as well as an extremely difficult multidisciplinary management problem for the physician. Probably no other problem in the category of neurologic diseases in infancy has been the source of greater dispute than that of the optimal management of the defective child who is afflicted with spina bifida cystica.

Pathology. Of the defects collectively termed *spina bifida cystica*, 75 per cent are meningomyeloceles and 25 per cent are meningoceles. A lumbar or lumbosacral defect is most common, being found in 69 per cent of infants with spina bifida cystica (Matson, 1969). The vast majority of these lesions are accompanied by hydrocephalus and Chiari malformations types 2 and 3. The type 2 malformation is composed of elongation and downward displacement of the pons and medulla, downward displacement of the cerebellar vermis, which protrudes through the foramen magnum, a beak-shaped deformity of the tectal plate, and enlargement of the massa intermedia (Fig. 78–3).

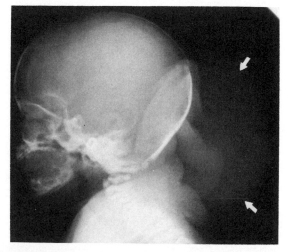

Figure 78–2. Occipital meningoencephalocele, lateral skull x-ray film. The large extracranial sac containing meningeal and brain tissue is outlined by white arrows. Surgical excision of the lesion was followed by progressive hydrocephalus, which required a shunting procedure.

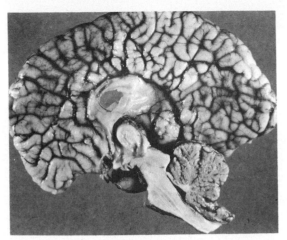

Figure 78–3. Arnold-Chiari malformation. Child with a thoracolumbar meningomyelocele. The Arnold-Chiari malformation consists of elongation of the lower brain stem with downward displacement of the inferior part of the vermis of the cerebellum. The tectal plate is "beaked," and the massa intermedia is enlarged. Polymicrogyria is present.

In 95 per cent of children with lumbar or lumbosacral meningomyelocele, the spinal cord demonstrates abnormalities of the cervical region. In 40 per cent of cases, there is hydromyelia, and in 20 per cent syringomyelia, diplomyelia, or other malformations (Mackenzie and Emery, 1971). A variety of gross and microscopic anomalies are also seen in the spinal cord and in the cerebral hemispheres (Yakovlev and Wadsworth, 1946). The most likely explanation for these anomalies is the presence of a teratogenic influence that accounts not only for the induction anomaly but also for the later malformations of cellular proliferation, migration, and architectonics (Gardner et al., 1975).

Most authors have accepted the concept that these defects are produced by an undetermined insult that prevents normal fusion and closure, although an alternative theory is that the neural tube becomes ruptured after closure, secondary to increased pressure within the central canal (Gardner, 1965). The discovery of myeloschisis in a human embryo only 5 mm long is supportive evidence for the failure of closure postulate (Lemire et al., 1965).

A number of mesodermal lesions accompany these ectodermal defects. These include splitting of the vertebral arches and other dysplasias of bone, such as double ribs and defects in the base of the skull, notably the posterior arch of the atlas (Blaauw, 1971).

Clinical Manifestations. The most common and clinically least significant form of spina bifida is spina bifida occulta, a mesodermal abnormality in which there is nonfusion of the vertebral laminar arches without external protrusion of the meninges. As isolated defects, most lesions are located at the first sacral or fifth lumbar vertebra. Occasionally, spina bifida occulta is accompanied by other congenital defects of the neuraxis. The most common are dermal sinuses and dimples (35 per cent), lipoid tumors (29 per

cent), and abnormalities of the filum terminale (24 per cent) (Anderson, 1975).

Spina bifida cystica is one of the commonest anomalies of the nervous system, with an incidence that ranges from 0.2 per 1000 livebirths in Japan to 4.2 per 1000 in Ireland (Laurence and Tew, 1971). A recurrence rate of 10 per cent is seen in affected families (Naggan, 1969). At birth, the defect may assume any one of a variety of appearances. These range from complete exposure of neural tissue to a flat, partially epithelialized membrane. In all instances, there is a laminar arch defect through which either meninges or meninges and neural elements protrude. Herniation of dura and arachnoid alone without neural components in the sac is called a

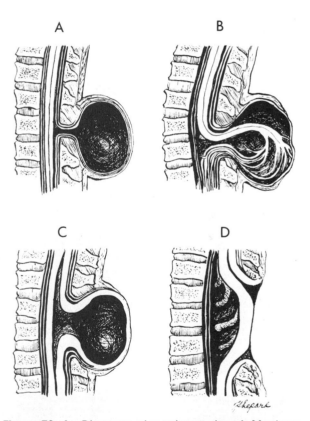

Figure 78–4. Diagram of meningoceles. *A,* Meningocele: Through the bony defect (spina bifida) the meninges herniate and form a cystic sac filled with spinal fluid. The spinal cord does not participate in the herniation and may or may not be abnormal. *B,* Myelomeningocele: Spina bifida with meningocele; the spinal cord is herniated into the sac and ends there or may continue in an abnormal way farther downward. *C,* Myelocystocele or syringomyelocele: The spinal cord shows hydromyelia; the posterior wall of the spinal cord is attached to the ectoderm and undifferentiated. *D,* Myelocele: The spinal cord is agraphic; a cystic cavity is in front of the anterior wall of the spinal cord. (From Benda, C. E.: Developmental Disorders of Mentation and Cerebral Palsies. New York, Grune & Stratton, Inc., 1952. Reprinted by permission.)

"meningocele." The soft, rounded mass on the back is usually skin-covered, although, infrequently, associated failure of ectodermal closure produces a sac covered by a delicate membrane that is susceptible to infection. Motor function in the legs is expected to be normal with this lesion unless there are other dysplastic changes of the spinal cord or brain. Meningomyeloceles (myeloceles, localized rachischisis) are 10 to 20 times more frequent than meningoceles and are of far greater consequence. The herniated sac contains meninges as well as neural tissue. (Fig. 78–4). Only infrequently does skin cover the lesion except in those patients in whom an associated lipoma overlies the defect, the so-called "lipomeningomyelocele" (Fig. 78–5). In most cases, the defect at birth is flat, consisting of poorly organized cord tissue lying exposed on the surface at the midline and surrounded by a pink or bluish, delicate, semitransparent membrane (Fig. 78–6). With the passage of time, fluid accumulation results in elevation of the lesion, giving rise to its cyst-like appearance of variable size (Fig. 78–7). The spinal cord superior to the surface lesion is frequently malformed, with the most common disturbance being hydromyelia.

The type and degree of neurologic deficit in a child with a meningomyelocele is determined by the location and size of the lesion, a matter succinctly reviewed by Stark in 1971. A large myelocele with the upper level extending to T_8 vertebral level creates denervation of the abdominal muscles bilaterally and of all muscle groups in the lower extremities. The

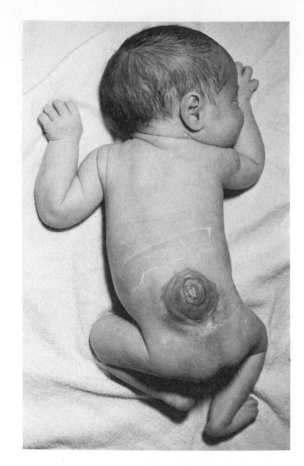

Figure 78–6. Lumbar meningomyelocele in a 3-day-old infant. There is moderate weakness of the proximal muscle groups and more extensive weakness of the distal musculature in the lower extremities. The lesion was flat at birth but began to elevate in the next 2 days.

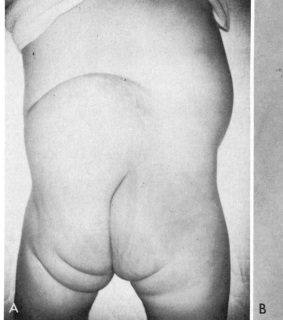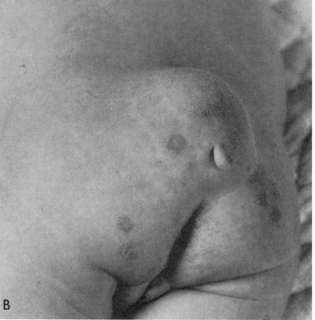

Figure 78–5. Two examples of lipomeningocele. Each presents in the left buttock as a firm, well-circumscribed, lobulated tumor that became tense when the infant cried. Over the surface of *B* are some macular erosions and a congenital skin tag and dimple. This last may be the pilonidal dimple displaced by the tumor.

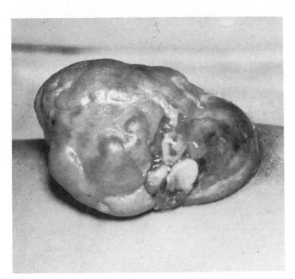

Figure 78–7. Close-up view of a lumbosacral myelomeningocele. The mass is covered with thin, transparent membrane. No well-differentiated nervous tissue can be distinguished with assurance.

abdomen bulges in the flank regions, and the legs are motionless and flaccid, without significant joint deformity if the entire spinal cord below the upper level is affected. The anal sphincter is patulous, and sensation is absent to the upper limits of the midline lesion. A low lumbar meningomyelocele with sparing of function down to L_4 results in sustained contraction of the hip flexors, quadriceps, and tibialis anterior muscles but paralysis of the hamstrings, gastrocnemius, and intrinsic musculature of the feet. The result is a striking deformity in which the lower limbs are held in flexion at the hips as well as extension of the knees and a calcaneovarus position of the feet. Several types of foot deformity may result with lumbosacral and sacral myeloceles, the position and posture being determined by which muscles retain innervation and which are paralyzed. Regardless of the upper level of the lesion, infants with clinical evidence of denervation of muscles supplied by S_{2-3-4} can be expected to have neurogenic bladder dysfunction.

Hydrocephalus only infrequently complicates spinal meningoceles but is a common complicating problem in the child with a meningomyelocele (Stein and Schut, 1979). It is generally stated that 85 to 90 per cent of infants with meningomyeloceles have hydrocephalus of one type or another (Lorber, 1961). The pathogenesis of hydrocephalus in these infants has been a matter of speculation for a number of years and remains unclear. Aqueductal obstruction of one of several types accounts for ventricular enlargement in some cases (Emery, 1974), although others have extraventricular obstructive (communicating) hydrocephalus. Blockage at the foramen magnum secondary to the Arnold-Chiari malformation, preventing access of cerebrospinal fluid to the intracranial subarachnoid space, has been stated to be a cause of communicating hydrocephalus in these cases but is doubted by some investigators (Drummond and Donaldson, 1974). Whatever the cause,

hydrocephalus of moderate degree is sometimes present in the neonate with meningomyelocele, even in the absence of abnormal suture separation or head enlargement.

An interesting but somewhat unusual clinical disturbance in the infant with a meningomyelocele and the Arnold-Chiari malformation is laryngeal stridor. Most reported patients have developed stridor a few weeks after birth, at a time when hydrocephalus was notably progressive. In some, stridor disappeared following shunt therapy or suboccipital craniectomy (Kirsch et al., 1968; Adeloye et al., 1970), but in others, relief of hydrocephalus had little influence on the respiratory difficulty (Fitzsimmons, 1965). Caudal displacement of the medulla, secondary to increased pressure above, resulting in traction on the vagus nerves has been suggested as an explanation for this disorder. Bilateral medullary hemorrhages involving the region of the nucleus ambiguus were found in the cases described by Morley in 1969.

Diagnosis. The presence of a meningomyelocele in the newborn infant is obvious in most instances. The small, skin-covered lesion accompanied by minimal motor deficits in the legs can present some initial diagnostic difficulties and rarely is not proved a defect in neural tube closure until operation is performed. More practical diagnostic issues in the infant with a meningomyelocele are whether or not hydrocephalus coexists or hydronephrosis is present. Measurement of head size, transillumination, and ultrasonographic and CT scanning will indicate the presence of hydrocephalus. Increased intracranial pressure is seen in only about 15 per cent of infants with myelomeningocele, and its absence, consequently, does not correlate with the absence of ventricular enlargement (Stein and Schut, 1979).

On roentgenographic examination of the skull most infants with myelomeningocele exhibit a characteristic defect, referred to as "lückenschädel," or "craniolacunia" (Fig. 78–8). This peculiar, honeycombed appearance of the skull is transient, disappearing in the early months after birth. It probably is the result of a defect in membranous bone formation and not secondary to in utero intracranial hypertension, as is often stated.

Treatment. Management of the child with a neural tube closure defect of the spinal region requires a multidisciplinary approach that involves several medical and surgical specialties. The spinal meningocele, which is covered only by a delicate membrane, is surgically corrected as early as possible because of the excellent potential outcome and the danger of infection until the lesion is removed. Those that are skin covered are also surgically excised, although the timing of the procedure is much less critical. Even

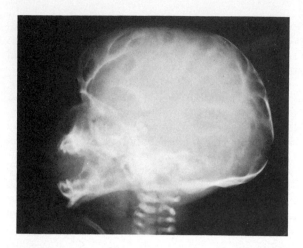

Figure 78—8. Lückenschädel, or craniolacunia. Honey-combed pattern of the skull in the newborn infant with meningomyelocele, usually associated with hydrocephalus.

when the meningocele appears uncomplicated, the child should be evaluated periodically following surgery to be certain that hydrocephalus is not developing and that bladder function remains normal.

Selection of methods of treatment for the child with an "open" meningomyelocele with neurologic bladder dysfunction, weakness of the legs, and hydrocephalus is far more controversial because established guidelines are available for only a small percentage. The infant who has a small lesion with minimal or mild neurologic deficits is a candidate for immediate or early surgical closure unless the sac is obviously infected or sepsis is evident. The child who has a large "open" lesion, especially if infected, total paralysis of the legs, and significant head enlargement due to advanced hydrocephalus at birth has little chance of survival and virtually no possibility of eventual reasonable intellectual or motor function. This condition is ordinarily not managed surgically in view of the limited accomplishments of this approach.

The child with a meningomyelocele between these two extremes of severity poses the current dilemma with regard to management. The choice of immediate aggressive therapy, delayed and stepwise surgical therapy, or totally conservative treatment should logically be partially based on the natural history of the condition. The available information about natural history has solved few problems in this country, where most affected infants receive at least partial therapy, such as antibiotics for acquired infections and shunts for hydrocephalus. In studies of infants who received no therapy except for conventional feeding and infant care, the majority, perhaps over 90 per cent, have died by 1 year of age (Hide et al., 1972; Lorber, 1972).

In the 1960s, the procedure of immediate surgical closure of the spinal lesion and early shunting therapy

for hydrocephalus was adopted in certain centers in Great Britain (Sharrard et al., 1963). This approach developed because of the recognition of dismal outcome among many in whom treatment was delayed and because of the belief that deterioration of motor function in the legs resulted from desiccation of the exposed neural tissue after birth. After some years' experience with immediate and aggressive surgical treatment, certain observers (Lorber, 1971) now believe a more conservative approach is warranted, with candidates for early operation selected on an individual basis. To this date, the best method of treatment of the infant with a meningomyelocele remains in question, and the ideal solution is clearly in the areas of prevention and prenatal detection.

OTHER DYSRAPHIC STATES

Diastematomyelia

The term *diastematomyelia* designates a split, or cleft, in a segment of the spinal cord; conventionally, however, it refers to a congenital anomaly in which the cord is transected by a bony or cartilaginous septum that extends from the posterior surface of a vertebral body to the dura or laminar arch dorsally. The etiology of this unusual malformation is unknown; however, it occurs more frequently in girls than boys and is usually associated with other defects that allow identification of its presence (Perret, 1957; Dale, 1969). In almost all cases, the lesion is in the lower thoracic or lumbar region and is associated with an overlying cutaneous abnormality in the form of a tuft of hair, a hemangioma, or a visible and palpable lipoma. The absence of such overlying cutaneous abnormalities has been described with diastematomyelia but is quite rare (Sedzimir et al., 1973). Except for the associated cutaneous lesions, detectable abnormalities in the newborn or early infant period are not common, but, when present, they consist of a unilateral foot deformity such as talipes varus or pes cavus or atrophy of one lower extremity, usually with a foot deformity. Two distinct clinical syndromes occur (Guthkelch, 1970). The first is a unilateral nonprogressive neural and mesodermal hypoplasia in which one hypoplastic lower extremity is enervated by the relevant hypoplastic segment of cord. The second, seen more commonly, is a progressive condition that either appears de novo, or is superimposed upon the first syndrome. Neurologic signs are not noted until after the child begins to ambulate, when a disturbance of gait becomes evident.

With suspicion aroused by cutaneous anomalies and hypoplasia of one extremity, one can almost always establish the diagnosis with tomographic studies of the lumbosacral spine or with myelography. The most consistent radiographic finding is interpedicular widening a few segments above and below the site of the bony or cartilagenous spur without erosion of pedicles. The midline septum, or spur, is radiographically visible in certain instances, but its absence on x-ray films does not exclude the diagnosis. Myelography establishes the diagnosis in most cases by demonstrating that the dye column is divided by the septum, producing a linear or circular midline defect.

Treatment consists of laminectomy with removal of the median septum, which traverses the cord. Past experience has indicated that surgical treatment is not followed by recovery of limb atrophy or foot deformity but that it can usually be expected to arrest further progression of neurologic deficits (Hendrick, 1971).

Sacral Agenesis

Agenesis of the sacrum and coccyx is usually associated with anomalous development of the lumbosacral cord and other major or minor dysraphisms. The defect is seen in approximately 1 per cent of offspring of diabetic mothers (Sarnat et al., 1976).

Neurodermal Sinus (Congenital Dermal Sinus)

The majority of dermal sinuses (e.g., the pilonidal sinus) do not connect with the central nervous system and are therefore of limited neurologic importance. Neurodermal sinuses are one of the most common occult spinal dysraphisms. They represent a communication lined by stratified squamous epithelium between skin and any portion of the neuraxis. Most commonly, the defects are in the lumbosacral and occipital regions. These two points represent the posterior and anterior neuropores, respectively.

The sinus is often surrounded by a small mound of skin, the dimple, or by other cutaneous lesions, such as tufts of hair or angiomas. It often overlies a spina bifida occulta. It may expand into an epidermoid or dermoid cyst at its proximal end, thus causing segmental neurologic deficits. The presence of an open sinus tract may allow drainage of cerebrospinal fluid or provide a portal of entry for bacterial infection. A neurodermal sinus is one of the most common causes of recurrent meningitis (Matson and Jerva, 1966).

These lesions require neurosurgical exploration with complete excision of the sinus (Matson, 1969).

CONGENITAL SCALP DEFECT

Congenital scalp defect, also known as aplasia cutis congenitalis, is an uncommon anomaly that occurs in either sex. It may occur in an otherwise normal child or may be associated with a wide variety of other cerebral or extracranial anomalies (Fowler and Dumars, 1973; Ruiz-Maldonado and Tamayo, 1974), including trisomy 13–15. Rarely, congenital scalp defects are associated with similiar cutaneous lesions elsewhere on the body. In many cases, congenital scalp defect occurs in sporadic fashion. It has also been observed in siblings (Hodgman et al.,

1965) and in both a parent and offspring (Johnsonbaugh et al., 1965).

The most common location of the defect is at the vertex, but, occasionally, paired lesions are found in the parietal regions. At birth, a congenital scalp defect is often ulcerated or crusted and may appear to be infected. Over the following weeks or months, the lesion becomes covered by a layer of epithelium and subsequently resembles a scarred area. The region of the defect remains devoid of hair thereafter.

In most cases, the underlying skull is intact; however, in some there are underlying skull defects of variable size that close spontaneously during the first few months after birth. Still others have associated oval or circular defects in the skull that persist into adulthood.

The pathogenesis of this anomaly has been debated for years and remains undetermined. Autosomal dominant inheritance has been suggested in certain cases. Treatment is conservative for most patients, especially for those with cerebral anomalies resulting in severe functional defects. Plastic repair has been recommended in certain instances (Kosnik and Sayers, 1975).

ANTERIOR MIDLINE DEFECTS

Holoprosencephaly

Whereas anencephaly is the most catastrophic dysraphism, holoprosencephaly is the most devastating of the anterior anomalies. It is caused by induction failure of three germ layers: cephalic mesoderm, adjacent neuroectoderm, and the entodermal anlage for facial structures. Like anencephaly, it is time-specific and stimulus-nonspecific. Associated chromosomal abnormalities are frequent, including nondisjunction leading most commonly to trisomy 13–15 and less often to trisomy 18. The malformation also is overrepresented in infants of diabetic mothers. It is likely that an environmental toxic stimulus accounts for both the embryonic failure and the chromosomal defects.

In essence, the defect is one of failure of the primary cerebral vesicle to cleave and expand bilaterally with associated midline facial defects (DeMyer, 1967; DeMyer, 1971). Various degrees of severity are recognized. In its most complete expression, the brain is characterized by a single large ventricular cavity. The thalamus remains undivided, the inferior frontal and temporal regions are often absent, and the remainder of the isocortex is rudimentary. In the less severe forms, partial or complete division of the hemispheres is evident, but the olfactory bulbs and tracts are absent or hypoplastic (arhinencephaly) (De Myer, 1971).

In the most extreme form, the infant's face is overwhelmed by cyclopia, a single median orbital fossa and eye with protruding noselike appendage above the orbit. Other constitutional dysplastic features include polydactyly, ventricular septal defect, and cardiac and digestive tract anomalies.

The less extensively malformed infant demonstrates hypotelorism, a median cleft lip, and a nose that lacks its bridge, columella, or septum.

The neurologic picture in these anomalies is highlighted by severe developmental retardation, seizures, rigidity, apnea, temperature imbalance, and, rarely, hydrocephalus. Diagnostic studies include skull and facial roentgenograms to demonstrate deformed anterior craniobasal bones, dermatoglyphics, and a CT scan. When the patient has many extracephalic anomalies, a chromosomal defect is likely, whereas in their absence the karyotype is usually normal. A minority of cases are familial, and a single gene defect with variable expressivity has been postulated.

Other Faciotelencephalopathies

A number of disorders are included in this group, all sharing the characteristics of median cleft lip and palate and various degrees of induction anomalies of the brain (DeMyer, 1971), which result in developmental defects of varying severity. CT scans will often delineate the nature and extent of the cerebral maldevelopment.

Disorders of Cellular Migration and Proliferation

Although it is recognized that disorders of induction will produce secondary migration or proliferation anomalies, this discussion is confined to those disorders of cellular migration that are unassociated with defects of embryogenesis.

MICROCEPHALY

Inasmuch as several of these developmental anomalies manifest themselves by microcephaly, this condition will be considered first.

Microcephaly is defined by a head circumference, as measured around the glabella and the occipital protuberance, that is more than two standard deviations below the mean for age, sex, race, and gestation. The expected normal head circumferences at birth and in the first few weeks can be obtained for term infants from the graphs compiled by Nellhaus, and those for premature infants from the data collected by Lubchenco and colleagues. Except for cases in which there is premature closure of the sutures (craniosynostosis), the small size of the skull

reflects a small brain. However, not all children with head circumferences below two standard deviations are mentally retarded (Avery et al., 1972; Martin, 1970). A child with "measurement microcephaly" who is of small stature because of familial factors or growth retardation secondary to malabsorption or cardiac disease is, therefore, not necessarily in the same category from the standpoint of CNS function as one with microcephaly resulting from organic brain disease.

An abnormally small brain either is caused by anomalous development during the first 7 months of gestation (primary microcephaly) or is the result of an insult incurred during the last 2 months of gestation or during the perinatal period (secondary microcephaly).

Primary microcephaly includes a variety of insults that cause anomalies of induction and migration. The condition may be transmitted as an autosomal recessive disorder (Robain and Lyon, 1972). Most infants with this condition are obviously abnormal at birth. They have not only a distinctly small head but also characteristic facial and cranial configurations. Their rounded heads with small or absent anterior fontanel and recessed or sloped forehead indicative of the shallow anterior cranial fossa readily identify them as infants with severe morphologic cerebral abnormalities. Some demonstrate immediate signs of neurologic dysfunction such as hypotonicity, hypertonicity, or an abnormal cry, whereas others function surprisingly normally for the first few months after birth. The type of pathology found in infants of this sort varies, but abnormalities of the gross configuration of the brain are usual.

Lissencephaly is near total or total absence of cerebral convolutions (agyria), reminiscent of the fetal brain during the second to fourth months of gestation (Miller, 1963).

Pachygyria appears to represent a developmental arrest of maturation and cell migration at a slightly later stage, with the result being abnormally broad, flat cerebral convolutions with a thick cerebral cortex. The ventricular system is usually mildly enlarged, and other anomalies, such as areas of gray matter heterotopia, are usually present in these types of malformed brains.

Polymicrogyria is more often associated with hydrocephalus than microcephaly and is characterized by either localized or generalized excessive and small cerebral convolutions. Whether microgyria is associated with an arrest of neuronal migration or is a result of an insult to the postmigratory cortex has not been entirely clarified (Richman et al., 1974). The clinical picture is generally one of mental retardation and spasticity, or hypotonia with active deep tendon reflexes ("atonic cerebral palsy").

Microcephaly is present in infants with certain chromosomal disturbances, such as trisomy 13–15 and trisomy 17–18. There are also at least 20 well-defined dysmorphic syndromes with grossly normal karyotypes that are associated with microcephaly.

The best known intrauterine acquired causes for

microcephaly include transplacentally transmitted infections such as rubella, cytomegalovirus disease, and toxoplasmosis. Maternal phenylketonuria with serum phenylalanine levels over 15 mg per 100 ml during pregnancy is another cause of microcephaly and intrauterine growth failure (Fisch et al., 1969; Frankenburg et al., 1968). Maternal irradiation exposure (Plummer, 1952) and certain drugs can possibly lead to brain damage and microcephaly.

A variety of insults—infectious, traumatic, metabolic, and anoxic—during the last part of the third trimester and the perinatal period cause destruction of brain with reduced brain growth and early closure of sutures. As a rule, when the injury has occurred in the perinatal period, the head circumference at birth is normal, and microcephaly only becomes apparent months later.

CRANIOSYNOSTOSIS

Craniosynostosis (craniostenosis) is a disorder in which premature closure of one or more cranial sutures results in a disturbance of the shape and configuration of the skull. In many instances, premature fusion of the sutures is the only evident abnormality the child exhibits; in others, craniosynostosis and other associated anomalies represent an identifiable syndrome, often genetically determined. These "primary" forms of premature cranial suture closure are in contrast with conditions in which early suture closure is a passive process resulting from lack of normal brain growth. This is observed in the infant with microcephaly and can occur subsequent to successful shunt procedures for advanced hydrocephalus. Abnormally rapid suture closure in early infancy can also occur in association with certain metabolic disturbances, the most notable being the rachitic disorders and idiopathic hypercalcemia (Reilly et al., 1964).

The etiology of primary craniosynostosis is not known. Most cases unassociated with other anomalies are sporadic, although repeated occurrence within a family has been described. Craniosynostoses consistently associated with certain other anomalies, such as Crouzon's disease or Apert's syndrome, may appear in sporadic fashion but are generally regarded to be inherited disorders (Cohen, 1975). An explanation for the type of deformity of the head resulting from premature closure of one or other cranial sutures was proposed by Virchow in 1851. He observed that inhibition of normal growth of the skull occurred in a direction perpendicular to the suture that is prematurely fused, resulting in compensatory enlargement in a direction parallel to the unyielding suture. The time at which cranial sutures normally achieve functional closure is quite variable, but abnormal sutural diastasis is commonly observed in children up to 10 or 12 years of age suffering increased intracranial pressure. The metopic suture differs from the other major sutures in that closure normally occurs in the first year of life. Trigonocephaly, therefore, occurs only when fusion of the metopic suture takes

place in fetal or very early postnatal life. In general, the most overt cranial deformities are the result of prenatal suture closure, regardless of which suture or sutures are affected (Ingraham et al., 1948). Since the brain reaches approximately 80 per cent of the adult weight by 3 to 4 years of age, individual suture closure at this time is a matter of little consequence.

Clinical Aspects. Certain types of craniosynostosis, such as sagittal suture synostosis (scaphocephaly), are more common in males than in females. Isolated closure of the sagittal suture, the most common variety of the disease, is the one least often associated with other defects. Premature closure of the coronal sutures can likewise occur as the only apparent abnormality but is more often associated with other congenital anomalies. Oxycephaly secondary to multiple cranial suture fusion represents the least common form of the condition and is the most severe type because of the resulting restriction of cerebral growth and subsequent increased intracranial pressure.

The newborn infant with sagittal craniosynostosis presents with an elongated but narrow head, often with a small or absent anterior fontanel (Figs. 78–9 and 78–10). The forehead is usually considerably broader than the occipital region. A palpable ridge is present, especially over the posterior portion of the fused suture. Although the sagittal suture may be closed along its total length, it is important to recognize that suture closure over even a short segment will effectively limit growth of the skull perpendicular to the entire length of that suture. In the absence of the other anomalies, the infant with scaphocephaly secondary to sagittal synostosis is not expected to have abnormal neurologic signs or signs of increased pressure. The signs are only those of distortion of head shape, since compensatory growth through other sutures permits normal brain growth. The problem is generally considered to be primarily cosmetic; however, examples are not rare of older children with uncorrected sagittal synostosis who subsequently developed visual disturbances or increased intracranial pressure (Andersson and Gomes, 1968; Anderson and Geiger, 1965).

Bilateral coronal synostosis results in a brachycephalic head shape in which the skull is broad anteriorly but shortened in the anteroposterior direction and elevated in the region anterior to the fontanel (Fig. 78–11). The forehead is broad and flattened, usually with a "pinched" appearance just above and lateral to the eyebrows. The eyes appear wide-set, and, in some cases, proptosis is present. Palpable ridges are sometimes present over fused coronal sutures but are rarely as definite as the ridging over a closed sagittal suture. Bilateral coronal craniosynostosis is frequently associated with other anomalies and is the most common type of suture closure in

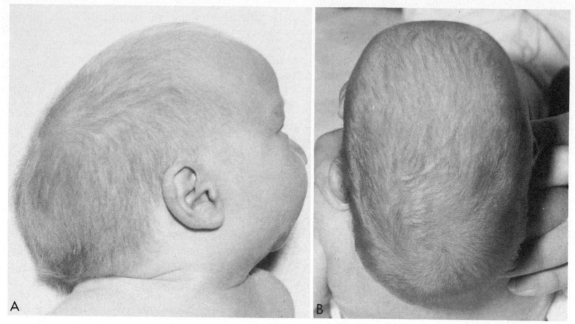

Figure 78–9. Three-week-old infant with sagittal craniosynostosis. *A*, Lateral view demonstrates the elongated head shape with tapering in the occipital region. Except for the abnormal configuration of the head, the child is developmentally normal for age. *B*, Vertex view reveals the characteristic long, narrow shape of the calvarium with premature closure of the sagittal suture.

children with familial craniosynostosis, including Crouzon's disease and Apert's syndrome. Unilateral coronal synostosis gives rise to an asymmetric cranial deformity called *plagiocephaly*. The forehead adjacent to the fused coronal suture is flattened or indented, the eyebrow is elevated, and the homolateral eye appears prominent. The ocular prominence re-

sults from the associated involvement of the orbit, which is shallower and more oblique than is normally the case.

Prenatal or early postnatal fusion of the metopic suture results in a narrow, triangularly shaped forehead, which has a palpable and visible ridge betraying the underlying closed suture. The orbits are oval-

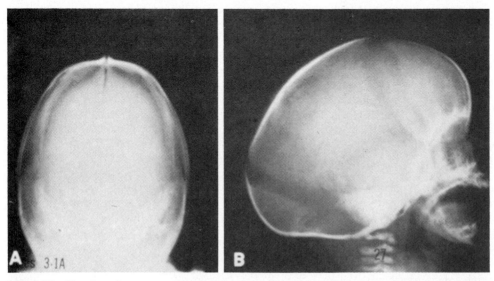

Figure 78–10. Roentgenographic findings in a 3-week-old child with sagittal craniosynostosis. *A*, Occipital view reveals the narrow configuration of the skull with "heaping up" of bone along the fused sagittal suture. *B*, Lateral view demonstrates the scaphocephalic shape of the skull with hyperostosis of the closed sagittal suture. The coronal and lambdoidal sutures are more separated than normal. (Hope, J. W., Spitz, E. B., and Slade, H. W.: Radiology *65*:183, 1955.)

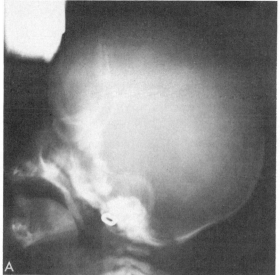

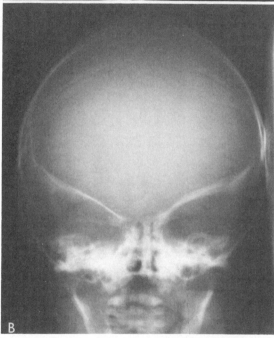

Figure 78–11. Roentgenographic findings in a newborn infant with a bilateral coronal craniosynostosis. *A*, Lateral view of the skull shows the short anteroposterior diameter and hyperostosis along both fused coronal sutures. *B*, The PA view of the skull demonstrates the elevated and oblique position of the sphenoid ridge on either side.

shaped and the eyes are abnormally closely approximated, a condition referred to as *hypotelorism*. The keel-shaped, angulated forehead of the infant with trigonocephaly is best observed by viewing the head from the vertex. Metopic suture synostosis occurs either in isolated fashion without other defects or associated with other, often significant, anomalies (Anderson et al., 1962). One associated pattern is the presence of midline facial clefts and arhinencephaly, or absence of the olfactory nerves and other parts of the rhinencephalon, in addition to a single anterior lateral ventricle with hypoplasia or absence of the corpus callosum (Currarino and Silverman, 1960).

The child with trigonocephaly and associated cerebral defects is expected to reveal early developmental retardation and eventual mental retardation.

Premature closure of the lambdoid sutures alone is very rare but can occur on occasion with sagittal synostosis or with total cranial suture fusion. Oxycephaly, or total suture synostosis, is an infrequent but severe form of craniosynostosis and is the only type of the disease in which the head circumference of the child may be significantly reduced. Inability of the brain to expand causes increased pressure symptoms and signs, both clinical and roentgenographic. Growth of the skull in such infants occurs in regions of least resistance, with the result being bilateral bulging of the temporal squama just about the ears and striking prominence at the bregma. Thinning of the calvarium and deeply convolutional markings are seen on radiographs in such cases. Visual loss, retardation, and seizures may later complicate this disorder, owing to the effects of chronic increased pressure on the immature brain.

In certain cases, premature cranial suture closure is part of a spectrum of anomalies giving rise to identifiable syndromes with eponymic designations. Crouzon's disease, or craniofacial dysostosis, is commonly inherited on a dominant basis, although some cases occur in the absence of a family history. Clinical features include cranial deformity, usually due to coronal synostosis, but other sutures may also be affected. In rare instances, all cranial sutures are fused at birth in the child with Crouzon's disease, leading to gross disturbances of the face and head and severe effects of increased pressure (Shiller, 1959). Facial abnormalities that are constantly present include a "parrot's beak" deformity of the nose, maxillary hypoplasia, protrusion of the mandible, and exophthalmos, often associated with divergent strabismus (Dodge et al., 1959). Untreated patients are susceptible to a variety of problems secondary to intracranial hypertension or compression of the orbital contents and optic nerves. A bizarre but rare disorder with features somewhat similar to those of Crouzon's disease is referred to as Kleeblattschädel, or cloverleaf skull (Angle et al., 1967; Feingold et al., 1969). Intrauterine synostosis of multiple or all cranial sutures in concert with hydrocephalus accounts for the grotesque characteristics of the child with this severe malformation. At birth, the infant exhibits advanced exophthalmos, hypertelorism, bulging in the areas of the closed anterior fontanel and the squamosal sutures, and downward displacement of the ears. In some cases, facial bone deformities are similar to those of Crouzon's disease, suggesting a possible relationship of Kleeblattschädel to hereditary craniofacial dysostosis (Hall et al., 1972). The anomaly has also been associated with the skeletal changes of thanatophoric dwarfism (Partington et al., 1971) and with other anomalies.

Apert's syndrome, or acrocephalosyndactyly, occurs in either sporadic or familial fashion and has been claimed to be related to increased paternal age. The pattern of suture closure varies to some degree, but bilateral coronal synostosis is by far the most common (Fig. 78–12). Syndactylism of the hands and feet is the distinguishing feature of this disorder, although other anomalies may also be found. Choanal atresia or stenosis has been observed in some and can create airway problems during certain diagnostic studies unless recognized. Related syndromes have received a variety of designations, such as Carpenter's syndrome and Chotzen's syndrome, depending on the combined anomalies (Table 78–1).

Diagnosis. Craniosynostosis in the newborn or young infant is usually suspected on the basis of an abnormality of the shape of the head. The distinctive palpable and sometimes visible ridge over the prematurely closed suture is an additional aid in identification of the condition. Roentgenographic examination is confirmatory in most instances but can be misleading unless one is familiar with the possible radiographic variations. For example, trigonocephaly may be obvious from the appearance of the child and the presence of a distinctive ridge, even though the metopic suture may appear patent on radiographic examination. The metopic suture is best observed by x-ray examination in which a modified Water's view or the submental-vertex view is used. Hyperostosis and "heaping up" of a synostosed suture, in addition to a generally abnormal configuration of the skull are the most dependable x-ray findings indicative of craniosynostosis. Unaffected sutures are often disproportionately separated, reflecting compensatory effects allowing brain growth.

Several conditions must be differentiated from craniosynostosis in the newborn and young infant.

Table 78–1. Classification of Premature Cranial Suture Closure

I. "Simple" craniosynostosis
  A. Scaphocephaly—premature closure of the sagittal suture.
  B. Brachycephaly—premature closure of the coronal sutures.
  C. Oxycephaly—premature closure of all cranial sutures.
  D. Trigonocephaly—premature closure of the metopic suture.
  E. Plagiocephaly—premature closure of one coronal or lambdoidal suture.
II. Craniosynostosis with associated anomalies
  A. Crouzon's disease (craniofacial dysostosis). Premature closure of coronal or other sutures, beaked nose, maxillary hypoplasia, prognathism, exophthalmos.
  B. Kleeblattschädel (cloverleaf skull). Multiple cranial suture synostosis with hydrocephalus. Facial dysostosis and long bone anomalies in some cases.
  C. Apert's syndrome (acrocephalosyndactyly). Premature closure of coronal or other sutures, syndactylism.
  D. Carpenter's syndrome (acrocephalopolysyndactyly). Acrocephaly, peculiar facies, brachysyndactyly of fingers, polysyndactyly of toes, mental retardation, other anomalies.
  E. Chotzen's syndrome. Acrocephalosyndactyly with hypertelorism, ptosis, mental retardation.
  F. Pfeiffer syndrome. Acrocephalosyndactyly with broad thumbs and great toes, normal intellect.
  G. Trigonocephaly with hypotelorism, arhinencephaly.
III. Secondary craniosynostosis
  A. Following shunts for hydrocephalus.
  B. Early, passive sutural closure with microcephaly.
  C. Associated with metabolic disease (rickets, idiopathic hypercalcemia of infancy, hypophosphatasia).

The infant's head is frequently asymmetric because of postural effects, a condition especially likely to occur when the child lies with his head turned in one direction. This is seen with torticollis and also in developmentally retarded children who remain relatively immobile longer than normal. The result is unilateral occipital flattening, usually with some degree of flattening of the forehead on the opposite side. A small or absent anterior fontanel in the first few weeks after birth raises concern regarding either the rate of brain growth or the patency of sutures. This anomaly can occur as a normal variation or can be the result of an accessory bone arising from a separate ossifi-

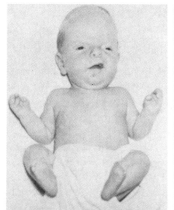 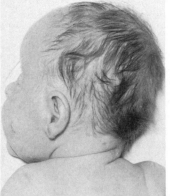 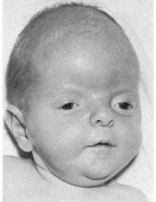

Figure 78–12. Apert's syndrome (acrocephalosyndactyly). Bilateral coronal synostosis results in a brachycephalic head shape with "high" forehead and shortened AP diameter of the skull. Note the bilateral syndactyly.

cation center in the anterior fontanel. This is called an anterior fontanel bone (Girdany and Blank, 1965) and is of no clinical significance. The size and shape of the head are normal in such infants, and sutures are patent radiographically. Microcephaly is the most commonly discussed differential diagnostic consideration with craniosynostosis but is usually easily differentiated on the basis of physical examination of the child and x-ray examination of the skull. Whereas the size of the head is abnormally small in the microcephalic child, it is the configuration that is disturbed in most cases of craniosynostosis. Microcephaly is characterized on skull radiographs by a relatively thick calvarium in many instances, without convolutional markings and with sutures that are approximated or overlapped but without bony fusion, at least in the newborn period.

Treatment. Debate has long existed about the advisability of surgical correction for craniosynostosis, the optimal time of its performance, the age at which it is no longer beneficial, and whether it is totally for cosmetic reasons or important in some cases to prevent visual loss, mental retardation, or other neurologic deficits. To some degree, the confusion is attributed to observations made years ago when craniosynostosis and microcephaly were not clearly distinguished prior to attempts at surgical intervention. Although since then certain authors have doubted the benefits of surgical treatment of craniosynostosis (Hemple, 1961; Freeman and Borkowf, 1962), the current consensus is that a properly performed linear craniectomy is of definite value if done sufficiently early (Shillito and Matson, 1968; Anderson and Geiger, 1965; Andersson and Gomes, 1968).

For the best cosmetic results, surgical treatment of craniosynostosis is usually recommended when the infant is between 4 and 8 weeks of age. Severe cases with total suture fusion and secondary increased intracranial pressure are often attacked even earlier. When surgery has not been done for either sagittal, metopic, or coronal synostosis by age 12 to 18 months, it is not likely that much can be achieved cosmetically. It is unclear whether surgery beyond 1 year of age is indicated to prevent future compromise of vision or increased intracranial pressure.

The accepted procedure for sagittal synostosis is bilateral parasagittal craniectomies and lining of the bony margins with some inert substance to prevent refusion of the edges. The procedure for a fused metopic suture is linear craniectomy through the suture itself. In addition, horizontal incisions of the frontal bone are performed across each supraorbital region from the temporal end of the coronal suture to the midline to allow expansion of the frontal bones. Fused coronal sutures are likewise attacked directly with bony excision at the site of the closed suture. When multiple synostoses are present, surgical correction is often staged, with the procedures done a week or more apart.

MEGALENCEPHALY

Megalencephaly is a disorder in which the head is enlarged because of abnormal enlargement of the brain. It occurs under a wide variety of circumstances, sometimes being present at birth but often not becoming evident until later in infancy. Megalencephaly is familial in some instances and can occur with or without other associated anomalies (Riley and Smith, 1960). Although it is frequently accompanied by developmental and mental retardation, hypotonia, or convulsions, it can occur in the absence of any evident neurologic deficit. In the newborn or young infant, megalencephaly is often difficult to differentiate from hydrocephalus by the clinical findings. However, in megalencephaly signs of increased intracranial pressure are absent, cranial sutures are not abnormally separated, and the anterior fontanel, although frequently large, is soft. Demonstration of normal or only slightly enlarged ventricles by CT scan or ultrasonographic studies will establish the diagnosis. Megalencephaly occurs in several recognized syndromes, most of which are diagnosed more readily in the older infant or child than in the neonate. In the newborn infant, megalencephaly may be associated with achondroplasia, cerebral gigantism, or the degenerative disorder referred to as "Canavan's disease." The Russell-Silver syndrome is a form of intrauterine growth retardation in which an abnormally large head is notably associated with a low birth weight (Szalay, 1963; Fuleihan et al., 1971) (Fig. 78–13). The striking discrepancy between head size and body size of children with this disorder raises the consideration of hydrocephalus, but the large head is the result of a relatively large brain. Other features often observed with the Russell-Silver syndrome include limb asymmetry, triangular shape of the face, and elevated urinary gonadotropins.

HYDROCEPHALUS

The term *hydrocephalus* includes a group of conditions associated with ventricular enlargement. The amount of cerebrospinal fluid (CSF) is increased and in most cases is under increased pressure. Hydrocephalus is usually the consequence of obstructed CSF drainage. The variation in the pathologic picture, including the nature and the extent of CSF pathway dilatation and the amount of brain damage, depends primarily on the site of obstruction, whereas the clinical evolution depends on the time at which obstruction develops.

An account of the embryology, physiology, and anatomy of CSF dynamics and ventricular and subarachnoid spaces is outside the scope of this text. The interested reader is referred to the 1980 review by Fishman.

Etiology and Pathology.   Hydrocephalus occurs whenever there is a disequilibrium between production and absorption of CSF. Any block in the CSF pathway from the foramina of Monro to the tubular arachnoid villi of the subarachnoid space results in CSF under increased pressure and dilation of ventricular and subarachnoid spaces. Therefore, with one possible exception, all hydrocephalic conditions are obstructive. Obstructive hydrocephalus is conventionally divided into noncommunicating and communicating types. In the former, the obstructive site is within the ventricular cavity, including the outlet foramina of the fourth ventricle. In the latter, the obstruction occurs distally to the fourth ventricle foramina (Magendie and Luschka), in the cisterns or cerebral subarachnoid spaces.

Regardless of the site of the obstruction, it is the arterial pulse thrust of the choroid plexus that is responsible for compressing the ventricular wall, enlarging the ventricular cavity, and producing parenchymal disruption. The pulse thrust increases with increasing mean CSF pressure and splits the ventricular ependymal lining (Milhorat, 1970). This allows free and continuing transependymal flow of CSF into white matter, producing a spongy, atrophic, and edematous dissolution of nerve fibers and swelling of gray matter neurons and astrocytes (Weller and Shulman, 1972; Rubin et al., 1976). It is still unclear to what extent normally nonfunctioning CSF drainage routes, including the choroid plexuses and the periventricular capillaries, become operative with increased CSF pressure and contribute to stabilization of pressure in the human hydrocephalic (Cutler et al., 1973). In the newborn, particularly the premature, the paucity of cerebral myelin and any preexisting asphyxial tissue damage frequently allow ventricular dilation to occur at normal CSF pressures (Hill and Volpe, 1981).

Noncommunicating hydrocephalus is most likely caused by abnormalities in which the pathways are most narrow, notably the aqueduct of Sylvius, the fourth ventricle, or the foramina of Monro (Table 78–2).

The most common site of intraventricular obstruction in infants with congenital hydrocephalus is within the aqueduct. The underlying pathology may be one of several types, separable in most instances only by histologic examination. Forking (''atresia'') of the aqueduct represents a nonpatent system in which the aqueduct at various levels consists of multiple channels lined by ependyma that may or may not communicate with one another and that are separated by neural tissue. This lesion may occur as an isolated abnormality causing hydrocephalus or may be associated with other anomalies, especially meningomyelocele and the Arnold-Chiari malformation.

In stenosis of the aqueduct, the aqueduct is his-

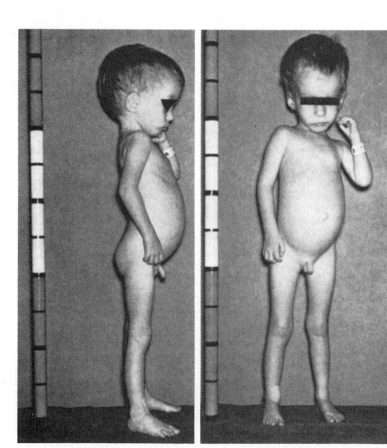

Figure 78–13.   Abnormally large head compared to body size in a child with the Russell-Silver syndrome. Such children are often erroneously suspected of having hydrocephalus but can be identified appropriately by the low birth weight for gestational age and the characteristic facial features. Striking limb asymmetry is often present. (Szalay, G. C.: J. Pediatr. *63*:622, 1963.)

Table 78–2. Classification and Types of Hydrocephalus

Noncommunicating (intraventricular obstructive)
1. Maldevelopments of the aqueduct (stenosis, forking ["atresia"], septal defects, gliosis).
2. Obstruction due to mass lesions (neoplasm, cyst, hematoma, aneurysm of the vein of Galen).
3. Obstruction secondary to exudate, hemorrhage, or parasites.
4. Obstruction of the fourth ventricle outlet foramina (Dandy-Walker syndrome, arachnoiditis).

Communicating (extraventricular obstructive)
1. Postinfectious, posthemorrhagic, or developmental adhesions of basilar cisterns or surface subarachnoid space.
2. Arachnoid villi obstruction by erythrocytes.
3. Communicating hydrocephalus with the Arnold-Chiari malformation.
4. Developmental failure of arachnoid villi (presumptive).
5. Hypovitaminosis A (experimental animals).

Communicating hydrocephalus due to excessive cerebrospinal fluid formation (choroid plexus papilloma)

tologically normal but abnormally small in caliber. There is an absence of excessive subependymal glia and of other evidence of an inflammatory reaction. Little is known of the origin of this disorder. It may represent a form of hydrocephalus that is slowly progressive or may even remain silent until later in childhood. Gliosis of the aqueduct is generally considered a postinflammatory process, perhaps secondary to an intrauterine viral infection. A variety of experimental viral infections have been shown to produce structural abnormalities of the aqueduct. In particular, Johnson and Johnson in 1968 were able to induce hydrocephalus due to aqueductal stenosis in hamsters by intracerebral injection of mumps virus. Fluorescent antibody staining indicated virus growth to be limited to the ependymal cells. That this observation may have applicability to the clinical situation was shown by the presence of a cell-mediated immune response to mumps virus in two infants with aqueductal stenosis and in one third of newborns with myelomeningoceles (Thompson and Glasgow, 1980).

Microscopic examination of the brain shows the aqueduct to be narrowed or occluded by overgrowth of ependymal cells and the ependymal lining to be replaced by gliosis. A variant, also postinflammatory in nature, appears as a septal obstruction at the caudal end of the aqueduct.

The Dandy-Walker syndrome is an unusual form of hydrocephalus in the newborn infant. Although head enlargement with this condition may be obvious at birth, in some cases it does not become apparent until months later. Speculation continues with regard to the pathogenesis of this type of malformation, but at present it is considered to represent a defect of neural tube closure at the cerebellar level, with atresia of the outlet foramina of Luschka and Magendie representing only one of several associated developmental defects (Friede, 1975; Hart et al., 1972).

The end result of these lesions is a marked cystic distention of the fourth ventricle with lateral displacement of the cerebellar hemispheres. The vermis of the cerebellum is hypoplastic, being represented by only a thin sheet of tissue roofing the distended fourth ventricle. Other cerebral anomalies are seen in some cases and include agenesis of the corpus callosum and porencephaly. The Dandy-Walker syndrome is suspected clinically in the infant with head enlargement in whom the greatest degree of enlargement is from the region of the external ears to the occiput. Diagnosis becomes more probable when an abnormal degree of transillumination is observed over the region of the posterior fossa but not elsewhere. The diagnosis is confirmed by CT scan.

The Chiari malformation alone or in combination with other anomalies accounts for 40 per cent of all cases of hydrocephaly in children (Laurence, 1959). Whether the obstruction is caused by fourth-ventricle block secondary to atresia of the outlet foramina, aqueductal stenosis, or herniation with obliteration of subarachnoid pathways around the brain stem or higher remains in dispute.

A variety of other lesions may cause noncommunicating hydrocephalus in the newborn or small infant (Table 78–2). These include neoplasms within the posterior fossa or of the choroid plexus, arachnoid cysts, aneurysms of the vein of Galen, and a posterior fossa subdural hematoma secondary to mechanical trauma of the infant (see Chapter 77).

Communicating hydrocephalus represents about 30 per cent of all cases of childhood hydrocephalus. Once the CSF leaves the foramina of the fourth ventricle and enters the cisterns, it must progress into the cerebral and cerebellar subarachnoid spaces. Drainage is jeopardized if the cisterns or the arachnoid villi over the cerebral cortex are obstructed by thickened arachnoid or meninges. This may be the result of intracranial hemorrhage or bacterial meningitis.

In premature infants, intraventricular hemorrhage is secondary to neonatal asphyxia. Subarachnoid hemorrhage is more commonly seen in term infants and is produced by mechanical trauma. The pathogenesis and pathology of these conditions are discussed more fully in Chapter 77. As a rule when hydrocephalus develops early following intracranial hemorrhage in the neonate, the site of obstruction is usually the aqueduct or, less fequently, the foramina of Monro (noncommunicating hydrocephalus). When the condition evolves later, it is related to an obliterative arachnoiditis that occurs most commonly in the posterior fossa, where the blood tends to collect (Larroche, 1972). Communicating hydrocephalus secondary to the congenital absence of arachnoid villi may be more common than has been reported (Guitierrez et al., 1975).

Infections, including toxoplasmosis, cytomegalovirus disease, and syphilis, account for congenital hydrocephalus in a small proportion of cases. Another small percentage of infants with hydrocephalus due to aqueductal stenosis inherit the disease as a sex-linked recessive trait (Bickers and Adams, 1949; Jansen, 1975; Edwards et al., 1961). Except for the clustering of affected males within a family and the maldevelopment of thumbs in many of the cases, this form of hydrocephalus is not distinguishable from many other types in the neonate.

Aside from this condition, which presents the only known example in humans of an isolated structural abnormality caused by a single gene, the genetic factors operative in the etiology of hydrocephalus have not been clarified. Among siblings of patients with primary congenital hydrocephalus without spine defects, the prevalence of anencephaly and spina bifida cystica has been estimated to be five times higher than the expected incidence in the general population (Lorber and De, 1970). The empirical risk of a major congenital malformation in subsequent offspring following the birth of a child with congenital hydrocephalus is approximately one in 25 (Lorber and De, 1970).

The only recognized exception to the rule that hydrocephalus results from obstruction either within or without the ventricular system occurs with the rare choroid plexus papilloma. Ventricular enlargement in infants with this tumor has been attributed to cerebrospinal fluid secretion from the lesion in excess of the system's absorptive capabilities (Matson and Crofton, 1960). Indeed, Eisenberg and coworkers found that the preoperative rate of CSF production in a child with such a tumor was about four times the normal rate, a value known to exceed normal absorptive capacity of the subarachnoid space (Mann et al., 1978). However, it has also been argued that hydrocephalus in this condition occurs as a consequence of arachnoidal adhesions, obstruction of the subarachnoid spaces secondary to an elevated CSF protein, and frequent bleeding from the tumor (Laurence et al., 1961).

Clinical Aspects. Symptoms and signs observed vary, depending on the age of the child, the acuteness of onset of hydrocephalus, and the rapidity of its progression. In the newborn period and in early infancy, the head grows at an abnormal rate, so that the infant is macrocephalic within 1 to 2 months, if not at birth. Occasionally, the head is so large at term that normal birth is impossible unless the head is decompressed by insertion of a needle into the ventricle. As a rule, infants with intraventricular obstructive hydrocephalus show more rapid progression of head enlargement and other clinical signs than do those with communicating hydrocephalus. In some instances, the baby shows no abnormality of behavior, feeds well, and progresses adequately in motor skills, with the only sign that a medical problem exists being the abnormally rapid rate of growth of the head. More often, the infant with congenital hydrocephalus is irritable, feeds poorly, has recurrent vomiting, and

shows inadequate weight gain. Seizures are not common in infants with hydrocephalus, and papilledema is infrequent, even in those with marked head enlargement. If the condition proceeds unarrested, optic atrophy may eventually develop. The infant with hydrocephalus resulting from aqueductal obstruction from compression by an aneurysm of the great vein of Galen may show signs of high-output cardiac failure. Heart failure in the absence of evidence of internal cardiac anomalies plus a loud bruit over the scalp suggest this unusual condition.

Developmental motor skills are occasionally delayed, but some hydrocephalic infants progress in a remarkably normal fashion during the first year. Hydrocephalus of mild degree does not account for profound developmental delay by 6 to 12 months of age unless the retardation is due to the disorder that caused the hydrocephalus. As hydrocephalus progresses, the disproportion between head size and size of the facial structures becomes more apparent. Distention of scalp veins and enlargement and bulging of the anterior fontanel reflect elevated intracranial pressure. Increased muscle tone and hyperreflexia in the lower limbs have been attributed to stretching of fibers arising in the parasagittal area that must project around the angle of the lateral ventricle to enter the internal capsule en route to supply the legs (Yakovlev, 1946). These fibers could be affected earlier, with progressive ventricular enlargement, than the descending fibers to the upper limbs, which arise more laterally on the motor strip. Late signs in hydrocephalic infants include the "setting sun" sign and the "cerebral cry," the latter being characterized by its brevity and high-pitched, shrill quality. The "setting sun" sign is believed to be due to pressure of the suprapineal recess of the third ventricle upon the mesencephalic tectum. The phenomenon may, however, also be elicited in normal infants under 4 weeks of age by a sudden change in the position of the head and in infants up to 20 or even 40 weeks of age by removal of a bright light that has been placed in front of their eyes (Cernerud, 1975). A variety of other ocular signs may occur in the infant with congenital hydrocephalus, although lack of cooperation and irritability make analysis difficult. Internal strabismus is occasionally observed, and limited vertical gaze may be present. Horizontal nystagmus also may be evident.

Diagnosis. The most important aspect of the physical examination of an infant who is believed to have hydrocephalus is accurate measurement of the occipitofrontal circumference of the head. A single measurement is useful and may strongly suggest the existence of some form of disease state; however, serial determinations at periodic intervals with results plotted on a graph are of greater value. Attention should be paid to any change in the rate of growth, especially any precipitous increase in head size.

Transillumination of the skull should be performed whenever hydrocephalus is considered (Shurtleff, 1975) (see Chapter 76). Abnormalities of transillumination in hydrocephalus indicate that the cerebral mantle is less than 1 cm in depth. In addition to indicating advanced hydrocephalus or "hydranencephaly," abnormal transillumination may be observed in infants with subdural effusions, scalp edema, or porencephaly. Arachnoid cysts over the convexity of the brain may also be demonstrable by transillumination (Anderson and Landing, 1966). An infant with the Dandy-Walker syndrome may exhibit abnormal transillumination adjacent to the dilated fourth ventricle. Care must be taken not to overinterpret the findings with small premature infants because of the extreme thinness of the skull overlying the subarachnoid space characteristic of such infants (Vyhmeister et al., 1977).

In the Chiari type 2 malformation, 50 per cent of neonates display craniolacunia on radiographic examination of the skull (Fig. 78–8). Roentgenograms of the spine are indicated in any evaluation of infantile hydrocephalus. These may reveal spina bifida occulta or abnormalities of the cervical vertebrae.

CT scans and ultrasonography have enormously simplified the evaluation of the hydrocephalic infant and are unassociated with patient morbidity and study failures inherent in air encephalography and angiography. A CT scan demonstrates not only the size and position of the ventricles but also the width of the subarachnoid spaces at the base of the brain and over its convexity. Aqueductal stenosis can be demonstrated by the dilation of the lateral and third ventricles and the presence of a normal-sized or small fourth ventricle. One can diagnose the Dandy-Walker syndrome by observing an enlarged fourth ventricle and a large posterior fossa cyst. Communicating hydrocephalus manifests itself by dilation of the entire ventricular system and the subarachnoid spaces at the base of the brain and over the lower portion of the convexity (Naidich et al., 1976). In contrast to diffuse cerebral atrophy (hydrocephalus ex vacuo), communicating hydrocephalus is usually associated with an absence or narrowing of the subarachnoid spaces over the higher portions of the convexity of the brain. The possibility of the presence of tumors or larger arteriovenous malformations can be excluded by a CT scan supplemented by intravenous injection of contrast material (Fig. 78–14).

Ultrasonography is of invaluable assistance in the diagnosis of hydrocephalus and, more importantly, in the evaluation of the *effectiveness* of surgery or other therapeutic measures (Shields and Manger, 1983).

Dynamic information concerning CSF clearance can be obtained by the use of walter-soluble, nonionic metrizamide. The dye is injected through the lumbar subarachnoid space, and CT scans are obtained immediately and after 24 hours. Normally, the dye clears from the ventricular and subarachnoid spaces within 24 hours by penetrating through the brain. In hydrocephalus, there is delayed brain penetration of the dye, evidenced by its persistence in ventricles and subarachnoid spaces beyond 24 hours (Drayer and Rosenbaum, 1978).

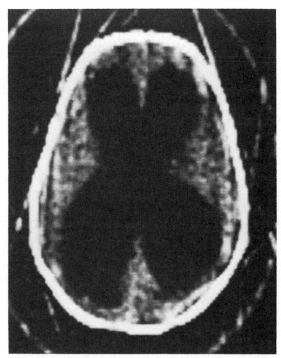

Figure 78–14. Computerized axial tomography (EMI scan). Advanced hydrocephalus in a 2-month-old infant. Horizontal plane with frontal portion of the skull at the top. The skull is dense white, and the lateral ventricles, which are almost symmetrically distended, are black.

Treatment. Despite remarkable advances in the comprehension of the physiology and pathology of hydrocephalus, our ability to provide consistently successful treatment has not yet been achieved. Medical therapy has offered relatively little, and the multitudinous surgical procedures that have been developed are evidence of the lack of complete acceptance of any single approach. Although an attitude of total pessimism is unwarranted, the currently available surgical treatment of the infant with progressive hydrocephalus must be recognized to be less than ideal and to be characterized by a variety of potentially frustrating and perplexing complications.

The desirability of surgical treatment for infants with congenital hydrocephalus for whom the cause cannot be removed requires consideration of the expected benefits from treatment when compared with the natural course of the illness. Laurence and Coates in 1962 studied 182 untreated patients reported over 20 years and found that 89 (48 per cent) had died and 81 (44 per cent) were considered to have arrested spontaneously. Of the "arrested" group, 38 per cent were judged to have IQ's of 85 or above. In 1963, Yashon reported 58 patients with unoperated infantile hydrocephalus, 23 of whom had a fatal outcome. Of the survivors, 31 were considered "arrested." The concept of spontaneous arrest of infantile hydrocephalus, however, is subject to varied meanings depending on how the term is defined and what methods are used to demonstrate its occurrence. To have significance, arrest of hydrocephalus should mean that further growth of the head does not occur, at least until the rest of the body has caught up with the head size from the relative standpoint. Furthermore, arrest of the process should allow restoration of the ventricular size toward normal, with re-establishment of the cerebral mantle. Assigning the designation of "arrested hydrocephalus" to a neurologically devastated child whose head has reached enormous proportions but then ceases to grow is artificial, is probably in error, and dilutes the potential meaning of "significant arrest." If reasonably rigid criteria are adhered to, spontaneous and permanent arrest of progressive hydrocephalus in infancy appears to be an infrequent event (Foltz and Shurtleff, 1963; Lorber and Zachary, 1968). In the series of Hemmer and Bohm, only 9 per cent of shunts placed in infants with communicating hydrocephalus or hydrocephalus associated with myelomeningoceles could be removed. In summary, when comparing the outcome of untreated infantile hydrocephalus patients with that of those managed surgically, there is little doubt that the results are better in the treated groups, in whom the immediate success rate for control of hydrocephalus is in the range of 70 per cent (Yashon, 1963).

When surgical treatment of the infant or child with progressive hydrocephalus is necessary, the method selected depends on many factors, including the site of the obstruction, certain characteristics of the ventricular fluid, and the experience with different surgical procedures. In some cases, procedures of a temporary nature are indicated when it is suspected that the more conventional shunt operations will be unsuccessful. For example, a child recovering from meningitis or subarachnoid hemorrhage complicated by communicating hydrocephalus can be maintained by the use of a ventriculostomy reservoir until a more permanent shunt can be inserted (Rickham and Penn, 1965). The high-protein–containing ventricular fluid often present in such cases will likely block the valves of the more permanent shunts, requiring repeated revisions. Regardless, treatment of infantile hydrocephalus must be assumed to be surgical in most cases because medical measures have not been adequate.

Surgical treatment of progressive hydrocephalus in infancy has included either one of the so-called "physiologic" operations of third ventriculostomy and choroid plexectomy or the more commonly used shunting procedures. The first widely recognized shunting procedure for hydrocephalus was developed by Torkildsen in 1939 and is known as ventriculocisternostomy. The Torkildsen shunt drains fluid from one lateral ventricle to the cisterna magna, and thus its use is restricted to hydrocephalus of the noncommunicating type. It remains of value for the older child or adult with an obstructive process in the posterior fossa, but, for technical reasons, it is not applicable to the infant. Shunts from the ventricle or spinal subarachnoid space to almost every conceivable body cavity have been designed. Currently, the treatment of choice is to drain the CSF from the lateral ventricle into the peritoneal cavity. For primary shunts in communicating and noncommunicating hydrocephalus in infants, this has been our exclusive recommendation. Complicating shunt-induced infections, such as meningitis and ventriculitis, appear in approximately 5 per cent of the cases. Their current treatment was reviewed by Rennels and Wald in 1980.

Several types of valves are widely used, and newer ones are under investigation (Sells and Shurtleff, 1977). The Holter valve consists of two stainless steel check valves connected by silicone tubing. The Pudenz-Heyer-Schulte valve is a plastic bubble pump placed under the scalp, with its distal end connected to the slit valve. The latter apparatus can be "pumped" to check for patency and to clear partial obstructions. The Holter valve can be attached to various types of reservoirs that are placed in the burr hole to measure ventricular pressure or to instill antibiotics.

In considering the prognosis of the shunted child in terms of mental development and neurologic sequelae, the primary pathology, the degree of hydrocephalus prior to shunting, and the postshunt course must all be borne in mind.

Ventriculoperitoneal shunts are applicable to either communicating or noncommunicating hydrocephalus but are plagued by the predisposition of the peritoneal end of the device to become repeatedly obstructed (Scott et al., 1955; Jackson and Snodgrass, 1955). Except for the need for periodic revision, ventriculoperitoneal shunts are far less often beset by complications than are the vascular shunts.

HYDRANENCEPHALY

Hydranencephaly is a purely descriptive term referring to a condition in which the greater portion of both the cerebral hemispheres and the corpus striatum are reduced to membranous sacs composed of glial tissue covered by intact meninges, encompassing a cavity filled with clear, protein-rich CSF. (Fig. 78–15). The basal ganglia, brain stem, and cerebellum are preserved but may reveal a variety of morphologic abnormalities.

There are at least four different pathogenic mechanisms involved in hydranencephaly. First, it has been argued that hydranencephaly is a type of hydrocephalus that has run its course in utero. The presence of preserved ependyma and aqueductal stenosis in some cases supports this as one possible mechanism. In other instances, hydranencephaly has been the consequence of intrauterine infections or

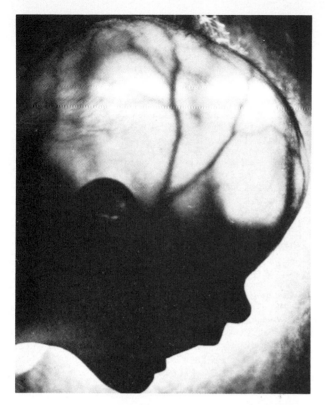

Figure 78–15. Hydranencephaly. Transillumination causes the skull to light up and to show the blood vessels in sharp relief. In this infant, the vault of the skull is not unduly enlarged. (From Laurence, K. M.: Congenital abnormalities in infancy. Oxford, Blackwell Scientific Publications, 1963.)

1978). If the child survives beyond 2 or 3 months, expected developmental landmarks are not achieved and the evidence of spasticity becomes more apparent. Autonomic dysfunction is sometimes manifested by wide swings in body temperature, in part related to the environmental temperature (Appenzeller et al., 1970). In most of these infants, electroencephalography reveals markedly depressed voltages or even a virtually flat tracing. Ventricular fluid may be clear and have a normal protein content or xanthochromic and show a marked increase in protein, again depending on the cause of the process. Many infants with these disorders characterized by severe cerebral destruction die early in infancy, whereas a few survive for remarkably long periods of time. Of 28 children with "hydranencephaly" reviewed by Hunziker, only nine survived beyond 3 months of age.

MÖBIUS SYNDROME

This condition, first described in 1887 by Chisholm, was delineated a year later by Möbius. It is characterized by congenital paralysis of the facial muscles and impairment of lateral gaze. The syndrome results from diverse causes. Pathologic lesions include complete or partial absence of the facial nuclei, dysplasia of the facial musculature, and hypoplasia of the facial nerve. The entity has also been seen in a variety of conditions in which there is progressive disease of muscle, anterior horn cell, or peripheral neurons. In other instances, there has been an absence, faulty attachment, or fibrosis of the extraocular muscles; electromyographic studies have suggested the added presence of a supranuclear lesion (Pitner et al., 1965).

Most cases of Möbius syndrome show a variable degree of unilateral or asymmetric or symmetric bilateral facial paralysis, with an inability to abduct the eyes beyond the midline (Henderson, 1939). Occasionally, the weakness may be restricted to portions (e.g., quadrants) of the face. Atrophy of the tongue, paralysis of the soft palate or masseters, congenital club foot, deafness, or a mild spastic diplegia may also be present. Because of bulbar deficits, the disorder in language communication is far greater than general intelligence would suggest (Meyerson and Foushee, 1978). The condition is nonprogressive but must be distinguished from myotonic dystrophy, or congenital muscular dystrophy (see Chapter 80).

other gestational insults. The condition may also develop as a genetically determined defect in vascular ontogenesis or as the outcome of vascular occlusion of both internal carotid arteries or their main branches. A small number of cases probably result from a severe developmental anomaly in which normal formation of the cerebral mantle has not occurred (Yakovlev and Wadsworth, 1946). Thus, hydranencephaly should not be considered a diagnostic entity but the end result of one of many destructive processes in the cerebrum occurring during the prenatal period or the birth process or even postnatally.

The clinical manifestations observed in infants with hydranencephaly are variable. Although children with these disorders may appear intact to the mother, careful examination by one familiar with neurologic activity of the neonate will reveal abnormalities in most. These include excessive sleepiness and irritability manifested by continuous crying during the waking state. Feeding problems are usual, often because of lethargy and poor sucking ability. Tremulousness of limbs and increased muscle tone are frequently observed along with enhanced deep tendon reflexes. Nystagmus may be excessive, and optic atrophy is common. The normal neonatal reflexes, such as the grasp, Moro, and stepping reflexes, can usually be elicited but become abnormal because of their persistence beyond the expected time of disappearance (Halsey et al., 1968; Aylward et al.,

REFERENCES

Adeloye, A., Singh, S. P., and Odeku, E. L.: Stridor, myelomeningocele, and hydrocephalus in a child. Arch. Neurol. *23*:271, 1970.

Alter, M.: Anencephalus, hydrocephalus, and spina bifida. Arch. Neurol. 7:411, 1962.

Anderson, F. M.: Occult spinal dysraphism. A series of 73 cases. Pediatrics 55:826, 1975.

Anderson, F. M., and Geiger, L.: Craniosynostosis. A survey of 204 cases. J. Neurosurg. 22:229, 1965.

Anderson, F. M., and Landing, B. H.: Cerebral arachnoid cysts in infants. J. Pediatr. 69:88, 1966.

Anderson, F. M., Gwinn, J. L., and Todt, J. C.: Trigonocephaly. Identity and surgical treatment. J. Neurosurg. 19:723, 1962.

Andersson, H., and Gomes, S. P.: Craniosynostosis. Review of the literature and indications for surgery. Acta Pediatr. Scand. 57:47, 1968.

Angle, C. R., McIntire, M. S., and Moore, R. C.: Cloverleaf skull: Kleeblattschädel-deformity syndrome. Am. J. Dis. Child. 114:198, 1967.

Appenzeller, O., Snyder, R., and Kornfeld, M.: Autonomic failure in hydrencephaly. J. Neurol. Neurosurg. Psychiatry 33:532, 1970.

Avery, G. B., Meneses, L., and Lodge, A.: The clinical significance of "measurement microcephaly." Am. J. Dis. Child. 123:214, 1972.

Aylward, G. P., et al.: Behavioral and neurological characteristics of a hydranencephalic infant. Dev. Med. Child. Neurol. 20:211, 1978.

Barr, M., Hanson, J. W., Currey, K., et al.: Holoprosencephaly in infants of diabetic mothers. J. Pediatr. 102:565, 1983.

Bickers, D. S., and Adams, R. D.: Hereditary stenosis of the aqueduct of Sylvius as a cause of hydrocephalus. Brain 72:246, 1949.

Blaauw, G.: Defect in posterior arch of atlas in myelomeningocele. Dev. Med. Child. Neurol. 25(Suppl.):113, 1971.

Black, P. McL.: Selective treatment of children with myelomeningocele. Neurosurgery 5:334, 1979.

Blumenfeld, R., and Skolnik, E. M.: Intranasal encephaloceles. Arch. Otolaryngol. 82:527, 1965.

Byrd, S. E., et al.: Computer tomography in the evaluation of encephaloceles in infants and children. J. Comp. Assist. Tomog. 2:81, 1978.

Cernerud, L.: The setting-sun eye phenomenon in infancy. Dev. Med. Child. Neurol. 17:447, 1975.

Chisholm, J. J.: Congenitale Lähmung des 6. and 7. Hirnnervenpaares bei einem Erwachsenen. Arch. f. Augenheilk. 17:414, 1887.

Coffey, V. P., and Jessop, W. J. E.: A study of 137 cases of anencephaly. Br. J. Prev. Soc. Med. 11:174, 1957.

Cohen, M. M.: An etiologic and nosologic overview of craniosynostosis syndromes. Birth Defects 11:137, 1975.

Collaborative Study. Amniotic fluid acetylcholinesterase electrophoresis as a secondary test in the diagnosis of anencephaly and open spina bifida in early pregnancy. Lancet 2:321, 1981.

Currarino, G., and Silverman, F. N.: Orbital hypotelorism, arhinencephaly, and trigonocephaly. Radiology 74:206, 1960.

Cutler, R. W., et al.: Overproduction of CSF in communicating hydrocephalus. Neurology 23:1, 1973.

Dale, A. J. D.: Diastematomyelia. Arch. Neurol. 20:309, 1969.

DeMyer, W.: The median cleft face syndrome. Neurology 17:961, 1967.

DeMyer, W.: Classification of cerebral malformations. Birth Defects Original Article Series. 7:78, 1971.

Dodge, H. W., Wood, M. W., and Kennedy, R. L. J.: Craniofacial dysostosis: Crouzon's disease. Pediatrics 23:98, 1959.

Donn, S. M., and Philip, A. G. S.: Early increase in intracranial pressure in preterm infants. Pediatrics 61:904, 1978.

Drayer, B. P., and Rosenbaum, A. E.: Pediatric metrizamide CT cisternography: cerebro-spinal fluid circulation and hydrocephalus. Neurology 28:71, 1978.

Drummond, M. B., and Donaldson, A. A.: Air, Myodil and Conray studies in the hydrocephalus of myelomeningocele. Dev. Med. Child. Neurol. 16(Suppl. 32):131, 1974.

Edwards, J. H., Norman, R. M., and Roberts, J. M.: Sex-linked hydrocephalus: report of a family with 15 affected members. Arch. Dis. Child. 36:481, 1961.

Eisenberg, H. M., McComb, J. G., and Lorenzo, A. V.: Cerebrospinal fluid overproduction and hydrocephalus associated with choroid plexus papilloma. J. Neurosurg. 40:381, 1974.

Emery, J. L.: Deformity of the aqueduct of Sylvius in children with hydrocephalus and myelomeningocele. Dev. Med. Child. Neurol. 16(suppl. 32):40, 1974.

Emery, J. L., and Kalhan, S. C.: The pathology of exencephalus. Dev. Med. Child Neurol. 12(suppl.):51, 1970.

Feingold, M., O'Connor, J. F., Berkman, M., and Darling, D. B.: Kleeblattschädel syndrome. Am. J. Dis. Child. 118:589, 1969.

Fisch, R. O., Doeden, D., Lansky, L. L., and Anderson, J. A.: Maternal phenylketonuria. Detrimental effects on embryogenesis and fetal development. Am. J. Dis. Child. 118:847, 1969.

Fishman, R. A.: Cerebrospinal Fluid in Diseases of the Nervous System. Philadelphia, W. B. Saunders Co., 1980.

Fitzsimmons, J. S.: Laryngeal stridor and respiratory obstruction associated with meningomyelocele. Arch. Dis. Child. 40:687, 1965.

Foltz, E. L., and Shurtleff, D. B.: Five-year comparative study of hydrocephalus in children with and without operation (113 cases). J. Neurosurg. 20:1064, 1963.

Fowler, G. W., and Dumars, K. W.: Cutis aplasia and cerebral malformation. Pediatrics 52:861, 1973.

Frankenburg, W. K., Duncan, B. R., Coffelt, R. W., Koch, R., Coldwell, J. G., and Son, C. D.: Maternal phenylketonuria: implications for growth and development. J. Pediatr. 73:560, 1968.

Freeman, J. M., and Borkowf, S.: Craniostenosis. Review of the literature and report of thirty-four cases. Pediatrics 30:57, 1962.

Friede, R. L.: Developmental Neuropathology. New York, Springer-Verlag, 1975.

Fuleihan, D. S., Der Kaloustian, V. M., and Najjar, S. S.: The Russell-Silver syndrome. Report of three siblings. J. Pediatr. 78:654, 1971.

Gardner, E., O'Rahilly, R., and Prolo, D.: The Dandy-Walker and Arnold-Chiari malfunction: clinical, developmental and teratological considerations. Arch. Neurol. 32:393, 1975.

Gardner, W. J.: Hydrodynamic mechanism of syringomyelia: its relationship to myelocele. J. Neurol. Neurosurg. Psychiatry 28:247, 1965.

Girdany, B. R., and Blank, E.: Anterior fontanel bone. Am. J. Roentgenol. 95:148, 1965.

Guitierrez, Y., Friede, R. L., and Kaliney, W. J.: Agenesis of arachnoid granulations and its relationship to communicating hydrocephalus. J. Neurosurg. 43:553, 1975.

Guthkelch, A. N.: Occipital cranium bifidum. Arch. Dis. Child. 45:104, 1970.

Hall, B. D., Smith, D. W., and Shiller, J. G.: Kleeblattschädel (cloverleaf) syndrome: Severe form of Crouzon's disease? J. Pediatr. 80:526, 1972.

Halsey, J. H., Jr., Allen, N., and Chamberlin, H. R.: Chronic decerebrate state in infancy. Neurologic observations in long surviving cases of hydranencephaly. Arch. Neurol. 19:339, 1968.

Hart, N. M., Malamud, N., and Ellis, W. G.: The Dandy-Walker syndrome: a clinicopathological study based on 28 cases. Neurology 22:771, 1972.

Hemmer, R., and Böhm, B.: Once a shunt, always a shunt? Dev. Med. Child. Neurol. 37(suppl.):69, 1976.

Hemple, D. J., Harris, L. E., Svien, H. J., and Holman, C. B.: Craniosynostosis involving the sagittal suture only: guilt by association? J. Pediatr. 58:342, 1961.

Henderson, J. L.: The congenital facial diplegia syndrome: clinical features, pathology and etiology. Brain 62:381, 1939.

Hendrick, E. B.: On diastematomyelia. Prog. Neurol. Surg. 4:277, 1971.

Hide, D. W., Williams, H. P., and Ellis, H. L.: The outlook for the child with a myelomeningocele for whom early surgery was considered inadvisable. Dev. Med. Child. Neurol. 14:304, 1972.

Hill, A., and Volpe, J. J.: Normal pressure hydrocephalus in the newborn. Pediatrics 68:623, 1981.

Hodgman, J. E., Mathies, A. W., and Levan, N. E.: Congenital scalp defects in twin sisters. Am. J. Dis. Child. 110:293, 1965.

Holtz, A., Borman, G., and Li, C. P.: Hydrocephalus in mice infected with polyoma virus. Proc. Soc. Exper. Biol. Med. 121:1196, 1966.

Hullin, D. A., et al.: Amniotic fluid cholinesterase measurement as a rapid method for the exclusion of fetal neural-tube defects. Lancet 2:325, 1981.

Hunziker, K.: Ueber einen Fall von Hydranencephalie. Mschr. Psychiat. Neurol. 114:129, 1974.

Ingraham, F. E., Alexander, E., and Matson, D. D.: Clinical studies in craniosynostosis; analysis of fifty cases and description of a method of surgical treatment. Surgery 24:518, 1948.

Jackson, I. J., and Snodgrass, W.: Peritoneal shunts in the treatment of hydrocephalus, 4 year study of 62 patients. J. Neurosurg. 12:216, 1955.

Jansen, J.: Sex-linked hydrocephalus. Dev. Med. Child. Neurol. 17:633, 1975.

Johnson, R. T., and Johnson, K. P.: Hydrocephalus following viral infection. The pathology of aqueductal stenosis developing after experimental mumps virus infection. J. Neuropathol. Exper. Neurol. 27:591, 1968.

Johnsonbaugh, R. E., Light, I. J., and Sutherland, J. M.: Congenital scalp defects in father and son. Am. J. Dis. Child. 110:297, 1965.

Kirsch, W. M., et al.: Laryngeal palsy in association with myelomeningocele, hydrocephalus and the Arnold-Chiari malformation. J. Neurosurg. 28:207, 1968.

Kosnik, E. J., and Sayers, M. P.: Congenital scalp defects: aplasia cutis congenita. J. Neurosurg. 42:32, 1975.

Larroche, J. C.: Post-haemorrhagic hydrocephalus in infancy: anatomical study. Biol. Neonate 20:287, 1972.

Laurence, K. M.: The pathology of hydrocephalus. Ann. Roy. Coll. Surg. Engl. 24:388, 1959.

Laurence, K. M., and Coates, S.: The natural history of hydrocephalus. Detailed analysis of 182 unoperated cases. Arch. Dis. Child. 37:345, 1962.

Laurence, K. M., Hoare, R. D., and Till, K.: The diagnosis of the choroid plexus papilloma of the lateral ventricle. Brain 84:628, 1961.

Laurence, K. M., and Tew, B. J.: Natural history of spina bifida cystica and cranium bifidum cysticum. Arch. Dis. Child. 46:127, 1971.

Lemire, R. J., Shepard, T. H., and Alvord, E. C.: Caudal myeloschisis (lumbo-sacral spina bifida cystica) in a five millimeter (horizontal XIV) human embryo. Anat. Rec. 152:9, 1965.

Lorber, J.: Systematic ventriculographic studies in infants born with meningomyelocele and encephalocele. Arch. Dis. Child. 36:381, 1961.

Lorber, J.: Spina bifida cystica. Results of treatment of 270 consecutive cases with criteria for selection for the future. Arch. Dis. Child. 47:854, 1972.

Lorber, J.: The prognosis of occipital encephalocele. Develop. Med. Child Neurol. 9(suppl.):75, 1967.

Lorber, J.: Results of treatment of myelomeningocele: analysis of 524 unselected cases, with special reference to possible selection for treatment. Dev. Med. Child Neurol. 13:279, 1971.

Lorber, J., and De, N. C.: Family history of congenital hydrocephalus. Dev. Med. Child Neurol. 12(suppl. 22):94, 1970.

Lorber, J., and Zachary, R. B.: Primary congenital hydrocephalus. Arch. Dis. Child. 43:516, 1968.

Lubchenco, L. O., Hansman, C., and Boyd, E.: Intrauterine growth in length and head circumference as estimated from live births at gestational ages from 26 to 42 weeks. Pediatrics 37:403, 1966.

Mackenzie, N. G., and Emery, J. L.: Deformities of the cervical cord in children with neurospinal dysraphism. Dev. Med. Child. Neurol. 25(suppl.):58, 1971.

Mann, J. D., et al.: Regulation of intracranial pressure in rat, dog, and man. Ann. Neurol. 3:156, 1978.

Martin, H. P.: Microcephaly and mental retardation. Am. J. Dis. Child. 119:128, 1970.

Matson, D. D.: Neurosurgery of Infancy and Childhood. 2nd ed. Springfield, Ill., Charles C Thomas, 1969.

Matson, D. D., and Crofton, F. D. L.: Papilloma of the choroid plexus in childhood. J. Neurosurg. 17:1002, 1960.

Matson, D. D., and Jerva, M. J.: Recurrent meningitis associated with congenital lumbosacral dermal sinus tract. J. Neurosurg. 25:288, 1966.

Mealey, J., Jr., Dzenitis, A. J., and Hockey, A. A.: The prognosis of encephaloceles. J. Neurosurg. 32:209, 1970.

Meyerson, M. D., and Foushee, D. R.: Speech, language and hearing in Moebius syndrome: a study of 22 patients. Dev. Med. Child Neurol. 20:357, 1978.

Milhorat, T. H., et al.: Structural, ultrastructural and permeability changes in the ependyma and surrounding brain favoring equilibration in progressive hydrocephalus. Arch. Neurol. 22:397, 1970.

Miller, J. Q.: Lissencephaly in 2 siblings. Neurology 13:841, 1963.

Milunsky, A.: Prenatal detection of neural tube defects. J.A.M.A. 244:2731, 1980.

Moebius, P. J.: Ueber angeborene doppelseitige Abducens-facialis Lähmung. Münch. Med. Wschn. 35:91, and p. 108, 1888.

Morley, A. R.: Laryngeal stridor, Arnold-Chiari malformation and medullary haemorrhages. Dev. Med. Child Neurol. 11:471, 1969.

Naggan, L.: The recent decline in prevalence of anencephaly and spina bifida. Am. J. Epidemiol. 89:154, 1969.

Naidlich, T. P., et al.: Evaluation of pediatric hydrocephalus by computed tomography. Radiology 119:337, 1976.

Nakano, K. K.: Anencephaly: a review. Dev. Med. Child Neurol. 15:383, 1973.

Nellhaus, G.: Head circumference from birth to eighteen years. Pediatrics 41:106, 1968.

Partington, M. W., Gonzales-Crussi, F., Khakee, S. G., and Wollin, D. G.: Cloverleaf skull and thanatophoric dwarfism. Arch. Dis. Child. 47:656, 1971.

Perret, G.: Diagnosis and treatment of diastematomyelia. Surg. Gynecol. Obstet. 105:69, 1957.

Pitner, S. E., Edwards, J. E., and McCormick, W. F.: Observations of pathology of Möbius syndrome. J. Neurol. Neurosurg. Psychiatry 28:362, 1965.

Plummer, G.: Anomalies occurring in children exposed in utero to the atomic bomb in Hiroshima. Pediatrics 10:687, 1952.

Pollock, J. A., Newton, T. H., and Hoyt, W. F.: Transsphenoidal and transethmoidal encephaloceles. Radiology 90:442, 1968.

Reilly, B. J., Leeming, J. M., and Fraser, D.: Craniosynostosis in the rachitic spectrum. J. Pediatr. 64:396, 1964.

Rennels, M. B., and Wald, E. R.: Treatment of Haemophilus influenzae type B meningitis in children with cerebrospinal fluid shunts. J. Pediatr. 97:424, 1980.

Richman, D. P., Stewart, R. M., and Caviness, V. S., Jr.: Cerebral microgyria in a 27-week fetus: an architectonic and topographic analysis. J. Neuropathol. Exper. Neurol. 33:374, 1974.

Rickham, P. P., and Penn, I. A.: The place of the ventriculostomy reservoir in the treatment of myelomeningocoeles and hydrocephalus. Dev. Med. Child Neurol. 7:296, 1965.

Riley, H. D., Jr., and Smith, W. R.: Macrocephaly, pseudopapilledema and multiple hemangiomata. Pediatrics 26:293, 1960.

Robain, O., and Lyon, G.: Familial micrencephalus due to cerebral malformation. Acta Neuropathol. 20:96, 1972.

Rubin, R. C., et al.: Hydrocephalus: I. Histological and ultrastructural changes in the preshunted cortical mantle. Surg. Neurol. 5:109, 1976.

Ruiz-Maldonado, R., and Tamayo, L.: Aplasia cutis congenita, spastic paralysis and mental retardation. Am. J. Dis. Child. 128:699, 1974.

Salmon, J. H., Hajjar, W., and Bada, H. S.: The fontogram: a non-invasive intracranial pressure monitor. Pediatrics 60:721, 1977.

Sarnat, H. B., Case, M. E., and Graviss, R.: Sacral agenesis: neurologic and neuropathologic features. Neurology 26:1124, 1976.

Scott, M., Wycis, H. T., Murtagh, F., and Reyes, U.: Observations on ventricular and lumbar subarachnoid peritoneal shunts in hydrocephalus in infants. J. Neurosurg. 12:165, 1955.

Sedzimir, C. B., Roberts, J. R., and Occleshaw, J. V.: Massive diastematomyelia without cutaneous dysraphism. Arch. Dis. Child. 48:400, 1973.

Sells, C. J., and Shurtleff, D. B.: Cerebrospinal fluid shunts. West. J. Med. 127:93, 1977.

Sharrard, W. J. W.: Meningomyelocele: prognosis of immediate operative closure of the sac. Proc. Roy. Soc. Med. 56:510, 1963.

Shields, D., and Manger, M.: Ultrasound evaluation of neonatal intraventricular hemorrhage. Perinatol. Neonatol. (In press, 1983.)

Shiller, J. G.: Craniofacial dysostosis of Crouzon. Pediatrics 23:107, 1959.

Shillito, J., Jr., and Matson, D. D.: Craniostenosis: a review of 519 surgical patients. Pediatrics 41:229, 1968.

Shurtleff, D. B.: Transillumination of skull in infants and children. Am. J. Dis. Child. 107:14, 1964.

Shurtleff, D. B., Kronmal, R., and Foltz, F. C.: Follow-up comparison of hydrocephalus with and without myelomeningocele. J. Neurosurg. 42:61, 1975.

Stark, G. D.: Neonatal assessment of the child with a myelomeningocele. Arch. Dis. Child. 46:539, 1971.

Stein, S. E., and Schut, L.: Hydrocephalus in myelomeningocele. Child's Brain 5:413, 1979.

Thompson, J. A., and Glasgow, L. A.: Intrauterine viral infection and the cell-mediated immune response. Neurology 30:212, 1980.

Torkildsen, A.: A new palliative operation in cases of inoperative occlusion of the Sylvian aqueduct. Acta Chir. Scand. 82:117, 1939.

Virchow, R.: Ueber den Cretinismus, namentlich in Franken, und ueber pathologische Schädelformen. Verh. phys-med. Ges. Würzburg 2:230, 1851.

Vogel, F. S.: The anatomic character of the vascular anomalies associated with anencephaly, with consideration of the role of abnormal angiogenesis in the pathogenesis of cerebral malformation. Am. J. Pathol. 39:163, 1961.

Vyhmeister, N., Schneider, S., and Cha, C.: Cranial transillumination norms of the premature infant. J. Pediatr. 91:980, 1977.

Weller, R. O., and Shulman, K.: Infantile hydrocephalus: clinical histological and ultrastructural study of brain damage. J. Neurosurg. 36:255, 1972.

Windham, G., and Edmonds, L. D.: Current trends in the incidence of neural tube defects. Pediatrics 70:333, 1982.

Yakovlev, P. I.: Paraplegias of hydrocephalus (clinical note and interpretation). Am. J. Ment. Defic. 51:561, 1947.

Yakovlev, P., and Wadsworth, R. C.: Schizencephalies. A study of the congenital clefts in the cerebral mantle. Part I. J. Neuropathol. Exper. Neurol. 5:116, 1946.

Yashon, D.: Prognosis in infantile hydrocephalus. J. Neurosurg. 20:105, 1963.

Yashon, D., Jane, J. A., and Sugar, O.: The course of severe untreated infantile hydrocephalus. J. Neurosurg. 23:509, 1965.

79

Paroxysmal Disorders

By John H. Menkes*

Seizures occur with a relatively high frequency during the neonatal period and present special problems in terms of their diagnosis and treatment. The basic mechanisms underlying seizures will not be discussed in this chapter. Instead, the interested reader is referred to reviews by Goldensohn and Niedermeyer that cover the genetic, biochemical, electrophysiologic, and neuropathologic factors involved in seizures.

Etiology. The factors inducing seizures in the newborn infant and their relative frequency as determined by autopsy are presented in Table 79–1. The most common identifiable causes are perinatal asphyxia and trauma, particularly when they result in subdural and intraventricular hemorrhage (Hopkins,

---

* This chapter includes portions written by Dr. William E. Bell that appeared in the 4th edition of this book.

1972). Developmental anomalies of the brain and metabolic disturbances are probably far more common than would appear from the autopsy studies of Craig and the composite series of Volpe, since a large proportion of these patients do not succumb to their illness. Characteristically, seizures due to perinatal asphyxia and its complications start within the first 24

Table 79–1. Major Autopsy Findings in Infants With Neonatal Seizures*

Infections	29	
E. coli		9
Developmental anomalies of CNS	14	
Trauma	97	
Subdural hemorrhage		30
Intraventricular hemorrhage		23
Venous congestion, edema		16
Subarachnoid hemorrhage		14
Multiple hemorrhages		6
Sinus thrombosis		4
Other		4
Extracerebral hemorrhages, shock	9	
Kernicterus	4	
No abnormalities (? metabolic)	9	

* After Craig, W. S.: Convulsive movements occurring in first 10 days of life. Arch. Dis. Child. 35:336, 1960.
(From Menkes, J. H.: Textbook of Child Neurology. 2nd ed. Philadelphia, Lea and Febiger, 1980.)

hours of life. According to the findings published by Volpe in 1981, 60 per cent of infants experienced the onset of spells within 12 hours of birth. Neonatal seizures due to developmental defects also start in the first 3 days of life; in fact, when seizures are first noted within 2 hours of birth they are unlikely to be caused by perinatal asphyxia (Brann and Dykes, 1977), and a developmental defect, metabolic disturbances, or drug withdrawal should be suspected.

Hypoglycemic and hypocalcemic convulsions are relatively common during the neonatal period. According to Keen, they account for 6 per cent and 34 per cent of neonatal seizures, respectively. Hypocalcemia of "early onset," occurring during the first 2 or 3 days after birth, is observed in the infant of low birth weight for gestational age, associated with perinatal complications, in infants of diabetic mothers, and in a variety of other stress situations. The reduced serum calcium in such infants may cause or contribute to the occurrence of convulsions; however, in some infants, correction of the calcium deficit does not alleviate the neurologic abnormalities. Hypocalcemia of "late onset" occurs late in the first week or early in the second week after birth and is usually attributed to the phosphate load in feedings in the presence of relative parathyroid and renal immaturity. Seizures due to this are rapidly abolished by elevation of the serum calcium level. It is important to remember that neonatal hypocalcemia that proves to be resistant to therapy may be secondary to maternal hyperparathyroidism (Mizrahi and Gold, 1964; Hartenstein and Gardner, 1966), idiopathic neonatal hypoparathyroidism (Smith and Zike, 1963), or the DiGeorge syndrome, in which congenital absence of the parathyroid and thymus glands is associated with other anomalies (Kretschmer et al., 1968). A curious and poorly understood disorder is a form of neonatal hypocalcemia that responds poorly to supplemental calcium: the reduction of the ion is secondary to primary hypomagnesemia (Paunier et al., 1968; Vainsel et al., 1970). Tetany, convulsions, and hypocalcemia characterize this condition; however, the reduced serum calcium cannot be corrected until the deficiency of serum magnesium is eliminated (Davis et al., 1973). In this disorder, the onset of seizures generally occurs in the neonatal period but can be delayed for several months after birth.

Neonatal hypoglycemia is another important metabolic cause of seizures as well as other abnormal neurologic signs. Hypoglycemia in the neonate is diagnosed when glucose levels are less than 30 mg per 100 ml in the full-term infant and less than 20 mg per 100 ml in the premature child. The infant of a diabetic mother, the infant stressed during parturition or in the newborn period, and the newborn infant with hyperviscosity are all susceptible to hypoglycemia, which may precipitate convulsions. Rarely, hyperinsulinism is caused by such lesions as islet cell hyperplasia and islet cell tumors. Symptoms may appear as early as 1 to 2 hours following birth, particularly in infants who are small for gestational age, but

Table 79–2. Time of First Seizures in Various Inborn Errors of Metabolism

Condition	Onset of Seizures
Phenylketonuria	1 to 18 months
Maple syrup urine disease	1 to 2 weeks
Urea cycle disorders	2 days to $2\frac{1}{2}$ years
Organic acidemias	
Propionic acidemia	First week
Methylmalonic acidemia	First week to first month
Pyruvic dehydrogenase defects	1 day or later
Isovaleric acidemia	First week
Galactosemia	First week
Pyridoxine dependency	3 hours to 7 days
Congenital amaurotic idiocy	2 weeks or later

as a rule they are delayed until 3 to 24 hours. In about 25 per cent of infants, hypoglycemia does not become symptomatic until after 24 hours. The clinical picture of symptomatic hypoglycemia is highlighted by tremors, apnea or tachypnea, cyanosis, convulsions, and lethargy (Raivio, 1968). Additional metabolic causes of neonatal seizures include hyponatremia, hypernatremia, and polycythemia with hyperviscosity (Gross et al., 1973; Wood, 1959). Hyponatremia in the newborn infant can be caused by excessive administration of salt-free fluids to the mother during labor or to the child after birth. It may also occur as the result of inappropriate secretion of antidiuretic hormone, resulting in water retention, or increased salt loss secondary to diarrhea. Neonatal hypernatremia has followed accidental substitution of salt for sugar in infant feedings and has occurred with severe diarrhea. In exceptional circumstances, inborn errors of metabolism may be responsible for neonatal convulsions (Berenberg and Kang, 1971; Kang et al., 1973; Carton et al., 1969) (Table 79–2) (see Chapter 58).

Although vitamin B_6, or pyridoxine, dependency is an even more unusual metabolic defect that causes neonatal or even intrauterine seizures (Bejšovec et al., 1967), it is important because of the availability of treatment. Infants with this familial inborn metabolic error require far more pyridoxine than the normal child and exhibit neonatal difficulties when it is not provided (Scriver, 1960; Waldinger and Berg, 1963). Respiratory dysfunction, neuromuscular hyperirritability, and convulsions that can lead to death unless treatment is instituted are the clinical hallmarks of this disorder.

Seizures are common events in newborn infants who have infections of various types, the most important being bacterial meningitis. Because of this possibility, lumbar puncture and cerebrospinal fluid examination are warranted whenever unexplained seizures occur in the young infant. Other infectious illnesses that may be associated with neonatal seizures are congenital rubella, cytomegalovirus encephalitis, toxoplasmosis, and disseminated infection with herpes simplex or Coxsackie B viruses.

The narcotic withdrawal syndrome in newborn infants of mothers who are narcotic addicts has been recognized with increased frequency in recent years (Naeye et al., 1973). Although convulsions are not common among these infants, they have been observed in those severely affected (Zelson et al., 1971; Herzlinger et al., 1977). The seizure incidence is somewhat higher in infants born to methadone-addicted mothers (Herzlinger et al.). Convulsions are even more likely to be encountered in infants of mothers taking barbiturates, particularly the shorter acting type, and in neonates passively addicted to alcohol (Pierog et al., 1977). Signs of neonatal withdrawal usually appear during the first or second day after birth but in exceptional cases can be delayed for several days (Kandall and Gartner, 1974). The offspring of addicted mothers are usually prematurely born or small for gestational age. The usual withdrawal signs include irritability, tremulousness, tachypnea, vomiting or diarrhea, and fever. The more severely affected infant may have sufficient fluid loss to become dehydrated, develop hypocalcemia, or exhibit frank generalized convulsions. Diagnosis might be anticipated when the mother admits to drug intake, has withdrawal symptoms herself, or attempts to leave the hospital with the infant against medical advice within 1 day after birth.

Intoxication of the infant by accidental injection of a local anesthetic, such as mepivacaine, into the scalp during caudal anesthesia of the mother is an additional possible cause of seizures soon after birth (Sinclair et al., 1965; Kim et al., 1979). Bradycardia is associated with respiratory depression, limpness, dilated pupils, and convulsions within the first 6 hours of birth (Hillman et al., 1979). The puncture wound, identifying the site of the injection into the fetal scalp, is visible in some cases. Gastric lavage and exchange transfusion have been recommended for this condition because of its life-threatening characteristics (Sinclair et al., 1965).

Lastly, one may also encounter an autosomal dominant syndrome of benign neonatal seizures (Quattlebaum, 1979).

Clinical Findings. Only a small percentage of newborn infants experience classic tonic-clonic convulsions, and neither petit mal nor pyschomotor attacks have been encountered in that age range. More commonly, one encounters a variety of fragmentary, or multifocal, clonic attacks (Rose and Lombroso, 1970; Volpe, 1973). These consist of asymmetric clonic jerking or shifting clonic movements that migrate from limb to limb in a disorderly manner. Strictly focal seizures involving one or both limbs on one side of the body are also common and in most instances do not indicate a localized cerebral disturbance. Generalized tonic seizures resembling episodes of decerebrate rigidity are also encountered and are usually accompanied by irregular respiratory patterns, ocular deviation, or pupillary abnormalities. This type of an attack often reflects severe underlying brain disease and, consequently, a poor prognosis.

Other seizure manifestations in the neonate, especially in the premature newborn, are much more subtle, and sometimes their nature is difficult to interpret. They include rhythmic eye movements, chewing or unusual rowing, or swimming or pedaling movements of arms or legs, abrupt changes in the respiratory pattern, and even apneic spells (Dreyfus-Brisac and Monod, 1964). These types of seizures undoubtedly reflect the immaturity of the nervous system of the newborn infant and its inability to propagate epileptic discharges.

Diagnosis. Episodic disturbances in the newborn that must be differentiated from convulsive activity include "jitteriness," which differs from seizures in its tendency to be provoked or aggravated by tactile stimulation and in its precipitation by placement of the body parts into certain positions. This author has encountered a familial syndrome of excessive jitteriness. It may well be related to familial quivering of the chin as described by Wadlington in 1958. This condition must be distinguished from the excessive jitteriness induced by the sequelae of neonatal asphyxia.

The intensely spastic infant may erroneously be assumed to be convulsing when clonus is provoked by certain exogenous stimuli. Such movements in the hypertonic child can usually be stopped promptly by altering the limb position.

The primary concern of the physician treating the neonate with seizures is the immediate identification of those causes that are amenable to some specific form of treatment. Therefore, the appropriate studies must be performed to exclude hypocalcemia, hypoglycemia, hypomagnesemia, hyponatremia, sepsis, and meningitis. Pyridoxine dependency can be added to this list, although it is a rare disorder. Diagnosis of seizures secondary to perinatal complications or congenital malformations of the brain can be accepted only after the aforementioned possibilities have been eliminated by the results of the laboratory examinations. In most cases, the infant who is convulsing because of hypoxic-ischemic injuries acquired during birth can be diagnosed on the basis of the history of perinatal distress, the presence of other abnormal neurologic signs, and the presence of an abnormal ultrasonographic or CT scan.

The diagnostic assessment should include a complete blood count and urinalysis, serum glucose, calcium, phosphorus, magnesium, and electrolytes. A rapid estimate of the blood sugar range can be made by a Dextrostix test. If the test indicates a low serum glucose, it is advisable to administer 25 per cent glucose intravenously, after blood is obtained for glucose determination.

Other indicated studies may include determinations of blood pH, serum ammonia, and serum amino acids. Serologic tests for rubella, cytomegalovirus, toxoplasmosis, and other infections may also be advisable, depending on the other laboratory findings. Blood culture and lumbar puncture for cerebrospinal fluid examination, as well as an ultrasonographic or CT scan, are additional valuable procedures.

An electroencephalogram is best obtained in the interictal period. This procedure, however, is a minor factor in the diagnosis and management of the patient. It is more valuable in helping one determine the prognosis for the newborn with a seizure disorder and, less often, in verifying whether a clinical phenomenon represents a seizure equivalent.

Treatment. When the underlying cause for seizures cannot be treated specifically, the physician will have to content himself with their symptomatic therapy.

Phenobarbital is the best anticonvulsant for use during the neonatal period. The drug is administered in an intramuscular loading dose of 15 to 20 mg/kg (Lockman et al., 1979; Fischer et al., 1981; Painter et al., 1978). It is clear that this dosage is required in order to achieve adequate anticonvulsant blood levels (15 to 30 µg/ml). Peak concentrations are reached within 1½ to 6 hours following the injection, and maintenance doses of 3 to 4 mg/kg/day are initiated once the blood barbiturate level drops below 15 to 20 µg/ml. Because of the very long half-life of the drug in the neonate, this usually does not occur until 5 to 7 days of age (Lockman et al., 1979). These dosages are not influenced by gestational age. Nevertheless, it is imperative that for optimal seizure control daily or twice daily barbiturate levels be secured.

We have not had much success in the control of neonatal convulsions using oral or parenteral phenytoin, but we have seen a number of toxic reactions when the latter route had been used. This may be due to the immaturity of the hepatic hydroxylating system responsible for phenytoin detoxification.

Diazepam has also been suggested as an anticonvulsant in the newborn. The drug, however, is no better than phenobarbital for the treatment of neonatal seizures (Volpe, 1973). However, its short duration of action makes it a poor drug for maintenance. Furthermore, one of the principal side effects of diazepam is respiratory depression, which is most likely to occur in infants receiving a combination of diazepam and phenobarbital. Finally, it must be stressed that whenever seizures are not controlled by adequate phenobarbital therapy, they respond poorly to other drugs, including diazepam and valproic acid.

Prognosis. The prognosis of neonatal seizures depends on their cause. In other words, the eventual outcome is heavily determined by the nature of the underlying brain disease or systemic disorder that triggers the convulsions.

Table 79–3. Follow-up of 278 Infants With Neonatal Seizures*

Normal	140	
Died within 3 months	63	
Cerebral hemorrhage		26
Cerebral edema		16
Malformation of CNS		3
Abnormal	75	
Mental retardation		17
Mental retardation and seizures		14
Seizures		5
"Cerebral palsy"		37

* After Prichard, J. S.: The character and significance of epileptic seizures in infancy. In Kellaway, P., and Petersen, I. (Eds.): Neurological and Electroencephalographic Correlative Studies in Infancy. New York, Grune & Stratton, 1964.
(From Menkes, J. H.: Textbook of Child Neurology. 2nd ed. Philadelphia, Lea and Febiger, 1980.)

Seizures due to hypocalcemia starting 5 to 10 days after birth in an otherwise normal infant are generally associated with an excellent prognosis. Conversely, the majority of infants who experience seizures as a result of cardiopulmonary disease die within a few months of birth. Those having convulsions as a consequence of perinatal asphyxia or malformations of the central nervous system have a better prognosis with respect to survival but not with respect to normal intellectual development and freedom from subsequent seizures (Dennis, 1978). Follow-up studies on infants with neonatal seizures are summarized in Table 79–3. These results, reported in 1964, are not significantly different from those recorded in more current publications (Volpe, 1981). In a significant proportion of children, seizures recur during the first 2 years of life, and some of these patients go on to suffer from infantile spasms.

An infant with neonatal convulsions has a relatively good prognosis with respect to normal development in the presence of the following findings:

1. Seizures subside within 24 hours.

2. The neurologic examination is normal and no abnormalities of eye movements can be observed.

3. The child returns to routine feeding schedule within 5 days.

4. The electroencephalogram, probably the most useful prognostic indicator, is normal. In the 1970 experience of Rose and Lombroso, neonates with seizures but a normal interictal electroencephalogram have an 86 per cent chance of normal development at age 4 years. The presence of multifocal spikes, or sharp waves, is a particularly ominous finding, and only 12 per cent of infants showing such a pattern achieve normal development.

When prognosis is classified according to causation of the seizures, one finds that 50 per cent of infants whose convulsions are due to an underlying asphyxial injury will develop normally. By contrast, less than 10 per cent of infants with intraventricular hemorrhage and none of those with congenital anomalies of the brain will escape intellectual deficits (Volpe, 1981).

There is much controversy but little data with respect to how long anticonvulsants should be given to an infant who has suffered seizures during the neonatal period.

Although experimental data derived from rats suggest an adverse effect of phenobarbital on the developing nervous system, the applicability of these results to the human whose brain is more mature at birth has not been demonstrated.

Nevertheless, we have made it a practice to maintain adequate phenobarbital blood levels for the first 3 months of life. Thereafter, in the face of normal development, continued freedom from seizures, and a normal electroencephalogram, we allow the infant to outgrow his phenobarbital dosage, so that when blood levels drop below 15 µg/ml the drug can be discontinued.

REFERENCES

Bejšovec, M., Kulenda, Z., and Ponca, E.: Familial intrauterine convulsions in pyridoxine dependency. Arch. Dis. Child. 42:201, 1967.

Berenberg, W., and Kang, E. S.: The congenital hyperammonemic syndrome. Dev. Med. Child Neurol. 13:355, 1971.

Brann, A. W., and Dykes, F. D.: The effects of intrauterine asphyxia on the full-term neonate. Clin. Perinatol. 4:149, 1977.

Carton, D., et al.: Argininosuccinic aciduria: neonatal variant with rapid fatal course. Acta Paediatr. Scand. 58:528, 1969.

Craig, W. S.: Convulsive movements occurring in first 10 days of life. Arch. Dis. Child. 35:336, 1960.

Davis, J. A., Harvey, D. R., and Yu, J. S.: Neonatal fits associated with hypomagnesaemia. Arch. Dis. Child. 40:286, 1973.

Dennis, J.: Neonatal convulsions: aetiology, late neonatal status and long-term outcome. Dev. Med. Child Neurol. 20:143, 1978.

Dreyfus-Brisac, C., and Monod, N.: Electro-clinical studies of status epilepticus and convulsion in the newborn. In Kellaway, P., and Petersen, I. (Eds.): Neurological and Electroencephalographic Correlative Studies in Infancy. New York, Grune & Stratton, Inc., 1964.

Fischer, J. H., et al.: Phenobarbital maintenance dose requirements in treating neonatal seizures. Neurology 31:1042, 1981.

Freeman, J. M.: Neonatal seizures—diagnosis and management. J. Pediatr. 77:701, 1970.

Goldensohn, E. S.: The Epilepsies. In Goldensohn, E. S., and Appel, S. H. (Eds.): Scientific Approaches to Clinical Neurology. Philadelphia, Lea & Febiger, 1977, pp. 654–692.

Gross, G. P., Hathaway, W. E., and McGaughey, H. R.: Hyperviscosity in the neonate. J. Pediatr. 82:1004, 1973.

Hartenstein, H., and Gardner, L. I.: Tetany of the newborn associated with maternal parathyroid adenoma. N. Engl. J. Med. 274:266, 1966.

Herzlinger, R. A., Kandall, S. R., and Vaughan, H. G.: Neonatal seizures associated with narcotic withdrawal. J. Pediatr. 91:638, 1977.

Hillman, L. S., Hillman, R. E., and Dodson, W. E.: Diagnosis, treatment, and follow-up of neonatal mepivacaine intoxication secondary to paracervical and pudendal blocks during labor. J. Pediatr. 95:472, 1979.

Hopkins, I. J.: Seizures in the first week of life. A study of aetiological factors. Med. J. Aust. 2:647, 1972.

Kandall, S. R., and Gartner, L. M.: Late presentation of drug withdrawal symptoms in newborns. Am. J. Dis. Child. 127:58, 1974.

Kang, E. S., Snodgrass, P. J., and Gerald, P. S.: Ornithine transcarbamylase deficiency in the newborn infant. J. Pediatr. 82:642, 1973.

Keen, J. H.: Significance of hypocalcemia in neonatal convulsions. Arch. Dis. Child. 44:356, 1969.

Kim, W. Y., Pomerance, J. J., and Miller, A. A.: Lidocaine intoxication in a newborn following local anesthesia for episiotomy. Pediatrics 64:643, 1979.

Kretschmer, R., Say, B., Brown, D., and Rosen, F. S.: Congenital aplasia of the thymus gland (DiGeorge's syndrome). N. Engl. J. Med. 279:1295, 1968.

Lockman, L. A., et al.: Phenobarbital dosage for control of neonatal seizures. Neurology 29:1445, 1979.

Mizrahi, A., and Gold, A. P.: Neonatal tetany secondary to maternal hyperparathyroidism. J.A.M.A. 190:155, 1964.

Naeye, R. L., Blanc, W., Leblanc, W., and Khatamee, M. A.: Fetal complications of maternal heroin addiction: abnormal growth, infections, and episodes of stress. J. Pediatr. 83:1055, 1973.

Niedermeyer, E.: Epileptic seizure disorders. In Niedermeyer, E., and Lopes da Silva, F. (Eds.): Electroencephalography. Baltimore, Urban & Schwarzenberg, 1982.

Painter, M. J., et al.: Phenobarbital and diphenylhydantoin levels in neonates with seizures. J. Pediatr. 92:315, 1978.

Paunier, L., Radde, I. C., Kooh, S. W., Connen, P. E., and Fraser, D.: Primary hypomagnesemia with secondary hypocalcemia in an infant. Pediatrics 41:385, 1968.

Pierog, S., Chandavasu, O., and Wexler, I.: Withdrawal symptoms in infants with the fetal alcohol syndrome. J. Pediatr. 90:630, 1977.

Prichard, J. S.: The character and significance of epileptic seizures in infancy. In Kellaway, P., and Petersen, I. (Eds.): Neurological and Electroencephalographic Correlative Studies in Infancy. New York, Grune & Stratton, Inc., 1964.

Quattlebaum, T. G.: Benign familial convulsions in the neonatal period and early infancy. J. Pediatr. 95:257, 1979.

Raivio, K. O.: Neonatal hypoglycemia. II. A clinical study of 44 idiopathic cases with special reference to corticosteroid hormones. Acta Paediatr. Scand. 57:540, 1968.

Rose, A. L., and Lombroso, C. T.: Neonatal seizure states. A study of clinical, pathological, and electroencephalographic features in 137 full-term babies with a long-term follow-up. Pediatrics 45:404, 1970.

Scriver, C. R.: Vitamin B6-dependency and infantile convulsions. Pediatrics 26:62, 1960.

Sinclair, J. C., Fox, H. A., Lentz, J. F., Fuld, G. L., and Murphy, J.: Intoxication of the fetus by a local anesthetic. N. Engl. J. Med. 273:1173, 1965.

Smith, F. G., Jr., and Zike, K.: Idiopathic hypoparathyroidism in neonatal period. Am. J. Dis. Child. 105:182, 1963.

Vainsel, M., Vandervelde, G., Smulders, J., Vosters, M., Hubain, P., and Loeb, H.: Tetany due to hypomagnesaemia with secondary hypocalcemia. Arch. Dis. Child. 45:254, 1970.

Volpe, J. J.: Neonatal seizures. N. Engl. J. Med. 289:413, 1973.

Volpe, J. J.: Neurology of the Newborn. Philadelphia, W.B. Saunders Co., 1981.

Wadlington, W. B.: Familial trembling of the chin. J. Pediatr. 53:316, 1958.

Waldinger, C., and Berg, R. B.: Signs of pyridoxine dependency manifest at birth in siblings. Pediatrics 32:161, 1963.

Wood, J. L.: Plethora in the newborn infant associated with cyanosis and convulsions. J. Pediatr. 54:143, 1959.

Zelson, C., Rubio, E., and Wasserman, E.: Neonatal narcotic addiction: 10 year observation. Pediatrics 48:178, 1971.

80

Diseases of the Motor Unit

By John H. Menkes

Because of the relative simplicity of the motor unit, the disorders discussed in this chapter have a limited means of clinical expression, and their diagnosis rests to a great extent on the proper application of laboratory techniques. An approach to the diagnostic evaluation of the hypotonic infant follows:

1. Establish whether hypotonia is due to central nervous system involvement, a systemic or metabolic disease, or a neuromuscular disorder. No details need to be given at this point, but there has been a recent tendency to underestimate the importance of a careful history and a good physical examination. One of the chief distinguishing features of a neuromuscular disorder is the appearance of alertness and responsiveness in the flaccid child with muscle disease as opposed to the lethargy and stupor that accompany cerebral birth insults.

2. Once the infant's difficulties have been shown to be the consequence of a neuromuscular disorder, perform laboratory studies to obtain further information.
   a. Evaluate serum enzymes. The most widely used enzyme assay in the assessment of muscle disease is serum creatine phosphokinase (CPK). An elevation in its level is seen in some infants with congenital muscular dystrophy but is also found in normal neonates for the first few days of life.
   b. Examine the cerebrospinal fluid. An elevated CSF protein is the hallmark of neonatal polyneuropathy.
   c. Obtain an electrocardiogram. The EKG is abnormal in glycogen storage disease, Type II (Pompe's disease), in some cases of congenital muscular dystrophy, and, less often, in congenital myotonic dystrophy. It is normal in spinal muscular atrophy (Werdnig-Hoffmann disease).
   d. Obtain an electromyogram. In the neonate, the quadriceps and deltoid muscles are best suited for this procedure. The EMG will provide information as to whether hypotonia is neurogenic—due to involvement of the anterior horn cells (e.g., in infantile spinal muscular atrophy) or the peripheral nerve—or myopathic. In most instances, the EMG will not provide an answer regarding the type of denervation or the nature of the myopathy. However, in myasthenia gravis and infantile botulism, special electrodiagnostic techniques will be diagnostic (Aminoff, 1980). Very little ad-

ditional information can be gathered from nerve conduction studies.

3. Perform a muscle biopsy. This procedure is essential to the diagnosis of most infants with neuromuscular diseases. The biopsy is performed on a muscle which has not been previously subjected to EMG, and the specimen is prepared for histology, histochemistry, and electron microscopy. Open and needle biopsy both have their proponents, and the interested reader is referred to Dubowitz and Brooke and to Edwards and coworkers for further discussion.

Diseases of the Motoneuron

SPINAL MUSCULAR ATROPHY (WERDNIG-HOFFMANN DISEASE)

In infants, spinal muscular atrophy is the principal disease affecting the motoneuron. This is a disease or group of diseases transmitted by an autosomal recessive gene and manifested by widespread muscular atrophy.

Although initial pathologic descriptions of the disease pointed to the conspicuous loss of anterior horn cells from spinal cord and brain stem (Byers and Banker, 1961), it is becoming evident that when carefully searched for, other areas of the central nervous system, notably the dorsal root ganglia, posterior columns, optic nerves, and cranial nerve nuclei are also involved (Probst et al., 1981). In the usual infant coming to necropsy, anterior horn cells are absent from the entire length of the spinal cord. Of the residual cells, some are in the process of degenerating or are being phagocytized by satellite cells. An unusual finding that may reflect the basic defect in this puzzling disease is the prominent glial proliferation at the proximal portion of the anterior spinal roots,

707

changes that are believed to start during fetal life (Chou and Nonaka, 1978).

In about one third of cases, the disease is present at birth. The infants present a classic picture of a neuromuscular disease. They are hypotonic or floppy, with a symmetric muscle weakness that is more extensive in the proximal part of the limbs. What little spontaneous movements are left can be found in the small muscles of the hands and feet. The affected muscles are atrophied, although this is concealed by the normal amounts of subcutaneous fat seen in the newborn. Muscles of the trunk, neck, and thorax are equally affected, and the infant assumes a characteristic "frog posture." Muscles of the face and diaphragm are commonly spared during the initial phases. Bulbar musculature is affected with consequent impairment of sucking and swallowing. Fasciculation may be noted in the tongue, but this finding is often difficult to obtain in the crying youngster. Deep tendon reflexes are nearly always reduced or absent. There are no sensory loss, no intellectual retardation, and no sphincter disturbances.

In most instances, the disease progresses rapidly, so that infants who are affected at birth rarely survive the first year of life. In some, neonatal respiratory distress may be fatal (Kyllerman, 1977).

Electromyographic findings help confirm the clinical impression of motoneuron disease. The finding most specific for this condition—and not observed in any other—is the presence of spontaneous, rhythmic muscle activity at a frequency of 5 to 15 per second, which can be activated by voluntary effort (Buchthal and Olsen, 1970). Still, muscle biopsy is the only certain way of determining the diagnosis (Dubowitz, 1980).

Neither the cause of this disease nor its treatment is known.

terior horn cells are markedly reduced, and the EMG findings are consistent with denervation. About 10 to 20 per cent of infants with spinal muscular atrophy will demonstrate contractures, especially of the distal portion of the limbs (Byers and Banker, 1961). In other instances, there are changes compatible with congenital muscular dystrophy, congenital myotonic dystrophy, fibrosis of the anterior spinal roots, or evidence of embryonic denervation and maturation arrest of the muscle.

An early and vigorous orthopedic program has been advocated. This is often of considerable benefit to infants with arthrogryposis of non-neuromuscular origin.

Of the various other conditions affecting the motoneuron of the neonate, only type II glycogen storage disease (Pompe's disease) and neonatal poliomyelitis occur with sufficient frequency to be mentioned at this point (Baskin et al., 1950).

Diseases of the Axon

Both acute and chronic polyneuropathies have been documented in neonates (Goebel et al., 1976; Kasman et al., 1976). We have seen two such cases in hypotonic infants in whom an elevated CSF protein in the absence of pleocytosis suggested the diagnosis. Occasionally, the polyneuropathy appears to be transmitted as a dominant trait with partial expressivity in one parent (Kasman et al., 1976).

Diseases of the Neuromuscular Junction

The disorders to be considered under this heading include myasthenia gravis, infantile botulism, and neonatal tetanus. The venoms of several reptiles and insects also affect the neuromuscular junction, but these conditions need not be considered in this text.

ARTHROGRYPOSIS

Arthrogryposis refers to multiple congenital contractures of limbs fixed in flexion or, less commonly, in extension accompanied by diminution and wasting of skeletal muscle. Other congenital malformations, particularly clubfoot and cerebral maldevelopment, are often part of the syndrome (Beckerman and Buchino, 1978). In one group of infants, the neuromuscular apparatus is normal, and arthrogryposis results from restricted intrauterine muscle movements. This can result from either a malformed uterus or oligohydramnios (e.g., Potter's syndrome). In another group of infants, the condition is due to one of at least three distinct neuromuscular syndromes. Probably the most common is one in which the an-

MYASTHENIA GRAVIS

Three forms of myasthenia gravis have been encountered in the neonatal period (Seybold and Lindstrom, 1981; Fenichel, 1978). All demonstrate muscular weakness responsive to anticholinesterase medication and display a decremental response to repetitive motor nerve stimulation. Neonatal myasthenia gravis is the most common of these disorders. It is seen in 10 to 15 per cent of infants born to myasthenic mothers. Congenital myasthenia gravis is a genetically transmitted disorder that occurs in infants born to nonmyasthenic mothers who demonstrate muscle weakness during the neonatal period. A third disorder, characterized by a defect in the assembly or attachment of acetylcholine esterase to the postsynaptic membrane, has been described by Engel and coworkers.

Juvenile myasthenia gravis designates a disorder that is similar to the one seen in adults. However, onset of this condition prior to 1 year of age has not yet been documented (Snead et al., 1980). In this condition, as in adult myasthenia, the pathophysiology has now been fairly well delineated. For as yet unknown reasons an autoimmune response, stimulated, possibly, by an infectious agent and selectively enhanced by thymus cells, is mounted against the postsynaptic acetylcholine receptors (Newson-Davis et al., 1981; Shore et al., 1979). The ensuing antibodies induce an increased degradation of these receptors, so that the number of functional receptors may be reduced to as little as 10 per cent of normal (Engel et al., 1977).

Neonatal myasthenia presumably results from the passive transfer of antiacetylcholine receptor antibodies across the placenta (Keesey et al., 1977). In this form of myasthenia, symptoms usually appear during the first 24 hours or, at the latest, by the third day of life. In all instances, there is a paresis of the lower bulbar muscles that results in a weak cry and difficulty in sucking or swallowing. Generalized hypotonia is found in about one half the infants. It may be severe enough to produce respiratory difficulty (Fenichel, 1978).

The clinical diagnosis is confirmed by administration of 0.1 mg of edrophonium chloride (Tensilon). In some infants, a positive response may be obscured by the response to the injection, and the longer acting neostigmine (Prostigmin) should be used. The latency of Prostigmin is greater than that of Tensilon, but it is sufficiently long-acting for one to determine muscle strength accurately. The diagnosis is further documented by repetitive nerve stimulation at 10 to 50/sec, which produces transmission fatigue (Wise and McQuillen, 1970). Serum antiacetylcholine receptor antibody levels are elevated in some asymptomatic newborns of myasthenic mothers.

Myasthenic symptoms usually respond promptly to anticholinesterase medication, and, even if the illness is untreated, its duration is generally less than 5 weeks. Exchange transfusion has been used to remove antibody in the most severely affected infants (Pasternak et al., 1981).

In about one half of patients with congenital myasthenia gravis, symptoms commence prior to 2 years of age, and more than one infant per family may be affected (Herrmann, 1971). In many instances, fetal movements are reduced, and during the neonatal period there may be feeding difficulties and a weak cry. As a rule, the initial symptoms in congenital myasthenia are not as severe as those in the neonatal variant, and the disease may consequently go undetected. Fenichel distinguishes a variant, known as "familial infantile myasthenia," that is characterized by severe respiratory and feeding difficulties at birth and differentiated from congenital myasthenia by the absence of impaired extraocular mobility in the former disorder. Antiacetylcholine receptor antibodies can be detected in but a small proportion of subjects with congenital myasthenia (Seybold and Lindstrom, 1981).

A few patients with congenital myasthenia have spontaneous remissions, but usually the course of the disease is protracted, with mild symptoms that are refractory to medical therapy.

INFANT BOTULISM

Botulism is a toxic condition induced by the ingestion of food in which *Clostridium botulinum* has grown and produced toxin.

Over the last few years a syndrome of infantile botulism has been delineated. It has its onset in infants between the ages of 3 and 18 weeks, and it is characterized by hypotonia, hyporeflexia, and weakness of the cranial nerve musculature. The infant often has a history of constipation, lethargy, and poor feeding. External ophthalmoplegia may be present, along with evidence of autonomic dysfunction. Cardiovascular symptoms are absent, and the EKG is normal. Almost all infants recover completely, with the illness lasting between 3 and 20 weeks.

On electromyograms, the motor unit action potentials are brief, of small amplitude, and excessive in number, a picture consistent with that observed in adult botulism (Oh, 1977). Type A and type B spores of *C. botulinum* have been found in stool. The cause of the illness is obscure. However, exposure to honey contaminated with *C. botulinum* has been documented in a high proportion of infants (Arnon et al., 1979).

Symptomatic therapy, including respiratory support and nasogastric feeding, must suffice.

NEONATAL TETANUS

This condition is caused by a clostridial infection of the umbilical stump. Although extremely rare in this country and limited to home-delivered infants (Adams et al., 1979), the condition is a major health hazard in some underdeveloped countries (Pinheiro, 1964). Trismus, with consequent inability to nurse, and striking nuchal rigidity are the initial symptoms in 70 per cent of infants. Generalized tetanic spasms occur less often and indicate a more severe form of the disease.

Treatment has been outlined by Adams and coworkers. It consists of supportive care, sedation, the administration of tetanus immune globulin, and treatment of the infected umbilical stump with penicillin.

Diseases of Muscle

THE MUSCULAR DYSTROPHIES

Of the various forms of muscular dystrophy only one entity, termed "congenital muscular dystrophy," is evident at birth. Duchenne muscular dystrophy, which is sex-linked and the most common of these conditions, does not produce obvious clinical symptoms until after the child begins walking.

The cause of congenital muscular dystrophy is unknown, but it undoubtedly differs from that responsible for the sex-linked form. Unlike the Duchenne form, it is transmitted as an autosomal recessive trait. Infants are markedly hypotonic and weak from birth on, with involvement of face and respiratory muscles. Sucking and swallowing difficulties are seen in about one half of patients. Sixty per cent of neonates have contractures, and some demonstrate the full clinical picture of arthrogryposis. Although most infants follow a normal mental development, severe retardation has been reported in some families.

Laboratory studies reveal an elevated CPK level during the early stages of the disease, and EKG abnormalities are found in about 20 per cent of patients (Donner et al., 1975). Electromyography usually elicits a myopathic pattern, although neurogenic changes have been recorded (McMenamin et al., 1982). Muscle biopsy demonstrates pathologic changes consistent with a dystrophic process (Dubowitz, 1980). As is the case for Duchenne muscular dystrophy, treatment is entirely supportive. Nevertheless, the clinical course is not inexorably downhill but remains more or less static.

MYOTONIC DISORDERS

A number of genetically distinct conditions share the clinical feature of myotonia of the voluntary muscles. Of these, congenital myotonic dystrophy is the only one liable to be encountered in the neonate.

The main features of the disease, as it expresses itself in infancy, are generalized hypotonia (involving principally the neck muscles), difficulty with sucking and swallowing, and, occasionally, severe respiratory difficulties (Harper, 1975). Arthrogryposis may be present at birth, and there may be a history of recurrent hydramnios. Myotonia is not demonstrable on clinical examination or by electromyography (Dubowitz, 1980).

The disease is transmitted as an autosomal dominant trait, but, for unknown reasons, the mother is the affected parent in some 90 per cent of infants (Dyken and Harper, 1973). Inasmuch as serum CPK values and electromyographic findings are usually normal during the neonatal period and muscle biopsy demonstrates only arrested maturation of fibers (Sarnat and Silbert, 1976), the diagnosis is best determined by eliciting myotonia on the electromyogram of the affected parent.

About one half of infants whose myotonic dystrophy is symptomatic during the neonatal period die before 1 year of age. The survivors show gradual improvement of their hypotonia and respiratory and feeding difficulties; in fact, many of them will learn to walk. However, mental retardation becomes apparent in some 80 to 90 per cent (Harper, 1975).

Only supportive treatment is available for the myotonic infant. Linkage of the locus for myotonic dystrophy with those of ABH secretion and Lutheran blood group has been established. Since the secretion status of an embryo can be determined at 9 weeks' gestation by detection of antigens in the amniotic fluid, prediction of the clinical status of the offspring is possible in some 15 per cent of couples with better than 90 per cent probability of being correct (Schrott et al., 1973).

CONGENITAL MYOPATHIES ("BENIGN CONGENITAL HYPOTONIAS")

For several years, the term "benign congenital hypotonia" has designated muscular weakness in an infant who, rather than getting progressively worse and finally dying of his condition (as is usually the case in infantile spinal muscular atrophy) may either improve with progressive muscular maturation or at least hold his own. Oppenheim's poorly described patients with amyotonia congenita would probably belong to this group, along with a number of those with new and pathologically well-defined muscular disorders (Table 80–1) (Brooke et al., 1979).

Clinical features characteristic of each entity are listed in Table 80–1. As a rule, these are not sufficient to establish the diagnosis, which must rest on the results of a muscle biopsy.

MUSCULAR HYPERTROPHY

Congenital muscular hypertrophy can be associated with several distinct conditions. A syndrome of generalized muscular enlargement, severe mental retardation with widespread porencephaly, was first described by de Lange in 1934. It is probably not too uncommon, for we have seen several such infants in whom severe developmental retardation was the consequence of perinatal asphyxia.

Hypothyroidism (Debré-Sémélaigne syndrome)

Table 80–1. Some Congenital Myopathies

Disease	Characteristic Clinical Features	Muscle Biopsy Abnormalities	Reference
Nemaline myopathy	Dominant or sporadic transmission; associated skeletal dysmorphism; respiratory problems	Rod-like expansions of Z band	Shafiq et al., 1967
Central core disease	Dominant or sporadic transmission; associated congenital dislocation of hip	Central area of fiber devoid of mitochondria; myofibril disruption variable	Armstrong et al., 1971
Myotubular myopathies	Ptosis; weak external ocular muscles; autosomal dominant and sex-linked forms	Small fibers, mostly type I, with central nuclei in chains	Raju et al., 1977
Mitochondrial myopathies	Extremely variable	Increased size or numbers of mitochondria, "ragged-red" fibers	DiMauro et al., 1980
Multicore (Minicore) disease	Nonprogressive proximal weakness; neck muscle weakness	Multiple small areas of severe filament disruption devoid of mitochondrial enzymes	Heffner et al., 1976
Congenital fiber type disproportion	Muscle contractures; congenital dislocation of hips	Type I fibers smaller than type II; increased variability in fiber diameter	Cavanagh et al., 1979
Fingerprint myopathy	Tremors; mental retardation	Subsarcolemmal; inclusions resembling fingerprints	Engel et al., 1977
Sarcotubular myopathy	None	Dilated and fragmented sarcotubules in type II fibers	Jerusalem et al., 1973
Zebra-body myopathy	None	Unique bodies on electron microscopy	Lake and Wilson, 1973
Reducing body myopathy	None	Inclusions rich in SH groups and ribonucleic acid	Brooke and Neville, 1972
Trilaminar myopathy	Rigidity of muscle tone gradually disappearing with age; increased serum CPK	Distinctive 3-zone fibers by histochemistry and electron microscopy	Ringel et al., 1978
Ullrich's disease	Marked contractures at birth; hyperflexibility of distal joints; myopathic EMG	Nonspecific myopathic changes	Nonaka et al., 1981
Cap disease	Flexion contractures	70% of muscle fibers lack ATP-ase peripherally; abnormally arranged myofibrils	Fidzianska et al., 1981
Type II fiber deficient myopathy	Myopathic facies; tented circumflex upper lip	Absence of type II, hypoplastic type I fibers	Dinn and O'Doherty, 1980
Cytoplasmic body myopathy	None	Cytoplasmic bodies in myofibrils	Goebel et al., 1976
Central nuclei myopathy	X-linked transmission; fatal during neonatal period	Small muscle fibers with central nuclei	Askanas et al., 1979

(From Menkes, J. H.: Textbook of Child Neurology. 2nd ed. Philadelphia, Lea and Febiger, 1980.)

and myotonic dystrophy are two rare causes of congenital muscular hypertrophy (Wilson and Walton, 1959). Finally, a syndrome (Beckwith-Wiedemann) of muscular hypertrophy, macroglossia, omphalocele or umbilical hernia, transient neonatal hypoglycemia, mental retardation, and microcephaly has been described by a number of authors (Sotelo-Avila et al., 1980).

OTHER MUSCULAR DISEASES

In addition to the disorders listed in Table 80–1, several disorders of glycogen metabolism can present during the neonatal period. Of these, glycogen storage disease, type II (Pompe's disease) is probably the most common. This condition presents with severe weakness and hypotonia and impaired swallowing and sucking. It can be distinguished clinically from the other muscular disorders by the associated presence of cardiomegaly, EKG abnormalities, and, occasionally, hepatomegaly. An excess of glycogen is apparent on muscle biopsy (Dubowitz, 1980) (see Chapter 59).

Glycogen storage diseases, type III (debrancher deficiency) and type V (McArdle's disease), have also been reported in early infancy (Dubowitz, 1980; DiMauro and Hartlage, 1978).

REFERENCES

Adams, J. M., Kenny, J. D., and Rudolph, A. J.: Modern management of tetanus neonatorum. Pediatrics 64:472, 1979.
Aminoff, M. J.: Electrodiagnosis in Clinical Neurology. London, Churchill-Livingstone, 1980.

Armstrong, R. M., et al.: Central core disease with congenital hip dislocation: Study of two families. Neurology 21:369, 1971.

Arnon, S. S., et al.: Honey and other environmental risk factors for infant botulism. J. Pediatr. 94:331, 1979.

Askanas, V., et al.: X-linked recessive congenital muscle fiber hypotrophy with central nuclei. Arch. Neurol. 36:604, 1979.

Baskin, J. L., Soule, E. H., and Mills, S. D.: Poliomyelitis of the newborn: pathologic changes in two cases. Am. J. Dis. Child. 80:10, 1950.

Beckerman, R. C., and Buchino, J. J.: Arthrogryposis multiplex congenita as part of an inherited symptom complex. Two case reports and a review of the literature. Pediatrics 61:417, 1978.

Brooke, M. H., Carroll, J. E., and Ringel, S. P.: Congenital hypotonia revisited. Muscle and Nerve 2:84, 1979.

Brooke, M. H., and Neville, H. E.: Reducing body myopathy. Neurology 22:829, 1972.

Buchthal, F., and Olsen, P. Z.: Electromyography and muscle biopsy in infantile spinal muscular atrophy. Brain 93:15, 1970.

Byers, R. K., and Banker, B. Q.: Infantile muscular atrophy. Arch. Neurol. 5:140, 1961.

Cavanagh, N. P. C., Lake, B. D., and McMeniman, P.: Congenital fibre type disproportion myopathy: a histological diagnosis with an uncertain clinical outlook. Arch. Dis. Child. 54:735, 1979.

Chou, S. M., and Nonaka, I.: Werdnig-Hoffmann disease: Proposal of a pathogenetic mechanism. Acta Neuropathol. 41:45, 1978.

de Lange, C.: Congenital hypertrophy of the muscles, extrapyramidal motor disturbances and mental deficiency. Am. J. Dis. Child. 48:243, 1934.

DiMauro, S., and Hartlage, P. L.: Fatal infantile form of muscle phosphorylase deficiency. Neurology 28:1124, 1978.

DiMauro, S., et al.: Fatal infantile mitochondrial myopathy and renal dysfunction due to cytochrome-C-oxidase deficiency. Neurology 30:795, 1980.

Dinn, J. J., and O'Doherty, N.: Congenital Type II fibre deficient myopathy. Irish J. Med. Sci. 149:53, 1980.

Donner, M., Rapola, J., and Somer, H.: Congenital muscular dystrophy: a clinico-pathological and follow-up study of 15 patients. Neuropädiatrie 6:239, 1975.

Dubowitz, V.: The Floppy Infant. Clin. Dev. Med. No. 76, London, William Heinemann, 1980.

Dubowitz, V., and Brooke, M. H.: Muscle Biopsy: A Modern Approach. Philadelphia, W.B. Saunders Co., 1973.

Dyken, P. R., and Harper, P. S.: Congenital dysmorphica myotonica. Neurology 24:465, 1973.

Edwards, R., et al.: Needle biopsy of skeletal muscle in the diagnosis of myopathy and the clinical study of muscle function and repair. N. Engl. J. Med. 302:261, 1980.

Engel, A. G., Lambert, E. H., and Gomez, M. R.: A new myasthenic syndrome with end plate acetylcholinesterase deficiency, small nerve terminals and reduced acetylcholine release. Ann. Neurol. 1:315, 1977.

Engel, A. G., et al.: Ultrastructural localization of the acetylcholine receptor in myasthenia gravis and in its experimental autoimmune model. Neurology 27:307, 1977.

Fenichel, G. M.: Clinical syndromes of myasthenia in infancy and childhood. Arch. Neurol. 35:97, 1978.

Fidzianska, A., et al.: "Cap disease": new congenital myopathy. Neurology 31:1113, 1981.

Goebel, H. H., Schloom, H., and Lenard, H. G.: Congenital myopathy with cytoplasmic bodies. Neuropediatrics 12:166, 1981.

Goebel, H. H., Zeman, W., and DeMyer, W.: Peripheral motor and sensory neuropathy of early childhood simulating Werdnig-Hoffmann disease. Neuropädiatrie 7:182, 1976.

Harper, P. S.: Congenital myotonic dystrophy in Britain. I. Clinical aspects. Arch. Dis. Child. 50:505, 1975.

Heffner, R., et al.: Multicore disease in twins. J. Neurol. Neurosurg. Psychiat. 39:602, 1976.

Herrmann, C., Jr.: The familial occurrence of myasthenia gravis. Ann. N. Y. Acad. Sci. 183:334, 1971.

Jerusalem, F., Engel, A. G., and Gomez, M. R.: Sarcotubular myopathy. Neurology 23:897, 1973.

Kasman, M., Bernstein, L., and Schulman, S.: Chronic polyradiculoneuropathy of infancy. Neurology 26:565, 1976.

Keesey, J., et al.: Anti-acetylcholine receptor antibody in neonatal myasthenia gravis. N. Engl. J. Med. 296:55, 1977.

Kyllerman, M.: Infantile spinal muscular atrophy (morbus Werdnig-Hoffmann) causing neonatal asphyxia. Neuropädiatrie 8:53, 1977.

Lake, B. D., and Wilson, J.: Zebra body myopathy: clinical, histochemical and ultrastructural studies. J. Neurol. Sci. 24:437, 1973.

McMenamin, J. B., Becker, L. E., and Murphy, E. G.: Congenital muscular dystrophy: a clinicopathological report of 24 cases. J. Pediatr. 100:692, 1982.

Newsom-Davis, J., Willcox, N., and Calder, L.: Thymus cells in myasthenia gravis selectively enhance production of anti-acetylcholine-receptor antibody by autologous blood lymphocytes. N. Engl. J. Med. 305:1313, 1981.

Nonaka, I., et al.: A clinical and histological study of Ulrich's disease (congenital atonic-sclerotic muscular dystrophy). Neuropediatrics 12:197, 1981.

Oh, S. J.: Botulism: electrophysiological studies. Ann. Neurol. 1:481, 1977.

Oppenheim, H.: Über allgemeine und lokalisierte Atonie der Muskulatur (Myotonia) im frühen Kindesalter. Monatsschr. Psychiat. Neurol. 8:232, 1900.

Pasternak, J. F., et al.: Exchange transfusion in neonatal myasthenia. J. Pediatr. 99:644, 1981.

Péña, C. E., et al.: Arthrogryposis multiplex congenita: report of two cases of a radicular type with familial incidence. Neurology 18:926, 1968.

Pinheiro, D.: Tetanus of the newborn infant. Pediatrics 34:32, 1964.

Probst, A., et al.: Sensory ganglioneuropathy in infantile spinal muscular atrophy. Neuropediatrics 12:215, 1981.

Raju, T. N. K., et al.: Centronuclear myopathy in the newborn period causing severe respiratory distress. Pediatrics 59:22, 1977.

Ringel, S., et al.: A new congenital neuromuscular disease with trilaminar muscle fibers. Neurology 28:282, 1978.

Sarnat, H. B., and Silbert, S. W.: Maturational arrest of fetal muscle in neonatal myotonic dystrophy. Arch. Neurol. 33:466, 1976.

Schrott, H. G., Karp, L., and Omenn, G. S.: Prenatal prediction in myotonic dystrophy: guidelines for genetic counselling. Clin. Genet. 4:38, 1973.

Seybold, M. E., and Lindstrom, J. M.: Myasthenia gravis in infancy. Neurology 31:476, 1981.

Shafiq, S. A., et al.: Nemaline myopathy. Report of a fatal case with histochemical and electron microscopic studies. Brain 90:817, 1967.

Shore, A., et al.: Identification of two serum components regulating the expression of T-lymphocyte function in childhood myasthenia gravis. N. Engl. J. Med. 301:625, 1979.

Snead, O. C., et al.: Juvenile myasthenia gravis. Neurology 30:732, 1980.

Sotelo-Avila, C., Gonzalez-Crussi, F., and Fowler, J. W.: Complete and incomplete forms of Beckwith-Wiedemann syndrome: their oncogenic potential. J. Pediatr. 96:47, 1980.

Wilson, J., and Walton, J. N.: Some muscular manifestations of hypothyroidism. J. Neurol. Neurosurg. Psychiat. 22:320, 1959.

Wise, G. A., and McQuillen, M. P.: Transient neonatal myasthenia. Arch. Neurol. 22:556, 1970.

81

Focal Intracranial Suppurative Lesions

Despite the frequent occurrence of bacterial sepsis and meningitis in the newborn and young infant, brain abscesses as well as other focal suppurative infections are unusual in this age group. When abscess within the cerebrum does occur in early infancy, it is usually secondary to septicemia. Because of its rarity and the nonspecific character of its clinical manifestations, the condition often goes unsuspected (Sanford, 1928; Butler et al., 1975; Munslow et al., 1975).

Vomiting, lethargy, convulsions, and signs of increased intracranial pressure are the most common features of brain abscess in the young infant. Tenseness of the anterior fontanel and rapidly progressive head enlargement have been present in most reported cases in early infancy (Hoffman et al., 1970). Fever is frequently absent, but peripheral blood leukocytosis is customary. Cerebral abscess formation in the infant is multiple in some cases but when solitary is likely to reach enormous proportions before causing death or until the lesion is identified by CT scans or ultrasonography. Treatment consists of appropriate antibiotic therapy and proper drainage of the lesion by one method or another. The mortality rate is high in this age group. Progressive hydrocephalus requiring shunting is a common complication among survivors.

Subdural empyema is a more common intracranial suppurative lesion than brain abscess in early infancy (Farmer and Wise, 1973). Suppuration may be either unilateral or bilateral, and most cases complicate gram-negative or staphylococcal meningitis. Either subdural empyema, epidural empyema, or meningitis may also complicate an infected cephalhematoma in the newborn child. Pus in the subdural space is poorly tolerated by the young infant and sometimes leads to cortical vein or venous sinus thrombosis. Signs due to the lesion are usually obscured by those of meningitis, and diagnosis is made by CT scans and confirmed by angiography (van Alphen and Dreissen, 1976). Subdural empyema represents a serious complication of meningitis in the infant and is associated with a high incidence of lasting sequelae.

Spinal Epidural Abscess

Spinal epidural suppuration is uncommon at any age but is especially rare in early infancy. Of the few reported cases in the young infant, most have been caused by *Staphylococcus aureus* and have resulted from hematogenous spread in the septic child. Con-genital dermal sinus in the low back can be complicated by epidural abscess formation, although this is infrequent, particularly in infancy.

Although symptoms are usually nonspecific, this condition should always be considered in an irritable infant who screams when moved or handled and in whom tenderness of the spine can be elicited.

Treatment of the condition includes intravenously administered antibiotics and surgical drainage of the lesion. The prognosis is far better in early recognized cases, and the greater the neurologic deficits, and the longer they persist before surgical drainage, the less the extent of expected recovery (Palmer and Kelly, 1972; Aicardi and Lepintre, 1967; Rushworth and Martin, 1958).

Miscellaneous Neurologic Disorders Presenting in the Newborn

By John H. Menkes*

Reye Syndrome

Reye syndrome is characterized by an acute, usually severe noninflammatory encephalopathy and impaired liver function with hypoglycemia and elevated glutamic oxalacetic transaminase and ammonia levels. It often follows a viral illness by several days. The pathogenesis remains obscure.

Although Reye syndrome is unusual in infancy, it has been described in at least three infants in the first month of life. In 1980, Sullivan-Bolyai and coworkers noted a high percentage of affected black males in their series and a more severe outcome when the disorder occurred in the first months of life.

Intracranial Venous Sinus Thrombosis

Thrombosis of the superior sagittal sinus or of multiple intracranial venous sinuses is a devastating insult

---

* This chapter includes portions written by Dr. William E. Bell that appeared in the 4th edition of this book.

in the infant, in part because of the cerebral damage from the disturbance of venous drainage, but also because of the other cerebral effects of the primary condition that causes it. The most widely recognized cause of dural sinus occlusion in early infancy is diarrhea with severe dehydration, especially of the hypernatremic type (Luttrell and Finberg, 1959). It may also complicate generalized sepsis or sepsis with meningitis or subdural empyema. Hyperviscosity secondary to cyanotic congenital heart disease, especially if associated with infection or dehydration, is another possible precipitating factor.

In the living infant, diagnosis of venous sinus thrombosis is difficult because the clinical signs are not specific and are usually combined with neurologic signs related to the underlying cause. Cerebral dysfunction in the infant with sinus thrombosis results from impairment of cortical venous drainage, with secondary cortical vein distention or occlusion giving rise to extensive hemorrhagic cerebral infarction. Bilateral signs, focal or generalized convulsions, coma, and signs of increased intracranial pressure are present in most (Yang et al., 1969). The cerebrospinal fluid is blood-tinged or xanthochromic as the result of subarachnoid bleeding, and the protein content is significantly increased. The mortality rate in infants with major dural sinus thrombosis is high, and survivors are left with neurologic deficits of variable degree.

Congenital Intracranial Aneurysms and Vascular Malformations

Saccular, or "berry," aneurysms, generally considered to be the result of localized congenital defects of the media of the arterial wall, rarely give rise to clinical illness in the childhood age group. They are usually located on major vessels at the base of the brain, and they give rise to symptoms and signs either by rupture with subarachnoid hemorrhage or by a mass effect with compression on adjacent structures. Clinical manifestations in the newborn period or in early infancy caused by aneurysms of this type are extremely rare but have been described (Pickering et al., 1970; Shucart and Wolpert, 1972; Lee et al., 1978). In the few neonatal cases described, spontaneous intracranial bleeding is characterized by an abrupt onset, irritability, vomiting, decreased alertness or coma, and findings indicative of sudden increase in intracranial pressure. Diagnosis before death depends on CT scans and angiographic examination.

A better known type of congenital aneurysm that can produce signs in the newborn infant is aneurysmal malformation of the great vein of Galen (Fig. 81–1). This lesion actually represents an arteriovenous

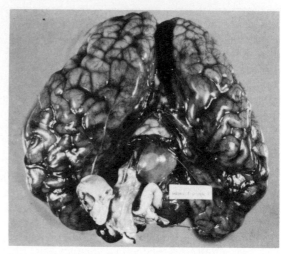

Figure 81–1. Aneurysm of the vein of Galen. Large, saccular mass is located just dorsal to the upper brain stem and, thus, in close proximity to the aqueduct of Sylvius. Initial clinical manifestations are caused by either aqueductal obstruction or high-output cardiac failure.

shunt of large volume. Signs appearing during the neonatal period are primarily those of congestive heart failure. Shunting of a large volume of blood results in decreased peripheral resistance and increased cardiac output. This produces a high output congestive heart failure with cardiomegaly and left axis deviation on EKG. A loud intracranial bruit, often heard without auscultation, a palpable thrill, and engorged scalp veins are other notable features (Gomez et al., 1963; Holden et al., 1972; Montoya et al., 1971; Stein and Wolpert, 1980; So, 1978). In some cases, obstruction of the aqueduct from the adjacent lesion gives rise to hydrocephalus with rapidly progressive head enlargement. Diagnosis of this type of vascular malformation is made on the basis of a CT scan, followed by cerebral angiography. Surgical treatment of aneurysm of the vein of Galen has been attempted (Morelli, 1968), although, when associated with cardiac failure, the lesion carries a poor prognosis in the infant.

Arteriovenous malformations in the cerebral parenchyma only rarely produce clinical signs in the newborn or young infant but can be a source of spontaneous bleeding or seizures (Beatty, 1974). Intraventricular hemorrhage, sometimes fatal, can occur in early infancy as well as in older persons from a cryptic hemangioma of the choroid plexus (Doe et al., 1972). Most described cases have been identified at necropsy.

Congenital Brain Tumors

Although certain types of intracranial tumors are believed to arise from congenital "rests," it is decidedly unusual for abnormal signs to be present in the neonatal period. Chordomas originate from notochord remnants but rarely become symptomatic until adulthood. It has been postulated that craniopharyngiomas develop from remains of the embryonic Rathke pouch but only infrequently cause abnormal signs in the young infant (Azar-Kia et al., 1975; Tabaddor et al., 1974).

Congenital brain tumors that do give rise to neurologic abnormalities in the newborn period are more often supratentorial (75 to 80 per cent of cases) and tend to present with increased intracranial pressure, enlarging head size, and, less often, intracerebral hemorrhage. Their histologic characteristics are generally unusual. A number of cases with cerebral teratomas have been described in newborn infants, sometimes with massive involvement of the brain by the neoplasm (Oberman, 1964; Greenhouse and Neubuerger, 1960; Finck and Antin, 1965). Meningiomas (Mendiratta et al., 1967), medulloblastomas (Kadin et al., 1970; Papadakis et al., 1971), and pontine gliomas (Luse and Teitelbaum, 1968) have also been reported in the neonate but have no characteristic clinical features that will aid in their recognition.

Papilloma of the choroid plexus sometimes will cause abnormal head enlargement in the early weeks of life and is an important lesion because of the possibility of its surgical removal (Matson and Crofton, 1960). Infants with this tumor are usually considered to have hydrocephalus due to the more common causes until an intraventricular mass is demonstrated by CT scan or ultrasonography.

Nasal glioma is a congenital tumor composed of connective tissue and neural elements. The lesion may present extranasally, as a firm nonpulsatile mass at the base of the nose or intranasally, in which case it is easily confused with a nasal polyp (Strauss et al., 1966; Katz and Lewis, 1971). The mass is benign and is generally regarded to be a glial heterotopia and not a brain tumor in the usual sense. Differential diagnosis includes dermoid cyst, nasal polyp, and nasal encephalocele.

Although more properly a concern of the physician dealing with neurologic problems of late infancy and childhood, the phakomatoses (neurocutaneous syndromes) occasionally are evident at birth.

Approximately 43 per cent of infants with neurofibromatosis exhibit physical signs at birth, usually multiple café-au-lait spots (Fienman and Yakovac, 1970). Symptoms of tuberous sclerosis can be present at birth or in early infancy. The characteristic depigmented nevi are sometimes visible at birth; in the experience of Pampiglione and Moynahan, reported in 1976, 12 per cent of their patients developed adenoma sebaceum prior to 1 year of age. Seizures may also be present during the neonatal period, and the CT scan demonstrates the multiple scattered calcium deposits at a time when plain radiographs of the skull are still negative (Kuhlendahl et al., 1977).

Sturge-Weber syndrome is readily diagnosable in the newborn by observation of the presence of a portwine vascular nevus on the upper part of the face involving at least one eyelid and the supraorbital region. CT scans or even plain skull films may show intracranial calcifications (Nellhaus et al., 1967).

Congenital Intraspinal Tumors

Intraspinal tumors, which are infrequent in early infancy, are less likely to be intramedullary in infants than they are in older children. Because of the rare occurrence of intraspinal masses in this age group, the difficulty in recognizing the progressive nature of the neurologic deficits and the relatively poor diagnostic value of neurogenic bladder and sensory disturbances, early identification of such lesions is often delayed. They are easily confused with, and erroneously diagnosed as, cerebral palsy, cervical cord birth injury, or brachial plexus stretch palsy.

Intraspinal lesions above the second lumbar vertebra cause signs of spinal cord dysfunction. The character of signs of cord involvement or compression is less predictable in infants than in older children. Although spastic signs are expected, the infant with a cervical or thoracic cord lesion can present with hypotonic limbs that exhibit enhanced deep stretch reflexes. Spinal rigidity, although not always present, is a finding that should suggest the possibility of some form of intraspinal mass, regardless of the age of the child. Intraspinal lesions below the second lumbar vertebra give rise to manifestations of cauda equina compression or to a combination of signs indicative of involvement of the conus medullaris and the cauda equina. Compression of the cauda equina results in hypotonic or flaccid legs, often asymmetrically so, with reflex loss and muscular atrophy in affected regions. A sensory level to pin stimulation usually indicates a spinal cord lesion but can also occur with intraspinal lesions below the termination of the spinal cord.

Although astrocytomas or ependymomas of the spinal cord can occur in infancy, they are unusual in the newborn period (Tachdjian and Matson, 1965). Signs of congenital neuroblastoma are usually those of metastatic disease and include hepatomegaly and cutaneous nodules (Schneider et al., 1965), but direct invasion to the intraspinal epidural space can also complicate these lesions. Direct extension from a primary adrenal tumor is likely to affect the mid-to-low thoracic cord, whereas that from a mediastinal neuroblastoma will involve the low cervical or upper thoracic portion of the spinal cord. Sarcomatous lesions of various types can either invade the epidural space from the retroperitoneal region or arise primarily within the spinal canal. Extramedullary compression of the spinal cord can also result from a variety of benign or malignant tumors of the vertebrae.

Probably the most frequently identified intraspinal tumor in the young infant is the intradural lipoma (Swanson and Barnett, 1962; Dubowitz et al., 1965). Most are found in the lumbar or lumbosacral region, although they can occur elsewhere. The presence of a lumbar intradural lipoma is usually signaled by the presence of an associated extradural lipomatous mass, which presents as a soft painless swelling on the midline of the low back. A cutaneous dermal sinus or hemangioma is frequently observed in the region of the superficial mass. Radiographs of the spine are diagnostically revealing in most cases because of the presence of widening of the pedicles with pedicular erosion. When the intradural mass extends into the lower part of the spinal canal, hypoplasia or destructive changes of the sacrum are often visualized. Neurologic signs caused by an intradural lipoma usually do not develop until the child is a few years of age.

In the infant with intradural lipoma, signs of denervation, when present, are usually in the form of a foot deformity and wasting of one lower limb, with associated deep reflex asymmetry. The advisability of surgical excision of the intradural lipoma is a controversial matter. Complete removal can usually not be accomplished because of the intimate relationship between the mass and the neural elements. Partial excision is recommended when there is evidence of progressive neurologic dysfunction, although every effort must be made not to produce additional deficits from the surgical procedure itself.

Diagnosis of an intraspinal tumor of any type is on the basis of the clinical findings, appropriate radiographs of the spine, and contrast myelography. The latter procedure is technically more difficult in the infant than in the older child and especially so if a lumbar puncture has been done within a few days preceding the study. For this reason, it is advisable to withhold a spinal fluid examination until the time of myelography if an intraspinal mass is suspected.

Heredodegenerative Diseases

Only a few of the heredodegenerative diseases affecting the nervous system occur in the newborn (Table 81–1). As a rule, these diseases are difficult to diagnose during the neonatal period. Their clinical manifestations (i.e., spasticity, hypotonia, seizures, unusual eye movements) are far more commonly the consequence of perinatal asphyxia or cerebral malformations. Thus, it is only when the infant's progressive deterioration becomes evident that their presence begins to be suspected.

A few clues, however, have been established. The presence of combined upper and lower motor neuron signs—the most common of which are seizures, hypotonia, and absent deep tendon reflexes—should alert the physician to a white matter degenerative disease. One can confirm the diagnosis by finding a striking elevation of CSF protein and characteristic pathologic alterations on a sural nerve biopsy.

The presence of kinky, poorly pigmented hair points to kinky hair disease or giant axonal neuropathy, whereas a hoarse cry suggests lipogranulomatosis, cretinism, or Cornelia de Lange syndrome.

Table 81–1. Heredodegenerative Diseases Apparent During the First Month of Life

Condition	Reference
Diffuse cerebral degenerative diseases	
White matter degenerations	
Globoid cell leukodystrophy (Krabbe's disease)	Schochet et al., 1969
Spongy degeneration of white matter (Canavan's disease)	Sacks et al., 1965
Metachromatic leukodystrophy	Bubis and Adlesburg, 1966
Pelizaeus-Merzbacher disease	Ulrich and Herschkowitz, 1977
Sudanophilic leukodystrophy	Sarnat and Adelman, 1973
Infantile neuroaxonal dystrophy	Janota, 1979
Alexander's disease	Nagao et al., 1981
Gray matter degenerations	
"Alper's disease" (lactic acidoses, mitochondrial myopathies)	Jellinger and Seitelberger, 1977
Kinky hair disease (Menke's syndrome)	Danks et al., 1972
Heredodegenerative diseases of the basal ganglia	
None	
Heredodegenerative diseases of cerebellum, brain stem, spinal cord, and peripheral nerve	
Hypertrophic interstitial polyneuropathy (Dejerine-Sottas disease)	Anderson et al., 1973
White matter hypoplasia	Chattha and Richardson, 1977
Giant axonal neuropathy	Mizuno et al., 1979
Familial dysautonomia	Perlman et al., 1979
Lipid storage diseases	
Congenital amaurotic idiocy	Hagberg et al., 1965
GM$_1$ gangliosidosis	O'Brien, 1978
GM$_3$ gangliosidosis	Maclaren et al., 1976
Lipogranulomatosis (Farber's disease)	Abul-Haj et al., 1962
I-cell disease	Spritz et al., 1978

Coarse facies is an early feature of I-cell disease and generalized GM_1 and GM_3 gangliosidoses. Macroglossia occurs in the neonate not only with cretinism but also with Beckwith-Wiedemann syndrome, GM_1 gangliosidosis, and GM_3 gangliosidosis. The diagnosis of the last two disorders depends on a biopsy of bone marrow or skin.

For a fuller discussion of these disorders, the reader is referred to texts of child neurology (e.g., Menkes, 1980).

FAMILIAL DYSAUTONOMIA (RILEY-DAY SYNDROME)

Familial dysautonomia is an autosomal recessive disorder confined to Jews of Eastern European descent. In the United States, the frequency of the carrier state in this group is one in 50.

The basic defect appears to involve an abnormality in β-nerve growth factor (NGF). Cells derived from patients with this condition produce normal amounts of an immunoreactive NGF protein that only has 10 per cent of normal biological activity (Schwartz and Breakefield, 1980).

Clinical signs of this condition are usually present soon after birth, although their nonspecific character makes early diagnosis extremely difficult. Diminished muscle tone, poor Moro response, difficulty with feeding because of inability to coordinate the suck and swallow mechanisms, and respiratory distress are the usual initial abnormalities in the neonatal and early infancy periods (Geltzer et al., 1964). Later, the dysautonomic child will demonstrate developmental retardation, episodic fever, absent deep tendon reflexes, diminished to absent lacrimation, scoliosis, excessive sweating, episodic hypertension, and relative indifference to pain stimulation. As the result of reduced pain sensation, older children frequently show the effects of recurrent traumatic lesions, such as corneal ulcerations, Charcot joints, or soft tissue scars or deformities of the fingers or toes.

The diagnosis of dysautonomia depends on the patient's history and genetic background and on the clinical features of the condition. Of the various tests designed to elicit autonomic dysfunction, the intradermal histamine test has been the most reliable in our experience. In normal subjects, intradermal injection of histamine phosphate (0.03 to 0.05 ml of a 1 : 1000 solution) produces a local wheal and a red erythematous flare extending 1 to 3 cm beyond the wheal. In dysautonomic patients, the flare response is absent. A similar response may be produced in atopic dermatitis and in some disorders of the spinal cord or peripheral nerves (e.g., progressive sensory neuropathy).

Treatment of the condition is purely symptomatic. Impaired swallowing as well as vomiting and abdominal distention may be relieved with bethanechol (Urecholine), a parasympathomimetic agent. (Axelrod, 1972).

REFERENCES

Abul-Haj, S. K., et al.: Farber's disease: report of a case with observations on its histogenesis and notes on the nature of the stored material. J. Pediatr. *61*:221, 1962.

Aicardi, J., and Lepintre, J.: Spinal epidural abscess in a 1-month old child. Am. J. Dis. Child. *114*:665, 1967.

Anderson, R. M., et al.: Hypertrophic interstitial polyneuropathy in infancy: clinical and pathological features in two cases. J. Pediatr. *82*:619, 1973.

Axelrod, F. B., and Bloom, J.: Caring for the Child with Familial Dysautonomia. (A Handbook for Patients.) New York, Dysautonomic Foundation, 1975.

Axelrod, F. B., et al.: Treatment of familial dysautonomia with bethanecol (Urecholine). J. Pediatr. *81*:573, 1972.

Azar-Kia, B., Krishnan, U. R., and Schechter, M. M.: Neonatal craniopharyngioma. J. Neurosurg. *42*:91, 1975.

Beatty, R. A.: Surgical treatment of a ruptured intracerebral arteriovenous malformation in a newborn. Pediatrics *53*:571, 1974.

Bell, W. E., and McCormick, W. F.: Reye's syndrome. *In* Neurologic Infections in Children. Philadelphia, W.B. Saunders Co., 1981.

Bubis, J. J., and Adlesburg, L.: Congenital metachromatic leukodystrophy: report of a case. Acta Neuropathol. *6*:298, 1966.

Butler, N. R., Barrie, H., and Paine, K. W. E.: Cerebral abscess as a complication of neonatal sepsis. Arch. Dis. Child. *32*:461, 1975.

Chattha, A. S., and Richardson, E. P.: Cerebral white-matter hypoplasia. Arch. Neurol. *34*:137, 1977.

Danks, D. M., et al.: Menkes' kinky hair syndrome: an inherited defect in copper absorption with widespread effects. Pediatrics *50*:188, 1972.

Doe, F. D., Shuangshoti, S., and Netsky, M. G.: Cryptic hemangioma of the choroid plexus. Neurology *22*:1232, 1972.

Dubowitz, V., Lorker, J., and Zachary, R. B.: Lipoma of the cauda equina. Arch. Dis. Child. *40*:207, 1965.

Farmer, T. W., and Wise, G. R.: Subdural empyema in infants, children and adults. Neurology *23*:254, 1973.

Fienman, N. L., and Yakovac, W. C.: Neurofibromatosis in childhood. J. Pediatr. *76*:339, 1970.

Finck, F. M., and Antin, R.: Intracranial teratoma of the newborn. Am. J. Dis. Child. *109*:439, 1965.

Geltzer, A. I., Gluck, L., Talner, N. S., and Polesky, H. F.: Familial dysautonomia. Studies in the newborn infant. N. Engl. J. Med. *271*:436, 1964.

Gomez, M. R., Whitten, C. F., Nolke, A., Bernstein, J., and Meyer, J. S.: Aneurysmal malformation of the great vein of Galen causing heart failure in early infancy. Pediatrics *31*:400, 1963.

Greenhouse, A. H., and Neubuerger, K. T.: Intracranial teratomata of the newborn. Arch. Neurol. *3*:718, 1960.

Hagberg, B. G., et al.: Congenital amaurotic idiocy. Acta Paediatr. Scand. *54*:116, 1965.

Hoffman, H. J., Hendrick, E. B., and Hiscox, J. L.: Cerebral abscess in early infancy. J. Neurosurg. *33*:172, 1970.

Holden, A. M., et al.: Congestive heart failure from intracranial arteriovenous fistula in infancy: clinical and physiological considerations in 8 patients. Pediatrics *49*:30, 1972.

Huttenlocher, P. R., and Trauner, D. A.: Reye's syndrome in infancy. Pediatrics *62*:84, 1978.

Janota, I.: Neuroaxonal dystrophy in the neonate. Acta Neuropathol. *46*:151, 1979.

Jellinger, K., and Seitelberger, F.: Spongy encephalopathies in infancy: spongy degeneration of CNS and progressive infantile poliodystrophy. *In* Goldensohn, E. S., and Appel, S. H. (Eds.): Scientific Approaches to Clinical Neurology. Philadelphia, Lea and Febiger, 1977, pp. 363–386.

Jellinger, K., and Sunder-Plassmann, M.: Connatal intracranial tumors. Neuropädiatrie *4*:46, 1973.

Kadin, M. E., Rubinstein, L. J., and Nelson, J. S.: Neonatal cerebellar medulloblastoma originating from the fetal external granular layer. J. Neuropathol. Exper. Neurol. 29:583, 1970.

Katz, A., and Lewis, J. S.: Nasal gliomas. Arch. Otolaryngol. 94:351, 1971.

Kuhlendahl, H. D., et al.: Cranial computer tomography in children with tuberous sclerosis. Neuropädiatrie 8:325, 1977.

Lee, Y. J., Kandall, S. R., and Ghali, V. S.: Intracerebral arterial aneurysm in a newborn. Arch. Neurol. 35:171, 1978.

Levine, O. R., Jameson, A. G., Nellhaus, G., and Gold, A. P.: Cardiac complications of cerebral arteriovenous fistula in infancy. Pediatrics 30:563, 1962.

Luse, S. A., and Teitelbaum, S.: Congenital glioma of brain stem. Arch. Neurol. 18:196, 1968.

Luttrell, C. N., and Finberg, L.: Hemorrhagic encephalopathy induced by hypernatremia. Arch. Neurol. Psychiatry 81:424, 1959.

Maclaren, N. K., et al.: GM$_3$ gangliosidosis: a novel human sphingolipodystrophy. Pediatrics 57:106, 1976.

Matson, D. D., and Crofton, F. D. L.: Papilloma of the choroid plexus in childhood. J. Neurosurg. 17:1002, 1960.

Mendiratta, S. S., Rosenblum, J. A., and Strobos, R. J.: Congenital meningioma. Neurology 17:914, 1967.

Menkes, J. H.: Textbook of Child Neurology. 2nd ed. Philadelphia, Lea and Febiger, 1980.

Mizuno, Y., et al.: Giant axonal neuropathy. Combined central and peripheral nervous system disease. Arch. Neurol. 36:107, 1979.

Montoya, G., Dohn, D. F., and Mercer, R. D.: Arteriovenous malformation of the vein of Galen as a cause of heart failure and hydrocephalus in infants. Neurology 21:1054, 1971.

Morelli, R. J.: Surgery of aneurysms of the great vein of Galen. Rocky Mountain Med. J. 65:41, 1968.

Munslow, R. A., Stovall, V. S., Price, R. D., and Kohler, C. M.: Brain abscess in infants. J. Pediatr. 51:74, 1975.

Nagao, H., et al.: Alexander disease: clinical, electrodiagnostic and radiographic studies. Neuropediatrics 12:22, 1981.

Nellhaus, G., Haberland, C., and Hill, B. J.: Sturge-Weber disease with bilateral intracranial calcification at birth and unusual pathologic findings. Acta Neurol. Scand. 43:314, 1967.

Oberman, B.: Intracranial teratoma replacing brain. Arch. Neurol. 11:423, 1964.

O'Brien, J. S.: The gangliosidoses. In Stanbury, J. B., Wyngaarden, J. B., Fredrickson, D. S., Goldstein, J. L., and Brown, M. S. (Eds.): The Metabolic Basis of Inherited Disease. 5th ed. New York, McGraw-Hill, 1983, pp. 945–972.

Palmer, J. J., and Kelly, W. A.: Epidural abscess in a 3-week-old infant: case report. Pediatrics 50:817, 1972.

Pampiglione, G., and Moynahan, E. J.: The tuberous sclerosis syndrome: clinical and EEG studies in 100 children. J. Neurol. Neurosurg. Psychiat. 39:666, 1976.

Papadakis, N., Millan, J., Grady, D. F., and Segerberg, L. H.: Medulloblastoma of the neonatal period and early infancy. J. Neurosurg. 34:88, 1971.

Perlman, M., Benady, S., and Saggi, E.: Neonatal diagnosis of familial dysautonomia. Pediatrics 63:238, 1979.

Pickering, L. K., Hogan, G. R., and Gilbert, E. F.: Aneurysm of the posterior inferior cerebellar artery. Rupture in a newborn. Am. J. Dis. Child. 119:155, 1970.

Rushworth, R. G., and Martin, P. B.: Acute spinal epidural abscess: a case in an infant with recovery. Arch. Dis. Child. 33:261, 1958.

Sacks, O., Brown, W. J., and Aguilar, M. J.: Spongy degeneration of white matter. Canavan's disease. Neurology 15:165, 1965.

Sanford, H. N.: Abscess of the brain in infants under twelve months of age. Am. J. Dis. Child. 35:256, 1928.

Sarnat, H. B., and Adelman, L. S.: Perinatal sudanophilic leukodystrophy. Am. J. Dis. Child. 125:281, 1973.

Schneider, K. M., Becker, J. M., and Krasna, I. H.: Neonatal neuroblastoma. Pediatrics 36:359, 1965.

Schochet, S. S., et al.: Krabbe's disease (globoid leukodystrophy): Electron microscopic observations. Arch. Pathol. 88:305, 1969.

Schum, T. R., et al.: Neonatal intraventricular hemorrhage due to an intracranial arteriovenous malformation: a case report. Pediatrics 64:242, 1979.

Schwartz, J. P., and Breakefield, X. O.: Altered nerve growth factor in fibroblasts from patients with familial dysautonomia. Proc. Natl. Acad. Sci. 77:1154, 1980.

Shucart, W. A., and Wolpert, S. A.: An aneurysm in infancy presenting with diabetes insipidus. J. Neurosurg. 37:368, 1972.

So, S. C.: Cerebral arteriovenous malformations in children. Childs Brain 2:242, 1978.

Spritz, R. A., et al.: Neonatal presentation of I-cell disease. J. Pediatr. 93:954, 1978.

Stein, B. M., and Wolpert, S. M.: Arteriovenous malformations of the brain. Arch. Neurol. 37:1, 1980.

Strauss, R. B., Callicott, J. H., and Hargett, I. R.: Intranasal neuroglial heterotopia. Am. J. Dis. Child. 111:317, 1966.

Sullivan-Bolyai, J., Nielson, D. B., Morens, D. M., et al.: Reye syndrome in children less than 1 year old: some epidemiological observations. Pediatrics 65:627, 1980.

Swanson, H. S., and Barnett, J. C., Jr.: Intradural lipomas in children. Pediatrics 29:911, 1962.

Tabaddor, K., Shulman, K., and Dal Canto, M. C.: Neonatal craniopharyngioma. Am. J. Dis. Child. 128:381, 1974.

Tachdjian, M. O., and Matson, D. D.: Orthopaedic aspects of intraspinal tumors in infants and children. J. Bone Joint Surg. 47A:223, 1965.

Thibault, J. H., and Manuelidis, E. E.: Tuberous sclerosis in a premature infant. Report of a case and review of the literature. Neurology 20:139, 1970.

Ulrich, J., and Herschkowitz, N.: Seitelberger's connatal form of Pelizaeus-Merzbacher's disease. Acta Neuropathol. 40:129, 1977.

Van Alphen, H. A., and Dreissen, J. J.: Brain abscess and subdural empyema. J. Neurol. Neurosurg. Psychiat. 39:481, 1976.

Yang, D. C., Sohn, D., and Anand, H. K.: Thrombosis of the superior longitudinal sinus during infancy. J. Pediatr. 74:570, 1969.

12 PART INFECTIONS

82

Immunology

By Robertson Parkman

General Considerations

The unique physiology of the neonatal immune system protects the normal infant against some pathogens to which older children are susceptible (chickenpox, measles, *Hemophilus influenzae*) while infections with organisms that give little difficulty later in life (enteric gram-negative bacteria, herpes simplex virus, cytomegalovirus, *Candida albicans*) occur. This chapter will focus on the unique aspects of the neonatal immune system and how they relate to the newborn's susceptibility to infectious disease.

At birth, the infant passes from a relatively pathogen-free environment to one containing a great variety of pathogens—bacterial, viral, fungal, or protozoan. The success of the infant in protecting himself against these pathogens depends on the capacity of his immune system to respond to the pathogens.

Male infants have an increased susceptibility to infections when compared with female infants. In 1965, Washburn and his collaborators reported that the enhanced susceptibility was more marked in newborn infants than in older ones. Bacterial meningitis occurred 1.8 times more frequently in male infants than in females; for septicemias, the ratio was 2.02:1. The basis of the increased susceptibility of male infants is not clear.

The defense mechanisms of the newborn infant can be divided into cellular and humoral components. Those mechanisms that require previous exposure to the specific pathogen to be effective are called "immune," and those components that require no prior exposure for their effectiveness are known as "nonimmune," or "general" (Table 82–1).

Table 82–1. Defense Mechanisms Against Infectious Pathogens

	Humoral Defense	Cellular Defense
General	Complement system Properdin system	Granulocytes Monocytes Reticuloendothelial system
Immune	Immunoglobulins	Lymphocytes

Specific Humoral Immunity

IMMUNOGLOBULINS

Immunoglobulins are the mechanisms by which specific humoral immunity is mediated. The immunoglobulin molecule is composed of four polypeptide chains: two light chains and two heavy chains. There are presently five known classes of immunoglobulins that are named according to their heavy chains, which are unique for each class: IgG, IgA, IgM, IgD, and IgE. The light chains are common to all the immunoglobulin classes (Merler and Rosen, 1966).

IgG

IgG is the predominant immunoglobulin (approximately 75 per cent) in adult life. Antibodies to viruses, bacterial toxins, and the encapsulated pyogenic bacteria are almost exclusively IgG. Maternal IgG molecules are actively transported across the placenta so that at birth infants have IgG levels equal to, if not slightly greater than, those of normal mothers. The IgG molecule has a specific combining site that permits it to attach to the placenta. The mechanism by which the IgG is transferred across the placenta is unknown; however, there may be some selectivity based on the fact that infants of hypergammaglobulinemic mothers have normal IgG levels and that infants may have smallpox hemagglutination inhibition titers significantly greater than those of their mothers. The transplacental transfer of IgG increases with increasing gestational age (Fig. 82–1). Since the majority of the antibody is transferred during the third trimester, cord IgG levels of premature infants are decreased when compared with those of full-term infants. Transplacentally derived maternal IgG is degraded by the newborn, with a half-life of 3 to 4 weeks; thus, biologically significant maternal IgG may be present in the infant's circulation for from 3 to 12 months, depending on the initial IgG levels, with the duration of protective antibody being least in premature infants (Washburn, 1966).

The full-term infant of a normal mother has a full complement of adult IgG antibodies; therefore, newborn infants are not susceptible to most common viral infections (measles, rubella, chickenpox) until the transplacentally acquired antibody titer drops to biologically nonprotective levels. The presence of the transplacental derived antibody is the reason that the immunization of children with MMR vaccine (measles, mumps, and rubella) is delayed until 14 months.

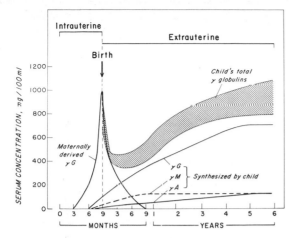

Figure 82–1. Schematic representation of fetal and neonatal immunoglobulin levels. (Adapted from Janeway, C. A. *In* Nelson, W. E., Vaughan, V. C., and McKay, R. J. [Eds.]: Textbook of Pediatrics. 9th ed. Philadelphia, W. B. Saunders Co., 1969).

The presence of passive antibody can lead to ineffective immunization (Provenzano et al., 1965). Passive antibody protection against the encapsulated pyogenic organisms (e.g., *Staphylococcus, Hemophilus influenzae, Streptococcus, Pneumococcus*) is present for the first several months. However, there are no transplacental antibodies to the somatic antigens of the enteric gram-negative organisms (Table 82–2).

At birth, the synthetic rate of IgG is less than that of adults. The lowered synthetic rate of IgG may continue for the first several months of life so that the total serum IgG level decreases to its minimal value at 3 to 4 months, after which time the serum IgG levels begin to rise in normal children. If there is a delay in the onset of increased IgG synthesis, the period of hypogammaglobulinemia may be prolonged (see discussion of agammaglobulinemia further on in this chapter).

Early onset group B streptococcal sepsis and meningitis demonstrate the dependence of the neonate on maternal transmission of antistreptococcal IgG. Infants of women who are colonized with group B streptococci are at risk for developing early onset disease. Colonized women with high antibody titers to the type III polysaccharide of the group B strepto-

Table 82–2. Antibodies Passively Acquired by the Fetus

Antigens to Which Antibodies in Cord Blood Are Equal to or Higher than Those in Maternal Blood	Antigens to Which Antibodies in Cord Blood Are Less than Those in Maternal Blood or at Times Absent
Tetanus	*Hemophilus influenzae*
Diphtheria	Blood group antigens
Streptococcus	*Shigella*
Staphylococcus	Poliomyelitis
Bordetella pertussis	*Salmonella* (O antigen)
Toxoplasma	*Escherichia coli* (H and O antigen)
Salmonella (H antigen)	

coccus transmit this IgG to the fetus transplacentally. Neonatal antibody titres to this organism are directly correlated with maternal levels. Colonized women whose infants remained healthy have been shown to have higher serum antistreptococcal antibody titers than colonized women whose infants developed early onset group B streptococcal disease (Baker et al., 1981). Investigations of the value of maternal immunization against group B streptococcus are currently in progress in a number of centers. A colonized woman who has had a child with early onset group B streptococcal disease may soon have access to a vaccine either prior to or during a subsequent pregnancy. For the infant with overwhelming group B streptococcal sepsis, early exchange transfusion of fresh, whole, irradiated blood from a donor with high antistreptococcal titers may be beneficial.

The transplacental transfer of maternal IgG may, in some cases, have a detrimental effect on the fetus or newborn. If the mother has either naturally occurring or immune IgG antibodies against red blood cell antigens (such as ABO, Rh, Kell, or Le) or platelet antigens present in the fetal cells, the antibody coated cells will be destroyed in the fetus, producing either erythroblastosis fetalis or neonatal isoimmunothrombocytopenia. Blood group A or B individuals usually produce naturally occurring isohemagglutinins of the IgM class that do not cross the placenta, whereas group O individuals may produce isohemagglutinins that are IgG. Thus, blood group A and B infants of blood group O mothers may receive naturally occurring IgG antibodies, transplacentally producing ABO-incompatible erythroblastosis.

IgM

IgM represents 15 per cent of normal adult immunoglobulin. Antibodies to gram-negative enteric organisms, blood group antigens, and some viral antigens are IgM. Since IgM is a large molecule that does not readily cross the placenta, little maternal IgM antibody is found in fetal or neonatal circulation. The IgM in cord blood, then, is fetal antibody. The absence of maternal IgM leaves the newborn without passively acquired protection against gram-negative enteric bacteria or viruses.

Synthesis of IgM by the fetus begins at 10 to 15 weeks of gestation (Lawton and Cooper, 1977). Little antibody synthesis occurs in utero, since the fetus is in an antigenically null environment. The presence of IgM levels of greater than 20 mg/ml at birth suggests increased in utero antigenic stimulation. Possible sources of this stimulation include transplacentally acquired maternal blood elements and congenital infections (cytomegalovirus, toxoplasmosis, rubella, herpes). Routine measurements of IgM and IgA levels to screen for congenital infection are not warranted. However, in the case of either the intrauterine growth—retarded infant or the infant with stigmata of intrauterine viral infection, the cord blood IgM level can be a rapid first test to determine whether or not the infant has been exposed to a viral infection. An elevated umbilical cord IgM level demands that specific viral titers (TORCH) be obtained from both the mother and infant. Elevated titers to any of the common intrauterine viruses requires repeat titers in 6 weeks. In the case of active viral infection, neonatal titers will be persistently elevated. If the elevated titers are simply due to passive transmission of antibody, these neonatal titers will decrease at the time of the second screen at 6 weeks of age.

IgA

IgA accounts for 10 to 15 per cent of normal adult serum immunoglobulin; however, its principal role is as the primary immunoglobulin in secretions, including those of the upper respiratory system and gastrointestinal tract and colostrum. Only about 10 per cent of secretory IgA is derived from serum; the rest is locally produced. IgA can be detected on the surface of fetal B cells from the twelfth week of gestation (Gatherings et al., 1977), but very little IgA is present in serum or secretions for the first 2 years of life. Since IgA does not cross the placenta, little IgA is usually found in the cord blood. A cord IgA of greater than 20 mg per 100 ml is a sign, as is increased IgM, of in utero antigenic stimulation. Normal infants have detectable serum IgA levels by the end of the first month of life, but adult levels are not achieved until the age of 10 years (Smith, 1969).

Colostrum has a high content of secretory IgA, with peak IgA levels present on postnatal day 3 in breast milk from mothers of both term and preterm infants. Gross and colleagues have shown that IgA levels are higher in breast milk from mothers of preterm infants (256 mg/gm protein) than in that from mothers of term infants (97 mg/gm protein). In breast-fed infants, IgA levels in tears and nasal secretions are higher than those of formula-fed controls. Ogra and colleagues have examined IgA metabolism in the newborn and suggest that IgA is absorbed in the neonatal gastrointestinal tract and subsequently eliminated from nasal and conjunctival mucosal surfaces.

Work by several investigators suggests that IgA-producing cells in Peyer's patches produce IgA directed specifically against antigens present in the maternal gastrointestinal tract. Some of these cells subsequently migrate to the lactating mammary gland, where this specifically stimulated IgA is released into colostrum and breast milk. Unlike other immunoglobulins, IgA is resistant to the proteolytic effects of gastric acid. Secretory IgA coats the gut mucosa, prevents bacterial adherence to mucosal surfaces, and inhibits invasion of the mucosa by enterobacteria and parasites (Walker and Isselbacher, 1977). Therefore, maternal colostral IgA may play a role in passive immunity to enterobacteria.

IgE

IgE antibodies do not cross the placenta in significant amounts. The most important biological activity of IgE immunoglobulin is its skin-sensitizing activity. Infants of mothers with significant allergic histories and symptoms do not give positive wheal-and-flare reactions to antigens to which their mothers are sensitive.

IgD

IgD globulins have no known specific biological activity. Although little IgD is found in cord blood, at least 50 per cent of cord blood lymphocytes contain IgD on their cell surface. Often these pre-B lymphocytes express surface IgM as well as IgD. The simultaneous expression of these two classes of immunoglobulin on the lymphocyte surface suggests that these are immature B lymphocytes (Conley and Cooper, 1981). As the cells are exposed to and stimulated by new antigens, they mature into functioning B lymphocytes. During this process, the frequency of IgD as a surface marker decreases.

Immune Reactivity

Initially, it was felt that the newborn infant was immunologically incompetent; that is, that the infant was incapable of specific humoral or cellular immune responses. However, it is now clear that the fetus and newborn can respond normally to a wide variety of antigens (Silverstein, 1964). Specific IgM antibody to intrauterine infections such as syphilis and rubella has been detected by 16 to 20 weeks of gestation, and IgG antibodies of fetal origin have been detected in the third trimester. After birth, the infant has his primary experience to most antigens, and antibodies to enterobacilli and skin bacteria soon appear in the circulation. The presence of maternal IgG may decrease the newborn's response to some antigens, contributing to the previous concept of the newborn's immunoincompetence.

Specific Cellular Immunity

LYMPHOCYTE ONTOGENY

Lymphocytes can be classified into three groups: (1) T, or thymus-derived, (2) B, or bone marrow—

derived, and (3) null (neither T nor B) lymphocytes (Raff, 1973). T lymphocytes from both adults and fetuses form rosettes with sheep red blood cells (E) and are responsible for protection against fungal, viral, and some enterobacillary infections and mediate homograft rejections. B lymphocytes are characterized by the presence of immunoglobulin on their cell surfaces and a surface receptor for the third component of the complement system (C3). Some circulating B lymphocytes after antigen exposure migrate to the lymph nodes, where they differentiate into plasma cells that synthesize much of the circulating immunoglobulin.

Whereas the newborn infant has significant passive humoral immunity due to transplacental maternal IgG, the infant's cellular immunity is totally in lymphocytes of fetal origin. Immunocompetent cells capable of responding to foreign lymphocytes in the mixed lymphocyte reaction are found in the fetal liver at 5 weeks' gestation. Prior to 8 weeks' gestation, the thymus is composed of only stromal and reticular elements (fetal thymus). After 8 weeks, T lymphocytes are found and lymphoid follicles and Hassall's corpuscles develop (adult thymus); by 12 to 14 weeks, T lymphocytes are found in the fetal spleen; by 15 to 20 weeks' gestation, the fetus has significant numbers of peripheral T lymphocytes (August et al., 1971).

Lymphocytes that stain with a fluoresceinated antiserum to IgM are first found in the fetal liver at 9 weeks and in the spleen at 11 weeks. Fetal spleen cells are capable of in vitro IgM synthesis at 11 weeks and IgG synthesis at 13 weeks. By 20 weeks' gestation, the fetus has the capacity to respond with specific antibody production to some antigenic stimuli.

At birth, the absolute number of T lymphocytes is increased as compared with adult levels, even though the percentage of T lymphocytes is lower than adult levels. The number of B lymphocytes as determined by the presence of a receptor for C3 is increased at birth in both absolute number and percentage. Adult values for T and B lymphocytes are found by 2 to 3 years of age (Fleisher et al., 1975).

Infants who are small for gestational age (SGA) or premature have decreased numbers of T lymphocytes with an equivalent decrease in mitogenic responsiveness. Premature infants normalize their T lymphocytes number by 1 month, whereas SGA infants have depressed T lymphocyte counts 12 months after birth. SGA infants have decreased levels of circulation thymic hormones, suggesting that their decrease in T lymphocyte number may be secondary to the lack of normal thymic endocrine function, since thymic involution has been associated with fetal growth retardation (Chandra, 1981).

Immunocompetent T lymphocytes function primarily by the release of mediators, such as migration inhibition factor (MIF) or interferon, following the specific stimulation of sensitized lymphocytes. Neonatal lymphocytes are capable of MIF production after stimulation with allogenic lymphocytes, and interferon production is normal after mitogenic and polyriboinosinic-cytidilic acid stimulation.

Because of the privileged nature of the uterus, the circulating neonatal T lymphocytes are virginal; thus, the infant displays no skin test reactivity to intra-

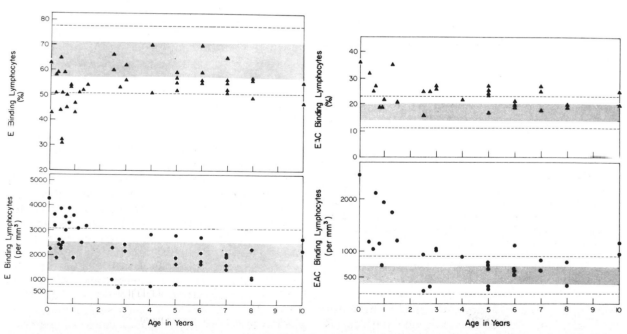

Figure 82–2. Scattergram demonstrating the percentage and absolute number of E-binding (T) lymphocytes (*A*) and EAC-binding lymphocytes (*B*) in infants and children. Shaded areas represent the normal adult levels ±1 S.D. (From Fleisher, T. A., et al.: Pediatrics 55:163, 1975.)

dermal skin testing and no in vitro production of MIF to specific antigenic stimulation. The infant's response to fungal and viral infections is a primary rather than a secondary response. The lack of immune T lymphocytes may explain the neonate's increased susceptibility to severe and sometimes fatal infections with viruses such as cytomegalovirus and herpes simplex. Before the infant is capable of a successful cellular immune response (5 to 10 days), death may have occurred. Thus, the normal cellular immune responses may not be of significant aid and the use of direct antiviral therapy, such as 8-cyclo-guanosine, should be considered. The lack of immune T lymphocytes is also the basis for the high frequency of oral and perineal moniliasis in infants. Moreover, recurrent moniliasis with adequate drug therapy (nystatin) should suggest a possible cellular immune defect. (For a review of host defenses see Miller, 1978.)

Although many of the newborn's lymphocytes appear to be qualitatively normal, there is some evidence that they can be made partially tolerant to foreign histocompatibility antigens. In 1960, Fowler and coworkers reported that infants given exchange transfusions with fresh blood showed increased survival of skin grafts from the blood donors but not from random individuals.

Under certain conditions normal infants may not be able to destroy allogenic lymphocytes they receive in transfusion of fresh blood or platelets. The infused lymphocytes may then attack the infants and produce graft-versus-host disease, which may be fatal.

CASE 82–1

A female infant of 36 weeks' gestation was born after receiving two intrauterine transfusions at 30 and 32 weeks' gestation for Rh erythroblastosis. After birth, two exchange transfusions were necessary for hyperbilirubinemia. All intrauterine and exchange transfusion blood was from male donors. At 12 days, the infant developed hepatosplenomegaly, a skin rash, and thrombocytopenia.

Bone marrow aspiration revealed spontaneously dividing male cells, and 25 per cent of peripheral blood lymphocytes demonstrated a male karyotype. The diagnosis of graft-versus-host disease was made. Although treatment with antithymocyte globulin was instituted, the patient died.

Comment. The spontaneously dividing male cells were from the first of the exchange transfusions. Since the patient had no demonstrable primary immunodeficiency, it was felt that she had been made partially tolerant to certain histocompatibility antigens because of the intrauterine transfusions. Because of the partial tolerance, she was unable to reject the lymphocytes from the exchange transfusion blood.

Graft-versus-host disease has also been observed in recipients of maternal platelets used to transfuse patients with isoimmune neonatal thrombocytopenia. Since mothers share one HLA haplotype with their infants, the capacity of the neonate to reject the maternal lymphocytes contaminating the platelets is reduced. Further, the maternal lymphocytes may be specifically sensitized to the paternal antigens as a consequence of pregnancy. The irradiation of exchange transfusion blood or maternal platelets with 5000 rads will eliminate the possibility of graft-versus-host disease (Parkman et al., 1974).

General Humoral Immunity

The complement system is a series of nine serum proteins that react in a sequential fashion with IgG or IgM antibody that has combined with circulating soluble antigens or the surface antigens of bacteria, cells, fungi, or protozoa. The activated complement components liberate protein mediators that can (1) increase vascular permeability, (2) attract granulocytes, (3) permit phagocytosis of antibody-coated microorganisms, or (4) cause lysis and death of the organisms. Individuals and animals with low or absent C1, C2, C3, C4, C5, C6, and C7 have been identified. Only those individuals with a low or absent C3 or C5 have had an increased susceptibility to infections.

The fetus is capable of synthesizing all normal serum proteins, even though the concentrations of some components are decreased as compared with adult values (i.e., alpha-lipoprotein, haptoglobin, ceruloplasmin, C3, and factor B). The concentration of the third component of the complement system, C3, determines the rate of phagocytosis of antibody-coated bacteria. The attachment of C3 to bacteria requires the previous fixation of C1, C4, and C2 after either IgM or IgG antibodies have reacted with the bacterial cell wall. Since the neonatal C3 level, 70 to 110 mg per 100 ml, is less than adult values of 100 to 200 mg per 100 ml, the opsonizing capacity of the neonate's serum is decreased, but the clinical importance of the decrease is not clear.

Because the neonate has very low levels of his own IgG and is only beginning to make significant amounts of IgM, another mechanism is necessary for the opsonization of bacteria to which the neonate has no antibody. The properdin system provides such an opsonic mechanism. The rate of phagocytosis mediated by the properdin system is controlled by the level of factor B. Since the concentration of factor B is low in most cord blood samples and absent in some, the capacity of neonatal serum to support phagocytosis by adult granulocytes of particles coated with gram-negative lipoprotein is markedly reduced and may account in part for the increased susceptibility of neonates to gram-negative enteric infections (Stossel et al., 1973).

GRANULOCYTE AND MONOCYTE FUNCTION

Granulocyte function in newborn infants appears to be generally normal as measured either in vitro or in vivo by cutaneous skin windows. Neonatal monocytes have decreased in vitro phagocytosis; however, the clinical significance of the observation is not known. Previous cases of in vitro defects of granulocyte phagocytosis may have been caused by the aforementioned serum defects rather than by primary granulocyte dysfunction. The chemotactic response of neonatal granulocytes to normal stimuli may be slightly decreased.

RETICULOENDOTHELIAL SYSTEM (RES)

The RES is composed of the fixed phagocytic cells of the spleen, liver, and other body tissues. Like the circulating granulocytes and monocytes, they are responsible for the removal of circulating pathogens and foreign particles. Maximal RES phagocytosis partially depends on serum factors that may be depressed in newborn serum. The absence of a significant proportion of the RES as in congenital hyposplenia increases the frequency of bacterial infections, presumably because of the decreased ability of the RES to clear the blood stream of bacteria (Kevy et al., 1968).

Specific Immune Deficiencies

AGAMMAGLOBULINEMIA

Certain humans are incapable of normal immunoglobulin production (Geha et al., 1974). The most severe deficiency is found in those patients who have X-linked agammaglobulinemia and who have an absolute absence of B lymphocytes with no significant immunoglobulin production of any class. Individuals with such a disorder suffer from recurrent infections with encapsulated pyogenic bacteria (*Staphylococcus, Streptococcus, Pneumonococcus, Meningococcus,* and *Hemophilus influenzae*). Since significant maternal IgG is present until at least 3 months of age, an increased incidence of bacterial infections due to agammaglobulinemia is not seen until after that time. In the case of an infant with a family history that is positive for agammaglobulinemia, one can establish the diagnosis at birth by noting the absence of circulating B lymphocytes in the infant's peripheral blood.

The common variable form of agammaglobulinemia is a sporadic disease of later onset in which B lymphocytes are present. In both forms of agammaglobulinemia, the number and the function of the T lymphocytes are normal.

Some patients in later life can suffer from selective lack of IgG subclasses or from dysgammaglobulinemia in which decreased IgG levels are associated with increased IgM or IgA levels, or both. However, the onset of recurrent infections with these syndromes starts in later life.

DiGEORGE SYNDROME

The DiGeorge syndrome is the consequence of a developmental abnormality involving the third and fourth pharyngeal pouches. The abnormalities include midline cardiac defects, absent parathyroid glands leading to neonatal tetany, an atypical facies including hypertelorism and high arched palate, auricular maldevelopment, and absence of the thymus gland (Fig. 82–3). Because the thymus gland is ab-

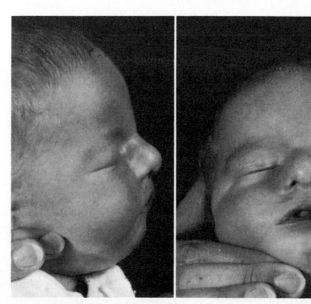

Figure 82–3. Typical facies of infant with DiGeorge's syndrome. Note the hypertelorism, shortened lip philtrum, and lowset, notched pinnae.

sent, significant T-lymphocyte maturation does not occur, although B lymphocytes appear in normal numbers. The infants suffer from recurrent fungal infections, especially moniliasis, and the common viral illnesses may be fatal. The triad of atypical facies, neonatal tetany, and lymphopenia should suggest the diagnosis. The lack of normal lymphocyte proliferation to stimulation by phytohemagglutinin and a decreased number of T lymphocytes are definitive proof of the diagnosis. The infant's immune defect can be corrected by the subcutaneous transplantation of a fetal thymus (August et al., 1970). Within 24 hours, immunocompetent T lymphocytes of recipient origin will appear. Because of the inability of these patients to destroy foreign cells, any fresh blood products given to such infants should be irradiated before administration in order to eliminate the possibility of graft-versus-host disease.

SEVERE COMBINED IMMUNE DEFICIENCY

Severe combined immune deficiency (SCID) is a syndrome in which affected infants have no functional T- or B-cell immunity. A variety of specific genetic defects can produce the SCID phenotype, including absence of the lymphoid stem cells, a block in normal peripheral T- and B-cell differentiation, and absence of a normal thymic endocrine function (Fig. 82–4). The affected children suffer from both viral and fungal infections (T-cell deficiency) and from infections with pyogenic bacteria (B-cell deficiency). The sine qua non of severe combined immune deficiency is the persistence of the fetal thymic archi-

tecture in which there are no lymphocytes. Therefore, in questionable cases, a thymic biopsy will establish the diagnosis of severe combined immune deficiency. Affected infants may be clinically well for the first 1 to 2 months and then present with recurrent diarrhea, oral moniliasis, pulmonary congestion, and recurrent pyogenic infections.

There are two genetic forms of the disease, an X-linked and an autosomal recessive, which have equal frequency. The male-to-female ratio is 3:1. Approximately 50 per cent of infants with the autosomal recessive form have a concomitant absence of normal adenosine deaminase (ADA) in their red cells and other tissues. The absence of ADA has allowed the prenatal diagnosis of SCID from cultured amnion cells (Hirschhorn et al., 1975).

Infants suspected of SCID because of a positive family history should be placed in protective isolation at birth. A chest radiograph should be obtained to determine the presence of a normal thymic shadow, and the capacity of the infant's lymphocytes for responding to phytohemagglutinin and allogenic lymphocytes (mixed lymphocyte culture) and to rosette with sheep red blood cells should be determined. The absence of T lymphocytes in the presence of a positive family history establishes the diagnosis. As in the case of DiGeorge syndrome, all blood products should be irradiated with 5000 rads prior to administration to infants suspected of suffering from SCID.

WISKOTT-ALDRICH SYNDROME

The Wiskott-Aldrich syndrome is an X-linked recessive disorder in which affected males have eczema, thrombocytopenia with platelets of reduced size, and decreased T-cell function with increasing age. The eczema and decreased T-cell function are

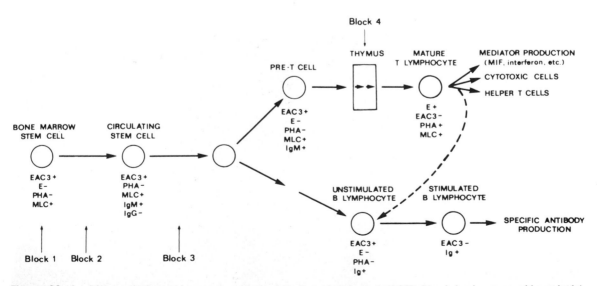

SITES OF DEFECTS IN SCID

Figure 82–4. Differentiation of immune system and sites of defects in SCID. Block 1, absence of lymphoid stem cell; Block 2, adenosine deaminase (ADA) deficiency; Block 3, peripheral differentiation block; Block 4, abnormal thymic epithelium.

usually not seen until several months to years of age; however, the thrombocytopenia with platelets of reduced size can be detected in the neonatal period and should be screened for in patients with a positive family history. Affected patients are prone to developing recurrent infections with viral, fungal, and bacterial organisms.

Bone Marrow Transplantation

Allogeneic bone marrow transplantation is an effective form of therapy for children with genetic disorders of the bone marrow, including severe combined immunodeficiency, the Wiskott-Aldrich syndrome, osteopetrosis, and primary granulocyte disorders (infantile agranulocytosis, chronic granulomatous disease, etc.). Bone marrow transplantation is currently possible only if an HLA-identical donor (usually a sibling) is available. Children with severe combined immune deficiency can be transplanted without any pretransplant immunosuppression, since they are devoid of any functioning immune system that might reject the infused bone marrow. The transplantation of 50×10^6 nucleated bone marrow cells per kilogram of recipient weight will uniformly engraft recipients with T and B lymphocytes of donor origin. However, no engraftment of donor hematopoietic cells occurs (Gatti et al., 1968; Parkman et al., 1975). Follow-up studies of SCID recipients 10 years after transplantation has revealed the persistence of normal immunity of donor origin.

Disorders of the hematopoietic stem cell, including the Wiskott-Aldrich syndrome and granulocyte disorders, require therapy prior to transplantation to eradicate the recipient's abnormal hematopoietic stem cells (Parkman et al., 1978). The attempted transplantation of individuals with abnormal hematopoietic stem cells following preparation with immunosuppressive drugs alone has not led to hematopoietic engraftment. The use of methods such as total body irradiation and administration of busulfan has eradicated the abnormal recipient hematopoietic stem cells and permitted both hematopoietic and lymphoid engraftment. Because of the adverse effects of total body irradiation on the development of the central nervous system, administration of busulfan may be the preferable method of preparing young infants; however, the long term effects of busulfan therapy on central nervous system development is presently unknown.

The primary limitation in bone marrow transplantation is the attack of donor immunocompetent cells against the recipient (i.e., graft-versus-host disease). The infused bone marrow is not irradiated to prevent graft-versus-host disease, since the irradiation would destroy the capacity of the bone marrow to engraft. Graft-versus-host disease following bone marrow transplantation is treated with immunosuppressant drugs (methotrexate, prednisone, and/or antithymocyte serum). Treatment of donor marrow with monoclonal antibodies to remove selected cells responsible for graft-versus-host disease provides a potentially useful mechanism for preventing the development of this reaction. Allogenic bone marrow transplantation is a potentially curative form of therapy for abnormalities of both lymphoid and hematopoietic stem cells. At present, it is used for severe combined immune deficiency, Wiskott-Aldrich syndrome, osteopetrosis, and granulocyte disorders. In the future, it may be used to treat genetic metabolic disorders, including Gaucher's disease and Hurler's and Hunter's syndromes as well as the hemoglobinopathies (thalassemia and sickle cell disease).

RECURRENT PYOGENIC INFECTIONS

Since neonates have adequate maternal IgG, recurrent infections with pyogenic bacteria cannot be due to decreased IgG levels but instead must be due to defects in the other components of the defense system (i.e., other humoral factors, especially C3, or primary defects of the granulocytes).

Primary defects in granulocyte function will predispose infants to recurrent pyogenic infections in the early neonatal period. Chronic granulomatous disease is a disorder in which the granulocytes of affected infants are able to phagocytize bacteria normally but are unable to produce the superoxide and related molecules necessary for the destruction of the organisms (Holmes et al., 1966). Primary abnormalities of the granulocyte membrane or granulocyte actin result in granulocytes that are unable to migrate or phagocytize normally (Boxer et al., 1974). The congenital absence of C3 will produce a markedly reduced rate of phagocytosis, predisposing the infant to pyogenic infections. All of these disorders are characterized by the early onset of recurrent bacterial infections with both gram-positive and gram-negative organisms.

Conclusions

The newborn infant may suffer severe infections from a spectrum of pathogens that are markedly different from the organisms causing disease in older children and adults. The infant has passive antibody protection against many of the common bacterial and viral pathogens and is thus protected. However, marginal defects including decreased serum C3 and factor B concentrations, decreased granulocyte chemotactic activity, and possible decreased RES function may contribute to the increased incidence of enterobacillary infections that is observed in neonates. The virgin state of the infant's T lymphocytes may lengthen the time period required before the newborn lymphocytes are able to control fungal and viral infections. Genetic disorders of both lymphoid and hematopoietic stem cells are potentially correctable by allogenic bone marrow transplantation.

REFERENCES

Alper, C. A., Colten, H. R., Rosen, F. S., et al.: Homozygous deficiency of the third component of complement (C3) in a patient with repeated infections. Lancet 2:1179, 1972.

August, C. S., Berkel, A. I., Driscoll, S., et al.: Onset of lymphocyte function in the developing human fetus. Pediatr. Res. 5:539, 1971.

August, C. S., Levey, R. H., Berkel, I., et al.: Establishment of immunological competence in a child with congenital thymic aplasia by a graft of fetal thymus. Lancet 1:1080, 1970.

Baker, C. J., Edwards, M. S., and Kasper, D. L.: Role of antibody to native type III polysaccharide of group B streptococcus in infant infection. Pediatrics 68:544, 1981.

Bazaral, M., Orgel, A., and Hamburger, R. N.: IgE levels in normal infants and mothers and an inheritance hypothesis. J. Immunol. 107:794, 1971.

Boxer, L. A., Hedley-Whyte, E. T., and Stossel, T. P.: Neutrophil actin dysfunction and abnormal neutrophil behavior. N. Engl. J. Med. 291:1093, 1974.

Brambell, F. W. R., and Hemmings, W.: The transmission of antibodies from mother to fetus. In Villee, C. A. (Ed.): The Placenta and Fetal Membranes. Baltimore, Williams & Wilkins, 1960, p. 71.

Brown, G., and Greaves, M. F.: Cell surface markers for human T and B lymphocytes. Eur. J. Immunol. 4:302, 1974.

Bruton, O. C.: Agammaglobulinemia. Pediatrics 9:722, 1952.

Carr, M. C., Stites, D. P., and Fudenberg, H. H.: Dissociation of response to phytohemagglutinin and adult allogeneic lymphocytes in human fetal lymphoid tissues. Nature (New Biol.) 241:279, 1973.

Chandra, R. K.: Serum thymic hormone activity and cell-mediated immunity in healthy neonates, preterm infants, and small-for-gestational age infants. Pediatrics 67:407, 1981.

Cohen, I. R., and Norins, L. C.: Antibodies of the IgG, IgM, and IgA classes in newborn and adult sera reactive with gram-negative bacteria. J. Clin. Invest. 47:1053, 1968.

Conley, M. E., and Cooper, M. D.: Immature IgA B cells in IgA deficient patients. N. Engl. J. Med. 305:495, 1981.

Cooper, M. D., Faulk, W. P., Fudenberg, H. H., et al.: Meeting report of the Second International Workshop on Primary Immunodeficiency Diseases in Man. Clin. Immunol. Immunopathol. 2:416, 1974.

DeKoning, J., Van Bekkum, D. W., Dicke, K. A., et al.: Transplantation of bone marrow cells and fetal thymus in an infant with lymphopenic immunological deficiency. Lancet 1:1223, 1969.

Dossett, J. H., Williams, R. C., and Quie, P. G.: Studies on interaction of bacteria, serum factors, and polymorphonuclear leukocytes in mothers and newborns. Pediatrics 44:49, 1969.

Fleisher, T. A., Luckasen, J. R., Sabad, A., et al.: T and B lymphocyte subpopulations in children. Pediatrics 55:162, 1975.

Forman, M. L., and Stiehm, E. R.: Impaired opsonic activity but normal phagocytosis in low-birth-weight infants. N. Engl. J. Med. 281:926, 1969.

Fowler, R., Jr., Schubert, W. K., and West, C. D.: Acquired partial tolerance to homologous skin grafts in the human infant at birth. Ann. N.Y. Acad. Sci. 87:413, 1960.

Gatherings, W. E., Lawton, A. R., and Cooper, M. D.: Immunofluorescent studies of the development of pre-B cells, B lymphocytes and immunoglobulin isotype diversity in humans. Eur. J. Immunol. 7:804, 1977.

Gatti, R. A., Allen, H. D., Meuwissen, H. J., et al.: Immunological reconstitution of sex-linked lymphopenic immunological deficiency. Lancet 2:1366, 1968.

Geha, R. S., Schneeberger, E., Merler, E., et al.: Heterogeneity of "acquired" or common variable agammaglobulinemia. N. Engl. J. Med. 291:1, 1974.

Gitlin, D., and Biasucci, A.: Development of gamma G, gamma A, gamma M, beta-1-c/beta-1-a, C′1 esterase inhibitor, ceruloplasmin, transferrin, hemopexin, haptoglobin, fibrinogen, plasminogen, alpha-1-antitrypsin, orosomucoid, beta-lipoprotein, alpha-2-macroglobulin, and pre-albumin in the human conceptus. J. Clin. Invest. 48:1433, 1969.

Gitlin, D., and Craig, J. M.: The thymus and other lymphoid tissues in congenital agammaglobulinemia. Pediatrics 32:517, 1963.

Gluck, L., and Silverman, W. A.: Phagocytosis in premature infants. Pediatrics 20:951, 1957.

Graham, C. W., Saba, T. M., Lolekha, S., et al.: Deficient serum opsonic activity for macrophage function in newborn infants. Proc. Soc. Exp. Biol. Med. 143:991, 1973.

Gross, S. J., Buckley, R. H., Wakil, S. S., McAllister, D. C., David, R. J., and Faix, R. G.: Elevated IgA concentration in milk produced by mothers delivered of preterm infants. J. Pediatr. 99:389, 1981.

Hirschhorn, R., Berates, N., Rosen, F. S., et al.: Adenosine deaminase deficiency in a child diagnosed prenatally. Lancet 1:69, 1975.

Holmes, B., Quie, P. G., Windhorst, D. B., et al.: Fatal granulomatous disease of childhood, an inborn error of phagocytic function. Lancet 1:1225, 1966.

Janeway, C. A.: Diagnosis of hypogammaglobulinemia. J.A.M.A. 180:320, 1962.

Kapoor, N., Kirkpatrick, D., Blaese, R. M., Oleske, J., Hilgartner, M. H., Chaganti, R. S. K., Good, R. A., and O'Reilly, R. J.: Reconstitution of normal megakaryocytopoiesis and immunologic functions in Wiskott-Aldrich syndrome by marrow transplantation following myeloablation and immunosuppression with busulfan and cyclophosphamide. Blood 57:692, 1981.

Keller, R., Dwyer, J. E., et al.: Intestinal IgA neutralizing antibodies in newborn infants following poliovirus immunization. Pediatrics 43:330, 1969.

Kempe, C. H., and Benenson, A. S.: Vaccinia: passive immunity in newborn infants. J. Pediatr. 42:525, 1953.

Kevy, S. V., Tefft, M., Vawter, G. F., et al.: Hereditary splenic hypoplasia. Pediatrics 42:752, 1968.

Kohler, P. F.: Maturation of the human complement system. J. Clin. Invest. 52:671, 1973.

Kornfeld, S. J., and Plaut, A. G.: Secretory immunity and the bacterial IgA proteases. Rev. Inf. Dis. 3:521, 1981.

Kretschmer, R., Say, B., et al.: Congenital aplasia of the thymus gland (DiGeorge's Syndrome). N. Engl. J. Med. 279:1295, 1968.

Lawton, A. R., and Cooper, M. D.: Two new stages of antigen independent B-cell development in mice and humans. In Cooper, M. D., and Dayton, D. H. (Eds.): Development of Host Defenses. New York, Raven Press, 1977, p. 43.

Lawton, A. R., Self, K. S., Royal, S. A., et al.: Ontogeny of B lymphocytes in the human fetus. Clin. Immunol. Immunopathol. 1:84, 1972.

Lepow, M. L., Warren, R. J., Gray, N., Ingram, V. G., and Robbins, F. C.: Effect of Sabin type I poliomyelitis vaccine administered by mouth to newborn infants. N. Engl. J. Med. 264:1071, 1961.

Merler, E., and Rosen, F. S.: The gamma globulins. I. Structure and synthesis of the immunoglobulins. N. Engl. J. Med. 275:480, 1966.

Miller, M. E.: Chemotactic function in the human neonate: Humoral and cellular aspects. Pediatr. Res. 5:487, 1971.

Miller, M. E.: Host Defenses in the Human Neonate. New York, Grune & Stratton, 1978.

Miller, M. J., Sunshine, P. J., and Remington, J. S.: Quantitation of cord serum IgM as a screening procedure to detect congenital infection: results in 5,006 infants. J. Pediatr. 75:1287, 1969.

Ogra, P. L., and Dayton, D. H. (Eds.): Immunology of Breast Milk. New York, Raven Press, 1980.

Ogra, S. S., Weintraub, D., and Ogra, P. L.: Immunologic aspects of human colostrum and milk: III. Fate and absorption of cellular and soluble components in the gastrointestinal tract of the newborn. J. Immunol. 119:245, 1977.

Osborn, J. J., Dancis, J., and Julia, J. F.: Studies of the immunology of the newborn infant. I. Age and antibody production. II. Interference with active immunization by passive transplacental circulating antibody. Pediatrics 9:736, 10:328, 1952.

Osborn, J. J., Dancis, J., and Rosenberg, B. F.: Studies of the immunology of the newborn infant. III. Permeability of the placenta to maternal antibody during fetal life. Pediatrics 10:450, 1952.

Parkman, R., Gelfand, E. W., Rosen, F. S., et al.: Severe combined immunodeficiency and adenosine deaminase deficiency. N. Engl. J. Med. 292:714, 1975.

Parkman, R., Mosier, D., Umansky, I., et al.: Graft-versus-host disease following intrauterine and exchange transfusions for hemolytic disease of the newborn. N. Engl. J. Med. 290:359, 1974.

Parkman, R., Rappeport, J., Geha, R., Belli, J., Cassady, R., Levey, R., Nathan, D. G., and Rosen, F. S.: Complete correction of the Wiskott-Aldrich syndrome by allogeneic bone marrow transplantation. N. Engl. J. Med. 298:921, 1978.

Propp, R. P., and Alper, C. A.: "C3" synthesis in the human fetus and lack of transplacental passage. Science 162:672, 1968.

Provenzano, R. W., Wetterlow, L. H., and Sullivan, C. L.: Immunization and antibody response in the newborn infant. I. Pertussis inoculation within 24 hours of birth. N. Engl. J. Med. 273:959, 1965.

Pyke, K. W., Dosch, H. M., Ipp, M. M., et al.: Intrathymus defect in severe combined immunodeficiency disease. N. Engl. J. Med. 293:424, 1975.

Raff, M. D.: T and B lymphocytes and immune responses. Nature 242:19, 1973.

Ray, C. G.: The ontogeny of interferon production by human leukocytes. J. Pediatr. 76:94, 1970.

Rosen, F. S., and Janeway, C. A.: Immunologic competence of the newborn infant. Pediatrics 33:159, 1964.

Silverstein, A. M.: Ontogeny of the immune response. Science 144:1423, 1964.

Smith, R. T., and Eitzman, D. V.: The development of the immune response. Pediatrics 33:163, 1964.

Stiehm, E. R., Ammann, A. J., and Cherry, J. D.: Elevated cord macroglobulins in the diagnosis of intrauterine infections. N. Engl. J. Med. 275:971, 1966.

Stossel, T., Alper, C. A., and Rosen, F. S.: Serum dependent phagocytosis of paraffin oil emulsified with bacterial lipopolysaccharide. J. Exp. Med. 137:690, 1973.

Walker, W. A., and Isselbacher, K. J.: Intestinal antibodies. N. Engl. J. Med. 297:767, 1977.

Warwick, W. J., Good, R. A., and Smith, R. T.: Failure of passive transfer of delayed hypersensitivity in the newborn human infant. J. Lab. Clin. Med. 56:139, 1960.

Washburn, T. C.: A longitudinal study of serum immunoglobulins in newborn premature infants. Bull. Johns Hopkins Hosp. 118:40, 1966.

Washburn, T. C., Medearis, D. N., and Childs, B.: Sex differences in susceptibility to infections. Pediatrics 35:57, 1965.

Yievin, R., Salzberger, M., and Olitzki, A. L.: Development of antibodies to enteric pathogens: placental transfer of antibodies and development of immunity in childhood. Pediatrics 18:19, 1956.

Bacterial Infections of The Newborn

By Kenneth McIntosh*

83

In this chapter we attempt to present pertinent information concerning commonly encountered bacterial infections of newborn infants. Emphasis is placed on pathogenesis, diagnosis, and management, and every effort has been made to discuss recent data. We begin with a section on antibiotic usage, since this is central to the management of all bacterial infections in the neonatal period.

Rational Antibiotic Usage in Neonates

Selection of antibiotic therapy in newborn infants must depend on (1) the historical experience with infections in the nursery, (2) the susceptibility of commonly encountered bacterial pathogens, and (3) familiarity with antibiotic pharmacokinetics in neonates. It is important for pediatricians to know which organisms cause disease most commonly in the nursery and intensive care unit and the current antimicrobial susceptibilities of these organisms. Moreover, it has been shown in many instances that the judicious use of antibiotics in the nursery setting can limit the emergence and spread of resistant bacteria.

The rapidly changing physiologic processes characteristic of the neonatal period may profoundly affect the pharmacology of antimicrobial agents. Absorption, distribution, metabolism, and excretion of drugs depend in part on the maturity and age of the infant. The dosage and frequency of administration schedule must be determined for infants of different gestational and chronological ages and cannot be extrapolated from studies of normal adults. Failure to take these physiologic and metabolic changes into account when administering antibiotics to neonates may result in either ineffective or toxic drug dosages.

* This chapter includes some contributions from previous authors, Drs. Alexander Schaffer, George H. McCracken, Jr., and Jorge B. Howard.

It is a general rule that as few antibiotics as possible should be used to treat individual infections and that, whenever possible, single drugs should be employed. Frequently, however, combining two drugs is good medical practice. This is true at the initiation of treatment, before culture and sensitivity data are available, in covering for the relatively wide variety of likely bacterial species in newborn sepsis, or, sometimes, after the organism has been identified to take advantage of antibiotic synergy in widespread and severe infections by bacteria difficult to eliminate with a single drug.

Often, bacterial sepsis is suspected in newborn infants because of nonspecific symptoms and signs, cultures are taken, and antibiotics are administered only to find that after 72 hours the cultures are all sterile. Not infrequently there is improvement in the child during this interval, coincident with the antibiotic treatment. At this time, the pediatrician must use clinical judgment. If the cultures were obtained from the proper sites in the proper way, and if the microbiology laboratory is reliable, it is usually wise to discontinue antibiotics at this point and re-evaluate the child at frequent intervals thereafter. Sometimes, culture results are difficult to interpret (*Staphylococcus epidermidis* from a blood culture; gram-negative organisms from a tracheal aspirate in a long-term occupant of the nursery). In these instances, a knowledge of the pathogenicity of these organisms in neonates should be combined with the clinical appearance of the infant and other laboratory data so that a plan that minimizes the unnecessary use of antibiotics can be developed.

Although antibiotics are commonly used in an attempt to prevent infection of neonates, their efficacy is limited to a few well-defined circumstances. A good example of one such circumstance is the use of topical 1 per cent silver nitrate, tetracycline, or erythromycin to prevent ophthalmia neonatorum. However, when antibiotics are used as "broad coverage" against many potential pathogens, they are rarely effective. This umbrella method of chemoprophylaxis encourages the emergence of resistant strains among previously susceptible bacteria and causes alteration of the normal bacterial flora of the gastrointestinal and respiratory tracts.

Table 83–1 is intended as a guide for treating neonatal bacterial diseases. Modification of these schedules may be necessary in certain specific infections and in patients with compromised hepatic or renal function.

Pathogenesis of Neonatal Infections

Throughout pregnancy and until the membranes rupture, the infant is usually well protected from microbes. Under normal circumstances, it is not until delivery and in the immediate neonatal period that the infant is exposed to many organisms, including aerobic and anaerobic bacteria, viruses, fungi, and protozoa. This encounter initiates colonization of the respiratory and gastrointestinal tracts. The vast majority of neonates establish their microbial flora without incident; however, an occasional infant develops disease caused by one of these organisms. The factors contributing to conversion from colonization to disease are not completely understood.

There appear to be four separate mechanisms by which bacteria reach the fetus or newborn to cause infection. First, certain bacteria (particularly *Treponema pallidum*, *Listeria monocytogenes*, and *Mycobacterium tuberculosis*) can reach the fetus through the maternal bloodstream, causing transplacental infection. This is an uncommon event and usu-

Table 83–1.   Dosage Regimens for Antibiotics Commonly Used in Newborn Infants

Drug	Route	Daily Dosage	
		Infants <1 Week of Age	*Infants 1–4 Weeks of Age*
Amikacin sulfate	IM, IV	15 mg/kg (2)*	15–20 mg/kg (2 or 3)
Ampicillin sodium†	IV, IM	50 mg/kg (2)	100 mg/kg (3)
Carbenicillin disodium	IV, IM	225–300 mg/kg (3 or 4)	400 mg/kg (4)
Chloramphenicol sodium succinate	IV, IM	25 mg/kg (1)	50 mg/kg (1 or 2)
Colistimethate sodium	IV, IM	5–8 mg/kg (2 or 3)	5–8 mg/kg (2 or 3)
Colistin sulfate	Oral	15 mg/kg (4)	15 mg/kg (4)
Gentamicin sulfate	IM, IV	5 mg/kg (2)	7.5 mg/kg (3)
Kanamycin sulfate	IM, IV	15–20 mg/kg (2)	20–30 mg/kg (2 or 3)
Methicillin sodium†	IV, IM	50–75 mg/kg (2)	75–100 mg/kg (3 or 4)
Nafcillin sodium†	IV, IM	50 mg/kg (2)	75–100 mg/kg (4)
Neomycin sulfate	Oral	100 mg/kg (3 or 4)	100 mg/kg (3 or 4)
Oxacillin sodium	IV, IM	50 mg/kg (2)	150–200 mg/kg (4)
Crystalline penicillin G potassium†	IV, IM	50,000 units/kg (2)	50,000–125,000 units/kg (3)
Penicillin G procaine	IM	50,000 units/kg (1)	50,000 units/kg (1)
Polymyxin B sulfate	IV, IM	3.5–5 mg/kg (2 or 3)	3.5–5 mg/kg (2 or 3)
Tobramycin sulfate	IM, IV	4 mg/kg (2)	4 mg/kg (2 or 3)
Vancomycin	IV	30 mg/kg (2)	45 mg/kg (3)

* Numbers in parentheses represent numbers of doses in which the daily dosage should be equally divided.

† For meningitis, double the recommended dosage.

ally leads either to congenital infection not unlike infections caused by certain viruses or *Toxoplasma* or to still-birth with overwhelming infection. Second, it seems likely that many "early-onset" group B streptococcal diseases are the result of infection that occurs immediately before delivery (Baker, 1978). The bacteria appear to travel up from the vagina or cervix through either ruptured or intact membranes, leading to amnionitis, pneumonitis, and premature delivery. Third, infection may occur during passage through the birth canal at the time of delivery. Gonococcal ophthalmia and most infections with *Escherichia coli* appear to develop in this manner. In some instances (e.g., late onset group B streptococcal infection) colonization occurs at the time of birth and may develop, by unknown mechanisms, into disease several days or even weeks later. Finally, bacteria can be introduced after birth from the environment surrounding the baby, either in the nursery or at home.

The two most common bacterial pathogens during the neonatal period are the group B streptococcus and *Escherichia coli*. These two organisms account for approximately 70 per cent of systemic neonatal bacterial diseases. Both organisms are usually acquired from the mother during the intrapartum period. The acute (early onset) septicemic form of group B streptococcal disease may be caused by any of the group B types (B_I, B_{II}, or B_{III}), and the specific B type causing disease is usually found also in the maternal vaginal tract. Epidemiologic studies have shown that from 5 to 30 per cent of pregnant women are vaginally or rectally colonized with group B streptococci. Approximately one half the infants of colonized mothers are themselves asymptomatically colonized at birth, and a similar number acquire the organism without disease from the environment (Siegel et al., 1980; Yow et al., 1979). The major infantile colonization sites are skin, nasopharynx, and rectum. The group B streptococcus will persist in the nasopharynx and rectum for weeks to months, whereas cutaneous infection usually disappears by several weeks of age. It has been estimated that for every 100 infants colonized with group B streptococci, one infant will develop disease caused by this organism (Baker and Barrett, 1973).

Group B streptococcal meningitis is caused almost exclusively by the B_{III} organisms. These organisms may be acquired from nonmaternal sites. Clusters of three or four cases of meningitis caused by group B streptococci occurred in nurseries during short time periods, suggesting nosocomial acquisition.

Certain studies have shown that approximately 80 per cent of *E. coli* strains causing neonatal meningitis possess a single, specific capsular polysaccharide antigen, designated K1 (Robbins et al., 1974). This is remarkable when one considers that there are over 100 recognized K antigens associated with *E. coli* strains. By contrast, approximately 40 per cent of *E. coli* strains causing neonatal septicemia possess K1 and only 10 to 15 per cent of strains causing septicemia and urinary tract infections in adults contain this antigen.

731

Bacterial Infections of the Newborn

The reason for this association between K1 antigen and *E. coli* strains causing neonatal meningitis and, to a lesser degree, septicemia is unknown. The K1 polysaccharide is chemically identical with that in the capsule of group B meningococci. Animal studies have demonstrated that *E. coli* possessing K1 are highly virulent for mice and that this lethal effect can be completely prevented by the pretreatment of mice with minute amounts of specific K1 antibody (Robbins et al., 1974). Furthermore, outcome from neonatal meningitis is directly correlated with the presence, concentration, and persistence of K1 antigen in cerebrospinal fluid and blood of these infants (McCracken et al., 1974).

Extensive epidemiologic studies have shown that approximately 20 to 30 per cent of newborn babies are colonized rectally with *E. coli* (Sarff et al., 1975). This percentage may rise to 50 during the second and third weeks of life (Peter and Nelson, 1978). Thirty to 40 per cent of normal infants and children have K1 organisms on rectal swab culture, as do nearly 50 per cent of women at the time of delivery. Approximately two thirds of babies born to K1-positive mothers will be colonized with the identical serotypes of *E. coli* K1. Vertical transmission of these organisms has been documented in 70 per cent of neonates with *E. coli* K1 meningitis and as the major route of neonatal gastrointestinal colonization. The colonization to disease ratio for *E. coli* K1 is similar to that observed for group B streptococci; that is, approximately, 100 to 200 : 1. Nosocomial infection with *E. coli* K1 has also been observed in our premature nurseries.

Although the pathogenesis of neonatal group B streptococcal and *E. coli* K1 disease has not been completely elucidated, a reasonable hypothesis can be advanced. Studies in children and adults have clearly demonstrated that protection from disease caused by pneumococci, meningococci, and *Hemophilus influenzae,* type B, is afforded by specific antibody directed against the capsular polysaccharides possessed by these organisms. A lack of B_{III} antibody in sera from infants and their mothers with neonatal group B_{III} streptococcal disease has been documented (Baker and Kasper, 1976.) It is possible, but by no means proved to date, that a lack of K1 antibody in sera of neonates predisposes them to *E. coli* K1 disease as well. The mouse protection studies lend credence to this contention.

Although this discussion has centered on only two organisms causing neonatal disease, there are considerable data supporting the importance of vertical transmission of other microorganisms during the intrapartum period. These include *Listeria monocytogenes,* anaerobic bacteria (Chow et al., 1974), *Chlamydia* (Frommell et al., 1979), *Candida albicans* (Kozinn et al., 1958), and such viruses as cytomegalovirus and herpesvirus hominis.

Septicemia

Sepsis neonatorum (Siegel and McCracken, 1981) is a disease of infants who are less than 1 month of age, are clinically ill, and have positive blood cultures. The presence of clinical manifestations distinguishes this condition from the transient bacteremia observed in some healthy neonates.

The incidence of sepsis neonatorum is approximately 1 and 4 cases per 1000 livebirths for full-term and premature infants, respectively. These incidence rates vary from nursery to nursery and depend on conditions predisposing to infection.

Predisposing Factors. A number of factors have been shown to predispose infants to neonatal bacterial diseases. These include age and parity of the mother, prenatal care, sex of the infant, gestational age, and associated congenital anomalies. Perinatal maternal complications such as abruptio placentae, placenta praevia, maternal toxemia, premature rupture of the membranes, and chorioamnionitis all increase the incidence of neonatal septicemia. Congenital anomalies that cause a breakdown of anatomical barriers or of the immunologic system predispose the infant to infection.

Septicemia seems to be more frequent in male than in female infants.

The development of ventilatory equipment, intravenous hyperalimentation, and monitoring devices has made it possible to treat severely ill infants more effectively. However, these apparatuses are potential sources of opportunistic organisms that can cause nosocomial infection. The frequency of these infections is variable. It may be difficult to recognize them because of the severe underlying illness requiring intensive therapy and the frequent usage of antimicrobial agents in these infants.

Clinical Manifestations. The early signs and symptoms of septicemia are nonspecific and are frequently recognized only by the mother or nurse. Early temperature imbalance with transient hyper- or hypothermia, tachypnea, bouts of apnea, tachycardia, lethargy, vomiting, or diarrhea, and unwillingness to breast-feed may be noted. Jaundice, petechiae, seizures, and hepatosplenomegaly are late signs and usually denote a poor prognosis.

Although it is tempting to recommend a work-up for septicemia in all infants with nonspecific clinical manifestations, this is both impractical and unnecessary in many instances. A complete history and physical examination, coupled with clinical experience, are the best guides in determining the extent of work-up. If doubt exists, a blood culture should be obtained.

Etiology. Through the years, there has been a shift in the microorganisms responsible for neonatal septicemia and meningitis. This is clearly illustrated by the experience at Yale–New Haven Hospital, documented in Table 83–2 (Freedman et al., 1981). During the 1930s, group A streptococci were the predominant organisms. In the 1950s staphylococci (largely of phage group I) became a major cause of nursery outbreaks throughout the world. *Pseudomonas* was prominent during the same decade, perhaps because of the introduction of respiratory support systems. From the late 1950s on, *E. coli* has been an important cause of neonatal sepsis. The dramatic rise in incidence of group B streptococcal infections is notable and has been reflected in other

Table 83–2. Organisms Responsible for Neonatal Septicemia at Yale–New Haven (Conn.) Hospital (YNHH) From 1928 to 1978, No. (%)

Organism	1928–1932	1933–1943	1944–1957	1958–1965	1966–1978*
β-Hemolytic *Streptococcus*	15 (38)	18 (41)	11 (18)	8 (11)	86 (36)
Group A		16	5	—	—
Group B		2	4	1	76 (32)
Group D					
Enterococci		—	1	7	6
Nonenterococci					
(*S. bovis*)		—	—	—	3
Group F		—	1	—	—
Nongroupable		—	—	—	1
Escherichia coli	10 (26)	11 (25)	23 (37)	33 (45)	76 (32)
Klebsiella-Enterobacter	—	—	—	8 (11)	28 (12)
Staphylococcus aureus	11 (28)	4 (9)	8 (13)	2 (3)	12 (5)
Pseudomonas	1 (3)	—	13 (21)	11 (15)	5 (2)
S. pneumoniae	2 (5)	5 (11)	3 (5)	2 (3)	2 (1)
Proteus	—	—	—	—	4 (2)
Hemophilus	—	—	—	1 (1)	9 (4)
Mixed	—	3 (7)	1 (2)	—	11 (5)
Other	—	3 (7)	3 (5)	7 (10)	6 (3)
Total	39	62	73	80	324

* Data from 1958 to 1978 are derived only from infants born at YNHH as discussed in the "Methods" section.
(From Freedman, R. M., et al.: Am. J. Dis. Child. *135*:140, 1981.)

centers as well. Finally, both group D streptococci and *Klebsiella* have been relatively recent pathogens, the latter accounting for a high proportion of antibiotic-resistant organisms that colonize and infect babies in neonatal intensive care units (Goldmann et al., 1978). The prevalence rates for a specific bacterial pathogen vary from nursery to nursery and may change rather abruptly in any one unit. Knowledge of the most commonly isolated bacteria in a nursery or intensive care unit, coupled with the antimicrobial susceptibilities of these organisms, is invaluable in treating suspected sepsis neonatorum.

Streptococcal Disease. The group B streptococcus is the most common gram-positive organism causing septicemia and meningitis during the first month of life. As indicated earlier in the discussion of the pathogenesis of neonatal infections, vertical transmission of this organism from mother to infant is the most common route of infection. Nosocomial acquisition of infection has been implicated in some nurseries and may be more common than heretofore recognized. The incidence of group B streptococcal disease has varied widely from place to place and from year to year. Even during the years since 1969 (the period of increased incidence, as reported by Freedman et al. in 1981), the annual incidence in Dallas has ranged from 0.6 to 3.7 per 1000 livebirths (Siegel et al., 1980).

The most common clinical manifestations of group B streptococcal infections are septicemia, pneumonia, and meningitis, but other more localized syndromes also occur, including osteomyelitis and septic arthritis, otitis media, cellulitis, and conjunctivitis (Howard and McCracken, 1974). Generalized disease takes two clinically and epidemiologically distinct forms (Franciosi et al., 1973), early and late onset. The early form by definition occurs in the first 4 to 7 days of life, often within hours of delivery. It is characterized by a high incidence of maternal complications, especially premature labor and prolonged rupture of membranes. Infants with the early form of the disease are usually desperately ill within hours of delivery and may exhibit unexplained apnea or tachypnea, respiratory distress with hypoxia, and shock. Chest roentgenograms reveal a diffuse pulmonary infiltrate similar to that seen following aspiration or may be indistinguishable from the findings characteristic of hyaline membrane disease. Pathologic examination of the lungs of babies who die after this early onset form of the disease indicates that the infection often dates from before delivery; it seems likely that in many instances in utero disease precipitated premature delivery (Baker, 1978). The mortality rate is 50 to 80 per cent. Pneumonitis is the primary finding on pathologic examination, and postmortem cultures of the lung, blood, and cerebrospinal fluid yield group B organisms. However, histologic evidence of meningitis is usually lacking.

The late onset meningitic form of disease presents at 1 to 12 weeks of age and is indistinguishable from the other forms of purulent meningitis. Group B streptococci are grown from cultures of blood and cerebrospinal fluid, and the mortality rate is 20 to 40 per cent. The type B_{III} organism appears to be the principal offender in this condition. The pathogenesis is uncertain, but failure to culture the B_{III} organism from the maternal cervix suggests that acquisition of the pathogen may be from other persons in the infant's environment.

Group A streptococcal disease is not as common now as in previous decades (Dillon, 1966). Disease caused by this organism varies from a low-grade, chronic omphalitis to fulminant septicemia and meningitis. Because of the explosive nature of outbreaks in nursery settings, surveillance for colonized infants is probably indicated at the time the organism is found or when infant infections are recognized (see the discussion of nosocomial infections further on).

GROUP D STREPTOCOCCAL DISEASE. Group D streptococci include the enterococci and several other species, particularly *S. bovis,* which have been found in neonatal infection. Enterococci tend to be resistant to penicillin, and therefore ampicillin, with or without an aminoglycoside such as kanamycin or gentamicin, should be used. For nonenterococcal strains, penicillin may be adequate. The incidence of these infections appears to have increased during the past few years in many centers, so that they are recognized as often as, or more often than, those caused by *E. coli* (Siegel and McCracken, 1978). The clinical pattern of the disease is remarkably similar to that seen with group B streptococci (Alexander and Giacoia, 1978) and is frequently associated with complicated deliveries. Prognosis with prompt and appropriate antibiotic therapy appears, however, to be somewhat better.

Staphylococcal Disease. In the 1950s, phage group I *Staphylococcus aureus* was the most common bacterial agent causing septicemia in neonatal units. Its unique invasive properties caused disseminated disease with widespread manifestations, including neonatal mastitis, furunculosis, septic arthritis, osteomyelitis, and septicemia. Because blood stream infection is usually secondary to local invasion, a careful search for the primary focus must be made in all septic babies. Microbial surveillance, intensified infection control measures and local skin care have reduced colonization and disease rates caused by the group I organism.

More recently, coagulase positive staphylococcal disease in nurseries has been caused by organisms of the phage II group (Melish and Glasgow, 1971). These organisms produce an exotoxin (exfoliatin) that causes intraepidermal cleavage through the granular cell layer due to disruption of desmosomes (Melish et al., 1972). Clinical disease may take one of several forms, which include bullous impetigo, toxic epidermal necrolysis, Ritter's disease, and nonstreptococcal scarlatina. The initial finding in Ritter's disease is intense, painful erythema not unlike a severe sunburn. Over the next hours, bullae may form that, when ruptured, leave a tender, weeping erythematous area. A characteristic desquamation of large epidermal sheets occurs approximately 3 to 5 days after onset of illness. A fine desquamation is commonly seen in the perioral region. Bullous impetigo has been the most common disease associated with nursery outbreaks of phage group II staphylococcal infections.

Coagulase negative staphylococci (*Staphylococcus epidermidis*) may be identified in blood cultures of babies and are frequently dismissed as contaminants. Repeated isolation of this organism from blood associated with clinical signs of septicemia should alert the physician to its pathogenic role. Coagulase negative staphylococci are frequently, but not always, associated with arterial or venous catheters or ventriculoperitoneal shunts. Eradication of infection usually requires removal of the catheter or prosthesis as well as appropriate antibiotic therapy. Approximately 80 per cent of these organisms are resistant to penicillin G, and 50 to 60 per cent are also resistant to methicillin.

The drug of first choice in treating such infections is vancomycin (Schaad et al., 1980), although methicillin or oxacillin may be substituted if the organism proves sensitive in vitro.

Listeria monocytogenes. *Listeria* is a small, motile gram-positive rod that grows slowly in the laboratory and that in Gram stains can be mistaken for either corynebacteria or streptococci. It is a facultative intracellular parasite that is found widely in the animal kingdom, and infections in man are sometimes seen as a result of contact with domestic animals. As with group B streptococcal infections, there are two forms, early and late onset. Early onset infections are often acquired transplacentally. In such instances, fetal death and abortion may result, or the child may be born with hepatosplenomegaly, disseminated disease, and granulomatous papules on the trunk and oral mucous membranes. It is this form of the disease that has been called "granulomatosis infantisepticum." Perinatal complications are common in this group, and the prognosis is often grave. Late-onset disease takes the form of meningitis (Visintine et al., 1977), occurring usually in the second week of life but as late as the fourth or fifth week. The cerebrospinal fluid is highly cellular, the glucose is almost always markedly depressed, and monocytes are often seen on smear, although they are usually not the predominant cell type. Interestingly, the early-onset type of listeriosis, as with group B streptococcal disease, reflects the maternal genital colonization and can be one of several serotypes. Meningitis, on the other hand, is almost always caused by type IV B and is usually acquired from the environment (Albritton et al., 1976). The prognosis of the meningitic form is relatively good with regard to both survival and

sequelae. Ampicillin plus gentamicin or kanamycin should be given for the first 5 to 7 days, followed by ampicillin alone to complete a 2-week course. The combination of ampicillin and an aminoglycoside has been shown to kill listeria more rapidly than either drug alone (Gordon et al., 1972).

Escherichia coli Disease. *E. coli* are the most common gram-negative bacteria causing septicemia during the neonatal period. Approximately 40 per cent of *E. coli* strains causing septicemia possess K1 capsular antigen, and strains identical with that in blood can usually be identified in the patient's nasopharynx or rectal cultures (see previous discussion of pathogenesis of neonatal infections). The clinical features of *E. coli* septicemia are generally similar to those observed in infants with disease caused by other pathogens.

Pseudomonas septicemia may present with a characteristic violaceous papular lesion or lesions that after several days develop central necrosis. Although this is most commonly observed in *Pseudomonas* infection, it may also be associated with other pathogens. The neonate who receives broad spectrum antibiotics while in an environment potentially contaminated by "water-bugs" (respirators, moist oxygen, etc.) is likely to develop disease caused by *Pseudomonas* species or other fastidious organisms.

Diagnosis. The diagnosis of septicemia can only be made by recovery of the organism from blood cultures. Blood should be obtained from a peripheral vein rather than from the umbilical vessels, the outer several millimeters of which are frequently colonized with bacteria. Femoral vein aspiration should be avoided both because of potential contamination with coliform organisms from the perineum and because of the danger of inadvertent penetration of the hip joint capsule. It is frequently helpful to obtain cultures of other sites prior to initiating antimicrobial therapy. For example, percutaneous bladder aspiration of urine for culture is frequently helpful in identifying the urinary tract as the focus of infection. Nasopharyngeal, skin, and rectal cultures are frequently positive in the early septicemic form of listeriosis and group B streptococcal disease, but it must be remembered that colonization of these sites occurs commonly. Microscopic examination of material obtained from gastric aspiration for leukocytes and bacteria has been advocated as a means to identify infants who are at risk of developing systemic bacterial disease. It should be pointed out that the leukocytes in the infant's stomach are of maternal origin, and the bacteria observed on stained smears are probably carried from the nasopharynx to the stomach upon intubation. Thus, a history of amnionitis and examination of a pharyngeal swab smear for bacteria are as meaningful as a study of gastric aspirates. All infants with suspected septicemia should have a cerebrospinal fluid examination and culture prior to therapy.

Measuring the peripheral white blood cell count and differential is probably the most useful nonspecific and rapid test available (Philip and Hewitt, 1980). If the total count is under 5000 or if the band-to-neutrophil ratio exceeds or is equal to 0.2, bacterial sepsis should be strongly considered. The normal range of white blood cell counts in neonates is variable, and this should be taken into account in interpreting the values. Other tests, such as sedimentation rate, C-reactive protein, haptoglobin concentration, and nitroblue tetrazolium have been extensively evaluated but are rarely more useful than, and certainly no substitute for, the white blood cell count, the history, and the physical examination.

Prevention. Reports that there are surprisingly low rates of early-onset group B streptococcal disease in institutions in which infants receive an intramuscular dose of penicillin G at birth have kindled considerable interest in this approach to prevention (Steigman et al., 1978). Others have screened women toward the end of pregnancy and treated carriers of group B streptococci with one or two intravenous doses of ampicillin to prevent transmission to the newborn (Yow et al., 1979). At the present time neither of these practices is recommended: Controlled studies are few, and the possibility exists that penicillin-resistant infections might increase to obliterate the benefit provided by a reduction in group B streptococcal disease (Siegel et al., 1980). Also, in many instances group B streptococcal infections begin before delivery, and it seems unlikely that a single dose of penicillin would prevent them (Baker, 1978).

Therapy. Before the definitive diagnosis of septicemia is made and prior to the availability of microbial susceptibility studies, antibiotic therapy should be initiated using a combination that includes a penicillin and an aminoglycoside. The choice of antibiotics must be based on the historical experience of the nursery and the antimicrobial susceptibilities of bacteria recently isolated from both sick and healthy neonates. As initial therapy, ampicillin in combination with either kanamycin or gentamicin is a reasonable choice. Ampicillin is active in vitro against *Listeria monocytogenes* and enterococci as well as against many *E. coli* strains. When the historical experience of the nursery or the physical findings suggest *Pseudomonas* infection, carbenicillin in combination with gentamicin should be used. Because of extensive clinical experience, kanamycin is the preferred aminoglycoside for susceptible coliform bacteria. Pharmacologic studies have shown that the currently recommended kanamycin dosage of 15 mg per kg per day given every 12 hours to all neonates be modified to 15 to 30 mg per kg per day in two or three divided doses, depending on the birth weight and chronologic age. Gentamicin has been used safely and effectively in the treatment of neonatal bacterial diseases. In order to retain its effectiveness, this drug should be reserved for therapy of infections caused by kanamycin-resistant coliforms and *Pseudomonas* species. Once the pathogen is identified and its antimicrobial susceptibilities known, the most effective and least toxic drug or combination of drugs should be used. The aminoglycosides tobramycin and amikacin should not be used except in therapy of disease caused by kanamycin and gentamicin resistant gram-negative organisms.

Both exchange transfusions (Vain et al., 1980; Courtney et al., 1979) and granulocyte infusions (Laurenti et al., 1981) have been used as adjuncts to other therapies for the treatment of infants with sepsis. The numbers of infants treated have been small, and although the approach appears promising, greater experience and carefully controlled trials will be necessary before it can be widely recommended.

Purulent Meningitis

The relative incidence of purulent meningitis of the newborn varies among institutions and is higher in those city hospitals in which prenatal care is suboptimal and in which complicated pregnancies and deliveries often result in high risk premature births. Incidence rates are approximately two to four cases per 10,000 livebirths and may be as high as one case per 1000 livebirths in some nurseries. Group B streptococci and *E. coli* strains account for about 70 per cent of all cases, and *Listeria monocytogenes* is seen in an additional 5 per cent of infants.

Infants with group B streptococcal meningitis usually present beyond the first several days of life, and the group B_{III} organism is the principal serotype encountered in these infants. The mortality is 20 to 40 per cent. Streptococcal disease occurring in the first 48 hours after delivery is usually manifested as acute respiratory distress with or without shock. Although the organism is frequently isolated from postmortem cerebrospinal fluid cultures from these infants, histologic evidence of meningeal inflammation is usually lacking (Franciosi et al., 1973).

Approximately 80 per cent of all *E. coli* causing meningitis possess K1 antigen. The O18 and O7 somatic types and H6 and H7 flagellar types are most commonly associated with K1 strains cultured from cerebrospinal fluid (Sarff et al., 1975). The presence, concentration and persistence of this capsular polysaccharide antigen in cerebrospinal fluid and blood of infants with meningitis correlate directly with outcome from disease. The current mortality rates for neonatal *E. coli* meningitis vary from 20 to 30 per cent in some centers to 50 and 60 per cent in others.

The epidemiology and clinical manifestations of *Listeria* meningitis have been described previously in the discussion of septicemia. Very rare cases of meningitis due to *Campylobacter fetus* subspecies *intestinalis* have also been described, with onset at 1 to 22 days of age (three cases reviewed by Torphy and Bond, 1979). In these reported cases, the disease closely resembled neonatal bacterial meningitis due to other organisms and was associated with a very poor prognosis for survival. Many of the infants had been born prematurely.

Pathology.   The pathologic findings are similar regardless of bacterial etiology. The most consistent findings at necropsy of babies dying of meningitis are purulent exudate of the meninges and of the ependymal surfaces of the ventricles associated with vascular inflammation. The inflammatory response of neonates is similar to that observed in adults with meningitis, with the exception that babies have a sparsity of plasma cells and lymphocytes during the subacute stage of meningeal reaction. Hydrocephalus and a noninfectious encephalopathy can be demonstrated in approximately 50 per cent of infants dying with meningitis. Subdural effusions occur rarely in neonates. In contrast, this complication of meningitis is common in infants 3 to 12 months of age. Varying degrees of phlebitis and arteritis of intracranial vessels can be found in all infants dying of meningitis. Thrombophlebitis with occlusion of veins may occur in the subependymal zones. K1 antigen has been demonstrated in brain tissue of infants succumbing to *E. coli* K1 infection.

Clinical Manifestations.   The early signs and symptoms of neonatal meningitis are frequently indistinguishable from those of septicemia. Specific findings such as stiff neck and Kernig and Brudzinski signs are rarely found. Lethargy, feeding problems, and altered temperature are the most frequent presenting complaints, and respiratory distress, vomiting, diarrhea, and abdominal distention are common findings. A bulging fontanel may be a late sign of meningitis. Seizures are observed frequently and may be caused by direct central nervous system inflammation or occur in association with hypoglycemia, hyponatremia, or hypocalcemia.

Diagnosis.   Interpretation of cerebrospinal fluid cell counts in newborn infants may be difficult (Naidoo, 1968; Sarff et al., 1976). During the first several days of life, as many as 32 white blood cells per mm^3 (mean, 8 cells per mm^3) may be found in cerebrospinal fluid of healthy or high risk, uninfected babies. Approximately 60 per cent of these cells are polymorphonuclear leukocytes. During the first week, the cell count slowly diminishes in full-term infants but may remain high or even increase in premature babies. Cell counts in the range of 0 to 10 cells per mm^3 are observed at 1 month of age. The cerebrospinal fluid protein concentration may be as high as 170 mg per 100 ml, and the cerebrospinal fluid glucose to blood glucose percentage ratio is 44 per cent to greater than 100 per cent in both preterm and term

infants. Thus, it is apparent that the total evaluation of the cerebrospinal fluid examination is necessary in order to make an early diagnosis of neonatal meningitis. Although the cerebrospinal fluid cell counts and protein and sugar concentrations from normal infants overlap with those from infants with meningitis, less than 1 per cent of babies with proved meningitis have a totally normal cerebrospinal fluid study on the initial lumbar tap (Sarff et al., 1976).

It is important to examine carefully stained smears of cerebrospinal fluid from every infant with suspected meningitis. Grossly clear fluid may contain few white blood cells and many bacteria. The stained smears from approximately 20 per cent of neonates with proved meningitis will be interpreted as showing no bacteria. As the name implies, *Listeria monocytogenes* commonly evokes a mononuclear cellular response in the cerebrospinal fluid.

Two techniques of rapidly diagnosing bacterial meningitis have been described. The first, counterimmunoelectrophoresis (CIE), is used to detect bacterial capsular antigens in cerebrospinal fluid. Studies to date indicate that antigen can be identified in cerebrospinal fluid of approximately two thirds of infants with *E. coli* K1, *H. influenzae* (type B), and pneumococcal and meningococcal meningitis (McCracken et al., 1974; Shackelford et al., 1974). If concentrated urine is examined for antigen, the diagnosis of *H. influenzae* and meningococcal disease can be established in most patients. Group B streptococcal antigen has also been measured in body fluids. Quantitation of antigen is helpful in the prognosis of infants with purulent meningitis.

The second method involves detection of endotoxin utilizing the limulus lysate assay. Endotoxin can be measured in cerebrospinal fluid of patients with meningitis caused by coliform bacteria, *H. influenzae* (type B), or *Meningococcus* (Nachum et al., 1973). Both the CIE and the limulus lysate techniques take less than 1 hour to run and can be established in most hospital laboratories. If both methods are used, approximately 80 per cent of neonates with coliform meningitis can be identified within an hour of the initial lumbar tap (McCracken and Sarff, 1974).

Blood and urine cultures should be obtained from every infant with suspected meningitis.

Therapy.   Selection of appropriate antibiotic therapy is based in part on the achievable cerebrospinal fluid levels of these drugs in relation to the susceptibility of the organisms causing disease. The highest kanamycin and gentamicin concentrations in cerebrospinal fluid are approximately 40 per cent of the peak serum levels and are only equal to or slightly greater than the minimal inhibitory concentrations for disease-causing coliforms. In contrast, cerebrospinal fluid penicillin and ampicillin concentrations may be only 10 per cent of the corresponding peak serum levels, but these values are usually 10- to 100-fold higher than the greatest minimal inhibitory concentrations for group B streptococci and *L. monocytog-*

enes. The ability to attain spinal fluid antimicrobial activity that is many times greater than is necessary to inhibit the pathogen may explain the rapid sterilization of spinal fluid cultures from infants with gram-positive meningitis. Delayed sterilization of cerebrospinal fluid cultures from neonates with gram-negative meningitis may likewise be due to the low inhibitory and bactericidal spinal fluid concentrations. As a result of these considerations, one may find it necessary in some infants with coliform meningitis to alter the therapeutic regimens by adding a second antibiotic, by selecting a different aminoglycoside, by using one of the newer cephalosporin derivatives, or by changing the route of administration.

At the present time, ampicillin and either gentamicin or kanamycin are recommended for initial therapy of neonatal meningitis. The dosages of ampicillin are 100 mg per kg per day in two divided doses during the first week of life and 200 mg per kg per day in three divided doses thereafter. The dosages for gentamicin and kanamycin are the same as those used for septicemia (Table 83–1). All infants should have a repeat spinal fluid examination and culture at 24 to 36 hours after initiation of therapy. If organisms are seen on methylene blue or Gram-stained smears of the fluid, modification of the therapeutic regimen should be considered.

The Neonatal Meningitis Cooperative Study Group was unable to demonstrate a significant improvement in morbidity and mortality rates for infants with gram-negative bacillary meningitis treated with intrathecal gentamicin (1 mg daily) compared with those treated with parenteral therapy only (McCracken and Mize, 1976). Most infants with delayed sterilization of spinal fluid have ventriculitis, and cultures of ventricular fluid yield the pathogen. Intravenous and even intrathecal antibiotics often fail to achieve high concentrations in the ventricles. For these reasons, the Neonatal Meningitis Cooperative Study Group next undertook a large controlled study of intraventricular gentamicin (McCracken et al., 1980). As with intrathecal therapy, however, no advantage was gained by the direct daily instillation of gentamicin into the ventricles. In fact, the study was terminated early because infants receiving intraventricular drug showed a higher mortality (43 per cent) than the control group (13 per cent). Despite this, there are those who feel that delivery of aminoglycosides to the ventricle, using a surgically placed reservoir, is a helpful addition to intravenous therapy in cases in which ventriculitis has been documented by ventricular tap on the second or third day of illness (Wright et al., 1980).

If intrathecal or intraventricular gentamicin is used, it is advisable to monitor cerebrospinal or ventricular fluid levels in order to be certain that the drug is present in therapeutic and safe concentrations. Intrathecal or intraventricular therapy is continued until the fluid is sterile.

Several newer antimicrobial agents offer the promise of achieving high bactericidal levels in the ventricular fluid of babies with gram-negative bacillary meningitis, although none of them has, at this writing, been fully evaluated in controlled trials. Two new cephalosporin derivatives, cefotaxime (Belohradsky et al., 1980) and Moxalactam (Schaad et al., 1981), diffuse well into the cerebrospinal fluid and show good or excellent activity against most gram-negative rods. Trimethoprim-sulfamethoxazole is a drug whose metabolism in the newborn has not been thoroughly investigated but that may be useful in unusual situations (Darby, 1976). All these drugs remain experimental in the neonatal period. Chloramphenicol, because of its capacity to diffuse readily into the cerebrospinal fluid, has also been used in neonatal meningitis, and with frequent measurement of blood levels it is relatively safe. Nevertheless, results have been disappointing (Heckmatt, 1976), and its use except in unusual situations is not recommended.

Once the pathogen has been identified and the susceptibility studies are available, the single drug or combination of drugs that is most effective should be used. In general, penicillin is preferred for group B streptococcal infection, ampicillin with or without kanamycin or gentamicin for *L. monocytogenes* and *Enterococcus*, ampicillin plus gentamicin or kanamycin for coliforms, and carbenicillin plus gentamicin for *Pseudomonas* infections. There is no precise method for determining duration of antimicrobial therapy. A useful guide is to continue therapy for approximately 2 weeks after sterilization of cerebrospinal fluid cultures or for a minimum of 2 weeks for gram-positive meningitis and of 3 weeks for gram-negative meningitis, whichever is longest.

Attention to general supportive therapy is of utmost importance in caring for infants with meningitis. Disturbances of fluid and electrolyte balance are common, particularly in the first several days of illness when inappropriate antidiuretic hormone secretion may lead to fluid retention and hyponatremia. Ventilatory assistance is frequently necessary, and blood pressures should be carefully monitored. During the course of illness, hemoglobin and hematocrit values should be checked frequently because infection may exaggerate and prolong the anemias of infancy, particularly in premature infants. As with sepsis, some authorities recommend transfusions with fresh whole blood or frozen plasma as a means of providing nonspecific factors of host resistance.

Prognosis. The mortality in neonatal meningitis is high. The overall mortality rate is approximately 20 to 50 per cent, depending on the etiologic agent, the high risk factors predisposing the infant to illness, and the ability of nursery personnel and physicians to provide general supportive care. Short- and long-term sequelae of neonatal meningitis are frequent. The acute complications include communicating or noncommunicating hydrocephalus, subdural effusions, ventriculitis, deafness, and blindness. Gross retardation may be obvious immediately. However, many infants will appear relatively normal at time of discharge, and only after prolonged and careful follow-up will perceptual difficulties, reading problems, or signs of minimal brain damage become apparent. Approximately 40 to 50 per cent of survivors will have some evidence of neurologic damage.

Otitis Media

Otitis media is infrequently diagnosed in neonates because of the paucity of clinical findings and the difficulty in examining the infant's tympanic membrane (Warren and Stool, 1971). The external canal is narrow and often filled with cheesy debris. Because the healthy baby's membrane may appear thickened and dull, mobility of the drum by pneumoscopy should be used as the single most reliable indicator of middle ear infection.

Neonatal otitis media occurs most often in premature infants and almost exclusively in bottle-fed babies. The exact incidence of this disease is unknown, but it has been estimated to occur in approximately 1 to 5 per cent of infants 0 to 6 weeks of age. The onset of illness is insidious, and the most common complaints are rhinorrhea, irritability, and failure to thrive. Fever greater than 38° C and tugging of the affected ear are unusual.

It is important that all neonates with suspected otitis media have needle aspiration of middle ear contents because the pathogens associated with disease may be different from those encountered in infants beyond the first several months of life (Bland, 1972). The material obtained from aspiration is cultured in suitable media, and a stained smear is prepared for direct visualization of bacteria. E. coli, Staphylococcus aureus, and Klebsiella pneumoniae are causative in approximately one fifth of cases. Diplococcus pneumoniae and H. influenzae are the most frequently encountered pathogens during the first 6 weeks of life, as they are during the entire infancy period. Those babies under 2 weeks of age with otitis media should be treated in the hospital with parenterally administered antibiotics. Selection of initial therapy is based on results of the gram-stained smear. If organisms are not observed, oxacillin and gentamicin should be started and continued until results of cultures and susceptibility studies are available.

The importance of establishing the diagnosis and etiology of otitis media in neonates and of employing appropriate therapy cannot be overemphasized. Missed diagnosis and improper therapy may result in a chronic course of middle ear disease throughout infancy and, occasionally, in extension of infection to adjacent structures such as the mastoid or central nervous system.

Diarrheal Disease

Diarrheal disease during the neonatal period is usually brief and self-limited. Brief episodes of loose stools secondary to alterations of diet and feeding pattern are common in young infants. Modern sterilization practices and increased emphasis on infection control measures have significantly reduced the incidence of bacterial diarrhea in nurseries.

Etiology and Pathogenesis. Infectious diarrhea in newborns may be caused by bacteria, yeast (Candida), and viruses, but the most frequent of these are several species of bacteria. The pathogenesis of bacterial diarrhea appears to be complex and to depend very much on the particular species involved. Escherichia coli strains are believed to cause diarrhea by one of two mechanisms (DuPont and Hornick, 1973; Rudoy and Nelson, 1975). The first involves colonization of the upper small bowel by an organism capable of producing enterotoxin, a bacterial exotoxin ("enterotoxigenic strains"). These bacteria attach to, but do not invade, the gut wall. The enterotoxin causes stimulation of cyclic-AMP, which in turn inhibits sodium and chloride transport across the intestinal wall. As a result, these salts are lost into the lumen of the upper bowel, followed passively by water, causing a net loss of high electrolyte-containing stools. Vibrio cholerae and Vibrio parahaemolyticus appear to produce diarrhea by the same mechanism.

The second mechanism by which certain strains of E. coli produce diarrhea is invasion of the intestinal mucosa ("enteroinvasive strains"). The pathogenesis of Shigella diarrhea also appears to occur by this mechanism. Colonic invasion and subsequent destruction of the mucosa cause an outpouring of polymorphonuclear cells, blood, and mucus, with resultant dysentery and diarrhea.

When it was first recognized that E. coli produced epidemics of diarrhea in nurseries, certain "enteropathogenic" strains were serologically identified that had been epidemiologically associated with outbreaks. It seems clear now that many of these strains were enterotoxigenic or enteroinvasive. It has been clearly shown since that time that many diarrhea-producing strains of E. coli were not included among the identified "enteropathogenic" serotypes (Boyer et al., 1975). Such strains have been recognized both through traditional epidemiologic studies and by laboratory measurement of enterotoxigenic or enteroinvasive properties. For some time it was thought that the old serotyping methods were therefore outmoded in identifying such organisms. Measuring pathogenic potential in E. coli directly, however, is outside the capability of most laboratories. Moreover, a number of strains have now been identified and tightly associated by epidemiologic methods with diarrheal outbreaks, for which no pathogenic mechanism has been measurable. Many authorities now, therefore, recognize the utility (as well as the limitations) of serologic identification and consider it a reasonable adjunct to more sophisticated measurement of toxin production or invasive capacity (if these tests are available).

Salmonellae produce diarrhea by mechanisms that are even less clearly understood (Rubin and Weinstein, 1977). Many species invade the mucosa without destroying it and set up an inflammatory reaction in the lamina propria. From here, particularly in neonates and young infants, the bloodstream may be invaded. Finally, in rare instances *Campylobacter fetus* subspecies *jejuni* (the form that most often causes diarrhea in older individuals) may sometimes be seen in neonates, in whom it produces bloody diarrhea. The outcome is usually favorable (Anders et al., 1981).

Clinical Manifestations. It is difficult to differentiate the causes of diarrhea in neonates on the basis of clinical findings only. As a general rule, diarrhea caused by enteropathogenic strains of *E. coli* is insidious in onset, is associated with seven to 10 green, watery stools a day, and is usually without blood or mucus. The infants do not appear acutely ill. Complications are rare and are related primarily to dehydration and electrolyte disturbances. *Salmonella* gastroenteritis is usually associated with five to 10 foul-smelling, loose green stools daily that rarely contain mucus or blood. Complications, which are unusual, include extraintestinal foci of infection such as septicemia, osteomyelitis, and septic arthritis, Shigellosis is rare in neonates, but, when encountered, it is an acute illness associated with a profuse, watery, nonodorous diarrhea frequently containing blood and mucus. The infants may be very toxic, and illness in a small number of patients will initially mimic meningitis or gram-negative shock. Suppurative complications are rare, but dehydration and electrolyte disturbances are common and need immediate and constant attention.

A useful procedure for differentiating enteroinvasive from enterotoxigenic diarrhea is examination of fecal material for polymorphonuclear cells. Feces from patients with dysentery show significant numbers of polymorphonuclear cells, while those from patients with enterotoxigenic disease show very few neutrophils. This test may be helpful in selecting appropriate antimicrobial therapy.

Therapy. The single most important aspect of therapy for infantile diarrhea is maintenance of hydration and electrolyte balance. As a rule, parenteral solutions containing appropriate electrolytes should be administered during the time of active diarrhea, and the infant should be examined and weighed frequently to ensure proper rehydration and prevention of complications. Estimation of fluid loss from diar-

rhea and vomiting should be carefully recorded and used as a basis for replacement therapy.

The selection of an antimicrobial agent depends in part on the mechanism of diarrhea. An absorbable antibiotic such as ampicillin or chloramphenicol is indicated for disease caused by invasive bacteria, whereas orally administered nonabsorbable drugs such as neomycin or colistin sulfate are used for noninvasive organisms that produce enterotoxin.

All nursery infants with enteropathogenic *E. coli* should receive neomycin or colistin sulfate orally, whether or not they are symptomatic. Neomycin is administered orally in a dosage of 100 mg per kg per day in three or four divided doses. Colistin sulfate is administered in a dosage of 15 to 17 mg per kg per day orally in four divided doses. The duration of therapy is 3 to 5 days. Longer periods of therapy are unnecessary and may result in neomycin-induced steatorrhea (Nelson, 1971). If enteropathogenic *E. coli* are isolated from stools of nonhospitalized, asymptomatic infants, it is usually not necessary to treat these infants with antimicrobial agents; however, they should be followed carefully.

All infants with *Salmonella* gastroenteritis should have blood cultures performed and be examined for development of disease at other sites, such as bones and joints. Neonates with symptomatic *Salmonella* infections should receive antimicrobial therapy if they are febrile or toxic or if their diarrhea is severe because of the greater potential for systemic infection in these patients. Older infants and children with *Salmonella* gastroenteritis and asymptomatic or minimally symptomatic neonates with positive stool cultures for *Salmonella* species should not receive antibiotics. In these patients, antimicrobial therapy may prolong gastrointestinal *Salmonella* carriage and does not significantly affect the clinical course of disease. When therapy is indicated in the neonate or young infant, ampicillin is the drug of choice and should be administered parenterally in a dosage of 50 to 100 mg per kg per day, divided in two or three doses. Therapy is continued for approximately 5 to 7 days.

Although shigellosis in the neonate is rare, it may be associated with significant morbidity and mortality. All neonates with symptomatic shigellosis should be treated with ampicillin in a dosage of 50 to 100 mg per kg per day, administered parenterally in two or three divided doses. Duration of therapy is approximately 5 days. In some hospitals a significant percentage of ampicillin-resistant *Shigella* strains have been encountered. In these centers, trimethoprim-sulfamethoxazole is the initial drug of choice. The dosage is 10 mg TMP and 50 mg SMZ per kg per day in two divided doses for 5 days.

Any infant with diarrhea must be isolated from the other babies in the nursery. Surveillance of other infants in the unit and institution of infection control measures are also indicated (see discussion of nosocomial bacterial disease).

Urinary Tract Infection

Improved methods of obtaining sterile specimens have made it possible to define more accurately the incidence of neonatal urinary tract infection. With bladder aspiration technique (Edelman et al., 1973), bacteriuria may be demonstrated in approximately 1 per cent of full-term infants and 3 per cent of premature infants. Urinary tract infections are more common in babies born to bacteriuric mothers and in males during the neonatal period. After this period, these infections are more common in females.

Etiology. *Escherichia coli* is the most common etiologic agent of urinary tract infections. Approximately 70 per cent of *E. coli* strains belong to one of eight common somatic antigen groups similar to those found in older patients. Renal parenchymal disease may be associated with one of several *E. coli* capsular types: K1, K2ac, K12, or K13 (Kaijser, 1972). *Klebsiella* and *Pseudomonas* species are encountered less frequently. *Proteus* species commonly cause urinary tract disease in infants with meningomyeloceles. Gram-positive bacteria, with the exception of enterococci, are rare causes of urinary tract infection.

The higher frequency of urinary tract infections in male infants suggests that the predominant pathogenesis at this age may differ from that in the older child or adult. Bacteremia, with seeding in a kidney that is in some way abnormal, may be responsible for at least some cases.

Clinical Manifestations. The majority of infants with significant bacteriuria are asymptomatic. When symptoms are present they are usually nonspecific and include poor weight gain, altered temperature, cyanosis or gray skin color, abdominal distention, with or without vomiting, and loose stools. Jaundice, hepatomegaly and thrombocytopenia may be observed in a few infants with urinary tract infection, and these findings are associated with septicemia or cholestatic hepatitis or both in some babies. Localizing signs suggesting urinary tract involvement are unusual; when present, they usually consist of a weak urinary stream on voiding or an abdominal mass from bladder distention or hydronephrosis.

The diagnosis of urinary tract infections is made by examination and culture of a properly obtained specimen of urine. At any age, but particularly in the neonatal period, during which diagnosis of urinary tract infection brings with it suggestions of renal or collecting system anomalies and bacteremia, the diagnosis is never made on the basis of urinalysis alone.

However, a culture of a "bag urine" sample is valuable *only* if it is sterile. The presence of bacteria, even in high numbers and in pure culture, may always be accounted for by contamination from the perineum.

At all ages, urinary tract infection may be present in the absence of leukocytes in the urine. The converse is also true, particularly when the urine is collected in a sterile plastic bag. Leukocytes or round epithelial cells (easily confused with leukocytes) are often found in "bag urine" samples, particularly after circumcision, in the absence of urinary tract infection. For these reasons, culture (or, for rapid screening, Gram stain) of a suprapubic bladder aspiration is the only certain means to diagnose urinary tract infection. In newborns, in whom restriction of fluid intake is not appropriate, greater than 10,000 organisms per mm^3 of a single species (rather than greater than 100,000 as is often thought) are diagnostic if the specimen is obtained by bladder puncture. Moreover, concern about whether an infection is in the upper or lower urinary tract is rarely justified in the neonate, since either one carries with it concerns about urinary tract anomalies and bacteremia.

Therapy. All infants with suspected or proved urinary tract infections should have blood and urine cultures obtained prior to initiation of therapy. In general, antimicrobial agents should initially be administered parenterally because septicemia may occur in association with urinary tract infection, and antibiotic absorption after oral administration may be erratic in neonates. Ampicillin plus kanamycin or gentamicin should be administered to symptomatic infants with bacteriuria prior to results of cultures and susceptibility studies. Final antibiotic selection is based on these studies.

A repeat urine culture taken 48 to 72 hours after initiation of appropriate therapy should be sterile or show a substantial reduction in the bacterial count. Infants with persistent bacteriuria should be evaluated for inappropriate therapy, obstruction, or possible abscess formation. In the uncomplicated patient, therapy is usually continued for a period of 10 to 14 days. Blood urea nitrogen and serum creatinine levels should be determined at initiation and completion of therapy. If there is evidence of renal failure, dosage and frequency of administration of these drugs, particularly the aminoglycosides, may need to be altered. Approximately 1 week after discontinuing therapy, a repeat urine culture is obtained. If the culture is positive, therapy is reinstituted and a thorough investigation of the urinary tract is made in order to rule out obstruction or abscess formation.

All infants with documented urinary tract infections should have radiologic or ultrasonic evaluation of the urinary tract. An excretory urogram is obtained at the outset of therapy to rule out the possibility of gross congenital abnormalities of the urinary system. If obstruction is demonstrated, urologic procedures to ensure proper drainage are mandatory if therapy is to be successful. Because of the possibility of ureteral reflux associated with bladder inflammation, many urologists prefer to obtain the voiding cystourethrogram several weeks after therapy has been completed.

Prognosis. It is the physician's responsibility to be certain that neonates with documented urinary tract infections do not have congenital abnormalities of the urinary system. In such patients, recurrent urinary tract infections are common, and physical growth may be retarded until definitive surgery has been performed. One must conduct careful, long-term follow-up studies in every patient in order to detect recurrent infections, many of which will be asymptomatic.

Septic Arthritis and Osteomyelitis

During the neonatal and infancy period, the epiphyseal plate is traversed by multiple small transepiphyseal vessels that provide a direct communication between the articular space and the metaphysis of the long bones (Ogden and Lister, 1975). Thus, infection of a metaphyseal site can spread across the growth plate to penetrate the epiphysis. Because these perforating vessels disappear at approximately 1 year of age, osteomyelitis is usually not associated with septic arthritis in older infants and children. There are two possible exceptions to this rule: osteomyelitis of the proximal femur and of the proximal humerus. The capsules of the hip and shoulder attach below the metaphysis of the femur and humerus, respectively. Infection of the epiphyseal cartilage may rupture through the periosteum and enter the joint space, producing purulent arthritis. Because the capsular articulations of the hip and shoulder are permanent, osteomyelitis and septic arthritis may coexist, making the origin of infection difficult to establish. Because the inflammatory process of osteomyelitis or of septic arthritis can occupy the epiphyseal and metaphyseal sides of the growth plate, ischemia and necrosis of the plate may occur, resulting in permanent damage.

Etiology. *Staphylococcus aureus* is the most common etiologic agent of neonatal musculoskeletal infections. Group B streptococci have been encountered with increasing frequency since the 1970s (Memon et al., 1979). Coliform organisms and *Pseudomonas* are infrequent pathogens (Weissberg et al., 1974; Dich et al.; 1975; Nelson, 1972). Antecedent trauma, umbilical vessel catheterization, respiratory tract disease, and femoral venipunctures have been implicated in the pathogenesis of these infections in some infants.

Clinical Manifestations. Initial signs and symptoms are usually nonspecific. Most infants are not brought to medical attention until local signs such as swelling, irritability, and decreased motion of an extremity become apparent. Physical examination reveals swelling, localized pain on palpation, and resistance to movement of the affected extremity.

Localized heat and fluctuance are late findings. Occasionally, the diagnosis is made unsuspectingly when purulent material is obtained on attempted aspiration of the femoral vein. In this instance, the needle enters the swollen hip capsule.

Although blood cultures are frequently positive, clinically the infants usually do not appear septic. An exception is Group A beta-hemolytic streptococcal infection, in which the infant appears gravely ill.

Diagnosis. Blood cultures should be obtained from all infants with suspected osteomyelitis or septic arthritis. In infants with septic arthritis, a percutaneous needle aspiration of intra-articular pus should be performed; in osteomyelitis, direct needle aspiration of the affected periosteum and bone is attempted. If pus is obtained, the material should be Gram stained and cultured. Preliminary identification of the pathogen from stained smears is helpful in the selection of initial antimicrobial therapy.

In patients with suspected septic arthritis, radiographs may be normal or show widening of the articular space and capsular swelling. Later in the course of disease, subluxation and destruction of the joint are common. In early osteomyelitis, the normal radiographic water markings of the deep tissues adjacent to the affected bone are obliterated, indicating inflammation. Lifting of the periosteum from the bone may also be observed, but cortical destruction is unusual before the second week of illness, and new bone formation is a late finding. Resolution of bone changes is considerably slower than clinical improvement (Weissberg et al., 1974). There is very little experience to date with scanning techniques of bone in newborn and young infants. This procedure offers the advantage of earlier diagnosis than can be achieved with ordinary radiographs.

Therapy. Selection of initial antimicrobial therapy is based on results of examination of stained smears of aspirated purulent material and on the presence of associated clinical findings such as furuncles or cellulitis. If gram-positive cocci are observed, oxacillin should be started. Either kanamycin or gentamicin is indicated if gram-negative organisms are noted. If no organisms are seen or if doubt exists regarding their identification, oxacillin plus gentamicin or kanamycin should be used until results of the cultures are available. Direct instillation of an antibiotic into the joint space is unnecessary because most drugs will penetrate the inflamed synovium, and adequate concentrations are achieved in purulent material (Nelson, 1971). This also applies to treatment of osteomyelitis; direct instillation of antibiotics into acutely inflamed bone is unwarranted.

As a general rule, infection of the joint space and bone should be drained either by repeated aspiration or by surgery. Septic arthritis of the hip and shoulder is best treated with incision and drainage in order to prevent vascular compromise or extension of infection into the metaphysis. Orthopedic consultation should be obtained for all patients.

Antimicrobial therapy of neonatal musculoskeletal infections caused by staphylococci or coliform organisms is continued for a minimum of 3 weeks. Group B streptococcal infection is treated with penicillin G for approximately 3 weeks. The use of oral antibiotics as a substitute for parenteral therapy during the second and third weeks of therapy is unwise because of the difficulty in assuring complete compliance on the part of the parents and the lack of experience with this route of administration in neonates. In general, systemic symptoms disappear within several days of initiating therapy, although local signs such as heat, erythema, and swelling may persist for 4 to 7 days. Full range of motion may not return to the involved limb for several months. Because of this, physical therapy should be instituted early in illness to prevent contractures. Complete resolution of the radiographic changes may take several months.

Prognosis.   Mortality from these diseases is rare. However, morbidity may be considerable, particularly when a weight-bearing joint such as the hip or knee is involved. Contractures and muscle damage may be permanent.

Ophthalmia Neonatorum (see also Chapter 105)

Paralleling the increased incidence of venereal disease in the general population, ophthalmia neonatorum is again being observed in some areas of the country (Snowe and Wilfert, 1973). *Neisseria gonorrhoeae* is acquired during passage through the infected birth canal when the mucous membranes come in contact with infected secretions. Infection usually becomes apparent within the first 5 days of life and is initially characterized by a clear, watery discharge, which rapidly becomes purulent. This is associated with marked conjunctival hyperemia and chemosis. Both eyes are usually involved but not necessarily to the same degree. Untreated gonococcal ophthalmia may extend to involve the cornea (keratitis) and the anterior chamber of the eye. This may eventuate in corneal perforation and blindness. Until the introduction of adequate prophylactic measures, ophthalmia neonatorum was the most frequent cause of acquired blindness in the United States. Any infant presenting with a conjunctival discharge should have the material stained and cultured for gonococcus and other bacterial agents. Demonstration of gram-negative intracellular diplococci on stained smear is an indication for immediate penicillin therapy prior to definitive laboratory diagnosis.

Differential Diagnosis.   Conjunctivitis occurring in the first days of life can be either chemical or bacterial in nature. Chemical irritants such as silver nitrate cause transient conjunctival hyperemia and a watery discharge, but this is not associated with a purulent discharge. Common bacterial agents associated with conjunctivitis in neonates are *S. aureus, N. gonorrhoeae,* and *P. aeruginosa.* It is important to determine the specific etiology in order to select appropriate therapy and to prevent permanent sequelae to the eye. Viral conjunctivitis in a single nursery infant is unusual.

Conjunctivitis during the second or third week of life may be caused by viral, bacterial, or chlamydial agents. Viral conjunctivitis is frequently associated with other symptoms of respiratory tract disease, such as rhinorrhea, cough, and sore throat, and several individuals in the family unit may have simultaneous disease. In general, the discharge in viral conjunctivitis is watery or mucopurulent, but rarely purulent. Preauricular adenopathy is common. Staphylococci, streptococci, and, occasionally, gonococci cause conjunctivitis in this age group. A smear of the purulent material is helpful in differentiating these etiologic agents. However, the presence of bacteria on a Gram-stained smear of material is not necessarily related etiologically to the conjunctivitis. Normal inhabitants of the skin and mucous membranes, such as staphylococci, diphtheroids, and *Neisseria catarrhalis* may be observed.

Conjunctivitis caused by *Chlamydia* (inclusion blennorrhea) is a venereally transmitted disease that is observed in infants 5 to 14 days of age (Goscienski, 1970). Clinical manifestations vary from mild conjunctivitis to intense inflammation and swelling of the lids associated with copious purulent discharge. Pseudomembrane formation and a diffuse "matte" injection of the tarsal conjunctiva are common. The cornea is rarely affected, and preauricular adenopathy is unusual. In the early stages of disease, one eye may appear more swollen and infected than the other, but both eyes are almost invariably involved. Diagnosis is made by scraping the tarsal conjunctiva and looking for typical cytoplasmic inclusions within epithelial cells, using Giemsa stain. These inclusions will not be seen on smears of purulent discharge, and cultures of the discharge yield various bacteria that are not related etiologically to the clinical disease. A simplified technique to cultivate *Chlamydia* has been described but is not generally available in most hospitals. Without treatment the acute inflammation continues for several weeks, merging into a subacute phase of slight conjunctival injection with scant purulent material. Occasionally, chronicity develops, some cases persisting for over a year.

Therapy.   Ophthalmia neonatorum due to *N. gonorrhoeae* should be treated with parenteral antimicrobial therapy. Crystalline penicillin G should be administered intravenously or intramuscularly in a dosage of 50,000 to 75,000 units per kg per day in two divided doses for infants under 1 week and in three divided doses for infants over 1 week of age. Duration of parenteral therapy is 7 to 10 days. In addition to systemic antibiotic therapy, the eyes should be washed immediately and at frequent intervals with saline solution followed by topical administration of chloramphenicol or tetracycline. Initially, local saline irrigations are given every 1 or 2 hours, and gradually the interval is increased to every 6 to 12 hours as clinical improvement is noted. Patients with ophthalmia neonatorum should be isolated, and strict handwashing techniques should be employed because of the highly contagious nature of the exudate. Conjunctivitis caused by other bacterial agents should be treated parenterally with the single most appropriate agent as judged by susceptibility testing of the organism.

Inclusion blennorrhea is treated by topical administration of 10 per cent sulfacetamide or 1 per cent tetracycline ointment applied every 3 to 4 hours for approximately 14 days. Marked reduction in swelling and discharge is observed within 24 hours of therapy. Antigonococcal prophylaxis at birth has little, if any, effect on chlamydial infection. Some authors recommend treating chlamydial conjunctivitis with oral erythromycin in order to prevent subsequent development of pneumonitis.

Ophthalmia neonatorum is a preventable disease. One per cent silver nitrate instilled in both eyes in the immediate neonatal period is 90 to 95 per cent effective in preventing gonococcal ophthalmia. Silver nitrate should not be irrigated with saline, as this may reduce efficacy. Ophthalmic ointments containing tetracycline or chloramphenicol are also effective prophylactic agents. Bacitracin ophthalmic ointment is not effective. Penicillin drops are effective and produce less conjunctivitis than does silver nitrate, but we do not recommend their routine use because of the possible risk of sensitization.

Cutaneous Infections

The most common bacteria causing skin infections during the neonatal period are *Staphylococcus aureus* and groups A and B streptococci. Disease caused by *S. aureus* can assume several clinical forms, the most common being pustular lesions. These tend to concentrate in the periumbilical and diaper areas and rarely become invasive except when extensive areas are involved or when monitoring devices, catheters, or other invasive procedures are necessary in gravely ill infants. A stained smear and a culture of an intact lesion are usually helpful in identifying the pathogen. The organisms should be phage typed (they usually belong to group I) so that if additional cases are encountered in the same nursery, these infants and others in the unit can be evaluated

for the possibility of a nosocomial staphylococcal outbreak. If these infections are caused by the same phage type of staphylococcus, prompt measures should be instituted to determine the source of infection and to prevent further colonization and disease.

Therapy of cutaneous staphylococcal disease depends on the extent of the lesions and the general clinical condition of the infant. One can manage small, isolated pustules by local care using a mild cleansing agent or an antiseptic such as hexachlorophene or povidone iodine. Infants with more extensive cutaneous involvement or systemic signs of infection or both should be treated with parenteral antimicrobial agents. A penicillinase-resistant penicillin should be used initially; continuation of this drug will depend on the results of susceptibility testing.

The second form of neonatal staphylococcal disease has been previously described (see discussion of septicemia) and is referred to as "the expanded scalded-skin syndrome."

Group A beta-hemolytic streptococci occasionally cause disease in the nursery (Dillon, 1966). The most common manifestation is a low-grade omphalitis characterized by a wet, malodorous umbilical stump with minimal inflammation. Disseminated disease occurs secondary to blood stream invasion or by direct extension to the peritoneal cavity by way of the umbilical vessels. Identification of one infant with group A streptococcal disease in a nursery necessitates cultural surveillance of the other infants and of the personnel in the unit. The organism is usually introduced into the nursery by asymptomatic nasopharyngeal infection of personnel or parents. When a nursery outbreak is suspected, specific M and T typing of the organism is useful in defining the source and spread of infection. Group B streptococci have been associated with cellulitis, impetiginous lesions, and small abscesses in a few neonates. Penicillin is the drug of choice for streptococcal infections.

Necrotizing fasciitis is an unusual disease of newborn infants. This disease is frequently associated with surgical procedures, birth trauma, or cutaneous infection (Wilson and Haltalin, 1973). Staphylococci, either alone or associated with streptococci, are usually causative, but other bacteria, including gram-negative enteric bacilli, can be cultured. In this condition, subcutaneous tissues, including muscle layers, are invaded and the organism spreads along the fascial planes. Overlying skin may appear violaceous and is edematous, which imparts a thick "woody" sensation on palpation. The borders of the lesion are usually indistinct when compared with those seen with erysipelas, which are raised and easily palpated. Extensive surgery involving resection of destroyed tissue is imperative in treating necrotizing fasciitis. Blood and tissue cultures should be obtained, and oxacillin and gentamicin are the drugs of choice for initial therapy. Necrotic, fatty tissue many combine with calcium, resulting in tetany and convulsions.

Breast Abscess. Breast abscesses are most frequently encountered during the second or third weeks of life and occur more commonly in females, particularly those over 2 weeks of age. The disease does not occur in premature infants, presumably because of underdevelopment of the mammary gland in these infants. Bilateral disease is rare.

The major presentation of neonatal breast abscess is localized swelling with or without accompanying erythema and warmth. Systemic manifestations are uncommon, and only 25 per cent of these infants will have low-grade fever. *Staphylococcus aureus* is the major pathogen; coliforms and group B streptococci are encountered in a few infants. The diagnosis of breast abscess is best made by needle aspiration of the affected site. The single most important aspect of management is prompt incision and drainage by a skilled surgeon. Oxacillin should be administered for approximately 5 days during the period of drainage. Experience with this condition in Dallas indicates that antimicrobial therapy plays a secondary role to adequate drainage (Rudoy and Nelson, 1975). Long-term follow-up studies suggest that some girls will have diminished breast tissue on the affected side.

Nosocomial Bacterial Infections

Hospital-acquired (nosocomial) infections have become a significant problem in most hospitals and may affect 2 to 5 per cent of all hospitalized patients. In nurseries, nosocomial bacterial infections are of particular importance because of the unusual susceptibility of small infants to severe illness. This applies both to routine, short-stay nurseries and to intensive care nurseries in which babies are frequently intubated and on respirators and require monitoring or feeding by means of central catheters. In short-stay nurseries, problems are most frequently due to gram-positive organisms, *Staphylococcus aureus* most commonly but also streptococci (groups A and B). In intensive care nurseries, many organisms may pose a threat: *S. aureus* remains important, but *S. epidermidis* is also pathogenic; gram-negative enteric bacilli are frequently a hazard, and are often highly resistant to antibiotics. Fungi, particularly *Candida albicans,* are also seen.

In neonatal intensive care units, surveys have shown that as many as 15 per cent of infants hospitalized over 48 hours acquire nosocomial infections from their environment, many of them more than once (Hemming et al., 1976). In one such survey, surface infections accounted for 40 per cent of the total, pneumonia for 29 per cent, bacteremia for 14

per cent, and surgical, urinary tract, and central nervous system infections for many of the remainder. Staphylococci and gram-negative enteric bacilli were responsible for more than 90 per cent of these infections (Hemming et al., 1976). It has been shown that scrupulous attention to such matters as staff-to-patient ratios, nursery design, and containment principles can assist in minimizing the infection rate (Goldmann et al., 1981). The American Hospital Association urges every hospital to establish an Infection Control Committee, the functions of which are principally two-fold: (1) routine surveillance and education of personnel in principles of infection control, and (2) prompt recognition and control of a nosocomial infection when it occurs. All hospitals should hire an infection control practitioner to supervise and coordinate the infection control and surveillance programs.

When an infectious disease caused by the same organism appears in several infants from the same nursery over a short period of time, a nosocomial epidemic should be suspected. The sick infants must be isolated and cultured in order to identify the pathogen. If a specific, single pathogen is responsible for the outbreak, epidemiologic investigations to determine the source and mode of transmission of infection are greatly facilitated. Specialized bacteriologic methods are frequently available to identify markers, such as phage-type or bacteriocin-type, for specific bacteria. Such techniques allow the systematic tracing of the spread of an organism. It is probably best for the infection control practitioner and the nursery director to obtain expert microbiologic assistance in these instances. The investigation of each outbreak and the consequent control procedures recommended are often matters that require multidisciplinary planning and coordination.

The following discussions of specific bacterial infections are intended to familiarize the reader with some of the more common nosocomial infectious problems encountered in nurseries. This section is not designed to be an exhaustive review of each or all nosocomial bacterial infections.

Staphylococcal Infection. Phage group I *Staphylococcus aureus* (phage types 29, 52, 52A, 79, and 80) caused significant hospital disease in the late 1950s and early 1960s. Disease ranging from pustules and omphalitis to pneumonia, septicemia, and meningitis occurred in neonates during this period. Although the majority of infants are colonized with the epidemic strain during a staphylococcal outbreak, disease occurs in only a small percentage of these infants. Epidemic disease caused by phage group I organisms is still an important problem in many nurseries. In some, the disease re-emerged after 3 per cent hexachlorophene bathing was dicontinued. Disease is apparently milder than it was in the 1960s, but it is still widespread.

Disease caused by phage group II *Staphylococcus aureus* (phage types 3A, 3B, 3C, 55, and 71) in newborn and young infants has been encountered with increasing frequency. Clinical manifestations caused by this organism have been broadly classified into the expanded scalded skin syndrome (Melish and Glasgow, 1971). Nursery epidemics of bullous impetigo caused by group II staphylococci have been reported (Anthony et al., 1972). The source of one outbreak was a member of the nursery staff, who was a carrier of the organism, whereas an infant reservoir of infection and a change in bathing technique may have contributed to the other outbreaks. Contamination of circumcision site may be an additional source of such infections (Annunziato and Goldblum, 1978).

When staphylococcal disease occurs in a nursery, the extent of infection must first be determined. All infants and personnel associated with the index patient are cultured, and a random sampling is taken of the other infants. Personnel in the labor and delivery areas should not be omitted from the survey. The nares and umbilicus of the infant and the anterior nares and skin of personnel should be cultured. Active skin lesions are cultured also. All staphylococcal isolates are tested for coagulase production and phage type. A change in the percentage of infants colonized with *S. aureus* and an increase in the carriage of the specific virulent strain (phage type) are usually observed during nursery staphylococcal epidemics. As a general rule, fomites play a relatively minor role in nosocomial staphylococcal disease. Organisms carried on the hands of personnel have been implicated in outbreaks in several nursery epidemics.

Personnel who are carriers in an epidemic situation and are implicated in spread should be treated. Bacitracin ointment is smeared on the mucosa of the anterior nares three times a day and hexachlorophene showers and shampoos should be taken daily for 3 days. If possible, carriers should be kept away from work until they are free of the organism.

It should be remembered that in short-stay nurseries staphylococcal infections are often clinically manifest only several days after the infants are discharged. For this reason, some reporting system that includes infants requiring care after discharge is essential.

It is often necessary for the physician to take certain precautionary measures before the results of the cultures and phage typing are available. Selection of the one or several measures necessary to control a nursery epidemic must be individualized (Sutherland, 1973). The measures commonly employed are as follows:

1. Isolation of all infants colonized with the virulent *Staphylococcus*. It is advisable to form a cohort system in the nursery for exposed but as yet noncolonized infants and for all new admissions to the nursery. These separate cohorts are cared for by separate nursery staff and are maintained until discharge of the infants. Infected infants are removed from the cohort and placed in isolation.

2. Enforcement of infection-control techniques such as gowning, limited access to the unit, and thorough handwashing before and after handling each patient.

3. Use of antimicrobial agents. Topical antimicrobial therapy may be used for minor skin infections (pustules); parenteral antistaphylococcal therapy should be used for systemic staphylococcal diseases.

4. Initiation of routine bathing with antistaphylococcal cleansing agents such as 3 per cent hexachlorophene (diluted 1:2 to 1:5) or application of triple dye to the umbilicus of all new admissions to the nursery.

5. If all else fails, closing of the nursery to further admissions until the problem has either been solved or spontaneously disappeared.

After an outbreak is controlled, it is sometimes helpful to monitor the activity of staphylococci for a limited period of time by routine culturing of umbilical stumps and noses of infants on discharge from the nursery. A postcard system of surveillance for clinical infections after discharge is also helpful.

Bacterial Diarrhea. The infection control practitioners should be aware of the limitation of designating *E. coli* strains as enteropathogenic on the basis of serotyping only. If, however, *Shigella*, *Salmonella*, or an enteropathogenic strain of *E. coli* is identified in a nursery infant, proper measures should be taken to prevent spread of this agent to other babies. The mother is frequently the source of infection for the index case; subsequent cases are usually transmitted from infant to infant by nursery personnel.

Any nursery infant with diarrhea should be suspected of having a potentially communicable disease and be treated accordingly. Handwashing and other routine infection control procedures should be tightened, and bacterial stool cultures taken. If a bacterial pathogen is isolated, the baby in whom it is found should be moved to a special isolation area, if one is available, and treated with appropriate antimicrobial therapy. If other infants develop watery stools, they should be cultured, placed in the same isolation room as the index infant, and appropriately treated. Culturing of asymptomatic babies and personnel is not always indicated but is appropriate if it is clear that simple isolation and treatment of symptomatic cases is not controlling an outbreak.

Group A Streptococcal Infection. Group A beta-hemolytic *Streptococcus* was a common cause of puerperal and neonatal sepsis in the 1930s and early 1940s. With the advent of penicillin and its frequent use in maternity and nursery units, neonatal infections caused by this organism have become relatively uncommon. The primary source of group A streptococci in nursery outbreaks is either an attendant (nurse or physician) working in the unit or the mother. Once group A streptococci are introduced into a nursery, many infants become colonized but few develop clinical disease. The most common clinical manifestation is a low-grade, granulating omphalitis that fails to heal despite local measures. However, more significant disease may occur, including extensive cellulitis, septicemia, and meningitis.

Identification of one neonate with group A streptococcal infection is enough to warrant epidemiologic investigations of the nursery. All infants in close contact with the index case, a random sampling of other infants, and all nursery personnel should be cultured. Nasopharyngeal and umbilical cultures from infants and nasopharyngeal and rectal cultures from personnel should be obtained. Because nursery and maternity personnel are frequently interchangeable, the epidemiologic work-up should be coordinated with the obstetric service of the hospital.

Infants with streptococcal disease should be treated with aqueous or procaine penicillin G. During nosocomial outbreaks, all asymptomatic infants colonized with group A streptococci should receive penicillin. The prophylactic use of penicillin for all new admissions to the nursery may also be indicated. Benzathine penicillin G has been used effectively as prophylaxis against group A streptococcal infection in several nursery outbreaks.

Gram-Negative Infections. Since the early 1970s, a number of nursery outbreaks caused by specific gram-negative bacteria have been described, and virtually all have occurred in long-stay intensive care nurseries. Among the organisms incriminated were *Klebsiella pneumoniae, Flavobacterium meningosepticum, Pseudomonas aeruginosa, Proteus mirabilis, Serratia marcescens,* and *Escherichia coli.* A common feature of these outbreaks is that the majority of colonized infants are asymptomatic; those who develop disease usually have pneumonia, septicemia, or meningitis.

Infected fomites represent a common source of nursery outbreaks caused by gram-negative bacteria. Contaminated faucet aerators, sink traps and drains, suction equipment, bottled distilled water, cleansing solutions, humidification apparatus, and incubators have been incriminated (Javett et al., 1956). In addition, healthy colonized infants or nursery personnel may act as a source of infection, the organism being transmitted among infants by way of hands or gowns of personnel. During epidemics, asymptomatic colonization of infants with the specific pathogen is variable, ranging from 0 to 90 per cent.

The general approach to nursery outbreaks caused by gram-negative organisms is similar to that for epidemics of *Staphylococcus aureus.* It is often helpful to use selective antibiotic-containing media for isolation of the organisms involved from carriers. In addition to the steps outlined in the discussion of staphylococcal outbreaks, the limitation or even prohibition of certain broad-spectrum antibiotics can contribute to long-term control of the problem, although such antibiotics may be essential in treatment of cases or carriers during the acute phase of the outbreak. Hexachlorophene is not active against gram-negative organisms, and hands of personnel should be washed with chlorhexidine or an iodophor such as Betadine.

REFERENCES

Albritton, W. L., Wiggins, G. L., and Feeley, J. C.: Neonatal listeriosis: distribution of serotypes in relation to age at onset of disease. J. Pediatr. *88*:481, 1976.

Alexander, J. B., and Giacoia, G. P.: Early onset non-enterococcal group D streptococcal infection in the newborn infant. J. Pediatr. *93*:489, 1978.

Anders, J. B., Lauer, B. A., and Paisley, J. W.: Campylobacter gastroenteritis in neonates. Am. J. Dis. Child. *135*:900, 1981.

Annunziato, D., and Goldblum, L. M.: Staphylococcal scalded skin syndrome. A complication of circumcision. Am. J. Dis. Child. *132*:1187, 1978.

Anthony, B., Giuliano, D., and Oh, W.: Nursery outbreak of staphylococcal scalded skin syndrome. Am. J. Dis. Child. *124*:41, 1972.

Baker, C. J.: Early onset group B streptococcal disease. J. Pediatr. *93*:124, 1978.

Baker, C. J., and Barrett, F. F.: Transmission of group B streptococci among parturient women and their neonates. J. Pediatr. *83*:919, 1973.

Baker, C. J., and Kasper, D. L.: Correlation of maternal antibody deficiency with susceptibility to neonatal group B streptococcal infection. N. Engl. J. Med. *294*:753, 1976.

Belohradsky, B. H., Bruch, K., Geiss, D., Kafetzis, D., Marget, W., and Peters, G.: Intravenous cefotaxime in children with bacterial meningitis. Lancet *1*:61, 1980.

Bland, R. D.: Otitis media in the first six weeks of life: diagnosis, bacteriology and management. Pediatrics *49*:187, 1972.

Boyer, K. M., Peterson, N. J., Farzaneh, I., Patterson, C. P., Hart, M. C., and Maynard, J. E.: An outbreak of gastroenteritis due to E. coli O142 in a neonatal nursery. J. Pediatr. *86*:919, 1975.

Chow, A. W., Leake, R. D., Yamauchi, T., Anthony, B. F., and Guze, L. B.: The significance of anaerobes in neonatal bacteremia: analysis of 23 cases and review of the literature. Pediatrics *54*:736, 1974.

Courtney, S. E., Hall, R. T., and Harris, D. J.: Effect of blood transfusions on mortality in early-onset group B streptococcal septicemia. Lancet *2*:462, 1979.

Darby, C. P.: Treating *Pseudomonas cepacia* meningitis with trimethoprim-sulfamethoxazole. Am. J. Dis. Child. *130*:1365, 1976.

Dich, V. Q., Nelson, J. D., and Haltalin, K. C.: Osteomyelitis in infants and children. A review of 163 cases. Am. J. Dis. Child. *129*:1273, 1975.

Dillon, H. C.: Group A streptococcal infection in a newborn nursery. Am. J. Dis. Child. *112*:177, 1966.

DuPont, H. L., and Hornick, R. B.: Clinical approach to infectious diarrheas. Medicine *52*:265, 1973.

Freedman, R. M., Ingram, D. L., Gross, I., Ehrenkranz, R. A., Warshaw, J. B., and Baltimore, R. S.: A half century of neonatal sepsis at Yale. Am. J. Dis. Child. *135*:140, 1981.

Frommell, G. T., Rothenberg, R., Wang, S. P., and McIntosh, K.: Chlamydial infections of mothers and infants. J. Pediatr. *95*:28, 1979.

Goldmann, D. A., Durbin W. A., Jr., and Freeman, J.: Nosocomial infections in a neonatal intensive care unit. J. Infect. Dis. *144*:449, 1981.

Goldmann, D. A., Leclair, J., and Macone, A.: Bacterial colonization of neonates admitted to an intensive care environment. J. Pediatr. *93*:288, 1978.

Gordon, R. C., Barrett, F. F., and Clark, D. J.: Influence of several antibiotics, singly and in combination, on the growth of Listeria monocytogenes. J. Pediatr. *80*:667, 1972.

Goscienski, P.: Inclusion conjunctivitis in the newborn infant. J. Pediatr. 77:19, 1970.

Hargiss, C., and Larson, E.: The epidemiology of *Staphylococcus aureus* in a newborn nursery from 1970 through 1976. Pediatrics 61:348, 1978.

Heckmatt, J. Z.: Coliform meningitis in the newborn. Arch. Dis. Child. 51:569, 1976.

Hemming, V. G., Overall, J. C., Jr., and Brill, M. R.: Nosocomial infections in a newborn intensive-care unit: results of forty-one months of surveillance. N. Engl. J. Med. 294:1310, 1976.

Howard, J. B., and McCracken, G. H.: The spectrum of group B streptococcal infections in infancy. Am. J. Dis. Child. 128:815, 1974.

Javett, S. N., Heymann, S., Mundel, B., et al.: Myocarditis in the newborn infant. J. Pediatr. 48:1, 1956.

Kaijser, B.: *E. coli* O and K antigens and protective antibodies in relation to urinary tract infection. Goteborg, Sweden, University of Goteborg Press, 1972.

Kozinn, P. J., Taschdjian, C. L., Wiener, H., Dragutsky, D., and Minsky, A.: Neonatal candidiasis. Pediatr. Clin. North Am. 5:803, 1958.

Laurenti, F., Ferro, R., Isacchi, G., et al.: Polymorphonuclear leukocyte transfusion for the treatment of sepsis in the newborn infant. J. Pediatr. 98:118, 1981.

Lee, E. L., Robinson, M. J., Thong, M. L., Puthucheary, S. D., Ong, T. H., and Ng, K. K.: Intraventricular chemotherapy in neonatal meningitis. J. Pediatr. 91:991, 1977.

McCracken, G. H., and Mize, S. G.: A controlled study of intrathecal antibiotic therapy in gram negative enteric meningitis of infancy. Report of the Neonatal Meningitis Cooperative Study Group. J. Pediatr. 89:66, 1976.

McCracken, G. H., and Sarff, L. D.: Current status and therapy of neonatal *E. coli* meningitis. Hosp. Pract. October, 1974, p. 57.

McCracken, G. H., Sarff, L. D., Glode, M. P., Mize, S. G., Schiffer, M. S., Robbins, J. B., Gotschlich, E. C., Orskov, I., and Orskov, F.: Relation between *Escherichia coli* K1 capsular polysaccharide antigen and clinical outcome of neonatal meningitis. Lancet 2:246, 1974.

McCracken, G. H., Jr., Mize, S. G., and Threlkeld, N.: Intraventricular gentamicin therapy in gram-negative bacillary meningitis of infancy: Report of the Second Neonatal Meningitis Cooperative Study Group. Lancet 1:787, 1980.

Melish, M., and Glasgow, L.: Staphylococcal scalded skin syndrome: the expanded clinical syndrome. J. Pediatr. 78:958, 1971.

Melish, M., Glasgow, L., and Turner, M.: The staphylococcal scalded-skin syndrome: isolation and partial characterization of the exfoliatin toxin. J. Infect. Dis. 125:129, 1972.

Memon, I. A., Jacobs, N. M., Yeh, T. F., and Libien, L. D.: Group B streptococcal osteomyelitis and septic arthritis. Am. J. Dis. Child. 133:921, 1979.

Nachum, R., Lipsey, A., and Siegel, S. E.: Rapid detection of gramnegative bacterial meningitis by the limulus lysate test. N. Engl. J. Med. 289:931, 1973.

Naidoo, B. T.: The cerebrospinal fluid in the healthy newborn infant. S. Afr. Med. J. 42:933, 1968.

Nelson, J.: Antibiotic concentrations in septic joint effusions. N. Engl. J. Med. 284:349, 1971.

Nelson, J.: The bacterial etiology and antibiotic management of septic arthritis in infants and children. Pediatrics 40:437, 1972.

Nelson, J. D.: Duration of neomycin therapy for enteropathogenic *Escherichia coli* diarrheal disease. Pediatrics 48:248, 1971.

Ogden, J. A., and Lister, G.: The pathology of neonatal osteomyelitis. Pediatrics 55:474, 1975.

Peter, G., and Nelson, J. S.: Factors affecting neonatal *E. coli* K1 rectal colonization. J. Pediatr. 93:866, 1978.

Philip, A. G. S., and Hewitt, J. R.: Early diagnosis of neonatal sepsis. Pediatrics 65:1036, 1980.

Robbins, J. B., McCracken, G. H., Gotschlich, E. C., Orskov, F., Orskov, I., and Hanson, L. A.: *Escherichia coli* K1 capsular polysaccharide associated with neonatal meningitis. N. Engl. J. Med. 290.1216, 1974

Rubin, R. H., and Weinstein, L.: Salmonellosis, Microbiologic, Pathologic and Clinical Features. New York, Stratton Intercontinental Medical Book, 1977.

Rudoy, R., and Nelson, J. D.: Enteroinvasive and enterotoxigenic *Escherichia coli*. Am. J. Dis. Child. 129:668, 1975.

Rudoy, R. C., and Nelson, J. D.: Breast abscess during the neonatal period: a review. Am. J. Dis. Child. 129:1031, 1975.

Sarff, L. D., McCracken, G. H., Schiffer, M. S., Glode, M. P., Robbins, J. B., Orskov, I., and Orskov, F.: Epidemiology of *Escherichia coli* K1 in healthy and diseased newborns. Lancet 1:1099, 1975.

Sarff, L. D., Platt, L. H., and McCracken, G. H.: Cerebrospinal fluid evaluation in neonates: comparison of high-risk infants with and without meningitis. J. Pediatr. 88:473, 1976.

Schaad, U. B., McCracken, G. H., Jr., and Nelson, J. D.: Clinical pharmacology and efficacy of vancomycin in pediatric patients. J. Pediatr. 96:119, 1980.

Schaad, U. B., McCracken, G. H., Jr., Threlkeld, N., and Thomas, M. L.: Clinical evaluation of a new broad-spectrum oxa-beta-lactam antibiotic, moxalactam, in neonates and infants. J. Pediatr. 98:129, 1981.

Shackleford, P. G., Campbell, J., and Feigin, R. D.: Countercurrent immunoelectrophoresis in the evaluation of childhood infections. J. Pediatr. 85:478, 1974.

Siegel, J. D., and McCracken, G. H., Jr.: Group D streptococcal infections. J. Pediatr. 93:542, 1978.

Siegel, J. D., and McCracken, G. H., Jr.: Sepsis neonatorum. N. Engl. J. Med. 304:642, 1981.

Siegel, J. D., McCracken, G. H., Jr., Threlkeld, N., et al.: Singledose penicillin prophylaxis against neonatal group B streptococcal infections: a controlled trial in 18,738 newborn infants. N. Engl. J. Med. 303:769, 1980.

Snowe, R., and Wilfert, C.: Epidemic reappearance of gonococcal ophthalmia neonatorum. Pediatrics 51:110, 1973.

Steigman, A. J., Bottone, E. J., and Hanna, B. A.: Intramuscular penicillin administration at birth: prevention of early-onset group B streptococcal disease. Pediatrics 62:842, 1978.

Sutherland, J.: Comment. Pediatrics 51(suppl.):351, 1973.

Torphy, D. E., and Bond, W. W.: *Campylobacter fetus* infections in children. Pediatrics 64:898, 1979.

Vain, N. E., Mazlumian, J. R., Swarner, O. W., and Cha, C. C.: Role of exchange transfusion in the treatment of severe septicemia. Pediatrics 66:693, 1980.

Visintine, A. M., Oleske, J. M., and Nahmias, A. J.: *Listeria monocytogenes* infection in infants and children. Am. J. Dis. Child. 131:393, 1977.

Warren, W. S., and Stool, S. E.: Otitis media in low-birth-weight infants. J. Pediatr. 79:740, 1971.

Weissberg, E. D., Smith, A. L., and Smith, D. H.: Clinical features of neonatal osteomyelitis. Pediatrics 53:505, 1974.

Wilson, H. D., and Haltalin, K.: Acute necrotizing fasciitis in childhood. Am. J. Dis. Child. 125:591, 1973.

Wright, P. F., Kaiser, A. B., Bowman, C. M., et al.: The pharmacokinetics and efficacy of an aminoglycoside administered into the cerebral ventricles in neonates: implications for further evaluation of this route of therapy in meningitis. J. Infect. Dis. 143:141, 1981.

Yow, M. D., Mason, E. D., Leeds, L. J., et al.: Ampicillin prevents intrapartum transmission of group B streptococci. J.A.M.A. 241:1245, 1979.

84

Other Specific Bacterial Infections

Revised by Kenneth McIntosh

Only a few bacterial infections will be discussed in this chapter. They have been chosen chiefly because their manifestations in the neonatal period differ in some respects from those of later life.

Tuberculosis

In 1925, Debré and LeLong demonstrated convincingly that tuberculosis is, in most instances at least, not inherited but acquired by contact. They separated newborns from their tuberculous mothers immediately and in a large series found that none of the offspring had been infected. Similarly, Ratner and coworkers, reviewing carefully 260 infants born to mothers with tuberculosis at Sea View Hospital, found not one case of congenital tuberculosis, even though 39 of the mothers died of the disease shortly after delivery. There are nevertheless a number of examples of newborns dying of tuberculosis so early that intrauterine infection must be accepted as the only possible mode of origin. In others, in whom evidence of illness became manifest somewhat later, even though mother and child had been separated promptly after delivery, it appears likely that infection was acquired during birth by inhalation of infected amniotic fluid or vaginal secretions.

Incidence. Beitzke laid down certain criteria that he believes indicate that tuberculous infection is truly congenital. *Mycobacterium tuberculosis* must be grown from the infant's tissues. A primary complex must be demonstrated in the liver, indicating that bacilli were carried to it by the umbilical vein, or tuberculous lesions must be discovered at birth or within a few days thereafter. On the basis of these criteria, Horley in 1952 found in the literature 83 acceptable cases of congenital tuberculosis plus 41 of bacillemia without visible lesions. Considering the great frequency of the disease among young adults within the past century, prenatal hematogenous transmission must be extremely rare. In 1980, Hageman and coworkers reviewed 26 cases of neonatal tuberculosis acquired either in utero or perinatally,

all dating from after the time isoniazid was first introduced.

Pathology. Hematogenous infection is manifested by enlargement and caseation of the glands at the porta hepatis plus disseminated tubercles throughout the liver, comprising the primary complex. In addition, tubercles are scattered through the lungs and spleen and other viscera; the serous surfaces often are studded with them, and their cavities contain clear yellow fluid. Brain and meninges may be similarly involved. When lesions are most prominent in the lungs and a primary complex cannot be found in and about the liver, it is possible that the disease originated from inhalation of infected amniotic or vaginal contents at or shortly before delivery. The tubercles belong to Rich's category of soft tubercles showing local necrosis with little cellular reaction, indicating overwhelming infection with little host resistance.

Diagnosis. Infants whose disease was acquired in utero may be ill at birth or may develop normally until fever, lethargy, hepatomegaly, and other signs or symptoms occur at several days to several weeks of life. At the time, the infection may be sudden and overwhelming or insidious and prolonged. Symptoms are typically nonspecific: poor feeding, listlessness, fever, hepatosplenomegaly, lymphadenopathy, and, later, respiratory distress. Because the liver is the primary site of bacterial replication, the chest radiograph is often normal until late in the disease at which time the pattern of involvement is often miliary. Skin lesions (erythematous papules) may be seen.

When the infection is acquired at birth, respiratory or gastrointestinal symptoms tend to appear first. The infant is normal at birth and until about age 6 to 8 weeks. At this time, nonspecific symptoms appear—respiratory distress, fever, abdominal distention, gastrointestinal bleeding, purulent ear discharge, and failure to thrive. Anemia is often profound. The chest radiograph is frequently abnormal.

In order to determine the specific diagnosis, one must find organisms either in biopsy tissue—liver, lymph nodes, bone marrow (usually not skin lesions)—or in tracheal or gastric aspirates. Acid-fast stains of such materials, even of gastric aspirates, are very helpful. The cerebrospinal fluid, although often abnormal, infrequently yields organisms on culture. The presence of granulomata in microscopic sections of biopsy material is also a useful finding, but they are also seen in other neonatal diseases such as listeriosis. The tuberculin test is rarely positive during the disease, but may become so later. Presence of demonstrated infection and disease in the mother is often the clue that leads one to the correct diagnosis of tuberculosis in the child.

Management

Congenital Tuberculosis. If the mother has *miliary disease*, untreated in the last part of pregnancy, the infant is at greatest risk of having congenital tuberculosis. Such an infant deserves careful clinical evaluation, including a chest film, smear and culture of gastric washings and urine, examination and culture of the spinal fluid, and drug sensitivities determined on any organism recovered. The tuberculin test may not become positive for approximately 3 to 5 weeks or longer in such an infant, so reliance on a negative test is unwarranted. The necessity of separating the infant from the mother, who would be hospitalized, is obvious, and institution of INH, 10 mg per kilogram per day, is appropriate in the absence of manifest disease. If the infant has manifest disease, whether acquired before or at birth, two-drug therapy is indicated. Isoniazid, 15 to 20 mg/kg/day in two divided doses, should be combined with either streptomycin (40 mg/dose, intramuscularly, administered every other day for several months) or rifampin (15 to 20 mg/kg/day, orally, in a single dose). Although the experience in newborns with rifampin is limited, it appears to have no unusual toxicities in this age group other than the well-recognized occasional problems of hepatotoxicity and allergy. Rifampin should be continued for 9 months to 1 year and isoniazid for 1 year or more. If the infant has tuberculous meningitis, triple drug therapy is indicated: isoniazid 20 mg/kg/day, rifampin 20 mg/kg/day, and streptomycin 40 to 50 mg/kg/day.

A study by Escobar and associates from Cali, Colombia, demonstrates the efficacy of prednisone at 1 mg/kg/day for the first 30 days of illness. Prednisone therapy should not be initiated until adequate blood levels of antituberculous drugs are achieved, presumably after about 48 hours of initiating treatment.

Infant of a Mother on Therapy for Pulmonary Tuberculosis. A more frequent event is pregnancy in a mother with pulmonary tuberculosis on therapy. If the mother is sputum-positive, the risk to the infant is of course greater than it is if she has been on treatment some months and is sputum-negative. It would seem reasonable to separate the infant from the mother as long as she remains sputum-positive. Once her sputum has converted to negative, and she is known to be taking her medication regularly, separation from the infant is not necessary. Such an infant remains at greater risk than normal, in part because of the likelihood of other unidentified cases of tuberculosis in the environment. It seems appropriate to consider such an infant a candidate for BCG or INH prophylaxis, whether or not separation from the mother occurs.

Infant of a Mother with Treated Tuberculosis. Finally, and perhaps most frequently, an infant may be born to a mother with a history of treated tuberculosis, off therapy for some years before pregnancy. The possibility of relapse in the mother would be greatest if her disease were arrested for less than 5 years. Since the risk to the infant of a mother with inactive tuberculosis depends on her likelihood of reactivation, careful and frequent examinations of the mother are essential. Indeed, a tuberculin test in all women during pregnancy and at the time of delivery would be desirable. A postpartum chest film and one 3 months and another 6 months later are indicated in tuberculin-positive mothers. The management of the infant is less clear under these circumstances. A minimal requirement would be a tuberculin test with 5 T.U. (0.1 ml intermediate PPD or 0.0001 mg) at three monthly intervals during the first year of life if BCG is withheld.

Role of BCG. The arguments for BCG are based in part on the experience gained from its wide use in many countries with a very low incidence of subsequent tuberculosis and minimal complications. One study relevant to its role in newborn infants in tuberculosis households included 231 vaccinated by multiple puncture techniques and 220 control infants studied over a period of 19 years (Rosenthal et al., 1961). The infants were returned to their respective homes only if the source case was "closed." Even so, the infectivity rate in the nonvaccinated controls was 36.5 per cent at 1 year, suggesting that the state of infectiousness of an adult cannot always be ascertained with accuracy. The results of the Rosenthal study showed that there were three cases of tuberculosis among the 231 vaccinated infants, and 11 cases among the 220 controls. The controls included four deaths and four cases of miliary disease or meningitis; no deaths or disseminated disease occurred among the vaccinated. The strongest argument for BCG is the advantage gained from protection given at one time instead of daily, as with chemoprophylaxis. Kendig advocates the two-site method of BCG immunization, giving the material in two sites of the deltoid at the same time.

Not all trials have demonstrated the protective effect found in Rosenthal's study, and there are many who doubt the usefulness of BCG. The efficacy varies in part because of different potencies of the antigen and variations in the physiologic state of the host. During recent years the problem of differing reactions to the vaccine has been lessened by the availability of a *freeze-dried preparation,** found to be comparable to the liquid Danish vaccine in testing on newborn infants (Griffiths and Gaisford, 1956). The immunizing dose is 0.1 ml by intradermal injection. A small red papule appears at the site of injection within 7 to 10 days and may increase in size over the next few weeks. It leaves a smooth or pitted white scar in approximately 6 months. A tuberculin test should be performed in 2 or 3 months, and the immunization

---

* Manufactured by Glaxo Laboratories, Ltd., Middlesex, England, and distributed by Eli Lilly and Co., Indianapolis, Indiana.

repeated if it is negative. Occasionally, local granulomas and regional adenitis ensue. Another problem is the possibility that use of BCG could negate the value of subsequent tuberculin testing in a vaccinated individual. In general, the tuberculin reaction becomes small 1 year after BCG, and thus an increase in reactivity or a large reaction indicates *Mycobacterium* tuberculosis infection. Individual differences in tuberculin sensitivity, however, make the distinction often unreliable.

A special consideration with respect to INH prophylaxis in infants in the first days of life concerns the possible effects of long-term pharmacologic agents, with respect to absorption and excretion, that have necessitated great care in matters of dosage and indications in infancy. Studies on INH blood levels in newborn infants and long-term follow-up of treated infants are not available. However, no adverse effects have been noted among infants treated with INH. Neurotoxicity in particular seems less common in children than adults. Some further reassurance comes from a study of the outcome of pregnancy in mothers on INH, including 50 on therapy at the time of conception. There was no increase in fetal loss or neonatal death and no cancer detected among the 644 children followed up to 13 years (Hammond et al., 1967).

NURSERY EXPOSURE TO TUBERCULOSIS

Experiences in control of possible spread of infection from nursery personnel to infants led Light and coworkers to propose 3 months of oral INH prophylaxis for all exposed infants. The arguments are that acquisition of fulminant disease may occur rapidly and in the absence of a tuberculin conversion. The time lag before effective immunity can be achieved with BCG makes this form of protection less desirable.

MULTIPLE PSEUDOCYSTIC TUBERCULOSIS OF BONES

A case described by de Pape is mentioned briefly at this point because it appears to be an instance of congenital tuberculosis of bone.

CASE 84–1

An American Indian infant was born of parents who, unfortunately for themselves as well as for the certainty of the diagnosis in this case, both had strongly positive Wassermann results. The infant was normal at birth except for a notably swollen right fifth metacarpal. He *soon became pale, weak, and irritable, and at 10 weeks chronic purulent nasal discharge began. Cough and cervical node enlargement followed, then swellings over the skull and many of the long bones and fusiform enlargement of some digits. Hepatosplenomegaly developed. His own Wassermann test result was negative, but his Kahn test was weakly positive. The Mantoux test result was strongly positive, and radiographs of the lungs were suggestive of tuberculosis. Acid-fast bacilli were found in the aspirate from a fluctuant swelling over the forehead. In spite of treatment with streptomycin he died at 10 months. Autopsy showed widespread tuberculosis of the viscera and multiple loci of osseous tuberculosis.*

Comment. Had the parents not had syphilis, one could be certain that this infant had acquired tuberculosis transplacentally. As it is, one cannot be sure that the original metacarpal lesion was not syphilitic and that the ultimate acid-fast infection was not a later superimposition. This reconstruction seems to be unlikely.

Diphtheria

The virtual disappearance of diphtheria from the scene in many metropolitan areas inevitably decreases the consideration this disease receives in differential diagnosis. In view of the recent resurgence of other presumed eliminated infections, we must be careful lest a new generation of physicians who have had no experience with it forget its characteristics and its hazards.

Incidence. In Baltimore, the incidence for all age groups diminished from 260 per 100,000 in 1900 to 0 in 1957. Not all communities in the United States can boast such an enviable record, but all show tremendous declines. Diphtheria was never common in the neonatal period and is now almost nonexistent in that age group. However, occasional outbreaks are still encountered in nurseries, and the odd case still appears.

A 1970 outbreak in Austin, Texas, resulted in 88 cases; three of the patients died (Zolma et al., 1970). The authors concluded that to forestall an epidemic in a community, an immunization level of more than 80 per cent is required, not 70 per cent as usually taught. Twenty-five per cent of the affected children were under 4 years of age, but no mention was made of the incidence, if any, among newborns. However, this does not guarantee that one will never encounter a case in a newborn infant.

Etiology and Epidemiology. *Corynebacterium diphtheriae*, generally of the gravis type, is the responsible organism. Its soluble toxin produces antitoxin in the host during the course of natural infection and may be used, modified to toxoid, as a potent antigen to stimulate the formation of antitoxin in inoculated persons. The antitoxic titer from either source persists for a variable number of years and is capable of being boosted by reinfection or by subsequent doses of toxoid. Many newborns receive no antitoxin from a mother whose natural or artificial antitoxin titer had diminished to the vanishing point over the course of years devoid of re-exposure either to *C. diphtheriae* or to stimulating injections. These infants are susceptible to diphtheria, and contact with an infected person or a healthy carrier may cause the disease.

Such was the situation in Curtin's case reported in 1953. The mother's level of antitoxin was less than 0.001 unit per ml. A level of 0.005 unit is generally considered protective. A brother was found to be harboring *C. diphtheriae* in his pharynx, and his antitoxin concentration was 10 units per ml; hence he was a healthy carrier. The infant became ill on the twentieth day of life.

Diagnosis. We shall not go into the matter of diagnosis in detail. It differs in no respects from that in the older child. *Faucial* diphtheria is recognized by the characteristic membrane, *nasal* diphtheria by persistent discharge, often sanguineous, and the *laryngeal* form by slowly progressive hoarseness and aphonia and laryngotracheal obstruction. All are without sharp constitutional reaction. In all forms, diagnosis depends on bacteriologic identification of *C. diphtheriae*. Complications, chiefly myocarditis and postdiphtheritic paralysis, have been similarly encountered in the newborn.

Treatment. Diphtheria antitoxin must be given, intravenously when the condition appears serious, intramuscularly if the situation is not urgent. Doses of 20,000 to 50,000 units on 2 or 3 successive days will be more than sufficient. Preliminary testing for sensitivity must be carried out. Since penicillin has bactericidal effect upon *C. diphtheriae*, it should be given in doses approximating 300,000 units every 8 to 12 hours. Erythromycin is effective in the event of penicillin sensitivity. Treatment of complications will be carried out as for those in older infants.

Tetanus Neonatorum

As knowledge of hygiene penetrates deeper and deeper into the more primitive corners of the world, tetanus of the newborn approaches ever more nearly its vanishing point. A disease with which many of us had to contend not at all infrequently 35 years ago has become a rarity in metropolitan areas. It remains an infrequent but still serious problem in less sophisticated rural communities in the United States and is still not uncommon in the hinterlands of Africa and Asia. La Force and coworkers found that there had been 507 patients with tetanus in the United States in 1965 and 1966. Of these, 54 were newborns. Marshall reviewed the experience with 2198 neonatal cases seen at the Hôpital Albert Schweitzer in Haiti between September, 1957 and May, 1966,

reporting an overall mortality of 53 per cent from the disease. A more recent report from the same hospital indicated that the mortality had dropped to 26 per cent (Garnier et al., 1975).

Etiology and Pathogenesis. The causative agent is the bacterium *Clostridium tetani*. This gram-positive, anaerobic spore-bearer produces a soluble toxin with a special affinity for nervous tissue. It is susceptible to penicillin and the tetracyclines. It gains entrance into the newborn's body by way of the stump of the umbilical cord that had been cut by an unsterile instrument or covered with an unclean dressing. Rarely, a vaccination wound produced by an unclean instrument or upon contaminated skin imperfectly cleansed constitutes a portal of entry. The organism is long-lived by virtue of its spore formation, is a normal inhabitant of the intestinal tract of many domestic animals, and hence abounds in the soil of many localities.

Immunity to tetanus depends on the presence in the blood of an adequate concentration of antibody to the toxin. This is efficiently stimulated by immunization with toxoid. The blood of the newborn contains roughly the amount of tetanus antitoxin that is present in his mother's blood, or a bit more. Peterson and colleagues believe that concentrations as low as 0.01 antitoxin unit per ml may be protective against the disease, and levels higher than this may persist for years in actively immunized persons. Of the 54 mothers reported by La Force, only three were sure they had received any form of tetanus toxoid immunization.

Diagnosis. Signs appear between the sixth and fourteenth days after birth, most often at the beginning of the second week. Restlessness, irritability, and difficulty in sucking are followed within a day or two by fever, muscle stiffness, and, finally, convulsions. The temperature often rises to between 40° and 41°C (104° and 106° F). Physical examination at this stage shows the characteristic trismus and risus sardonicus and the tenseness and rigidity of all muscles, including those of the abdomen. The fists are held tightly clenched and the toes rigidly fanned. Characteristic are the opisthotonic spasms plus clonic jerkings that follow sudden stimulation by touch or by loud noise.

Laboratory investigations are best held to a minimum, since any manipulation produces painful spasm. Diagnosis is clear from the clinical evidence alone, and studies of blood, urine and cerebrospinal fluid, in all respects normal, add nothing of value. Attempts should be made to cultivate the organism from the presumed portal of entry.

Tetany of the newborn should never be confused with tetanus. Infants with tetany appear well between their convulsive episodes. The infant who is generally rigid from birth trauma has shown evidences of brain injury from birth, before the first sign of tetanus could possibly appear. Extraocular palsies commonly are present and abdominal rigidity absent. Response to stimulation is depressed rather than increased.

Course. The infant may die within the week after onset from respiratory arrest during a convulsive episode. If he does not die, improvement will become manifest within 3 to 7 days by gradual decline of temperature, decrease in the number of episodes of spasm, and slow resolution of rigidity. Complete disappearance of all signs of illness may take as long as 6 weeks.

Treatment. The first requirement is for tetanus antitoxin to neutralize the circulating toxin not already bound to nerve tissue. Where tetanus immune globulin (human) is available, it should be given intramuscularly, in a dose of 500 units (McCracken et al., 1971). If this is not available, 10,000 units of equine or bovine tetanus antitoxin should be given intramuscularly.

Penicillin, which kills the vegetative form of the bacterium, should be given in a dose of 300,000 units every 12 hours. Tetracycline may be of value as an alternative drug. The consensus appears to be that wide excision of the umbilicus is hazardous and does not appreciably improve chances for recovery.

Every known sedative has been used to control spasm, and there is no general agreement as to which one or ones should be chosen. Magnesium sulfate, which received high marks in early treatment regimens, has since been increasingly replaced by agents with which pediatricians are now more familiar. Phenobarbital (8 to 16 mg, every 4 hours orally or one half this amount intramuscularly or intravenously), chloral hydrate (0.3 gm, every 3 to 6 hours by rectum), and chlorpromazine (1 mg every 4 to 6 hours) are considered useful agents. Diazepam (Valium) has become the mainstay of treatment of older children with tetanus (Garnier et al., 1975), and it is probably also of great value in the neonate (1 to 2 mg/kg/day in divided doses). One aims at the ideal result of controlling spasm without depressing respiration, and one must feel one's way in each case. When intensive care and respirators are available, neuromuscular blockade with pancuronium bromide (Pavulon, 0.05 to 0.1 mg/kg administered every 2 to 3 hours) for the duration of the spasms (up to 6 weeks) has proved successful therapy (Adams et al., 1979). Endotracheal tubes have largely replaced tracheostomy under these circumstances. Howard and deVere have used intramuscular administration of meprobamate with no diminution of mortality but with significant reduction in the number of days of spasms and of hospitalization.

Fluids are best given through an indwelling intra-venous catheter at first, later through an indwelling gastric tube. The infant should be under close observation in a darkened room and disturbed and stimulated as infrequently as possible. Active immunization with alum-precipitated or fluid toxoid should be begun as soon as the infant improves, since the disease itself immunizes poorly, if at all.

Infant Botulism

Although *Clostridium botulinum* is widely distributed in soil and water, reports of infant botulism were rare before 1976, when Pickett and coworkers described an outbreak in California. The incidence is unknown, since presumably it has not been sought with adequate laboratory procedures. Most of the cases described have been in California and Utah.

Etiology. Investigation of 81 cases by the Center for Disease Control identified a potential source in opened jars of honey that had been added to baby food or used to coat pacifiers. Vacuum cleaner dust was found contaminated with spores of *C. botulinum* in the household of one infected infant. In the study from Utah (Thompson et al., 1980) it was noted that digging or construction was common in the neighborhoods in which cases were reported.

Clinical Course. Infant botulism has been described in patients as young as 3 weeks of age, but the peak incidence occurs at the usual time of weaning, from 6 weeks to 6 months of age. The infants have usually been born at term and described as normal until constipation is noted. The infants may seem lethargic and slow to feed. Some have a more acute onset of feeding difficulties, pooling of secretions, diminished gag reflex, loss of head control, and generalized weakness. If the diagnosis is not made and appropriate supportive treatment initiated, death from respiratory arrest may occur. Some infants diagnosed as victims of sudden infant death syndrome may have died from unrecognized botulism.

Diagnosis. The diagnosis depends on recovery of *C. botulinum* with or without its toxin from the stool in the presence of a compatible clinical picture. Stool and serum specimens should be sent to a laboratory equipped to identify the organism and its toxin. Electromyography has been helpful in the clinical diagnosis. Brief small-amplitude motor reaction potentials have been described. Both *C. botulinum* and toxin have been found in the stools of normal infants (Thompson et al., 1980).

Treatment. Botulinal antitoxin has not been useful in infant botulism, perhaps because of absence of demonstrable toxin in the serum. Ampicillin has been used, although its value in eliminating the organism is uncertain. Aminoglycoside antibiotics are contraindicated because of possible potentiation of neuromuscular weakness (L'Hommedieu et al., 1979).

J. P. Crozer Griffith, one-time Professor of Diseases of Children at the University of Pennsylvania and one of the early great pediatric clinicians, wrote his first treatise on typhoid fever in young infants before the beginning of the twentieth century. He recognized not only that they could acquire the disease after birth but also that babies born of mothers suffering from typhoid might acquire the infection in utero.

Incidence. Typhoid fever attained epidemic proportions in the summer and fall of every year throughout most of the United States until the end of the 1920s. By 1902, Griffith was able to report in some detail on 18 patients below the age of $2\frac{1}{2}$ years whom he had observed personally and on 325 certain cases plus 92 somewhat doubtful ones that he had collected from the literature. Typhoid fever was still occurring with sufficient frequency in the early 1920s. Since that time, it has declined in frequency so that now we rarely encounter more than one or two cases a year among infants and children. In 1902 Griffith and Ostheimer found 23 examples of congenital typhoid fever among their collected cases. We have not seen one in a pediatric experience that dates from 1923.

Diagnosis. The following case history, first reported by Weech and Chen in 1929, illustrates the course and diagnosis of an infant with typhoid fever.

CASE 84–2

A male infant was born prematurely after an uncomplicated pregnancy. Five days post partum, his mother had fever that proved later to be severe typhoid. The infant became febrile at the age of 26 days, but fever dropped to normal by crisis after 24 hours. The spleen was enlarged. White blood cell count was 11,000 per cu mm. Culture of the blood revealed B. typhosus (Salmonella typhi in modern terminology). The next day a bright red papular eruption appeared over the entire body and lasted 2 days. The white cell count was now 17,000, of which 37 per cent were polymorphonuclears. He had no more fever for 3 weeks, and then low-grade elevation reappeared for a few days. Blood culture was still positive. Two weeks later it was negative. The only other symptom or sign was failure to gain. All other cultures, from stool and urine, remained consistently negative. Eleven Widal tests were performed throughout the course, and none was positive.

Comment. The authors note the extreme youth of their patient, the mildness of the disease and the lack of gastrointestinal symptoms, the generalized exanthem that bore no resemblance to rose spots, the leukocytosis so unlike the leukopenic response of older persons, and the total failure of agglutinins to develop.

Treatment. First chloramphenicol, then ampicillin, were found to be highly effective against *S. typhi*. In the very young newborn, the well-known hazard of chloromycetin would make ampicillin the preferable antibiotic.

As an aside, we might mention that Schaffer observed an epidemic of typhoid in northern Mexico in the early 1970s that was caused by a strain of *S. typhi* that was refractory to both chloramphenicol and ampicillin. It was widely assumed that this strain developed because of the great overuse of these antibiotics.

Prognosis. Nineteen of the 23 infants with congenital cases collected by Griffith died, three recovered, and the fate of one was not stated. This very grave outlook for the congenital form of typhoid fever did not apply to the postnatally acquired examples, as evidenced by the mildness of the case reported by Weech and Chen. However, only 23 of the infants below 1 year of age in Griffith's series survived, whereas 77 died. One would suppose that many milder cases with recovery were not diagnosed and recorded.

We can find no reports on series of cases of newborns treated with chloramphenicol or ampicillin.

REFERENCES

Adams, J. M., Kenny, J. D., and Rudolph, A. J.: Modern management of tetanus neonatorum. Pediatrics 64:472, 1979.

Avery, M. E., and Wolfsdorf, J.: Diagnosis and treatment: approaches to newborn infants of tuberculous mothers. Pediatrics 42:519, 1968.

Beitzke, H., cited by E. A. Harris, G. C. McCullough, J. J. Stone, and W. M. Brock (see further on).

Curtin, M.: Neonatal diphtheria. Arch. Dis. Child. 28:127, 1953.

Debré, R., and LeLong, M.: The infant born of tuberculous parents, separated before contamination: its growth and resistance to disease. Ann. Med. 18:317, 1925.

de Pape, A. J.: Multiple pseudocystic tuberculosis of bone. J. Bone Joint Surg. 36B:637, 1954.

Escobar, J. A., Belsey, M. A., Duenas, A., and Medina, P.: Mortality from tuberculous meningitis reduced by steroid therapy. Pediatrics 56:1050, 1975.

Garnier, M. J., Marshall, F. N., Davison, K. J., and Lepreau, F. J.: Tetanus in Haiti. Lancet 1:383, 1975.

Griffith, J. P. C., and Ostheimer, M.: Typhoid fever in children under two and a half years of age. Am. J. Med. Sci. 124:868, 1902.

Griffiths, M. I., and Gaisford, W.: Freeze-dried BCG. Vaccination of newborn infants with a British vaccine. Br. Med. J. 2:565, 1956.

Hageman, J., Shulman, S., Schreiber, M., Luck, S., and Yoger, R.: Congenital tuberculosis: critical reappraisal of clinical findings and diagnostic procedures. Pediatrics 66:980, 1980.

Hammond, E. C., Selikoff, I. J., and Robitzek, E. H.: Isoniazid therapy in relation to later occurrence of cancer in adults and in infants. Br. Med. J. 2:792, 1967.

Harris, E. A., McCullough, G. C., Stone, J. J., and Brock, W. M.: Congenital tuberculosis: a review of the disease with report of a case. J. Pediatr. *32*:311, 1948.

Horley, J. F.: Congenital tuberculosis. Arch. Dis. Child. *27*:167, 1952.

Howard, F. H., and de Vere, W.: Intramuscular meprobamate in the treatment of tetanus in infants and children. J. Pediatr. *60*:421, 1962.

Kendig, E. L., and Chernick, V.: Disorders of the Respiratory Tract in Children. 3rd. ed. Philadelphia, W. B. Saunders Co., 1977.

La Force, F. M., Young, L. S., and Bennett, J. V.: Tetanus in the United States (1965–1966). N. Engl. J. Med. *280*:569, 1969.

L'Hommedieu, L., Stough, R., Brown, L., Kettrick, R., and Polin, R.: Potentiation of neuromuscular weakness in infant botulism by aminoglycosides. J. Pediatr. *95*:1065, 1979.

Light, I. J., Saideman, M., and Sutherland, J. M.: Management of newborns after nursery exposure to tuberculosis. Am. Rev. Resp. Dis. *109*:415, 1974.

Marshall, F. N.: Tetanus of the newborn. *In* Levine, S. Z. (Ed.): Advances in Pediatrics. XV. Chicago, Year Book Medical Publishers, 1968.

McCracken, G. H., Jr., Dowell, D. L., and Marshall, F. N.: Double-blind trial of equine antitoxin and human immune globulin in tetanus neonatorum. Lancet *1*:1146, 1971.

Peterson, J. C., Christie, A., and Williams, W. C.: Tetanus immunization. XI. Study of the duration of primary immunity and the response to late stimulating doses of tetanus toxoid. A.M.A. J. Dis. Child. *89*:295, 1955.

Pickett, J., Berg, B., Chaplin, E., and Brunstetter-Shafer, M.: Syndrome of botulism in infancy: clinical and electrophysiologic study. N. Engl. J. Med. *295*:770, 1976.

Ratner, B., Rostler, A. E., and Salgado, P. S.: Care, feeding and fate of premature and full-term infants born of tuberculosis mothers. Am. J. Dis. Child. *81*:471, 1951.

Rosenthal, S. R., et al.: BCG vaccination against tuberculosis in Chicago. Pediatrics *28*:622, 1961.

Thompson, J. A., Glasgow, L. A., Warpinski, J. R., and Olson, C.: Infant botulism: clinical spectrum and epidemiology. Pediatrics *66*:936, 1980.

Weech, A. A., and Chen, K. T.: Typhoid fever: report of a case in an infant less than one month of age. Am. J. Dis. Child. *38*:1044, 1929.

Weinstein, L.: Current concepts: tetanus. N. Engl. J. Med. *289*:1293, 1973.

Weinstein, L., and Murphy, T.: The management of tuberculosis during pregnancy. Clin. Perinatol. *1*:395, 1974.

Zalma, V. M., Older, J. J., and Brooks, G. F.: The Austin, Texas, diphtheria outbreak: clinical and epidemiological aspects. J.A.M.A. *211*:2125, 1970.

85

Viral Infections of the Fetus and Newborn

Revised by Kenneth McIntosh

Congenital Infections: Introduction

The infant who is born with an infection acquired transplacentally during the first, second, or early third trimester may have what is termed "congenital infection." Although these infections are in rare instances due to herpes simplex virus, varicella-zoster virus, and possibly even *Mycobacterium tuberculosis*, the commonest causes are rubella virus, cytomegalovirus, *Toxoplasma gondii*, and *Treponema pallidum*. These four organisms are the so-called, and somewhat misnamed, "TORCH" group. The confusion generated by this acronym arises because "H," or herpes simplex, so rarely belongs to the group and because syphilis is omitted. Certain other organisms may cause intrauterine infection but are usually transmitted just before delivery. This pattern is characteristic of herpes simplex virus, enteroviruses, group B streptococci, *Listeria*, and others, but these intrauterine infections differ little from those caused by the same organisms when acquired either just after delivery or during the first week or so of extrauterine life. For this reason, they are usually classified as "perinatal" rather than "congenital" infections.

Despite the extraordinary biologic heterogeneity of the four organisms responsible for congenital infections, the syndromes they produce are remarkably similar. The literature was carefully reviewed by Overall and Glasgow in 1970, and the results of this survey appear in Figure 85–1. Congenital syphilis is not shown in this figure. The most common manifestations include hepatomegaly, splenomegaly, pneumonia, bone lesions, and anemia. Differentiating features will also be discussed in the discussions of the individual infections.

The rational approach to the diagnosis of congenital infection depends on knowledge of the biology, epidemiology, and disease manifestations of each infection. Once the suspicion is raised, therefore, the differences rather than similarities among these diseases should be the object of our own analysis.

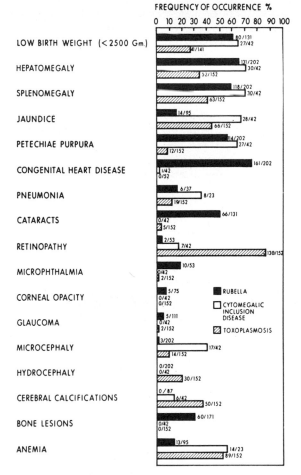

FREQUENCY OF OCCURRENCE %

0 10 20 30 40 50 60 70 80 90 100

LOW BIRTH WEIGHT (<2500 Gm.) — 80/131, 27/42, 41/141

HEPATOMEGALY — 131/202, 30/42, 52/152

SPLENOMEGALY — 118/202, 30/42, 63/152

JAUNDICE — 14/95, 28/42, 66/152

PETECHIAE PURPURA — 114/202, 27/42, 12/152

CONGENITAL HEART DISEASE — 161/202, 1/42, 0/52

PNEUMONIA — 6/37, 8/23, 19/152

CATARACTS — 66/131, 0/42, 5/152

RETINOPATHY — 2/53, 7/42, 138/152

MICROPHTHALMIA — 10/53, 0/42, 2/152

CORNEAL OPACITY — 5/75, 0/42, 0/152

GLAUCOMA — 5/111, 0/42, 2/152

MICROCEPHALY — 3/202, 17/42, 14/152

HYDROCEPHALY — 0/202, 0/42, 30/152

CEREBRAL CALCIFICATIONS — 0/87, 6/42, 50/152

BONE LESIONS — 60/171, 0/42, 0/152

ANEMIA — 13/95, 14/23, 89/152

■ RUBELLA
□ CYTOMEGALIC INCLUSION DISEASE
▨ TOXOPLASMOSIS

Figure 85–1. Manifestations of symptomatic congenital rubella, cytomegalic inclusion disease, and toxoplasmosis. (From Overall, J. C., and Glasgow, L. A.: Virus infections of the fetus and newborn infant. J. Pediatr. *77*:315, 1970.)

Congenital Rubella

Since 1941, when Gregg first made the association of maternal rubella and cataracts in infants, physicians have been aware of the teratogenicity of the rubella virus. Not until the epidemic of 1964 and 1965 in North America, however, were the multiple manifestations of the rubella syndrome fully appreciated and the later consequences well delineated. Since that time, the capacity to grow the virus in tissue culture has led rapidly to the development of vaccines and a reduction in incidence of congenital disease, at least in the United States. Occasional cases, however, continue to appear, and the disease unfortunately retains more than merely historic interest.

Etiology. Maternal rubella infection within a month before conception and through the second trimester may be associated with disease in the infant. The classic findings of congenital rubella predominate when the onset of maternal infection occurs during the first 8 weeks of gestation. Cataract occurs with maternal rubella before the sixtieth day after the first day of the last menstrual period; heart disease is

found almost exclusively when maternal infection is before the eightieth day (i.e., first trimester). Deafness, the most common manifestation, occurs, along with retinopathy, as a consequence of both first and second trimester maternal infections (Ueda et al., 1979). The incidence of congenital rubella defects following maternal rubella varies widely between series but is probably from 15 to 25 per cent throughout the first trimester, 5 to 7 per cent in the fourth month, and 1 to 2 per cent in the fifth month. The infant may excrete the virus for many months after birth despite the pressure of neutralizing antibody and thus pose a hazard to susceptible individuals in his environment. Only rarely can the virus be recovered by 1 year of age. An exception is the cataract, which has harbored virus for as long as 3 years.

Diagnosis. The infected infants are usually born at term but are of low birth weight. They may show only a few manifestations of the disease, such as glaucoma or cataracts, or they may have a systemic illness characterized by purpuric lesions, hepatosplenomegaly, cardiac defects, pneumonia, and meningoencephalitis. Table 85–1, from the study of Rudolph and coworkers in Houston, shows the distribution of findings in their extensive series. The skin lesions, which have been described as resembling a "blueberry muffin," are shown in Figure 85–2. These represent extramedullary hematopoietic tissue within the skin (Brough et al., 1967). Thrombocytopenia is commonly seen (Cooper et al., 1965). Osseous lesions include a large anterior fontanel and striking

Table 85–1. Clinical Findings in 81 Infants with Congenital Rubella Syndrome*

	Group 1: Expanded Rubella Syndrome	Group 2: Classic Rubella Syndrome	Group 3: History of Maternal Rubella, Presumably Normal Baby
Number of Infants	34	37	10
Sex { Male	26	23	7
Female	8	14	3
Mean gestational age (weeks)	40.1	39.8	39.8
Mean birth weight (gm)	2178	2533	3327
Purpura	78%	0	0
Thrombocytopenia (<140,000)	100%	0	0
Hepatomegaly	85%	81%	20%
Splenomegaly	76%	62%	10%
Cardiac defects	78%	86%	0
Eye defects	41%	54%	0
Full fontanel	69%	43%	0
Positive viral isolation	66%	25%	50%
Mortality	32%	8%	0

* Rudolph, A. J., et al.: Am. J. Dis. Child. *110*:416, 1965.

lesions in the long bones. Linear areas of radiolucency and increased density are found in the metaphyses (Fig. 85–2D). The provisional zones of calcification are also irregular. The changes in rubella are not pathognomonic of the disease but resemble those of other congenital infections, such as cytomegalic inclusion disease.

The cardiac lesions include patent ductus arteriosus, septal defects, and stenosis of the peripheral pulmonary arteries. Myocardial necrosis has been observed (Cooper et al., 1969).

Among the manifestations that may occur after the newborn period ("late-onset disease") are a generalized rash with seborrheic features that may persist for weeks, interstitial pneumonia (either acute or chronic) such as described by Phelan and Campbell, defective hearing from involvement of the organ of Corti or central auditory imperception, or even complete autism. Infants with "late-onset disease" not infrequently have immunologic abnormalities, with elevated total IgM and depressed total IgG (Soothill et al., 1966). They may be susceptible to infection with unusual organisms such as *Pneumocystis carinii* or to development of histiocytosis (Claman et al., 1970).

A few longitudinal studies of somatic growth reveal that most infants remain smaller than average through infancy but grow at a normal rate. Stunting

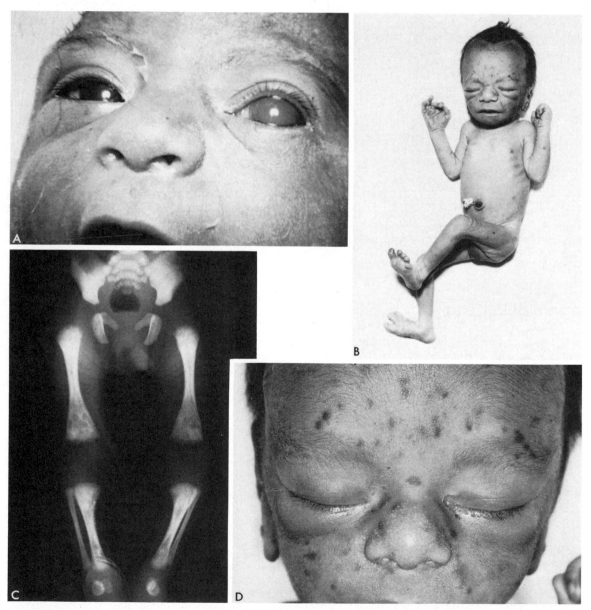

Figure 85–2. *A,* Note the prominence of the eyes and the clouding of the left eye typical of advanced congenital glaucoma. *B,* Term infant, underweight, with "blueberry muffin" rash over the face. *C,* Bone lesions in congenital rubella. The provisional zones of calcification are poorly defined. Multiple radiolucent defects are apparent. *D,* Closeup of rash shown in *B.* (Figure courtesy of Dr. A. J. Rudolph.)

of growth was more common after rubella in the first 8 weeks of pregnancy than after later infection. A higher than expected incidence of diabetes mellitus has been reported after congenital rubella.

Laboratory Findings. The laboratory diagnosis of congenital rubella must be made during the first year of life, unless one is fortunate enough to recover virus from an affected site such as the lens after that time. Both serology and virus isolation may be helpful. If antirubella titers are elevated at birth or shortly thereafter and remain high during the first year, the diagnosis of intrauterine infection is assured. Antirubella IgM may be found, but this determination can be confused by the presence of rheumatoid factor, found in many chronic infections. The presence of elevated total IgM in cord blood, once considered helpful in diagnosis of congenital infections, is now thought to be neither sensitive nor specific.

The virus is most often isolated from throat swabs but may also be found in the spinal fluid or urine. In "late-onset" disease, the virus is found in affected skin and lung.

Treatment. There is no specific therapy for congenital rubella. The infants may need blood transfusions, if bleeding, and general supportive measures.

The question of management of the pregnant woman who is exposed to or who herself contracts the disease should be answered after weighing the known risks. If, at the time of exposure, serum antibody is detectable, the fetus is probably completely protected. If the level is either undetectable or borderline, then a large dose of immune serum globulin (0.3 to 0.4 ml/kg) is advised, although the protective effect of this maneuver is in question. Decisions about interruption of pregnancy must be made only after maternal infection has been proved. A rise in antibody must be measured in two or more sera in the same laboratory on the same day; test variation may account for apparent antibody "rises" measured on different days.

Decisions concerning induced abortion should also take into account the risk of rubella-associated damage to the fetus. This is highest when maternal infection occurs in the first eight weeks of pregnancy.

Prognosis. The consequences of fetal rubella may not be evident at birth but may instead become apparent in subsequent months. Hardy and coworkers followed 123 infants with documented congenital rubella and found that 85 per cent of them were not clinically suspect until after discharge from the nursery. Communication disorders, hearing defects, some mental or motor retardation, and small heads by 1 to 3 years of age were among the major problems to present after the newborn period. A predisposition to inguinal hernias was also noted.

It is important to note that even in the absence of mental retardation, neuromuscular development is frequently abnormal. Desmond and coworkers, reporting in 1978, followed 29 children in this category and found 25 of them abnormal. Hearing loss, difficulties with balance and gait, learning deficits, and behavioral disturbances were found in more than one half the affected children.

An alarming report of chronic progressive panencephalitis with onset at age 11 years, after congenital rubella, appeared in 1975 by Weil and coworkers. The patient was small for age, with sensorineural hearing loss of 60 decibels at age 4 years. At age 11 years, he had the insidious onset of motor incoordination, ataxia, and myoclonic jerks, with progressive deterioration. Although this complication of congenital rubella must be rare, it emphasizes that the etiology of subacute sclerosing panencephalitis need not be restricted to the measles virus.

Prevention. Live attenuated rubella virus vaccine is now available, safe, and effective (Lepow et al., 1968), although the duration of immunity is uncertain. Given as a single subcutaneous injection, it is recommended for children between ages 1 year and puberty and for women of childbearing age with a negative hemagglutination inhibition antibody test. It should be given only if there is assurance that there is no likelihood of pregnancy for the next 2 months, because of potential hazard to the fetus.

Fortunately, follow-up studies of a large number of women inadvertently immunized during or just before pregnancy have indicated that although the fetus is sometimes infected there appear to be no or, at most, very rare adverse consequences (Hayden et al., 1980). Despite this, it appears advisable to administer vaccine only in the immediate postpartum period or when pregnancy can be avoided. A mild rubella-like illness is sometimes seen after immunization, with arthralgia occurring 10 days to 2 weeks after injection.

Cytomegalovirus

Although the final chapter on cytomegalovirus infections in utero and in the newborn period is still not written, much has been learned about this ubiquitous and often confusing virus since its first cultivation in vitro in 1955 and since the recognition that it caused the devastating syndrome called *cytomegalic inclusion disease* (Weller, 1971; Weller and Macauley, 1957). Cytomegalovirus infection at any age is usually asymptomatic. After a period of active replication, the virus usually becomes latent but retains the capability of reactivation under special circumstances. Such reactivation appears to occur frequently during pregnancy.

The fetus can be infected either by a newly acquired maternal infection (Davis et al., 1971) or by a reactivated maternal infection. The former, although less common than the latter, appears to carry a much higher risk of severe disease in the fetus. Indeed, in reactivated infections newborns are normal on examination, and if defects appear, they do not apparently do so until some time later in childhood. At the present time, however, follow-up studies of congenitally infected infants whose mothers were proved to be antibody-positive before pregnancy are incomplete, and the prognosis of such infections, although clearly better than that of primary infections, is uncertain.

A newborn without congenital infection can be infected by its mother, either at the time of delivery or through the breast milk, by acquisition from the nursery or home environment, or by transfusion of blood from a donor who is antibody-positive (i.e., latently infected). Perinatal or postnatal acquisition from the mother appears to be entirely benign and very common. Postnatal acquisition from the environment is probably less common and may be benign, although lower respiratory illness may occur under these circumstances (Stagno et al., 1981). Acquisition from blood transfusion often results in severe, sometimes fatal, generalized disease in a setting in which maternal antibody is lacking (Yeager et al., 1981).

Incidence. The proportion of children and adults with detectable cytomegalovirus antibody varies with age, geographical location, and socioeconomic status. In the United States, about 60 per cent of adult women have complement fixing antibody. The incidence of excretion in the cervix or urine appears to rise during pregnancy from 3 per cent in the first trimester to as much as 12 per cent at term, although such findings are extremely variable. The overall incidence of congenital infection is 1.0 to 1.5 per cent of livebirths (Starr et al., 1970). It is higher than this (3.4 per cent) among babies of mothers who were antibody-positive before pregnancy (Stagno et al., 1977), a finding that implies that most intrauterine infections result from reactivated maternal infections. Indeed, two babies infected in sequential pregnancies from a single mother were found to be excreting viruses that were identical by restriction endonuclease mapping (Stagno et al., 1977). The first of these infants had severe cytomegalic inclusion disease; the second, although excreting virus at birth, was normal.

The incidence of neonatal and postnatal infection is still higher. Approximately half the babies of mothers excreting virus at term will acquire infection in the first weeks of life (Reynolds et al., 1973). Many of these babies are infected through breast milk (Hayes et al., 1972). None, apparently, are affected adversely by the infection. All infants, regardless of which route they have been infected by, excrete virus for a prolonged period, usually 1 year or more (Emanuel and Kenny, 1966).

Etiology. Cytomegalovirus is a member of the herpes virus family. Although all strains are serologically related, there appear to be some variations in antigenicity, and it is not clear at present whether this heterogeneity is important with regard to the incidence of exogenous reinfections. The virus differs from herpes simplex and varicella viruses in that it lacks the enzyme thymidine kinase. This renders it resistant to those newer antivirals that depend on this enzyme for their action, such as Acyclovir.

As with rubella, it seems likely that the virus first infects the placenta and then the fetus and that the placenta functions as a relative barrier in this sequence.

Pathology. Characteristic multinuclear giant cells with both cytoplasmic and intranuclear inclusion bodies are found in many organs. Liver, lungs, brain, pancreas, and kidneys contain them in large numbers. Mononuclear cell infiltration and diffuse fibrosis may be intense. In the brain are areas of necrosis, often subependymal and periventricular, and glial overgrowth, containing heavy deposits of calcium. Petechiae and larger hemorrhages involve skin and serous surfaces.

Diagnosis. Infants infected with the virus are often prematurely delivered. In the classic form of the infection, cytomegalic inclusion disease, newborn infants have an acute progressive disseminating disease. They show petechiae and ecchymoses and are jaundiced at birth, or jaundice appears within a few hours and becomes intense. The liver and spleen are enlarged and firm from the start and may increase in size for a number of days. Skull radiographs usually show periventricular calcifications. Fever as high as 39°C (102° to 103° F) may be found. Tachypnea and moderate dyspnea suggesting pulmonary involvement may appear. Pallor may or may not be striking. Puncture wounds bleed for many minutes, and hemorrhage from internal organs may cause death.

Table 85–2. Newborn Clinical Findings in 34 Patients with Congenital CMV Infection, All of Whom Were Symptomatic by 2 Weeks of Age

Abnormality	Positive/Total Examined (%)
Petechiae	27/34 (79)
Hepatosplenomegaly	25/34 (74)
Jaundice	20/32 (63)
Microcephaly*	17/34 (50)
Small for gestational age†	14/34 (41)
Prematurity‡	11/32 (34)
Inguinal hernia	5/19§ (26)
Chorioretinitis	4/34 (12)

* Less than tenth percentile based upon Colorado Intrauterine Growth Charts, for premature newborns (Lubchenco et al.) or more than 2 SD below mean for term babies based upon data of Nellhaus.
† Weight less than tenth percentile for gestational age.
‡ Gestational age less than 38 weeks.
§ Boys.
(From Pass, R. F., et al.: Pediatrics 66:758, 1980).

It is clear from prospective studies that most congenital cytomegalovirus infections are asymptomatic at birth and that milder manifestations of infections are more common than the aforementioned classic syndrome. A chart describing the frequency of various clinical findings in 34 infants who were symptomatic by 2 weeks of age is shown in Table 85–2 (Pass et al., 1980). Petechiae, hepatosplenomegaly, and jaundice were the commonest signs at this age. Ten of this group of infants died of their disease, most of them before 3 months of age, and all primarily because of severe neurologic impairment. Although microcephaly was seen in only half the infants at birth, a number of additional children became microcephalic as they grew older. Still others developed hearing or visual impairment, so that the proportion of surviving infants with sensorineural handicaps increased to 91 per cent at the time the study was performed.

Uncommon findings at birth are cardiac defects and a number of gastrointestinal malformations. None of these has been systematically associated with cytomegalovirus infection, however. Musculoskeletal abnormalities also occur, with indirect inguinal hernia being the most common.

An example of one nonclassic form was reported by a group from the Babies' Hospital of New York and is described in the following case.

CASE 85–1

A premature infant was quite well at birth, showing only a slightly enlarged liver and spleen. At the age of 5½ weeks, after having gained from 1570 gm to 2200 gm, and after having behaved quite well in all respects, abdominal distention was noted. The liver and spleen were now very large. Blood was normal, platelets were not diminished, but cerebrospinal fluid was xanthochromic and contained an excess of red blood cells and protein. Skull radiographs revealed microcephaly and calcifications that appeared to outline dilated lateral ventricles. At 6½ weeks chorioretinitis was noted in one eyeground. The infant improved for a while, but he had to be readmitted to hospital at 3 months because of vomiting, fever, and the appearance of a petechial rash. At that time, his platelet count had fallen to 60,000 per cubic millimeter, and his liver and spleen had become huge. Inclusion bodies were found in the urine sediment, and the typical virus was grown from a specimen of urine. He was still alive at 1 year of age, retarded physically and mentally, and hydrocephalic. The Sabin dye tests and complement fixation tests for toxoplasmosis were negative in both mother and patient.

Comment. It is obvious that this form of cytomegalic inclusion disease is difficult to differentiate from congenital toxoplasmosis and that great reliance must be placed on laboratory studies.

Laboratory Investigations. The laboratory diagnosis of congenital cytomegalovirus infection can be made with absolute certainty only through detection of the virus in organs or culture specimens at birth or within the first 3 weeks of life. The most sensitive detection system is growth of the virus in tissue culture, but other methods, particularly observation of typical inclusion bodies in urine sediment cells or in biopsy specimens, are of value when viral culture facilities are not available. Serologic tests are often difficult to interpret. If no antibody is found in the infant's blood, then cytomegalovirus infection is ruled out. The presence of antibody, however, is not helpful, and even serial antibody titers cannot differentiate between congenital infection and perinatally acquired infection. Tests for IgM antibody to cytomegalovirus are often confused by the presence of rheumatoid factor.

A presumptive diagnosis may sometimes be made after several months of age if virus is found and the clinical syndrome is classic. Other causes of congenital infection must, of course, be ruled out, since there is such extensive overlap in symptomatology.

The principal laboratory test abnormalities seen in infants with symptomatic cytomegalovirus infection at birth are shown in Table 85–3. In addition to those features shown in this table, anemia (usually hemolytic) is common.

The urine usually contains bile, but no urobilin. Albumin is commonly present, as are some red and white blood cells. Sediment that has been dried, fixed, and stained with hematoxylin and eosin often demonstrates the characteristic inclusion bodies within desquamated renal epithelial cells (Fig. 85–3),

Table 85–3. Laboratory Abnormalities in Newborns with Symptomatic Congenital CMV Infection

Test	Abnormal/Total Examined (%)
Increased cord serum IgM (>20 mg/100 ml); range, 22–170	21/25 (84)
Atypical lymphocytosis (≥5%)*; range, 5%–42%	8/10 (80)
Elevated SGOT (>80 μU/ml)* range, 85–495	14/18 (79)
Thrombocytopenia (<100,000 platelets/cu mm)†; range, 3000–66,000	17/28 (61)
Conjugated hyperbilirubinemia (direct serum bilirubin >2 mg/100 ml)†; range, 3–21	19‡/31 (61)
Increased CSF protein (>120 mg/100 ml)†; range, 130–198	9/19 (47)

* Determinations during first month of life.

† Determinations during first week of life.

‡ One patient with jaundice had a maximum direct bilirubin of 1.2 mg/100 ml but was icteric within 24 hours of birth.

(From Pass, R. F., et al.: Pediatrics 66:758, 1980.)

so-called "owl's eye cells." Virus may be cultivated from the urine for an extraordinary length of time.

Treatment. All attempts to treat the viral infection have failed, including administration of idoxuridine, cytosine arabinoside, adenine arabinoside, Acyclovir, interferon, and interferon inducers. Transient reduction in the titer of virus excreted in the urine may be seen, but no clinical benefit has occurred. Corticosteroids and cytotoxic agents have been used without success. Transfusion is indicated for anemia. Exchange transfusion should be performed if the indirect-reacting bilirubin concentration approaches 20 mg per 100 ml.

Prognosis. Of infants who are symptomatic at birth, some 25 per cent will die within the first 3 months (Weller and Hanshaw, 1962; Pass et al., 1980). Of the remainder, 60 to 75 per cent will have intellectual or developmental impairment (Berenberg and Nankervis, 1970), about one third will have hearing loss, one third will have neuromuscular disorders (spasticity or seizures), and a smaller proportion will have visual impairment due to chorioretinitis. Only 10 to 25 per cent will be normal late in childhood, and these will inevitably be those who demonstrated minimal abnormalities at birth.

The fate of the congenitally infected infant who was normal at birth is still not entirely clear. Two published series (Hanshaw et al., 1976; Reynolds et al., 1974) indicate variable risks of deafness and reduction of I.Q. scores. In both instances, however, the case finding method was measurement of cord IgM level, and an increase in this value might be found only in more severely affected infants (possibly reflecting primary infection in the mother). In one other follow-up study (Kumar et al., 1973), the children were found to be normal at 4 years, but audiometric screening was not performed.

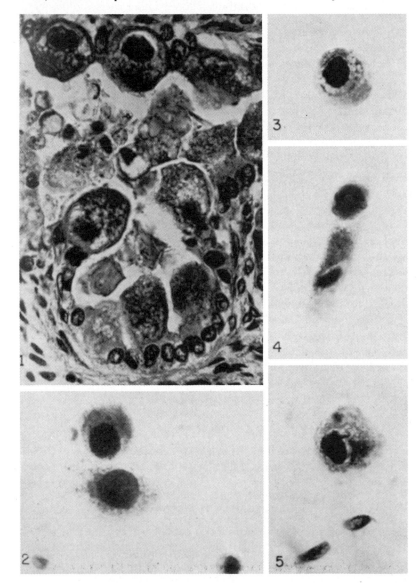

Figure 85–3. *1,* Renal tubule from a patient who died with cytomegalic inclusion disease. Note the intranuclear and intracytoplasmic inclusion bodies, with associated degeneration and desquamation of cells. Some of the necrotic cells appear as large masses of cytoplasm. *2, 3, 4,* Various types of cytomegalic cells observed in the urinary sediment from this infant. The shape of the cell in *3* suggests that it originated in the lower part of the collecting tubules or in the pelvis. In *4,* note the two small desquamated cells whose size corresponds to that of normal tubular cells. *5,* Cytomegalic cell and two normal cells from the gastric mucosa, observed in the sediment from a gastric washing. Hematoxylin and eosin, × 782. (Blanc, W. A.: Am. J. Clin. Pathol. *28*:46, 1957.)

The enteroviruses of humans include polioviruses, Coxsackie viruses A and B, and the echoviruses. Fortunately, poliovirus infection of neonates is now rare. According to early accounts, however, infants infected in the perinatal period developed severe, often fatal diseases, with a high incidence of paralysis in the survivors. Readers are referred to the 1955 review by Bates and to the 1976 chapter of Cherry for further information.

Since Coxsackie A virus infections have been described only rarely, we shall limit this review to a consideration of only those diseases associated with Coxsackie B and echoviruses.

Incidence. All enterovirus infections are seasonal, occurring most frequently during the late summer and early autumn in temperate climates. The incidence varies from year to year, with outbreaks sometimes caused by a single Coxsackie or echo serotype and sometimes by several. Disease in neonates is uncommon but reflects the broader picture of infections in the population at large. It seems likely that severe disease in neonates is seen with a frequency equal to or greater than that of perinatal herpes virus infection.

Etiology. It appears that any of the nonpolio enteroviruses can cause disease in the neonate. Coxsackie B viruses are associated primarily with myocarditis and aseptic meningitis or combinations of the two (Kibrick and Benirschke, 1958). Echoviruses, however, are seen more often with either severe nonspecific febrile illnesses with disseminated intravascular coagulation (Nagington et al., 1978), aseptic meningitis (Cramblett et al., 1973; Linnemann et al., 1974), or hepatitis (Modlin, 1980). With both groups of viruses, nonspecific febrile illnesses with or without rash are commonly seen.

Infection takes place either just before or just after birth. Because a number of infants have been delivered by cesarean section with intact membranes, it seems likely that transplacental infection occurs. Regardless of whether the mother or some other caretaker is the source, severe disease may result when the baby lacks antibody to the infecting strain. It is not clear at present why the newborn infant is so highly susceptible to overwhelming illness. Nursery outbreaks of both Coxsackie B (Javett et al., 1956) and echovirus infections (Cramblett et al., 1973; Nagington et al., 1978) have been reported in which severe, and sometimes fatal, illnesses have occurred.

Pathology. In Coxsackie B infections, myocardial necrosis and inflammation may be seen that is patchy or diffuse, with extensive infiltration by lymphocytes, mononuclear cells, histiocytes, and some polymorphonuclear leukocytes. Similar infiltrates are seen in the meninges in both Coxsackie and echovirus infections. When liver or adrenal glands are involved, there is usually extensive hemorrhage as well as inflammation and necrosis.

Diagnosis. When disease is acquired from the mother, an infant is characteristically well at birth, although premature delivery is more frequent in this group. The mother, however, may be febrile at this time. The baby develops fever, anorexia, and vomiting after an incubation period of 1 to 5 days. At that point, the clinical evolution depends on the infecting virus and the extent of involvement.

In most instances, the disease is mild and self-limited. Rash may appear in some infants and aseptic meningitis in others. If myocarditis is present, the liver rapidly enlarges, the heart dilates, and the sound becomes muffled. The echo- and electrocardiograms show diffuse myocardial inflammation. Not infrequently, disseminated intravascular coagulation, refractory hypotension, and death follow rapidly. However, in many infants myocardial involvement is temporary, and recovery occurs over the course of several weeks.

The severity of central nervous system infections is also quite variable. Enteroviruses can produce overwhelming meningoencephalitis, sometimes with cranial nerve signs. It is more common, however, to see a moderate or mild meningitis characterized by only temporary irritability, lethargy, fever, and feeding difficulty. Some infections, particularly those with echoviruses, are characterized by a rampant and overwhelming hepatitis (Modlin, 1980). Others present primarily as pulmonary disease, and still others manifest as diarrhea and even necrotizing enterocolitis (Lake et al., 1976). Disseminated intravascular coagulation develops in virtually all instances of widespread, fulminant involvement.

Treatment. The myocarditis and heart failure must be treated by digitalization, diuretics, and other measures. Both plasma infusions and exchange transfusions have been attempted in overwhelming enterovirus infections with little evidence of beneficial effect. The use of steroids should be discouraged unless there is a clear rationale.

Prognosis. By the time disseminated intravascular coagulation has developed, the prognosis is grave. On the other hand, many infants with Coxsackie B myocarditis survive, and prognosis in such instances is probably more closely related to the energy with which cases are sought by electrocardiogram and viral diagnostic measures. Few long-term follow-up studies have been published, but the available information suggests that recovery is complete in most instances.

The prognosis following central nervous system involvement is also not clear. Most do well. However, a number of studies of infants under 3 months of age with aseptic meningitis have suggested that there may be some impairment of intellectual development when compared with carefully selected control groups (Wilfert et al., 1981; Sells et al., 1975; Farmer et al., 1975).

The following case illustrates the fulminant disease caused by Coxsackie virus B-2.

CASE 85–2

A white male infant was born to a 35-year-old multipara after a difficult breech delivery but suffered no ill consequences. He breathed and cried spontaneously and seemed quite well. On the fourth postnatal day, his mother became febrile, a few rales were heard in her chest, and her white blood cell count was low. On the fifth day the infant's temperature rose to 101.8° F, and later that day tachypnea with cyanosis and grunting expiration were noted. Pulse rate was 198 per minute. Physical examination was unrewarding. Hemoglobin was 14.7 gm, white blood cells numbered 4700 per cubic millimeter, urine showed albumin, 1 +, blood culture proved sterile, and nasopharyngeal culture revealed no pathogens. He was given chloramphenicol, 100 mg every 8 hours orally, and penicillin, 300,000 units every 8 hours intramuscularly. On the sixth day, the temperature rose to 103° F, respiratory rate was 80, pulse rate 220, the color was grayish blue, and the liver edge had descended 1.5 cm below the right costal margin. The patient was digitalized with Cedilanid. Lumbar puncture produced fluid containing protein in excess (2 + Pándy) and 2500 red blood cells and 1200 white blood cells per cubic millimeter. Over the next few days, the infant's general condition improved slightly, but diarrhea developed with numerous blood-tinged, liquid, green stools. Stool cultures showed no pathogens. On the thirteenth day he went into severe shock, the temperature falling to 95.6° F, the extremities becoming cold and mottled blue. A few clicking rales were heard throughout the lungs. The liver was down 3 cm and was firm. He died soon thereafter.

Antemortem diagnosis leaned strongly toward a disseminated viral infection, with myocarditis, pneumonitis, and encephalomyelitis among its manifestations. Virus studies were made at the University Hospital of Baltimore (courtesy of Dr. Theodore Woodward) and were confirmed at the National Institutes of Health. Coxsackie virus B-2 was grown from cerebrospinal fluid, blood, throat washings, and brain.

Comment. The onset of a febrile illness in this 5-day-old infant coincided with a similar illness in his mother. Tachycardia and heart failure developing in a previously normal heart suggested primary myocarditis, and cerebrospinal fluid alterations suggested encephalomyelitis. The combination of these two indicated generalized infection, with either a virus or *Toxoplasma* the most likely pathogen. The former

appeared the more probable cause in view of the simultaneous maternal illness and the absence of jaundice, hepatosplenomegaly, and thrombocytopenia. (Since the appearance of this abstract in the first edition of this book, this case and one other have been reported in detail by Robino and coworkers.)

Herpes Simplex Infections

Herpes simplex viruses are classified into two types: Type 1 causes about 98 per cent of oral and labial infections and almost 100 per cent of encephalitis outside the newborn period; type 2 causes 90 per cent of genital herpes and most cases of aseptic meningitis (Nahmias and Roizman, 1973). Seventy to 85 per cent of neonatal herpes simplex infections are due to herpes type 2 (Nahmias and Visintine, 1976; Whitley et al., 1980). It is likely that most infections are acquired from the mother shortly before or at the time of delivery. Some, perhaps accounting for the slight excess of cases due to type 1 above the percentage found in the adult genital tract, must be acquired from other sources. Considering the extraordinary frequency of labial herpes in the adult population, however, acquisition of herpes simplex from such lesions must be an extremely rare event.

Incidence. Genital herpes infections have been increasing in incidence steadily since the 1970s. The frequency of neonatal disease has probably also increased, although it fortunately remains low. Nahmias estimates one detected case in every 7500 deliveries among an indigent population (Nahmias and Visintine, 1976). Approximately 120 cases are thought to occur in the United States each year.

Etiology and Pathogenesis. Most infants acquire the virus from the maternal genital tract at the time of delivery. Lesions have been reported at the site of intrapartum monitoring electrodes on the infant's scalp. A smaller number are infected several days before delivery and are born with clinically evident disease. There are a few cases described of infants with a syndrome more closely resembling congenital viral infection who were probably infected in utero during the first or second trimester (South et al., 1969; Florman et al., 1973). Cases proved to have been acquired from individuals other than the mother, or even from the mother at any time other than during delivery, are extremely rare (Linnemann et al., 1978).

A recent report suggests that severity of disease in the newborn is related to the level of circulating, placentally transmitted antibody to the infecting type (Yeager et al., 1981). This finding is consistent with the idea that primary genital infection in the mother at delivery is more hazardous to the baby than recurrent infection (Nahmias et al., 1971).

Pathology. Macroscopically, many viscera, but chiefly liver, lungs, and adrenals, are riddled with pale yellow, firm, necrotic nodules, measuring 1 to 6 mm in diameter. Under the microscope, massive coagulation necrosis is seen to involve the parenchyma, stroma, and vessels in these areas. Necrotizing, calcifying lesions of the brain may also be found. Intranuclear eosinophilic inclusions as well as multinucleated giant cells may be seen, both representing the individual cell's response to viral infection.

Diagnosis. Mothers of infants with neonatal herpes simplex infection are often young and primiparous. About one third of the babies are premature. Most are normal at birth and develop illness at 5 to 10 days of age. Overt herpetic disease in the maternal genital tract is evident in only about one third of patients (Whitley et al., 1980). In most of the remainder, the virus probably originates in an asymptomatic maternal genital infection.

The clinical manifestations of disease have been classified into two broad groups: disseminated and localized (Nahmias and Visintine, 1976). Within the former group, two categories are recognized—those with and those without central nervous system involvement. Localized infections include those involving the central nervous system alone and those with isolated skin or eye disease. Localized infections have, in general, the better outlook, and those with only skin involvement the best.

Disseminated disease usually begins in the first week of life. Skin vesicles may be the first or a later sign but do not appear at all in more than half. Systemic symptoms, although insidious in onset, progress rapidly. Poor feeding, lethargy, and fever may be accompanied by irritability or convulsions if the central nervous system is involved. These symptoms are followed rapidly by jaundice, hypotension, disseminated intravascular coagulation, apnea, and shock. This form of disease is indistinguishable at its onset from both neonatal enterovirus infection and bacterial sepsis.

Localized disease may begin somewhat later, with most cases appearing in the second week of life. When the central nervous system is the primary site of infection, the skin or eyes may or may not be involved; if not, then brain biopsy may, as with encephalitis in older subjects, be the only mode of diagnosis. The infants are lethargic, irritable, and tremulous, and seizures are frequent and difficult to control.

Eye infections usually take the form of keratoconjunctivitis or chorioretinitis. On the neonatal skin, herpes simplex virus produces the characteristic grouped vesicles seen in later life, although individual lesions may be large and even bullous, and late lesions are typically eroded, flat, irregular ulcers with an erythematous base.

In disseminated disease, there is usually chemical evidence of hepatocellular injury. If the central nervous system is involved, the spinal fluid usually contains white cells (mostly lymphocytes) and sometimes demonstrates erythrocytes, and the protein level is usually elevated. Except when encephalitis is the only manifestation of disease, as already mentioned, herpes simplex virus is readily recovered from clinical samples. In the disseminated form, virus is present in blood, CSF, conjunctivae, respiratory secretions, and urine. In the localized form, virus can be found at the site of disease. Scrapings of skin vesicles will show giant, multinucleated cells when stained with Wright or Giemsa stain (the Tzanck smear), typical of either herpes or varicella virus infection. Reagents are now available for identification of the virus by immunofluorescence in such scrapings. Definitive microbiologic diagnosis, however, requires growth of the virus in tissue culture. Fortunately, herpes simplex virus can be detected by its cytopathic effect in 24 to 48 hours in most instances. When herpes neonatorum is suspected, viral cultures of the throat, conjunctival and cerebrospinal fluid, blood, and urine should all be obtained, as well as scrapings of any suspicious skin lesions. Moreover, the mother's genital and respiratory tracts should also be sampled. Serologic assays are rarely helpful and are difficult to interpret in view of the cross-reactions between the two herpes serotypes.

Treatment and Prevention. If a mother has active genital herpes simplex infection at the time of delivery and if the membranes are either intact or have been ruptured for less than 4 hours, the baby should be delivered by cesarean section. The risk to the child is greatest if maternal infection is primary (i.e., if the mother has previously had no infection with either type 1 or type 2). Recurrences, however, with infectious virus recoverable from the genital area at the time of delivery also pose a hazard. A schema for the preventive measures to be taken in these complex situations is presented in the 1978 report of Visintine and coworkers.

When neonatal disease is suspected, every effort to establish a definitive diagnosis must be made as rapidly as possible. As soon as this diagnosis is ascertained, the infant should receive adenine arabinoside (Vidarabine), 20 mg/kg/day administered intravenously over a 12-hour period for 10 days. This treatment has been shown to be effective in all forms of the disease, reducing (but by no means eliminating) both mortality and sequelae. The survival results of the Collaborative Antiviral Study Group trials for infants with central nervous system or disseminated disease are shown in Figure 85–4 (Whitley et al., 1980). Mortality in infants with localized disease outside the central nervous system has always been close to zero. If cultures are negative, breast-feeding is safe (Grossman et al., 1981).

Prognosis. Even with antiviral treatment, the prognosis for survivors is not good. More than half de-

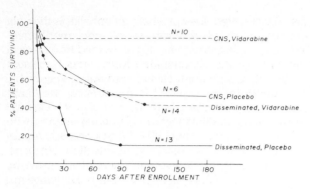

Figure 85–4. Outcome of herpes simplex virus infection in neonates according to type of disease and therapy. Points represent last death(s). (From Whitley, R. J., et al.: Pediatrics *66:*495, 1980.)

velop microcephaly, spasticity, paralysis, seizures, deafness, or blindness. Those with skin involvement often have recurrent crops of skin vesicles for several years of life.

The following case illustrates a typical severe generalized illness in an infant with disseminated disease.

CASE 85–3

A 5-day-old female infant was admitted to the Sinai Hospital of Baltimore because of fever, anorexia, and lethargy. The mother had herpetic lesions about the genitalia at the time of delivery. After normal pregnancy and labor and spontaneous delivery, the infant appeared quite well for the first 4 days, when a temperature of 102° F and anorexia were noted. On admission she was well developed, but a bit dehydrated, alert, with good cry. Temperature was 100.8° F, pulse rate 150, and respirations 40 to 50 per minute. A large pustular lesion was noted on the left cheek. The liver was felt 1.5 cm below the right costal margin; the spleen was not palpable. White blood cells numbered 5600 per cubic millimeter; 73 per cent were polymorphonuclear. Hemoglobin was 16.9 gm per 100 ml. Blood cultures were negative, and cultures of the skin lesions were sterile.

In spite of chloramphenicol and penicillin, the temperature remained elevated from 98° to 102° F. A few scattered skin lesions appeared during the fifth day, and more were visible on the seventh day. These latter ones appeared vesicular. On this day, a venipuncture wound bled for more than an hour, and platelets numbered 42,000 per cubic millimeter. The infant was given a transfusion. The liver and spleen gradually enlarged. The temperature became subnormal. The patient was given 100 ml of her mother's plasma in the hope that it might contain specific antibodies. Attacks of apnea and generalized convulsions followed. Death followed one of the apnea spells on the seventh hospital day, the twelfth day of life.

Autopsy showed extensive necrobiotic lesions characteristic of generalized herpes simplex in the liver, lungs, and adrenals. There was hemorrhagic infiltration of the lesions, and many inclusion bodies were clearly

visible within the cells. The brain was similarly involved. Hemorrhagic esophagitis was intense. Virus of herpes simplex was isolated from vesicles, blood, adrenals, lung, and liver. Neutralization tests of the mother's blood were negative, and those of the infant's blood were weakly positive and inconclusive.

Comment. This infant was undoubtedly infected during parturition by contact with the mother's genital herpes. Skin lesions appeared on the fourth day, and new vesicles developed during the course. Unlike in most instances of the disease, jaundice was never prominent. The liver and spleen enlarged, and thrombocytopenia with bleeding and evidences of brain damage appeared. The virus was identified. Neutralizing bodies were not found in appreciable quantities in the mother or child.

Varicella

There is some confusion about the term "congenital varicella" that would probably be best resolved by our reserving this term for the very rare cases transmitted to the fetus in the first or second trimester of pregnancy (Srabstein et al., 1974). Also called "congenital varicella" in the literature but probably better termed "neonatal varicella" are those cases of infant varicella beginning before or on the tenth day of life and therefore (because of the incubation period of the disease) acquired in utero. The two syndromes are thoroughly discussed in Gershon's 1975 report. Some cases (e.g., that described by Bai and John in 1979) fall somewhere in between.

Incidence. Gershon has found only six reported cases of the congenital varicella syndrome. Neonatal varicella, however, is considerably more common. In the same review, Gershon discusses 50 cases from the literature, all apparently acquired from maternal varicella developing at or near term.

Etiology and Pathogenesis. The congenital varicella syndrome is acquired during maternal varicella that occurs during the first or second trimester. The virus must be transmitted transplacentally during the viremia that precedes or accompanies the rash. Clearly, however, in most situations the fetus either is not infected at all or recovers fully in utero, since the syndrome itself is so rare and because varicella during pregnancy is not uncommon.

Neonatal varicella is also probably transplacentally acquired in most cases. Since the incubation period for varicella is between 10 and 21 days, those cases beginning in the first 10 days of life are considered to have been acquired in utero. The prognosis, however, differs markedly between those cases in which maternal illness began 5 or more days from delivery and those in which maternal illness occurred from 4 days before to 1 day after delivery. In the former group, neonatal disease usually begins within the first 4 days of life, and the prognosis is good. Of 27 cases cited by Gershon in her reviews, all survived. Presumably, maternal immunity has appeared before delivery and has been transferred to the baby before birth. In the latter group, neonatal disease begins between 5 and 10 days after delivery. Of the 23 cases described, seven (30 per cent) died of overwhelming varicella and two barely survived after severe disease. In those instances in which the infant's pre-illness antibody has been measured in severe disease, none has been found.

Presumably, the placenta acts as a partial barrier to infection at term as well as earlier during pregnancy. Only about one in six such maternal infections results in neonatal disease (Meyers, 1974).

Diagnosis. The rare cases of congenital varicella syndrome are characterized by the presence of unusual cicatrices, asymmetric muscular atrophy and limb hypoplasia, low birth weight, chronic encephalitis with cortical atrophy, and ophthalmitis (chorioretinitis, microphthalmia, atrophy, and cataracts).

Neonatal varicella follows typical maternal varicella and thus can usually be anticipated. When the disease appears in the infant during the danger period (from 5 to 10 days of age), it resembles closely varicella in the immunodeficient or immunosuppressed host. Recurrent crops of skin vesicles develop over a prolonged period of time, reflecting the neonate's inability to control the infection. Visceral dissemination is common, with involvement of the liver, lung, and brain. Secondary bacterial infection may occur.

Disease that is evident at birth or that appears in the first 4 days of life is usually mild, presumably owing to modification by maternal immunity.

The laboratory may be helpful in confirming the diagnosis. Scrapings of skin lesions, as with herpes simplex infections, show large multinucleated cells when stained with Wright or Giemsa stain (Tzanck smears). The virus can be grown in tissue culture from skin and visceral lesions.

Prevention and Treatment. Infants of mothers who develop varicella from 4 days before to one day after delivery should receive high-titered immune globulin as soon as possible. Such preparations (zoster immune globulin, or varicella-zoster immune globulin) have been shown to prevent chicken pox in exposed older children (Brunell et al., 1969) and are available through the Center for Disease Control in Atlanta, Georgia. If special globulin preparations are not available, then standard immune serum globulin (0.5 to 1.0 ml/kg) should be given.

If severe disease develops, antiviral chemotherapy might be considered, although there are no reports of controlled trials in this age group. Drugs that might be effective are adenine arabinoside (15 mg/kg/day) and acycloguanosine (Acyclovir).

Viral Hepatitis

Much has been learned about viral hepatitis (hepatitis A, hepatitis B, and non-A, non-B hepatitis) since the 1960s. Perhaps the most important finding to neonatologists pertains to the frequency with which hepatitis B is transmitted to infants at the time of birth and the short- and long-term consequences of these infections. This frequency in turn depends primarily on the prevalence of the hepatitis B carrier state among women of childbearing age.

In certain parts of the world and among certain ethnic groups, as many as 7 to 10 per cent of all infants acquire hepatitis B infections at the time of birth, and a high proportion of these infections are chronic. The possible relationship of these infections to chronic liver failure and hepatic carcinoma in adult life is becoming increasingly convincing.

Incidence. The incidence of neonatal hepatitis B infections depends on a number of factors. One of these is the carriage rate of hepatitis B surface antigen (HB_sAg) in mothers, which varies from 0.1 per cent in the United States and Europe to 15 per cent in Taiwan and parts of Africa, with intermediate rates in Japan, South America, and Southeast Asia. Another factor is the infectivity of the mother at the time of delivery. This is high if symptomatic acute disease is present (60 to 70 per cent transmission) (Gerety and Schweitzer, 1977) or, in carriers, if e antigen is present (80 to 95 per cent transmission) (Okada et al., 1976). Although HB_sAg has been found in breast milk, breast-feeding does not appear to have any influence, either positive or negative, upon the rate of transmission (Beasley et al., 1975).

Etiology and Pathogenesis. Hepatitis B virus is the only representative of a unique group of DNA-containing viruses that infects the human host. The virus localizes primarily in hepatic parenchymal cells but circulates in the bloodstream, along with several subviral antigens, for periods of time ranging from a few days to many years. It seems clear that despite either acute or persistent viremia in the mother, the virus rarely crosses the placenta and that infection in the neonatal period occurs at or shortly after birth, probably by means of virus carried in maternal blood.

Once infection has been established, the usual long incubation period of several weeks to 6 months passes before the infant develops antigenemia.

Diagnosis. Infants with hepatitis B infection do not show clinical or chemical signs of disease at birth. The usual pattern is the development of chronic antigenemia with mild and often persistent enzyme elevations, beginning at 2 to 6 months of age. Occasionally, the antigenemia is entirely missed, and the child is merely found to have antibody to the surface antigen at 6 to 12 months of age. Sometimes, the infection is clinically manifest, with jaundice, fever, hepatomegaly, and anorexia, followed by either recovery or chronic active hepatitis. Very rarely, fulminant hepatitis is seen.

The laboratory is essential in the diagnosis of hepatitis B infection. Evaluations of serum enzymes and of bilirubin reflect the extent of liver damage. There are now several helpful serologic tests that identify the virus involved. HB_sAg appears early, usually before liver disease is found, and may disappear or persist. Antibody to the hepatitis B core antigen (anti-HB_c) usually appears during or shortly after the acute disease and lasts for years. Last to appear, usually several weeks or even months after the illness (and never if HB_sAg persists) is antibody to the surface antigen, or anti-HB_s. It is very unusual for all three of these tests to be entirely negative in the presence of hepatitis B infection.

Prevention and Treatment. Possible preventive measures include passive immunization with high-titered human immune serum globulin (HBIG) and use of the newly developed hepatitis B vaccine. The former has now been shown to protect exposed infants in high-risk situations, reducing the long-term carrier rate from 91 per cent to 23 per cent in babies of e-antigen–positive mothers (Beasley et al., 1981), individually. HBIG at birth and at 3 and 6 months of age should be administered in situations in which the risk is highest: in the presence of e antigenemia in the mother or when birth takes place during or shortly before acute hepatitis B in the mother. The use of HBIG in infants of e-antigen–negative, asymptomatic mothers will hinge on its availability and cost and the results of controlled trials under these circumstances. The use of vaccine at the time of birth to prevent antigenemia has not been reported at this time.

Western Equine Encephalitis

As far as we can determine, only one instance in which the virus of Western equine encephalitis may have been transmitted from mother to fetus has been reported, and it is documented in the following case history.

CASE 85–4

Shinefield and Townsend cite the case of a mother who became ill 9 days after sleeping on an unscreened porch where she was repeatedly bitten by mosquitoes. The porch was contiguous to a yard in which there were forty chickens, a known reservoir host to the Western equine encephalitis virus. She had fever, lethargy, and severe headache. Her antibodies to this organism rose to 1:128. Three days after the onset of her illness she delivered twins, one of whom became ill on the fifth day, the other 12 hours later. They had high fever, twitching, stiff neck, bulging fontanels, cerebrospinal

fluid pleiocytosis of 700 cells, of which 58 per cent were polymorphonuclear, and protein of 240 mg per 100 ml. Cerebrospinal fluid sugar was not reduced. The fluid was sterile. Courses were stormy for 1 week, after which both infants recovered. Antibodies rose from 0 to 1:16 in one twin and from 0 to 1:128 in the other.

Comment. Since the incubation period of Western equine encephalitis is usually said to last from 4 to 21 days, and since the mother's own incubation period was clearly 9 days, the authors feel that the disease was almost surely acquired ante partum rather than at the moment of delivery. We cannot quarrel with this conclusion.

Nosocomial Viral Infections

Previous reference has been made to nursery outbreaks of enterovirus infections that cause diseases ranging from mild, benign febrile illness to aseptic meningitis, myocarditis, and overwhelming generalized infections with disseminated intravascular coagulation (Cramblett et al., 1973; Nagington et al., 1978; Javett et al., 1956). As was also mentioned, nursery-acquired herpes simplex infections are fortunately rare, and symptomatic nosocomial cytomegalovirus infections appear to be largely confined to recipients of latently infected blood who themselves lack antibody. Two other groups of viruses, however, previously unrecognized as important agents in the newborn period, appear to be responsible for a significant proportion of nursery-acquired viral infections. These are the respiratory and the diarrhea viruses.

RESPIRATORY VIRUSES

It seems likely that any member of the large number of respiratory viruses can cause symptomatic respiratory disease in newborn infants. The association has been described for rhinoviruses, adenoviruses, parainfluenza viruses, influenza virus, and respiratory syncytial virus. Adenovirus, rhinovirus, and parainfluenza virus infections are characterized by mild rhinorrhea under these conditions. Influenza virus infections are usually mild, but in the absence of maternally transmitted antibody they can be life-threatening, with extensive pneumonia and hypoxia and a prolonged course. The most extensive nursery outbreaks, however, have been caused by respiratory syncytial virus (Berkovich and Taranko, 1964; Hall et al., 1979).

Respiratory syncytial virus is the major cause of viral pneumonia and bronchiolitis in infants and children. In temperate climates, it causes large annual epidemics during the cold months. Nosocomial infections are frequent during these times, with illness in the hospital staff probably a major factor in spread from infant to infant. Several nursery outbreaks have been described. In one of these, cultures were obtained prospectively, so that a full picture of the viral pathogenicity and epidemiology could be drawn (Hall et al., 1979). Twenty-three of 66 infants hospitalized for 6 or more days and therefore at risk of nosocomial infection were infected. Only one was asymptomatic. Six had pneumonia, eight presented with upper respiratory infection, four had predominantly apneic spells, and four demonstrated nonspecific signs. Pneumonia and apnea were almost exclusively seen in those over 3 weeks of age, and nonspecific signs were most commonly observed in those under that age. Four (17 per cent) infants died, two unexpectedly, during their infections. Infants in isolettes did not seem to be protected against acquiring infection. Eighteen of the 53 nursery personnel were infected during the outbreak. Eighty-three per cent of these patients were symptomatic.

DIARRHEA VIRUSES

The best studied of the diarrhea viruses are the rotaviruses. This important group of viruses, with at least four serotypes, is responsible for a large proportion of significant and sometimes severe diarrhea in infants 6 to 24 months of age (Steinhoff, 1980). Nursery-acquired infections are extraordinarily frequent in parts of the world in which they have been looked for; surprisingly, however, they appear to be benign in the great majority of infected infants. In certain nurseries in Sydney, Australia, and in London, 30 to 50 per cent of 5-day-old babies excreted the virus (Murphy et al., 1977; Chrystie et al., 1978). However, more than 90 per cent of these infected infants were asymptomatic. The remainder had loose stools and vomiting, but this proportion was only slightly greater than that found among uninfected infants.

Much remains to be discovered about these infections. It is not known, for example, how long these infants excreted virus after discharge from the nurseries, what the mode of spread was, or why the infections were so harmless in these babies. Thus, at least for the time being, rotavirus infections in nurseries appear to be an interesting and surprisingly common oddity with only minor clinical consequences.

REFERENCES

Bai, P. V. A., and John, T. J.: Congenital skin ulcers following varicella in late pregnancy. J. Pediatr. 94:65, 1975.

Bates, T.: Poliomyelitis in pregnancy, fetus and newborn. A.M.A. J. Dis. Child. 90:189, 1955.

Beasley, R. P., Hwang, L.-Y., Lin, C.-C., et al.: Hepatitis B immune globulin (HBIG) efficacy in the interruption of perinatal transmission of hepatitis B virus carrier state. Lancet 2:388, 1981.

Beasley, R. P., Stevens, C. E., Shiao, I.-S., and Meng, H.-C.: Evidence against breast-feeding as a mechanism for vertical transmission of hepatitis B. Lancet 2:740, 1975.

Berenberg, W., and Nankervis, G.: Long-term follow-up of cytomegalic inclusion disease of infancy. Pediatrics 46:403, 1970.

Berkovich, S., and Taranko, L.: Acute respiratory illness in the premature nursery associated with respiratory syncytial virus infections. Pediatrics 34:753, 1964.

Brough, A. J., Jones, D., Page, R. H., and Mizukami, I.: Dermal erythropoiesis in neonatal infants. Pediatrics 40:627, 1967.

Brunell, P. A., Ross, A., et al.: Prevention of varicella by zoster immune globulin. N. Engl. J. Med. 280:1191, 1969.

Cherry, J. D.: Enteroviruses. In Remington, J. S., and Klein, J. O. (Eds.): Infectious Diseases of the Fetus and Newborn Infant. Philadelphia, W. B. Saunders Co., 1976, pp. 306–413.

Chrystie, I. L., Totterdell, B. M., and Banatvala, J. E.: Asymptomatic endemic rotavirus infections in the newborn. Lancet 1:1176, 1978.

Claman, H. N., Savatte, V., Githens, J. H., and Hathaway, W. E.: Histiocytic reaction in dysgammaglobulinemia and congenital rubella. Pediatrics 46:89, 1970.

Cooper, L. Z., Green, R. H., et al.: Neonatal thrombocytopenic purpura and other manifestations of rubella contracted in utero. Am. J. Dis. Child. 110:416, 1965.

Cooper, L. Z., Ziring, P. R., Ockerse, A. R., et al.: Rubella: clinical manifestations and management. Am. J. Dis. Child. 118:18, 1969.

Cramblett, H. G., Haynes, R. E., Azimi, P. H., Hilty, M. D., and Wilder, M. H.: Nosocomial infection with echovirus type II in handicapped and premature infants. Pediatrics 51:603, 1973.

Davis, L. E., Tweed, G. V., Stewart, J. A., et al.: Cytomegalovirus mononucleosis in a first trimester pregnant female with transmission to the fetus. Pediatrics 48:200, 1971.

Desmond, M. M., Fisher, E. S., Vorderman, A. L., et al.: The longitudinal course of congenital rubella encephalitis in nonretarded children. J. Pediatr. 93:584, 1978.

Dudgeon, J. A.: Congenital rubella. J. Pediatr. 87:1078, 1975.

Emanuel, I., and Kenny, G. E.: Cytomegalic inclusion disease of infancy. Pediatrics 38:957, 1966.

Farmer, K., MacArthur, B. A., and Clay, M. M.: A follow-up study of 15 cases of neonatal meningoencephalitis due to coxsackie virus B5. J. Pediatr. 87:568, 1975.

Florman, A. L., Gershon, A. A., Blackett, P. R., and Nahmias, A. J.: Intrauterine infection with herpes simplex virus: resultant congenital malformations. J.A.M.A. 225:129, 1973.

Gerety, R. J., and Schweitzer, I. L.: Viral hepatitis type B during pregnancy, the neonatal period, and infancy. J. Pediatr. 90:368, 1977.

Gershon, A. A.: Varicella in mother and infant: problems old and new. In Krugman, S., and Gershon, A. A. (Eds.): Infections of the Fetus and the Newborn Infant. New York, Alan R. Liss, Inc., 1975, pp. 79–95.

Gregg, N. M.: Congenital cataract following German measles in the mother. Tr. Ophthal. Soc. Austr. 3:35, 1941.

Grossman, J. H., Wallen, U. C., and Sever, J. L.: Management of genital herpes simplex virus infection during pregnancy. Obstet. Gynecol. 58:1, 1981.

Hall, C. B., Kopelman, A. E., Douglas, R. G., Jr., et al.: Neonatal respiratory syncytial virus infection. N. Engl. J. Med. 300:393, 1979.

Hanshaw, J. B., Scheiner, A. P., Moxley, A. W., et al.: School failure and deafness after "silent" congenital cytomegalovirus infection. N. Engl. J. Med. 295:468, 1976.

Hardy, J. B., Monif, G. R. G., and Sever, J. L.: Studies in congenital rubella. Baltimore 1964–65, II. Clinical and virologic. Bull. Hopkins Hosp. 118:97, 1966.

Hayden, G. F., Herrmann, K. L., Buimovici-Klein, E., et al.: Subclinical congenital rubella infection associated with maternal rubella vaccination in early pregnancy. J. Pediatr. 96:869, 1980.

Hayes, K., Danks, D. M., Gibas, H., and Jack, I.: Cytomegalovirus in human milk. N. Engl. J. Med. 287:177, 1972.

Javett, S. N., Heymann, S., Mundel, B., et al.: Myocarditis in the newborn infant. J. Pediatr. 48:1, 1956.

Kibrick, S., and Benirschke, K.: Severe generalized disease (encephalohepatomyocarditis) occurring in the newborn period due to infection with coxsackie virus, Group B. Pediatrics 22:857, 1958.

Kumar, M. L., Nankervis, G. A., and Gold, E.: Inapparent congenital cytomegalovirus infection: a follow-up study. N. Engl. J. Med. *288*:1370, 1973.

Lake, A. M., Lauer, B. A., Clark, J. C., Wesenberg, R. L., and McIntosh, K.: Enterovirus infections in neonates. J. Pediatr. *89*:787, 1976.

Lepow, M. L., Veronelli, J. A., Hostetler, D. D., et al.: A trial with live attenuated rubella vaccine. Am. J. Dis. Child. *115*:639, 1968.

Linnemann, C. C., Jr., Buchman, T. G., Light, I. J., et al.: Transmission of herpes simplex type 1 in a newborn nursery: identification of viral isolates by DNA "fingerprinting." Lancet *1*:964, 1978.

Linnemann, C. C., Steichen, J., Sherman, W. G., and Schiff, G. M.: Febrile illness in early infancy associated with ECHO virus infection. J. Pediatr. *84*:49, 1974.

Maupas, P., Chiron, J.-P., Barin, F., et al.: Efficacy of hepatitis B vaccine in prevention of early HB$_s$Ag carrier state in children: controlled trial in an endemic area (Senegal). Lancet *1*:289, 1981.

McCracken, G. H., Hardy, J. B., Chen, T. C., Hoffman, L. S., Gilkeson, M. R., and Sever, J. L.: Serum immunoglobulin levels in newborn infants. II. Survey of cord and follow up sera from 123 infants with congenital rubella. J. Pediatr. *74*:383, 1969.

Medovy, H.: Western equine encephalomyelitis in infants. J. Pediatr. *22*:308, 1943.

Meyers, J. D.: Congenital varicella in term infants: risk reconsidered. J. Infect. Dis. *129*:215, 1974.

Modlin, J. F.: Fatal echovirus II disease in premature neonates. Pediatrics *66*:775, 1980.

Murphy, A. M., Albrey, M. B., and Crewe, E. B.: Rotavirus infections in neonates. Lancet *2*:1149, 1977.

Nagington, J., Wreghitt, T. C., Gandy, G., Robertson, N. R. C., and Berry, P. J.: Fatal echovirus II infections in outbreak in special-care baby unit. Lancet *2*:725, 1978.

Nahmias, A. J., Josey, W. E., Naib, Z. M., et al.: Perinatal risk associated with maternal genital herpes simplex virus infection. Am. J. Obstet. Gynecol. *110*:825, 1971.

Nahmias, A. J., and Roizman, B.: Infection with herpes-simplex viruses 1 and 2. N. Engl. J. Med. *289*:667, 719, 781, 1973.

Nahmias, A. J., and Visintine, A. M.: Herpes simplex. *In* Remington, J. S., and Klein, J. O. (Eds.): Infectious Diseases of the Fetus and Newborn Infant. Philadelphia, W. B. Saunders Co., 1976, pp. 156–190.

Okada, K., Kamiyama, I., Inomata, M., et al.: e Antigen and anti-e in the serum of asymptomatic carrier mothers as indicators of positive and negative transmission of hepatitis B virus to their infants. N. Engl. J. Med. *294*:746, 1976.

Overall, J. C., and Glasgow, L. A.: Virus infections of the fetus and newborn infant. J. Pediatr. *77*:315, 1970.

Pass, R. F., Stagno, S., Myers, G. J., and Alford, C. A.: Outcome of symptomatic congenital cytomegalovirus infection: results of long-term longitudinal follow-up. Pediatrics *66*:758, 1980.

Phelan, P., and Campbell, P.: Pulmonary complications of rubella embryopathy. J. Pediatr. *75*:202, 1969.

Reynolds, D. W., Stagno, S., Hosty, T. S., Tiller, M., and Alford, C. A.: Maternal cytomegalovirus excretion and perinatal infection. N. Engl. J. Med. *289*:1, 1973.

Reynolds, D. W., Stagno, S., Stubbs, K. G., et al.: Inapparent congenital cytomegalovirus infection with elevated cord IgM levels: causal relation with auditory and mental deficiency. N. Engl. J. Med. *290*:291, 1974.

Robino, G., Perlman, A., et al.: Fatal neonatal infection due to coxsackie B2 virus. J. Pediatr. *61*:911, 1962.

Rudolph, A. J., Singleton, E. B., et al.: Osseous manifestations of congenital rubella syndrome. Am. J. Dis. Child. *110*:428, 1965.

Sells, C. J., Carpenter, R. L., and Ray, G. C.: Sequelae of central nervous system enterovirus infections. N. Engl. J. Med. *293*:1, 1975.

Shinefield, H. R., and Townsend, T. E.: Transplacental transmission of western equine encephalomyelitis in twins. J. Pediatr. *43*:21, 1953.

Soothill, J. E., Hayes, K., and Dudgeon, J. A.: The immunoglobulins in congenital rubella. Lancet *1*:1385, 1966.

South, M. A., Tompkins, W. A. F., et al.: Congenital malformation of the central nervous system associated with genital type (type 2) herpesvirus. J. Pediatr. *75*:13, 1969.

Srabstein, J. C., Morris, N., Larke, R. P. B., et al.: Is there a congenital varicella syndrome? J. Pediatr. *84*:239, 1974.

Stagno, S., Brasfield, D. M., Brown, M. B., et al.: Infant pneumonitis associated with cytomegalovirus, *Chlamydia*, Pneumocystis and Ureaplasma: a prospective study. Pediatrics *68*:322, 1981.

Stagno, S., Reynolds, D. W., Huang, E.-S., et al.: Congenital cytomegalovirus infection: occurrence in an immune population. N. Engl. J. Med. *296*:1254, 1977.

Starr, J. G., Bart, R. D., Jr., and Gold, E.: Inapparent congenital cytomegalovirus infection: clinical and epidemiological characteristics in early infancy. N. Engl. J. Med. *282*:1075, 1970.

Steinhoff, M. C.: Rotavirus: the first five years. J. Pediatr. *96*:611, 1980.

Ueda, K., Nishida, Y., Oshina, K., and Shepard, T. H.: Congenital rubella syndrome: correlation of gestational age at time of maternal rubella with type of defect. J. Pediatr. *94*:763, 1979.

Visintine, A. M., Nahmias, A. J., and Josey, W. E.: Genital herpes. Perinatal Care *2*:32, 1978.

Weil, M. L., et al.: Chronic progressive panencephalitis due to rubella virus simulating subacute sclerosing panencephalitis. N. Engl. J. Med. *292*:994, 1975.

Weller, T. H.: The cytomegaloviruses: ubiquitous agents with protean clinical manifestations. Part I, N. Engl. J. Med. *285*:203; Part II, *285*:267, 1971.

Weller, T. H., and Hanshaw, J. B.: Virologic and clinical observations on cytomegalic inclusion disease. N. Engl. J. Med. *266*:1233, 1962.

Weller, T. H., Macauley, J. C., et al.: Isolation of intranuclear inclusion producing agents from infants with illnesses resembling cytomegalic inclusion disease. Proc. Soc. Exp. Biol. Med. *94*:4, 1957.

Whitley, R. J., Nahmias, A. J., Soong, S.-J., et al.: Vidarabine therapy of neonatal herpes simplex virus infections. Pediatrics *66*:495, 1980.

Whitley, R. J., Nahmias, A. J., Visintine, A. M., Fleming, C. L., and Alford, C. A.: The natural history of herpes simplex virus infection of mother and newborn. Pediatrics *66*:489, 1980.

Wilfert, C. M., Thompson, R. J., Jr., Sunder, T. R., et al.: Longitudinal assessment of children with enteroviral meningitis during the first three months of life. Pediatrics *67*:811, 1981.

Yeager, A. S., Arvin, A. M., Urbani, L. J., and Kemp, J. A.: The relationship of antibody to outcome in neonatal herpes simplex infections. Infect. Immunol. *29*:532, 1980.

Yeager, A. S., Grumet, F. C., Hafleigh, E. B., et al.: Prevention of transfusion-acquired cytomegalovirus infections in newborn infants. J. Pediatr. *98*:281, 1981.

86

Coccidioidomycosis

Coccidioidomycosis is very rare in newborn infants but has been reported. In 1964, Ziering and Rockas described a 3-month-old infant whose initial symptoms appeared within the first month. In addition to the rare adult-to-infant transmission of coccidioidomycosis, it also appears that infants can be infected by porous fomites brought from an endemic area to one in which the disease is rare (Rothman et al.). This brief summary of the example described by Townsend and McKey will serve to illustrate the problems of diagnosis and treatment.

CASE 86–1

A 3-week-old white female infant had been well until 2 days before admission. The only pertinent fact in the family history was that the father had lived in the San Joaquin Valley for 12 years. The infant exhibited high fever, irritability and anorexia. She was acutely ill, with a temperature of 104° F, respirations 132 per minute. She was pale, and her neck was slightly stiff. Her fontanel was full but not tense. Hemoglobin was 12.3 gm and fell to 8.2 gm after 1 week. White blood cells numbered 71,800 and fell gradually to 19,800 with normal differential counts. Cerebrospinal fluid showed 700 cells, 80 per cent polymorphonuclears, 195 mg of protein, and 15 mg of sugar on admission. Cell count within the next month varied from 5 to 98, protein from 46 to 64 mg, and sugar from 34 to 49 mg. Cerebrospinal fluid cultures, negative on four occasions, finally became positive for C. immitis *one month after admission. The organism could never be grown from urine, blood, bone marrow, or gastric washings. Complement fixation was positive for* C. immitis, *4 +, in the first dilution.*

The patient seemed better 5 days after multiple antibiotic therapy had been started, but then her temperature began to spike. Radiographs showed patchy infiltration of both lungs. The spleen gradually became larger; infiltration of lungs spread. Rimifon, streptomycin, and para-aminosalicylic acid were given. In spite of this therapy, cervical nodes and spleen grew larger, a papular rash appeared over the trunk, and the infant grew steadily weaker and died 2 months after admission. Autopsy showed disseminated coccidioidomycosis.

Interesting and disturbing is the fact that repeated coccidioidin skin test results were never positive.

Comment. This 3-week-old infant did not live in, but was exposed to a father who had lived in, the circumscribed desert region in our Southwest in which coccidioidomycosis is endemic. The infection

Fungus Infections

Revised by Kenneth McIntosh*

manifested itself first as a meningoencephalitis, followed by progressing pneumonitis and disseminated lesions, producing splenomegaly, glandular enlargement, and an exanthem. No thrombocytopenia or purpura ever appeared. The skin test result never became positive. Cerebrospinal fluid cultures did not become positive for the fungus until 1 month after the onset. The complement fixation test gave the earliest confirmation of the diagnosis.

Ziering and Rockas achieved a notable success in treatment of their very ill patient, who had extensive pulmonary lesions plus subcutaneous abscesses, osteitis and periostitis, and iridocyclitis. The infant was given courses of amphotericin B over a period of 18 months without toxic effects. His complement fixation titer diminished and his skin test became positive, indications of marked improvement.

The first report of maternal-infant transmission was a fatal case found by Bernstein and coworkers in 1981. Their patient, born at 36 to 37 weeks' gestation to a mother who had cervical coccidioidomycosis and membranes that had been ruptured for 24 hours, was febrile at 5 days of age and had extensive pneumonia by 6 days. The organisms were seen on gram stain of the tracheal aspirate and confirmed in postmortem cultures. The course was fulminant, with death at 10 days of age.

Cryptococcosis

Cryptococcosis is caused by infection with *Torula histolytica* (*Cryptococcus neoformans*). It is important in the newborn because it invades the central nervous system, where it sets up a meningoencephalitis that closely resembles that produced by *Toxoplasma* and cytomegalovirus. Some of the earliest examples were reported by Neuhauser and Tucker in 1948. Emanuel and colleagues were able to find 23 affected children reported in the literature to 1961. Three definite and three almost certain cases involved illness within the first month of life.

Pathogenesis. *Cryptococcus* is an occasional inhabitant of the female genital tract, and it is believed

---

* This chapter includes some contributions from a previous author, Dr. Arnold Smith.

that the infant acquires infection during passage through the birth canal. Symptoms begin so promptly after birth in some cases that one is forced to think seriously that infection may be transmitted transplacentally. It is, however, of interest that strains of *C. neoformans* pathogenic for humans have been isolated from cow's milk, with or without concomitant bovine mastitis (Emmons, 1953; Pounder et al., 1952).

Diagnosis. The diagnosis and course of three patients with cryptococcosis who were reported by Neuhauser and Tucker are illustrated in the following case histories.

CASE 86–2

A 7-week-old male infant was admitted to hospital. He had been born after a precipitous delivery and was cyanotic after birth, requiring resuscitation. Twitchings and rigidity followed on the second day and did not entirely disappear for several weeks. He never ate well, and, despite tube-feeding, he did not gain weight. Upon admission he was emaciated and chronically ill. The head was a bit large, there were cataracts in both eyes, and the spleen and liver were large. Opisthotonos, ankle clonus, and positive Babinski reflex marked his neurologic examination. Cerebrospinal and subdural fluid contained an excess of protein and many red blood cells. Blood cell count was unremarkable, but no mention was made of platelets. He died suddenly after having been in hospital for 3 weeks. In this case it is difficult to date the onset, since many of the early symptoms might easily have stemmed from intracranial damage sustained at the time of birth.

CASE 86–3

The course of Neuhauser and Tucker's second patient began quite differently, the reason for admission on the nineteenth day of life being persistent, severe jaundice from birth. Abdominal enlargement was noted at 1 week; the urine was dark, and the stools were light. The spleen and liver were huge. Temperature never exceeded 100° F. He died 4 days after admission. No cause other than the patient's torula infection was found for the jaundice. Platelets were not mentioned. In this example, one wonders whether infection may not have begun before birth.

CASE 86–4

The third case of Neuhauser and Tucker again differed from the other two in mode of onset. The infant began to have convulsions and incessant crying at 2 weeks of age and was admitted to hospital 4 days later.

He was well at birth and until he was 2 weeks old. The head, heart, and lungs seemed normal on examination. The liver and spleen were very large. Neurologic examination showed only hyperactive reflexes. The platelets numbered only 66,000 per cubic millimeter. Otherwise the blood was normal, as was the urine. On the ninth hospital day, the infant had gross hematuria. Death occurred on the following day.

Comment. Radiographs of the skulls in all three cases showed spotty calcifications within the substance of the brain. In Case 86–4, interstitial pneumonitis, focal atelectasis, and a large granulomatous lesion in the right upper lobe were noted on the chest radiograph. Two infants showed chorioretinitis, and two showed physical signs of central nervous system involvement. All had hepatosplenomegaly. Fever was almost nonexistent in all. All showed hydrocephalus and diffuse areas of focal degeneration throughout their brains.

It is clear that Cases 86–2 and 86–4 are virtually indistinguishable from toxoplasmosis of early life on the basis of history and physical findings alone, whereas the story in Case 86–3, with the principal involvement in the liver, is highly suggestive of either cytomegalic inclusion disease or viral hepatitis. Diagnosis will depend on (1) exclusion of toxoplasmosis by Sabin's dye test and complement fixation studies, and (2) exclusion of cytomegalic inclusion disease by inability to demonstrate inclusion bodies in the cells or urinary sediment or of gastric washings and by virus culture. *Cryptococcus* has been seen in and cultivated from the cerebrospinal fluid of newborn infants five times, twice ante mortem and three times post mortem.

Treatment. Amphotericin B in a total intravenous dose of 30 mg per kilogram over a 3-week period may be adequate therapy for disseminated disease with meningoencephalitis. In treating serious systemic fungal diseases in infants and children, we first administer a test dose of amphotericin B (0.1 mg/kg) intravenously over a ½-hour period. If this is tolerated without rash, fever, or fall in blood pressure over the ensuing 3 hours, the maintenance dose is immediately begun (0.75 to 1.0 mg/kg/day in a single infusion over several hours intravenously). Gradually increasing the dose by increments over several days has, in our experience, not been necessary. In cases that progressively deteriorate or relapse, intrathecal therapy, in addition to the intravenous route, often produces a cure, particularly in the absence of underlying disease (Edwards et al. 1970; Sarosi et al., 1969). Since intrathecal therapy is often necessary over a protracted course, an intraventricular reservoir can facilitate this route if used with knowledge of the potential hazards (Diamond and Bennett, 1973). 5-Fluorocytosine (5-FC) should not be used alone, as the emergence of 5-FC–resistant strains has been a major cause of treatment failure with this drug (Block et al., 1973). This drug may have a role when used with amphotericin B because the combination is synergistic in vitro and in vivo (Medoff et al., 1971). Clinical trials with this combination are not available in adults or in children.

Disseminated Histoplasmosis

No very young infant has been observed who has suffered from the primary pulmonary form of histoplasmosis or from the localized granulomatous variety that involves skin, oropharynx, larynx, or other viscera. This brief discussion will be limited therefore to the general disseminated form.

Incidence. The disease is widespread in the United States and elsewhere, but certain areas seem to be heavily contaminated and their populations infected in large numbers. Cases are by no means confined to the broad central belt of high infection rate of which Tennessee appears to be the center. In the eastern United States, the shore counties of Maryland are the source of an appreciable number of histoplasma infections. Children below 2 years seem to be highly susceptible, and when they become infected, they almost always have the disseminated form. Cases developing within the first month of life are extremely uncommon, but many examples have been reported in the third month and later.

Etiology. The invading organism is a fungus, *Histoplasma capsulatum*. Depending on environmental conditions, the fungus may grow in a yeast-like phase or in a mycelial phase. It is found in the soil in the mycelial phase, and it is from the soil that most human infection appears to be derived.

Diagnosis. Infected infants become ill with fever that often spikes to high levels once a day accompanied by rapid enlargement of the spleen and liver, bronchopneumonic pulmonary infiltrations of nonspecific nature, progressive anemia, and thrombocytopenia. The disease resembles disseminated tuberculosis in some respects but differs from it in that histoplasmosis is associated with a greater degree of hepatosplenomegaly, has no miliary pulmonary involvement, and fails to invade the meninges. Its later appearance, the usual but not invariable absence of jaundice, and again its aversion to the central nervous system distinguish it from cytomegalic inclusion disease and toxoplasmosis. Differentiation from coccidioidomycosis and torulosis, which also make their appearance toward the end of the first month or later, may be impossible on clinical grounds alone. One will be influenced somewhat by geographic and epidemiologic considerations, but the final diagnosis will depend on laboratory investigations.

A positive histoplasmin skin test is of use, but the result may be negative in as many as half the early acute cases as well as in those patients who are severely ill with the disease. Histoplasmin reactions are not infrequently positive when other fungi are the responsible etiologic agents. By far the most reliable laboratory indication of the disease is growth of *Histoplasma capsulatum* from peripheral blood, liver biopsy, or bone marrow samples, especially the latter. The chief objection to this test is the length of time one must wait for the answer. Quickest and quite reliable confirmation can be obtained from demonstration of specific histoplasmosis (H) and mycelia (M) precipitin bands by the micro-Ouchterlony technique (Holland and Holland, 1966).

Treatment. Amphotericin B is the only effective therapy. Little and coworkers reported four cures in children, three of whom were 3, 5, and 8 months of age at the time treatment was begun. The drug is given intravenously, in a daily dosage of 0.25 to 1.0 mg per kilogram, dissolved in 5 per cent dextrose to a concentration not exceeding 1.0 mg per 10 ml. The infusion must be given slowly over a period of several hours. Infusions are continued for 4 to 8 weeks, daily at first, later every alternate day. Headache, nausea, vomiting, and, in some babies, anaphylactoid reactions are not uncommon side effects, but they need not contraindicate continuation of therapy. We achieved a notable success by this method in a nearly moribund 4-month-old baby.

Candidiasis (Moniliasis)

Oral and cutaneous candidiasis are discussed in Chapter 99 (see p. 881). We shall not provide a detailed consideration of this topic here but shall instead confine ourselves to a brief review of several of the complications of thrush that are of interest to the neonatologist.

Attention should be called to the demonstration that gentian violet in the 1 per cent aqueous solution commonly used to treat oral thrush can cause mucous membrane lesions (Slotkowsky, 1957).

DISSEMINATED CANDIDIASIS

This once rare disease is now becoming common in many nurseries. This is probably the result of the intensive use of broad-spectrum antibiotics in premature (and more vulnerable) infants and developmental, suboptimal leukocytic phagocytosis and killing of *Candida albicans* (Xanthou et al., 1975), but the most important factor is the use of central venous hyperalimentation. *Candida albicans* grows in all alimentation solutions in use, but the rate depends on composition and temperature (Goldmann and Maki, 1973). The organisms can reach densities of approximately 100,000 per ml, and yet the solution appears clear to the eye; further infection due to contaminated intravenous fluids produces an insidious infection. A description of a typical case, reported by Hill and coworkers, follows.

CASE 86–5

The patient was a 1928-gm infant born to a 33-year-old primigravida at approximately 32 weeks' gestation. The infant, who was delivered by cesarean section because of placenta previa, required intubation and resuscitation in the delivery room. Because of persistent respiratory distress and periods of apnea, the patient was transferred to the University of Minnesota Neonatal Intensive Care Unit at approximately 12 hours of age. Severe hyaline membrane disease necessitated the use of respiratory therapy, and an umbilical artery catheter was inserted to monitor blood gases.

On the fifth hospital day, apnea, acidosis, and questionable pneumatosis intestinalis observed on an abdominal radiograph prompted the institution and continuance of penicillin and kanamycin therapy, although blood, urine, and cerebrospinal fluid cultures remained sterile. Hyperalimentation through the umbilical arterial catheter was started on the sixth hospital day. On the ninth hospital day, a recurrence of apnea and acidosis prompted repeat cultures, and the antibiotic therapy was changed to ampicillin and gentamicin. The patient improved clinically, but after 4 days Candida albicans *grew out in the blood culture drawn on the ninth day. The catheter in the umbilical artery was removed and replaced 12 hours later with an internal jugular venous catheter, and amphotericin B therapy was initiated. Four days later, after three negative blood cultures and a negative cerebrospinal fluid culture were obtained, the amphotericin B was discontinued. Urine cultures continued to yield 7000 to 50,000 colonies of* C. albicans *per milliliter. On the twenty-sixth hospital day, 17 days after the initial positive blood cultures, edema of feet, ankles, and knees was observed. This was considered to have a vascular etiology, and the extremities were elevated.*

On the twenty-ninth hospital day, bilateral knee and ankle effusions developed and were accompanied by warmth and erythema. Synovial fluid contained numerous polymorphonuclear leukocytes (PMNs), but no organisms were seen on direct examination. Candida albicans *subsequently grew from fluid obtained from both knees and the left ankle. Repeat urine cultures yielded 100,000 colonies of* C. albicans *per milliliter, although blood cultures remained sterile. A cerebrospinal fluid specimen obtained on the twenty-ninth hospital day contained six PMNs and 22 monocytes with a glucose of 29 mg per 100 ml and protein of 84 mg per 100 ml. This specimen also yielded* C. albicans *on culture.*

Comment. This case illustrates several important principles in the diagnosis of disseminated candidiasis. The infection is septicemic, with blood cultures yielding the organism and the urine containing the organisms cleared by the kidney. Blood cultures obtained through the hyperalimentation catheter do sample infected thrombi adjacent to the tip but do not aid in differentiating between disease that will resolve with catheter removal (Ellis and Spivack, 1967) and life-threatening illness. Peripheral blood cultures obtained by venipuncture are a more reliable indicator of ongoing candidemia. In overwhelming infections the organisms can be seen in stained smears of buffy coat preparations (Silverman et al., 1973). Skin lesions can be seen (Bodey and Luna, 1973) that yield the organism on aspiration. Candida ophthalmitis is an occasional complication of candidemia (Fishman et al., 1972) and can serve as a focus for continued candidemia (Haring et al., 1973). Every infant in whom the diagnosis of candidal sepsis is suspected should have indirect funduscopic examination. Other manifestations of candidal sepsis in newborns are osteomyelitis (Freeman et al., 1974; Adler et al., 1972; Klein et al., 1972), meningitis, endocarditis (Joshi and Wang, 1973; Shapira et al., 1974), and arthritis.

Because of the importance of host factors, the course of disseminated candidiasis is unpredictable, making therapeutic generalizations impossible. If the infection is catheter related, the catheter should be removed. In most instances, amphotericin B is administered until it is clear that there are no occult foci. In patients with meningitis or progressive clinical deterioration, 5-fluorocytosine is used in combination with amphotericin B.

CONGENITAL CANDIDIASIS

Many examples of candidal infection acquired in utero have been reported by now. Dvorak and Gavaller's patient, reported in 1966, had a diffuse macular rash and respiratory distress at birth and died at 34 hours of age. Autopsy showed extensive bronchopneumonia, the sections filled with hyphae and spores. The placenta was also heavily infected with the fungus.

In these instances, ascending infection produces chorioamnionitis with dissemination to the fetus, which can lead to spontaneous abortion (Ho and Aterman, 1970). In most instances, the severity of disseminated candidiasis acquired in utero is such that the infant expires before therapy can be considered (Schirar et al., 1974).

On the one hand, cutaneous candidiasis, evident at the time of birth, can be seen in the absence of systemic involvement (Rhatigan, 1968; Aterman, 1968). On the other hand, cases of systemic candidiasis, probably acquired in utero, have been described in the absence of rash (Johnson et al., 1981). The rash, when it does occur, evolves from maculopapular to vesicular to pustular.

It thus appears that *Candida*, like bacteria, may infect the fetus by hematogenous dissemination from the umbilical vessels, leading to systemic infection, or be limited to cutaneous candidiasis.

Adams reported that five of eight infants who had oral thrush showed respiratory distress, cyanosis, and leukocytosis. They all had signs of pneumonitis. In one who died, it was found that *Candida* had invaded the pulmonary parenchyma, and the author believed this to have been an example of true thrush pneumonitis. Winter cannot accept Adams' autopsied case as one of mycotic pneumonia but believes that this complication has been demonstrated beyond doubt in a 1-year-old and in a number of older persons.

More recently it has become an unexpected finding at autopsies of newborn infants (Koenig, 1971). The course was not always fulminant, and there is little specificity to the roentgenographic picture. Infants with thrush and pneumonia should be suspected of having *Candida* as the infecting agent, particularly if they have been pretreated with broad spectrum antibiotics. Isolation of *Candida albicans* from the blood of such infants is strongly suggestive of bronchopulmonary candidiasis, but demonstration of hyphae in tracheal aspirates or pulmonary tissue is the best evidence of infection. This is often difficult and hazardous because of the concomitant thrush and problems of bronchoscopy in sick infants.

Beckmann and Navarro recorded the following case history.

CASE 86–6

A 4 pound 11 ounce (2125 gm) infant was discharged from the nursery on the tenth day of life, well except for thick deposits of thrush upon the tongue. Gentian violet and 2 per cent ferric chloride solution were used locally, but the lesion became ulcerative and spread to involve all the oral and buccal mucous membranes. Cyanosis during feeding appeared, and rales were heard throughout both lungs. At 3 months of age, the infant was admitted to hospital, weighing 5 pounds 6 ounces (2435 gm). His temperature was 98.6° F and never rose during his stay. He was malnourished, cyanotic, and critically ill. There were mucopurulent nasal and oral discharges. Radiographs showed patches of pneumonia, atelectasis, and emphysema. Attempted feeding caused choking and cyanosis. Intravenous fluid therapy, transfusion, penicillin, and Gantrisin failed to improve his condition. Mycostatin, 175,000 units orally every 6 hours, was begun. Within 48 hours his mouth was practically healed! The respiratory difficulty improved more slowly and was not gone until the second week.

Comment. The authors admit that the diagnosis of *C. albicans* pneumonitis was far from proved but believe that the response to the fungicidal antibiotic was striking enough to be highly suggestive.

THRUSH ESOPHAGITIS

A not inconsiderable number of cases have been reported in which oral thrush has advanced to involve the nasopharynx and the esophagus. When this occurs, swallowing becomes almost impossible, and during the attempts to swallow, much liquid appears to be aspirated into the tracheobronchial tree. Choking spells with cyanosis result.

Wolff and coworkers reported two examples from Birmingham, England. The first is described in the following case history.

CASE 86–7

A female infant weighed 6 pounds (2720 gm) at birth and seemed well until her sixteenth day, when anorexia and vomiting began. When she was admitted the next day, her general condition seemed good, but the tongue and buccal mucous membranes were covered with a white membrane from which C. albicans *was identified by smear. After 3 days of treatment with 1 per cent gentian violet locally and 0.01 per cent solution (4 ml, 3 times a day orally), there was no improvement. It did not respond to sulfonamide or, later, to penicillin. Profuse viscid discharge from the mouth and nose appeared. At this stage the infant could not swallow, and attempts led to repeated bouts of cyanosis. On the eighth day, hydroxystilbamidine was begun, 15 mg (5 mg per kilogram) in 0.75 ml of water injected slowly into the intravenous infusion tubing. This was repeated every 12 hours. A staphylococcus, coagulase-positive, was grown from the blood. Streptomycin was given in addition to the other drug. Improvement began while the infant was on hydroxystilbamidine alone. After 6 days, the intravenous drip was removed, and oral feedings were started. On the eighteenth day, barium swallow showed that incoordination of swallowing was still present, with much iodized oil entering the trachea during the act of deglutition. Gavage feedings were begun again and were able to be discontinued 1 week later.*

Comment. Such contiguous spread should be suspected in infants with thrush when swallowing becomes difficult and aspiration seems to be taking place. Not surprisingly, the contiguous spread can be more anterior and produce signs and symptoms of congenital stridor (Perrone, 1970).

ENTERIC CANDIDIASIS

Kozinn and Taschdjian deplore the tendency to forget the possibility of enteric candidiasis in the differential diagnosis of diarrhea in the young infant. They stress that it is a not uncommon complication of thrush and that it may lead to systemic invasion and death.

The diagnosis should be suspected whenever diarrhea complicates thrush or cutaneous candidiasis, especially if the infant has been on antimicrobial therapy. Direct examination of stools reveals in many cases the mycelial form of the fungus, a finding that is much more significant than visualization of yeast forms.

Good clinical response and disappearance of the organisms can be attained with nystatin in 80 per cent of cases. Amphotericin B may be helpful in severe cases.

REFERENCES

Adams, J. M.: A reevaluation of the pneumonias of infancy. J. Pediatr. 25:369, 85, 1944.

Adler, S., Randall, J., and Plotkin, S. A.: Candidal osteomyelitis and arthritis in a neonate. Am. J. Dis. Child. 123:595, 1972.

Ashcraft, K. W., and Leape, L. L.: Candida sepsis complicating parenteral feeding. J.A.M.A. 212:454, 1970.

Aterman, K.: Pathology of candida infection of the umbilical cord. Am. J. Clin. Pathol. 49:798, 1968.

Beckmann, A. J., and Navarro, J. E.: Pneumonia complicating oral thrush treated with mycostatin, a new antifungal antibiotic. J. Pediatr. 46:587, 1955.

Bernstein, D. I., Tipton, J. R., Schott, S. F., and Cherry, J. D.: Coccidioidomycosis in a neonate; maternal-infant transmission. J. Pediatr. 99:752, 1981.

Block, E. R., Jennings, A. E., and Bennett, J. E.: 5-Fluorocytosine resistance in Cryptococcus neoformans. Antimicrob. Agents Chemother. 3:649, 1973.

Bodey, G. P., and Luna, M.: Skin lesions associated with disseminated candidiasis. J.A.M.A. 229:1466, 1974.

Burry, A. F.: Hydrocephalus after intra-uterine fungal infection. Arch. Dis. Child. 32:161, 1957.

Diamond, R. D., and Bennett, J. E.: A subcutaneous reservoir for intrathecal therapy of fungal meningitis. N. Engl. J. Med. 288:186, 1973.

Dvorak, A. M., and Gavaller, B.: Congenital systemic candidiasis: report of a case. N. Engl. J. Med. 274:540, 1966.

Edwards, V. E., Sutherland, J. M., and Tyner, J. H.: Cryptococcosis of the central nervous system. J. Neurol. Neurosurg. Psych. 33:415, 1970.

Ellis, C. A., and Spivack, M. L.: The significance of candidemia. Ann. Intern. Med. 67:511, 1967.

Emanuel, B., Ching, E., Lieberman, A. D., and Golden, M.: Cryptococcus meningitis in a child successfully treated with amphotericin B, with a review of the literature. J. Pediatr. 59:577, 1961.

Emmons, C. W.: Cryptococcus neoformans, strains from an outbreak of bovine mastitis. Mycopathol. Mycol. Appl. 6:231, 1953.

Fishman, L. S., Griffin, J. R., and Sapico, F. L.: Hematogenous candida endophthalmitis: a complication of candidemia. N. Engl. J. Med. 286:675, 1972.

Freeman, J. B., Wienke, J. W., and Soper, R. T.: Candida osteomyelitis associated with intravenous alimentation. J. Pediatr. Surg. 9:783, 1974.

Goldmann, D. A., and Maki, D. G.: Infection control in total parenteral nutrition. J.A.M.A. 223:1360, 1973.

Haring, H., Johnston, R., and Touloukian, R.: Successfully treated candida endophthalmitis. Pediatrics 51:1027, 1973.

Heiner, D. C.: Diagnosis of histoplasmosis. Pediatrics 22:616, 1958.

Henderson, J. L.: Infection in the newborn. Edinburgh Med. J. 50:535, 1943.

Hill, H. R., Mitchell, T. G., Matsen, J. M., et al.: Recovery from disseminated candidiasis in a premature neonate. Pediatrics 53:748, 1974.

Ho, C. Y., and Aterman, K.: Infection of the fetus by candida in a spontaneous abortion. Am. J. Obstet. Gynecol. 106:705, 1970.

Holland, P., and Holland, N. H.: Histoplasmosis in early infancy: hematologic, histochemical and immunologic observations. Am. J. Dis. Child. 112:412, 1966.

Johnson, D. E., Thompson, T. R., and Ferrieri, P.: Congenital candidiasis. Am. J. Dis. Child. 135:273, 1981.

Joshi, W., and Wang, N. S.: Repeated pulmonary embolism in an infant with subacute candida endocarditis of the right side of the heart. Am. J. Dis. Child. 125:257, 1973.

Klein, J. D., Yamauchi, T., and Horlick, S. P.: Neonatal candidiasis meningitis and arthritis: observations and review of literature. J. Pediatr. 81:31, 1972.

Koenig, N. D.: Candida pneumonia in newborn infants. Dtsch. Med. Wochenschr. 96:818, 1971.

Kozinn, P., and Taschdjian, C. L.: Enteric candidiasis: diagnosis and clinical considerations. Pediatrics 30:71, 1962.

Little, J., Bruce, J., Andrews, H., Crawford, K., and McKinley, G.: Treatment of disseminated infantile histoplasmosis with amphotericin B. Pediatrics 24:1, 1959.

Medoff, G., Comfort, M., and Kobayoshi, G. S.: Synergistic action of amphotericin B and 5-fluorocytosine against yeast-like organisms. Proc. Soc. Exp. Biol. Med. 138:571, 1971.

Neuhauser, E. B. D., and Tucker, A.: The roentgen changes produced by diffuse torulosis in the newborn. Am. J. Roentgenol. 59:805, 1948.

Perrone, J. A.: Laryngeal obstruction due to Monilia albicans in a newborn. Laryngoscope 80:288, 1970.

Peterson, J. C., and Christie, A.: Histoplasmosis. Pediatr. Clin. North Am. 2:127, 1955.

Pounder, W. D., Amberson, J. M., and Jaeger, R. F.: A severe mastitis problem associated with Cryptococcus neoformans in a large dairy herd. Am. J. Vet. Res. 13:121, 1952.

Rhatigan, R. M.: Congenital cutaneous candidiasis. Am. J. Dis. Child. 116:545, 1968.

Rothman, P. E., Graw, R. G., and Harria, J. C.: Coccidioidomycosis—possible fomite transmission. Am. J. Dis. Child. 118:792, 1962.

Sarosi, G. A., Parker, J. D., Doto, I. L., and Tosh, F. E.: Amphotericin B in cryptococcal meningitis. Ann. Intern. Med. 71:1079, 1969.

Schirar, A., Rendu, C., Vielk, J. P., et al.: Congenital mycosis (Candida albicans). Biol. Neonate 24:273, 1974.

Shapira, Y., Drucker, M., Russell, A., et al.: Candida endocarditis and encephalitis in an infant. Clin. Pediatr. 13:542, 1974.

Shatai, T.: Neonatal coccidioidomycosis in premature twins. Am. J. Dis. Child. 132:634, 1978.

Silverman, E. M., Norman, L. F., and Goldman, R. T.: Diagnosis of systemic candidiasis in smears of venous blood stained with Wright's stain. Am. J. Clin. Pathol. 60:473, 1973.

Slotkowsky, E. L.: Formation of mucous membrane lesions secondary to prolonged use of one percent aqueous gentian violet. J. Pediatr. 51:652, 1957.

Townsend, T. E., and McKey, R. W.: Coccidioidomycosis in infants. Am. J. Dis. Child. 86:51, 1953.

Winter, W. G., Jr.: Candida (Monilia) infections in children. Pediatr. Clin. North Am. 2:151, 1955.

Wolff, O. H., Petty, B. W., Astley, R., and Smellie, J. M.: Thrush oesophagitis with pharyngeal incoordination treated with hydroxystilbamidine. Lancet 1:991, 1955.

Xanthou, M., Valassi-Adawn, E., Kintzonidou, E., et al.: Phagocytosis and killing ability of Candida albicans by blood leukocytes of healthy term and preterm babies. Arch. Dis. Child. 50:72, 1975.

Ziering, W. H., and Rockas, H. R.: Coccidioidomycosis: Long-term treatment with amphotericin B of disseminated disease in a three-month-old baby. Am. J. Dis. Child. 108:454, 1964.

87

One of the organisms that causes congenital infection of the human fetus, often presenting in the newborn period as a local or generalized disease, is *Toxoplasma gondii.* It is obscure why this agent, so different in its biology from cytomegalovirus, rubella, and *Treponema pallidum,* should present so similar a clinical picture. Differentiation from these other syndromes on clinical and laboratory grounds is essential to treatment and prognosis and depends on the extensive knowledge of its epidemiology, clinical behavior, and microbiology gained since the 1960s.

Incidence.   Inapparent infection with the protozoon is widespread throughout the world. Population samples indicate that the percentage of adults with antibody is increased at lower geographical latitudes. Feldman found approximately 10 per cent positives by complement fixation tests in Iceland, 30 per cent in New Orleans, and 65 per cent in Tahiti. However, latitude is by no means the only determining factor. The number of positive reactors in Paris, for instance, is unusually high and has been attributed to Parisians' fondness for raw or undercooked meat. With regard to congenital toxoplasmosis, Eichenwald was able to comment on the clinical findings in 75 infants and children, Feldman in 103, indicating that the disease cannot be considered rare.

Serum specimens from 23,000 pregnant women in the Collaborative Perinatal Research Project were studied by Sever for evidence of infection with *Toxoplasma.* Thirty-eight per cent of the women had evidence of toxoplasmosis at some time in the past. Five infants among the group had definite congenital toxoplasmosis. The most recent estimates of frequency of congenital infection in the United States range from 1 to 4 in 1000 livebirths.

Desmonts and Couvreur, reporting from Paris, found 183 women considered to have been infected during pregnancy. The overall rate of infection in their survey was 6.3 per 100 pregnancies. There were 11 abortions, seven stillbirths, and 59 patients with congenital toxoplasmosis. In this latter group, two infants died, seven had severe disease, 11 had mild disease, and 39 had no symptoms or signs at the time of the survey.

Etiology.   The disease is caused by infestation with a protozoon, *Toxoplasma gondii,* so named because it was first isolated in 1909 from a North African rodent called the "gondi." In addition to the large number of human beings who are infected, many domestic and wild animals and birds harbor the organism. The domestic cat is the only definitive host and is the reservoir of the infective oocysts that are

Protozoal Infections: Congenital Toxoplasmosis

Revised by Kenneth McIntosh

passed in the feces. Congenital toxoplasmosis is caused by invasion of the fetal blood stream by parasites during a stage of maternal parasitemia. It is likely that the parasitemia occurs only with initial infection and often in the absence of any maternal symptoms. Mothers whose infections become chronic and inapparent do not transmit the disease to subsequent fetuses. Desmonts and Couvreur describe infection of the fetus in 33 per cent of all maternal infections. This figure should, however, be considered only an estimate because many mothers in this study were treated. The proportion infected is high throughout pregnancy, although severe disease in the newborn is seen only with first and second trimester infections.

Postnatal infections also occur in children, but the youngest patient we have encountered in the literature is a 7-month infant who became ill with diarrhea at 3 months of age. The disease occurred 1 month after the institution of unpasteurized goat's milk feeding and was almost surely the result of that form of alimentation (Riemann et al., 1975).

Pathology.   The toxoplasma is a crescentic oval organism, 4 to 7 microns long, with a single, approximately central nucleus. In tissues it is intracellular, and small or large agglomerates are often seen. In later stages, the organism is often seen lying within a cystic space, especially in the brain and skeletal and heart muscle.

In the newborn, the principal locus of infection is the central nervous system. Lesions consist of areas of necrosis in which calcium is ultimately deposited and throughout which cysts or the naked parasite may be sparsely scattered. Similar lesions are less abundant in liver, lungs, myocardium, skeletal muscle, spleen, and other tissues. There is little cellular inflammatory reaction, consisting mostly of lymphocytes, monocytes, and plasma cells. The pathologic picture is not specific unless organisms or cysts can be demonstrated.

Diagnosis.   The majority of infants with congenital toxoplasmosis have no symptoms or apparent abnormalities at birth. In Desmonts and Couvreur's series, there were two subclinical cases for each clinical one. Such infants, however, usually develop disease as they grow older.

The so-called "classic triad" of congenital toxoplasmosis is present in only a small proportion of symptomatic cases. Chorioretinitis, hydrocephalus, and intracranial calcifications were present in 86, 20, and 37 per cent, respectively, of the large series of Eichenwald. Fever, hepatosplenomegaly, and jaundice are frequent signs, even in the absence of central nervous system or ocular findings. Rash and pneumonitis occasionally occur. The spinal fluid is often abnormal. Anemia is frequent, and thrombocytopenia and eosinophilia are occasionally seen. Cataracts, microphthalmia, and glaucoma, so common in rubella, are rare. Microcephaly is less common than hydrocephalus. Diarrhea is occasionally a prominent symptom.

Neurologic and ocular involvement frequently appear later if they are absent at birth. Convulsions, mental retardation, and spasticity are all common sequelae. A morphologically characteristic relapsing chorioretinitis is the commonest sequela of congenital toxoplasmosis, although involvement of the anterior uveal tract also occurs (O'Connor, 1974). It is also clear that most, if not all, cases of *Toxoplasma* chorioretinitis represent the sequelae of congenital infection. Treatment may change the rather grim prognosis of congenital disease, as discussed further on.

Although some infants are highly symptomatic at birth, the disease may also be insidious in onset.

In 1953, Beckett and Flynn reported two infants with toxoplasmosis. The first is described in the following case history.

CASE 87–1

An infant born at term seemed normal until the fifth day, when ptosis of one lid was noted. In the fourth week, vomiting and pallor developed; in the fifth week, high-pitched cry, enlargement of the head, and opisthotonos were noted. Examination at 6 weeks showed dehydration, pallor, sluggishness, hydrocephalus, bulging fontanel, separated sutures, and right facial nerve palsy. The liver and spleen were not large, purpura was absent, and platelets were normal. Cerebrospinal fluid was grossly abnormal and xanthochromic, containing 200 red blood cells per cubic millimeter and 2900 mg of protein per 100 ml. Skull radiographs showed fine scattered calcifications.

The epidemiology in this example was noteworthy. The antibody titer of the mother against Toxoplasma *registered 1:4906, whereas that of a pet dachshund that had had "brain fever" with residual paralysis of one leg at the time of the infant's conception was 1:256!*

Other more bizarre forms of the disease have been described. Silver and Dixon's case, described in the following paragraph, is one of the more remarkable ones, demonstrating how protean the manifestations of congenital toxoplasmosis can be.

CASE 87–2

This infant's course was one of increasing lethargy, poor appetite, and bleeding manifestations until admission in his sixth week. Facial nerve palsy, hepatosplenomegaly, lethargy, pupillary membranes, and cataracts were found. Cerebrospinal fluid was xanthochromic and contained a few white and red blood cells and 1000 mg of protein per 100 ml. Radiographs of the skull showed flaky calcific densities. This patient's course in hospital was characterized by hypothermia, persistent hypernatremia, and inability to concentrate urine except when treated with posterior pituitary extract. He also showed eosinophilia of the peripheral blood (30 per cent) and of the bone marrow.

Laboratory Findings. Since culture of the organism is tedious and expensive, laboratory diagnosis depends heavily on interpretation of various serologic tests. There are a number of valuable tests for antibody to *Toxoplasma gondii*. Although the Sabin-Feldman dye test was at one time the standard method, more recently several tests, easier to perform and of equal reliability, have supplanted it in many laboratories. These include particularly the indirect fluorescent antibody (IFA) and ELISA tests. Both tests can be adapted to measure IgM antibody. Complement fixation and indirect hemagglutination tests are also performed but are somewhat more difficult to interpret.

Antibody develops during acute infection in the mother and remains high or drops slowly over time. A single high antibody titer implies but does not prove recent infection. In the infant, the titer at birth equals or exceeds the mother's, regardless of whether or not the baby is congenitally infected. Over the first year in the uninfected infant, the titer drops with a half-life of about 30 days. In the infected infant, although the titer may drop somewhat for the first few months, it rises again to a high level by the first birthday. IgM anti-*Toxoplasma* antibody may be present at birth or at any time for the next few months. A negative *Toxoplasma* antibody titer in the infant's serum essentially excludes the diagnosis.

As with other congenital infections, false-positive IgM antibody titers may be caused by rheumatoid factor.

Treatment. Drug treatment of toxoplasmosis in various animal models is highly effective. There is unfortunately no convincing prospectively controlled study of the drug therapy in the acutely infected mother or in the infant. It is also likely that the various treatments available are effective against the proliferative form of toxoplasmosis but not against the encysted form and that eradication of organisms by chemotherapy is not possible. Despite these reservations, however, treatment of congenitally infected infants is recommended, and it is likely as well that mothers found to be acutely infected during pregnancy should also receive therapy.

The two most promising drug regimens are pyrimethamine plus sulfadiazine and Spiramycin. At the present time, Spiramycin is not available in the United States but may be purchased in Canada and Europe. Since pyrimethamine may have teratogenic effects, its use is not recommended during the first trimester.

Corticosteroids have been recommended as an adjunct to chemotherapy in the presence of active inflammation. In the newborn, this applies particularly to those infants with high cerebrospinal fluid protein levels, but there is again no evidence for their efficacy under these conditions. They should never be used alone.

The present recommendations, then, are summarized as follows (Remington and Desmonts, 1976):

In definite congenital infection, pyrimethamine (1 mg/kg/day orally once a day) and sulfadiazine (50 to 100 mg/kg/day orally in two doses) are given for 21 days, alternating with 30 to 45 day courses of Spiramycin (100 mg/kg/day orally in two doses) for the first year of life. Prednisone, 1 to 2 mg/kg/day in two doses, should be used during active ocular or central nervous system inflammation, and folinic acid (5 mg orally or intramuscularly twice a week) during pyrimethamine treatment.

If the diagnosis is not certain, then shorter courses of treatment are recommended. However, because of the prognosis for cerebral or ocular involvement even in the asymptomatic child, more prolonged treatment is considered warranted whenever congenital infection has been assured.

Prognosis.　It has been known for some time that the prognosis in untreated infants with overt disease at birth is poor (Eichenwald, 1960). Cerebral calcifications are a particularly ominous finding. More recently, prospective follow-up studies of congenitally infected infants asymptomatic at birth have shown that even in this group chorioretinitis is frequent and central nervous system involvement is not uncommon. In 1980, Wilson and coworkers found that 11 of 13 such infants developed chorioretinitis and that one developed, in addition, seizures and severe psychomotor retardation. In the same study, 11 other children were detected and followed because they presented with symptoms. All 11 had been asymptomatic at birth. In this group, three developed major neurologic sequelae, five were blind in both eyes, and three were blind in one eye. Ocular involvement may not begin until the end of the first decade.

Congenital Malaria

In spite of the high prevalence of malaria in many parts of the world, "congenital malaria," that is, malaria acquired either in utero or in the perinatal period, is a relatively uncommon disease. Maternal parasitemia is presumably frequent, but transmission to the fetus appears to be effectively prevented in the great majority of instances by a solid placental barrier. Disease acquired in utero is, consequently, rare. Transmission at the time of birth is somewhat more common and is probably a consequence of placental leak of infected erythrocytes during delivery combined with inadequate immunity at the time of transmission.

Etiology and Incidence.　More than 150 cases of congenital malaria have been described in the literature. These have involved all four species of *Plasmodium* infecting humans. The incidence in endemic areas has been estimated to be 0.3 per cent, with disease more likely when a mother acquires malaria for the first time during pregnancy.

Diagnosis.　The mother may or may not have symptomatic malaria during pregnancy, and cases have been described in which maternal disease was acquired not in an endemic area but through intravenous drug use or transfusion. In most instances, however, the history of exposure to malaria is clear. The child is usually normal at birth. Symptoms appear at 3 to 12 weeks of age. Fever is followed by hepatosplenomegaly, loss of appetite, listlessness, progressive hemolytic anemia, diarrhea, and jaundice.

The diagnosis is normally confirmed by demonstration of characteristic parasites on a thin or thick blood smear, and the particular species is determined by the morphology of the stained forms. Serologic studies can be used to confirm the diagnosis. If intrauterine transmission occurred, IgM antibody may be present in the cord blood (Thomas and Chit, 1980; Hindi and Azimi, 1980).

Treatment and Prognosis.　Congenital malaria, like transfusion-acquired malaria, has no exoerythrocytic (liver) stage. When the organism is chloroquine-sensitive, therefore, chloroquine alone (5 mg/kg of the base by mouth or gavage daily for 5 days) is adequate for treatment, and primaquine is not required. When chloroquine resistance is suspected, multiple drugs may be necessary.

Not every child of every mother with malaria requires treatment at birth, since most will not acquire the disease. When maternal malaria is recognized at parturition, the infant should be followed with care and treatment instituted if necessary.

Follow-up blood smears should confirm that treatment has been successful. In such instances, the prognosis is excellent.

REFERENCES

Beckett, R. S., and Flynn, F. J., Jr.: Toxoplasmosis: report of two new cases with a classification and with a demonstration of the organisms in the human placenta. N. Engl. J. Med. 249:345, 1953.

Desmonts, G., and Couvreur, J.: Cerebral toxoplasmosis, a prospective study of 378 pregnancies. N. Engl. J. Med. 270:1110, 1974.

Eichenwald, H.: Congenital toxoplasmosis. A study of one hundred fifty cases. Am. J. Dis. Child. 94:411, 1957.

Eichenwald, H.: A study of congenital toxoplasmosis. In Siim, J. C. (Ed.): Human Toxoplasmosis. Copenhagen, Munksgaard, 1960.

Feldman, H. A.: The clinical manifestations and laboratory diagnosis of toxoplasmosis. Am. J. Trop. Med. 2:420, 1953.

Feldman, H. A.: Toxoplasmosis. N. Engl. J. Med. 279:1370, 1431, 1968.

Hindi, R. D., and Azimi, P. H.: Congenital malaria due to Plasmodium falciparum. Pediatrics 66:977, 1980.

O'Connor, G. R.: Manifestations and management of ocular toxoplasmosis. Bull. N.Y. Acad. Med. 50:192, 1974.

Remington, J. S., and Desmonts, G.: Toxoplasmosis. In Remington, J. S., and Klein, J. O. (Eds.): Infectious Diseases of the Fetus and Newborn Infant. Philadelphia, W. B. Saunders Co., 1976.

Riemann, H. P., Meyer, M. E. et al.: Toxoplasmosis in an infant fed unpasteurized goat milk. J. Pediatr. 87:537, 1975.

Sever, J. L.: Perinatal infections affecting the developing fetus and newborn. In The Prevention of Mental Retardation Through Control of Infectious Disease. Proceedings of a Conference, June 9–11, 1966. U.S. Department of Health, Education and Welfare, Public Health Service Publication No. 1692.

Shabin, B., Papadopoulou, Z. L., and Jenis, H.: Congenital nephrotic syndrome associated with congenital toxoplasmosis. J. Pediatr. 85:366, 1974.

Silver, H. K., and Dixon, M. S., Jr.: Congenital toxoplasmosis: report of case with cataract, "atypical" vasopressin-sensitive diabetes insipidus, and marked eosinophilia. A.M.A. J. Dis. Child. 88:84, 1954.

Thomas, V., and Chit, C. W.: A case of congenital malaria in Malaysia with IgM malaria antibodies. Trans. Roy. Soc. Trop. Med. Hyg. 74:73, 1980.

Wilson, C. B., Remington, J. S., Stagno, S., and Reynolds, D. W.: Development of adverse sequelae in children born with subclinical congenital Toxoplasma infection. Pediatrics 66:767, 1980.

88

Infections with Spirochetal Organisms

Congenital Syphilis

Prior to 1945, the chapter on congenital syphilis in a textbook devoted to diseases of the newborn would have had to be the most important one in the section concerned with infections because of the great number of newborns affected and the broad variety of clinical syndromes produced. If this chapter had been omitted in the 1950s and 1960s, it would scarcely have been missed. In many parts of the United States a young pediatrician might have completed 3 years of residency in a large urban hospital without ever having encountered one case. Now the situation has changed. The disease is staging a modest comeback.

Incidence. During the 1930s and 1940s, in the congenital syphilis clinic of the Harriet Lane Home,

60 to 80 infants and children showed up each week for arsenical therapy. A great many more were lost to view before completing their 2- to 3-year course of treatment. It was an unusual week if we did not discover three or four new examples in the general outpatient department. Then for several decades, a year or more might pass without our seeing one. The curve of incidence has been rising since the early 1970s, however.

Etiology and Pathogenesis. The organism responsible for syphilis is the *Treponema pallidum*. This delicate, corkscrew-shaped, flagellated, highly motile spirochete is almost identical in appearance with *T. pertenue*, which causes yaws. These two diseases, like smallpox and cowpox, produce a cross-immunity for one another. This fact was established for us when, after having spent 2 years on yaws-infested Fiji and not having encountered one case of syphilis, we were transferred to yaws-free India, where syphilis became one of our main medical preoccupations (Schaffer).

Syphilis can be acquired by introduction of *Treponema* through an abrasion in the skin or mucous membrane or by transplacental transmission. Adults and some children become infected percutaneously, whereas young infants almost invariably receive their organisms from their mothers via the placenta and the umbilical vein. This crossing over may take place at any time beyond the fourth month of gestation but ordinarily occurs in its later stages. Fetuses infected early may die in utero, but the usual outcome is the birth of an apparently normal infant who becomes ill within the first few weeks of life.

Pathology. Since *Treponema* enters the fetal blood stream directly, the primary stage of infection is completely bypassed. There is no chancre and no local lymphadenopathy. Instead, the liver, the immediate target of the invasion, is flooded with organisms, which then penetrate all the other organs and tissues of the body to a lesser degree. Exactly where they take root and arouse local pathologic response, which in turn produces the presenting signs and symptoms, is unpredictable. Principal sites of predilection are the liver, skin, mucous membranes of the lips and anus, bones, and the central nervous system. If fetal invasion has taken place early, the lungs may be heavily involved in a characteristic *pneumonia alba,* but this condition is seldom compatible with life. *Treponema* may be found in almost any other organ or tissue of the body but seldom causes inflammatory and destructive changes in loci other than the ones named previously.

Under the microscope, the tissue alterations consist of nonspecific interstitial fibrosis with or without evidences of low-grade inflammatory response in the form of round cell inflammation. Necrosis follows fairly regularly in bone but only rarely in other tissues. Localization and gumma formation are not common in the neonate. Noteworthy is extensive extramedullary hematopoiesis in liver, spleen, kidneys, and other organs.

Diagnosis. The earliest sign of congenital syphilis is apt to be snuffles. The nose becomes obstructed and begins to discharge clear fluid at first and purulent or even sanguineous material later.

Cutaneous lesions appear at any time from the second week on. They are sparse or numerous and are copper-colored, round, oval, iris-shaped, circinate, or desquamative. Even more characteristic than their appearance is their distribution. Their favorite sites include perioral, perinasal, and diaper regions. Palms and soles are involved also, but there the rash is soon replaced by diffuse reddening, thickening, and wrinkling. In heavily infected infants, the rash may become generalized. Mucocutaneous junctions become involved in typical fashion. The lips become thickened and roughened and tend to weep. Radial cracks appear that traverse the vermilion zone up to and a bit beyond the mucocutaneous margins of the lips. These are the beginnings of the radiating scars that may persist for many years as rhagades. Similar mucocutaneous lesions involve the anus and vulva, but in these locations one also encounters, though less frequently, the white, flat, moist, raised plaques known as "condylomata."

Radiographs of the bones reveal characteristic osteochondritis and periostitis in more than 90 per cent of infants with congenital syphilis. In most the bone lesions are asymptomatic, but in a few, severe enough to lead to subepiphyseal fracture and epiphyseal dislocation, extremely painful pseudoparalysis of one or more extremities may supervene. Radiographic alterations include an unusually dense band at the epiphyseal ends, below which is a band of translucency whose margins are at first sharp but that later become serrated, jagged, and irregular. The shafts become generally more opaque, but spotty areas of translucency throughout them may give them a moth-eaten look. The periosteum of the long bones becomes more and more thickened. Epiphyses separate because the dense end plate breaks away from the shaft by fracture through the subepiphyseal zone of decalcification. This is exactly what happens in the pseudoparalysis of scurvy, although the reason for the weakening of the subepiphyseal bone is quite different. In syphilis, pseudoparalysis appears within the first 3 months; in scurvy, it seldom presents before 5 months.

Signs of visceral involvement include hepatomegaly, splenomegaly, and general glandular enlargement. Palpable epitrochlear nodes are not pathognomonic but are highly suggestive of congenital syphilis. The liver may be greatly enlarged, firm, and nontender. Associated with this may be jaundice, which appears in the second or third week, is seldom intense, and does not persist for many days. Anemia, probably indicative of bone marrow infection and hematopoietic suppression, may become severe. Lesions in the gastrointestinal tract and pancreas may occur and produce distention and delay in passage of meconium.

A small number of the cases of congenital nephrosis are caused by *T. pallidum.*

Clinical signs of central nervous system involvement seldom appear in the newborn, even though one third to one half of those infected suffer such involvement. This is demonstrated by CSF changes of increased protein content, by a mononuclear pleocytosis of up to 200 or 300 cells per cubic milliliter, or by positive VDRL test.

Diagnosis is confirmed by dark-field visualization of *Treponema* in scrapings from any lesion or from any body fluid, by characteristic bone changes on radiographs, and by positive serologic tests for syphilis. These tests must be interpreted with caution, however. Since the IgG portion of reagin is transmitted across the placenta, its finding in the baby's serum means no more than that the mother has or has had syphilis. She may have been cured during pregnancy and yet still have quantities of reagin in her blood or she may not have been treated at all and still not have passed the disease on to her fetus. A higher titer in the infant's blood than in the mother's is not evidence of fetal infection, nor is an elevated concentration of total IgM in the cord serum.

The most helpful specific test is a positive finding in the newborn's blood of IgM antibody against *T. pallidum,* IgM-FTA-ABS. This is fluorescent *Treponema* antibody from which antibodies from treponemes other than pallidum have been removed by absorption. If positive, this finding is usually an indicator of congenital syphilis, although in the presence of rheumatoid factor false-positive tests are occasionally seen. Even this test, however, is not always positive at first, even when infection is present in the infant, possibly because the infection had been acquired so late in pregnancy that specific antibodies had not had time to form.

Thus, when an infant's blood VDRL is positive at birth, one is not justified in making the diagnosis of congenital syphilis unless pathognomonic signs are also present. If they are not, serial determinations of reagin titer must be performed. If passively acquired, the titer will fall to zero within 4 to 12 weeks; it will slowly rise if the disease is actually present. If the IgM-FTA-ABS test is also positive at birth, treatment may be initiated. If the test is negative, however, it should be repeated several times at 3- or 4-week intervals.

Treatment. McCracken's studies have convinced him that we must treat infants with central nervous system involvement somewhat differently from those without this localization. One reason for this is that he was unable to find adequate levels of penicillin in the cerebrospinal fluid of infants given the drug in the form of benzathine penicillin. His recommendations for treating each group follow verbatim.

1. *Infants without central nervous system involvement.* Administration of either procaine penicillin G in a single daily dose of 50,000 units per kilogram for 10 days or benzathine penicillin G, 50,000 units per kilogram as a single dose intramuscularly is satisfactory therapy for patients with congenital syphilis without central nervous system involvement. The serum VDRL titer falls slowly after adequate microbial therapy; approximately 10 per cent of patients have reactive tests at 2 years of age.

2. *Infants with central nervous system involvement.* Administration of either crystalline penicillin G, 30,000 to 50,000 units per kilogram in two or three doses or procaine penicillin G, 50,000 units per kilogram in one daily dose, is recommended for all infants with central nervous system syphilis. Therapy should be continued for a minimum of 2 weeks and preferably for a total of 3 weeks. The spinal fluid cell count and protein content decrease slowly over a period of several months in the successfully treated patient.

Hardy and coworkers reported a case, rare in their and our experience, of an infant who died of congenital syphilis. His mother had received penicillin G 10 days before delivery, and he himself was given massive doses for 17 days after birth. In spite of all this, *T. pallidum* was recovered from the infant's eyes after his death.

Leptospirosis (Weil's Disease)

Lindsay and Luke reported the only case of congenital leptospirosis on record. It is briefly abstracted here because of its similarity to several of the other transplacentally transmitted infections.

CASE 88–1

A male infant's mother had been a waitress in a restaurant known to be infested with rats, but she had never become ill. The infant was born at term, weighing 7 pounds 13 ounces (3540 gm); vernix and amniotic fluid were brown, but the infant seemed well. Icterus appeared at 34 hours, and listlessness, cyanosis, dyspnea, and convulsions followed rapidly. The liver enlarged slightly. The blood was essentially normal, although platelets were not counted or mentioned. The urine contained bile. Cerebrospinal fluid was normal. The infant died at 48 hours.

Autopsy revealed heavy lungs with bloody, frothy fluid in the trachea and bronchi. There were numerous subpleural hemorrhages, and the parenchyma was congested, edematous, and hemorrhagic, but there was no inflammatory reaction. The enlarged liver showed extensive degenerative and necrotic changes with no evidence of bile stasis or regeneration. There were equally striking degenerative alterations of renal tubular epithelium, with protein and cellular casts within the tubules. Rare leptospirae were seen scattered throughout the liver sections stained by Dieterle and Levaditi stains. The mother's blood showed a high titer of agglutinins to L. icterohaemorrhagiae and L. canicola, which disappeared after a few months.

Comment. Weil's disease is contracted through contact with feces of infected rats. One cannot doubt that in this instance the mother acquired infection in this way but that it remained asymptomatic. Leptospirae crossed the placenta and produced disease of the fetus that became apparent on the second day of extrauterine life and quickly caused death. Such transplacental transmission has been observed in animals.

Neonatal Helminthiasis

It is worthy of passing mention, at least, that a few newborn infants with neonatal infestations of a variety of worms have been reported. Chu and coworkers encountered an infant of 8 months' gestational age, delivered by cesarean section because of prolonged labor and fetal distress, whose mother vaginally passed a mature worm. The infant was well on the second day but rectally passed a 30 cm mature

Ascaris lumbricoides and another on the sixth day. The worm almost surely had penetrated the fetus's intestinal tract after migration into the uterus and across the placenta.

The authors point out that similar migrations have been reported for *Schistosoma* (*Bilharzia*), *Taenia*, and *Enterobius* helminths.

REFERENCES

Alford, C. A., Polt, S. S., et al.: Gamma-M-fluorescent treponemal antibody in the diagnosis of congenital syphilis. N. Engl. J. Med. *280*:1086, 1969.

Chu, W-G., Chen, P-M., et al.: Neonatal ascariasis. J. Pediatr. *81*:783, 1972.

Hardy, J. B., Hardy, P. H., et al.: Failure of penicillin in a newborn with congenital syphilis. J.A.M.A. *212*:1345, 1970.

Lindsay, S., and Luke, J. W.: Fatal leptospirosis (Weil's disease) in a newborn infant. J. Pediatr. *34*:90, 1949.

McCracken, G. H., and Kaplan, M.: Penicillin treatment for congenital syphilis: a critical reappraisal. J.A.M.A. *228*:855, 1974.

Nelson, N. A., and Struve, V. R.: Prevention of congenital syphilis by treatment of syphilis in pregnancy. J.A.M.A. *161*:869, 1956.

Oppenheimer, E. H., and Hardy, J. B. H.: Congenital syphilis in the newborn: clinical and pathological observations in recent cases. Johns Hopkins Med. J. *129*:63, 1971.

Rosen, E. U., and Richardson, N. J.: A reappraisal of the value of the IgM fluorescent treponemal antibody absorption test in the diagnosis of congenital syphilis. J. Pediatr. *87*:38, 1975.

Scotti, A. T., and Logan, L.: A specific IgM antibody test in neonatal congenital syphilis. J. Pediatr. *73*:242, 1968.

Wilkinson, R. H., and Heller, R. H.: Congenital syphilis: resurgence of an old problem. Pediatrics *47*:27, 1971.

13 PART DISORDERS OF NUTRITION

89

Infant Nutrition

Revised with the assistance of
Elaine E. Farrell*

Probably no topic has been of greater interest and concern to those caring for newborn infants than infant feeding. The options have been many. For the normal infant born at term, breast-feeding has been viewed as optimal. The composition and volume of breast milk, the frequency of the infant's desire to nurse, and the amounts taken on the average are well documented. Almost all attempts at artificial feeding with modified cow's milk formulas have been tested against the standard of the results of successful breast-feeding. In this chapter, we will review the fundamentals of feeding of the newborn infant, providing a description of breast-feeding, a discussion of the use of modified formulas when breast-feeding is not feasible, and, finally, special considerations in feeding the preterm infant.

---

* This chapter is revised from the contributions of Dr. John R. Raye, which appeared in the 4th edition of this book.

Fundamentals

The basic purpose of all infant feeding is to provide appropriate nutrients in a manner that allows each individual to reach his or her full potential for cellular growth. Protein, fat, carbohydrate, minerals, and vitamins are required to meet these needs. Within each broad nutrient category, specific requirements also exist. Thus, the quality of each nutrient may be of equal importance to the total quantity. Too little of a required nutrient may result in growth restriction, whereas excess amounts of a specific nutrient may result in an inadequate or abnormal growth pattern.

Under normal circumstances, infants appear to regulate their daily volume intake on the basis of caloric intake. Fomon and coworkers have shown that as the caloric density of a formula is increased, ad lib intake decreases proportionally. For this reason, very high caloric density feedings may result in inadequate daily fluid intakes. Best estimates suggest that the normal term infant needs approximately 120 kcal per kilogram per day to achieve full growth potential during the first month of life. Water requirements necessitated by this caloric load are in the range of 150 ml per kcal, or 180 ml per kilogram, per day. In general, most infant formulas contain 67 kcal per 100 ml, and this caloric density (20 kcal per ounce) meets both fluid and caloric requirements. Provision of ad-

Table 89–1. Guidelines for Feeding

Weight	1200 gm*	1200–1500 gm*	1500–2000 gm*	
Feeding Interval:	q 2 hr	q 2–3 hr	q 3–4 hr	
Hours of Life	ml/feed	ml/feed	ml/feed	Type of Feeding†
4–8	1–2	2–3	5–15	Sterile water × 1
	1–2	2–3	5–15	D5W × 2‡
8–12	1–2	2–3	5–15	D5W: formula 1:1
12–24	2–4	4–6	5–15	D5W: formula 1:1
24–48	3–6	6–9	10–25	D5W: formula 1:1
48–72	4–8	8–12	15–35	D5W: formula 1:1
72+	5–10	10–15	20–45	Full strength formula
Increment per feed per day after 72 hrs	1–2	2–3	5–15	Formula

* Infants less than 1200 grams or larger infants in respiratory distress may require I.V. feeding until they can tolerate sufficient enteral intake. If this period is prolonged, I.V. protein ± fat solutions should be considered.

† Feedings should be increased only if the preceding step is well tolerated as measured by gastric aspirates of less than 2 to 4 ml, no abdominal distention, and no significant blood or sugar in stools.

‡ D5W = 5 percent dextrose in water.

Table 89–2. Percentage of Calories Obtained from Constituents of Feedings

Constituent	Desirable Range	Type of Milk		
		Human	*Prepared Formula*	*Cow's (Whole)*
Protein	6–12	7	9	20
Fat	30–55	55	48	50
Carbohydrate	35–55	37	42	29

equate calories does not necessarily result in adequate growth, however. A specific distribution of calories among nutrient subgroups is necessary as well. Table 89–2 outlines the desirable percentage of calories to be provided daily from protein, fat, and carbohydrate. It should be clear from this table, for example, why whole cow's milk is not ideal for infant feeding. It is apparent, however, that human breast milk and proprietary formula are similar both in caloric density and caloric distribution. Certain differences do exist, nevertheless, in the composition of the caloric sources.

Changing Trends in Breast-Feeding

The prevalence of breast-feeding varies from decade to decade and from community to community throughout the world. A survey in 1979, conducted with a questionnaire mailed to 46,648 mothers in the United States, brought a response rate of 57 per cent. The findings are illustrated in Tables 89–3 and 89–4.

A marked swing toward more breast-feeding practiced for a longer period characterized the 1970s. The reasons for this change are not known with certainty, although many physicians have become convinced that it remains the ideal method of feeding the normal newborn infant. Perhaps the emphasis on a more natural lifestyle has had an influence. Mother-infant bonding, thought to be enhanced by nursing, has been a topic of interest to physicians and parents

alike, as evidenced by books, newspaper articles, and television programs on the subject. The vanguard group of women among whom breast-feeding became most popular were college graduates and relatively affluent. The lowest incidence of breast-feeding remains among the poor in the rural South, particularly among the black population (Martinez and Nalezienski, 1981).

Human Milk and Modified Cow's Milk Formula

Nutritional Differences. Human milk differs from cow's milk in a number of aspects, as shown in Table 89–5. Importantly, the protein content is lower and the lactalbumin:casein ratio is much higher in human milk.

Räihä and colleagues, in comparing utilization of formula with whey to casein ratios of 60:40 and 18:82, did note increased renal losses of amino acids in the high casein group.

It has also been noted that human milk contains substantially more cystine and taurine than cow's milk. Although cystine is technically not an essential amino acid, the newborn infant has a relative deficiency in the ability to convert methionine to cystine. This results in a relative increase in the cystine requirement, which is more adequately met by breast milk.

Analysis of the qualitative differences in fat between breast and other milks again reveals significant

Table 89–3. Percentage of Infants at 1 Week of Age Receiving Different Milks and Formulas (1955 to 1979)

Year	Total Breast Milk*	Prepared Infant Formula	Evaporated Milk	Whole Cow's Milk	Total*
1955	29.2	23.2	45.9	4.1	102.4
1960	28.4	34.9	40.0	2.8	106.1
1965	26.5	59.0	17.3	1.5	104.3
1970	24.9	74.9	3.0	0.6	103.4
1975	33.4	69.2	0.7	0.3	103.6
1978	45.1	58.6	0.5	0.1	104.3
1979	49.7	54.7	0.3	0.1	104.8

* Total includes supplemental feeding (i.e., formula in addition to breast-feeding).

(From Martinez, G. A., and Nalezienski, J. P.: Pediatrics 67:260, 1981.)

Table 89–4. Percentage of Infants Receiving Different Milks and Formulas at Ages 5 to 6 Months*

Milk or Formula	1971	1978	1979	% Point Change 1978–1979	% Point Change 1971–1979	8-Year ARG†
Breast‡	5.5	20.5	23.0	2.5	17.5	19.6
WCM/EM§	68.1	32.9	25.2	(7.7)	(42.9)	(11.7)
Total prepared formulas	28.0	51.6	57.6	6.0	29.6	9.4
Without iron	14.6	14.6	17.3	2.7	2.7	2.1
With iron	13.4	37.0	40.3	3.3	26.9	14.8
Total‡	101.6	105.0	105.7			
N	2629	16,137	25,004			

* Includes infants 5 and 6 months of age.
† Average annual rate of gain. Values in parentheses indicate a loss (i.e., a decrease).
‡ Includes supplemental bottle feeding; totals may not be exact because of rounding.
§ Whole cow's milk/evaporated milk.
(From Martinez, G. A., and Nalezienski, J. P.: Pediatrics 67:260, 1981.)

differences. Although slightly higher in total fat content, the fatty acid composition of breast milk is such that fat absorption is superior to that of synthetic formula (Barnes et al., 1974). This is a result of increased concentrations of medium-chain triglycerides and monounsaturated fatty acids in human milk. Manufacturers of prepared formula have attempted to improve fatty acid absorption from their products

by the addition of polyunsaturated fatty acids, such as linoleic, to the saturated fatty acids of cow's milk. Although fat absorption has been improved, vitamin E absorption has been decreased. György has also called attention to the lipase content of human milk, which results in the liberation of well-absorbed free fatty acids.

Calcium absorption is superior with human milk

Table 89–5. Comparison of Human and Cow's Milk with Proprietary Formula

	Human Milk	Cow's Milk	Proprietary Formula*
Water (ml per 100 ml)	87	87	87–90
Protein (gm per 100 ml)	1.1	3.5	1.5
Lactalbumen:casein ratio	60:40	18:82	20:80
Lactose (gm per 100 ml)	6.8	4.9	7.0–7.2
Fat (gm per 100 ml)	4.5	3.7	3.6
Linoleic (percent of fat)	7	1	21–41
Calories (kcal per 100 ml)	67–75	67	67
Minerals			
Sodium (mEq per liter)	7	22	9–11
Potassium (mEq per liter)	13	35	19–20
Chloride (mEq per liter)	11	29	11–16
Calcium (mg per 100 ml)	34	117	55–58
Phosphorus (mg per 100 ml)	14	92	43–46
Magnesium (mg per 100 ml)	4	12	4–5
Iron (mg per 100 ml)	.05	.05	Trace–.15†
Copper (mg per 100 ml)	.04	.03	0.4–0.6
Total ash (gm per 100 ml)	0.2	0.7	0.3–0.4
Vitamins			
A (I.U. per liter)	1898	1025	1700–2500
Thiamine (µg per liter)	160	440	400–710
Riboflavin (µg per liter)	360	1750	630
Niacin (mg per liter)	1.5	0.9	4–8
Pyridoxine (µg per liter)	100	640	260–420
Pantothenate (mg per liter)	1.8	3.5	2–3.1
Folacin (µg per liter)	52	55	32–100
B_{12} (µg per liter)	0.3	4	1–2
C (mg per liter)	43	11	36–53
D (I.U. per liter)	22	14	400–422
E (I.U. per liter)	1.8	0.4	10–13
K (µg per liter)	15	60	19–69

(Adapted from data assembled by Fomon, S. J.: Infant Nutrition. 2nd ed. Philadelphia, W. B. Saunders Co., 1974.)
* Range of composition of commonly used proprietary formula, Enfamil, Similac.
† Iron-supplemented formula contains 12 mg per liter.

feedings, and seems to parallel fat absorption. The hypocalcemia seen after several days of cow's milk feedings is due to both decreased calcium absorption and the high phosphate load of cow's milk. This "nutritional disease" is not seen in newborn infants fed breast milk. As noted in Table 89–5, little improvement has been made in altering the calcium to phosphorus ratio or total phosphate content of standard proprietary formula. Specific low-solute formulas, however, are commercially available with improved calcium-to-phosphate ratios. Cow's milk contains only one half the human milk concentration of lactose, whereas commercial formulas have been supplemented with this sugar.

As noted in Table 89–5 the ash content of commercial formula is significantly higher than that of breast milk. This additional solute load must result in either increased water requirements, hyperosmolarity, or edema. Davies has documented an increase in serum osmolarity in formula-fed infants. She has suggested that this hyperosmolarity may be aggravated by improper dilution of formula. The effects of this chronic, mild hyperosmolarity are not known. Taitz has speculated on the possibility of an increased risk of hyperosmolar dehydration, with its central nervous system sequelae, following episodes of diarrhea and vomiting. Similarly, high neonatal solute intakes in some animal models have been associated with the development of hypertension in the adult.

All proprietary formulas are supplemented with adequate amounts of appropriate vitamins for the term infant; however, these supplements may not be adequate for the premature infant.

Since human milk is low in vitamins D and K, particularly if the maternal diet is marginal, supplemental vitamins are recommended once full feedings are established. The routine use of vitamin K, given in the form of intramuscular vitamin K_1 oxide shortly after birth, has eliminated hemorrhagic disease of the newborn. The iron content of breast milk is low but well absorbed by most infants. When maternal iron intake is adequate, nursing infants do not require supplemental iron for 4 to 6 months.

Although proprietary formulas that are not iron-fortified contain no additional iron, those formulas that are iron-fortified contain 12 to 13 mg per liter. Since the study of Andelman and Sered in 1966, which documented early storage and subsequent utilization of dietary iron, the American Academy of Pediatrics Committee on Nutrition has recommended supplementary iron for all infants. This universal form of supplementation, although somewhat controversial, has received much support for two reasons: (1) it is clear that iron deficiency during infancy is still widespread (Owen et al., 1974), and (2) it is known that an infant's intake of nonmilk iron-containing foods is not reliable (Dallman, 1974; Rios et al., 1975).

Human milk contains adequate amounts of fluoride when the maternal drinking water contains more than one part per million of fluoride. In areas in which the water content of fluoride is lower, breast-fed infants should receive 0.5 mg of fluoride daily. The same applies to those who are fed formulas diluted with water.

This brief comparison of the composition of human milk and proprietary formula should suggest that although total calories and caloric distribution are similar some fundamental qualitative nutritional differences do exist. Certain non-nutritional differences also exist.

Non-Nutritional Differences. The major non-nutritional advantages of breast-feeding fall into three areas: increased resistance to infection, development of mothering, and convenience.

Evaluation of the literature that suggests that breast-feeding is superior to formula in protecting the infant from various forms of infection is hazardous at best. A 1959 study by Mellander and coworkers clearly suggested that infants who were fed entirely on breast milk for the first 3 months of life had significantly fewer respiratory and diarrheal infections when compared with infants fed evaporated milk formula. In 1981, Narayanan and colleagues again showed that low birth weight infants fed breast milk were better protected against infection when compared with infants in a control group who were fed formula. There are, however, objective reasons that such differences might exist. Colostrum and, to a larger extent, transitional milk are both high in secretory IgA. This antibody is thought to be surface-active in the gastrointestinal tract and critical to the development of local gastrointestinal immunity. This IgA has been found unchanged in the stools of breast-fed infants and thus appears to be resistant to digestion and capable of local activity. Warren and others, for example, have documented that the presence of polio antibodies in breast milk may prevent infection by vaccine virus in the infant.

In breast milk, factors other than immunoglobulins have been thought to play some role in protecting the infant from enteric infections. Breast milk contains large amounts of lysozyme, which may have a direct bacteriocidal effect. Pitt and coworkers demonstrated in fresh breast milk high concentrations of macrophages that appeared capable of killing bacteria in vitro. In a rat model of necrotizing enterocolitis, these macrophages appeared to prevent development of disease. It is important to note that the antibacterial activity of these macrophages was diminished by either freezing or sterilizing the fresh milk but persisted with refrigeration up to 24 hours.

The presence in human milk of a factor that promotes growth of the bacterium *Lactobacillus bifidus* has also been noted. These bacteria are capable of producing lactic and acetic acids, resulting in an increased acidity of the stools of breast-fed infants when compared with those of infants who are formula-fed. The combination of a lower pH and overgrowth by *L. bifidus* appears to result in diminished enteric colonization by *E. coli* and perhaps other invasive bacteria.

It has been suggested that other bacterial "resistance" factors are also present in human milk, but the roles of these in the prevention of infection are even less clear. For example, human milk is rich in lactoferrin, an iron-binding protein that Bullen and coworkers have shown to inactivate *E. coli* both in vitro and in vivo. The addition of iron to this protein blocked this bacteriocidal ability. This latter finding has been suggested as an argument against routine iron supplementation of formula.

Thus, it appears that fresh human milk may play a direct role in protecting the gastrointestinal surface of the neonate. Many of these properties appear to be lost in processing or are completely lacking in proprietary formula. Excellent reviews of this material have been provided by Goldman and Smith and by Gerrard.

The close relationship fostered by the physical intimacy of breast-feeding has always been considered a positive factor in the development of a secure and happy child. There is, however, little proof of this. In animal work, particularly with primates, infants deprived of mothering appear to be less inquisitive and less secure, and they have difficulty developing sexual and family behavior as adults. Klaus and coworkers have attempted to gather objective data regarding the development of this mothering behavior. In their studies, extended physical contact between mother and infant in the first 4 days of life significantly increased certain measures of mothering behavior. These measures included questions to evaluate closeness of mother-child contact and observations of soothing and touching behavior. Duration of "en face" positioning was also evaluated (Fig. 89–1). Differences in mother-child interaction between the routine and extended contact groups persisted up to 11 months later. While bottle-feeding clearly does not preclude extended physical contact, breast-feeding seems to almost guarantee it and, in addition, supplies both physiologic and sensory feedback to the mother. There would be no disagreement, however, that the quality of the experience may be of as much importance as the quantity.

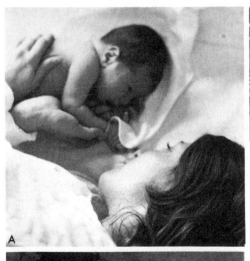

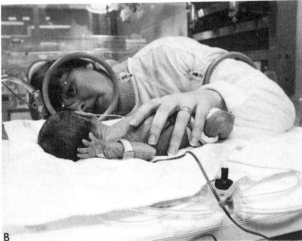

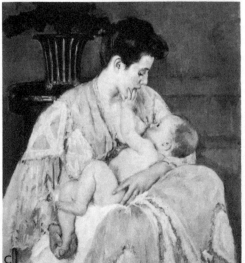

Figure 89–1. Mothers in the "en face" position. En face is defined as occurring when the mother's face is rotated such that her eyes and those of the infant meet full in the same vertical plane of rotation. *A*, A mother and her full-term infant. *B*, A mother and her premature infant. *C*, *Mother and Child*, by Mary Cassatt. (*A* and *B*, Klaus, M., and Kennell, J.: *In* The Care of the High-risk Neonate. Philadelphia, W. B. Saunders Company, 1973. *C*, Courtesy of the Art Institute of Chicago, Chicago, Illinois.)

Other objective evidence of the psychologic advantages of breast-feeding is not available. Newton has theorized that well-controlled studies are almost impossible because women who choose to breast-feed are different in some respects from those who do not (e.g., the former may be less rigid and more physical). He has also suggested that the suppression of cyclic hormonal changes for the first several months of breast-feeding, which also results in amenorrhea, may influence the consistency of mother-child interaction.

The speculative nature of some of the aforementioned data cannot be denied. It is clear, however, that breast-feeding is more economical than formula-feeding. This is true even when the cost of the additional maternal food intake is considered (McKigney, 1971). Breast-feeding is also more convenient—no bottles to wash, no formula to mix and warm, no opportunity to overconcentrate or dilute the milk. The risk of contamination of the milk by enteric pathogens is very low. This fact has been of major importance in certain underdeveloped areas of the world in which attempts to improve infant nutrition by provision of milk supplements resulted in increased mortality rates because of formula contamination by impure water supplies.

Although bacterial contamination of breast milk does not occur, contamination of human milk by maternally ingested drugs does. In certain circumstances, this fact provides a clear contraindication to breast-feeding. The extensive reviews by Knowles and O'Brien should be in the files of every pediatrician. In 1981, Berlin also reviewed this subject.

The list of maternal drugs that preclude breast-feeding appears to have shortened over the years (Table 89–6). It is important to differentiate between the excretion of a particular drug and the significance of the intake of that drug by the infant. It is not often necessary to curtail breast-feeding for this reason, particularly when alternative forms of maternal medication are available.

Concern has also arisen over the effect of breast-feeding on neonatal jaundice. As a general rule, breast-fed infants do not appear to become more icteric than infants fed commercial formula (Dahms et al., 1973; Maisels and Gifford, 1983). There does exist, however, a small group of infants who develop significant and prolonged hyperbilirubinemia in association with breast-feeding. In these infants, jaundice subsides rapidly on elimination of breast milk and returns on its reintroduction. It is thought that the presence of high concentrations of a steroid ($3\alpha 20\beta$-pregnanediol) in the milk of these mothers may be responsible for this clinical finding. This steroid appears to inhibit bilirubin conjugation in vitro in certain animal species. There appears to be some doubt, however, whether this observation is true in humans. (Adlard and Lathe, 1970). Furthermore, when Ramos and his coworkers fed this steroid to infants, no significant increase in hyperbilirubinemia was noted. More recent research implicates abnormal lipolytic activity with elevated nonesterified fatty acid concentrations in inhibitory breast milk. Regardless of the etiology, the clinical observation certainly is true. It is unlikely that this form of hyperbilirubinemia is responsible for clinical sequelae, and modest or prolonged icterus of this etiology is not a reason to terminate breast-feeding.

The advantages of fresh, human breast milk certainly seem to outweigh those of either proprietary formula or evaporated milk formula for term infants. At present, however, it is not possible to distinguish objectively between the end products of different feeding regimes. It is also true that breast-feeding is not for everyone. The working mother may find breast-feeding impossible and should not be made to feel guilty. The mother who is uncomfortable with the degree of physical intimacy involved in breast-feeding is unlikely to succeed. The same is true of those who resent the social intrusion. One should

Table 89–6. Drugs Contraindicated for the Nursing Mother

Drug or Condition	Reason
Lithium	Significant blood levels in the infant (0.33–0.5 maternal levels)
Antimetabolites	Anti-DNA activity
Radioactive pharmaceuticals	Radioactivity in breast milk
Very lipid-soluble drugs (hexachlorophene, PCBs, DDT, THC)	Only elimination route through milk; measure level if any doubt of maternal body burden
Phenindione	Bleeding in 1 case report with ↑ PT and ↑ PTT
Mothers homozygous for cystic fibrosis (sodium)	Sodium content of milk high: 132 to 280 mEq/liter
Chloramphenicol	Possible bone marrow depression
Isoniazid (INH)	Anti-DNA drug; metabolite (acetyl INH), which is thought responsible for liver toxicity, also secreted in milk

PCB = polychlorinated biphenyl; THC = tetrahydrocannabinol; PT = prolonged prothrombin time; PTT = prolonged partial thromboplastin time.
(Data from Berlin, C. M., Jr.: Obstet. Gynecol. *58*(Suppl.):175, 1981.)

never force a mother to breast-feed her infant, for little but frustration can be gained for mother, infant, and physician. For those who are undecided, however, we must enthusiastically provide the facts and develop their interest and confidence.

Unfortunately, the pediatrician usually sees the "maybe's" too late, that is, after delivery and after the administration of drugs to suppress lactation. At this point, in the midst of the turmoil of hospital routines, it is a rare woman who, without adequate preparation or inordinate desire, can suddenly make a go of it. Similarly, it is unusual to convince a woman to breast-feed an infant after previous children have been bottle-fed. It seems that the conversion must take place in prenatal classes for primigravidas.

Basics of Breast-Feeding

Perhaps the most important basis for breast-feeding, besides temperament, is a sound understanding of milk production. From this understanding comes the confidence to progress from a frustrating if not ticklish experience to successful and pleasurable feeding. Successful feeding requires two distinct physiologic processes on the mother's part. The first is milk production, which is mediated by prolactin, an anterior pituitary hormone. Milk production is stimulated by sucking and emptying the breast. The importance of emptying the breast in maintaining adequate milk production cannot be overemphasized. Little milk will be available to the infant, however, without adequate milk "let-down." This second process, mediated by oxytocin secreted by the posterior pituitary, results in contraction of myoepithelial cells, rupture of holocrine secretory cells, and transport of milk to the nipple area. The "let-down" process releases the "hind milk," which is higher in fat content (4 to 7 per cent) than that which is first available within the ductile system ("fore milk"). The importance of confidence and relaxation in stimulating milk "let-down" and milk production makes it crucial that the hospital environment be conducive to breast-feeding. The initial appearance of colostrum, followed by transitional milk, and finally the appearance of real milk at 3 to 7 days should be anticipated landmarks. Manual expression or the use of the breast pump should be explained as useful techniques. The importance of emptying the breast as well as the significance of ductile plugging ("caking") and breast abscesses should be carefully explained, along with other aspects of breast and nipple care. Woody and Woody as well as Applebaum have provided some excellent guidelines for support of the "lost art" of counseling mothers in these regards.

Breast-feeding should begin when both mother and infant are alert and ready. Normally, this would be at 4 to 8 hours of age. Initial feeds should be limited to 5 minutes per breast in order to stimulate but not irritate the nipples. The mother must be content with the dual role of this early nursing as stimulation for the initiation of milk production as well as a learning experience for both her and the infant rather than a nutritional "happening." Both must learn to relax and interact in a productive manner during these early sessions.

In the hospital, feedings should take place every 3 to 4 hours. They should be continued through the night in order to facilitate milk production and to avoid the discomfort of initial breast engorgement. As milk production increases and nipples become less irritated, the period of nursing is extended to 10 minutes on each breast. By the end of the first week, nursing should be well established, with the infant sucking on one breast for 15 minutes and finishing for 10 to 15 minutes on the second breast. At the next feeding, the pattern is reversed. Supplemental bottles are to be avoided until milk production and mother-infant interaction are well established. After that period, supplemental bottles may still result in decreased milk production, and their regular use should be discouraged.

Basics of Formula-Feeding

Occasionally, breast-feeding is not practical, in which event infants may require feeding with modified cow's milk.

Immediately following delivery, most infants are in a "quiet, alert" phase, in which they will suckle more avidly than in the next 3 to 6 hours. When the infant arouses, sterile water should be offered, and the response of the infant should be carefully observed. If sucking is vigorous and swallowing occurs, 10 to 20 ml are usually adequate. Coughing, regurgitation, drooling, or difficulty in swallowing should alert one to the possibility of a blind esophageal pouch or aspiration, and subsequent feedings must be withheld until the patency of the esophagus and absence of a fistula are established. Following this initial test feeding with water, regular feedings at intervals of 3 to 5 hours (or when the infant arouses and seems hungry) can be initiated. A typical feeding schedule for a normal term infant is as follows:

	Amount	Interval	Concentration
First 12 hours	15 ml	4 hrs	20 cal/30 ml
Second 12 hours	20 ml	4 hrs	20 cal/30 ml

Then increase by 15 ml every day as tolerated to 90 ml per feeding.

If prepared formulas are used, the vitamin content on the label should be noted. Usually, no further vitamin supplement is needed. If the formula does not contain vitamins, supplemental vitamins can be added at about 1 week of age to provide vitamin A (500 international units), vitamin C (50 mg), vitamin D (400 units), and vitamin E (15 to 25 international units daily). (See Appendix 2 for composition of some commercially available formulas.)

The pendulum of infant feeding programs varying from very rigid to completely unstructured now seems to lie halfway between those alternatives. A feeding schedule that results in the infant being fed every 3 to 5 hours upon waking and seeming hungry appears sensible. A longer period between feedings is to be encouraged at night, again with feeding delayed until some interest is demonstrated by the infant. Feedings should take place in a comfortable, relaxed atmosphere in which the attentions of both mother and infant can focus on each other. Attentiveness and physical closeness are essential. Over the first few weeks, a productive routine will be established consisting of 5 to 6 feedings a day.

Some attention should be paid to the present vogue of infant overfeeding. As noted previously, a total intake of 180 ml per kilogram of standard formula provides adequate intake of all nutrients for the normal infant. Fomon has noted that mean intakes are in considerable excess of this amount. Significantly larger amounts given as a show of love or in competition to raise the "All American Baby" lead to high caloric and solute loads. Storage of these additional calories as fat may stimulate the multiplication of adipocytes. Hirsch has speculated that this increase in the number of fat cells may increase the risk of obesity in adult life. Similarly high solute loads in infancy may be associated with an additional risk

of hypertension in subsequent years (American Academy of Pediatrics, Committee on Nutrition, 1974).

Introduction of Solid Foods

An increasing tendency toward the early introduction of solid foods has accompanied the transition from breast- to bottle-feeding. At the present time, many mothers introduce cereals as early as 2 to 3 weeks of age, followed shortly by fruits, vegetables, and, finally, meats. Although this practice is not clearly harmful, it does appear to increase the cost of infant feeding without any demonstrated advantage. Adequate nutrients in appropriate distribution are provided by either breast milk or cow's milk formula for the first 6 months of life. The high calorie and ash content of these supplemental foods again raises the question of long-term effects noted previously for overfed infants. Davies has documented significantly elevated serum osmolarities in infants fed milk plus supplemental foods when compared with those in breast- or formula-fed infants. For these reasons, it seems proper to discourage the introduction of solids prior to 4 to 6 months of age.

Feeding the Low Birth Weight Infant

The intrauterine environment is characterized by continuous transplacental transport of nutrients. Preterm birth produces a dramatic change in that the infant must receive nutrients through the gastrointestinal tract, by intravenous administration, or, often, by both routes. The past decades have been characterized by controversies surrounding the issues of the appropriate composition of formulas, techniques of feeding, intervals between feedings, and, more recently, approaches to intravenous alimentation. The reader is referred to Dr. Thomas Cone's "History of Infant and Child Feeding" for a review of past approaches to nutritional support of infants (Cone, 1981). This chapter will focus on current understanding of ways to feed low birth weight infants, with our full awareness that this will not be the last word on this important topic.

Body Composition

The body composition of the premature infant differs from that of the term infant in a number of ways. Although these differences have been detailed previously (see Chapter 4), certain of them have important nutritional implications and will be mentioned

here briefly. Total body water is significantly increased in premature infants. This appears to be due mainly to an increase in the extracellular fluid space and results in an increased risk of water imbalance. Energy stores in the form of glycogen and particularly fat are markedly reduced in the preterm infant. Fat, for example, is virtually absent in infants under 1500 grams. Similarly, transplacental transport and storage of specific minerals such as calcium and iron occur in late pregnancy, so that infants born prior to 34 to 36 weeks' gestation may lack the stores of these elements necessary for postnatal metabolic needs. In addition to these energy and mineral deficits, heat and water losses are increased because of the high relative surface area. Initial oxygen consumption, although slightly below that of the term infant on a per kilogram basis, rises gradually over the next several weeks, finally exceeding that of the term infant by 20 per cent (Sinclair et al., 1970).

The small for gestational age infant suffers from similar nutritional handicaps. Because of a relative decrease in transplacental transport of nutrients, energy stores are low. Cassidy has noted that as a manifestation of this intrauterine "starvation" the extracellular fluid space is large. Oxygen consumption, initially similar to that of the term infant, rises over the first 5 days of life and significantly exceeds that of the term infant over the next several weeks (Hill and Robinson, 1968).

Both types of low birth weight infants, then, suffer from low energy stores and high water turnover at a time when demands caused by rapid cellular multiplication are high. These facts, coupled with poor fat absorption and a gastrointestinal tract that may poorly tolerate the volume loads required to meet these metabolic demands, place the low birth weight infant in a precarious nutritional position.

Nutritional Requirements

The aim is to support a growth rate that approaches expected intrauterine growth in the third trimester without imposing excess loads on metabolic or excretory systems.

The quality and quantity of protein required by the low birth weight infant remain under study. Davidson and coworkers and Omans and colleagues found that their infants grew well on 3 to 4 gm of protein per kg per day, but Räihä and associates found that formulas containing 3 gm of protein per 100 ml could produce acidosis and hyperaminoacidemia. They suggested that a lactalbumin:casein ratio modified to a 60:40 ratio in a 3 per cent formula provides a reasonable rate of growth and serum protein levels. The mixture has sufficient aminoacids to provide adequate cystine and prevent excess intake of tyrosine, methionine, and phenylalanine.

Excessive protein intake can lead to elevation of phenylalanine and tyrosine in some low birth weight infants. Although no acute adverse effects were noted by Avery and coworkers, mild intellectual deficits were described by Mamunes and colleagues among children 5 years after they had had transient tyrosinemia. Their performance varied inversely with the duration of elevated tyrosine values in the first weeks of life.

Formulas with appropriate protein but high mineral content have resulted in the appearance of edema in low birth weight infants. Babson and Bramhall noted that when ash content of formula was high (0.87 gm per 100 ml) the additional weight gain

Table 89–7. Estimated Requirements for Calories in the Low Birth Weight Infant (< 1300 gm)

Item	Kcal per Kg per Day
Stool and urine losses	18.2
Basal metabolic rate	47.0
Intermittent activity	4.3
Thermal effect of food	11.3
Growth	67.8
Total	148.6

(Data from Reichman, B. C., et al.: Pediatrics 69:446, 1982.)

Table 89–8.

Day	Fluid Requirements (ml per kg per day)
1	80–100
2	100–120
3	120–140
>3	150–180

noted was not accompanied by a similar increase in linear growth.

Total fluid requirements for the low birth weight infant are generally in the range of 80 to 200 ml per kg per day, depending on age and environment (Table 89–8). These are basic requirements and must be increased appropriately in a number of situations. Phototherapy, for example, has been shown by Wu and Hodgman to increase insensible water losses by more than 100 per cent. This may result in an increase in daily water requirements in the range of 15 to 20 ml per kg per day. Even greater increases in daily water requirements are found in infants nursed under open radiant heat warmers (Williams and Oh, 1974). On a per kilogram basis, these additional losses increase as weight of the infant decreases. This is in part due to the higher relative surface area in proportion to the total weight of the smaller infants.

Gastrointestinal fat absorption is impaired in the preterm infant. To some extent, this is true in the small for gestational age infant as well. Prepared formulas that are high in saturated and polyunsaturated fats, especially linoleic, are absorbed particularly poorly. The addition of linoleic acid to the saturated fat of cow's milk in an attempt to improve total fat absorption may result in clinically significant vitamin E deficiency (see Chapter 90). Tantibhedhyangkul and Hashim as well as Roy and coworkers have documented improved fat absorption in the preterm infant with medium-chain triglycerides. Nitrogen absorption was significantly enhanced as well under these conditions.

A large fraction of transplacental mineral transport takes place in the last few weeks of gestation. The preterm infant who is born prior to this period has significantly decreased total body content of most minerals, most importantly of calcium and iron. Impaired transplacental transport may result in similar deficits, particularly of calcium, in the small for gestational age infant. Hypocalcemia may be seen in the neonatal period, whereas the effects of iron deficiency are not evident for 8 to 10 weeks. Thus, calcium should be supplied to the low birth weight infant in a utilizable form, that is, not in formulas high in phosphate and unsaturated fatty acids.

Modified Formulas

Although the last word on modified formulas for the low birth weight infant is surely not in and despite the probability that they will require considerable individualization, formulas developed according to current understanding of nutritional needs are commercially available. The composition of these formulas is such that they provide 47 per cent of calories from fat, 42 per cent from carbohydrates and 11 per cent from protein in a 60:40 whey:casein ratio. The water intake is 130 ml/kg/day when caloric intake is 120 cal/kg/day. Vitamins and minerals are added in amounts estimated to meet daily requirements. These formulas are useful for the growing low birth weight infant but should be started in a dilute strength to establish tolerance.

Human Milk

Human milk, from an infant's own mother, has many advantages for the low birth weight infant. When mothers are able to express their milk, it can be kept in sterile containers in a refrigerator for the use of their infant. Pooled breast milk is not advised, since some samples have been found to contain cytomegalovirus, and other viruses are probably present as well. An infant should be at less risk from microorganisms in his own mother's milk but could lack antibodies to milk from other mothers.

Milk from mothers who deliver preterm infants may be 15 to 20 per cent higher in total protein and 20 to 30 per cent higher in total energy and lipid levels than that of mothers who deliver at term. After the first week, lactose is lower in milk from mothers of preterm infants. If the infant can tolerate 150 to 200 ml/kg, nutritional requirements may be met by breast milk (Anderson et al., 1981). It is not evident that human milk is adequate in amounts of all trace minerals required by rapidly growing infants, since zinc deficiency symptoms have been noted in immature infants who are fed breast milk alone. Supplemental calcium and vitamin D are probably indicated in infants who are fed only breast milk.

The major limitation of breast milk alone is that many immature infants cannot tolerate the volumes required to meet nutritional needs. Also, studies other than those of Anderson and coworkers have shown less significant differences in composition (Sann et al., 1981). The addition of medium-chain triglycerides and simple sugars to breast milk can increase caloric density (Roy et al., 1975).

The addition of glucose to breast milk will increase caloric content but also raise the osmolarity. Breast milk alone is 286 mOsm/kg on the average, compared with 290 to 300 mOsm/kg of a lactose-containing 20 cal/30 ml formula. We have used Polycose as an additive because it is a mixture of medium-chain glucose polymers with minimal branching. It appears to be metabolized on cell surfaces and does not increase intraluminal osmolality. An isosmolar formula with 8 gm of carbohydrate/100 ml, 50 per cent as lactose and 50 per cent as Polycose, seems well tolerated (Brans, 1974; Kien, 1980). Further studies

are needed to see if this approach will result in less glucose intolerance (hyperglycemia) than has been reported with oral glucose.

Timing

Calorie, protein, and water intake by the low birth weight infant should begin as soon as possible following birth. Both the true premature and particularly the small for gestational age infant are at risk for developing significant hypoglycemia, as meager energy stores are depleted if a reliable ongoing source of calories is not available. In general, the more severe the growth limitation, the higher the risk of hypoglycemia, so that premature infants under 1500 grams and those with birth weights under the third weight percentile for gestational age should receive parenteral calories until an adequate gastrointestinal supply is achieved. Larger preterm infants benefit from early feedings, as do term infants; these feedings result in significant elevations of mean blood sugar, less neonatal weight loss, improved intestinal motility, and less subsequent hyperbilirubinemia (Wu et al, 1967; Rabor et al., 1968).

Methods of Nutrient Supply

MAJOR DECISIONS

One must first decide whether or not the gastrointestinal tract can tolerate the introduction of nutrient materials. This decision should be based on an assessment of the adequacy of intestinal motility judged by bowel sounds, normal stooling patterns, and lack of abdominal distention. Anatomic obstruction or decreases in motility can result from congenital malformations of the intestinal tract, hypoxia, hypokalemia, or gastrointestinal disease processes such as meconium ileus, meconium plugging, Hirschsprung's disease, and necrotizing enterocolitis. Increased intestinal transit times have been noted in very small infants without other obvious pathology. In the presence of signs of functional or anatomic intestinal obstruction, nutrients must be provided by the parenteral route.

If intestinal motility appears adequate, a second decision must be made regarding the level at which nutrients can be most safely delivered into the gut. Should one introduce feedings by mouth, directly into the stomach, or beyond the pylorus? This decision must involve an evaluation of the adequacy and coordination of the sucking and swallowing mechanisms. Gryboski has demonstrated that these processes are not well developed until 34 to 36 weeks' gestation. She has also noted that their coordination and efficiency tend to improve with post-natal age. Thus, it does not appear logical to attempt initial nipple feedings of infants who are less than 34 weeks' gestation or who exhibit depression of these reflexes for other reasons.

The adequacy of gastric emptying must also be considered prior to nipple or direct intragastric feedings. The best way to do this is by evaluation of gastric residuals after a trial feeding. Gastric emptying is significantly more rapid when the infant is placed in the right-lateral or prone position, and these positions should be used to facilitate emptying in most low birth weight infants. Cavell observed gastric emptying times in healthy term infants between 1 and 6 months of age and noted that those on human milk emptied one half the volume in 48 minutes. By contrast, those on a modified cow's milk formula of equal osmolality and lactose content required 78 minutes.

It is also necessary to decide whether the infant can tolerate relatively low volume, intermittent feedings as his only caloric supply. Appropriately grown infants, who are greater than 34 weeks' gestation, usually have energy stores that, although meager, will suffice for the delay between 3-hour feedings. Severely small for gestational age infants, however, although physically able to ingest larger volumes of formula, may not have adequate energy stores to tolerate the period between feedings. These infants will require either parenteral caloric supplementation in addition to oral feedings or one of the continuous nonparenteral feeding techniques reviewed in the following discussion. This is also true, in general, for infants of less than 34 weeks' gestation.

Infants who are tachypneic, with respiratory rates over 60 to 70, are also poor candidates for oral feedings. It is important to realize that the introduction of oral feedings introduces a second peak of morbidity and mortality (the first peak being birth itself). For this reason, it is important that risks other than those associated with feedings be minimal or at least well defined before oral feedings are instituted.

NONPARENTERAL METHODS OF NUTRIENT SUPPLY

Oral. If, in the larger low birth weight infant, oral feedings seem to be the technique of choice, as in the term infant, distilled water seems a reasonable fluid for the first feeding. This is followed by proprietary formula at a concentration of 20 to 24 calories per ounce. No advantage of either more dilute or more concentrated formula has been demonstrated. In fact, certain "elemental" high solute formulas have been associated with an increased incidence of necrotizing enterocolitis (Book et al., 1974).

Volumes. The volume of liquid that can be tolerated depends on the stomach's capacity and emptying time. For vigorous infants who can suckle and who have no contraindication to oral feedings, it is appropriate to provide 2 ml/kg birth weight per feeding on the first day. The amounts can be increased by 2 to 3 ml/kg birth weight each day for the first 10 days of life. Before each increase in feeding, it is useful for one to ascertain whether the stomach contains residual formula from the last feeding by inserting a feeding tube into the stomach and attempting to aspirate milk.

Intermittent Gavage. For infants who are not able to tolerate breast-feeding but who have adequate gastrointestinal function, gavage feedings may be instituted. Whenever gavage feedings are given, the infant should be provided with a pacifier to permit sucking during the feeding. Bernbaum and coworkers provided convincing evidence of accelerated maturation of the sucking reflex and better weight gain in association with decreased intestinal transit time when infants were given pacifiers during gavage feedings. A feeding catheter is passed either orally or nasally into the stomach. One confirms its position by injecting a small bolus of air while listening over the stomach. Residual gastric fluid is measured, and formula is allowed to flow in by gravity. Forcing formula in under pressure increases the likelihood of gastric distention, regurgitation, and aspiration.

Rates of gastric emptying are similar in term premature or small for gestational age infants (Yu, 1975). In the infant under 1200 to 1500 gm, however, small gastric volumes may result in inadequate water and caloric supplies. In these circumstances supplemental parenteral fluid and calories may be necessary to provide for the infant's nutritional requirements. In fact, in the very small infant, 24 to 48 hours of parenteral fluids may be required prior to the institution of gavage feedings.

One problem with gavage feedings is the occasional appearance of bradycardia noted on tube passage. This problem has been detailed by Hassel-meyer and Hon, who found that most reflex bradycardia occurred when the tip of the tube was 5 cm from the anterior nares and occurred immediately on introduction of the tube. In some small infants, this vagal response may cause considerable consternation. Generally, once the tube is in place the bradycardia is not persistent. In these sensitive infants, it may be advisable to leave the gavage tube in place between feedings. In most circumstances, however, feeding tubes should be removed between feedings to prevent partial withdrawal of the catheter into the esophagus, nasal ulcerations, gastric irritation, and increased nasal airway resistance. If the tube is to be left in between feedings, the proximal end should be left open to allow for gastric decompression and to prevent regurgitation of gastric contents into the esophagus.

Continuous Gavage. An alternate method for supplying fluids by gavage is continuous infusion. This method utilizes an infusion pump to supply formula at an initial rate of 1 to 2 ml per hour, with increments until required volumes are achieved. Gastric residuals are checked every 1 to 2 hours. This technique may result in higher daily feeding volumes than achieved by intermittent gavage feedings, particularly in the first few days of life. Postfeeding hypoxia may also be minimized by this technique. It does not eliminate the risks of development of significant gastric residuals or catheter dislodgment, however, and requires careful observation of the infant.

Transpyloric. Another constant infusion technique has received considerable attention over the past few years, that of infusion of formula beyond the pylorus, or continuous nasojejunal (or nasoduodenal) feeding. Following placement of the catheter in the stomach, the infant is placed on his right side, and the catheter is allowed to pass through the pylorus to the distal duodenum or jejunum. Transpyloric positioning of the catheter can be documented by aspiration of bile or alkaline material or with radiographs. If distal duodenal or jejunal positioning is achieved, isosmolar formula is infused at a rate of 60 to 80 ml per kilogram the first day with gradual increases each subsequent day to meet all daily fluid and caloric requirements. Initially, the tube is aspirated every hour to confirm placement and the adequacy of gastrointestinal motility.

The major advantage of transpyloric feeding is the low risk of gastric pooling of formula and associated regurgitation and aspiration. Even with more proximal duodenal placement, significant gastric reflux of formula occurs in less than 15 per cent of patients. Thus, this technique can even be used on very sick infants with poor gastric emptying; for example, very adequate fluid and caloric intakes can be rapidly achieved in infants on respirators.

The gravity of the complications associated with this feeding technique (e.g., duodenal perforation) requires that transpyloric feedings not be used routinely or without meticulous attention to technical details. When other oral feeding methods do not place an infant at jeopardy, they should be used initially. Nevertheless, the value of nasojejunal feeding cannot be overestimated in certain well-defined clinical situations. Among these situations one might include infants on ventilators, infants with intermittent apnea requiring bag and mask ventilation, and other circumstances in which delays in gastric emptying preclude adequate gastric caloric intake. Wells and Zachman demonstrated significant increase in rates of weight gain when nasojejunal feeding was compared with intermittent gavage feedings. However, no benefit of transpyloric feedings compared with gastric gavage feedings could be demonstrated in a prospective controlled trial in preterm infants under 33 weeks' gestation reported by Pereira and Lemons in 1981.

Gastrostomy. Brief mention should be made here about the use of gastrostomy as a method of feeding small infants. Although some controversy raged during the early 1960s regarding the role of this method of feeding, a controlled study published by Vengusamy and coworkers in 1969 clearly demonstrated that the routine use of gastrostomy for feeding low birth weight infants was associated with increased morbidity and mortality. At the present time, gastrostomy should be used only prior to or following gastrointestinal surgery, where it plays an important role in preventing subsequent gastric distention as well as in providing a route for feeding.

The techniques of nipple, gavage, continuous intragastric, and transpyloric feedings provide the basis for the great majority of nutrient supply to the low birth weight infant. Parenteral feeding techniques, however, should be considered in situations in which adequate nutrition cannot be provided by nonparenteral means.

PARENTERAL METHODS OF NUTRIENT SUPPLY

The initial use of 10 per cent dextrose solutions in many low birth weight infants has become routine. In the immature infant, glucose solutions will safely provide partial daily water and calorie needs until the time at which adequate volume and calories can be provided nonparenterally. These requirements are outlined in Tables 89–7 and 89–8. It is recommended that all infants who weigh less than 1750 grams be maintained on these simple solutions, starting by 6 hours of age and continuing until adequate amounts of nutrients are provided by alternate means. As the volume of nonparenteral feedings is increased, one should concomitantly reduce the parenteral glucose solutions. In normal circumstances, maintenance sodium (2 to 4 mEq per kg per day) and potassium (2 to 3 mEq per kg per day) are added on the second day. This form of supplementation should not be required after the third or fourth day. It is important to note that in very small infants, even this glucose load may be excessive and may result in significant hyperglycemia and glycosuria. For this reason frequent urine sugar testing should be done with an eye to decreasing glucose input. In general, the infusion site should be a peripheral vein unless an umbilical arterial catheter is required for blood sampling or pressure monitoring. The use of umbilical venous catheters is to be discouraged because of the risk of infection and thrombosis.

Partial Parenteral Nutrition. According to the 1971 report of Benda and Babson, when longer delays occur before achieving adequate volumes of nonparenteral feeding, a source of amino acids (2 gm per 100 ml) should be added to the standard 10 per cent glucose solution. In their report, these authors also advocated additional calories in the form of ethanol (7 cal per gm). However, the use of ethanol has been discouraged since the 1973 report by Peden and coworkers of ethanol intoxication in a significant number of infants who were followed with plasma alcohol levels. Although the osmolality of these amino acid and glucose solutions is quite high (900 to 1200 mOsm per kg), some success has been achieved in maintaining peripheral venous infusion sites. Controlled studies by Pildes and coworkers and by Brans and colleagues have demonstrated modest increases in rates of weight gain in infants whose oral feedings were supplemented with glucose and amino acid solutions compared with those of infants whose feedings were supplemented with simple glucose solutions. Complications of hyperglycemia, hyperosmolarity, hyponatremia, and metabolic acidosis were noted frequently in Brans' series.

Total Parenteral Nutrition.   One of the most exciting advances of the late 1960s was the demonstration by Dudrick that the use of parenteral solutions containing an amino acid source, glucose, minerals, and vitamins could by itself support adequate long-term growth in both experimental animals and humans. Since that time, many modifications have been made in the composition of the infusate. Heird and Winters published an excellent review of "the state of the art," and the composition of their infusate is shown in Table 89–9. Originally, the nitrogen source was a hydrolysate of either casein or fibrin, but a mixture of pure crystalline amino acids at present appears to offer certain advantages. It should be noted that the nitrogen source, although contributing only 10 per cent of the total calories, is an essential factor in providing substrate for continued cellular multiplication.

The osmolality of this mixture is extremely high,

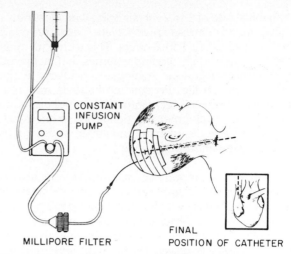

Figure 89–2. Schematic depiction of the infusion technique for total parenteral nutrition. (From Heird, W. C., and Driscoll, J. M., Jr.: Clin. Perinatol. 2:309, 1975.)

in the range of 1800 mOsm per kg water. (Normal serum osmolality is 300 mOsm per kg water.) One of Dudrick's major contributions, in fact, was the demonstration that an infusate of this type could be tolerated without marked elevations in serum osmolality when infused slowly into a central vein. His technique of superior vena cava placement through the jugular vein remains the most widely used technique of administration. The use of a distant cutaneous exit site (Fig. 89–2) seems to minimize the development of local thrombophlebitis with prolonged vessel catheterization.

The successful use of total parenteral nutrition depends in large part on meticulous attention to the technical details of infusate preparation and use. It should not be attempted where protocols for its preparation, administration, and constant monitoring of its metabolic results have not been developed. It is beyond the scope of this work to detail the technical aspects of this form of parenteral nutrition. In general, the initial infusate contains significantly less glucose and protein than the amounts noted in Table 89–9, and concentrations are increased only in the absence of hyperglycemia, metabolic acidosis, and hyperammonemia. Thus, since most of the calories are in the form of glucose, initial caloric intakes may be low. Close attention must be paid to alterations in fluid and electrolyte balance of the patient so that appropriate modifications may be made in the infusate composition. Because the infusate itself is an excellent culture medium for both bacteria and yeasts, every precaution must be taken to prevent contamination of both infusate and infant. Use of the central venous line for the sampling of blood or the injection of medication is to be avoided.

In spite of the most careful metabolic and microbiologic surveillance, the list of complications is long and the rate is moderately high. When the central venous lines are used only for infusions and when

Table 89–9.   Composition of Total Parenteral Nutrition Infusate

Constituent	Amount
Nitrogen source	2.5 gm per kg per day
Glucose	25 to 30 gm per kg per day
Sodium (NaCl)	3 to 4 mEq per kg per day
Potassium	2 to 3 mEq per kg per day
Calcium (Ca gluconate)	0.5 mEq per kg per day
Magnesium (MgSO$_4$)	0.25 mEq per kg per day
Vitamins	
MVI	1 ml per day
Vitamin B$_{12}$	5 to 10 μg per day
Folic acid	50 to 75 μg per day
Vitamin K$_1$	250 to 500 μg per day
Total volume	130 ml per kg per day

(From Heird, W. C., and Driscoll, J. M., Jr.: Clin. Perinatol. 2:309, 1975.)

Table 89–10. Common Complications of Total Parenteral Nutrition

Metabolic
  Hyperglycemia/hypoglycemia
  Azotemia
  Metabolic acidosis
  Hyperammonemia
  Abnormalities of liver function
  Abnormal serum amino acids

Catheter related
  Infection
  Dislodgment
  Erosion

meticulous attention is given to prevent infection, the infection rate remains relatively low, about 5 to 6 per cent in our hands. Generalized fungal infections due to *Candida albicans* have been a particular problem. Major common complications are listed in Table 89–10. In view of the seriousness of these problems, total parenteral alimentation should not be used when safer methods of nutrient supply are available. It is clear that this form of nutrition is essential in infants who have major abnormalities of the gastrointestinal tract (e.g., major intestinal resection, short bowel syndromes, omphaloceles and gastroschisis, chronic diarrhea). Whether this technique has significant advantages in other situations is at present a matter of some controversy. Its use in very low birth weight infants has been advocated by some, although Driscoll and coworkers in a careful analysis of their data have suggested that its routine use in this circumstance is not warranted.

Intravenous Lipid. After fairly extensive use in Europe and Scandinavia, intravenous lipid solution was approved for use in the mid 1970s in the United States and has been virtually the single factor enabling us to consider the peripheral alimentation approach with respect to long-term nutritional therapy. These solutions are emulsions consisting of 10 per cent (and frequently 20 per cent) soybean oil, 1.2 per cent egg lecithin, and 2.5 per cent glycerol, which deliver an isosmotic, chylomicron-sized particle to the circulation. The caloric content is 1.1 kcal/ml, and up to 50 per cent of the daily caloric intake may be supplied by fat without causing ketosis. With increased experience, new potential hazards continue to be described. These include the relatively rare acute allergic reactions of rash, fever, respiratory distress and vomiting, cholestatic jaundice, decreased platelet adhesiveness, and hyperlipidemia, with a possible displacement of unconjugated bilirubin from albumin by free fatty acids. Decreased macrophage function and diminished neutrophil chemotactic activity have been described, and the reports of Levene and coworkers and of Friedman and colleagues showing lipid deposits in the pulmonary capillary advise its cautious use in preterm infants with pulmonary disease.

CHOLESTASIS ASSOCIATED WITH INTRAVENOUS ALIMENTATION. Because the use of intravenous alimentation has become increasingly widespread, benefits and hazards are now in sharper focus. Touloukian and others noted evidence of cholestasis among infants on prolonged alimentation as early as 1973, but the full description of the pathology awaited later reports, such as those by Bernstein and coworkers and by Dahms and Halpin.

Incidence. The incidence must vary among centers as a function of the types of infants given alimentation, the duration of the therapy, and, probably, the nature of the solutions used. In one prospective study by Vileisis and coworkers of 43 infants who received intravenous alimentation for more than 2 weeks, about one third of them developed evidence of cholestasis. The infants in this study were given either 2.5 gm/kg protein or 4.0 gm/kg protein in the form of Aminosyn, which is a crystalline aminoacid solution. Dextrose was given in amounts of about 15 gm/kg/day, and Intralipid was administered in dosages that averaged 2.5 gm/kg/day. When the high-protein and the low-protein groups were compared, the frequency of cholestatic jaundice was similar, but the onset was earlier in the high-protein group. When jaundiced infants were compared with nonjaundiced ones on alimentation, a higher dextrose intake was found in the jaundiced infants. Thus, both aminoacid and dextrose intakes correlate with hepatic changes.

Diagnosis. Most neonatologists consider a direct (conjugated) bilirubin value of over 2 mg/dl or greater than 10 per cent of the total bilirubin concentration as evidence of hepatic dysfunction. Levels of direct bilirubin up to 10 mg/dl have been seen. Alkaline phosphatase levels may be elevated, and bile salts and serum enzymes (SGOT and SGPT) may be increased.

Clinical course. Abnormalities in liver function are uncommon within the first 2 weeks of intravenous alimentation. Elevated bilirubin levels persist as long as alimentation is continued but usually resolve within 2 weeks of its cessation. Some abnormalities in liver function tests may persist for months, but they eventually return to normal.

In one study with serial biopsies, Dahms and Halpin found bile stasis early and later discovered periportal inflammation and bile duct proliferation. Biopsies after clinical recovery showed minimal periportal fibrosis.

Treatment. A difficult clinical decision arises when the infant is dependent on intravenous alimentation and has abnormal liver function tests. It seems logical to lower the concentration of both aminoacids and dextrose to the minimal amounts required for maintenance in order to avoid further injury to the liver.

REFERENCES

Adlard, B. P. F., and Lathe, G. H.: Breast milk jaundice: effect of $3_\alpha 20_\beta$-pregnanediol on bilirubin conjugation by human liver. Arch. Dis. Child. 45:186, 1970.

American Academy of Pediatrics, Committee on Nutrition: Iron-fortified formulas. Pediatrics 47:786, 1971.

American Academy of Pediatrics, Committee on Nutrition: Salt intake and eating patterns of infants and children in relation to blood pressure. Pediatrics 53:115, 1974.

American Academy of Pediatrics, Committee on Nutrition: Nutritional needs of low birth weight infants. Pediatrics 60:519, 1977.

American Academy of Pediatrics, Committee on Nutrition: Nutrition and Lactation. Pediatrics 68:435, 1981.

Andelman, M. B., and Sered, B. R.: Utilization of dietary iron by term infants. Am. J. Dis. Child. 111:45, 1966.

Anderson, G. H., Atkinson, S. A., and Bryan, M. H.: Energy and macronutrient content of human milk during early lactation from mothers giving birth prematurely and at term. Am. J. Clin. Nutr. 34:258, 1981.

Andrew, G., et al.: In vivo effect of intralipid intravenous feeding on serum lipids and bilirubin in the neonate. Pediatr. Res. 9:362, 1975.

Applebaum, R. M.: The modern management of successful breast feeding. Pediatr. Clin. North Am. 17:203, 1970.

Avery, M. E., Clow, C. L., Menkes, J. H., et al.: Transient tyrosinemia of the newborn: dietary and clinical aspects. Pediatrics 39:378, 1967.

Babson, S. G., and Bramhall, J. L.: Diet and growth in the premature infant. J. Pediatr. 74:890, 1969.

Barnes, L. A., Morrow, G., III, et al.: Calcium and fat absorption from infant formulas with different fat blends. Pediatrics 54:217, 1974.

Bell, E., Weinstein, M., and Oh, W.: Heat balance in premature infants: comparative effects of convectively heated incubator and radiant warmer, with and without plastic heat shield. J. Pediatr. 96:460, 1980.

Benda, G. I., and Babson, S. G.: Peripheral intravenous alimentation of the small premature infant. J. Pediatr. 79:494, 1971.

Berlin, C.: Pharmacologic considerations of drug use in the lactating mother. Obstet. Gynecol. 58(suppl.):17, 1981.

Bernbaum, J. C., Pereira, G. R., Watkins, J. B., and Peckham, G. J.: Nonnutritive sucking during gavage feeding enhances growth and maturation in premature infants. Pediatrics 71:41, 1983.

Bernstein, J., Chang, C. H., Brough, A. J., and Heidelberger, K. P.: Conjugated hyperbilirubinemia in infancy associated with parenteral alimentation. J. Pediatr. 90:361, 1977.

Book, L. S., et al.: Necrotizing enterocolitis in infants fed on elemental formula. Pediat. Res. 8:379, 1974.

Boros, S. J., and Reynolds, J. W.: Duodenal perforation: complication of neonatal nasojejunal feeding. J. Pediatr. 85:107, 1974.

Brans, Y. W., et al.: Feeding the low birth weight infant: orally or parenterally? Preliminary results of a comparative study. Pediatrics 54:15, 1974.

Brans, Y. W.: Meeting carbohydrate needs. In Sunshine, P. (Ed.): Feeding the Neonate Weighing Less Than 1500 Grams—Nutrition and Beyond. Columbus, Ohio, 79th Ross Conference, Ross Laboratories, 1980, p. 23.

Bullen, J. J., Rogers, H. J., and Leigh, L.: Iron-binding proteins in milk and resistance to Escherichia coli infection in infants. Br. Med. J. 1:69, 1972.

Cashore, W. J., et al.: Nutritional supplements with intravenously administered lipid, protein hydrolysate and glucose in small premature infants. Pediatrics 56:8, 1975.

Cassady, G.: Body composition in intrauterine growth retardation. Pediatr. Clin. North Am. 17:79, 1970.

Cavell, B.: Gastric emptying in infants fed human milk or infant formula. Acta Paediatr. Scand. 70:639, 1981.

Chen, J. W., and Wong, P. W. K.: Intestinal complications of na-

sojejunal feeding in low-birth-weight infants. J. Pediatr. 85:109, 1974.

Cone, T. E., Jr.: History of infant and child feeding: from the earliest years through the development of scientific concepts. In Bond, J. T., Filer, L. J., Jr., Leveille, G. A., et al. (Eds): Infant and Child Feeding. New York, Academic Press, 1981, pp. 3–34.

Dahms, B. B., and Halpin, T.C., Jr.: Serial liver biopsies in parenteral nutrition–associated cholestasis of early infancy. Gastroenterology 81:136, 1981.

Dahms, B. B., Krauss, A. N., et al.: Breast feeding and serum bilirubin values during the first 4 days of life. J. Pediatr. 83:1049, 1973.

Dallman, P. R.: Iron, vitamin E, and folate in the preterm. J. Pediatr. 85:742, 1974.

Davidson, M., et al.: Feeding studies in low-birth-weight infants. J. Pediatr. 70:695, 1967.

Davies, D. P.: Plasma osmolarity and feeding practices in healthy infants in first 3 months of life. Br. Med. J. 2:340, 1973.

Drillien, C. M.: Aetiology and outcome in low-birth weight infants. Dev. Med. Child Neurol. 14:563, 1972.

Drillien, C. M.: Abnormal neurologic signs in the first year of life in low birth weight infants: possible prognostic significance. Dev. Med. Child Neurol. 14:575, 1972.

Driscoll, J. M., Jr., et al.: Total intravenous alimentation in low-birth-weight infants: a preliminary report. J. Pediatr. 81:145, 1972.

Dudrick, S. J.: Long term total parenteral nutrition with growth, development and positive nitrogen balance. Surgery 64:134, 1968.

Dweck, H. S.: Feeding the prematurely born infant. Clin. Perinatol. 2:183, 1975.

Dweck, H. S., and Cassady, G.: Glucose intolerance in infants of very low birth weight. I. Incidence of hyperglycemia in infants of birth weights 1100 grams or less. Pediatrics 53:189, 1974.

Ehrenkranz, R. A.: Continuous and bolus techniques for alimentation of the low birth weight infant. In Sunshine, P. (Ed.): Feeding the Neonate Weighing Less Than 1500 Grams—Nutrition and Beyond. Columbus, Ohio, 79th Ross Conference, Ross Laboratories, 1980, p. 74.

English, D., Roloff, J., Lukens, J., et al.: Intravenous lipid emulsions and human neutrophil function. J. Pediatr. 99:913, 1981.

Finberg, L.: Human milk feeding and vitamin D supplementation—1981. J. Pediatr. 99:228, 1981.

Fisher, G., Wilson, S., et al.: Diminished bacterial defenses with intralipid. Lancet 2:819, 1980.

Fitzhardinge, P. M., and Steven, E. M.: The small-for-date infant, 1. Later growth patterns. Pediatrics 49:671, 1972.

Fomon, S. J.: Infant Nutrition. 2nd ed. Philadelphia, W. B. Saunders Co., 1974.

Fomon, S. J.: What are infants fed in the United States? Pediatrics 56:350, 1975.

Fomon, S. J., Filer, L. J., Jr., et al.: Influence of formula concentration on caloric intake and growth of normal infants. Acta Pediatr. Scand. 64:172, 1975.

Friedman, Z., Marks, K., Maisels, M., et al.: Effect of parenteral fat emulsion in the pulmonary and reticuloendothelial systems in the newborn infant. Pediatrics 61:694, 1978.

Gerrard, J. W.: Breast-feeding: second thoughts. Pediatrics 54:757, 1974.

Goldman, A.: Immunologic factors and leukocytes in human milk. In Selected Aspects of Perinatal Gastroenterology: Mead Johnson Symp. Perinat. Dev. Med. 11:49, 1977.

Goldman, A. S., and Smith, C. W.: Host resistant factors in human milk. J. Pediatr. 82:1082, 1973.

Gresham, E. L.: Unpublished data.

Gross, S., Geller, J., and Tomarelli, R.: Composition of breast milk from mothers of pre-term infants. Pediatrics 68:490, 1981.

Gryboski, J. D.: Suck and swallow in the premature infant. Pediatrics 43:96, 1969.

György, P.: The uniqueness of human milk: biochemical aspects. Am. J. Clin. Nutr. 24:970, 1971.

Hasselmeyer, E. G., and Hon, E. H.: Effects of gavage feeding of premature infants on cardiorespiratory patterns. Military Med. 136:252, 1971.

Heird, W. C., and Driscoll, J. M., Jr.: Newer methods of feeding low birth weight infants. Clin. Perinatol. *2*:309, 1975.

Heird, W. C., and Winters, R. W.: Total parenteral nutrition. The state of the art. J. Pediatr. *86*:2, 1975.

Hill, J. R., and Robinson, D. C.: Oxygen consumption in normally grown, small-for-dates and large-for-dates new-born infants. J. Physiol. *199*:685, 1968.

Hirsch, J.: Adipose cellularity in relation to human obesity. Adv. Intern. Med. *17*:289, 1971.

Kien, C. L., Sumners, J. E., Heimler, R., and Grausz, J. P.: Carbohydrate energy absorption in premature infants. Pediatr. Res. *14*(abstr.):502, 1980.

Klaus, M., Jerauld, R., and Kreger, N.: Maternal attachment: Importance of the first postpartum days. N. Engl. J. Med. *286*:460, 1972.

Klaus, M., and Kennell, J.: Care of the mother. *In* Klaus, M., and Fanaroff, A. (Eds.): Care of the High risk Neonate. Philadelphia, W. B. Saunders Co., 1973, pp. 98–118.

Klaus, M., and Kennell, J.: Care of the parents. *In* Klaus, M., and Fanaroff, A. (Eds.): Care of the High Risk Neonate. 2nd ed. Philadelphia, W. B. Saunders Co., 1979, pp. 146–164.

Knowles, J. A.: Excretion of drugs in milk—a review. J. Pediatr. *66*:1068, 1965.

Lawrence, R.: Breast Feeding: A Guide for the Medical Profession. St. Louis, C. V. Mosby, 1980.

Levene, M., Desai, R., and Wigglesworth, J.: Pulmonary fat accumulation after intralipid infusion in the pre-term infant. Lancet *2*:815, 1980.

Lloyd-Still, J. D., et al.: Intellectual development after severe malnutrition in infancy. Pediatrics *54*:306, 1974.

Maisels, M. J., and Gifford, K.: Breast feeding, weight loss and jaundice. J. Pediatr. *102*:117, 1983.

Mamunes, P., Prince, P. E., Thornton, N. H., et al.: Intellectual deficits after transient tyrosinemia in the term neonate. Pediatrics *57*:675, 1976.

Martinez, G. A., and Nalezienski, J. P.: 1980 Update: the recent trend in breast-feeding. Pediatrics *67*:260, 1981.

Martinez, G. A., and Dodd, D. A.: 1981 milk feeding patterns in the United States. *71*:166, 1983.

McKigney, J.: The uniqueness of human milk: Economic aspects. Am. J. Clin. Nutr. *24*:1005, 1971.

Mellander, O., et al.: Breast feeding and artificial feeding; a clinical, serological and biochemical study of 402 infants, with a survey of the literature. The Norbotten Study. Acta Paediatr. Scand. *48*(Suppl 116), 1959.

Naeye, R. L.: Structural correlates of fetal undernutrition. *In* Waisman, H. A., and Kerr, G. (Eds.): Fetal Growth and Development. New York, McGraw-Hill Book Co., 1970, p. 241.

Narayanan, I., Prakash, K., et al.: The value of human milk in the prevention of infection in the high-risk low-birthweight infant. J. Pediatr. *99*:496, 1981.

Newton, N.: The uniqueness of human milk: psychologic differences between breast and bottle feeding. Am. J. Clin. Nutr. *24*:993, 1971.

O'Brien, J. E.: Excretion of drugs in human milk. Am. J. Hosp. Pharm. *844*, 1974.

Ogra, S. S., Weintraub, D., and Ogra, P. L.: Immunologic aspects of human colostrum and milk. III. Fate and absorption of cellular and soluble components in the gastrointestinal tract of the newborn. J. Immunol. *119*:245, 1977.

Olson, M.: The benign effects on rabbits' lungs of the aspiration of water compared with 5 per cent glucose or milk. Pediatrics *46*:538, 1970.

Omans, W. B., et al.: Prolonged feeding studies in premature infants. J. Pediatr. *59*:951, 1961.

Owen, G. M., Kram, K. M., et al.: A study of nutritional status of preschool children in the United States, 1968–1970. Pediatrics *53*:597, 1974.

Peden, V. H., et al.: Intravenously induced infantile intoxication with ethanol. J. Pediatr. *83*:490, 1973.

Pereira, G. R., and Lemons, J. A.: Controlled study of transpyloric and intermittent gavage feeding in the small preterm infant. Pediatrics *67*:68, 1981.

Pildes, R. S., et al.: Intravenous supplementation of L-amino acids and dextrose in low-birth-weight infants. J. Pediatr. *82*:945, 1973.

Pitt, J., Barlow, B., et al.: Macrophages and the protective action of breast milk in necrotizing enterocolitis. Pediatr. Res. *8*:384, 1974.

Poland, R. L., Schultz, G., et al.: High milk lipase activity associated with breast milk jaundice. Pediatr. Res. *14*:1328, 1980.

Rabor, I. F., et al.: The effects of early and late feeding of intrauterine fetally malnourished (IUM) infants. Pediatrics *42*:261, 1968.

Räiha, N., Rassin, D., et al.: Milk protein quality and quantity. Pediatr. Res. *4*:370, 1975.

Räihä, N. C., Heinonen, K., Rassin, D. K., et al.: Milk protein quantity and quality in low-birth-weight infants. I. Metabolic responses and effects on growth. Pediatrics *57*:659, 1976.

Ramos, A., Silverberg, M., and Stern, L.: Pregnanediols and neonatal hyperbilirubinemia. Am. J. Dis. Child. *111*:353, 1966.

Rassin, D. K., Gaull, G. E., Räihä, N. C. R., et al.: Milk protein quantity and quality in low-birth-weight infants. IV. Effects on tyrosine and phenylalanine in plasma and urine. J. Pediatr. *90*:356, 1977.

Reichman, B. C., Chessen, P., Putet, G., et al.: Partition of energy metabolism and energy cost in the very low birth weight infant. Pediatrics *69*:446, 1982.

Rhea, J. W., et al.: Nasojejunal feeding: an improved device and intubation technique. J. Pediatr. *82*:951, 1973.

Rios, E., Hunter, R. E., et al.: The absorption of iron as supplements in infant cereal and infant milk. Pediatrics *55*:687, 1975.

Rogers, H. J., and Singe, C.: Bacteriostatic effect of human milk on *Escherichia coli*: the role of IgA. Immunology *34*:19, 1978.

Roy, C. C., et al.: Correction of the malabsorption of the preterm infant with a medium-chain triglyceride formula. J. Pediatr. *86*:446, 1975.

Roy, R. N., and Sinclair, J. C.: Hydration of the low-birth-weight infant. Clin. Perinatol. *2*:393, 1975.

Sann, L., Bienvenue, F., Lahet, C., et al.: Comparison of the composition of breast milk from mothers of term and preterm infants. Acta Paediatr. Scand. *70*:115, 1981.

Simhon, A., and Mata, L.: Anti-rotavirus antibody in human colostrum. Lancet *1*:39, 1978.

Sinclair, J. C., and Silverman, W. H.: Intrauterine growth in active tissue mass of the human fetus, with particular reference to the undergrown baby. Pediatrics *38*:48, 1966.

Sinclair, J. C., et al.: Supportive management of the sick neonate. Pediatr. Clin. North Am. *17*:863, 1970.

Sun, S. C., et al.: Duodenal perforation: A rare complication of neonatal nasojejunal tube feeding. Pediatrics *55*:371, 1975.

Taitz, L. S.: Overfeeding in infancy. Proc. Nutr. Soc. *33*:113, 1974.

Tantibhedhyangkul, P., and Hashim, S. A.: Medium-chain triglyceride feeding in premature infants: Effects on fat and nitrogen absorption. Pediatrics *55*:359, 1975.

Touloukian, R. J., and Downing, S. E.: Cholestasis associated with long-term parenteral hyperalimentation. Arch. Surg. *106*:58, 1973.

Valman, H. B., et al.: Continuous intragastric milk feeds in infants of low birth weight. Br. Med. J. *3*:547, 1972.

Vengusamy, S., et al.: A controlled study of feeding gastrostomy in low birth weight infants. Pediatrics *43*:815, 1969.

Vileisis, R. A., Inwood, R. J., and Hunt, C. E.: Prospective controlled study of parenteral nutrition—associated cholestatic jaundice: effect of protein intake. J. Pediatr. *96*:893, 1980.

Walker, W. A.: Development of intestinal host defense mechanisms and the passive protective role of human milk. *In* Selected Aspects of Perinatal Gastroenterology: Mead Johnson Symp. Perinat. Dev. Med. *11*:39, 1977.

Warren, R. L., Lepow, M. L., et al.: The relationship of maternal antibody, breast feeding and age to the susceptibility of newborn infants to infection with attenuated poliovirus. Pediatrics *34*:4, 1964.

Welsh, J. K., and May, J. T.: Anti-infective properties of breast milk. J. Pediatr. 94:1, 1979.

Wilkinson, A., and Yu, V. Y. H.: Immediate effects of feeding on blood-gases and some cardiorespiratory functions in ill newborn infants. Lancet 1:1083, 1974.

Williams, P. R., and Oh, W.: Effects of radiant warmer on insensible water loss in newborn infants. Am. J. Dis. Child. 128:511, 1974.

Williams, N., and Oski, S.: Vitamin E status of infants fed formula containing medium-chain triglycerides. J. Pediatr. 96:70, 1980.

Woody, N. C., and Woody, H. B.: Management of breast feeding. J. Pediatr. 68:344, 1966.

Wu, P. Y. K., and Hodgman, J. E.: Insensible water loss in preterm infants: Changes with postnatal development and nonionizing radiant energy. Pediatrics 54:704, 1974.

Wu, P. Y. K., et al.: "Early" versus "late" feeding of low birth weight neonates. Pediatrics 39:733, 1967.

Yu, V. Y. H.: Effect of body position on gastric emptying in the neonate. Arch. Dis. Child. 50:500, 1975.

90

Disorders of Vitamins and Trace Minerals*

General Considerations

In the United States, vitamin deficiency conditions are rarely seen or even considered in a general pediatric practice. These deficiency syndromes are even rarer in the neonatal period. Blood levels of vitamins B and C are higher on the fetal than on the maternal side of the placenta, so that extreme deficiency states in the mother are required for reduction of neonatal stores. The striking progress in increasing survival of the very small premature infant has brought with it a reassessment of "adequacy" of vitamin stores. Clinical and laboratory evidence of both vitamin and mineral deficiency states indicative of the preterm infant's reduced stores or increased requirements or both have been documented.

Methods of prolonged parenteral nutrition that require consideration of specific vitamin and mineral needs remind us of the many lessons learned during the development of various proprietary formulas. The 1950s and 1960s abounded with examples of new formulas and new processing techniques, each of which reduced concentrations of vitamins previously found adequate in breast or condensed cow's milk. For the first time, in many instances, neonatal vitamin deficiency syndromes were recognized in the absence of severe maternal deficiency states. We must continually be chagrined at these iatrogenic diseases caused by "advances" in neonatal care.

Faddism, too, must bear its responsibility for iatrogenic disease. The use of high doses of vitamin A ("if

a little is good . . .") has merited as many case reports as deficiency of the vitamin. Dietary fads such as the severely deficient Zen macrobiotic diet must be watched with caution as they pass through their era of popularity. Similarly, one must continue to be aware that certain ethnic groups, by reason of dietary customs or lack of availability of nutritious foods, are at risk for specific vitamin deficiency syndromes.

Vitamin dependency syndromes representing alterations in vitamin requirements of specific individuals have assumed great practical and theoretical importance. In general, these are hereditary diseases involving specific biochemical abnormalities. Symptoms develop in the face of a normal body pool of the vitamin but are ameliorated when increased concentrations of the vitamin are present.

It is clear, therefore, that neither our increasing knowledge of neonatal medicine nor the wide use of proprietary formula, with its "full" complement of vitamin and mineral supplements, has yet made this chapter superfluous.

Vitamin A Deficiency

Incidence. Frank vitamin A deficiency, as evidenced by its pathognomonic corneal signs, Bitot's spots, and xerophthalmia, has not been reported within the first month of life. Chemical findings compatible with subclinical deficiency, however, are present in some mature and many premature infants. Prolonged intake of inadequate amounts of vitamin A may result in chemical evidence of deficiency appearing by 4 months of age. For these reasons, a brief discussion of the syndrome will be presented. Infants with problems in dietary fat absorption, such as those with cystic fibrosis described by Keating and Fergin, are also at increased risk.

Etiology. One of the fat-soluble vitamins, dietary vitamin A is obtained both as carotenoids and as vi-

---

* This chapter contains contributions from previous authors, Drs. Alexander J. Schaffer and John R. Raye.

tamin A. Ingested vitamin A goes through a series of interconversions in the gut mucosa and liver. Carotenes are converted to a form of vitamin A in the intestinal mucosa during absorption. Increases in dietary fat and protein may increase daily vitamin requirements.

The mechanism of action of vitamin A, other than in retinal pigment formation, is unknown. It has been suggested that the vitamin is important for cell growth and membrane stability. Certainly, the major pathologic finding in vitamin A deficiency is squamous metaplasia of epithelial surfaces, with accumulation of keratinized cells.

In early pregnancy, maternal vitamin A levels are low. At 16 weeks, levels begin to rise gradually (Gal and Parkinson, 1972), achieving values 1.5 times normal by term. Cord blood levels of vitamin A at term are not significantly different from maternal levels, although fetal carotenoid levels are significantly lower than the mother's. Mean cord levels are 23.6 µg per 100 ml of vitamin A and 12.5 µg per 100 ml of carotenoids. In general, serum vitamin A levels less than 20 mg per 100 ml have been accepted as evidence of low body stores. In term infants, levels then rise gradually over the first months of life. Premature infants, however, may be handicapped with respect to vitamin A acquisition for a number of reasons. Henley and coworkers found low liver stores of vitamin A in infants who weighed less than 2500 grams who died on the first day of life. With respect to absorption of a test dose of vitamin, premature infants again fared less well than term infants. Decreased absorption of the vitamin seemed to correlate with the decreased ability of the small premature infant to absorb dietary fat. At 3 weeks of age, one fourth of the preterm infants in their study who were not on vitamin A supplements had serum vitamin A levels below 20 µg per 100 ml. No infant on vitamin supplements fell below that level. Thus, adequate dietary vitamin supplementation is required to allow development of adequate body stores in the preterm infant.

Diagnosis. Although clinical vitamin A deficiency has not been clearly identified in the first month of life, by 3 months of age the full-blown deficiency syndrome may be seen in infants on inadequate vitamin intake.

The following case of Bass and Fisch is an excellent example of this course, which is marked by growth failure, anemia, epithelial metaplasia, and increased intracranial pressure.

CASE 90–1

A female infant was born at term by spontaneous delivery. Birth weight was 7 pounds (3175 gm). Because of a history of milk allergy in siblings, the infant was immediately put on a soy milk diet without vitamin supplement. At the age of 3½ months, the infant was brought to the physician's office because of marked enlargement of the breasts. No diagnosis was made. In 2 weeks, the infant had become extremely irritable and had a temperature of 100.5° F. The child appeared pale and extremely restless but did not look acutely ill. The breasts were still enlarged. There was marked bulging of the fontanel. The child had received no drugs. Lumbar puncture revealed bloody fluid under high pressure. Culture of the fluid showed no growth. Vitamin A deficiency was suspected. Urine could not be examined because the urethral opening could not be located, owing to excessive cornified epithelium. Penicillin was administered without improvement. Vitamin A was then given daily. In one day, the child's disposition had improved and the fontanel was softer. The next day the child was well. During the next few weeks, the gynecomastia gradually improved.

May and coworkers have suggested in a less well-documented case that the evidence of vitamin A deficiency in the premature may consist of failure to gain weight, hypoproteinemia, and peripheral edema.

The clinical diagnosis of vitamin A deficiency can be confirmed by the finding of low serum vitamin levels and by clinical response to vitamin supplementation.

Treatment. Fomon has estimated the daily vitamin A requirement as 250 I.U. per day and suggested an advisable intake of 500 I.U. per day (Tables 90–1 and 90–2). Breast milk and standard formula contain approximately three times this amount per liter. Treatment of the deficiency state should be achieved by 5000 I.U. over a period of several days followed by maintenance therapy of 1500 per day. It should be remembered that vitamin A overdosage is in itself harmful and to be avoided.

Table 90–1. Advisable Intakes of Vitamins

Vitamin	Daily Intake
A	500 I.U.
D	400 I.U.
E	4 I.U.*
K	15 µg
C	20 mg
Thiamin	0.2 mg
Riboflavin	0.4 mg
Niacin†	5 mg
B₆	0.4 mg
Folacin	50 µg

* Greater intakes may be desirable for infants receiving formulas supplying more than 15 per cent of calories from polyunsaturated fatty acids (e.g., formulas in which approximately one half of the fat is supplied from corn oil or soy oil).

† Including nicotinamide equivalents (60 mg tryptophan = 1 mg niacin).

(From Fomon, S. J.: Infant Nutrition. 2nd ed. Philadelphia, W. B. Saunders Co., 1974.)

Table 90–2. Estimated Requirements for Vitamins

Vitamin	Requirement
A	250 I.U./day
D	100–200 I.U./day
E	0.4 mg/gm PUFA*
K	5 μg/day
C	10 mg/day
Thiamin	0.2 mg/1000 kcal
Riboflavin	<0.5 mg/1000 kcal
Niacin†	4.4 mg/1000 kcal
B₆	9 μg/gm protein
Folacin	<50 μg/day

* Polyunsaturated fatty acid.

† Including nicotinamide equivalents (60 mg tryptophan = 1 mg niacin).

(From Fomon, S. J.: Infant Nutrition. 2nd ed. Philadelphia, W. B. Saunders Co., 1974.)

Vitamin A Excess

Excessive vitamin A intake is capable of causing both an acute and a chronic form of toxicity. The chronic form, presenting with growth failure, hyperostosis, and craniotabes, manifests itself only after months of overdosage and shall not be considered further here. The acute form, however, may be seen following a single massive dose of the vitamin and will be considered briefly. Also of interest is a report by Bernhardt and Dorsey that suggested the possible teratogenic effects of large doses of vitamin A in early pregnancy. Similar findings have been observed in animal studies.

Incidence.   No case of vitamin A toxicity has been reported in the first month of life. Marie and Sée reported one infant at 8 weeks of age, and Knudson and Rothman reported another at 7 weeks. Since symptoms have been noted following a single dose of the vitamin, it is probable that instances will be observed within the neonatal period. Of some interest is the extremely high vitamin A content of polar bear liver (18,000 I.U. per gm). Arctic explorers who have ignored eskimo taboos and sampled it have developed severe symptoms of acutely increased intracranial pressure.

Etiology.   The mechanism by which vitamin A causes its toxic effects is not known. It is interesting that toxicity is noted only following ingestion of vitamin A, not of carotenes. Ingestion of the latter substances results only in benign carotenemia.

Diagnosis.   The major symptoms following the ingestion of high doses of vitamin A appear to be related to an acute increase in intracranial pressure. Vomiting, irritability or lethargy, and a bulging fontanel are seen.

Vitamin B₁ Deficiency, Beriberi

Deficiency of vitamin B₁ affects infants in two age groups. A congenital form develops within the first few days of life, and an infantile form is seen from 2 to 3 months after birth.

Incidence.   Although beriberi is common in Asian countries, where polished rice is the main dietary staple, both its forms are extremely rare in this country. The congenital type, not reported in the United States since 1944, occurs only in infants born to mothers who are B₁-deficient. The infantile form has been reported at 2 to 7 months of age, following prolonged breast-feeding by mothers who suffer from malnutrition. It has also been seen following feedings of improperly supplemented prepared formula, particularly some early soybean products.

Etiology.   Thiamine, vitamin B₁, is indispensable in the human economy. It acts as a coenzyme in the conversion of pyruvic acid to acetaldehyde, one of the intermediate steps in the metabolism of carbohydrates. In the adult, withdrawal of thiamine from the diet produces symptoms within a week. B₁, however, seems to be actively transported across the placenta, and Slobody and coworkers have reported that mean cord levels are twice maternal levels. This fact may well explain the rarity of congenital beriberi except in circumstances of extreme maternal deprivation.

Fomon has suggested that the daily requirement of thiamine for infants is 0.2 mg per 1000 kcal per day. This amount is adequately supplied in both cow's milk and human milk. Human milk, however, is not rich in thiamine. In thiamine-deficient breast-feeding mothers, the relatively low margin of safety of B₁ supply to the infant may be inadequate over a period of months and may result in the appearance of infantile beriberi. Fehily has called attention to another possible form of vitamin B₁ deficiency in the breast-fed infant that is associated with the rapid onset of central nervous system depression and that progresses to coma and death. She has suggested that this disease may be due both to inadequate intake of thiamine and to the accumulation of toxic byproducts in the milk of deficient women.

Diagnosis.   Congenital beriberi presents within the first 3 to 4 days of life, usually within hours of birth. Rapid progression with congestive heart failure, convulsions, and coma may be seen.

Case 90–2

Van Gelder and Darby's case is one of the best-documented examples of neonatal beriberi. A mother had only mild edema and numbness and tingling of the hands and feet to show for her deficiency state. A 7 pound 5 ounce (3300 gm) infant was born after normal labor and delivery but was cyanotic and needed resus-

citation. For 3 hours he appeared well but then again became blue. Examination revealed cyanosis, a few crackling rales at both bases behind, extreme tachycardia, and an increased area of cardiac dullness. The liver edge was just palpable. Radiographs showed the heart to be very large (Fig. 90–1). Cyanotic spells recurred throughout the first day and were more frequent on the second. On this day, the cry became feeble and hoarse. At 30 hours head retraction appeared, followed by convulsions and rigidity of the extremities. Without further diagnostic efforts, 50 mg of thiamine hydrochloride was given subcutaneously at 42 hours and repeated at 50 hours. Convulsions and rigidity disappeared at 46 hours, but cyanosis persisted. By 62 hours improvement was dramatic. Thiamine was kept up, 50 mg every 8 hours, for 11 days. Heart rate and size steadily diminished. An electrocardiogram on the fourth day showed evidences of myocardial disease but was normal after 7 weeks.

Infantile beriberi, unlike the congenital form, has an insidious onset. Symptoms of anorexia and lethargy are first noted at 2 to 3 months of age. Vomiting develops, and the infant may then rapidly deteriorate with congestive heart failure (misnamed the "pneumonic" phase). This is followed by a meningeal phase, with bulging fontanel, opisthotonos, coma, and death. Cochrane and coworkers have suggested that autopsy findings of degeneration of nerve cells and increased gliosis in pons, midbrain, and medulla, with striking endothelial hyperplasia, may strongly support this diagnosis in the undernourished infant.

Treatment. As has been indicated, thiamine administration is the only therapeutic agent required. A dose of 10 mg every 6 to 8 hours should be sufficient. Supportive measures for the congestive heart failure should be provided. Seizures generally respond promptly to thiamine administration without need of other anticonvulsant therapy. Clearly, the mother of the infant with either congenital beriberi or the infantile form secondary to breast-feeding requires vitamin B_1 therapy as well.

Pyridoxine Deficiency and Dependency

The active form of vitamin B_6 plays an important role as a coenzyme for a broad variety of reactions in amino acid, glycogen, and short chain fatty acid metabolism. Clinical manifestations of body pool depletion of the coenzyme result in a clinically defined deficiency syndrome. Another form of B_6 "insufficiency" known as pyridoxine dependency is, however, of more immediate interest. In this form, the apoenzyme with which B_6 combines in its coenzyme function is modified so that unusually high concentrations of the coenzyme must be present to facilitate the enzymatic reaction and prevent either accumu-

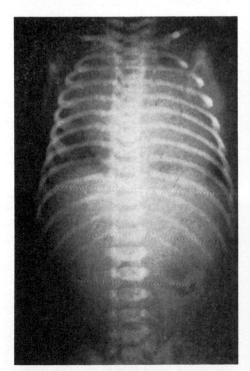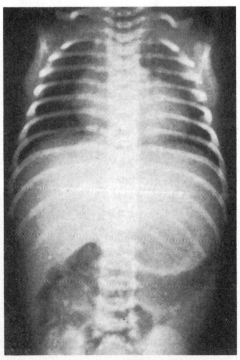

Figure 90–1. *A*, Roentgenogram of an infant 18 hours old with congenital beriberi, before thiamine therapy was instituted, showing an enlarged cardiac shadow. *B*, Roentgenogram of the child 11 days after administration of the first dose of thiamine, showing reduction in size of the cardiac shadow. (Van Gelder, D. W., and Darby, F. U.: J. Pediatr. *25*:226, 1944.)

lations of substrate or deficiency of products of the reaction. As noted previously, B_6 acts broadly as a coenzyme and hence there are several forms of B_6 dependency.

Incidence. True pyridoxine deficiency is extremely rare. It does not occur at birth but is a result of inadequate B_6 intake over the first months of life. In the early 1950s, a modification in the processing of a particular prepared formula led to inactivation of the vitamin. This B_6-deficient formula resulted in an epidemic of seizures, which occurred at 6 weeks to 4 months of age in infants fed exclusively on this formula. The "epidemic" was elegantly reported in May's 1954 report. In general, and under normal conditions, both unprocessed cow's and human milk contain adequate amounts of the vitamin. It has been suggested, however, that breast-feeding by severely malnourished B_6-deficient mothers may result in a deficiency state in the infant. Both malabsorption and vitamin inhibition by drugs such as isoniazid and penicillamine have resulted in deficiency states in older children, but similar effects have not been noted in neonates.

The most common form of pyridoxine dependency in the neonatal period also presents with seizures not unlike those occurring with the deficiency syndrome. This form of vitamin dependency, however, is not due to a diminished transplacental or neonatal supply of the vitamin but rather to an increased vitamin requirement by specific individuals. More than 50 documented cases of pyridoxine-dependent neonatal seizures have been reported from many parts of the world. As noted by Hunt in 1954, this abnormality of pyridoxine metabolism appears to be genetically determined and is inherited as an autosomal recessive. Other forms of B_6 dependency are associated with cystathioninuria, xanthurenicaciduria, homocystinuria, and hyperoxaluria. All are hereditary. These forms have been reviewed by Scriver and Rosenberg and will not be discussed further.

Etiology. The naturally occurring forms of pyridoxine are widely distributed in nature in grains, meat, and dairy products. These forms are converted in the body to pyridoxal-5'-phosphate, which, as noted previously, acts as a coenzyme for a broad variety of enzymatic reactions, particularly in amino acid metabolism. Heller and associates have noted the common occurrence of low pyridoxine levels in pregnant women. No abnormalities of maternal or fetal outcome, however, were found to correlate with low maternal B_6 levels. Brophy and Sriteri, however, reported low levels of pyridoxal phosphate in preeclamptic mothers, as well as evidence of decreased placenta transfer of the vitamin in these women. Con-

tractor and Shane as well as Brophy and Sriteri confirmed the low vitamin levels in pregnant women but noted that fetal cord blood levels at term were several times greater than maternal levels. These latter observations suggest active transport of the vitamin across the placenta and provide an explanation for absence of symptoms of the deficiency state in the immediate neonatal period. A group of premature infants studied by Reinken and Mangold, however, had low cord levels of pyridoxal-5'-phosphate at birth. These data may suggest that active transport of the vitamin occurs primarily late in pregnancy and that the premature infant may be at higher risk for development of the deficiency state.

In animals, pyridoxine deficiency leads to severe growth limitations, anemia, changes in skin and hair, and seizures. In the infant, the major expression of either the deficiency or dependency state is seizures. It is felt that this manifestation is a result of decreased production of gamma-aminobutyric acid (GABA), a central nervous system inhibitory neurotransmitter. The active form of the vitamin appears to cocatalyze the conversion of glutamic acid to GABA with the apoenzyme glutamic acid decarboxylase. As noted by Scriver, deficiency of GABA predisposes the brain to hyperirritability and seizures. In the deficiency state, reduced amounts of the coenzyme pyridoxal-5'-phosphate are present. In the dependency state, the apoenzyme glutamic acid decarboxylase is altered so that markedly increased amounts of the coenzyme are required for the normal production of GABA. It is important to re-emphasize that in the dependency state tissue vitamin levels are normal in the face of clinical symptoms. Why this particular enzyme system of all those affected by the vitamin seems to dominate the neonatal presentation of vitamin insufficiency is not known.

Diagnosis. In May's original report of the 1953 deficiency "epidemic," extreme central nervous system irritability was the only early symptom of B_6 deficiency. As the degree of deficiency progressed, owing to lack of adequate vitamin intake, the onset of brief tonic-clonic seizures was noted at 1 to 4 months of age. Anemia and growth failure were not observed, although in 1950 Snyderman and coworkers reported both in retarded infants subjected to experimental vitamin deficiency. Rare subsequent reports of true deficiency states confirm seizures as the predominant clinical symptom.

In pyridoxine dependency, irritability and seizures are the sole symptoms. In the dependency state, however, seizures may start in utero, as reported by Bejsovec and colleagues. In this report, three siblings appeared to have a severe form of the disease, and all had intrauterine seizures beginning between the fifth and seventh month of gestation. It is interesting that in the third infant seizures were controlled by high maternal doses of B_6.

In the majority of cases, however, seizures are noted in the first hours after delivery. The following case, described by Swaiman and Milstein, is typical.

The patient, a girl, was born at term and weighed 6 pounds, 10 ounces (3260 gm). The delivery was uncomplicated. There was no family history of seizures or neurologic disease. During her pregnancy, the mother did not receive supplemental pyridoxine.

The child appeared healthy until 3 hours of age, when she began having generalized major motor clonic seizures. The blood calcium was 8.5 mg per 100 ml, and blood sugar was 73 mg per 100 ml. The subdural space did not contain fluid, and the results of a spinal fluid examination were normal. Although the patient received phenobarbital, she had intermittent generalized seizures throughout the first day. The seizures gradually decreased in frequency during phenobarbital therapy, and, by the seventh day of life, she no longer needed the drug. She was fed a commercial milk formula containing 0.3 mg pyridoxine per quart. No other vitamins were given.

At 17 days of age, the patient had another seizure, and daily phenobarbital therapy was resumed. She appeared overly sensitive to noise but otherwise was normal.

Subsequently, the patient had three generalized tonic major motor seizures. Administration of anticonvulsants, calcium, and glucose failed to control the seizures, which continued intermittently for the next few days, until she received 100 mg of pyridoxine intramuscularly. The seizures stopped within an hour. Twitching began again 6 days later and was controlled with 10 mg of pyridoxine. She then remained seizure free on 25 mg of pyridoxine a day.

Occasionally, as in a case reported by Gentz, seizures may begin as late as 3 weeks of age, although some increase in muscle tone was noted earlier. In most cases, seizures have been brief and tonic-clonic in nature. An interesting feature is the inability of anticonvulsants to control this seizure disorder in contrast to the rapid control achieved by a single dose of 50 mg of pyridoxine. This feature has been considered of some diagnostic use. Frequently, a single dose of pyridoxine is given to the neonate during a seizure in an early effort to rule out this diagnostic possibility. It has been widely suggested that this therapeutic trial is even more meaningful when performed with EEG running. Control of seizures and reversion of EEG to normal within minutes after receiving the vitamin have been considered the ultimate in diagnostic orchestration. Iinuma and co-workers have tempered this approach slightly by suggesting that, although seizure control may be achieved rapidly, it may require up to 24 hours before the EEG returns to full normality.

Long-term follow-up of B_6-dependent children with seizures suggests normal development in those treated early and aggressively. Children whose diagnosis is delayed, with seizures persisting for weeks, or children who periodically experience inadequate B_6 supplements do not seem to fare as well.

The early onset and high continuing vitamin requirements should allow for clear differentiation of deficiency and dependency states. The tryptophan loading test, although normal in dependency states, results in an increase in xanthenurenic acid in true deficiency states. This is a result of the importance of B_6 as a coenzyme in the further breakdown of tryptophan and has been used to confirm the differentiation of these clinical entities.

Treatment. Prevention of the deficiency state requires only adequate vitamin B_6 supplementation. In general, 0.03 mg of pyridoxine a day is thought adequate for the neonate, and this amount is provided by proprietary formulas. Treatment of deficiency would simply require replenishment of the body pool and could be accomplished by daily 50 to 100 mg doses for several days.

Dependency states vary in vitamin B_6 requirements. In general, 25 to 100 mg of the vitamin are required daily to prevent irritability and seizures. This requirement apparently continues for life, although no long-term follow-up studies are available at present.

Vitamin C Deficiency

Scurvy affects the newborn so rarely that a detailed discussion of the effects of vitamin C deficiency is not warranted. Of some interest, however, is the role of vitamin C in a form of transient tyrosinemia seen in premature infants.

Incidence. Since the reports of Jackson and Park in 1935 and Ingalls in 1938, no subsequent cases of scurvy in the immediate neonatal period have been detailed. Jackson and Park's patient was an infant born to a woman who in all probability also had the disease. This fact is of some interest following the report of Sherlock and Rothschild of scurvy appearing in a woman on a Zen macrobiotic diet. This diet has gained some popularity in certain health-food circles and well may eventually account for other neonatal cases in the literature.

Etiology. It appears that neonatal scurvy must be associated with maternal vitamin C deficiency. Whether preterm infants are more susceptible because of decreased transplacental acquisition of the vitamin is not known. Ingalls' three patients were all premature, but no concomitant description is given of maternal health. These infants were fed pooled breast milk, which is thought to contain enough ascorbic acid to prevent development of disease (43 mg per liter). It is interesting that cow's milk contains very little ascorbic acid and that the calf, unlike the human, can synthesize the vitamin. Humans, apparently along with the Indian fruit bat and the guinea pig, have lost this ability. Although in this country all formula is now adequately supplemented with vitamin C, Grewar has had considerable experience with infants as young as 5 months who developed scurvy on diets consisting exclusively of unfortified formula.

Ascorbic acid is essential for normal collagen synthesis by hydroxylation of proline as well as for normal function of osteoblasts and fibroblasts. In the preterm infant, interaction between ascorbic acid, protein intake, and the enzymatic conversion of tyrosine to parahydroxyphenylpyruvic acid is of some importance. High protein intakes, over 5 gm per kilogram per day, lead to an accumulation of tyrosine that tends to inhibit its own enzymatic conversion. Ascorbic acid tends to reverse this inhibition and decrease serum and urine levels of tyrosine. Transient tyrosinemia appears to be a relatively common occurrence in premature infants and occurs occasionally in term infants fed high protein diets. The sig-

nificance of the transient elevation of blood tyrosine and transient tyrosinuria, which tends to peak at the end of the first week of life, is not clear. In general, this form of vitamin C dependence is thought to be a transient development defect and of no long-term significance. Menkes and colleagues, however, have suggested that severe transient tyrosinemia may have some long-term central nervous system residua. This subject and the differentiation of this entity from hereditary tyrosinemia have been reviewed by Scriver and Rosenberg.

Diagnosis. Because of the rarity of neonatal scurvy, few conclusions can be drawn regarding its clinical presentation. Jackson and Park's infant presented with only weight loss and extreme irritability. Ingalls' patients were symptomatic. The classic signs of infantile scurvy, detailed by Grewar, of irritability, tenderness of lower limbs, weakness, fever, and gingival hemorrhages would be expected. Swelling of costochondral cartilages was prominent in his series. Radiographs of the long bones show the characteristic findings of generalized osteoporosis, with thickening of the zone of provisional calcification, spur

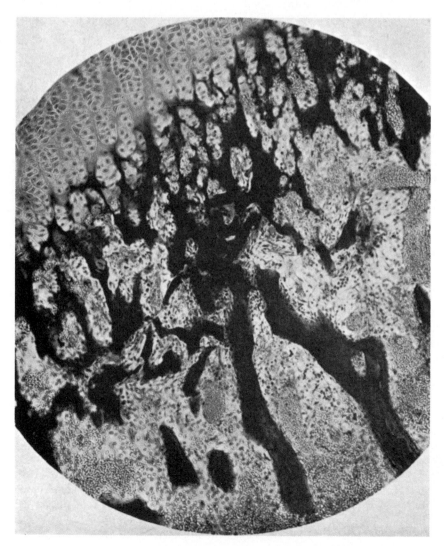

Figure 90–2. Photomicrograph of histologic section from upper end of humerus to show typical scorbutic lesion. Above is the proliferative cartilage. The black network is the scorbutic lattice. Note how it is fractured. In the center, the fragments are driven together into an impacted mass; to the left and right, they lie crosswise but appear to be free. To the histologist, it is at once evident that the lattice is bare; i.e., no bone has formed on its surface. The supporting connective tissue of the marrow (*Gerüstmark*) is beautifully shown. Around the fragments of the lattice are osteoblasts. They surround the fragments loosely as swarms of bees surround the head of the person whom they are attacking. Under normal conditions they lie in orderly rows against the surfaces of the trabeculae. The blood vessels are full of red blood cells, but no hemorrhages are visible. (Jackson, D., and Park, E. A.: J. Pediatr. 7:741, 1935.)

formation at the cartilage-shaft junction, and sub-periosteal hemorrhages. Caffey has noted the occasional difficulty in differentiating the radiographic picture of early scurvy from that seen in congenital syphilis. Neonatal copper deficiency may present a somewhat similar radiologic appearance (see p. 810).

Treatment. The recommended daily intake of ascorbic acid for neonates is 35 to 50 mg. In infants on high-protein diets, as much as 100 mg per day may be required to cause reduction of elevated blood tyrosine levels. For the treatment of scurvy in infants, Grewar has recommended doses of vitamin C up to 1000 mg per day. By 5 days, improvement is seen and the dose may be reduced.

Vitamin D Deficiency

The full spectrum of sequelae of fetal and neonatal vitamin D deficiency is still not clear. In 1930, Maxwell described classic rickets present at birth. Several recent reports have emphasized the appearance of rickets in small premature infants on inadequate vitamin D supplementation. Other reports have suggested that neonatal hypocalcemia with or without associated convulsions and late dental hypoplasia also may well be results of inadequate maternal or fetal vitamin D metabolism.

Incidence. Certainly, florid rickets presenting in the neonatal period is extremely rare. Few cases have been added to Maxwell's original reports. Ford and coworkers as well as Moncrieff and Fadahunsi described congenital rickets in infants born of Asian immigrants with osteomalacia, and they suggested careful observation of this population. Interestingly enough, Maxwell's original patients were also infants of Asian mothers with a form of osteoporosis thought to represent nutritional rickets. Of perhaps more immediate interest is the report of Lewin and colleagues, who noted that almost all their surviving infants who weighed less than 1000 grams at birth developed radiologic evidence of rickets at 2 to 3 months of life. These infants were not given supplemental vitamin D in addition to that supplied by commercial formula.

A resurgence of rickets in infants at 1 to 2 years of age has been reported among infants who have been maintained on prolonged breast-feeding and among those whose parents provide a diet low in vitamin D. Breast milk alone does not usually provide adequate amounts of vitamin D for the first year of life.

Etiology. Present knowledge suggests that vitamin D undergoes conversion to 25-hydroxyvitamin D in the liver and a second subsequent hydroxylation to 1,25-hydroxyvitamin D in the kidney. This later metabolite appears to be the active form of the vitamin that is responsible for absorption of calcium from the gut and remodeling of bone. Vitamin D and 25-hy-droxyvitamin D appear to cross the placenta by diffusion or facilitated diffusion (Hillman and Haddad, 1975). Fetal and cord levels, therefore, reflect maternal serum levels. In the term infant following birth, levels are well maintained, whereas levels are low at birth and may fall over several weeks in premature infants with or without supplementary vitamin D (Hillman and Haddad, 1975). In the absence of adequate amounts of the active form of the vitamin, decreased calcium availability may occur. This may result in neonatal hypocalcemia, as noted by Rosen and coworkers, but certainly is not the only etiologic factor in this common disorder. Decreased calcium availability also leads to ineffective calcification of bone and teeth as a manifestation of vitamin D deficiency (Fig. 90–3).

The prevalence of osteopenia and even rickets in low birth weight infants is not explained by deficiency of the active form of vitamin D, except in populations in which maternal D deficiency exists. Glorieux and coworkers speculate that in some infants transplacental mineral supply is limiting because they found that even 1200 I.U. of vitamin D_3 did not alter the course of hypocalcemia in the first 5 days of life. Previous studies had established that the vitamin is absorbed in the gut and hydroxylated in the liver after 32 weeks' gestation.

Diagnosis. At the present time, neonatal rickets is most often a purely radiologic diagnosis. Typical rarefaction and irregular fraying of the zone of provisional calcification of the radius and ulna, with some splaying of the metaphyses, is noted. Thickening of the costochondral junctions resulting in the "rachitic rosary" may be seen. Clinically, softening of cranial bones, craniotabes, and fractures occur. Hypoplasia of dental enamel, particularly of incisors, may appear much later (Purvis and coworkers, 1973).

Biochemical alterations consist of low or normal serum calcium and phosphorus levels and high alkaline phosphatase levels. Vitamin D levels can be obtained. The association of some neonatal hypocalcemic seizures with vitamin D deficiency has been suggested by Roberts and colleagues. Whether or not this is a common event is unknown.

Treatment. Vitamin D supplementation of infant formula is clearly the basis of both prevention and treatment. The recommended daily requirement, 400 I.U., appears to be adequate for both. In general, milk supplementation in the United States is based on the addition of 400 I.U. per quart. A small premature who may need less than 180 ml a day of formula to meet nutritional requirements will receive less than 80 I.U. of vitamin D a day. As detailed by Lewin and coworkers and by Tulloch, this degree of supplementation may lead to the development of bony changes by 2 months of age. Thus, it is rec-

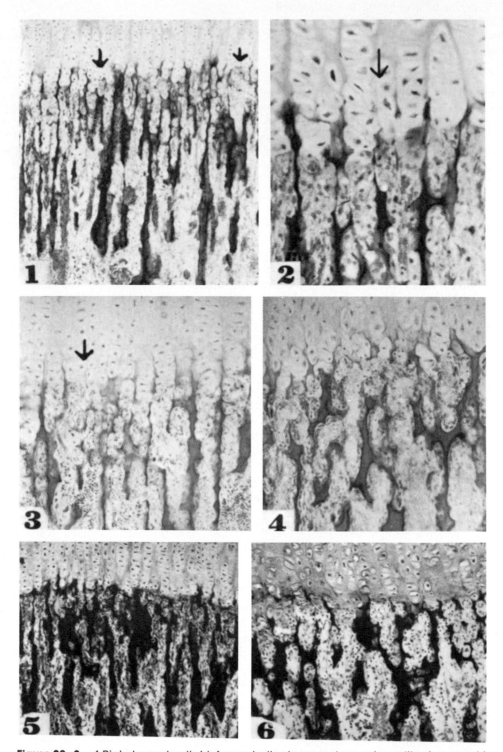

Figure 90–3. *1,* Rickets, acute, slight. Arrows indicate several areas in cartilaginous matrix between hypertrophic cells where disposition of inorganic materials is lacking (as indicated by failure to stain with hematoxylin). *2,* Rickets, acute, slight. Higher power to show area in matrix between several rows of hypertrophic cells where deposition of inorganic materials is faulty. *3,* Rickets, acute, slight. Focus of defective calcification in cartilage. *4,* Rickets, acute, moderate. Large focus of defective calcification in cartilage. *5,* Rickets, acute, severe. Except for a few areas, there is virtual cessation of lime salt deposition in provisional zone of calcification. *6,* Rickets, acute, severe. Sudden and complete cessation of deposition of inorganic materials in areas of hypertrophic cells. The suddeness is evidenced by the adequacy (dark staining materials) beneath. (Follis, R. H., Park, E. A., and Jackson, D.: Bull. Johns Hopkins Hosp. *91:*480, 1952.)

ommended that the preterm infant receive a full 400 I.U. of vitamin D daily regardless of size. It is interesting that Tulloch has suggested that the smallest infants may have increased daily requirements (800 I.U.), perhaps based on liver or renal enzymatic immaturity with regard to conversion of vitamin D to its active forms. Wolf and colleagues have made similar recommendations based on a comparison of alkaline phosphatase levels in premature infants given 500 or 1000 I.U. daily for the first 50 days of life. As yet this increased requirement has not been documented, although Hillman and Haddad noted little or no increase in the low serum levels of vitamin D in some premature infants given 400 I.U. daily either orally or intravenously over the first 5 to 6 weeks of life (see Chapter 53).

Vitamin E Deficiency

The syndrome in the premature infant that we now recognize as vitamin E deficiency was delineated as recently as the mid 1960's by Hassan, Oski, Ritchie, and their respective coworkers. Prior to that time biochemical vitamin E deficiency, recognized for many years, was an interesting biochemical finding in search of a "disease" (see Chapter 103).

Incidence. Another disease of progress, clinical vitamin E deficiency probably does not occur in breast-fed infants. This is exclusively a disease of the small premature infant, and both the processing of cow's milk to create our current proprietary formula and the supplementation of this formula with iron have increased the risk of clinical sequelae. In fact, in 1968 Ritchie's group noted some evidence of vitamin E–responsive clinical or biochemical abnormalities in two thirds of the infants under 1500 grams whom they investigated. This figure is undoubtedly high and perhaps has been reduced by alterations in infant formula since that time. Nevertheless, in dealing with small prematures one must continuously keep this clinical entity in mind.

Etiology. Vitamin E, a fat-soluble vitamin (alpha-tocopherol), crosses the placenta, but fetal serum levels are less than one fourth of those of the mother (Leonard et al., 1972; Mino and Nishino, 1973). Leonard has suggested that fetal levels change little during the course of pregnancy, although earlier studies by Dju and coworkers reported sharply reduced serum levels in the premature infant. After birth, vitamin E must be absorbed from the gastrointestinal tract. Bell and coworkers studied 28 infants, ranging in weight from 0.68 to 1.45 kg, and demonstrated that they could maintain adult levels of tocopherol after orogastric administration. Two aspects of vitamin E absorption are of critical importance. Linoleic and other polyunsaturated fatty acids (PUFA) common in the vegetable oils, which are used to supplement many commercial formulas, decrease vitamin E absorption. Thus, as the amount of PUFA in the diet increases, the amount of vitamin E

required to maintain an adequate serum level also increases. This has been documented by Williams and coworkers. Breast milk, which is low in PUFA, has a high E/PUFA ratio and hence is ideal to promote vitamin E absorption. E/PUFA ratios greater than 0.6 are thought adequate for vitamin E absorption. In this regard, the advantages of breast milk have been clearly demonstrated by Lo and colleagues.

Melhorn and Gross have documented the ability of dietary iron supplements to block vitamin E absorption and increase hemolysis. The mechanism of this iron effect is not clear but is thought to be associated with the ability of iron to catalyze the non-enzymatic auto-oxidation of unsaturated fatty acids. Gross and Melhorn have suggested that this iron effect may not be a problem when using new water-soluble vitamin E preparations.

The small premature infant then, in whom poor vitamin E absorption is aggravated by a diet high in PUFA and by the presence of supplemental iron, is at high risk for subsequent vitamin E deficiency. Cord levels of vitamin E tend to be in the range of 0.2 to 0.3 mg per 100 ml, a level below the 0.5 mg per 100 ml thought to be associated with metabolic defects. Normal levels are achieved in the term infant within 2 weeks, but, in the premature without appropriate E supplementation, levels may continue to fall over the first 6 to 8 weeks. In a study by Williams and coworkers, there appeared to be no increased absorption of vitamin E as measured in very low birth weight infants who were fed diets containing 50 per cent of the fat content as medium-chain triglycerides. This again probably reflects the limiting effect of iron in the formula.

Although muscle necrosis and sterility may be seen in vitamin E–deficient experimental animals and in severe vitamin E deficiency associated with prolonged steatorrhea outside the neonatal period, the major effect of vitamin E deficiency in the neonate seems to be on red cell membrane stability. It is well known that the tocopherols are antioxidants, and it has been assumed that vitamin E contributes to stability of RBC membrane by preventing oxidation of lipids and sulfhydryl groups (Jacob and Lux, 1968).

More recent work has suggested that vitamin E–selenium complexing may be an important step in stabilizing the red cell membrane. Regardless of mechanism, the vitamin E–deficient red cell is subject to in vivo hemolysis and to hydrogen peroxide stimulated hemolysis in vitro.

Diagnosis. The classic work of Oski and Barness established the association of vitamin E deficiency and hemolytic anemia in the premature infant. In their patients, the diagnosis was made between 6 and 8 weeks of age. Anemia accompanied by a mild reticulocytosis and pyknocytosis was found to correlate with low serum tocopherol levels. Red cell survival was significantly shortened to a half life of 11 to 15 days. No other clinical signs were observed, and the anemia responded promptly to vitamin E administration. Ritchie and coworkers, following the earlier work of Hassan's group, noted similar hematologic findings. In addition, they observed thrombocytosis with platelet counts as high as 600,000 per cubic milliliter. They also found that the patients often had subcutaneous edema of the legs and genitalia with puffiness of the eyelids. Serum proteins and electrolytes were normal. Occasionally, a papular erythematous rash was present. All findings disappeared within 2 to 3 weeks following vitamin E administration.

A major problem is the differentiation of this mild hemolytic anemia from the physiologic anemia of prematurity. The mild elevation of the reticulocyte count (5 to 8 per cent) in the face of a continuing fall in hemoglobin has been suggested by Dallman to be a helpful differentiating feature. The appearance of pyknocytes and thrombocytosis may also be useful. Vitamin E levels may be obtained, and serum levels less than 0.5 mg per 100 ml are considered low. The peroxide hemolysis test after the first 2 weeks of life is helpful. The increase in hemolysis seems to correlate well with the degree of E deficiency, although the test is not entirely specific for this vitamin effect. A normal peroxide hemolysis test, however, would make vitamin E deficiency very unlikely.

Treatment. When vitamin E deficiency has been demonstrated, treatment with 75 to 100 I.U. of alpha-tocopherol daily should be instituted. A response is seen within 2 weeks in the hematologic indices. Improved RBC survival and a decrease in peroxide hemolysis are seen within a few days. After a week, the dose of alpha-tocopherol may be reduced to maintenance levels.

Most standard formulas contain 10 to 13 I.U. per liter of alpha-tocopherol and have an adequate E/PUFA ratio. This appears to be adequate supplementation for prevention of E deficiency in most infants over 2000 grams. Smaller infants, especially those on supplementary iron, require higher doses of vitamin E, in the range of 15 to 25 I.U. daily. Gross and Melhorn have presented data showing more effective absorption of a water solution form of the vitamin, which at 25 I.U. daily achieved "sufficient" serum levels and prevented clinical evidence of deficiency in all infants studied.

PROPHYLAXIS AGAINST RETROLENTAL FIBROPLASIA

Infants who are premature and who require increased inspired oxygen to maintain adequate arterial oxygen tensions are at risk of retrolental fibroplasia (RLF). In recent years, with ever smaller infants living longer with the support of neonatal intensive care, the number of infants with retrolental fibroplasia is increasing. Even room air may be toxic to very immature retinal vessels (see Chapter 103).

The possibility that vitamin E deficiency may be an etiologic factor was considered by Owens and Owens in the late 1940s, who demonstrated protection from alpha-tocopheryl acetate among infants in a controlled trial. Others failed to confirm the relationship, probably because at that time the confounding factor of oxygen administration had not been clarified. Once the central role of oxygen in pathogenesis of RLF became clear, further studies with vitamin E were discontinued until 1974, when Johnson and coworkers reported benefit from intramuscular vitamin E. The rationale for resumption of studies is that vitamin E is a biologic antioxidant, and premature infants are relatively deficient in it.

The most convincing clinical demonstration of efficacy of vitamin E was reported on a group of 101 preterm infants, all less than 1500 grams at birth. Hittner and colleagues showed that infants who were given 100 mg/kg of vitamin E orally per day had less severe RLF than those who received only 5 mg/kg/day. Because of these positive clinical findings, we recommend starting vitamin E within the first 24 hours in infants who will require increased concentrations of oxygen because of cardiopulmonary disease and continuing the high-dose prophylaxis for the duration of oxygen therapy.

Vitamin K Deficiency

Without parenteral vitamin K supplementation to the newborn or parturient mother, vitamin K deficiency would rank as the most common deficiency syndrome of all. This disorder and its pathogenesis have been discussed in an earlier section and will not be reconsidered here (see Chapter 64).

Copper Deficiency

An X-linked recessive disorder of copper metabolism, Menkes' disease is discussed in Chapter 63.

Following reports of metabolic sequelae in copper-deficient animals, a clinical syndrome associated with low serum levels of copper has been recognized in infants.

Incidence. This entity seems to occur particularly in the small premature infant. It is interesting that two of the three cases of copper deficiency reported by Griscom and coworkers occurred in severely undergrown members of premature twin pregnancies. Small prematures maintained for prolonged periods on parenteral alimentation following bowel surgery also appear to be at risk. Clinical findings have not been reported prior to 2 months of age.

Etiology. Copper is an essential nutrient combining with a number of proteins in the body. Copper-containing enzymes such as cytochrome oxidase are required for cellular respiration. The precise mechanism by which copper deficiency results in its characteristic symptoms, however, is unknown.

During fetal life, copper seems to be concentrated in the fetal liver. Levels are very high, exceeding those of the adult after 20 weeks' gestation (Widdowson et al., 1972). Deficiency after birth appears to be the result of very low postnatal copper intake coupled with prematurity. In the premature, although hepatic copper concentrations may be high initially, the total amount of the element available during the period of rapid neonatal growth may be inadequate. Hillman and coworkers showed that full-term infants had low cord serum copper and ceruloplasmin levels that increased to adult levels by 1 month of age, whereas very low birth weight infants required up to 4 months to achieve normal levels, despite increased copper content in their formula. This may represent a maturational delay in the liver production of ceruloplasmin.

Diagnosis. A sideroblastic anemia, neutropenia, and bone abnormalities are among the most commonly reported findings in neonatal copper deficiency. The following case, reported by Griscom and coworkers, is typical.

CASE 90–4

This infant was a 680-gram member of a twin pair, born at 31 weeks' gestation. Initial hospital course was uneventful without any respiratory distress. At 66 days of age, irritability and a low-grade fever developed. A chest film showed irregularity of aeration with a distribution suggestive of aspiration. Healing fractures of the anterolateral portions of many ribs were evident; this led to a skeletal survey that showed separation of the left proximal humeral epiphyseal cartilage, severe systemic osteoporosis, poorly mineralized subperiosteal new bone along the shafts of the long bones, enlargement of the costochondral cartilages, and metaphyseal cupping. The hematocrit was 17 per cent, with a 1.3 per cent reticulocyte count. Neutropenia was noted. Vitamin intake, particularly of vitamins C and D, was adequate. At 71 days of age, the infant suffered a cardiorespiratory arrest. Pathologic examination of the bones revealed findings compatible with copper deficiency, and a measurement of liver copper content was very low.

Bone lesions, as noted previously, may include rib fractures and beading of costochondral cartilages. Osteoporosis, metaphyseal cupping and irregularities, epiphyseal separations, and periosteal new bone formation may be seen. At times, these findings may mimic those seen in scurvy.

Diagnosis is based on finding low serum copper

levels and low serum ceruloplasmin. The reticulocyte response to copper administration should be rapid. Disappearance of the bone lesions and neutropenia should follow within 2 weeks. Serum, calcium, phosphorus, and alkaline phosphatase levels should be normal.

Treatment. Ashkenazi and associates have recommended a dietary intake of copper between 100 and 500 μg per day. Their treatment program for older infants with full-blown deficiency states consisted of 1 to 3 mg of oral copper sulfate for several days, followed by maintenance dietary copper. In Menkes' syndrome, because of the defect in copper absorption, high daily oral doses of copper must be used.

Zinc Metabolism

With the introduction of total parenteral nutrition, zinc deficiency states have been identified before the addition of supplemental zinc. For these reasons, it seems important to review some of the findings of zinc deficiency.

Sources of Zinc. The major dietary sources of zinc are meat, fish, poultry, eggs, and dairy products. The recommended allowances for infants are 3 to 5 mg/day, for children 10 mg/day, and for adults 15 to 25 mg/day.

Zinc Deficiency. The clinical findings include fever and lesions of the skin and mucous membranes, sometimes secondarily infected. Occasionally, there is unremitting diarrhea and alopecia is common. Kay and Tasman-Jones reported these findings in 1975 in infants in the fourth week of total parenteral nutrition. They were treated with zinc sulfate, 1 to 2 mg/kg/day, with dramatic improvement within a few days.

In older individuals, disorders of taste and smell, mental change, and cerebellar dysfunction have been associated with a low serum zinc concentration and have improved with the administration of zinc.

Laboratory Diagnosis. Serum zinc levels are higher in infants under 35 weeks' gestation than in those born nearer to term. Postnatally, zinc levels in serum fall from about 150 μg/dl in the first week to levels of about 100 μg/dl by 2 months postnatal age (Sann et al., 1980). A demonstration of a plasma level of less than 65 μg/dl or hair concentrations of less that 70 μg/gm of hair are considered diagnostic. Sometimes, there is a decrease in serum alkaline phosphatase. The diagnosis is established by a clinical response to dietary zinc supplementation.

REFERENCES

Ashkenazi, A., Levin, S., et al.: The syndrome of neonatal copper deficiency. Pediatrics 52:525, 1973.

Avery, M. E., Clow, C. L., et al.: Transient tyrosinemia of the newborn: dietary and clinical aspects. Pediatrics 39:378, 1967.

Bass, M. H., and Fisch, G. R.: Increased intracranial pressure with bulging fontanel. Neurology 11:1091, 1961.

Bejsovec, M., Kulenda, Z., and Ponca, E.: Familial intrauterine convulsions in pyridoxine dependency. Arch. Dis. Child. 42:201, 1967.

Bernhardt, I. B., and Dorsey, D. J.: Hypervitaminosis A and congenital renal anomalies in a human infant. Obstet. Gynecol. 43:750, 1974.

Brophy, M. H., and Siiteri, P. K.: Pyridoxal phosphate and hypertensive disorders of pregnancy. Am. J. Obstet. Gynecol. 121:1075, 1975.

Caffey, J.: Pediatric X-ray Diagnosis. 6th ed. Chicago, Year Book Medical Publishers, 1972, pp. 1237–1243.

Cochrane, W. A., Collins-Williams, C., and Donohue, W. L.: Superior hemorrhagic polioencephalitis occurring in an infant—probably due to thiamine deficiency from use of a soybean product. Pediatrics 28:771, 1961.

Committee on Nutrition, American Academy of Pediatrics: Zinc. Pediatrics 62:408, 1978.

Contractor, S. F., and Shane, B.: Blood and urine levels of vitamin B_6 in the mother and fetus before and after loading of the mother with vitamin B_6. Am. J. Obstet. Gynecol. 107:635, 1970.

Dallman, P. R.: Iron, vitamin E and folate in the preterm infant. Pediatrics 85:742, 1974.

DeLuca, H. F.: Vitamin D: the vitamin and the hormone. Fed. Proc. 33:2211, 1974.

Dju, M. Y. et al.: Vitamin E (tocopherol) in human fetuses and placentae. Etud. Neonat. 1:1, 1952.

Farrell, P. M.: Vitamin E deficiency in premature infants. J. Pediatr. 95:869, 1979.

Fehily, L.: Human milk intoxication due to B_1 avitaminosis. Br. Med. J. 2:590, 1944.

Fomon, S. J.: Infant Nutrition. 2nd ed. Philadelphia, W. B. Saunders Co., 1974.

Ford, J. A., Davidson, D. C., et al.: Neonatal rickets in Asian immigrant population. Br. Med. J. 3:211, 1973.

Gal, I., and Parkinson, C. E.: Variations in the pattern of maternal serum vitamin A and carotenoids during human reproduction. Int. J. Vitamin Nutr. Res. 42:565, 1972.

Gentz, J., Hemfelt, S., et al.: Vitamin B metabolism in pyridoxine dependency with seizures. Acta Pediatr. Scand. 56:17, 1967.

Glorieux, F. H., Salle, B. L., Delvin, E. E., and David, L.: Vitamin D metabolism in preterm infants: serum calcitriol values during the first five days of life. J. Pediatr. 99:640, 1981.

Gordon, E. F., Gordon, R. C., and Passal, D. B.: Zinc metabolism: basic, clinical, and behavioral aspects. J. Pediatr. 99:341, 1981.

Grewar, D.: Infantile scurvy. Clin. Pediatr. 4:82, 1965.

Griscom, N. T., Craig, J. N., and Neuhauser, E. B. D.: Systemic bone disease developing in small premature infants. Pediatrics 48:883, 1971.

Gross, S., and Melhorn, D. K.: Vitamin E-dependent anemia in the premature infant. III. Comparative hemoglobin, vitamin E and erythrocyte phospholipid responses following absorption of either water-soluble or fat-soluble d-alpha tocopheryl. J. Pediatr. 85:753, 1974.

Hassan, H., Hashim, S. A., et al.: Syndrome in premature infants associated with low plasma vitamin E levels and high polyunsaturated fatty acid diet. Am. J. Clin. Nutr. 19:147, 1966.

Heller, S., Salkeld, R. M., and Körner, W. F.: Vitamin B_6 status in pregnancy. Am. J. Clin. Nutr. 26:1339, 1973.

Henley, T. H., Dann, M., and Golden, W. R. C.: Reserves, absorption and plasma levels of vitamin A in premature infants. Am. J. Dis. Child. 68:257, 1944.

Hillman, L. S., and Haddad, J. G.: Human perinatal vitamin D metabolism. I.: 25-hydroxyvitamin D in maternal and cord blood. J. Pediatr. 84:742, 1974.

Hillman, L. S., and Haddad, J. G.: Perinatal vitamin D metabolism. J. Pediatr. 86:928, 1975.

Hillman, L.: Seroserum copper concentrations in premature and SGA infants during the first three months of life. J. Pediatr. 98:305, 1981.

Hillman, L., Martin, L., and Fiore, B.: Effect of all copper supplementation on serum copper and ceruloplasmin concentrations in premature infants. J. Pediatr. 98:311, 1981.

Hittner, H. M., Godio, L. B., Rudolph, A. J., et al.: Retrolental fibroplasia: efficacy of vitamin E in a double-blind clinical study of preterm infants. N. Engl. J. Med. 305:1365, 1981.

Hunt, A. D., Stokes, J., Jr., et al.: Pyridoxine dependency: report of a case of intractable convulsions in an infant controlled by pyridoxine. Pediatrics 13:140, 1954.

Iinuma, K., Narisawa, K., et al.: Pyridoxine dependent convulsion: effect of pyridoxine therapy on electroencephalograms. Tohoku J. Exp. Med. 105:19, 1971.

Ingalls, T. H.: Ascorbic acid requirements in early infancy. N. Engl. J. Med. 218:872, 1938.

Jackson, D., and Park, E. A.: Congenital scurvy: a case report. J. Pediatr. 7:741, 1935.

Jacob, H. S., and Lux, S. E.: Degradation of membrane phospholipids and thiols in peroxide hemolysis: studies in vitamin E deficiency. Blood 32:549, 1968.

Johnson, L., Schaffer, D., and Boggs, T. R.: The premature infant, vitamin E deficiency and retrolental fibroplasia. Am. J. Clin. Nutr. 27:1158, 1974.

Kay, R. G., and Tasman-Jones, C.: Acute zinc deficiency in man during intravenous alimentation. Aust. N.Z. J. Surg. 45:325, 1975.

Keating, J. P., and Fergin, R. D.: Increased intracranial pressure associated with probable vitamin A deficiency in cystic fibrosis. Pediatrics 46:41, 1970.

Knudson, A. G., Jr., and Rothman, P. E.: Hypervitaminosis A. Am. J. Dis. Child. 85:316, 1953.

Leonard, P. J., Doyle, E., and Harrington, W.: Levels of vitamin E in the plasma of newborn infants and of the mothers. Am. J. Clin. Nutr. 25:480, 1972.

Lewin, P. K., Reid, M., et al.: Iatrogenic rickets in low birth weight infants. J. Pediatr. 78:207, 1971.

Lo, S. S., Frank, D., and Hitzig, W. H.: Vitamin E and haemolytic anaemia in premature infants. Arch. Dis. Child. 48:360, 1973.

Marie, J. and Sée, G.: Hydrocéphalie aigüe bénigne du nourisson après ingestion d'une dose massive unique de vitamines A et D. Sem. Hôp. Paris 27:1744, 1951.

Maxwell, J. P.: Two cases of foetal rickets. J. Pathol. Bacteriol. 33:327, 1930.

Maxwell, J. P., Hu, C. H., and Turnbull, H. M.: Foetal rickets. J. Pathol. Bacteriol. 35:419, 1932.

May, C. D., et al.: Clinical studies of vitamin A in infants and in children. Am. J. Dis. Child. 59:1167, 1940.

May, C. D.: Vitamin B_6 in human nutrition: a critique and an object lesson. Pediatrics 14:269, 1954.

Melhorn, D. K., and Gross, S.: Vitamin E-dependent anemia in the premature infant. I. Effects of large doses of medicinal iron. J. Pediatr. 79:569, 1971.

Melhorn, D. K., and Gross, S.: Vitamin E-dependent anemia in the premature infant. II. Relationships between gestational age and absorption of vitamin E. J. Pediatr. 79:581, 1971.

Menkes, J. H., Welcher, D. W., et al.: Relationship of elevated blood tyrosine to ultimate intellectual performance of premature infants. Pediatrics 49:218, 1972.

Mino, M., and Nishino, H.: Fetal and maternal relationship in serum vitamin E level. J. Nutr. Sci. Vitaminol. 19:475, 1973.

Moncrieff, M., and Fadahunsi, T. O.: Congenital rickets due to maternal vitamin D deficiency. Arch. Dis. Child. 49:810, 1974.

Moynahan, E. J.: Acrodermatitis enteropathica: a lethal inherited human zinc–deficiency disorder. Lancet 2:399, 1974.

Oski, F. A., and Barness, L. A.: Vitamin E deficiency: A previously unrecognized cause of hemolytic anemia in the premature infant. J. Pediatr. 70:211, 1967.

Owens, W. C., and Owens, E. U.: Retrolental fibroplasia in premature infants. II. Studies on the prophylaxis of the disease: The use of alpha tocopherol acetate. Am. J. Ophthal. 32:1631, 1949.

Purvis, R. J., Barrie, W. J., et al.: Enamel hypoplasia of the teeth associated with neonatal tetany: a manifestation of maternal vitamin D deficiency. Lancet 2:811, 1973.

Reinken, L., and Mangold, B.: Pyridoxal phosphate values in premature infants. Int. J. Vitam. Nutr. Res. 43:472, 1973.

Ritchie, J. H., Fish, M. B., et al.: Edema and hemolytic anemia in premature infants. N. Engl. J. Med. 279:1185, 1968.

Roberts, S. A., Cohen, M. D., and Forfar, J. O.: Antenatal factors associated with neonatal hypocalcaemic convulsions. Lancet 2:809, 1973.

Rosen, J. F., Roginsky, M., et al.: 25-Hydroxyvitamin D plasma levels in mothers and their premature infants with neonatal hypocalcemia. Am. J. Dis. Child. 127:220, 1974.

Sann, L., Rigal, D., Galy, G., et al.: Serum copper and zinc concentration in premature and small-for-date infants. Pediatr. Res. 14:1040, 1980.

Scriver, C. R.: Vitamin B$_6$ deficiency and dependency in man. Am. J. Dis. Child. 113:109, 1967.

Scriver, C. R., and Rosenberg, L. E.: Amino Acid Metabolism and Its Disorders. Philadelphia, W. B. Saunders Co., 1973.

Shaw, J. C. L.: Trace elements in the fetus and young infant. I. Zinc. Am. J. Dis. Child. 133:1260, 1979.

Sherlock, P., and Rothschild, O.: Scurvy produced by a Zen macrobiotic diet. J.A.M.A. 199:130, 1967.

Slobody, L. B., Willner, M. M., and Mestern, J.: Comparison of vitamin B levels in mothers and their newborn infants. Am. J. Dis. Child. 77:736, 1949.

Snyderman, S. W., Carretero, R., and Holt, E., Jr.: Pyridoxine deficiency in the human being. Fed. Proc. 9:371, 1950.

Swaiman, K., and Milstein, J.: Pyridoxine dependency and penicillamine. Neurology 20:78, 1970.

Tulloch, A. L.: Rickets in the premature. Med. J. Aust. 1:137, 1974.

Van Gelder, D. W., and Darby, F. U.: Congenital and infantile beriberi. J. Pediatr. 25:226, 1944.

Widdowson, E. M., Chan, H., et al.: Accumulation of Cu, Zn, Mn, Cr, and Co in the human liver before birth. Biol. Neonate 20:360, 1972.

Williams, M. L., Shott, R. J., et al.: Role of dietary iron and fat in vitamin E deficiency anemia of infancy. N. Engl. J. Med. 292:887, 1975.

Wolf, H., et al.: Der Bedarf an Vitamin D und an 25-Hydroxycholecalciferol bei frühgeborenen Kindern während der ersten Lebenszeit. Klinische Pädiatrie 187:331, 1975.

PART 14. DISORDERS OF THE SKELETAL SYSTEM

We have discussed in other sections of this book some of the disorders of the skeletal system. Craniostenosis, microcephaly, encephalocele, myelocele, and others have been discussed in the section concerning disorders of the nervous system; osteomyelitis is considered in the discussion of infections. Rickets and scurvy are reviewed with the vitamin deficiency diseases. There remains a miscellaneous group of disorders, some of which involve bone alone, some joints alone, and the remainder both bone and other tissues.

91

The Branchial Arch Syndromes and Cleft Lip and Cleft Palate

Revised by F. Clarke Fraser

The clinical features of mandibulofacial dysostosis were first described by Treacher Collins in 1900. Pierre Robin later lumped together hypoplasia of the mandible, glossoptosis, and cleft palate into a syndrome that bears his name. McKenzie groups them under the all-inclusive title of "the first arch syndrome," although the second branchial arch and temporal bone primordia are also involved in the developmental disturbance. More recently, a number of other branchial arch syndromes have been identified, and McKenzie's grouping is certainly an oversimplification (Cohen, 1976).

Incidence. Although each member of the group is comparatively rare, their sum total is not inconsiderable.

Etiology and Pathogenesis. The first and second branchial arch syndromes involve an array of defects that include underdevelopment of the external ear, the middle ear ossicles, the condyle and ramus of the mandible, the zygomatic arch, the malar bone, and, often, the temporal bone except for the petrous portion housing the inner ear. A group of syndromes share these features. Some are sufficiently different in the spectrum of defects displayed and in their genetic pattern to be considered separate entities. They can be grouped into those that are predominantly unilateral, such as hemifacial microsomia and oculoauriculovertebral dysplasia (Goldenhar syndrome) and those that are bilateral, including mandibulofacial dysostosis (Treacher Collins syndrome) and oculomandibulodyscephaly (Hallermann-Streiff-François syndrome).

Mandibulofacial Dysostosis (Treacher Collins Syndrome)

Etiology and Pathogenesis. Extrapolating from an animal model, Poswillo in 1975 suggested that the basic defect is reduction in the mesencephalon and in the preotic neural crest tissue destined to reinforce the mesodermal core of the first two branchial arches, with consequent disturbance of the spatial arrangement of the eye and ear. The inheritance is autosomal dominant, but with reduced penetrance and variable expressivity. About 60 per cent of cases are sporadic, and presumably fresh mutations, but near relatives

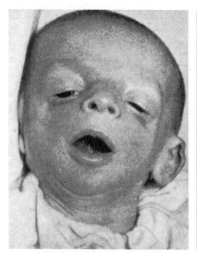 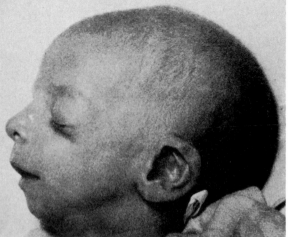

Figure 91–1. Typical Treacher Collins syndrome, or mandibulofacial dysostosis. *A,* Anterior view of the face shows the characteristic slanting, downward from within outward, of the lid slits. Also characteristic is the notching at the junction of the middle and outer thirds of the lower eyelid and the sharp angulation of the lid at that point. *B,* Lateral view, showing the receding jaw and the low-set, soft, slightly deformed external ear. (This example is one of those reported by McKenzie and Craig: Arch. Dis. Child. *30:*391, 1955. Photograph reproduced with the permission of the senior author.)

should be examined carefully for minor signs of the syndrome before one assumes that a patient is a sporadic case.

Diagnosis. A fully developed mandibulofacial dysostosis includes defective eyes, ears, and mandible. The ocular fissures are slanted downward from within out. There is a notch at the junction of the outer and middle thirds of the lower eyelid in about 75 per cent of cases, and from this point the lid angles sharply upward toward the outer canthus. Eyelashes are absent or sparse in the outer two thirds of the lower lids. The mandible is small, the chin receding, the degree of overbite considerable. There is great variability in the amount of micrognathia. The zygomatic bones are often hypoplastic. The ears may be malformed in a number of different ways: the auricles either hypoplastic or large, floppy, and low-set (Fig. 91–1), the external meatus stenotic or atretic (over one third have conductive deafness), with skin tags, fistulas, or flame-shaped areas of hypertrichosis between the tragus and the corner of the mouth. Associated defects such as high-arched palate, choanal atresia, and others are occasionally present. Mental deficiency is not a feature of the syndrome.

Diagnosis may be obvious at a glance, or attention may be called to the infant by the nurse's report that it has considerable difficulty in sucking and swallowing. She may also note that there appears to be excessive mucus in the mouth and pharynx. Intermittent spells of cyanosis, as in the Pierre Robin syndrome, are not infrequent.

The differential diagnosis includes Goldenhar syndrome (oculoauriculovertebral dysplasia), which is rarely familial, almost always unilateral, involves notching of the upper rather than the lower lid, and epibulbar dermoids. The basic defect may be the formation of a hematoma during the formation of the anastomosis that leads to the development of the stapedial arterial system. Hemifacial microsomia (unilateral microtia, macrostomia, and failure of the mandibular ramus and condyles to form) may be a variant of this. In the Nager acrofacial dysostosis, mandibulofacial dysostosis occurs with preaxial reduction defects of the upper limbs. Inheritance is autosomal recessive.

Treatment. The first problems may be those concerned with feeding difficulties and the intermittent cyanosis and respiratory distress associated with micrognathia and glossoptosis. When this is overcome, one should look carefully into the matter of hearing disability. If any is present, the appropriate steps should be taken early. These may involve surgical correction of an atretic or stenotic external auditory meatus or the use of a hearing aid and will surely call for special education. Finally, plastic surgery may be indicated to improve the child's appearance.

Micrognathia and The Pierre Robin Syndrome

Hypoplasia of the mandible, micrognathia, is encountered in a few infants as a solitary defect. More

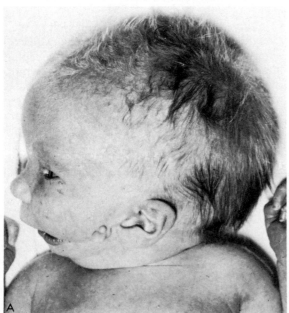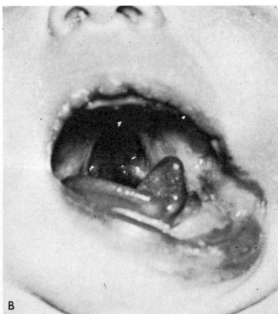

Figure 91–2. *A,* Lateral view of face shows low-set malpositioned ear and extreme degree of micrognathia. In addition, a linear skin defect including several accessory skin tags runs from the ear to the corner of the mouth. *B,* With the mouth open, a large midline cleft in the posterior half of the palate is visible. This combination of defects is more than is to be expected in the Treacher Collins syndrome or the Pierre Robin syndrome. It represents a more complicated error in development of the first visceral arch. This example was culled from the files of the Harriet Lane Home.

often, it is part of a group of signs that, described first by Robin as a clinical entity, has since borne his name. The Robin triad of micrognathia, cleft palate, and glossoptosis leads to retraction of the sternum, cyanosis, and malnutrition.

Micrognathia is also one of the numerous congenital anomalies that combine to make up the trisomy 18 (E, 16–18) syndrome. Associated congenital anomalies, most commonly talipes equinovarus, are present in about one half the infants (Davies, 1973).

Etiology. As already mentioned, some students of the problem believe the Robin syndrome to be one manifestation of faulty development of the first branchial arch. Pruzansky and Richmond call attention to an older theory that points out that mandibular micrognathia is a physiologic phenomenon in early intrauterine life and that at this time the tongue blocks the pharyngeal spaces and occupies part of the nasal cavity. If for some reason micrognathia persists, the tongue cannot fall out of the nasal cavity. Its presence there may prevent the palate from fusing, and cleft palate results.

Most cases are sporadic. Most of the reported familial cases appear to represent cases of the Stickler syndrome, which may also account for the reported association with eye problems (severe myopia, retinal detachment). Thus the family history, in cases of the Robin syndrome, should include inquiry into the presence in near relatives of joint problems, eye problems, and deafness.

Diagnosis. The pediatrician does not have the equipment needed to make precise anthropometric measurements, nor are these necessary in order to arrive at a diagnosis of isolated micrognathia. A mandible that is so small that it imparts to its owner a "bird face," or, as Dennison prefers to call it, a "shrew face" cannot be overlooked. Lesser degrees of micrognathia need not cause concern unless bouts of cyanosis, due to glossoptosis, occur. In this event, lateral radiographs of the skull should suffice to show whether the tongue is displaced posteriorly and upward enough to encroach upon the airway. The severer grades lead to noisy, difficult breathing, and may indeed cause death. If not, it is apt to produce sternal cupping (pectus excavatum) and the Harrison's groove deformity of the lower ribs. There may also be such difficulty in swallowing that high degrees of malnutrition ensue, which may also be responsible for death. If cleft palate is associated, the Robin syndrome is complete. Associated congenital heart disease is not uncommon. Indeed heart failure without congenital defect has also been reported (Jeresaty et al., 1969). In this case failure, with cor pulmonale and pulmonary edema, resulted from the severe respiratory obstruction, similar in all respects to that which follows the hypoxia caused by hypertrophied tonsils and adenoids.

Treatment. Robin himself thought that postural treatment, so-called "orthostatic nursing," sufficed in most cases. The infant was to be fed while lying on his abdomen with his chest elevated by a small pillow. The upward and outward reaching for the bottle that this position entailed would hasten the mandible's forward growth. At the outset, if respiratory distress is severe, tube-feeding is useful and may have to be continued for several weeks.

No completely satisfactory approach to management has been described. Most infants who survive with severe deformity owe their lives to their skilled nurses. In the most obstructed infants, tracheostomy is warranted. Some will require gastrostomy. Optimizing respiratory function and nutrition allows growth to work toward ameliorization of the deformity.

Harelip

Harelip, or cleft lip, represents a failure of proper merging and fusion of the facial swellings that form the upper lip. The cleft may be no larger than a barely perceptible dent in the vermilion border or it may extend into the nostril; it may be unilateral or bilateral or midline. Most often, it is unilateral and left-sided. It may or may not be associated with cleft palate; if it is, the palate defect appears to be a secondary consequence of the developmental disturbance resulting from the failure of lip closure. Other congenital defects may coexist. Additional congenital deformities need not, however, be confined to this area.

Etiology. Harelip, with or without cleft palate, occurs 40 times as often in siblings and children of the affected individual as in the general population (i.e., in about 4 per cent). Its incidence is seven times the expected in aunts, uncles, nieces and nephews and about three times the expected in first cousins (Carter, 1969). The risk for other malformations is not increased unless a genetic syndrome is involved.

It occurs in about 0.1 per cent of all births and nearly twice as often in males as in females. The majority of cases of cleft lip or palate can be attributed to the interaction of several genes and several environmental factors.

There are now over 150 recognized syndromes that include harelip or cleft palate or both. Over 50 per cent are manifestations of mutant genes; about half of these are autosomal dominant, half are autosomal recessive, and a few are X-linked. The remainder do not seem to be familial. Although the deformity can be produced experimentally in animals by maternal dietary deficiencies as well as by teratogens, only a few instances in humans can be related to agents such as thalidomide, diphenylhydantoin, or rubella. Others in the nonfamilial groups are associated with chromosomal aberrations, notably D trisomy.

Diagnosis. This presents no difficulty.

Treatment. Cleft lips may be operatively repaired as soon as the surgeon desires. One need wait only until the initial weight loss has been regained and the nutritional state is satisfactory. Seldom does uncomplicated cleft lip, even if bilateral, cause any difficulty in feeding, except possibly in the immediate postoperative period. Genetic counseling is helpful in allaying guilt and fears of recurrence but preferably after the initial period of shock and adjustment.

Cleft Palate

Imperfect closure of the palate, as of the lip, may vary from simple cleavage of the uvula and soft palate to the most grotesque and serious malformations. Palatal clefts may be single and midline and unassociated with harelip. At their worst, they are double clefts running from the soft palate forward to either side of the nose, continuous with widely spread cleft lip on each side, leaving the isolated intermaxillary process and the nose projecting upward between gaping slits in the face. As with cleft lip, other congenital defects often coexist.

Etiology. As with cleft lip, some cases are associated with syndromes that may result from mutant genes or chromosomal aberrations; a minority are caused by environmental insults, and most have a multifactorial basis. However, the genetic basis for isolated cleft palate appears to be different from that for cleft lip. Thus the sibs of a child with cleft palate have an increased risk (about 2 per cent) of having a cleft palate (but not a cleft lip), whereas the sibs of a child with cleft lip have an increased risk of having a cleft lip (with or without cleft palate) but not an isolated cleft palate.

Treatment. The pediatrician's most important task when confronted with a newborn with a severe form of this disorder is to comfort the parents and relatives and to reassure them, no matter how dreadful the situation seems to be at that moment, that with clever plastic surgery a fairly good result can be anticipated. They must be told, not all at once, that a number of operations will have to be done, that feeding will present some difficulties, that speech training will be required, and that excellent dentistry and orthodontia will be needed. In most medical centers, teams of specialists in these various fields collaborate in supervising the child's progress; the final, and a very important, member of the team is a child psychiatrist. Through his efforts, not only the child but also the parents will be assisted in surmounting the distressing years of reconstruction. In smaller communities—and often in large cities—the pediatrician has to undertake this function.

When the palatal malformation is severe, orthodontic appliances may be helpful in promoting improved alignment. They may be inserted during the first days of life (Oliver, 1969). Feeding has in our experience not been too difficult. In spite of their inability to create suction, these infants feed sufficiently well from a dropper or syringe. There is often some regurgitation through the nose, but this too is not excessive. For a time they may require a liquid concentrated feeding until they learn to manage solid foods. The palate will be repaired at 18 months or later.

REFERENCES

Carter, C. O.: Genetics of common disorders. Br. Med. Bull. 25:52, 1969.

Cohen, M. M., Jr.: Dysmorphic syndromes with craniofacial manifestations. In: Stewart, R. E., and Prescott, G. H. (Eds.): Oral Facial Genetics, St. Louis, C. V. Mosby Co, 1976.

Cohen, M. M., Jr.: Syndromes with cleft lip and cleft palate. Cleft Palate J. 15:306, 1978.

Davies, P.: Management of the Pierre Robin syndrome. Devel. Med. Child. Neurol. 15:359, 1973.

Dennison, W. M.: The Pierre Robin syndrome. Pediatrics 36:336, 1965.

Fazen, L. E., Elmore, J., and Nadler, H. L.: Mandibulo-facial dysostosis (Treacher Collins syndrome). Am. J. Dis. Child. 117:700, 1969.

Fonkalsrud, E. W., and Jones, M.: Pierre Robin syndrome in infancy. Nasoesophageal intubation. Am. J. Dis. Child. 124:79, 1972.

Fraser, F. C.: The genetics of cleft lip and cleft palate. Am. J. Hum. Genet. 22:336, 1970.

Goldberg, M. H., and Eckblom, R. H.: The treatment of the Pierre Robin syndrome. Pediatrics 30:450, 1962.

Grabb, W. C., Rosenstein, S. W., and Bzoch, K. R. (Eds.) Cleft Lip and Palate. Surgical, Dental, and Speech Aspects. Boston, Little, Brown and Co., 1971.

Jeresaty, R. M., Huszar, R. V., and Basu, S.: Pierre Robin syndrome: cause of respiratory obstruction, cor pulmonale, and pulmonary edema. Am. J. Dis. Child. 117:710, 1969.

Nisenson, A.: Receding chin and glossoptosis; a cause of respiratory difficulty in the infant. J. Pediatr. 32:397, 1948.

Nora, J. J., and Fraser, F. C.: Medical Genetics: Principles and Practice. 2nd ed. Philadelphia, Lea and Febiger, 1981.

Oliver, H. T.: Construction of orthodontic appliances for the treatment of newborn infants with clefts of the lip and palate. Am. J. Orthodont. 56:468, 1969.

Poswillo, D.: The pathogenesis of the first and second branchial arch syndrome. Oral Surg. 35:302, 1973.

Poswillo, D.: The pathogenesis of the Treacher Collins syndrome (mandibulofacial dysostosis). Br. J. Oral Surg. 13:1, 1975.

Pruzansky, S., and Richmond, J. B.: Growth of mandible in infants with micrognathia; clinical implications. A.M.A. J. Dis. Child. 88:29, 1954.

92

The Chondrodystrophies

By F. Clarke Fraser

The chondrodystrophies, or, more appropriately, the osteochondrodysplasias, are a heterogeneous group of disorders of cartilage and bone growth that result in disproportionate short stature. A discussion or even a listing of all the distinct entities is beyond the scope of this text. A selected list of them appears in Table 92–1.

According to Rimoin, the approach to evaluation of the dwarfed patient begins with assignment to a general category: Most patients with disproportionate short stature have a skeletal dysplasia, whereas those with proportionate short stature more likely have endocrine, nutritional, cytogenic, or intrauterine growth retardation. Within the disproportionate group, is the problem short-limb or short-trunk dwarfism? If short-limb, is it rhizomelic (proximal segment), mesomelic (middle), acromelic (distal), or some combination? Are there extraskeletal abnormalities? Answers to these questions will considerably reduce the differential diagnosis, if not determine the diagnosis. A complete skeletal survey is the next step. The family history may be helpful, as is histologic examination in some cases. Even in the lethal types, making the diagnosis is important for proper counseling of the parents, particularly with respect to the risk of recurrence (which may be anywhere from 50 per cent to virtually 0) and the possibility of prenatal diagnosis.

Achondroplasia

Achondroplasia is the most common of the chondrodystrophies, with an incidence of 1:10,000. It shows autosomal dominant inheritance, but about 80 per cent of these infants are born of normal parents and presumably represent fresh mutations. Thus, the recurrence risks for sibs of these "sporadic" cases is very low, but each offspring has a 50:50 chance of being affected. Care must be taken to distinguish this from similar chondrodystrophies that are recessively inherited, with a 1 in 4 recurrence risk for "sporadic" cases. Hypochondroplasia, a milder form, also shows autosomal dominant inheritance and may be an allelic mutant.

The classic phenotype includes short limb rhizomelic (affecting the proximal segment most severely) dwarfism, a normally proportioned trunk, large head

with bulging forehead, depressed nose bridge, and relatively prominent mandible. The foramen magnum is small, and mild ventricular dilatation is common; internal hydrocephalus develops occasionally. The infant's limbs are covered with fatty folds of skin, and the hands extend only to about the hip joint. The hands are short and broad, with "trident" fingers, and there is limited extension and pronation of the elbows. Infants may be hypotonic and slow in motor development but are usually normal in this respect by the age of 2 years. Radiographs show the characteristic short, broad long bones, with flaring metaphyses, short, broad pelvis with horizontal acetabular roofs, and narrow, deep sacrosciatic notches, vertebral interpediculate distances decreasing from L1 to L5, narrow spinal canal, and short skull base. Histologically (contrary to older reports), endochondral ossification is regular and well organized. Periosteal ossification is relatively increased, and it may be that the basic defect is a decrease in rate of endochondral ossification, with normal rate of membranous ossification, resulting in short, squat bones with cupped ends.

Treatment is of no avail. The psychologic aspects of the unhappy situation must be handled with delicacy and care. No benefit is gained by withholding the details of diagnosis and prognosis from the parents. So far, prenatal diagnosis is not possible at a time when therapeutic abortion is still possible.

Achondrogenesis

The term "achondrogenesis" has been used inconsistently in the literature; Rimoin suggests the following classification:

Parenti-Fraccaro Type. This recessively inherited severe form of chondrodystrophy causes stillbirth or

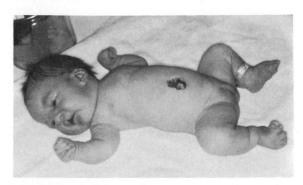

Figure 92–1. Newborn infant with classic achondroplasia. Note the relatively long trunk and very short extremities.

death early in life. The babies are small (25 to 29 cm, 900 to 1800 gm), the neck is very short, the arms are extremely short and stubby, and the thoracic cavity is small and barrel-shaped. The membranous bones of the skull are variably ossified, rendering the skull soft; the vertebral column shows total lack of ossification of the vertebral bodies, but ossification centers for the pedicles and arches are present. The ribs are short, narrow, and expanded at the costochondral junction. There are no ossification centers in the sternum, and the pelvis is poorly ossified. The long bones are extremely short and bowed and are expanded at the metaphyses, with longitudinally projecting spurs.

Histologically, there is orderly cellular maturation until the hypertrophic zone, but calcification and ossification are disorderly, with haphazard capillary penetration.

Langer-Saldino Type. This form of achondrogenesis is also recessively inherited and results in severe dwarfism and in stillbirth or early neonatal death. The head is very large in relation to the body, the neck is short and hidden in skin folds, the trunk is short and squared, with distended abdomen, and the limbs are very short. Ossification is much reduced in the lumbar vertebrae, sacrum, pubis, and ischium, and the sacrum and pubic bones are not seen. The long bones are short but usually not bowed, and the metaphyseal margins are irregular, with bony spurs. Histologically, the epiphyseal cartilage appears lobulated and mushroomed, with increased vascularity. Resting

Table 92–1. Selected Constitutional Disorders of Bone

I. OSTEOCHONDRODYSPLASIAS (abnormalities of cartilage/bone growth and development)
A. Defects of growth of tubular bones and/or spine
   1. Achondrogenesis type I (Parenti-Fraccaro)
   2. Achondrogenesis type II (Langer-Saldino)
   3. Thanatophoric dysplasia
   4. Thanatophoric dysplasia with clover-leaf skull
   5. Short rib polydactyly syndrome type I (Saldino-Noonan)
   6. Short rib polydactyly syndrome type II (Majewsky)
   7. Chondroplasia punctata
      a. rhizomelic type
      b. dominant type
      c. other types (not including conditions with stippling such as Zellweger syndrome, warfarin embryopathy)
   8. Campomelic dysplasia
   9. Other dysplasias with congenital bowing of the long bones
   10. Achondroplasia
   11. Diastrophic dysplasia
   12. Metatropic dysplasia
   13. Chondroectodermal dysplasia (Ellis–van Creveld)
   14. Asphyxiating thoracic dysplasia (Jeune)
   15. Spondyloepiphyseal dysplasia congenita (Spranger-Wiedemann)
   16. Other spondyloepiphyseal dysplasias recognizable at birth
   17. Kniest dysplasia
   18. Mesomelic dysplasia
      a. of Nievergelt
      b. of Langer
      c. of Robinow
      d. of Reinhardt
      e. other types
   19. Acromesomelic dysplasia
   20. Cleidocranial dysplasia
   21. Larsen syndrome
   22. Otophalatodigital syndrome

II. DYSOSTOSES (malformation of individual bones, singly or in combination)
A. Dysostoses with cranial and facial involvement
   1. Craniosynostosis (several types)
   2. Craniofacial dysostosis (Crouzon)
   3. Acrocephalosyndactyly (Apert) and others
   4. Acrocephalopolysyndactyly (Carpenter) and others
   5. Mandibulofacial dysostosis
      a. Treacher Collins type
      b. other types
   6. Oculomandibulofacial syndrome (Hallerman-Streiff-François)
   7. Nevoid basal cell carcinoma syndrome
B. Dysostoses with predominant axial involvement
   1. Vertebral segmentation defects (including Klippel-Feil)
   2. Cervico-oculoacoustic syndrome (Wildervanck)
   3. Sprengel anomaly
   4. Spondylocostal dysostosis
      a. dominant form
      b. recessive forms
   5. Oculovertebral syndrome (Weyers-Thier)
   6. Osteo-onychodysostosis (nail-patella syndrome)
   7. Cerebrocostomandibular syndrome
C. Dysostoses with predominant involvement of limbs
   1. Acheiria
   2. Apodia
   3. Ectrodactyly syndrome
   4. Aglossia-adactyly syndrome
   5. Congenital bowing of long bones (several types)
   6. Familial radioulnar synostosis
   7. Brachydactyly (several types)
   8. Symphalangism
   9. Polydactyly (several types)
   10. Syndactyly (several types)
   11. Polysyndactyly (several types)
   12. Camptodactyly
   13. Poland syndrome
   14. Rubinstein-Taybi syndrome
   15. Pancytopenia-dysmelia syndrome (Fanconi)
   16. Thrombocytopenia absent radius (TAR) syndrome
   17. Orodigitofacial syndrome
      a. Papillon-Léage and Psaume type
      b. Mohr type
   18. Cardiomegalic syndrome (Holt-Oram and others)
   19. Femoral-facial syndrome
   20. Multiple synostoses (includes some forms of symphalangism)
   21. Scapuloiliac dysostosis (Kosenow-Sinios)
   22. Hand-foot-genital syndrome
   23. Focal dermal hypoplasia (Goltz)

III. IDIOPATHIC OSTEOLYSES
A. Phalangeal (several forms)
B. Tarsocarpal
   1. Including François type and others
   2. With nephropathy
C. Multicentric
   1. Several types, including Winchester type
   2. Hajdu-Cheney type

cartilage is markedly hypercellular, with little matrix. Cellular column formation is absent at the growth plate, and there is complete disorganization of endochondral ossification. The primary defect may affect matrix synthesis, with secondary disorganization of ossification.

The recurrence risk for sibs in both these types of achondrogenesis is 1 in 4, making it very important not to confuse them with infants with achondroplasia or thanatophoric dwarfism. Prenatal diagnosis has been accomplished in the second trimester.

The term "achondrogenesis" has also been applied (inappropriately) to a nonlethal form of short-limb dwarfism, in which the limbs and hands are extremely short, the effect increasing distally so that the fingers are so short they may be functionless. About half these infants have polydactyly. There are varying degrees of aplasia or hypoplasia of the bones of the limbs. Until the pathogenesis of this disorder is known, Rimoin suggests that the condition be known as "Grebe disease."

Campomelic Dwarfism

This short-limbed dwarfism mainly affects the lower limbs and is associated with relatively long slender bones and anterior bending of the femur and tibia. A large calvaria, small face, lowset ears, hypertelorism, a depressed nasal root, and micrognathia are characteristic. Cleft palate is frequent. The ribs are narrow and wavy, the clavicles slender, the pelvis high and narrow with hypoplasia of the rami and vertically oriented ischia. Death usually occurs in the neonatal period. There is an apparent excess of affected females, with a number of these presenting as chromosomal males (46XY) with female external genitalia and no HY antigen. Some patients have ambiguous genitalia. The recurrence risk is low, although affected sibs have been reported.

Thanatophoric Dwarfism

This lethal form of dwarfism is characterized by markedly shortened extremities, more rhizomelic than that of achondroplasia, a narrow thorax, and a relatively large head, with bulging forehead, prominent eyes, and depressed nose bridge. The thorax is

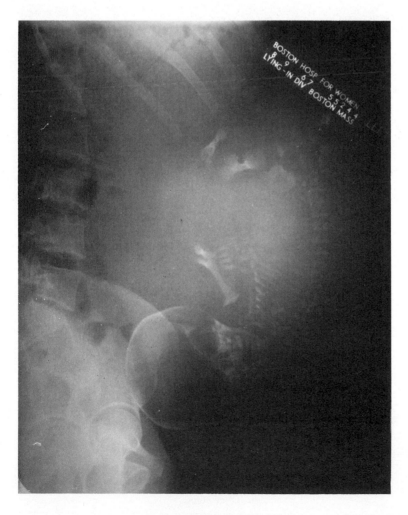

A

Figure 92–2. *A,* Achondroplastic fetus in the uterus of a normal woman.

very narrow in all dimensions and is pear-shaped with very short ribs; respiratory distress contributes to early death. The short extremities, which are covered by numerous skin folds, are held extended from the body. Hydrocephalus may be severe. Radiographic examination reveals short long bones with marked bowing and irregular metaphyseal flaring and spicule-like cupping. The pelvis is small, with flat acetabulae, and with bony spicules projecting upward and downward from the medial surfaces of the ischium. Vertebral bodies are poorly developed and decreased in height; there is a lumbar stenosis, and, on frontal projection, the lumbar vertebrae have an inverted-U appearance (Fig. 92–3). Histologically, there is generalized disruption of endochondral ossification.

There is no well-documented familial case, according to Rimoin, and the most likely cause seems to be a dominant mutation.

Diastrophic Dwarfism

Diastrophic dwarfism was formerly classified as achondroplasia but shows autosomal recessive, rather than dominant, inheritance. It is a rhizomelic, short-limb dwarfism associated with club feet (metatarsus varus and equinus, very resistant to therapy),

ulnar deviation of broad, short hands with limitation of finger flexion, and a proximally inserted, hypermobile thumb held in abduction—a "hitchhiker thumb"—and cleft palate in about 25 per cent of cases. In the first few weeks of life, most patients develop an acute inflammation of the ear pinnae that subsides, leaving a thick, firm ear with patches of calcification or even ossification eventually. Joint contractures and progressive scoliosis can be a problem.

The basic defect seems to be a generalized disease of cartilage, perhaps in the metabolism of the chondrocyte, leading to early cell death.

Chondrodysplasia Punctata

This heterogeneous group of disorders is also known by several other names, two of which are "chondrodystrophia calcificans congenita" and "congenital stippled epiphyses." The condition is characterized by radiographic stippling of the epiphyses and extraepiphyseal cartilage. Stippling of the

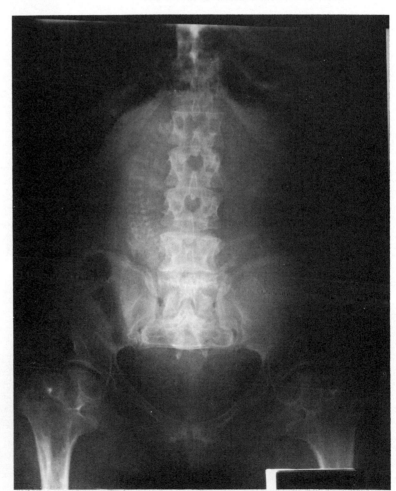

B

Figure 92–2. *Continued. B,* Achondroplastic mother with a normal fetus in uterus. (Courtesy of Drs. R. Wilkinson and N. T. Griscom, Boston Hospital for Women.)

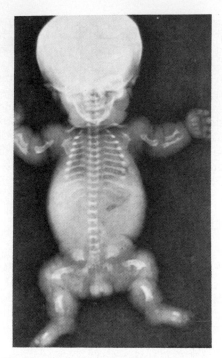

Figure 92–3. X-ray view of entire skeleton of newborn infant showing great shortening of all the extremities, great distortion in size and shape, and irregularities of the epiphyseal ends of the long bones. The head appears somewhat large in contrast to the face. (Aegerter, E., and Kirkpatrick, J. A., Jr.: Orthopedic Diseases. 3rd ed. Philadelphia, W. B. Saunders Co., 1968.)

epiphyses can also be found in several other diseases, including the cerebrohepatorenal syndrome, multiple epiphyseal dysplasia, GM₁ gangliosidosis, Smith-Lemli-Opitz syndrome, trisomies 18 and 21, maternal warfarin embryopathy, and cretinism.

The *rhizomelic* type of chondrodysplasia punctata is recessively inherited and shows severe rhizomelic shortening of the limbs, joint contractures, cataracts (about 75 per cent), ichthyosiform erythroderma with alopecia, and a peculiar, coarse facies with depressed nose bridge. Many die in infancy, and those who survive are at risk for mental retardation, microcephaly, and spastic paresis.

The *Conradi-Hunerman* type is less severe than the rhizomelic type, and many infants show autosomal dominant inheritance, although there may be a recessive type and an X-linked dominant type, lethal in males. The dwarfing is not rhizomelic and may be asymmetric. Cataracts are less frequent (18 per cent), and intelligence is not impaired. The epiphyseal calcifications may disappear.

Metatropic Dwarfism

This autosomal recessive disorder has frequently been confused with Morquio's disease. Affected infants have short limbs and normal body length, but kyphoscoliosis develops, resulting in short-trunk dwarfism. Although death may occur in infancy, survival to adulthood is common. Radiographs demonstrate marked platyspondyly and short long bones with irregular expanded metaphyses and flattened irregular epiphyses.

The Kniest syndrome, another form of short-trunk dwarfism, although radiologically similar to metatropic dwarfism, appears to be a separate entity, according to Rimoin. The condition may be associated with cleft palate, hearing loss, myopia, and limited joint movement. The genetics in this condition are unclear.

Chondroectodermal Dysplasia

Otherwise known as the Ellis–van Creveld syndrome, this recessively inherited short-limb dwarfism is characterized by associated postaxial polydactyly,

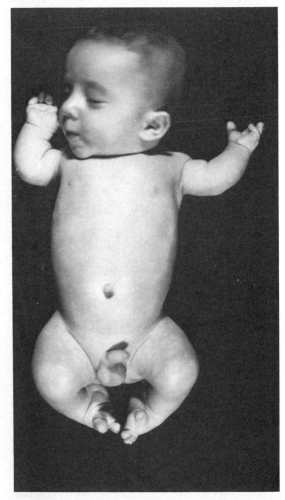

Figure 92–4. Diastrophic dwarfism. Note the normal head and face except for low-set ears with thickened pinnae, modest shortening of the trunk, and severe limb shortening. The club feet are resistant to treatment. The "hitch-hiker thumb" can be seen on the left hand. The great toe has a similar configuration. (Courtesy of Dr. Robert Wilkinson, Children's Hospital, Boston.)

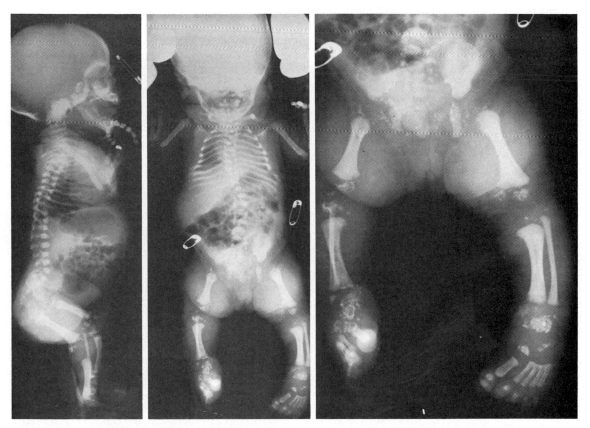

Figure 92-5. Roentgenograms of skeletal system of an example of chondrodysplasia punctata, rhizomelic, reported by Savignac. Note the short, broad bones, especially evident in the femora and tibiae. The ends of the long bones are somewhat distorted but less so than is usual in classic achondroplasia. Most striking of all is the irregular, stippled calcification of the carpal and tarsal regions and in the neighborhood of all the joints. (Reproduced with the kind permission of the author, Dr. E. M. Savignac.)

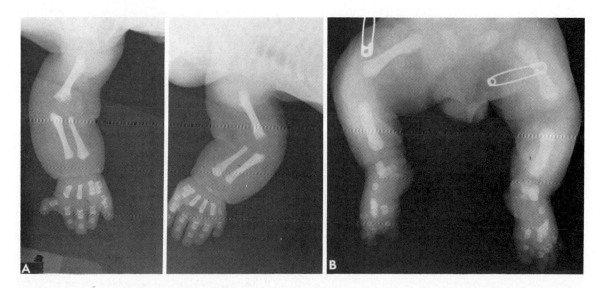

Figure 92-6. Roentgenograms of upper extremities (*A*) and lower extremities (*B*) show shortening and broadening of the long bones, rounding and blunting of the ends of most, and wedging and irregularities of the ends of the humeri and of the upper ends of the ulnae.

This dwarfed, 1-month-old infant showed, in addition to the dyschondroplasia, polydactylism, syndactylism, and absence of fingernails and toenails. This combination of defects constitutes the Ellis–van Creveld syndrome. The films were discovered in the x-ray files of the Harriet Lane Home.

dystrophic nails and teeth, congenital heart disease in about 50 per cent of patients (usually atrial septal defect), varying degrees of fusion of the inner surface of the upper lip to the gingival margin, and, occasionally, epispadias or hypospadias. The shortening of the limbs is mesomelic, becoming more extreme distally, with short, squat bones having expanded metaphyses. The phalanges are short and have cone-shaped epiphyses. The acetabular roof of the pelvis has a trident configuration. The mutant gene has a high frequency in certain Amish groups but also occurs in other populations. The recurrence risk is 1 in 4, and prenatal diagnosis is possible.

Asphyxiating Thoracic Dysplasia

Somewhat similar to chondroectodermal dysplasia is asphyxiating thoracic dysplasia, or Jeune syndrome. It too is a recessively inherited short-limbed dwarfism, with similar radiologic findings in the pelvis and the short tubular bones of the hand. Polydactyly occurs less frequently, however, and ectodermal defects are rare. The thorax is extremely small, with shortened ribs, and respiratory death in infancy is common. Those who survive may have only a mild reduction in height as adults although some develop progressive renal disease (see pp. 197 and 198).

Spondyloepiphyseal Dysplasia Congenita

This autosomal dominant form of spondyloepiphyseal dysplasia is a short-trunk dwarfism in which the child has a dysplastic spine and epiphyses, an unusual round face, and an extremely short neck. Growth retardation may not appear until 1 to 2 years of age. With time, dorsal kyphosis and lumbar lordosis exaggerate the disproportion, and the child may be diagnosed as having Morquio's disease. The limbs show some rhizomelic shortening. Cleft palate and clubfoot may occur, and over 50 per cent of patients have severe myopia or retinal detachment or both. In the newborn, there is retarded ossification of the epiphyseal centers, especially of hips, knees, and ankles. Further genetic heterogeneity probably remains to be clarified.

REFERENCES

Beighton, P.: Inherited Disorders of the Skeleton. New York, Churchill-Livingston, 1978.

Bergsma, D. (Ed.): Birth Defects Compendium. 2nd ed. New York, Alan Liss, 1979.

Curran, J. P., Sigmon, B. A., and Opitz, J.: Lethal forms of chondrodysplastic dwarfism. Pediatrics 53:76, 1974.

Gefferth, K.: Metatropic dwarfism. In Kaufman, H. J. (Ed.): Intrinsic Diseases of Bone. Prog. Pediatr. Radiol. 4:137, 1973.

Golbus, M. S., and Hall, B. D. (Eds.): Diagnostic Approaches to the Malformed Fetus, Abortus, Stillborn, and Deceased Newborn. Birth Defects: Original Article Series XV. No. 5A. New York, Alan Liss, 1979.

Jequier, S., and Dunbar, J. S.: The Ellis-van Creveld syndrome. In Kaufman, H. J. (Ed.): Intrinsic Diseases of Bone. Prog. Pediatr. Radiol. 4:167, 1973.

Kozlowski, K., Maroteaux, P., Silverman, F., Kaufmann, H., and Spranger, J.: Classification des dysplasies osseuses. Ann. Radiol. 12:965, 1969.

Langer, L. O.: Thoracic-pelvic-phalangeal dystrophy: Asphyxiating thoracic dystrophy of the newborn, infantile thoracic dystrophy. Radiology 91:447, 1968.

McKusick, V.: Mendelian Inheritance in Man. 5th ed. Baltimore, The Johns Hopkins University Press, 1978.

Murdoch, J. L., Walker, B. A., and Hall, J. G.: Achondroplasia—a genetic and statistical survey. Ann. Hum. Genet. 33:227, 1970.

Rimoin, D. L.: In Harris, H., and Hirschhorn, K. (Eds.): Advances in Human Genetics. Vol. 5. New York, Plenum Press, 1975.

Saldino, R. M.: Lethal short-limbed dwarfism: achondrogenesis and thanatophoric dwarfism. Am. J. Roentgenol. 112:185, 1971.

Silverman, F. N.: Achondroplasia. In Kaufman, H. J. (Ed.): Intrinsic Diseases of Bone. Prog. Pediatr. Radiol. 4:94, 1973.

Spranger, J. W., Langer, L. O., and Wiedemann, H. R.: Bone Dysplasias; An Atlas of Constitutional Disorders of Skeletal Development. Philadelphia, W. B. Saunders Co., 1974.

Walker, B. A., Scott, C. J., Hall, J. G., Murdoch, J. L., and McKusick, V. A.: Diastrophic dwarfism. Medicine 51:1, 1972.

93

Marfan Syndrome

Marfan syndrome is a hereditary disorder of connective tissue with many somatic manifestations including very long fingers, and it was therefore formerly called "arachnodactyly" (spider fingers). Since several other syndromes show arachnodactyly, the term should not be used as a synonym for Marfan syndrome.

Inheritance is autosomal dominant, but those who carry the gene show great differences in the severity and variety of features expressed (variable expressivity) and occasionally fail to show any manifestations of the mutant gene (reduced penetrance), making counseling difficult. About 15 per cent or less do not have an affected relative and presumably represent fresh mutations. Since many of the features are not present at birth, the condition is often difficult to diagnose at this stage unless there is an affected near relative.

Pathogenesis. Many of the pathologic alterations in Marfan syndrome can be attributed to an abiotrophy of connective tissue (i.e., to its imperfect structure leading to precocious weakening under stress). In the eye, this leads to subluxation of the lens; in the musculoskeletal system, to hyperextensibility of joints, kyphoscoliosis, and inguinal hernia; in the great vessels, to cystic medial necrosis that often terminates in dissecting aneurysm; and in the lungs to emphysema (Bolande and Tucker, 1964).

Diagnosis. In addition to the long thin fingers and toes (present in about 90 per cent of cases), other skeletal deviations from the normal may be seen: long, slender arms and legs, dolichocephaly (long, narrow head), high-arched palate, joint laxity, kyphoscoliosis, and pectus excavatum or carinatum. The upper to lower segment ratio is usually more than two standard deviations below the mean, arm span is greater than height, the hand to height ratio is greater than 11 per cent, the foot to height ratio is greater than 15 per cent, and the metacarpal index (length to width) is increased. Over the course of months or years, abnormalities of other organs and systems may or may not appear. These include joint laxity, eye defects (of which myopia and dislocation of the lens—usually upward—are the ones most frequently met), and cardiac disorders. These last are often mistaken for rheumatic heart disease, since the valves and chordae tendineae are involved in a fibrous thickening that produces murmurs similar to those of rheumatic endocarditis. The terminal event in many of these patients, rarely in infancy (one aged

Other Congenital Defects Involving Bones

Revised by F. Clarke Fraser

9 months has been reported), more often in late childhood or early adulthood, is the growth and rupture of an aortic aneurysm. Pathologically, the great vessels will be seen to have undergone a gradual but relentless progression of cystic medial necrosis.

The disorder will be looked for carefully in infants in a family in which the diagnosis of Marfan syndrome has been made in a parent or other near relative. It may be suspected if the newborn has inordinately long, thin, tapering fingers and toes, especially if these are accompanied by dolichocephaly, joint laxity, myopia, and the aforementioned skeletal disproportions. Echocardiography usually reveals a characteristic picture. Increased aortic compliance, measured by Doppler ultrasonography, is a most valuable diagnostic sign (Child et al., 1981). One does not expect to find the cardiac and severe ocular abnormalities to be fully developed within the first months of life, but they have been seen this early.

The differential diagnosis includes *homocystinuria* (autosomal recessive), which can be ruled out by the absence of excess homocystine in the urine, and *congenital contractural arachnodactyly*, also dominantly inherited, in which the arachnodactyly is accompanied by multiple joint contractures and large, floppy ears. The distinction is important as these patients do not develop the severe ocular and cardiac complications of Marfan syndrome, and the contractures improve with age.

Treatment. Treatment is symptomatic. The use of propranolol to reduce the probability of aortic aneurysm is under investigation. Preliminary results are discouraging.

Prognosis. Prognosis is variable, depending on whether or not cardiac and vascular complications supervene; there is no way of predicting which children will ultimately show these manifestations. Murdoch and coworkers have calculated the life expectancy of persons with Marfan syndrome. The average age at death was 32 years. This rather dismal outlook may improve with increased awareness of the condition and continuing progress in management of the cardiovascular complications. Improved methods of measuring aortic compliances are leading to earlier diagnosis (Child et al., 1981).

CASE 93–1

(This is case J. G. of Bolande and Tucker, abstracted and reprinted here with the permission of the senior author.)

This 1-month-old white male infant was admitted with a diagnosis of congenital Marfan syndrome. During breech extraction of the 3.5 kg baby, the left femur was fractured. Both mother and father are unusually tall and slender. On examination, the infant measured 58 cm and weighed 3.5 kg. The head was narrow and long, the ears were soft and floppy, and there was an entropion of the right eye. A grade I systolic murmur

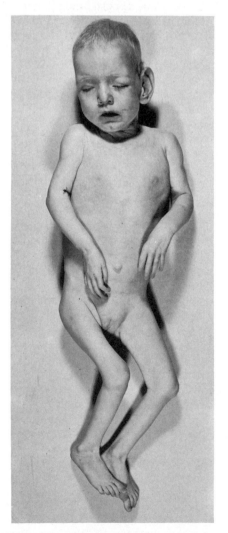

Figure 93–1. Photograph of infant with Marfan's syndrome. Note the extremely long arms and hands, legs and feet, the long, narrow skull, the very large ears, and the dropped left wrist.

was heard in the third left intercostal space. The extremities were long and thin, with extremely long hands, fingers, feet, and toes, and a flail wrist on the left. Bilateral inguinal hernias were visible. Deep tendon reflexes were absent (Fig. 93–1).

Fluoroscopy revealed cardiac enlargement and pulmonary vascular congestion. The murmur became louder and harsher, cardiac failure ensued, dislocation of the right lens became obvious, the lungs became emphysematous, and the infant died after about 5 weeks in hospital.

Comment. This is an example of Marfan syndrome that was diagnosable shortly after birth, with many of the associated visceral lesions by the time of death, before the infant was 3 months of age. One wonders whether this was a homozygote for the Marfan gene.

Osteogenesis Imperfecta (OI)

Osteogenesis imperfecta is a heterogeneous group of diseases involving bone fragility. The nosology will become clearer as recombinant DNA technology clarifies the genetics of collagen. At present, four major groups are recognized (Sillence et al., 1979), but there is undoubtedly heterogeneity within them. Only cases in groups 2 or 3 are likely to be problems in the neonatal period.

Dominant OI With Blue Sclerae (Group 1). In this type, often referred to as "OI tarda," brittle bones and blue sclerae usually appear after birth, although fractures occasionally occur prenatally. About 40 per cent of adults have severe hearing impairment. It has a frequency of about one per 28,000 births. About 15 per cent of patients have a negative family history and probably represent fresh mutations. The natural history is well described by Sillence and colleagues.

Lethal Perinatal OI (Group 2). This is the classic OI congenita, but since other types can occasionally manifest themselves before birth, the terminology is confusing. Shortening and bowing of the upper and lower limbs are present at birth, and radiographs show characteristic crumpling of the femora, marked angulation of the tibiae and sometimes the femora, fractures of the long bones, beaded ribs, and poor ossification of the vault and base that resembles a membranous bag of bones. The sclerae are usually blue. The affected infants expire in the newborn period, perhaps from damage to the poorly protected brain. The condition has been detected in utero in the second trimester, so prenatal diagnosis is possible.

The frequency is about one in 62,000 births. Inheritance is autosomal recessive in a majority of families, but the segregation ratio seems to be less than 1 in 4, suggesting genetic heterogeneity. At least one subgroup has a decreased proportion of type 1 to type 3 collagen in the skin.

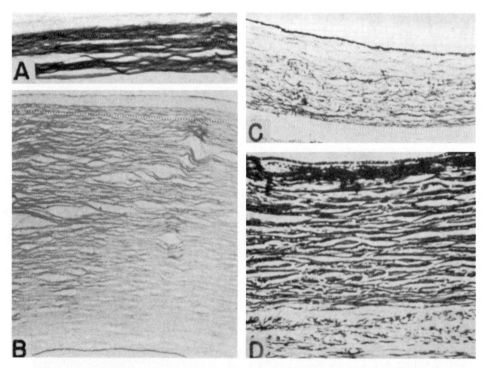

Figure 93–2. (*A* and *C* are from the patient; *B* and *D* are controls.) *A* and *B*, Corneas from infant with osteogenesis imperfecta and from control stained with periodic acid–Schiff technique. In addition to showing a great difference in width, the former stains red, while the latter is almost colorless. *C* and *D*, Scleras from infant with osteogenesis imperfecta and from normal infant. These exemplify difference in thickness and thin reticulum found in former (silver stain). (Follis, R. H., Jr.: J. Pediatr. *41*:713, 1952.)

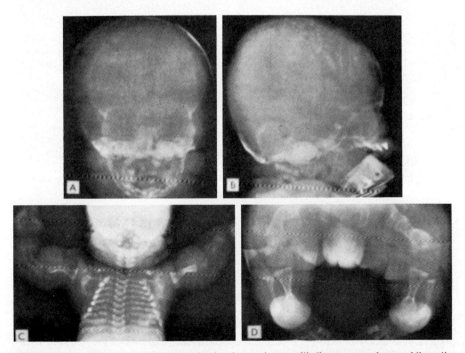

Figure 93–3. Osteogenesis imperfecta. A newborn with the severe form of the disease. In *A* and *B*, note the inadequate mineralization of the cranial bones, the wide sutures, and multiple centers of ossification. Multiple fractures of the extremities and rib cage as well as "crumpling" of the femora are evident in *C* and *D*. The cortices are thin, and the spongiosa is deficient. (Aegerter, E., and Kirkpatrick, J. A., Jr.: Orthopedic Diseases. 3rd ed. Philadelphia, W. B. Saunders Co., 1968.)

only in the last month of gestation. Dentinogenesis imperfecta is common, but deafness is not.

Progressively Deforming OI With Normal Sclerae (Group 3). This is the group that causes the most diagnostic confusion. Fractures are often present at birth, but the bones do not show the crumpled appearance evident in group 2. The sclerae are usually not blue. There is a marked reduction in frequency of fractures between 5 and 10 years of age but a progressive deformity of the limbs during childhood and of the spine during late childhood and adolescence. There is marked ligamentous laxity, and about one in four children show easy bruising. About half the patients have dentinogenesis imperfecta. The frequency is about one in 200,000 births. Most cases are sporadic, but some families show an autosomal recessive pattern. The skin collagen is unstable.

Dominant OI Without Blue Sclerae (Group 4). This type resembles group 1 except for the lack of blue sclerae. Also, type 4 OI is much rarer than type 1. Occasionally, fractures occur before birth, and at least one case has been diagnosed prenatally, but

Cleidocranial Dysostosis

Cleidocranial dysostosis is a rare autosomal dominant developmental disorder in which deformity of the skull and absence of clavicles are manifest in most cases, but either or both of these defects may be absent. Penetrance is high, but, because of variable expressivity, the condition cannot be ruled out without a thorough radiologic examination. About one case in three appears to be a fresh mutation.

Diagnosis. The defect most often noted first is extreme softness of the skull. The fontanels may be huge, the major sutures widely patent, and the metopic suture widely separated. Very little membranous calvarial bone has been laid down before birth. There are other defects of facial bones of great variety. The clavicles may be completely absent, or one or two thirds of each may be missing or not joined. When both clavicles are absent, extraordinary mobility of the shoulders is possible to the point of ap-

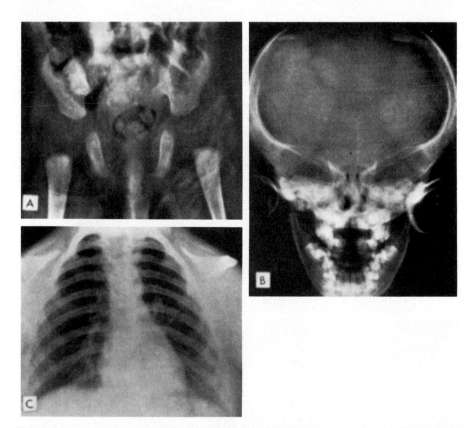

Figure 93–4. Cleidocranial dysostosis. A and B, Radiographs of the pelvis and skull of a male infant age 6 months. The pubic bones are underdeveloped; only a small portion of the body of each is evident. The epiphyseal centers for the heads of the femora are tiny. The radiograph of the skull (B) shows widely patent sutures and fontanels, numerous centers of ossification in the cranial bones, and an increase in the biparietal diameter. The facial bones are small. This child has no clavicles, and the radiograph of his mother's chest (C) reveals absence of clavicles. (Aegerter, E., and Kirkpatrick, J. A., Jr.: Orthopedic Diseases. 3rd ed. Philadelphia, W. B. Saunders Co., 1968.)

proximating the acromial processes beneath the chin. Deformities, nonjunction, and underdevelopment of the bones of the pelvis and of almost any other of the skeletal parts may coexist. The characteristic defects from which the disorder derives its name are shown in Figure 93–4. The soft skull of the newborn may be confused with that of infants with osteogenesis imperfecta or hypophosphatasia.

Prognosis. The cranium completes its ossification slowly, the fontanels and metopic sutures often remaining open until adult life. The sutures generally remain depressed, leaving the frontal and parietal areas prominently bossed in "hot-cross-bun" fashion. The permanent teeth may be late in erupting and may have enamel hypoplasia, retention cysts, and malformed roots. Morbidity and mortality are not increased by cleidocranial dystrophy.

Treatment. There is none available.

Hemihypertrophy

This is a rare disorder that may occur as an isolated finding or as a feature of several syndromes, including Russell-Silver syndrome (see further on) and Beckwith syndrome. There is little evidence that it is genetically transmitted, since, in the 135 cases reported up to 1961, it had recurred in two generations only a few times and in three generations only once. Some deviation from the normal process of twinning has been suggested as its cause.

Since about 1950, a large body of information has accrued concerning the association of congenital defects with malignancies of early life. Hemihypertrophy stands high on the list of those found with unusual frequency in the presence of Wilms' tumor and adrenal carcinoma. This matter is discussed more fully in Chapter 107.

Diagnosis. Some or all of the structures on one side of the body are noted to be larger than the corresponding ones on the other side. The time at which this inequality becomes apparent depends on the degree of hemihypertrophy, which may vary within wide limits. The leg and arm of the affected side are larger in both length and girth, and measurements of the long bones by radiographic study show them to be longer than the contralateral ones. Growth continues for several years, making the discrepancy more noticeable, but toward puberty excessive growth ceases. By then, one leg may be an inch or two longer than the other.

Treatment. Several methods have been used in the attempt to slow down excessive growth of the leg so that both the limp and the scoliosis that result from discrepancy in leg length can be minimized. Stapling a growing end is probably the most satisfactory method.

Syndrome of Congenital Hemihypertrophy, Intrauterine Dwarfism, and Elevated Urinary Gonadotropins

Tanner's excellent study has shown that there is no justification for separating cases of this nature with hemihypertrophy (Silver syndrome) from those without it (Russell syndrome). The asymmetry is usually present in infancy and may involve one side or only the face, trunk, or limbs. The face is triangular and small with a broad forehead and small chin. The head thus may appear large but in fact tends to have a circumference somewhat below average. The mouth is often thin-lipped with down-turned corners. Clinodactyly is frequent, and syndactyly, café-au-lait spots, muscle weakness, and cryptorchidism may be present. Elevation of urinary gonadotropins may sometimes occur in both males and females, but, contrary to previous claims, puberty is usually normal. Familial occurrence has been reported occasionally, but most cases are sporadic.

Defects of Radius and Thumb

The skeletal dysplasias are so numerous and varied that their description is beyond the scope of this book (Bergsma's Atlas and Compendium is a useful reference.) However, defects of the radius are part of so many syndromes that their presence in the infant should lead the physician to look for associated abnormalities, since identifying the syndrome is important for both prognosis and genetic counseling. Radial dysplasias may range from complete absence of the radial ray to minimal hypoplasia of a low-set thumb. They may be sporadic or may be a feature of the following syndromes.

GENETIC SYNDROMES

Holt-Oram Syndrome. Varying degrees of radial dysplasia occur in association with congenital heart malformations, usually atrial septal defect but sometimes ventricular septal defect, transposition of the great vessels, or single coronary artery. Some patients also manifest the Duane syndrome (a defect of ocular adduction). The inheritance is autosomal dominant.

Fanconi's Anemia. Various combinations of anomalies including microcephaly, kidney malformations, and skeletal defects (often including radial dysplasias) are present at birth, and a pancytopenic anemia develops later. The diagnosis can be confirmed by the presence of an excessive number of chromosome breaks in peripheral lymphocyte cultures. The inheritance is autosomal recessive.

Thrombocytopenia—Absent Radius Syndrome.
Also showing autosomal recessive inheritance, this syndrome is distinguished by the fact that the thumb is present, contrary to the findings in Fanconi's anemia. There is amegakaryocytosis, but this may be transient; if the infant survives the first year, the prognosis is relatively good.

Craniosynostosis—Radial Aplasia Syndrome.
This very rare syndrome has been reported in sibs and may be recessively inherited.

IVIC Syndrome. Variable radial ray defects are associated with mixed congenital hearing loss, strabismus, and (in 10 per cent) imperforate anus in this autosomal dominant condition.

"SPORADIC" SYNDROMES

The VATER, or VACTEL, Syndrome. This is a syndrome of unidentified etiology (although maternal ingestion of certain drugs is suspected) in which radial dysplasia is associated with vertebral anomalies, anal atresia, tracheoesophageal fistula, and cardiac defects.

The Thalidomide Syndrome. This is really a series of syndromes, depending on the time of ingestion of the drug, and may "copy" several of the aforementioned genetic syndromes. One hopes that this syndrome will not be seen again by neonatologists.

Acrofacial Dysostosis (Nager). This syndrome includes (besides absence of thumbs or radii or both)

cleft palate, micrognathia, gastroschisis, and a rudimentary phallus.

CHROMOSOMAL SYNDROMES

Absence or hypoplasia of the thumb may occur in patients with a deletion of chromosome 13 long arm.

REFERENCES

Aegerter, E., and Kirkpatrick J. A.: Orthopedic Diseases: Physiology, Pathology, Radiology. 4th ed. Philadelphia, W. B. Saunders Co., 1975.

Bergsma, D. (Ed.): Birth Defects Atlas and Compendium. National Foundation March of Dimes. 2nd ed. Baltimore, Williams & Wilkins Co., 1979.

Bolande, R. P., and Tucker, A. S.: Pulmonary emphysema and other cardiorespiratory lesions as part of the Marfan abiotrophy. Pediatrics 33:356, 1964.

Carson, N. A. J., et al.: Homocystinuria: clinical and pathological review of ten cases. J. Pediatr. 66:565, 1965.

Child, A. H., et al.: Aortic compliance in connective tissue disorders affecting the eye. Ophthal. Paediatr. Genet. 1:59, 1981.

Follis, R. H., Jr.: Osteogenesis imperfecta congenita: a connective tissue diathesis. J. Pediatr. 41:713, 1952.

Gellis, S. S., and Feingold, M.: Picture of the month: congenital hemihypertrophy and adrenal carcinoma. Am. J. Dis. Child. 115:445, 1968.

Gordon, R. J., and Meskin, L. H.: Congenital hemihypertrophy: a review of literature and report of a case, with special emphasis on oral manifestations. J. Pediatr. 61:870, 1961.

Holmes, L. B., Moser, H. W., Halldorsen, S., Mack, C., Pant, S. S., and Matzilevich, B.: Mental Retardation. An Atlas of Diseases with Associated Physical Abnormalities. New York, Macmillan, 1972.

Kalter, H., and Warkany, J.: Congenital malformations. N. Engl. J. Med. 308:424, 1983.

Murdoch, J. L., Walker, B. A., Halpern, B. L., Kuzma, J. W., and McKusick, V. A.: Life expectancy and causes of death associated in the Marfan syndrome. N. Engl. J. Med. 286:804, 1972.

Pyeritz, R. E., and McKusick, V. A.: The Marfan syndrome: diagnosis and management. N. Engl. J. Med. 300:772, 1979.

Remigio, P. A., and Grinvalsky, H. T.: Osteogenesis imperfecta congenita associated with conspicuous extraskeletal connective tissue dysplasias. Am. J. Dis. Child. 119:524, 1970.

Sillence, D. O., Senn, A., and Danks, D. M.: Genetic heterogeneity in osteogenesis imperfecta. J. Med. Genet. 16:101, 1979.

Tanner, J. M., Lejarraga, H., and Cameron, N.: The natural history of the Silver-Russell syndrome: a longitudinal study of thirty-nine cases. Pediatr. Res. 9:611, 1975.

Warkany, J.: Congenital Malformations. Notes and Comments. Chicago, Year Book Medical Publishers, 1971.

94

Congenital Dislocation of The Hip

Congenital Defects Involving Joints

Revised by F. Clarke Fraser

The hip joint is only rarely completely dislocated at birth or within the first month of life. The more common lesion is subluxation, that is, a dislocatable hip with nearly stable reductions and an Ortolani click.

Incidence.   Estimates of frequency vary with the nature of the population and the intensity of screening. Surveys of infants in the first few days of life have provided figures ranging from 4 to 7 per 1000 livebirths. The likelihood of recurrence in sibs varies with sex of both proband and sib, ranging from roughly 5 per cent for the brothers of an affected female to about 20 per cent for the sisters of an affected male. These figures are for neonatal diagnosis; the proportion that would progress to overt dislocation is considerably less.

Etiology.   Females are affected much more often than males, the overall reported ratio being eight females to one male. Whites outnumber blacks by 50 to 1. Noteworthy is the disproportion of breech positions among the affected babies. One of about five of them has presented in the breech position, whereas overall only one of about 40 fetuses is a breech presentation. In order to explain the disproportion between females and males, Andren and others have looked for an endocrine factor in addition to the mechanical one in breech presentation. It is possible that maternal progesterone induces the fetal uterus to produce relaxin, which affects the tensile stength of the ligaments about the hip adversely. Formerly, most authors considered dysplasia of the joint the primary factor, followed by subluxation and dislocation resulting from muscular pull and, eventually, weight bearing. The dysplastic joint is an imperfectly ossified one with a shallow acetabulum and a capsule that is soft and less elastic and strong than is normal. There appear to be genetic predisposing factors, including a polygenic system influencing acetabular conformation and a major locus influencing joint laxity.

Diagnosis.   The diagnosis of actual dislocation of the femoral head out of the acetabular cavity is not difficult. However, this is only rarely present at birth and may not become obvious for several months after birth. When present, at any age, it produces apparent shortening of the dislocated limb. One can discern shortening by pressing the knees flatly and firmly against the table top while holding the pelvis rigidly straight, that is, not tilted to one side or the other. The position of the soles should match per-

fectly. An additional sign of shortening is asymmetry of the creases of the thigh. In some infants, all the creases of one thigh will appear to be higher than those of the other. In many, one will see not only this finding but also an extra crease or two in the seemingly shortened side. However, an extra crease or two on one side is seen frequently in infants who have no other signs of dislocation of the hip and who grow up without ever exhibiting them.

The cardinal sign of subluxation, with or without actual dislocation, is inability to abduct the affected thigh. One can demonstrate this by flexing the thighs to a right angle with the infant lying supine and attempting to bring them outward and downward, one at a time, until they lie upon the table top. When a sharp click can be felt and heard consistently on one side (Ortolani's sign) and when the difference in ease of abduction between the two thighs is striking, one can be fairly certain that subluxation is present (Fig. 94–1). Minor differences or inconstant ones may not be considered diagnostic. This is especially true in the first week or two of life, when the newborn prefers to maintain vigorously his fetal "position of comfort." The leg on the affected side often is kicked less freely than the other. It may be held constantly in a position of slight internal rotation and flexion.

Radiographs of the dislocated hip show upward

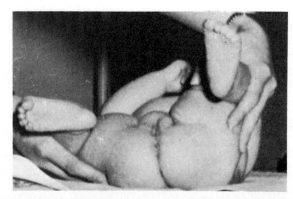

Figure 94–1.   Infant with subluxation of left hip. The nurse is able to abduct the right but not the left thigh down to the level of the table. (Pray, L. G.: Pediatrics 9:94, 1952.)

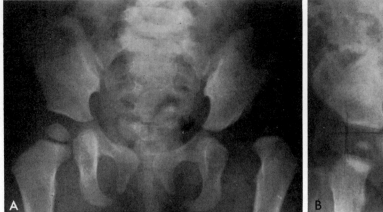
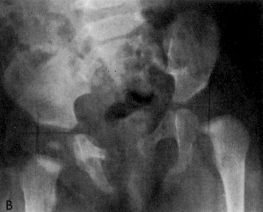

Figure 94–2. *A,* X-ray view of hips shows the right femoral head to be in its proper position with respect to its acetabulum. The left femur is placed farther from the pelvis than is the right, its epiphyseal center and its acetabulum are less well developed, and its long axis projected runs lateral to the edge of the ilium. *B,* The left femoral head is displaced slightly upward and outward, the acetabulum is shallow, and the epiphyseal center is poorly developed. (Pray, L. G.: Pediatrics 9:94, 1952.)

and outward malposition of the femoral head. The acetabular angle is generally greater than 30 degrees, whereas that of normal infants is generally below 30 degrees. There is unfortunately a fair amount of overlap. In the newborn, delay in ossification of the epiphysis of the femoral head is of no help, since this does not ordinarily occur until 6 weeks of age in the normal child. However, absence of any acetabular cupping, widening of the space between femur and pelvis, and lateral displacement of the projected line of the long axis of the femur may be notable. This points, in normal hips, directly toward the position of the acetabulum, whereas in the dysplastic ones it misses the lateral margin of the ilium.

Treatment. Treatment is successful and simple in inverse proportion to the age at which it is begun. When diagnosed early, many subluxated hips can be prevented from ever dislocating by some simple device that holds the affected leg abducted and laterally rotated (e.g., a Pavlik harness). Generally, splinting can be discontinued before the end of the third month. Cases diagnosed later may require longer splinting and, at times, more drastic forms of intervention. The pediatrician in any case will not take it upon himself to detail the therapeutic measures needed.

Genu Recurvatum

This is a comparatively rare deformity, characterized by abnormal hyperextensibility of the knee joint.

Etiology. The number of females who are affected is significantly greater than the number of males.

Many more babies with genu recurvatum present by the breech than is to be expected. Both these statistical observations have been documented for congenital dislocation of the hip. They lend credibility to the hormonal-postural theory of pathogenesis of both these disorders—that is, that maternal progesterone induces, via the fetal uterus, the production of relaxin and that the abnormal stresses of the breech position distort one or both of the abnormally relaxed joints. The disorder may also occur as a feature in a number of disorders, such as the Ehlers-Danlos, Marfan, Klinefelter, and Turner syndromes.

Diagnosis. The extended leg or both legs describe a concave arc when hyperextended at the knee (Fig. 94–3). Hyperextensibility is mild or severe; that is,

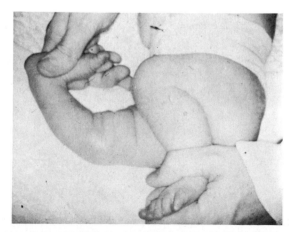

Figure 94–3. Genu recurvatum, right. The condition is unusually severe, with actual posterior dislocation of the knee.

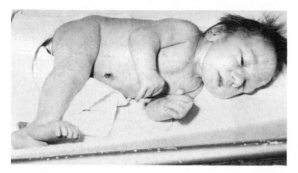

Figure 94–4. Arthrogryposis congenita, distal, type I. One can see clearly the rigid extremities, the lower ones in extension, the upper ones in flexion, and the tightly balled fists.

the arc is shallow or deep. In severe cases, there may be actual posterior dislocation of the knee.

Prognosis. Spontaneous improvement is the rule.

Treatment. Nothing need be done for cases of mild or moderate severity. Posterior splinting or, rarely, casting for 2 to 4 weeks is indicated for the most severe forms.

Arthrogryposis Multiplex Congenita

The term *arthrogryposis multiplex congenita* describes a highly heterogeneous group of conditions manifesting fixation of the joints. The common factor is restriction of joint movement in utero, which can have a neurogenic or myogenic basis or result from mechanical restriction (e.g., oligohydramnios). Hall, in her excellent 1982 review, has identified a number of specific entities among the myriad of conditions that fall into this group.

Category 1 includes cases with primarily limb involvement, excluding the distal arthrogryposes. The associated appearance is characteristic. The limbs are usually in extension or mild flexion, with internal rotation of shoulders, talipes equinovarus, flexion of wrist and hand, and amyoplasia of limb and limb

girdle muscles. Intelligence is normal. The contractures are resistant to physical therapy. The condition appears to be nonfamilial. Category 2 is heterogeneous and includes the distal arthrogryposes. Limbs are usually in flexion. The muscles may be doughy or woody. Autosomal dominant and recessive types have been distinguished. In category 3, severe mental retardation, often with microcephaly, is seen. The limbs are always flexed and may be spastic. The recurrence risk appears low.

Distal arthrogryposis type 1 affects only the joints. The hand is always affected; the fingers are clenched and overlapping, as in trisomy 18, but the contractures respond well to stretching exercises. The feet are usually involved, often with calcaneovalgus or equinovarus deformity. There may be varying degrees of flexion contracture at elbows, knees, and hips. Inheritance is autosomal dominant. There is much variability, both between and within families. Response to physical therapy is generally good.

Distal arthrogryposis type 2 includes cases with anomalies besides those of the joints, including various combinations: kyphoscoliosis, vertebral anomalies, short neck with sloping shoulders, trismus, ptosis, short stature, cleft palate and/or lip, borderline intelligence, and an unusual hand configuration with hyperextension at the metacarpophalangeal joint. Five subtypes can be identified: (1) the Gordon syndrome—autosomal dominant clubfoot, cleft palate, and camptodactyly; (2) autosomal dominant short stature, short neck, ptosis, and smooth, shiny, tapering fingers with mild camptodactyly; (3) distal contractures with cleft lip (there is vertical transmission, but the mode of inheritance is not clear); (4) distal contractures with ''idiopathic'' scoliosis, autosomal dominant; and (5) trismus camptodactyly with hyperextension of the metacarpophalangeal joints and variable distal contractures of hands and feet, knees, elbows, shoulders, and (in all cases) hips. Vertical

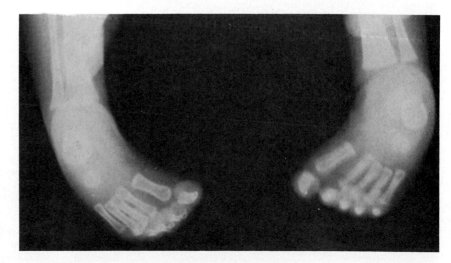

Figure 94–5. Arthrogryposis in twins. Roentgenograms show the bones to be normal, but the soft tissues of the joint regions appear to be thickened and opacified. (Lipton, E. L., and Morgenstern, S. H.: A.M.A. J. Dis. Child. *89*:233, 1955.)

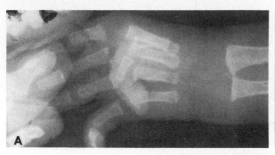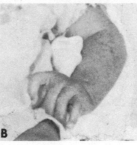

Figure 94–6. Arthrogryposis in twins. *A,* Roentgenogram of wrist of second twin. *B,* Photograph of arm shows the wrist fixed in dorsiflexion and the fingers tightly flexed. (Lipton, E. L., and Morgenstern, S. H.: A.M.A. J. Dis. Child. *89:*233, 1955.)

transmission is seen in some cases. Micrognathia, scoliosis, small tongue, facial asymmetry, and low-normal intelligence may be seen.

In addition there are a number of well-recognized syndromes involving distal contractures, including the whistling-face (Freeman-Sheldon) syndrome, the trismus pseudocamptodactyly syndrome, and congenital contractural arachnodactyly.

In general, the prognosis for patients with distal arthrogryposis is quite good if proper management (stretching exercise, appropriate orthopedic procedures) is followed from birth.

Gout

Gout strikes children rarely, young infants even more infrequently. It has, however, been described in a 5-week-old infant, and a recurrence was reported in an infant in whom the onset was at or before 3 weeks of age.

CASE 94–1

This case, reported by Rosenthal and coworkers, deserves brief summarization. It concerns a white male

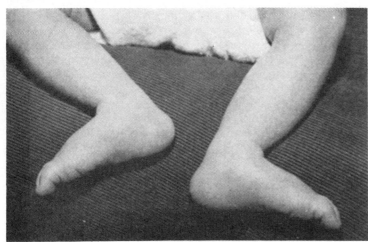

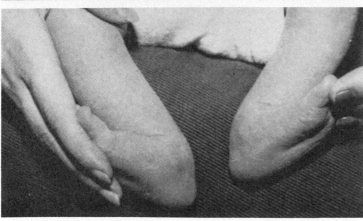

Figure 94–7. Calcaneovalgus deformity. *A,* Feet at rest. *B,* Same feet under test. (Miller, W. R.: J. Pediatr. *51:*527, 1957.)

infant, born after normal pregnancy, labor, and delivery, who weighed 4.2 kg at birth. At 3 weeks, his mother noted reddish-brown solid material on his diaper. At 7 weeks weight gain had been poor, and projectile vomiting began. The reddish-brown material increased in quantity in the diapers and accumulated on the penis.

At 3 months, the infant was hospitalized for continued vomiting and dehydration. Weight was now ½ ounce above birth weight. He was pale and undernourished, but the rest of the examination revealed nothing abnormal. Urine pH was 4.5, specific gravity 1.008, albumin and sugar negative. Hemoglobin was 10.0 gm; white blood cells numbered 12,250 per cubic millimeter, with a normal differential. The blood nonprotein nitrogen level was 60 mg per 100 ml.

The reddish-brown material in the urine was identified as uric acid. Serum uric acid concentration was 18.6, urea nitrogen 67, and creatinine 2.3 mg per 100 ml.

The diagnosis of gout plus secondary renal insufficiency seemed justified.

Fluids were forced, and 1.0 gm of sodium citrate was given by mouth every 4 hours. As the pH of the urine rose, the precipitate disappeared. The blood uric acid level fell to 8.0 mg per 100 ml, where it remained. At 18 months, the baby seemed well and weighed 11.82 kg. His urine was alkaline (he was still taking sodium citrate, 1.0 gm 4 times a day), his serum urea nitrogen was 21 mg, and his uric acid was 8.3 mg per 100 ml.

There was a strongly positive family history for gouty diathesis in the family. A 15-year-old half-brother had urinary calculi, joint pains, and a high uric acid level. He was improved by probenecid. The father also had renal calculi and an elevated blood uric acid level. The maternal grandmother had a high blood uric acid level.

Disorders of the Feet

A thorough discussion of congenital malformations of the feet is beyond the scope of this test. We shall compromise by describing briefly three conditions that demand vigorous treatment soon after birth.

PES CALCANEOVALGUS

This is the absolutely flat and sometimes slightly convex foot that often lies at rest dorsiflexed at an acute angle to the foreleg. When gentle pressure is

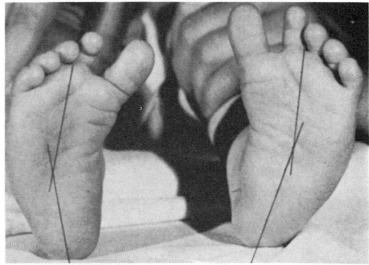

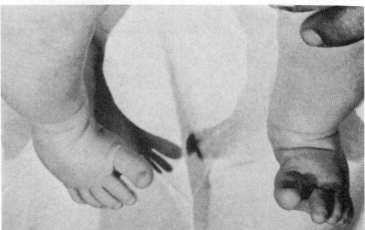

Figure 94–8. Metatarsus varus. (Miller, W. R.: J. Pediatr. *51*:527, 1957.)

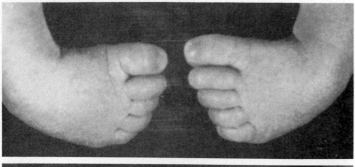

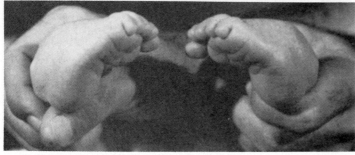

Figure 94–9. Congenital clubfeet. (Miller, W. R.: J. Pediatr. *51*:527, 1957.)

applied to the sole of the foot, dorsiflexion increases easily until its dorsal surface lies in contact with the shin (Fig. 94–7).

These feet should be casted in the equinovarus position for 4 to 6 weeks, and this therapy should be repeated several times if necessary. Continued treatment with tarsosupinator shoes and, perhaps, with the Denis Browne bar will probably be needed for several years.

PES METATARSOVARUS

In this condition the heel and posterior half of the foot appear normal, but the forefoot angulates sharply inward. Thus, the outer border of the foot is convex, whereas its inner border is concave (Fig. 94–8).

If the foot can be straightened by gentle traction, with the thumb held firmly over the apex of the convexity, no immediate treatment is needed. If, however, the angulation is difficult or impossible to overcome, casting is probably indicated. Later use of corrective shoes may or may not be necessary.

PES EQUINOVARUS

This is the classic clubfoot with sharp and tight hyperextension and incurving of the entire foot (Fig. 94–9). It is often a solitary defect but not infrequently it is associated with congenital dislocation of the hip, myelomeningocele, arthrogryposis, or other defects.

It requires immediate and long-term orthopedic care. Most cases can be corrected by casting and subsequent shoe corrections. A few will require open operation.

REFERENCES

Andren, L., and Borglin, N. E.: Disturbed urinary excretion pattern of oestrogens in newborns with congenital dislocation of the hip. Acta Endocrinol. *37*:423, 1961.

Browne, D.: Congenital deformities of mechanical origin. Arch. Dis. Child. *30*:37, 1955.

Dickerson, R. C.: Congenital dislocation of the hip. Pediatrics *41*:977, 1968.

Hall, J. G. In Bergsma, D. (Ed.); Birth Defects Compendium. 2nd ed. New York, A. R. Liss, 1979, p. 121.

Hall, J. G., Reed, S. G., and Green, G.: The distal arthrogryposes: delineation of new entities—review and nosologic discussion. Am. J. Med. Genet. *11*:185, 1982.

Miller, W. R.: Observations on the examination of children's feet. J. Pediatr. *51*:527, 1957.

Rosenmann, A., and Arad, I.: Arthrogryposis multiplex congenita: neurogenic type with autosomal recessive inheritance. J. Med. Genet. *11*:91, 1974.

Rosenthal, J. M., Gaballah, S., and Rafelson, M. E.: Gout in infancy manifested by renal failure. Pediatrics *33*:251, 1964.

Sherk, H. H., Pasquariello, P. S., and Watters, W. C.: Congenital dislocation of the hip. Clin. Pediatr. *20*:513, 1981.

von Rosen, S.: Diagnosis and treatment of congenital dislocation of the hip in the newborn. J. Bone Joint Surg. *44B*:284, 1962.

Warkany, J.: Congenital Malformations. Notes and Comments. Year Book Medical Publishers, Chicago, 1971.

Wynne-Davies, R.: A family study of neonatal and late diagnosis, congenital dislocaton of the hip. J. Med. Genet. *7*:315, 1970.

95

Congenital Bowing and Angulation of Long Bones (Congenital Kyphoscoliotic Tibia, Congenital Pseudoarthrosis of the Tibia)

As the name implies, this disorder consists in abnormal curvature of one or more bones that has developed in utero. We exclude syndromes that include tibial angulation as a feature (e.g., camptomelic dwarfism).

Incidence.   The condition is rare.

Etiology.   The condition is not familial. However, many patients have been reported to have family histories of neurofibromatosis or stigmata of neurofibromatosis (Gwinn and Barnes), possibly as a result of bone erosion by a neurofibroma.

The cause is believed by some to lie in abnormal mechanical pressure upon the growing limb, although the not infrequent coexistence of other congenital malformations casts doubt upon this hypothesis. In Angle's case, the "position of comfort" of the newborn infant seemed to consist of the soles of the feet being placed in the midportion of the convexity

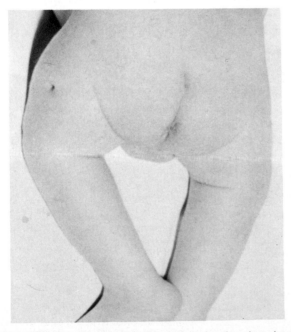

Figure 95–1. Photograph of lower limbs showing shortening and angulation of the femora. That of the left femur is seen clearly, and the characteristic dimple at the apex of the convexity is obvious. (Angle, C. R.: Pediatrics 13:257, 1954.)

Miscellaneous Disorders of the Skeletal System

Revised by F. Clarke Fraser

of the opposite femur. Angle inferred that the foot applied right angular pressure to the femur and acted as the fulcrum against which intrauterine forces acted.

Diagnosis.   The tibia is by far the most frequently affected bone, some being angulated anteriorly, some posteriorly. Males are involved more often than females. Multiple osseous angulation is not too uncommon. Characteristically, a deep dimple overlies the apex of the convexity. On radiographs, the cortex is thickened on the concave side and thinned on the convex side. Radiolucent cystic areas are not infrequently seen on radiographs within the mass of angulated bone. Actual fracture may take place at this point. When it does, nonunion (i.e., pseudoarthrosis) often follows. This makes the prognosis for ultimate cure very gloomy.

Treatment.   Treatment consists in orthopedic correction. This may necessitate operative fracture and casting.

Congenital Lumbar Hernia

Lee and Mattheis recalled to attention this unusual malformation. We have encountered a case identical in all respects. As an acquired phenomenon, lumbar hernia, following accidental or surgical trauma, is not uncommon, but only a dozen of the congenital variety have been reported.

Etiology.   This is plainly a developmental defect arising early in gestation. The lower ribs are distorted, hemivertebrae of the lower dorsal and upper lumbar region are usually found, and the fascial and muscle coats are thinned. Some muscles may indeed be missing. Its occurrence is inexplicable on embryologic grounds, since, as Nastin said, "Nothing in the development of the abdominal wall can account for the formation of a gap in the lumbar region."

Diagnosis.   At birth, the entire lumbar area on one side is seen to protrude. The mass is soft and com-

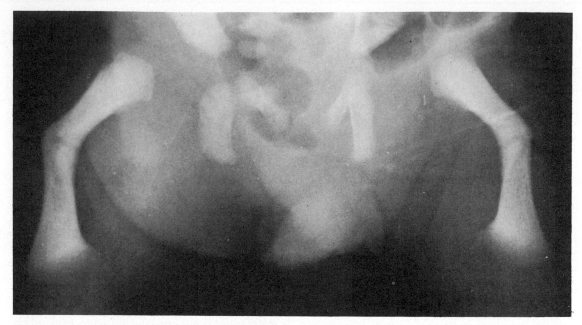

Figure 95–2. Roentgenogram of the femurs shows bilateral angulation and fracture. (Angle, C. R.: Pediatrics *13*:257, 1954.)

pressible, and within it no discrete tumor can be palpated. The only associated malformation in the case reported by Lee and Mattheis was an undescended testis on the same side.

Treatment. Treatment is surgical. The defect is closed by imbrication of muscles, fasciae, and aponeuroses.

Fractures Sustained During Delivery

Simple and depressed fractures of the skull have been discussed previously (*see* Chapter 77). Pathologic fractures sustained in utero are encountered in newborns with osteogenesis imperfecta (*see* Chapter 93).

The clavicles are the bones most often fractured

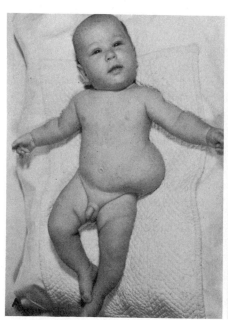

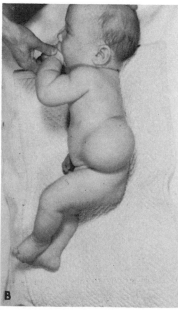

Figure 95–3. Photographs of an infant in the anteroposterior (*A*) and lateral (*B*) views show a grapefruit-sized mass projecting from the left flank. (Lee, C. M., Jr., and Mattheis, H.: Arch. Dis. Child. *32*:42, 1957.)

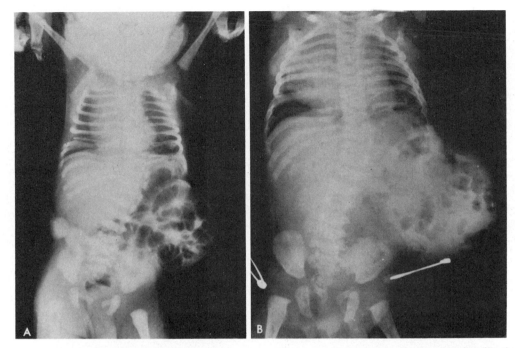

Figure 95–4. Anteroposterior roentgenograms of the same infant show the mass to be filled with apparently normal bowel. Several of the lower thoracic vertebrae are deformed. (Lee, C. M., Jr., and Mattheis, H.: Arch. Dis. Child. *32:*42, 1957.)

during delivery. Shoulder dystocia, probably the commonest cause of prolonged and difficult delivery, calls for vigorous, often violent, manipulation of the arm and shoulder. Resulting fracture of one clavicle may be incomplete (i.e., greenstick) or complete. In the first instance no disability or pain need be present, and the first intimation that the accident occurred may be the discovery of a large callus in the second week of life. Complete fractures are manifest immediately after birth by the infant's refusal to move the affected arm, by crying as though in pain whenever the arm is moved, by tenderness and, at times, visible angulation or hematoma over the fracture site, and by hypermobility of the bone. The Moro response is absent on that side. Radiographic examination verifies the diagnosis.

Less often, the humerus and, even more rarely, the femur can be fractured during delivery. Diagnosis of these conditions is not difficult and is made by eliciting their conventional signs, and it is verified by radiographic examination.

It must be remembered that the discovery of a fractured clavicle or humerus does not automatically rule out concomitant brachial plexus or peripheral nerve injury. Indeed, their presence augments the likelihood of the concomitance of one of these neurologic traumas. When a fracture is found, evidences of upper, lower, or combined brachial palsy and of diaphragmatic paralysis will be sought out.

With improved methods estimating fetal size (e.g., ultrasonography) and a greater willingness among physicians to deliver infants in the breech position by cesarean section, we rarely see traumatic fractures inflicted during delivery.

Epiphyseal Injuries in Breech Delivery

Shulman and Terhune summarized knowledge of this disorder in 1951. That it is not excessively uncommon is indicated by the fact that they had observed four cases themselves.

Etiology. Firstborns are affected almost exclusively because the relatively rigid primiparous musculature necessitates greater force during extraction of the infant. Breech presentations requiring manual extraction or version and extraction are most liable to this type of injury, but it may occur in any delivery in which vigorous pulling is done. The upper epiphysis of the femur is the site most commonly involved, with the upper epiphysis of the humerus in the second numerical position. The usual traumatic result is separation of the epiphysis without dislocation.

Diagnosis. Clinical signs do not become apparent until the second day. Then, if it is the upper femoral epiphysis that has been injured, the infant assumes the batrachian (froglike) position, and the soft tissues over the upper thigh become full, tense, and reddened. Pressure and passive motion cause pain. Low fever and much irritability may be present. All symptoms and signs clear within 1 to 2 weeks.

Radiographs show nothing until the end of the first week. At that time, excessive subperiosteal calcification makes its appearance about the injured site. Dislocation of the epiphysis may be visualized.

CASE 95–1

Shulman's fourth case is of especial interest. On the tenth day of life, this male infant had great swelling and tenderness of the lower third of both thighs. Radio-graphs showed considerable subperiosteal calcification in these areas (Fig. 95–5), and the infant's blood calcium level was 8.7 mg per 100 ml. Five days later, he had three generalized convulsions, and his calcium level had fallen to 5.6 mg. The logical assumption was that hypocalcemic tetany had followed withdrawal of calcium from the circulating blood during the phase of calcification of the callus.

Treatment. No treatment is needed unless there is dislocation. If there is dislocation, a cast may have to be applied.

Klippel-Feil Syndrome

This syndrome, or malformation association, of short neck, low hairline, and limited cervical mobility was first described by Klippel and Feil in 1912. A web neck and torticollis are often present. Roentgenograms almost always show fusion of two or more bodies or arches of cervical vertebrae.

Associated defects include spina bifida, other axial

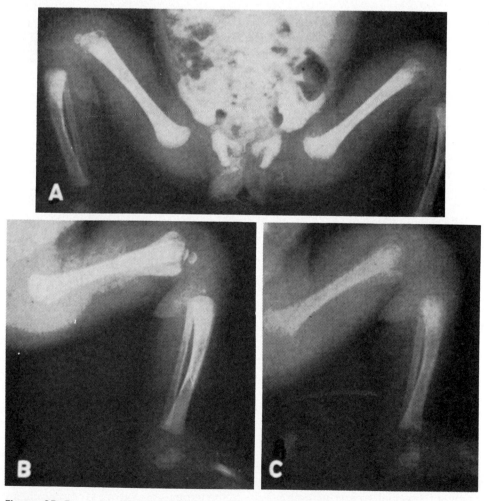

Figure 95–5. *A,* Roentgenogram at 11 days of age showing osteochondritis and slight subperiosteal changes of lower third of both femora. *B,* Left, and *C,* right, on sixteenth day of life, showing definite subperiosteal calcification of both lower femora. (Shulman, B. H., and Terhune, C. B.: Pediatrics *8*:693, 1951.)

skeletal deformities, deafness in as many as 30 per cent of patients, and congenital heart defects in nearly 50 per cent. Major neural tube defects including syringomyelia may be present.

The malformation is usually sporadic, although isolated parent-child and sib-sib combinations have been reported. Fortunately, the syndrome is rare, estimated to occur in one per 42,000 births. Sixty-five per cent of patients are female.

REFERENCES

Angle, C. R.: Congenital bowing and angulation of long bones. Pediatrics 13:257, 1954.

Baird, P. A., Robinson, G. C., and Buckler, W. St. J.: Klippel-Feil syndrome: A study of mirror movement detected by electromyography. Am. J. Dis. Child. 113:546, 1967.

Bound, J. P., Finlay, H. V. L., and Rose, F. C.: Congenital anterior angulation of the tibia. Arch. Dis. Child. 17:179, 1952.

Gwinn, J. L., and Barnes, G. R.: Radiological case of the month. Am. J. Dis. Child. 114:401, 1967.

Lee, C. M., Jr., and Mattheis, H.: Congenital lumbar hernia. Arch. Dis. Child. 32:42, 1957.

Nastin, cited by Lee and Mattheis.

Palant, D. J., and Carter, B. L.: Klippel-Feil syndrome and deafness. Am. J. Dis. Child. 123:218, 1972.

Shulman, B. H., and Terhune, C. B.: Epiphyseal injuries in breech delivery. Pediatrics 8:693, 1951.

Smith, D. W.: Recognizable Patterns of Human Malformation. 3rd ed. Philadelphia, W. B. Saunders Co., 1982.

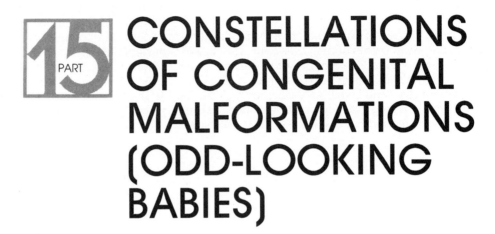

PART 15

CONSTELLATIONS OF CONGENITAL MALFORMATIONS (ODD-LOOKING BABIES)

Repeatedly one sees babies born with various associated congenital malformations of such striking similarity of facies and other characteristics that one would expect a single teratogenic factor to be responsible for them all. In some, such a factor can be assigned, but more often it cannot.

Described elsewhere in this volume are the visible features that stigmatize the following:

1. Hormonal deprivation or excess
   a. Cretinism
   b. Hypopituitarism
   c. Hyperadrenocorticism
   d. Infants of diabetic mothers
   e. Hypoparathyroidism
2. Errors of metabolism, for the most part inborn
   a. Phenylketonuria
   b. Homocystinuria
   c. Idiopathic hypercalcemia
3. Maternal drug ingestion
   a. Androgenic substances
   b. Thalidomide
   c. Fetal alcohol syndrome
   d. Dilantin syndrome
   e. Tridione syndrome
4. Exposure to radiant energy
   a. Microcephaly

Others are discussed in the sections devoted to disorders of the system that is most obviously involved in their deviation from the normal. Examples are the Pierre Robin syndrome, Treacher Collins syndrome, the dyschondroplasias, and acrocephalosyndactylism. There remain others whose manifestations are so widespread that they cannot be classified by system. The reader is referred to Smith's Recognizable Patterns of Human Malformation for a more complete discussion.

96

Gross Chromosomal Aberrations

Revised by F. Clarke Fraser

Not until 1956 was it established that the modal number of chromosomes in human cells is 46. This diploid number represents 22 pairs of autosomes and two sex chromosomes, either two X's or an X and a Y. Spermatocytes and oocytes undergo meiosis in which the resulting cells (spermatids or oocytes) receive only one member of each pair. Thus, the sper-

matozoon and the unfertilized ovum contain the haploid number of chromosomes, 22 autosomes and either an X or a Y. Fertilization means restoration of the chromosome number to 46 in the new individual so created.

It is not unexpected that mishaps occur during these complicated maneuvers. When errors in number, size, or configuration result, visible under the microscope in properly prepared specimens, they are termed "gross chromosomal aberrations," in contradistinction to the invisible alterations in single DNA nucleotides that result in the mutations underlying the inborn errors of metabolism.

A typical normal karyotype is shown in Figure 96–1. The 44 autosomes are divided into groups A (three pairs, 1, 2, 3), B (two pairs, 4, 5), C (seven pairs, 6, 7, 8, 9, 10, 11, 12), D (three pairs, 13, 14, 15), E

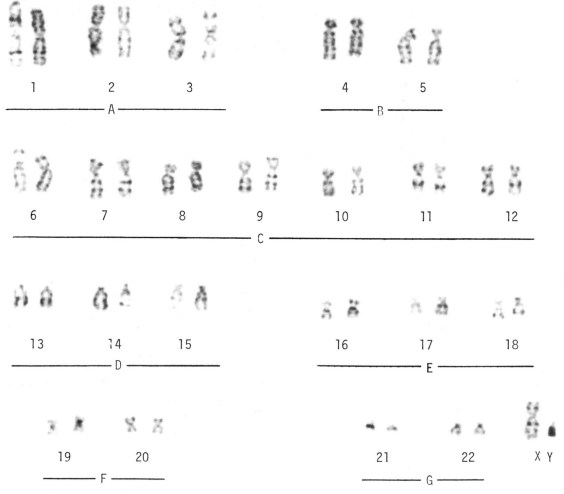

Figure 96–1. Karyotype of normal male showing banding produced by trypsin treatment of Seabright (1972). (Courtesy of Dr. Hope Punnett.)

(three pairs, 16, 17, 18), F (two pairs, 19, 20) and G (two pairs, 21, 22). These are distinguished from one another by size and by position of the centromere, which divides each chromosome into two arms (arms equal, metacentric; somewhat unequal, submedian; or with constriction almost at the end, acrocentric).

Furthermore, since the early 1970s, innovations in staining techniques have revealed patterns of bands along the chromosomes so that each chromosome, as well as specific regions of a chromosome, can be individually identified. Study of prophase chromosomes, before they have fully contracted to the metaphase state, permits even finer resolution of structure. Thus, it is possible to detect much more subtle aberrations (deletions and rearrangements) than was previously possible. Figure 96–1 shows a karyotype prepared after G banding with a modified Giemsa staining technique. These techniques have greatly increased the discrimination and precision of cytogenic diagnosis, and the number of recognizable syndromes resulting from chromosomal aberrations is rapidly increasing. A convention has been adopted whereby the short arm of a chromosome is labeled "p" and the long arm "q." Each band has a specific number. The relations between abnormalites in specific chromosomes and resultant alterations in phenotype are only just beginning to be understood.

Chromosomes may be abnormal in number, size, or configuration. Such abnormalities are brought about by failure of a pair of chromosomes to segregate during meiosis (*nondisjunction*) or by breakage and subsequent rearrangements (*deletions, inversions, translocations,* and others). A few individuals are *mosaics*; that is, their body is made up of two or more cell lines, with different karyotypes.

From the data accumulated to the present time, the following generalizations can be made:

1. Loss of any one entire autosome is almost always incompatible with life.

2. At least one X chromosome is essential to life and development.

3. The Y chromosome is the male-determining chromosome. In its absence, life and development may proceed, but in the female developmental pathway and, when there is only one X, far from perfectly.

4. Excesses of chromatin material, in the form of extra entire chromosomes or of translocations or insertions of portions of chromosomes, are often compatible with continued life and development.

5. Gross autosomal aberrations are associated with multiple congenital structural defects.

6. Mosaicism may exist in individuals (a) who are phenotypically normal, (b) who have all the characteristics associated with their abnormal karyotype, or (c) who have some intermediate phenotype.

7. At least 10 well-defined clinical syndromes have been identified to date that are analogous with corresponding alterations in one autosome group (trisomies 13, 18, 21, and 22; deletion of the short arm of 4, 5, and 9; deletion of the long arm of 13, 18, 21, and 22). Other syndromes resulting from "partial trisomy" or deletion of specific segments of autosomes (e.g., 4p, 8p, 9p) are gradually being delineated. Yunis and colleagues have prepared a useful list of the abnormal features occurring in the more recently recognized syndromes. Most of them are difficult to diagnose reliably by phenotype; if there is any suspicion of a chromosomal syndrome, it is best to confirm it by karyotyping.

8. Two well-defined clinical syndromes result from specific aberrations of sex chromosomes (Turner, XO, and Klinefelter, XXY). A third is by no means uncommon (XYY), but at least one of the behavioral abnormalities ascribed to it has become the subject of heated controversy. A host of other aberrations of sex chromosomes have been encountered, but the constellations of congenital defects that they produce are not so well defined.

The frequency of autosomal aberrations has been established as about five per 1000 births. However, the use of modern banding techniques will undoubtedly increase this number considerably. Sex chromosome aberrations account for about two per 1000 births. As many as 60 per cent of spontaneous abortions are associated with a chromosomal aberration according to the meticulous studies of Boué and Lazar.

The recent advances in cytogenic techniques have also increased greatly the precision of prenatal diagnosis of chromosomal aberrations (see Chapter 3).

Dermatoglyphics

The study of ridge patterns on fingers and palms and of crease patterns on palms and digits dates back to the 1892 observations of Sir Francis Galton. The variations from the normal have been utilized increasingly more often in recent years for the diagnosis of syndromes, especially those associated with chromosomal aberrations.

These cannot be discussed in detail here, but they have been reviewed by Preus and Fraser in their 1972 report. The most important patterns looked for are the following:

1. Fingerprints. These are conventionally classified as arches, loops, or whorls, and loops are commonly designated as radial or ulnar, depending on the orientation of their open end.

2. Transverse palmar lines. There should be two of these. When there is only one or when the two are joined by a distinct bridge, the resulting line is known as a "simian crease." If the proximal transverse line extends to the ulnar border of the hand, it is called a "Sydney line."

3. Position of axial triradius. In normal individuals, the axial triradius is found to lie near the proximal border of the palm. Displacement distally, that is, toward the center of the palm, occurs in normal indi-

viduals but more frequently appears with a variety of syndromes. Its height can be measured as a percentage of the height from the distal wrist crease to the proximal crease at the base of the third digit. If this is greater than 40 per cent, the axial triradius is referred to as t″. Bilateral t″ occurs in 80 per cent of children with Down syndrome or trisomy 13, in roughly 20 per cent of children with trisomy 18, de Lange syndrome, and Rubinstein-Taybi syndrome, and in 3 per cent of normal children.

Baird has observed a family, thirteen of whose twenty-four members in three generations show complete absence of dermal ridges. This defect appeared to be transmitted as a dominant, non—sex-linked trait with variable penetrance.

Trisomy 21 (Down Syndrome, Mongolism)

Trisomy 21 is an association of congenital anomalies that imparts to its subjects a characteristic facies. These children are by no means identical, but facies and body build are so similar that they bear a strong family resemblance. A common basic defect is reduced intellectual capacity, but even this is variable in degree.

Incidence. Down syndrome accounts for 15 to 20 per cent of cases of severe mental retardation. In the United States, the incidence is about 0.9 per 1000 livebirths. Variations in incidence depend on demographic factors such as fertility rates in women over age 35 years, the accessibility of prenatal diagnosis, and the option of abortion.

The risk of an affected infant increases with maternal age. At age 35 years, the risk is one in 300 births; at age 40 years, it is one in 100 births. By age 45 years, the frequency of Down syndrome is one in 25 births (Hook and Lindsjo, 1978). About 25 per cent of children with Down syndrome receive an extra chromosome from their fathers. The relationship to paternal age is not nearly as clear as the relationship to maternal age.

Etiology. The frequency of Down syndrome is greatest in infants of mothers near the end of the child-bearing period, although this tendency appears to be decreasing.

In 1959, two teams of observers reported almost simultaneously the finding of an extra chromosome in the karyotypes of Down syndrome children. The forty-seventh chromosome seemed to fit into group G (21, 22); hence the disorder was termed "trisomy 21." The mechanism responsible for the extra chromosome was believed to be nondisjunction during meiosis, a "mistake" in the segregation of the chromosomes. This appeared to explain the observation that many of these infants were born to older mothers, since geneticists have long been aware that nondisjunction is a more frequent accident in their aging laboratory subjects than in the young. It also explains why the disorder is sporadic and not familial in most cases.

It soon became clear that not all Down syndrome children were trisomic for 21. A minority had the normal number of chromosomes, with two pairs of acrocentric autosomes in group G, but one atypical chromosome in another group. To take a frequent example, one of pair 14 may be missing but replaced by a chromosome that appears to consist of the long arms of 14 and 21. These chromosomes arise by "robertsonian" translocation, in which the centromeres of 21 and 14 have fused; the short arms are lost, but their absence does not seem to have any effect. Hence, these individuals possess a superabundance of 21 chromatin, just as those with trisomy 21 do. These karyotypes are termed "46, translocation 14/21." Translocations of 21 to other chromosomes have been reported less commonly.

Translocations of this nature, unlike trisomies, are sometimes found in a balanced form in one parent and in other close relatives of the affected infant; hence, this rearrangement is familial and heritable, transmitted from one generation to others as an autosomal dominant. In these cases, the association with increased maternal age does not appear. Such translocations do not produce abnormalities if they are "balanced"—that is, if they have one 21, one 14, and the 14/21 translocation chromosome—so there is no excess chromosomal material. However, balanced carriers may produce unbalanced gametes, and spontaneous abortion or chromosomal syn-

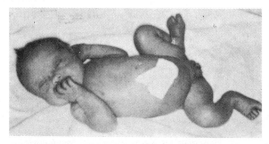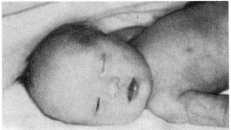

Figure 96–2. *A,* Overall view of Down syndrome infant made on the second day of life. General hypotonia is suggested by the relaxed appearance in what appears to be an awkward position. *B,* Head and face of the infant show the round, short skull, well-developed epicanthus, slanting of lid slits upward from within outward, and shallow orbits.

dromes in the offspring may result. Fortunately, such carriers may now take advantage of prenatal diagnosis (see Chapter 2).

The trisomic individual, although himself or herself the result of a sporadic aberration, is capable of transmitting the condition as a dominant. Fortunately, few have produced offspring.

Finally, there have by now been reported a number of infants who are mosaics for trisomy 21 or translocations 14/21 or 21/22. Some have manifested all the defects of Down syndrome; some have presented with only a few of them. Some members of this subgroup have attained an intellectual capacity within the range of normal. Mosaicism may explain the heretofore mystifying stories about children who had many of the stigmata of the syndrome but who were able nevertheless to keep up with and at times excel their peers in scholastic performance.

Diagnosis. Most infants with Down syndrome can be diagnosed at birth or at first glance. In a few, the diagnosis may remain in doubt. A diagnostic index based on dermatoglyphic and other features can make or exclude the diagnosis reliably in over 97 per cent of patients (Rex and Preus, 1982). If there is a reasonable suspicion of Down syndrome, one should request a karyotype in order to establish whether there is a regular trisomy or a translocation. If the latter, the parents should be karyotyped, and, if they are translocation carriers, other family members should be studied so that those at increased risk can be identified. There are a number of characteristics that become manifest only later in life, but usually enough are sufficiently obvious from the moment of birth to allow one to make the diagnosis with assurance (Figs. 96–2 and 96–3). These signs may include (and it must be remembered that not all children with Down syndrome demonstrate *all* the anatomic defects of the syndrome) the following:

Small Size. Twenty per cent are prematurely born. Very few are as large as expected for their gestational ages.

Globular Brachycephalic Skull. The suboccipitobregmatic circumference is generally small; the skull is short and round with a flat occiput.

Characteristic Eyes. The eyes slant upward from within outward. There is a prominent epicanthic fold involving the inner half of the upper eyelid. This is associated with a flat nose-bridge and tends to disappear as the child gets older. The eyeball is not recessed, giving rise to the flat face (flache Gesicht) noted by observers long ago. The iris may be speckled with a ring of round, grayish (Brushfield's) spots, but this sign is rapidly obscured if the iris is darkly pigmented.

Red Cheeks. This sign may not be prominent immediately after birth, but it becomes increasingly so with the passage of months.

Narrow and Short Palate. (Shapiro et al., 1967).

Short, Flat-bridged Retroussé Nose.

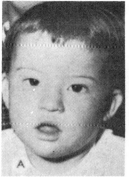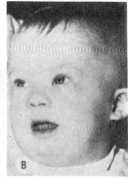

Figure 96–3. Photographs of two siblings with Down Syndrome caused by a translocation, not trisomy 21. (Warkany, J., et al.: Pediatrics *33*:290, 1964.)

Protruding Tongue. Later, the dorsum of the tongue becomes dry, wrinkled, and fissured, features of the so-called "scrotal tongue."

Loose Skin Covering the Lateral and Dorsal Aspects of the Neck.

Characteristic Hands. The fingers are short; the hands appear square. The thumb is low-set and separated a bit more than usual from the second finger. The fifth finger is apt to be short and incurved, to have but one transverse crease, and to show absence or hypoplasia of its middle phalanx on radiographs. The two usual transverse palmar creases are often replaced by a single deep one, the simian crease.

Umbilical Hernia. This feature is often present.

Characteristic Feet. The great toe is separated from the second toe. Between these toes a deep crease begins and continues in an arc around the thenar eminence to the medial edge of the sole.

Muscular Hypotonia. This, associated with laxity of ligaments, permits extraordinary malleability. The great toe can easily be placed in the infant's mouth and the hand hyperextended until it lies flat against the dorsal aspect of the forearm.

Narrow Acetabular Angle, Iliac Index (II), and Broadened Iliac Bones. These can be determined by radiographic study.

Retarded Psychomotor Development. This cannot be determined in the neonatal period but will become manifest soon.

Congenital Heart Defect. A common associated malformation (found in 50 per cent of patients) is an interventricular septal defect, characteristically a persistent ostium primum or atrioventricular canal.

Duodenal Atresia. This congenital malformation is present in trisomy 21 children many times more often than it is in normals.

Leukemia and Leukemoid Reactions. A great many more trisomy 21 children have these blood dyscrasias than do normal children, although the absolute frequency is fairly low.

Prognosis. The hazards to life confronting children with Down syndrome are fairly numerous. They include coexisting severe congenital defects, to which these children are inordinately liable. Among infants born with esophageal atresia, duodenal atresia and imperforate anus are found in a large number with Down syndrome. Many such cases have been reported among series of examples of annular pancreas. Congenital heart defects are common concomitants of the syndrome. Many of these turn out to be simple high interventricular septal defects (e.g., persistent ostium primum), which do little more than produce a loud murmur, but some are more complicated and more serious. Patients with Down syndrome are extremely liable to upper respiratory tract infections, which, in preantibiotic days, often became lower respiratory tract infections and were responsible for many deaths. Few infants die for this reason now.

The outlook for these children with respect to physical and mental development is discouraging, but the picture may not be nearly as bleak as the parents imagine. In a discussion limited to newborns, this concerns us only because it has direct bearing on the advice one has to give the parents. Almost all the signposts of development will appear late—in some moderately late, in others extremely so. In a study of the variability of trisomy 21, Levinson and coworkers pointed out that whereas a few affected infants learned to sit alone between 6 and 8 months, most could not sit until they were over a year. A few learned connected speech, that is, sentence formation, by about 3 years of age, but most could not form sentences until they were more than 6 years old, and some never learned how. The best equipped will fall into the classification of low-grade morons, but most will have to be designated as imbeciles. Practically none are truly idiots. (However, these observations were based largely on children who were raised in institutions and may be unduly pessimistic.) They are almost without exception pleasant, lovable, nondestructive children who love music and are educable to a point far beyond that which we used to think possible. Smith and Wilson have prepared a well-illustrated book that provides useful information about the characteristics of children with Down syndrome, which parents of such children will find helpful.

Trisomy 22

This syndrome has been clearly defined only since the advent of modern banding techniques. The features include growth retardation, mental retardation, microcephaly, micrognathia, preauricular skin tags or sinuses, low-set, abnormal ears, cleft palate, congenital heart disease, and digitalized or malopposed thumbs. The so-called "cat-eye" syndrome appears to result from partial trisomy or tetrasomy of the short arm of chromosome 22. The main features are colobomas, hypertelorism, down-slanted (antimongoloid) palpebral fissures, anal atresia, and many features of full-blown trisomy 22, excluding cleft palate.

Trisomy 18

The second most common autosomal trisomy syndrome results from an extra chromosome in group E (16–18), now known to be 18. It has a frequency of one in 3500 births or less.

Etiology. Nondisjunction appears to account for the majority of these cases. But, exactly as in trisomy 21, other defects in the karyotype were soon observed to be associated with the same clinical syndrome. Identical babies have been reported to have partial trisomy, translocations, or mosaicisms (10 per cent of cases). The same conditions of familial incidence and heredity as those cited for Down syndrome apply to this syndrome.

Diagnosis. One should note the following representative signs in the constellation of obstetric and congenital abnormalities that earmark children with these defects (remembering that, as in trisomy 21, not all the babies of this genre will manifest all the deviations from normal) (Fig. 96–4): (1) advanced parental age; (2) low birth weight after term gestation; (3) low-set, abnormal ears; (4) micrognathia (and microstomia); (5) mental retardation; (6) characteristically flexed fingers, with flexion contraction of the two middle digits, which are overlapped by the flexed

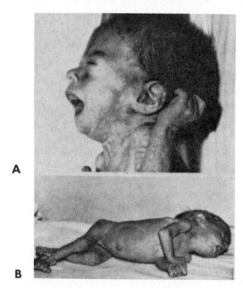

Figure 96–4. *A,* Photograph of head of newborn infant with trisomy E. This shows well the low-set large ears and micrognathia. In *B,* a high degree of malnutrition, arthrogryposis, and characteristic flexion deformities of the fingers are demonstrated. (Hecht, F., et al.: J. Pediatr. *63:*605, 1963.)

thumb and index and little fingers; (7) congenital heart defect, almost always a ventricular septal defect, often coupled with patent ductus arteriosus; (8) rocker-bottom feet.

In addition to exhibiting these almost universal abnormalities, many affected children have ptosis of one or both eyelids, syndactyly, an abnormally jutting occiput, genitourinary defects, hernias, and other scattered imperfections. About one of four show the typical simian palmar crease, and dermatoglyphic studies reveal a striking preponderance of arch patterns. Arches on seven or more fingers occur in 80 per cent of cases, and less than six arches or more than two whorls is reason to be very skeptical of the diagnosis.

Prognosis. Most of these babies die in early infancy, generally from heart failure, but occasional survival into childhood is reported. One patient was living at 20 years at the time his report appeared. His karyotype was that of a translocation.

Treatment. Each defect must be treated individually. Clearly, one can look forward to little benefit from therapy. One should offer the parents prenatal diagnosis for subsequent pregnancies, since the increased risk in such situations is assumed to be about 1 or 2 per cent.

Trisomy 13

Trisomy of one of the group D autosomes, number 13, and mosaicisms of this aberration are much less common than those of group E.

Diagnosis. D trisomies have several defects in common with E trisomies. These are (1) psychomotor retardation, (2) malformed ears, (3) flexion deformities of wrist, hand, and fingers, (4) congenital heart defects (in 90 per cent, usually ventricular septal defect, patent ductus arteriosus, or rotational anomalies), (5) rocker-bottom feet, and (6) simian creases.

In addition, these children manifest abnormalities that are not characteristic of trisomy E. Such abnormalities are eye defects (microphthalmos, colobomata of iris, cataracts); broad, flattened nose; failure of fusion of maxillary and palatal processes (harelip, cleft palate); postaxial polydactyly; umbilical defects (hernia, omphalocele); abnormalities of the genitals (in the female, bicornuate or septate uterus; in the male, cryptorchidism, small, anteriorly placed scrotum); polycystic kidneys; cutaneous hemangiomas; gross defects of the brain (arhinencephaly and others); tendency to grand mal seizures, myoclonic jerks, and severe breath-holding spells; skin defects of the scalp; and characteristic dermatoglyphics (radial loops and arches, single palmar creases— in 60 per cent—and thenar exit of the A line).

These children have assumed additional impor-

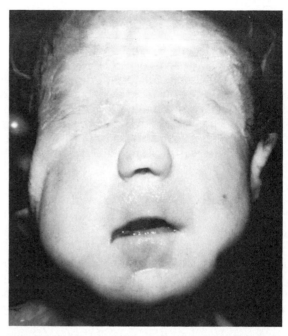

Figure 96–5. Photograph of a newborn infant with the trisomy D syndrome. Note microphthalmos and the bizarre nose with (in this case) a single centrally placed nostril. The ears are also low-set and malformed. (We are grateful to Dr. Barbara Migeon for this illustration.)

tance because of the finding in most of them of several hematologic abnormalities. They have increased fetal hemoglobin (HbF), Bart's hemoglobin (gamma-4), and, possibly, embryonic hemoglobins (Gower, type II).

Prognosis. Death in early infancy is usually the rule, although some children survive for several years.

Treatment. Harelip and cleft palate may be repaired, and other defects amenable to surgical correction may be given appropriate therapy.

Trisomy 8

About half the cases of trisomy 8 are mosaic. There is an excess of affected males. Mental retardation is mild to moderate. Skeletal anomalies are common and include ankylosed large joints, clubfoot, absent patella, arachnodactyly, and brachydactyly. Deep grooves in the palms and soles are characteristic in infancy. The facies is reminiscent of that appearing with Williams syndrome, with a prominent, pouting lower lip and micrognathia. Less than half the patients have a congenital heart malformation—ventricular septal defect, atrioseptal defect, or patent ductus arteriosus.

Trisomy 9p

The severity depends on the amount of extra chromosomal material present. The facies is characterized by eccentric pupils, hypertelorism, prominent lower epicanthic fold, antimongoloid palpebral fissures, and a worried look. The palms of the hands are disproportionately long, with a single palmar crease and an increased frequency of arches. About half the patients have a heart malformation, usually ventricular septal defect.

Le Cri du Chat (Cat's Cry) 5P – Syndrome

Lejeune observed three cases in which a deletion of the short arms of chromosome 5 was associated with a consistent and characteristic constellation of malformations. This was the first autosomal deletion syndrome to be defined. As one would expect, the phenotypes described in these syndromes are quite variable, presumably depending on the extent and location of the deletion.

All his patients demonstrated microcephaly, micrognathia, epicanthus, oblique (antimongoloid) palpebral fissures, hypertelorism, low-set ears, severe mental retardation, and *a peculiar cry resembling that of a cat*. However, the facies is not as strikingly characteristic as it is in the trisomy syndromes. There is an excess of affected females.

The karyotype in all cases showed 46 chromosomes, but autosome 5 in the B group was lacking part of the short arm. The frequency is about one in 50,000 births.

The 4P – Syndrome

A second deletion syndrome in the B group has been identified as involving the short arm of chromosome 4. The main features are low birth weight, profound psychomotor retardation, microcephaly, hypertelorism with a prominent glabella and broad nose, coloboma iridis, low-set, simple ears, a carplike mouth, cleft lip and palate, and hypospadias in males. The dermatoglyphic features include ridge dissociation, increased arches and decreased whorls, and an increased frequency of bilateral simian creases in 30 per cent.

13Q – Syndrome

Patients with deletions of the long arm of 13 usually show severe mental retardation, microcephaly, trigonocephaly, broad nasal root and bridge, hyper-

telorism, coloboma or microphthalmia, large low-set ears, webbing of the neck, heart malformations (50 per cent), imperforate anus (occasionally), and hypospadias. Retinoblastoma is a frequent finding when band q14 is missing.

The 18Q – Syndrome

Infants with deletions of the long arm of 18 are characterized by microcephaly, hypotonia, mental and physical retardation, midface hypoplasia, hypertelorism, coloboma of iris, retinal defects, large ears with a small canal, carplike mouth, long, tapering fingers, heart malformations (40 per cent), cryptorchidism, clubfoot, an excess of dermatoglyphic whorl patterns, and dimpled knuckles, elbows, and knees.

The 21Q – Syndrome

This syndrome, which before "banding" was available was known as "G deletion syndrome I," is characterized by microcephaly, psychomotor retardation, down-slanting (antimongoloid) palpebral fissures, a prominent nose bridge, large low-set ears, dolichocephaly, and hypertonia.

The 22Q – Syndrome

This syndrome, formerly called "G deletion syndrome II," is characterized by microcephaly, psychomotor retardation, low-set ears, epicanthal folds, flat nasal bridge, ptosis, bifid uvula, clinodactyly, and syndactyly.

Gross Aberration of Sex Chromosomes

These are described in detail in the discussion of abnormalities of sexual differentiation (see Chapter 56).

Small Deletion Syndromes

The advent of extended prophase banding led to the identification of very small deletions that involve only one band and that are associated with several syndromes previously of unknown etiology, some of which are described elsewhere in this volume. Because the association is not (so far) constant and the information is preliminary, we will not discuss these syndromes in this chapter but will simply list them here, along with the location of the deletion:

Langer-Giedion (trichorhinophalangeal type II) syndrome: 8q22 deletion.
Aniridia-Wilms syndrome: 11p13 deletion.
Retinoblastoma–mental retardation syndrome: 13q14 deletion.

Prader-Willi syndrome: 15q11 — 12 deletion.
Sipple syndrome (multiple endocrine neoplasia type II): 20p — deletion.
DiGeorge syndrome: 22q11 deletion.

REFERENCES

General

Bergsma, D. (Ed.): Birth Defects Atlas and Compendium. 2nd ed. Baltimore, Williams & Wilkins Company, 1979.

Bersu, E. T.: Anatomical analysis of the developmental effects of aneuploidy in man: the Down syndrome. Am. J. Med. Genet. *5*:399, 1980.

Boué, A., and Lazar, P.: Retrospective and prospective epidemiological studies of 1500 karyotyped spontaneous human abortions. Teratology *12*:11, 1975.

de Grouchy, J., and Turleau, C.: Clinical Atlas of Human Chromosomes. New York, John Wiley & Sons, 1977.

Forbes, A. P.: Fingerprints and palm prints (dermatoglyphics) and palmar flexion creases in gonadal dysgenesis, pseudoparathyroidism and Klinefelter's syndrome. N. Engl. J. Med. *270*:1268, 1964.

Friedman, J. M.: Genetic disease in the offspring of older fathers. Obstet. Gynecol. *57*:745, 1981.

Galton, F.: Finger Prints. London, MacMillan and Co., 1892.

Hecht, F., Bryant, J. S., et al.: The nonrandomness of chromosomal abnormalities: association of trisomy 18 and Down's syndrome. N. Engl. J. Med. *271*:1081, 1964.

Jacobs, P. A.: Recurrence risks for chromosomal abnormalities. Birth Defects. Original Article Series 15(5C): 71, 1979.

Jacobs, P. A., Aitken, J., Frackiewickz, A., Law, P., Newton, M. S., and Smith, P. G.: The inheritance of translocations in man. Ann. Hum. Genet. *34*:119, 1970.

Kaback, M. M. (Ed.): Genetic Issues in Pediatric and Obstetric Practice. Chicago, Year Book Medical Publishers, 1981.

Nitowsky, H., Sindhavananda, N., et al.: Partial 18 monosomy in the cyclops malformation. Pediatrics *37*:260, 1966.

Nora, J. J., and Fraser, F. C.: Medical Genetics: Principles and Practice. 2nd ed. Philadelphia, Lea and Febiger, 1981.

Penrose, L. S., and Smith, G. F.: Down's Anomaly. Boston, Little, Brown and Company, 1966.

Preus, M., and Fraser, F. C.: Dermatoglyphics and syndromes. Am. J. Dis. Child. *124*:933, 1972.

Smith, D. W.: Recognizable Patterns of Human Malformation. 3rd ed. Philadelphia, W. B. Saunders Co., 1982.

Warkany, J., Weinstein, D., Soukup, S. W., Rubinstein, J. H., and Curless, M. C.: Chromosome analyses in a children's hospital. Selection of patients and results of studies. Pediatrics *33*:290, 454, 1964.

Yunis, J. J. (Ed.): New Chromosomal Syndromes. New York, Academic Press, 1977.

Down Syndrome

Armendares, S., Urrusti-Sanz, J., and Diaz-del-Castillo, E.: Iliac index in newborns: Comparative values at term, in prematurity and in Down's syndrome. Am. J. Dis. Child. *113*:229, 1967.

Caffey, J., and Ross, S.: Pelvic bones in infantile mongolism. Am. J. Roentgenol. *80*:458, 1958.

Carr, J.: Mental and motor development in young mongol children. J. Ment. Def. Res. *14*:205, 1970.

Conen, P. E., and Erkman, B.: Combined mongolism and leukemia. Am. J. Dis. Child. *112*:429, 1966.

Dicks-Mireaux, M.: Mental development of infants with Down's syndrome. Am. J. Ment. Def. 77:26, 1972.

Holmes, L. B.: Genetic counseling for the older pregnant woman: new data and questions. N. Engl. J. Med. *298*:1419, 1978.

Hook, E. B., and Lindsjo, A.: Down syndrome in livebirths by single year maternal age interval in a Swedish study: comparison of results from a New York study. Am. J. Hum. Genet. *30*:19, 1978.

Jacobs, P. A., Baikie, A. G., Brown, W. M. C., and Strong, J. A.: The somatic chromosomes in mongolism. Lancet *1*:710, 1959.

Levinson, A., Friedman, A., and Stamps, F.: Variability of mongolism. Pediatrics *16*:43, 1955.

Nicolis, F. B., and Sacchetti, G.: Nomogram for the x-ray evaluation of some morphological anomalies of the pelvis in the diagnosis of mongolism. Pediatrics *32*:1074, 1963.

Penrose, L. S., and Smith, G. F.: Down's anomaly. Boston, Little, Brown and Co., 1966.

Rex, A. P., and Preus, M.: A diagnostic index for Down syndrome. J. Pediatr. *100*:903, 1982.

Shapiro, B. L., Gorlin, R. J., et al.: The palate and Down's syndrome. N. Engl. J. Med. *276*:1460, 1967.

Smith, D. W., and Wilson, A. A.: The Child with Down's Syndrome (Mongolism). Philadelphia, W. B. Saunders, 1973.

Weinstein, E. D., and Warkany, J.: Maternal mosaicism and Down's syndrome. J. Pediatr. *63*:599, 1963.

Wilson, R. G., et al.: Decreasing mosaicism in Down's syndrome. Clin. Genet. *17*:335, 1980.

E Trisomy

Hodes, M. E., et al.: Clinical experience with trisomies 18 and 13. J. Med. Genet. *15*:48, 1978.

Rohde, R. A., Hodgman, S. E., and Cleland, R. S.: Multiple congenital anomalies in the E trisomy (group 16–18) syndrome. Pediatrics *33*:258, 1964.

Uchida, J. A., Lewis, A. J., Bowman, J. M., and Wang, H. C.: A case of double trisomy no. 18 and triple-X. J. Pediatr. *60*:498, 1962.

Weber, F. M., and Sparks, R. S.: Trisomy E (18) syndrome: clinical spectrum in 12 new cases, including chromosome radioautography in 4. J. Med. Genet. 7:363, 1970.

D Trisomy

Miller, J. Q., Picard, E. H., Alkan, M. K., Warner, S., and Gerald, P. S.: A specific congenital brain defect (arhinencephaly) in 13–15 trisomy. N. Engl. J. Med. *268*:120, 1963.

Smith, D. W., Patau, K., Therman, E., Inhorn, S. L., and DeMars, R. J.: The D_1 trisomy syndrome. J. Pediatr. *62*:326, 1963.

Walzer, S., Park, G. S., et al.: Hematologic changes in the D_1 trisomy syndrome. Pediatrics *38*:419, 1966.

Wilson, M. G., and Melnyk, J.: Translocation—normal mosaicism in D_1 trisomy. Pediatrics *40*:842, 1967.

Cri du Chat Syndrome

Dumars, K. W., Jr., Gaskill, C., and Kitzmiller, N.: Le cri du chat (crying cat) syndrome. Am. J. Dis. Child. *108*:533, 1964.

Hijmans, J. C., and Shearin, D. B.: Partial deletion of short arms of chromosome no. 5: report of a case in a fraternal twin. Am. J. Dis. Child. *109*:85, 1965.

Lejeune, J., et al.: Deletion partielle du bras court du chromosome 5: individualisation d'un nouvelle état morbide. Sem. Hôp. Paris *25*:1069, 1964.

MacIntyre, M. N., Staples, W. I., LaPolla, J., and Hempel, J. M.: The "cat cry" syndrome. Am. J. Dis. Child. *108*:538, 1964.

97

Some Multiple Malformation Syndromes Not Caused by Gross Chromosomal Aberrations

Revised by F. Clarke Fraser

The title of this chapter perhaps should read a bit differently, with the words "known to be" inserted before "caused by gross chromosomal aberrations." We say this because continuing improvements in cytogenic techniques may eventually lead to the detection of small deletions, duplications, or other aberrations consistently associated with some of these syndromes (see, for instance, the section at the end of Chapter 96). In the meantime, their causes remain obscure.

As is true in all areas of neonatology, growth in this field has been extremely rapid. The late David W. Smith identified 221 recognizable patterns of human malformation in the second edition of his monograph on this subject, published in 1976. In the third edition, published in 1982, 355 different syndromes are recognized. We do not propose to compete with him but shall limit our discussion to a few of the most common malformations and the ones that, for historic and other reasons, interest us most. However, it should be pointed out that a not inconsiderable number of such constellations have been described in other sections (i.e., in the discussions of cretinism, the first and second arch syndromes, the various dyschondroplasias, phocomelia, renal agenesis, and many others).

Nuclear Agenesis (Möbius Syndrome)

Facial nerve palsy is most often unilateral and unassociated with other congenital palsies or defects. When it is bilateral or when other congenital abnormalities of cranial nerves or of the osseous system of the face or extremities are present concomitantly, the syndrome may fall into the category of nuclear agenesis.

Incidence. The condition is infrequent, but not extremely rare. Many instances have been misinterpreted as pseudobulbar palsies resulting from birth injury.

Etiology and Pathology. Both dominant transmission and an increased frequency of consanguineous parents (favoring autosomal recessive inheritance) are recorded, but most cases are isolated. According to Baraitser, if the diagnosis of Möbius syndrome is considered to include skeletal defects, the risk of recurrence is low (2 per cent); if there is only facial diplegia, with or without eye muscle involvement, the diagnosis may eventually become one of the known, genetically determined primary muscle or anterior horn cell disorders. The pathologic evidence is difficult to interpret, but there seems to be aplasia of the nuclei of the facial nerves and of adjacent cranial nerve nuclei. This was considered to be the primary defect by Möbius, but some observers have felt that the failure of development of nuclei might be secondary to a primary defect of mesenchyma causing imperfect development of nerves. Evans, in his brilliant analysis of all possible etiologic factors, suggested that all the lesions found might be traced to leakage of cerebrospinal fluid down the branchial arches and limb buds shortly after the seventh week of gestation.

Diagnosis. The sine qua non is facial nerve palsy. If it is bilateral, no other abnormalities must coexist to make Möbius syndrome a strong diagnostic possibility. If the palsy is unilateral, however, it is more likely to stem from an obstetric injury than from nuclear agenesis unless other congenital lesions coexist. These include one or more additional cranial nerve palsies, chiefly of extraocular movement, and of the palate, tongue, and masseters. Micrognathia, high arched palate, syndactylism, Klippel-Feil deformity, and club feet are some of the associated skeletal abnormalities.

The presenting sign is the extraordinary immobility of the face, as notable in the first few days of life as it is in later life. The facies mirrors no emotion, pleasant or unpleasant. This leads to the incorrect assumption of mental incompetence that will plague these afflicted children throughout life.

Treatment. Nothing can be done for the facial nerve palsy. Some of the associated defects are susceptible to treatment, and each of these deserves the best available therapy.

Leprechaunism

The name for this complex and vaguely defined disorder was suggested by the elfin facies of the affected infants. They also manifest physiologic and pathologic deviations from the normal, pointing toward a complicated endocrine disturbance. It is extremely rare, probably recessively inherited.

Diagnosis. The babies are small and develop slowly, both physically and mentally, often succumbing in the first few months. They have a grotesque, "elfin" facies with a flat nose bridge, flaring nostrils, thick lips, large low-set ears, hirsutism, enlarged breasts, large penis in males, prominent clitoris in females, deficiency of subcutaneous tissues, motor and mental retardation, and severe failure to thrive. Abnormalities of carbohydrate metabolism regulation are suggested by hypoglycemia, hyperinsulinism, decreased blood sugar response to epinephrine and glucagon, and hyperplasia of the islands of Langerhans, but no basic defect has been identified.

Treatment. Complications, particularly infections, should be treated. Gastrostomy feedings have been of temporary benefit in some cases.

The Oral-Facial-Digital Syndrome (OFD I Syndrome)

As the name indicates, this constellation of multiple congenital defects involves structures within the oral cavity, of the face, and of the extremities.

Etiology. The disease is strongly familial and is almost entirely confined to females. The consensus appears to be that the OFD I syndrome is an X-linked dominant condition, almost always lethal in males.

Diagnosis. The oral lesions include partial clefts or lobulations of the tongue, thick mucobuccal bands binding the tongue to the cheeks and gums, and palatal clefts and other anomalies of the palate. Facial

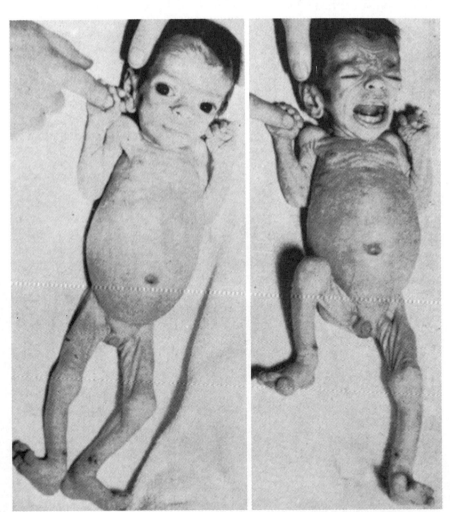

Figure 97–1. Note the extreme malnutrition, the huge ears, large eyes with black irises, the upturned nose, large mouth and pointed chin, and very large hands and feet.

Treatment. Plastic procedures are indicated for cleft lip and cleft palate and for freeing the tongue as much as is possible.

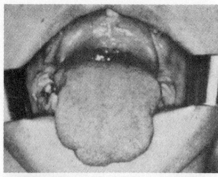

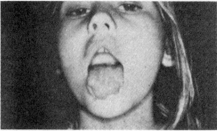

Figure 97–2. Photograph showing one of the characteristic tongue malformations in the oral-facial-digital syndrome. Note the irregular multifidity associated with this syndrone. (Ruess, A. L., et al.: Pediatrics *20*:985, 1962.)

deformities include shortness of alar cartilages and columella, median cleft of the lip, and hypertelorism. At times, there are alopecia and coarse hair and dry skin. Brachydactyly, clinodactyly, and syndactyly may involve the digits. About half the affected patients are mentally retarded.

The OFD II (Mohr) syndrome is similar but includes conductive hearing loss and postaxial polydactyly. Inheritance is autosomal recessive.

Oculoauriculovertebral Dysplasia (Goldenhar Syndrome)

In this constellation, congenital defects of the eyes, ears, face, mandible, and vertebral column are found. Patients with this syndrome resemble those with mandibulofacial dysostosis (Treacher Collins syndrome) in several ways but have, in addition, epibulbar dermoids, notching of the upper (rather than lower) lid, and a higher frequency of vertebral defects. Hemifacial microsomia may be a variant.

Incidence. The condition is very rare.

Etiology. The chromosomal pattern has been studied in a few examples, and no aberrations have been found. It is rarely a familial disease. The pathogenesis of the disorder therefore is not known.

Diagnosis. Epibulbar dermoid cysts, colobomata of the upper lid, iris, and choroid, and, at times, microphthalmos characterize the eyes of these patients. The eyes do not commonly slant downward, nor is the lower lid notched, as is the case in mandibulofacial dysostosis. The external and middle ear may be absent, displaced downward, or malrotated, or there may be one or more ear tags. Asymmetric facial and mandibular hypoplasia are typical. Hemivertebrae are common. Associated defects of heart, lungs (agenesis), and extremities are not infrequent. Mental deficiency occurs in only 10 to 15 per cent of cases.

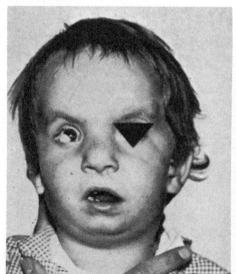

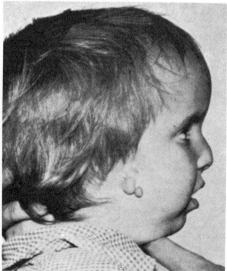

Figure 97–3. Note the epibulbar dermoid cyst of the right eye, and the virtually absent right external ear, its place taken by several rudimentary tags. This is typical oculoauriculovertebral dysplasia. (Gorlin, R. J., et al.: J. Pediatr. *63*:991, 1963.)

Treatment. Conductive deafness is a major concern if both external auditory canals are incompletely developed, in which case a hearing aid should be used from infancy. Plastic surgery is indicated for dermoids and ear tags; occasionally, an external auditory canal can be created.

Congenital Ectodermal Dysplasia of the Face

This is a unique combination of an extraordinary facial conformation with skin and hair abnormalities confined to the face.

Incidence. Setleis and coworkers have encountered five such infants and children. They were unable to find any others reported.

Etiology. The five children were members of three families of Puerto Ricans. The authors concluded that the disorder was transmitted as an autosomal recessive. No gross chromosomal aberrations were found in these children.

Diagnosis. The facies appears aged and leonine, the eyebrows sweep sharply upward and laterally,

the nose is prominent with a rubbery, fleshy tip, and the mouth is large and arched downward. All these children had skin defects over the region of the temples, and one had a similar linear scarlike lesion on his lower lip and chin. The eyelashes were missing from either both lids or only the lower lids, with multiple rows of lashes on the upper lids.

Treatment. None is indicated.

De Lange Syndrome (Typus Degenerativus Amstelodamensis)

In 1933, de Lange described a group of infants whose resemblances were so marked that she thought they constituted a discrete entity.

Diagnosis. The infants and children are remarkable chiefly for their facial appearance and their unusual extremities. The facies is striking because of an unruly mop of coarse hair, a low irregular hairline

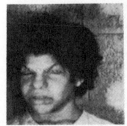
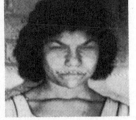

Figure 97–4. *A,* This newborn with congenital ectodermal dysplasia of the face shows two rows of eyelids on the upper lid, fleshy tip of nose and chin, symmetrical, round temporal skin defects, and a linear defect involving the lower lip and chin. *B,* At a later age, a heavy mop of scalp hair has developed, and the eyebrows have grown out in the characteristic upward and outward sweep. (Setleis, H., et al.: Pediatrics *32:*540, 1963.)

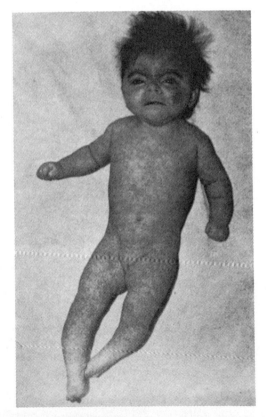

Figure 97–5. Notable are the coarse mop of hair growing low on the forehead, the eyebrows that cross the bridge of the nose to meet the midline, the short upward-tilted nose, and the "carp mouth." The extremities are short and taper strikingly. (Ptacek, L. J., et al.: J. Pediatr. *63:*1000, 1963.)

resulting in a narrow forehead, thick eyebrows that meet in the midline, long eyelashes, flat nasal bridge and short upturned nose with forward-tilting nostrils, a long upper lip, a crescentic mouth that curves downward, and a small mandible (Fig. 97–5). The extremities are short and tapering, the digits particularly so, with incurved fifth finger.

In addition, these children are much smaller than average, both in height and weight, and their heads are small and brachycephalic. The ears are often low-set, and the neck is short and webbed. Simian creases are not uncommonly present. In the male the genitals are small, the testes hypoplastic. In their 1963 report, Ptacek and colleagues commented on the fact that the nipples and umbilicus are tiny in these children. Much lanugo hair grows over the shoulders, back, and extremities of some of these infants. All are mentally retarded.

Pathology and Pathologic Physiology. Ptacek's autopsied 17-month-old female infant showed extremely small, immature organs, a bicornuate uterus, virtual absence of germ cells in the ovaries, and lack of myelinization of the brain. The thymus was tiny (0.8 gm). Two of Schlesinger's babies showed at postmortem examination microcephalic brains with grossly normal pituitary glands that, however, contained no basophilic cells. The thyroids revealed poor colloid formation in glands lined with low cuboidal epithelium. In one of his cases, no lipoid could be demonstrated in the zona fasciculata of the adrenals.

In vivo studies of endocrine function have shown low protein-bound iodine and poor radioactive iodine uptake in some cases, but not all, persistently low blood sugar level after insulin sensitivity test, and poor response of 17-hydroxysteroids after ACTH administration.

In sum, microcephaly, cortical atrophy, and evidences of multiple endocrine deficiency, especially of trophic hormones of anterior pituitary origin, seem to be the main pathologic findings.

Etiology. Familial occurrence is the exception and the risk of recurrence in a sib is probably considerably less than 5 per cent. Partial trisomy of chromosome 3q presents a similar picture.

Virtually all the newborns are short and small at birth relative to their gestational age, possibly indicating placental insufficiency.

Prognosis. Many feed poorly, gain slowly, and die during infancy. Most of the survivors are institutionalized later because of severe mental defect.

Treatment. There is no effective therapy.

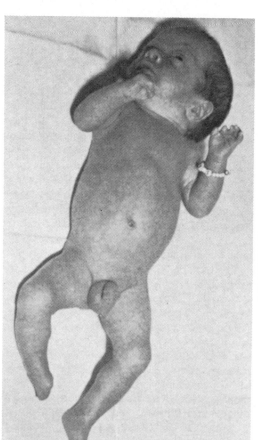
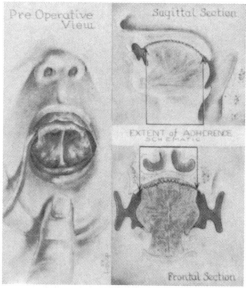

Figure 97–6. *A,* Photograph showing an infant who is well proportioned except for an extensive amputation of the right foot and more distal amputations of the toes of the left foot and the fingers of both hands. *B,* Diagrammatic sketch of the adhesion of almost the entire length of the dorsum of the tongue to the palate. (Wilson, R. A., et al.: Pediatrics *31:*1051, 1963.)

Ankyloglossia Superior

This is an unusual association of an oral lesion consisting of an extensive adhesion of the tongue to the palate with deformities of the extremities.

Incidence. The disorder is rare.

Etiology. Buccal mucosal smears and chromosomal analyses have thus far revealed no aberrations. There is no increased familial incidence. No maternal drug ingestion has been implicated. The pathogenesis is unknown.

Diagnosis. The tongue is firmly adherent to the palate, rendering sucking and swallowing impossible. The tongue may be hypoplastic, the palate highly arched and, at times, cleft. The most common malformations of the extremities are distal amputations of the digits or of the limbs a bit more proximally.

Treatment. Wilson and coworkers were able to free the tongue from the palate by blunt dissection. Little more can be done.

Seckel's Bird-Headed Dwarfism

Seckel's name has become the eponym for a remarkable subgroup of microcephalic dwarfs. These infants are born small, with small heads in which sutures synostose prematurely. These findings plus large eyes, beaked noses, micrognathia and low-set, malformed ears give these children an extraordinary and characteristic appearance. They are likely to have simian creases and clinodactyly. Associated congenital malformations often coexist.

The affected infants are usually undersized for gestational age, with birth weights at term of under 2 kg. They grow very slowly and seldom attain an adult height of more than $3\frac{1}{2}$ feet; mental development is equally slow. Their cerebrums are small, with a simple convolutional pattern resembling that of the chimpanzee.

The defect appears to be transmitted as an autosomal recessive.

Genetic Counseling

Genetic counseling deals with situations in which someone is concerned with the possibility that a disorder known or suspected to be genetic will occur in the family. In the present context, the persons receiving counsel are usually the parents of a newborn child with a malformation, syndrome, or disease who are concerned about the possibility of recurrence in a future child. The aim is to help the parents and family comprehend the medical facts, the way heredity contributes to the disorder, the risk of recurrence, and the options for dealing with the risk of recurrence as well as to assist them in both choosing the course of action that seems appropriate to them and acting accordingly.

However, the genetic evaluation of the family begins well before the genetic counseling process. When prenatal diagnosis is involved, genetic evaluation may begin in early pregnancy. In the newborn nursery, the genetic work-up is directed primarily toward diagnosis.

Genetic Evaluation of the Infant

The approach to genetic evaluation can be formulated as a series of questions:

1. Does the baby have a disease of clearly nongenetic origin, such as infection or birth trauma? Microcephaly, cataracts, retinopathy, heart defects, and other abnormalities should raise the question of prenatal infection with rubella, toxoplasma, cytomegalovirus, herpesvirus, or other teratogenic organisms. A

TORCH screening should be done in such cases—in 6 months it may be too late to verify the diagnosis. Does the mother have a disease with teratogenic implications, such as diabetes mellitus or hyperphenylalaninemia? Did the mother take any drugs suspected of being teratogenic? It is useful to inquire about nonmedical drugs such as LSD and marijuana at this point. With the exception of alcohol, there is no evidence that these are teratogenic, but parents who have taken them may fear that this was the cause of the baby's disorder and may need reassurance. The teratogenicity of maternal alcoholism is now well established, and this should be inquired about in cases of microcephaly, low birth weight, seizures, or malformations, particularly if the characteristic facies is present. Heavy smoking is also harmful to the fetus.

2. Does the baby have a disease of clearly genetic etiology, such as hemophilia, an inborn error of metabolism, or a chondrodystrophy (see Table 97–1 for examples)? The family history may be useful here, but the clinical and laboratory features will obviously provide the most important diagnostic information. Biochemical screening of serum and urine may detect unusual metabolites that will reveal the diagnosis in an otherwise puzzling comatose, seizing, vomiting, or acutely ill infant. Genetic heterogeneity should be kept in mind, that is, that conditions with similar clinical features may be genetically distinct. For instance, the Hurler form of mucopolysaccharidosis shows autosomal recessive inheritance, whereas the Hunter form is X-linked, and achondroplasia has an autosomal dominant mode of inheritance, while achon-

Table 97–1. Selected List of Mendelian Disorders Presenting in the Newborn Period*

Acrocephalopolysyndactyly (Noack). AD
Acrocephalosyndactyly (Apert). AD
Adrenogenital syndrome. AR
Albinism (several types). AR
Albinism, ocular. XR; occasionally AR
Albinism, partial, with deafness. XR
Albinism with platelet defect (Hermansky-Pudlak). AR
Aniridia. AD
Anonychia with poly-, syn- or adactyly. AD
Aortic stenosis, supravalvular. AD (in a few families)
Arachnodactyly (Marfan). AD
Asphyxiating thoracic dystrophy (Jeune). AR
Atrial septal defect. AD (in a few families)
Cataract. AD, AR, XR
Cataract, acidosis, hypotonia, etc. (Lowe). XR
Cataract with microcornea. XR
Cerebrohepatorenal syndrome (Zellweger). AR
Chondrodystrophia calcificans congenita, Conradi type. AD
Chondrodystrophia calcificans congenita, rhizomelic type. AR
(severe) or AD (mild)
Cleft lip/palate with lip pits. AD
Cleft lip with lobster claw defect, etc. (EEC syndrome). AD
Cleft lip with popliteal web. AD
Cleft palate with face and digit anomalies—OFD I. XD
Cleft palate with face and digit anomalies—OFD II. AR
Cleft palate; deafness, characteristic facies, bone dysplasias (otopalatodigital). AR
Cleidocraniodysostosis. AD
Craniocarpal-tarsal dystrophy (whistling face). AD
Craniofacial dysostosis (Crouzon). AD
Cretinism, goitrous. AR (some cases)
Cutis laxa. AR; less severe form. AD
Cutis hyperelastica (Ehlers-Danlos). AD, AR, and XR forms
Deafness, congenital, severe. AD, AR, XR
Deafness with ECG conduction defects, freckles, etc. (Leopard). AD
Deafness with preauricular pits or branchial sinus ± renal malformations. AD
Diabetes insipidus, ADH deficient. AD
Diabetes insipidus, nephrogenic. XR
Dislocations, multiple; flat facies, etc. (Larsen). AR
Dwarfism, achondrogenesis. AR
Dwarfism, achondroplasia. AD
Dwarfism, bird-headed (Seckel). AR
Dwarfism, diastrophic. AR
Dwarfism, mesomelic dyschondrosteosis (Leri). AD
Dwarfism, metatropic. AR
Dwarfism, pyknodysostosis. AR
Dwarfism, with cataracts, marble epiphyses, etc. (Cockayne). AR
Dwarfism, with fine, sparse hair (cartilage-hair hypoplasia). AR
Dwarfism, with polydactyly, tooth and nail defects (Ellis–van Creveld). AR
Dwarfism, with spherophakia (Weil-Marchesani). AR
Dwarfism, with spondyloepiphyseal dysplasia congenita. AD
Dwarfism, with telangiectasias, chromosome breaks (Bloom). AR
Dysautonomia (Riley-Day). AR
Ectodermal dysplasia, anhidrotic. XR
Ectodermal dysplasia, hidrotic (Clouston). AD
Epidermolysis bullosa; simplex and dystrophic. AD
Epidermolysis bullosa lethalis. AR

Eyelids, displaced inner canthi, deafness, white forelock (Waardenburg). AD
Facial diplegia ± various anomalies (Möbius). Minority are AD or AR
Focal dermal hypoplasia (Goltz). XR
Hemangiomatosis of von Hippel-Lindau. AD
Hydrocephalus with aqueductal stenosis. XR (some)
Hypospadias, dysphagia (G) syndrome. XD
Hypospadias-hypertelorism (BBB) syndrome. AD
Ichthyosiform erythroderma. AR
Ichthyosis sauroderma. AR
Ichthyosis vulgaris. XR
Incontinentia pigmenti. XR
Iridocorneal mesodermal dysgenesis, hypodontia (Rieger). AD
Iris hypoplasia with glaucoma. XR
Kinky-hair syndrome (Menkes). XR
Laurence-Moon-Biedl syndrome (postaxial polydactyly at birth). AR
Leprechaunism. (AR)
Lymphedema (Milroy). AD (some)
Mandibulofacial dysostosis (Treacher-Collins). AD
Megalocornea, ± cataracts. XR, some AR or AD
Microphthalmia/anophthalmia. Usually sporadic, occasionally AD, AR, XR
Microphthalmia with digital anomalies. XR (some)
Muscular atrophy, progressive, spinal (Werdnig-Hoffman). AR
Myopathy, nemaline. AD (?)
Myopia, retinal detachment, joint degeneration (Stickler). AD
Myotonic dystrophy (Steinert). AD
Nail-patella syndrome. AD
Nephrosis, congenital. AR (one type)
Neurofibromatosis. AD
Noonan syndrome. AD
Oculodentodigital dysplasia. AD
Optic atrophy, congenital (Behr). AR
Osteogenesis imperfecta lethalis. AR (few)
Osteogenesis imperfecta tarda. AD, occasionally AR
Osteomalacia from hypophosphatasemia. AR
Osteopetrosis, mild form. AD
Osteopetrosis, severe form. AR
Pachyonychia congenita. AD
Polycystic kidney disease, infantile. AR
Polycystic kidneys, microcephaly, polydactyly, cleft palate, etc. (Meckel). AR
Polydactyly, postaxial. AD (some)—also see various syndromes
Pseudoglioma retina (Norrie). XR
Ptosis, congenital. AD (reduced penetrance)
Ptosis, external ophthalmoplegia, myopia. XR
Radial absence with thrombocytopenia. AR
Radial defect with cardiac malformation (Holt-Oram). AD
Radial defect with other malformations, pancytopenia (Fanconi). AR
Radioulnar synostosis. AD
Retinal aplasia. AD or AR
Smith-Lemli-Opitz syndrome. AR
Spastic diplegia, ichthyosis, mental retardation (Sjögren-Larsson). AR
Syndactyly. AD (often)—see also various syndromes
Tibial absence, polydactyly. AD
Tuberous sclerosis. AD
Xanthomatosis, calcified adrenals, hepatosplenomegaly (Wolman). AR

* A = autosomal; D = dominant; R = recessive; X = X-linked (inborn errors of metabolism are excluded).

drogenesis is autosomal recessive. If the disease does have a mendelian basis, a recurrence risk can be calculated according to the mode of inheritance of the disorder and the family history in the present case.

3. If the baby's disorder does not fall into either of the aforementioned categories, does the baby have features that suggest a syndrome? If so, the subsequent investigation and management will depend on the nature of the syndrome. Some syndromes are well known to pediatricians; others are so rare as to be "once-in-a-lifetime" events for the neonatologist, and one must resort to appropriate compendia, atlases, and catalogues or to consultation with a clinical geneticist experienced in syndromology, if available. It should be recognized, however, that many children with combinations of dysmorphic features so unusual, and a facies so striking, that one feels sure they have a syndrome, nevertheless defy classification by even the most experienced syndromologists. Furthermore, many dysmorphic features are age-dependent, and an infant who, as he grows older, will develop the facies associated in the physician's mind with a particular syndrome may have a quite different appearance at birth. Conversely, in some children, collections of minor anomalies that may lead one to suspect a syndrome may simply represent the "family facies," or be normal variants, and may even disappear in childhood.

4. When a syndrome cannot be identified, one must consider what further investigations are necessary. Is examination of the chromosomes indicated? The indications for karyotyping have continued to expand as improved methods of staining have allowed detection of progressively more subtle deletions, duplications, and rearrangements of chromosomal material. Except in cases in which a specific, nonchromosomal syndrome has been identified, karyotyping should be considered in the baby who has multiple malformations, ambiguous genitalia, or hypospadias of moderate or severe degree or who exhibits unexplained small size or failure to thrive, especially when these are accompanied by dysmorphogenic features, including dermatoglyphic abnormalities.

5. In any case, the family history should be screened for clues to the possible genetic basis for the baby's problem. Taking a detailed family history is usually neither feasible nor justified at the time of admission. On the other hand, following the time-honored practice of asking whether there are any relatives with "diseases of hereditary tendency," such as allergy, cancer, epilepsy, heart disease, insanity, or tuberculosis, is not likely to be rewarding.

The most useful question to ask when taking the family history is whether problems similar to the present one have occurred in other members of the family. The answer will usually be negative, even when the disease is clearly genetic (since those dominantly inherited diseases that present in the newborn nursery are usually the result of new mutation, and recessive ones have only a one in four probability of recurrence), but when it is positive, it can be very

helpful. For example, a little girl was admitted in coma, following a measles infection. The fact that she had been acidotic was noted on the previous discharge summary, but its significance was not realized until review of the family history uncovered the fact that a sib had died in acidotic coma. The parents had been told (in another country) that this was caused by renal tubular acidosis, which was stated (incorrectly) to be nongenetic. Investigation of this clue led to the correct diagnosis, methylmalonic aciduria.

When surgery is contemplated, it is also wise to inquire about relatives with bleeding tendencies or unusual reactions to anesthetics.

The patient's sibs should be listed by age and sex, and their state of health noted. Data about abortions and stillbirths should also be included in the report. The main reason for this is that parents sometimes do not recognize what constitutes a "similar problem," as the preceding example demonstrates. The causes of any deaths in sibs should be established. For example, the mother of a child admitted for "cerebral palsy" told me that a previous child had died of "pneumonia," but she did not mention that the underlying cause was Tay-Sachs disease, which the second child also had.

If ancestors or collateral relatives are found to have diseases causing problems similar to that of the patient, a pedigree should be constructed so that the mode of inheritance can be evaluated.

Finally, one should ask about the possibility of parental consanguinity, since this can be a clue that the baby's problem may be caused by a recessively inherited disease and lead one to consider recessively inherited diseases that fit the clinical picture. If the baby's disease is unusual, the possibility of a hitherto unrecognized recessive disorder, with a one in four recurrence risk for sibs, should be kept in mind, particularly when there is parental consanguinity, even if no specific disease can be identified.

Counseling the Family

It is difficult for anyone who has not had the experience to imagine the feeling of the parents of a baby who is born defective. They are shocked, bewildered, scared, and often angry. Counseling at this point is directed largely to explaining the nature of the baby's disorder and the short-term prognosis and to providing as much emotional support as possible. This can, and probably should, be done by the family physician or pediatrician, who knows the parents, although it is sometimes left to the genetic counselor, particularly in cases of chromosomal problems and inborn errors of metabolism, in which the geneticist is involved in making the diagnosis. During this initial stage, the cause of the disorder is not the most important worry of the parents, except that they will often feel that the child's defect is a sign that they themselves are defective in some way and may benefit by airing these feelings. This is usually not the time to go deeply into the question of recurrence risks for future children, for in most cases the parents will not be listening. They should be made aware, however, that such information will be available later.

When the initial crisis is over and the parents become aware of the long-term significance of their baby's defect, they may begin to wonder more about the cause of the child's disease and, in particular, whether it might happen again. At this time, the specifically *genetic* counseling should be given. Again, this may be provided by the physician who cares for the patient, but referral to a medical geneticist may be helpful if the genetic aspects are at all complex— which they are, more often than not. If it is delayed too long, the parents may have either already started another pregnancy, unaware of the high risk or burden, or taken irreversible measures to prevent subsequent pregnancies, unaware that the risk and burden are low. To inform the parents that there is a risk of recurrence is particularly important if prenatal diagnosis is possible. Even if prenatal diagnosis is not possible, parents still must be made aware of what the risks are so that they will neither be shocked by an unforeseen recurrence nor be deterred from having children when the risk is negligible, but be able to make an informed decision. It should not be assumed that they will actually do so; some parents are not helped by knowledge of the risk figures in choosing whether or not to have another baby and, in fact, enter a prolonged state of indecision in which they "let things take their course." Nevertheless, they should be given the information, since even these parents are usually able to recall the precentage risk quite accurately, and one cannot distinguish, in advance, those who will use the information in making their decision from those who will not. The genetic counselor should write a letter to the family for future reference and to the referring doctor for reasons of courtesy and, in these litigious days, to document the fact that the parents have been informed, particularly when prenatal diagnosis is appropriate.

DETERMINING THE RECURRENCE RISK

In order to determine the recurrence risk, it is useful to assign the disorder in question to one of four etiologic categories: those due to an environmental agent, to a chromosomal aberration, to a multifactorial interaction, or to a mutant gene. To do this, it is necessary, of course, to be certain that the diagnosis is correct, keeping in mind the possibility of genetic heterogeneity.

Defects due to environmental agents will recur in sibs only if the environmental agent recurs. Maternal alcoholism, diphenylhydantoin (phenytoin), and warfarin are the main teratogens with which recurrence may be a problem. Congenital cytomegalovirus has been reported in sibs, but the probability of recurrence is not known and is therefore probably small (see Chapter 1).

Defects Due to Chromosomal Aberrations

The recurrence risks here depend upon the nature of the aberration. For simple trisomies, one can explain to the parents that the baby's extra chromosome arose as the result of a mistake in the pairing and separation of the chromosomes during formation of the sperm or egg, that it was an "accident" and is not likely to happen again, the empiric risk being about 1 or 2 per cent for subsequent babies. This, however, is a high enough risk to justify the monitoring of subsequent pregnancies by amniocentesis.

When a translocation is involved, the risk cannot be estimated precisely, since it probably varies according to where the translocation segments are and how they affect pairing and separation of the chromosomes. One can say only that if the translocation is present in one of the parents, the risk of a subsequent baby having a possibly harmful chromosomal aberration is higher than it is for a simple trisomy but probably not as high as the theoretical expectation on the basis of random segregation; the important thing is to emphasize that the parents *can* have normal children but that amniocentesis is available if they want to be certain that there will be no recurrence. The only exception is translocation of one chromosome to its homologue, in which case the outcome is certain to be an unbalanced complement for every offspring.

Defects of Multifactorial Causation

In these conditions, which include most of the common malformations (e.g., neural tube defects, cleft lip, cleft palate, many congenital heart malformations, pes equinovarus, and congenital hip dislocation), the recurrence risks have been determined empirically and can be provided by the counselor for the particular defect and family history. For normal parents with only one affected child, the risk is usually approximately 2 to 5 per cent. For more complicated situations, one should consult the literature or a genetic counselor. It is important to inform parents of a child with a neural tube defect (anencephaly, spina bifida cystica, or multiple vertebral anomalies) of the recurrence risk, since subsequent pregnancies can be monitored by ultrasonography and alpha-fetoprotein measurements.

Here the recurrence risk depends on the mode of inheritance of the disorder and the family history. There are three major patterns of mendelian inheritance and a fourth fairly rare one.

Autosomal Dominant Inheritance. Autosomal simply means not sex-linked. Dominant mutant genes are those that manifest their presence even when the other gene of the pair is normal; that is, every carrier of a disease-causing mutant gene has the disease. Such diseases are rare, and an affected person therefore almost always carries one mutant and one normal member of that pair; each offspring will receive either one or the other, and thus will have a 50:50 chance of being affected with the disease. Similarly, the affected person must have received the gene from somewhere, so that one parent should also be affected.

A certain amount of confusion can be caused by the fact that some individuals with dominantly inherited conditions represent fresh mutations, so that they do not have an affected parent. The family history is negative, thus the mutant individual is a "sporadic" case. The sibs of such a sporadic case will have a very low risk, but the offspring will have the usual 50:50 chance of being affected.

The more severe the effects of the mutant gene are, the greater will be the proportion of cases that are sporadic. To take an extreme example, a mutant gene that causes early death or sterility will always result in a sporadic case, since there will be no opportunity to transmit the gene. An example is the Apert type of acrocephalosyndactyly, in which few affected subjects have had offspring, so that almost all cases are sporadic. At the other extreme is the hydrotic type of ectodermal dysplasia, in which virtually all affected subjects have an affected parent. About 80 per cent of cases of achondroplasia are sporadic, indicating an intermediate degree of severity.

Another complication is the phenomenon of reduced penetrance. In certain conditions showing dominant inheritance, some carriers of the mutant gene do not show any overt manifestations of the disease. Various explanations can be advanced: Examination has failed to detect subtle signs that are actually present, a developmental threshold has not been reached, or (in diseases of variable age of onset) the signs of the disease have not yet appeared—and in some cases no explanation is known. The important thing is to recognize which diseases may do this (they include Marfan syndrome, neurofibromatosis, retinoblastoma, and Treacher Collins syndrome), since in a "sporadic" case a parent may actually carry the gene but not manifest it, and the risk for sibs will not be as low as it would for a new mutation. Thus the situation is complicated, and consultation with a genetic counselor may be useful.

Autosomal Recessive Inheritance. In this condition, the mutant gene does not produce disease when the other member of the pair (allele) is normal, but only when the other member is also mutant. The affected child must therefore inherit a mutant gene from each of the parents, who are themselves normal because they each carry a normal gene of that pair as well as the mutant allele. The child has one chance in two of getting the mutant gene from each parent, and therefore $\frac{1}{2} \times \frac{1}{2} = \frac{1}{4}$ chance of getting the mutant gene from both parents and thus of being affected. Similarly, any subsequent child of these parents will also have one chance in four of being affected.

If parents are related, it is more likely that they will both carry the same mutant gene. This is why the frequency of cousin marriages is increased in the parents of children with rare, recessively inherited diseases.

These diseases are likely to result from enzyme deficiencies, and an increasing number are eligible for prenatal diagnosis.

X-Linked Recessive Inheritance. In females, recessive genes on the X chromosome behave as they do on the autosomes: There are two X chromosomes, and the mutant gene, being rare, will usually have a normal allele to mask its effect. (An exception resulting from X chromosome inactivation will be mentioned shortly.) In the male, however, there is only one X chromosome, so a "recessive" gene will be expressed. Thus, a female carrier of one gene for, say, hemophilia A will not be a "bleeder." Each of her sons will receive either the X chromosome carrying the mutant gene or the one carrying the normal allele, and will thus have an equal chance of being affected or unaffected. Offspring of affected males will receive either the mutant-bearing X and be carrier females or the Y and be unaffected sons.

The situation is complicated a little by the phenomenon of lyonization, that is, the condition in which in each cell of a female, one X chromosome is inactivated, so a female carrying a gene for, say, X-linked muscular dystrophy (Duchenne) is a mosaic (mixture) composed of some cells in which the X carrying the mutant is active and other cells in which the X carrying the normal allele is active. This is presumably why carrier females often show dystrophic patches in their muscles. Since inactivation occurs early in development and is random with respect to which chromosome gets inactivated, occasionally, in a great majority of the cells of a carrier female, the X carrying the normal allele may be inactivated. This may account for the occasional carrier female who manifests the disease. It also explains why tests for carrier females usually do not detect all carriers—in the great majority of the cells of some carrier females, the X carrying the mutant allele may be inactivated.

The most difficult situation to counsel for X-linked recessive diseases is the "sporadic" case. When there are no affected relatives, one must decide whether the affected son represents a fresh mutation, in which case the mother is not a carrier, and the risk for future sons is low. Alternatively, the mutation may have occurred farther back in the family but not have yet been transmitted to a male, in which case the mother will be a carrier, and the risk for future sons will be one in two. For some diseases, tests are available that will detect some carrier females, but usually not all, because of lyonization. Thus, for Duchenne muscular dystrophy, for example, an elevated creatine phosphokinase level is strong evidence that the mother is a carrier, but a normal level is not conclusive evidence that she is not.

The geneticist can estimate the probability that the mother of a sporadic case is a carrier on the basis of the available information. To begin with the simplest case, a first-born affected male with no maternal uncles, it can be calculated from the principles of population genetics that if the disease in question is lethal (as for Duchenne dystrophy), the probabilities are two out of three that the mother is a carrier and one out of three that she is not. The probability of not being a carrier increases with the number of unaffected sons born, with the number of unaffected brothers of the mother, although not so much, and with how far into the normal range the tests for carrier detection fall, so probability must be calculated for each case. The important thing for the physician to realize is that *even if there are no affected relatives, one should not assume that the mother is not a carrier.*

X-Linked Dominant Inheritance. This pattern of inheritance is relatively rare, but examples do exist, for instance, vitamin-D–resistant hypophosphatemic rickets. The distinguishing feature is that men carrying the dominant mutant gene on the X chromosome will transmit it to all their daughters, who will be affected, but to none of their sons.

REACHING A DECISION

Now that parents have some appreciation of the nature of their baby's disease and of the burden that it will impose upon the family as well as information concerning the risk of recurrence, it will be necessary for them to decide whether they want other children, and, if not, what to do about it. Some geneticists maintain that the genetic counselor's role is simply to provide the facts in a nondirective way and let the parents decide what to do with them. Others feel that the parents will appreciate help in reaching a decision from someone they regard as having had experience in helping others to manage similar problems. It is difficult for the counselor to be completely nondirective in this situation. Certainly, the counselor should never tell parents that they should or should not have children. Every case is unique and is influenced by

a great many factors besides the scientific facts. The counselor may be able to provide helpful support while the parents talk through their problems. He should also be ready to refer them to appropriate sources, whether it be a cleric, social worker, psychiatrist, gynecologist, or urologist, where indicated. Again, the pediatrician may be the best person to help the family at this stage, but the specialist in genetic counseling often seems to play the major role, perhaps by default. If so, he should take pains to inform the referring doctor of his findings and his evaluation of the family's response, especially in situations in which long-term follow up may seem desirable.

REFERENCES

Baraitser, M.: Genetics of Moebius syndrome. J. Med. Genet. *14*:415, 1977.

Berg, J. M., et al.: The de Lange syndrome. Oxford, Pergamon Press, 1970.

Doege, T. C., Thuline, H. C., et al.: Studies of a family with the oral-facial-digital syndrome. N. Engl. J. Med. *271*:1073, 1964.

Evans, P. R.: Leprechaunism. Arch. Dis. Child. *30*:479, 1955.

Evans, P. R.: Nuclear agenesis: Möbius syndrome: the congenital facial diplegia syndrome. Arch. Dis. Child. *30*:237, 1955.

Gorlin, R. J., Pindborg, J. J., and Cohen, M. M.: Oculoauriculovertebral dysplasia. In Syndromes of the Head and Neck. 2nd ed. New York, McGraw-Hill, 1976.

Henderson, J. L.: The congenital facial diplegia syndrome: clinical features, pathology and aetiology. A review of 61 cases. Brain *62*:381, 1939.

Jervis, G. A., and Stimson, C. W.: De Lange syndrome: the "Amsterdam type" of mental defect with congenital malformation. J. Pediatr. *63*:634, 1963.

McKusick, V. A., Mahloudji, M., et al.: Seckel's bird-headed dwarfism. N. Engl. J. Med. *277*:279, 1967.

Nisenson, A., Isaacson, A., and Grant, S.: Mask-like facies with associated congenital anomalies (Möbius syndrome): report of 3 cases. J. Pediatr. *46*:255, 1955.

Ptacek, L. J., Opitz, J. M., Smith, D. W., Gerritsen, T., and Waisman, H. A.: The Cornelia de Lange syndrome. J. Pediatr. *63*:1000, 1963.

Ruess, A. L., Pruzansky, S., Lis, E. F., and Patau, K.: The oral-facial-digital syndrome: a multiple congenital condition of females with associated chromosomal abnormalities. Pediatrics *20*:985, 1962.

Salmon, M. A., and Webb, J. N.: Dystrophic changes associated with leprechaunism in an infant. Arch. Dis. Child. *38*:530, 1963.

Schlesinger, B., Clayton, B., Bodian, M., and Jones, K. V.: Typus degenerativus amstelodamensis. Arch. Dis. Child. *38*:349, 1963.

Setleis, H., Kramer, B., Valcarcel, M., and Einhorn, A. H.: Congenital ectodermal dysplasia of the face. Pediatrics *32*:540, 1963.

Silver, H. K.: The de Lange syndrome. Am. J. Dis. Child. *108*:523, 1964.

Smith, D. W.: Recognizable Patterns of Human Malformation: Genetic, Embryologic, and Clinical Aspects. 3rd ed. Philadelphia, W. B. Saunders Co., 1982.

Summitt, R. L.: Leprechaunism. In Bergsma, D. (Ed.): Birth Defects Compendium. 2nd ed. New York, A. R. Liss, 1979.

Townes, P. L., Wood, B., and McDonald, J.: Further heterogeneity of the oral-facial-digital syndromes. Am. J. Dis. Child. *130*:548, 1976.

Wahrman, J., Berant, M., et al.: The oral-facial-digital syndrome: A male-lethal condition in a boy with 47/XXY chromosomes. Pediatrics *37*:812, 1966.

Wilson, R. A., Kliman, M. R., and Hardyment, A. F.: Ankyloglossia superior (palato-glossal adhesion in the newborn infant). Pediatrics *31*:105, 1963.

Bergsma, D. (Ed.): Birth Defects Atlas and Compendium. National Foundation March of Dimes. Baltimore, Williams & Wilkins Co., 1973.

Bonaitie-Pellié, C., and Smith, C.: Risk tables for genetic counselling in some common congenital malformations. J. Med. Genet. *11*:374, 1974.

Fraser, F. C.: Genetics as a health-care service. N. Engl. J. Med. *295*:486, 1976.

Holmes, L. B.: Current concepts in genetics. Congenital malformations. N. Engl. J. Med. *295*:204, 1976.

Holmes, L. B., Moser, H. W., Halldorsen, S., Mack, C., Pant, S. S., and Matzilevich, B.: Mental Retardation. An Atlas of Diseases with Associated Physical Abnormalities. New York, The Macmillan Co., 1972.

Lippman-Hand, A., and Fraser, F. C.: Genetic counseling: provision and reception of information. Am. J. Med. Genet. *3*:113, 1979.

Lynch, H. T.: International Directory of Genetic Services. The National Foundation March of Dimes, White Plains, New York, 6th ed. 1980.

McKusick, V.: Mendelian Inheritance in Man. 5th ed. Baltimore, The Johns Hopkins University Press, 1978.

Nora, J. J., and Fraser, F. C.: Medical Genetics: Principles and Practice. 2nd ed. Philadelphia, Lea and Febiger, 1981.

Smith, D. W.: Recognizable Patterns of Human Malformation. 3rd ed. Philadelphia, W. B. Saunders Co., 1982.

Stevenson, A. C., and Davison, B. C. C.: Genetic Counselling, London, Heinemann, 1970.

Yunis, J. J. (Ed.): New Chromosomal Syndromes. New York, Academic Press, 1977.

PART 16

DISORDERS OF THE SKIN

No attempt has been made in this section to describe all the skin conditions that may be met in the neonatal period. We have preferred to limit consideration to those disorders that represent congenital defects, to infections that are unique to or have special char- acteristics in the neonatal period, to skin tumors that are encountered at birth or within the first month, and to skin lesions that appear to result from toxic agents or hypersensitization in this age group.

98

Congenital and Hereditary Disorders of the Skin

By Nancy B. Esterly and
Lawrence M. Solomon

Numerous heritable disorders may be apparent in the newborn infant and may cause diverse aberrations of pigmentation, texture, elasticity, and structural integrity of the integument. Some of these entities are confined to the skin, but others produce anomalies of several organ systems. Although, fortunately, most of these disorders are relatively uncommon, we have included the more frequently encountered, particularly those that have a prominent cutaneous component.

The Ichthyoses

HARLEQUIN FETUS

This severe type of congenital ichthyosis should not be confused with harlequin color change. This rare disorder may represent the extreme form of lamellar ichthyosis (nonbullous congenital ichthyosiform erythroderma) and is inherited as an autosomal recessive trait. Although the molecular defect is not known, x-ray diffraction analysis performed on the horny layer of one harlequin fetus demonstrated an abnormal cross-B fibrous protein as the major keratinous component (Craig et al., 1970). Another such infant was found to have elevated levels of cholesterol and triglyceride in the upper epidermis as well as evidence of excess lipid deposits on electron microscopy of the skin (Buxman et al., 1979).

The earliest known description of harlequin fetus in English was written by a clergyman, the Reverend Oliver Hart of Charleston, South Carolina, in 1750, and is as accurate as any in the medical literature:

The skin was dry and hard and seemed to be cracked in many places, somewhat resembling the scales of a fish. The mouth was large and round and wide open. It had no external nose, but two holes where the nose would have been. The eyes appeared to be lumps of coagulated blood, turned out, about the bigness of a plum, ghastly to behold. It had no external ears, but holes where the ears should be. The hands and feet appeared swoln, were crumpt up, and felt quite hard. The back part of its head was much open. It made a strange kind of noise, very low, which I cannot describe. It lived about eight and forty hours and was alive when I saw it.

The appearance and consistency of the skin of these infants has inspired innumerable metaphors. It has been likened to baked apple, tree bark, a loosely built wall, elephant or rhinoceros skin, a coat of mail, and Moroccan leather. The skin is hard, brown, cracked, and rigid, flattening the nose, ears, and digits. Chemosis of the conjunctivae obscures the globes, the lips are gaping, and the nails and hair are hypoplastic or absent. The viscera are usually normal. No treatment can be offered except humidity, lubrication and attempts to provide a temperature-controlled environment and electrolyte balance in the blood, but these infants almost inevitably succumb to the disease because of inability to feed and ventilate adequately. Survival beyond 6 weeks is extremely unusual. Genetic counseling for the families of these infants is mandatory.

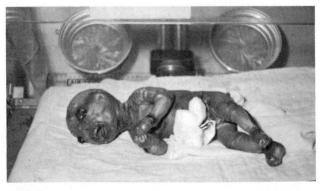

Figure 98–1. Harlequin fetus. (Photograph reproduced with the kind permission of Dr. Marvin Cornblath.)

Collodion babies also occur uncommonly, although not as rarely as the harlequin fetus. The infant is born tightly encased in a shiny membrane resembling parchment or oiled silk, which is perforated by scalp and lanugo hair. To some observers, the infant looks as if he has been varnished or lacquered. The tautness of the membrane holds the face immobile and distorts the features. Motion of the limbs is restricted. Within a day or two, the membrane begins to fissure and peel, especially about the thorax and joints. In some instances, the skin beneath the membrane has a beefy-red color, and it may continue to scale or form a new membrane.

The collodion baby probably represents a phenotype for several genotypes. Most of these infants develop lamellar ichthyosis, but membranes have also been observed in patients with X-linked ichthyosis and, possibly, epidermolytic hyperkeratosis. Occasional infants appear to have perfectly normal skin subsequent to shedding of the membrane. No abnormality of the internal organs has been associated, and the mortality rate for these infants is low in contrast to that of the harlequin fetus (Esterly, 1968). A prolonged period of observation may be required to determine the outcome and prognosis. As soon as a secure diagnosis has been made, genetic counseling should be provided.

Treatment consists of humidity and lubrication with a bland ointment until the membrane has been desquamated. Cutaneous infections from gram-positive organisms and *Candida albicans* are a common problem; however, overzealous administration of antibiotics may lead to gram-negative infections and subsequent septicemia.

MAJOR TYPES OF ICHTHYOSIS

Six distinct types of ichthyosis have been delineated on the basis of their clinical and histologic features and their patterns of genetic transmission (Solomon and Esterly, 1973). Most of these disorders are apparent at birth. They can be outlined briefly as follows:

Ichthyosis Vulgaris. This is the most common form of ichthyosis and is inherited as an autosomal dominant trait. Onset is usually after the first 3 months of life. Scaling spares the flexural areas but affects the palms and soles.

X-linked Ichthyosis. This variant affects males only and may be present at birth. The scales are large and dark and prominent on the neck and limbs, with sparing of the palms and soles and variable sparing of the flexural areas. A deep corneal dystrophy may be detected by slit-lamp examination but usually is not apparent until late childhood or adolescence. Patients with this disorder have been shown to lack steroid sulfatase (Elliott, 1979); absence of this enzyme's activity has been demonstrated in leukocytes, hair bulbs, stratum corneum, and cultured fibroblasts and keratinocytes.

Lamellar Ichthyosis (nonbullous congenital ichthyosiform erythroderma). Inherited as an autosomal recessive trait, this disorder is present at birth and is characterized by an erythroderma and large yellowish-brown scales over the entire body, with involvement of all of the flexures as well as the palms and soles. Ectropion may be present and is progressive in severely affected individuals.

Epidermolytic Hyperkeratosis (bullous congenital ichthyosiform erythroderma). Also affected at birth, these patients have a generalized erythroderma and small, thick, yellow, shotty scales. Scaling is accentuated in the flexural areas, and the palms and soles may be involved. The eruption of bullae, most frequently on the lower legs, is characteristic of the disease in infancy and childhood. Transmission is by an autosomal dominant gene.

Ichthyosis Linearis Circumflexa. This is a rare dermatosis, present at birth and transmitted as an autosomal recessive disorder. It is characterized by

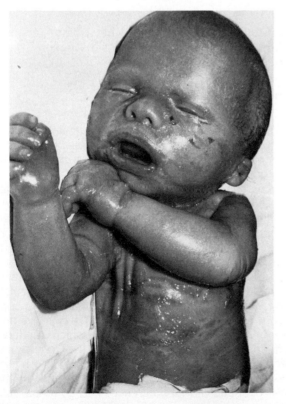

Figure 98–2. Collodion baby. Note the ectropion, eclabium, and areas of rupture in the membrane over the anterior thorax.

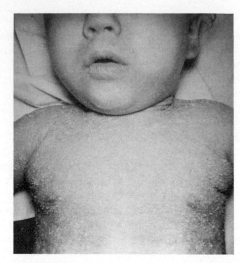

Figure 98–3. Infant with lamellar ichthyosis. Generalized scaling of the trunk with relative sparing of the face. The scales are finer and lighter in color than those in older children with this disease.

migratory, polycyclic lesions with a peripheral double-edged scale and hyperkeratosis of the flexural areas.

Erythrokeratodermia Variabilis. This type of ichthyosis is also very rare; it is inherited in an autosomal dominant fashion and can be detected in infancy. Affected individuals have transient migratory areas of discrete macular erythema as well as fixed hyperkeratotic plaques.

It is important to distinguish the various forms of ichthyosis so that the physician can offer a prognosis and appropriate genetic counseling to the family. Frequently, the clinical picture and pedigree data provide sufficient information on which to base a diagnosis; however, at times a period of observation beyond the first 4 weeks of life is required to assess the situation accurately. A skin biopsy may help solve a diagnostic dilemma, as all types of ichthyosis have a fairly characteristic histologic pattern (Solomon and Esterly, 1973).

Therapy is restricted to topical preparations. Hydration of the stratum corneum is important and can be accomplished by bathing with a water dispersible bath oil. Lubrication with a bland adherent emollient such as petrolatum, Aquaphor, or Eucerin should be provided immediately following the bath and whenever necessary throughout the day. Urea-containing emollients (10 to 20 per cent) are also effective preparations. Other available modalities such as vitamin A acid (0.1 per cent), lactic acid in petrolatum (5 per cent), and preparations containing propylene glycol are not required in early infancy and should be reserved for older patients. Irritating soaps and detergents should be avoided. Extremes in temperature and excessively dry indoor heating also impose undue hardship on these individuals.

Studies using orally administered aromatic derivatives of retinoic acid have shown promising results in the management of several types of ichthyosis (Fritsch, 1981). However, these drugs are still under experimental study, and we must await the results to ascertain whether the risks will in fact be less than the benefits before we recommend their use.

The prognosis is related to the severity of the condition and the type of ichthyosis.

SYNDROMES WITH ICHTHYOSIS AS A FEATURE

Several syndromes, identifiable in infants, have ichthyosis as a major feature (Solomon and Esterly, 1973). Brief descriptions of five of these follow:

Netherton's Syndrome. Ichthyosis (lamellar or linearis circumflexa), hair shaft defects, and atopic diathesis.

Sjögren-Larsson Syndrome. Lamellar ichthyosis, spastic diplegia, and mental retardation.

Rud's Syndrome. Ichthyosis, epilepsy, mental retardation, sexual infantilism.

Conradi's Syndrome. Patterned scaling, stippled epiphyses, cataract, bony anomalies, transient scaling.

KIO Syndrome. Atypical ichthyosiform erythroderma, vascularizing keratitis, sensorineural deafness, nail and hair abnormalities.

Albinism

Oculocutaneous albinism is a congenital defect of pigmentation that is clinically manifest by hypopigmentation of the skin, hair, and eyes, with associated photophobia and nystagmus. It is a disease that affects all races; estimates of gene frequency vary depending on the population under consideration. As with many genetic disorders, the incidence of affected individuals is increased in certain racial isolates in which there is a high percentage of consanguineous marriages.

Oculocutaneous albinism is inherited in an autosomal recessive fashion. The presence of genetic heterogeneity has been well documented for this condition. The characteristic pigmentary changes are due to a defect in tyrosinase formation, which interferes with melanin synthesis. Three types of oculocutaneous albinism—tyrosinase-negative, tyrosinase-positive, and yellow—can be distinguished on the basis of subtle clinical differences and by a hair bulb tyrosine test (Witkop et al., 1971). Oculocutaneous albinism should be distinguished from simple ocular albinism, which is transmitted in a sex-linked manner.

Affected infants, whatever their race, have a marked decrease in skin pigment and yellow or white hair. The irides are bluish gray or pink in reflected light. Photophobia and nystagmus of variable degree are present, depending on the type of albinism. Visual acuity is almost always impaired. Patients with tyrosine-negative oculocutaneous albinism have the most severe form of visual impairment. Associated abnormalities may include hemorrhagic diathesis (Hermansky-Pudlak syndrome), small stature, and defective mentation. Deafness can occur in association with oculocutaneous albinism as well as with a number of other pigmentary disorders (Konigsmark, 1972).

In patients with the tyrosinase-positive and yellow forms of albinism, some pigment may accumulate with increasing age. Concomitant with the development of pigment in the irides, visual acuity may improve significantly. There is no treatment for the albinism, but sunscreen preparations should be provided to protect against excessive exposure to sunlight. Such patients are predisposed to sun-induced carcinogenesis.

Partial Albinism (Piebaldism)

Although there are few reported families with this disorder, the disease is believed to be more common than the literature would indicate. Partial albinism is a heritable disorder transmitted by an autosomal dominant gene. Ultrastructural studies show absence of melanocytes in the depigmented areas of skin and normal melanocytes in the uninvolved skin (Comings and Odland, 1966). A genetic defect in melanoblast differentiation has been proposed to account for these findings.

Partial albinism is present at birth but may be relatively inconspicuous if the infant is very fair-skinned. The amelanotic areas predominate on the ventral skin, with relative sparing of the dorsal surface. A favored site of involvement is the central forehead, where a triangular or diamond-shaped defect extends to the scalp to produce a white forelock. Similar areas may be found on the eyebrows, chin, trunk, midarm, and midleg. This disorder is readily differentiated from albinism, in which the absence of pigment is uniform. Vitiligo may have a similar appearance, but it is not congenital and usually does not remain fixed. Waardenburg's syndrome may also cause confusion. Occasional families may have associated defects such as sensorineural deafness and mental retardation (Telfer et al., 1971). The defects remain constant throughout life and are not amenable to treatment, although adequate cosmetic results may be achieved

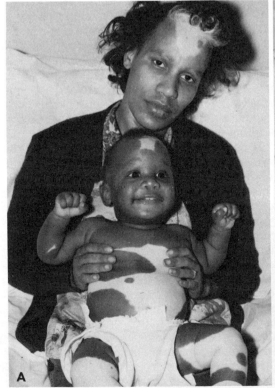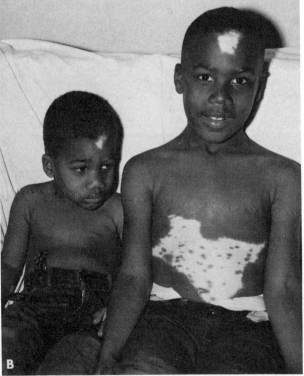

Figure 98–4. *A,* Mother and child with partial albinism. Both have patches on the forehead, although of different sizes and shapes. The areas of nonpigmentation on the infant's trunk and extremities are unusually extensive. *B,* Siblings with different degrees of partial albinism. (Jahn, H. M., and McIntire, M. S.: A.M.A. J. Dis. Child. *88:*481, 1954.)

with the use of hair dyes and cosmetics (e.g., Covermark).

Aplasia Cutis Congenita (Congenital Absence of Skin)

Congenital absence of skin is a rare developmental anomaly that occurs most often on the scalp but that also may involve the skin of the trunk and extremities. The defects are usually along the midline of the scalp in the parietal or occipital areas and may be solitary or multiple, measuring up to several centimeters in diameter. Multiple defects, particularly those on the trunk and extremities, may be strikingly symmetric in distribution (Levin et al., 1980). The lesion is sharply marginated, often oval or round, and can be ulcerated, bullous, cicatricial, or covered with a tough membrane. The depth of the base can vary from the level of the dermis to that of the arachnoid, with defects in the calvarium and dura.

Histologic examination of tissue from the defect demonstrates an absent epidermis and a diminished number of appendageal structures and dermal elastic fibers or, in deeper lesions, absence of all layers of the integument. No evidence of inflammation or pathogenic organisms is usually detectable.

Although most instances of aplasia cutis are sporadic, there are several well-documented pedigrees demonstrating autosomal dominant transmission of the defect (Fisher and Schneider, 1973). Association with other developmental abnormalities, such as cleft lip and palate, syndactyly, clubbing of hands and feet, congenital heart disease, vascular lesions, and malformations of the brain, also have been recorded in

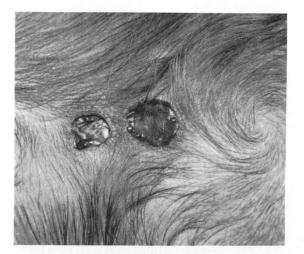

Figure 98–5. Two sharply punched-out ulcers on the scalp of a normal newborn male infant whose mother's labor and delivery were normal. The defects extended to the subcutaneous tissue and healed in 3 weeks with the formation of thin, white atrophic scars.

occasional patients (Fowler and Dumars, 1973; Ruiz-Maldonado and Tamayo, 1974). In addition, scalp defects are frequently found in infants with trisomy 13.

The cause of aplasia cutis congenita is unknown. Incomplete closure of the neural tube has been offered as an explanation for midline scalp lesions but does not serve to explain defects elsewhere on the body surface. The findings of a twin fetus papyraceus or a placental infarct or both have suggested vascular thrombosis as a cause in infants with lesions on the trunk and limbs (Levin et al., 1980). Healing of the lesions is usually uneventful, resulting in an atrophic or hypertrophic scar, which is always hairless. The repair process takes weeks to months, during which time little treatment is required. Secondary infections will respond to compresses and topical antibiotic ointment; if there is an associated bony defect, the patient must be observed for the possibility of a complicating meningitis. Those lesions that fail to heal or produce cosmetically unacceptable scars can be excised with primary closure (Kosnik and Sayers, 1975). Punch-graft hair transplant or scalp reduction for larger lesions may be attempted as an alternative procedure.

Incontinentia Pigmenti

Also known as the Bloch-Sulzberger syndrome, incontinentia pigmenti is now widely recognized as a multisystem disease affecting structures of both ectodermal and mesodermal origin. The disorder is restricted almost exclusively to females, although a few affected males have been reported. The abnormal gene is believed to be transmitted on the X chromosome, with a dominant effect in females and a lethal effect in males. Several well-documented pedigrees demonstrating mother-daughter transmission have been recorded; an increased incidence of spontaneous abortions has been noted in these kindreds (Gordon and Gordon, 1970).

The most striking feature of this disorder is the bizarre skin eruption that, in most patients, can be divided into three stages. The bullous phase, which generally lasts for the first 3 to 4 months, is characterized by widespread inflammatory vesicular lesions in a linear distribution on the scalp, trunk, and extremities. The infant is otherwise well, although a peripheral eosinophilia as high as 50 per cent may be associated. The vesicular phase is superseded by the verrucous phase, in which warty lesions appear in roughly the same distribution as the blisters but are most pronounced on the hands and feet. The third stage, most familiar to pediatricians, consists of macular gray or brown pigmentation in whorls, stripes, and feathered patterns that are independent of the sites of previous lesions. The pigmentary lesions are usually permanent. In an occasional infant, the typical pigmentary changes are present at birth, and the first two stages are never evident (Lerer et al., 1973).

It is important to recognize the particular anomalies that accompany the skin changes in about 80 per

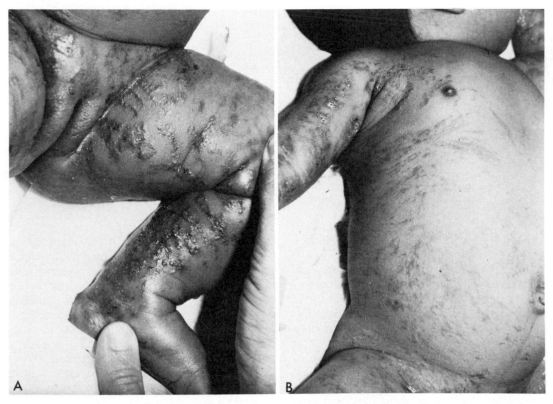

Figure 98–6. Incontinentia pigmenti. *A,* Inflammatory vesicular and crusted lesions on the legs. *B,* Whorled pigmentation developing on the trunk of a 1-month-old infant who still has inflammatory lesions on the limbs.

cent of affected individuals. Central nervous system aberrations include seizures, microcephaly, retardation, and spastic paralysis. Patchy alopecia, defective dentition, ocular abnormalities, and, less commonly, cardiac and bony defects have all been documented repeatedly in affected children (Carney, 1976).

Differential diagnosis sometimes poses a serious problem during the neonatal period. Although the linear blisters are often so characteristic that they permit instant recognition of the disorder, at times certain procedures must be performed to exclude other bullous abnormalities (Solomon and Esterly, 1973). Skin biopsy during the bullous phase, although not pathognomonic, will show intraepidermal vesicles filled with eosinophils. Alterations in the epidermal melanocytes and dermal deposits of melanin are apparent in the later phases of the disease (Guerrier and Wong, 1974).

Treatment of the skin lesions is not necessary. Occasionally, vesicular lesions become extremely inflamed or secondarily infected. In the latter instance, cool tap water compresses and antibiotic therapy may be required. If other anomalies are present, on-going care should be provided by the appropriate specialists.

Cutis Laxa

Cutis laxa is a rare, genetically determined disorder in which the skin hangs in pendulous folds, producing a lugubrious facies and a grotesque, prematurely aged appearance. Both autosomal dominant and autosomal recessive forms have been described (Beighton, 1972). Males and females are affected equally. An X-linked form has also been delineated (Byers, 1980). It should be noted that cutis laxa can be found in many disorders (e.g., combined immunodeficiency disease and the Prader-Willi and the Langer-Giedion syndromes).

The facies of a patient with cutis laxa is characteristic, with hooked nose, everted nostrils, a long upper lip, and sagging cheeks. The infant may have a strikingly hoarse cry due to redundant laryngeal tissue. Individuals with the autosomal dominant form of cutis laxa suffer few ill effects, apart from their

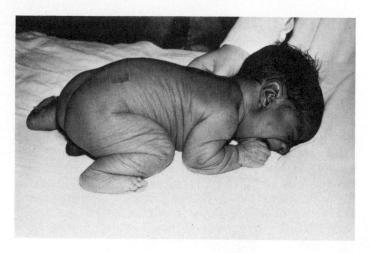

Figure 98–7. Newborn infant with dwarfism and cutis laxa.

altered appearance, and enjoy good health and a normal life span. Pulmonary and cardiovascular manifestations are absent or minimal. In contrast, patients with the recessive form of the disorder are often seriously compromised and may die in childhood of pulmonary or cardiovascular complications. Systemic manifestations include diverticula of the gastrointestinal and urogenital tracts, rectal prolapse, multiple hernias, pulmonary emphysema, and cardiac disease (Mehregan et al., 1978). A few infants have been reported who manifested additional defects, such as skeletal anomalies, dislocation of the hips, and intrauterine growth retardation.

Although the basic defect is unknown, all the manifestations are attributable to abnormalities of the elastic tissue. Elastic fibers are diminished in the papillary and upper dermis, whereas those in the lower dermis undergo fragmentation and granular degeneration (Mehregan et al., 1978). Similar changes occur in the elastic tissue of affected viscera. Plastic surgery can improve the physical appearance of these patients. The internal manifestations are not amenable to therapy. In the X-linked form of the disorder, defective cross-link formation in collagen is attributed to decreased lysyl oxidase activity (Byers et al., 1980).

Ehlers-Danlos Syndrome

In contrast to patients with cutis laxa, those with Ehlers-Danlos syndrome have skin that is hyperextensible rather than loose-fitting and that, when stretched, snaps back into place readily. Fragility of the skin is also characteristic, leading to easy bruising and bleeding; minor trauma may produce gaping wounds, which heal with cigarette-paper–like scars that are often detectable over the forehead, knees, elbows, and anterior lower legs. These patients tolerate surgical procedures poorly because of difficulty

in healing and frequent dehiscence of surgical wounds. Other cutaneous findings include redundant skin on the palms and soles, molluscoid pseudotumors over pressure points, and small, lipid-containing cysts that may calcify and that are identifiable radiologically as subcutaneous. Hypermobility of the joints with skeletal deformity and ocular manifestations such as epicanthal folds, blue sclerae, microcornea, retinal detachment, and subluxation of the lens are frequently present. Although diverticula and hernias can occur, they are by no means as common as in cutis laxa (McKusick, 1972).

Genetic heterogeneity has been well established for Ehlers-Danlos syndrome; eight forms have been delineated on the basis of differences in clinical findings (Hollister, 1978). It has been postulated that all forms of the Ehlers-Danlos syndrome are due to a defect in the biogenesis of collagen of the skin and

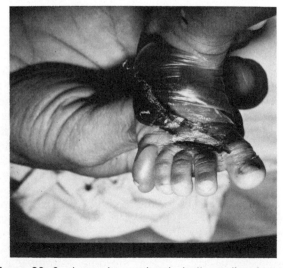

Figure 98–8. Large hemorrhagic bulla on the dorsum of the foot and small tense clear blister on the fifth toe of an infant with a scarring form of epidermolysis bullosa.

other affected organs. A biochemical defect, deficiency of lysyl hydroxylase, has been demonstrated in type VI (Pinnell et al., 1972). Type IV Ehlers-Danlos syndrome is characterized by a type III collagen deficiency, type V by lysyl oxidase deficiency, and type VII by procollagen peptidase deficiency (Hollister, 1978). These specific defects have been identified by culture of dermal fibroblasts from a simple skin biopsy.

Epidermolysis Bullosa

This group of diseases, all characterized by vesiculobullous lesions that arise in response to minimal trauma or shearing force to the skin, are most easily classified by the presence or absence of scarring (Bauer and Briggaman, 1979). Most authors recognize at least five distinct types of epidermolysis bullosa, separable on the basis of clinical and histologic features, although a few families have been described with variants of the well-known forms of this disorder. The five subgroups are as follows:

EPIDERMOLYSIS BULLOSA SIMPLEX

This disorder, inherited as an autosomal dominant trait, is present at birth or early in infancy. Bullae arise most frequently over pressure points such as the elbows and knees, as well as on the legs, feet, and hands. Mucous membrane involvement is minimal or absent. The extensive erosions that sometimes result from the trauma of birth may be mistaken for cutis aplasia. Nails may be lost but almost always regrow. The level of cleavage in the blister is in the basal layer of the epidermis, and, for this reason, the disease does not cause scarring. The prognosis is relatively good, and the propensity to blister may decrease with age.

WEBER-COCKAYNE DISEASE

The blisters in this disease are usually limited to the hands and feet, although they occasionally occur elsewhere on the body. This type of epidermolysis bullosa, which is inherited in an autosomal dominant fashion, usually does not occur during the neonatal period. Cytolysis of the suprabasilar cells and marked dyskeratosis are the characteristic biopsy findings; healing proceeds without the formation of scars.

EPIDERMOLYSIS BULLOSA LETALIS (HERLITZ TYPE)

Although the designation "letalis" implies an ominous prognosis, patients with this disorder exhibit varying degrees of severity as with other forms of epidermolysis bullosa, and not all patients die within the first year or two of life. The disorder is transmitted

as an autosomal recessive trait. Bullae and moist erosions occur on the scalp, in the perioral area, and over pressure points elsewhere on the body. Some of these erosions become the sites of vegetating granulomas. The hands and feet are relatively spared, and digital fusion, inevitable in the recessive dystrophic type of epidermolysis bullosa, does not occur. Nails are affected and may be lost permanently. Mucous membrane erosions are inconspicuous and rarely cause distress of any significance; however, defective dentition is the rule. These patients grow poorly, appear malnourished, and have a chronic recalcitrant anemia. The cleavage plane in the skin lesions occurs between the plasma membrane of the basal cell and the basement membrane. The hemidesmosomes responsible for attachment of the basal cells to the basement membrane are reduced in number and abnormally structured. Since the separation does not involve the dermis, uncomplicated blisters heal without scarring.

RECESSIVE DYSTROPHIC EPIDERMOLYSIS BULLOSA

This type of epidermolysis bullosa is inherited as an autosomal recessive trait and, as might be expected, consanguineous marriages are frequent in affected kindreds. These infants often have extensive denuded lesions at birth and during the neonatal period. Bullae may be hemorrhagic and occur on all surfaces, including the hands and feet; loss of nails is usual. Over subsequent years the mobility of the fingers and toes becomes severely restricted, as fusion of digits, bone resorption and the inevitable mitten-like deformity of the hands and feet ensue. Mucous membrane involvement may be severe, resulting in esophageal strictures and serious impairment of nutrition due to the restriction of oral intake. These bullae are subepidermal, and always eventuate in scarring. On electron microscopy, there are diminished or absent anchoring fibrils associated with marked degeneration of collagen in the papillary portion of the dermis. Also evident is excess abnormal collagenase in fibroblast cultures.

DOMINANT DYSTROPHIC EPIDERMOLYSIS BULLOSA

These two variants of epidermolysis bullosa (Cockayne-Touraine and Pasini variants) are less severe than the recessive dystrophic type. Of the two, the Pasini variant tends to be more severe. Although the bullae are subepidermal and heal with scarring, the disease may be relatively mild, involving mainly hands, feet, and skin over bony protuberances. Nails

may be indicated from early infancy (Hruby and Esterly, 1973).

may be lost. Milia are common and may appear in profusion in the soft, wrinkled scars; pigmentary changes are also usual. Mucous membrane lesions, if present, are mild, and general health may be unimpaired. The appearance of albopapuloid lesions on the trunk during adolescence is a unique feature of the Pasini variant.

Diagnosis. The diagnosis of infants with this group of diseases is not always easy. Bullous impetigo is probably the most commonly confused entity. A positive culture may indicate either secondary infection of epidermolysis bullosa or impetigo. Absence of organisms is suggestive of epidermolysis bullosa. The distribution of the lesions may be a diagnostic aid. Those of impetigo more often begin in the diaper region and spread peripherally; in epidermolysis bullosa, the earliest lesions occur on extremities and those points that make closest contact with the crib sheets, such as the heels, wrists, knees, and sacrum. The fluid within the bullae is more likely to be clear or hemorrhagic in epidermolysis bullosa, but turbid contents do not positively gainsay this diagnosis. A careful family history for blistering diseases should, of course, be taken. A biopsy of an induced blister for light and electron microscopy also may help confirm the diagnosis.

Treatment. There is no specific therapy for this group of disorders. Systemic corticosteroids have been ineffective except in the prevention of severe stricture formation in the esophagus from lesions of the recessive dystrophic type. Oral administration of vitamin E, which has been advocated by some physicians, has been found by us to be ineffective in most cases. The infant should be protected from trauma as much as possible. Cribs, highchairs, and infant seats should be well padded, and only soft toys offered for play. Clothing with metal closures should be avoided. If mucous membrane is involved, soft nipples, bulb syringes, and devices used for feeding infants with cleft palates should be employed. Bathing may have to be restricted to avoid excessive handling. Compresses with normal saline or 0.25 to 0.5 per cent silver nitrate for eroded areas may be helpful in some instances. Hot water should never be used, since warm temperatures are said to increase the tendency to blister. Petrolatum or nonsensitizing topical antibiotic ointments such as Polysporin should be applied to oozing or crusted areas to prevent adherence of the skin to clothing and sheets. Adhesive tape should never be applied, as large areas of epidermis may be torn off with its removal.

Every attempt should be made to ensure adequate nutrition, but growth may be impaired despite these efforts. Anemia should be anticipated in patients with severe disease, and high doses of supplemental iron

Lupus Erythematosus

Infants born to mothers with acute, subacute, and clinically latent systemic lupus erythematosus or other tissue disorders can manifest transient hematologic abnormalities, congenital complete heart block, and serologic evidence of lupus erythematosus during the first few months of life. Characteristic lesions of discoid lupus may be present with or without evidence of systemic disease (Draznin et al., 1979; Hardy et al., 1979). The lesions are usually localized to the scalp, face, and shoulders and are erythematous, scaly, sharply demarcated, depressed areas with the characteristic carpet-tack scale. A skin biopsy from one of these lesions can be diagnostic; hyperkeratosis, follicular plugging, epidermal atrophy with degeneration of the basal cell layer, and a periappendageal and perivascular lymphocytic infiltrate are present as typical histologic features. Direct immunofluorescent studies on a snap-frozen biopsy specimen should demonstrate the deposition of immunoglobulin, most often IgG, and complement at the dermal-epidermal junction. Appropriate tests for the collagen disorders should be performed on infant *and mother* (Vonderheid et al., 1976; Draznin et al., 1979; Franco et al., 1981).

During the spring and summer months, affected infants should be protected from undue exposure to sunlight by application of one of the many available sunscreen preparations. The activity of the skin lesions may be controlled by local treatment with a fluorinated corticosteroid cream. The skin lesions are thought to be self-limited; however, good prognostic studies are not available, so a predictable outcome cannot be assured.

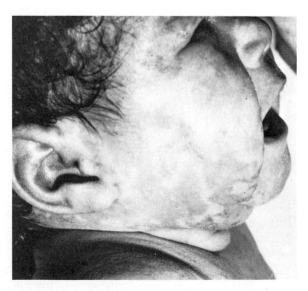

Figure 98–9. Newborn infant with cutaneous lesions of neonatal lupus erythematosus.

The term "ectodermal dysplasia" has been used traditionally to designate two particular disorders, hidrotic and anhidrotic ectodermal dysplasia. The term connotes abnormalities of the skin and its appendages, the sweat gland, the sebaceous gland, and the hair follicle, but it has been applied to disease entities by many authors in instances in which abnormalities of nails, hair, or teeth are a prominent feature of a particular syndrome. This practice has caused some confusion in the literature, and, for this reason, we believe it is most helpful to define or qualify the type of ectodermal defect, if possible, when describing a particular entity (Solomon and Keuer, 1980). Although a number of entities might thus be included under this heading, we will confine our discussion to three: hidrotic ectodermal dysplasia, anhidrotic ectodermal dysplasia, and the EEC syndrome.

HIDROTIC ECTODERMAL DYSPLASIA

Sweating response is normal in this form of ectodermal dysplasia. Hypoplasia, absence or dystrophy of the nails, sparse hair, and hyperkeratosis of the palms and soles are characteristic. The teeth are usually normal but may be small and subject to decay. The disorder is inherited as an autosomal dominant trait.

ANHIDROTIC ECTODERMAL DYSPLASIA

The anhidrotic form of this disorder is probably of greater interest to the neonatologist and pediatrician, as it may cause difficulties during the first year of life. The most serious disturbance is the absence of sweating, due to rudimentary or absent eccrine sweat glands, which results in marked heat intolerance and episodes of hyperpyrexia during infancy (Richards and Kaplan, 1969). If the possibility of this disorder is not considered, such infants may undergo numerous hospitalizations and tests until the true nature of the problem is appreciated.

Patients with anhidrotic ectodermal dysplasia have several identifiable features that, although sometimes difficult to appreciate in a small infant, should permit the physician to make the diagnosis. The skin is pale, thin, and dry, with a prominent venous pattern over most of the body, but hyperpigmented and wrinkled in the periorbital area. The facies is characteristic, with frontal bossing, depression of the central face, saddle nose, thick protruding lips, and a prominent chin. The hair is sparse and usually blond and has an unruly appearance. The changes in dentition cannot, of course, be appreciated until late infancy. Hypodontia with conical, poorly formed teeth is the rule; these changes can be detected on radiographs of the jaws prior to eruption of the teeth. Atrophic rhinitis, diminished lacrimation, hoarseness, and hypoplastic or

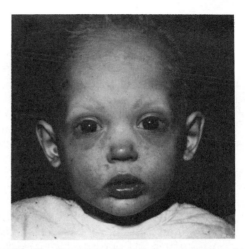

Figure 98–10. Female with fully expressed anhidrotic ectodermal dysplasia. Note the sparse, wispy hair, hyperpigmentation around the eyes, depressed nasal bridge, and protruding lips and ears.

absent mucous glands in nasotracheobronchial passages are frequent findings in these patients (Reed et al., 1970). If the diagnosis is in doubt, a skin biopsy will demonstrate the absence of eccrine sweat glands. Techniques used to elicit sweating, such as pilocarpine iontophoresis or examination of the sweat pores on the palm with o-phthalaldehyde, can also be utilized to demonstrate the defect (Esterly et al., 1973). Atopic dermatitis occurs almost universally in these children (Reed et al., 1970), as well as a decrease in T-cell function (Davis and Solomon, 1976).

In most families, the disorder is transmitted as an X-linked recessive, with the fully expressed disease appearing only in males. Carrier females may be detected by minor clinical stigmata or by decreased sweat pore counts and abnormal dermatoglyphic findings (Crump and Danks, 1971; Esterly et al., 1973). However, females with the complete syndrome have been carefully documented, and, in these families, an autosomal recessive gene appears to be operating (Gorlin et al., 1970).

Once the diagnosis is made, it is important to educate parents so that these children are protected from overexertion and undue exposure to heat. Defective lacrimation can be palliated by the use of artificial tears. The nasal mucosa should be treated with saline irrigations for removal of adherent crusts, followed by application of petrolatum. Regular dental evaluations should be started early in life and prostheses constructed, if necessary, for maintenance of good nutrition and improvement in the appearance of the child prior to his starting school. Some of these children also require a wig and reconstructive procedures later in life to improve facial configuration.

EEC SYNDROME

The EEC syndrome consists of ectodermal dysplasia (E), ectrodactyly (E), and cleft lip and palate (C). This syndrome affects both ectodermal and mesodermal tissues and is probably an inherited disorder, although the genetic transmission is not well defined. The cutaneous and appendageal anomalies include diffuse hypopigmentation affecting both skin and hair, scanty scalp hair and eyebrows, dystrophic nails and small teeth with enamel hypoplasia. Sweating appears to be intact, and sweat glands are present on skin biopsy. The clefting of the lip is usually complete and bilateral, and the palate has a median cleft. Dry granulomatous lesions in the corners of the mouth consistently yield *Candida albicans* on culture. Anomalies of the hands and feet include lobster claw deformity, syndactyly, and clinodactyly. Other findings include scarred lacrimal ducts, blepharitis and conjunctivitis, xerostomia, conductive hearing loss, and, occasionally, retardation. Although incomplete forms of this syndrome have been documented, the fully developed EEC syndrome should not be confused with other types of ectodermal dysplasia (Pries et al., 1974).

REFERENCES

Bauer, E. A., and Briggaman, R. A.: The mechanobullous diseases (epidermolysis bullosa). *In* Fitzpatrick, T. B., et al. (Eds.): Dermatology in General Medicine. New York, McGraw-Hill, 1979.

Beighton, P.: The dominant and recessive forms of cutis laxa. J. Med. Genet. *9*:216, 1972.

Buxman, M., Goodkin, P. E., Fahrenbach, W. H., and Dimond, R. L.: Harlequin ichthyosis with epidermal lipid abnormality. Arch. Dermatol. *115*:189, 1979.

Byers, P. H., Siegel, R. C., Holbrook, K. A., Narayanan, A. S., Bernstein, P., and Hall, J. G.: X-linked cutis laxa. N. Engl. J. Med. *303*:61, 1980.

Carney, R. G., Jr.: Incontinentia pigmenti. A world statistical analysis. Arch. Dermatol. *112*:535, 1976.

Comings, D. E., and Odland, G. F.: Partial albinism. J.A.M.A. *195*:519, 1966.

Craig, J. M., Goldsmith, L. A., and Baden, H. P.: An abnormality of keratin in the harlequin fetus. Pediatrics *46*:437, 1970.

Crump, J. A., and Danks, D. M.: Hypohidrotic ectodermal dysplasia. J. Pediatr. *78*:466, 1971.

Davis, J. R., and Solomon, L. M.: Cellular immunodeficiency in anhidrotic ectodermal dysplasia. Acta Derm. Venereol. *56*:115, 1976.

Draznin, T. N., Esterly, N. B., Furey, N. L., and Debofsky, H.: Neonatal lupus erythematosus. J. Am. Acad. Dermatol. *1*:437, 1979.

Elliott, S. T.: X-linked ichthyosis: a metabolic disease. J. Am. Acad. Dermatol. *1*:139, 1979.

Esterly, N. B.: The ichthyosiform dermatoses. Pediatrics *42*:990, 1968.

Esterly, N. B., Pashayan, H. M., and West, C. E.: Concurrent hypohidrotic ectodermal dysplasia and X-linked ichthyosis. Am. J. Dis. Child. *126*:539, 1973.

Fisher, M., and Schneider, R.: Aplasia cutis congenita in three successive generations. Arch. Dermatol. *108*:252, 1973.

Fowler, G. W., and Dumars, K. W.: Cutis aplasia and cerebral malformation. Pediatrics *52*:861, 1973.

Franco, H. L., Weston, W. L., Peebles, C., Forstot, L., and Phanuphank, P.: Autoantibodies directed against sicca syndrome antigens in the neonatal lupus syndrome. J. Am. Acad. Dermatol. *4*:67, 1981.

Fritsch, P.: Oral retinoids in dermatology. Intern. J. Dermatol. *20*:314, 1981.

Gordon, H., and Gordon, W.: Incontinentia pigmenti: Clinical and genetical studies of two familial cases. Dermatologica *140*:150, 1970.

Gorlin, R. J., Old, T., and Anderson, V. E.: Hypohidrotic ectodermal dysplasia in females. A critical analysis and argument for genetic heterogeneity. Z. Kinderheilkd. *108*:1, 1970.

Guerrier, C. J. W., and Wong, C. K.: Ultrastructural evolution of the skin in incontinentia pigmenti (Bloch-Sulzberger). Dermatologica *149*:10, 1974.

Hardy, J. D., Solomon, S., Barwell, G. S., Beach, R., Wright, V., and Howard, F. M.: Congenital complete heart block in the newborn associated with maternal systemic lupus erythematosus and other connective tissue disorders. Arch. Dis. Child. *54*:7, 1979.

Hollister, D. W.: Heritable disorders of connective tissue: Ehlers-Danlos syndrome. Pediatr. Clin. North Am. *25*:575, 1978.

Hruby, M. A., and Esterly, N. B.: Anemia in epidermolysis bullosa letalis. Am. J. Dis. Child. *125*:696, 1973.

Konigsmark, B.: Hereditary childhood hearing loss and integumentary system disease. J. Pediatr. *80*:909, 1972.

Kosnik, E. J., and Sayers, M. P.: Congenital scalp defects: aplasia cutis congenita. J. Neurosurg. *42*:32, 1975.

Lerer, R. J., Ehrenhranz, R. A., and Campbell, A. G. M.: Pigmented lesions of incontinentia pigmenti in a neonate. J. Pediatr. *83*:503, 1973.

Levin, D. L., Nolan, K. S., and Esterly, N. B.: Congenital absence of skin. J. Am. Acad. Dermatol. *2*:203, 1980.

McKusick, V. A.: Heritable Disorders of Connective Tissue. St. Louis, C.V. Mosby Co., 1972.

Mehregan, A. H., Lee, S. C., and Nabai, H.: Cutis laxa (generalized elastolysis). A report of four cases with autopsy findings. J. Cutan. Pathol. *5*:116, 1978.

Morgan, J. D.: Incontinentia pigmenti (Bloch-Sulzberger syndrome). Am. J. Dis. Child. *122*:294, 1971.

Pinnell, S. R., Krane, S. M., Kenzora, J., and Glimcher, M. J.: A new heritable disorder of connective tissue with hydroxylysine-deficient collagen. N. Engl. J. Med. *286*:1013, 1972.

Pries, C., Mittleman, D., Miller, M., Solomon, L. M., Pashayan, H. M., and Pruzansky, S.: The EEC syndrome. Am. J. Dis. Child. *127*:840, 1974.

Reed, W. B., Lopez, D. A., and Landing, B.: Clinical spectrum of anhidrotic ectodermal dysplasia. Arch. Dermatol. *102*:134, 1970.

Richards, W., and Kaplan, M.: Anhidrotic ectodermal dysplasia: an unusual cause of hyperpyrexia in the newborn. Am. J. Dis. Child. *117*:597, 1969.

Ruiz-Maldonado, R., and Tamayo, L.: Aplasia cutis congenita, spastic paralysis and mental retardation. Am. J. Dis. Child. *128*:699, 1974.

Solomon, L. M., and Esterly, N. B.: Neonatal Dermatology. Philadelphia, W. B. Saunders Co., 1973.

Solomon, L. M., and Keuer, E. J.: The ectodermal dysplasias. Arch. Dermatol. *116*:1295, 1980.

Telfer, M. A., Sugar, A., Jaeger, E. A., and Mulchay, J.: Dominant piebald trait (white forehead and leukoderma) with neurological impairment. Am. J. Hum. Genet. *23*:383, 1971.

Vonderheid, E. C., Koblenzer, P. J., Ming, P. M. L., and Burgoon, C. T., Jr.: Neonatal lupus erythematosus, Arch. Dermatol. *112*:698, 1976.

Witkop, C. J., Jr., White, J. G., Nance, W. E., Jackson, C. E., and Desnick, S.: Classification of albinism in man. Clinical Delineation of Birth Defects, Part XII, Skin, Hair and Nails. Baltimore, Williams & Wilkins, 1971, p. 13.

99

Infections of the Skin

By Nancy B. Esterly and
Lawrence M. Solomon

The newborn skin may be the site of a variety of lesions of infectious origin. Some types represent localized disease, whereas others are a reflection of generalized disease. Although certain systemic infections such as disseminated herpes simplex (see Chapter 83), varicella-zoster (see Chapter 83), and *Pseudomonas* sepsis produce characteristic skin lesions, these lesions have been described in the appropriate chapter as a feature of the total clinical pictures. Other systemic infections, such as cytomegalic inclusion disease, toxoplasmosis, and rubella, cause less distinctive lesions that are not specific for the particular disease entity; these, also, are described elsewhere. In this chapter, we will confine our discussion to those infections that are primarily cutaneous in nature.

Bullous Impetigo

Impetigo is one of the most common infections that plague the infant and neonatologist. The disease may occur sporadically in an individual infant, or it may involve a number of infants simultaneously or sequentially in an epidemic form. Although usually not life-threatening, the possibility of bacteremic spread to visceral organs should not be overlooked. Constant surveillance of nursing techniques in the nursery is essential to preventing the initiation of epidemics. The appearance of a single case demands immediate investigation and possible revision of these techniques.

The number of cases originating in a given nursery is related to the physical facilities and adequacy of care in handling the infants. Overcrowding, insufficient nursery personnel, carelessness in the simple matters of washing and gowning on the part of both

nurses and physicians, and other infractions of elementary rules of hygiene may lead to an increased incidence of impetigo. This is particularly true now that hexachlorophene bathing has been abandoned as standard nursery procedure because of the potential neurotoxicity of the compound if it is absorbed. If modern nursery procedures are fastidiously observed, however, the recommendations for skin care proposed by the Committee on the Fetus and Newborn (1974) should be adequate to prevent the occurrence of impetigo. Furthermore, it appears that enforced aseptic techniques actually may be more effective in preventing superficial skin infection than is the routine use of hexachlorophene bathing (Gehlbach et al., 1975).

Bullous impetigo is caused by a coagulase-positive hemolytic *Staphylococcus aureus.* Most often, the organism can be classified as one of the group 2 phage types (Albert et al., 1970), although occasional infections can be attributed to organisms in other phage groups. (Curran and Al-Salihi, 1980). In contrast to the lesions of some of the congenital blistering diseases, those of bullous impetigo usually appear during the latter part of the first week or as late as the second week of life. The diaper region is the one most frequently involved, but bullae may arise anywhere on the body surface. The blisters may vary considerably in size and may spread to contiguous areas, often forming arcs or circles, but they usually do not exhibit the characteristic grouping in grapelike clusters seen in the cutaneous eruptions of herpes simplex infection. Staphylococcal bullae are flaccid, filled with straw-colored or turbid fluid, and rupture easily, leaving a red, moist, denuded base, which then becomes covered by a thin varnish-like crust. These lesions are very superficial, re-epithelialize rapidly, and do not result in scars.

The diagnosis is suggested by the demonstration of gram-positive cocci on smears of the blister fluid and confirmed by identification of the organism on culture of material from the blister.

Treatment should be instituted promptly, and strict isolation maintained until the lesions have resolved. Compresses with sterile water, normal saline, or Burow's solution applied every few hours will cause ma-

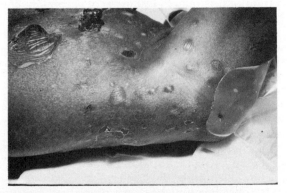

Figure 99–1. Bullous impetigo. Multiple intact and ruptured bullae on the abdomen, hip, and thigh of a newborn infant. No underlying erythema is present.

ceration, rupture, and drying of blisters. Extremely limited infections may be treated with a topical antibiotic ointment, preferably Polysporin. More extensive lesions require a systemically administered antibiotic that will effectively eradicate a penicillinase-producing strain of *Staphylococcus*. Ultimately, the sensitivities of the organism cultured should determine the choice of antibiotics.

Staphylococcal Scalded Skin Syndrome (Ritter's Disease)

Traditionally called Ritter's disease when it occurs in the newborn infant, the exfoliative form of this disorder is now included with nonstreptococcal scarlatiniform eruption and bullous impetigo in the discussion of staphylococcal scalded skin syndrome (Melish and Glasgow, 1971; Elias et al., 1977). Although a somewhat similar cutaneous reaction pattern may result from drug hypersensitivity in the older child or adult, scalded skin syndrome in the infant is virtually always a staphylococcal disease. As might be expected because of their common origin, all three forms of the scalded skin syndrome may be seen simultaneously in a nursery epidemic of staphylococcal disease.

Although initial reports suggested that all patients with Ritter's disease were infected with group 2 phage

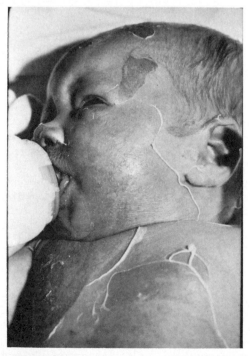

Figure 99–2. Staphylococcal scalded skin syndrome (Ritter's disease). Intense erythema and peeling of large areas of epidermis.

type staphylococci (Melish and Glasgow, 1971; Albert et al., 1970; Anthony et al., 1972), later evidence suggests that strains in other phage groups are also capable of causing scalded skin syndrome (Curran and Al-Salihi, 1980). These organisms produce an erythrogenic exotoxin called *exfoliatin,* which causes the intraepidermal separation responsible for the clinical manifestations of blistering and exfoliation of large sheets of skin. The toxin has been isolated, purified, and partially characterized (Kondo et al., 1973) and has been studied extensively in the murine model (Melish and Glasgow, 1970; Elias et al., 1974).

The onset of scalded skin syndrome is often abrupt, and the disease may progress with astonishing rapidity. Affected infants have an intense, generalized erythema that most often starts on the face and spreads to the contiguous skin. Facial edema may be quite striking. Oozing from the conjunctival area and crusting around the nose and mouth give the infant a characteristic "sad mask" appearance. The reddened skin is exquisitely sensitive to touch, and the formation of flaccid bullae may precede widespread exfoliation in which the skin peels in large sheets, leaving a moist, red, denuded surface. The denudation, which can be induced by light stroking with the examining finger, is called "Nikolsky's sign," and it can always be elicited in the exfoliative form of the disease. Separation usually occurs first on the face and in the flexural areas and may be incomplete, leaving a rolled edge of epidermis at the junction of the unpeeled and desquamated areas. The skin over the hands and feet may be shed in a glovelike fashion. Infants with scalded skin syndrome may be toxic or appear relatively well, but fluctuations in body temperature, poor feeding, and irritability due to skin tenderness are usual manifestations of the infection. With rapid, widespread denudation, fluid balance may become a serious problem. Conjunctivitis, omphalitis, or other localized inflammatory lesions may be prominent, depending on the portal of entry of the organism.

Approximately 2 to 3 days after onset, the denuded areas become dry, and a flaky desquamation ensues. Resolution occurs in another 3 to 5 days, leaving no residual lesions. Since the intraepidermal cleavage plane is at the level of the granular layer, scarring occurs only in instances of secondary complications.

The infant with the less severe form of this disease, the scarlatiniform eruption, also exhibits a generalized erythema, but Nikolsky's sign is absent. The skin has a sandpaper-like texture similar to that of the skin of the patient with streptococcal scarlet fever; however, the palatal enanthem, strawberry tongue, and perioral pallor are lacking. Instead, perioral erythema with subsequent fissuring and crusting result in the rather characteristic facial appearance. A dry, flaky desquamative phase also occurs at the end of the first week in this form of the disease.

The only helpful laboratory procedures are bacterial cultures. Blood cultures should be obtained, since sepsis, although uncommon, may supervene. In the exfoliative form, fluid from intact bullae is sterile; however, exudate from denuded or crusted areas may yield the organism. Purulent drainage from any area, such as the conjunctival sac, is also a good source of *Staphylococcus,* as are nasopharyngeal and throat cultures. Phage typing is of interest and should be obtained if possible. Gram stains of material obtained for culture may be used to confirm the clinical diagnosis if clumps of gram-positive cocci can be demonstrated. Polymorphonuclear leukocytes may be sparse or absent on smear. The presence of a peripheral leukocytosis is not a reliable indication of infection.

The differential diagnosis includes severe seborrheic dermatitis, C_5 dysfunction syndrome, epidermolytic hyperkeratosis (bullous congenital ichthyosiform erythroderma), epidermolysis bullosa, erythema multiforme, and diffuse cutaneous mastocytosis. Further studies, including a skin biopsy, may be required in confusing situations, but the clinical picture of scalded skin syndrome is usually sufficiently characteristic to make the diagnosis. Although extremely uncommon, it should be appreciated that boric acid poisoning in the young infant causes a clinical picture indistinguishable from that of scalded skin syndrome. Appropriate toxicology studies must be performed for confirmation of this diagnosis (Rubenstein and Mesher, 1970).

Since most of the staphylococcal strains that cause this syndrome are penicillinase-producing organisms, systemic administration of a penicillinase-resistant penicillin is the therapy of choice. Corticosteroids are not indicated. Fluid and electrolyte replacement and measures for maintenance of normal body temperature may be required. Crusted and denuded areas may be treated with compresses of Burow's or normal saline solution. Application of a bland emollient may accelerate the return to normal during the flaky desquamative phase.

Other Staphylococcal Skin Lesions

Staphylococci may also cause superficial pustulosis, folliculitis, or localized cutaneous abscesses. Superficial lesions, if limited, may respond to compresses and topical antibiotic therapy. Deeper lesions will require systemic antibiotic therapy and, occasionally, surgical intervention. Procedures such as fetal monitoring may induce abscess formation and associated osteomyelitis. Although usually not a pathogen, *Staphylococcus epidermidis* also has been implicated in this type of lesion (Overturf and Balfour, 1975).

Candidiasis

Candidal infections during the neonatal period are most often manifest as mucosal lesions (thrush) or as localized or generalized dermatitis. Rarely, umbilical cord granulomas or a widespread systemic mycosis may occur. The relatively high incidence of localized mucosal or cutaneous lesions can be attributed to the acquisition of *Candida albicans* as normal flora in the oral cavity and gastrointestinal tract by a significant number of infants (Kozinn et al., 1957). One longitudinal study of infants from birth through 1 year of age demonstrated a maximal isolation peak in infants 4 weeks of age, when 82 per cent of infants were found to have *Candida* in the mouth (Russell and Lay, 1973). *Candida albicans* is not a saprophyte of normal skin. In infants, the yeast is deposited on the surface of the integument via the saliva and feces. The original source of the yeast, in most instances, is the mother, who may be a vaginal or intestinal

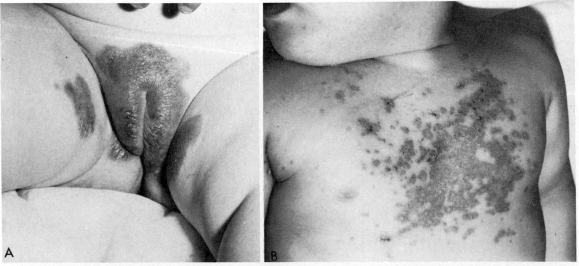

Figure 99–3. *A,* Sharply demarcated erythematous scaly candidal rash in the groin. *B,* Candidal eruption on the central chest of an infant.

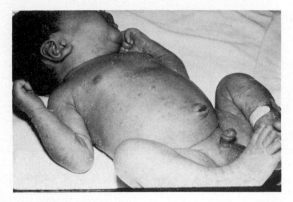

Figure 99–4. Infant of 10 days with generalized vesicopustular, scaly eruption sparing only the face and scalp. Oral mucosa was not involved. Hyphae and budding yeasts were seen on KOH preparation, and *Candida albicans* was cultured from the lesions. The infant's mother had a candidal vaginitis during the pregnancy.

carrier of the organism or who may have had overt disease during her pregnancy.

The peak incidence of thrush occurs during the beginning of the second week of life. The lesions are readily recognized as plaques of white, friable, pseudomembranous material on an erythematous base distributed over the tongue, palate, buccal mucosa,

and gingivae. Both yeast and mycelial fungal elements can be demonstrated on a potassium hydroxide preparation of material removed from a typical lesion. The diagnosis may be confirmed by identification of the organism on culture. Oral lesions usually respond promptly to a course of nystatin suspension 100,000 to 200,000 units administered by mouth four times daily for 10 to 14 days.

Localized candidal infections of skin are also common in infants. Intertriginous areas, particularly the diaper area, are most commonly affected, but even facial eruptions can occur, presumably by the infant's acquiring the organism while passing through the vagina. Multiple tiny vesicopustules erode and merge, forming bright, erythematous, scaly plaques, often with a scalloped edge bordered by a fringe of epithelium. Scattered satellite vesicopustules develop beyond the margins of the plaque and are one of the hallmarks of cutaneous candidiasis. Diaper area eruptions usually result from contamination of the perineal skin with feces containing *C. albicans*; therefore, it is usual to have involvement of perirectal skin. The moisture and maceration of the diaper and flexural areas encourage proliferation of the yeast; pruritus and burning associated with the dermatitis may cause extreme discomfort.

When involving the perineal skin, cutaneous candidiasis may be confused with superficial staphylococcal infection or with a primary irritant diaper dermatitis. Potassium hydroxide preparations of scrapings from involved skin will disclose budding yeasts and mycelia, confirmatory evidence of yeast

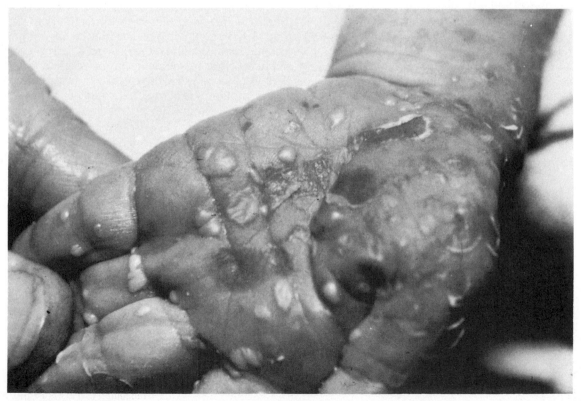

Figure 99–5. Congenital cutaneous candidiasis—pustular stage—in a 6-day-old infant. A maculopapular rash was present at birth. (Courtesy of P. J. Kozinn, N. Rudolf, A. A. Tariq, M. R. Reale, and P. K. Goldberg.)

infection. Localized cutaneous candidiasis should be treated with a specific candidicidal agent, nystatin, miconazole, clotrimazole, or amphotericin B in a cream, ointment, lotion, or powder. Generally, ointments are the most soothing and best tolerated.

Occasionally, a widespread cutaneous dermatitis occurs either as a result of spread from an untreated localized plaque or by contamination of the entire integument during the process of birth. Superficial vesicopustules rupture, leaving a denuded surface with a ring of detached epidermis. The lesions spread peripherally, forming confluent plaques of dermatitis with generalized scaling. Mucous membrane involvement may be associated. Extensive cutaneous lesions may occur in normal newborns, in infants with an underlying dermatologic disease, such as acrodermatitis enteropathica or ichthyosis, in patients with immunodeficiency disease, or in those with chronic mucocutaneous candidiasis and endocrinopathies. Confusion with other types of infection, including congenital syphilis and seborrheic dermatitis, is possible, and the presence of yeast should be confirmed by potassium hydroxide preparation and culture. Normal infants respond rapidly to application of anticandidal topical agents; patients with underlying disease may be refractory to therapy.

Intrauterine infection with *C. albicans* may result in lesions of the placenta and fetal membranes and characteristic granulomas of the umbilical cord (Schirar et al., 1974). The cord lesions are multiple yellowish-white papules, usually measuring 1 to 3 millimeters in diameter. A mixed inflammatory cell infiltrate and fungal elements are demonstrable on histologic sections of the cord lesions prepared with the appropriate stains. Although most of these infants have been born prior to term, premature or prolonged rupture of the membranes is extremely rare. Some affected infants have been delivered by cesarean section. Ascending infection from a vaginal or cervical focus is believed to be the route of invasion. The amniotic fluid is often positive for *Candida albicans* when it is smeared and cultured.

In addition to involvement of the cord and fetal adnexa, there is often generalized cutaneous candidiasis but sparing of the mucous membranes (Kam et al., 1975; Rudolph et al., 1977). Rarely, disseminated infection has occurred in the lungs and gastrointestinal tract, presumably as the result of aspiration or swallowing of infected amniotic fluid. Hematogenous spread has not been documented. Infants without visceral involvement respond rapidly to therapy with standard topical anticandidal agents.

Streptococcal Infections

Cutaneous streptococcal infections occur in the newborn but are less common than staphylococcal infections. *Group A streptococci* may cause disease of epidemic proportions (Dillon, 1966; Peter et al., 1975) following introduction of the organism into the nursery by maternal carriers or nursery personnel.

The umbilicus is a frequent site of infection, which is manifested by seropurulent drainage from the umbilical stump and erythema and pustules on the contiguous abdominal skin. Conjunctivitis, paronychia, vaginitis, and an erysipelas-like eruption have also been described (Geil et al., 1970; Dillon, 1966). Since sepsis and meningitis may result, infected infants should be treated promptly and strict isolation instituted. As with staphylcoccocal infection, serious efforts should be made to identify the source of the organism. These infections respond readily to penicillin, which should be administered for a 10-day course.

Group B streptococci are now one of the most frequently encountered pathogens in the newborn nursery. Early-onset disease (first week of life), probably acquired in utero or during delivery, is most commonly manifested as septicemia with respiratory distress and shock. Late-onset disease (after the first week of life) is acquired post partum and more often takes the form of meningitis. Patients with early-onset disease may harbor the organism on the skin. One report suggests that the group B streptococcus should be included in the list of organisms capable of causing impetigo neonatorum. In 1975, Belgaumkar reported a term infant with widespread superficial ulcerations and crusted lesions noted at birth. Membranes had ruptured 22 hours prior to delivery, but the lochia was negative for group B streptococci on culture. Rapid healing followed a course of parenteral penicillin. With the emergence of this organism as a primary pathogen in the newborn infant, it is possible that cutaneous disease due to group B streptococci will become a more common phenomenon in the nursery population.

REFERENCES

Albert, S., Baldwin, R., Czekajewski, S., van Soestbergen, A., Nachman, R., and Robertson, A.: Bullous impetigo due to group II *Staphylococcus aureus*. Am. J. Dis. Child. *120*:10, 1970.

Anthony, B. F., Giuliano, D. M., and Oh, W.: Nursery outbreak of staphylococcal scalded skin syndrome. Am. J. Dis. Child *124*:41, 1972.

Belgaumkar, T. K.: Impetigo neonatorum congenita due to group B beta-hemolytic streptococcus infection. J. Pediatr. *86*:982, 1975.

Committee on Fetus and Newborn. Skin care of newborns. Pediatrics *54*:682, 1974.

Curran, J. P., and Al-Salihi, F. L.: Neonatal staphylococcal scalded skin syndrome: massive outbreak due to an unusual phage type. Pediatrics *66*:285, 1980.

Dillon, H. C., Jr.: Group A Type 12 streptococcal infection in a newborn nursery. Am. J. Dis. Child. *112*:177, 1966.

Elias, P. M., Fritsch, P., and Epstein, E. H., Jr.: Staphylococcal scalded skin syndrome. Clinical features, pathogenesis, and recent microbiological and biochemical developments. Arch. Dermatol. *113*:207, 1977.

Elias, P. M., Mittermayer, H., Tappeiner, G., Fritsch, P., and Wolff, K.: Staphylococcal toxic epidermal necrolysis (TEN): The expanded mouse model. J. Invest. Dermatol. *63*:467, 1974.

Gehlbach, S. H., Gutman, L. T., Wilfert, C. M., Brumley, G. W., and Katz, S. L.: Recurrence of skin disease in a nursery: Ineffectuality of hexachlorophene bathing. Pediatrics 55:422, 1975.

Geil, C. C., Castle, W. K., and Mortimer, E. A., Jr.: Group A streptococcal infections in newborn nurseries. Pediatrics 46:489, 1970.

Kam, L. A., and Giacoia, G. P.: Congenital cutaneous candidiasis. Am. J. Dis. Child. 129:1215, 1975.

Kondo, I., Sakurai, S., and Sarai, Y.: Purification of exfoliatin produced by Staphylococcus aureus of bacteriophage group II and its physicochemical properties. Infect. Immun. 8:156, 1973.

Kozinn, P. J., Taschdjian, C. L., Dragutsky, D., and Minsky, A.: Cutaneous candidiasis in early infancy and childhood. Pediatrics 20:827, 1957.

McCracken, G. H., Jr.: Group B streptococci: The new challenge in neonatal infections. J. Pediatr. 82:703, 1973.

Melish, M. E., and Glasgow, L. A.: Staphylococcal scalded skin syndrome: The expanded clinical syndrome. J. Pediatr. 78:958, 1971.

Melish, M. E., and Glasgow, L. A.: Staphylococcal scalded skin syndrome—development of an experimental model. N. Engl. J. Med. 282:1114, 1970.

Overturf, B. D., and Balfour, G.: Osteomyelitis and sepsis: Severe complications of fetal monitoring. Pediatrics 55:244, 1975.

Peter, G., and Hazard, J.: Neonatal group A streptococcal disease. J. Pediatr. 87:454, 1975.

Rubenstein, A. D., and Mesher, D. M.: Epidemic boric acid poisoning simulating staphylococcal toxic epidermal necrolysis of the newborn infant: Ritter's disease. J. Pediatr. 77:884, 1970.

Rudolph, N., Tariq, A. A., Reale, M. R., Goldberg, P. K., and Kozinn, P. J.: Congenital cutaneous candidiasis. Arch. Dermatol. 113:1101, 1977.

Rudolph, R. I., Schwartz, W., and Leyden, J. J.: Treatment of staphylococcal toxic epidermal necrolysis. Arch. Dermatol. 110:559, 1974.

Russell, C., and Lay, K. M.: Natural history of Candida species and yeasts in the oral cavities of infants. Arch. Oral Biol. 18:957, 1973.

Schirar, A., Rendu, C., Vielh, J. P., and Gautray, J. P.: Congenital mycosis (Candida albicans). Biol. Neonate 24:273, 1974.

100

Nevi and Cutaneous Tumors

By Lawrence M. Solomon and
Nancy B. Esterly

There is no universally accepted or even satisfying definition of the word "nevus." By common usage, it has come to mean a cutaneous malformation of the skin represented by a localized collection of cells in a considerably advanced state of differentiation. The distinction between hamartoma and nevus is not clear. In a nevus, the aggregation of cells in the skin may originate from any tissue normally found in skin and may attempt to become functional (i.e., produce pigment or keratin) or may form imperfect versions of their destined structures (i.e., abortive hair follicles, blood vessels, sebaceous glands).

In 1969, Pinkus and Mehregan reported that nevi are derived from pluripotential epithelial germ buds in the basal layer of the epidermis that undergo aberrant development. It is possible that a disturbance in tissue growth factors may also play a significant role in their genesis.

The clinical forms of cutaneous nevi are extremely numerous, and a discussion of each would be beyond the scope of this chapter. For this reason, we have summarized the spectrum of nevi to be found in Table 100–1. We will discuss the most common and important nevi in the following pages.

Hemangiomas and Other Vascular Malformations

Localized vascular malformations, also known as vascular nevi, or hemangiomas, occur extremely frequently in the pediatric population. The incidence of all vascular nevi is probably about 6 to 25 per cent. We believe that for the numbers to be more accurately considered they should be separated into cavernous hemangiomas (about 5 to 10 per cent) and nevus flammeus (about 30 per cent) (Harris et al., 1975). Hemangiomas may be superficial (about 65 per cent), subcutaneous (15 per cent), or mixed (20 per cent) (Rook, 1972). The clinical appearance of the lesion often does not correspond exactly to the histopathologic classification (Wade, 1978). Two types of hemangiomas have been described: capillary and cavernous. Capillary hemangiomas consist of dilated vessels, often associated with endothelial proliferation, and develop fibrotic changes as they resolve. Cavernous hemangiomas have, in the lower dermis, large irregular spaces filled with blood, lined by a single layer of endothelial cells and by a fibrous wall of varying thickness. Both pathologic changes may be found in different portions of many hemangiomas. It is important to note that a biopsy and pathologic study of a section will often not distinguish the

Table 100–1. Spectrum of Nevi

Epidermal
Keratinocytic (Epidermal) Nevi
Nevus unius latens
Systematized verrucous nevi
Small verrucous nevi
Ichthyosis hystrix
Unilateral congenital ichthyosiform erythroderma
Epidermal nevus syndrome
Benign congenital acanthosis nigricans
Porokeratosis of Mibelli
Inflammatory linear verrucous epidermal nevus (Ilven)

Appendageal (Organoid) Nevi
Sebaceous nevi ⎫
Hair follicle nevi ⎬ comedo nevi
Apocrine duct nevi ⎭
    (nevus syringocystadenoma papilliferus)

Melanocytic Nevi

Dermal
Melanocytic Nevi
Vascular Nevi
Connective Tissue Nevi
Collagen
Elastic tissue
Digital fibroma
Juvenile fibromatosis
Osteoma cutis
Nervous Tissue Nevi
Nasal glioma
Meningioma

Subcutaneous Tissue
Lipoma
Nevus lipomatosis superficialis
Michelin tire baby
Encephalocraniocutaneous lipomatosis

Mixed
Benign teratomas (dermoids)

(From Solomon, L. M., and Esterly, N. B.: Neonatal Dermatology. Philadelphia, W. B. Saunders Co., 1973.)

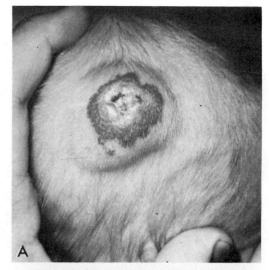

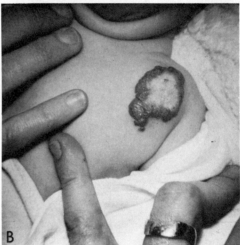

Figure 100–1. *A*, Mixed capillary and cavernous hemangioma with small central ulceration on the scalp of an infant, *B*, Involuting strawberry hemangioma with central gray fibrotic area.

differences between congenital and acquired vascular nevi, nor between nevi and other reactive vascular phenomena (Pinkus and Mehnegan, 1981). Clinically, one can classify cutaneous hemangiomas in the neonatal period into two types: flat telangiectatic hemangiomas (nevus flammeus, port-wine stain) and raised angiomas (capillary, cavernous, or mixed). A second useful consideration is whether the lesions are strictly cutaneous or are associated with other abnormalities. Thirdly, the rate of endothelial mitosis may be the most important distinguishing feature among hemangiomas (Mulliken and Glowacki, 1982).

TELANGIECTATIC NEVI

These lesions are among the most frequent abnormalities of the skin of the newborn infant. They are designated "nevus flammeus" as a group but may be subdivided into "salmon patch," "nuchal nevus," and "port-wine stain." The typical lesion is flat and bright to dark red and has a sharp border. Those found at the base of the skull tend to remain with increasing age. A paler variety of nevus flammeus may be found over the eyelids, between the eyes, and on the mid-forehead (salmon patch). Hemangiomas in these sites tend to be less visible as the skin becomes less translucent, and they usually fade completely. However, in moments of anger or during intense exercise or flushing, the lesion may become visible. Telangiectatic nevi on other sites, such as the cheeks, usually do not fade but instead acquire a purplish hue, which suggests the term "port-wine stain." Port-wine stains occur much less frequently than nuchal nevi but are more often associated with ocular complication when they are located in the area of the ophthalmic portion of the trigeminal nerve. In 1980, Bartsky and coworkers found glaucoma to occur in 10 per cent of such patients. Nevus flammeus may, in fact, be found almost anywhere on the body or on any mucosal surface.

Macular telangiectatic nevi occur in the following conditions with varying frequency: trisomy 13, Rubinstein-Taybi syndrome, Beckwith-Wiedemann syndrome, pseudothalidomide syndrome (SC syndrome), Wyburn-Mason syndrome, and the epidermal nevus syndrome.

STURGE-WEBER SYNDROME

A nevus flammeus affecting that area of skin innervated by the ophthalmic portion of the trigeminal nerve may be a sign of Sturge-Weber syndrome (Alexander and Norman, 1960). This syndrome represents a congenital malformation (not hereditarily transmitted) of the vessels of the skin, meninges, and, frequently, the ocular orbit. The malformation is most often unilateral, but bilateral involvement is not rare (about one in 10 cases). The clinical features are port-

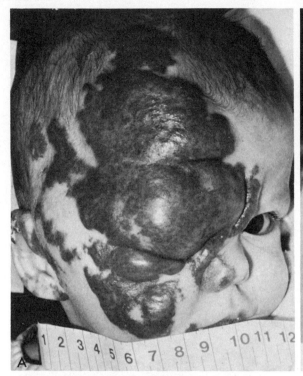
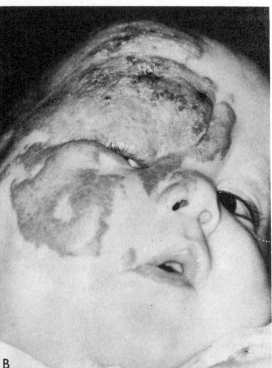
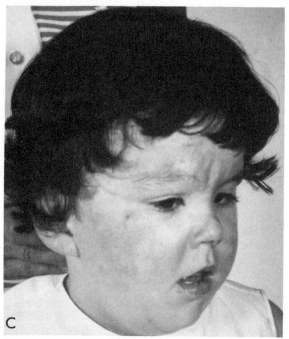

Figure 100–2. *A*, A flat hemangioma was noted at birth and by 3 weeks of age had expanded, as shown in the figure. After 11 weeks of prednisone (20 mg per day), the lesion had regressed, as shown in *B*. *C*, Nearly complete regression is evident by age 4 years. She is a normally intelligent child whose only residual problem is strabismus.

wine nevus, perimeningovascular calcification, seizures, hemiparesis, and mental retardation. Ocular complications include glaucoma, buphthalmos, choroidal angiomas, and optic atrophy. The hemangioma may also involve the mouth, tongue, and buccal mucosa. Nevus flammeus is also frequently present elsewhere on the body.

Careful neurologic and ophthalmologic examinations and electroencephalographic studies should be performed during infancy as a basis for future evaluations. Periodic assessment of intelligence and behavior and radiographic examination of the skull not only may confirm the diagnosis but, more importantly, may also indicate the degree of severity of the process. In some patients only minimal central nervous system involvement will occur, whereas in others the disorder may cause profound retardation and frequent seizures. Longitudinal observation of the patient is required before an appropriate prognosis can be made. The radiographic finding of double-contoured ("tram-line") calcification in the cerebral cortex is not seen during infancy but develops during childhood; therefore, CAT scans of the skull should be done at an early age, even if the skull radiographs are normal in appearance. Unilateral depression of cortical activity and episodes of spike discharges are the most characteristic EEG changes.

Treatment measures include anticonvulsant drugs, management of glaucoma and a masking screen (Covermark) for the skin lesions. Laser treatment of the cutaneous lesions may be feasible in the older child if the lesion is not too large. In severely affected infants neurosurgical procedures aimed at removal of abnormal meningeal and cortical tissue have been palliative (Peterman et al., 1958). Plastic repair of gingival overgrowth due to either hemangioma or anticonvulsant therapy also may be indicated.

CAVERNOUS AND STRAWBERRY HEMANGIOMAS

These hemangiomas may be single or multiple. The lesions are raised and may be felt as a mass in the skin or deeper tissues. The borders can be either well or poorly defined. Superficial lesions are bright red, lobulated, and somewhat compressible. Deeper lesions may have a bluish hue or be flesh-toned if the overlying skin is not significantly involved. Histologic examination of these lesions usually is not helpful, since they often have a mixed picture. About one fourth of the lesions are present at birth (Simpson, 1959; Rook, 1972) as an area of blanched skin with a few superficial dilated vessels. Approximately 1 per cent of newborn infants are affected (Hidano and Nakajima, 1972), with a somewhat higher incidence in preterm infants (Harris et al., 1975).

Evolution. Most of these lesions increase in size during the first 3 to 6 months of life. A subsequent stationary interval is followed by involution, which may take a variable period of time. The vast majority

of hemangiomas resolve by 7 to 9 years of age without treatment (Margileth, 1971). Involution of an individual strawberry hemangioma is heralded by the appearance of gray fibrotic plaques on the surface, a change in color to a darker hue, and softening of the mass. As healing progresses, the skin may return to normal color or be streaked by a few telangiectatic vessels. The texture of the healing skin is flabby at first but improves with time. Those patients we have followed whose hemangiomas have been allowed to involute spontaneously have achieved a more successful cosmetic result than those subjected to surgical or radiologic intervention.

Complications. The following complications may occur in cavernous and capillary hemangiomas:

1. Local: necrosis, ulceration, hemorrhage, and infection.

2. Impingement on particular structures: obstruction of vision, interference with respiration, hearing impairment, and interference with nutrition.

3. Systemic: hemangiomas in internal organs, congestive heart failure, thrombocytopenia, and disseminated intravascular coagulation.

4. Complications following treatment with radiation, surgery, or injection of sclerosing agents: scarring, ulceration, damage to internal organs, and local impairment of growth.

5. Psychological and social problems.

Treatment. For uncomplicated hemangiomas, the treatment of choice is patient observation. The lesion should be measured regularly and its growth recorded and followed. In our experience, parents inevitably show signs of anxiety and a need for constant reassurance. Before-and-after photographs of involuted lesions in other children often alleviate parental concern. Local compression of accessible lesions has been advocated (Mangus, 1973) and is helpful.

1. Treatment of local complications: Massive hemorrhage is rare. Minor episodes of bleeding will respond to compression. Necrotic, ulcerated, and infected areas should be cultured and treated with appropriate antibiotics, either topically or systemically. The ulcers will heal, but scarring may result.

2. When large hemangiomas interfere with vital functions or sight, surgical intervention or the use of systemically administered corticosteroids (prednisone, 2 mg per kg in a single daily morning dose or an alternate-day regimen) for 6 to 12 weeks may halt expansion and initiate involution of the lesion (Fost and Esterly, 1968; Brown et al., 1972).

3. Hemangiomatous involvement of internal organs such as the liver, gastrointestinal tract, and bladder, high output congestive heart failure, and Kasabach-Merritt syndrome (see further on) are life-

threatening conditions that require active intervention (Berman and Lim, 1978). Prednisone in large doses has been helpful in some infants, but unfortunately not all patients respond.

4. The prime complication of therapy is scarring. Regrowth after surgery is not uncommon. All one can do in such instances is to wait for involution and follow with plastic repair and cosmetic screens such as Covermark.

5. A small number of hemangiomas simply will not resolve in spite of all one may do. For this reason, an unequivocally certain prognosis of resolution may be premature. The subsequent psychologic and social problems of these individuals require constant support from the physician and social agencies. We have found that if patients are willing to express their feelings openly, they seem to cope with the issue somewhat better. On rare occasions, psychiatric help should be sought.

KLIPPEL-TRENAUNAY-WEBER SYNDROME

A vascular nevus may involve an entire limb or large area and cause hypertrophy of skin, subcutaneous tissue, muscle, and bones. The cutaneous lesion, which is usually visible at birth, affects boys more often than girls (Mullins et al., 1962). Associated deformities include venous varicosities, capillary or cavernous hemangiomas, and, rarely, arteriovenous fistulas. Treatment is not very effective, and surgical repair and occasionally amputation may have to be considered, owing to severe deformity and functional loss of a limb.

DIFFUSE NEONATAL HEMANGIOMATOSIS (DISSEMINATED HEMANGIOMATOSIS, VISCERAL HEMANGIOMATOSIS, MILIARY HEMANGIOMATOSIS)

Numerous cutaneous lesions may be present at birth or develop within the first few weeks of life. The most commonly involved organ systems are the central nervous system, liver, gastrointestinal tract, and lungs, although any organ may be involved. Affected infants may develop high-output congestive failure, pulmonary obstruction, neurologic deficit, or gastrointestinal hemorrhage leading to early death (Holden and Alexander, 1970; Burman et al., 1967). In 1978, Berman and Lim reviewed the literature and found that untreated patients had a mortality rate of 81 per cent, whereas treated patients had a mortality rate of 29 per cent.

The cutaneous lesions are small, dome-shaped, and red or dark blue. The presence of a profusion of hemangiomas in the skin should alert the physician to search for internal involvement (rarely, visceral involvement is not found). Systemic corticosteroid therapy is the treatment of choice (Brown et al., 1972). The prognosis is improving with carefully individualized therapy.

KASABACH-MERRITT SYNDROME

During the first few months of life (Shim, 1968) a rapidly expanding cavernous hemangioma may be complicated by the development of thrombocytopenia. A few infants have developed this complication with lesions as small as 5 or 6 centimeters in diameter. Thrombocytopenia can be followed by bleeding and anemia. Bleeding is believed to be caused by a trapping of platelets in the hemangioma and a depletion of circulating clotting factors (Konstras et al., 1963; Rodriguez-Erdmann et al., 1971). Hypofibrinogenemia and decreased factors II, V, VII, and VIII may be found. Fibrin split products are elevated, an indication of the consumption coagulopathy. Red blood cell and platelet survivals are also shortened. The prognosis of Kasabach-Merritt syndrome is serious, and the results of various forms of treatment are difficult to evaluate. Administration of systemic corticosteroids, compression of the lesion, and surgical extirpation have been followed by improvement in the hematologic status. A severe consumption coagulopathy may require heparin for control. Aspirin and other antiplatelet drugs have also been advocated. Radiation to the hemangioma has been effective in some cases, but the hazards of such therapy must be carefully weighed.

CUTIS MARMORATA TELANGIECTATICA CONGENITA (CONGENITAL GENERALIZED PHLEBECTASIA)

This label may describe several clinically similar diseases. In its most common form, a lower limb and part of the trunk demonstrate vascular reticulation in a bluish-red network (Mizrahi and Sachs, 1966; Way et al., 1974). Nodules that are dark and thrombosed lesions lead to superficial ulceration that then undergoes healing and leaves a scarred defect with a net-like distribution. Although this disease occurs in the newborn period, it has none of the characteristics of nevi. It does resemble a localized area of vasculitis or thrombosis with healing. Overall, the prognosis is fairly good. Most children recover from the disorder with minimal cutaneous dysfunction; a few suffer some associated anomalies, but these latter represent a more diffuse involvement and are rarely seen in the localized form.

Improvement in appearance is usual but is not always pleasing to the observer. If hypertrophy of a limb results, it is difficult to distinguish from Klippel-Trenaunay-Weber syndrome.

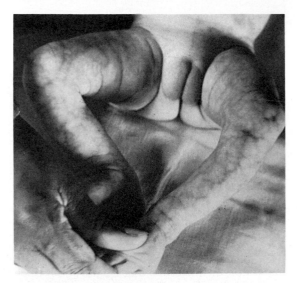

Figure 100–3. Cutis marmorata telangiectatica congenita. Note the striking network of dilated vessels most distinct over the extremities. (Humphries, J. M.: J. Pediatr. 40:486, 1952.)

CIRSOID ANEURYSM (ARTERIOVENOUS FISTULAR MALFORMATION)

This rare lesion may be found anywhere on the body but is usually located on the scalp. The lesion may be several centimeters in size, is elevated and warm, and often pulsates. A murmur may be auscultated in the area of involvement. Angiography may identify one or more central feeding vessels. These vessels should be tied or the lesion surgically extirpated at some time during early childhood. A fistulous aneurysm may complicate a cavernous hemangioma.

BLUE RUBBER BLEB NEVUS SYNDROME

This interesting and extremely rare syndrome (Fretzin and Potter, 1965) consists of multiple cavernous hemangiomas of skin, mucous membrane, bowel, and, less frequently, spleen, liver, and central nervous system. Numerous lesions may be present at birth. They range in size from 1 millimeter to several centimeters and have three peculiar characteristics: They look like blue nodules and resemble the blueberry muffin lesions seen in other rare disorders, they are tender to palpation, and they are surmounted by droplets of sweat. Treatment is restricted to resection of involved areas of bowel. Blue rubber bleb hemangiomas do not resolve spontaneously.

RARE VASCULAR NEVI

Other rare vascular tumors that may occur in the newborn include linear verrucous hemangioma, benign juvenile hemangioendothelioma, hemangiopericytoma, and multiple glomus tumors.

LOCALIZED MALFORMATIONS OF THE LYMPHATIC VESSELS

Localized nevoid tumors of lymphatic vessel origin (lymphangiomas) are less common than hemangiomas in infants. A mixed tumor consisting of lymphatics and blood vessels may also occur; however, at times it is difficult to distinguish the tissue of origin of a vascular tumor, especially if bleeding into a lymphatic bleb has occurred. Four morphologic forms of lymphangioma have been distinguished. The histologic features of all are basically quite similar: They consist of dilated lymph channels forming cystic structures of varying size that are lined by a simple endothelium, characteristic of a lymphatic vessel.

Lymphangioma Circumscriptum. Lymphangioma circumscriptum is the most common variant of lymphangioma encountered in the infant (Peachy et al., 1970). It is usually located on the upper portion of the limbs, in the axillary or inguinal folds, and on the oral mucosa. The lesion consists of a grapelike cluster of very thin-walled translucent vesicles filled with a clear or somewhat bloody fluid. The surrounding skin may have a red to wine color and be somewhat verrucous. Although most of the lesions appear to be very superficial, there is most often an associated anomaly of the deeper vessels. Biopsy or incision of a group of vesicles may result in chronic drainage that may be repaired only by excision of the entire lesion and application of full-thickness grafts. This form of lymphangioma may recur even after extensive surgery.

Simple Lymphangioma. The simple lymphangioma is extremely rare and occurs as a skin-colored nodule on the head, thorax, or oral mucosa. Chronic drainage and recurrence following surgical excision may complicate management.

Diffuse Lymphangioma. The diffuse lymphangioma is a large, ill-defined, soft tissue mass involving skin, subcutaneous tissue, and muscle on the trunk, extremities, face, lips, or tongue. Marked enlargement of the affected area may result from invasion by the cystic lymphatics complicated by stasis and infection. Surgical intervention is often extremely difficult to perform in these cases but may be the only alternative if oral lesions interfere with feeding.

Cystic Hygroma (Cavernous Lymphangioma). More localized, but in many ways similar to diffuse lymphangioma, the hygroma is a large, multiloculated, translucent lesion that may involve any part of the body but most frequently affects the face, trunk, and shoulder-girdle area. It expands rapidly. Surgery may be curative (Saijo et al., 1975), and an attempt at excision should be made before the lesion reaches unmanageable proportions.

Lymphedema. Lymphedema is swelling as a result of lymphatic stasis. A wide-spread defect (or aplasia) of lymphatic channels may result in the characteristic brawny edema. Females are affected more frequently than males. The lower limbs are the sites of predilection, but other sites may also be involved, and, rarely, chylothorax or ascites may be present. When the legs are involved and autosomal dominant transmission can be demonstrated, the eponym "Milroy's disease" may be applied. Patients with diffuse lymphatic malformations require extensive radiologic contrast studies for adequate evaluation and lifetime vascular supportive treatment to the affected areas. It should be stressed that the underlying defect in many of the lymphedemas is unclear, and that arteriovenous dysfunction may also be involved in the pathogenesis of the swelling. Lymphedema of the legs occurs in the Turner (XO) syndrome.

Pigmented Nevi

There are fewer pigmented lesions in the skin of the newborn than in the adult. Pigmented lesions may be caused by hyperactivity of the pigment-forming cells (melanocyte) in the epidermis, by collections of cells of melanocytic origin in the basal areas of the epidermis and high in the dermis (melanocytic nevus cells), or by collections of spindle-shaped melanocytic cells deep in the dermis (dermal melanocytes). The location of the melanocytic cells in the skin, the degree of melanin production, and the numbers of cells present are the variables that determine the size, shape, surface, and color of the nevus.

Not all known types of melanocytic lesions occur in the newborn. Some of them are described in the following paragraphs.

CAFÉ-AU-LAIT SPOTS

Café-au-lait spots are flat lesions of light brown color in whites and of darker brown color in blacks. They vary in size from a couple of centimeters in their largest diameter to much larger lesions that cover a significant portion of the surface anatomy. The surface is usually uniform in color, but minor variations may occur. Single small lesions (under 3 cm) are found in 19 per cent of normal newborn infants (Whitehouse, 1966). Much larger lesions or the presence of six or more café-au-lait spots (Crowe et al., 1956) connote an existing underlying pathologic condition, usually neurofibromatosis or the Albright syndrome (McCune-Albright syndrome).

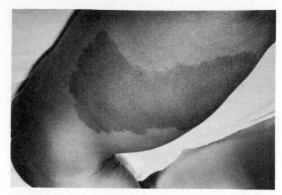

Figure 100–4. Large cafe-au-lait spot on the trunk of a newborn infant.

Neurofibromatosis. Neurofibromatosis is an autosomal dominant disease that occurs about once in 3000 livebirths. The cutaneous manifestations in the newborn infant are limited to the presence of a few café-au-lait spots, which become more numerous as the child grows. The presence of more than five café-au-lait spots (≥ 0.5 cm in diameter) in a child under 5 years of age is highly suggestive of neurofibromatosis. Axillary freckling is an almost invariable feature of the syndrome as well. The protuberant cutaneous tumors, consisting of perineural elements, usually appear in late childhood and adolescence. Neurofibromatosis is a complex disease with multiorgan involvement, and these patients should be carefully observed for other manifestations of the disease (Crowe et al., 1956). The physician faced with the need to discriminate between the café-au-lait spots of neurofibromatosis and those of other conditions is often in a quandary. Overall assessment of the results of the clinical examination as well as light and electron microscopic study of a biopsy from such a macule will often yield an accurate decision. Besides an increased number of melanocytes within the lesion, the keratinocytes and melanocytes may (but not invariably) contain large melanin organelles (macromelanosomes) (Johnson and Charneco, 1970). These changes are found in most patients with neurofibromatosis and only rarely in Albright's syndrome. However, macromelanosomes are also found in a wide variety of other conditions; therefore, one must not consider their presence as a diagnostic feature (Eady et al., 1975; Ortonne et al., 1980). Café-au-lait spots may also be found in, among other disorders, the Bloom syndrome, the Russell-Silver syndrome, the epidermal nevus syndrome and the Leopard syndrome. Perhaps it is also wise to remember that up to 2 per cent of black infants may have 1 to 3 café-au-lait spots that are of no significance (Alper et al., 1979).

There is a need for an in-vitro test to further our means of making the diagnosis in the small infant. Bidot-Lopez and Frankel (1983) have found skin fibroblasts to undergo viral transformation in neurofibromatosis patients nine times more readily than in controls. If these studies retain some specificity, we may soon have a tool to meet our clinical needs.

Albright's Syndrome (McCune-Albright Syndrome). Albright's syndrome (Albright et al., 1937) consists of polyostotic fibrous dysplasia, endocrine dysfunction, sexual precocity (in females), and large café-au-lait spots. The café-au-lait lesions in this syndrome may be unilateral, have irregular borders, are elongated and very large, and usually contain melanocytes with normal-appearing melanosomes.

FLAT MELANOCYTIC NEVI (JUNCTIONAL NEVI)

Flat, dark-brown to black, sharply demarcated melanocytic nevi are found in about 2 per cent of newborn infants (Pack and Davis, 1956; Alper, 1979). They vary in size and grow proportionately with the infant. Most frequently, one may find one or two lesions in normal infants, but more numerous melanocytic nevi are found in a number of syndromes, such as the epidermal nevus syndrome and accompanying giant nevus. The presence of these lesions in profusion, either at birth or within the first month of life, usually signifies a more widespread disorder. Flat nevi have a characteristic histologic appearance. They consist of nests of cuboidal cells clustered at the base of the epidermis, at the junction with the dermis. For this reason, flat melanocytic nevi are called "junctional nevi."

The differential diagnosis of junctional nevi may include urticaria pigmentosa, postinflammatory hypopigmentation, and juvenile lentigines. Freckles are not seen at birth or during the first few months of life. The lentiginous spots found in the leopard syndrome appear after the first year of life, and those in the Peutz-Jeghers syndrome appear at about puberty. In generalized hereditary lentiginosis, an autosomal dominant disease with mental retardation and nystagmus, the numerous lentigines are present at birth.

The treatment of melanocytic nevi depends, in part, on their location and the age at which they appear. The most frequent concern of parents and pediatricians is the lesions' potential for malignant transformation. The risk for small lesions (1 to 2 cm) is probably small but greater for *congenital* lesions than for lesions that appear after birth (Solomon, 1980; Rhodes and Melski, 1982; Rhodes et al., 1982). For this reason, there is increasing tendency to remove congenital melanocytic nevi by surgical excision. The pediatrician can best advise at what stage of growth the infant can best tolerate the procedure physically and psychologically.

MONGOLIAN SPOTS, BLUE NEVI, NEVI OF OTA AND ITO

More than 90 per cent of black and Oriental infants but less than 5 per cent of white children (Pratt, 1953) are born with mongolian spots, deep-brown to slate-gray or blue-black, large macular areas of varying size located over the lumbosacral area. Although the buttocks area is the most frequent site, multiple lesions involving the lower limbs, back, flanks, and shoulders are not uncommon.

Mongolian spots represent collections of spindle-shaped melanocytes located deep in the dermis. Most mongolian spots gradually fade during the first few years of life, but some may remain for a lifetime as a slate-gray discoloration.

Nevus of Ota is a blue or black discoloration involving the orbital and zygomatic area. The sclera and fundus on the affected side also may appear to be stained black. When the lesion is located in the deltotrapezius area, it is called "nevus of Ito." A biopsy is not necessary, since the lesion is clinically quite characteristic. Treatment of nevus of Ota is only of concern after the child starts school and should include an adequate cosmetic cover (such as Covermark) for the affected area. When the eye itself is involved, periodic examination by an ophthalmologist is suggested.

RAISED MELANOCYTIC NEVI

Blue Nevi. Blue nevi are so called because of their deep Prussian blue color and are, on occasion, found at birth (Lund and Kraus, 1962) on the scalp, face, arms, or buttocks. These are oval, dome-shaped tumors, which protrude above the skin surface, in contrast to the flat bluish nevi described in the preceding paragraphs. Two types of blue nevi have been histologically described: in one, the melanocytic component is similar to that found in mongolian spot, and in the second, the melanocytes take the form of cuboidal cells with a pale vacuolated cytoplasm.

Giant Nevi. Giant nevi are, from the perspective of the neonatologist, the most important of the con-

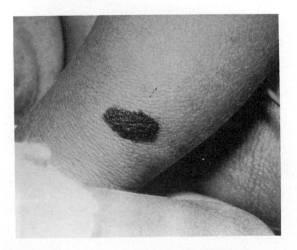

Figure 100–5. Dark brown irregular congenital nevus on the limb of an infant.

genital pigmented nevi. This is true because of their more than occasional propensity toward malignant degeneration (Reed et al., 1965; Greeley et al., 1965). These nevi vary in size from lesions of several centimeters to massive deformities covering half the body, usually in the thoracic area. Extremely large lesions involving the back, thorax, and abdomen are called "bathing-trunk nevi." The lesion is invariably noticed at birth, is raised, fleshy, brown or black, and has a leathery or cerebrate surface. Also, the pigment may appear to spill over, staining the surrounding skin with a junctional halo. Coarse hair grows in the area in many children but may not be apparent until childhood. Histologically, the lesion consists of a plethora of melanocytic nevus cells. These cells may be pigment-laden or clear and cuboidal or spindle-shaped and invade the entire cutis, subcutaneous tissue, and even muscle, fascia, and periosteum. The meninges may also be involved, resulting in central nervous system disorders and leptomeningeal melanocytosis (Reed et al., 1965; Hoffman and Freeman, 1967).

About 10 to 15 per cent of patients with giant pigmented hairy nevi of the bathing trunk type develop malignant melanoma. For this reason, it is desirable to remove these lesions surgically. The postoperative course in patients undergoing extensive procedures may be very difficult, but the dangers inherent in giant nevi warrant a drastic surgical approach.

Dysplastic Nevus Syndrome. Familial (B-K mole) or sporadic malignant melanoma may occur in some patients with acquired (postnatal) nevi. These usually slowly appear during adolescence (Elder et al., 1980).

White Macules

Localized areas of hypopigmentation on the skin of the newborn infant are prognostically significant. A distinction must first be made between vitiligo (or complete depigmentation) and hypopigmentation. The vitiliginous lesion is dead white when fully developed, and may be seen in ordinary daylight, even in fair skinned infants. The hypopigmented lesion is slightly lighter in color than the surrounding skin and, in fair-skinned children, may require exposure of the skin to a Wood's light to be made apparent. Simple hypopigmented macular plaques may be seen as an innocent unchanging localized defect in melanocyte function (achromic nevus), in congenital giant halo nevi containing a flat junction nevus surrounded by an area of hypopigmentation (Berge and Voorhees,

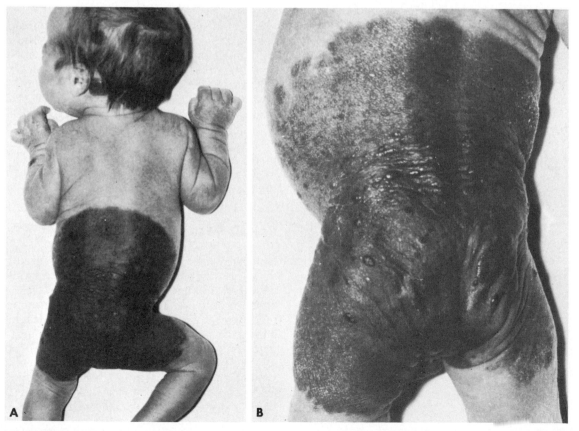

Figure 100–6. A, Newborn infant with large black nevus covering the "bathing trunk" area. The closer view (B) permits visualization of the nodular surface typical of giant nevi.

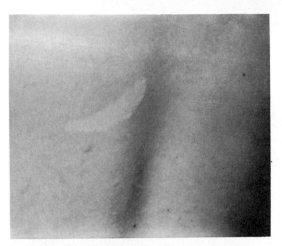

Figure 100–7. White leaf macule on the back of a patient with tuberous sclerosis.

1971), as a result of postinflammatory hypopigmentation, as a pale vascular anomaly called "nevus anemicus" (Greaves et al., 1970), or as evidence of an incipient hemangioma.

Small oval areas of hypopigmentation, often in the shape of a European–mountain-ash leaflet, are found at birth on the thorax and limbs of 90 per cent or more of infants with tuberous sclerosis, especially if the skin is carefully examined under a Wood's light (Mosher et al., 1979). The number of white spots may be quite variable, but their presence should alert the pediatrician to the need for a careful genetic history and thorough examination of the infant and all members of the family for further evidence of tuberous sclerosis. When a question exists about the nature of a hypopigmented macule, a biopsy specimen taken from it and prepared for electron microscopic examination may help resolve the issue. In vitiligo and partial albinism, a few or no melanocytes may be found. Melanocytes are present in the white macule of tuberous sclerosis, but the melanosomes are poorly pigmented.

Tuberous sclerosis is an autosomal dominant disease characterized by the development of multiple fibroangiomas, which ultimately may affect the skin (digital fibromas, adenoma sebaceum); the central nervous system (intercerebral tubers), leading to intracerebral calcification and seizure disorders; and the eye (retinal glial tumors). Moderate to severe mental retardation and seizures may be associated. The prognosis depends on the number of organs involved and the extent of fibroangiomatous involvement of individual organs. Serious complications of tuberous sclerosis include hamartomas of the lung and kidney and rhabdomyomas of the heart.

EPIDERMAL NEVI

Epidermal (epithelial, verrucous) nevi represent congenital disturbance of cells involved in keratin production and hypertrophy of the epidermis. These lesions may be present at birth and continue to spread during the first or second decade of life. Less frequently, they appear after the neonatal period. A spectrum of epidermal lesions may be seen on different anatomic areas of the same patient. The lesions may be deeply or slightly pigmented, be well or poorly demarcated, and have either a unilateral or bilateral distribution. Affected skin varies from warty to scaly. Given the morphologic variability of epidermal nevi, it is not surprising to find a host of Latin names describing them. Until evidence is accumulated to distinguish these lesions on other than strictly morphologic grounds, we prefer to consider epidermal nevi as a group. A brief description of some of the common morphologic variants follows:

1. *Nevus Unius Lateris:* A linear, highly verrucous lesion that streaks across a variable portion of the anatomy. The lesion may be strictly unilateral on one surface and cross the midline on another surface of the body. If the limbs are affected, nail deformity is frequent. When the scalp, face, or neck is involved, the adnexal tissues, such as the sebaceous glands, may participate by becoming enlarged. If a large part of the body is affected, the process may be referred to as "systematized epithelial nevus." When the sebaceous gland element on the scalp is very prominent, some authors prefer the term "linear nevus sebaceous."

2. *Verrucous nevus:* A more localized form that consists of a short (6 to 10 cm) warty streak across the thorax, arm, or abdomen. Occasionally (in the neck or axilla), the warty element is so localized as to result in a narrow string of small, soft tumors that resemble seborrheic keratoses but that are fleshier in consistency. Smaller epidermal nevi may be represented by a 2- to 3-centimeter linear lesion on the scalp or face, frequently mistaken for a melanocytic nevus.

3. *Ichthyosis Hystrix:* A scaly eruption often involving both sides of the body but in some areas stopping abruptly at the midline. The patterns formed

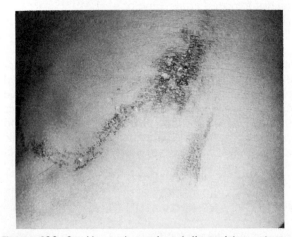

Figure 100–8. Linear hyperkeratotic epidermal nevus on the back and lateral thorax.

result in an appearance of marbling, feathery streaks, sheets, or whorls of colored thickenings of the skin.

Histopathology.   Two distinct forms of epidermal disorder may be seen:

1. Hyperkeratosis, papillomatosis, and a decrease in the granular layer.

2. Hyperkeratosis and vacuolization (ballooning) of the cells, which may give rise to microvesicles in the epidermis.

The former description is more often seen in nevus unius lateris and the latter in ichthyosis hystrix; however, we have seen both histologic pictures in biopsies taken from different areas in the same patient or in different stages of a single lesion.

Epidermal Nevus Syndrome.   The epidermal nevus syndrome (Solomon and Esterly, 1975) consists of widespread epidermal nevi (any of the aforementioned types); bony abnormalities, including kyphoscoliosis, hemihypertrophy, discordance in limb length and vertebral anomalies; central nervous system disorders, including seizures, mental retardation, and hemiplegia; and vascular disorders, primarily hemangiomas of skin and of the central nervous system. We have seen one case of Wilms' tumor with epidermal nevus but without hemihypertrophy. Other malignancies also occur in this syndrome with a greater than expected frequency, both in the affected skin and in other organ systems such as the brain, salivary glands, and kidney.

Treatment.   The optimal treatment of epidermal nevi of small dimension is simple excision down to the subcutaneous tissue. Lesions recur if underlying dermis is not removed. Since malignant degeneration (usually basal cell epitheliomas) may occur at a later date (Swint and Klaus, 1970), it is preferable to excise smaller lesions, but large lesions are difficult to treat surgically and it may be impractical to attempt surgery in all but exposed areas. One of us (LMS) has treated such severely affected adults with 13-cis-retinoic acid with modest success.

Prognosis.   Epidermal nevi in any other area except the scalp and face are unpredictable. Continued spread may persist until well after puberty. We have seen none resolve spontaneously. Affected infants should have a thorough physical examination and appropriate radiologic and electroencephalographic studies if defects in bony structure or neurologic function are detected.

JUVENILE XANTHOGRANULOMA

About one fifth of infants with juvenile xanthogranuloma have visible lesions at birth (Helwig and

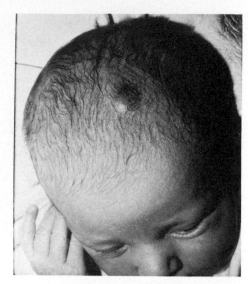

Figure 100–9.   Solitary juvenile xanthogranuloma on the scalp, a typical site for these lesions.

Hackney, 1954), and in two thirds they are present by 6 months of age (Nomland, 1959). Xanthogranulomas are benign tumors of fat-laden histiocytic cells and Touton giant cells associated with a chronic inflammatory process. In the majority of affected infants, the lesions are confined to the skin of the upper half of the body. Usually, they are firm, red-yellow papules; macules, nodules, and confluent lesions are rare (Esterly et al., 1972). Most of the lesions resolve spontaneously within 6 to 12 months of onset but may leave residual pigmentary or atrophic changes. The vast majority of infants are otherwise healthy and have no abnormalities of serum lipids. In 1979, Crocker reported that an increased incidence of familial café-au-lait spots and neurofibromatosis occurs in infants with juvenile xanthogranuloma.

Ocular involvement is the only complication of concern. Cellular infiltrates may invade the iris, ciliary body, episclera, or entire orbit. The ocular tumors may precede, coincide with, or follow the onset of skin lesions, and they may present as unilateral glaucoma, hyphema, uveitis, heterochromium iridis, or proptosis (Zimmerman, 1965; Gaynes and Cohen, 1967). Treatment of ocular lesions by x-irradiation or systemically administered corticosteroids may be necessary for prevention of serious sequelae (Gaynes and Cohen, 1967; Smith and Ingram, 1968). Very rarely, lesions have developed in the lung, testis, or pericardium. The cutaneous lesions do not require treatment.

MASTOCYTOSIS (URTICARIA PIGMENTOSA)

Mastocytosis is a disease of undetermined origin. Although pedigrees of affected individuals have been carefully studied (Selmanowitz et al., 1970), the question of genetic transmission remains unresolved. Mast cells may infiltrate the skin and result in a variety

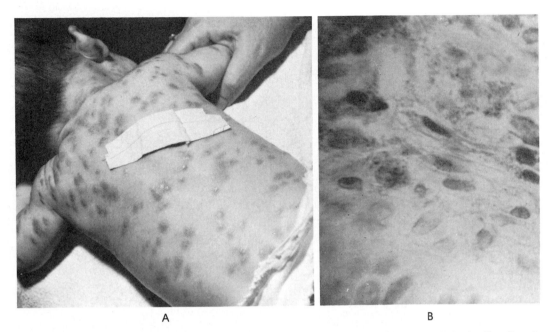

A   B

Figure 100–10. *A,* Deeply pigmented nodules and macules on the back of an infant with urticaria pigmentosa. A group of vesicles is visible just below the bandage that covers the biopsy site. *B,* Microscopic section from biopsy of patient stained with Giemsa. The mast cells can be identified as spindle-shaped cells containing granules that are located in the upper dermis.

of lesions of differing prognostic significance. Infants may have solitary lesions, a generalized maculopapular eruption, or, rarely, diffuse thickening of the skin (Sagher and Evan-Paz, 1967; Solomon and Esterly, 1973).

The solitary tumor may be discovered at birth or may develop shortly thereafter. The lesion is often oval, pink, yellow, or light brown, and it measures under 6 centimeters in length. It is raised, has a pebbly surface, and feels rubbery, and it may appear anywhere on the body surface. If rubbed or traumatized, mastocytomas develop a wheal (Darier's sign), and in the newborn infant they may blister or become hemorrhagic. A blister may be the sole presenting sign of a localized mast cell infiltrate.

All forms of the disease are due to an infiltrate of mast cells in the dermis that may be demonstrated by Giemsa stain. Symptoms are due to release of histamine from the mast cells. Itching is usual, and, with widespread lesions and occasionally with solitary lesions, massive histamine release may result in episodes of flushing, irritability, tachycardia, respiratory distress, and hypotension. Coagulopathy may occur rarely. In the systemic form of the disease, the liver, spleen, lymph nodes, bone marrow, and gastrointestinal tract may show evidence of mast cell invasion (Sagher and Evan-Paz, 1967).

Solitary cutaneous lesions usually have no systemic component and may be treated conservatively without recourse to extensive studies and with every expectation that the lesion will resolve spontaneously within a few years. The maculopapular form also has a relatively good prognosis in childhood. Systemic involvement carries a poor prognosis.

In patients with any form of mastocytosis, the following should be avoided: trauma to the lesions, hot showers, excessive rubbing, aspirin, codeine, polymyxin B, and procaine (all histamine releasers). Cyproheptadine hydrochloride in regular doses may offer some relief when symptoms become bothersome. Oral disodium cromoglycate has helped relieve symptoms in adults.

REFERENCES

Albright, I., Butler, A. M., Hampton, A. O., and Smith, P.: Syndrome characterized by osteitis fibrosis disseminata, areas of pigmentation and endocrine dysfunction with precocious puberty in females. N. Engl. J. Med. *216*:727, 1937.

Alexander, G. L., and Norman, R. M.: The Sturge-Weber Syndrome. Bristol, John Wright and Sons, 1960.

Alper, J., Holmes, L. B., and Mihm, M. C.: Birthmarks with serious medical significance: nevocellular nevi, sebaceous nevi, and multiple café au lait spots. J. Pediatr. *95*:696, 1979.

Bartsky, S. H., Rosen, S., Geer, D. E., et al.: The nature and evolution of port wine stains: a computer assisted study. J. Invest. Dermatol. *74*:154, 1980.

Berger, R. S., and Voorhees, J. J.: Multiple congenital giant nevocellular nevi with halos. Arch. Dermatol. *104*:515, 1971.

Berman, B., and Lim, H. W. P.: Concurrent cutaneous and hepatic hemangiomata in infancy. Report of a case and a review of the literature. J. Cutan. Surg. Oncol. 4:869, 1978.

Bidot-Lopez, P., and Frankel, J. W.: Enhanced viral transformation of skin fibroblasts from neurofibromatosis patients. Ann. Clin. Lab. Med. 13:27, 1983.

Brown, S. H., Jr., Neerhout, R. C., and Fonkalsrud, E. W.: Prednisone therapy in the management of large hemangiomas in infants and children. Surgery 71:168, 1972.

Burman, D., Mansell, P. W. A., and Warin, R. P.: Miliary hemangiomata in the newborn. Arch. Dis. Child. 42:193, 1967.

Crocker, A. L.: The histiocytosis syndromes. In: Fitzpatrick, T. B., Eisen, A. Z., Wolff, K., Freedberg, I. M., and Austen, K. F.: Dermatology in General Medicine. 2nd ed. McGraw-Hill, 1979, p. 1171.

Crowe, F. W., Schull, W. J., and Neel, J. V.: A Clinical, Pathological and Genetic Study of Multiple Neurofibromatosis. Springfield, Charles C Thomas, 1956.

Eady, P. A. J., Sparrow, G. P., and Grice, K.: Naevoid pigmentation with giant melanosomes. Two cases. Proc. Roy. Soc. Med. 68:759, 1975.

Elder, D. E., Goldman, L. I., Goldman, S. C., Greene, M. H., and Clark, W. H., Jr.: Dysplastic nevus syndrome. Cancer 46:1787, 1980.

Esterly, N. B., Sahihi, T., and Medenica, M.: Juvenile xanthogranuloma: an atypical case with study of ultrastructure. Arch. Dermatol. 105:99, 1972.

Fost, N. C., and Esterly, N. B.: Successful treatment of juvenile hemangiomas with prednisone. J. Pediatr. 72:351, 1968.

Fretzin, D. F., and Potter, B.: Blue rubber bleb nevus. Arch. Intern. Med. 116:924, 1965.

Gaynes, P. M., and Cohen, G. S.: Juvenile xanthogranuloma of the orbit. Am. J. Ophthalmol. 63:755, 1967.

Greaves, M. W., Birckett, D., and Johnson, C.: Nevus anemicus: a unique catecholamine dependent nevus. Arch. Dermatol. 102:172, 1970.

Greeley, P. W., Middleton, A. G., and Curtain, J. W.: Incidence of malignancy in giant pigmented nevi. Plast. Reconstr. Surg., 36:26, 1965.

Harris, L. E., Stayura, L. A., Ramirez-Talavera, P. F., and Annegers, J. F.: Congenital and acquired abnormalities observed in live born and stillborn neonates. Mayo Clin. Proc. 50:85, 1975.

Helwig, E., and Hackney, V. C.: Juvenile xanthogranuloma. Am. J. Pathol. 30:625, 1954.

Hidano, A., and Nakajima, S.: Earliest features of the strawberry mark in the newborn. Br. J. Dermatol. 87:138, 1972.

Hoffman, H. J., and Freeman, A.: Primary leptomeningeal melanoma in association with giant hairy nevi. Report of two cases. J. Neurosurg. 26:62, 1967.

Holden, K. R., and Alexander, R.: Diffuse neonatal hemangiomatosis. Pediatrics 46:411, 1970.

Johnson, B. L., and Charneco, D. R.: The café-au-lait spot in neurofibromatosis and normal individuals. Arch. Dermatol. 102:442, 1970.

Kontras, S. G., Green, O. C., King, L., and Diran, R. J.: Giant hemangioma with thrombocytopenia. Am. J. Dis. Child. 105:188, 1963.

Lund, H. A., and Kraus, J. M.: Melanotic tumors of the skin. Fascicle 3, Atlas of Tumor Pathology. Armed Forces Institute of Pathology. Washington, D. C., 1962.

Mangus, D. J.: Continuous compression therapy of hemangiomas: evaluation in two cases. Plast. Reconstr. Surg. 49:490, 1973.

Margileth, A. M.: Developmental vascular abnormalities. Med. Clin. North Am. 18:773, 1971.

Mizrahi, A. M., and Sachs, P. M.: Generalized congenital phlebectasia. Am. J. Dis. Child. 112:72, 1966.

Mosher, D. B., Fitzpatrick, T. B., and Ortonne, J. P.: Abnormalities of pigmentation. In: Fitzpatrick, T. B., Eisen, A. Z., Wolff, K., Freedberg, I. M., and Austen, K. F.: Dermatology in General Medicine, 2nd ed. New York, McGraw-Hill, 1979, p. 594.

Mulliken, J. B., and Glowacki, J.: Hemangiomas and vascular malformations in infants and children: a classification based on endothelial characteristics. Plast. Reconstr. Surg. 69:421, 1982.

Mullins, J. F., Naylor, D., and Pedetski, J.: The Klippel-Trenaunay-Weber syndrome (nevus vasculosus osteohypertrophicus). Arch. Dermatol. 86:202, 1962.

Nomland, R.: Nevoxanthogranuloma. J. Invest. Dermatol. 22:207, 1959.

Ortonne, J. P., et al.: Valeur diagnostique des taches café-au-lait (TCL). Ann. Dermatol. Venereol. (Paris) 107:313, 1980.

Pack, G. T., and Davis, J.: Moles. N.Y. State. J. Med. 56:3998, 1956.

Peachy, R. D. G., Lim, C. C., and Whimster, J. W.: Lymphangioma of skin. A review of 65 cases. Br. J. Dermatol. 83:519, 1970.

Peterman, A. F., Hayles, A. B., Dockerty, M. B., and Love, J. G.: Encephalotrigeminal angiomatosis (Sturge-Weber disease): clinical study of 35 cases. J.A.M.A. 167:2169, 1958.

Pinkus, H., and Mehnegan, A. H.: A Guide to Dermatohistopathology. New York, Appleton-Century-Crofts, Inc., 1969, pp. 352–354.

Pinkus, H., and Mehnegan, A. H.: A Guide to Dermatohistopathology. 2nd ed. New York, Appleton-Century-Crofts, Inc., 1981, pp. 495–496.

Pratt, A. G.: Birthmarks in infancy. Arch. Dermatol. 67:302, 1953.

Reed, W. B., Becker, S. W., Sr., Becker, S. W., Jr., and Nickel, W. R.: Giant pigmented nevi, melanoma and leptomeningeal melanocytosis. Arch. Dermatol. 91:100, 1965.

Rhodes, A. R., and Melski, J. W.: Small congenital nevocellular nevi and the risk of cutaneous melanoma. J. Pediatr. 100:219, 1982.

Rhodes, A. R., Sober A. J., Day, C. L., Melski, J. W., Harrist, T. J., Mihm, M. C., and Fitzpatrick, T. B.: The malignant potential of small congenital nevocellular nevi: an estimate of association based on a histologic study of 234 primary cutaneous melanomas. J. Am. Acad. Dermatol. 6:620, 1982.

Rodriguez-Erdmann, F., Button, L., Murray, J. E., and Moloney, M.: Kasabach-Merritt syndrome: coagulo-analytical observations. Am. J. Med. Sci. 261:9, 1971.

Rook, A.: Angiomatous nevi. In Rook, A., Wilkinson, D. S., and Ebling, F. J. G. (eds.): Textbook of Dermatology. 2nd Ed. Blackwell Scientific Pub., London, 1972, p. 140.

Sagher, F. and Evan-Paz, Z.: Mastocytosis and the Mast Cell. Chicago, Year Book Medical Publishers, 1967.

Saijo, M., Munroe, I. R., and Mancer, K.: Lymphangioma: long-term follow-up study. Plast. Reconstr. Surg. 56:642, 1975.

Sanchez, N. P., Rhodes, A. R., Mandell, F., and Mihm, M. C.: Encephalocraniocutaneous lipomatosis: a new syndrome. Br. J. Dermatol. 104:89, 1981.

Selmanowitz, V. J., Orentreich, N., Tiangco, C. C., and Demis, D. J.: Uniovular twins discordant for cutaneous mastocytosis. Arch. Dermatol. 102:34, 1970.

Shim, W. K. T.: Hemangiomas of infancy complicated by thrombocytopenia. Am. J. Surg. 116:896, 1968.

Simpson, J. R.: Natural history of cavernous hemangiomata. Lancet 2:1057, 1959.

Smith, J. L. S., and Ingram, R. M.: Juvenile oculodermal xanthogranuloma. Br. J. Ophthalmol. 52:696, 1968.

Solomon, L. M.: The management of congenital melanocytic nevi. Arch. Dermatol. 116:1017, 1980.

Solomon, L. M., and Esterly, N. B.: Neonatal Dermatology. Philadelphia, W. B. Saunders Co., 1973.

Solomon, L. M., and Esterly, N. B.: Epidermal and other congenital organoid nevi. Curr. Probl. Pediatr. Nov. 1975.

Solomon, L. M., Fretzin, D. F., and De Wald, R. L.: The epidermal nevus syndrome. Arch Dermatol. 97:273, 1968.

Swint, R. B., and Klaus, S. W.: Malignant degeneration of an epithelial nevus. Arch. Dermatol. 101:56, 1970.

Wade, T. R., Kamino, H., and Ackerman, A. B.: A histologic atlas of vascular lesions. J. Dermatol. Surg. Oncol. 4:845, 1978.

Way, B. H., Herrmana, J., Gilbert, E. F., Johnson, S. A. M., and Opitz, J. M.: Cutis marmorata telangiectatica congenita. J. Cutan. Pathol. 1:10, 1974.

Whitehouse, D.: Diagnostic value of the café-au-lait spot in children. Arch. Dis. Child. 41:316, 1966.

Zimmerman, L. C.: Ocular lesions of juvenile xanthogranuloma. Am. J. Ophthalmol. 60:1011, 1965.

101

In this chapter, we will discuss a number of mysterious cutaneous disorders that cause concern to the physician or mother. Most of these disorders are self-limited, some are quite serious, and the pathogenesis of only one of them (miliaria) is understood. They share one common characteristic: All may be diagnosed with certainty, and, for this reason, a clear concept of the clinical process and the requisites for establishing a diagnosis are essential for pediatricians.

Miscellaneous Skin Disorders

By Lawrence M. Solomon and Nancy B. Esterly

Seborrheic Eczema

Definition. Perhaps a word about terminology is appropriate because of the commonly expressed bewilderment about what the terms "eczema," "dermatitis," and "seborrhea" mean. Some authors consider the term "eczema" to be synonymous with "dermatitis." For the purposes of discussion, we would like to consider this term to represent a "family" of diseases, whereas "eczema" may be considered a "genus" and "atopic eczema" a "species" of cutaneous disorder. The qualifying adjective "seborrheic" describes a type of inflammatory skin disease that has a particular appearance and evolution and is therefore fairly specific (Solomon and Rostenberg, 1978).

Appearance. Seborrheic eczema is a common disorder having two peaks of occurrence in early infancy. It appears during the first week or two of life as "cradle cap," or "milk crust," and then again from the end of the first month to the third month, this time as a more widespread process involving the scalp, ears, forehead, and flexural areas, including the perineum (Beare and Rook, 1972).

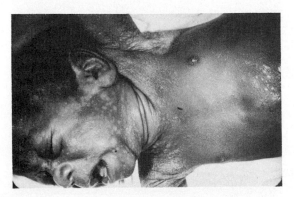

Figure 101–1. Infant with seborrheic eczema on the face and neck and in the axillae. Note the scaling and hypopigmentation. Temporary hypopigmentation is common in black infants with this disorder.

The primary lesion of seborrheic eczema is a greasy, yellow, flaky scale on an erythematous base. The scales coalesce to form patches that may, in flexural areas such as the ear folds, erode and leave fissures that weep and become infected. Other areas that may become involved are the neck folds, arm and leg folds, and the diaper area.

Etiology. The cause of seborrheic eczema is unknown, but it is one of the group of eczemas that appear to be endogenous in origin, as opposed to the exogenous eczemas caused by, for example, primary irritants, infections, or topical allergens. There has been considerable speculation as to the relationship of seborrheic eczema to atopic eczema, a disease that occurs in the older infant. Certainly, the cutaneous lesions and distribution in both conditions are often similar. Furthermore, occasional cases of seborrheic eczema diagnosed with assurance when first seen in the month-old infant may, on prolonged observation, evolve into typical atopic eczema. It is almost impossible on strictly morphologic grounds to say that any one child with seborrheic eczema will not develop atopic eczema. Some observers consider the greasy, scaling eruption of seborrhea as an early stage of atopic eczema.

Evaluation. Most infants with seborrheic eczema seem perfectly well except for the dermatitis.* The eruption may last 3 to 6 weeks or longer and then heal and never reappear, or it may, as mentioned previously, evolve into atopic dermatitis. In the rare infant, seborrheic eczema may become a generalized process with full-blown exfoliative erythroderma, or *Leiner's disease.* Familial cases of Leiner's disease have an ominous prognosis (Jacobs and Miller,

---

* The presence of purpura and systemic manifestations, such as listlessness, poor feeding, failure to thrive, recurrent fever, mouth lesions, or hepatosplenomegaly, should alert the physician to the possibility that the eczematous process may be a manifestation of a serious underlying illness, such as Wiskott-Aldrich syndrome or histiocytosis (Solomon and Esterly, 1973; Fitzpatrick, 1981).

1972). It has recently become apparent that familial Leiner's disease may be a manifestation of a functional defect of the fifth component of complement (C5). The administration of plasma was life-saving for the infants studied (Jacobs and Miller, 1972).

Treatment.   For cradle cap: Frequent shampooing is the secret to effective management of the condition. Sebulex shampoo or Fostex cream or (in the winter months) a tar shampoo should control the problem and may be used daily or two or three times a week, depending on the severity of the scaling. When the scaling persists, 1 per cent salicylic acid or 3 per cent sulfur in cold cream may be applied to the scalp following the shampoo.

For seborrheic eczema in flexures or diaper area: Bathe the infant with *tepid* water containing a little Alpha Keri oil (advise the mother to expect a slippery infant). Any soap, such as Dove soap, will do. Dress in cotton clothing, avoiding wool, nylon, or abrasive synthetic fabrics. Absorbent, disposable diapers are acceptable but should be changed frequently. The perineum may be protected with simple zinc oxide paste.* The soiled paste can be removed with mineral oil at each diaper change, then fresh paste can be applied. One per cent hydrocortisone cream may be used up to four times a day for brief periods, periodically (8 to 14 days), to accelerate resolution. It is frequently wise to culture the perineal area, where pustules or ulceration may herald supervening infection with *Candida* or pathogenic bacteria. Appropriate treatment should be instituted if pathogenic organisms are identified. The infant's room should be humidified in winter and air-conditioned in summer, since infants with widespread dermatitis may have difficulty tolerating extremes of heat, dryness, or humidity.

Harlequin Color Change

This condition is not to be confused with an entirely different disorder called harlequin fetus. Harlequin color change, first described by Neligan and Strang in 1952, is characterized by reddening of one half of the body and simultaneous blanching of the other half. A sharp line of demarcation runs from the center of the forehead, down the nose and chin and trunk, very nearly in the midline. Occasionally, the line of demarcation may be incomplete, sparing the face and genitalia. Harlequin color change occurs most frequently in low birth weight infants, but the color change may be seen in about 10 per cent of other-

wise normal infants on the third and fourth days of life, and occasionally earlier or later. Apparently the color change is accentuated by gravitational force, since turning the body from one side to the other induces blanching of the upper half and reddening of the lower half. The total duration of these episodes may vary from a few minutes to several hours. Harlequin color change occurs most often during the first 4 days of life (Mortensen and Stougard-Andresen, 1959), but some infants may still experience such episodes up to 3 weeks of age. There is no accompanying change in respiratory rate, pupillary reflexes, muscle tone, or response to external stimuli. Harlequin color change probably represents a state of vascular instability related to temporary inadequacy of the autonomic nervous system. It has no pathologic significance, requires no treatment, and can be expected to disappear no later than the third week of life.

Acne Neonatorum

Acne neonatorum is usually a self-limited process, but has most interesting physiologic, genetic, and pathologic implications. The lesions can be found at birth or may not be noticed until several weeks postnatally. They appear in crops on the cheeks, nose, chin, and, occasionally, forehead. Individually, each lesion may be an open comedo (a blackhead), a closed comedo (a granular, pale papule), or an inflammatory papule. Cystic lesions very rarely occur. The patients in this age group are almost always boys. In infantile acne, which occurs after 3 months of age, there is only a small preponderance of males over females.

Acne neonatorum is, surprisingly, sometimes difficult to distinguish at first examination from other common conditions found in the newborn. The differential diagnosis and discriminating features include the following:

1. Erythema toxicum—there are lesions on the trunk. The process usually resolves in 72 hours. The

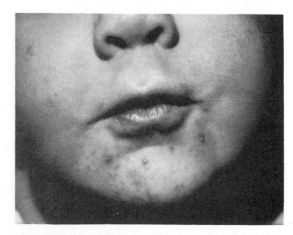

Figure 101–2. Papules, pustules, and comedones (acne) on the chin and cheeks of an infant male.

* Zinc oxide 30 per cent, talc 30 per cent, petrolatum 40 per cent.

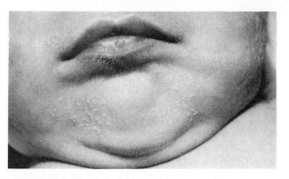

Figure 101–3. Numerous grouped milia on the chin of a newborn infant.

classic "flea bite" appearance of the lesion connotes much inflammation in erythema toxicum.

2. Milia*—the lesions are smaller, uniform in appearance, and not inflammatory. Comedones are absent.

3. Miliaria rubra—the lesions tend to be vesiculopustular and widespread, mostly involving intertriginous areas.

4. Sebaceous gland hyperplasia—these are uniform, pinpoint, yellow, noninflammatory papules without comedones.

5. Candidiasis—scrapings for potassium hydroxide (KOH) preparations and cultures from the lesions should resolve this possible source of confusion.

6. Follicular eczema in the older infant may closely mimic the changes seen in acne. The presence of eczema elsewhere on the body should alert the astute observer to the diagnosis.

7. An acneiform eruption of the forehead and face may be caused by excessive use of petrolatum, oils, or creams.

8. Keratosis pilaris—this disorder frequently affects the cheeks of infants and may be very difficult to distinguish from an acneiform eruption. Often only time helps permit adequate evolution and destruction of the two disorders.

The cause of acne neonatorum has not been elucidated, but certain elements that may contribute to the process have been studied. In most instances, the infant does not suffer from an endocrine disturbance, since the urinary excretion of 17-ketosteroids is normal (Tromovitch et al., 1963). There is, however, a strong genetic component to the process, since a familial tendency for acne is frequently present (Hellier, 1954). The fact that infants with infantile acne tend to develop severe acne later in life (Hellier, 1954) suggests that the acnegenic process in the infant is related to a genetically determined end-organ (pilosebaceous unit) hyperresponsiveness to androgens, possibly those of the mother, that have crossed the placental barrier. Androgens produced by the male infant are probably also contributory factors. It is also interesting to note that infants with the feminizing testis syndrome, who are unable to respond to testosterone, never develop infantile (or adolescent) acne.

In most instances, given the self-limited nature of the process, no special treatment of neonatal acne is required. In severe cases, a mild salicylic acid or sulfur-containing lotion, such as lotio alba or Komed lotion, will suffice. Alternatively, a mild water-based benzoyl peroxide is also helpful. Creams, ointments, and topical steroids should be avoided. The face may be washed with plain soap and water or Fostex soap. Caution is necessary in using irritant scrubs or lotions (such as retinoic acid or benzoyl peroxide) on infants with very fair skin, since one may stimulate more of an inflammatory reaction than one bargained for. Similarly, irritants used on black skin may cause unwanted hyper- or hypopigmentation at the site of treatment.

Milia and Sebaceous Gland Hyperplasia

Milia are formed in about 40 per cent of full-term infants (Gordon, 1959). They are multiple (single lesions are called "milium"), 1- to 2-millimeter keratin-filled white lesions that occur on the face of the newborn. The sites of predilection are the cheeks, nasolabial folds, forehead, nose, ears, chin, and periorbital areas. Large milia (more than 2 mm) are found in the orofaciodigital (OFD) syndrome (Solomon et al., 1970). Rarely, milia may occur in unusual sites, such as on the arms and legs or the penis.

Histologically, a milium represents a defect in pilosebaceous formation in which an invagination of epidermal tissue forms a keratin-producing pocket that eventually may lose its canalicular attachment to the surface and, thereby, become a cyst lined by several layers of keratin-producing cells. The expressed contents of milial cysts resemble tiny white pearls and consist mostly of keratin.

The most frequent confusion in diagnosis stems from the resemblance of milia to the lesions of sebaceous gland hyperplasia, which occur in the same areas. The papules of sebaceous gland hyperplasia are smaller (pinpoint) lesions that are more yellow, and sebaceous material can be expressed from them. Milia usually exfoliate within a few weeks without scarring. Even the large milia of the OFD syndrome exfoliate in 3 to 4 months, but these lesions do leave pitted scars.

EPSTEIN'S PEARLS

These tiny cystic lesions occur in about 85 per cent of newborn infants. The lesions are usually grouped,

---

* A rare exception is the giant milia found on the face and ears in the orofaciodigital syndrome. These cystic lesions are usually very striking, and examination of the mouth, hair, and hands should resolve the diagnostic dilemma.

firm, and movable, and they are opaque white, in contrast to mucinous and alveolar cysts, which are larger, translucent, and somewhat firmly adherent to the alveolar ridge tissue. Epstein's pearls are also self-limited but may take several months to resolve (Solomon and Esterly, 1973).

Erythema Toxicum Neonatorum

Erythema toxicum is an inflammatory cutaneous disease of unknown origin that affects about half of all full-term newborns. It occurs more frequently among term-weight infants (2 kg and more) and less frequently among preterm infants (Harris and Schick, 1956; Taylor and Bondurant, 1957; Carr et al., 1966). Lesions are occasionally present at birth. In the majority of infants, the lesions develop at between 24 and 48 hours but may occur as late as 2 weeks postpartum. No predilection of the disease for race, sex, season, or geographic location has been noted.

The basic lesion in erythema toxicum is a small (1 to 3 mm) papule that becomes a sterile vesicle, usually white and firm and surrounded by a prominent halo of erythema and some edema. An entire lesion may measure about 1 to 3 centimeters across. The number of lesions present may vary from a few to dozens. The areas most frequently involved are the chest and back, but the arms, legs, buttocks, and face may not be spared. Individual lesions may last only a few hours, but the eruption usually lasts 3 to 6 days, disappearing spontaneously. Recurrence is rare. There is no evidence of systemic manifestations accompanying the process, other than peripheral blood eosinophilia of varying degree.

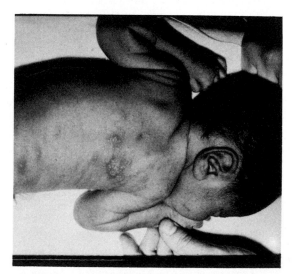

Figure 101–4. Florid lesions of erythema toxicum on the back of a newborn infant. The pustules are large and surrounded by an erythematous halo. Smears of the pustular contents showed only eosinophils.

On examination of histologic secretions prepared from a lesion of erythema toxicum, one finds eosinophil-filled intraepidermal vesicles and an intradermal inflammatory component, also heavily infiltrated with eosinophils but containing other polymorphonuclear leucocytes and a few lymphocytes. These cells, usually accompanied by edema, tend to localize around superficial blood vessels, and especially around the superficial portion of the pilosebaceous organ. The eosinophilic infiltrate has suggested to some authors that erythema toxicum is a disease of hypersensitivity, but studies attempting to incriminate chemical or microbiologic substances, acquired either transplacentally or vaginally from mother, drugs, topical irritants, sebum, or milk, have failed to provide support for this hypothesis. At present, all that can be said with certainty is that erythema toxicum is a benign inflammatory disease of unknown cause.

The differential diagnosis of erythema toxicum may occasionally raise some troublesome doubts. Entities that may be considered as possible alternatives to the diagnosis include transient neonatal pustular melanosis, miliaria rubra, pyoderma, and candidiasis. Miliaria rubra usually affects the flexures, face, arms, and legs, and it rarely disappears as rapidly without treatment as does erythema toxicum. Moreover, the vesicles do not contain eosinophils in abundance. Pyoderma and cutaneous candidiasis may be identified by gram stain and KOH preparation and culture of the pustular contents. Furthermore, polymorphonuclear leukocytes predominate in the pustule of pyoderma. A useful diagnostic procedure when the diagnosis is in doubt consists of preparation of a Wright- or Giemsa-stained smear from the intralesional contents. The presence of large numbers of eosinophils may be considered strong evidence to support a diagnosis of erythema toxicum if the infant is otherwise well.

Erythema toxicum requires no treatment, since it resolves spontaneously within a brief period. Not infrequently, however, a mother may worry about the eruption, and reassurance should be provided.

Miliaria

Miliaria is a cutaneous eruption caused by a functional or morphologic disturbance in sweat secretion. In the days before air-conditioned nurseries were commonplace, miliaria was a frequent occurrence; however, with the advent of environmental humidity and temperature control, it has decreased sharply in frequency. Lately, with the use of phototherapy for hyperbilirubinuria, we are once more observing an increase in this minor cutaneous nuisance. This recrudescence is probably brought about by the heat generated by the lights placed over the incubators and inadequate air flow in the crib or incubator.

Miliaria takes two principal clinical forms, depending on the site of obstruction in the sweat duct. The less serious form, *miliaria crystallina*, consists of small, very superficial, clear, thin-walled, noninflammatory vesicles, resulting from sweat retention localized in the epidermis just below the stratum corneum. *Miliaria rubra* consists of small, erythematous, grouped papules and results from rupture of the intraepidermal portion of the sweat duct. The resultant vesicle is found at the level of the basal layer of the epidermis and may be surrounded by many inflammatory cells. The papules may become pustular if the inflammatory component is prominent.

The distribution of miliaria is usually accentuated in the intertriginous areas, but it is common to find the face, scalp, and shoulders also involved.

During the first few days of life, the differential diagnosis of miliaria includes erythema toxicum, candidal infection, and early pyoderma. Culture, gram stain, and KOH preparation of vesicular contents should resolve the question regarding the presence of yeast or bacteria. The vesicles of erythema toxicum are usually full of eosinophils. Treatment of miliaria should be conservative. The infant may be placed in a cooler, less humid environment, and the application of calamine lotion to the body folds should result in resolution of the lesions in several days.

Sclerema Neonatorum

Sclerema neonatorum is a serious, uncommon cutaneous change occurring in the first or, less commonly, second week of life in debilitated or preterm newborns. It results in widespread stone-hard, nonpitting induration of the skin. The affected infant is immobilized and feels cold to the touch. The face is

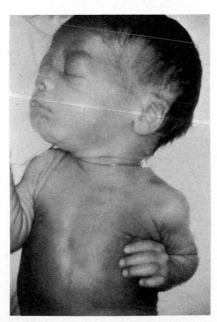

Figure 101–5. Sclerema neonatorum. Note the masklike expression on the face, "pseudotrismus" of the partially immobilized mouth, and thickening of the skin over the face, arms, and hands. (From the Collection of the American Academy of Pediatrics. Reproduced with permission of the officers of the Academy.)

fixed in a masklike expression; the joints are stiff. The skin change is a manifestation of a systemic process that may include sepsis, pneumonia, gastroenteritis, and, occasionally, multiple congenital anomalies. Body temperature and blood pressure are unstable, feeding is poor, and apneic spells are common. Complications such as central nervous system depression, cyanosis, respiratory distress, and convulsions frequently supervene. Changes in blood urea nitrogen and potassium and decrease in blood carbon dioxide (Levin and Milunsky, 1965) may reflect the severe constitutional stress.

The mechanism responsible for the sclerema is unknown, but biochemical and crystalline changes in the subcutaneous fat of affected infants have suggested a shift in its composition toward an increase in triglycerides (Horsefield and Yardley, 1965) and in the ratio of saturated to unsaturated fats. Specifically, palmitin and stearin were found to be increased, with abnormal excess formation of a large crystalline structure of these substances in the subcutaneous fat (Kellum, 1968).

The histologic changes in sclerema are not highly specific; surprisingly little inflammation is evident. On examination of sections from biopsies, one usually sees edema and thickening of the interlobular septa of the fat panniculus.

The treatment of sclerema neonatorum is essentially that of management of a very sick infant. Maintenance of normal body temperature, control of infection, adequate nutrition, and balance of fluid and electrolytes are required. Corticosteroid therapy has been advocated for this disorder, but controlled studies have not shown steroids to be effective in altering the mortality rate (Levin et al., 1961), which approaches 50 per cent.

Subcutaneous Fat Necrosis

The lesions of subcutaneous fat necrosis are very similar to those of sclerema neonatorum, and the pathogenesis leading to the two diseases may be identical. However, the former process is highly localized, whereas the latter is diffuse; the infant with sclerema is usually very sick, whereas subcutaneous fat necrosis may be a benign self-limited process. Subcutaneous fat necrosis is usually discovered within the first 2 weeks of life, most frequently between the fifth and tenth days, but may be found as early as the second or as late as the twenty-fourth day. The lesions are sharply circumscribed nodules or plaques, hard, and of a dusky reddish-purple hue. Most often, they are found in areas in which a fat pad is present: cheeks, buttocks, back, arms, and thighs. The affected area may have an uneven surface and a sharp margin delineating it from surrounding normal skin. The lesions may become the site of

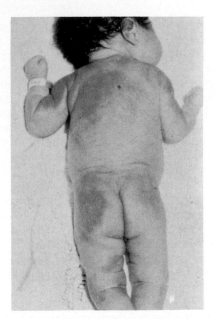

Figure 101–6. Rear view of newborn showing several large discolored areas of subcutaneous fat necrosis. They were irregular in size and shape, felt firm, and were not hot or tender.

dystrophic subcutaneous calcification, and rarely, hypercalcemia may accompany the process. When cutaneous calcification is present, radiographic examination of the skin may provide supportive evidence for the diagnosis. Extensive calcification may lead to extrusion and drainage of a liquefied material from the discharging lesion. The drainage site (usually sterile) often heals with scarring.

Although most infants appear to suffer few systemic complications of subcutaneous fat necrosis, a few vomit, fail to thrive, become irritable, develop fever, and refuse to feed. Rarely, visceral calcification may supervene (Sharlin and Koblenzer, 1970).

Numerous causes have been ascribed to subcutaneous fat necrosis. Most prominent among these are obstetric trauma, intrauterine asphyxia (Chen et al., 1981), and hypothermia. Obstetric trauma is commonly observed without the consequences of fat necrosis, and the maintenance of normal body temperature is a common problem in healthy preterm infants, so one must take a reserved attitude toward these suppositions. It is probable that if these factors contribute to fat necrosis, they do so only in infants susceptible to the disease.

The management of subcutaneous fat necrosis depends on the severity of the process, the presence of drainage ulcerations, and systemic complications. In all cases, *warm or hot packs to the lesions should be avoided.* In most infants, the process is self-limited and resolution occurs over a period of a few weeks to months without much residual atrophy or scarring. Where fluctuant areas are present, careful needle as-

piration may reduce scarring. In infants with hypercalcemia or visceral calcification, restriction of oral calcium intake, decrease in vitamin D intake, and administration of corticosteroids systemically may aid in resolution of the process.

Transient Neonatal Pustular Melanosis

This benign disorder occurs relatively frequently in the newborn and is most apparent at birth in blacks. Characteristic lesions consist of small, superficial pustules that rupture easily, leaving a collarette of fine scale and hyperpigmented macules that are often discernible at the sites of unroofed pustules. The macules are seen more commonly at birth and may represent end-stage lesions of pustules that have ruptured in utero. The lesions may be profuse or sparse and can involve all body surfaces, including the palms, soles, and scalp. Areas of predilection are the forehead, anterior neck and submental area, lower back, and shins.

The cause of the eruption is unknown. Affected infants are otherwise well. Gram stains and bacterial cultures obtained from intact pustules uniformly fail to disclose the presence of organisms. Wright-stained smears of pustular fluid contain cellular debris, polymorphonuclear leukocytes, and few or no eosinophils. The differential diagnosis includes erythema toxicum, candidiasis, and staphylococcal pyoderma, which can usually be distinguished with the aforementioned studies. The pustules last about 48 hours; the macules may persist for up to 3 months. The

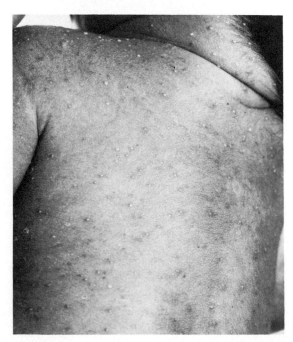

Figure 101–7. Numerous superficial pustules on the neck and back of a 1-day-old infant. A few pustules have ruptured, leaving a collarette of scale.

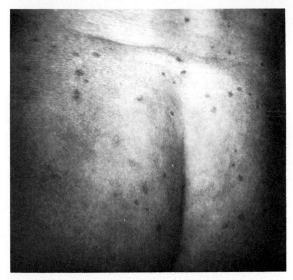

Figure 101–8. Transient neonatal pustular melanosis. Hyperpigmented macules on the lower back and buttocks, some of which are encircled by scale. (From Ramamurthy, R. S., Reveri, M., Esterly, N. B., Fretzin, D. F., Pyati, S. P., Sethupathy, R., and Pildes, R. S.: Transient neonatal pustular melanosis. J. Pediatr. *88*:831, 1976.)

disorder is transient and self-limited and requires no therapy.

REFERENCES

Beare, J. M., and Rook, A.: The newborn. *In* Rook, A., Wilkinson, D. S., and Ebling, F. J. G. (Eds.): Textbook of Dermatology. 2nd ed. Philadelphia, F. A. Davis Co., 1972, p. 168.

Carr, J. A., Hodgeman, J. E., Freedman, R. J., and Levan, N. E.: Relationship between toxic erythema and infant maturity. A.M.A. J. Dis. Child. *112*:129, 1966.

Chen, T. H., Shewmake, S. W., Hansen, D. D., and Lacey, H. L.: Subcutaneous fat necrosis of the newborn. Arch. Dermatol. *117*:36, 1981.

Fitzpatrick, R., Rapaport, M. S., and Silva, D. G.: Histiocytosis X. Arch. Dermatol. *117*:253, 1981.

Gordon, J.: Miliary sebaceous cysts and blisters in the healthy newborn. Acta Obstet. Gynaecol. Scand. *38*:352, 1959.

Harris, J. R., and Schick, B.: Erythema neonatorum. A.M.A. J. Dis. Child. *92*:27, 1956.

Hellier, F. F.: Acneiform eruptions in infancy. Br. J. Dermatol. *66*:25, 1954.

Horsefield, G. J., and Yardley, H. J.: Sclerema neonatorum. J. Invest. Dermatol. *44*:326, 1965.

Jacobs, J. C., and Miller, M. E.: Fatal familial Leiner's disease: a deficiency of the opsonic activity of serum complement. Pediatrics *49*:225, 1972.

Kellum, R. E., Ray, T. L., and Brown, G. R.: Sclerema neonatorum. Report of case analysis of subcutaneous and epidermaldermal lipids by chromatographic methods. Arch. Dermatol. *97*:372, 1968.

Levin, S. E., Bakst, C. M., and Isserow, L.: Sclerema neonatorum treated with corticosteroids. Br. Med. J. *2*:1533, 1961.

Levin, S. E., and Milunsky, A.: Urea and electrolyte levels in the serum in sclerema neonatorum. J. Pediatr. *67*:812, 1965.

Mortensen, O., and Stougard-Andresen, P.: Harlequin color change in the newborn. Acta Obstet. Gynecol. Scand. *38*:352, 1959.

Neligan, G. W., and Strang, L. B.: A "harlequin" colour change in the newborn. Lancet *2*:1005, 1952.

Sharlin, D. N., and Koblenzer, P.: Necrosis of subcutaneous fat with hypercalcemia. A puzzling and multifaceted disease. Clin. Pediatr. *9*:290, 1970.

Solomon, L. M., and Esterly, N. B.: Eczema in Neonatal Dermatology. Philadelphia, W. B. Saunders Co., 1973, p. 125.

Solomon, L. M., and Esterly, N. B.: Transient Cutaneous Lesions in Neonatal Dermatology. Philadelphia, W. B. Saunders Co., 1973, p. 43.

Solomon, L. M., Fretzin, D., and Pruzansky, S.: Pilosebaceous dysplasia in the oral-facial-digital syndrome. Arch. Dermatol. *102*:596, 1970.

Solomon, L. M., and Rostenberg, A., Jr.: Atopic dermatitis and infantile eczema. *In* Samter, M., Talmadge, D. W., Rose, B., Austen, F. K., and Vaughan, J. H. (Eds.): Immunological Diseases. 3rd ed. Boston, Little, Brown and Co., 1978, p. 953.

Solomon, L. M., Fretzin, D., and Pruzansky, S.: Pilosebaceous dysplasia in the oral-facial-digital syndrome. Arch. Dermatol. *102*:596, 1970.

Taylor, W. B., and Bondurant, C. P.: Erythema neonatorum allergicum. Arch. Dermatol. *76*:591, 1957.

Tromovitch, T. A., Abrams, A. A., and Jacobs, P. H.: Acne in infancy. A.M.A. J. Dis. Child. *106*:230, 1963.

17 PART

DISORDERS OF THE EYE

102

Disturbances of Motility

By David L. Guyton

There are only a few ophthalmic disorders that demand immediate attention in the neonatal period. Even when one of these is present, it is the consulting ophthalmologist rather than the pediatrician who almost always will direct or carry out treatment. Nevertheless, the pediatrician should have sufficient knowledge in this field to know when it is safe and proper to mark time, and when he must act with all possible speed in order to save vision and, possibly, life. Opportunities to save life will be limited to early recognition of malignancy and the immediate institution of appropriate therapy. There are more chances to save sight. For example, a large eye or hazy cornea should raise a suspicion of congenital glaucoma. Although congenital glaucoma is rare, a few days delay in recognition may mean the difference between good and bad vision for life. Early surgery for congenital cataract is mandatory if it is significant enough to produce visual deprivation, which leads to permanent impairment of sight. A constantly deviating eye in congenital strabismus is also deprived of normal sensory development, and treatment should not be delayed.

Retrolental fibroplasia will be discussed in Chapter 103 (see p. 909); xerophthalmia is noted under vitamin deficiencies (see p. 800).

Strabismus

A great many infants and children manifest strabismus (misalignment of the eyes) when focusing (accommodating) to overcome farsightedness. Because newborns make little or no attempt to accommodate, one is not concerned with this form of strabismus in them. Attention in this age period is limited to the paralytic form, to congenital strabismus (usually crossed eyes—congenital esotropia) and to pseudostrabismus.

PARALYTIC STRABISMUS

When the stormy period of a severe episode of birth cerebral damage subsides, a cranial nerve palsy that appeared during its active stage may persist.

Also, if a newborn survives a bout of meningoencephalitis caused by *Toxoplasma,* cytomegalic inclusion virus, or another organism, the strabismus that accompanied it may not disappear. If it does not disappear after several months, there is either a permanent cranial nerve palsy or a permanent strabismus caused by a preceding contraction of opposing extraocular muscles.

Differential diagnosis of paralytic strabismus is usually straightforward because there is generally a history of other neurologic problems. Advice as to treatment is less simple, however, for the following two reasons:

1. The amount of brain damage in other fields may be so great that repair of the relatively unimportant deviating eye seems unwarranted.

2. Surgical correction of paralytic strabismus may be difficult. One cannot return function to a paralyzed muscle. It is usually possible, however, to improve the position of the eye somewhat by recessing or weakening opposing muscles. A transposition of part or all of the vertical rectus muscles is occasionally used for a paralytic lateral rectus muscle, but full improvement cannot be expected.

CONGENITAL ESOTROPIA

This form of strabismus is considerably more frequent than is the paralytic form. Crossed eyes are sometimes noted at birth, but more often the pediatrician first becomes aware of the problem at the first or second monthly examination. Diagnosis is complicated in the neonatal period by the fact that the baby may not reliably fix and follow a light until age 3 months. Until that time, alignment may only be judged by inspection. One may evaluate eye movements by noting the responses made to noises or by rolling the infant's head from side to side, eliciting the vestibulo-ocular reflex. The infant's outward turning eye should rotate all the way to the outer canthus when one performs this "doll's head" maneuver.

Children with congenital esotropia usually alternate fixation from one eye to the other and often show "crossed fixation," using the left eye to look to the right and the right eye to look to the left. If one eye turns in constantly (Fig. 102–1), amblyopia of that eye is almost certain, and appropriate therapy should be instituted without delay.

Although an eye that cannot rotate all the way to the outer canthus suggests a paretic lateral rectus muscle (sixth cranial nerve), contracture of the medial rectus muscle on congenital esotropia may produce the same effect. The two problems are usually dis-

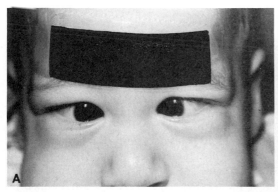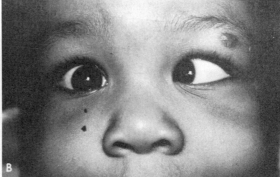

Figure 102–1. Strabismus. *A,* Congenital esotropia with alternating fixation. *B,* Congenital esotropia with constant in-turning of the left eye. There is also a hemangioma of the left upper eyelid. At surgery, the medial rectus muscles in cases of congenital esotropia are often somewhat tight, presumably not because of a defect in the muscle, but rather from physiologic contracture. (From the collection of Dr. Arnall Patz.)

tinguished by history, with sixth nerve pareses most commonly caused by hydrocephalus.

If the infant's eyes are not straight by age 3 to 5 months, the child should be referred promptly to the ophthalmologist. Most pediatric ophthalmologists now believe that surgical correction of congenital esotropia must be completed by age 18 to 24 months in order for the infant to have any significant binocular vision.

PSEUDOSTRABISMUS

It is often difficult to tell whether an infant's eyes are straight or not. Parents and pediatricians alike confuse pseudostrabismus with true strabismus. Simply an appearance of crossed eyes does not necessarily signify strabismus (Fig. 102–2). Many children have broad nasal bridges and epicanthal folds of skin covering over the nasal sclera. With the nasal sclera hidden, the child's eyes may appear to turn inward, particularly in certain gaze directions. The presence

of pseudoesotropia rather than true esotropia may be confirmed by observation of the epicanthal folds of skin and by careful attention to the position of the corneal light reflexes. If the infant fixes on a handlight held between the examiner and the infant, the reflections of the handlight in the cornea will appear as bright points of light falling just nasal to the center of each pupil if both eyes are indeed directed toward the light. When true strabismus is present, the light reflexes will be located asymmetrically. If only pseudostrabismus is present, reassurance of the parents is all that is necessary.

Congenital Ptosis

Inability to raise one or both upper eyelids is encountered as a solitary congenital defect or as an anomaly associated with inability to rotate the eye

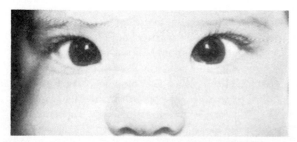

Figure 102–2. Child with pseudoesotropia. Note wide bridge of nose and prominent epicanthal folds simulating esotropia. Flashbulb reflection is centered in each pupil, showing that the eyes are indeed straight. (From Patz, A.: Md. State Med. J. *8:*600, 1959.)

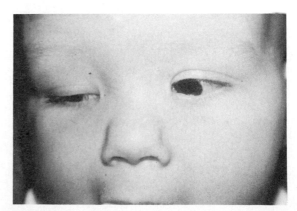

Figure 102–3. Unilateral congenital ptosis. (From the collection of Dr. Arnall Patz.)

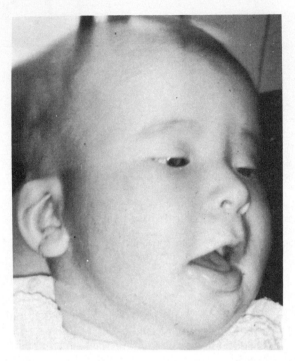

Figure 102–4. Bilateral congenital ptosis of the upper lids.

upward. The combination stems from incomplete development of the superior rectus muscle and the related elevator of the lid, the levator palpebrae superioris. Isolated ptosis is usually a failure of development of only the levator muscle. Isolated ptosis may be unilateral or bilateral (Figs. 102–3 and 102–4).

Congenital ptosis should not be confused with upper facial nerve palsy in which the main disability is that of closing the eye tightly rather than opening it widely. Drooping lids, common in myasthenia gravis of older patients, are seen only occasionally as a sign of myasthenia of the newborn.

Congenital ptosis is generally hereditary, and this isolated defect of the levator palpebrae superioris is usually transmitted as a dominant trait.

Treatment of congenital ptosis consists of a plastic surgical procedure performed well after the neonatal period has passed. If the ptosis is severe enough to cover the pupil, however, the lid should be raised early in infancy to avoid permanent deprivation amblyopia.

Nystagmus

Nystagmus that is present at birth may result from decreased central vision ("sensory type") or from a primary defect in the ocular motor system in the brain stem ("motor type"). Sensory nystagmus may result from opacification of the lens (cataract), from hazing of the cornea (glaucoma and other causes), from dragging of the retina (retrolental fibroplasia), from macular scarring due to chorioretinitis, from retinoblastoma, or from hereditary defects such as a hypoplastic fovea in some forms of albinism.

Motor nystagmus is often seen without any other associated defects, but the nystagmus itself prevents full development of visual acuity. Visual acuity does not worsen in later years, however, and many patients make a satisfactory adjustment to the visual difficulties that this defect involves.

Nystagmus that is acquired during the neonatal period is rare and usually associated with an underlying structural intracranial defect or a systemic metabolic abnormality.

Although head nodding may be present with congenital nystagmus, it much more typically accompanies the fine rapid nystagmus of spasmus nutans, a benign condition that is not present at birth but that develops and disappears during the first year or two of life. Spasmus nutans usually does not prevent the eventual development of normal visual acuity.

REFERENCES

Harley, R. (Ed.): Pediatric Ophthalmology. Philadelphia, W. B. Saunders Co., 1975.

Helveston, E. M., and Ellis, F. D.: Pediatric Ophthalmology Practice. St. Louis, C. V. Mosby, 1980.

von Noorden, G. K., and Maumenee, A. E.: Atlas of Strabismus. 3rd ed. St. Louis, C. V. Mosby, 1977.

103

Retinopathy of Prematurity

By John W. Payne

Retinopathy of prematurity (ROP), or retrolental fibroplasia, was first identified in 1941 by Terry. With the increased availability of oxygen after World War II and its liberal use in closed incubators, the incidence of ROP reached epidemic proportions by 1950. Indeed, it became the leading cause of blindness in children in the United States. It is estimated that over 25 per cent of premature newborns were identified as affected. The actual incidence was probably much higher, since the indirect ophthalmoscope, which allows one to detect early stages of the disease in the peripheral retina, was not yet in use.

In 1951, Campbell published an uncontrolled clinical study that first suggested intensive oxygen therapy as an important etiologic factor. Subsequently, the first controlled nursery study by Patz and coworkers and the experimental production of ROP by Ashton and colleagues strongly implicated oxygen. Other reports (Gyllensten and Hellström, 1952; Lanman et al., 1954; Patz et al., 1953) and the cooperative study by Kinsey verified these early observations. Oxygen administration consequently was radically curtailed by the mid-1950s, and the incidence of ROP decreased dramatically. By the 1960s, however, pediatricians (Avery et al., 1960; McDonald, 1963; Warley and Gairdner, 1962) recognized an increased mortality and morbidity from hyaline membrane disease associated with this rigid restriction of the use of oxygen in the premature nursery.

Incidence. Since the mid-1960s, the incidence of ROP in the premature population has risen again (Fig. 103–1). Three factors are probably involved. First, the use of the indirect ophthalmoscope allows milder forms of the acute disease, previously overlooked, to be identified. Secondly, pediatricians are aware of the increased mortality and/or brain damage resulting from severe limitation of the use of oxygen in the premature population and consequently have been more liberal in the use of oxygen in high-risk premature infants. Finally, with modern medical techniques, pediatricians are saving smaller high-risk infants who rarely survived before. Phelps estimated that the survival rate of infants with birth weights under 1000 gm has risen from 8 per cent to approximately 35 per cent (about 50 per cent in 1981 in Brigham and Women's nurseries).

Reports (e.g., Doray and Orquin, 1981; Gunn et al., 1980; Hittner et al., 1981) from many of the intensive care units here and abroad indicate that the actual incidence of ROP, although variable, is quite high (Table 103–1). In survivors having birth weights of 1500 gm or less, it ranges from 4 to 65 per cent. In survivors having birth weights of 1000 gm or less, it ranges from 40 to 77 per cent. Cicatricial sequelae are most common in the lower birth weight infants and probably occur in 20 to 40 per cent of those affected (Bauer, 1978; Kinsey et al., 1977; Petersen, 1981; Phelps, 1981). Blindness probably occurs in about 5 per cent or less of those with active ROP. However, even with conservative estimates, 250 to

Table 103–1. Incidence of Retinopathy of Prematurity (ROP) in Survivors

	Total survivors ≤1500 gm birth weight	ROP (%)	Total survivors ≤1000 gm birth weight	ROP (%)
Kinsey et al. (1977)	86*	37	—	—
Kingham (1977)	521†	16	—	—
Gunn et al. (1980)	80	34	—	—
Doray and Orquin (1981)	270	4	—	—
Hittner et al. (1981)	51	65	—	—
Kalina and Karr (1981)	882	14	129	40
Palmer (1981)	87	36	37‡	65
Petersen (1981)	1104§	10	—	—
Procianoy et al. (1981)	138	49	31	77
Yamanouchi et al. (1981)	111	18	24	63

* <1200 gm birth weight.
† "High risk infants," not by birth weight.
‡ <1100 gm birth weight.
§ Also includes those of any birth weight on mechanical ventilation or 30 per cent O₂ for 12 hours or more.

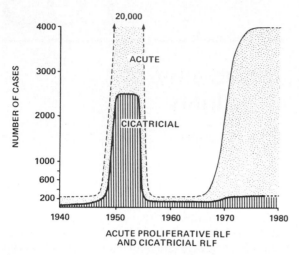

Figure 103-1. Incidence of acute proliferative and cicatricial RLF in the USA. Mild acute proliferative RLF for the most part remained undiagnosed during the epidemic years, and approximately 20,000 new cases occurred annually (Kinsey, 1956). Most of the increased incidence of RLF in this past decade is due to acute proliferative cases, most of which undergo spontaneous remission.

500 infants are blinded from ROP annually in the United States.

There seems to be an irreducible minimum incidence of ROP, in spite of the most careful arterial Pa_{O_2} monitoring (Kinsey et al., 1977). Therefore, an immature retina is fundamental to the development of the disease, and excess oxygen alone can be considered the major precipitating factor. Many other factors increase the risk of developing the disease in the premature infant and will be discussed later.

Pathogenesis

Immaturity of the Retinal Vasculature. The normal retina is unique in that it contains no blood vessels until the fourth month of gestation. Vascularization begins at the optic disc and then proceeds slowly toward the peripheral retina. The nasal retina is fully vascularized at about 8 months' gestation, but the wider temporal retina is not fully vascularized until after full-term delivery (Fig. 103–2). Consequently, at any stage of prematurity, the temporal retina is much more susceptible to ROP. This process may explain the occasional case of ROP in the premature without a history of oxygen therapy or in the full-term infant.

Primary and Secondary Effects of Oxygen on the Immature Retina. The primary effect of oxygen on the infant or experimental animal with an incompletely vascularized retina is retinal vasoconstriction, which, if sustained, is followed by some degree of vascular closure (Fig. 103–3). Damage to the capillary endothelium follows, and, ultimately, complete closure of the immature portions of the vascular bed occurs.

After removal to ambient air, new vessel formation occurs at the area of retinal capillary damage and obliteration. These new vessels erupt through the surface of the retina to proliferate into the vitreous, an event similar to that seen in advanced stages of diabetic and sickle cell retinopathy.

Later Findings. Ashton has demonstrated in the developing retina that cords and sheets of mesenchymal tissue grow out from the optic disc, beginning

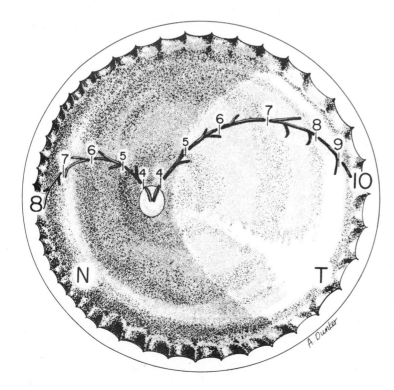

Figure 103-2. Schematic drawing of the posterior segment of the eye. The retina is avascular until 4 months' gestation, at which time vessels start from the optic nerve, reaching nasal periphery at 8 months' gestation. Temporal periphery is not vascularized until 1 month after birth of the *full-term* infant. This explains predilection of temporal periphery for RLF and occasional cases of RLF in full-term infants.

OXYGEN IN RLF

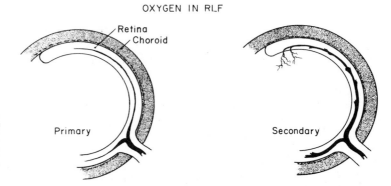

Figure 103–3. Schematic diagram showing initial, primary, vasoconstrictive effect of oxygen and the secondary proliferation following removal to room air. During primary constriction, destruction of more anterior, immature vessel complexes occurs.

at 16 weeks' gestation, and are the immediate precursors of the premature capillaries that follow behind. Flynn and coworkers have postulated that these newly formed vessels are exquisitely sensitive to high levels of oxygen and constrict. The mesenchymal tissue then ceases to migrate peripherally and forms a mesenchymal shunt resembling the appearance of a hepatic sinusoid. This shunt then separates the vascularized retina from peripheral avascularized retina. Adjacent to the areas of capillary closure, neovascularization occurs (Flynn et al., 1977) (Fig. 103–4). Patz and others have postulated that ischemic retina may be producing some factor that induces vasoproliferation. Glaser and coworkers have already demonstrated vasoproliferative activity in extracts of mammalian retina. Such a factor may be the common denominator linking ischemia and the vasoproliferation seen in other retinal diseases such as diabetes and sickle cell disease.

Flower and coworkers have studied the influence of the prostaglandin system on the production of ROP. Preliminary animal data suggest the possibility that the prostaglandin mechanism may be involved in the response of the immature retinal vessels. Flower and his group have also carefully investigated the possible role of Pa_{CO_2} on the immature retinal vasculature.

Clinical Classification. Although the basic classification of ROP remains the same, various authors (Kingham, 1977; Kingham et al., 1981; McCormick, 1977; Uemura and Akiyama, 1981) have made revisions, attempting to develop a classification that better reflects modern understanding of the multitude of steps in the progression of the disease. This has led to a widespread confusion in the literature. Consequently, an expanded standardized classification is presently being developed that, it is hoped, will be universally used. In the meantime, the following is the Patz version of Terry's original classification, which is still widely used:

Acute Stages. The earliest signs of acute ROP are vasoconstriction and vascular closure during the time the infant is receiving excessive oxygen. This is rarely observable, owing to the hazy media in these very young, often very sick, infants (Cantolino et al., 1971).

Stage I: Early peripheral vasoproliferation—beginning of a visible demarcation line between vascular and more peripheral avascular retina.

Stage II: More advanced peripheral changes with prominent mesenchymal shunt at the demarcation line. Secondary dilatation and tortuosity of vessels in posterior pole.

Stage III: Retinal vasoproliferation with extension into the vitreous. Vitreal retinal traction or vitreous hemorrhage or both.

Stage IV: Advanced proliferation with localized retinal detachment.

Stage V: Total retinal detachment.

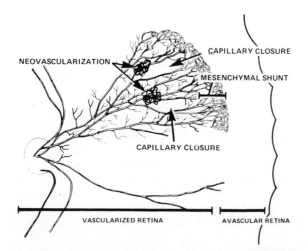

Figure 103–4. Schematic diagram of acute RLF. Note the mesenchymal shunt at the border between vascular and avascular retina. Areas of capillary closure and adjacent neovascularization are seen posterior to the mesenchymal shunt.

Spontaneous Regression. Spontaneous regression takes place in approximately 80 per cent of infants with stage I or stage II disease. Residual scarring may be minimal or imperceptible, and no loss of vision occurs. Regression can occur in later stages of the disease, but usually some cicatricial changes remain.

Cicatricial Grades. The following five categories of cicatricial findings range from minor (grade I) to serious (grade V) changes:

Grade I: Minor peripheral retinal scarring and vascular abnormalities. Preretinal fibrosis. High myopia is common. Vision correctible to normal.

Grade II: Disc distortion with dragging of vessels temporally. Temporal traction on the macula may occur (heterotropia). If so, vision usually ranges between 20/40 and 20/200.

Grade III: Temporal retinal fold and traction. Vision often ranges between 20/200 and 5/200.

Grade IV: Incomplete temporal retinal mass. Often localized traction detachment of retina. Vision ranges from the ability to see and count fingers to perception of hand motions.

Grade V: Complete retrolental mass. Organized retinal detachment. Vision deteriorates to no light perception. Cataracts, secondary glaucoma, and/or phthisis may ensue.

Diagnosis. Because the primary stage of vasoconstriction of retinal vessels is difficult to observe, the ophthalmologist has no role in the premature nursery in monitoring Pa$_{O_2}$ levels (Cantolino et al., 1971). However, the examination can and should be performed with an indirect ophthalmoscope when the infant is between 4 and 8 weeks of age (Palmer, 1981). In 1974, the American Academy of Pediatrics made the following recommendation:

A person experienced in recognizing retrolental fibroplasia (retinopathy of prematurity) should examine the eyes of all infants born at less than 36 weeks' gestation or weighing less than 2000 grams (4.2 lbs.) who have received oxygen therapy. This examination should be made at discharge from the nursery and at three to six months of age.

If at examination the far temporal periphery is difficult to visualize, the examination should be repeated in several weeks to make certain that ROP is not present. Presently, some premature infants are being discharged on nasal oxygen. These infants are clearly still at risk and should have ophthalmoscopic examination at 3 to 4 weeks after the supplemental oxygen is discontinued. If early disease is detected, the authors usually examine the infant every 2 to 3 weeks during the active phase. *We urge all pediatricians to see that infants in the suspect group be examined by ophthalmologists without delay.* Irate parents are usually those to whom the possibility of eye disease has not been mentioned or whose children have not had an ophthalmologic consultation until obvious problems are apparent.

Management

Acute Proliferative Disease. The experimental treatment of acute stage III ROP using laser therapy or cryotherapy or both to the peripheral retina has been studied (Payne and Patz, 1972). Since then, there have been numerous reports on the efficacy of such treatment (Hindle and Leyton, 1978; Kingham, 1978; Nagata and Tsuruoka, 1972; Sasaki et al., 1976). Others have been enthusiastic about retinal detachment surgery in the acute stages (McPherson and Hittner, 1979). Unfortunately, the disease is often asymmetric, and its progression can suddenly stop at any stage. Therefore, at the present time the efficacy of any treatment of the acute disease is unproven and awaits the results of a controlled multicentered study. It is hoped that such a study is forthcoming.

Vitrectomy also has been tried in advanced cicatricial disease without much success (Michels, 1981; Merritt et al., 1981; Treister and Machemer, 1977). However, in 1981 Charles reported encouraging results in total traction retinal detachment (grade V) using vitrectomy with an approach through the ciliary body. He has been able to achieve a successful anatomic reattachment of the retina in 14 of 23 cases and presently recommends the surgery at 4 to 8 months of age. He reports promising visual results in some cases, but further follow-up is needed. This surgery is still experimental, and he is operating on one eye only.

Late Cicatricial Changes. As children who had acute ROP grow up, late ocular complications of the disease are being seen in older age groups (Kalina, 1980). Myopia is frequently associated with ROP, particularly when cicatrization occurs. This myopia is of a multifactorial nature and not due solely to the axial length of the eye. It is usually related to the severity of the cicatricial changes and is frequently greater than six diopters (Tasman, 1979). Retinal pigmentation, microvascular abnormalities, and vitreous membranes are often seen in asymptomatic patients. Dragging of the retina temporally is common with heterotopia of the fovea. This may lead to strabismus, amblyopia, or a pseudoesotropia. Late retinal detachments can occur at any age and are more frequent in the highly myopic group (Tasman, 1970). Late vitreous hemorrhage from persistent neovascularization has been reported and successfully treated with focal laser therapy (Payne and Patz, 1979). As a multitude of ocular problems can occur at any age, children with a history of the acute disease should be followed regularly by an ophthalmologist.

Prevention

Risk Factors. A multicentered cooperative study reported by Kinsey and coworkers in 1977 and supported by the National Eye Institute tried to establish an arterial oxygen saturation level above which ROP occurred more frequently. However, the results revealed no relation between the incidence of ROP and Pa_{O_2} as presently sampled. No safe level of arterial oxygen saturation was determined. The cooperative study did identify low birth weight, length of time in oxygen, and oxygen concentration as risk factors for the development of the disease. Other studies have identified gestational age, apnea requiring bag and mask resuscitation with oxygen, septicemia, degree of illness, blood transfusion, intraventricular hemorrhage, and mechanical ventilation as additional risk factors (Bossi et al., 1981; Gunn et al., 1980; Procianoy et al., 1981; Shahinian and Malachowski, 1978). All these risk factors occur more frequently in low birth weight infants; consequently, it is unlikely that ROP will be totally eliminated from the premature population as long as these risk factors are present.

Transcutaneous Monitoring. Transcutaneous continuous monitoring of arterial oxygen saturation levels has become an invaluable adjunct to the management of the fragile premature infant in many nurseries. There are still technical problems to be overcome to enhance its accuracy and effectiveness. It is hoped that such careful regulation of the arterial oxygen level will lower the incidence and severity of ROP. However, the 1981 report of Yamanouchi and colleagues still shows a high incidence of ROP in low birth weight infants in spite of the use of transcutaneous continuous monitoring of oxygen levels.

Vitamin E. In the epidemic years, Owens and Owens reported encouraging results using vitamin E in treating prematures. After identification of hyperoxia as a primary contributing factor in the pathogenesis of ROP, interest in vitamin E waned. The 1977 animal studies by Phelps and Rosenbaum and the 1974 preliminary nursery reports by Johnson and coworkers also suggest that vitamin E may play a role.

Preliminary studies by Kretzer and Hittner have shown basic changes in the ultrastructure of spindle cells in high-risk preterm infants. They studied the eyes of six premature infants from the control group and the eyes of seven premature infants from the groups treated with vitamin E. The spindle cells in retinas of preterm infants given continuous oxygen because of respiratory distress showed an increase in gap junctions. It is postulated that these increased gap junctions halt the normal vasoformative process. In the group treated with vitamin E, the increase in gap junctions was suppressed. This exciting work opens up vast areas that now must be investigated in vitro and in vivo.

Hittner and colleagues reported in 1981 that vitamin E does reduce the severity but not the incidence of ROP in their nursery population. The report consisted of 101 infant survivors having birth weights of less than 1500 gm. The incidence of ROP in both the control and treated groups was 65 per cent. This unusually high incidence of the disease and the multivariate analysis of the statistics leave the conclusions of this study open to question. Several other clinical trials on the efficacy of vitamin E therapy are still in progress. It seems prudent to withhold final conclusions until all the reports are in.

Summary. At the present time, there appears to be an irreducible minimum incidence of ROP, in spite of the most meticulous arterial oxygen monitoring in our best neonatology units. Close cooperation between the pediatrician and ophthalmologist is essential to identification and management of infants affected by this potentially blinding disease. Only further research will clarify the possibilities of prevention.

REFERENCES

Ashton, N.: Oxygen and the growth and development of retinal vessels. In vivo and in vitro studies. Am. J. Ophthalmol. *62*:412, 1966.

Ashton, N.: Oxygen and the growth and development of retinal vessels. The XX Francis I. Proctor Lecture. *In* Kimura, S. J., and Caygill, W. N., (Eds.): Vascular Complications of Diabetes Mellitus. St. Louis, C. V. Mosby, 1967, pp. 3–32.

Ashton, N., Ward, B., and Serpell, G.: Role of oxygen in the genesis of retrolental fibroplasia: a preliminary report. Br. J. Ophthalmol. *37*:513, 1953.

Avery, M. E., and Oppenheimer, E. H.: Recent increase in mortality from hyaline membrane disease. J. Pediatr. *57*:553, 1960.

Bauer, C. R.: The occurrence of retrolental fibroplasia in infants of birth weight 1000 grams and less. Clin. Res. *26*:824A, 1978.

Bossi, E., Koerner, F., and Zulauf, M.: Retinopathy of prematurity (ROP): Risk factors—a statistical analysis with matched pairs. Syllabus: Retinopathy of Prematurity Conference. Vol. II: Washington, D.C., Dec. 4–6, 1981, p. 536.

Brockhurst, R. J., and Chishti, M. I.: Cicatricial retrolental fibroplasia: its occurrence without oxygen administration and in full term infants. Albrecht von Graefes Arch. Klin. Exp. Ophthalmol. *195*:113, 1975.

Campbell, K.: Intensive oxygen therapy as a possible cause of retrolental fibroplasia: a clinical approach. Med. J. Aust. *2*:48, 1951.

Cantolino, S. J., O'Grady, G. E., Herrera, J. A., et al.: Ophthalmoscopic monitoring of oxygen therapy in premature infants: fluorescein angiography in acute retrolental fibroplasia. Am. J. Ophthalmol. *72*:322, 1971.

Charles, S.: Vitreous surgery for retinopathy of prematurity (ROP). Syllabus: Retinopathy of Prematurity Conference. Vol. II. Washington, D.C., Dec. 4–6:858, 1981.

Doray, B. H., and Orquin, J.: Incidence of retinopathy of prematurity. Syllabus: Retinopathy of Prematurity Conference. Vol. I. Washington, D.C., Dec. 4–6, 1981, p. 477.

Flower, R. W.: A new perspective on the pathogenesis of retrolental fibroplasia: the influence of elevated arterial pCO_2. Syllabus: Retinopathy of Prematurity Conference. Vol. II. Washington, D.C., Dec. 4–6:20, 1981.

Flower, R. W., and Blake, D. A.: Retrolental fibroplasia. Evidence for a role of the prostaglandin cascade in the pathogenesis of oxygen-induced retinopathy in the newborn beagle. Pediatr. Res. *15*:1293, 1981.

Flynn, J. T., O'Grady, G. E., Herrera, J., Kushner, B. J., et al.: Retrolental fibroplasia. I. Clinical observations. Arch. Ophthalmol. *95*:217, 1977.

Foos, R. Y.: Acute retrolental fibroplasia. Albrecht von Graefes Arch. Klin. Exp. Ophthalmol. *195*:87, 1975.

Glaser, B. M., D'Amore, P. A., Michels, R. G., Patz, A., and Fenselau, A.: Demonstration of vasoproliferative activity from mammalian retina. J. Cell. Biol. *84*:298, 1980.

Gunn, T. R., Easdown, J., Outerbridge, E. W., and Aranda, J. V.: Risk factors in retrolental fibroplasia. Pediatrics *65*:1096, 1980.

Gyllensten, O. J., and Hellström, B. E.: Retrolental fibroplasia—Animal experiments; effect of intermittently administered oxygen on postnatal development of eyes of fullterm mice. Preliminary report. Acta. Paediatr. *41*:577, 1952.

Hindle, N. W., and Leyton, J.: Prevention of cicatricial retrolental fibroplasia by cryotherapy. Can. J. Ophthalmol. *13*:277, 1978.

Hittner, H. M., Godio, L. B., Rudolph, A. J., et al.: Retrolental fibroplasia: efficacy of vitamin E in a double-blind clinical study of preterm infants. N. Engl. J. Med. *305*:1365, 1981.

Johnson, L., Schaffer, D., and Boggs, T. R.: The premature infant, vitamin E deficiency and retrolental fibroplasia. Am. J. Clin. Nutr. *27*:1158, 1974.

Kalina, R. E.: Treatment of retrolental fibroplasia. Therapeutic review. Surv. Ophthalmol. *24*:229, 1980.

Kalina, R. E., and Karr, D. J.: Retrolental fibroplasia—experience over two decades in one institution. Syllabus: Retinopathy of Prematurity Conference. Vol. I. Washington, D.C. Dec. 4–6, 1981, p. 328.

Kingham, J. D.: Acute retrolental fibroplasia. Arch. Ophthalmol. *95*:39, 1977.

Kingham, J. D.: Acute retrolental fibroplasia. II. Treatment by cryosurgery. Arch. Ophthalmol. *96*:2049, 1978.

Kingham, J. D., Hittner, H., Patz, A., Kalina, R., Tasman, W., Mousel, D., and Foos, R.: The classification of acute retrolental fibroplasia. Syllabus: Retinopathy of Prematurity Conference. Vol. I. Washington, D.C., Dec. 4–6, 1981, p. 264.

Kinsey, V. E.: Retrolental fibroplasia: cooperative study of retinal fibroplasia and the use of oxygen. Arch. Ophthalmol. *56*:481, 1956.

Kinsey, V. E., Arnold, H. J., Kalina, R. E., Stern, L., Strahlman, M., Odell, G., Driscoll, J. M., Jr., Elliott, H., Payne, J. W., and Patz, A.: Pa$_{O_2}$ levels and retrolental fibroplasia: a report of the cooperative study. Pediatrics *60*:655, 1977.

Kretzer, F., and Hittner, H., Johnson, A., et al.: Vitamin E and retrolental fibroplasia: ultrastructural support of clinical efficacy. Ann. N.Y. Acad. Sci. *393*:145, 1982.

Kushner, B. J., Essner, D., Cohen, I. J., and Flynn, J. T.: Retrolental fibroplasia. II. Pathologic correlation. Arch. Ophthalmol. *95*:29, 1977.

Lanman, J. U., Guy, L. P., and Dancis, J.: Retrolental fibroplasia and oxygen therapy. J.A.M.A. *155*:223, 1954.

McCormick, A. Q.: Retinopathy of prematurity. Curr. Probl. Pediatr. 7:11, 1977.

McDonald, A. D.: Cerebral palsy in children of very low birth weight. Arch. Dis. Child. *38*:579, 1963.

McPherson, A., and Hittner, H. M.: Scleral buckling in 2½- to 11-month-old premature infants with retinal detachment associated with acute retrolental fibroplasia. Ophthalmology *86*:819, 1979.

Merritt, J., Eifrig, D., Lawson, E., and Sprague, D.: Lensectomy-vitrectomy for stage V cicatricial retrolental fibroplasia. Ophthal. Surg. *13*:300, 1982.

Michels, R. M.: Personal communication, 1981.

Nagata, M., and Tsuruoka, Y.: Treatment of acute retrolental fibroplasia with xenon arc photocoagulation. Jpn. J. Ophthalmol. *16*:131, 1972.

Owens, W. C., and Owens, E. U.: Retrolental fibroplasia in pre-

mature infants. II. Studies on the prophylaxis of the disease: the use of alpha tocopheryl acetate. Am. J. Ophthalmol. *32*:1631, 1949.

Palmer, E. A.: Natural history of retinopathy of prematurity. Syllabus: Retinopathy of Prematurity Conference. Vol. II. Washington, D.C., Dec. 4–6, 1981, p. 441.

Palmer, E. A.: Optimal timing of examination for acute retrolental fibroplasia. Ophthalmology *88*:662, 1981.

Patz, A.: Friedenwald memorial lecture. I. Studies on retinal neovascularization II. Jonas S. Friedenwald, Man of Science. Invest. Ophthalmol. Vis. Sci. *19*:1127, 1980.

Patz, A., Eastham, A., Higginbotham, D. H., et al.: Oxygen studies in retrolental fibroplasia in experimental animals. Am. J. Ophthalmol. *36*:1511, 1953.

Patz, A., Hoeck, L. E., and de la Cruz, E.: Studies on the effect of high oxygen administration in retrolental fibroplasia: I. Nursery observations. Am. J. Ophthalmol. *35*:1248, 1952.

Payne, J. W., and Patz, A.: Treatment of acute proliferative retrolental fibroplasia. Trans. Am. Acad. Ophthalmol. Otolaryngol. 76:1234, 1972.

Payne, J. W., and Patz, A.: Current status of retrolental fibroplasia. The retinopathy of prematurity. Review article. Ann. Clin. Res. *11*:205, 1979.

Petersen, R. A.: Six years of experience with retrolental fibroplasia in the joint program for neonatology at Harvard Medical School. Syllabus: Retinopathy of Prematurity Conference. Vol. I. Washington, D.C., Dec. 4–6, 1981, p. 346.

Phelps, D. L.: Retinopathy of prematurity: an estimate of vision loss in the United States—1979. Pediatrics *67*:924, 1981.

Phelps, D. L.: Vision loss due to retinopathy of prematurity. Letter to editor. Lancet *1*:606, 1981.

Phelps, D. L., and Rosenbaum, A. L.: The role of tocopherol in oxygen-induced retinopathy: kitten model. Pediatrics *59*(suppl.):998, 1977.

Procianoy, R. S., Garcia-Prats, J. A., Hittner, H. M., Adams, J. M., and Rudolph, A. J.: An association between retinopathy of prematurity and intraventricular hemorrhage in very low birth weight infants. Acta. Paediatr. Scand. *70*:473, 1981.

Sasaki, K., Yamashita, Y., Mackawa, T., and Adachi, T.: Treatment of retinopathy of prematurity and active stage of cryocautery. Jpn. J. Ophthalmol. *20*:384, 1976.

Shahinian, L., Jr., and Malachowski, N.: Retrolental fibroplasia. A new analysis of risk factors based on recent cases. Arch. Ophthalmol. *96*:70, 1978.

Tasman, W.: Vitreo-retinal changes in cicatricial retrolental fibroplasia. Trans. Am. Ophthalmol. Soc. *68*:548, 1970.

Tasman, W.: Late complications of retrolental fibroplasia. Ophthalmology *86*:1724, 1979.

Terry, T. L.: Extreme prematurity and fibroblastic overgrowth of persistent vascular sheath behind each crystalline lens. I. Preliminary report. Am. J. Ophthalmol. *25*:203, 1942.

Treister, G., and Machemer, R.: Results of vitrectomy for rare proliferative and hemorrhagic disease. Am. J. Ophthalmol. *84*:394, 1977.

Uemura, Y., and Akiyama, K.: Classification of active retinopathy. Syllabus: Retinopathy of Prematurity Conference. Vol. II. Washington, D.C., Dec. 4–6, 1981, p. 253.

Warley, M.A., and Gairdner, D.: Respiratory distress syndrome of the newborn. Principles in treatment. Arch. Dis. Child. *37*:455, 1962.

Yamanouchi, I., Igarashi, I., and Ouchi, E.: Incidence and severity of retinopathy of prematurity in low birth weight infants monitored by continuous transcutaneous oxygen monitoring. Syllabus: Retinopathy of Prematurity Conference. Vol. II. Washington, D.C., Dec. 4–6, 1981, p. 505.

104

Congenital Cataracts

True congenital cataracts occurring in the neonatal period are rare. Such cataracts that do occur at this time are frequently so inconspicuous that they are not noticed until later in life with slit-lamp examination. Congenital cataracts are frequently inherited as an autosomal dominant trait, although sporadic congenital cataracts have also been reported. Maternal rubella in the first trimester of pregnancy may frequently lead to the appearance of congenital cataracts, as can various congenital syndromes (e.g., Lowe's syndrome). The occurrence of congenital cataracts should also initiate a search for an enzyme deficiency such as galactosemia.

The observation of a white pupil (leukocoria) (Fig. 104–1) should prompt an early and complete ocular examination for exclusion of such conditions as retinoblastoma, persistent hyperplastic primary vitreous, and congenital cataracts. In children with congenital cataracts, apart from those with some of the congenital syndromes and those with the rubella complex, the eye is generally of normal size, and the pupil will dilate well. In early, less dense cataracts, one may perceive the changes only by using the direct ophthalmoscope with a +8 to +12 lens at a distance of 6 to 12 inches from the eye and by identifying opacities at the level of the lens with retroillumination against the red reflex of the retina. Occurrence of a pendular nystagmus or strabismus in a neonate should also initiate a careful examination for ocular media opacities such as congenital cataracts.

Most cataracts in neonates can safely be observed without intervention if total occlusion of the pupil is not present. In the past, bilateral congenital cataracts were usually treated surgically, with extracapsular cataract extraction performed with an aspiration technique; dense monocular cataracts were usually associated with a poor prognosis for visual recovery,

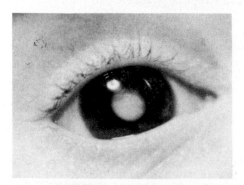

Figure 104–1. Congenital cataract. The opaque lens stands out sharply. (From the collection of Dr. Arnall Patz.)

Other Neonatal Disorders of the Eye

By Lawrence W. Hirst

and cataract extraction was not attempted. The poor visual prognosis in those cases was usually considered to be due to the association of other congenital ocular anomalies with the anisometropia and resultant amblyopia. Results of later small series involving surgical removal of unilateral congenital cataracts suggest that the prognosis is slightly more optimistic if surgery is performed early, within the first 2 to 3 months of life. This more radical approach has yet to be confirmed in larger series, but with the modern development of microsurgical techniques early intervention may offer a better prognosis for dense monocular and binocular cataracts.

Refractive Problems in Neonates

The incidence of myopia and anisometropia in premature infants is higher than that in full-term babies. Over 70 per cent of premature infants have more than one diopter of astigmatism, and it appears that the incidence of severe myopia and astigmatism becomes greater with increasing prematurity. Very premature infants should be refracted after the first few months of life, once their condition is stable, so that one can determine whether large refractive errors that could hinder maturation of visual function are present.

Unilateral congenital myopia is frequently present at birth and may result in development of amblyopia in the involved eye. Suspicion of this condition may be heightened by apparent unilateral proptosis that, on closer examination, is actually an enlarged globe. Care should be taken in these children to exclude unilateral congenital glaucoma.

Infantile Glaucoma

Glaucoma occurring in the neonate is a potentially blinding disease and requires emergency treatment. It is considered to be of a multifactorial inheritance pattern, although there are certain congenital anomalies (e.g., Sturge-Weber syndrome, aniridia, and

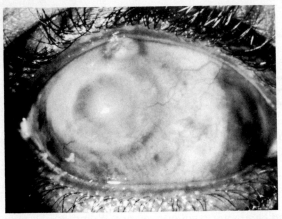

Figure 104–2. Late congenital glaucoma. Note the unusual breadth of the cornea and its diffuse haziness. Pericorneal vascular congestion is striking. (From the collection of Dr. Richard Hoover, Baltimore.)

mesodomal dysgenesis, including Rieger's anomaly, Peter's syndrome, and Weill-Marchesani syndrome) that have a definite inheritance pattern, usually autosomal dominant. The incidence of infantile glaucoma is said to range from 0.01 per cent to 0.048 per cent. Of these cases, 40 per cent will be present at the time of birth. The male-to-female ratio is 2 to 1 at birth, and in most cases the defect is bilateral, although there is frequently asymmetric involvement. Commonly associated ocular anomalies are myopia,

Table 104–1. Causes of Corneal Opacities at Birth

1. Congenital glaucoma
2. Birth trauma to cornea
3. Intrauterine keratitis (e.g., rubella, syphilis)
4. Mucopolysaccharidoses (e.g., Hurler's syndrome)
5. Neonatal keratoconjunctivitis (e.g., gonococcal)
6. Corneal dystrophies (e.g., congenital hereditary endothelial dystrophy, posterior polymorphous endothelial dystrophy)
7. Tumors (e.g., corneal dermoids)
8. Chemical injury to eye (inappropriate silver nitrate administration)

anisometropia, and nystagmus, all of which may contribute to the rather disappointing overall long-term prognosis for vision, which is rarely better than 20/50.

In the first 5 days of life, the most common presenting signs and symptoms are hazy cornea (88 per cent) (Fig. 104–2), photophobia (44 per cent), increased corneal size (31 per cent) (Fig. 104–3), and increased ocular size (25 per cent). One other commonly noted symptom is epiphora. Despite a wide variety of other conditions (Table 104–1) that may also cause corneal opacities at birth, all infants with opaque or cloudy corneas should be treated as emergencies and examined carefully both at the bedside and under general anesthesia.

A careful history should be obtained from the parent, with particular attention given to a possible familial trait. The presence of aniridia should initiate a search for possible Wilm's tumor.

Assessment of this congenital glaucoma primarily involves examining the infant under anesthesia with applanation tonometry (influenced considerably by the depth and type of anesthesia), gonioscopy, and

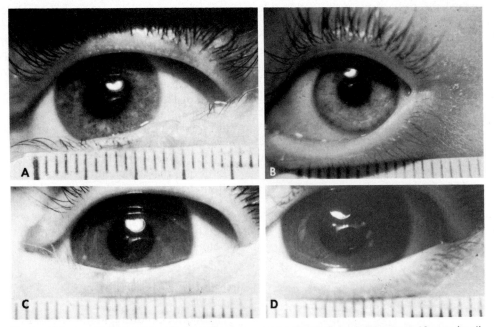

Figure 104–3. *A,* Normal eyeball with cornea of normal size. It measures 10 mm in diameter. *B,* Small eyeball with microcornea, measuring 6.5 mm across. This photograph is included for comparison and contrast. *C,* Early glaucoma, without hazing of cornea or tearing of Descemet's membrane. The cornea is 13.5 mm wide. *D,* Early glaucoma; cornea is 14.0 mm in diameter. (From the collection of Dr. Arnall Patz.)

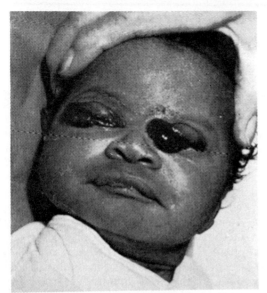

Figure 104—4. At 10 days of life, note the marked edema of both conjunctivae of the upper lids while the eversion of the lids has practically returned to normal. (Stillerman, M. L., Emanuel, B., and Padorr, M. P.: J. Pediatr. 69:656, 1966.)

optic disc drawings and photography (for evaluation of the fundus). Corneal diameter measurements are also imperative. Unfortunately, two of the principal parameters in adult glaucoma either cannot be obtained or are not reliable in congenital infantile glaucoma. First, the cup-to-disc ratio in the eye may be greater than 1:3 in normal children and the disc is frequently not grossly excavated until advanced glaucoma is present. Second, visual field testing cannot be performed in young infants. A generally accepted upper level of intraocular pressure, as measured by applanation tonometry, is 17 mm Hg in neonates.

Treatment of this condition is primarily surgical. Goniotomy is the principal mode of operative therapy and is aimed at increasing the facility of outflow of aqueous humor through the angle structures, since obstruction of this flow is thought to be the primary cause of the glaucoma. Whether this blockage is due to an abnormal membrane across the angle of the eye or to developmental anomalies such as abnormal insertions of ciliary muscles remains unclear.

Children with this form of glaucoma will require careful and frequent follow-up examinations performed after administration of repeat general anesthesia. Of those children tested after the age of 5 years, approximately 40 per cent will obtain better than 20/40 vision if pressure is satisfactorily controlled. Early surgical therapy would appear to control the pressure in 85 per cent of children in whom the diagnosis is made and in whom treatment is initiated before the age of 1 year.

Eversion of the Eyelids

The eyelids of the newborn may be everted at birth secondarily, that is, in the presence of microphthalmos, buphthalmos, lid defects, or other abnormalities of the eyes. Primary eversion, without discoverable contributing cause, has been reported only a few times. The tarsal conjunctivae, facing outward, are chemotic and hyperemic (Fig. 104—4). There is no history of obstetric difficulties or other ocular abnormalities. The lids return to normal in a few weeks, following the application of an ophthalmic ointment and moist, sterile gauze dressings.

REFERENCES

Barkan, O.: Surgery of congenital glaucoma. Review of 196 eyes operated by goniotomy. Am. J. Ophthalmol. 36:1523, 1953.

Beller, R., Hoyt, C. S., Marg, E., and Odom, J. V.: Good visual function after neonatal surgery for congenital monocular cataracts. Am. J. Ophthalmol. 91:559, 1981.

Costenbader, F. D., and Kwitko, M. L.: Congenital glaucoma. An analysis of seventy-seven consecutive eyes. J. Pediatr. Ophthalmol. 4:9, 1967.

Dominguez, A., Banos, M. S., Alvarez, M. G., Contra, G. F., and Quintela, F. B.: Intraocular pressure measurement in infants under general anesthesia. Am. J. Ophthalmol. 78:110, 1974.

Fulton, A. B., Manning, K., Salem, D., and Petersen, R. A.: Cycloplegic refractions of premature infants. Am. J. Ophthalmol. 91:490, 1981.

Haas, J. S.: Congenital glaucoma: end results of treatment. Trans. Am. Acad. Ophthalmol. Otolaryngol. 59:333, 1955.

Merin, S., and Morin, D.: Heredity of congenital glaucoma. Br. J. Ophthalmol. 56:414, 1972.

Owens, W. C., and Hughes, W. F.: Results of surgical treatment of congenital cataract. Arch. Ophthalmol. 39:339, 1948.

Radtke, N. D., and Cohan, B. E.: Intraocular pressure measurement in the newborn. Am. J. Ophthalmol. 78:501, 1974.

Richardson, K. T., Jr.: Optic cup symmetry in normal newborn infants. Invest. Ophthalmol. 7:137, 1968.

Richardson, K. T., Jr., Ferguson, W. J., Jr., and Shaffer, R. N.: Long-term functional results in infantile glaucoma. Trans. Am. Acad. Ophthalmol. Otolaryngol. 71:833, 1967.

Rogers, G. L., Tishler, C. L., Tsou, B. H., Hertle, R. W., and Fellows, R. R.: Visual acuities in infants with congenital cataracts operated on prior to 6 months of age. Arch. Ophthalmol. 99:999, 1981.

Ryan, S. J., Blanton, F. M., and von Noorden, G. K.: Surgery of congenital cataract. Am. J. Ophthalmol. 60:583, 1965.

Scheie, H. G.: The management of infantile glaucoma. A.M.A. Arch. Ophthalmol. 62:35, 1959.

Shaffer, R. N.: New concepts in infantile glaucoma. Canad. J. Ophthalmol. 2:243, 1967.

von Noorden, G. K., Ryan, S. J., and Maumenee, A. E.: Management of congenital cataracts. Trans. Am. Acad. Ophthalmol. Otolaryngol. 74:352, 1970.

Weiss, D. I.: Congenital mesodermal anomalies and glaucoma. Invest. Ophthalmol. 7:123, 1968.

105

Infections of the Eye

By Lawrence W. Hirst

Neonatal Conjunctivitis (Ophthalmia Neonatorum)

Prophylaxis. During the years following Credé's introduction of silver nitrate prophylaxis for ophthalmia neonatorum, the use of topical silver nitrate has been under considerable investigation and controversy. The occurrence of a mild self-limited chemical conjunctivitis, most prominent within the first 6 hours of life in 90 per cent of infants treated with topical silver nitrate, has led to the reappraisal of this method of prophylaxis. Examination of the routine use of silver nitrate has revealed that it is effective against *Neisseria gonorrhoeae,* resulting in a decrease in the incidence rate from 10 per cent to approximately 0.5 per cent. In vitro testing has confirmed its activity not only against *Neisseria gonorrhoeae* but also against *Staphylococcus aureus* and *Escherichia coli* at concentrations of 0.1 per cent. Despite this in vitro and in vivo effectiveness, a survey has shown that perhaps 20 per cent of maternity hospitals are no longer using this method of prophylaxis. The reasons for this are principally (1) the mild transient chemical conjunctivitis noted in most infants treated with this method, (2) the occasional severe keratoconjunctivitis reported as a result of inappropriate silver nitrate use, for example, silver nitrate elution from a silver nitrate stick, and (3) the known failure of this method of prophylaxis against other causes of neonatal conjunctivitis, principally chlamydial infection.

These problems have led to the current reappraisal of the overall prophylaxis for neonatal conjunctivitis and the following recommendations by the Committee on Infectious Diseases, American Academy of Pediatrics:

Children born to mothers with no evidence of chlamydial or gonococcal genital disease should be treated with 1 per cent silver nitrate solution in single-dose wax ampoules (in order to prevent the severe chemical keratoconjunctivitis associated with the inadvertent use of either silver nitrate sticks or concentrated solution that forms following evaporation from other silver nitrate containers). One places two drops of 1 per cent silver nitrate solution from a sealed wax ampoule into the lower cul-de-sac while holding the patient's eyelids open and allowing the solution to run into the conjunctival sac and remain in situ for at least 30 seconds. There is evidence to suggest that irrigation of the conjunctival sac after prophylaxis does *not* prevent the almost 100 per cent occurrence of a mild chemical conjunctivitis during the first 24 hours and therefore should not be performed. Alternative regimens for prophylaxis in children of apparently noninfected mothers can include the use of 1 per cent tetracycline in oil drop or 0.5 per cent erythromycin drops. Infants delivered by cesarean section should also be given ocular prophylaxis. The choice of treatment of children born to mothers known to be affected by the chlamydial or gonococcal infections will be discussed later.

Incidence. Although a wide variety of conjunctival flora may be grown within the first 48 hours after birth, most organisms disappear from the conjunctival sac by that time. These organisms include all aerobic bacteria, *Hemophilus, Streptococcus* (including the enterococcus group), *Staphylococcus epidermidis, Escherichia coli, Corynebacterium, Neisseria, Bacillus,* and *Micrococcus* species as well as a wide variety of anaerobic bacteria. Despite these many conjunctival species and the common continuing presence of bacterial flora even after the use of silver nitrate prophylaxis, the incidence of bacterial conjunctivitis in neonates born to noninfected mothers is probably no higher than approximately 8 per cent. The most common responsible bacterial agents are *Staphylococcus aureus, Streptococcus viridans, Escherichia coli,* and *Staphylococcus epidermidis.* However, with between 2.4 and 12.7 per cent of puerperal women being infected with genital strains of *Chlamydia trachomatis* and approximately 44 per cent of their infants developing clinical chlamydial conjunctivitis, this form of neonatal infection has become the most common form of conjunctivitis, affecting approximately 3 per cent of all newborns.

Differential Diagnosis. Despite attempts to differentiate etiologic agents by the time of onset of the conjunctivitis after delivery and to distinguish the clinical features associated with each individual conjunctivitis, the common forms of neonatal conjunctivitis may occur at any time from 24 hours to 4 weeks without any clinical features that characteristically differentiate one type from another. The early red eye and slight mucous discharge that occur within the first 10 to 12 hours and that resolve within 24 hours are almost always associated with the use of silver nitrate prophylaxis. The onset of a florid mucopurulent conjunctivitis within the first 2 to 4 days is characteristic of gonococcal infections but is by no means pathognomonic. Although it was shown in one series that chlamydial conjunctivitis is most common within the first week, other authors have found that the onset can occur as late as the first 6 weeks of life. The slightly later onset of herpes simplex II infection does not assist in the diagnosis of this condition, although the occurrence of either corneal epithelial dendrites or a herpes simplex skin eruption is pathognomonic of this condition.

Pseudomembrane formation is not uncommon and therefore cannot be used to differentiate the etiologic agent. Because there is considerable overlap regarding the onset and clinical findings, the differentiation of the etiologic agents of the various forms of neonatal conjunctivitis depends primarily on the history of proved genital infection of the mother and on adequate examination of the neonate by conjunctival scrapings and cultures.

Methods of Scrapings and Cultures. The use of topical anesthetic should be avoided if possible, but, if necessary, proparacaine (0.5 per cent) should be used.

For bacteria and fungi, a Kimura spatula dipped in Trypticase soy broth (Minitip) should be passed across the inferior fornix, inferior tarsal plate, and superior tarsal plate and inoculated onto chocolate agar, blood agar, Sabouraud agar, and a liquid nutrient medium. Separate specimens should be taken from the right and left sides.

For viral collection, a calcium alginate swab should be passed across the inferior fornix, inferior tarsal plate, and superior tarsal plate and placed in recently thawed viral transport medium.

For chlamydial cultures, the cultures are preferably taken after scrapings of the conjunctival surface for smears. A dry calcium alginate swab is passed across the inferior fornix, inferior tarsal plate, and superior tarsal plate, and it is then placed into recently thawed chlamydial transport medium. Separate cultures should be taken from right and left sides.

SPECIFIC FORMS OF NEONATAL CONJUNCTIVITIS

Chlamydial Conjunctivitis (Inclusion Blennorrhea)

This condition has been reported to occur in as many as 2.8 per cent of all newborns or, more importantly, 35 per cent of neonates born to genitally infected mothers. The causative agent is *Chlamydia trachomatis* serotypes D, E, F, G, H, I, J, and K. This infection occurs despite silver nitrate prophylaxis, anytime from the first week through from 4 to 6 weeks after delivery but rarely within the first 2 or 3 days. It is associated with a unilateral or bilateral mucopurulent discharge, generally clear corneas early in the course, and occasional pseudomembrane formation. Later in the course, superior and inferior micropannus may appear on the cornea if the infection persists for a number of weeks. At the same time, conjunctival follicles may become evident after the first 6 weeks (there is no lymphoid tissue in the newborn conjunctiva, so earlier development of follicles is not possible). The history of symptomatic genital infection in the mother should alert the clinician to the possibility of chlamydial infection. Chlamydial cultures should be taken prior to the use of local topical anesthetic drops. Calcium alginate swab sampling from the inferior conjunctival fornix and superior tarsal conjunctival plate rather than from the mucous discharge is performed. The inoculation of this onto McCoy cells may yield a positive culture in excess of 50 per cent of all chlamydial conjunctivitis. A complete assessment for chlamydial infection should also include cultures taken from the mother's cervix and from the child's nasopharynx and throat. Conjunctival epithelial scrapings taken with a Kimura spatula after instillation of a topical anesthetic (proparacaine 0.5 per cent) and staining of the resultant scrapings with the microimmunofluorescent technique may be expected to yield in excess of 90 per cent positive results. Giemsa staining for intracytoplasmic inclusions and for mixed acute and chronic inflammatory cells is helpful. Serology for chlamydial antibodies may reveal diagnostic titers. Although initial clearing of the clinical conjunctivitis may be obtained by the use of topical erythromycin or tetracycline only, it is generally considered appropriate to use systemic antibiotics because of the known propensity of *Chlamydia* to infect the nasopharynx, ears, lungs, and genital tract of infants with chlamydial conjunctivitis. Also, the use of topical tetracycline alone for 4 weeks has been shown to be associated with a reisolation of *Chlamydia trachomatis* in 75 per cent of treated infants. These facts, together with the development of corneal changes of inadequately treated chlamydial conjunctivitis, support the use of other systemic antibiotics. The oral administration of erythromycin succinate, 40 mg per kg daily for 21 days in the infants, together with topical 1 per cent tetracycline ointment four times a day for the same length of time, should be supplemented by treatment of the mother and, if necessary, the father with systemic septrin. Careful observation of the infant after completion of the treatment is required for the early diagnosis of persistence or recurrence of chlamydial infection. Similar treatment should be considered for infants who are free of conjunctivitis but born to mothers with known chlamydial infection.

Gonococcal Conjunctivitis

The incidence of gonococcal conjunctivitis is difficult to assess, with few cases reported to date. The

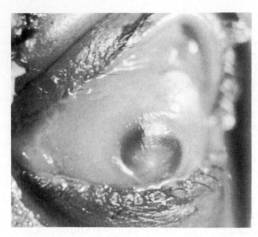

Figure 105–1. Advanced case of gonorrheal ophthalmia. Note the intense panophthalmitis with reddening and thickening of both the bulbar and the tarsal conjunctivae and ulceration of the cornea and sclera. (From the collection of Dr. Arnall Patz.)

usual agent, *Neisseria gonorrhoeae,* is transmitted from maternal genital infection. Pseudogonococcal infection has been reported with *Branhamella catarrhalis.* The onset of this infection generally occurs within the first 2 or 3 days and usually before 5 days with early lid swelling, lid edema, and serosanguineous exudate, followed by mucopurulent discharge. If untreated, spontaneous healing can occur within 7 to 10 days, but usually corneal ulceration and final perforation with loss of the eye occur (Fig. 105–1). Investigation should include conjunctival cultures taken, prior to topical anesthesia administration, from the conjunctival epithelial surface rather than from exudate with a Kimura spatula and inoculated onto chocolate blood agar and held in 20 per cent carbon dioxide. Similar cultures should be taken from the mother's cervix. Transport of the specimen may be also performed with Stuart's medium. Conjunctival scrapings, taken after topical anesthetic application, are smeared and stained with gram stain to reveal gram-negative intracellular diplococci. Treatment of children with this form of conjunctivitis should include isolation, careful hygiene of mucus from the lids, and intravenous crystalline penicillin G, 50,000 units per kg of body weight daily in two divided doses for 7 days. The use of topical agents appears ineffective. Treatment of the mother should proceed concurrently. The occurrence of beta-lactamase–producing *Neisseria gonorrhoeae* should be suspected in recalcitrant cases, and the use of kanamycin or cefuroxime should be considered.

Herpes Simplex Keratoconjunctivitis

The incidence of this agent in neonatal conjunctivitis is low but becoming greater with the increasing incidence of genital herpes infection. The herpes simplex virus type 2 responsible for this conjunctivitis may result in unilateral or bilateral conjunctivitis (nonfollicular in the neonate) that may be associated with lid vesicles and corneal epithelial dendritic figures. The occurrence of either of the latter two should establish the clinical diagnosis, which may be supported by demonstration of cytopathic effects on cell cultures inoculated by a cotton tip drawn across the conjunctival surface and transported immediately in viral transport media to the laboratory. Scrapings taken from the conjunctival surface may reveal giant cells with intracytoplasmic inclusions. Sequential serology may reveal a rising neutralizing antibody titer. Treatment should consist of administration of 3 per cent vidarabine ointment five times per day for 10 days or idoxuridine ointment five times per day for 10 days or 1 per cent trifluorothymidine drops every 2 hours, seven doses per day, for 10 days. The association of recurrent corneal herpetic disease following a primary follicular conjunctivitis with herpes simplex virus type 2 infection is unclear.

Staphylococcal Conjunctivitis

This infection, which is usually nosocomially acquired, may occur within the first postnatal week and is usually manifested by profuse mucoid discharge and conjunctival hyperemia and chemosis. Treatment should include strict isolation and close observation of other neonates for similar infection. Treatment consists of lid hygiene and 0.5 per cent erythromycin ophthalmic ointment or bacitracin eye ointment applied six times per day for 2 weeks. Despite the usually innocuous course of this conjunctivitis, corneal infection following mild corneal epithelial trauma may lead to rapid corneal perforation. The scalded skin syndrome has been reported following staphylococcal conjunctivitis.

Coliform Conjunctivitis

This conjunctivitis may be indistinguishable from the staphylococcal form and is treated with 0.5 per cent neomycin ointment or 1 per cent tetracycline eye drops used six times per day for 2 weeks.

Other Forms of Neonatal Conjunctivitis

Other forms of neonatal conjunctivitis may be caused by *Pneumococcus, Streptococcus, Hemophilus,* and *Pseudomonas.* The use of 0.5 per cent erythromycin ointment is appropriate for the infections caused by *Pneumococcus, Streptococcus,* and *Hemophilus;* topical gentamicin or tobramicin should be used for *Pseudomonas* infections. Occasional cases of *Candida* conjunctivitis have been reported. This type of infection should respond to a 3-week course of natamicin drops given six times per day. A

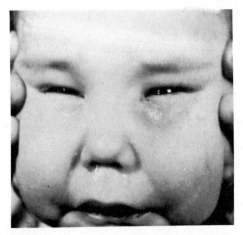

Figure 105–2. Acute dacryocystitis. Note the swollen, reddened lower lid and the cystic swelling in the angle between the eye and the bridge of the nose. (From the collection of Dr. Arnall Patz.)

rare nonmicrobial conjunctivitis, ligneous conjunctivitis, has been reported in neonates. It is characteristically a bilateral membranous conjunctivitis with mucoid polysaccharide deposition within the membrane. The treatment of this infection, including the reported use of hyaluronidase, remains speculative.

Lacrimal Outlet Obstruction (Dacryostenosis, Dacryocystitis)

The etiology of lacrimal outlet obstruction is obscure, but in some cases it has reportedly followed an autosomal dominant inheritance pattern. There appears to be a local developmental abnormality at 4 to 6 months' gestation.

Despite the high rate of early nasal lacrimal duct obstruction (>50 per cent nonfunctional nasolacrimal ducts in 1- to 5-day-old infants), acute infection (dacryocystitis) as evidenced by swelling in the inner canthal region, redness and tenderness over this area, and mucopurulent discharge from the eye is extremely rare in neonates (Fig. 105–2). However, when such infection does occur, systemic antibiotics effective against *Streptococcus, Staphylococcus,* and *Hemophilus* should be instituted. Resolution is usually swift, and external drainage of the lacrimal sac is rarely necessary. Persistent postinfection epiphora may occur that may necessitate attempted probing of the nasal lacrimal duct.

More than 80 per cent of congenitally blocked nasolacrimal ducts will have spontaneously opened by 3 months of age. If acute infections have not occurred but epiphora continues beyond 6 months of age (indicating probable dacryostenosis), gentle probing of the nasal lacrimal system under general anesthesia should be performed. One may need to perform repeat probing in order to establish patency. The most frequent obstruction occurs at the nasal mucosal end of the duct.

One should also perform careful nasal examination with the infant under general anesthesia in order to exclude turbinate pathology. If surgical bypass of the obstruction is required, one usually undertakes dacryocystorhinostomy or insertion of a Jones tube or both (depending on the site of lacrimal outlet obstruction).

Orbital Cellulitis

This fortunately rare infection, presenting with reduced ocular motility, proptosis, chemosis of conjunctiva, and pain should initiate a radiologic search for sinus infection. Systemic antibiotics should be administered, and drainage of sinus mucocele, if present, should be performed as a matter of urgency.

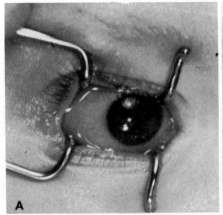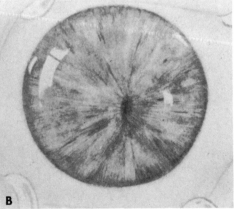

Figure 105–3. *A,* Photograph of the eye of a newborn who had suffered uveitis during gestation. *B,* Artist's conception of the resulting lesion. The pupil resembles a tightly closed camera shutter. This is the contracted fibrosed iris, firmly bound down to the lens and fixed. (From the collection of Dr. Arnall Patz.)

Uveitis

The fetal eye manifests an extraordinary susceptibility to chorioretinitis. Many infections acquired transplacentally, as well as a few acquired postnatally, localize in this situation. Toxoplasmosis, cytomegalic inclusion disease, disseminated herpes virus infection, rubella, and syphilis are some of the diseases in which chorioretinitis may be one sign. Involvement of the iris and ciliary body, iridocyclitis, is extremely uncommon.

REFERENCES

Brook, I., Martin, W. J., and Finegold, S. M.: Effect of silver nitrate application on the conjunctival flora of the newborn, and the occurrence of clostridial conjunctivitis. J. Pediatr. Ophthalmol. Strabismus 15:179, 1978.

Cassady, J. V.: Developmental anatomy of nasolacrimal duct. Arch. Ophthalmol. 47:141, 1952.

Chandler, J. W., Alexander, E. R., Pheiffer, T. A., Wang, S., Holmes, K. K., and English, M.: Ophthalmia neonatorum associated with maternal chlamydial infections. Trans Am. Acad. Ophthalmol. Otolaryngol. 83:302, 1977.

Cohen, K. L., and McCarthy, L. R.: Haemophilus influenzae ophthalmia neonatorum. Arch. Ophthalmol. 98:1214, 1980.

Committee on Drugs, Committee on Fetus and Newborn, and Committee on Infectious Diseases: Prophylaxis and treatment of neonatal gonococcal infections. Pediatrics 65:1047, 1980.

Credé: Reports from the obstetrical clinic in Leipzig. Prevention of eye inflammation in the newborn. Am. J. Dis. Child. 121:3, 1971.

Firat, T.: Ligneous conjunctivitis. Am. J. Ophthalmol. 78:679, 1974.

Fox, K. R., and Golomb, H. S.: Staphylococcal ophthalmia neonatorum and the staphylococcal scalded skin syndrome. Am. J. Ophthalmol. 88:1052, 1979.

Grossman, T. H., and Putz, R.: Uber die angeborene Tranengangstenose der Neugeborenen, ihre Anatomie, ihre Folgen und Behandlung. Klin. Monatsbl. Augenheilkd. 160:563, 1972.

Hammerschlag, M. R., Chandler, J. W., Alexander, E. R., English, M., Chiang, W. T., Koutsky, L., Eschenbach, D. A., and Smith, J. R.: Erythromycin ointment for ocular prophylaxis of neonatal chlamydial infection. J.A.M.A. 244:2291, 1980.

Hornblass, A.: Severe silver nitrate ocular damage in newborn nursery. N.Y. State J. Med. 76:1875, 1976.

Johnson, D., and McKenna, H.: Bacteria in ophthalmia neonatorum. Pathology 7:199, 1975.

Jones, D. B., Liesegans, T. J., and Robinson, N. M.: Laboratory Diagnosis of Ocular Infections. Cumitech 13, American Society for Microbiology, May 1981.

Korchmaros, I., Szalay, E., Fodor, M., and Fedak, L.: Probable etiology of the non-opened lacrimal pathway. In Yamaguchi, M. (Ed.): Recent Advances on the Lacrimal System. Tokyo, Asahi Evening News, 1980. pp. 23–29.

Korchmaros, I., Szalay, E., Fodor, M., and Jablonszky, E.: Spontaneous opening rate of congenitally blocked nasolacrimal ducts. In Yamaguchi, M. (Ed.): Recent Advances on the Lacrimal System. Tokyo, Asahi Evening News, 1980. pp. 30–35.

Liesmaa, M., and Vannas, S.: Rise in congenital anomalies of the lacrimal passages in southern Finland since 1959. Acta Ophthalmol. 43:85, 1969.

Nishida, H., and Risemberg, H. M.: Silver nitrate ophthalmic solution and chemical conjunctivitis, Pediatrics 56:368, 1975.

Ostler, H. B.: Oculogenital disease. Surv. Ophthalmol. 20:233, 1976.

Persson, K., Rönnerstam, R., Svanberg, I., and Holmberg, L.: Maternal and infantile infection with Chlamydia in a Swedish population. Acta Paediatr. Scand. 70:101, 1981.

Prentice, M. J., Hutchinson, G. R., and Taylor-Robinson, D.: A microbiological study of neonatal conjunctivae and conjunctivitis. Br. J. Ophthalmol. 61:601, 1977.

Rees, E., Tait, I. A., Hobson, D., Byng, R. E., and Johnson, F. W. A.: Neonatal conjunctivitis caused by Neisseria gonorrhoeae and Chlamydia trachomatis. Br. J. Vener. Dis. 53:173, 1977.

Rees, E., Tait, I. A., Hobson, D., Karayiannis, P., and Lee, N.: Persistence of chlamydial infection after treatment for neonatal conjunctivitis. Arch. Dis. Child. 56:193, 1981.

Rowe, D. S., Aicardi, E. Z., Dawson, C. R., and Schachter, J.: Purulent ocular discharge in neonates: significance of Chlamydia trachomatis. Pediatrics 63:628, 1979.

Schachter, J., Hold, J., Goodner, E., Grossman, M., Sweet, R., and Mills, J.: Prospective study of chlamydial infection in neonates. Lancet 2:377, 1979.

Spark, R. P., Dahlberg, P. W., and LaBelle, J. W.: Pseudogonococcal ophthalmia neonatorum. Branhamella (Neisseria) catarrhalis conjunctivitis. Am. J. Clin. Pathol. 72:471, 1979.

Tumors of the Eye and Orbit

By William R. Green and Arnall Patz

The overall number of tumors of the eye that appear within the neonatal period is small. Most of them are hamartomas or choristomas, and the most common of these are dermoids and hemangiomas. The one malignant neoplasm of utmost importance in this age period is retinoblastoma. It is imperative that this diagnosis be made promptly and that therapy be instituted without delay. An apparent neoplasm that must be differentiated from tumor in this location is encephalocele, presenting either in the orbit or in the angle between the eye and the bridge of the nose.

Hemangioma

As has been indicated earlier (see Chapter 100), the upper lids are a common site for the port-wine stains of nevus flammeus. These may be faint or extremely prominent. When present, one or more of the same type can be expected to be located over the nuchal region. The faint ones fade within a few months, the more deeply colored ones within a few years. They need no treatment.

Hemangiomas not infrequently involve the palpebral conjunctivae. These may take the form of nevus flammeus also, imparting a deeper purplish color to a portion of the conjunctiva and thickening it slightly. Alternatively, as in the skin, the tumors may be more deeply seated cavernous hemangiomas producing visible bulges within the eyelid that protrude into the conjunctival sac (Fig. 106–1). Not infrequently, hemangiomas of the conjunctiva are accompanied by similar nevi elsewhere. In one of our pa-

tients thick, deep angiomas covered the lower lid, conjunctiva, the pharyngeal wall, and the tonsil on one side. Thin, superficial nevi in this location require no treatment. Deeper ones may have to be treated because of their sheer size and the irritation they may inflict upon the eyeball. We prefer surgical excision to x-irradiation. Prior to either procedure, cortisone probably deserves a trial for 10 days to 2 weeks.

Hemangiomas may also be present within the orbit. These may be of sufficient size to produce proptosis and disturbances of extraocular movement. They almost invariably project out of the orbit into an eyelid, where they are visible beneath the tarsal conjunctiva. Like hemangiomas everywhere, their natural tendency is toward ultimate shrinking and disappearance. One should allow them plenty of opportunity to subside. If either proptosis or fixation of the eyeball is serious or if the tumor seems to be growing, some form of treatment is indicated. A course of prednisone should be tried first. A dose of 2 to 3 mg per kilogram per day for 10 to 14 days will allow assessment of its effect. If the hemangioma has regressed, the steroids can be tapered until the lowest dose needed to prevent growth is ascertained. We have maintained some infants on low doses of prednisone for many months and then stopped medication with no recurrence. Occasionally, steroids are ineffective, and careful x-irradiation or intralesional steroid injection in capable hands is indicated.

Choristomas

Epibulbar choristomas include dermoids, dermolipomas, complex choristomas, dermis-like choristomas, ectopic lacrimal gland tissue, and osseous choristomas (Elsas and Green, 1975).

Dermoids are the most commonly encountered epibulbar lesions in the newborn and usually are located near or straddling the limbus temporally and slightly inferiorly (Fig. 106–1). Fine hairs emanate from the surface, and an arc of lipid may be present in the cornea after a clear zone. Surgery for such lesions is for cosmetic purposes only. Difficulties may

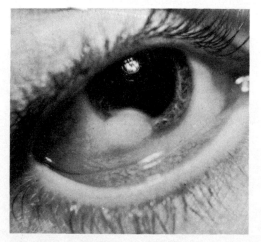

Figure 106–1. Dermoid of the eye. There is a dead-white cyst arising at the limbus and overlying portions of both the cornea and the conjunctiva. (From the collection of Dr. Arnall Patz.)

be encountered at surgery for several reasons: No cleavage plane exists between the lesion and the eye; rare intraocular extension is observed; and, occasionally, a scleral staphyloma may be encountered in association with the dermoid.

Limbal dermoids occurring in association with aural fistulas or extra-auricular appendages may be features of the oculoauricular vertebral dysplasia syndrome of Goldenhar.

The cystic types of dermoids are congenital lesions encountered most frequently in the upper lid or in the orbit superotemporally or in both areas. These cysts may be very small at birth but continue to enlarge throughout life. Only 20 to 25 per cent are clinically evident at birth.

Histopathologically, the solid dermoid of the limbus consists of a dermis-like connective tissue in which pilosebaceous apparatus are present. The dermoid cyst is filled with keratinous debris, contains a variable number of hair shafts and sebaceous material, and is lined by keratinized stratified squamous epithelium and a dense corium-like connective tissue in which pilosebaceous units are present and have continuity with the cyst lumen.

Dermolipomas consist of a dermis-like connective tissue and adipose tissue and are most frequently encountered superotemporally in the conjunctiva, giving the lid a fullness. Surgery for these lesions is strictly cosmetic; complications can be encountered, especially if overzealous excision is attempted. If removal is done, only the superficial portion or enough to correct the cosmetic defect should be excised. There is no clear cleavage plane between the lesion and subjacent tissue, and there may be deeper orbital extension and connections with the fascial sheaths of the superior and lateral rectus muscles. The lesion may also involve the five to seven orifices and ducts of the lacrimal gland.

Retinoblastoma

Once uniformly fatal, retinoblastoma, the most common intraocular malignancy of childhood, can now be detected and treated successfully enough to preserve both life and vision. Retinoblastoma occurs with a frequency of one case per 17,000 to 34,000 livebirths. The tumor may be present at birth; however, the diagnosis is most frequently made between the ages of 1½ and 2 years.

Pathology. The tumor arises in the retina and may extend in a mound-like fashion internal to the retina (endophytic) or external to the retina (exophytic). Multiple sites of origin in the same and fellow eye are common and do not necessarily arise simultaneously. The tumor tends to undergo necrosis, giving a char-

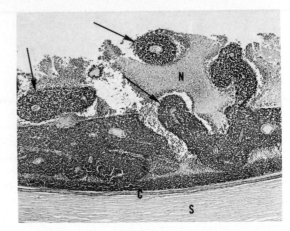

Figure 106–2. Characteristic pattern of retinoblastoma with extensive necrosis (N) and a collarette of viable tumor cells around blood vessels (arrows). (S = sclera; C = choroid.) Hematoxylin and eosin (×45).

acteristic pattern of collarettes of viable tumor around blood vessels, separated by necrotic areas, that often develop calcification (Fig. 106–2).

The tumor may extend into the vitreous as nonvascularized seedings. According to Ellsworth, such vitreous seeding of the tumor is a sign of poor prognosis. Extension of the tumor into the anterior chamber may produce signs of inflammation or glaucoma or both, either of which may mask the underlying neoplasm and result in delays in diagnosis and therapy. The most common route of extraocular extension is along the optic nerve, by which the tumor gains access to the subarachnoid space and intracranial cavity.

Invasion of retinoblastoma into the vascular choroid is a potential source of hematogenous spread of the tumor. In advanced cases, direct extension through the sclera into the orbit may occur.

Three forms of cytodifferentiation have been recognized. The first is the Homer-Wright rosette, which consists of a ring of tumor cells around a central area containing fibrillar material and no acid mucopolysaccharide. This pattern of tumor cells is also seen in neuroblastoma and medulloblastoma. Flexner-Win-

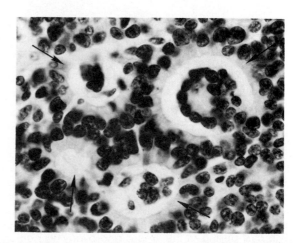

Figure 106–3. Flexner-Wintersteiner rosettes of retinoblastoma (arrows). Hematoxylin and eosin (×750).

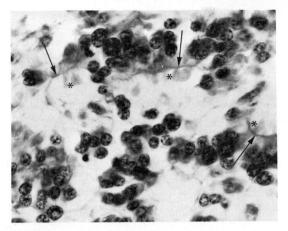

Figure 106–4. Fleurettes of retinoblastoma containing a structure analogous to the external limiting membrane of the retina (arrows) and rudimentary photoreceptors (asterisks). Hematoxylin and eosin (× 850).

tersteiner rosettes (Fig. 106–3) are specific for retinoblastoma and consist of a ring of low columnar cells with basally located nuclei around a lumen in which a hyaluronidase-resistant acid mucopolysaccharide is present. Filamentous cytoplasmic projections of the tumor cells extend into the lumen and have rudimentary photoreceptor differentiation. T'so and coworkers have described clusters of cells (fleurettes) (Fig. 106–4), which have more definite photoreceptor differentiation.

Heredity. Approximately 6 per cent of retinoblastoma cases are familial. The mode of transmission is autosomal dominant, with penetrance varying between 20 and 95 per cent but most frequently stated to be 80 per cent. In 1969, Ellsworth reported that both familial and sporadic retinoblastoma are due to germinal mutations but that penetrance is low in unilateral sporadic cases and high in bilateral sporadic cases. The probability of bilateral retinoblastoma in sporadic cases ranges from 18 to 31 per cent, whereas in hereditary cases it is between 92 and 95 per cent if a parent is affected, 83 per cent if two or more siblings are affected, and 60 per cent if a distant relative is affected.

Partial deletions of the long arm of chromosome 13 have been reported in at least 72 instances of hereditary retinoblastoma. The likelihood of chromosome 13q − deletions is greatest in the presence of associated severe malformations such as microcephaly, mental retardation, and skeletal anomalies. With special banding techniques, the deletions have been located on chromosome 13q 31-32 and 13q 33-34. In some instances, the deletion has been at 13q 14; when in that location, less severe malformations have been reported. It seems prudent to examine chromosomes in all cases of retinoblastoma.

Genetic Counseling. In cases of established hereditary retinoblastoma, the gene is generally transmitted to 50 per cent of offspring. Normal parents with one affected child and with no prior family his-

tory will have a 4 to 7 per cent probability of producing a second offspring with retinoblastoma. Normal parents with two or more affected children will have a 50 per cent probability of producing a genetically affected offspring, with the incidence of retinoblastoma depending on penetrance. A survivor of bilateral sporadic retinoblastoma or a patient with multiple lesions in one eye has the inherited type and will produce clinically affected offspring in 50 per cent of cases, whereas a survivor of unilateral sporadic retinoblastoma will produce clinically affected children in 10 per cent of offspring.

Diagnosis. The most frequent sign, observed in about 56 per cent of patients with retinoblastoma (Ellsworth, 1969), is leukocoria (white pupil). The white reflex in the pupil is frequently observed by the child's mother.

The presence or onset of strabismus is the second most common sign (20 per cent). This sign is particularly important, since the general physician may be the first to examine such a patient. We believe infants and children with strabismus should have an ophthalmoscopic examination to rule out the possibility of retinoblastoma. Often, this can be accomplished by wide dilation of the pupil, restraint of the child, and examination with an indirect ophthalmoscope. If such is not possible, examination should be performed under sedation or anesthesia.

Other, less common presenting signs and symptoms include a red, painful eye with glaucoma (7 per cent); orbital cellulitis (3 per cent); unilateral mydriasis (2 per cent); heterochromia (1 per cent); and

Table 106–1. Diagnosis in 265 Patients with Lesions Simulating Retinoblastoma

Diagnosis	Per Cent of Total
Persistent hyperplastic primary vitreous	19.0
Retrolental fibroplasia	13.5
Posterior cataract	13.5
Coloboma of choroid or disc	11.5
Uveitis	10.0
Nematode endophthalmitis	6.5
Congenital retinal fold	5.0
Coats' disease	4.0
Old vitreous hemorrhage	3.5
Retinal dysplasia	2.5
Tumor other than retinoblastoma	1.5
White-with-pressure sign	1.0
Juvenile xanthogranuloma	1.0
Retinoschisis	1.0
Tapetoretinal degeneration	1.0
Endophthalmitis	1.0
Persistent tunica vasculosa lentis	1.0
Miscellaneous	3.5
	100.0

(From Howard, G. M., and Ellsworth, R. M.: Am. J. Ophthalmol. 60:610, 1965.)

Table 106–2. Prognosis Based on Size and Extent of Tumor

Group I— very favorable, 95 per cent cure
      A. Solitary tumor, less than 4 disc diameters in size, at or behind the equator
      B. Multiple tumors, none over 4 disc diameters in size, all at or behind the equator
Group II— favorable, 87 per cent cure
      A. Solitary tumor, 4 to 10 disc diameters in size, at or behind the equator
      B. Multiple tumors, 4 to 10 disc diameters in size, behind the equator
Group III— doubtful, 67 per cent cure
      A. Any lesion anterior to the equator
      B. Solitary tumors larger than 10 disc diameters and behind the equator
Group IV— unfavorable, 69 per cent cure
      A. Multiple tumors, some larger than 10 disc diameters
      B. Any lesion extending anterior to the ora serrata
Group V— very unfavorable, 34 per cent cure
      A. Massive tumors involving over half of retina
      B. Vitreous seeding

(From Ellsworth, R. M.: Trans. Am. Ophthalmol. Soc. 67:462, 1969.)

hyphema (1 per cent). In 3 per cent of cases, the retinoblastoma was observed at the time of a routine examination.

Other conditions can be confused clinically with retinoblastoma. These conditions are listed in Table 106–1.

Prognosis. Both clinical and histopathologic features have been found to be of some help in prognosticating the course of retinoblastoma. If distant metastases are demonstrated, the disease is invariably fatal, despite current modes of chemotherapy and radiation.

The size and extent of disease within the globe has been found useful in determining therapy and prognosis (Ellsworth, 1969). Table 106–2 lists five clinical categories. Histopathologic criteria in estimating prognosis include optic nerve invasion, choroid invasion, scleral extension, epibulbar extension, and degree of cytodifferentiation.

Treatment. Enucleation of the eye is the treatment of choice in patients who have large tumors in one eye and no family history of retinoblastoma (groups IV and V; Table 106–2). Children with small, unilateral tumors (groups I, II and III; Table 106–2) that are diagnosed early because of the onset of strabismus or because of a family history or detection at a routine ophthalmologic examination are treated primarily with radiotherapy rather than enucleation. In bilateral cases, tumor is usually more advanced in one eye. Such patients are treated by enucleation of the more severely affected eye and by radiation ther-

apy, with or without chemotherapy, for the other eye. Ellsworth generally restricts chemotherapy to those patients in groups IV and V.

Bilateral advanced tumors in groups IV and V are treated by irradiation and chemotherapy. Selected cases of small residual or new tumor growth can be treated by other techniques, such as cryotherapy, photocoagulation, radon-seed implantation, and cobalt-60 application.

Some authorities have stressed focal techniques, such as localized betatron therapy from the side, cobalt plaques, photocoagulation, and cryosurgery, in the treatment of single or multiple tumors of 10 mm or less (Bedford, 1975). Tumors larger than 10 mm would appear to be best treated by whole-eye irradiation.

Some authors (Bedford, 1975) appear to be moving away from the opinion that the most seriously affected eye or, in unilateral cases, the involved eye should be treated by enucleation. It would appear that the only indication for enucleation is the clinical suspicion that the optic nerve may be involved because of tumor at or adjacent to the disc.

REFERENCES

Bedford, M. A.: Treatment of retinoblastoma. Adv. Ophthalmol. 31:2, 1975.

Doxanas, M. T., Green, W. R., Arentsen, J. J., and Elsas, F. J.: Lid lesions of childhood: a histopathologic survey at the Wilmer Institute (1923–1974). J. Pediatr. Ophthalmol. 13:5, 1976.

Ellsworth, R. M.: The practical management of retinoblastoma. Trans. Am. Ophthalmol. Soc. 67:462, 1969.

Elsas, F. J., and Green, W. R.: Epibulbar tumors in childhood. Am. J. Ophthalmol. 79:1001, 1975.

Fost, N. C., and Esterly, N. B.: Successful treatment of juvenile hemangiomas with prednisone. J. Pediatr. 72:351, 1968.

Howard, G. M., and Ellsworth, R. M.: Differential diagnosis of retinoblastoma. A statistical survey of 500 children. I. Relative frequency of the lesions which simulate retinoblastoma. Am. J. Ophthalmol. 60:610, 1965.

Knudson, A. G., Meadows, A. T., Nichols, W. W., and Hill, R.: Chromosomal deletion and retinoblastoma. N. Engl. J. Med. 295:1120, 1976.

Kolata, G. B.: Genes and the story of Wilms' tumor. Science 207:970, 1980.

Kushner, R. J.: Intralesional corticosteroid injection for infantile adnexal hemangioma. Am. J. Opthalmol. 93:496, 1982.

Iliff, C. E., and Ossofsky, H. J.: Tumors of the Eye and Adnexa in Infancy and Childhood. Springfield, Ill., Charles C Thomas, 1962.

Nicholson, D. H., and Green, W. R.: Tumors of the eye, lids, and orbit in children. In Harley, R. D. (Ed.): Pediatric Ophthalmology. Philadelphia, W. B. Saunders Co., 1975.

Sparkes, R. S., Murphree, A. L., Lingua, A., et al.: Gene for hereditary retinoblastoma assigned to human chromosome 13 by linkage to esterase D. Science 219:971, 1983.

T'so, M. O. M., Fine, B. S., and Zimmerman, L. E.: The Flexner-Wintersteiner rosettes in retinoblastoma. Arch. Pathol. 88:664, 1969.

T'so, M. O. M., Zimmerman, L. E., and Fine, B. S.: The nature of retinoblastoma. I. Photoreceptor differentiation: a clinical and histopathologic study; II. Photoreceptor differentiation: an electron microscopic study. Am. J. Ophthalmol. 69:339, 350, 1970.

Yunis, J. J., and Ramsay, W.: Retinoblastoma and sub-band deletion of chromosome 13. Am. J. Dis. Child. 132:161, 1978.

PART 18 MISCELLANEOUS DISORDERS

107

Congenital Malignant Disorders

By Allen D. Schwartz

Many tumors peculiar to individual organs and specific localities of the body are discussed in their appropriate sections. Thus, retinoblastoma is discussed among the disorders of the eye, and teratoma is considered in the chapters devoted to various anatomic areas. Here we will discuss the more common malignant disorders that may occur in the neonate without including an exhaustive list of case reports of every congenital tumor recorded in the literature.

Incidence and Mortality. A study of death certificates by Fraumeni and Miller during the 5-year period ranging from 1960 to 1964 revealed that the death rate from malignant diseases in infants under 28 days of age was 6.24 per one million livebirths (Table 107–1). Over one half of cancer deaths in the neonatal period occurred in the first week of life, and over one third occurred on the first day (Table 107–2).

Basing their report on the Third National Cancer Survey (1969–1971), Bader and Miller found the incidence of malignant neoplasms in the United States to be 183.4 per one million livebirths in infants younger than 1 year and 36.5 per one million livebirths in newborns younger than 29 days. The cancer incidence in those under 1 year was almost 3.5 times greater than mortality determined from death certificates from 1960 to 1969. When mortality of infants under age 1 year is used as an indicator of frequency, leukemia appears to be the most common cancer followed by neuroblastoma, CNS tumors, and renal tumors. When ranked by incidence, neuroblastoma is most common, followed by leukemia, renal tumors, sarcomas, retinoblastomas, and CNS tumors. Because retinoblastoma is so often cured, the incidence is 159 times greater than the mortality. Among newborns, the incidence of neuroblastoma is more than ten times greater than the mortality for this tumor, whereas the incidence of leukemia is less than two times greater than its mortality. Thus, a study of mortality differs markedly from one of incidence, since certain malignancies are rapidly fatal, others lead to death beyond the neonatal period, and a large number are curable or undergo spontaneous regression. Data from the Third National Cancer Study indicate that approximately 653 cancers are diagnosed annually in infants in the United States and that 130 of these cancers are found in newborns. A summary of incidence, mortality, and types of malignancies seen in the neonate and infant is shown in Table 107–3.

Pathogenesis

TRANSPLACENTAL TUMOR PASSAGE

Malignant disease in the mother is very seldom transmitted across the placenta to the fetus. Wells

Table 107–1. Mortality from Malignant Neoplasms in United States Children Under 5 Years as Compared with Those Under 28 Days of Age, 1960 to 1964

| Neoplasms | No. Deaths under 5 years | Deaths under 28 Days | | |
		No.	Rate Per 10^6 Livebirths	Per Cent*
Leukemia	4592	44	2.11	1.0
Neuroblastoma	1049	27	1.30	2.6
Brain tumor	1035	7	0.34	0.7
Wilms' tumor	696	9	0.43	1.3
Liver cancer, primary	196	10	0.48	5.1
Teratoma	111	9	0.43	8.1
Sarcoma, type specified	1940	12	0.58	1.2
Other		12	0.58	
Total	9619	130	6.25	1.4

* Percentage of neonatal deaths among type-specific cancers in patients under 5 years of age (e.g., for leukemia = (44 × 100)/4592 = 1.0).

(From Fraumeni, J. F., and Miller, R. W.: Am. J. Dis. Child. *117*:186, 1969.)

Table 107–2. Deaths from Neonatal Cancer According to Specific Diagnosis, Age, and Sex

		Age		Sex	
Neoplasms	<24 hr	<6 days	1–4 weeks	Male	Female
Leukemia	10	9	25	21	23
Neuroblastoma	13	2	12	15	12
Sarcoma	7	1	4	7	5
Liver cancer, primary	4	3	3	6	4
Wilms' tumor	1	6	2	6	3
Teratoma	7	1	1	4	5
Brain tumor	3	1	3	4	3
Other	6	5	1	4	8
Total	51	28	51	67	63

(From Fraumeni, J. F., and Miller, R. W.: Am. J. Dis. Child. *117*:186, 1969.)

accepted as certain only four examples of such occurrences. Two were melanosarcomas that caused death of the children, in one instance at 8 months with metastasis to the liver, and in the other at 10 months with disseminated disease. In both instances, the placenta had extensive metastases. A maternal lymphosarcoma was discovered in one infant's liver, and a bronchogenic carcinoma had metastasized to the skin of the knee of a fourth fetus.

A small number of cases of malignant melanomas of the mother with spread to the fetus have been reported since Wells' 1940 review (Holland, 1949; Cavell, 1963; Brodsky et al., 1965). The infant reported by Cavell recovered from the metastatic disease. Kasdon recorded two instances of Hodgkin's disease occurring in infants of mothers with the disorder. Maternal virilizing tumors have resulted in fetal virilization due to transplacental passage of androgens secreted by the neoplasm, but the tumors have not spread to the fetus (Haymond and Weldon,

1973). Multiple myeloma has been reported in a small number of pregnant women (Lergier et al., 1974). In two instances, no abnormal myeloma protein was found in the infants, but a transient abnormal protein thought to be passively transferred from the mother was demonstrated in two others. None of the infants had evidence of disease.

Leukemia has not been found in newborn infants of women with this malignancy, although two children of affected mothers developed the disease at 5 and 9 months of age. In these instances, both mothers and children had acute lymphoblastic leukemia (Cramblett et al., 1958; Bernard et al., 1964). Although leukemia in mice can be transmitted to their offspring by viruses in breast milk, there is no evidence that leukemia is passed to the human infant in this manner.

The development of choriocarcinoma in an infant as a complication of placental choriocarcinoma is rare. In at least four instances, both mother and infant have been affected. This represents tumor transmission from the fetus to the mother because the trophoblast, the site of origin, is composed of fetal rather than maternal tissue. In all the recorded cases, summarized by Witzleben and Bruninga, there was either a recognized placental choriocarcinoma or absence of a primary site in the infants with disseminated malignancy. These authors stressed the characteristic presentation of hematemesis or hemoptysis, anemia, hepatomegaly, and pulmonary metastasis in the infant. The diagnosis is established by the demonstration of elevated urinary or plasma gonadotropin levels.

Table 107–3. Incidence and Mortality of Malignant Tumors in United States Neonates and Infants

	Incidence				Mortality				
	<29 Days		<12 Mos.		<29 Days		<12 Mos.		
Tumor Type	No.	Rate*	No.	Rate* (A)	No.	Rate*	No.	Rate* (B)	Ratio (A/B)
Leukemia	5	4.7	34	31.8	101	2.6	807	20.8	1.5
Neuroblastoma	21	19.7	67	62.7	70	1.8	302	7.8	8.0
CNS	1	0.9	15	14.0	12	0.3	257	6.6	2.1
Kidney	5	4.7	21	19.7	21	0.5	141	3.6	5.4
Reticuloendotheliosis	0	0	3	2.8	7	0.2	131	3.4	—
Sarcoma	4	3.7	19	17.8	29	0.7	129	3.3	5.4
Liver	0	0	8	7.5	15	0.4	99	2.6	2.9
Lymphoma	1	0.9	2	1.9	2	<0.1	60	1.5	1.3
Teratoma	0	0	3	2.8	11	0.3	28	0.7	4.0
Carcinoma	1	0.9	6	5.6	6	0.2	18	0.5	11.2
Germ cell, excluding teratoma	0	0	0	0	0	0	6	0.2	—
Retinoblastoma	0	0	17	15.9	1	<0.1	4	0.1	159.0
Other	1	0.9	1	0.9	20	0.5	62	1.6	—
Total	39	36.4	196	183.4	295	7.6	2044	52.7	3.5

* Per one million livebirths per year.

(From Bader, J. I., and Miller, R. W.: Am. J. Dis. Child. *133*:157, 1979. Copyright 1979, American Medical Association.)

ENVIRONMENTAL FACTORS

The review by Fraumeni and Miller showed no significant annual variation or aggregation of cases of neonatal cancers in the United States. Children exposed prenatally to the atomic bombs in Hiroshima and Nagasaki have no significant excess of mortality from leukemia or other cancers. A number of authors have reported that abdominal radiation to the mother during pregnancy increases the risk of the child in utero of subsequently developing leukemia (Diamond et al., 1973), whereas others do not substantiate the existence of a relationship between prenatal x-ray exposure and childhood cancer (Totter and MacPherson, 1981).

In 1971, Herbst and coworkers reported that large doses of diethylstilbestrol (DES) given to pregnant women were related to the development of adenocarcinoma of the vagina in their daughters of that pregnancy from 14 to 22 years later. A relationship between exposure in utero to stilbestrol and its close synthetic analogs during the first half of pregnancy with the later development of clear-cell adenocarcinoma of both vagina and cervix is now well-established. According to the 1977 calculations of Herbst and colleagues, the risk of developing such tumors is approximately 0.14 to 1.4 per 1000 DES-exposed females up until the age of 24 years. The tumors are rare in females under 14 years of age, but the frequency rises rapidly to a peak at 19 years, after which there is a precipitous drop. In addition to neoplastic changes, several nonmalignant epithelial and structural alterations of the lower genital tract have been noted (Robboy et al., 1979), as have deformities of the endometrial cavity (Kaufman et al., 1977). Other authors have reported an increased risk of unfavorable outcome of pregnancy in DES daughters. Detailed studies of males exposed in utero to DES showed increased frequencies of testicular hypoplasia, cryptorchidism, epididymal cysts, microphallus, increased abnormal sperm forms, and lowered sperm counts. An estimated 30 per cent of the males studied

are probably infertile (Bibbo et al., 1977; Gill et al., 1979). A small number of males have been found to have seminomas (Conley et al., 1983).

A number of other agents known to cross the placenta may possibly be carcinogenic to the offspring. In utero exposure to phenytoin (diphenylhydantoin) is associated with a syndrome in the newborn that includes hypoplasia of the midface, tapering of the fingers and toes, and hypoplasia or aplasia of the nails. At least five children with fetal hydantoin syndrome have been reported to have neuroblastoma (Ehrenbard and Chaganti, 1981; Jiminez et al., 1981), and one has been found to have an extrarenal Wilms' tumor (Taylor et al., 1980). One young adult with a history of exposure in utero to phenytoin has developed a malignant mesenchymoma (Blattner et al., 1977).

The fetal alcohol syndrome, a disorder occurring in the children of mothers who consume excessive amounts of alcohol, is characterized by developmental delay, growth deficiency, and multiple minor anomalies. One child with this syndrome has been reported with neuroblastoma (Kinney et al., 1980), a second with hepatoblastoma (Khan et al., 1979), and a third with adrenocortical carcinoma (Hornstein et al., 1977). One child with neuroblastoma has had both the fetal alcohol and hydantoin syndromes (Seeler et al., 1979).

Jick and associates noted an increase in pregnancies ending in spontaneous abortion and in congenital anomalies in live infants born to women presumed to have used vaginal spermicides near the time of conception. Two of the children were found to have neoplasms shortly after birth. Gold and coworkers found that more children with brain tumors than normal children or children with other cancers were exposed to barbiturates in utero or during early childhood. This finding may be relevant in light of the reported association of maternal ingestion of barbiturates during pregnancy with microcephaly in infants (Spiedel and Meadow, 1972).

Agents implicated in childhood neoplasia following in utero exposure also often have teratogenic effects (Table 107–4). In the case of DES and, possibly, phenobarbital, the same organ appears to be at risk for both the oncogenic and teratogenic effects of the

Table 107–4.   Drugs Associated with Teratogenic and Carcinogenic Disorders Following In Utero Exposure

Drug	Teratogenic Effects	Carcinogenic Effects
DES	Structural alterations on genital tract	Vaginal and cervical adenocarcinoma
Phenytoin (diphenylhydantoin)	Fetal hydantoin syndrome	Neuroblastoma Wilms' tumor*
Alcohol	Fetal alcohol syndrome	Neuroblastoma* Hepatoblastoma* Adrenocortical carcinoma*
Vaginal spermicides	Limb reduction deformities* Chromosomal abnormalities* Hypospadias*	Medulloblastoma* Nesidioblastosis*
Phenobarbital	Microcephaly*	Brain tumors*

* Present data are only suggestive of an etiologic association.

drug. It is of interest that phenytoin exposure in the adult has been associated with the development of lymphomas, whereas exposure in utero has been associated with neuroblastomas. Thus, an agent may have various teratogenic or oncogenic effects, depending on the susceptibility of the target organ at the time of exposure, prenatally or well into adult hood. The same toxic agent has been shown in animals to be teratogenic to the fetus in the second quarter of pregnancy and carcinogenic in the latter half of pregnancy (Napolkov, 1973). Experimental evidence in animals suggests that maternal chemical carcinogen exposure may result in an increased incidence of tumors not only in the offspring but also in later generations of untreated descendants (Tomatis, 1979).

HOST FACTORS

Certain host factors seem to predispose an individual to the development of neoplastic disease. There is an increased incidence of leukemia in persons with Down syndrome, Fanconi's aplastic anemia, and Bloom syndrome and of leukemia and lymphoreticular malignancies in individuals born with immunodeficiency disorders such as ataxia-telangiectasia, Wiskott-Aldrich syndrome, and congenital thymic alymphoplasia. Of interest are the observations that phenytoin depresses immune function (Sorrell et al., 1971) and that immune deficiency occurs in children with the fetal alcohol syndrome (Johnson et al., 1981). Miller found Down syndrome to be more common than usual among siblings of children with leukemia. Both Down syndrome and leukemia occur more frequently among children of older mothers. Borges and coworkers found cytogenic variants of prezygotic origin in four of 25 nonmongoloid children with acute leukemia and suggested that the aneuploid cell might be more susceptible to malignant change.

Although the risk of developing leukemia is increased slightly in a dizygotic twin or other sibling of a child who has the disease, the chance of developing leukemia is greatest in a monozygotic twin. If one monozygotic twin has leukemia, the cotwin has approximately a 25 per cent chance of developing leukemia, usually within weeks or months of the diagnosis in the sibling.

A small number of well-defined hereditary disorders such as neurofibromatosis, tuberous sclerosis, and basal-cell carcinoma syndrome are associated with an increased incidence of certain neoplasms. The neoplastic diseases, however, seldom present during infancy. Kindreds have been reported in which multiple members developed the types of malignant diseases that usually occur in sporadic fashion. Although the number of such families is small, it is hard to escape the conclusion that, at least in some instances, heredity plays an important role in the development of malignancy.

CONGENITAL DEFECTS

An unexpectedly large number of childhood tumors occur in association with certain congenital defects. Children with Wilms' tumor have an increased incidence of congenital aniridia. Aniridia is a rare anomaly, found in only one of 75,000 individuals. It is about 1000 times more likely to occur in children with Wilm's tumor (one in 75). The association with a deletion in chromosome 11 has been described in at least 20 patients. From the clinical perspective, if an infant has aniridia, chromosome analysis should be undertaken. If a deletion of chromosome 11 is found, the child should be monitored for Wilms' tumor with serial ultrasonographic studies of the kidneys.

Other problems associated with Wilms' tumor include anomalies of the genitourinary tract. Congenital hemihypertrophy occurs excessively with Wilms' tumor, adrenocortical neoplasia, and hepatoblastoma, and it is also associated with hamartomas and with the visceral cytomegaly syndrome described by Beckwith. Hamartomas occur commonly in children with Wilms' tumor and adrenocortical neoplasia. One child has been reported with hepatoblastoma and Wilms' tumor; another, with congenital hemihypertrophy, had an adrenocortical adenoma and years later developed a Wilms' tumor. Of interest is the fact that Beckwith's visceral cytomegaly syndrome affects the kidney, adrenal cortex, and liver, the three organs that develop the malignancies associated with hemihypertrophy. These relationships among hemihypertrophy, visceral cytomegaly syndrome, hamartomas, and malignancy have been reviewed by Miller. The associations of congenital anomalies with childhood neoplasias again emphasize the close relationship between oncogenesis and teratogenesis.

Congenital Leukemia

Leukemia rarely occurs during the first month of life. Most of the neonatal cases reported have been acute myelogenous leukemia, in contrast to the predominance of acute lymphoblastic leukemia found in later childhood. To date, no child born to a mother with leukemia has been found to have the disease during the neonatal period. Instances of familial neonatal leukemia must be extremely rare. Campbell and coworkers described male and female siblings who died at 10 and 8 weeks of age of myelogenous leukemia and a third female in the family who died at 4 weeks of age with a clinical course similar to that of her siblings, although a definite diagnosis was not made.

Congenital leukemia is occasionally associated with a number of congenital anomalies (Miller et al., 1969) and with chromosomal disorders such as

Down syndrome, trisomies D and E, and a number of nonspecific chromosomal abnormalities. Subtle cytogenic abnormalities may occur more commonly than previously believed in affected infants and their parents when studied with newer cytogenic techniques (Goh et al., 1980).

Diagnosis. The clinical manifestations of leukemia may be evident at birth, with hepatosplenomegaly, petechiae, and ecchymoses. Leukemic cell infiltration into the skin, leukemia cutis, results in nodular fibroma-like masses. These tumors are freely movable over the subcutaneous tissue and result in a blue or gray discoloration of the overlying skin (Fig. 107–1). Such cutaneous lesions are commonly found when the disease appears at birth and have been noted in stillborn premature infants with leukemia. They may be the first clinical signs of the disease. At birth, many of the infants have respiratory distress due to either leukemia infiltration in the lungs or atelectasis. The author has seen one leukemic infant who developed severe respiratory difficulty soon after birth from a fatal pulmonary hemorrhage, presumably secondary to thrombocytopenia.

In those infants who develop signs of the disease within the first month but in whom no detectable signs of leukemia were noted at birth, the symptoms are often ill defined, with low-grade fever, diarrhea, hepatomegaly, and failure to gain weight. Hemorrhagic manifestations are often the first signs of the disease, and leukemia cutis is uncommon.

Hemoglobin levels are often normal at first, but they soon fall to low levels. Total white blood cell counts may be within normal limits or diminished, but leukocytosis is usually present. White cell counts of 150,000 to 250,000 per mm^3 or more are not unusual, and counts as high as 1,300,000 per mm^3 have been recorded. Leukocyte counts often rise progressively before death. There is usually a predominance of blast cells and immature granulocytes. Auer rods may be present in the blast cells (Fig. 107–2). These intracellular inclusions are composed of lysosomes and are considered to be pathognomonic of acute myelogenous leukemia.

Differential Diagnosis. A number of newborn infants reported in the earlier literature who were originally thought to have leukemia were later found to have other diseases. The predominance of myelogenous leukemia in this age group has contributed to the difficulty in differentiating the disorder from leukemoid reactions. Confusion with infections such as congenital syphilis, cytomegalovirus infection, toxoplasmosis, and bacterial septicemia may occur because of the leukocytosis, organomegaly, and thrombocytopenia that may accompany these diseases. The low platelet counts and leukemoid reactions reported in infants with congenital amegakaryocytic thrombocytopenia may also lead to an incorrect diagnosis of leukemia, but the absence of radii commonly seen in these children is a major clue to the correct diagnosis.

Several infants who were reported to have leukemia were later discovered to have severe erythroblastosis fetalis. Such infants usually have hepatosplenomegaly, large numbers of nucleated erythroblasts in the peripheral blood, and, occasionally, thrombocytopenia. Small infiltrates of extramedullary erythropoiesis may appear in the skin and superficially resemble leukemia cutis.

Infants with neonatal neuroblastoma often have hepatomegaly and may also have discolored tumor nodules in the subcutaneous tissue. Their blood counts are usually normal, and specimens of bone marrow, if involved, reveal small clusters of neuroblastoma cells. Although these cells may resemble leukemic blast cells, their tendency to occur in clumps in an otherwise normal bone marrow distinguishes them from leukemic cells, which usually completely replace the normal bone marrow.

A marked leukemoid reaction may occur in a newborn infant following in utero exposure to betamethasone (Bielawski et al., 1978). Lack of the usual clinical and laboratory findings of leukemia and history of maternal drug exposure usually exclude the diagnosis of leukemia.

Pathology. Biopsy or autopsy shows heavy infiltration of many immature leukocytes into extrahe-

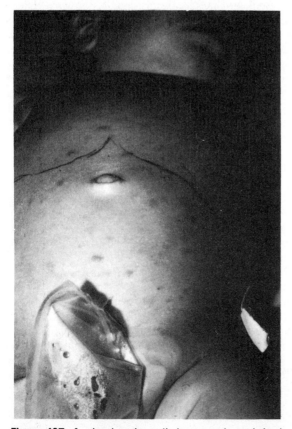

Figure 107–1. Leukemia cutis in a newborn infant.

matopoietic tissues. The bone marrow is hypercellular, with a marked predominance of the immature cells of the series affected, either myeloid or lymphoid. Cirrhosis of the liver has been noted at autopsy in several infants.

Therapy and Prognosis.   The course of the disease is usually one of rapid deterioration and death from hemorrhage or infection. Although the length of survival has been significantly prolonged in children with leukemia, there has been little successful experience in treating the neonate. The author is aware of one newborn infant with acute lymphoblastic leukemia who experienced a remission for a year following the use of multiple chemotherapeutic agents. Drugs used in the treatment of myelogenous leukemia in older children and adults may be of value, but reports of the use of such agents in treating neonatal leukemia have been anecdotal, with the infant usually experiencing a poor or short response. Exchange transfusions may cause clinical improvement by rapidly decreasing an extremely high white blood cell count; unfortunately, however, the response is usually transient (Warrier et al., 1981). Spontaneous remissions, which occur in Down syndrome infants with leukemia, are rarely experienced by the normal child. One infant with a normal karyotype has been reported to have a transient spontaneous remission that lasted until the age of 9 months, when the child finally had a relapse and died of acute myelogenous leukemia (Van Eys and Flexner, 1969). A second infant with acute lymphocytic leukemia had two spontaneous remissions later responded to chemotherapy and was in remission at age 48 months (Chu et al., 1983).

LEUKEMIA WITH DOWN SYNDROME

An increased incidence of acute leukemia in children with Down syndrome is now well recognized. A review of the world literature by Rosner and Lee revealed 227 children with both disorders; 31 per cent had acute myeloblastic leukemia, and 69 per cent had acute lymphoblastic leukemia. Among 47 newborn mongoloids with leukemia, 58 per cent had myeloblastic leukemia, and 42 per cent had lymphoblastic leukemia. Eighteen additional Down syndrome infants who had a transient disorder initially indistinguishable from acute myelogenous leukemia experienced complete clinical and hematologic recovery. In those with "transient leukemia" who died of other causes, no evidence of leukemia could be found at postmortem examination. It has been suggested by Ross and associates that the transient disorder is due to a defect in the regulation of granulocyte multiplication and maturation, possibly related to the chromosomal abnormality. The increased incidence of neonatal polycythemia in Down syndrome patients observed by Weinberger and Oleinick have led these investigators to propose that the abnormality in the regulation of hematopoiesis is not limited to granulocyte production. However, a number of mongoloid infants with transient leukemia have had recurrence of their disease leading to death, indicating that the disorders of marrow dysfunction and neonatal leukemia may not be separate entities but intimately related.

The high incidence of spontaneous remission of leukemia in infants with Down syndrome makes it difficult to interpret their response to antileukemic therapy. It may be most prudent to withhold the use of chemotherapeutic agents in this unusual group of neonates unless the clinical course is one of rapid deterioration.

Neuroblastoma

Neuroblastoma is the most common malignant tumor in infancy. The neoplasm originates from neural crest cells that normally give rise to the adrenal

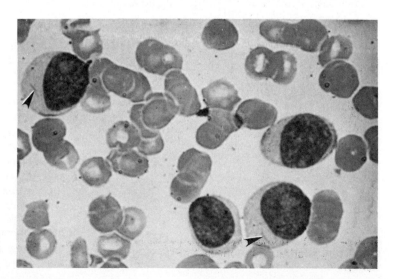

Figure 107–2. Malignant blast cells with Auer rods (arrows) present in cytoplasm diagnostic of acute myelogenous leukemia.

medulla and sympathetic ganglia. In infancy, the first clinical manifestations are usually due to the presence of metastatic disease rather than the primary tumor. Yet despite the occurrence of widespread disease, the prognosis in the neonate is remarkably good.

Clinical Manifestations. Neuroblastoma may present as a tumor mass anywhere sympathetic neural tissue normally occurs. Over half of affected children have the primary tumor within the abdomen, arising in the adrenal medulla or a sympathetic ganglion. The tumor may arise in the posterior mediastinum, and because of bronchial obstruction the symptoms may be either increasing dyspnea or pulmonary infection. The neoplasm may also arise in the neck or pelvis. Involvement of the stellate ganglion may result in Horner syndrome, which includes sinking in of the eyeball, ptosis of the upper eyelid, slight elevation of the lower lid, constriction of the pupil, narrowing of the palpebral fissure, and anhidrosis (Fig. 107–3). The neoplasm arising from a paravertebral sympathetic ganglion has an unusual tendency to grow into the intervertebral foramina, causing spinal cord compression and resultant paralysis. Careful periodic neurologic evaluation should be carried out on the child with a neuroblastoma arising from this location, since the onset of cord compression may necessitate emergency neurosurgical intervention. The late diagnosis of this complication has resulted in permanent paraplegia.

Metastatic lesions, especially of the skin and liver, are common presenting findings during the neonatal period. Often the primary site cannot be discovered. Hawthorne and coworkers found that the skin nodules first become erythematous for 2 or 3 minutes after palpation and then blanch, presumably owing to vasoconstriction from release of catecholamines from the tumor cells. They consider this to be a diagnostic sign of subcutaneous neuroblastoma.

The liver often bears the brunt of metastatic dis-

semination, becoming studded with innumerable foci of tumor growth. The tumor commonly presents in the newborn as a rapidly growing hepatic neoplasm. Rarely, stippled calcifications occur in the liver metastases. Hagstrom reported a fetus that could not be delivered intact because the abdomen contained a nodular 700-gm liver, resulting in dystocia. The abdomen had to be opened and much of the liver cut away piecemeal before delivery could be accomplished. The right adrenal gland was entirely replaced by a neuroblastoma. An infant reported by Larimer was delivered easily, but severe respiratory difficulty and cyanosis, apparently due to abdominal distention, were noted at birth. The child lived only 9 hours. Autopsy showed a huge 425-gm liver filled with bulging spherical nodules, a right adrenal gland weighing 83 gm filled with neuroblastoma, and metastatic involvement of mesenteric lymph nodes and the left adrenal gland.

Neuroblastomas arising from sympathetic ganglia lower in the abdomen give rise to the clinical pictures consistent with their locations. Thus presacral neuroblastomas may simulate presacral teratomas and be distinguished from them only by biopsy. Hepler's case is an instructive example. A 3-week-old male infant had been unable to void from birth, and an indwelling catheter had been passed into his bladder. A tumor of the lower part of the abdomen could be felt. The mass was palpable rectally, filling the hollow of the sacrum and extending forward to the symphysis. A cystogram showed the bladder to be displaced upward and to the left. A preoperative diagnosis of presacral teratoma was made. At operation, most of the tumor was removed and proved to be a neuroblastoma. Postoperatively, 1260 roentgens of x-irradiation were given over a 2-month period. The remainder of the tumor disappeared, and the child was well 4 years later.

Several children with neuroblastoma have been reported whose sole presenting symptom was persistent, intractable diarrhea. Green and colleagues described two patients with chronic diarrhea who were discovered to have chest masses and a third who had a mass in the region of the left adrenal gland that contained stippled calcifications. The children were thought to have had either cystic fibrosis or celiac syndrome before the roentgenographic discoveries were made. Their symptoms dramatically abated following surgical removal of their tumors. It is believed that such symptoms are due to excessive excretion by the tumor of an enterohormone, vasoactive intestinal peptide (Swift et al., 1975).

The association of acute myoclonic encephalopathy and neuroblastoma has been described by numerous authors. This usually consists of rapid multidirectional eye movements (opsoclonus), myoclonus, and truncal ataxia in the absence of increased intracranial pressure. In many instances, neurologic improvement occurred once the tumor had been removed. Despite the fact that it has been suggested that the encephalopathy is due to toxic neurologic effects of catecholamine catabolites, at

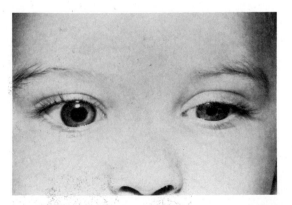

Figure 107–3. Horner's syndrome in an infant with neuroblastoma arising from the left cervical sympathetic ganglion.

least one child has been described who developed neurologic symptoms 19 months after removal of the tumor and return to normal of the previously elevated levels of urinary catecholamines. It has been proposed that an immune factor, possibly an antibody, reacts with an antigen common to both neuroblastoma and cerebellar cells, resulting in cerebellar damage (Bray et al., 1969). The excellent prognosis for survival of children with opsomyoclonus suggests that such a mechanism may not only cause the neurologic damage but also result in cure.

A report from the Netherlands suggests that there may be signs and symptoms in mothers whose fetuses have neuroblastoma. Voûte and coworkers reported six women who had sweating, pallor, headaches, palpitations, hypertension, and tingling in the feet and hands during the eighth and ninth months of pregnancy. All the women delivered children who were diagnosed as having neuroblastoma shortly after birth or during the first few months of life. Because the mothers' symptoms disappeared postpartum, the authors proposed that they were caused by fetal catecholamines entering the maternal circulation. It is not known how commonly this syndrome occurs.

Occasionally, a newborn infant with congenital neuroblastoma may be thought to have erythroblastosis. The infant reported by Falkinburg and Kay developed severe jaundice and, because of hepatosplenomegaly, was mistakenly thought for a time to have hemolytic disease of the newborn. An increase of nucleated red cells was noted in the child's blood. Anders and coworkers described two newborn infants with congenital neuroblastoma that had metastasized to the liver and placenta who were thought to have hydrops fetalis. In one, the diagnosis was established by histologic examination of the placenta.

Melanotic neuroectodermal tumors of infancy are uncommon neoplasms derived from cells of the neural crest. These melanin-containing tumors usually are diagnosed between 1 and 8 months of age and most commonly appear overlying the maxilla. With few exceptions, the tumor behaves in a benign manner (Cutler et al., 1981).

In summary, abdominal neuroblastoma of the newborn most commonly manifests itself by enlargement of the liver alone. An additional mass, the primary tumor, sometimes may be palpable. Otherwise unexplained persistent diarrhea occasionally may be the only symptom of the tumor. Metastases to lungs, bones, skull, and orbit are rare in the neonate, although clumps of tumor cells are often found if one carefully examines bone marrow aspiration specimens (Fig. 107–4). In 1965, Schneider and coworkers reported on 56 cases of neonatal neuroblastoma recorded in the English literature since 1940. Fifty-two per cent had metastases at the time of the original diagnosis, but only 3 per cent had metastasized to bone. The liver was involved in 65 per cent, and subcutaneous metastases were seen in 32 per cent. These figures differ strikingly from those for older infants and children (Table 107–5).

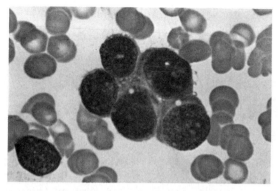

Figure 107–4. Clump of neuroblastoma cells found in bone marrow aspiration.

Biochemical Features. In 1957, Mason and colleagues reported an increased excretion of pressor amines in the urine of an infant with neuroblastoma. Subsequent studies in children with neuroblastoma have shown elevated levels of norepinephrine as well as its biochemical precursors and their metabolites in the urine, including dopa, dopamine, normetanephrine, homovanillic acid (HVA), and vanillylmandelic acid (VMA). According to Williams and Greer, 95 per cent of patients have an elevated urinary excretion of VMA or HVA or both. In occasional cases, however, there is no elevation of catecholamines. It is therefore important to measure urinary catecholamines in a child prior to surgical removal of a neuroblastoma or initiation of therapy in order to determine whether or not it is a catecholamine-producing tumor. This unique property of the neoplasm can be used not only as a diagnostic aid but also as a useful means of assessing the response to therapy or detecting the recurrence of tumor. Laug and coworkers reported that the prognosis of patients with dissem-

Table 107–5. Incidence of Metastases in the Newborn with Neuroblastoma

Site	Number	Percentage	All Ages (per cent)
Liver	20	64.6	24.3
Subcutaneous	10	32.3	2.6
Marrow	3	9.7	
Lung	2	6.5	13.2
Spleen	2	6.5	2.0
Kidney	2	6.5	2.0
Pancreas	2	6.5	
Brain	2	6.5	15.8
Bone	1	3.2	47.4
Nodes	1	3.2	32.2
Pleura	1	3.2	
Myocardium	1	3.2	
Periadrenal	1	3.2	

(From Schneider, K. M., Becker, J. M., and Krasna, I. H.: Pediatrics *36*:359, 1965.)

inated disease correlated directly with VMA/HVA ratio—the higher the value, the better the prognosis.

Urinary excretion of cystathionine is detectable in most patients with neuroblastoma but is found in a number of childhood neoplasms (Helson et al., 1972). Plasma carcinoembryonic antigen (CEA) levels are also elevated in many cases, but this finding also is nonspecific. CEA levels, however, may be of value in monitoring response to therapy (Frens et al., 1976). Serum lactic dehydrogenase levels increase with advanced disease, fall with remission, and rise with recurrence. The degree of initial elevation may have prognostic significance in patients with advanced disease (Quinn et al., 1980).

Pathology. The most primitive histologic subgroup of this tumor, the neuroblastoma, is very cellular and is composed of small round cells with scant cytoplasm. The ganglioneuroma, its more benign counterpart, is composed of large, mature ganglion cells with abundant cytoplasm, whereas the ganglioneuroblastoma is intermediate in the degree of cellular differentiation. However, the histologic appearance of an individual tumor may show various degrees of cellular maturation. Although attempts have been made to correlate prognosis with histologic grading, there appears to be a much better correlation between prognosis and both clinical staging of the disease and the patient's age at the time of diagnosis. Thus, most oncologists have not found the finer points of histologic grading to be a major factor in influencing therapy or determining prognosis.

Prognosis. It has been known that the chance of survival of a patient with neuroblastoma is inversely correlated with the age of the child at the time of diagnosis. The infant who has widespread disease appears to have a better chance of survival than the older child with a lesser degree of tumor dissemination.

The site of origin also has been considered to be a factor influencing survival, and a more favorable prognosis has been observed in children with mediastinal neuroblastoma. Coldman and associates found patients with nonadrenal tumors to have a greater probability of survival than those with adrenal tumors, a factor they found to be independent of age and degree of tumor dissemination.

Evans and coworkers proposed a clinical staging for children with neuroblastoma that is helpful in predicting the ultimate prognosis. Children with stage I disease have tumor limited to the organ of origin; those with stage II have regional tumor spread that does not cross the midline; stage III tumors extend across the midline; and stage IV disease includes patients with distant metastases to lymph nodes, lung, brain, or bone. Those with a greater degree of spread

Table 107–6. Two Year Survival of 234 Children with Neuroblastoma

Age (months)	Stage					Total
	I	II	III	IV	IV-S	
<12	10/11	14/15	2/4	4/17	18/20	48/67
12–23	4/5	5/8	3/7	0/26	1/1	13/47
≥24	2/3	4/12	3/13	3/88	2/4	14/120
Total	16/19	23/35	8/24	7/131	21/25	75/234

(From D'Angio et al.: Lancet 1:1046, 1971.)

tend to have a poorer prognosis, and in those with stage IV disease the malignancy is usually fatal.

One unique group of patients with disseminated disease has such a good prognosis, however, that a separate category called stage IV-S was proposed to distinguish them from other patients with widespread involvement. This special group of children have remote spread of tumor involving the liver, skin, and/or bone marrow without roentgenographic evidence of skeletal metastases. This pattern occurs most commonly in infancy. Eighteen of 20 infants under the age of 1 year with stage IV-S disease reported by D'Angio and associates were cured of their disease. The 2-year survival rate of all of those with stage IV-S disease was 84 per cent as compared with 5 per cent survival in those with stage IV disease. This association between age at the time of diagnosis, clinical staging, and survival is shown in Table 107–6. Recently, biologic differences have been demonstrated between stages IV-S and IV neuroblastoma. Hann and coworkers found elevated serum ferritin levels in the majority of children with stage IV disease but not in those with stage IV-S neuroblastoma. E-rosette inhibitory factor was present frequently in the serum of stage IV patients but was seldom present in the serum of stage IV-S patients. Elevated serum ferritin and E-rosette inhibition therefore appear to be associated with an unfavorable prognosis.

A number of children have experienced spontaneous tumor regression despite the presence of metastases. In other instances, malignant neuroblastomas have apparently undergone maturation into benign ganglioneuromas. The following case history is an example of spontaneous regression.

CASE 107–1

A 2-month-old white female infant was referred to the Children's Memorial Hospital of Chicago with a chief complaint of "lumps in the skin" since birth. The lesions were purple, and they blanched when pressure was applied. A biopsy of one of the skin lesions was diagnostic of neuroblastoma. Results of a bone marrow examination, liver-spleen scan, and roentgenograms of the chest and skeleton were normal. An intravenous pyelogram revealed lateral displacement of the left ureter, suggesting a left paravertebral mass. Urinary VMA excretion was elevated to 90 μg per mg of creatinine (normal: 20 μg per mg of creatinine or less). A diagnosis of disseminated neuroblastoma was made, the primary tumor probably arising from a left paravertebral sympathetic ganglion in the abdomen. No therapy was administered. The skin lesions completely resolved by 4 months of age (Fig. 107–5), at which time a repeat of intravenous pyelogram showed no evidence of the paravertebral mass. The urinary excretion of VMA decreased to 8 μg per mg of creatinine. At 7 years of age, the child was well and had no evidence of neuroblastoma.

The diagnosis of neuroblastoma was made before the age of 6 months in 21 of 29 cases collected by Everson and Cole in which spontaneous regression occurred. The remainder were diagnosed between 6 and 24 months of age. This relationship of spontaneous regression to age has also been noted by Evans and coworkers, who found that the majority of those with tumor regression were under 6 months of age and were usually those with stage II or stage IV-S disease. Stage I patients, however, could not be evaluated because the tumor was usually completely resected.

The incidence of spontaneous regression of neuroblastoma may be more common than is clinically evident. Beckwith and Perrin detected the presence of microscopic clusters of neuroblastoma cells, termed "neuroblastoma in situ," in the adrenal glands of a significant number of infants under the age of 3 months with no clinical evidence of tumor upon whom postmortem examinations were performed. They estimated the incidence of neuroblastoma in situ to be about 40 times greater than the number of cases of clinically diagnosed disease. Basing their theory on these findings, they proposed that the great majority of these tumors either degenerated or underwent differentiation to normal tissue. Turkel and Itabashi, however, believe that such neuroblastic nodules represent normal changes in the developing adrenal gland and noted their presence in 100 per cent of 169 fetal adrenal glands they examined. Whether or not neuroblastoma in situ is a true neoplasm, it completely disappears after 3 months of life under normal circumstances.

Treatment. The unpredictable course of neuroblastoma, with its occasional spontaneous maturation or regression, not only makes the tumor unusual but also causes difficulty in evaluating therapy. The cases reported by Bodian suggested that massive doses of vitamin B_{12} led to cure, but subsequent evaluation of the collected experiences of others failed to confirm these observations. One likely explanation for Bodian's successful results was that his series was heavily weighted with young patients who experi-

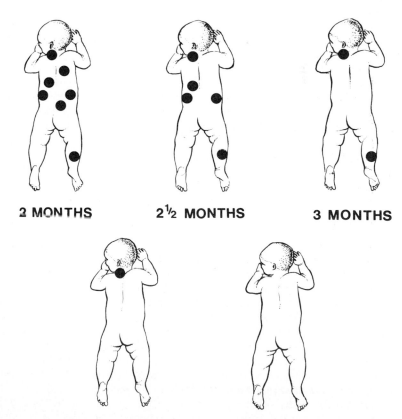

2 MONTHS **2½ MONTHS** **3 MONTHS**

3½ MONTHS **4 MONTHS**

Figure 107–5. Spontaneous regression of skin lesions of disseminated neuroblastoma. (Schwartz, A. D., et al.: J. Pediatr. *85*:760, 1974.)

enced spontaneous remission. Reports that surgical assault on the primary tumor may influence regression of distant metastases must also be interpreted with caution in view of the natural history of the disease.

The response of neuroblastoma to chemotherapy is often dramatic, with the most impressive results occurring in children under the age of 1 year. Yet, despite well-documented initial regression of tumor, the use of a variety of drugs has done little to improve survival in this disease, as shown by the data collected by Leikin and coworkers. The tumor is radio-responsive and radiation therapy has been successfully used to shrink large tumor masses and relieve symptoms of pain and spinal cord compression. However, its routine use for eradication of residual tumor after surgery has not been conclusively demonstrated to affect ultimate survival.

The policy of most oncologists is to resect completely, if possible, the stage I neuroblastoma. Available data can support no specific treatment regimen in view of the lack of influence of chemotherapy on the ultimate prognosis of those with stage III or IV disease. There is some evidence that irradiation is of benefit in patients with stage III disease, but it appears to be unrelated to survival in stage I, II, and IV disease (Koop and Schnaufer, 1975). The extremely high fatality rate in older children with regional extension or disseminated disease warrants an aggressive approach with further evaluation of newer therapeutic agents. The observations by the Hellstroms that neuroblastoma is capable of evoking both cell-mediated and humoral-immune responses in the host may eventually lead to effective forms of immunotherapy. It has been suggested that the infant with the special pattern of metastases classified as stage IV-S disease be observed for a period of time before the decision is made to initiate therapy because the high cure rate in this group may be due to spontaneous tumor regression.

Wilms' Tumor

Wilms' tumor, or nephroblastoma, the most common intra-abdominal tumor of childhood, was first described as a clinical entity in 1899. In contrast to neuroblastoma, this neoplasm, with optimal treatment, is associated with an increasing rate of cure that has been one of the dramatic success stories in the field of cancer therapy. The National Wilms' Tumor Study, established in 1969, has helped in the rapid accumulation of information regarding the prognosis and therapy of this tumor, which results in death if untreated.

Clinical Manifestations. The majority of children with Wilms' tumor have either an abdominal mass or an increase in abdominal size noted as the first clinical evidence of disease. This is often first discovered by a parent and brought to the attention of the physician. The tumor lies deep in the flank, is attached to the kidney or is part of it, and is usually firm and smooth. It seldom extends beyond the midline, even though it may grow downward beyond the iliac crest. In about 5 to 10 per cent of all cases, tumors involve both kidneys. Gross hematuria is a rare presenting symptom, but microscopic hematuria is found in approximately one fourth of the cases. According to Sullivan and coworkers, hematuria in Wilms' tumor is not a poor prognostic sign, as it is in adults with hypernephroma. Hypertension, occasionally noted in older infants and children, has not been observed in the newborn. The tumor may sometimes present with abdominal pain and be discovered at laparotomy (Rosenfeld et al., 1977). Occasionally, acute hemorrhage into the tumor may result in a rapidly enlarging mass, usually associated with anemia and fever (Ramsey et al., 1977).

Wilms' tumor is seldom diagnosed at birth or during the neonatal period, although several renal tumors have been so large as to have caused dystocia during delivery. Wells reported five certain cases and 11 probable ones in this age group. Hartenstein found seven more cases that were diagnosed in the neonatal period and added one of his own. Of the 77 children treated at the M. D. Anderson Hospital and Tumor Institute over a period of 18 years, only one was diagnosed during the first month of life (Sullivan et al., 1973).

Rare cases of Wilms' tumor associated with polycythemia have been reported. This finding is secondary to an increased production of erythropoietin by the neoplasm. The demonstration of elevated plasma erythropoietin levels in five of eight nonpolycythemic children with Wilms' tumor studied preoperatively by Murphy and colleagues led these investigators to suggest that this test may be useful in the diagnosis and evaluation of response to therapy.

Hereditary Associations and Congenital Anomalies. The association among Wilms' tumor, hemihypertrophy, congenital aniridia, hamartomas, and genitourinary defects has been discussed earlier in this chapter. The finding of hemihypertrophy should alert the physician to observe the child for the possible development of Wilms' tumor, adrenal cortical tumor, or hepatoma. Some of these patients may have incomplete forms of the Beckwith-Wiedemann syndrome (Sotelo-Avila et al., 1980). A number of cases of pseudohermaphroditism, nephron disorders, and Wilms' tumor have also been reported. Occasionally, certain members of a family may have the congenital anomaly and another have the neoplasm. Meadows and coworkers reported one family in which a mother had congenital hemihypertrophy, three of the children had Wilms' tumor, and a fourth had a urinary tract anomaly. Aniridia is usually inherited in an autosomal dominant pattern with high penetrance and little variability of phenotypic expression. The child with aniridia who has Wilms' tumor does not have this usual inheritance pattern but has sporadic congenital aniridia. Pilling reported 26 children with aniridia, 20 of whom had the sporadic type. Seven of the 20 developed Wilms' tumor. It appears that the risk of developing Wilms' tumor is higher if the sporadic aniridia is accompanied by a major genitourinary tract anomaly, severe mental retardation or both. The Wilms' tumor–aniridia syndrome, a combination of mental retardation, microcephaly, bilateral aniridia, anomalies of the pinna, Wilms' tumor, and ambiguous genitalia, is associated with a small deletion of chromosome 11. Although usually sporadic, this syndrome may occasionally be familial (Yunis and Ramsay, 1980). Rarely, affected persons may demonstrate all the findings except the Wilms' tumor (Riccardi et al., 1978). There are two reports of aniridia in monozygous twins in which only one member of each pair developed Wilms' tumor (Maurer et al., 1979; Miller, 1979). Reports of tumors occurring in siblings, identical twins, parent-child pairs, and cousins with no malformations indicate that hereditary factors at times may play a major role in the development of this neoplasm (Knudson and Strong, 1972).

Prognostic Factors. Three factors seem to influence the response to therapy and ultimate prognosis of the child with Wilms' tumor: the histologic pattern, the age of the patient at the time of diagnosis, and the extent of disease (Breslow et al., 1978). Tumors with better differentiation, showing glomeruloid and tubular formation, indicate a better chance for survival than those with anaplastic and sarcomatous patterns. Those under 2 years of age at diagnosis have fewer relapses, especially to distant sites, than older children. Age, however, seems to be of little prognostic significance regarding mortality. Specimens weighing over 250 grams and positive regional lymph nodes, however, are important predictors of both relapse and mortality.

The most common staging system now in use is that devised by the National Wilms' Tumor Study Group and is being used for the Third National Wilms' Tumor Study. This staging system is as follows:

Stage I: Tumor limited to the kidney and completely resected.
Stage II: Tumor extending beyond the kidney but completely resected. The tumor may have been biopsied, or there may have been local spillage.
Stage III: Residual nonhematogenous tumor confined to the abdomen. Lymph node involvement in the abdomen. Diffuse peritoneal spillage or tumor growth that has penetrated the peritoneal surface.
Stage IV: Hematogenous metastases. Lymph node involvement beyond the abdominal cavity.
Stage V: Bilateral renal involvement at diagnosis.

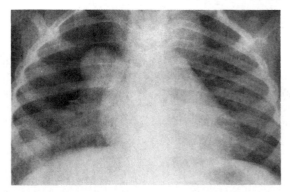

Figure 107–6. Pulmonary metastases of Wilms' tumor.

The clinical staging is an important factor in predicting survival; those with more extensive spread have a poorer prognosis. Therefore, adequate evaluation of the extent of tumor involvement is essential and should include at the minimum an intravenous pyelogram and a roentgenographic evaluation of the lungs, the most commonly involved area of hematogenous spread (Fig. 107–6). Other commonly involved sites of metastatic spread are the liver, retroperitoneum, peritoneum, mediastinum, and pleurae. Children with Wilms' tumor having a sarcomatous pattern not only have a high rate of recurrence but also develop bony and brain metastases.

Therapy and Prognosis. Prior to 1950, the two major modalities of therapy for Wilms' tumor, surgical removal and radiation therapy, resulted in cure rates approaching 50 per cent. The advantage of treatment with the chemotherapeutic agent actinomycin D was demonstrated in 1966 by Farber, who reported an 89 per cent survival rate in children who had no evidence of metastatic disease at the time of diagnosis and who were followed for at least 2 years and a 53 per cent survival rate in those presenting with evidence of metastatic disease. The drug therapy appeared to prevent clinical hematogenous metastases following surgical removal and radiation to the tumor bed by presumably destroying nondetectable, microscopic tumor foci, especially in the lungs. Vincristine sulfate also has striking activity against Wilms' tumor and appears to be at least as effective as actinomycin D. Other agents shown to have activity against this tumor include adriamycin, cyclophosphamide, and bleomycin.

Results of the first two National Wilms' Tumor Studies show that treatment with vincristine and actinomycin is superior to treatment with either drug alone. Postoperative radiation therapy adds little benefit to those with totally excised tumors, and 6 months of therapy with two drugs appears to be as effective as 15 months of therapy in such patients. Patients with more advanced disease fared better following treatment with three drugs (actinomycin, vin-

Miscellaneous Disorders

cristine, doxorubicin) than with two (actinomycin, vincristine). Patients with unfavorable histology had a significantly poorer prognosis than those with favorable histology, as did those with positive nodes (D'Angio et al., 1971). Thus, Wilms' tumor, a neoplasm that is fatal if untreated, presently has a cure rate approaching 90 per cent. The use of newer therapeutic agents may continue to improve these remarkably successful results.

Neoplasms Related to Wilms' Tumor

A number of neonatal renal tumors have been confused with the typical Wilms' tumor in the past. Now that these neoplasms have been recognized as separate entities, they are more commonly diagnosed during the neonatal period than is the classic nephroblastoma, which very rarely occurs during the first month of life.

MESOBLASTIC NEPHROMA

The congenital mesoblastic nephroma, or fetal mesenchymal hamartoma, was clearly distinguished from Wilms' tumor in 1967 by Bolande and coworkers, who emphasized its benign nature. The involved kidney is usually greatly enlarged and distorted by the tumor, but, contrary to the findings with Wilms' tumor, there is usually no lobulation, necrosis, hemorrhage, or discrete capsule between neoplasm and compressed kidney (Fig. 107–7). The histologic picture is of a preponderance of interlacing bundles of spindle-shaped cells within which dysplastic tubules and glomeruli are irregularly scattered. Extrarenal infiltration is common, especially into the perihilar connective tissues. Polyhydramnios and pre-

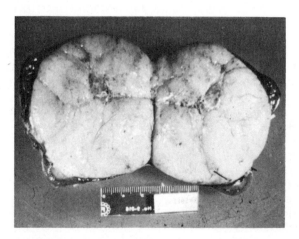

Figure 107–7. Congenital mesoblastic nephroma compressing and nearly totally replacing the kidney.

mature labor occur with increased frequency in women whose infants have mesoblastic nephroma. The tumor may be diagnosed prenatally with ultrasonography (Blank et al., 1978).

The vast majority of patients have been cured by nephrectomy alone. It has been suggested that the previous confusion with Wilms' tumor might account for the excellent survival rates reported in infants. There is good evidence that more patients with mesoblastic nephroma have died as a result of aggressive chemotherapy and irradiation than from the tumor itself. Nephrectomy is the treatment of choice; however, in very rare instances the tumor has been unusually aggressive. Because of the occasional case in which there is recurrence, it is now recommended that when the surgical margins are involved or uncertain or when the typical appearance of congenital mesoblastic nephroma is not present, additional therapy is indicated in addition to removal of the involved kidney.

PERSISTENT RENAL BLASTEMA

Accumulations of immature renal tissue are not normally found beyond 36 weeks' gestation, the time at which nephrogenesis normally ceases. Nodular renal blastema is characterized by microscopic nests of primitive cells in the subcapsular renal cortex resembling the blastemal cells of Wilms' tumor but lacking mitoses. Although benign, these nodules are thought to have the potential for neoplastic transformation. They are found in one of every 200 to 400 postmortem examinations of infants under 4 months of age, but they are discovered in the kidneys of children over 4 months of age only in cases of Wilms' tumor. When nodular renal blastema becomes massive and confluent and replaces the cortex, it is referred to as "nephroblastomatosis" (Bove and McAdams, 1976). Kumar and associates reported the nodular renal blastema–nephroblastomatosis complex in eight of 118 patients (6.8 per cent) with Wilms' tumor. Five of these eight patients had bilateral tumors. Children with this disorder may also have the congenital anomalies associated with Wilms' tumor. The fact that nodular renal blastema is rarely found in older children suggests that the majority of these lesions regress, a situation analogous to the course of neuroblastoma in situ. It is believed that those that persist give rise to Wilms' tumor, whereas a small number progress to diffuse nephroblastomatosis. Complete progression of nodular renal blastema to nephroblastomatosis to Wilms' tumor has been documented (Kulkarni et al., 1980). Children with massive bilateral involvement will often respond to therapy used for Wilms' tumor (deChadarévian et al., 1977; Telander et al., 1978). Although persistent renal blastema is not a true malignancy, it probably has been confused with Wilms' tumor in the past, and it appears in many instances to be a precursor of this malignancy.

A renal neoplasm in infants is known by a variety of names: polycystic nephroblastoma, benign multilocular cystic nephroma, well-differentiated polycystic Wilms' tumor, and cystic partially differentiated nephroblastoma. It is a cystic encapsulated tumor occurring before 2 years of age. The cysts are lined by epithelium and show a mixture of partially differentiated and undifferentiated metanephrogenic blastema, that differentiates this lesion from multilocular cysts of the kidney. The tumor appears to have a benign course, and nephrectomy is the treatment of choice (Joshi et al., 1977). These neoplasms probably represent a differentiated form of nephroblastoma (Gallo and Penchansky, 1977).

Hepatic Malignancies

Primary malignant tumors of the liver are uncommon in infants and children. The most common hepatic malignant neoplasm in infancy is, in fact, metastatic neuroblastoma. The two major histologic types of hepatomas are hepatoblastoma and hepatocellular carcinoma. Hepatoblastomas usually occur in infants and are rarely seen after 3 years of age. Of the 129 cases reported by Exelby and coworkers, almost half were 18 months or younger, 11 were under 6 weeks of age, and 3 were newborns. Hepatocellular carcinomas, however, appear to have a bimodal age distribution, occurring either in very young children below 4 years or in patients between the ages of 12 and 15 years. Both types of tumors occur more commonly in males.

The most common presenting symptoms of hepatic tumors are an upper abdominal mass and an enlarging abdomen. Anorexia, weight loss, and pain also frequently occur. Laboratory studies of liver function are rarely helpful in establishing a diagnosis and are usually normal. Alpha-fetoprotein, an alpha-1 globulin that occurs normally in the fetus and disappears in the first few weeks of life, is often present in the serum of the child with hepatic malignancy. A number of children with hepatoblastoma have elevated levels of the amino acid cystathionine in their urine. If present, cystathioninuria may allow one to differentiate among hepatoblastoma and a number of benign and malignant disorders, but this finding also occurs in about 50 per cent of patients with neuroblastoma.

Hepatic calcification is demonstrated in 20 per cent of cases on the plain abdominal roentgenogram. Radioisotopic liver scanning usually demonstrates the presence of a neoplasm and is useful in following regeneration of the liver after hepatic lobectomy and in diagnosing tumor recurrence. Angiography is useful in determining whether both lobes of the liver are involved. If one lobe is free of malignancy and there is no evidence of distant metastatic disease, a lobectomy of the involved portion of the liver should be performed despite the high operative mortality. At the present time, surgery appears to be the only means for cure. In the aforementioned large series, there was no evidence that radiation therapy or chemotherapy controlled disease that could not be totally resected. When incomplete excision was performed no patient survived, but 60 per cent of those with hepatoblastoma and 33 per cent with hepatocellular carcinoma were cured if the tumor could be completely excised. However, a number of cases have been reported in which initially inoperable tumors could be removed and the patient cured by a second surgical procedure following reduction in tumor size by the use of chemotherapy and radiation therapy. Chemotherapy after total gross tumor resection may increase survival rates (Hermann and Lonsdale, 1970; Ikeda et al., 1979; Shafer and Selinkoff, 1977; Evans et al., 1982).

In addition to hepatomas, a variety of very rare liver tumors have been reported in infants. Angiosarcomas are thought to be the malignant form of infantile hemangioendotheliomas. One interesting case occurred in a 20-month-old child following in utero exposure to arsenic (Falk et al., 1981), a toxin implicated in hepatic angiosarcomas in adults. Seventeen cases of hepatic teratomas have been reported in children, the majority occurring in females less than 3 years of age (Todani et al., 1977). About one half of hepatic teratomas are malignant, and approximately one half are benign.

Sacrococcygeal Teratomas

Teratomas are neoplasms that contain derivatives of more than one of the three primary germ layers of the embryo. Although these tumors are often benign, one or more of the germ layer derivatives may develop malignant characteristics. Teratomas arise in a wide variety of locations of the body but usually occur along the axial midline during early childhood.

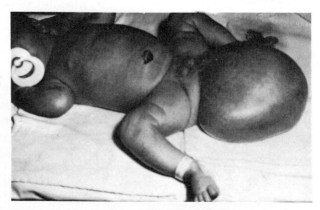

Figure 107–8. Large sacrococcygeal teratoma in a newborn girl.

After puberty, teratomas most frequently occur in the gonads, particularly the ovary.

The sacrococcygeal region is the most common site of teratomas in the first year of life, and the sacrococcygeal teratoma is the most common solid tumor in the newborn. Females are affected two to four times more frequently than males. Most tumors present as a mass protruding between the coccyx and rectum and may be quite large (Fig. 107–8). About 10 per cent are found by rectal examination. Nearly all arise at the tip or inner surface of the coccyx and can be diagnosed early in life by the pediatrician who makes the rectal examination a routine part of the physical examination.

Sacrococcygeal teratomas may be confused with meningomyeloceles, rectal abscesses, pelvic neuroblastomas, pilonidal cysts, and a variety of very rare neoplasms that may occur in this region. The majority of benign teratomas in this area produce no functional difficulties, even when marked intrapelvic extension is present. Thus, bowel or bladder dysfunction, painful defecation, and vascular or lymphatic obstruction suggest that the lesion is malignant.

Treatment of sacrococcygeal tumors is primarily surgical and has been described in detail by Donnellan and Swenson and by Gross and associates. They should be excised as soon as possible because small, undifferentiated foci may proliferate and become aggressive. They are attached to the coccyx, and therefore removal of the entire coccyx is a necessary part of the surgical procedure. Failure to remove the coccyx results in a 30 to 40 per cent risk of local recurrence.

The incidence of malignancy for sacrococcygeal teratomas diagnosed before 2 months of age is approximately 10 per cent. After this age, the incidence of malignancy rises to 67 per cent for males and 48 per cent for females. In the series of 398 cases reported by Altman and associates, 60 per cent of the patients with malignant tumors died within 10 months of surgery, 21 per cent were alive with residual disease, 11 per cent were alive without apparent disease, and 9 per cent were lost to followup. These findings contrast markedly with the mortality rate reported for children with benign lesions, which was approximately 5 per cent.

TYPE I

Predominantly external with minimal presacral component

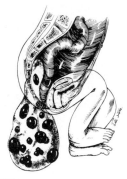

Frequency 46.6%
Metastatic rate 0%
Mortality rate 11%

TYPE II

Presenting externally, but significant intrapelvic extension

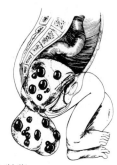

Frequency 34.6%
Metastatic rate 6%
Mortality rate 18%

TYPE III

Predominant mass pelvic with extension into abdomen

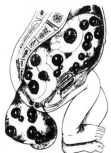

Frequency 8.8%
Metastatic rate 20%
Mortality rate 28%

TYPE IV

Entirely presacral with no external presentation

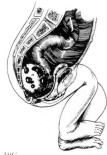

Frequency 10%
Metastatic rate 8%
Mortality rate 21%

Figure 107–9. Location of sacrococcygeal teratomas in 398 patients. (After Altman, R. P., et al.: Pediatr. Surg. 9:389, 1974. Reprinted by permission.)

A topographic classification for sacrococcygeal tumors appears valuable in predicting potential for metastatic behavior and survival (Fig. 107–9). An internal location predisposes the tumor to metastatic behavior, possibly because the delay in diagnosis is associated with a greater risk of malignant transformation. Therapy for children with malignant sacrococcygeal teratoma is far from optimal. Even those who have localized tumor that is grossly completely excised usually have recurrence. The tumor may respond to combination chemotherapy and radiation therapy, and occasional cures, even in those patients with unresectable disease, have been reported. Unfortunately, some children have died from the complications of the intensive therapy (Raney et al., 1981).

Disorders of Uncertain Origin

Letterer-Siwe Disease (Acute Disseminated Histiocytosis X)

The eponymic title seems preferable to the awkward descriptive name "acute nonlipid disseminated reticuloendotheliosis." This disease demonstrates many similarities to eosinophilic granuloma and Hand-Schüller-Christian disease, and the three are usually classified as reticuloendothelioses or histiocytoses. In the full-blown case of Letterer-Siwe's disease, the patient develops fever, hepatosplenomegaly, lymphadenopathy, skin rash, destructive bone lesions, anemia, thrombocytopenia, and recurring secondary infections.

Incidence. This rare form of histiocytosis X has been reported in newborn infants but more often presents with rashes and hepatosplenomegaly in the first months of life. By 1970, Juberg and coworkers identified the disorder in twins (both twins in three of four monozygotic pairs). In an analysis of occurrence in sibships, they proposed a single gene manifest as a recessive and located on an autosome.

Etiology and Pathology. Theories as to etiology range from those of specific infection, nonspecific tissue response to a variety of infective agents, tissue reaction as an abnormal immunologic response through tumor, to some kind of hereditary defect.

The pathognomonic lesions are microscopic aggregations of large, pleomorphic mononuclear cells that contain no lipoid material. An admixture of plasma cells, lymphocytes, a few eosinophils, and neutrophils is usually present. At times, focal necrosis occurs; at other times, proliferative fibrous tissue changes are present. These lesions may be found in skin, liver, spleen, lungs, lymph nodes, and other organs and tissues.

Diagnosis. The onset may be noted as early as the first day of life or at any time during the first year. In the Vanderbilt series, two infants had skin manifestations at birth, and one was lethargic from birth. In one, abdominal enlargement due to enlargement of the liver and spleen was seen at 3 weeks. Onset in the 11 other cases was noted after the neonatal period. The authors made the point that evidences of infection were more prominent in infants with early onset than in those whose first manifestations appeared later. In some infants, infection (chiefly respiratory and often complicated by discharging otitis media) preceded for some weeks the signs suggesting reticuloendotheliosis; in others, the infections were clearly secondary.

Hepatosplenomegaly appears early in virtually all cases. General glandular enlargement of moderate degree is usual but not universal. Rash may herald the disease or may develop later. This ordinarily resembles and is mistaken for seborrheic dermatitis, since it appears first in the scalp and hairline and is more pronounced in the skin folds before becoming generalized, and because the individual maculopapules composing it have greasy, scaly surfaces. Bone lesions are not encountered in all cases. When present, they are often overlaid by visible and palpable fluctuant swellings. These lesions in the skull and long bones are the sharply defined destructive ones characteristic of eosinophilic granuloma and generalized xanthomatosis. Pulmonary infiltration, found post mortem in all cases in the form of interstitial pneumonitis with infiltration of large mononuclear cells, may in a few infants become obvious clinically and be visualized on radiographs. One infant who failed to thrive from birth was found to have pulmonary infiltrates throughout both lungs, with diffuse histiocytic infiltration, and no other signs whatsoever.

The course is rapidly or slowly progressive, in general more rapid in those whose onsets are earlier. It is marked by fever, anorexia, failure to gain and grow, and gradual fall of hemoglobin content and platelet count. Hemorrhagic manifestations may appear.

Treatment and Prognosis. Letterer-Siwe disease was at one time generally believed to be invariably fatal. Bierman, in 1966, was able to list eight cases of infants who improved after, and almost surely because of, antibiotic therapy.

More recent therapeutic efforts have bypassed antibiotics, utilizing instead vinblastine or 6-mercaptopurine, with or without prednisone. Lahey reviewed the outcomes in 83 patients, of whom 65 were less than 2 years old. Their diagnoses included the three varieties of histiocytosis, Letterer-Siwe disease, Hand-Schüller-Christian disease, and eosinophilic granuloma. Of these 65 infants, treated with either vinblastine, vinblastine and prednisone, or 6-mercaptopurine and prednisone, between 44 and 64 per cent achieved either good or complete remission.

Familial Erythrophagocytic Lymphohistiocytosis

MacMahon and coworkers warn us not to confuse this entity with Letterer-Siwe disease. These infants also become ill within the first few months of life, with fever, anorexia, and wasting. The liver and spleen become very large, pallor progresses, and the blood shows increasing anemia, granulopenia, and thrombocytopenia. Bone marrow reveals erythroid and myeloid hyperplasia and paucity of polymorphonuclear leukocytes. Some infants have nuchal rigidity, and their spinal fluids show a number of lymphocytes and histiocytes. Their downhill course may be temporarily halted by splenectomy.

The liver, spleen, and at times the central nervous system reveal at biopsy or autopsy striking infiltration of lymphocytes and histiocytes that phagocytose erythrocytes greedily.

Several of the reported cases have involved two members of the same sibship. MacMahon believes that the disease resembles a primary proliferative state of the reticuloendothelial system more than a proliferative response to some antigenic stimulus.

REFERENCES

Allen, J. E.: Teratomas in infants and children. In Holland, J. F., and Frei, E., III. (Eds.): Cancer Medicine. Philadelphia, Lea and Febiger, 1973.

Alpert, M. E., and Seeler, R. A.: Alpha fetoprotein in embryonal hepatoblastoma. J. Pediatr. 77:1058, 1970.

Altman, R. P., Randolph, J. G., and Lilly, J. R.: Sacrococcygeal teratomas: American Academy of Pediatrics Surgical Section Survey—1973. J. Pediatr. Surg. 9:989, 1974.

Anders, D., Kindermann, G., and Pfeifer, U.: Metastasizing fetal neuroblastoma with involvement of the placenta simulating fetal erythroblastosis. J. Pediatr. 82:50, 1973.

Aron, B. S.: Wilms' tumor—a clinical study of eighty-one patients. Cancer 33:637, 1974.

Bader, J. L., and Miller, R. W.: U.S. cancer incidence and mortality in the first year of life. Am. J. Dis. Child. 133:157, 1979.

Barnes, A. B., Colton, T., Gundersen, J., Noller, K. L., Tilley, B. C., Strama, T., Townsend, D. E., Hatab, P., and O'Brien, P. C.: Fertility and outcome of pregnancy in women exposed in utero to diethylstilbestrol. N. Engl. J. Med. 302:609, 1980.

Beckwith, J. B.: Mesenchymal renal neoplasms of infancy revisited. J. Pediatr. Surg. 9:803, 1974.

Beckwith, J. B., and Perrin, E. V.: In situ neuroblastoma: a contribution to the natural history of neural crest tumors. Am. J. Pathol. 43:1089, 1963.

Bell, R. J. M.: Fetal virilisation due to maternal Krukenberg tumour. Lancet 1:1162, 1977.

Bernard, J., Jacquillat, C., Chavalet, F., Boiron, M., Stoitchkov, Y., and Tanzer, J.: Leucémie aiguë d'une enfant de 5 mois née d'une mère atteinte de leucémie aiguë au moment de l'accouchement. Nouv. Rev. Franc. Hémat. 4:140, 1964.

Bibbo, M., Gill, W. B., Azizi, F., Blough, R., Fang, V. S., Rosenfield, R. L., Schumacher, G. F. B., Sleeper, K., Sonek, M. G., and Wield, G. L.: Follow-up study of male and female offspring of DES-exposed mothers. Obstet. Gynecol. 49:1, 1977.

Bielawski, D., Hiatt, I. M., and Hegyi, T.: Betamethasone-induced leukaemoid reaction in pre-term infant. Lancet 1:218, 1978.

Blank, E., Neerhout, R. C., and Burry, K. A.: Congenital mesoblastic nephroma and polyhydramnios. J.A.M.A. 240:1504, 1978.

Blattner, W. A., Henson, D. E., Young, R. C., and Fraumeni, J. F., Jr.: Malignant mesenchymoma and birth defects, prenatal exposure to phenytoin. J.A.M.A. 238:334, 1977.

Bodian, M.: Neuroblastoma: an evaluation of its natural history and the effects of therapy, with particular reference to treatment by massive doses of vitamin B_{12}. Arch. Dis. Child. 38:606, 1963.

Bolande, R. P.: Congenital and infantile neoplasia of the kidney. Lancet 2:1497, 1974.

Bolande, R. P., Brough, A. J., and Izant, R. J.: Congenital mesoblastic nephroma of infancy: a report of eight cases and the relationship to Wilms' tumor. Pediatrics 40:272, 1967.

Borges, W. H., Nicklas, J. W., and Hamm, C. W.: Prezygotic determinants in acute leukemia. J. Pediatr. 70:180, 1967.

Bove, K. E., and McAdams, A. J.: The nephroblastomatosis complex and its relationship to Wilms' tumor: a clinicopathologic treatise. Perspect. Pediatr. Pathol. 3:185, 1976.

Bray, P. F., Ziter, F. A., Lahey, M. E., and Myers, G. G.: The coincidence of neuroblastoma and acute cerebellar encephalopathy. J. Pediatr. 75:983, 1969.

Breslow, N. E., Palmer, N. F., Hill, L. R., Buring, J., and D'Angio, G. J.: Wilms' tumor: prognostic factors for patients without metastases at diagnosis. Cancer 41:1577, 1978.

Brodsky, I., Baren, M., Kahn, S. B., Lewis, G., Jr., and Tellum, M.: Metastatic malignant melanoma from mother to fetus. Cancer 18:1048 1965

Campbell, W. A. B., Macafee, A. L., and Wade, W. G.: Familial neonatal leukaemia. Arch. Dis. Child. 37:93, 1962.

Cavell, B.: Transplacental metastasis of malignant melanoma. Acta Paediatr. Suppl. 146:37, 1963.

Chu, J., O'Connor, D. M., Gale, G. B., and Silverstein, M. J.: Congenital leukemia: two transient regressions without treatment in one patient. Pediatrics 71:277, 1983.

Coldman, A. J., Fryer, C. J. H., Elwood, J. M., and Sonley, M. J.: Neuroblastoma: influence of age at diagnosis, stage, tumor site, and sex on prognosis. Cancer 46:1896, 1980.

Conklin, J., and Abell, M. R.: Germ cell neoplasm of sacrococcygeal region. Cancer 20:2105, 1967.

Conley, G. R., Sant, G. R., Ucci, A. A., and Mitcheson, H. D.: Seminoma and epididymal cysts in a young man with known diethylstilbestrol exposure in utero. J.A.M.A. 249:1325, 1983.

Cramblett, H. G., Friedman, J. L., and Najjar, S.: Leukemia in an infant born of a mother with leukemia. N. Engl. J. Med. 259:727, 1958.

Cutler, L. S., Chaudry, A. P., and Topazian, R.: Melanotic neuroectodermal tumor of infancy: an ultrastructural study, literature review, and reevaluation. Cancer 48:257, 1981.

D'Angio, G. J., Evans, A. E., and Koop, C. E.: Special pattern of widespread neuroblastoma with a favorable prognosis. Lancet 1:1046, 1971.

D'Angio, G. J., Evans, A., Breslow, N., Beckwith, B., Bishop, H., Farwell, V., Goodwin, W., Leape, L., Palmer, N., Sinks, L., Sutow, W., Tefft, M., and Wolff, J.: The treatment of Wilms' tumor: results of the second National Wilms' Tumor Study. Cancer 47:2302, 1981.

deChadarévian, J., Fletcher, B. D., Chatten, J., and Rabinovitch, H. H.: Massive infantile nephroblastomatosis: a clinical, radiological, and pathological analysis of four cases. Cancer 39:2294, 1977.

Delalieux, C., Ebinger, G., Maurus, R., and Sliwowski, H.: Myoclonic encephalopathy and neuroblastoma. N. Engl. J. Med. 292:46, 1975.

Diamond, E. L., Schmerler, H., and Lilienfeld, A. M.: The relationship of intrauterine radiation to subsequent mortality and development of leukemia in children: a prospective study. Am. J. Epidemiol. 97:283, 1973.

Donnellan, W. A., and Swenson, O.: Benign and malignant sacrococcygeal teratomas. Surgery 64:834, 1968.

Ehrenbard, L. T., and Chaganti, R. S. K.: Cancer in the fetal hydantoin syndrome. Lancet 2:97, 1981.

Engel, R. R., Hammond, D., Eitzman, D. V., Pearson, H., and Krivit, W.: Transient congenital leukemia in 7 infants with mongolism. J. Pediatr. 65:303, 1964.

Evans, A. E., D'Angio, G. J., and Randolph, J.: A proposed staging for children with neuroblastoma. Cancer 27:374, 1971.

Evans, A. E., Gerson, J., and Schnaufer, L.: Spontaneous regression of neuroblastoma. J. Natl. Cancer Inst. Monogr. 44:49, 1976.

Evans, A. E., Land, V. J., Newton, W. A., et al.: Combination chemotherapy (vincristine, adriamycin, cyclophosphamide, and 5-fluorouracil) in the treatment of children with malignant hepatoma. Cancer 50:821, 1982.

Everson, T. C., and Cole, W. H.: Spontaneous Regression of Cancer: A Study and Abstract of Reports in the World Medical Literature and of Personal Communications Concerning Spontaneous Regression of Malignant Disease. Philadelphia, W. B. Saunders Company, 1966, pp. 88–163.

Exelby, P. R., Filler, R. M., and Grosfeld, J. L.: Liver tumors in children in particular reference to hepatoblastoma and hepatocellular carcinoma: American Academy of Pediatrics Surgical Section Survey—1974. J. Pediatr. Surg. 10:325, 1975.

Falk, H., Herbert, J. T., Edmonds, L., Heath, C. W., Jr., Thomas, L. B., and Popper, H.: Review of four cases of childhood hepatic angiosarcoma: elevated environmental arsenic exposure in one case. Cancer 47:382, 1981.

Falkinburg, L. W., and Kay, M. N.: A case of congenital sympathogonioma (neuroblastoma) of the right adrenal simulating erythroblastosis fetalis. J. Pediatr. 42:462, 1953.

Farber, S.: Chemotherapy in the treatment of leukemia and Wilms' tumor. J.A.M.A. 108:826, 1966.

Fleming, I., and Pinkel, D.: Clinical staging of Wilms' tumor. J. Pediatr. 74:324, 1969.

Fraumeni, J. F., and Miller, R. W.: Cancer deaths in the newborn. Am. J. Dis. Child. 117:186, 1969.

Frens, D. B., Bray, P. F., Wu, J. T., and Lahey, M. E.: The carcinoembryonic antigen assay: prognostic value in neural crest tumors. J. Pediatr. 88:591, 1976.

Gallo, G. E., and Penchansky, L.: Cystic nephroma. Cancer 39:1322, 1977.

Geiser, C. F., Baez, A., Schindler, A. M., and Shih, V. E.: Epithelial hepatoblastoma associated with congenital hemihypertrophy and cystathioninuria: presentation of a case. Pediatrics 46:66, 1970.

Gill, W. B., Schumacher, G. F. B., Bibbo, M., Straus, F. H., II, and Schoenberg, H. W.: Association of diethylstilbestrol exposure in utero with cryptorchidism, testicular hypoplasia, and semen abnormalities. J. Urol. 122:36, 1979.

Goh, K., Lee, H., and Klemperer, M.: Evidence of clastogens in acute leukemia: chromosomal abnormalities in healthy parents of congenital leukemic patients. Cancer 46:109, 1980.

Gold, E., Gordis, L., Tonascia, J., and Szklo, M.: Increased risk of brain tumors in children exposed to barbiturates. J. Natl. Cancer Inst. 61:1031, 1978.

Green, M., Cooke, R. E., and Lattanzi, W.: Occurrence of chronic diarrhea in three patients with ganglioneuromas. Pediatrics 23:951, 1959.

Gross, L.: Transmission of mouse leukemia virus through milk of virus-infected C3H female mice. Proc. Soc. Exp. Biol. Med. 109:830, 1962.

Gross, R. E., Clatworthy, H. W., Jr., and Meeker, I. A., Jr.: Sacrococcygeal teratomas in infants and children. A report of 40 cases. Surg. Gynecol. Obstet. 92:341, 1951.

Hagstrom, H. T.: Fetal dystocia due to metastatic neuroblastoma of the liver. Am. J. Obstet. Gynecol. 19:673, 1930.

Haicken, B. N., and Miller, D. R.: Simultaneous occurrence of congenital aniridia, hamartoma, and Wilms' tumor. J. Pediatr. 78:497, 1971.

Hann, H. L., Evans, A. E., Cohen, I. J., and Leitmeyer, J. E.:
Biological differences between neuroblastoma stages IV-S and IV: Measurement of serum ferritin and E-rosette inhibition in 30 children. N. Engl. J. Med. 305:425, 1981.

Hartenstein, H.: Wilms' tumor in a newborn infant: report of a case with autopsy studies. J. Pediatr. 35:381, 1949.

Hawthorne, H. C., Nelson, J. S., Witzleben, C. L., and Giangiacomo, J.: Blanching subcutaneous nodules in neonatal neuroblastoma. J. Pediatr. 77:297, 1970.

Haymond, M. W., and Weldon, V. V.: Female pseudohermaphroditism secondary to a maternal virilizing tumor: case report and review of the literature. J. Pediatr. 82:682, 1973.

Hellstrom, K. E., and Hellstrom, I.: Immunity to neuroblastoma and melanomas. Ann. Rev. Med. 23:19, 1972.

Helson, L., Fleisher, M., Bethune, V., Murphy, M. L., and Schwartz, M. K.: Urinary cystathionine, catecholamine, and metabolites in patients with neuroblastoma. Clin. Chem. 18:613, 1972.

Hepler, A. B.: Presacral sympathicoblastoma in an infant causing urinary obstruction. J. Urol. 49:777, 1943.

Herbst, A. L., Ulfelder, H., and Poskanzer, D. C.: Adenocarcinoma of the vagina: association of maternal stilbestrol therapy with tumor appearance in young women. N. Engl. J. Med. 284:878, 1971.

Herbst, A. L., Cole, P., Colton, T., Robboy, S. J., and Scully, R. E.: Age-incidence and risk of diethylstilbestrol-related adenocarcinoma of the vagina and cervix. Am. J. Obstet. Gynecol. 128:43, 1977.

Hermann, R. E., and Lonsdale, D.: Chemotherapy, radiotherapy, and hepatic lobectomy for hepatoblastoma in an infant: report of a survival. Surgery 68:383, 1970.

Holland, E.: A case of transplacental metastases of malignant melanoma from mother to fetus. J. Obstet. Gynaecol. Brit. Emp. 56:529, 1949.

Hornstein, L., Crowe, C., and Gruppo, R.: Adrenal carcinoma in child with history of fetal alcohol syndrome. Lancet 2:1292, 1977.

Ikeda, K., Suita, S., and Nakagawara, A.: Preoperative chemotherapy for initially unresectable hepatoblastoma in children. Arch. Surg. 114:203, 1979.

Jablon, S., and Kato, H.: Childhood cancer in relation to prenatal exposure to atomic-bomb radiation. Lancet 2:1000, 1970.

Jick, H., Walker, A. M., Rothman, K. J., Hunter, J. R., Holmes, L. B., Watkins, R. N., D'Ewart, D. C., Danford, A., and Madsen, S.: Vaginal spermicides and congenital disorders. J.A.M.A. 245:1329, 1981.

Jiminez, J. F., Brown, R. E., Seibert, R. W., Seibert, J. J., and Char, F.: Melanotic neuroectodermal tumor of infancy and fetal hydantoin syndrome. Am. J. Pediatr. Hematol./Oncol. 3:9, 1981.

Johnson, S., Knight, R., Marmer, D. J., and Steele, R. W.: Immune deficiency in fetal alcohol syndrome. Pediatr. Res. 15:908, 1981.

Joshi, V. V., Banerjee, A. K., Yadav, K., and Pathak, I. C.: Cystic partially differentiated nephroblastoma. Cancer 40:789, 1977.

Joshi, V. V., Kay, S., Milstein, R., Koontz, W. W., and McWilliams, N. B.: Congenital mesoblastic nephroma of infancy: report of a case with unusual clinical behavior. Am. J. Clin. Pathol. 60:811, 1973.

Kasdon, S. C.: Pregnancy and Hodgkin's disease. Am. J. Obstet. Gynecol. 57:282, 1949.

Kaufman, R. H., Binder, G. L., Gray, P. M., Jr., and Adam, E.: Upper genital tract changes associated with exposure in utero to diethylstilbestrol. Am. J. Obstet. Gynecol. 128:51, 1977.

Kersey, J. H., Spector, B. D., and Good, R. A.: Cancer in children with primary immunodeficiency diseases. J. Pediatr. 84:263, 1974.

Khan, A., Bader, J. L., Hoy, G. R., and Sinks, L. F.: Hepatoblastoma in child with fetal alcohol syndrome. Lancet 1:1403, 1979.

Kinney, H., Faix, R., and Brazy, J.: The fetal alcohol syndrome and neuroblastoma. Pediatrics 66:130, 1980.

Knudson, A. G., Jr., and Strong, L. C.: Mutation and cancer: a model for Wilms' tumor of the kidney. J. Natl. Cancer Inst. 48:313, 1972.

Koop, C. E., and Schnaufer, L.: The management of abdominal neuroblastoma. Cancer 35:905, 1975.

Kulkarni, R., Bailie, M. P., Bernstein, J., and Newton, B.: Progression of nephroblastomatosis to Wilms' tumor. J. Pediatr. 96:178, 1980.

Kumar, A. P. M., Pratt, C. B., Coburn, T. P., and Johnson, W. W.: Treatment strategy for nodular renal blastema and nephroblastomatosis associated with Wilms' tumor. J. Pediatr. Surg. 13:281, 1978.

Larimer, R. C.: Neuroblastoma (sympathogonioma) of the adrenal in a newborn infant. J. Pediatr. 34:365, 1949.

Laug, W. E., Seigel, S. E., Shaw, K. N. F., Landing, B., Baptista, J., and Gutenstein, M.: Initial urinary catecholamine metabolite concentrations and prognosis in neuroblastoma. Pediatrics 62:77, 1978.

Leikin, S., Evans, A., Heyn, R., and Newton, W.: The impact of chemotherapy on advanced neuroblastoma. Survival of patients diagnosed in 1956, 1962, and 1966–68 in Children's Cancer Study Group A. J. Pediatr. 84:131, 1974.

Lergier, J. E., Jiménez, E., Maldonado, N., and Veray, F.: Normal pregnancy in multiple myeloma treated with cyclophosphamide. Cancer 34:1018, 1974.

MacMahon, B., and Levy, M. A.: Prenatal origin of childhood leukemia—evidence from twins. N. Engl. J. Med. 270:1082, 1964.

Martin, E. S., and Griffith, J. F.: Myoclonic encephalopathy and neuroblastoma. Am. J. Dis. Child. 122:257, 1971.

Mason, G. A., Hart-Mercer, J., Millar, E. J., Strang, L. B., and Wynne, N. A.: Adrenaline-secreting neuroblastoma in an infant. Lancet 2:322, 1957.

Maurer, H. S., Pendergrass, T. W., Borges, W., and Honig, G. R.: The role of genetic factor in the etiology of Wilms' tumor: two pairs of monozygous twins with congenital abnormalities (aniridia; hemihypertrophy) and discordance for Wilms' tumor. Cancer 43:205, 1979.

Meadows, A. T., Lichtenfeld, J. L., and Koop, C. E.: Wilms' tumor in three children of a woman with congenital hemihypertrophy. N. Engl. J. Med. 291:23, 1974.

Miller, D. R., Newstead, G. J., and Young, L. W.: Perinatal leukemia with a possible variant of Ellis–van Creveld syndrome. J. Pediatr. 74:300, 1969.

Miller, R. W.: Down's syndrome (mongolism), other congenital malformations and cancers among the sibs of leukemic children. N. Engl. J. Med. 268:393, 1963.

Miller, R. W.: Persons at exceptionally high risk of leukemia. Cancer Res. 27:2420, 1967.

Miller, R. W.: Relation between cancer and congenital defects: an epidemiologic evaluation. J. Natl. Cancer Inst. 40:1079, 1968.

Miller, R. W.: Discordance for Wilms' tumor in MZ twins with aniridia. Childhood Cancer Etiol. Newsletter No. 56, 1979.

Moe, P. G., and Nellhaus, G.: Infantile polymyoclonia–opsoclonus syndrome and neural crest tumors. Neurology 20:756, 1970.

Murphy, G. P., Mirand, E. A., Johnston, G. S., Gibbons, R. P., Jones, R. L., and Scott, W. W.: Erythropoietin release associated with Wilms' tumor. Johns Hopkins Hosp. Bull. 120:26, 1967.

Napalkov, N.: In Tomatis, L., Mohr, U., and Davis W. (Eds.): Transplacental Carcinogenesis. International Agency for Research on Cancer Scientific Publication No. 4, 1973.

Perez, C., Kaiman, H. A., Keith, J., Mill, W. B., Vietti, T. J., and Powers, W. E.: Treatment of Wilms' tumor and factors affecting prognosis. Cancer 32:609, 1973.

Pierce, M. I.: Leukemia in the newborn infant. J. Pediatr. 54:691, 1959.

Pilling, G. P.: Wilms' tumor in seven children with congenital aniridia. J. Pediatr. Surg. 10:87, 1975.

Quinn, J. J., Altman, A. J., and Frantz, C. N.: Serum lactic dehydrogenase, an indicator of tumor activity in neuroblastoma. J. Pediatr. 97:89, 1980.

Ramsey, N. K. C., Dehner, L. P., Coccia, P. F., D'Angio, G. J.,

and Nesbit, M. E.: Acute hemorrhage into Wilms' tumor. J. Pediatr. 91:763, 1977.

Raney, R. B., Jr., Chatten, J., Littman, P., Jarrett, P., Schnaufer, L., Bishop, H., and D'Angio, G. J.: Treatment strategies for infants with malignant sacrococcygeal teratoma. J. Pediatr. Surg. 16:573, 1981.

Reimann, D. L., Clemmens, R. L., and Pillsbury, W. A.: Congenital acute leukemia: skin nodules, a first sign. J. Pediatr. 46:415, 1955.

Riccardi, V. M., Sujansky, E., Smith, A. C., and Francke, U.: Chromosomal imbalance in the aniridia-Wilms' tumor association: 11p interstitial deletion. Pediatrics 61:604, 1978.

Robboy, S. J., Kauffman, R. H., Prat, J., Welch, W. R., Gaffey, T., Scully, R. E., Richart, R., Fenoglia, C. M., Verata, R., and Tilley, B. C.: Pathologic findings in women enrolled in the National Cooperative Diethylstilbestrol Adenosis (DESAD) Project. Obstet. Gynecol. 53:309, 1979.

Rosenfeld, M., Rodgers, B. M., and Talbert, J. L.: Wilms' tumor with abdominal pain. Arch. Surg. 112:1080, 1977.

Rosner, F., and Lee, S. L.: Down's syndrome and acute leukemia: myeloblastic or lymphoblastic? Report of forty-three cases and review of the literature. Am. J. Med. 53:203, 1972.

Ross, J. D., Moloney, W. C., and Desforges, J. F.: Ineffective regulation of granulopoiesis masquerading as congenital leukemia in a mongoloid child. J. Pediatr. 63:1, 1963.

Sawitsky, A., and Desposito, F.: A survey of American experience with vitamin B_{12} therapy of neuroblastoma. J. Pediatr. 67:99, 1965.

Schneider, K. M., Becker, J. M., and Krasna, I. H.: Neonatal neuroblastoma. Pediatrics 36:359, 1965.

Schwartz, A. D., Dadash-Zadeh, M., Lee, H., and Swaney, J. J.: Spontaneous regression of disseminated neuroblastoma. J. Pediatr. 85:760, 1974.

Seeler, R. A., Israel, J. N., Royal, J. E., Kaye, C. I., Rao, S., and Abulaban, M.: Ganglioneuroblastoma and fetal hydantoin-alcohol syndrome. Pediatrics 63:524, 1979.

Shafer, A. D., and Selinkoff, P. M.: Preoperative irradiation and chemotherapy for initially unresectable hepatoblastoma. J. Pediatr. Surg. 12:1001, 1977.

Sorrell, T. C., Forbes, I. J., Burness, F. R., and Rischbieth, R. H. C.: Depression of immunological function in patients treated with phenytoin sodium (sodium diphenylhydantoin). Lancet 2:1233, 1971.

Sotelo-Avila, C., Gonzalez-Crussi, F., and Fowler, J. W.: Complete and incomplete forms of Beckwith-Wiedemann syndrome: their oncogenic potential. J. Pediatr. 96:47, 1980.

Spear, G. S., Hyde, T. P., Gruppo, R. A., and Slusser, R.: Pseudohermaphroditism, glomerulonephritis with the nephrotic syndrome and Wilms' tumor in infancy. J. Pediatr. 79:677, 1971.

Speidel, B. D., and Meadow, S. R.: Maternal epilepsy and abnormalities of the fetus and newborn. Lancet 2:839, 1972.

Stark, C. R., and Mantel, N.: Effects of maternal age and birth order on the risk of mongolism and leukemia. J. Natl. Cancer Inst. 37:687, 1966.

Sukarochana, K., and Kiesewetter, M. B.: Wilms' tumor: factors influencing long-term survival. J. Pediatr. 69:747, 1966.

Sullivan, M. P., Hussey, D. H., and Ayala, A. G.: Wilms' tumor. In Sutow, W., Vietti, T., and Fernbach, D. (Eds.): Clinical Pediatric Oncology. St. Louis, The C. V. Mosby Co., 1973, p. 359.

Swift, P. G. F., Bloom, S. R., and Harris, F.: Watery diarrhea and ganglioneuroma with secretion of vasoactive intestinal peptide. Arch. Dis. Child. 50:896, 1975.

Taylor, W. F., Myers, M., and Taylor, W. R.: Extrarenal Wilms' tumour in an infant exposed to intrauterine phenytoin. Lancet 2:481, 1980.

Telander, R. L., Gilchrist, G. S., Burgert, E. O., Jr., Kelalis, P. P., and Goellner, J. R.: Bilateral massive nephroblastomatosis in infancy. J. Pediatr. Surg. 13:163, 1978.

Todani, T., Tabuchi, K., Wantanabi, Y., and Tsutsumi, A.: True hepatic teratoma with high alpha fetoprotein in serum. J. Pediatr. Surg. 12:591, 1977.

Tomatis, L.: Prenatal exposure to chemical carcinogens and its effect on subsequent generations. Natl. Cancer Inst. Monogr. 51:159, 1979.

Totter, J. R., and MacPherson, H. G.: Do childhood cancers result from prenatal X-rays? Health Physics 40:511, 1981.

Transplacental carcinogenesis (editorial). Lancet *1*:1425, 1973.

Turkel, S. B., and Itabashi, H. H.: The natural history of neuroblastic cells in the fetal adrenal gland. Am. J. Pathol. *76*:225, 1974.

Van Eys, J., and Flexner, J. M.: Transient spontaneous remission in a case of untreated congenital leukemia. Am. J. Dis. Child. *118*:507, 1969.

von Studnitz, W., Käser, H., and Sjoerdsma, A.: Spectrum of catecholamine biochemistry in patients with neuroblastoma. N. Engl. J. Med. *269*:232, 1963.

Voorhess, M. L.: Neuroblastoma with normal urinary catecholamine excretion. J. Pediatr. *78*:680, 1971.

Voûte, P. A., Jr., Wadman, S. K., and van Putten, W. J.: Congenital neuroblastoma: symptoms in the mother during pregnancy. Clin. Pediatr. *9*:206, 1970.

Warrier, R. P., Ravindranath, Y., Emami, A., and Lusher, J.: Exchange transfusion for hyperleukocytosis, anemia, and metabolic abnormalities in leukemia. J. Pediatr. *98*:338, 1981.

Weinberger, M. M., and Oleinick, A.: Congenital marrow dysfunction in Down's syndrome. J. Pediatr. *77*:273, 1970.

Wells, H. G.: Occurrence and significance of congenital malignant neoplasms. Arch. Pathol. *30*:535, 1940.

Williams, C., and Greer, M.: Homovanillic acid and vanilmandelic acid in diagnosis of neuroblastoma. J.A.M.A. *183*:836, 1963.

Witzleben, C. L., and Bruninga, G.: Infantile choriocarcinoma: a characteristic syndrome. J. Pediatr. *73*:374, 1968.

Wolff, J. A.: Advances in the treatment of Wilms' tumor. Cancer *35*:901, 1975.

Wolff, J. A., D'Angio, G., Hartmann, J., Krivit, W., and Newton, W. A.: Long-term evaluation of single versus multiple courses of actinomycin D therapy of Wilms' tumor. N. Engl. J. Med. *290*:84, 1974.

Yunis, J. J., and Ramsay, N. K. C.: Familial occurence of the aniridia–Wilms' tumor syndrome with deletion 11p 13-14.1. J. Pediatr. *96*:1027, 1980.

Disorders of Uncertain Origin

Altman, A. J., and Schwartz, A. D.: Malignant Diseases of Infancy, Childhood and Adolescence. 2nd ed. Philadelphia, W. B. Saunders Co., 1983, pp. 334–337.

Batson, R., Shapiro, J. L., Christie, A., and Riley, H. D., Jr.: Acute nonlipid disseminated reticuloendotheliosis. A.M.A.J. Dis. Child. *90*:323, 1955.

Bierman, H. R.: Apparent cure of Letterer-Siwe disease. Seventeen-year survival of identical twins with nonlipoid reticuloendotheliosis. J.A.M.A. *196*:368, 1966.

Cederbaum, S. D., Niwayama, G., et al.: Combined immunodeficiency presenting as the Letterer-Siwe syndrome. J. Pediatr. *85*:466, 1974.

Gotoff, J. P., and Esterly, N. B.: Editorial: Histiocytosis. J. Pediatr. *85*:592, 1974.

Greenberger, J. S., Crocker, A. C., Vawter, G., et al.: Results of treatment of 127 patients with systemic histiocytosis (Letterer-Siwe syndrome, Schüller-Christian syndrome, and multifocal eosinophilic granuloma). Medicine *60*:311, 1981.

Hertz, C. G., and Hambrick, G. W.: Congenital Letterer-Siwe disease: a case treated with vincristine and corticosteroids Am. J. Dis. Child. *116*:553, 1968.

Juberg, R. C., Kloepfer, H. W., and Oberman, H. A.: Genetic determination of acute disseminated histiocytosis X (Letterer-Siwe syndrome). Pediatrics *45*:753, 1970.

Lahey, M. E.: Histiocytosis X: comparison of three treatment regimens. J. Pediatr. *87*:179, 1975.

Lanzkowsky, P.: Histiocytosis syndromes. *In* Lanzkowsky, P. (Ed.): Pediatric Oncology. New York, McGraw-Hill Book Co., 1983.

Lucaya, J.: Histiocytosis X. Am. J. Dis. Child. *121*:289, 1971.

MacMahon, H. E., Bedizel, M., and Ellis, C. A.: Familial erythrophagocytic lymphohistiocytosis. Pediatrics *32*:868, 1963.

McClure, P. D., Strachan, P., and Saunders. E. F.: Hypofibrinogenemia and thrombocytopenia in familial hemophagocytic reticulosis. J. Pediatr. *85*:67, 1974.

Miller, D. R.: Familial reticuloendotheliosis: Concurrence of disease in five siblings. Pediatrics *38*:986, 1966.

Schoeck, V. W., Peterson, R. D. A., and Good, R. A.: Familial occurrence of Letterer-Siwe disease. Pediatrics *32*:1055, 1963.

PART 19 NEONATAL PHARMACOLOGY

108

Principles of Neonatal Pharmacology

By Robert J. Roberts*

General Concepts

INTRODUCTION

A 1500-gm premature infant born in North America is exposed to about 20 prescribed drugs between conception and discharge from the nursery. On the average, four to 10 medications are given to the mother and reach the fetus or infant transplacentally or through breast milk; after birth, the low-birth-weight infant is usually exposed to about seven agents by nursery routine (e.g., vitamin K, triple-dye, and penicillin opthalmic ointment) and seven drugs prescribed for specific indications. Total xenobiotic exposure is substantially greater since over-the-counter medications, alcohol, nicotine, caffeine, and environmental pollutants such as heavy metals and polycyclic hydrocarbons must be considered. The extent of exposure is emphasized by the presence of salicylate, hexachlorophene, and caffeine in many random cord plasma samples. Even benzyl alcohol, used as a preservative in intravenous saline solutions, has been associated with toxicity in premature infants. Common chemicals such as these can affect the developing mammal.

The current trend of fetal and neonatal exposure to drugs is complex. Widespread knowledge of the tragic consequences of early exposure to thalidomide, for example, has prompted a cautious approach to other drugs by physicians and patients. The tendency to limit exposure in the population at large, however, has been offset by the progressive regionalization of high-risk perinatal care and the coincident emergence of an attitutde of aggressive diagnostic and therapeutic intervention. This attitude has added new dimensions to drug utilization, with respect to benefit and potential risk for the infant before, during, and after birth.

The scope of treatment before birth expands rapidly with reports of the use of propranolol, vitamin B$_{12}$, and, especially, agents such as glucocorticoids designed to accelerate the lung maturation. During birth, interpretation of sophisticated cardiopulmonary data gathered from the fetus during monitoring now requires an awareness of the modification of these functions by drugs. Finally, the breadth of current neonatal therapeutics is emphasized by a recent drug utilization survey conducted in the Neonatal Intensive Care Unit of the Montreal Children's Hospital, wherein it was found that more than 70 different drugs were prescribed for 320 infants (Table 108–1). Many specific medications have been discussed

Table 108–1. Frequency of Drug Exposure in the Newborn, 1977–1979

No.	Drug	No. of Patients (Frequency)	Per Cent
1	Calcium gluconate	116	52.7
2	Gentamicin injectable	95	43.2
3	Sodium bicarbonate	94	42.7
4	Ampicillin	93	42.3
5	Glycerine suppositories	70	31.8
6	Konakion (vitamin K)	55	25.0
7	Penicillin	54	24.5
8	Furosemide	53	24.1
9	Kanamycin	41	18.6
10	Infantol (vitamin)	35	15.9
11	Potassium chloride	33	15.0
12	Fer-In-Sol	33	15.0
13	Nitrous oxide	29	13.2
14	Medium-chain triglyceride	28	12.7
15	d-Tubocurarine	26	11.8
16	Phenobarbital	25	11.4
17	Cloxacillin	24	10.9
18	Sodium chloride	24	10.9
19	Digoxin	23	10.4
20	Aquasol E (vitamin E)	23	10.4
21	Halothane	21	9.5
22	Diazepam	19	8.6
23	Caffeine	19	8.6
24	Mycostatin	19	8.6
25	Chloramphenicol	16	7.3
26	Adrenalin	16	7.3
27	Atropine	15	6.8
28	Prostigmine	13	5.9
29	Neosynephrine	12	5.4
30	Insulin	10	4.5
31	Hydrochlorothiazide	10	4.5
32	Cyclogel	10	4.5
33	Spironolactone	10	4.5
34	Vitamin B$_{12}$	09	4.1
35	Tobramycin	09	4.1
36	Priscoline (α-tolazoline)	09	4.1
37	Bacitracin	08	3.6
38	Meperidine	08	3.6
39	Edecrin	08	3.6
40	Methicillin	08	3.6

(From Aranda et al.: Ther. Drug Monitoring 2:39, 1980.)

* This chapter includes some contributions of previous authors, Drs. Allen H. Neims, Jacob V. Aranda, and Peter M. Loughnan.

elsewhere; this chapter has been organized to include the broad overview of general pharmacologic principles important to drug management of newborn disease, and a review of selected drugs which are currently being utilized in the treatment of newborn disease.

PRINCIPLES OF NEONATAL THERAPEUTICS

For neonates, in contrast to adults, there is a paucity of information regarding drug disposition (absorption, distribution, metabolism, and excretion). Disastrous experiences such as chloramphenicol-induced "gray baby" syndrome are dramatic illustrations of the importance of understanding the fundamental principles involved in drug disposition and action in neonates.

Drug Absorption. Absorption of drugs from the gastrointestinal tract of neonates should be expected to be under the same influences as those in older infants, children, and adults. The basic mechanism for drug absorption is diffusion. Major factors that can alter the rates and extent of drug absorption include gastrointestinal mobility, pH, and contents, including bacterial flora. Rane points out the importance of considering the physiologic developmental changes that occur with these factors in the neonate. Unfortunately, few studes have examined questions of drug bioavailability and rate of absorption in neonates. One exception is the report by Bell and co-workers, which dispels the notion that the premature infant absorbs vitamin E poorly from the intestinal tract. Absorption of drug from intramuscular injection sites depends largely on vascular perfusion surrounding the site of injection. Inflammation with vasconstriction, avascular tissue, and shock can drastically modify both rate of absorption and bioavailability. It is important to recognize that not all drugs are suitable for intramuscular administration because of tissue insolubility problems (local precipitation) with agents such as phenytoin or because of significant pain on administration of drugs such as digoxin.

Distribution. This is the process that leads to the partition of drugs between the various body organs and tissues (compartments). The distribution of a drug is determined by several factors including blood flow, pH and composition of body fluids and tissues, physical/chemical properties of the drug (lipid solubility, ionization constant), and extent of drug-binding to plasma or other body proteins. The binding of many drugs (e.g., digoxin, theophylline, phenytoin, phenobarbital, salicylate, and penicillins) to plasma protein is diminished in the newborn compared with that in the nonpregnant adult. It is generally accepted that the binding of drugs to plasma proteins can be a modulating factor not only in distribution of drugs in the body but also in dose-response relationships and the rate of elimination of drugs from the body. Figure 108–1 illustrates this important concept. The

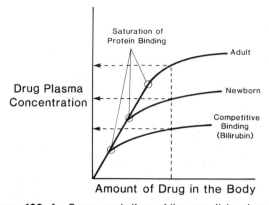

Figure 108–1. Representation of the possible changes in plasma protein binding of drugs with changes in the actual amount of plasma protein (newborn vs. adult) or as a consequence of changes in available binding sites for drug (competitive binding). Note the changing relationship between the concentration of drug in the plasma and the amount of drug in the body.

influence of different amounts of plasma protein (newborn versus adult) or number of available protein-binding sites for drug (competitive binding, i.e., by bilirubin or other drugs) on the distribution of drug between plasma and the remainder of the body is represented by the three theoretical curves in this figure. The changing slope of each curve means that there is not a fixed relationship between the concentration of drug in the plasma and the amount of total drug in the body. The major change in the relationship occurs as a consequence of saturation of plasma protein binding sites. If the changing equilibrium between plasma concentration and total body content of drug as depicted in Figure 108–1 is not appreciated, serious problems can result. For example, the dotted lines illustrate how differences in protein-binding can result in a different plasma drug concentration for each curve despite equivalent amounts of total drug in the body (i.e., equal doses administered). If drug doses are increased in the newborn in an attempt to achieve the "effective" plasma drug concentration shown for the adult, the total amount of drug in the newborn body will be greater, possibly leading to toxicity or an exaggerated response. Since protein-bound drug is in equilibrium with free (unbound) drug in the plasma, this fraction (free drug) is typically increased under conditions of reduced quantity or decreased binding capacity of plasma protein. Because free drug is generally believed to be the pharmacologically active fraction, there may not be any necessity to increase the plasma drug concentration to achieve equal pharmacologic effect in the situation of reduced protein binding. As an illustration, in adults with asthma, increasing bronchodilation is observed over the plasma concentration range of total theophylline, 5 to 20 µg/ml, but toxicity becomes more likely above 20 µg/ml. Let us assume tentatively the applicability to apneic newborns of this upper limit of desired concentration, since it is determined by toxicity, not efficacy. At the theophylline plasma concentration of 17 µg/ml, 56 per cent of the drug is affixed to protein in adult plasma. The therapeutic plasma concentration range in adults of 10 to 20 µg/ml, therefore, corresponds to 4.4 to 8.8 µg/ml of unbound theophylline. Only 36 per cent of theophylline is bound to protein in full-term newborn cord plasma. The concentration limits for unbound drug of 4.4 to 8.8 µg/ml would, therefore, correspond to a plasma concentration range for total theophylline of 6.9 to 13.8 µg/ml. This computed range for theophylline is remarkably similar to that (6.6 to 11.0 µg/ml) found appropriate by Shannon and colleagues during treatment of premature infants with apnea. Thus, decreased plasma protein binding of drug may not require alteration of dosing requirements despite the existence of differing plasma drug concentrations. However, decreased plasma protein binding may influence the ability to translate from the ideal therapeutic plasma concentration in the adult to those in the newborn.

The possible influence of competitive protein-binding by endogenous substrates such as bilirubin or other drugs on drug distribution (drug plasma—to—tissue concentration relationships) is also illustrated in Figure 108–1. Competitive binding causes drug to be displaced from plasma protein, which results in greater amounts of free (unbound) drug in plasma and a shift in equilibrium that drives drug into tissues. Thus, the result is the same as if the actual amount of plasma-protein was reduced. It is important to recognize that there can be a changing relationship between the plasma concentration and amount of endogenous material (bilirubin) in tissue occurring as well in these competitive binding situations. The drug could displace bilirubin from protein binding sites, and this "released" bilirubin would redistribute to tissue. The less rapid rate of rise in the curve means that a large change in total body bilirubin content could be occurring in the face of smaller changes in plasma bilirubin concentration. This has been offered as an explanation of how some highly protein-bound drugs may predispose an infant to the development of kernicterus. Important in this regard is the actual amount of drug present in the plasma (nanograms versus milligrams). Table 108–2 lists the plasma protein binding percentages of several drugs in the newborn. The wide range of values observed reflects not only the relative affinity of the drug for the available protein binding sites but also the concentration of drug found in the plasma following therapeutic doses.

The cause (or causes) of the deficient plasma protein binding of drugs at birth is not yet fully defined. It is in part due to decreased plasma albumin concentrations (also applicable to the gravid woman at term), but competition by endogenous ligands or qualitative differences in neonatal plasma protein or

Table 108–2. Plasma Protein Binding of Drugs in the Neonate

Drug	Per Cent Protein Bound
Ampicillin	7–12
Diazepam	84–98
Digoxin	14–26
Furosemide	94
Indomethacin	95
Methicillin	65
Phenobarbital	30–50
Phenytoin	70–90
Sulfasoxazole	65–70
Theophylline	36

both remain possible contributors. The postnatal age at which adultlike binding is attained is unknown, since most studies have been restricted to cord plasma samples. With phenytoin, most of the deficiency has disappeared before the age of 3 months.

Metabolism. A large number of drugs undergo metabolic conversion prior to elimination from the body. Biotransformation of a drug in general results in a more polar, less lipid-soluble molecular species that can be expected to be more rapidly eliminated than the parent compound by renal excretion or other routes. There are two major categories of drug biotransformation: (1) the nonsynthetic reactions, including oxidation, reduction, and hydrolysis, and (2) the synthetic or conjugation reactions. Although the liver is regarded as the major organ responsible for biotransformation of drugs, many other organs in the body possess considerable potential to metabolize drugs.

Both the relative deficiency in the capacity to oxidize a drug at birth and the rate of maturation of that capacity vary with the drug. Each of these characteristics also exhibits marked individual variability. Most drugs, including phenytoin, phenobarbital, diazepam, amobarbital, tolbutamide, nortriptylene, mepivacaine, theophylline, and caffeine, exhibit prolonged half-lives or low body clearance rates or both shortly after birth (Morselli et al., 1980). Even among those drugs poorly disposed of, there are quantitative differences; for example, elimination of the methylxanthines is substantially slower than that of phenytoin, both relative to adult values.

The influences of gestational age and birth per se on metabolism of drugs are not clearly defined. The capacities to oxidize antipyrine and diazepam are more deficient in premature infants than in their full-term counterparts. There is good evidence in guinea pigs and some evidence in human beings that birth in itself does initiate maturation of drug oxidative function, although the rate of maturation may be slower in infants of very low birth weights. The aspect of birth that triggers maturation is undefined. The 2- to 4-fold deficiency in body clearance rates associated with most oxidized drugs at birth correlates well with fetal hepatic concentrations of cytochrome P-450 mono-oxygenase activity observed midgestationally. The influences of specific illness, general condition, hypoxemia, nutritional state, drug interactions (e.g., prenatal treatment with glucocorticoid) and other factors on oxidative drug capacity remain virtually unexplored.

Certain important conjugative processes, especially glucuronidation, are also diminished in newborns compared with those in older neonates and infants. Chloramphenicol-induced "gray baby" syndrome has been explained by reduced rate of glucuronide conjugation resulting in an unexpected rate of accumulation of toxic amounts of the drug. Most of the previous comments regarding oxidation apply as well to the processes of glucuronidation. Sulfation, as distinct from glucuronidation, is active in the neonate, as evidenced by metabolite patterns of acetaminophen (Miller and Roberts, 1976). Acetylation, glutathione conjugation, mercapturic acid formation, and conjugation with amino acids are processes likely to be somewhat deficient at birth. Maturational characteristics of hepatic blood flow, transport of drugs into hepatocytes, intracellular binding of drugs, and biliary secretion, alone or in combination, are likely to influence the disposition of certain drugs and have been extensively reviewed in the literature (Rane, 1980).

Excretion. The dominant pathway for drug elimination from the body is renal excretion. The most important characteristics of the neonatal renal function relative to drug elimination include a low glomerular filtration rate, glomerular preponderance, nephron heterogeneity, low effective renal blood flow, and low tubular function compared with adult functions. The deficient glomerular filtration and renal tubular secretion in the neonate merits great concern, since many drugs in clinical use are eliminated by the kidney through these mechanisms. Neonatal glomerular filtration rate is about 30 per cent of the adult rate expressed per unit surface area. The plasma disappearance rates of aminoglycosides, kanamycin, and gentamicin, which are eliminated mainly by glomerular filtration, reflect these changes in GFR. The dosage schedules recommended for these drugs have taken this into account. Renal blood flow may influence the rate at which drugs are presented to and eliminated by the kidney. The average values for effective renal plasma flow, as measured by the para-aminohippurate clearance (C_{PAH}), is 15 per cent of that of the adult in the neonate less than 12 hours of age, assuming complete extraction of PAH. The rate at which renal clearance matures appears to vary not only among infants but also among drugs. Urinary pH also can influence the rate of renal excretion of drugs that are subject to nonionic diffusion.

Summary. Drug disposition may be significantly altered by a variety of disease states that affect the respective organ systems involved in drug absorption, distribution, metabolism, and excretion. The major observations of altered drug disposition have involved congestive heart, liver, or renal failure and the pathophysiologic states of hypoxemia and acidoses. These observations have been thoroughly reviewed by Rane.

PRINCIPLES OF NEONATAL PHARMACOKINETICS

Designing an optimal therapeutic program requires not only a thorough understanding of the pharmacology of the drug under consideration but also a rigorous and thoughtful examination of the patient's physiologic and biochemical status. The reason for these requirements relate to the fact that the ultimate outcome of drug therapy represents a continued interplay among (1) the intrinsic pharmacology of the drug, (2) the organ, cellular and/or subcellular responses to the drug, and (3) the effect of the disease process on these events. The ability to anticipate the therapeutic outcome is further compromised by biologic variations and variability among patients.

One of the more useful management methods that aids the physician in dealing with these complex pharmacologic, biochemical, and physiologic circumstances (drug pharmacodynamics) is the use of quantitative measurements of drug concentrations in serum or plasma (drug pharmacokinetics). The basic rationale for measuring drug concentrations in biologic samples relates to the fact that the onset, intensity, and reversibility of drug effects are proportional to the concentration of the drug at the site of action and that the concentration at the site of action is relatable to the level in the biologic sample examined. The therapeutic goal of the physician is to achieve and maintain a drug concentration at the site of action that will produce the maximum desired effect with a minimal risk of toxicity. This is the so-called "target concentration concept." By understanding and appropriately applying pharmacokinetics, the physician is able to predict the concentrations of the drug in the blood at any time after dose or series of doses. In other words, the physician can predetermine the ideal dosing requirements for each patient. Again, the critical assumption is that the intensity of action of the drug is directly proportional to its concentration in the blood. The following material will introduce some of the basic concepts and terms used in drug pharmacokinetics.

The Body Compartments. Single-compartment pharmacokinetics is considered the least complex situation in drug movements in the body. The basic assumption is that after the drug is introduced into the blood, it rapidly equilibrates with the tissues of the body so that the rate at which the blood concentration changes reflects the rate at which concentrations of drug change in most tissues of the body.

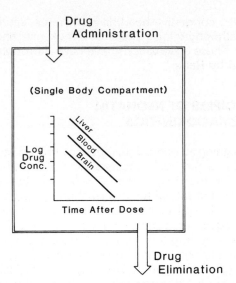

Figure 108–2. Representation of single compartment drug disappearance curves.

Thus, if we were to look at drug concentration in blood and tissues at various times after injection, the pattern of drug decline in all major tissues would be parallel.

Even though the concentrations in various tissues are different at any one time, the rate at which the tissue and blood concentrations decline is equivalent (Fig. 108–2). This similarity in drug flux in all major tissues indicates that the body may be considered as a single compartment. With single-compartment kinetics, the movement of drugs follows the laws of first-order kinetics, meaning that the instantaneous rate at which the amount of drug changes within the body depends on the amount of drug present at that time.

Volume of Distribution. The relationship between plasma concentration of the drug (Cp) and the total amount of drug in the body (Ab) is shown in the following equation:

$$Cp = \frac{Ab}{Vd}$$

In this formula, Vd is the volume of distribution of the drug in the body. The volume of distribution (Vd) is a mathematic term relating Ab and Cp and has no physiologic identity. It is very useful, however, in predicting the plasma concentration of drug resulting from a given dose. For example:

$$
\begin{aligned}
\text{Gentamicin Vd} &= 0.4 \text{ l/kg} \\
Ab^0 &= 2.5 \text{ mg/kg} \\
Cp^0 &= \frac{2500 \ \mu g/kg}{400 \ ml/kg} \\
&= 6.25 \ \mu g/ml \text{ at zero} \\
&\quad \text{time after administration}
\end{aligned}
$$

Also note that if the dose is doubled, the plasma concentration will double. Thus, dosage adjustment with drugs that follow first-order single-compartment kinetics is straightforward with a predictable result if one knows the plasma concentration resulting from a given dose.

Drug Half-Life. The half-life of a drug in the blood or body is the time required for any given concentration in the blood (or any given amount in the body) to decline to one half of the initially selected value. For example, if it takes 1 hour for the plasma level of a drug to decline from 6 $\mu g/ml$ to 3 $\mu g/ml$, the half-life is 1 hour. The relationship between half-life (T½) and the first-order rate constant for elimination (Ke) is represented in the following equation:

$$T\frac{1}{2} = \frac{0.693}{Ke}$$

The values for Ke, half-life, and the volume of distribution are assumed to be constant in an individual

Table 108–3. Serum Half-Lives and Therapeutic Levels of Drugs Employed in the Treatment of Neonatal Disease

Drug	T½ (range in hr)	Therapeutic Range (μg/ml)	Recommended Sampling Time After Dose (hr)
Gentamicin	2–12	Peak 5–8	1–2
Tobramycin	2–12	Trough 1–2	6–12
Kanamycin	4–18	Peak 15–25	1–2
		Trough 2–4	6–12
Chloramphenicol	10–24	Peak 15–20	1–3*
		Trough 5–10	4–8
Digoxin	20–180	1–3	>8
Phenobarbital	36–144	10–30	>6
Phenytoin	15–105	10–20	>8
Caffeine	37–231	7–20	>4†
Theophylline	12–64	Peak 20	1
		Trough 10	>4†

* May have delayed hydrolysis of ester (Kauffman et al., 1981).
† See Table 108–8.

after any given dose of any one drug. One can say, therefore, that for drugs with first-order single-compartment kinetics, these values are independent of the drug dose. However, for any given drug these values may vary among individuals in the population. Disease states in particular can cause these values to change, and it is necessary to appreciate these possible fluctuations when an unexpected intensity of drug response is observed. In addition, individual drugs have distinct physical properties, and each is handled uniquely in the body. Pharmacokinetic parameters, therefore, vary widely among different drugs. Table 108–3 is a partial listing of drugs frequently employed in neonates that can be usefully monitored. It can be noted from this table that half-lives differ widely among the various drugs.

Multicompartment Distribution. Many drugs distribute in the body as if there were more than one compartment. After administering an I.V. dose, one would observe the plasma concentration curve to have the shape depicted in Figure 108–3 when it is plotted on semilog paper. The accelerated portion of the disappearance curve at the earlier times after the dose (α phase) indicates that the drug is distributing out of the plasma into tissues. In other words, more than one process is operating to remove the drug from the blood compartment. During the linear phase (β phase), all tissues are saturated, and the drug levels in the blood are declining through metabolism or excretion or both. During the β phase, the drug may re-enter the central compartment from the peripheral compartment because of lower plasma levels favoring diffusion of drug out of tissues as opposed to going into tissues during the early (α phase) high-plasma concentration. Ordinarily, the half-lives of drugs following two-compartment pharmacokinetics are determined during the linear, or β, phase.

Zero-Order Kinetics. The pharmacokinetics of the drug are said to be dose-dependent (or concentration-dependent) when the half-life of the drug changes with increasing doses (or levels of drug in the blood). This dependency of half-life on drug dose or drug concentration usually arises because elimination processes (e.g., metabolism or excretion or both) become saturated when large amounts of the drug are present in the body. For some drugs, elim-

Table 108–4. Drugs that Demonstrate Saturation Kinetics with Therapeutic Doses in Neonates

Caffeine
Chloramphenicol
Diazepam
Furosemide
Indomethacin
Phenytoin

ination processes appear to be saturated at low, therapeutic doses, and dose-dependent kinetics therefore prevail at all regular therapeutic doses. Once saturation of elimination occurs, the drug is eliminated at a constant rate (e.g., mg/hr), exhibiting zero-order, or saturation, kinetics. Thus, the rate of decline of the drug in the body is a constant and is not proportional to the amount of drug in the body as is the case with first-order kinetics. Many drugs exhibit zero-order kinetics when high concentrations are present in the body, but after the drug levels fall because of existing elimination processes, first-order kinetics prevail. As a result, one observes progressively shorter half-lives as the concentration of drug in the blood decreases. Some examples of drugs that show saturation-type kinetics are provided in Table 108–4. The plasma disappearance curve for such situations is shown in Figure 108–4.

Multiple Doses and The "Plateau Principle." During the typical course of drug therapy, many doses of drug are ordinarily administered. Each additional dose is usually given prior to complete elimination of the previous dose (or doses) from the body, resulting in the addition of more drug to that already present in the body. With repeated administration, the levels of drug in the body increase for a time, but the rate of drug elimination also increases. Steady-state, or plateau, levels will be reached when the elimination of drug increases to equal the amount of

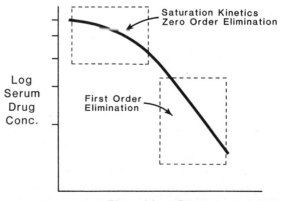

Log Serum Drug Conc.

Saturation Kinetics Zero Order Elimination

First Order Elimination

Time After Dose

Figure 108–4. Representation of saturation, or zero-order (serum concentration dependent), and first-order (serum concentration independent) pharmacokinetics.

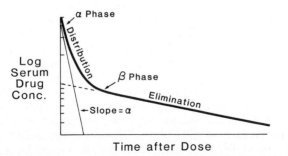

α Phase

Distribution

Log Serum Drug Conc.

β Phase

Elimination

←Slope = α

Time after Dose

Figure 108–3. Representation of multicompartment serum drug disappearance curve.

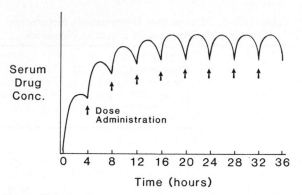

Figure 108–5. Representation of multiple dosing with accumulation of serum drug levels to steady-state concentration.

drug administered at each dosing interval. Careful examination of the hypothetical blood level curve shown in Figure 108–5 reveals important principles that one should consider when selecting a dosage regimen for therapy. The curve in Figure 108–5 represents the changes that occur when an oral dose of a drug with a half-life of 4 hours is given every 4 hours. Note that (1) four half-lives (16 hours in the example case) are needed for the drug to reach what is essentially steady-state, or plateau, level; (2) during the interval between doses, blood levels fluctuate owing to drug absorption and elimination; (3) once steady state has been reached (approximately four half-lives) the maximum and minimum blood levels are the same after each dose; and (4) after giving a drug repeatedly using an interval of one half-life, one can expect a maximum (or minimum) blood level to be reached at steady state that is 1.4 times larger than that reached after the first dose. The objective of the multiple-dose regimen should be to maintain the patient's blood level within a maximum state of concentration and the minimum effective concentration. If the dosage interval is too short, accumulation of drug above a maximum safe concentration will result. If the dosage interval is too long, a subtherapeutic level will occur.

Loading Dose. In order to minimize the time required to achieve therapeutic levels of selected drugs, particularly those with a half-life of more than 12 hours, one can sometimes use loading doses of the drug. The loading dose required for a drug will be determined by the volume and rate of distribution. Loading doses can be hazardous, particularly with drugs that are distributed slowly into extravascular tissues or that are preferentially absorbed by certain tissues, thereby producing toxic levels. Digoxin is one drug that can cause the latter situation, and it is therefore necessary for one to divide the total loading dose (digitalization) into two or three smaller doses in order to reduce toxicity.

Continuous Infusion of Drugs (First-Order Kinetics). Elimination of the fluctuations in blood levels between doses can be achieved by constant infusion of the drug. Upon infusion, the drug will accumulate (assuming loading doses are not employed) to a plateau level, at which time the rate of elimination will equal the rate of infusion. After the infusion is discontinued, blood level decline will occur according to first-order kinetics.

Clinical Application of Drug Concentration Measurements. The various motivating factors that can be considered as justification for a pharmacokinetic evaluation of a patient's therapeutic program have been reviewed by Aranda and coworkers. Drugs that have a narrow therapeutic window (i.e., toxic levels close to therapeutic levels) such as aminoglycosides, chloramphenicol, digoxin, and theophylline can be more ideally managed with individual blood level monitoring. Clinical evidence of therapeutic failure or toxicity is also strong rationale for blood level monitoring of drugs. Monitoring for better patient motivation or compliance, change of the dosage form or product, and modification of the dosage regimen are additional acceptable criteria. Certain drug/drug interactions may modify the pharmacologic effect of the involved medications that can be associated with alteration of drug concentration. Impaired elimination of drug through hepatic or renal dysfunction frequently results in substantial and/or unpredictable alterations in drug clearance. One can more readily optimize drug dosing under these circumstances with therapeutic monitoring. Unfortunate accidents with overdose can be documented and followed by drug blood level measurements. However, there are drugs whose serum concentration is irrelevant because of the common employment of large doses that are known to be essentially without toxicity (penicillins and cephalosporins) and drugs that can be more easily quantitated by clinical parameters (antihypertensives) than by blood level measurements. The effect of some drugs such as furosemide simply do not correlate with blood levels because the concentration at the locus of effect is not in constant equilibrium with the blood (see discussion of furosemide).

Problems In Clinical Use of Drug Concentration Measurements. Lack of awareness of and/or attention to critical aspects of clinical monitoring of drug concentrations can potentially lead to disasters, even in the face of sophisticated analytical methodology. Kauffman has reviewed in detail the various factors that one must consider in order to ensure appropriate therapeutic drug monitoring technique. To summarize, the physician must recognize that the drug concentrations in the blood are not static (except with constant infusion), as are most endogenous substances such as electrolytes. Therefore, the timing of samples relative to drug administration must be accurate. In this regard, Roberts has reviewed the unique problems of I.V. drug delivery in the neonate that can contribute to the difficulties of accurate timing of blood samples. The most striking observation relates to the delay in administration of the drug to the patient. Failure to appreciate this delay can obviously result in mistiming of peak and/or trough blood level samples obtained for purposes of optimizing drug therapy. Adjustment of drug dosages based on such data could easily place the patient at risk either for toxicity due to overdosage (in response to low drug blood level) or for therapeutic failure due to underdosage (in response to high blood level). Of additional concern is loss of drug dosage as a consequence of routine turnover of intravenous sets as a procedure for minimizing problems of bacterial contamination. It was determined through study of dosing times and intravenous replacement times in the neonatal unit at University of Iowa Hospitals and Clinics that approximately 36 per cent of the total daily dose of various intravenous medications was unknowingly lost in the discarded intravenous sets. Drug delivery systems have been devised to minimize these problems (Leff and Roberts, 1981).

Most importantly, drug plasma concentrations must be interpreted in the context of the complete clinical picture. Drug dosage regimens should be designed to treat the patient, not the drug concentration (Kauffman, 1981). Table 108–3 provides a summary of blood level values for drugs that have been monitored in a meaningful and useful fashion during neonatal therapy.

Selected Drugs

The following discussion of selected drugs represents an effort to summarize the critical pharmacologic and therapeutic aspects of those drugs for which there is reasonable evidence regarding their potential therapeutic efficacy. Other drugs that are effective therapeutic agents have been discussed adequately in other chapters. Obviously, a large number of drugs remain that have had experience in neonates. Their absence from this discussion or other chapters represents the tentative nature of the evidence favoring their use in treatment of neonatal disease.

CARDIOVASCULAR DRUGS

Dopamine is an inotropic agent that has been employed in the treatment of shock in adults and, more recently, for myocardial dysfunction in asphyxiated neonates. Because the experience with dopamine in neonates is limited and largely uncontrolled, its value in the treatment of the wide variety of clinical conditions in which cardiovascular decompensation is pronounced remains unproved (Driscoll et al., 1978; Volkman, 1979).

Dopamine possesses a number of dose-dependent pharmacologic effects, perhaps accounting for some of the divergent clinical experiences. In low doses (less than 2 µg/kg/min) specific dopaminergic effects result in decreased vascular resistance in mesentery, renal, coronary, and cerebral vessels. Infusion of such low doses of dopamine has been associated with an increase in glomerular filtration, renal blood flow, and sodium excretion in adults. Because of these effects, dopamine is especially useful in the management of cardiogenic, traumatic, and hypovolemic shock, in which increases in sympathetic activity may result in compromise of renal function. More moderate doses of dopamine (less than 10 µg/kg/min) result in a positive inotropic effect on the myocardium. This inotropic effect of dopamine is believed to result from a direct effect on B_1 receptors in the myocardium and from the capability of dopamine to cause the release of norepinephrine from nerve terminals located in the myocardium. During the administration of high doses (greater than 10 µg/kg/min), dopamine has a stimulatory effect on alpha-adrenergic receptors (Goldberg et al., 1977). Several different investigators have shown that the alpha-adrenergic receptor agonist activity of dopamine is less than that of epinephrine and norepinephrine. Dopamine has been shown to have less effect on heart rate compared with *isoproterenol* when doses employed of each produce equivalent increases in cardiac output. Also, isoproterenol, although a potent peripheral vasodilator, does not routinely produce an increase in renal blood flow because of redistribution of blood flow to skeletal muscle, especially if there is no change or a decrease in blood pressure. Myocardial efficiency is improved by dopamine as measured by increases in coronary arterial blood flow with relatively less increase in myocardial oxygen consumption. Thus, the pharmacologic property of greatest value with dopamine appears to be selected dilation of renal, mesenteric, cerebral, and coronary vessels (low dose) coupled with an increase in cardiac output (moderate doses).

Dopamine appears to be a safe drug when used in conjunction with meticulous monitoring of the patient and is effective in increasing systemic blood pressure and urine production with minimal adverse effects. The dosage should be a continuous infusion individualized to each patient's needs, starting with low to moderate doses (2 to 5 µg/kg/min). Dopamine should be considered the drug of choice in myocardial dysfunction, particularly if tachycardia is to be avoided. Because isoproterenol produces a stronger inotropic effect than dopamine in the isolated neonatal canine myocardium, it has been proposed as the drug of choice for increasing cardiac output (Driscoll et al., 1978). The fact that isoproterenol can cause a shunting of blood away from critical organs (kidneys, gut, brain, liver) as a consequence of potent vasodilation effects in the skin and skeletal muscle as well as cause myocardial necrosis should limit its use to very select situations requiring an increase in heart rate as a means of improving cardiac output. Adverse effects resulting from the use of dopamine in neonates have been minimal. In one case, an accidental bolus dose of dopamine (675 μg/kg) produced an increase in systemic pressure but little effect on pulmonary pressure (Drummond et al., 1981).

Tolazoline is classified as an alpha-adrenergic blocker that directly affects cardiac and smooth muscle by three mechanisms: (1) sympathomimetic effect, including cardiac stimulation; (2) parasympathomimetic effect, including stimulation of the gastrointestinal tract that can be blocked by atropine; and (3) "histamine-like" effect, including stimulation of gastric secretion and peripheral vasodilation. With usual doses of tolazoline, very little alpha-adrenergic blockade is produced. Direct vasodilation and cardiac stimulation commonly occur with the blood pressure response varying depending on the relative contributions of these two effects.

The major clinical use of tolazoline in neonates has been in the treatment of pulmonary hypertension, or persistent fetal circulation. Considerable clinical experience has accumulated with tolazoline alone or in combination with dopamine (Bloss et al., 1980; Drummond et al., 1981; Sumner and Frank, 1981). The efficacy of tolazoline is difficult to judge because additional interventions have often been involved, including dopamine, neuromuscular paralysis, and/ or volume expansion. In addition, many studies have failed to include a comparable control group. Variation in individual patient response to tolazoline has been characterized as representative of the multiple pharmacologic effects of tolazoline, the variability in endogenous histamine stores present in the lung of the infant (Drummond et al., 1981), and/or the status of pulmonary vascular resistance in the patient at the time tolazoline is administered (Lock et al., 1979). The alpha-adrenergic blocking action of tolazoline probably is not involved in tolazoline's lowering of elevated pulmonary vascular resistance (Goetzman and Milstein, 1979). The patients who appear to respond most ideally to tolazoline administration are those who are maintained in an optimal status of cardiac output and systemic pressure with volume expansion and/or dopamine in conjunction with the specific efforts to decrease pulmonary vascular resistance with tolazoline. The ideal dosing program for tolazoline is 1 to 2 mg/kg I.V. bolus followed by a constant infusion of 1 to 2 mg/kg/hr via a scalp vein.

In contrast to dopamine, tolazoline is associated with a multitude of complications, which are listed in Table 108–5. Stevens and coworkers note that many, if not all, of the reported side effects for tolazoline could be ascribed to the infant's underlying disease state. There are obvious differences among reports of the complications associated with tolazoline, which may again reflect the wide variety of disease pathophysiology involved in these studies. Pharmacologically, it is possible to identify certain of these side effects, such as the gastrointestinal hemorrhage (histamine release) and the hypotension (direct peripheral vascular smooth muscle relaxation), as being specific to tolazoline.

The use of *vasodilators* in the management of infants who have evidence of myocardial dysfunction is the subject of a 1980 commentary by Lees. The basis for vasodilator therapy first proposed for treatment in adults by Sarnoff and Berglund in 1952 is based on the fact that when ventricular filling pressure is adequate, a substantial increase in cardiac output can be achieved with arteriolar vasodilation with a negligible change in arterial blood pressure. A wide variety of pharmacologically active vasodilators are available for such use, a few of which have been evaluated in neonates. The rationale and use of the various vasodilators have been reviewed by Lakier and colleagues. The traditional management for cardiac failure has included digitalis and diuretics and buffer or ventilatory support (Bucciarelli et al., 1977), along with the use of individual inotropic agents such as isoproterenol and dopamine (Cabal et al., 1980). Dillon and coworkers reported in 1980 on the use of nitroprusside in six patients ranging from 6 months to 28 years who had severe congestive heart failure. Four of these six patients showed improvement with vasodilator therapy. Although vasodilator therapy holds great promise for treatment of myocardial dysfunction, these investigators appropriately conclude that these drugs should not be used indiscriminately because of the experimental nature of the approach and the limited experience with their use in neonates and older children.

The major pharmacologic action of the *digitalis glycosides* is an increase in the force of myocardial contraction (inotropic effect). They also appear to affect myocardial conduction, refractory period, excitability, and automaticity, which are represented by electrocardiographic changes including shortening of the Q–T interval, decreased amplitude of T wave, S–T segment changes, prolongation of the P–R interval, and slowing of the heart rate.

Infants who demonstrate signs and symptoms comparable with heart failure remain the primary

Table 108–5. Side Effects of Tolazoline

Side Effects	Estimated Per Cent Occurrence in Various References*
Erythema	60
Oliguria	42, 30, 15, 11
Hypotension	67, 50, 20, 19
Thrombocytopenia	45, 31, 6, 4
Gastric bleeding	55, 33, 12, 8, 4
Increased gastric secretion	100, 36
Pulmonary hemorrhage	12, 2

* Goetzman et al., 1976; Purohit et al., 1978; Stevenson et al., 1979; Bloss et al., 1980; Johnson et al., 1980; Stevens et al., 1980.

benefactors of the pharmacologic actions of the digitalis glycosides. Although digoxin remains the mainstay with or without concomitant diuretic therapy, major conceptual advances such as the use of vasodilators and selected inotropic agents have challenged digoxin's role as the leading therapeutic agent. The use of digoxin in infants with left-to-right shunts as the sole means of therapy has also been seriously challenged in several reports (White and Lietman, 1978; Warburton et al., 1980). Extracardiac effects of digoxin may be important in this regard, as Milstein and coworkers demonstrated in newborn lambs that digoxin increased pulmonary vascular resistance, a beneficial feature with left-to-right ductal shunts but a detrimental effect in cases of pulmonary hypertension.

An excellent review on the clinical pharmacokinetics of digoxin in infants was published by Wettrell and Andersson in 1977. Although the variation in overall absorption of oral dosage forms of digoxin appears to be of minor importance, there are important differences in rates of absorption from patient to patient. Digoxin appears in the blood within 5 minutes of oral intake and reaches peak concentrations between 30 minutes and 3 hours. In pediatric patients with severe congestive heart failure, the amount of digoxin absorbed after oral administration may be reduced. Both pain and incomplete and erratic absorption of digoxin after muscular injection have been repeatedly demonstrated, and, therefore, the agent should not be administered in this manner. The plasma protein binding of digoxin is low and in the same range as that found in adults (20 to 30 per cent). No significant interaction between digoxin and other protein-bound endogenous compounds such as bilirubin and other drugs occurs. The predominant mechanisms of digoxin elimination are metabolism and renal and biliary excretion. The major mechanism is renal excretion of unchanged digoxin by glomerular filtration and tubular secretion. In patients with diminished renal function, care must be taken to avoid toxic accumulation of digoxin. The body clearance of digoxin, which takes into account all drug elimination processes, appears to be lower during the first week of life than during the following month. Only small amounts of digoxin can be anticipated to be removed by exchange transfusion (less than 6 per cent of the previously administered dose), even if the exchange transfusion is performed shortly after drug administration because of the two-compartment distribution (Wettrell and Andersson, 1977).

Although there has traditionally been an understanding that infants are more tolerant to digoxin toxicity than older patients, there can be no question that infants of any age or size can respond to digoxin therapy with toxic reactions (Halkin et al., 1978). In full-term neonates and infants, serum concentrations exceeding 3.5 ng/ml during maintenance therapy are in most cases associated with some evidence of toxicity. Serum concentrations exceeding 3.5 ng/ml should be considered extremely hazardous, and infants should be vigorously monitored and steps to reduce the dose of digoxin should be taken unless very critical clinical states dictate a continuation of the regimen. In this regard, it should be recognized that the inotropic effect of digoxin in infants has been shown to occur at lower doses of digoxin than previously recommended (Pinsky et al., 1979). In addition, a greater number of electrocardiographic abnormalities were found in premature infants than in term neonates and infants receiving similar doses of digoxin.

Dose recommendations. A variety of doses of digoxin have been recommended over the years. Whether there is truly any efficacy associated with digitalization as opposed to initiation of a maintenance dose of digoxin remains to be established in preterm and full-term neonates. There is evidence that the amount of digoxin given to pediatric patients during acute digitalization based on most of the older prevailing dosage schedules loads the body with a potentially toxic dose of digoxin. It would seem most valid to utilize the data generated from serum concentrations obtained during the maintenance therapy in infants to arrive at optimal inotropic digoxin dosage recommendations. Using such criteria, Nyberg and

Table 108–6. Recommended Oral Digoxin Doses in Premature and Full-Term Neonates and Infants

Dose*	Prematures (μg/kg)	Full-Term (μg/kg)	Infants (1–12 mo.) (μg/kg)
Digitalization	10–30	30	35
Maintenance:			
given every 12 hours	2.5–5	5	7–12

* Digitalization dose is administered in three equally divided doses or in three unequally divided doses (one half, one fourth, one fourth) every 8 hours. The first maintenance dose should not be given before 12 hours after the last of the digitalizing doses. Intravenous doses are generally 70 to 80 per cent of the oral dose because of the assumed bioavailability differences.

References: Prematures—Berman et al.; Pinsky et al., 1979; Warburton et al., 1980; Nyberg and Wettrell, 1980. Full-Term—Wettrell and Andersson, 1977; Nyberg and Wettrell, 1980. Infants (1 to 12 mo.)—Nyberg and Wettrell, 1980.

Wettrell arrived at dosage recommendations that are supported by the studies published by Berman and coworkers, Pinsky and colleagues, Halkin and associates, and Warburton and coauthors. These dosage recommendations are shown in Table 108–6.

It must be remembered that these are computed dosage schedules based on pharmacokinetic parameters for the *average* patient in each age group. Differences in distribution or receptor sensitivity or both among individuals can alter the relationship between serum concentration and effect. One must therefore consider individual variability along with the digoxin serum concentration measurements and the clinical observations to arrive at the optimal maintenance dose for each patient. Close scrutiny of renal function is also imperative because of its importance in digoxin elimination. A simple but general rule is that patients with one half the normal renal clearance should receive one half the maintenance dose of digoxin.

Digitalization. It would appear upon review of the literature that many cases of digoxin intoxication occur in infants who are being digitalized or who were recently digitalized. Such experience has lead to the recommendation that loading (digitalization) be eliminated except in those rare cases in which conditions demand immediate full therapy.

Digoxin toxicity. The development of toxicity represents the most serious limitation to the clinical use of digoxin. Reported rates of cardiac toxicity vary from 8 to 35 per cent. Although the basis for the cardiotoxicity remains in doubt, three main components are believed to be involved: (1) an action of the adrenergic nervous system producing nonuniform neural activity, (2) an action on the adrenal medulla, and (3) a direct action on the cardiac tissue. These mechanisms have been reviewed in detail by Lathers and Roberts. At least three studies fail to support the postulate of an increased tolerance to high digoxin doses and to high serum concentrations of digoxin in infants. Serum digoxin concentrations obviously neither determine the diagnosis of digoxin toxicity nor negate it. The elements of individual sensitivity to the drug, the pharmacokinetic variability between individual patients, and the overlap between the nontoxic and toxic range of digoxin discouraged the selection of a maximal threshold serum digoxin concentration for toxicity.

It is generally agreed, however, that if therapeutic effect (assuming digoxin is unquestionably the drug of choice) is not satisfactory, even if serum concentrations of digoxin are optimal (less than 2 ng/ml), the dose can be increased with careful monitoring for evidence of digoxin toxicity. Careful monitoring of serum potassium and calcium should be accomplished as well because of the known aggravation of digoxin toxicity. Serum digoxin levels in excess of 3.5 ng/ml have been frequently associated with toxicity and, therefore, should generally be avoided.

The arrhythmias associated with digoxin are similar to those reported for older infants and children, consisting chiefly of sinoatrial node depression with associated ectopic supraventricular beats and rhythms and atrioventricular conduction disturbances. The electrocardiogram has been found by most investigators to be the most reliable guide in determining digitalis intoxication in young infants.

Appropriate treatment of hypertension in the neonate is best managed by determination of the mechanism of the hypertension coupled with selection of the appropriate pharmacologic agent. Although many drugs possess the capability of lowering blood pressure, the mechanism for this effect varies considerably. Pruitt in 1981 and Bailie and Mattioli in 1980 published excellent reviews of the pharmacology of *antihypertensives.* Unfortunately, very little literature exists regarding the use of antihypertensives in neonates despite the fact that they are a very important part of therapeutic management of neonatal disease. In a 1978 review, Adelman reported experience with various antihypertensives in neonates with hypertension. The drugs are listed in Table 108–7 with published dosage recommendations.

Table 108–7. Antihypertensive Agents Used in the Management of Neonates with Hypertension ¯

| Drug* | Recommended Dosage† | | |
	Dose	Frequency of Administration	Route
Chlorothiazide	10–25 mg/kg/dose*	q 12 hr	P.O.
Furosemide	1–2 mg/kg/dose‡	6–24 hr	I.V.
Hydralazine	0.4–0.8 mg/kg/dose	4–12 hr	I.M., I.V.
Diazoxide	2 mg/kg/dose§	q 10–15 min to effect	I.V.
Propranolol	0.025 mg/kg/dose	q 6 hr	I.V.
	0.25 mg/kg/dose	q 6 hr	P.O.
Nitroprusside	0.5–8.0 µg/kg/min.		I.V.

* Drugs listed are from Adelman, 1978.
† Recommended doses for neonates are from Pruitt, 1981, except as noted.
‡ From Peterson, 1980.
§ From Boerth and Long, 1977.

Nitroprusside, which is a direct-acting vasodilator, has been used in children (Gordillo-Paniagua et al., 1975). *Diazoxide,* a nondiuretic benzothiadiazine derivative, has been used as an effective antihypertensive in infants and children. There has been a controversy in the literature regarding the influence of rate of administration of diazoxide on the magnitude of antihypertensive response. Boerth and Long concluded from their work in children with secondary hypertension that acute therapeutic reduction of diastolic blood pressure can be obtained more safely and effectively by titration with 2 mg/kg intravenous injections of diazoxide repeated at 10- to 15-minute intervals.

Oberfield and coworkers and Friedman and colleagues reported the use of *captopril,* an orally effective inhibitor of angiotensin I–converting enzyme in severe childhood hypertension. This agent is effective in lowering blood pressure in essential and renovascular hypertension as well as in the hypertension associated with advanced renal disease (Gavras et al., 1978). Hypertensive conditions associated with excessive renin levels in neonates (renovascular disease accounts for 93 per cent of reported cases of hypertension in neonates, according to Adelman) may be particularly suitable to treatment with angiotensin I–converting enzyme inhibition if refractory to more standard modes of antihypertensive therapy. Reported side effects in adults include hypotension, fever, and rash. The possible pathophysiologic consequences of hyperreninemia and elevation of angiotensin I as well as suppression of aldosterone have not been addressed (Friedman et al., 1980).

PHARMACOLOGIC MANAGEMENT OF THE DUCTUS ARTERIOSUS

The identification of factors responsible for control and regulation of the state of constriction or relaxation of the ductus arteriosus has been largely responsible for the evolution of pharmacologic manipulation of the ductus arteriosus. The use of *indomethacin,* a prostaglandin synthetase inhibitor, as a means of pharmacologically closing the ductus arteriosus has increased, particularly since less toxic but effective doses have been established and also because it has been recognized that digitalis and diuretics in the very small premature infant have little or no beneficial effect on the hemodynamic deterioration (Clyman and Heymann, 1981).

A substantial number of clinical studies employing indomethacin for purposes of closing patent ductus arteriosus have shown it to be effective, but with varying degrees of success. Success rates vary from 18 to 89 per cent. Three double-blind controlled trials of indomethacin and ductal closure have been reported (Yeh et al., 1981; Yanagi et al., 1981; Nestrud et al., 1980). These controlled studies allow comparison of indomethacin effect with the natural course of ductal patency. In these studies, a significant effect of indomethacin was observed compared

with that in control subjects in all three studies (58 per cent vs. 18 per cent, 89 per cent vs. 22 per cent, and 85 per cent vs. 11 per cent, respectively). The reasons for lack of indomethacin responsiveness of ductus include (1) lack of sufficient sensitivity of the ductus to indomethacin, (2) independent factors that influence the ductus or drug activity, and (3) failure to reach adequate levels of indomethacin for inhibition of the critical prostaglandin synthesis.

The oral absorption of indomethacin is believed to be quite variable. Once absorbed, indomethacin is highly protein bound (95 per cent), but in normal therapeutic levels, it does not displace bilirubin from albumin-binding sites. Indomethacin is metabolized but is also excreted in the urine unchanged (Morselli et al., 1980). Although variations in hepatic drug metabolism or in renal excretion or in both could be major contributing factors to the observed pharmacokinetic differences among neonates, it is worth noting that enterohepatic recirculation of indomethacin can be substantial, as Kwan and coworkers found in their study that an average of 50 per cent of an intravenous, oral, or rectal dose of indomethacin underwent biliary recirculation. Recirculation to the biliary system could result in an "apparent" prolonged plasma disappearance of the drug.

Because of the variable pharmacokinetics of indomethacin in neonates and the dose-related renal dysfunction experienced particularly in the early studies, it is important to examine carefully the existing experience with dosage regimens. The most frequently employed dose is 0.2 to 0.3 mg/kg given orally or intravenously (no commercial I.V. product available). Subsequent doses are generally given at 8- to 24-hour intervals if evidence of ductal patency persists to provide a maximum dosage of 0.6 mg/kg. Authors employing these dosages have reported only transient and reversible decrease in renal function and gastrointestinal disturbance (Yeh et al., 1981; Yanagi et al., 1981); or no toxicity (Yaffe et al., 1980). Recurrence of the hemodynamically significant ductal murmur within 1 or 2 weeks after initial dosing has been reported to be responsive to additional doses of indomethacin. An intravenous preparation of indomethacin is currently under development that will, it is hoped, reduce the difficulties with drug stability and unpredictability of oral absorption. Continued investigations will be necessary to determine whether a true reduction in overall morbidity and mortality can be accomplished with early indomethacin intervention for patent ductus arteriosus.

A number of clinical studies have reported successful employment of E-type prostaglandins in neonates for maintenance of the patency of the ductus arteriosus. PGE_1 has become one of the most valuable pharmacologic tools in the acute management of a variety of cyanotic congenital cardiac malformations in which patency of the ductus arteriosus is mandatory for life-sustaining pulmonary or systemic blood flow (Heymann, 1981). Although surgical procedures exist for successful palliation of many of these cardiac malformations, mortality risks are great because of the unpredictable development of acute deterioration in oxygenation as a result of spontaneous reduction in ductal-dependent pulmonary or aortic blood flow. PGE_1 infusion can result in significant improvement in systemic oxygenation, perfusion, and acidemia resulting from such cyanotic congenital heart abnormalities and thereby potentially influence any morbidity or mortality that might otherwise develop during diagnostic and/or surgical procedures. Elliot and coworkers first reported the successful employment of PGE_1 for maintenance of ductal patency in babies with severe congenital heart disease. Numerous reports on the successful use of PGE_1 therapy in a wide variety of congenital heart disease have subsequently appeared in the literature (Heymann, 1981; Olley and Coceani, 1980). The clinical improvement in these infants has been attributed both to an increase in blood flow through the ductus secondary to the PGE_1-induced dilation and to a decrease in peripheral vascular resistance (systemic or pulmonary or both).

PGE_1 has been used in the treatment of the following cyanotic congenital heart malformations: aortic arch interruption and coarctation, pulmonary artery atresia or stenosis (with or without ventricular septal defect), severe tetralogy of Fallot, transposition of the great arteries, and tricuspid valve anomalies (atresia or insufficiency). Although PGE_1 can be effective in neonates with hypoplastic left heart syndrome, inoperable features of this anomaly preclude the continued infusion once diagnosis and inoperable circumstances are confirmed. In most infants, any beneficial effects of PGE_1 are obvious clinically and biochemically (Pa_{O_2}) within minutes of the start of infusion. Failure to respond may be due to unresponsive ductus arteriosus, hypoplastic pulmonary arteries, inappropriate positioning of the infusion catheter (which results in lack of delivery of PGE_1 to the ductus arteriosus), or erroneous diagnosis.

The recommended initial dose of PGE_1 is 0.05 μg/kg/min, given as a continuous infusion (diluted in saline or dextrose solution). By monitoring Pa_{O_2}, preferably with a transcutaneous oxygen electrode, one can determine the ideal infusion dose. Once the maximum Pa_{O_2} has been reached, the rate of PGE_1 infusion can often be reduced without a subsequent deterioration in Pa_{O_2}.

The side effects associated with PGE_1 infusion in neonates were reviewed by Lewis and coworkers in 1981. In this study, approximately 20 per cent of infants receiving PGE_1 encountered reactions that were felt to be either definitely or probably related

to the drug. The PGE_1-induced side effects included cutaneous vasodilation (flushing), hypotension, respiratory depression (apnea), fever, jitteriness, and seizures. Individual dosing adjustments along with appropriate supportive care (respiratory ventilation for apnea, volume expansion for hypotension) help minimize the impact of these side effects on the patient's wellbeing.

NEUROMUSCULAR BLOCKERS

Despite the frequent use of neuromuscular blockers in the respirator care of neonates, few systemic studies have explored their consequence on the clinical status of this patient population. Stark and coworkers studied 35 infants who were mechanically ventilated and who received *pancuronium* for control of respiration. In about half the patient population, arterial oxygenation improved 6 hours following paralysis. The authors were unable to define a specific group of patients in whom paralysis would be beneficial. Henry and coworkers and Crone and Favorito reported a more uniform improvement in their respective patient populations of neonates with respiratory disease. Finer and Tomney also reported dramatic reduction in periods of hypoxia and hyperoxia in 10 low birth weight neonates. In all the aforementioned studies, pancuronium appeared to be well tolerated, with no serious untoward effects attributable to its administration. Nugent and coworkers, in an eloquent review of the pharmacology of muscle relaxants in infants and children, point out that there are significant clinical differences in the neuromuscular blockers. *D-Tubocurarine* has an association with hypotension that is probably due to a combination of factors including histamine release, sympathetic blockade with peripheral dilation, and direct myocardial depression reducing cardiac output. Pancuronium does not result in significant histamine release and can cause an increase in cardiac output and blood pressure. These later results have been attributed to either a vagolytic or a sympathomimetic effect (Roizen and Feeley, 1978). Since histamine has been proposed to play a role in attempts to dilate the pulmonary vascular bed pharmacologically in neonates with pulmonary hypertension or vasospasm, it would seem important for one to evaluate critically pancuronium versus d-tubocurarine in neonates with pulmonary hypertension. These two neuromuscular blocking agents have been variably employed in conjunction with the use of tolazoline. Bennett and coworkers have shown age-dependent dosage requirements for pancuronium and d-tubocurarine in neonates. The potency ratio of pancuronium is approximately nine times that of d-tubocurarine at 1 day of age, and this ratio decreases progressively to a ratio of 8:1 at 1 week, 7:1 at 2 weeks, and 6:1 at 4 weeks. Prematurity, acidosis, and hypoxemia all tend to decrease dosing requirements. Whether or not there are clinically significant differences in efficacy among these neuromuscular blockers or other agents with less neonatal experience such as metocurine (Henry et al., 1979) remains to be determined.

THEOPHYLLINE AND CAFFEINE THERAPY OF NEONATAL APNEA

One of the more frustrating clinical problems in the neonatal intensive care unit is apnea in the premature infant. Its role in morbidity and mortality in the low birth weight infant has been a factor in the development of aggressive preventive and therapeutic approaches. In 1973, Kuzemko and Paala found a decrease in the frequency of apneic attacks in neonates treated with *theophylline*. Since publication of that report, many investigators have confirmed the effect of theophylline in decreasing the frequency or abolishing the occurrence of apneic spells. More recently, *caffeine* has been shown to have similar efficacy and has become the drug of choice in the treatment of apnea, despite the lack of control trials in support of this position. The potential advantages of employing caffeine in the treatment of apnea are substantial. Caffeine appears to have a much wider therapeutic index than theophylline, and there is no metabolic conversion of caffeine to theophylline to confuse the interpretation of the pharmacologic effect (and also less need for therapeutic drug monitoring), less fluctuation in plasma concentrations, and fewer peripheral (non-CNS) effects.

An excellent review by Aranda and colleagues presents the pharmacologic data on the methylxanthines. Both theophylline and caffeine can increase cardiac contractility, although their effect on heart rate is unpredictable because they are able to increase heart rate as the result of direct effects on the myocardium as well as decrease heart rate as a result of direct stimulation of medullary vagal nuclei. With large doses, however, myocardial stimulation usually predominates, and tachycardia is manifest. Although the methylxanthines have been shown to dilate the pulmonary, coronary, and systemic blood vessels, cerebral blood vessels have been shown to constrict in response to theophylline. Since these findings have been largely from adult studies, it would be important to establish whether similar effects occur in premature infants who are undergoing therapy with methylxanthines for apnea. Hyperglycemia, glycosuria, and ketonuria have been reported in caffeine- and theophylline-intoxicated infants. Significant increases in serum glucose and insulin have been reported with therapeutic doses of theophylline and caffeine (Srinivasan et al., 1981). Whether these effects relate to the ability of the methylxanthines to affect catecholamines, metabolism, or the endocrine system is unclear. Some changes in renal function associated with minor fluid and electrolyte disturbances have been reported to occur with theophylline, but similar studies of caffeine have not been conducted.

Among the most fascinating methods of drug metabolism in neonates is that of theophylline. Several investigators have demonstrated that theophylline undergoes methylation to produce caffeine. The mean ratio of caffeine to theophylline in plasma in neonates treated with theophylline is about 0.3, although caffeine plasma levels may reach up to 50 per cent of the theophylline plasma level. The obvious implication is that the pharmacologic data on theophylline in the neonate must take into account the possible contribution of caffeine, which in some neonates is present in significant quantities. In infants, caffeine is largely excreted unchanged (80 to 90 per cent). Since caffeine remains the major molecular constituent in urine for at least 3 months postnatally, neonatal capacity to metabolize caffeine appears to be markedly deficient.

Numerous pharmacokinetic studies in neonates have been accomplished with both theophylline and caffeine. A summary of these pharmacokinetic studies is shown in Table 108–8. The relatively shorter plasma half-life for theophylline in older premature infants compared with that in neonates has been interpreted to represent maturational changes in theophylline elimination. Attainment of adult rates of theophylline elimination has been observed by 6 months of age. Caffeine plasma half-life in premature and full-term newborn infants is approximately 16 times longer than that in adults (100 hours versus 6 hours). The changes in caffeine elimination with postnatal age have not been systematically studied, al-

Table 108–8. Pharmacokinetic Profile and Dosage Recommendations for Theophylline and Caffeine in Neonates

Drug	Half-Life Hr* (range)	Clearance* ml/kg/hr	Recommended Dose†	
			Loading	*Maintenance*
Theophylline	30 (12–64)	23.4 (4–68)	5 mg/kg	1 mg/kg/8 hr to 3.6 mg/kg/12 hr
Caffeine	100 (37–231)	8.8 (2.5–16.8)	10 mg/kg	2.5 mg/kg/24 hr

* Values represent mean of reported literature values, with the range of reported values shown in parentheses (Aranda et al., 1981).
† Dosage recommendations are for the free base administered P.O. or I.V.

though it has been estimated that adult rates of elimination are attained at about 3 to 5 months.

Based on these pharmacokinetic and metabolic findings, rational dose guidelines for theophylline and caffeine have been proposed (Table 108–8). Although there is no definitive study showing ideal plasma concentration of theophylline and caffeine for the treatment of apnea, the data available suggest that apnea control without toxicity can be obtained at theophylline levels between 5 and 15 μg/ml. For caffeine, Aranda recommends plasma concentrations between 5 and 20 μg/ml. Doses required to attain these levels are also shown in Table 108–8. A loading dose of theophylline of 5.5 to 6.2 mg/kg (active free base) could be expected to produce a plasma concentration of about 10 μg/ml. Maintenance doses of theophylline should range between 1 mg/kg every 8 hours and 3.6 mg/kg every 12 hours. Care must be taken in assessing the actual percentage of theophylline (free base) in various theophylline-containing preparations. The dosing recommendations for caffeine as proposed by Aranda include a loading dose of 10 mg/kg of active caffeine base with a maintenance dose of 2.5 mg/kg every 24 hours.

ANTICONVULSANTS

The importance of early recognition and definitive treatment of neonatal seizures has been emphasized in Chapter 79 as well as in other reports (Volpe, 1977). The drug employed for treatment of neonatal seizures has generally been *phenobarbital,* especially because of the frequent occurrence of hypoxic-ischemic encephalopathy and the proposed role of barbiturates in decreasing cerebral metabolic rate. A loading dose of 10 mg/kg is given intravenously over several minutes followed by a second loading dose (5 to 10 mg/kg) if seizure activity persists. Pharmacokinetic studies by Painter and coworkers and by Lockman and colleagues have demonstrated that a loading dose of phenobarbital of at least 15 to 20 mg/kg must be given to achieve blood levels in the therapeutic range (20 μg/ml). For maintenance therapy, phenobarbital is administered in a dose of approximately 2.5 mg/kg/dose every 12 hours. No significant differences in absorption have been reported for oral versus intramuscular administration (Boreus et al., 1975). Studies by Painter and colleagues suggest that the plasma half-life of phenobarbital becomes progressively shorter with age, which, for the individual neonate, may necessitate appropriate increases in dose to maintain seizure control. They observed mean T½ values ranging between 50 and 100 hours, with plasma levels between 15 and 40 μg/ml. In general, plasma disappearance rate is faster in infants than in newborns and adults (Morselli, 1976).

Phenytoin has been recommended as an additional drug for those patients who continue to exhibit seizure activity despite appropriate treatment with phenobarbital. As with phenobarbital, loading doses are recommended (10 mg/kg I.V., which can be repeated if necessary) followed by a maintenance dose of 2.5 mg/kg given every 12 hours. Oral administration of phenytoin has been shown by Painter and coworkers to be ineffective in establishing adequate blood levels, and intramuscular phenytoin is known to be poorly absorbed. In a study of neonates, Loughnan and colleagues observed a rapidly changing and variable elimination of phenytoin after birth. Combining their data with existing literature, they determined the mean phenytoin plasma half-lives to be 80, 15, and 6 hours for the age groups 0 to 2, 3 to 14, and 15 to 150 days, respectively. One can, therefore, anticipate changing maintenance dosage requirements for neonates according to age. Only 30 to 50 per cent of phenobarbital is protein-bound, so interactions based on displacement of other drugs or bilirubin from proteins is uncommon. In contrast, phenytoin is highly protein-bound (70 to 90 per cent in the neonate versus approximately 90 per cent in adults, according to Rane and coworkers). The decreased protein binding of phenytoin in neonates is extremely important, since the result is a higher concentration of unbound (active) fraction. Thus, a therapeutic concentration in a neonate (extrapolating from children and adult experience) would be approximately 6 to 14 μg/ml rather than 10 to 20 μg/ml. Definitive studies relating anticonvulsant effect and serum concentration in neonates have not been accomplished for either phenobarbital or phenytoin.

Metabolism of phenobarbital and phenytoin is an extremely important factor, accounting for a significant portion of the aforementioned variable pharmacokinetics. Boreus and coworkers reported 70 per cent of the urinary output of phenobarbital in neonates to be unchanged drug in the first 48 hours of life, decreasing to 35 to 40 per cent by the fifth to sixth day of life. Only a very small percentage (<5 per cent) of phenytoin is excreted unchanged in the urine in adults, the remainder being metabolized by the liver prior to excretion. The metabolism of phenytoin is generally saturated at therapeutic blood levels, although very little work regarding this has been done with neonates.

Phenobarbital is a relatively nontoxic drug, with minimal side effects reported with its use in neonates. The effects of prolonged administration on the developing nervous system remain unclear. In contrast to phenobarbital, phenytoin has an extensive history of drug interactions, many of which result in altered phenytoin pharmacokinetics. A dementing encephalopathy with few other signs has been observed in chronically intoxicated children (Logan and Freeman, 1969). High levels of phenytoin (>20 μg/ml) have also been associated with increased seizure frequency, cerebellar damage, and peripheral neuropathy (Johnson and Freeman). Allergic and hematologic reactions unrelated to dose have also been reported.

Diuretics are extremely useful and effective drugs that are capable of removing excess extracellular fluid in a wide variety of pathophysiologic states. Rational use of this class of drugs in neonates requires a basic understanding of developmental renal function and physiology as well as the mechanism of action of the various diuretics and their clinical pharmacology. Renal physiology and its developmental aspects have been reviewed by Hook and Bailie.

The effectiveness of *furosemide* in neonates with cardiac and renal disease has been well documented. In general, doses of 1 mg/kg given intravenously have produced a significant increase in renal excretion of sodium, chloride, potassium, calcium, aldosterone, and PGE and PGF 2α. The onset of diuretic activity occurs within 1 hour of parenteral administration but is delayed with oral administration. Peterson and co-workers found that the bioavailability of oral furosemide may be less than 20 per cent, mandating that larger doses be employed when administered orally. The plasma clearance of furosemide in the neonate is remarkably slow, correlating with the delay to peak effect (1 to 3 hours) and the longer duration of action (approximately 6 hours) compared with that in the adult. This delayed effect of furosemide in the neonate is consistent with the slow elimination of furosemide into the tubule lumen, where it exerts its pharmacologic effect. Plasma furosemide concentrations do not correlate with the diuretic or saluretic effect. The reported half-life of furosemide ranges from between 1.0 and 7.1 hours (Aranda et al., 1978) to 19.9 ± 3 hours (Peterson et al., 1980). There does appear to be a good correlation between furosemide plasma clearance and postnatal age (Peterson et al., 1980). This variable but prolonged clearance of furosemide suggests that the appropriate interval for administration be established for each neonate based on clinical need and the temporal characteristics of the diuretic response. Considering the prolonged plasma elimination of furosemide, Peterson and co-workers have expressed concern regarding drug accumulation with too frequent dosing intervals and the occurrence of ototoxicity (plasma levels associated with ototoxicity in adults equal 25 μg/ml).

Furosemide is highly bound to plasma protein (> 90 per cent), which largely explains the small volume of distribution (0.24 ± 0.3 l/kg, Peterson et al., 1980). Despite being highly protein bound, furosemide does not alter the reserve albumin binding capacity at plasma levels observed with a single therapeutic dose (approximately 2 μg/ml). Levels of 6.2 to 25.6 μg/ml have been reported to displace bilirubin in vitro (Aranda et al., 1978; Wennberg et al., 1977).

Considerable controversy exists regarding the use of furosemide in neonates with hyaline membrane disease and/or patent ductus arteriosus. Unlike Moylan and coworkers, who administered furosemide to patients between 2 and 14 days of age, Marks and colleagues could not demonstrate an improvement in the clinical status of their patients, who were given furosemide within 36 hours of age. Furosemide has generally been useful in treatment of interstitial pulmonary edema in more chronic lung states such as bronchopulmonary dysplasia and certainly should be considered as a valuable adjunct in the treatment of acute pulmonary edema associated with fluid overload.

The *thiazide* diuretics have also been used extensively in neonates. Although a variety of claims have been made regarding the efficacy and sodium-to-potassium excretion ratios of the various thiazide derivatives, there are no practical differences. The thiazides are more useful as antihypertensives than furosemide is. Furosemide should be considered a potentially more effective diuretic than any of the thiazides, but the actual extent of diuresis with any diuretic depends primarily on the dose administered and the extent of excess body fluid. The displacement of bilirubin from albumin is similar for furosemide and chlorothiazide, but the larger doses required for chlorothiazide place this drug at a greater theoretical risk for elevating the extent of body burden of free bilirubin. The recommended dosage for chlorothiazide is 5 to 10 mg/kg/dose P.O. or I.V. every 12 hours or as required.

The toxicities associated with furosemide and the other diuretic agents primarily reflect their major influences on fluid and electrolyte balance. Influences on calcium do differ, however: Furosemide proportionally increases the excretion of sodium and calcium; the thiazides decrease the renal excretion of calcium relative to sodium. Both increase the excretion of magnesium. Chronic administration of furosemide in neonates with chronic lung disease can result in hypochloremic alkalosis (secondary bicarbonate retention with serum CO_2 elevation), which can confuse the clinical interpretation of patient lung status.

OPIOID AND OPIOID ANTAGONISTS

The experience with opioids in neonates is primarily limited to those situations in which morphine-like drugs are inadvertently administered to the fetus when they are given to the mother during pregnancy or labor or both. Opioids have been useful in managing "narcotic withdrawal" in the neonate as well as for control of pain. The use of opioids such as *morphine* as a means of sedating infants mandates appreciation of the wide range of other pharmacologic effects that simultaneously occur, especially if chronic administration is a possibility. Therapeutic doses in humans depress all aspects of respiratory activity, including rate, minute, and tidal volume. Way and coworkers have reported that infants are more sensitive to the respiratory depressant effects of morphine than are adults. However, in studies in which equianalgesic doses are used, the same degree of respiratory depression occurs with morphine as with other opioids, including *meperidine*. Gastric emptying and propulsive contractions in the small and large intestine are diminished or abolished after administration of morphine and meperidine. Except for peripheral arteriolar and venous dilation, little effect is exerted on the cardiovascular system. Less obvious effects on the CNS include diminished stress-induced release of ACTH, suppression of the secretion of LH and thyrotropin, and enhanced release of prolactin and ADH. The use of opioids for sedation in pain-free patients should be strongly discouraged.

Because of significant metabolism of opioids by the gastrointestinal tract and liver, oral administration of morphine and other opioids, including meperidine, results in a lower response than that associated with parenteral administration. Morphine is metabolized primarily by conjugation with glucuronic acid, with very little unmetabolized drug being excreted in urine. Less than 10 per cent of administered morphine is excreted via the bile. Meperidine undergoes hydrolysis or *N*-demethylation and hydrolysis followed by conjugation. Very little meperidine is excreted unchanged. The respective ranges for plasma half-life and duration of action for morphine and meperidine are approximately 2 to 4 hours and 2 to 6 hours. The dose for morphine in infants is 0.1 to 0.2 mg/kg/dose (S.C., I.M., or I.V.), with the dose repeated as required. The dose for meperidine is 1 to 1.5 mg/kg/dose (S.C., I.M., or I.V.).

Naloxone is useful for reversal of narcotic-induced depression in the newborn infant. In contrast to nalorphine and levallorphan, naloxone appears to have almost no agonistic effects and produces no discernible subjective effects with recommended doses. Naloxone acts as a specific antagonist against morphine-like opioids and also against some nonopioid drugs. Care must be exercised in neonates of narcotic-dependent mothers, since a moderate-to-severe withdrawal syndrome can be induced. Indiscriminate use in all depressed newborns must also be discouraged. With intravenous administration, the antagonistic effects of naloxone should be immediate. The duration of action of naloxone may be variable (minutes to hours), depending on the quantity of drug present (agonist and antagonist) and the rate of metabolism and elimination. The usual duration of action for naloxone is 1 to 4 hours, with a plasma half-life of 1 hour. The recommended dose for naloxone is 0.01 mg/kg I.M. (I.V. if vascular perfusion is poor), which is repeated in 3 to 5 minutes if there is no response. Moore and coworkers realistically point out that since naloxone is comparatively safe and since it acts by competing for receptor sites occupied by the opioid, doses of 0.1 mg/kg of naloxone can be considered appropriate in known or probable cases of serious narcotic intoxication.

Conclusion

Because the field of neonatal pharmacology is wide and complex, a full discussion of this subject is beyond the scope of this text. For some topics, the reader can refer to other chapters in this book or to reports on subjects such as the use of vitamin E in the premature infant (Roberts, 1980) and drugs in breast milk (Wilson et al., 1980). There are some topics that are considered experimental or investigational and, therefore, not suitable for a practical neonatology text. A review of the available relevant literature supports the conclusion that considerable voids exist in our understanding and application of neonatal pharmacology and therapeutics. Progress in filling these voids will undoubtedly be a part of future research, but one must not overlook the fact that this progress will be greatly aided by ongoing conscientious re-examination of existing rational and effective therapy.

REFERENCES

General Pharmacology and Pharmacokinetics

Aranda, J. V., Turmen, T., and Cote-Boilean, T: Drug monitoring in the perinatal patient: uses and abuses. Ther. Drug Monitoring 2:39, 1980.

Bell, E. F., Brown, E. J., Milner, R., Sinclair, J. C., and Zipursky, A.: Vitamin E absorption in small premature infants. Pediatrics 63:830, 1979.

Brown, W. I., Buist, N. R. M., Gipson, H. T. et al.: Fatal benzyl alcohol poisoning in a neonatal intensive care unit. Lancet 1:1250, 1982.

Kauffman, R. E.: The clinical interpretation and application of drug concentration data. Pediatr. Clin. North Am. 28:35, 1981.

Leff, R. D., and Roberts, R. J.: Methods for intravenous drug administration in the pediatric patient. J. Pediatr. 98:631, 1981.

Lovejoy, F. H.: Fatal benzyl alcohol poisoning in neonatal intensive care units. Am. J. Dis. Child. 136:974, 1982.

Miller, R. P., and Roberts, R. J.: Acetaminophen elimination kinetics in neonates, children, and adults. Clin. Pharmacol. Ther. 19:284, 1976.

Morselli, P. L.: Clinical pharmacokinetics in neonates. Clin. Pharmacokinet. 1:81, 1976.

Morselli, P. L., Franco-Morselli, R., and Bossi, L.: Clinical pharmacokinetics in newborns and infants. Clin. Pharmacokinet. 5:485, 1980.

Rane, A.: Basic Principles of Drug Disposition and Action in Infants and Children. *In* Yaffe, S. J. (Ed.): Pediatric Pharmacology. New York, Grune & Stratton, 1980, p. 7.

Roberts, R. J.: Intravenous administration of medication in pediatric patients: problems and solutions. Pediatr. Clin. North Am. 28:23, 1981.

Dopamine

Driscoll, D. J., Gillette, P. C., Ezrailson, E. G., and Schwartz, A.: Inotropic response of the neonatal canine myocardium to dopamine. Pediatr. Res. 12:42, 1978.

Driscoll, D. J., Gillette, P. C., and McNamara, D. G.: The use of dopamine in children. J. Pediatr. 92:309, 1978.

Drummond, W. H., Gregory, G. A., Heymann, M. A., and Phibbs,

R. A.: The independent effects of hyperventilation, tolazoline, and dopamine on infants with persistent pulmonary hypertension. J. Pediatr. *98*:603, 1981.

Goldberg, L. I., Hsieh, Y., and Resnekov, L.: Newer catecholamines for treatment of heart failure and shock: an update on dopamine and a first look at dobutamine. Prog. Cardiovasc. Dis. *19*:327, 1977.

Volkman, P. H.: Use of dopamine for shock in neonates. J. Pediatr. *94*:852, 1979.

Tolazoline

Bloss, R. S., Turmen, T., Beardmore, H. E., and Aranda, J. V.: Tolazoline therapy for persistent pulmonary hypertension after congenital diaphragmatic hernia repair. J. Pediatr. *97*:984, 1980.

Drummond, W. H., Gregory, G. A., Heymann, M. A., and Phibbs, R. A.: The independent effects of hyperventilation, tolazoline, and dopamine on infants with persistent pulmonary hypertension. J. Pediatr. *98*:603, 1981.

Goetzman, B. W., and Milstein, J. M.: Pulmonary vasodilator action of tolazoline. Pediatr. Res. *13*:942, 1979.

Goetzman, B. W., Sunshine, P., Johnson, J. D., Wennberg, R. P., Hackel, A., Merten, D. F., Bartoletti, A. L., and Silverman, N. H.: Neonatal hypoxia and pulmonary vasospasm: response to tolazoline. J. Pediatr. *89*:617, 1976.

Johnson, G. L., Cunningham, M. D., Desai, N. S., Cottrill, C. M., and Noonan, J. A.: Echocardiography in hypoxemic neonatal pulmonary disease. J. Pediatr. *96*:716, 1980.

Lock, J. E., Coceani, F., and Olley, P. M.: Direct and indirect pulmonary vascular effects of tolazoline in the newborn lamb. J. Pediatr. *95*:600, 1979.

Purohit, D. M., Pai, S., and Levkoff, A. H.: Effect of tolazoline on persistent hypoxemia in neonatal respiratory distress. Crit. Care Med. *6*:14, 1978.

Stevens, D. C., Schreiner, R. L., Bull, M. J., Bryson, C. O., Lemons, J. A., Gresham, E. L., Grosfeld, J. L., and Weber, T. R.: An analysis of tolazoline therapy in the critically ill neonate. J. Pediatr. Surg. *15*:964, 1980.

Stevenson, D. K., Kasting, D. S., Darnall, R. A., Ariagno, R. L., Johnson, J. D., Malachowski, N., Beets, C. L., and Sunshine, P.: Refractory hypoxemia associated with neonatal pulmonary disease: the use and limitations of tolazoline. J. Pediatr. *95*:595, 1979.

Sumner, E., and Frank, J. D.: Tolazoline in the treatment of congenital diaphragmatic hernias. Arch. Dis. Child. *56*:350, 1981.

Vasodilators

Bucciarelli, R. L., Nelson, R. M., Egan, E. A., II, Eitzman, D. V., and Gessner, I. H.: Transient tricuspid insufficiency of the newborn: a form of myocardial dysfunction in stressed newborns. Pediatrics *59*:330, 1977.

Cabal, L. A., Devaskar, U., Siassi, B., Hodgman, J. E., and Emmanouilides, G.: Cardiogenic shock associated with perinatal asphyxia in preterm infants. J. Pediatr. *96*:705, 1980.

Dillon, T. R., Janos, G. G., Meyer, R. A., Benzing, G., III, and Kaplan, S.: Vasodilator therapy for congestive heart failure. J. Pediatr. *96*:623, 1980.

Lakier, J. B., Khaja, F., and Stein, P. D.: Rationale and use of vasodilators in the management of congestive heart failure. Am. Heart J. *97*:519, 1979.

Lees, M. H.: Perinatal asphyxia and the myocardium. J. Pediatr. *96*:675, 1980.

Sarnoff, S. J., and Berglund, E.: Neurohemodynamics of pulmonary edema: IV. Effect of systemic vasoconstriction and subsequent vasodilation on flow and pressure in systemic and pulmonary vascular beds. Am. J. Physiol. *170*:588, 1952.

Digoxin

Berman, W., Jr., Dubynsky, O., Whitman, V., Friedman, Z., and Maisels, M. J.: Digoxin therapy in low-birth-weight infants with patent ductus arteriosus. J. Pediat. *93*:652, 1978.

Halkin, H., Radomsky, M., Blieden, L., Frand, M., Millman, P., and Boichis, H.: Steady state serum digoxin concentration in relation to digitalis toxicity in neonates and infants. Pediatrics *61*:184, 1978.

Lathers, C. M., and Roberts, J.: Digitalis cardiotoxicity revisited. Life Sci. *27*:1713, 1980.

Milstein, J. M., Goetzman, B. W., and Bennett, S. H.: Pulmonary vascular response to digoxin. Pediatr. Res. *15*:468, 1981.

Nyberg, L., and Wettrell, G.: Pharmacokinetics and dosage of digoxin in neonates and infants. Eur. J. Clin. Pharmacol. *18*:69, 1980.

Pinsky, W. W., Jacobsen, J. R., Gillette, P. C., Adams, J., Monroe, L., and McNamara, D. G.: Dosage of digoxin in premature infants. J. Pediatr. *96*:639, 1979.

Warburton, D., Bell, E. E., and Oh, W: Pharmacokinetics and echocardiographic effects of digoxin in low-birth-weight infants with left-to-right shunting due to patent ductus arteriosus. Dev. Pharmacol. Ther. *1*:189, 1980.

Wettrell, G., and Andersson, K. E.: Clinical pharmacokinetics of digoxin in infants. Clin. Pharmacokinet. *2*:17, 1977.

Wettrell, G., Anderson, K. E., Bertler, A., and Lundstrom, N. R.: Concentrations of digoxin in plasma and urine in neonates, infants, and children with heart disease. Acta Paediatr. Scand. *63*:705, 1974.

White, R. D., and Lietman, P. S.: Commentary: a reappraisal of digitalis for infants with left-to-right shunts and "heart failure." J. Pediatr. *92*:867, 1978.

Antihypertensives

Adelman, R. D.: Neonatal hypertension. Pediatr. Clin. North Am. *25*:99, 1978.

Bailie, M. D., and Mattioli, L. F.: Hypertension: relationships between pathophysiology and therapy. J. Pediatr. *96*:789, 1980.

Boerth, R. C., and Long, W. R.: Dose-response relation of diazoxide in children with hypertension. Circulation *56*:1062, 1977.

Friedman, A., Chesney, R. W., Ball, D., and Goodfriend, T.: Effective use of captopril (angiotensin I–converting enzyme inhibitor) in severe childhood hypertension. J. Pediatr. *97*:664, 1980.

Gavras, H., Brunner, H. R., Turini, G. A., Kershaw, G. R., Tofft, C. P., Cuttelod, S., Gavros, I., Vukovich, R. A., and McKinstry, D.: Antihypertensive effect of the oral angiotensin converting enzyme inhibitor SW 14225 in man. N. Engl. J. Med. *298*:991, 1978.

Gordillo-Paniagua, G., Velasquez-Jones, L., Martini, R., and Valdez-Bolanos, E.: Sodium nitroprusside treatment of severe arterial hypertension in children. J. Pediatr. *87*:799, 1975.

Oberfield, S. E., Case, D. B., Levine, L. S., Rapaport, R., Rauh, W., and New, M. I.: Use of the oral angiotensin I–converting enzyme inhibitor (captopril) in childhood malignant hypertension. J. Pediatr. *95*:641, 1979.

Pruitt, A. W.: Pharmacologic approach to the management of childhood hypertension. Pediatr. Clin. North Am. *28*:135, 1981.

Indomethacin

Clyman, D. I., and Heymann, M. A.: Pharmacology of the ductus arteriosus. Pediatr. Clin. North Am. *28*:77, 1981.

Kwan, K. C., Breault, G. D., and Umbenhauer, E. R.: Kinetics of indomethacin absorption, elimination and enterohepatic circulation in man. J. Pharmacokinet. Biopharm. *4*:225, 1976.

Nestrud, R. M., Hill, D. E., Arrington, R. W., Beard, A. G., Dungan, W. T., Lau, P., Norton, J. B., and Readinger, R. I.: Indomethacin treatment in patent ductus arteriosus. Dev. Pharmacol. Ther. *1*:125, 1980.

Yaffe, S. J., Friedman, W. F., Rogers, D., Lang, P., Ragni, M., and Saccar, C.: The disposition of indomethacin in preterm babies. J. Pediatr. *97*:1001, 1980.

Yanagi, R. M., Wilson, A., Newfeld, E. A., Aziz, K. U., and Hunt, C. E.: Indomethacin treatment for symptomatic patent ductus arteriosus: a double-blind control study. Pediatrics *67*:647, 1981.

Yeh, T. F., Luken, J. A., Thalji, A., Raval, D., Carr, I., and Pildes, R. S.: Intravenous indomethacin therapy in premature infants with persistent ductus arteriosus—a double-blind controlled study. J. Pediatr. 98:137, 1981.

Prostaglandin E₁

Elliott, R. B., Starling, M. B., and Netze, J. M.: Medical manipulation of the ductus arteriosus. Lancet 1:140, 1975.

Heymann, M. A.: Pharmacologic use of prostaglandin E₁ in infants with congenital heart disease. Am. Heart J. 101:837, 1981.

Lewis, A. B., Freed, M. D., Heymann, M. A., Roehl, S. L., and Kensey, R. C.: Side effects of therapy with prostaglandin E₁ in infants with critical congenital heart disease. Circulation 64:893, 1981.

Olley, P. M., and Coceani, F.: Use of prostaglandins in cardiopulmonary disease of the newborn. Semin. Perinatol. 4:135, 1980.

Neuromuscular Blockers

Bennett, E. J., Ramamurthy, S., Dalal, F. Y., and Salem, M. R.: Pancuronium and the neonate. Br. J. Anaesthesiol. 47:75, 1975.

Crone, R. K., and Favorito, J.: The effects of pancuronium bromide on infants with hyaline membrane disease. J. Pediatr. 97:991, 1980.

Finer, N. N., and Tomney, P. M.: Controlled evaluation of muscle relaxation in the ventilated neonate. Pediatrics 67:641, 1981.

Henry, G. W., Stevens, D. C., Schreiner, R. L., Grosfeld, J. L., and Ballantine, T. V. N.: Respiratory paralysis to improve oxygenation and mortality in large newborn infants with respiratory distress. J. Pediatr. Surg. 14:761, 1979.

Nugent, S. K., Laravuso, R., and Rogers, M. C.: Pharmacology and use of muscle relaxants in infants and children. J. Pediatr. 94:481, 1979.

Roizen, M. F., and Feeley, T. W.: Pancuronium bromide. Ann. Intern. Med. 88:64, 1978.

Stark, A. R., Bascom, R., and Frantz, I. D., III: Muscle relaxation in mechanically ventilated infants. J. Pediatr. 94:439, 1979.

Theophylline and Caffeine

Aranda, J. V., Grondin, D., and Sasyniuk, B. I.: Pharmacologic considerations in the therapy of neonatal apnea. Pediatr. Clin. North Am. 28:113, 1981.

Aranda, J. V., and Turmen, T.: Methylxanthines in apnea of prematurity. Clin. Perinatol. 6:87, 1979.

Kuzemko, J. A., and Paala, J.: Apnoeic attacks in the newborn treated with aminophylline. Arch. Dis. Child. 48:404, 1973.

Shannon, D. C., Gotay, F., Stein, I. M., Rogers, M. C., Todres, I. D., and Moylan, F. B. M.: Prevention of apnea and bradycardia in low-birth-weight infants. Pediatrics 55:589, 1975.

Srinivasan, G., Pildes, R. S., Jaspan, J. B., Singh, J., Shankar, H., Yeh, T. F., and Tiruvury, A.: Metabolic effects of theophylline in preterm infants. J. Pediatr. 98:815, 1981.

Anticonvulsants

Boreus, L. O., Jalling, B., and Kallberg, N.: Clinical pharmacology of phenobarbital in the neonatal period. In Morselli, P. L., Gar-
attini, S., and Sereni, F. (Eds.): Basic and Therapeutic Aspects of Perinatal Pharmacology. New York, Raven Press, 1975, pp. 331–340.

Johnson, M. V., Freeman, J. M.: Pharmacological advances in seizure control. Pediatr. Clin. North Am. 28:179, 1981.

Lockman, L. A., Kriel, R., Zaske, D., Thompson, T., and Virnig, N.: Phenobarbital dosage for control of neonatal seizures. Neurology 29:1445, 1979.

Logan, W. J., and Freeman, J. M.: Pseudodegenerative disease due to diphenylhydantoin intoxication. Arch. Neurol. 21:631, 1969.

Loughnan, P. M., Greenwald, A., Purton, W. W., Aranda, J. V., Watters, G., and Neims, A. H.: Pharmacokinetic observations of phenytoin disposition in the newborn and young infant. Arch. Dis. Child. 52:302, 1977.

Painter, M. J., Pippenger, C., MacDonald, H., and Pitlick, W.: Phenobarbital and diphenylhydantoin levels in neonates with seizures. J. Pediatr. 92:315, 1978.

Rane, A.: Urinary excretion of diphenylhydantoin metabolites in newborn infants. J. Pediatr. 85:543, 1974.

Rane, A., Lunde, P. K. M., Jalling, B., Yaff, S. J., and Sjoqvist, F.: Plasma protein binding of diphenylhydantoin in normal and hyperbilirubinemic infants. J. Pediatr. 78:877, 1971.

Volpe, J. J.: Neonatal seizures. Pediatr. Clin. North Am. 4:43, 1977.

Diuretics

Aranda, J. V., Perez, J., Sitar, D. S., Collinge, J., Portuguez-Malavasi, A., Duffy, B., and Dupont, C.: Pharmacokinetic disposition and protein binding of furosemide in newborn infants. J. Pediatr. 93:507, 1978.

Hook, J. B., and Bailie, M. D.: Perinatal renal pharmacology. Ann. Rev. Pharmacol. Toxicol. 19:491, 1979.

Marks, H. K., Berman, W., Friedman, Z., et al.: Furosemide in hyaline membrane disease. Pediatrics 62:785, 1978.

Moylan, F. M. B., O'Connell, K. C., Todres, I. D., et al.: Edema of the pulmonary interstitium in infants and children. Pediatrics 55:783, 1975.

Peterson, R. G., Simmons, M. A., Rumack, B. H., Levine, R. L., and Brooks, J. G.: Pharmacology of furosemide in the premature newborn infant. J. Pediatr. 97:139, 1980.

Wennberg, R. P., Rasmussen, L. F., and Ahlfors, C. E.: Displacement of bilirubin from human albumin by three diuretics. J. Pediatr. 90:647, 1977.

Opioid and Opioid Antagonists

AAP Committee on Drugs. Naloxone use in newborns. Pediatrics 65:667, 1980.

Moore, R. A., Rumack, B. H., Conner, C. S., and Peterson, R. G.: Naloxone. Underdosage after narcotic poisoning. Am. J. Dis. Child. 134:156, 1980.

Way, W. L., Costley, E. C., and Way, E. L.: Respiratory sensitivity of the newborn infant to meperidine and morphine. Clin. Pharmacol. Ther. 6:454, 1965.

Miscellaneous References

Roberts, R. J.: Drugs and the newborn infant in pediatric pharmacology. In Yaffee, S. J. (Ed.): New York, Grune & Stratton, 1980, p. 149.

Wilson, J. T., Brown, D. R., Cherek, D. R., Dailey, J. W., Hilman, B., Jobe, P. C., Manno, B. R., Manno, J. E., Redetzki, H. M., and Stewart, J. J.: Drug excretion in human breast milk. Clin. Pharmacokinet. 5:1, 1980.

Appendices

Appendix 1

Pharmacopeia for the Newborn Period

Compiled with the assistance of Robert Roberts and Celeste Marx.

ABBREVIATIONS:
P.O.—by mouth I.M.—intramuscularly
I.V.—intravenously S.C.—subcutaneously
P.R.—by rectum Top.—locally

Drug	Route and Dose	Special Hazards
ACTH	I.M.; 3–5 units/kg/day, in 4 divided doses	
Adrenalin	*See* Epinephrine	
Albumin, 5%	I.V.; 1.0 gm/kg slowly	Hypervolemia; heart failure
Amikacin	I.V., I.M.; 7.5 mg/kg q 8–12 hr	Nephrotoxicity; ototoxicity; blood level monitoring recommended (desirable levels 10–25 µg/ml)
Amphotericin B	I.V.; 0.25–1.0 mg/kg/day, diluted and infused in 1–6 hr I.V. fluid volume	Nephrotoxicity; fever; flushing; anemia
Ampicillin	Neonates <7 days: 25–50 mg/kg q 12 hr I.M. or I.V.; >7 days: 25–50 mg/kg q 8 hr I.M. or I.V.	
Ascorbic acid	*See* Vitamin C	
Atabrine	P.O.; approximately 5 mg/kg b.i.d. or t.i.d.	
Atropine	S.C. 0.01 mg/kg; repeat q 2 hr p.r.n.	Hyperthermia
Bacitracin	I.M. only; 125 units/kg q 6 hr	Nephrotoxicity; less toxic drugs preferred
	Top.; as ointment (500 units/gm), q 4–8 hr	
Belladonna tincture	P.O.; 0.1 ml (0.03 mg atropine) q 4 hr a.c., increasing cautiously to flushing	Hyperthermia
Blood (packed cells)	I.V.; 5 ml/kg; repeat p.r.n.	
Blood (whole)	I.V.; 10 ml/kg; repeat p.r.n.	
Caffeine	P.O., I.V.; loading dose: 10 mg/kg; maintenance dose: 2.5 mg/kg q 24 hr (doses are for the free base)	
Calcium gluconate (10%; each ml contains 9 mg calcium)	Acute: 1–2 ml (9–18 mg Ca)/kg/dose I.V. for acute hypocalcemia; repeated 3 times (maximum)	Bradycardia if injected too quickly; necrosis from extravascular leakage; gastric necrosis and calcification if too concentrated
	Chronic: 3–9 ml/kg/day in 2–4 divided doses P.O. (30–80 mg Ca).	
Calcium lactate (13% calcium)	P.O.; 0.5 gm/kg/day in divided doses	*See* Calcium gluconate
Carbenicillin	I.V.; neonates <7 days: 100 mg/kg q 12 hr; >7 days: 100 mg/kg q 6–8 hr	
Cephalothin (Keflin)	I.V., I.M., 20 mg/kg q 8–12 hr	
Chloral hydrate	P.O.; 10–30 mg/kg dose q 6–8 hr p.r.n. Max. daily dose is 50 mg/kg/day.	Irritation; requires caution with cardiac or pulmonary disease
Chloramphenicol	P.O., I.V.; loading dose: 20 mg/kg; maintenance dose: neonates <14 days, 2.5 mg/kg q 6 hr; neonates >14 days, 5 mg/kg q 6 hr	Blood level monitoring mandatory (usual therapeutic level 10–25 µg/ml) hematologic, cardiac toxicity; "gray baby" syndrome
Chloromycetin	*See* Chloramphenicol	
Chlorothiazide (Diuril)	P.O.; 10–20 mg/kg/q 12 hr	Hypokalemia; hyponatremia
Chlorpromazine (Thorazine)	P.O., I.M., I.V.; 0.5 mg/kg q 6 hr	Extrapyramidal symptoms; potentiates hypnotics and narcotics
Cimetidine (Tagamet)	P.O., I.V.; 2.5–10 mg/kg q 6 hr	H_2 antagonist with little experience in neonates
Cortisone	P.O.; 0.5–2 mg/kg/day, in 4 equal doses, reduced slowly to minimal effective dose, withdrawn cautiously	*See* Hydrocortisone
Desoxycorticosterone acetate (DOCA)	I.M.; 2 mg the first day, then 0.5–1 mg/day	
Dexamethasone	I.M., I.V.; loading dose: 0.5–1.0 mg; maintenance dose: .05–0.1 mg/kg q 6 hr	

Drug	Route and Dose	Special Hazards
Diamox (Acetazolamide)	I.V., P.O.; 5 mg/kg/day as a single dose (diuretic) or divided into 3 equal doses (glaucoma)	Acidosis (chronic therapy)
Diazepam (Valium)	P.O., I.V., I.M.; sedative: 0.02–0.3 mg/kg q 6–8 hr; seizure: 0.3–0.75 mg/kg slow I.V. push	Diluted injection may precipitate; poor absorption following I.M. injection; respiratory depression; hypotension
Digoxin	Digitalization dose (TDD); I.M., P.O.:	

Digoxin digitalization:

		Weight	Dose
	Prematures	500–1000 gm	20 µg/kg
		1000–1500 gm	20–30 µg/kg
		1500–2000 gm	30 µg/kg
		2000–2500 gm	30–40 µg/kg
	Full-term to 1 month		60 µg/kg
	1 month to 2 years		60–80 µg/kg

I.V. dose is 75% of I.M. or P.O. dose; TDD is given in 3–4 divided doses over 24 hr
Maintenance dose:
(Begun 12 hours after last digitalization dose)
25 per cent of TDD in 2 divided doses (q 12 hr); usually 2.5 to 5 µg/kg q 12 hr

Drug	Route and Dose	Special Hazards
Diphenhydramine (Benadryl)	P.O.; 5 mg/kg/day, divided into 4–6 equal doses, a.c.	
Diphenylhydantoin sodium (phenytoin) (Dilantin)	Intravenous loading dose: 8–10 mg/kg P.O., I.V.; 3–5 mg/kg/day divided into 3 doses; increased cautiously after second week up to 10 mg/kg/day	Therapeutic blood level monitoring indicated (desirable level 5–15 µg/ml)
Diphtheria antitoxin	I.M., I.V.; 20,000–50,000 units/day for 2–3 successive days	Hypersensitivity reaction
DOCA	See Desoxycorticosterone acetate	
Dopamine	I.V. 2 to 20 µg/kg/min	Extravasation may lead to necrosis (Regitine is an antidote)
Epinephrine	S.C.: 1:1000 injection, 0.01 ml/kg; may be repeated every 15 min for 3–4 doses, then every 4 hours as needed
I.V.: 1:10,000 (1 ml 1:1000 may be diluted with 9 ml saline) 1 to 2 ml, repeated as needed	
Erythromycin (ethylsuccinate) (lactobionate)	P.O., I.V.; 10 mg/kg q 6 hr	I.V. administration painful
Ethacrynic acid (Edecrin)	I.V.; 1.0 mg/kg; diluted with 5% dextrose and water and given over a 5-min period	Ototoxicity
Fibrinogen	I.V.; 50 mg/kg; repeated p.r.n. as determined by clotting time	
Fludrocortisone (Florinef)	P.O.; 0.025–0.2 mg/day	Mineralocorticoid replacement
Folic acid	I.M.: 5 mg; repeated in 7–14 days
P.O.: 1 mg weekly for premature infants; 50 µg/day for term newborns	
Furosemide (Lasix)	P.O., I.V.; 1.0 mg/kg/dose up to 2 mg/kg/day	Hypokalemia; hyponatremia; hypochloremia
Gamma globulin	I.M.: preventive: 0.22 ml/kg; attenuating: 0.05 ml/kg; for agammaglobulinemia, 1 ml/kg, repeated every 2–4 weeks	
Gentamicin	I.V., I.M.; 2.5 mg/kg q 8 to 12 hr	Blood level monitoring indicated (desirable levels 2–8 µg/ml)
Gentian violet	Top: as 1–2% aqueous solution, b.i.d. (skin); as 1% aqueous solution, b.i.d. (mouth)	
Glucagon	I.M., I.V.; 30–100 µg/kg; may be repeated after 6–12 hr; infant of diabetic mother may require 300 µg/kg	Maximum dose 1 mg; higher doses possibly toxic
Heparin	Initial dose: I.V.; 50 units/kg; maintenance dose: 100 units/kg q 4 hr I.V.; dose titrated to yield 20–30 minute clotting time or 2–3 times pre-heparin clotting time	Intractable bleeding (reversible with protamine)
Hydralazine (Apresoline)	P.O., I.M., I.V.; 0.15 mg/kg every 6 hours; increased as needed in 0.1 mg/kg increments up to 4 mg/kg/day	
Hydrochlorothiazide (Hydrodiuril)	P.O.; 2.0–2.5 mg/kg every 12 hours	
Hydrocortisone	Adrenal crisis: P.O., I.M., I.V.; 3–10 mg/kg/day; physiologic replacement: P.O.; 1 mg/kg/day or 15–25 mg/m²/day	Suppression of immune response; elevation of white blood count
Indomethacin (Indocin)	P.O., I.V.; 0.1–0.2 mg/kg q 8–24 hr, maximum 0.6 mg/kg	Transient renal dysfunction; decreased platelet aggregation
Insulin	For diabetic acidosis, 1 unit/kg initially, then 1/2–1 unit/kg q 1–3 hr p.r.n.	
Iron	P.O.; 6 mg/kg/day elemental iron	
Isoniazid	P.O.; 10 mg/kg/day, single dose	
Isoproterenol (Isuprel)	I.V.; 0.05–0.1 µg/kg/min; increased to maximum 1.5 µg/kg/min	

Table continued on following page

Drug	Route and Dose	Special Hazards
Kanamycin	I.M., I.V.; 7.5–10 mg/kg q 8–12 hr	Nephrotoxicity; ototoxicity; monitoring of blood levels useful
Kayexalate	P.O.: 1 gm/kg; P.R.: 1.0–1.5 gm/kg; administered approximately every 6 hours	Given as a solution with 20% sorbitol to prevent intestinal obstruction; may decrease serum calcium or magnesium
Levothyroxine (Synthroid)	P.O.; 0.025–0.05 mg/kg/day	
Lidocaine	I.V.; 1–2 mg/kg infused over 5–10 min; may be repeated in 10 min as necessary	
Magnesium sulfate	I.M.; 0.2 ml/kg/dose 50% sol. q 4–8 hr (for tetanus neonatorum or other repeated convulsions)	Hypotension
Mecholyl	S.C.; 0.2 mg/kg; increased by 25% and repeated q 15 min until desired effect occurs (for paroxysmal tachycardia)	Cardiac arrest (atropine is an antidote)
Meperidine (Demerol)	P.O., I.M.; 1.0–1.5 mg/kg/dose q 4 hr p.r.n.	Respiratory depression reversible with naloxone
Methicillin (Staphcillin)	Neonate <7 days: 25–50 mg/kg q 8–12 hr; >7 days: 25–50 mg/kg q 6–8 hr	
Methyldopa (Aldomet)	P.O.; 5 mg/kg every 12 hr; increased as needed at 2-day intervals; maximum dosage 65 mg/kg/day	May cause false-positive Coombs' test; monitoring for hemolysis and leukopenia recommended
Methylene blue	I.V.; 0.1–0.2 mg/kg of 1% solution for methemoglobinemia, infused slowly	
Methylprednisolone (Solu-Medrol)	I.V., I.M.; in severe shock: 30 mg/kg every 6 hr	Hydrocortisone preferred for physiologic replacement
Morphine sulfate	I.V., I.M., S.C.; 0.1–0.2 mg/kg/dose q 6 hr p.r.n.	Respiratory depression reversible with naloxone
Moxalactam	I.V., I.M.; 50 mg/kg every 12 hr (<1 week); 8 hr (1–4 weeks); 6 hr (>4 weeks)	In gram-negative meningitis, a loading dose of 100 mg/kg is given prior to institution of this maintenance dose
Mycostatin	P.O.; 100,000–200,000 units q 6 hr Top.; as 2% ointment (in liquid petrolatum 95%, polyethylene 5%) 3–4 times daily	
Naloxone HCl (Narcan)	I.V., I.M., S.C.; 0.01 mg/kg/dose; may be repeated as necessary	
Neo-Calglucon (calcium glubionate)	P.O.; Calcium supplementation: begun in small amounts (0.1–0.2 ml) in each feeding; increased as tolerated to bring calcium intake from formula and supplement to 150 mg/kg/day; therapeutic dosage: 500 mg/kg/day	1 ml contains 23 mg elemental calcium; high osmotic load of syrup may cause diarrhea
Neomycin	P.O.; 10–25 mg/kg q 6 hr Top.; 0.5% ointment, 3–4 times daily	Renal toxicity and ototoxicity
Neostigmine (Prostigmin)	P.O.; 2 mg/kg/day, divided into 4–8 doses	Cardiac arrhythmia (atropine should be kept available)
Neutra-Phos-K	P.O.; used to supplement formula phosphorus intake to 75 mg/kg/day; diluted solution contains 250 mg phosphorus in 75 ml	Large amounts may cause catharsis; should be increased gradually to full supplementation
Nicotinic acid	6 mg/day	
Nitroprusside (Nipride)	I.V.; begun in dose of 1.0 μg/kg/min and increased as needed to control blood pressure	Profound hypotension possible, requires arterial line to monitor B.P; thiocyanate toxicity with long-term use
Nystatin	*See* Mycostatin	
Oxacillin (prostaphlin)	*See* Methacillin	
Oxytetracycline	*See* Tetracyclines	
Pancreatin	P.O.; 0.3 to 0.5 gm with each feeding P.R. and into colostomy; 0.3–0.5 gm in sufficient liquid (for meconium ileus)	
Pancuronium (Pavulon)	I.V.; 0.02 mg/kg/dose q 1–4 hr p.r.n.	Edema common
Paraldehyde	P.O., P.R., I.M.; 0.15 ml/kg; repeated q 4–6 hr	I.M. may cause sterile abscess
Penicillin G	I.M., I.V.; aqueous solution 20,000–50,000 units/kg q 6–12 hr I.M.; 20,000 units/kg/divided over 3–15 days (for treatment of congenital syphilis) Top; 50,000 units/gm (for prevention of gonorrheal ophthalmia) For treatment of gonococcal ophthalmia 50,000 units/kg/day for 7 days, plus local drops Up to 250,000 units/kg/day for Group B streptococcal infection	

Drug	Route and Dose	Special Hazards
Pentobarbital (Nembutal)	P.O., I.M.; 2–3 mg/kg q 8 hr p.r.n.	
Phenobarbital	Anticonvulsant: loading dose: 10–20 mg/kg, slow I.V. push; maintenance dose: 2–4 mg/kg q 12 hr; sedation: 2–3 mg/kg q 8–12 hr p.r.n.	Therapeutic blood level monitoring helpful with chronic therapy (therapeutic range 15–40 μg/ml)
Pitressin (aqueous)	S.C.; 1–3 ml/day, divided into 3 equal doses	
Plasma	I.V.; 10–20 ml/kg; repeated p.r.n.	Volume overload
Prednisone	P.O.; 1–3 mg/kg/day, divided into 4 doses	
Priscoline (Tolazoline)	Loading dose: 2 mg/kg I.V. push; maintenance dose: 2 mg/kg/hr I.V.	Hypotension; gastrointestinal and pulmonary bleeding; renal dysfunction
Procainamide (Pronestyl)	I.V.; 1.5–2.5 mg/kg infused over 10–30 min; may be repeated in 30 minutes if needed	
Propranolol (Inderal)	I.V.; 0.05–0.15 mg/kg infused over 10 min; may be repeated in 10 min then given every 8 hr	Relatively contraindicated in low-output congestive heart failure and patients with bronchospasm
Propylthiouracil	P.O.; 10 mg q 8 hr	
Protamine sulfate	I.V.; 1.0 mg for each 100 units heparin in previous 4 hr	
Pyridoxine	See Vitamin B$_6$	
Quinidine gluconate	P.O., I.M., I.V.; 2–10 mg/kg per dose; repeated q 2–6 hr until desired effect or toxicity occurs	Check electrocardiogram before each dose; discontinue if QRS interval increases by 0.02 second or more
Silver nitrate	For gonorrheal ophthalmia prophylaxis, 1 drop 2% solution in each eye	
Sodium bicarbonate	1–2 mEq/kg/dose I.V. (diluted to half strength)	Infused slowly
Solu-Cortef	I.M., I.V.; See Hydrocortisone	
Spironolactone (Aldactone)	P.O.; 0.25–1.0 mg/kg every 6–8 hr, up to 3 mg/kg/day	Onset of action delayed; active metabolite must be formed
Staphcillin	See Methicillin	
Streptomycin	I.M.; 5–20 mg/kg q 12 hr	
Sulfisoxazole (Gantrisin)	P.O., I.V.; 25 mg/kg q 6 hr	In prematures or in presence of jaundice, may lead to kernicterus
Tensilon	S.C., I.M.; 0.1 ml (as test for myasthenia gravis)	
Terramycin	See Tetracyclines	
Tetanus antitoxin	I.M., I.V.; 10,000–20,000 units on 2 successive days	
Tetanus immune globulin	I.M.; 3000–6000 units	For neonatal tetanus; optimal dosage not established
Tetracyclines	P.O., I.M., I.V.; 50 mg/kg/day in 4 divided doses orally; 2–3 divided doses I.M.	Rarely used; may stain teeth permanently
THAM (TRIS) (trishydromethylamino-methane)	Total dose (ml) = kg of body weight × base deficit; ¼ dose given over 2–5 min; rest according to response; maximum dose (24 hr) 40 ml/kg	Hypoglycemia
Theophylline	P.O., I.V.; loading dose: 5 mg/kg; maintenance dose: 1 mg/kg q 8 hr to 3.6 mg/kg q 12 hr	Blood level monitoring valuable in preventing toxicity (therapeutic range 4–15 μg/ml).
Thiamine	See Vitamin B$_1$	
L-Thyroxine	P.O.; starting dose 10 μg/kg/day (round off to nearest 12.5, 25.0, or 37.5 to coincide with pill size)	Average values only; adjusted by clinical response and T4 and TSH blood levels
Tobramycin	See Gentamicin	
Vancomycin	I.V., P.O.; 15 mg/kg q 8–12 hr	Nephrotoxicity; ototoxicity
Verapamil	I.V.; 0.1–0.2 mg/kg, infused slowly over 2 min; if response is inadequate, may be repeated in 30 min	Used in supraventricular tachycardia; during infusion EKG should be continuously monitored for signs of sinus bradycardia, AV blockade, or asystole
Vitamin A	P.O.; preventive, 600–1000 units/day	
Vitamin B$_1$ (thiamine)	P.O.; preventive 0.5–1.0 mg q.d. I.M.; therapeutic, 10 mg q 6–8 hr	
Vitamin B$_6$ (pyridoxine)	P.O.; preventive, 100 μg/l of ingested formula; therapeutic, 2–5 mg/day Test dose for dependency, 50 mg I.V.	
Vitamin C	P.O.; preventive, 25–50 mg/day, 100 mg/day for premature infants P.O. or I.M.; therapeutic 100 mg q 4 hr	
Vitamin D	P.O.; preventive, 400 I.U. daily	
Vitamin E	25 I.U. daily in premature infants for 2–3 months	
Vitamin K$_1$ oxide	I.M.; preventive, 1.0 mg, one dose only; therapeutic, 2.5–5.0 mg q 6–12 hr, titrated by prothrombin time	With thrombocytopenia, slow intravenous infusion at same dose

Appendix 2

Composition of Frequently Used Formulas

Infant Formula Product Comparison

| Formula | Nutrient Source | | | Kcal/oz | Gm/100 ml* | | | mEq/liter | |
	Protein	CHO	Fat		Protein	CHO	Fat	Ca++	P+
Breast milk	Lactalbumin 65% Casein 35% (% total N₂)	Lactose	High in olein Low in volatile fatty acids	22 13.4–35.8	1.1 0.7–2.0	7.0 4.9–9.5	4.5 1.3–8.3	17.2 8.6–30.5	9.1 4.4–17.3
Cow's milk	Lactalbumin 19% Casein 81% (% total N₂)	Lactose	Butter fat	20	3.2	4.7	3.8	68.5	58.7
Regular Similac (Ross)†	Nonfat milk	Lactose	Coconut oil: 53% Soy oil: 47%	20	1.5	7.2	3.6	25	25
Enfamil (M.J.)†	Nonfat milk	Lactose	Coconut oil: 20% Soy oil: 80%	20	1.5	7.0	3.7	26	28
Concentrated regular Similac 24‡ (Ross)	Nonfat milk	Lactose	Coconut oil: 60% Soy oil: 40%	24	2.2	8.5	4.3	36	36
Diluted regular Similac 13 (Ross)	Nonfat milk	Lactose	Coconut oil Soy oil	13	1.2	4.6	2.3	20.5	20.6
Low birth weight Similac LBW	Nonfat milk	Lactose: 50% Corn syrup solids: 50%§	MCT: 50%‖ Coconut oil Soy oil	24	2.2	8.5	4.5	36	36
Special Care (Ross)	Nonfat milk, demineralized whey (whey: casein, 6:4)	Lactose: 50% Corn syrup solids: 50%§	MCT: 50%‖ Corn oil: 30% Coconut oil: 20%	24	2.2	8.6	4.4	72	46.4
Enfamil Premature (M.J.)	Nonfat milk, demineralized whey (whey: casein, 6:4)	Lactose: 40% Corn syrup solids: 60%§	MCT: 40%‖ Corn oil: 40% Coconut oil: 20%	24	2.4	8.9	4.1	47	30.2
SMA "Preemie" (Wyeth)	Nonfat milk, demineralized whey (whey: casein, 6:4)	Lactose: 50% Maltodextrins: 50%	Coconut oil Oleo oil Safflower oil Soybean oil (13% MCTs)‖	24	2.0	8.6	4.4	37.5	25.8

Infant Formula Product Comparison (*Continued*)

mEq/liter			mOsm/kg H₂O	RSL mOsm/l	Indications for Use/Rationale
Na+	K+	Cl−			
7.5	13	10.6	280	75	Mean values
2.8–19	9.6–16.3	2.5–20.7	—	—	Range of values: 15 days–15 mo postpartum Preferred feeding for term infant. *Note*: Compositional variations due to stage of lactation may be a consideration when breast milk is provided to premature or high-risk infants with increased nutritional needs.
33.4	37.9	30.4	280	230	Not recommended under 8 mo unless modified. Avoid skim in babies 1 yr or younger.
11	20	15	290	108	Normal infant feeding. Sick infants without nutritional problems. Supplement for breast-fed infants.
10	17	13	278	105	
14.3	27.4	20.8	360	150	Compensation for a limited volume intake. Recovery from an illness-induced period of malnutrition.
9.6	14.9	11.5	190	85	Conservative initial 24- to 48-hr feedings for newborns and infants who have not been fed enterally for several days to weeks. *Note*: Inadequate in nutrients and calories.
16	25.6	24.8	290	160	Modified to meet the needs of premature infants. ↑ Ca, P, Na levels, modified fat blend, using MCT ↓ Lactose with corn syrup solids
15.2	25.6	18.3	300	147	

MINERAL AND VITAMIN DIFFERENCES (VALUES/LITER)

	Similac LBW	Special Care	Enfamil Premature	SMA "Preemie"
Iron (mg)	3	2.5	1.25	—
Zinc (mg)	8	10	8	—
Cu (mg)	8	1.7	.7	—
Vit. A (I.U.)	3000	4580	2500	3200
C (mg)	100	250	68	70
D (I.U.)	480	1000	500	510
E (I.U.)	18	25	15	15
K (µg)	—	83	75	70
Thiamine (mg)	1.0	1.7	.6	.8
Riboflavin (mg)	1.2	4.2	.7	1.3
Niacin (mg equiv.)	8.4	20	10	6.3
Folic acid (mg)	.1	.25	.24	.1
B₁₂ (µg)	2.0	3.7	2.5	2.0

The Na+/K+/Cl− rows aligned with the vitamin table:

Na+	K+	Cl−	mOsm/kg H₂O	RSL mOsm/l
13.6	22.7	19.1	300	152
13.9	19.2	14.9	268	175

Note: All formulations are intended for rapidly growing premature infants. Manufacturers recommend diluted initial feedings, with progression to full strength made over several days. With very low birth weight prematures, progression from half strength should be more gradual and cautious.

Table continued on following page

Infant Formula Product Comparison (*Continued*)

Formula	Nutrient Source			Kcal/oz	Gm/100 ml*			mEq/liter	
	Protein	*CHO*	*Fat*		*Protein*	*CHO*	*Fat*	*Ca++*	*P+*
Electrodialyzed									
SMA (Wyeth)	Nonfat milk, demineralized whey (whey: casein, 6:4)	Lactose	Coconut oil Oleo oil Safflower oil Soybean oil	20	1.5	7.2	3.6	22	21
PM 60/40 (Ross)	Demineralized whey Calcium Sodium caseinate	Lactose	Coconut oil Corn oil	20	1.6	7.6	3.5	20	13
Soy-based									
Isomil (Ross)	Soy protein isolate	Corn syrup sucrose	Coconut oil Soy oil	20	2	6.8	3.6	35	32
Prosobee (M.J.)	Soy protein isolate	Corn syrup solids§	Coconut oil Soy oil	20	2	6.9	3.6	31	31.9
Nursoy (Wyeth)	Soy protein isolate	Sucrose	Coconut oil Oleo oil Safflower oil Soybean oil	20	2.1	6.9	3.6	31.2	21.9
RCF (Ross)	Soy protein isolate	—	Coconut oil: 50% Soy oil: 50%	20 (with 7% CHO addition)	2	7	3.6	35	32.2
Hydrolyzed protein									
Nutramigen (M.J.)	Hydrolysed casein	Sucrose Modified tapioca starch	Corn oil	20	2.2	8.8	2.6	31	30
Pregestimil (M.J.)	Hydrolysed casein L-tryptophan L-cysteine L-tyrosine	Corn syrup solids§ Modified tapioca starch	Corn oil: 60% MCT oil: 40%‖	2.0	1.9	9.1	2.7	31	27

Infant Formula Product Comparison (*Continued*)

mEq/liter			mOsm/kg H₂O	RSL mOsm/l	Indications for Use/Rationale
Na+	*K+*	*Cl−*			
6.4	14.2	10.3	300	91	For both electrodialysed formulas, Na and K levels are lower than those of regular formulas; useful with decreased cardiovascular function. For both, lactalbumin: casein ratio is closer to that of human milk.
7	14.9	12.7	260	90	*Note:* Differences in Ca:P ratios. FM 60/40 is the preferred formula with decreased renal function. Low mineral content does not meet needs of rapidly growing prematures.
13	18.2	14.9	250	126	Isomil and Prosobee useful in cases of milk intolerance, lactase deficiency, and galactosemia and during the recovery stage following mild to moderate diarrhea.
12.4	20.8	15.2	200	130	
8.3	18.7	10.3	296	172	
13	18.2	14.9	Varies with CHO choice	126	Used in cases of CHO intolerance; CHO of choice (corn syrup solids recommended) to be added in stepwise progression to 7% total calories.

CHO Conc. (%)	Cal/oz
—	12
2	14
3	15
4	17
5	18
6	19

Note: 2% conc. with adequate intake usually prevents hypoglycemia and ketosis. If no oral CHO is tolerated, adequate glucose must be provided I.V.

mEq/liter			mOsm/kg H₂O	RSL mOsm/l	Indications for Use/Rationale
13.6	17.3	13.2	479	132	Used in cases of intact protein intolerance, lactase deficiency and galactosemia and during the recovery stage following mild to moderate diarrhea with soy intolerance.
13.6	18.7	16.1	348	124	Used in cases of malabsorption short gut syndrome, cystic fibrosis, celiac diseases, and intact protein intolerance with sensitivity to hyperosmolar solutions. Less palatable than Nutramigen. Also used as interim formula during transition from hyperalimentation to normal oral intake and during recovery stage following prolonged diarrhea

Table continued on following page

Infant Formula Product Comparison (*Continued*)

| Formula | Nutrient Source | | | Kcal/oz | Gm/100 ml* | | | mEq/liter | |
	Protein	*CHO*	*Fat*		*Protein*	*CHO*	*Fat*	*Ca++*	*P+*
Altered fat Portagen (M.J.)	Sodium caseinate	Corn syrup solids: 75%§ Sucrose: 25%	MCT oil: 86%‖ Corn oil: 11% Soy lecithin: 3%	20	2.4	7.8	3.2	31	30
Meat-based Meat Base Formula (Gerber)	Beef hearts	Sucrose Modified tapioca starch	Sesame oil	20	2.6	6.2	3.4	49	42
Controlled amino acids Lofenalac (M.J.)	Hydrolyzed casein with most phenylalanine removed L-tyrosine L-tryptophan L-histidine L-methionine	Corn syrup solids§ Modified tapioca starch	Corn oil	20	.35 (total N_2 equiv. 2.2)	8.8	2.7	31.2	30.2
Water Electrolyte Maintenance Pedialyte (Ross)	—	Glucose	—	6	—	5	—	4	—
Lytren (M.J.)	—	Corn syrup solids§ Glucose	—	9	—	7.6	—	4	5
5% glucose	—	Glucose	—	6	—	5	—	—	—
10% glucose	—	Glucose	—	12	—	10	—	—	—

Infant Formula Product Comparison (*Continued*)

Na+	K+	Cl−	mOsm/kg H₂O	RSL mOsm/l	Indications for Use/Rationale
	mEq/liter				
13.6	21.4	16.3	236	150	For cases in which minimal lactose content <.15%. Also for cases of fat malabsorption due to decreased pancreatic lipase, decreased bile salt production, or defect in fat transport.
11.8	13.7	13.6	—	143	For milk, lactose, or soy intolerance
13.6	17.4	13.2	356	132	PKU *Note*: When serum phenylalanine has reached acceptable levels (2–10 mg/100 ml) breast milk or infant formula should be added to meet growth requirements. Normal dilution of Lofenalac with no added sources of phenylalanine should not be used when phenylalanine levels cannot be monitored daily.
30	20	30	405	—	Pedialyte and Lytren used in cases of mild to moderate diarrhea for maintanance or replacement of water and electrolytes. Also used in cases of severe diarrhea in I.V. supplement.
30	25	25	290		
—	—	—	276	—	5% glucose used as initial oral feed after NPO.
—	—	—	552	—	

* Interconversion 100 ml → 100 Kcal; divide quantity/100 ml by: .67 (20 cal/oz); .81 (24 cal/oz); .44 (13 cal/oz).
† Available with and without added iron: 1.2 mg/100 ml.
‡ Available with and without added iron: 1.5 ml/100 ml.
§ Corn syrup solids: glucose polymers derived from hydrolysis of cornstarch.
‖ MCT: medium chain triglyceride oil. Contains triglycerides of primarily C_8 and C_{10} fatty acids that are readily hydrolyzed in absence of bile salts or pancreatic lipase or both.
References:
George, D. E., and Lebenthal, E.: Human milk/cow's milk comparisons. *In* Textbook of Gastroenterology and Nutrition, New York, Raven Press, 1981.
Gerber Professional Communications: Nutrient Values, 1981.
M.J. Products: Product Handbook, 1981.
Ross Products: Product Handbook, 1981.
Wyeth Products: Product Handbook, 1981.
(From Gotchell, F. [Ed.]: Physician's Handbook for Dietary Nutrition Services. Boston, Children's Hospital Medical Center, 1982.)

Estimated Daily Requirements of Premature Infants*

	| Growth and Nongrowth Body Weight Intervals (gm)								
	750–1000	1000–1250	1250–1500	1500–1750	1750–2000	2000–2250	2250–2500	2500–2750	2750–3000
Energy									
Growth (kal)	21	46	68	79	93	104	114	111	108
Nongrowth (kcal)	71	94	117	133	156	180	204	215	239
Total (kal/kg)	105	124	127	130	133	133	134	124	121
Protein									
Growth (gm)	1.78	3.45	4.44	4.79	4.85	4.90	4.68	4.27	3.77
Nongrowth (gm)	0.87	1.12	1.37	1.62	1.87	2.12	2.37	2.62	2.87
Total (gm/kg)†	3.02	4.06	4.22	3.94	3.58	3.30	2.96	2.62	2.30
Sodium									
Growth (mEq)	0.95	1.68	2.10	2.21	2.21	2.21	2.10	1.89	1.57
Nongrowth (mEq)	0.18	0.23	0.28	0.34	0.39	0.44	0.49	0.55	0.60
Total (mEq/kg)	1.29	1.69	1.73	1.56	1.38	1.24	1.09	0.92	0.75
Potassium									
Growth (mEq)	0.31	0.73	1.05	1.15	1.26	1.36	1.36	1.36	1.15
Nongrowth (mEq)	0.20	0.26	0.32	0.38	0.43	0.49	0.55	0.61	0.66
Total (mEq/kg)	0.58	0.88	0.99	0.94	0.90	0.87	0.80	0.75	0.63
Calcium									
Growth (mg)	148	317	442	530	592	632	660	627	592
Nongrowth (mg)	—	—	—	—	—	—	—	—	
Total (mg/kg)	169	282	321	326	316	300	278	239	206
Phosphorus									
Growth (mg)	49	110	148	172	188	197	202	194	177
Nongrowth (mg)	12	27	37	43	47	49	50	49	44
Total (mg/kg)	70	121	135	132	125	116	106	93	77
Magnesium									
Growth (mg)	9.0	18.5	25.2	30.0	33.5	35.5	37.0	35.5	32.5
Nongrowth (mg)	—	—	—	—	—	—	—	—	—
Total (mg/kg)	10.3	16.4	18.6	18.5	17.8	16.7	15.6	13.5	11.3

* Assuming extent of intestinal absorption as follows: energy: 75 per cent absorption for infants weighing 750 to 1500 gm, 80 per cent for those weighing 1500 to 2500 gm, and 85 per cent for those weighing more than 2500 gm; protein: 75 per cent absorption at 750 to 1250 gm, 77 per cent at 1250 to 1500 gm, 80 per cent at 1500 to 2250 gm, 83 per cent at 2250 to 2500 gm, and 85 per cent above 2500 gm; sodium and potassium: 95 per cent absorption throughout; calcium: 40 per cent throughout; phosphorus: 80 per cent throughout; magnesium: 20 per cent throughout.

† Based on arithmetic mean weight for the weight interval. (Data of O'Donnell, A. M., Ziegler, E. E., and Fomon, S. J., reproduced with permission of Dr. Fomon.)

NEWBORN MATURITY RATING
and
CLASSIFICATION

ESTIMATION OF GESTATIONAL AGE BY MATURITY RATING
Symbols: X - 1st Exam   O - 2nd Exam

NEUROMUSCULAR MATURITY

	0	1	2	3	4	5
Posture						
Square Window (Wrist)	90°	60°	45°	30°	0°	
Arm Recoil	180°		100°-180°	90°-100°	< 90°	
Popliteal Angle	180°	160°	130°	110°	90°	< 90°
Scarf Sign						
Heel to Ear						

PHYSICAL MATURITY

	0	1	2	3	4	5
SKIN	gelatinous red, transparent	smooth pink, visible veins	superficial peeling &/or rash, few veins	cracking pale area, rare veins	parchment, deep cracking, no vessels	leathery, cracked, wrinkled
LANUGO	none	abundant	thinning	bald areas	mostly bald	
PLANTAR CREASES	no crease	faint red marks	anterior transverse crease only	creases ant. 2/3	creases cover entire sole	
BREAST	barely percept.	flat areola, no bud	stippled areola, 1–2 mm bud	raised areola, 3–4 mm bud	full areola, 5–10 mm bud	
EAR	pinna flat, stays folded	sl. curved pinna, soft with slow recoil	well-curv. pinna, soft but ready recoil	formed & firm with instant recoil	thick cartilage, ear stiff	
GENITALS Male	scrotum empty, no rugae		testes descending, few rugae	testes down, good rugae	testes pendulous, deep rugae	
GENITALS Female	prominent clitoris & labia minora		majora & minora equally prominent	majora large, minora small	clitoris & minora completely covered	

Gestation by Dates _____ wks

Birth Date _____ Hour _____ am / pm

APGAR _____ 1 min _____ 5 min

MATURITY RATING

Score	Wks
5	26
10	28
15	30
20	32
25	34
30	36
35	38
40	40
45	42
50	44

SCORING SECTION

	1st Exam=X	2nd Exam=O
Estimating Gest Age by Maturity Rating	_____ Weeks	_____ Weeks
Time of Exam	Date _____ Hour _____ am/pm	Date _____ Hour _____ am/pm
Age at Exam	_____ Hours	_____ Hours
Signature of Examiner	_____ M.D.	_____ M.D.

(Scoring system: From Ballard, J. L., et al.: A simplified assessment of gestational age. Pediatr. Res. *11*:374, 1977. Figures: Adapted from Sweet, A. Y.: Classification of the low-birth-weight infant. *In* Klaus, M. H., and Fanaroff, A. A. [Eds.]: Care of the High-Risk Infant. 2nd ed. Philadelphia, W. B. Saunders Co., 1979, p. 79.)

CLASSIFICATION OF NEWBORNS —
BASED ON MATURITY AND INTRAUTERINE GROWTH
Symbols: X - 1st Exam   O - 2nd Exam

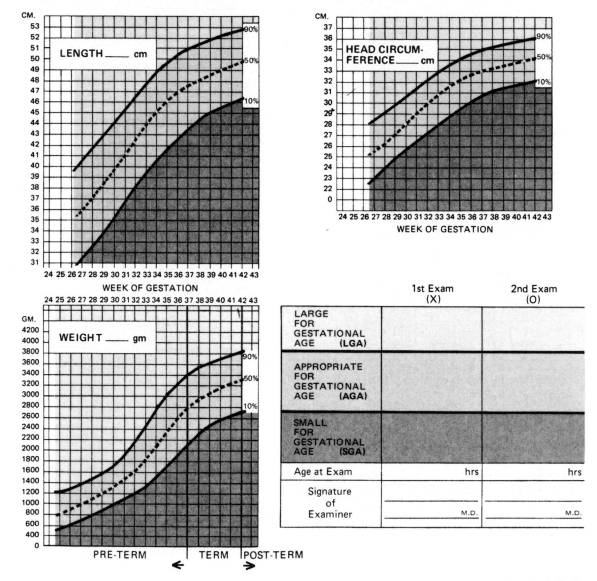

(Adapted from Lubchenco, L. C., Hansman, C., and Boyd, E.: Pediatrics *37*:403, 1966; Battaglia, F. C., and Lubchenco, L. C.: J. Pediatr. *71*:159, 1967.)

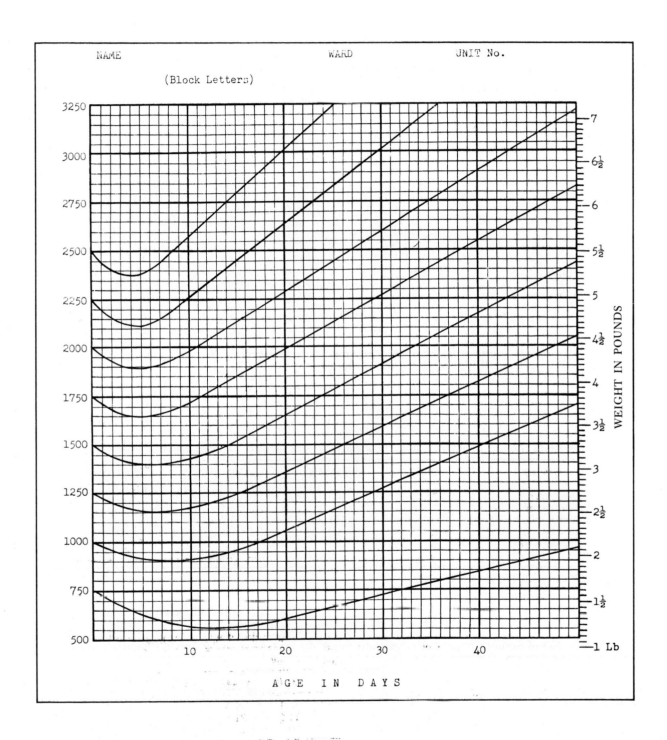

Normal Blood Chemistry Values, Term Infants

Determination	Sample Source	Cord	1–12 hr	12–24 hr	24–48 hr	48–72 hr
Sodium, mEq/l*	Capillary	147	143	145	148	149
		(126–166)	(124–156)	(132–159)	(134–160)	(139–162)
Potassium, mEq/l		7.8	6.4	6.3	6.0	5.9
		(5.6–12)	(5.3–7.3)	(5.3–8.9)	(5.2–7.3)	(5.0–7.7)
Chloride, mEq/l		103	100.7	103	102	103
		(98–110)	(90–111)	(87–114)	(92–114)	(93–112)
Calcium, mg/100 ml		9.3	8.4	7.8	8.0	7.9
		(8.2–11.1)	(7.3–9.2)	(6.9–9.4)	(6.1–9.9)	(5.9–9.7)
Phosphorus, mg/100 ml		5.6	6.1	5.7	5.9	5.8
		(3.7–8.1)	(3.5–8.6)	(2.9–8.1)	(3.0–8.7)	(2.8–7.6)
Blood urea, mg/100 ml		29	27	33	32	31
		(21–40)	(8–34)	(9–63)	(13–77)	(13–68)
Total protein, gm/100 ml		6.1	6.6	6.6	6.9	7.2
		(4.8–7.3)	(5.6–8.5)	(5.8–8.2)	(5.9–8.2)	(6.0–8.5)
Blood sugar, mg/100 ml		73	63	63	56	59
		(45–96)	(40–97)	(42–104)	(30–91)	(40–90)
Lactic acid, mg/100 ml		19.5	14.6	14.0	14.3	13.5
		(11–30)	(11–24)	(10–23)	(9–22)	(7–21)
Lactate, mm/l†		2.0–3.0	2.0			

* Acharya, P. T., and Payne, W. W.: Arch. Dis. Child. *40*:430, 1965.
† Daniel, S. S., et al.: Pediatrics *37*:942, 1966.

Normal Blood Chemistry Values, Low Birth Weight Infants, Capillary Blood, First Day

Determination	<1000	1001–1500	1501–2000	2001–2500
Sodium, mEq/l	138	133	135	134
Potassium, mEq/l	6.4	6.0	5.4	5.6
Chloride, mEq/l	100	101	105	104
Total CO$_2$, mEq/l	19	20	20	20
Urea, mg/100 ml	22	21	16	16
TSP, gm/100 ml	4.8	4.8	5.2	5.3

(Data from Pincus et al.: Pediatrics *18*:39, 1956.)

Mean ± SD of Serum Copper Concentrations (µg/dl) by Postconceptional Age in Premature Infants

	Weeks of Postconceptual Age										
	25–28	*29–30*	*31–32*	*33–34*	*35–36*	*37–38*	*39–40*	*41–42*	*43–44*	*45–46*	*47–60*
M	28.6	27.1	31.5	36.4	39.2	47.2	52.1	59.6	70.2	65.3	81.8
SD	17.1	14.9	17.5	14.6	13.8	24.1	11.6	21.1	28.1	15.8	18.0
N	16	27	35	43	33	22	20	18	18	9	4

(From Hillman, L. S.: J. Pediatr. *98*:305, 1981.)

Normal Values for Cerebrospinal Fluid*

	Prematures	Term Babies
Color	Xanthochromic mostly	Clear or xanthochromic
White cell count	8–10 (range 0–44)	6–8 (range 0–34)
Protein	180 mg per 100 ml (range 40–180)	45 mg per 100 ml (range 30–102)

Protein content, highest on the first day, tends to be under 50 mg per 100 ml by 1 month.
Sugar and chlorides must be compared with values in blood.

* Data from Samson: Ergebn. d. inn. Med. u. Kinderh. *41*:553, 1931; Otilia: Acta Paediatr. *35*:Suppl. 8, 1948; Bauer, C. H., et al.: J. Pediatr. *66*:1017, 1965; Wolf, H., and Hoepffuer, L.: World Neurol. *2*:871, 1961; and Widell, S.: Acta Paediatr. *47*:Suppl *115*, 1958.

Hematologic Values*

		1–3 days	4–7 days	2 weeks	4 weeks	6 weeks	8 weeks
<1200 gm birth weight	Hgb	15.6	16.4	15.5	11.3	8.5	7.8
	Retic	8.4	3.9	1.9	4.1	5.4	6.1
	Plat	148,000 ±61,000	163,000 ±69,000	162,000	158,000	210,000	212,000
	Leuk	14,800 ±10,200	12,200 ±7000	15,800	13,200	10,800	9900
	Seg	46	32	41	28	23	23
	Band	10.7	9.7	8.0	5.9	5.8	4.4
	Juv	2.0	3.9	5.3	3.6	2.6	2.0
	Lymph	32	43	39	55	61	65
	Monos	5	7	5	4	6	3
	Eos	0.4	6.2	1.0	3.7	2.0	3.8
	Nuc/RBC	16.7	1.1	0.1	1.0	2.7	2.0
>1200–1500 gm birth weight	Hgb	20.2	18.0	17.1	12.0	9.1	8.3
	Retic	2.7	1.2	0.9	1.0	2.2	2.7
	Plat	151,000 ±35,000	134,000 ±49,000	153,000	189,000	212,000	244,000
	Leuk	10,800 ±4000	8900 ±2900	14,300	11,000	10,500	9100
	Seg	47	31	33	26	20	25
	Band	11.9	10.5	5.9	3.0	1.4	2.1
	Juv	5.1	2.4	2.7	1.8	1.7	1.6
	Lymph	34	48	52	59	69	64
	Monos	3	6	3	4	5	5
	Eos	1.3	2.2	2.5	5.1	2.6	2.3
	Nuc/RBC	19.8	0.8	0	0.4	1.4	1.0

* Wolff and Goodfellow: Pediatrics *16*:753, 1955.

TERM NEWBORN

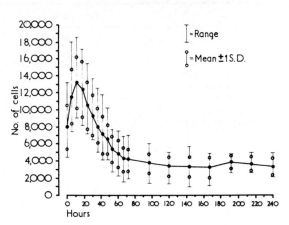

Means, ranges, and means ± 1 SD of neutrophils on 15 full-term healthy babies during the first 10 days of life.

PREMATURES

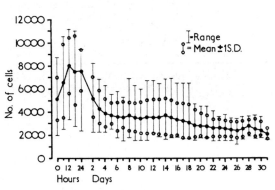

Means, ranges, and means ± 1 SD of neutrophils of 14 healthy babies during the first month of life (13 premature + 1 small for dates).

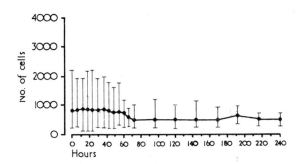

Means and ranges of the eosinophils of full-term babies during the first 10 days of life.

(Data of Xanthou, M.: Arch. Dis. Child. *45:*242, 1970.)

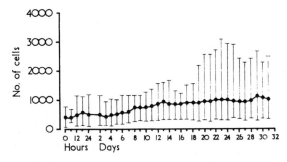

Means and ranges of eosinophils of low birth weight babies during the first month of life.

TERM NEWBORN

PREMATURES

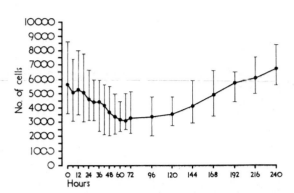

Means and ranges of lymphocytes of full-term babies during the first 10 days of life.

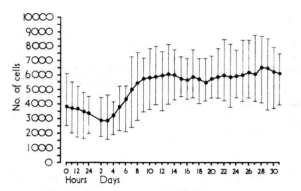

Means and ranges of lymphocytes of low birth weight babies during the first month of life.

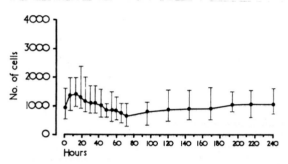

The mean and range of the monocytes of healthy full-term babies during the first 10 days of life.

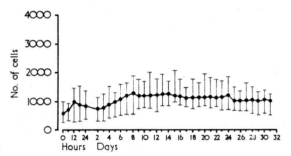

Means and ranges of monocytes of low birth weight babies during the first month of life.

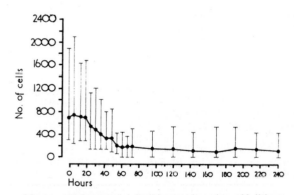

Means and ranges of metamyelocytes of full-term babies during the first 10 days of life.

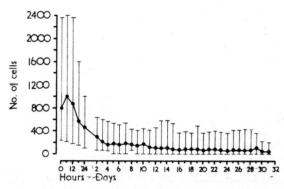

Means and ranges of metamyelocytes of 14 healthy babies during the first month of life.

(Data of Xanthou, M.: Arch. Dis. Child. 45: 242, 1970.)

Average Systolic, Diastolic, and Mean Blood Pressures during the First 12 Hours of Life in Normal Newborn Infants Grouped According to Birth Weight*

Birth Weight	Hour	1	2	3	4	5	6	7	8	9	10	11	12
1001 to 2000 gm	Systolic	49	49	51	52	53	52	52	52	51	51	49	50
	Diastolic	26	27	28	29	31	31	31	31	31	30	29	30
	Mean	35	36	37	39	40	40	39	39	38	37	37	38
2001 to 3000 gm	Systolic	59	57	60	60	61	58	64	60	63	61	60	59
	Diastolic	32	32	32	32	33	34	37	34	38	35	35	35
	Mean	43	41	43	43	44	43	45	43	44	44	43	42
Over 3000 gm	Systolic	70	67	65	65	66	66	67	67	68	70	66	66
	Diastolic	44	41	39	41	40	41	41	41	44	43	41	41
	Mean	53	51	50	50	51	50	50	51	53	54	51	50

* Kitterman, J. A., et al.: Pediatrics *44*:959, 1969.

Electrocardiographic Standards in Neonates*

Parameter	Age			
	0–24 hours	*1–2 days*	*3–6 days*	*7–30 days*
Number of patients	189	179	181	119
Heart rate (beats/min)	123 (99–148)	123 (97–149)	129 (101–161)	148 (115–177)
QRS axis (degree)	137 (91–185)	134 (93–190)	132 (91–186)	110 (76–151)
PR duration II (sec)	0.11 (.08–.14)	0.11 (.09–.13)	0.10 (.08–.13)	0.10 (.08–.13)
QRS duration V_5 (sec)	0.051 (.034–.069)	0.048 (.035–.060)	0.049 (.034–.063)	0.053 (.037–.076)
QT duration V_5 (msec)	0.29 (.22–.36)	0.28 (.24–.33)	0.27 (.23–.31)	0.26 (.23–.29)
P amplitude II (mvolts)	0.16 (.08–.25)	0.16 (.05–.25)	0.17 (.08–.27)	0.19 (0.09–0.29)
R amplitude V_{3R} (mvolts)	1.10 (0.42–1.86)	1.20 (0.53–2.00)	1.05 (0.16–1.82)	0.85 (0.28–1.60)
R amplitude V_1 (mvolts)	1.38 (0.62–2.36)	1.44 (0.64–2.45)	1.29 (0.50–2.14)	1.06 (0.44–1.88)
R amplitude V_5 (mvolts)	1.02 (0.25–1.88)	1.08 (0.45–1.98)	1.18 (0.45–1.94)	1.40 (0.61–2.09)
R amplitude V_6 (mvolts)	0.42 (0.03–0.96)	0.45 (0.05–0.98)	0.52 (0.08–1.05)	0.76 (0.31–1.38)
S amplitude V_{3R} (mvolts)	0.43 (0.04–1.18)	0.50 (0.04–1.20)	0.33 (0.03–0.79)	0.20 (0.02–0.55)
S amplitude V_1 (mvolts)	0.84 (0.09–1.85)	0.91 (0.14–1.90)	0.65 (0.06–1.48)	0.41 (0.04–0.95)
S amplitude V_5 (mvolts)	0.99 (0.35–1.78)	0.97 (0.20–1.58)	0.94 (0.38–1.67)	0.80 (0.26–1.35)
S amplitude V_6 (mvolts)	0.32 (0.03–0.78)	0.30 (0.03–0.75)	0.35 (0.04–0.80)	0.34 (0.04–0.84)
R/S amplitude V_{3R}	1.5 (0.3–4.8)	1.6 (0.3–4.2)	1.9 (0.2–5.8)	1.9 (0.2–4.5)
R/S amplitude V_1	2.24 (0.32–7.03)	1.96 (.31–5.31)	2.71 (0.40–7.43)	2.85 (1.11–6.37)
R/S amplitude V_5	0.7 (.0–7.0)	1.0 (0–5.0)	1.5 (0–5.0)	2.0 (0–5.1)
R/S amplitude V_6	1.97 (0.27–7.04)	2.49 (0.3–9.04)	2.15 (0.28–8.05)	3.29 (0.31–9.24)

* Mean with 5 per cent and 95 per cent values in parentheses.
(From Davignon, A., et al: Normal ECG standards for infants and children. Pediatr. Cardiol. *1*:123, 1979/80.)

Representative Values in Normal Infants at Term

	Umbilical vein	Arterial Blood					Reference
		30 min	1–4 hr	12–24 hr	24–48 hr	96 hr	
pH	7.33		7.30	7.30	7.39	7.39	
P_{CO_2} mm Hg	43		39	33	34	36	Reardon et al., 1960
HCO_3 mEq/l	21.6		18.8	19.5	20	21.4	Oliver et al., 1961
P_{O_2} mm Hg	28 ± 8		62 ± 13.8	68	63–87		Nelson et al., 1962,
O_2 saturation			95%	94%	94%	96%	1963
Crying vital capacity ml (for 3-kg infant)		77 (range, 56–110)			92 (69–128)	100	Sutherland and Ratcliff, 1961
Functional residual capacity, ml/kg		22 ± 8	25 ± 8	21 ± 1	28 ± 7	39 ± 9	Klaus et al., 1962
Lung compliance ml/cm H_2O/kg		1.5 ± 0.05		2.0 ± 0.4		1.7	Cook et al., 1957
Lung compliance/FRC ml/cm H_2O/ml			0.04 ± 0.10	.053 ± 0.009		0.065	Chu et al., 1964 Cook et al., 1957
Right to left shunt as percentage cardiac output			22% (range 11–29%)	24% (17–32%)			Prod'hom et al., 1964

		Comment	Reference
Respiratory frequency	34/min. range 20–60	1–2 days 1–11 days	Cook et al., 1955 Cross, 1949
Resistances cm H_2O/l/sec	29, 26 18 ± 6/3	Total lung resistance Airway resistance	Cook et al. 1949; Swyer et al., 1960; Polgar, 1962
Flow rates ml/sec	48–37 161–106	Max. insp., max. exp. rest crying	Swyer et al., 1957; Long and Hull, 1961
Ventilation ml/kg/min	200		Cook et al., 1955; Nelson et al., 1962
Dead space ml	4.4–9.2	Term infants	Nelson et al., 1962; Cook et al., 1955; Strang, 1961
Alveolar ventilation ml/kg/min	120–145	First 3 days of life	Nelson et al., 1962
O_2 consumption ml/kg/min	6.2	At neutral temperature	Oliver and Karlberg, 1963
CO_2 production ml/kg/min	5.1	At neutral temperature	Oliver and Karlberg, 1963
Alveolar-arterial O_2 differences mm Hg	28 ± 10, room air 311 ± 70, 100% O_2	Age 7 hr to 42 days Age 6 to 58 hr, 3 infants	Nelson et al., 1963
Arterial-alveolar CO_2 differences mm Hg	1.8 ± 3.8	Age 3 to 74 hours	Nelson et al., 1962

(From Avery, M. E., and Normand, C.: Anesthesiology 26: 510, 1965.)

Correlations Between Gestational Length and Embryonic and Fetal Bodily Dimensions

Week of Gestation	Crown-rump Length (cm)	Weight (gm)	Biparietal Diameter (cm)
6	0.5		
7	0.8	0.07	
8	1.5	0.22	
9	2.5	0.88	
10	3.5	3.5	
11	4.6	6.0	
12	5.7	11.0	
13	6.8	19.0	
14	8.1	33.0	
15	9.4	55.0	
16	10.7	80.0	
17	12.1	120.0	3.7
18	13.6	170.0	4.0
19	15.3	253.0	4.4
20	16.4	316.0	4.8
21	17.5	385.0	5.2
22	18.6	460.0	5.5
23	19.7	542.0	5.75
24	20.8	630.0	5.95
25	21.8	723.0	6.1
26	22.8	823.0	6.2
27	23.8	930.0	6.35
28	24.7	1045.0	6.5
29	25.6	1174.0	6.65
30	26.5	1323.0	6.85
31	27.4	1492.0	7.1
32	28.3	1680.0	7.3
33	29.3	1876.0	7.6
34	30.2	2074.0	7.8
35	31.1	2274.0	8.1
36	32.1	2478.0	8.35
37	33.1	2690.0	8.6
38	34.1	2914.0	8.9
39	35.1	3150.0	9.2
40	36.2	3405.0	9.55
41		3600.0	9.8
42		3650.0	9.85
		3750.0	10.0
		3900.0	10.2
		4000.0	10.3
		4200.0	10.6

(Data based on the study of Bartolucci, L.: Am. J. Obstet. Gynecol. *122*:439, 1975. Courtesy of Iffy, L., et al.: Pediatrics *56*;173, 1975.)

Temperature Equivalents

Celsius	Fahrenheit	Celsius	Fahrenheit
34.0	93.2	38.6	101.4
34.2	93.6	38.8	101.8
34.4	93.9	39.0	102.2
34.6	94.3	39.2	102.5
34.8	94.6	39.4	102.9
35.0	95.0	39.6	103.2
35.2	95.4	39.8	103.6
35.4	95.7	40.0	104.0
35.6	96.1	40.2	104.3
35.8	96.4	40.4	104.7
36.0	96.8	40.6	105.1
36.2	97.1	40.8	105.4
36.4	97.5	41.0	105.8
36.6	97.8	41.2	106.1
36.8	98.2	41.4	106.5
37.0	98.6	41.6	106.8
37.2	98.9	41.8	107.2
37.4	99.3	42.0	107.6
37.6	99.6	42.2	108.0
37.8	100.0	42.4	108.3
38.0	100.4	42.6	108.7
38.2	100.7	42.8	109.0
38.4	101.1	43.0	109.4

To convert Celsius to Fahrenheit:

$9/5 \times$ Temperature $+ 32$

Example: To convert 40° Celsius to Fahrenheit
$9/5 \times 40 = 72 + 32 = 104°$ Fahrenheit

To convert Fahrenheit to Celsius

(Temperature minus 32) $\times 5/9$

Example: To convert 98.6° Fahrenheit to Celsius
$98.6 - 32 = 66.6 \times 5/9 = 37°$ Celsius

Conversion of Pounds and Ounces to Grams

Ounces	1 lb	2 lb	3 lb	4 lb	5 lb	6 lb	7 lb	8 lb
	Grams							
0	454	907	1361	1814	2268	2722	3175	3629
1	482	936	1389	1843	2296	2750	3204	3657
2	510	964	1418	1871	2325	2778	3232	3686
3	539	992	1446	1899	2353	2807	3260	3714
4	567	1021	1474	1928	2381	2835	3289	3742
5	595	1049	1503	1956	2410	2863	3317	3771
6	624	1077	1531	1985	2438	2892	3345	3799
7	652	1106	1559	2013	2466	2920	3374	3827
8	680	1134	1588	2041	2495	2948	3402	3856
9	709	1162	1616	2070	2523	2977	3430	3884
10	737	1191	1644	2098	2552	3005	3459	3912
11	765	1219	1673	2126	2580	3033	3487	3941
12	794	1247	1701	2155	2608	3062	3515	3969
13	822	1276	1729	2183	2637	3090	3544	3997
14	851	1304	1758	2211	2665	3119	3572	4026
15	879	1332	1786	2240	2693	3147	3600	4054

Body Composition of the Reference Fetus

Gestational Age (weeks)	Body Weight (gm)	per 100 gm body weight				per 100 gm fat-free weight							
		Water (gm)	Protein (gm)	Lipid (gm)	Other (gm)	Water (gm)	Protein (gm)	Ca (mg)	P (mg)	Mg (mg)	Na (meq)	K (meq)	Cl (meq)
24	690	88.6	8.8	0.1	2.5	88.6	8.8	621	387	17.8	9.9	4.0	7.0
25	770	87.8	9.0	0.7	2.5	88.4	9.1	615	385	17.6	9.8	4.0	7.0
26	880	86.8	9.2	1.5	2.5	88.1	9.4	611	384	17.5	9.7	4.1	7.0
27	1010	85.7	9.4	2.4	2.5	87.8	9.7	609	383	17.4	9.6	4.1	6.9
28	1160	84.6	9.6	3.3	2.4	87.5	10.0	610	385	17.4	9.4	4.2	6.9
29	1318	83.6	9.9	4.1	2.4	87.2	10.3	613	387	17.4	9.3	4.2	6.8
30	1480	82.6	10.1	4.9	2.4	86.8	10.6	619	392	17.4	9.2	4.3	6.8
31	1650	81.7	10.3	5.6	2.4	86.5	10.9	628	398	17.6	9.1	4.3	6.7
32	1830	80.7	10.6	6.3	2.4	86.1	11.3	640	406	17.8	9.1	4.3	6.6
33	2020	79.8	10.8	6.9	2.5	85.8	11.6	656	416	18.0	9.0	4.4	6.5
34	2230	79.0	11.0	7.5	2.5	85.4	11.9	675	428	18.3	8.9	4.4	6.4
35	2450	78.1	11.2	8.1	2.6	85.0	12.2	699	443	18.6	8.9	4.5	6.3
36	2690	77.3	11.4	8.7	2.6	84.6	12.5	726	460	19.0	8.8	4.5	6.1
37	2940	76.4	11.6	9.3	2.7	84.3	12.8	758	479	19.5	8.8	4.5	6.0
38	3160	75.6	11.8	9.9	2.7	83.9	13.1	795	501	20.0	8.8	4.5	5.9
39	3330	74.8	11.9	10.5	2.8	83.6	13.3	836	525	20.5	8.7	4.6	5.8
40	3450	74.0	12.0	11.2	2.8	83.3	13.5	882	551	21.1	8.7	4.6	5.7

(Data of Ziegler, E. E., et al.: Iowa City, University of Iowa, 1975.)

Infant Age at First Tooth Eruption

Group	Gestational Age (wk)	No. of Infants	Chronologic Age (wk)		Postconceptual Age (wk)	
			Mean ± SD	Median	Mean ± SD	Median
1	26–28	8	44.6 ± 13.7	44.0	70.2 ± 13.8	70.0
2	29–31	24	41.7 ± 8.7	42.0	69.8 ± 8.6	70.0
3	32–34	50	34.9 ± 8.5	34.5	66.2 ± 8.3	66.5
4	35–37	47	34.2 ± 9.2	35.0	68.3 ± 9.1	69.0
5	38–40	38	31.9 ± 8.1	30.5	69.4 ± 8.1	67.5

(From Golden, N. L., Takieddine, F., and Hirsch, V. J., Jr.: Am. J. Dis. Child. 135:903, 1981.)

Conversion of Inches to Centimeters

Inches	cm	Inches	cm	Inches	cm
10	25.40	15	38.10	20	50.80
10½	26.67	15½	39.37	20½	52.07
11	27.94	16	40.64	21	53.34
11½	29.21	16½	41.91	21½	54.61
12	30.48	17	43.18	22	55.88
12½	31.75	17½	44.45	22½	57.15
13	33.02	18	45.72	23	58.42
13½	34.29	18½	46.99	23½	56.69
14	35.56	19	48.26	24	60.96
14½	36.83	19½	49.53		

Concentration of Various Drugs in Maternal Blood and Breast Milk Under Normal pH Conditions

Drug Administered (Therapeutic Dosage)	Drug Levels (unit/100 ml)		Administered Drug Appearing in Milk (%/day)
	Plasma or Serum (pH 7.4)	Milk (pH 7.0)	
Aspirin	1–5 mg	1–3 mg	0.5
Bishydroxycoumarin	11–16.5 mg	0.2 mg	0.5
Chloral hydrate	0–3 mg	0–1.5 mg	0.6
Chloramphenicol	2.5–5 mg	1.5–2.5 mg	1.3
Chlorpromazine	0.1 mg	0.03 mg	0.07
Colistin sulfate	0.3–0.5 mg	0.05–0.09 mg	0.07
Cycloserine	1.5–2 mg	1–1.5 mg	0.6
Diphenylhydantoin	0.3–4.5 mg	0.6–1.8 mg	1.4
Erythromycin	0.1–0.2 mg	0.3–0.5 mg	0.1
Ethanol	50–80 mg	50–80 mg	0.25
Ethyl biscoumacetate	2.7–14.5 mg	0–0.17 mg	0.1
Folic acid	3 μg	0.07 μg	0.1
Imipramine hydrochloride	0.2–1.3 mg	0.1 mg	0.1
Iodine 131	0.002 μc	0.13 μc	2–5
Isoniazid	0.6–1.2 mg	0.6–1.2 mg	0.75
Kanamycin sulfate	0.5–3.5 mg	0.2 mg	0.05
Lincomycin	0.3–1.5 mg	0.05–0.2 mg	0.025
Lithium carbonate	0.2–1.1 mg	0.07–0.4 mg	0.12
Meperidine hydrochloride	0.07–0.1 mg	trace (<0.1 mg)	<0.1
Methotrexate	3 μg	0.3 μg	0.01
Nalidixic acid	3–5 mg	0.4 mg	0.05
Novobiocin	1.3 5.2 mg	0.3–0.5 mg	0.15
Penicillin	6–120 μg	1.2–3.6 μg	0.03
Phenobarbital	0.6–1.8 mg	0.1–0.5 mg	1.5
Phenylbutazone	2–5 mg	0.2–0.6 mg	0.4
Pyrilamine maleate	–	0.2 mg	0.6
Pyrimethamine	0.7–1.5 mg	0.3 mg	0.3
Quinine sulfate	0.7 mg	0.1 mg	0.05
Rifampin	0.5 mg	0.1–0.3 mg	0.05
Streptomycin sulfate	2–3 mg	1–3 mg	0.5
Sulfapyridine	3–13 mg	3–13 mg	0.12
Tetracycline hydrochloride	80–320 μg	50–260 μg	0.03
Thiouracil	3–4 mg	9–12 mg	5

(Modified from Vorherr, H.: The Breast: Morphology, Physiology, and Lactation. New York, Academic Press, Inc., 1974.)

Note: Page numbers in *italics* refer to illustrations; references to tables include the designation *t*.

Index

Abdomen, assessment of, in newborn, 59
distention of, in intestinal obstruction, 350
Abdominal mass, 447
renal, differential diagnosis of, 447–451
Abdominal musculature, absence of, 414–417, *415*
Abdominal wall, defect of, 377, 378, *378*
Abducens nerve, birth injury of, 667
ABO incompatibility, hemolysis with, 593
clinical and laboratory features of, *591t*
Abortion, spontaneous and induced, complications of, 14
Abscess, brain, 713
breast, neonatal, 744
spinal epidural, 713
Acetazolamide, route and dose for, 971
Achalasia, 339
cricopharyngeal, 339
Achondrogenesis, 820–822
Achondroplasia, 820, *820*
Acid-base disturbances, in neonatal period, 49
Acidemia
argininosuccinic, 545
isovaleric, 549
methylmalonic, 551
propionic, 549–551, *550*
pyruvic, 551
Acidosis, metabolic, in acute renal failure, 460
renal tubular, distal, 400
proximal, 399
Aciduria, glutaric, 551–552
Acne neonatorum, 898–899, *898*
Acrocephalosyndactyly, 692, *692*, 692t
Acrofacial dysostosis, Nager, 817, 832
ACTH, route and dose for, 970
Adenoma, islet cell, hypoglycemia with, 520
Adenomatoid dysplasia, hypoglycemia with, 520
Adenomatoid malformation, cystic, of lung, 204
Adenosine deaminase (ADA) deficiency, in severe combined immune deficiency, 726, *726*
Adhesions, peritoneal, intestinal obstruction and, 367
preputial, 402
Adrenal glands
disorders of, 479–490
hemorrhage of, 481–482, *482*
hyperplasia of, congenital, 483
newborn screening for, 66
virilization due to, 509
hypoplasia of, 483
insufficiency of, hypercalcemia with, 474
transient, 482–483
overactivity of, 487
Adrenalin, route and dose for, 970
Aerobacter, pneumonia due to, 177

Afterload reduction, in congestive heart failure, 240
Agammaglobulinemia, 725
Aganglionosis, congenital, 368–371
intestinal obstruction and, 349
Age, gestational. See *Gestational age.*
maternal, effect on fetus/newborn, 9
prenatal cytogenetics and, 25
Aglossia congenita, 320
Agranulocytosis, congenital, 578
Air leak and trapping, 154–161
Airway pressure, continuous distending (CDAP), 217–218
optimal level of, 217, *217*
Albinism, 870–871
partial, 871–872, *871*
Albright's syndrome, 891
Albumin, in urine, 396
route and dose for, 970
Alcohol, maternal intake of, newborn abnormalities and, 13, *13*
teratogenic and carcinogenic effects of, 930t, 932
Aldactone, route and dose for, 973
Aldomet, route and dose for, 972
Aldosterone, end-organ unresponsiveness to, hyponatremia and, 488
Alimentary tract, normal rotation of, 347, *348*
Allantois, formation of, 378, *378*
Alpha$_1$-antitrypsin deficiency, hyperbilirubinemia with, conjugated, 645
Alpha-fetoprotein
analysis of, in amniotic fluid, 29
in maternal serum, 27, 30
methodology of, 29
problems of, 33
elevated, conditions associated with, 29t
levels of, as function of gestational age, 29, *30*
Alpha thalassemia, 602, 603t
Altitude, fetal size and, 95
Alveolar proteinosis, pulmonary, 188
Amikacin, route and dose for, 970
Amino acids, evaluation of levels of, in renal function, 399
inborn errors of metabolism of, 536–548
Amniocele, 375–376, *375, 376*
Amniorrhexis, 15–16
Amniotic fluid, 18
alpha-fetoprotein analysis of, 29
bilirubin estimation of, in hemolytic disease, 592, *592*
constituents of, 18t
fetal surfactant lipids in, tests for, 41, *42*
noninvasive sampling of, 31
sample acquisition of, risk of, 24
Amphotericin B, route and dose for, 970
Ampicillin, route and dose for, 970
Androgens, maternal overproduction of, virilization of female fetus by, 508

Anemia
approach to, general, 584–586
blood transfusions in, 586
Fanconi's, 572, 831
hemolytic, 589, 589t
acquired, 594
hereditary, 594–605
immune. See *Hemolysis, immune.*
vitamin E deficiency and, 809
hemorrhagic, 586–589, 587t
hypoplastic, 605–606
in hiatus hernia, 329
laboratory evaluation of, 584, 584t
of prematurity, 606–608
iron supplementation in, 608t
vitamin E supplementation in, 608t
physiologic, of infancy, 606
sickle cell, 604
Anencephaly, 680
Anesthesia, during childbirth, 21
Aneurysm, cirsoid, 889
intracranial, congenital, 714, *714*
Angiocardiography, 235–238
angled views in, 237t
Angiosarcoma, of liver, 941
Aniridia, with Wilms' tumor, 930, 938
chromosome deletion in, 852
Anisometropia, 915
Ankyloglossia superior, 318, *858*, 859
Anorchia, 406, 509
Anorexia, 317
Antibiotics, dosage regimens for, 730t
rational usage of, in neonate, 729–730
Antibody, passively acquired by fetus, 721t
Anticonvulsants, 705, 964
Antidiuretic hormone, inappropriate secretion of, hyponatremia and, 488
Antigen K1, neonatal meningitis and, 731
septicemia due to, 734
Antihypertensive agents, 445, 445t, 960, 960t
Antimetabolites, teratogenic effects of, 12
Antithrombins, 561
Anus, congenital deformities of, 356–358
imperforate, urogenital abnormalities and, 413
Aorta
ascending, systemic hypertension in, 237
coarctation of, 267–270, *268, 269*
differential diagnosis of, 287, 288
pressures in, normal, 237t
Aortic arch, anomalies of, 125
interrupted, 270–272, *271*
differential diagnosis of, 287
Aortic atresia, with hypoplastic left ventricle, 274–276, *274, 275*
Aortic stenosis, 272–274, *273*
differential diagnosis of, 287, 288
Aortopulmonary window, vs. patent ductus arteriosus, 288
Apert's syndrome, 692, *692*, 692t
Apgar scoring system, 103, 103t, 111
management based on, 105t

Aplasia cutis congenitalis, 687, 872, *872*
Apneic spells, 116
   neurologic dysfunction and, 676
   sleep states related to, 116, 116*t*
   theophylline and caffeine therapy of,
     963, 963*t*
Appendicitis, acute, 388
Apresoline, route and dose for, 971
Apt test, 316, 562
Arachnodactyly, congenital contractural,
   vs. Marfan syndrome, 827
Argininemia, 546
Argininosuccinic acidemia, 545
Arnold-Chiari malformation,
   hydrocephaly and, 695
   with meningomyelocele, *683*
Arrhythmia, sinus, 304
Arteriovenous fistular malformation, 889
   congestive heart failure and, 284, *285*,
     287
Arteritis, umbilical, septic, 374
Artery(ies). See names of specific arteries.
Arthritis, septic, 741–742
Arthrogryposis, 708
Arthrogryposis multiplex congenita, 835–
   836, *835, 836*
Ascites, chylous, 388–389
   fetal/neonatal, 386–391
   with posterior urethral valve, 432
Ascorbic acid, deficiency of, 805–807,
   806
   route and dose for, 970
Ask-Upmark kidney, 422
Asphyxia, neonatal, clinical findings in,
   588*t*
   treatment of, 104–107
   perinatal, neurologic consequences of,
     662, 669–679
Asphyxiating thoracic dysplasia, 197,
   198, 826
Aspiration, 128–133
   after birth, 131
   in utero, 129
   lung pathology in, 128, *129*
   meconium, 129
     suctioning of, 107, 129
   pneumonia due to, 173–174
Aspirin, abnormal platelet function and,
   573
   concentration of, in maternal blood
     and breast milk, 993
Asplenia, 265, *266*
Astigmatism, 915
Asymmetric crying facies, 667
Atabrine, route and dose for, 970
Atria, mean pressure elevation in, 236
   normal pressures in, 237*t*
Atrial flutter, 306, *306*
Atrioventricular block, 306–308, *307*
Atrioventricular canal, complete, 282,
   282, 283
Atropine, for resuscitation of newborn,
   106
   route and dose for, 970
Audiometry, brain-stem–evoked
   response, 659
Auditory response, neonatal, 72
Autosomal inheritance, dominant and
   recessive, 863
   disorders of, prenatal diagnosis of,
     28

Axial triradius, position of, 847
Axon, diseases of, 708

Bacitracin, route and dose for, 970
Back, assessment of, in newborn, 59
Bacterial infection, 729–747, 748–754
   nosocomial, 744–746
Bacterial peritonitis, 387–388
Bacteriuria, 740–741
Balloon atrial septostomy, in transposition
   of great arteries, 248
Basal ganglia, lesions of, due to perinatal
   asphyxia, 672
BCG, role of, in newborns, 749
Beckwith's syndrome, 320–321
   hypoglycemia with, 520
Behavior, neonatal, 68–82
   evaluation of, 77–78
   heart rate as measure of, 74–75
   intrauterine influences on, 68–69
   motor, organization of, 69–70
   sensory, 70–74
   social, 78–79
   state of, 68, 75–77
     breathing patterns in, 114, *115,*
     116
Belladonna tincture, route and dose for,
   970
Benadryl, route and dose for, 971
Beriberi, 802–803, *803*
Beta thalassemia, 603
Betamethasone, in utero exposure to,
   leukemoid reaction to, 933
Bile peritonitis, 388
Bile-plug syndrome, 646
Biliary atresia, liver biopsy in, *638,* 639
   obstructive jaundice due to, 637–641
   of intrahepatic ducts, 640
Bilirubin
   amniotic fluid levels of, in hemolytic
     disease, 592, *592*
   fetal metabolism of, 624
   formation and excretion of, 622–624,
     622, 623
   serum, concentrations for exchange
     transfusion, 628*t*
     highest total of, in newborns, 625*t*,
     626*t*
     in anemia, 586
    levels of, factors influencing, 626–
     627
Biopterin synthetase deficiency, *537,* 539
Birth injury
   abnormal presentation and, 19, 20*t*
   due to asphyxia, *662,* 669–679
   due to perinatal trauma, 661–669
   epiphyseal, in breech delivery, 841–
     842, *842*
   fractures, 840–841
Birth weight
   genetic regulation of, 45, 47*t*
   low. See also *Prematurity.*
     feeding of infant with, 791–797
     for gestational age, 45
     normal blood chemistry values for,
     984
     nutrient supply in, methods of, 793–
     797
     nutritional requirements of, 792
   maternal conditions related to, 16*t*
   measurement of, 56
   ultrasonographic estimation of, 37, 38
Bishydroxycoumarin, concentration of, in
   maternal blood and breast milk, 993

Blackfan-Diamond syndrome, 605
Bladder
   diverticula of, hydronephrosis and, 431
   exstrophy of, 411–413, *412*
   neurogenic, 431
   outlet obstruction of, 431–434
Blastema, renal, persistent, 940
Bleeding. See *Hemorrhage.*
Bleeding time, 562, 563*t*
Blennorrhea, inclusion, 919
Block-Sulzberger syndrome, 872–873,
   873
Blood
   clotting factors in. See *Clotting factors.*
   disorders of, 559–619
   fetal, oxygen content of, 225, *225*
     vs. maternal, Apt test for, 316, 562
   maternal, drug concentrations in, 993
   oxygen saturation of, after birth, 226,
     226
     fetal, 225, *225*
   packed cells, route and dose for, 970
   whole, route and dose for, 970
Blood chemistry values, normal, 984
Blood pressure, average, during first 12
   hours in newborn, 988
   measuring of, in neonate, 228
   normal newborn values of, 56
Blood smear, peripheral, 585
Blood sugar, newborn levels of, 514–
   515, *515*
   normal values for, 984
Blood transfusion. See *Transfusion.*
Blood urea, normal values for, 984
Blood vessels, disorders of, 559–619
Blood volume, placental/neonatal, factors
   determining, 20*t*
Blue diaper syndrome, 473
Blue nevi, 891
Blue rubber bleb nevus syndrome, 889
B lymphocyte, 723
Body compartments, pharmacokinetic,
   953, *954*
Body composition, fetal, 46, *47,* 48*t*, 991
   of premature infant, nutritional
     implications of, 791–792
Bohn's nodules, 318
Bone
   chondrodystrophies of, 820–826, 821*t*
   congenital defects involving, 827–832
   long, congenital bowing and angulation
     of, 839, *839, 840*
   tuberculosis of, multiple pseudocystic,
     750
Bone marrow, hypoplasia of,
   thrombocytopenia due to, 572
   transplantation of, 727
Bone metabolism, disorders of, 464–479
Botulism, infant, 709, 752
Bowel. See *Intestine.*
Bowing reflex, in anencephalics, 680
Brachial plexus palsy, due to birth injury,
   667–669, *668*
Brachycephaly, 692*t*
Bradycardia, sinus, 304
Brain
   abscess of, 713
   cystic degeneration of, 670, *671*
   damage of, due to perinatal asphyxia,
     662, 669–679
   periventricular leukomalacia of, 671,
     671
   tumor of, congenital, 714–715
   watershed pattern of, 671, *671*
Brain stem, circulatory lesions of, due to
   perinatal asphyxia, 672

Brain-stem–evoked response audiometry, 659
Branchial arch, anomalous developments of, 321
Branchial arch syndromes, 816–818
Breast abscess, neonatal, 744
Breast-feeding
  basics of, 790
  drugs contraindicated for, 789t
  hyperbilirubinemia and, 627, 789
  non-nutritional advantages of, 787–790
  trends in, 785, 785t, 786t
Breast milk
  calories from, 785t
  composition of, 974
  drug concentrations in, 993
  for low birth weight infant, 793
  nutritional differences of, vs. cow's milk and formula, 785–787, 786t
Breathing
  apneic, 116
  fetal, 111
  initial respiratory effort of, 111, 112, 113
  patterns of, 114–116
  periodic, 114
Breech delivery, complications associated with, 18, 18t
  epiphyseal injuries in, 841–842, 842
  vs. vertex vaginal, neonatal problems in, 18t
Bronchial stenosis, 124
Bronchogenic cyst, 206–208, 207, 208
Bronchopulmonary dysplasia, 148–149, 149
  with mechanical ventilation, 141, 142, 220
Burn, severe, hyponatremia and, 488

Café-au-lait spots, 890, 890
Caffeine, for neonatal apnea, 963, 963t
  half-life and therapeutic levels of, 954t
  route and dose for, 970
Calcaneovalgus deformity, 836, 837
Calcitonin, control of calcium and phosphate metabolism by, 464
  parathyroid hormone and, 465
Calcium
  concentration of, in acute renal failure, 460
  estimated daily requirements of, in premature, 980
  metabolism of, endocrine control of, 464–465
  perinatal, 465–466
  normal blood chemistry values for, 984
Calcium glubionate, route and dose for, 972
Calcium gluconate, route and dose for, 970
Calcium lactate, route and dose for, 970
Calories, percentage obtained from feedings, 785t
  requirements for, in low birth weight infant, 792t
Campomelic dwarfism, 822
Candidiasis, 771–774, 881–883, 881, 882
  congenital, 772
  conjunctival, 920
  disseminated, 771
  enteric, 773
  vs. acne neonatorum, 899

Cap disease, 711t
Captopril, 961
Caput medusae, 380, 380
Caput succedaneum, 662, 663
Carbamyl phosphate synthetase (CPS) deficiency, 545
Carbenicillin, route and dose for, 970
Carbohydrate metabolism, disorders of, 514–523
  inborn errors of, 529–536
Carcinoma, hepatocellular, 941
Cardiac catheterization, 235–238
Cardiomyopathy, 291–303
  hypertrophic, of infant of diabetic mother, 298–299
Cardiorespiratory conversion, hemodynamics of, 101, 226, 227
Cardiothoracic ratio, 231
Cardiovascular drugs, 957–961
Cardiovascular system, disorders of, 223–308
  evaluation of, in neonate, 227–238
Carpenter's syndrome, 692t
Casts, in urinary tract disorders, 397
Cataract, congenital, 915, 915
Cat-eye syndrome, 850
Catheterization, cardiac, 235–238
Cat's cry syndrome, 852
CDAP (continuous distending airway pressure), 217–218
  optimal level of, 217, 217
Cellulitis, orbital, 921
Centimeter, conversion of inches to, 993
Central core disease, 711t
Cephalhematoma, 662–664, 663
Cephalothin, route and dose for, 970
"Cerebral cry," in hydrocephalus, 696
Cerebrospinal fluid, examination of, in meningitis, 736
  in newborn, 656–658
  normal values for, 985
Cerebrospinal fluid–to-ureter shunting, hyponatremia and, 488
Cesarean section, effects on fetus/newborn, 16–18
  hyaline membrane disease risk with, 135
  neonatal respiratory problems and, 17, 17t
Chediak-Higashi syndrome, 580
Chemotaxis, 575, 576
Chest, assessment of, in newborn, 58
Chest wall, disorders of, 197–199
Childbirth, anesthesia during, 21
Chlamydia, conjunctivitis caused by, 742, 919
Chlamydia trachomatis pneumonia, 177
Chloral hydrate, concentration of, in maternal blood and breast milk, 993
  route and dose for, 970
Chloramphenicol, concentration of, in maternal blood and breast milk, 993
  half-life and therapeutic levels of, 954t
  route and dose for, 970
Chloride, normal blood chemistry values for, 984
Chloromycetin, route and dose for, 970
Chlorothiazide, as antihypertensive, 960t
  route and dose for, 970
Chlorpromazine, concentration of, in maternal blood and breast milk, 993
  route and dose for, 970
Choanal atresia, bilateral, 120
  unilateral, 120
Choledochal cyst, 640–641

Cholestasis, 644
  with intravenous alimentation, 797
Chondrodysplasia punctata, 823–824, 825
Chondrodystrophies, 820–826, 821t
Chondroectodermal dysplasia, 824–826, 825
Choriocarcinoma, transplacental passage of, 929
Choristoma, 923–924, 923
Choroid plexus, hydrocephalus in, 696
  papilloma of, 715
Chotzen's syndrome, 692t
Christmas disease, 566
Chromosomal aberrations, gross, 9, 846–853
  maternal age and, 25
  recurrence risk of, 862
Chromosomal rearrangement, balanced, prenatal diagnosis of, 26, 27
Chromosome, "fragile X," prenatal screening for, 29
Chromosome deletion syndromes, 852–853
Chylothorax, 213
Chylous ascites, 388–389
Cilia, immotile syndrome of, 188
Cimetidine, route and dose for, 970
Circulation
  fetal, 101
  neonatal cardiovascular changes and, 224–227
  persistent, 102, 161–164
  transitional, 226–227
Circulatory system, conversion of, at birth, 101, 226, 227
Circumcision, surgical, 401–402
Cirsoid aneurysm, 889
Citrullinemia, 545
Clavicles, fracture of, during delivery, 840
Cleft, laryngotracheoesophageal, 336–337
Cleft lip, 818–819
Cleft palate, 819
Cleidocranial dysostosis, 830–831, 830
Cloacal exstrophy, 413
Clotting factors, 561t
  concentrates of, 563
  hereditary deficiencies of, 564–566
  in newborn, 563t
Cloverleaf skull, 691, 692t
Clubfeet, congenital, 838, 838
Coagulation
  disseminated intravascular (DIC), 566–568, 567t
  hemolytic component of, 594
  localized intravascular, 568
  of newborn, 563t
Coccidioidomycosis, 769
Cockayne-Touraine variant, of epidermolysis bullosa, 875
Coliform conjunctivitis, 920
Colistin sulfate, concentration of, in maternal blood and breast milk, 993
Collodion baby, 869, 869
Colon. See also Intestine.
  atresia of, 355
  cyst of, 356
  duplication of, 356
  function of, 314
Complement system, 724

Congenital malformation, 9
  constellations of, 845–865
  involving bones, 827–832
  involving joints, 833–838
  malignant, 928–947
  recurrence risk of, determining of, 862–864
Conjunctivitis, 918–921
  chlamydial, 742, 919
  coliform, 920
  differential diagnosis of, 742
  gonococcal, 742, 919, *920*
  herpes simplex, 920
  ligneous, 921
  staphylococcal, 920
  streptococcal, 920
Conradi-Hunerman chondrodysplasia punctata, 824
Conradi's syndrome, ichthyosis with, 870
Constipation, 316
Convulsions, in newborn, 676
Coombs' test, 586
Copper, deficiency of, 810–811
  serum concentrations of, in premature infants, 984
Corneal opacity, causes of, at birth, 916t
Coronal synostosis, bilateral, 689, *691*
Coronary artery, anomalous left, vs. glycogen storage disease of heart, 300
Cortisone, route and dose for, 970
Coumadin, teratogenic effects of, 12
Counterimmunoelectrophoresis, in diagnosis of bacterial meningitis, 736
Cow's milk, calories from, 785t
  composition of, 974
  nutritional differences of, vs. breast milk and formula, 785–787, 786t
Coxsackie B virus infection, 761
Cradle cap, treatment of, 898
Cranial nerves, birth injuries to, 666
  sixth, paresis of, vs. congenital esotropia, 906
Cranial sutures, premature closure of, 689–693
  classification of, 692t
  with radial aplasia, 832
Craniofacial dysostosis, 691, 692t
Craniolacunia, 685, *686*
Craniosynostosis, 689–693
  classification of, 692t
  with radial aplasia, 832
Cranium bifidum, with encephalocele, 681, *681, 682*
Creatinine clearance, 396t, 398
Cricopharyngeal achalasia, 339
Cricopharyngeal incoordination, 338–339
Cri du chat 5p− syndrome, 852
Crigler-Najjar syndrome, 631, 632t
Crouzon's disease, 691, 692t
Cryptococcosis, 769–771
Cryptorchidism, 405–406
Culture, conjunctival, methods of, 919
Cutaneous. See *Skin*.
Cutis laxa, 873–874, *874*
Cutis marmorata telangiectatica congenita, 888, *889*
Cyanosis
  as manifestation of cardiac disease, 228, 241
  central, 241

Cyanosis (*Continued*)
  differential, 228
  differential diagnosis of, 286, 286t
  methemoglobinemia and, 610t
Cycloserine, concentration of, in maternal blood and breast milk, 993
Cyst
  balloon, vs. pneumothorax, 203
  branchial, 321, *322*, 323
  bronchogenic, 206–208, *207, 208*
  colonic, 356
  enterogenous, 208–209
  esophageal, 208–209
  gastrogenic, 208–209, 340–341, *341*
  genital, external, 410
  intraluminal, of intestine, 347
  laryngeal, 126
  of small intestine, *362, 363*
  omphalomesenteric duct, 383–384
  oral, 318
  ovarian, 409
  pseudocholedochal, 641
  pulmonary, 199–213
    air-containing, 199–204
    fluid-filled, 204–212
  rectal, 356
  renal, 423–426
  thyroglossal duct, spherical mass of, 323
  urachal, 379–380, *379*
  vitelline, 383–384
Cystathioninemia, *541*, 543
Cystic adenomatoid malformation, of lung, 204
Cystic fibrosis, 556–557
  jaundice with, 645
  newborn screening for, 66
  risk of producing child with, 556t
Cystourethrogram, voiding, 397
Cytogenetics, 25–26
Cytomegalic inclusion disease, 758
  inclusion bodies in, 759, *760*
  manifestations of, *755*
Cytomegalovirus infection, 757–760
  clinical findings in, 758t
  due to blood transfusion, 586
  laboratory abnormalities in, 759t
Cytoplasmic body myopathy, 711t

Dacryocystitis, 921, *921*
Dacryostenosis, 921, *921*
Dandy-Walker syndrome, 695
"Debrancher" disease, 535
Defense mechanisms, against infectious pathogens, 720, 720t
Deformation, 8, 9
De Lange syndrome, 857–858, *857*
Delivery
  birth injury due to. See *Birth injury*.
  breech, complications associated with, 18, 18t
  epiphyseal injuries in, 841–842, *842*
  fractures sustained during, 840–841
Delivery room, resuscitation in, 100–108
  equipment for, 106t
Demerol, route and dose for, 972
Depressor anguli oris muscle, congenital hypoplasia of, 667
Dermal sinus, congenital, 687
Dermatoglyphics, 847–848
Dermoid, of eye, 923, *923*
Dermolipoma, 924
DES, fetal exposure to, 12
  teratogenic and carcinogenic effects of, 930, 930t, 931

20,22-Desmolase deficiency, 486
Desoxycorticosterone acetate, route and dose for, 970
Dexamethasone, route and dose for, 970
Diabetes
  maternal, congenital anomalies in offspring of, 15
    hyaline membrane disease and, 135
    hypertrophic cardiomyopathy of infant of, 298–299
    hypoglycemia of infant of, 517, *517*
    perinatal complications in, 14t
    prenatal considerations for, 14
  pregnancy and, White classification of, 15t
Diabetes insipidus, nephrogenic, 555–556
Diabetes mellitus, transient, in neonate, 521
Dialysis therapy, in acute renal failure, 461
Diamox, route and dose for, 971
Diaphragm
  accessory, 196
  agenesis of, 196
  disorders of, 189–196
  eventration of, 193–196, *194, 195*
  paralysis of, 192–193
Diaphragmatic hernia, congenital, 189–192, *190–192*
  lung hypoplasia with, 186
Diarrhea, 316
  bacterial, 738–740
    nosocomial, 745
  conditions associated with, 316t
  viral, nosocomial, 767
Diastematomyelia, 686
Diastolic murmur, 229
Diastrophic dwarfism, 823, *824*
Diazepam, route and dose for, 971
Diazoxide, as antihypertensive, 960t, 961
Diethylstilbestrol (DES), fetal exposure to, 12
  teratogenic and carcinogenic effects of, 930, 930t, 931
DiGeorge syndrome, 725, *725*
  chromosome deletion in, 853
Digitalis glycosides, 958–960
  in treatment of congestive heart failure, 239
Digitalization, 960
  route and dose for, 971
Digoxin, 959
  dose recommendations for, 959, 959t
  half-life and therapeutic levels of, 954t
  in treatment of congestive heart failure, 239
  route and dose for, 971
  toxicity of, 960
Dihydropteridine reductase deficiency, *537*, 539
Dilantin, route and dose for, 971
Diphenhydramine, route and dose for, 971
Diphenylhydantoin, concentration of, in maternal blood and breast milk, 993
  route and dose for, 971
  teratogenic effect of, 11
Diphtheria, 750–751
Diphtheria antitoxin, route and dose for, 971
Disruption, 8
Diuretics, 965
  in treatment of congestive heart failure, 240
Diuril, route and dose for, 970

Diverticulum
  Meckel's, 384–385, *384*
  of bladder, hydronephrosis and, 431
  of urethra, male, 404
  pharyngeal, 321
DNA, genetic variation of, prenatal
    detection of, *32*, 33
DOCA, route and dose for, 970
Dopamine, 957
  route and dose for, 971
Down syndrome. See *Trisomy 21.*
Drugs
  absorption of, 951
  carcinogenic, following in utero
      exposure, 930, 930*t*
  cardiovascular, 957–961
  concentration of, in maternal blood
      and breast milk, 993
    measurements of, 956
  contraindicated for nursing mother,
      789*t*
  distribution of, 951, *951*
    multicompartment, 955, *955*
    single compartment, 953, *954*
    volume of, 954
  excretion of, 953
  first-order kinetics of, *955*, 956
  half-life of, 954, 954*t*
  immune hemolysis and, 594
  infusion of, continuous, 956
  loading dose of, 956
  maternal ingestion of,
      thrombocytopenia secondary to,
        572
      virilization of female fetus by, 508,
        508
  metabolism of, 952
  multiple doses of, 955, *956*
  neonatal exposure to, frequency of,
      950, 950*t*
  neonatal therapeutics of, principles of,
      951–953
  pharmacokinetics of, 953–957
  plasma protein binding of, 951, *951*,
      952*t*
  renal failure and, 460*t*, 461
  teratogenic, 11, 11*t*
    following in utero exposure, 930,
        930*t*
    susceptibility to, *11*
  therapeutic levels of, 954*t*
  zero-order kinetics of, 955, *955*
D trisomy, 851, *851*
Dubin-Johnson syndrome, 644
Ductus arteriosus
  hemodynamically significant, criteria
      for, 281*t*
  normal closure of, 226
  patent, 143, 278–281
    vs. aortopulmonary window, 288
  pharmacologic management of, 961
Duodenum
  atresia of, 351–352, *352*
    vs. hypertrophic pyloric stenosis, 343
  peptic ulcer of, 344
  stenosis of, 352–353
  stricture of, vs. hypertrophic pyloric
      stenosis, 343
Duplication
  esophageal, 327, *327*
  gastric, 340–341, *341*
  of colon, 356
  of penis, 402–403
  of rectum, 356
  of renal collecting system, 418–419,
      418
  of small intestine, *362*, 363

Dwarfism
  campomelic, 822
  diastrophic, 823, *824*
  intrauterine, with congenital
      hemihypertrophy and elevated
      urinary gonadotropins, 831
  metatropic, 824
  Seckel's bird-headed, 859
  thanatophoric, 822–823, *824*
Dysautonomia, familial, 717
  esophageal abnormalities in, 339
Dysostoses, 821*t*
Dysplasia, 8
Dysplastic nevus syndrome, 892
Dysrhythmia, cardiac, 304–308
  in utero, congestive heart failure and,
      287

Eagle-Barrett syndrome, 414
Ears, assessment of, in newborn, 58
Ebstein's anomaly, 259–261, *260*
  chest radiograph in, *232*
  differential diagnosis of, 286
Echocardiography, *233, 234, 234.* See
      also *Ultrasonography.*
  normal values for, in newborn, 235*t*
Echovirus infection, 761
Ectodermal dysplasia, 877–878
  anhidrotic, 877, *877*
  congenital, of face, 857, *857*
  EEC syndrome of, 878
  hidrotic, 877
Eczema, follicular, vs. acne neonatorum,
      899
  seborrheic, 897–898, *897*
Edecrin, route and dose for, 971
Edema, generalized, vs. Milroy's disease,
      390
  with neonatal tetany, 469
EEC syndrome, 878
Ehlers-Danlos syndrome, 874–875
18q– syndrome, 852
Ejection click, aortic, 228
  systolic, 228
  variable, 229
Ejection murmur, 229
Electrocardiography, 229–231
  in premature infant, 231
  normal, in term infant, 229, 230*t*
  standards of, in neonates, 988
Electroencephalography, in assessment of
      neonate, 658
Elephantiasis, 389
Elliptocytosis, hereditary, *596*, 598
Ellis–van Creveld syndrome, 824–826,
      825
Emphysema
  diagnosis of, 154
  interstitial, 158, *158*
  lobar, 159–161
    types of, 160*t*
  mediastinal, *156*, 157
    diagnosis of, 154
  obstructive, diagnosis of, 154
Empyema, subdural, 713
Encephalitis, Western equine, 766
Encephalocele, differential diagnosis of,
      682
  with cranium bifidum, 681, *681, 682*
Encephalopathy, acute myoclonic,
      neuroblastoma with, 934
Endocardial cushion defects, 281–284,
      282, 283
  differential diagnosis of, 288

Endocardial fibroelastosis, 295–298, *296,
      297*
  differential diagnosis of, 288
  vs. glycogen storage disease, 298, 300
  vs. myocarditis, 294
Endocrine deficiencies, multiple, severe
      hypoglycemia with, 519
Endocrine pancreas, development of,
      514
Endocrine system, disorders of, 463–523
Endonuclease recognition, in DNA, *32*,
      33
Endotoxin, limulus lysate assay of, in
      bacterial meningitis, 736
Endotracheal intubation, of newborn,
      104
Energy requirements, infant, 49, 50*t*
  in premature, 980
  of undersized infant, 96
"En face" position, 788, *788*
Enfamil, composition of, 974
Enterocolitis, necrotizing, 364–366, *365*
Enterogenous cyst, 208–209
Enteroumbilical fistula, 382, *383*
Enterovirus disease, 761–762
Enzyme abnormalities, of red blood cells,
      598–601
Eosinophilia, in premature infants, 580
Eosinophils, means and ranges of, *986*
Epidermal nevi, 893, *893*
Epidermal nevus syndrome, 894
Epidermolysis bullosa, *874*, 875–876
Epidural abscess, spinal, 713
Epignathus, 319, *319*
Epimerase deficiency, *531*, 534
Epinephrine, route and dose for, 971
Epiphysis(es), congenital stippled, 823,
      825
  injuries to, in breech delivery, 841–
      842, *842*
Epispadias, *403*, 404
Epithelial nevus, systematized, 893
Epstein's pearls, 318, 899
Epulis, congenital, 319
Equine encephalitis, Western, 766
Equinovarus, 838, *838*
Erb-Duchenne paralysis, 668
Erythema toxicum neonatorum, 900, *900*
Erythroblastosis fetalis, 590–593
  clinical and laboratory features of, 591*t*
  hypoglycemia with, 517
  vs. leukemia, 933
  vs. neuroblastoma, 935
Erythrocyte. See *Red blood cells.*
Erythroderma, ichthyosiform, 869
Erythrokeratodermia variabilis, 870
Erythromycin, concentration of, in
      maternal blood and breast milk, 993
  route and dose for, 971
Erythropoiesis, fetal, 581, 582*t*
Erythropoietic stimulating factor (ESF),
      581
Erythropoietin, 581
Escherichia coli, causing diarrhea, 738
  meningitis due to, 731
  septicemia due to, 734
Esophagitis, thrush, 773
Esophagoscopy, in hiatus hernia, 329
Esophagus
  absence of, 324
  acquired lesions of, 327–331

Esophagus (*Continued*)
  atresia of, with tracheoesophageal
    fistula, 332–335, *333, 334*
  compression of, by neighboring
    structures, 326–327
  congenital anomalies of, 324
  cyst of, 208–209
  disorders of, 324–331
  duplications of, 327, *327*
  erosions of, 330
  function of, 310
  neuromuscular control of, disorders of,
    338–340
  rupture of, 331
  stenosis of, 324–326, *325*
  stricture of, due to hiatal hernia, 330
Esotropia, congenital, 906, *907*
Estriol excretion, maternal, in fetal
    assessment, 39
  low or falling, causes of, *39t*
Estrogen, exogenous, fetal exposure to,
    12
  maternal ingestion of, male
    pseudohermaphroditism and, 510
Ethacrynic acid, route and dose for, 971
Ethanol, concentration of, in maternal
    blood and breast milk, 993
Ethyl biscoumacetate, concentration of, in
    maternal blood and breast milk, 993
E trisomy, 850–851, *850*
Euthyroid sick (low T$_3$) syndrome, 499
Exfoliatin, 880
Exomphalos, 375–376, *375, 376*
Exomphalos-macroglossia-gigantism
    (EMG) syndrome of Beckwith-
    Wiedemann, hypoglycemia with, 520
Exstrophy, cloacal, 413
  of bladder, 411–413, *412*
Extremities, assessment of, in newborn,
    59
Eye(s)
  assessment of, in newborn, 57
  disorders of, 905–926
  infections of, 918–922
  motility disturbances of, 906–908
  tumors of, 923–926
Eyelids, eversion of, 917, *917*
Eye movements, evaluation of, in
    neurologic examination, 654

Face, ectodermal dysplasia of, congenital,
    857, *857*
Facial nerve, birth injuries to, 666
  palsy of, bilateral, 854
Factor VIII deficiency, 565
Factor IX deficiency, 566
Factor XI deficiency, 566
Factor XIII deficiency, 566
Fallot, tetralogy of, 249–251, *249–251*
  differential diagnosis of, 286
  with pulmonary atresia, 251–253,
    252
Familial dysautonomia, 717
  esophageal abnormalities in, 339
Fanconi's anemia, 572, 831
Fasciitis, necrotizing, 743
Fat necrosis, subcutaneous, 901–902,
    902
  with neonatal hypercalcemia, 473

Feeding
  breast. See *Breast-feeding.*
  calories from, 785t
  formula, basics of, 790–791
  guidelines for, 784t
  of low birth weight infant, 791–797
  solid foods, introduction of, 791
Feet, disorders of, 837–838, *837, 838*
Feminization, testicular, 510
Fetal alcohol syndrome, 13
  neoplasia associated with, 932
Fetal circulation, 101
  neonatal cardiovascular changes and,
    224–227
  persistent, 102, 161–164
Fetal death, 3
  rate of, *4*
Fetal hydantoin syndrome, neoplasia
    associated with, 932
Fetomaternal hemorrhage, 587
Fetus
  antibodies passively acquired by, 721t
  ascites in, 386–391
  body composition of, 46, 47, 48t, 991
  breathing by, 111
  exogenous agents affecting, 11–13
  female, virilization of, 508
  genital development of, 503–505, *504*
  growth of, 43–48. See also *Growth,
    intrauterine retardation of.*
  harlequin, 868, *868*
  hemorrhage of, 587
    clinical findings in, 588t
  immunoglobulin levels in, *721*
  lung of, 110
    maturity assessment of, 41
  male, undervirilization of, 509
  maternal conditions affecting,
    9–11, 14–15
  risk assessment of, in third trimester,
    36–43
    tests for, 37t
  stress test of, 39, 39t
  viral infection of, 754–768
    manifestations of, *755*
Fiber deficient myopathy, Type II, 711t
Fiber type disproportion, congenital, 711t
Fibrin split product (FSP), 562
Fibrinogen, determination of, 562
  route and dose for, 971
Fibrinolysis, 561, *561*
Fibroelastosis, endocardial. See
    Endocardial fibroelastosis.
Fibrosarcoma, of lung, 210
Fingerprint myopathy, 711t
Fingerprints, 847
Fistula
  arteriovenous, 889
    congestive heart failure and, 284,
      285, 287
  branchiogenous, 321
  enteroumbilical, 382, *383*
  tracheoesophageal, types of, 332, *332*
    with esophageal atresia, 332–335,
      333, 334
    without esophageal atresia, 335–
      336, *336*
5p − syndrome, 852
Fleurette, of retinoblastoma, 925, *925*
Flexner-Wintersteiner rosette, 924, *924*
Florinef, route and dose for, 971
Fludrocortisone, route and dose for, 971
Fluid balance, in neonate, 48
Fluid maintenance, in renal failure, acute,
    459

Fluid requirements, of low birth weight
    infant, 792, 792t
Fluoroscopy, in hiatus hernia, 329
Folic acid, concentration of, in maternal
    blood and breast milk, 993
  route and dose for, 971
Fontanel, abnormal size of, disorders
    associated with, 57, 58t
Fontanel bone, anterior, 693
Foramen of Morgagni, hernia of, *191*
Formula
  calories from, 785t
  composition of, 974–979
  modified, for low birth weight infant,
    792–793, 974
  nutritional differences of, vs. human
    and cow's milk, 785–787, 786t
Formula-feeding, basics of, 790–791
4p− syndrome, 852
Fracture, skull, in newborn, 664, *664*
  sustained during delivery, 840–841
Fructose intolerance, hereditary, 535–
    536
Fructosuria, essential benign, 535
Fungus infection, 769–774
Furosemide, as antihypertensive, 960t
  as diuretic, 965
  route and dose for, 971
Fusion, labial, 408
  of oral cavity, congenital, 318

Galactokinase deficiency, *531,* 534
Galactose tolerance test, 532, *532*
Galactosemia, 529–534
  laboratory tests of, 531
  metabolic pathway of, 530, *531*
  newborn screening for, 63
  variants of, 529t
Galen, vein of, aneurysm of, 714, *714*
Gamma globulin, 720–722
  fetal and neonatal levels of, *721*
  route and dose for, 971
Gamma thalassemia, 603
Ganglion cells, *371*
Ganglioneuroblastoma, 936
Ganglioneuroma, 936
Gangliosidosis, GM$_1$, 553
Gantrisin, route and dose for, 973
Gastric. See also *Stomach.*
Gastric acid secretion, postnatal
    development of, 311, 311t
Gastric contents, aspiration of, neonatal
    pneumonia due to, 173–174
Gastroesophageal acid reflux, due to
    myotomy, 339
  hiatus hernia and, 327–330
Gastrogenic cyst, 208–209, 340–341,
    341
Gastrointestinal tract, development of,
    310t
  disorders of, 309–391
  symptoms of, 315–317
Gastroschisis, 377
Gastrostomy, in feeding of low birth
    weight infant, 795
Gaucher's disease, 553
Gavage feeding, of low birth weight
    infant, continuous, 794
  intermittent, 794
Gene, defective, 9
  mutant, recurrence risks of defects due
    to, 863
Genetic counseling, 859–864
  evaluation of infant in, 859–861
  of family, 861–864

Genetic diagnosis, prenatal, 24–36, *24t*
  indications for, 24, *24t*
  methodology of, 29–33
    of cytogenetic abnormalities, 25–26
    of neural tube defects, 26–28
    of single-gene disorders, 28–29
    problems of, 33–34
Genital area, assessment of, in newborn, 59
Genital development, fetal, 503–505, *504*
Genitalia
  ambiguous, evaluation of, 511–512, *511*
    steroidal biochemical findings in, 485, 512
  external, cysts of, 410
  malformations of, defects associated with, 511
Genital tract, abnormalities of, 401–411
Genitourinary tract, anomalies of, neoplasias associated with, 931
  congenital malformations of, 411–420
  disorders of, 393–462
Gentamicin, half-life and therapeutic levels of, *954t*
  route and dose for, 971
Gentian violet, route and dose for, 971
Genu recurvatum, 834–835, *834*
Gestation
  length of, correlated with embryonic and fetal bodily dimensions, 990
    perinatal mortality related to, 45, *45*
  prolonged, 97–98
Gestational age
  alpha-fetoprotein levels and, 29, *30*
  assessment of, 56, 655–656
    by extremity muscle tone, *95*, 656, *657*
    by maturity rating, *981*
    external characteristics for, *655t*
    reflex responses in, *656t*
  classification of, *982*
  intrauterine growth charts for, 45, *46*, *982*
  low birth weight for, 45
Giant nevi, 891, *892*
Gilbert's disease, 631, *632t*
Glanzmann's thrombasthenia, 573
Glaucoma, infantile, 915–917, *916*
Glioma, nasal, 715
Glomerular filtration rate, clinical evaluation of, *396t*, 397
Glomerulonephritis, 451–453
  extramembranous, 454
Glomerulonephropathy, membranous, 454
Glomerulosclerosis, congenital, 454
  focal, 454
Glucagon, deficiency of, hypoglycemia from, 519
  route and dose for, 971
Glucocorticoids, biosynthetic pathway of, *480*
  prenatal administration of, lung maturity and, 144
Glucose
  administration of, to asphyxiated newborn, 106
  blood, newborn levels of, 514–515, *515*
    normal values for, 984
  evaluation of levels of, in renal function, *396t*, 399
  for infant feeding, 978

Glucose-6-phosphate dehydrogenase deficiency, *597*, 598–600, *598, 599*
Glutaric aciduria, 551–552
Glycogen storage diseases, 534–535
  of heart, 299–301, *300, 301*
    vs. anomalous left coronary artery, 300
    vs. endocardial fibroelastosis, 298, 300
Glycogenosis, generalized, 535
Glycosuria, renal defects with, 399
GM₁ gangliosidosis, 553
Goiter, 323
  with inborn errors of thyroid synthesis, 496, *496*
  with transient hypothyroidism, 497
Goldenhar syndrome, 856–857, *856*
  vs. Treacher Collins syndrome, 817
Gonadal differentiation, disorders of, 505–509
Gonadal dysgenesis, pure, 507
  XY syndrome of, 509
Gonadotropins, elevated urinary, with congenital hemihypertrophy and intrauterine dwarfism, 831
Gonococcal conjunctivitis, 742, 919, *920*
Gordon syndrome, 835
Gout, 836–837
Graft-versus-host disease, 724
  following bone marrow transplantation, 727
  with intrauterine blood transfusion, 586
Gram, conversion of pounds and ounces to, 992
Gram-negative infection, nosocomial, 746
Granulocyte(s)
  function of, 725
    primary defects in, pyogenic infection and, 727
  physiology of, neonatal infection and, 576–577
    normal, 575–576, *575*
Granuloma, umbilical, 374
  candidal, 883
  vs. omphalomesenteric sinus, 383
  vs. umbilical polyp, 382
Granulomatosis infantisepticum, 734
Granulomatous disease, chronic, 579
  pyogenic infection and, 727
Graves' disease, maternal, neonatal thyrotoxicosis with, 500
Great arteries, anomalies of, 125–126
  transposition of, complete, 245–249, *246–248*
    differential diagnosis of, 286, 288
Grebe disease, 822
Growth
  genetic regulation of, 45
  intrauterine retardation of, 92–100
    conditions associated with, *93*
    long-term effects of, 96, *97t*
    pathologic findings in, *96*
    of fetus, 43–48
Growth charts, intrauterine, 45, *46, 982*
Gums, fusion of, congenital, 318
Guthrie bacterial assay, for PKU, 62, *62*

Hamartoma, of lung, 210
Haptoglobin, 586
Harelip, 818–819
Harlequin color change, 898
Harlequin fetus, 868, *868*
Head
  assessment of, in newborn, 57
  on neurologic examination, 654

Head (*Continued*)
  circumference measurement of, 56
  molding of, 662
Heart
  catheterization of, 235–238
  congenital malformations of, 243–290
    acyanotic, 267–285
    cineangiography of, angled views in, *237t*
    cyanotic, 245–267
      differential diagnosis of, 286, *286t*
    embryology of, 245
    etiology of, 244
    fetal hemodynamics with, 225
    incidence of, 243, *244t, 245t*
    vs. myocarditis, 294
  dysrhythmias of, 304–308
    in utero, congestive heart failure and, 287
  position of, 231
  size of, radiographic evaluation of, 231
  tumors of, 301–303, *301, 302*
Heart beat, ectopic, 304–305
Heart block, 306–308, *307*
  congenital complete, with maternal SLE, 618
Heart disease. *See also* Heart, *congenital malformations of.*
  differential diagnosis of, 285–288
  manifestations of, 238–242
Heart failure, congestive, 238–241
  differential diagnosis of, 287, *287t*
Heart murmurs, 229
  as manifestation of cardiac disease, 242
Heart rate
  as measure of neonatal attention and habituation, 74–75
  fetal monitoring of, during labor, 39, *40*
    prior to labor, 39, *39t*
  normal resting, 229, *230t*
  of normal newborn, 56
Heart rhythm, normal, 229
Heart sounds, 228
Heinz bodies, with G6PD deficient hemolysis, *597*, 599
Helminthiasis, neonatal, 780–781
Hemangioma, 884–890
  capillary, 884
  cavernous, 884, 887
  giant, thrombocytopenia with, 571
  of eye and orbit, 923
  strawberry, *885*, 887
Hemangiomatosis, diffuse neonatal, 888
Hematemesis, 316–317
Hematocrit, effect of viscosity, blood flow, and oxygen transport on, 609, *609*
  gestational values of, 582, *582t*
  values for, 584, *585t*
Hematologic values, 985
Hematoma, intracerebral, due to intraventricular hemorrhage, 673, *674*
  perirenal, 440
Hematuria, 396–397
Hemihypertrophy, 831
  congenital, with intrauterine dwarfism and elevated urinary gonadotropins, 831

Hemodialysis, in acute renal failure, 461
Hemoglobin
    changes in, during first year of life,
        606t
    cord blood, composition of, 601, *601*
    disorders of, hemolysis due to, 601–
        605
    function of, fetal and neonatal, 582,
        583, 584
    gestational values of, 582, 582t
    production of, fetal and neonatal, 601,
        601
    values for, 584, 585t
Hemoglobin H disease, 602
Hemoglobin M disorders, 611
Hemolysis
    due to hemoglobin disorders, 601–605
    immune, 590–594
        amniotic fluid bilirubin levels in, 592,
            592
        clinical and laboratory features of,
            591t
        drug-induced, 594
        due to ABO incompatibility, 593
        due to maternal disease, 594
        due to Rh disease, 590–593
        infant death rates from, *593*
Hemolytic disease. See *Anemia,
    hemolytic.*
Hemolytic-uremic syndrome, 568
Hemophilia A, 565
Hemophilia B, 566
Hemophilia C, 566
Hemophilus, conjunctivitis due to, 920
Hemorrhage
    due to platelet abnormalities, 569–573
    fetal, 587
        clinical findings in, 588t
    hemostatic abnormalities with, 573
    intracranial, 672t
        due to perinatal asphyxia, 673, *673*
        hydrocephalus following, 695
    neonatal, 560–575
        approach to infant with, 561–563
        blood components in therapy of,
            563
        laboratory evaluation of, 561, 562t
        vs. maternal, Apt test for, 316, 562
    of peptic ulcer, 344
    periventricular-intraventricular, 673,
        673
        intracerebral hematoma and, 673,
            674
        treatment of, 676
        ventricular dilation due to, 673, *674*
    pre- or intrapartum, resuscitation in,
        108
    postpartum, anemia due to, 589
    pulmonary, 214–216
    subdural, 665
    with liver disease, 568–569
Hemorrhagic anemia, 586–589, 587t
Hemorrhagic disease, of newborn, 563–
    564
Hemostasis, normal, physiology of, 560–
    561, *560*
Heparin, route and dose for, 971
Hepatitis
    neonatal, 641–643
        liver biopsy in, *638, 639*

Hepatitis (*Continued*)
    "toxic," 645–646
    viral, 765–766
Hepatoblastoma, 941
Hepatocellular carcinoma, 941
Heredodegenerative diseases, 716–717,
    716t
Herlitz type of epidermolysis bullosa, 875
Hermaphroditism, true, 507
Hernia
    diaphragmatic, congenital, 189–192,
        190–192
        lung hypoplasia with, 186
    hiatus, gastroesophageal acid reflux
        and, 327–330
    inguinal, 360–361
        vs. hydrocele, 360, 407
    lumbar, congenital, 839–840, *840,
        841*
    umbilical, 377–378
    umbilical cord, 375, *375*
Herpes simplex infection, 762–764
    conjunctival, 920
    survival results of, *764*
Heterotaxy syndromes, 265–267
Hiatus hernia, gastroesophageal acid
    reflux and, 327–330
Hips, assessment of, in newborn, 59
    dislocation of, congenital, 833–834
    subluxation of, 833, *833*
Hirschsprung's disease, 368–371
Histamine test, intradermal, for familial
    dysautonomia, 717
Histidinemia, 547
    newborn screening for, 67
Histiocytosis X, acute disseminated, 943
Histoplasmosis, disseminated, 771
History, newborn, 54, 54t
Holoprosencephaly, 687
Holt-Oram syndrome, 831
Holter valve, 698
Homer-Wright rosette, 924
Homocystinuria, *541*, 542
    newborn screening for, 64
    vs. Marfan syndrome, 827
Hormones, fetal growth and, 94
Horner's syndrome, with neuroblastoma,
    934, *934*
Host factors, in development of
    neoplastic disease, 930
Human milk. See *Breast milk.*
Hyaline membrane disease, 133–147
    differential diagnosis of, 137t
    mechanical ventilation in, 217–221
    observations in, 134t
    prenatal diagnosis of, 139, *140*
Hydralazine, as antihypertensive, 960t
    route and dose for, 971
Hydramnios, conditions associated with,
    18, *19*, 19t
Hydranencephaly, 698, *699*
Hydrocele, 406–407, *406*
    vs. inguinal hernia, 360, 407
Hydrocephalus, 693–698
    classification and types of, 695t
    with meningomyelocele, 685
Hydrochlorothiazide, route and dose for,
    971
Hydrocolpos, 408
Hydrocortisone, route and dose for, 971
Hydrodiuril, route and dose for, 971
Hydrogen ion concentration, in
    evaluation of renal function, 399
Hydrometra, 408
Hydrometrocolpos, 408, *409*

Hydronephrosis, 427–436
    categories of, 427, 428t
    differential diagnosis of, 450
Hydrops, 602
    nonimmune, 390–391
Hydrops fetalis, 635–636
    causes of, 636t
Hydroureteronephrosis, 428t
11-Hydroxylase deficiency, 486–487
17α-Hydroxylase deficiency, 487
21-Hydroxylase deficiency, 483–486
3β-Hydroxysteroid dehydrogenase
    deficiency, 486
18-Hydroxysteroid dehydrogenase
    deficiency, 487
Hygroma, cystic, 889
    of neck, *322, 323*
Hyperaminoaciduria, due to
    galactosemia, 532
Hyperbilirubinemia
    breast-feeding and, 627, 789
    conjugated, 644–646
        disorders with, 644t
    exchange transfusion in, indications for,
        628t
    phototherapy of, 590, 628–630, 628t
    unconjugated, 630–632
        clinical syndromes of, 632t
        pathologic causes of, 631t
Hypercalcemia, 470–476
    familial hypocalciuric, primary
        hyperparathyroidism and, 471
    idiopathic, 472, *473*
    phosphate depletion with, 474
    with adrenal insufficiency, 474
    with subcutaneous fat necrosis, 473
Hypercholesterolemia, familial, 553
Hyperglycemia, temporary idiopathic
    neonatal, 521
Hyperglycinemia, 546–547
    "ketotic," 546
    nonketotic, 546
Hyperinflation, 154–161
Hyperinsulinemia, 519–521
Hyperkalemia, in renal failure, acute, 459
Hyperkeratosis, epidermolytic, 869
Hyperlipidemia, familial, 552–553
    newborn screening for, 67
Hypermagnesemia, 476
Hypermethioninemia, 541, *541*
    newborn screening for, 64
Hypernatremia, 487
    seizures due to, 703
Hyperparathyroidism, maternal, neonatal
        hypocalcemia with, 467
    neonatal, primary, 471
        with maternal hypoparathyroidism,
            472, *472*
Hyperphenylalaninemia, 539–540
Hypertension, 441–447
    causes of, in infancy, 441, 442t
    in renal failure, acute, 460
    pharmacologic treatment of, 960, 960t
    pulmonary, persistent, 102
    ventricular, systolic, 237
Hyperthermia, maternal, effect on fetus/
    newborn, 13
Hyperthyroidism, 500–501, *500*
Hypocalcemia, 466–470
    clinical findings in, 469
    early, 466
    late, 467
    secondary to congenital
        hypoparathyroidism, 469
    seizures with, 703
    treatment of, 469

Hypocalcemia (*Continued*)
  with hypomagnesemia, 468
  with maternal hyperparathyroidism, 467
Hypoglycemia, 515–521
  classic transient, 518
  early transitional, 516–518
  in low birth weight infant, 793
  pathogenic factors in, 515, 516t
  secondary, 518
  seizures with, 703
  severe recurrent or persistent, 517t, 519–521
Hypomagnesemia, with hypocalcemia, 468
Hyponatremia, 488
  seizures due to, 703
Hypoparathyroidism, congenital, 469
  maternal, with neonatal hyperparathyroidism, 472, 472
Hypoperfusion, acute renal failure and, 456
  vs. parenchymal injury, urinary indices of, 457t, 458
Hypophosphatasia, 555
Hypopigmentation, 892
Hypoplastic anemia, 605–606
Hypoplastic left heart syndrome, 274–276, 274, 275
  differential diagnosis of, 287, 288
Hypospadias, 403–404, 403
  pseudovaginal perineoscrotal, 510
Hypotelorism, with metopic suture synostosis, 691
Hypothalamic-pituitary-thyroid system, 490–492
Hypothyroidism
  congenital, 493–499
    hyperbilirubinemia with, 631
    newborn screening for, 62, 63, 498
  transient, 497
Hypotonia, 676
  benign congenital, 710, 711t
  diagnostic evaluation of, 707

I-cell disease, 554
Ichthyosis, 868–870
  major types of, 869
  syndromes with, 870
Ichthyosis hystrix, 893
Ileum, atresia of, 353–355, 354
Ileus, meconium, 316, 355–356, 355
  intestinal obstruction and, 347
Imipramine hydrochloride, concentration of, in maternal blood and breast milk, 993
Immotile cilia syndrome, 188
Immune deficiency, 725–727
  severe combined (SCID), 726, 726
Immune reactivity, 722
Immunity
  cellular, general, 725
    specific, 722–724
  humoral, general, 724
    specific, 720–722
Immunoglobulins, 720–722
  fetal and neonatal levels of, 721
  route and dose for, 971
Immunology, 720–729
Impetigo, bullous, 879–880, 879
  vs. epidermolysis bullosa, 876
Inclusion blennorrhea, 919
Inclusion bodies, of cytomegalovirus infection, 759, 760

Incontinentia pigmenti, 872–873, 873
Inderal, route and dose for, 973
Indocin, route and dose for, 971
Indomethacin, for closure of ductus arteriosus, 281, 961
  route and dose for, 971
Infant. See *Neonate.*
Infection, 719–781
  bacterial, 729–747, 748–754
  defense mechanisms against, 720, 720t
  fungal, 769–774
  gram-negative, nosocomial, 746
  granulocyte physiology and, 576–577
  hemolytic anemia with, 594
  increased resistance to, with breast-feeding, 787
  nosocomial, 177
    bacterial, 744–746
    viral, 766–767
  of eyes, 918–922
  of lower respiratory tract, persistent or recurrent, 329
  of skin, 879–884
    bacterial, 743–744
  of urinary tract, 740–741
    without reflux, hydronephrosis and, 431
  pathogenesis of, 730–731
  protozoal, 775–778
  pyogenic, recurrent, 727
  seizures due to, 703
  staphylococcal, 733
    cutaneous, 743, 879–881
  streptococcal. See *Streptococcal disease.*
  thrombocytopenia with, 571
  umbilical, 373–374
    streptococcal, 883
  viral, 754–768
    manifestations of, 755
  with spirochetal organisms, 778–781
Ingestion, by neutrophil, 576, 576
Inguinal hernia, 360–361
  vs. hydrocele, 360, 407
Inheritance, mendelian patterns of, 863
Inotropic agents, in treatment of congestive heart failure, 240
Inspection, of newborn, 56–59
Insulin, route and dose for, 971
Intensive care facilities, perinatal-neonatal, regionalization of, 2
Intestine. See also *Colon.*
  evagination of, with patent omphalomesenteric duct, 382
  malrotation of, 349
    with volvulus, 358–360, 359–360
  nonrotation of, 349
  obstruction of, 346–351
    acquired, 364–368
    congenital, 351–364
    extrinsic, etiology of, 347
    hyperbilirubinemia with, 630
    intrinsic, etiology of, 347
    neurogenic, 349
  postnatal development of, in premature infant, 312–314, 312–314
    in term infant, 311–312
  reversed rotation of, 349
  rotation of, errors in, 347, 349
    normal, 347, 348
  rupture of, 358–359
  small, duplication of, 362, 363
Intracardiac pressure, elevated, 236
  normal, 237t

Intracellular killing, in phagocytosis, 576, 576
Intracranial aneurysm, congenital, 714, 714
Intracranial hemorrhage, 672t
  due to perinatal asphyxia, 673, 673
  hydrocephalus following, 695
Intracranial lesions, focal suppurative, 713
Intracranial thrombosis, venous sinus, 713–714
Intrahepatic bile ducts, atresia of, 640
Intraspinal tumors, congenital, 715–716
Intrathoracic tumors, 204–212
Intrauterine dwarfism, with congenital hemihypertrophy and elevated urinary gonadotropins, 831
Intrauterine growth charts, 45, 46, 982
Intrauterine growth retardation. See *Growth, intrauterine retardation of.*
Intrauterine pneumonia, 165–172
Intravascular coagulation syndromes, 566–568
Intravenous alimentation, cholestasis associated with, 797
Intrinsic factor secretion, postnatal development of, 311, 311t
Intussusception, 366–367
Inulin clearance, 396t, 398
Iodine 131, concentration of, in maternal blood and breast milk, 993
Iodothyronines, synthesis of, 490
Iron, route and dose for, 971
  supplementation of, in anemia of prematurity, 608t
Islet cell adenoma, hypoglycemia with, 520
Islets of Langerhans, endocrine cell types of, 514
Isomil, composition of, 976
Isoniazid, concentration of, in maternal blood and breast milk, 993
  route and dose for, 971
Isoproterenol, 957
  route and dose for, 971
Isovaleric acidemia, 549
Isuprel, route and dose for, 971
Ito, nevus of, 891
IVIC syndrome, 832

Jaundice, 621–650
  approach to, 649
  beginning within first 24 hours, laboratory tests in, 648t
  differential diagnosis of, 646–650
  breast-feeding effect on, 627, 789
  obstructive, 637–643
    due to biliary atresia, 637–641
    due to hepatitis, 641–643
  physiologic, 625–630
    criteria ruling out, 626t
    diagnosis and management of, 628–630
    factors producing, 627t
Jaw, size of, in newborn, 58
Jejunum, atresia of, 353–355
Jeune syndrome, 826
Joints, congenital defects involving, 833–838
Junction nevi, 891, 891

K1 antigen, neonatal meningitis and, 731
    septicemia due to, 734
Kanamycin, concentration of, in maternal
    blood and breast milk, 993
    half-life and therapeutic levels of, 954t
    route and dose for, 972
Karyotype, normal, 846, 846
Kasabach-Merritt syndrome, 888
Kawasaki's disease, 615
Kayexalate, route and dose for, 972
Keflin, route and dose for, 970
Keratoconjunctivitis, herpes simplex, 920
Keratosis pilaris, 899
Kernicterus, 633–635, 633
    with hemolytic disease, 590
Ketoaciduria, branched-chain, 540–541
Kidney(s). See also entries beginning
    Renal.
    agenesis of, bilateral, 416, 417–418,
        417
    congenital malformations of, 420–427
        renal failure and, acute, 457
    cysts of, 423–426
    dysplasia of, 421–422
    ectopic, 423
        differential diagnosis of, 450
    embryology of, 394
    enlarged, differential diagnosis of, 447–
        451
    horseshoe, 422
    hypoplasia of, 420
        segmental, 422
    normal, length of, 421
    multicystic, 423, 424
        differential diagnosis of, 450
    multiloculated cysts of, 423
    parenchymal injury in, 457
        urinary indices of, 457t, 458
    physical examination of, 448
    polycystic, 425
    solitary cysts of, 423
Kinetics, first-order, 955, 956
    zero-order, 955, 955
Kinky-hair syndrome, 554
KIO syndrome, ichthyosis with, 870
Klebsiella, pneumonia due to, 177
Kleeblattschädel, 691, 692t
Klinefelter syndrome, 505
Klippel-Feil syndrome, 842–843
Klippel-Trenaunay-Weber syndrome, 888
Klumpke's paralysis, 668
Kniest syndrome, 824
Kyphoscoliosis, congenital, of tibia, 839

Labia, fusion of, 408
Labor, onset of, mechanisms of, 84
    tocolytic agents for, 84, 84t
        dosage regimens for, 85t
Lacrimal outlet obstruction, 921, 921
Lactate, normal blood chemistry values
    for, 984
Lactic acid, normal blood chemistry
    values for, 984
Lambdoid suture, premature closure of,
    691
Langer-Giedion syndrome, 852
Langer-Saldino achondrogenesis, 821
Laryngeal stridor, 122–128
    with meningomyelocele, 685
Laryngotracheoesophageal cleft, 336–
    337

Larynx
    atresia of, congenital, 124
    congenital anomalies of, anatomic
        classification of, 122t
    cysts of, 126
    neoplasms of, 126
    stenosis of, congenital, 123
    stridor of, simple congenital, 122–123
    webs of, 123
Lasix, route and dose for, 971
Lazy leukocyte syndrome, 579
Lead, as teratogen, 12
Lecithin-sphingomyelin ratio, as index of
    lung maturity, 139, 140
Left heart syndrome, hypoplastic, 274–
    276, 274, 275
    differential diagnosis of, 287, 288
Leiner's disease, 897
Length, measurement of, in newborn, 56
Leprechaunism, 855
Leptospirosis, 780
Letterer-Siwe disease, 943
Leucine sensitivity, hypoglycemia and,
    521
Leukemia
    congenital, 931–933, 931, 932
        neutropenia due to, 579
        transplacental passage of, 929
        with Down syndrome, 933
Leukemoid reaction, in hemolytic
    disease, moderate, 591
Leukocoria, 915, 915
    with retinoblastoma, 925
Leukocyte, disorders of, 575–581
    functional, 579–580
    values of, in term and premature
        infants, 577t
Leukomalacia, periventricular, 671, 671
Levothyroxine, route and dose for, 972
Lidocaine, route and dose for, 972
Limbus, dermoids of, 924
Limulus lysate assay, in bacterial
    meningitis, 736
Lincomycin, concentration of, in maternal
    blood and breast milk, 993
Lip, cleft, 818–819
Lipids, fetal surfactant in amniotic fluid,
    tests for, 41, 42
    intravenous, 797
    metabolism of, inborn errors of, 551–
        554
Lipoma, lumbar intradural, 715
Lipomeningocele, 684, 684
Lissencephaly, 688
Listeria monocytogenes disease, 734
Lithium carbonate, concentration of, in
    maternal blood and breast milk, 993
Livebirth, 3
Liver
    biopsy of, in obstructive jaundice, 638,
        639
    in neuroblastoma, 934
    disease of, bleeding associated with,
        568–569
    malignant tumors of, 941
Liver function tests, in galactosemia, 532
Loading dose, 956
Lobar emphysema, 159–161
    types of, 160t
Lofenalac, composition of, 978
Low birth weight infant. See Birth weight,
    low.
Lucey-Driscoll syndrome, 631
Lückenschädel, 685, 686

Lumbar hernia, congenital, 839–840,
    840, 841
Lumbar puncture, 656–658
Lung(s). See also entries beginning
    Pulmonary.
    accessory lobes of, 211, 212
    agenesis of, 183–186
        survival rates in, 184, 184
    clearance of, at birth, 101
    cystic adenomatoid malformation of,
        204
    fetal, 110
    fibrosarcoma of, 210
    hamartoma of, 210
    hyperinflated, 154–161
    hypoplastic, 186–187
    in aspiration syndromes, 128, 129
    in hyaline membrane disease, 135,
        136
    liquid-filled, persistent, 183
    maturity of, fetal assessment of, 41
        lecithin-sphingomyelin ratio as index
        of, 139, 140
    sequestered lobes of, 210
Lupus erythematosus, 876, 876
    systemic, 617–618
Lymphangiectasis, pulmonary, congenital,
    187–188
Lymphangioma, 889
Lymphatic vessels, nevoid tumors of,
    localized, 889
Lymphedema, 890
    hereditary, 389–391
Lymph node, mucocutaneous syndrome
    of, 615, 616
    diagnostic criteria for, 616t
Lymphocyte, means and ranges of, 987
    ontogeny of, 722–724
    peripheral differentiation block of, in
        severe combined immune deficiency,
        726, 726
Lymphohistiocytosis, familial erythro-
    phagocytic, 943–944
Lymphoid stem cell, absence of, in
    severe combined immune deficiency,
    726, 726
Lyonization, 863
Lysosomal storage disease, 553–554
Lytren, composition of, 978

Macroglossia, congenital, 320
Macromelanosome, 890
Macule, white, 892–894, 893
Magnesium, estimated daily requirements
    of, in prematures, 980
    metabolism of, 476–477
    route and dose for, 972
Malaria, congenital, 777–778
Malformation, 8
    congenital. See Congenital
        malformation.
    epidemiology of, 8
    etiology of, 8t
    incidence and sex ratio of, 9t
Mandibulofacial dysostosis, 816–817,
    816
Maple syrup urine disease, 540–541
    newborn screening for, 64
Marfan syndrome, 827–828, 828
Mastocytosis, 894–895, 895
Maternal age, effect on fetus/newborn, 9
    prenatal cytogenetics and, 25
Maternal blood, drug concentrations in,
    993
    vs. fetal blood, Apt test for, 316, 562

Maternal conditions, affecting fetus, 9–11, 14–15
   related to perinatal death and birth weight, 16t
Maternal estriol excretion, in fetal assessment, 39
   low or falling, causes of, 39t
Maternal nutrition, effect on fetus/newborn, 10
Maturity rating, 981
   classification of newborns by, 982
McCune-Albright syndrome, 891
Meat Base Formula, composition of, 978
Meatitis, ulcerative, 402
Meatus, atresia of, 404–405
   stenosis of, 402
Mecholyl, route and dose for, 972
Meckel's diverticulum, 384–385, 384
Meconium, normal passage of, 350
Meconium aspiration, 129
   suctioning of, 107, 129
Meconium ileus, 316, 355–356, 355
   intestinal obstruction and, 347
Meconium peritonitis, 386–387, 386
Meconium plug, intestinal obstruction and, 347
Mediastinal air, 156, 157
   diagnosis of, 154
Mediastinum, neuroblastoma in, 205–206, 205, 206
   teratoma in, 210, 211
Megacolon, congenital, 368–371
Megacystis, 435
Megaesophagus, 339
Megalencephaly, 693
Megalopenis, 402
Megaloureter, congenital, 435
Melanocytic nevi, flat, 891, 891
   raised, 891, 892
Melanosis, pustular, transient neonatal, 902–903, 902, 903
Melena, 316–317
Melituria, laboratory tests for, 531
Membranes, premature rupture of, 15–16
   prolonged rupture of, pneumonia following, 165
Mendelian disorders, presenting in newborn period, 860t
Mendelian inheritance, patterns of, 863
Meningitis
   bacterial, seizures due to, 703
   E. coli strains causing, 731
   purulent, 735–738
   streptococcal, 733
     group B, pathogenesis of, 731
Meningocele, 682–686, 683–685
Meningomyelocele, 682–686, 683–685
Menkes' steely hair disease, 551, 555
Meperidine, 966
   concentration of, in maternal blood and breast milk, 993
   route and dose for, 972
Mercury, as teratogen, 12
Mesangial sclerosis, diffuse, 454
Mesenchymal dysplasia syndrome, 414
Mesenteric thrombosis, 367–368
Metabolic acidosis, in renal failure, acute, 460
Metabolic defects, hyperbilirubinemia with, conjugated, 644–645
   newborn screening for, 60–66
Metabolism
   inborn errors of, 525–558
     clinical signs of, in neonatal period, 528t
     diagnosis of, 528–529

Metabolism (Continued)
   inborn errors of, genetic origin of, 526–528, 526, 527
     seizures due to, 703, 703t
Metamyelocyte, means and ranges of, 987
Metatarsus varus, 837, 838
Metatropic dwarfism, 824
Methemoglobin, screening test for, 611
Methemoglobinemia, 610–612
Methicillin, route and dose for, 972
Methionine, elevations of, newborn screening for, 64
   remethylation defects of, 541, 542
   transsulfuration in metabolic pathway of, 541, 541
Methotrexate, concentration of, in maternal blood and breast milk, 993
Methyldopa, route and dose for, 972
Methylene blue, route and dose for, 972
Methylmalonic acidemia, 551
Methylprednisolone, route and dose for, 972
Metopic suture synostosis, 690
Metric equivalent charts, 992, 993
Microcephaly, 688
   vs. craniosynostosis, 693
Microcolon, 350, 358
Microcystic disease, infantile, 453
Microgastria, congenital, 340
Micrognathia, 817–818
Microphallus, 402
Midline defects, anterior, 687
Milia, 899–900
Miliaria, 900–901
Miliaria crystallina, 900
Miliaria rubra, 901
   vs. acne neonatorum, 899
Miliary disease, maternal untreated, congenital tuberculosis and, 749
Milroy's disease, 389, 890
   vs. edema, 390
Mineral(s), metabolism of, disorders of, 464–479
   trace, disorders of, 800, 810–811
Mineralocorticoids, biosynthetic pathway of, 480
Mitochondrial myopathy, 711t
Mitral atresia, with hypoplastic left ventricle, 274–276, 274
Möbius syndrome, 699, 854
Mohr syndrome, 856
Mongolian spots, 891
Mongolism. See Trisomy 21.
Moniliasis. See Candidiasis.
Monitors, for SIDS, 118
Monocyte, function of, 725
   means and ranges of, 987
Morgagni, foramen of, hernia of, 191
Moro response, 654, 654t
Morphine, 965
   route and dose for, 972
Mosaicism, 507
Motoneuron, diseases of, 707–708
Motor unit, diseases of, 707–712
Mouth, assessment of, in newborn, 58
   disorders of, 318–324
Moxalactam, route and dose for, 972
Mucocutaneous lymph node syndrome (MLNS), 615, 616
   diagnostic criteria for, 616t
Müllerian ducts, persistence of, 510
Multicore (Minicore) disease, 711t
MURCS anomaly, 414
Murmur, heart, 229
   as manifestation of cardiac disease, 242

Muscle, diseases of, 710–711
Muscle tone, evaluation of, 653
   gestational age assessment by, 95, 656, 657
Muscular atrophy, spinal, 707
Muscular dystrophy, congenital, 710
   newborn screening for, 66
Muscular hypertrophy, 710
Mutant genes, recurrence risks of defects due to, 863
Myasthenia gravis, 708
   neonatal, 556
Mycostatin, route and dose for, 972
Myelocele, 682–686, 683–685
Myelocystocele, 683
Myocardial ischemia, transient, 291–292
   differential diagnosis of, 287
Myocarditis, 292–295, 293, 294
   differential diagnosis of, 287, 288
Myopathy, congenital, 710, 711t
Myopia, 915
Myotonia, 710
Myotubular myopathy, 711t

NADH-methemoglobin reductase deficiency, 611
Nager acrofacial dysostosis, 817, 832
Nail-patella syndrome, 454
Nalidixic acid, concentration of, in maternal blood and breast milk, 993
Naloxone, 966
   route and dose for, 972
Narcan, route and dose for, 972
Narcotic withdrawal syndrome, of newborn, seizures due to, 704
Nasal glioma, 715
Nasal obstructions, 120–121
Nasopharyngeal tumors, 319–320
Neck, assessment of, in newborn, 58
   disorders of, 318–324
Necrosis, renal cortical and medullary, 439–440
   subcutaneous fat, 901–902, 902
   with neonatal hypercalcemia, 473
Neisseria gonorrhoeae, ophthalmia neonatorum due to, 742, 919, 920
Nemaline myopathy, 711t
Nembutal, route and dose for, 973
Neo-Calglucon, route and dose for, 972
Neomycin, route and dose for, 972
Neonatal death
   birth-weight specific statistics for, 104t
   early, 4
   from hyaline membrane disease, 134t
   gestational length related to, 45, 45
   in-hospital, 3t, 5
   late, 5
   maternal age and, 9, 10
   maternal conditions related to, 16t
   rate of, 4
Neonatal pharmacology, 950–968. See also Drugs.
Neonate
   as social being, 78–79
   attention and habituation of, heart rate as measure of, 74–75
   asphyxiated, treatment of, 104–107
   behavior of, 68–82. See also Behavior, neonatal.

Neonate (*Continued*)
cardiorespiratory conversion in, hemodynamics of, 101, 226, *227*
cardiovascular evaluation of, 227–238
classification of, by maturity and intrauterine growth, *982*
delivery room assessment of, 103
energy requirements of, 49, 50*t*
fluid balance in, 48
genetic evaluation of, 859–861
hemorrhagic disease of, 563–564
history of, 54, 54*t*
infection of, pathogenesis of, 730–731
immunoglobulin levels in, *721*
maternal conditions affecting, 9–11, 14–15
maturity rating of, *981, 982*
mortality and morbidity of, 3*t*, *4, 5, 5t*. See also *Neonatal death*.
motor behavior of, organization of, 69–70
neurologic evaluation of, 652–661
normal, 54–60
pharmacopeia for, 970–973
physical examination of, 55–59
physiological adaptations of, 48–52
premature, 44. See also *Prematurity*.
respiratory evaluation of, 111–112
in distress, priorities in, 141*t*
screening of, 60–67
follow-up, 65
specimen collection for, 61, *61*, 65
sensory capacities of, 70–74
size at term, 43, *44*
state of consciousness of, 68, 75–77
breathing patterns in, 114, *115*, 116
temperature regulation of, 50, 50*t*
term. See *Term infant*.
weight loss in, 48
Neonatology, aims of, 1–6
ethical dilemmas in, 1
Neoplasm. See *Tumor*.
Neostigmine, route and dose for, 972
Nephritis, interstitial, 454
Nephroblastoma. See also *Wilms' tumor*.
cystic, partially differentiated, 941
Nephroblastomatosis, 940
Nephrogram, 449
Nephroma, mesonephric, 940, *940*
Nephronophthisis, juvenile, 424
Nephropathies, 451–455
Nephrotic syndrome, infantile, 453–455, 453*t*
minimal lesion, 454
Nerve. See names of specific nerves.
Nervous system
central, malformations of, 680–702
of cellular migration and proliferation, 688–699
of embryogenic induction, 680–688
disorders of, 651–702
ontogenesis of, 652
Nesidioblastosis, hypoglycemia of infancy with, 519
Netherton's syndrome, ichthyosis with, 870
Neural tube defects, 680–688
prenatal genetic diagnosis of, 26–28
Neuroblastoma, 933–938, *934, 935*
congenital, 715

Neuroblastoma (*Continued*)
mediastinal, 205–206, *205, 206*
metastases with, incidence of, 935*t*
spontaneous regression of, 936, *937*
vs. leukemia, 933
Neurodermal sinus, 687
Neurodiagnostic procedures, 656–660
Neuroectodermal tumor, melanotic, 935
Neurofibromatosis, 890
Neurogenic stridor, 126–127
Neurologic examination, of neonate, 652–655
Neuromuscular blockers, 962
Neuromuscular junction, diseases of, 708–710
Neuromuscular maturity, newborn rating of, *981*
Neutra-Phos-K, route and dose for, 972
Neutropenia
cyclic, 578
due to leukemia, 579
idiopathic congenital, 578
isoimmune, 578
persistent, diagnostic evaluation of, 577*t*
secondary to drugs, 578
with maternal disease, 578
Neutrophil, ingestion by, 576, *576*
means and ranges of, *986*
Neutrophil muscular dystrophy, 579
Nevus(i), 884–896
of Ota, 891
pigmented, 890–892
spectrum of, 885*t*
vascular, 884–890
Nevus flammeus, 885
Nevus sebaceous, linear, 893
Nevus unius lateris, 893
Newborn. See *Neonate*.
Nicotinic acid, route and dose for, 972
Niemann-Pick disease, 553
Nikolsky's sign, 880
Nitroprusside, as antihypertensive, 960*t*, 961
in congestive heart failure, 958
route and dose for, 972
Nonstress test, of fetus, 39, 39*t*
Nose, assessment of, in newborn, 58
glioma of, 715
obstruction of, 120–121
Nosocomial infections, 177
bacterial, 744–746
viral, 766–767
Novobiocin, concentration of, in maternal blood and breast milk, 993
Nuclear agenesis, 854–855
Nuclei myopathy, central, 711*t*
Nursery, tuberculosis exposure in, 750
Nursoy, composition of, 976
Nutramigen, composition of, 976
Nutrition
disorders of, 783–813
in acute renal failure, 460
infant, 784–800. See also *Feeding* and *Breast-feeding*.
maternal, effect on fetus/newborn, 10
parenteral, 795–797. See also *Parenteral nutrition*.
Nystagmus, 908
Nystatin, route and dose for, 972

Oculoauriculovertebral dysplasia, 856–857, *856*
vs. Treacher Collins syndrome, 817
Oculomotor nerve, birth injury of, 667

Olfactory response, neonatal, 73
Oligohydramnios, 18
lung hypoplasia with, 186
Oligomeganephronia, 421
Omphalitis, 373–374
Omphalocele, 375–376, *375, 376*
Omphalomesenteric duct, congenital malformations of, 381–385
cyst of, 383–384
patent, 382, *383*
Omphalomesenteric sinus, 383
vs. urachal sinus, 379
Ondine's curse, 116
Onycho-osteodysplasia, hereditary, 454
Ophthalmia neonatorum, 742–743, 918–921
Opioids and opioid antagonists, 966
Opsonization, 576, *576*
Optic nerve, birth injury of, 667
Oral-facial-digital syndrome, 855–856, *856*
Oral feeding, of low birth weight infant, 794
Orbit, cellulitis of, 921
tumors of, 923–926
Organic acids, inborn errors of, 549–552
Ornithine transcarbamylase (OTC) deficiency, 545
Osteochondrodysplasia, 821*t*
Osteogenesis imperfecta, 828–830, *829*
Osteolysis, idiopathic, 821*t*
Osteomalacia, 474
Osteomyelitis, 741–742
Osteopenia, in prematures, 474–476
Osteoporosis, 474
Ota, nevus of, 891
Otitis media, 738
Ovary, cyst of, 409
embryologic differentiation of, 503, *504*
"Owl's eye cells," 760, *760*
Oxacillin, route and dose for, 972
Oxycephaly, 691, 692*t*
Oxygen
effects of, on immature retina, 910, *911*
hemoglobin affinity for, 583, *583, 584*
saturation of, after birth, 226, *226*
in fetal blood, 225, *225*
on cardiac catheterization, 236
therapy, 104, 217
transcutaneous monitoring of, 913
Oxytetracycline, route and dose for, 972
Oxytocin challenge test, 39

Pachygyria, 688
PAH (para-amino hippurate) clearance, 396*t*, 398
Palate, cleft, 819
Palmar grasp response, 654*t*, 655
Palmar lines, transverse, 847
Pancreas, annular, 361–363
intestinal obstruction and, 349
endocrine, development of, 514
Pancreatin, route and dose for, 972
Pancuronium, 962
route and dose for, 972
Panencephalitis, chronic progressive, complicating congenital rubella, 757
Papilloma, of choroid plexus, 715
hydrocephalus in, 696
Para-amino hippurate (PAH) clearance, 396*t*, 398
Paraldehyde, route and dose for, 972

Parathyroid hormone, calcitonin and, 465
  control of calcium and phosphate
    metabolism by, 464
  urinary indices of, 457t, 458
Parenteral nutrition, 795–797
  partial, 795
  total, 796, 796
    complications of, 797t
    infusate composition of, 796t
Parenti-Fraccaro achondrogenesis, 820
Parotitis, suppurative neonatal, 321
Paroxysmal disorders, 702–706
Pasini variant, of epidermolysis bullosa,
  875
Pavulon, route and dose for, 972
Pectus excavatum, 197
Pedialyte, composition of, 978
Penicillin, concentration of, in maternal
  blood and breast milk, 993
Penicillin G, route and dose for, 972
Penis, absence of, 402
  duplication of, 402–403
  torsion of, 403, 403
Pentobarbital, route and dose for, 973
Peptic ulcer, 344
Perforation, gastric, 344–345
  of peptic ulcer, 344
Perinatal asphyxia, neurologic
  consequences of, 662, 669–679
Perinatal mortality. See Neonatal death.
Perinatal-neonatal intensive care facilities,
  regionalization of, 2
Perinatal period, 2
Perinatal trauma, neurologic
  consequences of, 661–669
Perinatology, diagnostic and therapeutic
  advances in, 3t
Peripheral nerves, birth injuries to, 667
Peripheral pulses, evaluation of, 229
Perirenal hematoma, 440
Peritoneal adhesions, intestinal
  obstruction and, 367
Peritoneal dialysis, in acute renal failure,
  461
Peritonitis, 386
  bacterial, 387–388
  bile, 388
  meconium, 386–387, 386
Pes calcaneovalgus, 836, 837
Pes equinovarus, 838, 838
Pes metatarsovarus, 837, 838
Pfeiffer syndrome, 692t
Phagocytosis, 575, 576
Pharmacokinetics, neonatal, principles of,
  953–957
Pharmacology, neonatal, 950–968. See
  also Drugs.
Pharmacopeia, for newborn period, 970–
  973
Pharynx, diverticulum of, 321
  pseudodiverticulum of, 321
Phenobarbital
  concentration of, in maternal blood
    and breast milk, 993
  for neonatal seizures, 964
  half-life and therapeutic levels of, 954t
  route and dose for, 973
  teratogenic and carcinogenic effects of,
    930, 930t
Phenylalanine, hydroxylation pathway of,
  537
  increased blood concentration of,
    metabolic disorders with, 538t
Phenylbutazone, concentration of, in
  maternal blood and breast milk, 993

Phenylketonuria(PKU), 537–539
  "atypical," 539
  genetic origin of, 526, 526
  Guthrie bacterial assay for, 62, 62
  maternal, 540
  newborn screening for, 63
Phenytoin
  for neonatal seizures, 964
  half-life and therapeutic levels of, 954t
  route and dose for, 971
  teratogenic and carcinogenic effects of,
    930, 930t, 932
Phimosis, 401
Phlebectasia, congenital generalized, 888,
  889
Phosphate, depletion of, with
  hypercalcemia, 474
  evaluation of levels of, in renal
    function, 399
  metabolism of, endocrine control of,
    464–479
Phosphorus, concentration of, in renal
  failure, acute, 460
  estimated daily requirements of, in
    premature, 980
  normal blood chemistry values for, 984
Phototherapy, of hyperbilirubinemia,
  590, 628–630, 628t
Phrenic nerves, absent, lung hypoplasia
  with, 186
Physical examination, of newborn, 55–59
Physical maturity, newborn rating of, 981
Piebaldism, 871–872, 871
Pierre Robin syndrome, 817–818
Pigtail sign, of Hirschsprung's disease,
  369, 369
Pitressin, aqueous, route and dose for,
  973
Pits, branchiogenous, 321
Pituitary gland, hypoplasia of, 483
PiZZ genotype, hyperbilirubinemia with,
  conjugated, 645
PKU. See Phenylketonuria.
Placenta
  blood loss from, 588
  blood volume at birth, factors
    determining, 20, 20t
  examination of, 20
  growth of, 94
  viral transmission through, 166, 167
Plagiocephaly, 690, 692t
Plasma, fresh frozen, 563
  route and dose for, 973
Plasma flow, renal, clinical evaluation of,
  396t, 398
Plasma protein binding, of drugs, 951,
  951, 952t
Plateau principle, in drug therapy, 955,
  956
Platelet abnormalities, bleeding due to,
  569–573
Platelet count, 561, 563t
Platelet transfusion, 563
PM 60/40, composition of, 976
Pneumococcus, conjunctivitis due to, 920
Pneumocystis carinii pneumonia, 179–
  180
Pneumonia, 165–181
  acquired during birth, 172
  aspiration, 173–174
  Chlamydia trachomatis, 177
  complicating oral thrush, 773
  congenital, radiographic patterns of,
    168, 169–171
  incidence of, 165

Pneumonia (Continued)
  intrauterine, 165–172
  Klebsiella-Aerobacter, 177
  Pneumocystis carinii, 179–180
  postnatally acquired, 173–174
  prematurity incidence with, 173t
  Pseudomonas, 177–178
  staphylococcal, 174–176
  streptococcal, Group B, 176–177
  viral, 178–179
  with multiple pathogens, 180
Pneumopericardium, 158–159, 159
Pneumothorax, 155–157, 155–158
  vs. balloon cyst, 203
  with mechanical ventilation, 220
Polyarteritis nodosa, infantile, 615–617,
  615t
Polycystic renal disease, adult type, 426
  differential diagnosis of, 450
  infantile type, 425
Polycythemia, 608–610, 609t
  Wilms' tumor with, 938
Polyhydramnios, 18
Polymicrogyria, 688
Polyp, umbilical, 382–383
Polysplenia, 267
Pompe's disease, 535
Portagen, composition of, 978
Port-wine stain, 885
Postmaturity, 97–98
Postpartum hemorrhage, anemia due to,
  589
Post-term, 4
Potassium, estimated daily requirements
  of, in premature, 980
  normal blood chemistry values for, 984
Potter's syndrome, 416, 417–418, 417
P–R interval, 230, 230t
Prader-Willi syndrome, chromosome
  deletion in, 853
Prednisone, route and dose for, 973
Preeclampsia, fetal effect of, 14
Pregestimil, composition of, 976
Pregnancy, diabetes and, White
  classification of, 15t
  duration of, distribution curve of, 44
  multiple, fetal size and, 96
Prematurity, 44, 83–92
  anemia of, 606–608
    iron supplementation in, 608t
    vitamin E supplementation in, 608t
  behavior of, 69
  body composition of, nutritional
    implications of, 791–792
  clinical criteria for, 2, 94t
  electrocardiogram in, 231
  eosinophilia in, 580
  estimated daily requirements of, 980
  incidence of, 83
  intestinal development in, 312–314,
    312–314
  long-term outcome of, 87–91, 89, 90t
  mortality associated with, 86, 86–88,
    88t
  osteopenia in, 474–476
  patent ductus arteriosus with, 279–281
  pathophysiology of, 83–86
  perinatal approach to, 89t
  physical examination in, 59

Prematurity (*Continued*)
  pulmonary insufficiency of, chronic, 152, *152*
  retinopathy of, 909–914
    incidence of, 909, 909*t*, *910*
    vitamin E prophylaxis for, 810, 913
  T$_4$ levels in, transient low, 498
  thyroid function in, *492*, 493, *493*
  viability limits of, 86–87
  weight chart for, *983*
Prenatal care, effect on fetus/newborn, 10
  in diabetes, 14
Prenatal diagnosis, genetic. *See Genetic diagnosis, prenatal.*
  of hyaline membrane disease, 139, *140*
  of sexual differentiation abnormalities, 512
Preputial adhesions, 402
Preterm, 3. *See also Prematurity.*
Priscoline, route and dose for, 973
Procainamide, route and dose for, 973
Progestins, exogenous, fetal exposure to, 12
  maternal ingestion of, male pseudohermaphroditism and, 510
Pronestyl, route and dose for, 973
Properdin system, 724
Propionic acidemia, 549–551, *550*
Propranolol, as antihypertensive, 960*t*
  route and dose for, 973
Propylthiouracil, route and dose for, 973
Prosobee, composition of, 976
Prostaglandins, E-type, ductal patency and, 279, 961
Prostaphlin, route and dose for, 972
Prostigmin, route and dose for, 972
Protamine sulfate, route and dose for, 973
Protein
  plasma, drug binding in, 951, *951*, 952*t*
  requirements of, in low birth weight infant, 792
    in premature, 980
  total, normal blood chemistry values for, 984
Proteinosis, pulmonary alveolar, 188
Proteinuria, 396
  due to galactosemia, 532
Prothrombin time, 562, 563*t*
Protozoal infection, 775–778
"Prune belly," 414
Pseudoarthrosis, congenital, of tibia, 839
Pseudocholedochal cyst, 641
Pseudodiverticulum, pharyngeal, 321
Pseudohermaphroditism, male, 510
Pseudohypoaldosteronism, hyponatremia and, 488
Pseudomonas pneumonia, 177–178
Pseudomonas septicemia, 734
Pseudoparalysis, of congenital syphilis, 779
Pseudostrabismus, 907, *907*
Ptosis, congenital, 907–908, *907, 908*
Puddenz-Heyer-Schulte valve, 698
Pulmonary. *See also Lung(s).*
Pulmonary alveolar proteinosis, 188
Pulmonary artery pressure, elevated, 236
  normal, 237*t*

Pulmonary atresia
  tetralogy of Fallot with, 251–253, *252*
  with intact ventricular septum, 253–255, *253, 254*
    differential diagnosis of, 286
  with ventricular septal defect, differential diagnosis of, 286
Pulmonary cyst, 199–213
  air-containing, 199–204
  fluid-filled, 204–212
Pulmonary disorders, 181–189
Pulmonary dysfunction, persistent, 152
Pulmonary hemorrhage, 214–216
Pulmonary hypertension, persistent, 102
Pulmonary insufficiency, of prematurity, chronic, 152, *152*
Pulmonary lymphangiectasis, congenital, 187–188
Pulmonary plethora, 234
Pulmonary sequestration, 210
Pulmonary stenosis, with intact ventricular septum, 255
  differential diagnosis of, 286
Pulmonary tuberculosis, infant of mother on therapy for, 749
Pulmonary vascularity, radiographic assessment of, 232–234, *232*
Pulmonary venous return, total anomalous, 263–265, *263–265*
  differential diagnosis of, 286, 288
  with obstruction, chest radiograph in, *232*
Pulse, peripheral, evaluation of, 229
P wave, 230
Pyelography, antegrade, 450
  intravenous, 397
Pyelonephritis, vs. glomerulonephritis, 452
Pylorus, atresia of, 341–342
  hypertrophic stenosis of, 342–343, *343*
    vs. duodenal atresia or stricture, 343
Pyogenic infection, recurrent, 727
Pyridoxine, deficiency and dependency of, 803–805
  neonatal seizures due to, 703
  route and dose for, 973
Pyrilamine maleate, concentration of, in maternal blood and breast milk, 993
Pyrimethamine, concentration of, in maternal blood and breast milk, 993
Pyruvate kinase deficiency, hemolytic anemia due to, 600
Pyruvic acidemia, 551
Pyuria, 397

QRS complex, 230, 230*t*
Q–T interval, 230*t*, 231
Quinidine gluconate, route and dose for, 973
Quinine sulfate, concentration of, in maternal blood and breast milk, 993

Radiation, fetal exposure to, 12
Radiograph, chest, 231–234
  skull, 658
Radius, bilateral absence of, thrombocytopenia and, 572
  defects of, 831–832
Ranula, 318
RCF, composition of, 976

Rectal biopsy, normal, *371*
Rectal manometry, normal, *370*
  with Hirschsprung's disease, 369, *370*
Rectum, congenital deformities of, 356–358
Recurrence risk, of congenital defects, determining of, 862–864
Red blood cells
  disorders of, 581–615. *See also Anemia.*
  enzyme abnormalities of, 598–601
  gestational values of, 582, 582*t*
  hereditary disorders of, 594–598
  physiology of, normal, in fetus and neonate, 581–583
Red blood cell count, 584, 585*t*
Reducing body myopathy, 711*t*
5α-Reductase deficiency, 509
Reflexes, neonatal, evaluation of, 654, 654*t*
Reflux, gastroesophageal acid, hiatus hernia and, 327–330
Refractive errors, in neonates, 915
Regurgitant murmur, 229
Renal. *See also Kidney(s).*
Renal agenesis, bilateral, *416*, 417–418, *417*
Renal blastema, persistent, 940
Renal collecting system, duplication of, 418–419, *418*
Renal dysplasia, 421–422
  differential diagnosis of, 450
Renal failure, acute, 456–462
  etiologies of, 456, 456*t*
  drugs and, 460*t*, 461
Renal function, clinical evaluation of, 396*t*, 397–400
  embryological development of, 394
Renal mass, differential diagnosis of, 447–451
  distribution of, 448*t*
Renal necrosis, cortical and medullary, 439–440
Renal plasma flow, clinical evaluation of, 396*t*, 398
Renal scan, 397, 449
Renal thrombosis
  arterial, 439
  cortical and medullary necrosis due to, 439–440
  venous, 437–438
    differential diagnosis of, 450
Renal tubular acidosis, distal, 400
  proximal, 399
Renal tubular function, evaluation of, 396*t*, 399
Renin-angiotensin system, in hypertension, 442–446
Renogram, 397
Respiration. *See Breathing.*
Respiratory distress. *See also Hyaline membrane disease.*
  causes of, 113*t*
  cesarean section related to, 17, 17*t*
  clinical findings in, 588*t*
  diagnosis of, clues to, 114*t*
  evaluation of, priorities in, 141*t*
  frequency of, 112
  "late onset," 137
Respiratory rates, normal newborn, 56
Respiratory syncytial virus, nursery outbreaks of, 766
  pneumonia due to, 178–179
Respiratory system, disorders of, 109–164

Respiratory tract infection, lower
persistent or recurrent, 329
viral, nosocomial, 766
Resuscitation, delivery room, 100–108
equipment for, 106t
Reticular dysgenesis, 578
Reticulocyte, gestational values of, 582t
Reticulocyte count, 585, 585t
Reticuloendothelial system (RES), 725
Retina, vascular immaturity of, retrolental
fibroplasia and, 910, 910
Retinoblastoma, 924–926, 924, 925
Retinoblastoma–mental retardation
syndrome, 852
Retinopathy, of prematurity, 909–914
incidence of, 909, 909t, 910
vitamin E prophylaxis for, 810, 913
Retrolental fibroplasia. See Retinopathy,
of prematurity.
Reye syndrome, 713
Rh hemolytic disease, 590–593
clinical and laboratory features of, 591t
Rhabdomyoma, cardiac, 301, 301, 302
Rheumatic disorders, 615–619
Rickets, 474–476, 807–809, 808
Rifampin, concentration of, in maternal
blood and breast milk, 993
Riley-Day syndrome, 717
Ritter's disease, 880–881, 880
Robertsonian translocations, 26
Rosette, of retinoblastoma, 924, 924
Rotaviruses, nursery-acquired infection
with, 767
Rotor syndrome, 644
Rubella, congenital, 755–757, 756
clinical findings in, 755t
manifestations of, 755
Rud's syndrome, ichthyosis with, 870
Russell-Silver syndrome, 693, 694

Sacral agenesis, 687
Sacrococcygeal teratomas, 941–943,
941, 942
Sagittal suture synostosis, 689, 690
Salivary glands, inflammation of, 321
Salmonella gastroenteritis, 739
Salt wasting, with virilization, in 21-
hydroxylation defect, 484
Sarcotubular myopathy, 711t
Scalded skin syndrome, staphylococcal,
880–881, 880
Scalp defect, congenital, 687
Scalp pH, fetal, 41
Scaphocephaly, 689, 690, 692t
Sciatic nerve palsy, due to birth injury,
669
Sclerae, blue, with osteogenesis
imperfecta, 828
Sclerema neonatorum, 901, 901
Sclerosis, mesangial diffuse, 454
tuberous, 715, 893
cardiac rhabdomyoma with, 302,
303
white macule of, 893
Scraping, conjunctival, methods of, 919
Screening, newborn, 60–67
follow-up, 65
specimen collection for, 61, 61, 65
Screening laboratory, 61, 66
Screening tests, 61, 62t
confirmatory tests for, 62

Scrotum, hernia of, vs. inguinal hernia,
360
Scurvy, neonatal, 805–807, 806
Sebaceous gland hyperplasia, 899–900
Seborrheic eczema, 897–898, 897
Seckel's bird-headed dwarfism, 859
Seizures, 702–706
anticonvulsants for, 705, 964
Sepsis, hyperbilirubinemia with,
conjugated, 645
Sepsis neonatorum, 732–735
Septicemia, 732–735
Septostomy, balloon atrial, in
transposition of great arteries, 248
Sequestration, pulmonary, 210
"Setting sun" sign, in hydrocephalus,
696
Sex steroids, biosynthetic pathway of,
480
Sexual differentiation, abnormalities of,
503–513
classification of, 505t
prenatal diagnosis of, 512
Shigellosis, 739
Sialadenitis, 321
Sickle cell, genetic variants of, 604, 604
Sickle cell anemia, 604
Sickle cell disease, newborn screening
for, 64
SIDS, 117–118
apneic spells in, 116
"near miss," 117
Silver nitrate, route and dose for, 973
Simian crease, 847
Similac, composition of, 974
Sinus
dermal, congenital, 687
intracranial venous, thrombosis of,
713–714
neurodermal, 687
omphalomesenteric, 383
urachal, vs. omphalomesenteric, 379
Sinus arrhythmia, 304
Sinus bradycardia, 304
Sinus rhythm, normal, 229
Sinus tachycardia, 304
Sipple syndrome, chromosome deletion
in, 853
Sjögren-Larsson syndrome, ichthyosis
with, 870
Skeletal system, disorders of, 815–843
Skin
absence of, congenital, 872, 872
at birth, 57
disorders of, 867–903
congenital and hereditary, 868–878
infections of, 879–884
bacterial, 743–744
nevi of, 884–896
tumors of, 884–896
Skin tag, branchiogenous, 321
Skull, cloverleaf, 691, 692t
fractures of, in newborn, 664, 664
radiographs of, 658
SMA, composition of, 976
"Premie," 974
Smoking, maternal, fetal size and, 94
perinatal mortality and complications
with, 96t
Sodium, estimated daily requirements of,
in premature, 980
metabolism of, disorders of, 479–490
normal blood chemistry values for, 984
Sodium balance, in renal failure, acute,
459

Sodium bicarbonate, administration of, to
asphyxiated newborn, 104
route and dose for, 973
Solid foods, introduction of, 791
Solu-Cortef, route and dose for, 973
Solu-Medrol, route and dose for, 972
Special Care, composition of, 974
Spermatic cord, torsion of, 407
Spermicides, vaginal, teratogenic and
carcinogenic effects of, 930, 930t
Spherocytosis, hereditary, 594–598, 596
Spina bifida cystica, 682–686, 683–685
Spinal cord, perinatal trauma to, 665
Spinal epidural abscess, 713
Spinal muscular atrophy, 707
Spirochetal organisms, infection with,
778–781
Spironolactone, route and dose for, 973
Spondyloepiphyseal dysplasia congenita,
826
Staphcillin, route and dose for, 972
Staphylococcal conjunctivitis, 920
Staphylococcal disease, 733
cutaneous, 743, 879–881
nosocomial, 744
Staphylococcal pneumonia, 174–176
Staphylococcal scalded skin syndrome,
880–881, 880
State, of neonate, 68, 75–77
breathing patterns in, 114, 115, 116
Status marmoratus, 672, 672
Sternal cleft, upper, 197
Sternomastoid tumor, 322
Sternum, complete separation of, 197
Steroids, adrenal production of, 479–
481, 480
enzymatic defects in, 483–487, 484t
Stillbirth, 3
Stomach
aberrant umbilical, 374–375
disorders of, 340–346
duplication of, 340–341, 341
emptying of, delay in, 342
function of, 311
hypoplasia of, 340
obstruction of, intrinsic, 341–342
peptic ulcer of, 344
perforation of, 344–345
supradiaphragmatic, 327, 328
teratoma of, 345
Strabismus, 906–907, 907
paralytic, 906
with retinoblastoma, 925
Streptococcal conjunctivitis, 920
Streptococcal disease, 733
cutaneous, 743, 883
group A, 733
nosocomial, 745
group B, 733
cutaneous, 883
early onset, 731
maternal transmission of IgG and,
721
pathogenesis of, 731
group D, 733
Streptococcal pneumonia, Group B,
176–177
Streptomycin, route and dose for, 973
concentration of, in maternal blood
and breast milk, 993
Stress test, of fetus, 39, 39t

Stridor(s), 122–128
laryngeal, simple congenital, 122–123
neurogenic, 126–127
String sign, in pyloric stenosis, 343, *343*
Sturge-Weber syndrome, 715
nevus flammeus as sign of, 886
Subdural empyema, 713
Subdural hemorrhage, 665
Subdural taps, 658
Subglottic stenosis, acquired, 124
congenital, 124
Submaxillary glands, suppuration of, 321
Sucking, in newborn, 73
Suctioning, of newborn, 104
in meconium aspiration, 107, 129
Sudden infant death syndrome, 117–118
apneic spells in, 116
"near miss," 117
Sugar, blood, newborn levels of, 514–
515, *515*
normal blood chemistry values for,
984
888Sulfapyridine, concentration of,
in maternal blood and breast milk,
993
Sulfisoxazole, route and dose for, 973
Sulfur amino acid abnormalities, 541–
543, *541*
Suprabulbar paresis, congenital, 667
Surfactant, fetal lipid, in amniotic fluid,
tests for, 41, *42*
in hyaline membrane disease,
deficiency of, 136
replacement of, 143
Sydney line, 847
Synthroid, route and dose for, 972
Syphilis, congenital, 778–780
membranous glomerulonephropathy
due to, 452–454
Syringomyelocele, *683*

T_3, low, euthyroid sick syndrome of, 499
serum, alterations in, secondary to
alterations in TBG, 499
synthesis and secretion of, 490
T_4. See *Thyroxine.*
Tachycardia
paroxysmal, supraventricular, *304,*
305, *305*
vs. myocarditis, 295
sinus, 304
ventricular, 306
Tachypnea, transient, of newborn, 181–
183, *182*
Tactile sensitivity, of newborn, 73
Tagamet, route and dose for, 970
Tamm-Horsfall protein, in urine, 396
Taste, newborn response to, 73
Tay-Sachs disease, 553
prenatal diagnosis of, 28
TBG alterations, serum T_4 and T_3
alterations secondary to, 499
Teeth, eruption of, first, infant age at,
991
natal and neonatal, 318
Telangiectatic nevi, 885, *886*
Temperature
assessment of, in newborn, 55
body regulation of, in neonate, 50, *50t*

Temperature (*Continued*)
environmental, oxygen consumption
related to, *50,* 51
regulation of, in hyaline membrane
disease, 143
Temperature equivalents, 992
Tensilon, route and dose for, 973
Teratogens, 11, *11t*
in utero exposure to, 930, *930t*
susceptibility to, *11*
Teratoma
gastric, 345
mediastinal, 210, *211*
of neck, 323
sacrococcygeal, 941–943, *941, 942*
Term infant, 4
blood chemistry values of, normal, 984
electrocardiogram in, normal ranges of,
229, *230t*
representative values in, 989
size of, 43, *44*
thyroid function in, 492, *492, 493*
Testicular feminization, 510
Testis(es)
embryologic differentiation of, 503,
504
hydrocele of, 406–407, *406*
vs. inguinal hernia, 360, 407
undescended, 405–406
unresponsiveness of, to HCG and LH,
510
vanishing, syndrome of, 509
Testosterone, end-organ insensitivity to,
509–510
synthesis of, defects in, 509
Tetanus antitoxin, route and dose for,
973
Tetanus immune globulin, route and
dose for, 973
Tetanus neonatorum, 709, 751–752
Tetany, neonatal, 469
acute, emergency treatment of, 469
late, dietary factors for, 470
Tetracyclines, concentration of, in
maternal blood and breast milk, 993
route and dose for, 973
Tetrahydrobiopterin deficiency, *537,* 539
Tetralogy of Fallot, 249–251, *249–251*
differential diagnosis of, 286
with pulmonary atresia, 251–253, *252*
Thalassemia syndromes, 601–604
Thalidomide syndrome, 832
THAM, route and dose for, 973
Thanatophoric dwarfism, 822–823, *824*
Theophylline, for neonatal apnea, 116,
118, 963, *963t*
half-life and therapeutic levels of, *954t*
route and dose for, 973
Thiamine, deficiency of, 802–803, *803*
route and dose for, 973
Thiazide diuretics, 965
Thiouracil, concentration of, in maternal
blood and breast milk, 993
13q – syndrome, 852
Thoracic dysplasia, asphyxiating, 197,
198, 826
Thorazine, route and dose for, 970
Thrombasthenia, Glanzmann's, 573
Thrombocytopenia
complicating cavernous hemangioma,
888
due to bone marrow hypoplasia, 572
hereditary, 572
immune, due to drug-induced maternal
thrombocytopenia, 571
secondary to maternal disease, 570

Thrombocytopenia (*Continued*)
isoimmune, 569
with absent radius, 832
with giant hemangiomas, 571
with infection, 571
Thromboplastin time, activated partial,
562, *563t*
Thrombosis, intracranial venous sinus,
713–714
mesenteric, 367–368
renal. See *Renal thrombosis.*
Thrush, 882
oral, pneumonia complicating, 773
Thrush esophagitis, 773
Thumb, defects of, 831–832
Thymus, 205
abnormal epithelium of, in severe
combined immune deficiency, 726,
726
as tracheal mass, *322,* 323
enlarged, 210
Thyroglossal duct cyst, spherical mass of,
323
Thyroid, lingual and sublingual, 321
Thyroid function, neonatal, 492–493,
492, 493
Thyroid gland, disorders of, 490–502
dysgenesis of, 493–496, *494*
Thyroid hormones, secretion of, 490–
492
synthesis of, inborn errors of, 496
Thyroid-stimulating hormone, deficient
secretion or effect of, 496
Thyrotoxicosis, neonatal, 500
Thyroxine
radioimmunoassay for, as screening
test, 62
serum, alterations in, secondary to
alterations in TBG, 499
route and dose for, 973
synthesis and secretion of, 490
transient low levels of, in preterm
infants, 498
Thyroxine-binding globulin, alterations in,
serum T_4 and T_3 alterations
secondary to, 499
Tibia, kyphoscoliotic, congenital, 839
pseudoarthrosis of, congenital, 839
T lymphocyte, 723
Tobramycin, half-life and therapeutic
levels of, *954t*
route and dose for, 973
Tocolytic agents, 84, *84t*
dosage regimens for, *85t*
Tolazoline, 958
route and dose for, 973
side effects of, *958t*
Tomography, computed, in neurologic
evaluation of newborn, 659
Tongue, disorders of, 318–324
Tongue tie, 318
Tonic neck response, *654t,* 655
Torticollis, 322
Toxoplasmosis, congenital, 775–778
manifestations of, *755*
Trachea, compression of, by extrinsic
masses, 124
stenosis of, 124
Tracheoesophageal fistula, types of, 332,
332
with esophageal atresia, 332–335,
333, 334
without esophageal atresia, 335–336,
336

Transfusion
  blood, in anemia, 586
  cytomegalovirus infection and, 586
  exchange, in hyperbilirubinemia, 590,
    628t
    partial, in polycythemia, 609
  graft-versus-host disease due to, 724
  intrauterine, 592
    graft-versus-host disease following,
      586
  platelet, 563
  twin-twin, 588
Transillumination, 656
Translocation, of chromosome 21, 848,
    849
  Robertsonian, 26
Transplantation, bone marrow, 727
Transpyloric feeding, of low birth weight
    infant, 795
Trauma, perinatal, neurologic
    consequences of, 661–669
Treacher Collins syndrome, 816–817,
    816
Triad syndrome, 414–417, 415
Tricuspid atresia, 256–259, 257, 258
  differential diagnosis of, 286, 288
Tricuspid valve, Ebstein's anomaly of,
    259–261, 260
  chest radiograph in, 232
  differential diagnosis of, 286
Trigonocephaly, 691, 692t
Trilaminar myopathy, 711t
Trishydromethylaminomethane (THAM),
    route and dose for, 973
Trisomy, autosomal, maternal age and,
    25, 26
Trisomy 8, 851
Trisomy 9p, 852
Trisomy 13, 851, 851
Trisomy 18, 850–851, 850
Trisomy 21, 848–850, 848, 849
  karyotype of cell with, 25
  leukemia with, 933
  maternal age dependence of, 25, 26
Trisomy 22, 850
Truncus arteriosus, 261–263, 262
  differential diagnosis of, 288
Tryptophan, defect in intestinal transport
    of, 473
TSH, deficient secretion or effect of, 496
Tuberculosis, 748–750
  multiple pseudocystic of bones, 750
  nursery exposure to, 750
Tuberous sclerosis, 715, 893
  cardiac rhabdomyoma with, 302, 303
  white macule of, 893
d-Tubocurarine, 962
Tumor(s). See also names of specific
    tumors.
  brain, congenital, 714–715
  cutaneous, 884–896
  intraspinal, congenital, 715–716
  intrathoracic, 204–212
  malignant, congenital, 928–947
    congenital defects associated with,
      930
    host factors in, 930
    incidence of, 928, 929t
    mortality of, 928, 928t, 929t
    pathogenesis of, 928–931
    transplacental passage of, 928–930
  nasopharyngeal, 319–320
  neuroectodermal, melanotic, 935
  of eye and orbit, 923–926
  of heart, 301–303, 301, 302
  of larynx, 126

Tumor(s) (Continued)
  of liver, malignant, 941
  sternomastoid, 322
  Wilms', 938–940, 939
    congenital defects with, 930, 938
    neoplasms related to, 940–941
Turner syndrome, 505–507, 506
T wave, 230
21q– syndrome, 852
22q– syndrome, 852
Typhoid fever, 753
Tyrosinemia, 543–544
  transient, role of vitamin C in, 806
Tyrosinosis, 544

UDPG-4-epimerase deficiency, 531, 534
Ulcer, meatal, 402
  peptic, 344
Ulegyria, 672
Ullrich's disease, 711t
Ultrasonography
  in assessment of fetus, 31, 31, 36–39
  in cardiac evaluation, 233, 234, 234
  in neurologic evaluation, 659, 659
  renal, 397, 449
Umbilical artery, infection of, 374
  single, 373
Umbilical cord
  bleeding of, 588
  clamping of, timing of, 20
  delay in separation of, 374
  examination of, 20
  granuloma of. See Granuloma,
    umbilical.
  hernia of, 375, 375
  in postmaturity, 98, 98
  length of, 372
  looped, 372, 372, 373
  screening of blood of, 64
  velamentous insertion of, 372, 372
Umbilical stomach, aberrant, 374–375
Umbilicus
  disorders of, 372–381
  granuloma of. See Granuloma,
    umbilical.
  hernia of, 377–378
  infection of, 373–374
    streptococcal, 883
  polyp of, 382–383
Urachal cyst, 379–380, 379
Urachal sinus, vs. omphalomesenteric
    sinus, 379
Urachus, 378–380
Urea, blood, normal values for, 984
Urea cycle disorders, 544–546
Ureteral obstruction, 430
Ureterocele, 430–431
Ureteropelvic junction, obstruction of,
    429–430, 429
Ureterovesical obstruction, 430
Urethra, male, diverticulum of, 404
Urethral obstruction malformation
    complex, 414
Urethral valve, posterior, 431–434
Uridine diphosphate galactose-4-
    epimerase deficiency, 531, 534
Urinalysis, 395–396
Urinary gonadotropins, elevated, with
    congenital hemihypertrophy and
    intrauterine dwarfism, 831
Urinary tract, embryology of, 394
  infection of, 740–741
    without reflux, hydronephrosis and,
      431

Urine
  examination of, in newborn, 395
  fetal, 394
  formed elements in, in galactosemia,
    532
  newborn screening of, 65, 65
  pH of, 399
  volume of, in term infant, 395
Urogenital abnormalities, imperforate
    anus and, 413
Urography, intravenous, 397, 449
Uropathy, obstructive, 434–435
Urticaria pigmentosa, 894–895, 895
Uveitis, 921, 922

VACTEL syndrome, 832
VACTERL anomaly, 414
Vagina, agenesis of, 409–410
Vaginal delivery, vs. breech, neonatal
    problems in, 18, 18t
Vaginal spermicides, teratogenic and
    carcinogenic effects of, 930, 930t
Valium, route and dose for, 971
Vancomycin, route and dose for, 973
Varicella, 764–765
Vascular malformations, 714
Vasodilators, in myocardial dysfunction,
    958
VATER anomaly, 413, 832
Ventilation
  automatic control of, failure of, 116
  mechanical, 217–221
    complications of, 220
    in hyaline membrane disease, 140–
      143
    techniques of, 218–219
Ventilator, weaning from, 219–220
Ventricle(s)
  dilation of, due to intraventricular
    hemorrhage, 673, 674
  hypoplastic left, with aortic or mitral
    atresia or stenosis, 274–276, 274,
    275
  pressures in, elevated, 237
    normal, 237t
  single left, differential diagnosis of, 288
Ventricular hypertension, systolic, 237
Ventricular overload, in newborn, criteria
    for, 231t
Ventricular septal defects, 276–278, 277,
    278
  chest radiograph of, 232
  differential diagnosis of, 288
  with pulmonary atresia, differential
    diagnosis of, 286
Ventricular septum
  intact, with pulmonary atresia, 253–
    255, 253, 254
    differential diagnosis of, 286
  with pulmonary stenosis, 255
    differential diagnosis of, 286
Ventricular shunting procedures, for
    hydrocephalus, 698
Verapamil, route and dose for, 973
Verrucous nevi, 893
Vesicoureteral reflux, with bladder outlet
    obstruction, 432
Viral hepatitis, 765–766

1012

INDEX

Viral infection. See also names of specific viruses.
  nosocomial, 766–767
  of fetus and newborn, 754–768
  manifestations of, 755
Viral pneumonias, 178–179
Virilization, 508
  by androgen overproduction, maternal, 508
  by maternal drugs, 508, 508
  in 21-hydroxylation defect, 484
Viruses, myocarditis due to, neonatal, 292
  placental transmission of, 166, 167
Vital signs, newborn assessment of, 55
Vitamins, daily intake of, advisable amounts of, 801t
  disorders of, 800–813
  estimated requirements for, 802t
Vitamin A, deficiency of, 800–801
  excess of, 802
  route and dose for, 973
Vitamin B$_1$, deficiency of, 802–803, 803
  route and dose for, 973
Vitamin B$_6$, deficiency and dependency of, 803–805
  neonatal seizures due to, 703
  route and dose for, 973
Vitamin C, deficiency of, 805–807, 806
  route and dose for, 973

Vitamin D
  control of calcium and phosphate metabolism by, 464
  deficiency of, 807–809, 808
  metabolism of, perinatal, 465
  route and dose for, 973
Vitamin E
  deficiency of, 809–810
    hemolysis of erythrocytes in, 607, 607
    in anemia of prematurity, 607
    response to, 607t
    supplemental, 608t
  in prophylaxis of retinopathy of prematurity, 810, 913
  route and dose for, 973
Vitamin K, deficiency of, 810
  hemorrhagic disease of newborn and, 563
Vitamin K$_1$ oxide, route and dose for, 973
Vitelline cyst, 383–384
Vitelline duct, congenital malformations of, 381–385
  embryology of, 381, 382
Vitiligo, vs. hypopigmentation, 892
Vocal cords, paralysis of, 127
Volvulus, with intestinal malrotation, 358–360, 359–360
Vomiting, 315
Von Gierke's disease, 534
Von Willebrand's disease, 565

Water intoxication, hyponatremia and, 488

Watershed pattern, of cortical brain damage, 671, 671
Web, laryngeal, 123
Weber-Cockayne disease, 875
Weight, birth. See Birth weight.
Weight chart, premature, 983
Weil's disease, 780
Werdnig-Hoffmann disease, 707
Western equine encephalitis, 766
Williams elfin facies syndrome, 473, 473
Wilms' tumor, 938–940, 939
  congenital defects with, 930, 938
  neoplasms related to, 940–941
Wilson-Mikity syndrome, 149–152, 151
Wiskott-Aldrich syndrome, 572, 726
Wolff-Parkinson-White syndrome, electrocardiographic pattern of, 305, 305
Wolman's disease, 554

Xanthochromia, of cerebrospinal fluid, 657
Xanthogranuloma, juvenile, 894, 894
X-linked inheritance, disorders of, prenatal diagnosis of, 28
  dominant, 864
  recessive, 863

Zebra-body myopathy, 711t
Zero-order kinetics, 955, 955
Zinc, metabolism of, 811

Your Connected Quizzing access code.
Inprove your learning outcomes through
formative assessments with powerful reporting

CQST263318783383

Please note, after redeeming your access code,
you will be required to enter a Class Code
provided by your Professor

Professional Responsibility in Focus

Get started with your **Connected Casebook**

Redeem your code below to access the **e-book** with search, highlighting, and note-taking capabilities; a **study center** complete with practice questions, explanations, and videos; **case briefing** and **outlining** tools to support efficient learning; and more.

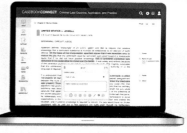

1. Go to www.casebookconnect.com
2. Enter your access code in the box and click **Register**
3. Follow the steps to complete your registration and verify your email address

If you have already registered at CasebookConnect.com, simply log into your account and redeem additional access codes from your Dashboard.

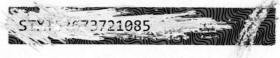

ACCESS CODE: STYW73721085

Scratch off with care.

Is this a used casebook? Access code already redeemed? Purchase a digital version at **CasebookConnect.com/catalog**.

If you purchased a digital bundle with additional components, your additional access codes will appear below.

"I liked being able to search quickly while in class."

"Being able to highlight and easily create case briefs was a fantastic resource and time saver for me!"

"I loved the practice exercises and study questions; they really helped me learn the material!"

10053479-0002

Focus Casebook Series

PROFESSIONAL RESPONSIBILITY IN FOCUS

Second Edition

John P. Sahl

Joseph G. Miller Professor of Law and Director of
The Joseph G. Miller and William C. Becker Center for Professional Responsibility
University of Akron School of Law

R. Michael Cassidy

Professor of Law and Dean's Distinguished Scholar
Boston College Law School

Benjamin P. Cooper

Senior Associate Dean, Professor of Law, and
Frank Montague, Jr. Professor of Legal Studies and Professionalism
University of Mississippi School of Law

Margaret C. Tarkington

Professor of Law and Dean's Fellow
Indiana University Robert H. McKinney School of Law

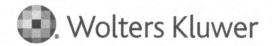

Published by Wolters Kluwer in New York.

Wolters Kluwer Legal & Regulatory U.S. serves customers worldwide with CCH, Aspen Publishers, and Kluwer Law International products. (www.WKLegaledu.com)

To contact Customer Service, e-mail customer.service@wolterskluwer.com, call 1-800-234-1660, fax 1-800-901-9075, or mail correspondence to:

> Wolters Kluwer
> Attn: Order Department
> PO Box 990
> Frederick, MD 21705

Printed in the United States of America.

1 2 3 4 5 6 7 8 9 0

ISBN 978-1-5438-0927-5

Library of Congress Cataloging-in-Publication Data

Names: Sahl, Jack P., author. | Cassidy, R. Michael, author. | Cooper,
   Benjamin P., author. | Tarkington, Margaret C., 1976- author.
Title: Professional responsibility in focus / John P. Sahl, Joseph G.
   Miller Professor of Law and Director of The Joseph G. Miller and William
   C. Becker Center for Professional Responsibility, University of Akron
   School of Law; R. Michael Cassidy, Professor of Law and Dean's
   Distinguished Scholar, Boston College Law School; Benjamin P. Cooper,
   Senior Associate Dean, Professor of Law, and Frank Montague, Jr.
   Professor of Legal Studies and Professionalism University of Mississippi
   School of Law; Margaret C. Tarkington, Professor of Law, Indiana
   University, Robert H. McKinney School of Law.
Description: Second edition. | New York : Wolters Kluwer, [2021] | Series:
   Focus casebook series | Includes bibliographical references and index. |
   Summary: "Law school casebook for courses on professional
   responsibility" — Provided by publisher.
Identifiers: LCCN 2020047426 (print) | LCCN 2020047427 (ebook) |
   ISBN 9781543809275 (hardcover) | ISBN 9781543831207 (ebook)
Subjects: LCSH: Legal ethics — United States. | LCGFT: Casebooks (Law)
Classification: LCC KF306 .S24 2021 (print) | LCC KF306 (ebook) |
   DDC 174/.30973 — dc23
LC record available at https://lccn.loc.gov/2020047426
LC ebook record available at https://lccn.loc.gov/2020047427

About Wolters Kluwer Legal & Regulatory U.S.

Wolters Kluwer Legal & Regulatory U.S. delivers expert content and solutions in the areas of law, corporate compliance, health compliance, reimbursement, and legal education. Its practical solutions help customers successfully navigate the demands of a changing environment to drive their daily activities, enhance decision quality and inspire confident outcomes.

Serving customers worldwide, its legal and regulatory portfolio includes products under the Aspen Publishers, CCH Incorporated, Kluwer Law International, ftwilliam.com and MediRegs names. They are regarded as exceptional and trusted resources for general legal and practice-specific knowledge, compliance and risk management, dynamic workflow solutions, and expert commentary.

Summary of Contents

Table of Contents   xi
Preface   xxv
Acknowledgments   xxvii

PART I: INTRODUCTION TO THE LEGAL PROFESSION 1

Chapter 1.   The Role and Responsibility of Lawyers   3

Chapter 2.   The Regulation of the Legal Profession   43

PART II: THE ATTORNEY-CLIENT RELATIONSHIP 99

Chapter 3.   The Attorney-Client Relationship   101

Chapter 4.   Competence — The Lawyer's Indispensable Duty   181

Chapter 5.   Confidentiality, the Attorney-Client Privilege, and
                  Work-Product Immunity   245

Chapter 6.   Conflicts of Interest   309

PART III: LAWYER AS ADVOCATE 369

Chapter 7.   Fairness in Adjudication   371

Chapter 8.   Special Ethical Issues in Criminal Practice   419

PART IV: DELIVERY OF LEGAL SERVICES
AND ACCESS TO JUSTICE 471

Chapter 9.   Practicing Law: Issues in Group Lawyering and the
                  Unauthorized Practice of Law   473

Chapter 10.   Marketing Legal Services   513

Chapter 11.   Access to Justice and Pro Bono Services   543

PART V: THE JUDICIARY 565

Chapter 12.   Judicial Ethics   567

Glossary   609
Table of Cases   617
Table of Rules   623
Index   629

Table of Contents

Preface   *xxv*
Acknowledgments   *xxvii*

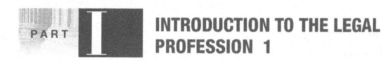

PART I INTRODUCTION TO THE LEGAL PROFESSION 1

Chapter 1: The Role and Responsibility of Lawyers   3

A. The Role of the Lawyer in the System of Justice   3

   1. Guardians of Due Process   4

   2. Self-Regulation and the Protection of Our Public Good   6

B. Law and Moral Responsibility   7

       Oliver Wendell Holmes, *The Path of the Law*   8

   1. Impact and Critique of the Bad Man Perspective   9

       Alexander Meiklejohn, *What of the Good Man?*   13

   2. Communication, Moral Dialogue, and Role Morality   15

       Spaulding v. Zimmerman   18

   3. Cultivating Moral and Professional Judgment   24

       Neil Hamilton, *Professionalism Clearly Defined*   25

C. Professional Responsibilities in Litigating, Advising, and Transactional Planning   30

   1. Shaping Client Conduct   31

   2. Providing Advice Outside of the Checks of the Adversary System   35

Chapter Summary   38

Applying the Rules   39

Professional Responsibility in Practice   40

Chapter 2: The Regulation of the Profession   43

A. Lawyer Regulation   **44**
   1. Regulatory Powers of State Courts   44
   2. Bar Associations and Lawyer Ethics (Conduct) Codes   45

B. Admission to the Bar   **48**
   1. Educational Requirements   49
   2. Character and Fitness   50
      Other Character Examples—Immigration Status, Bigotry,
      Financial Neglect   53
      In re Glass   **55**

C. Lawyer Discipline   **62**
   1. Misconduct Defined   62
      Drug and Alcohol Abuse   64
      Financial Misconduct   65
      Falsehoods and Other Deceptions   65
   2. The Disciplinary Process   66
   3. Sanctions — Aggravating and Mitigating Factors   68
   4. Disciplinary Authority; Choice of Law   69
   5. Reciprocal Discipline   70
   6. Lawyers' Duty to Report Misconduct   71
      In re Himmel   **74**

D. Legal Malpractice   **80**
   1. Background   80
   2. Lawyer Negligence and Legal Malpractice   81
      West Bend Mutual Insurance Co. v. Schumacher   **84**
   3. Legal Malpractice and Breach of Fiduciary Duty   88
      Burnett v. Sharp   **89**
   4. Minimizing Liability for Legal Malpractice   92

Chapter Summary   **94**

Applying the Rules   **95**

Professional Responsibility in Practice   **96**

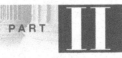

PART II   THE ATTORNEY-CLIENT RELATIONSHIP 99

Chapter 3: The Attorney-Client Relationship   101

A. Forming an Attorney-Client Relationship   **101**

1. Implied Attorney-Client Relationships   102
   Togstad v. Vesely, Otto, Miller & Keefe   *103*
2. Prospective Clients   108
   In re Marriage of Perry   *109*

B. Allocation of Attorney and Client Authority   **115**

1. Basic Allocation of Authority   115
   Red Dog v. Delaware   *117*
2. Counseling or Assisting the Client in Crime or Fraud   120
   Iowa Supreme Court Attorney Disciplinary
   Board v. Engelmann   *122*

C. Understanding the Identity of the Client   **124**

1. Organizational Clients   124
   Yablonski v. United Mine Workers of America   *126*
   "Mirandizing" the Organization's Constituents   *131*
   Reporting Up and Out   *134*
   Pang v. International Document Services   *136*
2. Government Clients   142
3. Insureds   143
   Obligations of a Lawyer Representing an Insured
   Who Objects to a Proposed Settlement Within Policy
   Limits, ABA Formal Opinion 96-403 (1996)   *144*
4. Clients with Diminished Capacity   146

D. Attorney as Fiduciary   **147**

1. Fees   147
   Communicating the Fee to the Client   *147*
   Contingent Fees   *148*
   A Reasonable Fee   *148*
   Sallee v. Tennessee Board of Professional Responsibility   *150*
   Fraudulent Fees   *156*
2. Safeguarding Client Funds and Property   159
   Segregation   *159*
   In re Sather   *161*
   Record Keeping   *167*
   Notification, Delivery, and Accounting   *168*
   Disputes over Property Held by the Attorney   *168*
3. Terminating the Representation   169
   In re Kiley   *170*
   Mandatory Withdrawal   *174*

        Permissive Withdrawal   *175*

        Duties Owed to the Client After Termination   *176*

Chapter Summary   **177**

Applying the Rules   **178**

Professional Responsibility in Practice   **179**

Chapter 4: Competence—The Lawyer's Indispensable Duty   181

A. The Competent Attorney   **182**

   1. Legal Knowledge and Skill   183

      Dahl v. Dahl   ***184***

   2. Inexperienced Lawyers   189

      Attorney Grievance Commission of Maryland v. Kendrick   ***190***

   3. Thoroughness and Preparation   192

   4. Competence and Technology   194

      Use of Cloud Computing Services, Ohio State Bar Association Informal Advisory Opinion 2013-03   *195*

   5. Diligence   197

      In re Disciplinary Action Against Howe   ***199***

   6. Communication   202

      Disclosing Potential Malpractice to a Client, North Carolina State Bar Ethics Opinion (2015)   *205*

      Martin Cole, *The Hardiest Perennials*   *207*

      Utah Bar Journal, *Discipline Corner*   *209*

B. Ineffective Assistance of Criminal Defense Counsel   **210**

   1. The Constitutional Test for Ineffective Assistance of Counsel   213

      Strickland v. Washington   ***214***

   2. *Strickland*'s First Prong: Deficient Performance   221

      Failure to Investigate   *222*

      Failure to Communicate   *223*

      Helmedach v. Commissioner of Correction   ***224***

      Deportation Consequences of a Plea   *228*

   3. *Strickland*'s Second Prong: Prejudice   229

C. When Incompetence Is Not Your Fault   **231**

Ethical Obligations of Lawyers Who Represent Indigent Criminal Defendants When Excessive Caseloads Interfere with Competent and Diligent Representation, ABA Formal Opinion 06-441 (2006) *231*

Ohio v. Jones **234**

D. Competence, Mental Health, and Substance Abuse **237**

Above the Law, *The Struggle* *240*

Chapter Summary **241**

Applying the Rules **242**

Professional Responsibility in Practice **243**

Chapter 5: Confidentiality, the Attorney-Client Privilege, and Work-Product Immunity   245

A. The Duty of Confidentiality **246**

    Purcell v. District Attorney for the Suffolk District **252**

B. The Attorney-Client Privilege **258**

  1. Introduction 258

    Attorney-Client Privilege Elements Defined *258*

  2. Scope of the Privilege 259

    The Confidential and Privileged Relationship *259*

    Communications for the Purpose of Legal Advice *259*

    Mixed Communications *261*

    No Privilege for Preexisting Client Documents and Underlying Facts *262*

    Entity Clients and the Privilege *262*

    Upjohn Co. v. United States **263**

    Government Lawyers and the Privilege *267*

    Common Interest Doctrine *268*

    Schaeffler v. United States **274**

  3. Waivers 279

    Protecting the Privilege in Adversarial Proceedings and During Representation *280*

    Selective Waiver *280*

    In re Pacific Pictures Corp. **282**

    Partial Disclosures and Subject Matter Waivers *286*

    Inadvertent Disclosures: Limiting Attorney-Client Privilege and Work-Product Waivers *288*

Ardon v. City of Los Angeles   *289*

    4. Exceptions   291

       Crime-Fraud Exception   *291*

       In re Grand Jury Investigation   **293**

       Joint-Clients Exception   *296*

       Self-Defense Exception   *296*

C. Work-Product Immunity   **297**

    1. Two Types of Work Product: Ordinary and Opinion   298

    2. Waivers and Exceptions to Work-Product Immunity   298

       Schaeffler v. United States   **299**

Chapter Summary   **303**

Applying the Rules   **305**

Professional Responsibility in Practice   **307**

Chapter 6: Conflicts of Interest   **309**

A. Current-Client Conflicts and Client Waivers   **310**

    1. Directly Adverse and Material Limitation Conflicts   310

       W. Bradley Wendel, *Conflicts of Interest Under the*
         Revised Model Rules   *311*

       Cinema 5, Ltd. v. Cinerama, Inc.   **314**

       Multiple/Joint Representation Conflicts   *318*

       Criminal Cases   *320*

       Civil Cases   *322*

B. Lawyer Personal-Interest Conflicts with Clients   **325**

    1. Business Transactions and Using Client Information   325

       In re Disciplinary Proceedings Against Creedy **327**

    2. No Gift Solicitations (or Writing Testimonial Bequests to Yourself)   330

    3. Literary Rights and Financial Assistance   331

    4. Aggregate Settlements   333

    5. No Prospective Malpractice Limitations   334

    6. No Proprietary Interest in Client Matter   335

    7. Sexual Relations with Clients   336

    8. Prospective-Client Conflicts and Advance Waivers   337

    9. Advocate-Witness Conflict   338

C. Former-Client Conflicts of Interest   **340**

       Western Sugar Coop. v. Archer-Daniels-Midland Co.   *343*

D. Imputation of Client Conflicts   351
    Goldberg v. Warner/Chappell Music, Inc.   356

E. Conflicts of Interests for Current and Former Lawyers in
   Government Service   362

F. Specific Conflicts Rules: Judges, Arbitrators, and Others   363

Chapter Summary   364

Applying the Rules   365

Professional Responsibility in Practice   367

PART III   LAWYER AS ADVOCATE 369

Chapter 7: Fairness in Adjudication   371

A. Meritorious Claims and Expediting Litigation   371
    In re Olsen   373

B. Obligation to Be Truthful   376
  1. Candor to the Court   376
    In re Richards   378
  2. Failure to Disclose Adverse Facts in *Ex Parte* Proceedings   380
  3. Failure to Disclose Controlling Legal Authority   380
    In re Thonert   381
  4. Client or Other Witness Giving False Testimony in Civil Litigation 383
    Committee on Professional Ethics v. Crary   385
    Limitations on a Lawyer's Participation in the Preparation
     of a Witness's Testimony, D.C. Bar Legal Ethics Committee
     Formal Opinion 79 (1979)   389

C. Fairness to the Opposing Party and Counsel   390
  1. Obstruction, Alteration, or Destruction of Evidence   390
  2. Discovery Obligations   392

D. Trial Tactics   393
  1. Disruption   393
  2. Civility   394

E. Maintaining the Impartiality of the Tribunal   395

F. Public Comment on Pending Civil Litigation   397
    Maldonado v. Ford Motor Co.   399

G. **Communicating with Represented Persons**   402

   Messing, Rudavsky & Weliky, P.C. v. President and
      Fellows of Harvard College   *404*

H. **Communicating with Unrepresented Persons**   408

I. **Truthfulness in Statements to Others**   409

   In re Crossen   *411*

Chapter Summary   415

Applying the Rules   416

Professional Responsibility in Practice   417

Chapter 8: Special Ethical Issues in Criminal Practice   419

A. **The Prosecutor**   419

   1. Who Do You Represent?   419

      Fred Zacharias, *Structuring the Ethics of Trial Advocacy*   420

   2. Quantum of Proof Necessary for Charging   424

      Benjamin Weiser, *Doubting Case, a Prosecutor Helped the Defense*   425

   3. Disclosure of Exculpatory Evidence   429

      Brady v. Maryland   **431**

      Prosecutor's Duty to Disclose Evidence and Information
         Favorable to the Defense, ABA Formal Opinion 09-454 (2009)   433

   4. Contact with Represented Suspects   437

      United States v. Lopez   **439**

   5. Statements to the Media   444

B. **The Criminal Defense Lawyer**   446

   1. Taking Possession of Physical Evidence   446

      The "Buried Bodies Case": Client's Confidences and Secrets;
         Past Crimes Disclosed to Lawyer; Plea Bargaining, New York
         State Bar Association Formal Opinion 479 (1978)   448

   2. Putting Your Client on the Stand   453

      Nix v. Whiteside   **454**

   3. Cross-Examining a Truthful Witness   463

      John Mitchell, *Reasonable Doubts Are Where You Find Them:*
         A Response to Professor Subin's Position on the
         Criminal Lawyer's "Different Mission"   463

Chapter Summary   469

Applying the Rules   469

Professional Responsibility in Practice   470

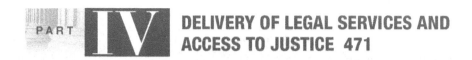

PART IV DELIVERY OF LEGAL SERVICES AND ACCESS TO JUSTICE 471

Chapter 9: Practicing Law: Issues in Group Lawyering and the Unauthorized Practice of Law   473

A. Law Firms and Associations   474
   1. Responsibility of Supervisors   474
   2. Responsibility of Junior Lawyers   475
      Davis v. Alabama State Bar   477
B. The Lawyer's Independence   481
   1. Independence from Non-Lawyers in Practicing Law   484
      Multidisciplinary Practice   485
      Sharing Fees with Non-Lawyers   485
      Ethical Considerations Relating to Participation in Fixed Fee Limited Scope Legal Services Referral Programs, Pennsylvania Bar Association Legal Ethics and Professional Responsibility Formal Opinion 2016-200 (2016)   486
      Non-Lawyer Ownership or Direction of Law Firms   491
   2. Restrictions on Lawyer's Practice   492
      In re Truman   493
   3. Sale of a Law Practice   496
C. Unauthorized Practice of Law (UPL)   497
   1. Justifications for the Professional Monopoly   497
   2. Defining the Practice of Law   498
D. Multijurisdictional Practice (MJP)   501
      Birbrower, Montalbano, Condon & Frank v. Superior Court   502
Chapter Summary   510
Applying the Rules   511
Professional Responsibility in Practice   512

Chapter 10: Marketing Legal Services   513

A. Communications vs. Solicitation   514
B. Regulation of Lawyer Advertising   514
   1. Constitutional Limits on the Bar's Power to Restrict Advertising   514
      Florida Bar v. Went For It, Inc.   517

2. Rules Governing Communications Concerning a Lawyer's Services   524

    False or Misleading Communications   525

    Required Disclosures   528

3. Social Media and Other Forms of Electronic Advertising   528

    Do the Advertising Rules Apply to Social Media?   529

    State Bar of California Standing Committee on Professional Responsibility and Conduct Formal Opinion 2012-186   529

    Unique Dangers of Social Media and Other Forms of Electronic Advertising   530

C. **Regulation of Solicitation**   532

1. Constitutional Limits on the Bar's Power to Limit Solicitation   532

    Ohralik v. Ohio State Bar Association   532

2. Rules Governing Solicitation   538

Chapter Summary   539

Applying the Rules   540

Professional Responsibility in Practice   541

Chapter 11: Access to Justice and Pro Bono Services   543

A. **"Civil Gideon"**   544

    Turner v. Rogers   545

B. **The Justice Gap**   552

C. **Possible Solutions**   555

1. Simplifying Court Procedures   555

2. Mandatory Pro Bono   556

3. Technology   556

4. Unbundled Legal Services   558

5. Regulatory Changes   559

    Non-Lawyers Delivering Legal Services   559

    Alternative Business Structures (ABS)   561

Chapter Summary   562

Applying the Rules   563

Professional Responsibility in Practice   563

PART **V** THE JUDICIARY 565

Chapter 12: Judicial Ethics 567

A. Performance of Judicial Duties 568
B. Extrajudicial Activities 570
C. Judicial Disqualification 572
    1. Disqualification Under the Code 572
        Cheney v. United States District Court for the District of Columbia 575
        Lawrence J. Fox, *I Did Not Sleep with That Vice President* 583
    2. Judges' Use of Social Media 590
    3. Constitutional Dimensions of Disqualification 591
D. Judicial Campaigns and Other Political Activity 594
    1. Fundraising 594
    2. Other Political Activity 596
        Republican Party of Minnesota v. White 598

Chapter Summary 605

Applying the Rules 606

Professional Responsibility in Practice 607

Glossary 609
Table of Cases 617
Table of Rules 623
Index 629

The Focus Casebook Series

Help students reach their full potential with the fresh approach of the **Focus Casebook Series**. Instead of using the "hide the ball" approach, selected cases illustrate key developments in the law and show how courts develop and apply doctrine. The approachable manner of this series provides a comfortable experiential environment that is instrumental to student success.

Students perform best when applying concepts to real-world scenarios. With assessment features, such as Real Life Applications and Applying the Concepts, the **Focus Casebook Series** off ers many opportunities for students to apply their knowledge.

Focus Casebook Features Include:

Case Previews and Post-Case Follow-Ups — To succeed, law students must know how to deconstruct and analyze cases. Case Previews highlight the legal concepts in a case before the student reads it. Post-Case Follow-Ups summarize the important points.

Case Preview

Brady v. Maryland

The petitioner in this case, Brady, and his companion, Boblit, were separately convicted of first degree murder and sentenced to death. At his trial, Brady did not deny playing a role in the murder but, seeking to avoid the death penalty, testified that Boblit did the actual killing. While on death row, Brady moved for a new trial after discovering statements made by Boblit — in which Boblit admitted to doing the actual killing — that had previously been withheld by the prosecutor.

As you read the *Brady* decision, ask yourself:

1. Is the withholding of ex
   sentation of perjured te

Post-Case Follow-Up

Attorney Francis Belge, the attorney who was the subject of this formal opinion, was also criminally charged under two sections of the New York Public Health statute making it a misdemeanor to fail to report the death of someone who died without medical assistance. Although Belge was subsequently exonerated by the trial judge in that criminal matter, the public outcry over the choices he made in the Buried Bodies case undercut his standing in the small-town community and ultimately his law practice. His life was ruined in many ways for "stepping up" to take on a difficult case, and then making a very courageous and unpopular decision within the context of that case.

Defendant Garrow in the Buried Bodies case was actually represented by two attorneys — Francis Belge and Frank Armani. Armani was not present when Belge observed and photographed one of the bodies, so he escaped indictment. In interviews after the Garrow prosecution, both attorneys explained that one of their motivations for checking to see if the bodies were located where the client said they would be was that they thought their client had mental health issues and might be fabricating the other crimes. Is this the sort of "preparation" contemplated by Rule 1.1?

The Focus Casebook Series

Real Life Applications—

Every case in a chapter is followed by Real Life Applications, which present a series of questions based on a scenario similar to the facts in the case. Real Life Applications challenge students to apply what they have learned in order to prepare them for real-world practice. Use Real Life Applications to spark class discussions or provide them as individual short-answer assignments.

Ohio v. Jones: Real Life Applications

1. A junior public defender is assigned nearly twice as many cases as she can handle. According to ABA Formal Opinion 06-441, what can and should the public defender do?

2. Sandra is an attorney who has just opened her own solo practice. She wants to bring in clientele, so she participates in a Groupon deal of the day. Under the deal, Sandra sells for $50 the first ten hours of legal work on any family law matter. She pledges to complete the work within a month of the purchase of the deal. One hundred people buy the deal on the day it is promoted, meaning that Sandra has to complete 1,000 hours of legal work within the month (there are only 744 hours in the month). What should Sandra do? What should she have done to avoid this problem if she wanted to participate in the Groupon deal of the day?

Applying the Concepts/Rules and Civil Procedure in Practice

These end-of-chapter exercises encourage students to synthesize the chapter material and apply relevant legal doctrine and code to real-world scenarios. Students can use these exercises for self-assessment or the professor can use them to promote class interaction.

Applying the Rules

1. In its opinion above, the California Bar determined that examples 2, 3, and 4 constitute advertising within the meaning of the Rules of Professional Conduct. Do those statements violate the rules?

2. Your law firm has been hired to represent two personal injury lawyers.

   a. The first
      Hamme
   b. The secc
      ing as "

Professional Responsibility in Practice

1. Eli comes to you asking you to represent him in slip and fall case against his neighbor, Cyrus, for an incident that occurred ten months ago. You meet with him for a half hour, but decide you do not want to take his case. Draft an appropriate declination letter to Eli.

2. Same facts as above, only this time you decide to take Eli's case and want to charge a one-third contingency fee. Draft a contingency fee agreement that complies with Rule 1.5.

3. Research whether an in-house attorney has a cause of action for wrongful discharge when fired for complying with mandatory rules of professional conduct in the state where you plan to practice or are attending law school.

4. Select a state that has decided to legalize marijuana. Research the ethics opinions in that state to see how that state approaches the problem of compliance

Preface

Ensure student success with the Focus Casebook Series.

THE FOCUS APPROACH

In a law office, when a new associate attorney is being asked to assist a supervising attorney with a legal matter in which the associate has no prior experience, it is common for the supervising attorney to provide the associate with a recently closed case file involving the same legal issues so that the associate can see and learn from the closed file to assist more effectively with the new matter. This experiential approach is at the heart of the *Focus Casebook Series*.

Additional hands-on features, such as Real Life Applications, Applying the Rules, and Professional Responsibility in Practice, provide more opportunities for critical analysis and application of concepts covered in the chapters. Professors can assign problem-solving questions as well as exercises on drafting documents and preparing appropriate filings.

CONTENT SNAPSHOT

The Second Edition of *Professional Responsibility in Focus* offers a comprehensive, updated exposition of the law governing lawyers. It incorporates more than a dozen new cases and other recent developments — such as the amended advertising and solicitation rules — in an expanded, practice-oriented text with new and revised footnotes. The casebook begins with an introduction to the legal profession and follows with concise, well-written chapters on the attorney-client relationship, covering competence, confidentiality, and conflicts of interest. The book also discusses the lawyer as advocate; special issues in criminal practice; issues concerning the delivery of legal services in general; access to justice; and judicial ethics. The first chapter on the moral responsibility of lawyers helps to situate and contextualize the rule-centric discussion of legal ethics that follows, by inviting students to appreciate the various roles that lawyers play in the legal system, their responsibilities to multiple stakeholders, and competing values at play in professional regulation.

ORGANIZATION

This second edition retains the popular, user-friendly format. We believe our problem-based approach to learning engages students and helps them to hone their skills at issue-spotting and problem-solving, while facilitating a greater understanding of the law of professional responsibility. For example, bulleted lists at the beginning of each chapter highlight that chapter's "Key Concepts," providing students with a helpful construct for developing a course outline. The second edition continues to provide a "Case Preview" of each key case in the chapter with several questions to help students to more efficiently and fully examine it. After each case, there is a brief "Post-Case Follow-Up" that informs students about noteworthy developments concerning the case and "Real Life Application" problems and questions. Our discussion problems are often based on real cases and offer students the opportunity to apply the rules in real-life scenarios.

Each chapter closes with three sections. The first, the "Chapter Summary," provides students with a helpful, albeit brief, explanation of the chapter's key concepts and take-aways. The next section, "Applying the Rules," containing problems, sometimes involving multiple issues and rules, provides students with another opportunity to review and apply the chapter's concepts. The third section, "Professional Responsibility in Practice," challenges students to creatively consider and apply some of the chapter's key concepts and principles in the real world of daily practice.

RESOURCES

The book is well-suited for either in-person or online instruction. The problems in the text may be used as breakout sessions for small group interaction, either in the classroom or on a remote platform. The PowerPoint slides and multiple-choice review questions developed for each chapter and contained in the expanded Teacher's Manual will guide instructors in creating their course content and assessment instruments. At the beginning of each chapter in the Teacher's Manual, we highlight some of the new materials to alert professors to the differences between the two editions.

Other resources to enrich your class include: Supplementary material such as *Examples & Explanations for Professional Responsibility, Sixth Edition* by W. Bradley Wendel. Ask your Wolters Kluwer sales representative or go to WKLegaledu.com to learn more about building the product package that's right for you.

Acknowledgments

I wish to thank my research assistants, David Belfiglio, Bridget Brenner, and Lindsay Casile, for their patience, hard work, and valuable contributions to this second edition. In addition, I am grateful to Susan Altmeyer of the University of Akron School of Law Library for her helpful research and support.

I also want to acknowledge the excellent work of my former research assistants, Dakota Perez, Tristan Serri, Patricia Ochman, and Cynthia Menta, for their very special help with the first edition. Other persons warranting particular recognition regarding the first edition include the University of Akron law librarians, Kyle Passmore and Susan Altmeyer, who provided significant research and support; and former Yale Law School Librarian Teresa Miguel-Sterns and her colleagues, Michael VanderHeijden and Jordan Jefferson, who provided noteworthy assistance while I was teaching summer classes at Yale. Finally, I am indebted to Art Garwin, the former Director of the ABA Center for Professional Responsibility, for his helpful suggestions and valuable guidance. JS

I am enormously grateful for the advice and guidance of Mary Ann Neary of the Boston College Law Library, and for the research and editing assistance of Mitchell Perne (BC Law '18), Matthew Sawyer (BC Law '19), and Taylor Vitelli (BC Law '22). MC

Thank you to Abigail Abide (University of Mississippi School of Law '17) for research assistance on the first edition, and to McKenna Raney-Gray (University of Mississippi School of Law '20) and Melanie Greer (University of Mississippi School of Law '22) for their help on the second edition. I am also grateful to the Legal Profession students I have taught over the last 13 years — your insightful comments and class participation helped shape this book. BC

A special thanks to my father, Jim Robertson, for reviewing and making insightful comments on the drafts of my chapters; and also thanks to my children, Joseph, Eli, Maisy, Cy, and Hal, for their patience and support during my work on this book. MT

We would like to thank the following for permission to reprint the identified material:

The American Bar Association (ABA) for:

ABA Formal Opinion 06-441 (2006). © 2006 by the American Bar Association.
ABA Formal Opinion 09-454 (2009). © 2009 by the American Bar Association.

ABA Formal Opinion 93-379 (1993). © 1993 by the American Bar Association.

ABA Formal Opinion 96-403 (1996). © 1996 by the American Bar Association.

"I Did Not Sleep with That Vice President," Professional Lawyer (2004). © 2004 by the American Bar Association.

"Joint Representation Checklist from 'The Ethics of Joint Representation,'" 40 Litigation Journal 1 (Fall 2013). © 2013 by the American Bar Association.

"Professionalism Clearly Defined," 18 Professional Lawyer 1, 4-5 (2008). © 2008 by the American Bar Association.

Select Excerpts from the ABA Model Rule of Judicial Conduct. © 2020 by the American Bar Association.

Select Excerpts from the ABA Model Rules of Professional Conduct. © 2020 by the American Bar Association.

Above excerpts reprinted with permission. All rights reserved.

AP Images for:

Photo of Joseph Yablonski by Henry Borroughs, May 29, 1969.

Photo of Tony Boyle by Bill Ingraham, February 18, 1978.

Photo of Samuel Leibowitz and the Scottsboro boys, AP file photo.

Photo of Spiderman DC Comics by Ed Bailey.

Photo of Claus von Bülow with his lawyer Alan Dershowitz by Charles Krupa, April 29, 1985.

William Bergmann, Julianne M. Hartzell, Elizabeth Ann Morgan, and Preston K. Ratliff from the Intellectual Property Owners Association. Sample Joint Defense and Common Interest Agreement, from Best Practices in Multi-Defendant Litigation, 2010 IPO Annual Meeting. Reprinted with permission.

Minnesota State Bar Association. Martin Cole, "The Hardiest Perennials," Bench & Bar of Minnesota, Vol. 64 (2007). Copyright © 2007.

The District of Columbia Bar. Limitations on a Lawyer's Participation in the Preparation of a Witness's Testimony, D.C. Bar Legal Ethics Committee Formal Opinion 79 (1979). Copyright © 1979.

Food Fight Films, LLC. Food Fight: Inside the Battle for the Market Basket.

Georgetown University Law Center. John B. Mitchell, "Reasonable Doubts Are Where You Find Them: A Response to Professor Subin's Position on the Criminal Lawyer's 'Different Mission,'" Georgetown Journal of Legal Ethics, Vol. 1 (1987). Reprinted with permission from the publisher.

Alexander Meiklejohn, *Free Speech and Its Relation to Self-Government* (1948). Harper Collins. Copyright © 1948.

Alexander M. Meiklejohn and D. Stuart Meiklejohn, for the photo of Alexander Meiklejohn.

New York State Bar Association. "Client's Confidences and Secrets; Past Crimes Disclosed to Lawyer; Plea Bargaining," New York State Bar Association Formal Opinion 479 (1978).

The New York Times. Benjamin Weiser, "Doubting Case, a Prosecutor Helped the Defense," June 23, 2008. Copyright © 2008 The New York Times Company. All rights reserved. Used under license.

North Carolina State Bar. "Disclosing Potential Malpractice to a Client," North Carolina State Bar 2015 Formal Ethics Opinion 4.

Ohio State Bar Association. "Use of Cloud Computing Services," Ohio State Bar Association Informal Advisory Opinion 2013-03. Copyright © 2013.

Pennsylvania Bar Association. "Ethical Considerations Relating to Participation in Fixed Fee Limited Scope Legal Services Referral Programs," Pennsylvania Bar Association Legal Ethics and Professional Responsibility Formal Opinion 2016-200 (2016). Copyright © 2016.

The State Bar of California. The State Bar of California's Committee on Professional Responsibility and Conduct, Formal Opinion No. 2012-186 (2017). Reprinted with permission.

Utah State Bar. "Discipline Corner," Utah Bar Journal (April 27, 2007). Reprinted with permission.

Vanderbilt Law Review. Fred Zacharias, "Structuring the Ethics of Trial Advocacy," Vol. 44 (1991). Vanderbilt University Law School. Copyright © 1991.

W. Bradley Wendel, "Conflicts of Interest Under the Revised Model Rules," Nebraska Law Review, Vol. 81 (2003). University of Nebraska College of Law. Reprinted with permission from the author.

Staci Zaretsky, "The Struggle: Will Alcoholism Treatment Affect Your Character and Fitness Review?" Abovethelaw.com, Aug. 22, 2016. Reprinted with permission from the author.

Professional Responsibility in Focus

Introduction to the Legal Profession

The Role and Responsibility of Lawyers

Lawyers play an important role in the United States justice system. It is through lawyers that individuals are able to gain access to government power in the protection of their lives, liberty, and property. This primary, and constitutional, role of lawyers in our justice system carries with it significant responsibilities. The lawyer has a responsibility to her client to protect life, liberty, and property. The lawyer has a responsibility to the integrity of the justice system, constitutional guarantees, and the rule of law. The lawyer has a responsibility to those affected by her actions. And the lawyer has a responsibility to herself — to her own integrity and moral identity.

A. THE ROLE OF THE LAWYER IN THE SYSTEM OF JUSTICE

Lawyers play a significant role in the administration of justice in the United States. A license to practice law renders the lawyer an instrument of government power — the lawyer's actions directly affect the extent of government power to be imposed in favor of or against people and their property. Despite this significant power over people's lives, lawyers are largely self-regulated with substantial autonomy from outside control. Yet self-regulation necessitates the undertaking of correlative duties to protect public goods, particularly justice and due process.

Key Concepts

- The role of the lawyer in the United States justice system
- The lawyer's social contract with the public
- Lawyer and client moral responsibility
- Moral dialogue and ascertaining client purposes
- Understanding and cultivating professionalism
- The differing responsibilities of lawyers as litigators, advisors, and transactional planners

3

1. Guardians of Due Process

Unlike other professions, the lawyer's work is directly tied to individual access to and protection from government power. Lawyers alone provide individuals meaningful access to an entire branch of government — the judiciary, which itself is composed almost entirely of lawyers. In addition, lawyers constitute a major component of the executive branch through the prosecutorial function. For those facing criminal charges, defense lawyers are constitutionally guaranteed to help protect the life, liberty, and property of the accused from government deprivation and overreaching.

Lawyers also provide meaningful access to law itself. Through litigation and other processes, lawyers enable people to enforce their rights against government and societal actors. Lawyers correlatively enable individuals, governments, and corporate or associative actors to mitigate and avoid purported liability. Notably, in transactional and non-litigation settings, lawyers assist people in creating legally binding contracts, business associations and structures, wills, trusts, and a manifold of other agreements and arrangements. If executed correctly, these agreements will have the force of law — meaning that the agreement will be backed by the full weight of government power should a breaching party be brought to court to enforce it. This access to the force of law is made available to individuals primarily through legal counsel. Even in the advice context, lawyers assist individuals in understanding what the law requires. This advice allows individuals to structure their conduct to avoid or invoke government power in the protection of life, liberty, and property.

Thus, in our justice system, lawyers should recognize their principal professional responsibility as guardians of due process.[1] It is through lawyers' actions that individuals are able to avoid or invoke government power to protect their lives, liberty, and property. This is true in civil, criminal, transactional, and advice contexts. Correspondingly, lawyers are also the primary mechanism through which law is enforced against individuals both civilly and criminally, thus depriving people of life, liberty, and/or property. Through lawyers' actions people may be sentenced to death or imprisonment; may be convicted of a crime and with that conviction face a host of legal and social consequences; may lose custody of their children; may have their property seized and sold, their wages garnished, their homes foreclosed on, or their savings and assets depleted — to name a few examples. Lawyers are instruments of state power. And attorneys who abuse their powers, act unethically, and work to deprive people unjustly of life, liberty, and property become instruments of state oppression.

A potent example is found in prosecutors who hide exculpatory evidence, resulting in the conviction of an innocent person. In Connick v. Thompson, 563 U.S. 51 (2011), several prosecutors colluded in hiding multiple pieces of exculpatory evidence that proved the accused defendant was innocent. Lab testing revealed that the perpetrator's blood was type B, yet Thompson, who was charged with the

---

1. *See* Geoffrey C. Hazard, Jr., *The Future of Legal Ethics*, 100 YALE L.J. 1239, 1246 (1991) ("The legal profession's basic narrative is a defense of due process. The lawyer's work consists of resistance to government intervention in the lives, liberty, or property of private parties.").

crime, had type O blood. Prosecutors failed to disclose the existence of the evidence or the lab results to the defense. Thompson was imprisoned for crimes he did not commit for 18 years, 14 of them on death row. His execution was stayed when an "eleventh-hour" effort by a private investigator uncovered a microfiche copy of the lab report identifying the perpetrator's blood type.[2] These prosecutors were instruments of state oppression, using their license to practice law to deprive Thompson of his liberty and Thompson's children (aged 4 and 6 at the time of his arrest) of being raised by their father.[3] No one can restore the 18 years of lost time and lost experiences to Thompson or his family.

As the instrument through which law is accessed and enforced, lawyers owe special duties to the integrity of the system of justice, the rule of law, and the rights and obligations of individuals. In the American adversary system, it is important that lawyers are committed to "a core of basic rights that recognize and protect the dignity of the individual in a free society."[4] As Monroe Freedman and Abbe Smith have noted, these rights include "personal autonomy, the effective assistance of counsel, equal protection of the laws, trial by jury, the rights to call and to confront witnesses, the right against involuntary self-incrimination, the right to require the government to prove guilt beyond a reasonable doubt, [] the right to petition the government for redress of grievances . . . and other rights [that] are also included in the broad and fundamental concept that no person may be deprived of life, liberty, or property without due process of law."[5] Lawyers thus exhibit an amplified devotion to professional duties associated with the protection of these rights, including confidentiality, loyalty, competence, communication, and complete knowledge.

Lawyers also understand the importance to any system of justice of creating and maintaining procedures that allow individuals to vindicate their rights. Lawyers thus often possess a strong commitment to adherence to procedures, especially those procedures that are created specifically to preserve a client's rights, such as the rights to call and confront witnesses. Nevertheless, complicated procedural requirements can also frustrate access to justice, resulting in a default of client rights and creating a trap for the unwary or the unrepresented.

By protecting the rights of their clients, lawyers in theory protect the overall adversary system and thus the rights of society as a whole. Behind the recognition of every major constitutional right is a lawyer whose ingenuity and perseverance on behalf of a specific client made it possible for the court to formally recognize the right. Indeed, the Supreme Court has indicated that the right to a lawyer is perhaps the most important right because it is essential to the protection of every other right.[6] However, the theory that society is protected by partisan lawyering is only accurate to the extent that both sides to a controversy have access to competent and ethical legal counsel. There are many people in the United States who have little or no access to legal counsel, and generally the divide between those with access and those without is attributable to the relative wealth or poverty of the

---

2. Connick v. Thompson, 563 U.S. 51, 87 (2011) (Ginsburg, J., dissenting).
3. *See* John Thompson, *The Prosecution Rests, But I Can't*, N.Y. Times, Apr. 9, 2011, Op-Ed.
4. Monroe H. Freedman & Abbe Smith, Understanding Lawyers' Ethics 15 (4th ed. 2010).
5. *Id.* at 15-16.
6. *Id.* at 16 (quoting United States v. Cronic, 466 U.S. 648, 654 (1984)).

individuals. This wealth-based allocation of access to legal counsel — and of one's ability thereby to invoke or avoid government power — undermines the basic fairness that should exist in a system of justice.

2. Self-Regulation and the Protection of Our Public Good

The legal profession is generally considered a self-regulated profession. The notion that attorneys are self-regulated is overstated: lawyers are indeed subject to external regulation, including any regulations imposed by federal and state legislatures or administrative agencies, or applicable to attorneys through constitutional law or international treaties. Indeed, the United States Supreme Court has made clear that traditional self-regulation is not a shield from valid external regulation — lawyers can be and are regulated by Congress and other external entities.[7]

Nevertheless, in large part, lawyers' rules of professional conduct can be viewed as a form of self-regulation. Generally, the legal profession in each state is governed by that state's judiciary — with the state's supreme court acting as the ultimate authority for professional governance. Judiciaries are primarily made up of attorneys, so regulation of lawyers by the judiciary can be considered a form of self-regulation. State supreme courts in turn delegate professional governance duties to the state bar and/or other state agencies — although retaining their status as the final authority governing the profession. Further, nearly every state, through its supreme court and state bar designees, has adopted some form of the Model Rules of Professional Conduct as the primary codified law governing lawyers in that jurisdiction. The **Model Rules of Professional Conduct** (Model Rules) are drafted by the American Bar Association (ABA), which is also composed of lawyers. Thus, the rules governing the profession are proposed by lawyers and adopted and enforced by lawyers (state supreme courts, state bars, and their designees) — which is why lawyering can be viewed as a self-governing profession.

But self-regulation comes with some responsibilities. Like other traditional self-regulating professions, lawyers have a social contract with the public. Neil Hamilton has explained that "[t]he public grants a profession autonomy to regulate itself through peer review, expecting the profession's members to control entry into and continued membership in the profession, to set standards for how individual professionals perform their work so that it serves the public good in the area of the profession's responsibility, and to foster the core values and ideals of the profession."[8]

As Hamilton explains, the public good committed to the care of the legal profession is justice.[9] If the legal profession safeguards that public good and polices its members, then the public will continue to allow the legal profession to largely govern itself, as outlined above. If, however, the legal profession fails to demonstrate its commitment to its public good or fails to punish erring members, then

---

7. Milavetz, Gallop & Milavetz v. United States, 559 U.S. 229, 237 (2010).
8. Neil Hamilton, *Professionalism Clearly Defined*, 18 PROF. LAW. 1, 4-5 (2008).
9. *Id.* at 8.

the public can revoke the social contract, which it does by enacting legislation that regulates lawyers externally. For example, in the fallout of the Enron and Worldcom corporate scandals, it became clear that lawyers played a major role in the law-breaking and cover-up of massive fraud that adversely affected the entire United States economy. Consequently, Congress enacted the Sarbanes-Oxley Act, which required attorneys to "report up" regarding potential violations of the securities laws and directed the SEC to create "minimum standards of professional conduct for attorneys appearing and practicing" before the SEC.[10] Congress and the SEC appropriated the task of professional governance of lawyers when it became clear that lawyers were not doing it themselves. When lawyers fail to fulfill their duty to safeguard justice — when they act unethically and undermine public confidence that they can be trusted to regulate themselves — legislatures and other governmental entities can and will supplant the profession's traditional self-regulation.

So how does the legal profession fulfill its public duty to safeguard justice? Hamilton explains that in return for the ability to self-regulate, "each member of the profession and the profession as a whole agree to meet certain correlative duties to the public." Lawyers are obliged to maintain "high standards of minimum competence and ethical conduct, to serve [justice,] the public purpose of the profession, and to discipline those who fail to meet these standards."[11] As will be covered in Chapter 4, incompetent attorneys impair and even nullify their clients' legal rights. It is imperative that in performing self-government, the legal profession insist on minimum levels of competence and ethical conduct so that clients and third parties are not unjustly deprived of their lives, liberty, and property through lawyers acting as agents of state power. Protecting the public good of justice is precisely compatible with lawyers acting as guardians of due process.

B. LAW AND MORAL RESPONSIBILITY

In *The Path of the Law*, Oliver Wendell Holmes forged the path of the legal realists with an audacious analytical device for understanding law. This device, often referred to as the "bad man perspective," boldly proposed the separation of law from morality. Holmes's hypothetical client, "the bad man," does not care at all about doing what is morally good — yet he still cares about avoiding government-enforced consequences for breaking laws. Holmes invites lawyers to take the view of this hypothetical "bad man." Under Holmes's view, the practice of law is concerned with predicting the actual monetary and

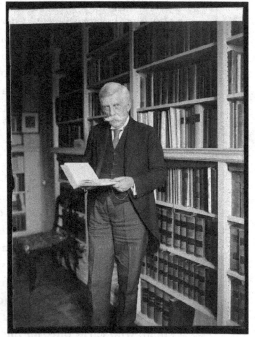

Oliver Wendell Holmes
Library of Congress Prints & Photographs Division, Washington, D.C.

10. 15 U.S.C. §7245 (2002).
11. Hamilton, *supra* note 8, at 5.

physical consequences for breaking the law, and, correspondingly, the practice of law is not concerned with the moral implications of those laws or with the morality of the client's or the lawyer's actions.

Oliver Wendell Holmes, The Path of the Law
10 Harv. L. Rev. 457 (1897)

When we study law we are not studying a mystery but a well known profession. We are studying what we shall want in order to appear before judges, or to advise people in such a way as to keep them out of court. The reason why it is a profession, why people will pay lawyers to argue for them or to advise them, is that in societies like ours the command of the public force is intrusted [sic] to the judges in certain cases, and the whole power of the state will be put forth, if necessary, to carry out their judgments and decrees. People want to know under what circumstances and how far they will run the risk of coming against what is so much stronger than themselves, and hence it becomes a business to find out when this danger is to be feared. The object of our study, then, is prediction, the prediction of the incidence of the public force through the instrumentality of the courts.

. . .

The primary rights and duties with which jurisprudence busies itself again are nothing but prophecies. One of the many evil effects of the confusion between legal and moral ideas, about which I shall have something to say in a moment, is that theory is apt to get the cart before the horse, and to consider the right or the duty as something existing apart from and independent of the consequences of its breach, to which certain sanctions are added afterward. But, as I shall try to show, a legal duty so called is nothing but a prediction that if a man does or omits certain things he will be made to suffer in this or that way by judgment of the court;—and so of a legal right.

. . .

I take it for granted that no hearer of mine will misinterpret what I have to say as the language of cynicism. The law is the witness and external deposit of our moral life. Its history is the history of the moral development of the race. The practice of it, in spite of popular jests, tends to make good citizens and good men. When I emphasize the difference between law and morals I do so with reference to a single end, that of learning and understanding the law. For that purpose you must definitely master its specific marks, and it is for that that I ask you for the moment to imagine yourselves indifferent to other and greater things.

. . . If you want to know the law and nothing else, you must look at it as a bad man, who cares only for the material consequences which such knowledge enables him to predict, not as a good one, who finds his reasons for conduct, whether inside the law or outside of it, in the vaguer sanctions of conscience. The theoretical importance of the distinction is no less, if you would reason on your subject aright. The law is full of phraseology drawn from morals, and by the mere force of language continually invites us to pass from one domain to the other without perceiving it, as we are sure to do unless we have the boundary constantly before our minds. The law talks about rights, and duties, and malice, and intent, and negligence, and so forth, and nothing is easier, or, I may say, more common in legal reasoning, than to take these words in their moral sense, at some stage of the argument, and so to drop into fallacy.

. . .

Take the fundamental question, What constitutes the law? You will find some text writers telling you that it is something different from what is decided by the courts of Massachusetts or England, that it is a system of reason, that it is a deduction from principles of ethics or admitted axioms or what not, which may or may not coincide with the decisions. But if we take the view of our friend the bad man we shall find that he does not care two straws for the axioms or deductions, but that he does want to know what the Massachusetts or English courts are likely to do in fact. I am much of his mind. The prophecies of what the courts will do in fact, and nothing more pretentious, are what I mean by the law.

Take again a notion which as popularly understood is the widest conception which the law contains; — the notion of legal duty, to which already I have referred. We fill the word with all the content which we draw from morals. But what does it mean to a bad man? Mainly, and in the first place, a prophecy that if he does certain things he will be subjected to disagreeable consequences by way of imprisonment or compulsory payment of money. . . . You see how the vague circumference of the notion of duty shrinks and at the same time grows more precise when we wash it with cynical acid and expel everything except the object of our study, the operations of the law.

. . .

I hope that my illustrations have shown the danger, both to speculation and to practice, of confounding morality with law, and the trap which legal language lays for us on that side of our way. For my own part, I often doubt whether it would not be a gain if every word of moral significance could be banished from the law altogether, and other words adopted which should convey legal ideas uncolored by anything outside the law. We should lose the fossil records of a good deal of history and the majesty got from ethical associations, but by ridding ourselves of an unnecessary confusion we should gain very much in the clearness of our thought.

1. Impact and Critique of the Bad Man Perspective

Holmes's view in fact redefined the path of the law. His article became one of the defining statements of both legal realism and positivism. Even today, although lawyers may not recognize that their legal perspectives trace back to Holmes, the fact is that much of the teaching and practice of law adopts Holmes's view. Students and lawyers are trained and expected to decipher what the operation of law is or will be upon their clients and to lessen any negative impacts — without much, or perhaps any, attention to the morality of the actions of the client and the effect of those actions on others. Even the Model Rules are primarily stated in ways that avoid wording containing moral implications; instead, the rules are written as purely law with defined consequences. Thus, the Rules of Professional Conduct themselves are written to be disassociated from morality—precisely what Holmes proposed and desired in order to grasp his, and the bad man's, "clear" picture of the law.

William Simon critiqued the bad man perspective, noting that many lawyers adopt the perspective by imputing certain basic ends — the ends of the hypothetical bad man — to their clients at the outset of a representation. In other words, lawyers work from the assumption that their clients are Holmes's bad man; they impute to their clients the selfish ends of the bad man and then work to achieve those ends. "The specific ends most often imputed are the maximization of freedom of movement and the accumulation of wealth." Simon says: "Of course, in practice lawyers often do not even go through the motion of presenting critical questions to the client as occasions for choice. They decide the questions unilaterally in terms of the imputed ends of selfishness."[12] Roger Cramton similarly explains: "Lawyers have a terrible habit of fitting client objectives into a simplified framework—an assumed world in which clients are governed only by selfish concerns—and then deciding matters for them as if the clients were moral ciphers."[13] Further, Simon argues that many clients, particularly those unfamiliar with the legal system, acquiesce in this redefinition of themselves:

> Confronted with the need to act in this strange situation, the client must make sense of it as best he can. The lawyer puts himself forth quite plausibly as the client's best hope of mastering his predicament. If he is to avoid being overwhelmed by chaos, he must acquiesce in his lawyer's definition of the situation. He must think in a manner which gives coherence of the advice he is giving. He may begin to do this quite unconsciously. If he is at all aware of the change, he is likely to see it as a defensive posture forced on him by the hostile intentions of opposing parties. . . . His only strategy of survival requires that he see himself as the lawyers and the officials see him, as an abstraction, a hypothetical person with only a few crude, discrete ends. He must assume that his subtler ends, his long-range plans, and his social relationships are irrelevant to the situation at hand. . . .
>
> The role of the bad man, conceived [by Holmes] as an analytical device for the lawyer becomes, under pressure of circumstances, a psychological reality for the client.[14]

Importantly, and as Simon reiterates, the "vague, crudely drawn psychological assumption" of the bad man "cannot begin to do justice to the specific complexity" of actual clients and their actual ends. Unlike "hypothetical" people, actual clients do not have "just a few, discrete ends, but rather many ends which are interrelated in a complex fashion . . . and are set in a social context in which the individual's fulfillment depends on his relations with others."[15]

It is not surprising that lawyers often see their clients in terms of the Holmesian bad man. Their bread-and-butter training in law school teaches them to view the law through the lens of the bad man — to see law sanitized of morality and often of

---

12. William H. Simon, *The Ideology of Advocacy: Procedural Justice and Professional Ethics*, 1978 WIS. L. REV. 29, 56-57.

13. Roger C. Cramton, Spaulding v. Zimmerman *Revisited: Confidentiality and Its Exceptions*, in LEGAL ETHICS: LAW STORIES 182 (Deborah L. Rhode & David J. Luban eds., 2006).

14. Simon, *supra* note 12, at 55-56.

15. *Id.* at 54-55.

societal ends. Law students are taught to think of law through hypothetical situations and borderline cases where making creative arguments to better a client's individual position is prized and rewarded. As Eli Wald and Russell Pearce have lamented regarding legal education, "the law itself is taught as a morally-free zone, a body of abstract principles subject to manipulation, in which the public interest is nothing more than an aggregate of clients' private interests, and in which a lawyer's role is to pursue aggressively her client's autonomous self-interest."[16] Moreover, imputing clear-cut ends is easier than taking the time and effort to know one's individually complex client. As Roger Cramton has explained, "[i]mputing selfish goal[s] simplifies the lawyer's work by allowing her to shirk the hard work of client counseling" because counseling requires that a lawyer "tak[e] the client seriously as a person, communicating with and advising the real client, not a client stereotype, and engaging in a moral dialogue in which lawyer and client can learn from each other."[17]

Indeed, Wald and Pearce argue that the Holmesian bad man ideal has carried over into the formation of professional identity because students are taught in law school to adopt an "autonomous self-interest professional ideolog[y]."[18] **Autonomous self-interest** "views clients as individualistic and atomistic entities whose goal is to pursue and maximize their self-interest aggressively without regard to others." In contrast, Wald and Pearce promote focusing student and lawyer professional ideology on "**relational self-interest**." They explain: "Relationally self-interested professionalism understands clients as attempting to pursue and maximize their self-interest in relation to others."[19] Both the attorney and the client have self-interests that are dependent upon their relationships with others, the long-term stability of such relationships, and the success of the overall economy and society in which they live. In fact, no one is solely autonomously self-interested. Everyone has relational self-interests precisely because we are human beings; humans are social creatures[20] whose happiness and success are often dependent upon the happiness and success of others. Thus, even the most selfish and materialistic individuals will still care about certain relationships with others, both personal and business, and about a stable economy and government because such are essential to their own personal success. Neither attorneys nor clients have to be altruistic, selfless people to recognize that considering their own relational self-interests is wise and likely to lead to better results for all affected in a circumstance warranting legal advice or action.

Wald and Pearce urge students and lawyers to help clients perceive their relational self-interests in dealing with a legal or ethical problem. Unfortunately, as Wald and Pearce thoroughly reveal, law students are generally taught "to understand their clients as autonomously self-interested, and to pursue their clients' autonomous self-interest *at the expense* of their clients' relational self-interest in considering the interests of opposing parties, third parties, the public good, and the spirit of the law."[21] Good lawyers when advising clients—whether in litigation or

---

16. Eli Wald & Russell G. Pearce, *Making Lawyers Good*, 9 U. St. Thomas L.J. 403, 415 (2011).
17. Cramton, *supra* note 13, at 182, 183.
18. Wald & Pearce, *supra* note 16, at 411.
19. *Id.*
20. Aristotle, Politics ("Man is by nature a social animal.").
21. Wald & Pearce, *supra* note 16, at 415.

transactions—will assist their clients in recognizing and then taking into account their clients' relational self-interests. It disserves clients when lawyers fail to consider interests that in the long term are important to the client and to the client's success.

But above and beyond the fact that everyone has relational self-interests that a competent lawyer should take into account, what about the client who simply does not fit into the self-centered Holmesian bad man mold? There are good people in the world. There are people who care deeply about helping others and about the welfare of society or of a specific community. How should a lawyer proceed for such a client? Imputing bad man ends to such a client is unwarranted and may entirely undermine the client's actual goals and desires.

Irrespective of the client, if the lawyer perceives law from the point of view of the Holmesian bad man, is that a desirable or accurate picture of what the law and justice system are, of what they should be, and of the appropriate role of the lawyer in the United States justice system? Alexander Meiklejohn criticized the bad man perspective as distorting the purposes of law and of our justice system. Taking his vantage from constitutional theory, Meiklejohn explored the democratic social contract created by the Constitution whereby "We, the People of the United States" established a government through which we could govern ourselves. Meiklejohn explained that under our system of government, all citizens have the privilege and responsibility of participating in government and all agree to abide by the laws thus created. Our governmental structure has "one basic purpose that the citizens of this nation shall make and shall obey their own laws, shall be at once their own subjects and their own masters."[22] Meiklejohn contended that Holmes's bad man construction of law—while a useful analytical device—is inconsistent with these basic constitutional purposes and social ends, "upon which the legal procedure depends for life and meaning." Meiklejohn viewed the Constitution and the democratic theory underlying our government as "an expression of human goodness"— an indication of faith in humanity to be able to govern themselves, to do so justly on the whole, and to choose what is best for society.[23] For Meiklejohn, law in the United States should be understood and interpreted through the lens of this democratic theory.

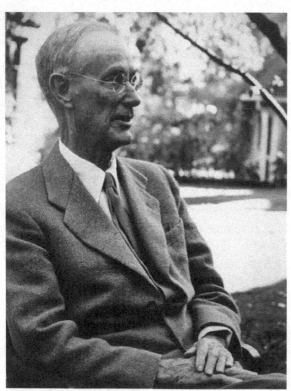

Alexander Meiklejohn
Courtesy of Alexander M. Meiklejohn and D. Stuart Meiklejohn

---

22. ALEXANDER MEIKLEJOHN, FREE SPEECH AND ITS RELATION TO SELF-GOVERNMENT 15-16 (1948).
23. *Id.* at 74-79.

Alexander Meiklejohn, What of the Good Man?
Free Speech and Its Relation to Self-Government 73-77 (1948)

As a student of philosophy, Mr. Holmes was, of course, deeply interested in the relation between the machinery of the law and the moral purpose of justice. His reflections upon that relation, though partial, were keen and incisive. With the zest of a good craftsman, he was, in legal theory, a mechanist. The activities of legislatures and courts he sees, from this point of view, simply as a play of forces which are in conflict. And he delights in the technical game of the manipulation of those forces. He follows the ups and downs of the contests of the law with lively interest and, at times, it must be said, with ironical glee. Human living is, he tells us, "a roar of bargain and battle." And though, as a dispassionate spectator, he is convinced that there is little, if anything, to be gained by the fighting except the fun of the fighting itself, Mr. Holmes, as a good soldier, plunges gloriously into the conflict.

That Mr. Holmes is a mechanist in legal theory is shown by his fascinating description of "The Path of the Law," in a speech given at the Boston University School of Law in 1897. "If you want to know the law and nothing else," he said, "you must look at it as a bad man, who cares only for the material consequences which such knowledge enables him to predict, not as a good one, who finds his reasons for conduct, whether inside the law or outside of it, in the vaguer sanctions of conscience." And again, "But, as I shall try to show, a legal duty so-called is nothing but a prediction that if a man does or omits certain things he will be made to suffer in this way or that by judgment of the court — and so of a legal right." And still again, "People want to know under what circumstances and how far they will run the risk of coming against what is so much stronger than themselves, and hence it becomes a business to find out when this danger is to be feared. The object of our study, then, is prediction, the prediction of the incidence of the public force through the instrumentality of the courts."

With the exception of the phrase, "the vaguer sanctions of conscience," these statements are impressive, both in their audacity and in their validity. As a technician, Mr. Holmes strips "the business of the law" of all "moral" implications. Legal battles he finds to be fought in terms of the conflict of interests, individual and social. Their results are the victories and defeats of forces and counterforces. And they are, for the technician, nothing else, except, it may be, a source of revenue. This is magnificent, clearheaded legal technology.

But there is a philosophic weakness in this mechanistic theory which can be stated in two different ways. First, being partial, it gives no adequate account of the deeper social ends and ideas upon which the legal procedure depends for life and meaning. These battles of which Mr. Holmes speaks are not fought in a jungle, in a moral vacuum. They are fought in the legislatures and courts which have been established by a self-governing society. They are not mere conflicts of interest. They are conflicts under laws which define a public interest. They are, therefore, fought by agreement as well as by difference — an agreement which is accepted by both sides. That agreement provides judges and juries whose duty it is to determine not merely what is going to happen, but what, under our plan of life, should happen. The fighting goes on under a Constitution in which We, the People, have formulated and made authoritative our deepest convictions concerning the welfare of men and of society. And Mr. Holmes' description of the legal machinery, valid as it is technologically, provided these deeper and wider meanings be given assured control, is utterly invalid if it be taken as an account of the total legal process. On this basis it seems fair to say that, as he interprets the freedom of speech which the Constitution protects, the one thing to which Mr. Holmes, the mechanist, does not pay attention is the Constitution itself. One finds in his arguing little reference to the fact that we of the United States have decided to be a self-governing community. There is not much said about a fundamental agreement among us to which we have pledged "our Lives, our Fortunes, and our sacred Honor." We are for the argument merely a horde of fighting individuals, restrained or supported by laws which "happen" to be on the books.

The same conclusion will be reached if we examine carefully what Mr. Homes says about "the vaguer sanctions of conscience," the demands and principles of morality. As we read his words about law and morality we must recognize that it is not strictly accurate to say that he takes no account whatever of the moral factor. It would be more true to say that he is troubled by it, that he does not know where to place it. As he studies legislation and litigation, morality constantly thrusts itself forward as a disturbing influence which threatens to clog the legal machinery. Mr. Holmes has told us that one cannot understand the law unless one looks at it as a bad man. But meanwhile, he is aware that men are, in some respects, good, even when they are dealing with the law. In the very midst of the conflicting forces of interest Mr. Homes finds "other things" such as "a good man's reason for conduct," revealing themselves and claiming relevance. In his statement of the mechanistic theory he says, ". . . I ask you for the moment to imagine yourselves indifferent to other and greater things." But the account of those other things when Mr. Holmes, in other moments, comes back to them, is vague, unclear, and shifting. As contrasted with the sharp and skillful phrases which describe the battles of the courts, the descriptions of morality are neither sharp nor skillful. The mind of Mr. Holmes deals easily, and even merrily, with the "bad man." But the "good man," as an object of philosophical inquiry, mystifies and confuses him. The bad man is clear — too clear to be true. He wants to know what he can get away with. He wants a prediction of the differing consequences of law-breaking, and of law-observance, so that he may have a ground for choosing between them. He hires a lawyer to tell him. The lawyer does what he is paid to do. And Mr. Holmes delights in beating them both at their own game. But meanwhile, what of the good man? What does he want? What is he trying to find out when, if ever, he goes to his lawyer? To those questions Mr. Holmes has no ready answer. His thought has very great difficulty in piercing through the legal machinery to discover those elements of human fellowship and virtue for the sake of which good men [and women] have established and maintained, against the assaults of bad men and their legal advisers, the laws and the Constitution of the United States. As against the dogma of Mr. Holmes, I would venture to assert the counterdogma that one cannot understand the basic purposes of our Constitution as a judge or a citizen should understand them, unless one sees them as a good man, a man who, in his political activities, is not merely fighting for what, under the law, he can get, but is eagerly and generously serving the common welfare.

2. Communication, Moral Dialogue, and Role Morality

How are attorneys to ascertain their clients' moral ends? Is a particular client Holmes's bad man or Meiklejohn's good man — or a complex mix of various desires, moral experiences, and ends? Robert Vischer has emphasized the importance of engaging in **moral dialogue** with the client to determine the client's actual desires and moral ends. He contends that "lawyers should openly discuss with their clients moral considerations, including their own moral views, that bear on the representation."[24]

Model Rule 2.1 expressly permits (but does not require) a lawyer to refer "not only to law, but to other considerations such as moral, economic, social and political factors, that may be relevant to the client's situation." Comment [2] explains that "it is proper for a lawyer to refer to moral and ethical considerations" precisely because "moral and ethical considerations impinge upon most legal questions and may decisively influence how the law will be applied."

Moral dialogue with the client should not interfere with the autonomy of the client. As will be explored in Chapter 3, Model Rule 1.2 explains that "a lawyer shall abide by a client's decisions concerning the objectives of representation." Thus, the attorney takes on a **role morality** where the lawyer acts as an agent for the client's purposes. Indeed, Rule 1.2(b) emphasizes that the "lawyer's representation of a client . . . does not constitute an endorsement of the client's political, economic, social or moral views or activities." This role morality of the lawyer is important in the system of justice precisely because lawyers are the guardians of due process and it is lawyers who provide individuals with access to government power. Such access to government power "should not be denied to people . . . whose cause is controversial or the subject of popular disapproval."[25] The United States bar has a long and honored tradition of lawyers who have represented people despite disagreement with their clients' causes or actions. At the inception of our country, John Adams agreed to represent the British soldiers involved in the Boston Massacre, thus ensuring that these unpopular clients were afforded a fair process. As Margaret Tarkington has explained:

> Adams the revolutionary aligned himself with British soldiers for legal representation precisely to preserve the legitimacy of the United States' emerging justice system. He did not agree with the British soldiers' actions or beliefs, but he did understand the need for due process, for the fair administration of the law, and for exertion of government power to be based on evidence (which he found wanting in this prosecution) — rather than being based on "[s]uspicions and prejudices," a hallmark of tyrannical legal systems. Attorneys today continue to recognize that the legitimacy of our justice system is not based solely on what process and protection is provided to the clearly innocent, deserving, or popular, but especially to the accused and to the unpopular. Consequently, despite their client's alleged bad acts, attorneys associate with

---

24. Robert K. Vischer, *Legal Advice as Moral Perspective*, 19 GEO. J. LEGAL ETHICS 225, 272 (2006).
25. Model Rule 1.2 cmt. [5].

clients to provide legal advice, assistance, and representation to lawfully protect life, liberty, and property — and thereby promote the legitimacy of our justice system.[26]

The comments to Model Rule 6.2 remind lawyers of this responsibility to the integrity of the justice system to accept "a fair share of unpopular matters or indigent or unpopular clients."

Thus, as comment [1] to Model Rule 1.2 expounds, the client has "the ultimate authority to determine the purposes to be served by legal representation." Nevertheless, there are limits to the lawyer's role morality: the client's purposes must be "within the limits imposed by law and the lawyer's professional obligations." The lawyer cannot advise or assist a client in conduct "the lawyer knows is criminal or fraudulent." *See* Model Rule 1.2(d). Further, lawyers have moral and professional obligations to the system of justice, the rule of law, and ultimately to their own moral identity. The Model Rules allow a lawyer to withdraw from a representation on the basis that "the client insists on taking action that the lawyer considers repugnant or with which the lawyer has a fundamental disagreement." *See* Model Rule 1.16(b)(4). Further, lawyers "ordinarily" are "not obliged to accept a client whose character or cause the lawyer regards as repugnant." *See* Model Rule 6.2 cmt. [1]. Such provisions recognize that lawyers have their own moral moorings on which they can rely in fulfilling their obligations as agents for individuals who seek access to or avoidance of government power.

By engaging in moral dialogue — by discussing the moral issues that are relevant to a representation — the attorney can ascertain the client's actual ends and moral interests rather than working from the lawyer's assumption or guessing at those interests and ends. Most often this will allow for greater client input into the representation. Further, where the lawyer and client disagree as to the morality of a situation, that disagreement will be known and considered rather than obscured. When lawyers ignore moral issues or impute bad man ends to clients, the lawyers avoid moral responsibility by relying on their role morality as agents and placing any moral blame with the client, whose assumed (but actually unascertained) interests the lawyer claims to be protecting. At the same time, without moral dialogue, clients may acquiesce in the lawyer's amoral framing of the issues, assuming that the lawyer's legalistic recommendations indicate a moral permissibility to the course of conduct. Thus, neither the lawyer nor the client are taking moral responsibility for the ensuing conduct or legal strategy. This dual shifting of moral accountability creates latitude for moral failure. Moral dialogue between the attorney and client — discussing relevant moral issues, including any negative effects on third parties, public interests, or society — results in the identification of the moral stakes pertinent to a representation and requires the attorney and client to consider their own moral moorings and responsibilities.

The crux of the matter is that even considering the role morality inherent in lawyering, the lawyer cannot escape being a moral agent.[27] It is part of what it means

---

26. Margaret Tarkington, *Freedom of Attorney-Client Association*, 2012 UTAH L. REV. 1071, 1116 (2012).

27. "The fact of [moral] pluralism, without more, cannot be used to squeeze out freestanding moral advice from the attorney-client relationship because an attorney remains a moral agent when acting in a professional capacity." W. Bradley Wendel, *Legal Ethics and the Separation of Law and Morals*, 91 CORNELL L. REV. 67, 111 (2005).

to be a human being and to live in society.[28] Thus, "the autonomy of the client is not some kind of moral trump card over the lawyer's own moral agency."[29] Lawyers' advice and actions have consequences that affect their clients, opposing parties, third parties, the larger community, the system of justice, and their own personal and professional identity. As Deborah Rhode puts it, "[l]awyers must assume personal moral responsibility for the consequences of their professional actions."[30] She contends that "the critical question is not by what right do lawyers impose their [moral] views, but by what right do they evade the responsibility of all individuals to evaluate the normative implications of their acts?"[31]

Case Preview

Spaulding v. Zimmerman

The *Spaulding* case presents a poignant framework for understanding the concepts discussed above. It revolves around the tragic story of 20-year-old David Spaulding, who was seriously injured as a passenger in a car wreck — he was unconscious for three days, suffered a severe brain concussion, broke both clavicles and multiple ribs, and had a "crushed chest." David was from a poor family who could not afford the "staggering" medical bills. The Spaulding family decided to sue the drivers and owners of the two cars, the Zimmerman and Ledermann families, in hopes of being able to obtain compensation from the car insurance policies. Both the Zimmerman and Ledermann families had lost a child in the same wreck. David worked for the Zimmermans, who ran a small road construction business, and had been getting a ride home from work with the Zimmermans at the time of the wreck. The Zimmermans' attorney, Norman Arveson, hired a medical expert to examine David's injuries. The defense medical expert, Dr. Hewitt Hannah, discovered something that none of the doctors treating and examining David had previously seen: in addition to his other serious injuries, the wreck had caused an aneurysm in David's aorta, which could rupture at any moment and cause David's immediate death unless surgically repaired. Dr. Hannah's report detailing this fact was given to Arveson, who shared it with the defense attorney for the Ledermanns, Chester Rosengren. David's attorney (negligently) failed to request the defense expert medical report. And neither of the defense attorneys nor Doctor Hannah told David about the fatal condition affecting him. The case was settled and, because David was still a minor, the trial court approved the settlement — without David (or the court) ever learning of the aneurysm. Over the next two and a half years David experienced severe chest pains; fortunately, he then had a physical examination as part of his army reserve status that revealed the aneurysm. He was sent to Minneapolis for immediate surgery, which

---

28. Vischer, *supra* note 24, at 273 ("Moral claims are part of human understanding, regardless of what attorneys would like to believe about the appropriate limit of their professional role.").
29. W. Bradley Wendel, *Professionalism as Interpretation*, 99 Nw. U. L. Rev. 1167, 1181 (2005).
30. Deborah L. Rhode, *Ethical Perspectives on Legal Practice*, 37 Stan. L. Rev. 589, 643 (1985).
31. *Id.* at 623.

took ten hours. The aneurysm had grown significantly over the two years such that the doctors had to sacrifice the recurrent laryngeal nerve to save David's life. David lost most of his speaking voice as a direct consequence of the delay in treatment.[32]

As you read *Spaulding v. Zimmerman*, look for the following:

1. Did the Minnesota Supreme Court view the law surrounding professional responsibility as informed by morality or, as Holmes recommended, as separated from ordinary morality?
2. Why didn't the defense lawyers or the Zimmermans/Ledermanns tell David Spaulding about the aneurysm? Were the attorneys required by their duty of confidentiality to keep the information secret?
3. What approach did the defense lawyers take in this case? Did they impute bad man ends to their clients? Did they consider the relational self-interests of their clients (whether the Zimmermans/Ledermanns or the insurance companies)?
4. What did the defense risk by not telling Spaulding or the court about the aneurysm?

Spaulding v. Zimmerman
116 N.W.2d 704 (Minn. 1962)

Appeal from an order of the District Court of Douglas County vacating and setting aside a prior order of such court dated May 8, 1957, approving a settlement made on behalf of David Spaulding on March 5, 1957, at which time he was a minor of the age of 20 years; and in connection therewith, vacating and setting aside releases executed by him and his parents, a stipulation of dismissal, an order for dismissal with prejudice, and a judgment entered pursuant thereto.

The prior action was brought against defendants by Theodore Spaulding, as father and natural guardian of David Spaulding, for injuries sustained by David in an automobile accident, arising out of a collision which occurred August 24, 1956, between an automobile driven by John Zimmerman, in which David was a passenger, and one owned by John Ledermann and driven by Florian Ledermann.

On appeal defendants contend that the court was without jurisdiction to vacate the settlement solely because their counsel then possessed information, unknown to plaintiff herein, that at the time he was suffering from an aorta aneurysm which may have resulted from the accident, because (1) no mutual mistake of fact was involved; [and] (2) no duty rested upon them to disclose information to plaintiff which they could assume had been disclosed to him by his own physicians. . . .

After the accident, David's injuries were diagnosed by his family physician, Dr. James H. Cain, as a severe crushing injury of the chest with multiple rib fractures; a severe cerebral concussion, probably with petechial hemorrhages of the brain; and bilateral fractures of the clavicles. At Dr. Cain's suggestion, on January 3, 1957, David

---

32. *See* Timothy W. Floyd & John Gallagher, *Legal Ethics, Narrative, and Professional Identity: The Story of David Spaulding*, 59 MERCER L. REV. 941, 944-52 (2008); Roger Cramton, *supra* note 13, at 175-76, 179-81.

was examined by Dr. John F. Pohl, an orthopedic specialist, who made X-ray studies of his chest. Dr. Pohl's detailed report of this examination included the following:

> ". . . The lung fields are clear. The heart and aorta are normal."

Nothing in such report indicated the aorta aneurysm with which David was then suffering. On March 1, 1957, at the suggestion of Dr. Pohl, David was examined from a neurological viewpoint by Dr. Paul S. Blake, and in the report of this examination there was no finding of the aorta aneurysm.

In the meantime, on February 22, 1957, at defendants' request, David was examined by Dr. Hewitt Hannah, a neurologist. On February 26, 1957, the latter reported to Messrs. Field, Arveson, & Donoho, attorneys for defendant John Zimmerman, as follows:

> The one feature of the case which bothers me more than any other part of the case is the fact that this boy of 20 years of age has an aneurysm, which means a dilatation of the aorta and the arch of the aorta. Whether this came out of this accident I cannot say with any degree of certainty and I have discussed it with the Roentgenologist and a couple of Internists. . . . Of course an aneurysm or dilatation of the aorta in a boy of this age is a serious matter as far as his life. This aneurysm may dilate further and it might rupture with further dilatation and this would cause his death.
>
> It would be interesting also to know whether the X-ray of his lungs, taken immediately following the accident, shows this dilatation or not. If it was not present immediately following the accident and is now present, then we could be sure that it came out of the accident.

Prior to the negotiations for settlement, the contents of the above report were made known to counsel for defendants Florian and John Ledermann.

The case was called for trial on March 4, 1957, at which time the respective parties and their counsel possessed such information as to David's physical condition as was revealed to them by their respective medical examiners as above described. It is thus apparent that neither David nor his father, the nominal plaintiff in the prior action, was then aware that David was suffering the aorta aneurysm but on the contrary believed that he was recovering from the injuries sustained in the accident.

On the following day an agreement for settlement was reached wherein, in consideration of the payment of $6,500, David and his father agreed to settle in full for all claims arising out of the accident.

Richard S. Roberts, counsel for David, thereafter presented to the court a petition for approval of the settlement, wherein David's injuries were described as:

> ". . . severe crushing of the chest, with multiple rib fractures, severe cerebral concussion, with petechial hemorrhages of the brain, bilateral fractures of the clavicles."

Attached to the petition were affidavits of David's physicians, Drs. James H. Cain and Paul S. Blake, wherein they set forth the same diagnoses they had made upon completion of their respective examinations of David as above described. At no time was there information disclosed to the court that David was then suffering from an aorta aneurysm which may have been the result of the accident. Based upon the petition for settlement and such affidavits of Drs. Cain and Blake, the court on May 8, 1957, made its order approving the settlement.

Early in 1959, David was required by the army reserve, of which he was a member, to have a physical checkup. For this, he again engaged the services of Dr. Cain. In this checkup, the latter discovered the aorta aneurysm. He then reexamined the X rays which had been taken shortly after the accident and at this time discovered that they disclosed the beginning of the process which produced the aneurysm. He promptly sent David to Dr. Jerome Grismer for an examination and opinion. The latter confirmed the finding of the aorta aneurysm and recommended immediate surgery therefor. This was performed by him at Mount Sinai Hospital in Minneapolis on March 10, 1959.

Shortly thereafter, David, having attained his majority, instituted the present action for additional damages due to the more serious injuries including the aorta aneurysm which he alleges proximately resulted from the accident. As indicated above, the prior order for settlement was vacated. In a memorandum made a part of the order vacating the settlement, the court stated:

> The facts material to a determination of the motion are without substantial dispute. The only disputed facts appear to be whether . . . Mr. Roberts, former counsel for plaintiff, discussed plaintiff's injuries with Mr. Arvesen, counsel for defendant Zimmerman, immediately before the settlement agreement, and, further, whether or not there is a causal relationship between the accident and the aneurysm.
>
> Contrary to the . . . suggestion in the affidavit of Mr. Roberts that he discussed the minor's injuries with Mr. Arvesen, the Court finds that no such discussion of the specific injuries claimed occurred prior to the settlement agreement on March 5, 1957.
>
> . . . the Court finds that [] the aneurysm now existing is causally related to the accident . . . , which, so far as the Court can find from the numerous affidavits and statements of fact by counsel, stands without dispute.
>
> The mistake concerning the existence of the aneurysm was not mutual. For reasons which do not appear, plaintiff's doctor failed to ascertain its existence. By reason of the failure of plaintiff's counsel to use available rules of discovery, plaintiff's doctor and all his representatives did not learn that defendants and their agents knew of its existence and possible serious consequences. Except for the character of the concealment in the light of plaintiff's minority, the Court would, I believe, be justified in denying plaintiff's motion to vacate, leaving him to whatever questionable remedy he may have against his doctor and against his lawyer.
>
> That defendants' counsel concealed the knowledge they had is not disputed. The essence of the application of the above rule is the character of the concealment. Was it done under circumstances that defendants must be charged with knowledge that plaintiff did not know of the injury? If so, an enriching advantage was gained for defendants at plaintiff's expense. There is no doubt of the good faith of both defendants' counsel. There is no doubt that during the course of the negotiations, when the parties were in an adversary relationship, no rule required or duty rested upon defendants or their representatives to disclose this knowledge. However, once the agreement to settle was reached, it is difficult to characterize the parties' relationship as adverse. At this point all parties were interested in securing Court approval. . . .
>
> When the adversary nature of the negotiations concluded in a settlement, the procedure took on the posture of a joint application to the Court, at least so far as the facts upon which the Court could and must approve settlement is concerned. It is here that the true nature of the concealment appears, and defendants' failure to

act affirmatively, after having been given a copy of the application for approval, can only be defendants' decision to take a calculated risk that the settlement would be final. . . .

To hold that the concealment was not of such character as to result in an unconscionable advantage over plaintiff's ignorance or mistake, would be to penalize innocence and incompetence and reward less than full performance of an officer of the Court's duty to make full disclosure to the Court when applying for approval in minor settlement proceedings.

1. The princip[le]s applicable to the court's authority to vacate settlements made on behalf of minors and approved by it appear well established. With reference thereto, we have held that the court in its discretion may vacate such a settlement, even though it is not induced by fraud or bad faith, where it is shown that in the accident the minor sustained separate and distinct injuries which were not known or considered by the court at the time settlement was approved; and even though the releases furnished therein purported to cover both known and unknown injuries resulting from the accident. The court may vacate such a settlement for mistake . . . as to the nature and extent of the minor's injuries, [] where it is shown that one of the parties had additional knowledge with respect thereto and was aware that neither the court nor the adversary party possessed such knowledge when the settlement was approved. . . . "Equity will prevent one party from taking an unconscionable advantage of another's mistake for the purpose of enriching himself at the other's expense."

2. From the foregoing it is clear that in the instant case the court did not abuse its discretion in setting aside the settlement which it had approved on plaintiff's behalf while he was still a minor. It is undisputed that neither he nor his counsel nor his medical attendants were aware that at the time settlement was made he was suffering from an aorta aneurysm which may have resulted from the accident. The seriousness of this disability is indicated by Dr. Hannah's report indicating the imminent danger of death therefrom. This was known by counsel for both defendants but was not disclosed to the court at the time it was petitioned to approve the settlement. While no canon of ethics or legal obligation may have required them to inform plaintiff or his counsel with respect thereto, or to advise the court therein, it did become obvious to them at the time, that the settlement then made did not contemplate or take into consideration the disability described. This fact opened the way for the court to later exercise its discretion in vacating the settlement and under the circumstances described we cannot say that there was any abuse of discretion on the part of the court in so doing under Rule 60.02(6) of Rules of Civil Procedure.

. . .

4. It is also suggested that the settlement made on behalf of the minor was in part at least dependent upon insurance limitations relating to plaintiff's injuries; and that these having been a factor should constitute a bar to the court's exercise of its discretion in vacating such settlement. No decisions are cited in support of this contention. There are, however, numerous decisions holding that insurance limitations have no part in the trial of actions relating to personal injuries or property damage; and it would seem fairly clear that the principles governing this rule would be equally applicable here. . . .

Affirmed.

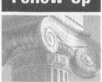

Post-Case Follow-Up

Spaulding is a striking example of professional and moral failure in a Holmesian framework where law and morality are entirely separated. The incompetence and amorality of those in the legal profession risked David's life — and actually caused him two and a half years of severe pain and the permanent loss of his natural speaking voice. Who failed David? David's lawyer was incompetent in failing to request the defense medical report. But what of the defense lawyers and their hired expert? What of the Minnesota trial court and supreme court? Note the extreme legalistic tone of both court opinions. Both courts skirt the high-stakes moral issue raised in the case by relying on the letter of the professional responsibility rule regarding confidentiality that existed at that time. According to the court, defense counsel acted in "good faith" because "no rule required or duty rested upon defendants or their representatives to disclose this knowledge." The rules of professional conduct appear to be the beginning and end of the court's moral discussion — without even acknowledging the life-or-death drama at issue.

But did the defense lawyers act in "good faith" — did they fulfill their professional responsibilities to their clients, to the justice system, to third parties, and to themselves? As will be discussed in a later chapter, a lawyer's duty of confidentiality is nearly sacrosanct with only a few limited exceptions; and while the Model Rules today would permit a lawyer to disclose confidences to "prevent reasonably certain death," the rule existing at the time of the *Spaulding* case only permitted disclosure where the lawyer was "accused by his client" or to protect others from "[t]he announced attention of a client to commit a crime."[33]

Nevertheless, the defense lawyers utterly failed in their duties to communicate to and counsel with their own clients. Neither the Zimmermans nor the Ledermanns were informed of David's aneurysm, and it appears that the Zimmermans' insurance company was also left uninformed.[34] Apparently, the lawyers imputed bad man ends to their clients, assuming that their clients wanted the least liability at all costs — even the cost of David's life. But is that actually what their clients wanted? The defense lawyers failed to treat their clients as human beings with their own moral moorings; and they failed to consider that their clients had relational self-interests and may have cared about third parties in the community in which they lived. What is the likelihood that the Zimmermans, who employed and knew David personally, would want to let him die of an aneurysm caused by the car wreck? The Zimmermans and Ledermanns both lost a family member in the car wreck and personally knew the pain of such loss — would they want to inflict that pain on a neighbor in their community? If the defense lawyers were only considering the interests of the insurance company, then they were acting under a conflict of interest, as they owed loyalty to the individual clients.[35] But even to the extent that it was proper to protect the interests of the insurance companies, would the insurance

---

33. ABA, Canon of Professional Ethics 37.
34. *See* Cramton, *supra* note 13, at 180.
35. *See id.* at 179.

companies (made up of actual people) want to risk David's life to save a few thousand dollars on the payout of a policy?[36] If David had died, could the individual defendants or the insurance companies have been held liable for an even larger amount? If it came out that the insurance companies had let David die to save them part of a policy payout, could that affect the insurance company's public relations and corporate value? The defense lawyers did not even discuss these issues with their clients. Similarly, Dr. Hannah, the medical expert, was so loyal to his role as a defense witness that he did not tell David. What happened to his Hippocratic Oath?

The defense lawyers also failed in their responsibility to the trial court—to inform the court of the aneurysm when making a joint application to the court regarding the extent of David's injuries for settlement. Lawyers have a duty of candor to the court and cannot present false statements of fact or law to the court. This misstep by defense counsel is the only one acknowledged by the court. The court says the defense lawyers thereby took an unjustified "calculated risk" that the settlement would be invalidated—yet the court makes no mention of the "calculated risk" taken as to David's life.

What about the defense lawyers' responsibility to themselves and their own moral identity? If you let a person die of something curable by withholding information from that person, could you look yourself in the mirror? Do not forget to ask yourself who you are becoming and whether that is the person you want to be. Richard Pemberton argued the *Spaulding* case on behalf of the defense to the Minnesota Supreme Court. He was a new lawyer and believed he was asked to do it because the senior lawyers were concerned about facing the justices in light of their actions. In hindsight, Pemberton has this to say about the case:

> When I briefed and argued the *Spaulding* case in the Supreme Court, I was within the first few months of legal practice and was attempting to defend a senior partner's handling of the matter in the trial court. After twenty years of practice, I would like to think that I would have disclosed the aneurysm of the aorta as an act of humanity and without regard to the legalities involved, just as I surely would now. You might suggest to your students in the course on professional responsibility that a pretty good rule for them to practice respecting professional conduct is to do the decent thing.[37]

David's Voice

In 2000, Timothy Floyd and John Gallagher located and interviewed David Spaulding.[38] David was in college studying to be a teacher at the time of the 1956 accident. He received a teaching certificate after the surgery to fix the aneurysm. However, as a direct result of the delay in treatment, he explained, "I didn't have much of a voice for teaching. I talked in a very high pitch." He was unable to find work as a permanent teacher, although he worked for three years as a regular substitute. With a "thin and reedy" voice, "I just couldn't survive in the classroom." He used the last money from the settlement to get a master's degree in school psychology and "was a school psychologist for about thirty-one years." As he

---

36. *See id.* at 182 ("Most people do the right thing under such circumstances and insurance personnel who adjust and settle liability claims are ordinary people doing ordinary work. Why do law students and lawyers assume that corporate actors are only interested in company profits and are totally lacking in moral sensitivity?").

37. *See id.* at 201.

38. *See* Floyd & Gallagher, *supra* note 32, at 933 & nn.8 & 15.

explained, "[w]ith this psychology business, it is just one-to-one." He ultimately had Teflon put on his left larynx, which lowered his vocal range to an appropriate pitch. Even so, Floyd and Gallagher note that "[o]nly when he speaks very quietly, emotionlessly, and with a steady control, can he say what is on his mind." In David's words, "People do not know what it is like to go through a life without a voice. If I try to shout, nothing comes out. If I talk like this [quiet, emotionlessly, and controlled], then I can talk. But if I try to increase my volume, it just comes out in a squeal. You know, we are in a coffee klatch, and the thing is, I'll start talking, and somebody else will take over the conversation. And there is nothing I can do. So I back away. Even when I am with four or five of my men friends and I will feel it's my turn to come in and start talking, I'll start to talk and then somebody just takes over." Floyd and Gallagher summarize: "It seemed to David Spaulding that all those people who might have saved him from more than two-and-a-half years of severe pain and the permanent loss of his natural voice had betrayed him. All of his assumptions about how decent people behave and how the system might support people's welfare had been dashed."[39]

Spaulding v. Zimmerman: Real Life Applications

1. What if the aneurysm had ruptured and David Spaulding had died? Who, if anyone, could have been held liable?

2. You work for Down & Out, a personal injury plaintiffs' law firm. Jane slips and falls in Leah's driveway. Jane and Leah are neighbors. Jane comes to you and asks about filing suit against Leah, but Jane believes that Leah's homeowners' insurance will actually be paying any sums in the lawsuit. You file suit against Leah on Jane's behalf. Not long thereafter, the homeowners' insurance company denies coverage for the slip and fall under Leah's policy, saying that the incident does not fall within the policy Leah purchased. As filed, Jane's lawsuit will proceed against Leah without insurance. What do you need to do?

3. You are hired to represent Zyg Bikes Inc. in a dispute with Tubular Co., the component manufacturer of the tubes that are incorporated into Zyg bicycles. You examine the documents in the matter, which show that Tubular failed to ship 10,000 tire tubes to Zyg in breach of their contract. In correspondence, Tubular claims that it shipped the tubes, and that Zyg must bear the loss if for some reason they did not arrive. Zyg disagrees. Assume that Tubular makes the best tire tubes in the industry, which is important to Zyg for the types of bikes it sells. In representing Zyg and deciding how to proceed, what interests are at stake that you should identify and discuss with your client?

3. Cultivating Moral and Professional Judgment

One of the lessons of *Spaulding* is that rules are not the beginning and end of the lawyer's moral and professional responsibilities. In this course and casebook, you will learn — and you must know — the rules of professional conduct. But the rules are the floor — the point below which you cannot go without risking discipline.

---

39. *See id.* at 951-52.

Moreover, as every lawyer knows, there is always some level of ambiguity in written rules — whether because of the language itself, the scope of application to particular facts, or the state's exercise of discretion in enforcing the rule. Lawyers are trained to see such ambiguity in written codes, and can use those skills to game and manipulate the Model Rules themselves to excuse unethical conduct. Many of the Model Rules are underenforced.[40] Moreover, the Model Rules are largely stripped of moral directives. Marianne M. Jennings criticizes lawyers for having "shaped a profession governed by rules and devoid of morality."[41] Whenever "the code, rules, or an opinion sanction an activity," or can be construed to sanction an activity, "we separate our own consciences from the behavior, label the behavior ethical and march forward with [] full confidence."[42] The situation is perhaps worse when the rules are silent on a matter. She quips: "If it ain't written down, it can and will be done."[43] If the rules fail to expressly prohibit an activity, does that make the activity ethical?

While knowing the rules is essential to becoming a lawyer and to avoiding discipline, compliance with the rules does not make one an exemplar of professionalism. Good lawyers aspire beyond the floor of the rules and the risk of discipline. As Floyd and Gallagher posit in their article telling David Spaulding's story, "[e]thics is more than rules, principles, and obligations, it's about how we live our lives and the kind of persons we are."[44] So what is professionalism, and how can one start down the path of cultivating moral and professional judgment?

The American Bar Association (ABA) and the Conference of Chief Justices (CCJ) have commissioned reports and plans to increase attorney professionalism. Synthesizing these reports and building on moral psychology, Neil Hamilton has offered the following five principles of professionalism.

Neil Hamilton, Professionalism Clearly Defined
18 Prof. Law. 4 (2007)

A. FIVE PRINCIPLES OF PROFESSIONALISM

[P]rofessionalism means that each lawyer:

1. Continues to grow in personal conscience over his or her career;
2. Agrees to comply with the ethics of duty — the minimum standards for the lawyer's professional skills and ethical conduct set by the Rules;

---

40. *See* Fred C. Zacharias, *The Future Structure and Regulation of Law Practice: Confronting Lies, Fiction, and False Paradigms in Legal Ethics Regulation*, 44 Ariz. L. Rev. 829, 861 (2002) ("many rules simply go unenforced or are patently underenforced").

41. Marianne M. Jennings, *The Model Rules and the Code of Professional Responsibility Have Absolutely Nothing to Do with Ethics: The Wally Cleaver Proposition as an Alternative*, 1996 Wis. L. Rev. 1223, 1238 (1996).

42. *Id.* at 1226.

43. *Id.* at 1238.

44. *See* Floyd & Gallagher, *supra* note 32, at 943.

3. Strives to realize, over a career, the ethics of aspiration — the core values and ideals of the profession including internalizing the highest standards for the lawyer's professional skills and ethical conduct;

4. Agrees both to hold other lawyers accountable for meeting the minimum standards set forth in the Rules and to encourage them to realize core values and ideals of the profession; and

5. Agrees to act as a fiduciary where his or her self-interest is overbalanced by devotion to serving the client and the public good in the profession's area of responsibility: justice.

   a. Devotes professional time to serve the public good, particularly by representing pro bono clients; and

   b. Undertakes a continuing reflective engagement, over a career, on the relative importance of income and wealth in light of the other principles of professionalism.

B. FURTHER ANALYSIS OF THE PRINCIPLES

1. Personal Conscience

Personal conscience, the first principle of professionalism, is an awareness of the moral goodness or blameworthiness of one's own intentions and conduct together with a feeling of obligation to be and to do what is morally good. Personal conscience in this definition includes (1) awareness that the person's conduct is having an effect on others, (2) a reasoning process to determine the moral goodness or blameworthiness of the person's intentions or conduct, and (3) a sense of obligation to be and to do what is morally good.

Personal conscience is the foundation on which a law student or practicing lawyer builds an ethical professional identity. Without this foundation, the remaining four principles of professionalism will collapse into a calculus of simple self-interest, including gaming the Rules of Professional Conduct themselves for self-advantage.

a. The Importance of Self-Scrutiny and Feedback from Others

The [ABA's] MacCrate and the Haynsworth Reports and the CCJ National Action Plan note the importance over a career of self-scrutiny along with feedback from and moral dialogue with others to contribute to a lawyer's professional growth. . . .

b. The Four Component Model and Personal Conscience

Moral psychology also offers a useful analytical framework with which to explore and understand personal conscience. Personal conscience involves awareness of a moral issue, a reasoning process to determine the moral goodness or blameworthiness of alternative courses of conduct, and a sense of obligation to do what is morally good. Similarly the moral psychology literature starts with the question, "what must we suppose happens psychologically in order for moral behavior to take place?" Morality in this meaning focuses on the social condition that humans live in groups and what one person does can affect others. In light of our understanding that what one person does can affect others, morality asks what do we owe others?

What are our duties to them? What rights can they claim? Scholars posit that four distinct capacities, called the Four Component Model, are necessary in order for moral behavior to occur:

1. Moral Sensitivity. "Moral sensitivity is the awareness of how an individual's actions affect other people. It involves being aware of different possible lines of action and how each line of action could affect the parties concerned. It involves imaginatively constructing possible scenarios and knowing cause-consequence chains of events in the real world; it involves empathy and role-taking skills."[66] Moral sensitivity requires the understanding of one's own intuitions and emotional reactions.

2. Moral Judgment. "Once the person is aware of possible lines of action and how people would be affected by each line of action (Component 1), then Component 2 judges which line of action is more morally justifiable — which alternative is just, or right."[68] It involves deliberation regarding the various considerations relevant to different courses of action and making a judgment regarding which of the available actions would be most morally justifiable. It entails integrating both shared moral norms and individual moral principles.

Shared moral norms and an individual's moral principles — what philosophy calls normative ethics — flow from one of two general sources. A rational approach uses analysis and logic in any situation to reason out right conduct from a set of first ethical principles. This "ethics of principle" approach can be derived from (1) faith or religious teachings, (2) cultural norms, or (3) moral philosophy like Kant's categorical imperative or Mills's utilitarianism. A second general source emphasizes the virtues and good habits of character in any situation and is more intuitive about the right conduct that a virtue or habit of character demands in the situation. Some people using this "ethics of character" approach find the relevant virtues or habits of character in faith or religious teachings. Others look to moral philosophy or cultural norms.

3. Moral Motivation and Commitment. Moral motivation and commitment have "to do with the importance given to moral values in competition with other values. Deficiencies in Component 3 occur when a person is not sufficiently motivated to put moral values higher than other values — when other values such as self-actualization or protecting one's organization replace concern for doing what is right."[72]

It is not only competing values that can halt moral action at this point, but competing drives and emotional states. For example, if someone must choose between having a steady paycheck to ensure her family has food on the table, with acting on her moral values, the drive to care for basic needs may override all else. . . .

4. Moral Character and Implementation. "This component involves ego strength, perseverance, backbone, toughness, strength of conviction, and courage. A person may be morally sensitive, may make good moral judgments, and may place a high priority on moral values, but if the person wilts under pressure, is easily distracted or discouraged, is a wimp and weak-willed, then moral failure occurs because of

---

66. James Rest & Darcia Narvaez, Moral Development in the Professions 23 (1994).
68. *Id.* at 23-24.
72. *Id.* at 24.

deficiency in Component 4 (weak character)."[74] Problem-solving skills including fig-
uring out the necessary sequence of concrete actions and working around impediments and unexpected difficulties as well as interpersonal skills are important.
Component 4 includes the knowledge, skills and abilities to manage conflicts, communicate effectively and minimize polarization.

Lawrence Walker notes that, "Moral failure can be a consequence of a deficiency
in any component: being blind to the moral issues in a situation, being unable to formulate a morally defensible position, failing to accord priority to moral concerns, or
being unable or unwilling to implement action."[76] It is important therefore to attend
to development of all four components. . . .

. . .

The greatest concern about "personal conscience in a professional context" as
the foundation of professionalism is the fear that a lawyer's personal conscience
will limit client autonomy and client equal access to justice. The lawyer's personal
conscience will trump client choices that are lawful. The central point of "personal
conscience in a professional context" is that the lawyer's personal conscience is now
informed and guided also by the role morality of the lawyer's function in the justice
system. That role morality calls on the lawyer who accepts a representation to honor
principles of client autonomy and equal access to justice. In the counseling role, for
example, the lawyer's duty is to help the client think through the client's best interests in the situation *from the client's shoes including the client's morality*. The lawyer
is not to impose the lawyer's morality on the client. This duty includes fairly and
completely presenting the law applicable to the client's situation. However a lawyer
who develops over a career in any of the capacities of the Four Component Model
should be a better counselor for all clients and should better understand adversaries.
For example, a lawyer whose own moral reasoning is at an early stage of development
will be limited in his or her ability to counsel a client who is at a more developed
stage of moral reasoning. The lawyer simply will not understand the client well. If the
reverse is true, the lawyer will understand the moral reasoning of the client and can
help the client think through the client's best interests from the client's shoes.

2. The Ethics of Duty

. . . The ethics of duty—the obligatory and disciplinary elements of the
Rules—state the minimum floor of competence and ethical conduct below which
the profession will impose discipline. An ethical professional identity requires each
law student and practicing lawyer to understand and internalize the ethics of duty.

3. The Ethics of Aspiration—The Core Values and Ideals of the Profession

The ethics of aspiration call on each law student and practicing lawyer, over the
course of a career, both to internalize and to strive to realize the core values and

---

74. Muriel Bebeau & Verna Monson, *Guided by Theory, Grounded in Evidence: A Way Forward for Professional Ethics Education, in* HANDBOOK ON MORAL AND CHARACTER EDUCATION (D. Narvaez & L. Nucci eds., in press).
76. Lawrence J. Walker, *The Model and the Measure: An Appraisal of the Minnesota Approach to Moral Development,* 31 J. OF MORAL EDUC. 353, 355 (2002).

ideals of the profession [as taken from the Model Rules of Professional Conduct and the ABA Reports and CCJ Action Plan on professionalism].

a. The Core Values of the Profession

- Competent Representation Including Reasonable Diligence and Reasonable Communication with the Client
- Loyalty to the Client
- Confidentiality of Client Information
- Zealous Advocacy on Behalf of the Client Constrained by the Officer of the Legal System Role
- Independent Professional Judgment
- Public Service to Improve the Quality of Justice, Particularly to Maintain and Improve the Quality of the Legal Profession and to Ensure Equal Access to the Justice System
- Respect for the Legal System and All Persons Involved in the Legal System

b. Ideals of the Profession

- Commitment to Seek and Realize Excellence at the Principles of Professionalism and the Core Values and Ideals of the Profession
- Integrity
- Honesty
- Fairness

4. *The Duty of Peer-Review*

. . . The Model Rules and the ABA Reports tend to focus on the requirement that peers report misconduct below the floor of the Rules. This is important, but the creation of strong ethical cultures emphasizing excellence at the skills, core values, and ideals of the profession is even more important. As the recent corporate scandals in corporations with well-drafted written ethics codes but corrupt cultures demonstrated, unethical culture will trump rules.

. . .

5. *The Duty to Restrain Self-Interest to Some Degree to Serve the Client and the Public Purpose of the Profession*

. . . The public good served by the legal profession is justice. The peer-review professions have always been about making a satisfactory living in addition to serving the client's interest and the public good. . . . A lawyer owes a client the fiduciary duties of safeguarding confidences and property, avoiding impermissible conflicts of interest, dealing honestly with the client, adequately informing the client, following the instructions of the client, and not employing adversely to the client powers arising from the attorney-client relationship. . . .

[In addition,] a lawyer is an agent and fiduciary not just for the client, but also for the legal system, the purpose of which is justice. The first sentence of the Preamble to the Model Rules in effect states this concept by providing that a lawyer is "a representative of clients, an officer of the legal system and a public citizen having special responsibility for the quality of justice." . . .

a. The Duty to Give Professional Time to Serve the Public Good, Particularly Pro Bono Assistance to the Disadvantaged

. . . [The] duty to provide pro bono or low fee assistance to the disadvantaged is uniquely compelling for the legal profession in comparison with the other peer-review professions. The moral justification for the work of the other peer-review professions depends to a much lesser degree on the proper functioning of the system within which the work is done than is the case with the moral justification for the work of the legal profession. A physician for example can serve the major public purpose of the profession, the health of individual patients, without significant concern that others will be negatively affected. . . . However a lawyer in litigation will serve the major public purpose of the profession, justice, only when the adversary system is working properly. The adversary system is the society's best approximation of justice only with (1) a competent neutral decision maker and (2) competent representation for all affected persons. . . .

b. The Duty to Reflect on How Much Is Enough

A common failing of all the definitions of professionalism is that they do not address adequately on the business aspects of the profession that may create tension between a lawyer's personal goals of income and wealth and the correlative duties, core values and ideals of the profession. The Stanley Commission Report states "All segments of the bar should . . . resist the temptation to make the acquisition of wealth a primary goal of law practice." . . .

While two ABA professionalism reports and the Preamble raise the question how much is a satisfactory living, that question is actually part of a larger question posed by the steadily increasing time demands of professional life in our culture. The larger question is how much life energy should be devoted to meeting professional duties (including making a satisfactory living) in comparison with the life energy devoted to other duties as a parent, spouse, adult child in support of elderly parents, friend, contributing member of non-professional communities and a whole person with dimensions other than work? . . .

C. PROFESSIONAL RESPONSIBILITIES IN LITIGATING, ADVISING, AND TRANSACTIONAL PLANNING

A major critique of the traditional law school curriculum is that it is primarily focused on training students for litigation as opposed to training them for transactional planning or for advising and counseling clients as to prospective client conduct. Indeed, to some extent this critique can be made of the Model Rules themselves. The Model Rules do not address transactional planning or counseling work to the same extent that they address litigation issues. Yet there are some major differences between these contexts that should be recognized and that should shape the lawyer's professional responsibilities in these roles.

Unfortunately, lawyers in practice often do not appreciate these differences — thus the issue is not solely one of training that will be completed upon graduation from law school. Many lawyers in practice approach transactional planning and providing legal advice about prospective client conduct in precisely the same way as they would approach legal analysis in litigation. So what are the differences between these contexts and how do those differences call for a correspondingly different approach to one's professional responsibilities?

1. Shaping Client Conduct

The first major difference — and one that almost cannot be overstated — is that in the advising and transactional planning scenarios, often the client has not yet acted. In the litigation context, the client has usually already acted and the question is how to mitigate liability or maximize compensation in light of those completed actions. But when a lawyer is asked to advise a client about prospective conduct or to perform transactional work, the client has yet to act. Thus, the attorney's interpretation of the law will most likely shape client conduct, which in turn will shape the consequences for all affected by that conduct, including both third parties and the client's own long-term interests and exposure to civil or criminal liability for those actions. In the transactional context, the lawyer's assistance is often needed to make the client's actions legally effective. Thus, lawyers are needed for bona fide, true sale, nonconsolidation, and other legal certifications in order for transactions to close and take legal effect. Consequently, the lawyer is not solely advising the client, but is assisting the client in effectuating whatever conduct the client is engaged in.

Importantly, Model Rule 1.2(d) prohibits a lawyer from either counseling a client to engage or assisting clients "in conduct that the lawyer knows is criminal or fraudulent." The rule refers to conduct that the lawyer "knows" is criminal or fraudulent, and the rules in turn define knowledge to require "actual knowledge," but such knowledge "may be inferred from the circumstances," as stated in Model Rule 1.0(f). Lawyers who provide certifications that they know are false in order to close a deal are assisting their clients in fraud, and in some cases, in criminal conduct.

For example, in the fallout of the Enron and Worldcom scandals, it became evident that the lawyers assisted in the fraud. As Susan Koniak has described, lawyers showed corporate executives and constituents how to break the law by "structuring bogus deals, vouching for nonexistent 'sales,' writing whitewash reports to keep the sheriff fooled and away."[45] Koniak claims that "lawyers were central, even more central than accountants to the corporate fraud at Enron." She notes that one major aspect of Enron's fraud was in "money-go-round" deals where "Enron made money and other assets go round in circles to inflate its profits." Koniak explains that "[a]ccountants cannot book such circles as 'sales'" — which is how they were

---

45. Susan P. Koniak, *When the Hurlyburly's Done: The Bar's Struggle with the SEC*, 103 COLUM. L. REV. 1236, 1237 (2003).

booked — "instead of 'loans' without two legal opinions, a 'true sale' opinion and a 'nonconsolidation' opinion." Thus, the accountants "could not act without the lawyers vouching for these deals." She states:

> Vinson [& Elkins] apparently issued "true sales" opinions in a number of these transactions, although it was surely not the only [law] firm to do so. More importantly, each of the banks [who made these deals with Enron] had their [own] lawyers who helped the banks with their part of the sham. The banks' lawyers set up puppet SPEs [special purpose entities] to allow the banks to funnel loans to Enron disguised as trades or sales. The lawyers also helped the banks to protect themselves from the prospect that Enron would go belly-up from the weight of all this undisclosed debt. . . . How many major law firms were helping banks in what appear to be fraudulent transactions? The Texas court denied motions to dismiss charges of securities fraud in connection with Enron's shady deals against Citigroup, J.P. Morgan, Credit Suisse First Boston, and Merrill Lynch. I have no doubt that those banks were represented by the "best" legal talent in this country — law firms considered to be of the highest caliber. And none of those lawyers noticed anything amiss? . . . Are we [] to believe that all the lawyers who worked on these deals were incapable of grasping just what it was they were doing? I rest my case.[46]

Why does the law require that lawyers be part of closing such transactions — that lawyers must issue true sale, bona fide, nonconsolidation, and other legal opinions for transactions to close? Because the lawyers, even as advocates, are supposed to maintain some level of gatekeeping for the rule of law. W. Bradley Wendel posits that lawyers have a moral obligation to the law itself when engaged in legal counseling and planning. Wendel notes that "citizens are obligated to treat the law as legitimate," and so too must lawyers, who are acting as agents of those citizens in their dealings with society; consequently, "lawyers are prohibited from manipulating legal norms to defeat the substantive meaning of these norms."[47] If lawyers engage in such instrumental manipulation, they "can commit a moral wrong vis-à-vis their obligation to serve as custodians or trustees of the law." Wendel recognizes the relational self-interests at issue in transactional planning:

> [The lawyer] must be concerned about the effective functioning of the law, because without it, neither she nor her client could realize their own interests. The market economy presupposes a background of stable law, custom, and enforcement that enforces private ordering. Even if a lawyer and client were concerned only with pursuing their own narrow interests, paradoxically it is only possible to behave self-interestedly within a framework of other-regarding obligations. A lawyer might evade regulatory requirements by aggressive structuring of transactions in one case, but cause long-run damage by eroding the capability of the legal system to facilitate the functioning of financial markets.[48]

---

46. *Id.* at 1242-43.
47. Wendel, *supra* note 27, at 72.
48. Wendel, *supra* note 29, at 1209.

Under Model Rule 1.2, lawyers are allowed to advise a client regarding "the legal consequences of any proposed course of conduct" and "the validity, scope, meaning or application of the law." This generally allows attorneys to advise clients to walk up to the edge of what is legal, but the rule expressly prohibits lawyers from advising or assisting clients to cross that line into what is illegal, false, and fraudulent. The Enron lawyers crossed that line. If we didn't need someone to vouch for the legal validity of transactions, we simply wouldn't need lawyer involvement. With that in mind, what if Enron's lawyers at Vinson & Elkins or the lawyers for the banks had refused to issue true sales opinions, had refused to structure the deals that hid Enron's debt, had told their client, "No, we cannot do that for you, it's a violation of securities laws and a fraud upon shareholders"? If the lawyers had refused, the transactions would not have closed, Enron (once a stable company) may not have gone bankrupt, the public would not have been duped into buying Enron's inflated stock (which sold at $90.75 in August 2000 and reduced to $0.67 in January 2002),[49] thousands of people would not have lost their jobs, and thousands more would not have lost billions of dollars in their life savings and 401k accounts.

And what of the executives who apparently wanted the lawyers to structure these deals and hide Enron's actual debt to inflate share prices? Many of the executives — Jeffrey Skilling, Kenneth Lay, Andrew Fastow, Richard Causey, Lea Fastow — were convicted of crimes for their roles in the massive fraud, serving various prison sentences, and J. Clifford Baxter, former Enron vice chairman, committed suicide.[50] The lawyers certainly did not serve their corporate client — Enron and its shareholders — well. But did they even provide good service to the non-client executives? How much of a favor is it to those executives to help them do something that ended up putting them in prison? The lawyers' actions shaped client conduct — had they said "no," things might very well have gone differently. Had they refused to issue fraudulent opinions and refused to structure bogus deals — which they were professionally required to refuse to do under Rule 1.2(d) — the drastic consequences for their client, their client's employees and shareholders, the executives, and the U.S. economy may have been avoided. The transactions could not have closed without lawyer help. Lawyers shaped the conduct and the resultant consequences.

Another striking example of shaping client conduct is found in the advising context. In the wake of the events of September 11, 2001, the Bush administration sought advice regarding legal restraints on the use of coercive interrogation techniques against detainees captured in Afghanistan. The Office of Legal Counsel (OLC) issued memos (now universally dubbed the "Torture Memos") narrowly construing the definition of "torture" as prohibited in the 1984 Convention Against Torture and the implementing federal statute, 18 U.S.C. §2340(A), which makes it a federal crime to engage in torture. As Wendel details:

> Lawyers in the OLC [] sought to construe the operative term, torture, as narrowly as possible. Torture is defined in the [federal] statute as an "act . . . specifically intended

---

49. CNN, *Enron Fast Facts, available at* http://www.cnn.com/2013/07/02/us/enron-fast-facts/.
50. The sentences ranged from one year to 14 years. Kenneth Lay was convicted of conspiracy and fraud, but died of a heart attack in Aspen, Colorado less than two months after his conviction. *See id.*

to inflict severe physical or mental pain or suffering," and severe pain and suffering is further defined as the prolonged harm caused by one of several enumerated acts. By focusing on the specific intent requirement and the element of severe pain or suffering, the lawyers created an implausibly restrictive definition of torture: "[T]he victim must experience intense pain or suffering of the kind that is equivalent to the pain that would be associated with serious physical injury *so severe that death, organ failure or permanent damage resulting in a loss of significant body function will likely result.*" Despite the plain meaning of the statutory language to the contrary, burning detainees with cigarettes, administering electric shocks to their genitals, hanging them by the wrists, submerging them in water to simulate drowning, beating them, and sexually humiliating them would not be deemed "torture" under this definition.[51]

Further, the lawyers in the OLC advised the administration that they could rely on "[s]tandard criminal law defenses of necessity and self-defense" to avoid liability for engaging in torture. As Milan Markovic explains, "[t]here is nothing 'standard' about this argument" because the statute "mentions no defenses, and the Convention Against Torture specifically states, 'No exceptional circumstances whatsoever, whether a state of war or a threat of war, internal political instability or any other public emergency, may be invoked as a justification of torture.'"[52] Thus, the advice regarding defenses was patently erroneous.

Importantly, the administration's purpose in seeking this advice—and the effect of the lawyers giving it—was to insulate the interrogators engaging in such techniques from prosecution for violating the laws against torture. Jack Goldsmith, who subsequently headed the OLC, characterized advice in the memos as a "golden shield," "get-out-of-jail-free card," or an "advance pardon" in order to "immunize officials from prosecutions for wrongdoing."[53] Daniel Pines explains that "in virtually every situation, government employees who rely on an [OLC] opinion in taking action will likely be absolved from any legal sanction."[54] Thus, as Markovic concludes, "[t]he Torture Memo's impact cannot be overstated. It was the basis for coercive techniques used against several high-ranking detainees" and ultimately led to "a list of aggressive interrogation procedures to be used at Guantanamo Bay that eventually migrated to Iraq."[55]

Why are executive employees who rely on OLC opinions immune from prosecution? Is it so that the executive branch can successfully avoid the purposes, restraints, and punishments created by law—as happened with the Torture Memos? Exactly the opposite. The purpose behind providing such immunity is to enable the proper functioning of law and government—specifically, to encourage the executive branch to seek legal advice so that the rule of law can be upheld, even when complex or unclear, and to encourage government officials to fulfill their government duties without being hindered by the prospect of prosecution or

---

51. Wendel, *supra* note 27, at 80-81.
52. Milan Markovic, *Can Lawyers Be War Criminals?*, 20 Geo. J. Legal Ethics 347, 352 (2007).
53. Office of Professional Responsibility Final Report, *available at* http://nsarchive.gwu.edu/news/20100312/OPRFinalReport090729.pdf.
54. Daniel L. Pines, *Are Even Torturers Immune from Suit? How Attorney General Opinions Shield Government Employees from Civil Litigation and Criminal Prosecution*, 43 Wake Forest L. Rev. 93, 97 (2008).
55. Markovic, *supra* note 52, at 348.

liability.[56] But in order for these purposes to be realized, lawyers as advisors (especially government advisors) must not construe and stretch the law to mean that anything a government actor wants to do is "legal." Otherwise the constraints and public purposes of law are eviscerated. Lawyers as advisors are to be gatekeepers and must show fidelity, not only to their clients, but also to the existence, meaning, and rule of law.

As in the transactional context, the Torture Memos were integral to the client's ultimate conduct. Had the lawyers refused to give them the green light, so to speak — had they advised their client that the activities the client wanted to engage in were likely torture under the Convention Against Torture and the implementing federal statute and that the Convention had a clear non-derogation rule that prohibited reliance on criminal law defenses or the extent of the national emergency — then the administration could not have engaged in the extreme interrogation techniques without risking prosecution. The interrogators likely would have decided not to engage in such conduct and, consequently, detainees would not have been tortured. Again, the attorneys' advice shaped both the client's conduct and the resultant consequences for third parties — in this case being tortured.

2. Providing Advice Outside of the Checks of the Adversary System

In law school, students are taught how to make creative arguments regarding the meaning of law or application to a given fact pattern; indeed, students are rewarded for their ability to recognize and make creative arguments. Such creativity, and the ability to see the malleability of law, is an essential skill of lawyering. But do legal advising and planning require a more tempered approach to creativity and legal interpretation than what is appropriate in litigation?

In the litigation context, lawyers can exercise significant creativity in proffering interpretations of the law because that creative interpretation will always be challenged by checks inherent in the adversary system. First, the opposing party will provide a competing interpretation of the law. Second, the judge — as the authority constitutionally established to do so — will determine the actual meaning of the law given the circumstances at hand, and a jury or judge will determine any questions of fact. Further, lawyers in litigation have duties of candor to the court; they are required to disclose controlling adverse authority and cannot make false statements of law or fact.[57] Similarly, in alternative dispute resolution processes, an arbitrator or other third-party neutral will make a decision about what should happen after hearing from both sides.

Thus, even if a lawyer advocates a farfetched interpretation of the law, that interpretation will be countered and then can only be accepted if the judge or third-party neutral agrees with it. Notably, the existence of an opposing party and

---

56. Pines, *supra* note 54, at 152-53.
57. Model Rule 3.3(a); Wendel, *supra* note 29, at 1172-73.

a third-party neutral can in fact cabin lawyer creativity in the first place. Litigators take into account the fact of opposition and the need to create an interpretation that the judge will be able to select as the authoritative interpretation of the law; they are wary of proffering arguments that the opposing party can mock as laughable or that will elicit the derision of the judge. Moreover, the opposing party and the judge will consider the effects of the client's actions on others and on the system of justice, as well as the meaning or public purpose behind the law. Thus, good litigators will also take such countervailing and relational interests into account in framing their arguments — even while advocating zealously for their clients — because doing so represents the most promising chance of success.

Much of lawyer training focuses on how to make creative arguments when these safeguards of the adversary system are in place, but when lawyers are acting in an advisory or transactional role, there are no such safeguards. Indeed, the attorney will often provide the only point of view to the client as to what the law means and what third-party and public interests are at stake before the client acts.[58] Wendel explains that advising and transactional planning "are distinctive precisely because there is no impartial referee to resist the lawyer's client-centered construction of the law." As "the sole legal interpreter," the "lawyer has the power to shape the law for good or for ill."[59]

Model Rule 2.1 requires lawyers as advisors to "exercise independent professional judgment" and "render candid advice." Comment [1] elaborates that "[a] client is entitled to straightforward advice expressing the lawyer's honest assessment," which may include "unpleasant facts and alternatives that a client may be disinclined to confront." Wendel argues that a good measure for evaluating whether advice and transactional planning is candid is whether the lawyers' interpretations of the law "could be publicly justified to other members of the relevant community."[60]

Both the Enron and the Torture Memos debacles provide potent examples of problematic advising. One Enron employee infamously reported:

> Say you have a dog, but you need to create a duck on the financial statements. Fortunately, there are specific accounting rules for what constitutes a duck: yellow feet, white covering, orange beak. So you take the dog and paint its feet yellow and its fur white and you paste an orange plastic beak on its nose, and then you say to your accountants, "This is a duck! Don't you agree that it's a duck?" And the accountants say, "Yes, according to the rules this is a duck." Everyone knows that it is a dog, not a duck, but that does not matter because you have met the rules for calling it a duck.[61]

The lawyers at Enron were the ones who actually structured the deals and wrote legal opinions vouching for their bona fide and legally compliant nature — essentially they were dressing up the dog and then verifying that it was in fact a duck. As Koniak reports, transactional lawyers, like those involved in the Enron scandal,

---

58. *See* Wendel, *supra* note 29, at 1173 ("In counseling and transactional representation, the only constraint on the assistance the lawyer may provide to the client is provided by the law itself, as interpreted by the lawyer on whose client the law is expected to act as a constraint.").
59. *Id.* at 1199.
60. *Id.* at 1210.
61. *Id.* at 1171.

don't need "to discover what the client is up to; they know, because they are drafting the scripts, structuring the transactions. They are in, if you will, on the ground floor. The problem is not so much knowing what the client is doing; it is respecting that the law has limits that apply to one's client."[62]

Similarly, with the Torture Memos, the lawyers came up with their implausibly narrow definition of torture[63] by relying on and misconstruing an unrelated health care benefits statute that contained the term "severe pain." The statute had absolutely nothing to do with defining torture, but dealt with what constitutes an "emergency condition" for health care benefits. As Wendel summarizes:

> The statute is plainly not setting out a definition of severe pain in terms of organ failure or dysfunction, but using severe pain as one symptom among many — including organ failure or dysfunction — which might reasonably lead a prudent layperson to conclude that a person is in need of immediate medical attention. A lawyer conscientiously applying the plain meaning rule could not in good faith conclude that severe pain is limited to cases threatening organ failure or dysfunction. The lawyers also downplayed cases arising under statutes in more closely analogous contexts, such as the Torture Victim Protection Act.[64]

Further, the OLC lawyers advised their clients of the availability of common law defenses such as necessity and self-defense, despite the fact that the Convention Against Torture has a clear non-derogation principle disavowing the availability of such defenses. The likely explanation for this shoddy work from "some of the ablest lawyers in government" is that the OLC lawyers were reverse engineering their legal advice: starting with the legal conclusion that their clients wanted them to reach and then working backwards to concoct a legal interpretation to support it — "in effect adopting the attitude that they would make the law say what they wanted it to say."[65]

Lawyers understand the indeterminacy of many laws; law is often malleable and can be shaped through interpretation and application. Yet, unlike the judiciary, lawyers simply lack the constitutional power to make authoritative determinations as to "what the law is" and how it will be applied in a given case.[66] At best, lawyers' creative interpretations of the law are mere predictions of what the law may be once a judge has ruled in that regard.[67] And at worst, their creative interpretations are one-sided manipulations calculated to excuse or mitigate client bad acts — and such "interpretations" have zero chance of representing or ever becoming law. Consequently, as David Luban reminds us, the lawyer's duty under Model Rule 2.1 is "to provide 'independent' and 'candid' advice about what the law requires, not advice

---

62. Koniak, *supra* note 45, at 1280.
63. Again, the OLC lawyers defined torture thus: "[T]he victim must experience intense pain or suffering of the kind that is equivalent to the pain that would be associated with serious physical injury so severe that death, organ failure, or permanent damage resulting in a loss of significant body function will likely result." *See* Wendel, *supra* note 27, at 81.
64. *Id.* at 81-82.
65. Wendel, *supra* note 29, at 1172.
66. Marbury v. Madison, 5 U.S. 137, 177 (1803).
67. Oliver Wendell Holmes, *The Path of the Law*, 10 Harv. L. Rev. 457 (1897) ("The object of our study, then, is prediction, the prediction of the incidence of the public force through the instrumentality of the courts.").

spun to say whatever the client wants."[68] Even if the client doesn't want to hear it, the lawyer's duty is clear. As comment [1] to Model Rule 2.1 states, "a lawyer should not be deterred from giving candid advice by the prospect that the advice will be unpalatable to the client."

Importantly, lawyers often disserve their clients when they act as yes-men and provide unqualified approvals of prospective client conduct based on creative and aggressive interpretations of the law. Clients need an "honest assessment" of the law — one that will notify them of nontrivial chances of liability, prosecution, or sanctions. As Wendel explains, "[t]here is nothing necessarily wrong with advancing creative arguments as long as they are clearly identified as such, with weaknesses and counterarguments candidly noted," but "a lawyer who does not flag creative and aggressive arguments as such violates her fiduciary duty to her client by providing purportedly neutral advice without the caveat that the lawyer's interpretation may not accurately represent the applicable law."[69] Further, in the fallout of any deal or advice gone bad that results in litigation or criminal prosecution, the opposing party and the judge, jury, or other third-party neutral will consider the countervailing interpretations of the law as well as the effects of the client's actions on others. It is absolutely in the client's best interest to have been informed of such considerations before the client has acted on the attorney's advice.

In addition to these duties to their clients, lawyers acting as advisors and transactional planners serve "as custodians or trustees of the law."[70] In examining the Enron scandal, Koniak criticized "lawyers [who] believe it is their duty to contort all law to meet the client's ends. And here is the crux of the matter. In such a world, law is no longer possible. Law, in such a world, does not affect behavior at all, it just recharacterizes it. If lawyers tear down all our laws, where shall we stand? What will protect us then?"[71] If the Enron and OLC lawyers had provided their clients with candid advice, an "honest assessment" of what the law means,[72] the laws and the public interests underlying them — including a stable economy and international norms prohibiting torture and inhumane treatment of people — may have been upheld.

Chapter Summary

■ Lawyers play a significant role in the administration of justice in the United States. A license to practice law makes the lawyer an instrument of government power and a guardian of due process — the lawyer's actions directly affect the

---

68. David Luban, *Torture and the Professions*, 26 CRIM. JUST. ETHICS 2, 60 (2007).
69. Wendel, *supra* note 27, at 85; *see also* Milan Markovic, *Advising Clients After Critical Legal Studies and the Torture Memos*, 114 W. VA. L. REV. 109, 157 (2011) ("[A]n attorney cannot fulfill his or her duty qua advisor by offering only his or her own view of what the law is" — rather, "lawyers should convey not only their own views of the law but also countervailing considerations because the law does not dictate any one outcome.").
70. Wendel, *supra* note 27, at 72-73.
71. Koniak, *supra* note 45, at 1280.
72. Model Rule 2.1 cmt. [1].

extent of government power to be imposed in favor of or against people and their property.

■ Lawyers owe professional responsibilities to their clients, to the system of justice and the rule of law, to third parties, and to their own integrity and moral identity.

■ The legal profession is generally considered a self-regulated profession because lawyers create and enforce the rules of professional conduct. Self-regulation implies a social contract with the public whereby the legal profession agrees to police its members, maintain high standards of conduct, and to safeguard its public good: justice.

■ As agents for their clients' purposes, lawyers engage in role morality, which is important to preserve equal access to government power for people who are unpopular or have limited means.

■ Lawyers should engage in moral dialogue with their clients to determine their clients' actual ends and desires instead of imputing bad man ends to them. Lawyers should recognize that their clients are complex human beings with varying desires and ends and that they have relational self-interests that can be negatively affected and should be taken into account in any legal representation.

■ Lawyers cannot escape being moral agents and must assume moral responsibility for their actions. Lawyers should introspectively examine the person they are becoming and strive to cultivate moral and professional judgment.

■ Lawyers' professional responsibilities are different when they are acting in an advising or planning role, as opposed to as litigators in the adversary system. In the advising and planning role, the lawyer's legal advice will shape client conduct and must be candid, providing an honest assessment of the law.

Applying the Rules

1. Hal practices family law and is assisting Gary in a divorce from his wife, Ann. The court issues a custody order giving Ann full custody of their minor son, James, and giving Gary biweekly visitation. Gary learns that a police report has been filed against Ann alleging that she punched James. Gary picks up James for visitation. He asks Hal whether he can disregard the custody order and not return James in light of the allegations of abuse by Ann. Hal advises Gary to not return James, and files an application for emergency custody with the court. The court denies the application, reaffirming custody with Ann. Nevertheless, Gary believes that Ann is abusive. Can Hal advise or assist Gary in continuing to keep James with him? What should Hal do?

2. Makayla is a transactional lawyer. She becomes aware that the financial statements for her client, Toys Inc., are inaccurate as they fail to properly disclose all of Toys Inc.'s debt. Makayla confronts Toys Inc.'s chief financial officer (CFO) about the inaccuracies. The CFO responds that he is aware of the inaccuracies, and that he will be sure to fix them by the next reporting period. Toys Inc. is

in the process of merging with Wild Child Inc. At the closing, Makayla checks the financial statements and realizes the inaccuracies have not been fixed or disclosed to Wild Child Inc. Can Makayla close the deal? What actions might she take?

3. Paulina works for the law firm Hunter & Shell. John Hunter, the senior partner, asks Paulina to write a letter for a client, Food Corp., advising it regarding whether it can unilaterally revoke accrued paid vacation of its employees with no compensation. Hunter stresses to Paulina that Food Corp. is planning on taking this action and wants her to write a letter advising Food Corp. that it legally can revoke the accrued paid vacation, so that it can show the letter to employees who object. Paulina researches the issue and determines that in the relevant state accrued paid vacation is considered wages and cannot be revoked without compensation; indeed, should Food Corp. take such action it could be liable for treble damages and may be sanctioned by the Department of Labor. How should Paulina advise Food Corp.? What should she tell John Hunter?

4. Johanna is in-house lawyer for Car Co. Xavier brings a personal injury case against Car Co., alleging that he was seriously injured because of faulty brakes in his car. When Johanna investigates the claim, it becomes evident that the faulty brakes are not solely a problem for Xavier's car, but derive from a design defect that affects hundreds of thousands of cars that Car Co. has already sold and/or are on the market. Car Co. asks Johanna for advice on whether to recall the car — which it believes will be somewhat more expensive than settlement payouts for injuries, even serious injuries, to consumers. How might Johanna advise Car Co.? Think about relational self-interests, as well as moral, economic, and legal concerns.

Professional Responsibility in Practice

1. What are your responsibilities as a member of the legal profession? Articulate your personal understanding of your professional obligations to your clients, the system of justice, third parties, and yourself.

2. In the Four Component Model for Personal Conscience discussed by Neil Hamilton, the first component is Moral Sensitivity — the awareness that one's actions affect others and the ability to trace through the consequences for different possible courses of action. Assume that you are Zimmerman's lawyer and decide to meet with Zimmerman to discuss the existence of Spaulding's aneurysm. Outline the possible different courses of action and the potential consequences of each.

3. Consider the OLC's expansive definition of torture. If you were representing someone who was being prosecuted for allegedly violating the federal statute implementing the Convention Against Torture by engaging in enhanced interrogation techniques, could you ethically argue that the OLC's interpretation is correct and should be adopted by the court? Is there any reason you might not do so?

The Regulation of the Legal Profession

The law governing lawyers is increasingly fragmented and no longer neatly accessible in one source.[1] The "traditional duo of courts and bar associations" historically provided the source of law governing lawyers, and it was primarily contained in professional ethics or conduct codes.[2] This duo of courts and bar associations and their conduct codes still play a leading role in the regulation of lawyers but today state and federal legislators, administrators, and others increasingly create additional duties for lawyers.[3] As we noted in Chapter 1, for example, Congress authorized the Securities and Exchange Commission (SEC) to create standards governing lawyer conduct in the securities field. The SEC has expanded lawyers' reporting duties beyond ABA Model Rule 1.13 to require lawyers to report any material breach of securities law to an organization's general counsel or CEO, whereas

Key Concepts

- Each state's highest court generally has inherent authority to regulate the legal profession
- Many federal courts adopt lawyer conduct rules patterned after state rules
- Government organizations may also regulate lawyers
- Applicants must show good character and fitness for bar admission
- Each state's highest court generally disciplines lawyers; federal courts usually adopt the state court's discipline
- Lawyers and clients have an agency relationship creating fiduciary duties
- Lawyers are professionally liable for breach of contract, breach of fiduciary duties, and negligent representation

---

1. John Leubsdorf, *Legal Ethics Falls Apart*, 57 Buff. L. Rev. 959 (2009) ("Nowadays, a lawyer's duties . . . are likely to vary with the lawyer's specialty, the tribunal or agency before which the lawyer practices, the state or states in which the lawyer is acting, and other factors.").
2. *See* Jack P. Sahl, *Cracks in the Profession's Monopoly Power*, 82 Fordham L. Rev. 2635-37 (2014) (quoting Leubsdorf, *supra* note 1, at 961).
3. *See* Leubsdorf, *supra* note 1, at 959-62; James M. Fischer, *External Control over the American Bar*, 19 Geo. J. Legal Ethics 59, 108 (2006).

Rule 1.13 requires reporting to higher authority in the organization only if the violation will result in substantial injury to the organization.[4]

In addition to the increasing fragmentation of the law governing lawyers, dramatic changes in the legal services market promise new challenges for lawyer regulation.[5] For example, the increasing cross-border practice of lawyers to meet client needs that traverse state and national boundaries and involve different legal systems, major law firm consolidations and closures, and the development of new technologies that promote a quick-paced and often stressful practice all potentially enhance the risk of lawyer mistakes and abuses. As a result of this changing landscape, lawyer regulation will continue to be an important concern of the profession. Regulators will need to be proactive and creative in this changing landscape to protect the public and the courts from lawyer misconduct and to maintain the integrity of the legal profession — the traditional goals of lawyer regulation.

A. LAWYER REGULATION

1. Regulatory Powers of State Courts

In general, each state's high court, usually its supreme court, possesses the authority to regulate the legal profession.[6] Some state constitutions expressly provide this regulatory authority to the courts, but in most states the supreme courts assert inherent and exclusive regulatory power based on the separation of powers doctrine.[7] In some states, the legislature and the courts share authority to establish rules regulating the profession with the courts having the ultimate authority over regulation.[8] This means there are at least 50 different regulatory regimes governing the legal profession and the delivery of legal services in the United States, presenting a regulatory compliance challenge for lawyers given the increase in cross-border practice.

The state supreme courts adopt professional conduct codes and regulate many aspects of practice ranging from bar admission and defining the practice of law to establishing continuing legal education and professional discipline standards. The

---

4. 17 C.F.R. §205.3(d)(2). Sarbanes-Oxley also established minimum practice standards for lawyers appearing before the SEC. 15 U.S.C. §7245 (2006). Leubsdorf, *supra* note 1, at 1018.

5. Samantha Stokes, *'Revolutionary Changes' Coming to Legal Industry, Report Finds*, THE AMERICAN LAWYER, LAW. COM (Jan. 6, 2020), https://www.law.com/americanlawyer/2020/01/06/revolutionary-changes-coming-to-legal-industry-report-finds/ (reporting law firms need to adapt to the changing landscape of technology and the shift from traditional firms to alternative legal service providers (ALSPs)); *but see* Lyle Moran, *How the Washington Supreme Court's LLLT Program Met Its Demise*, A.B.A. J. (July 9, 2020), *available at* https://www.abajournal.com/web/article/how-washingtons-limited-license-legal-technician-program-met-its-demise (reporting the Washington Supreme Court decided to sunset its Limited Licensed Legal Technician (LLLT) Program, an ALSP effort begun by the court in 2012, because of limited public interest in the program and its cost to the bar).

6. The idiosyncratic nature of lawyer regulation in the United States is reflected, in part, in New York, where the state legislature has vested regulatory control of the bar with four appellate divisions of the state supreme courts instead of with its high court, the New York Court of Appeals. *See* ABA/BNA Law. Man. on Prof'l Conduct at 201:101-02 (1996) (citing N.Y. Jud. Law §90 (2013)) [hereinafter ABA/BNA Man.].

7. *See id.* at 201:102. *But see* N.Y. Jud. Law §90 (2013) (where legislature authorized regulatory authority).

8. In re Garcia, 315 P.3d 117, 124 (Cal. 2014) (acknowledging the legislature and the California Supreme Court possess authority to create rules regulating admission to the bar but that the court "bears the ultimate responsibility" to determine admission and regulate law practice under its inherent powers).

state ethics codes and related rules generally track in whole or in part ABA model codes and standards, such as the ABA Model Rules of Professional Conduct for lawyers and the **ABA Standards for Imposing Lawyer Sanctions**. These courts rely on a system of administrative offices, such as a professional conduct board or a **continuing legal education** (CLE) office, to handle the actual regulatory work. Annual lawyer registration fees, reinstatement fees, and other funds, such as cost reimbursements from disciplined lawyers and civil penalties, help fund this regulatory framework.

State bar associations often provide valuable assistance to state supreme courts concerning lawyer and judicial regulation, for example, by recommending changes to ethics or conduct standards, issuing advisory opinions interpreting ethics rules, establishing task forces to examine the role of lawyers, and staffing fee dispute and discipline panels. Such assistance occurs irrespective of whether the bar is an "**integrated**" or "unified" state bar association (where the high court requires bar membership to practice law) or a "**non-integrated**" or "non-unified" bar, where bar association membership is voluntary.[9]

In addition to adopting lawyer and judicial ethics codes, each state's high court promulgates related rules for the internal governance of the bar and courts, such as rules concerning admission, CLE, lawyer discipline, and certification as a specialist. For example, the Florida Supreme Court adopted two amendments to the Rules Regulating the Florida bar, making it the first state to require technology-related CLE courses for lawyers.[10]

2. Bar Associations and Lawyer Ethics (Conduct) Codes

Bar associations arose in the American colonial period as a result of lawyers' social gatherings and eating clubs, where lawyers shared professional concerns.[11] Although the significance of bar associations declined in the early nineteenth century, by the 1870s they spearheaded an effort to professionalize the legal community and enhance its reputation by increasing training and admission standards while highlighting the profession's goal of promoting the administration of justice and upholding the honor of the profession.[12] In 1870, the landmark founding of the City Bar of New York was soon followed by the creation of other local bar associations, and ultimately, the establishment of a national bar association in 1878,

---

9. CHARLES W. WOLFRAM, MODERN LEGAL ETHICS 37-39 (1986) (noting integrated bars existed in 33 states and the District of Columbia by the 1980s and that they do not violate the First Amendment's freedom of speech or association principles (discussing Lathrop v. Donohue, 367 U.S. 820 (1961)). The Supreme Court held in Keller v. State Bar of California, 496 U.S. 1 (1990), that the integrated bar's mandatory dues may support matters that benefit all members of the bar, for example, supporting the lawyer disciplinary process or CLE. However, bar dues may not be used to support unrelated political or ideological issues that do not benefit the general membership, such as lobbying for legislation to ban armor-piercing ammunition. *Id.* at 15.

10. ABA/BNA MAN., *supra* note 6, at 620-21. The Amendment to Rule 6-10.3 (Minimum Continuing Legal Education Standards) increased Florida's CLE requirement beginning in 2017 from 30 to 33 hours over a three-year period with the additional three hours being in technologically related CLE.

11. WOLFRAM, *supra* note 9, at 34.

12. Allison Marston, *Guiding the Profession: The 1887 Code of Ethics of the Alabama State Bar Association*, 49 ALA. L. REV. 471, 473-75 (1998).

the American Bar Association.[13] These bar associations promoted their members' economic and social status, in part, by controlling admission to the profession and assisting in the regulation of the practice of law.[14]

In 1887, the Alabama State Bar Association promulgated the first code of ethics for lawyers in the United States and it became the basis for the ABA's first ethics code in 1908, the Canons of Legal Ethics.[15] There were originally 32 canons that provided general guidance for lawyer behavior in hope of promoting public "confidence in the integrity and impartiality" of the administration of justice. For example, Canon 1, The Duty of the Lawyer to the Courts, provided, in part: "[i]t is the duty of the lawyer to maintain towards the Courts a respectful attitude, not for the sake of the temporary incumbent of the judicial office but for the maintenance of its supreme importance."[16] Other canons addressed different aspects of practice in general terms such as directing lawyers to avoid abusing a client's trust for personal gain and to be candid and fair when dealing with the courts and other lawyers.[17] Twenty-two states adopted the canons by 1910, and the ABA ultimately issued 47 canons.[18]

In 1969, the ABA issued a new ethics code, the **Model Code of Professional Responsibility**. It consisted of nine canons that addressed broad principles of lawyer behavior with each canon followed by multiple ethical considerations (ECs) or aspirational statements that discussed those principles in greater detail. ECs were followed by Disciplinary Rules (DRs) that identified minimum standards of lawyer behavior. To illustrate, Canon 6 stated, "A Lawyer Should Represent a Client Competently," and EC 6-5 added the aspirational statement "[a] lawyer should have pride in his professional endeavors." DR 6-101, titled "Failing to Act Competently," warned that "[a] lawyer shall not: . . . [n]eglect a legal matter entrusted to him." A lawyer was subject to professional discipline for violating a DR but not for violating a canon or an EC.

In the summer of 1977, the ABA appointed the **Commission on the Evaluation of Professional Standards**, commonly known as the Kutak Commission in honor of its chair, Robert J. Kutak. It was charged with "evaluating whether existing standards of professional conduct provided comprehensive and consistent guidance for resolving the increasingly complex ethical problems in the practice of law."[19] As a result of the Kutak Commission's work, the ABA created a new ethics code, the Model Rules of Professional Conduct, adopted on August 2, 1983.

---

13. Mary M. Devlin, *The Development of Lawyer Disciplinary Procedures in the United States*, 17 J. PROF. LAW. 364-66 (1994) (reporting that "Jacksonian democracy's anti-elitist ethos, combined with the elimination of formal training requirements made admission to the bar relatively easy" causing, in part, the creation of local bar associations by the 1870s to establish professional control).

14. WOLFRAM, *supra* note 9, at 34.

15. Marston, *supra* note 12, at 471.

16. ABA CANONS OF PROFESSIONAL ETHICS, CANON 1.

17. *Id.* CANONS 11 & 22, at 426 & 429.

18. M. LOUISE RUTHERFORD, THE INFLUENCE OF THE AMERICAN BAR ASSOCIATION ON PUBLIC OPINION AND LEGISLATION 89 (1937).

19. COMMISSION ON EVALUATION OF THE RULES OF PROFESSIONAL CONDUCT, CHAIR'S INTRO. ("ETHICS 2000"), ABA MODEL RULES OF PROFESSIONAL CONDUCT, ABA COMPENDIUM OF PROFESSIONAL RESPONSIBILITY RULES AND STANDARDS 11 (2015) [hereinafter ABA RULES COMPENDIUM].

The Model Rules adopted a new format, consisting of rules and comments. The Model Rules' Preamble explains that some rules are partly obligatory and disciplinary in nature, usually stated as imperatives — "a lawyer shall or must" act a certain way or be subject to discipline. Some rules, however, are more permissive, stating "a lawyer may or should" act a certain way, giving the lawyer some discretion over his conduct. Yet other rules simply describe the relationship between the lawyer and the client or others.

The comments provide explanations and illustrations for each rule, and help guide lawyers and regulators in interpreting the rules. Failure to comply with a comment does not subject the lawyer to potential discipline, whereas noncompliance with a rule does create the risk of discipline.

Review of the Model Rules is a continual process and is part of the charge of the ABA Standing Committee on Ethics and Professional Responsibility. As a result, the Model Rules have been amended periodically. In 1997, the ABA established an **Ethics 2000 Commission** to conduct the first comprehensive review of the Model Rules since its creation in 1983.[20] A primary impetus for Ethics 2000 involved the desire to better understand the reasons for the lack of uniformity among the states' ethics codes based on the ABA Model Rules. Although 42 states and Washington, D.C. had adopted versions of the ABA Model Rules, there was "an undesirable lack of uniformity" among the versions.[21] A few states, like Ohio, still followed the old 1969 Code of Professional Responsibility, and California retained a separate regulatory system. Another impetus that would resurface in future ABA ethics reviews concerned the impact of technological developments on the delivery of legal services. The ABA House of Delegates, its legislative body, adopted the Ethics 2000 Commission's Report in August 2002 after some earlier modifications. Some of the Ethics 2000 changes included strengthening the lawyer's duty to communicate with a client and clarifying the lawyer's obligations to the tribunal and justice system.[22]

After Ethics 2000, the ABA conducted two more studies to determine what, if any, possible changes were necessary to the Model Rules or the regulation of the profession in general given developments in the legal services market. In 2009, the ABA appointed the **Ethics 20/20 Commission** to examine the impact of globalization and technology on the legal profession. The 20/20 Commission ultimately submitted ten resolutions to the ABA House of Delegates in 2012 and 2013 and all were adopted, albeit with some changes.[23]

---

20. The ABA has traditionally created commissions to consider possible reforms to its ethics code. They include the Kutak Commission (1977), the **Multidisciplinary Practice Commission** (2000), and the **Multijurisdictional Practice Commission** (2002). These commissions have met with varying degrees of success. *See* James E. Moliterno, *Ethics 20/20 Protected, Preserved, and Maintained*, 47 Akron L. Rev. 151, 158-60 (2014) (arguing that various ABA commissions' reform proposals fail due to the ABA's self-interest in protecting and maintaining the status quo, or fending off outside challengers and cultural change).

21. ABA Rules Compendium, *supra* note 19, at 15.

22. *Id.* at 17.

23. The resolutions covered such topics as Technology and Confidentiality; Technology and Client Development; Outsourcing; Practice Pending Admission (easing the burden on lawyers moving to a new jurisdiction by permitting practice after applying for admission and awaiting final approval); Admission by Motion (reducing the recommended years in practice prerequisite for motion admission); and Model Rule 1.6, Detection of Conflicts of Interest (permitting some disclosure of client information when a lawyer changes firms to avoid a conflict of interest). Laurel S. Terry, *Globalization and the ABA Commission on Ethics 20/20: Reflections on Missed Opportunities and Roads Not Taken*, 45 Hofstra L. Rev. 95, 98-100 (2014).

Ethics 20/20 provided some new ethics duties and concepts for lawyers, for example, requiring lawyers to keep abreast of technological changes, mandating an affirmative duty to communicate with clients, and clarifying which jurisdiction's conflict of interest rules apply to lawyers who are engaged in cross-border practice.[24] Two of the final four resolutions addressed the ability of foreign lawyers to practice in the United States as in-house counsel; a third resolution added foreign lawyers to the ABA's Model Rules on **Pro Hac Vice Admission**, and the final one addressed the "predominant effects" test for resolving which jurisdiction's conflict of interests rules apply in the transnational context.[25]

In 2014, the ABA created the **Commission on the Future of the Legal Services** (Futures Commission) in hope of improving both the delivery of and access to legal services. The Futures Commission Report issued 12 recommendations, with many containing multiple subsections or comments. For example, Recommendation 2 urged courts to consider regulatory innovations to promote greater access to legal services, such as authorizing new service providers like Washington's Triple LTs (Limited Licensed Legal Technicians) and alternative business structures (ABS) that might allow non-lawyers to own entities delivering legal services. Recommendation 5 also encouraged courts to be accessible and user-friendly to all litigants by providing forms in plain English, multilingual written materials, and physical and virtual access to everyone. Recommendation 6 called for the establishment of an innovation center to develop new and creative ways to address critical needs in the legal sector.

While there have been many changes to the Model Rules, they continue to highlight the fundamental notion that "lawyers play a vital role in the preservation of society" because of their training and special privilege to deliver legal services.[26] They assist clients and others in resolving their problems and obtaining access to justice. Lawyers are also officers of the court and owe it special duties, for example, to avoid unnecessary delay and misrepresentations. In short, lawyers occupy a unique place in our society and government, functioning as gatekeepers in the administration of justice with a special responsibility to promote access to justice.

B. ADMISSION TO THE BAR

Like other professions, the legal profession has historically cited its members' specialized training and their obligation to follow a code of ethics that highlights their commitment to deliver high-quality service to the public as reasons to exercise strict control over entry into the profession and the delivery of legal services. However, some observers contend the profession's "behavioral norms and implementation of

---

24. Rule 1.1 cmt. [8]; Rule 1.4 cmt. [3]; Rule 8.5 cmt. [5].
25. Terry, *supra* note 23, at 98-99.
26. ABA RULES COMPENDIUM, *supra* note 19, at 21. The ABA's willingness to review and change the rules is poignantly illustrated in recent amendments to the marketing rules. ABA, MODEL RULES OF PROFESSIONAL CONDUCT 7.1-7.5 (2018), *available at* https://www.americanbar.org/groups/professional_responsibility/committees_commissions/ethicsandprofessionalresponsibility/mrpc_rule71_72_73_74_75/. *See* Chapter 10, *infra*, *Marketing Legal Services* (discussing the marketing rules amendments adopted on Aug. 6, 2018).

discipline are self-serving."[27] As you proceed in this chapter, you should consider whether the current regulatory regime effectively promotes the public interest in access to legal services and justice.

The United States Supreme Court has rejected some bar admission decisions and regulations as violative of the United States Constitution. For example, in Supreme Court of New Hampshire v. Piper, 470 U.S. 274 (1985), the Court held a New Hampshire court rule limiting bar admission to only state residents violated the **Privileges and Immunities Clause** of Article IV of the United States Constitution.[28] The New Hampshire Supreme Court defended its rule by arguing that nonresident lawyers will be less likely to become familiar with local rules and procedures, to behave ethically, to be available for court proceedings, and to do pro bono work. The Court found no evidence to support the belief that nonresident lawyers will not keep abreast of rules and procedures, behave ethically, and attempt to perform pro bono work. The Court acknowledged that a nonresident might find it more difficult to attend meetings on short notice but that this reason was insufficient to justify the exclusion of nonresidents. Also, the state could protect its interests with less restrictive means by requiring the distant, nonresident lawyer to retain a local lawyer to be available for unscheduled meetings.[29]

1. Educational Requirements

In most states, admission to the practice of law requires applicants to complete a special course of study at law school and then to pass a multiday bar examination. Seven states still permit students to take the bar examination after completing a period of apprenticeship instead of attending law school.[30] Wisconsin is the only "diploma privilege" state where graduates of Wisconsin law schools are admitted to the bar without taking Wisconsin's bar examination.[31] Graduates of ABA-accredited

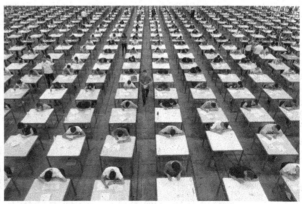

In most states, admission to the bar requires applicants to pass a multiday bar examination.
bibiphoto/Shutterstock.com

---

27. *See, e.g.*, Fred C. Zacharias, *The Myth of Self-Regulations*, 93 Minn. L. Rev. 1147, 1150-51 (1999).
28. *See also* Supreme Court of Virginia v. Friedman, 487 U.S. 59, 67 (1988) (declaring unconstitutional under the Privileges and Immunities Clause a rule requiring experienced lawyers waiving into Virginia to maintain a residence in the state).
29. 470 U.S. at 279-80.
30. Comprehensive Guide to Bar Admission Requirements 2019, Nat'l Conf. of Bar Exam. & ABA Sec. of Legal Ed. & Admission to the Bar 9-11 (identifying the seven "apprenticeship" states as California, Vermont, Virginia, Washington, Maine, New York, and West Virginia, the last three requiring a combination of apprenticeship and law school); *see Persons Taking and Passing the 2019 Bar Examination by Source of Legal Education*, The Bar Exam'r, https://thebarexaminer.org/2019-statistics/persons-taking-and-passing-the-2019-bar-examination-by-source-of-legal-education/ (last updated July 26, 2020) (reporting that only 38 of the 67,435 persons who took the bar examination in 2019 were "law office readers" or apprentices).
31. Wiesmueller v. Kosobucki, 571 F.3d 699 (7th Cir. 2009).

law schools are eligible to take the bar examination in any state. Graduates of non-ABA or state-only accredited law schools are limited to taking the bar examination in the state where the school is accredited. For example, California has a significant number of state-only accredited law schools and graduates of these schools are eligible to take only the California bar examination. The different treatment concerning bar examination eligibility may stem, in part, from the belief that ABA accreditation standards are sufficiently rigorous to promote any state's interest in protecting the public from unqualified persons practicing law.[32]

Many states permit "admission on motion." This approach permanently admits experienced lawyers in good standing in another state bar without requiring them to take a bar examination or only requiring a partial examination. States may limit admission on motion to those lawyers applying from states that offer a similar policy. To illustrate, state A waives its bar examination requirement and admits experienced lawyers from state B if state B reciprocates or similarly waives its bar examination requirement and admits experienced lawyers from state A. Courts have upheld these "reciprocity agreements."[33]

Section 2 of the Restatement (Third) of the Law Governing Lawyers (Restatement) notes that each federal district court, court of appeals, specialized federal court, and the Supreme Court have separate bars that require a separate admission and ongoing registration compliance to remain in good standing for each. It further notes admission to these bars is routine on application and may require lawyers to be admitted to a local bar. Section 2 reports some federal administrative agencies also have bars; admission to a state bar generally "suffices . . . to practice before almost all federal agencies."

2. Character and Fitness

The lawyer-client relationship is a fiduciary one with the lawyer acting as the agent for the benefit of the client-principal. Clients repose great trust in their lawyers to help them resolve their problems. The lawyer's knowledge and training give the professional significant power in the lawyer-client relationship and provides corrupt lawyers with the opportunity to harm clients and diminish public confidence in the justice system.

Given this potential for harm, bar admission applicants must typically demonstrate by clear and convincing evidence that they possess the requisite character, fitness, and moral qualifications to practice law. Some states only require the

---

32. ABA Accreditation Standard 301(a) provides that "[a] law school shall maintain a rigorous program of legal education that prepares its students, upon graduation, for admission to the bar and for effective, ethical, and responsible participation as members of the legal profession." A recent, controversial provision requires law schools to also publish "learning outcomes designed to achieve these objectives." Standard 301(b). ABA Section on Legal Education and Admissions, 2019-2020 STANDARDS AND RULES OF PROCEDURE FOR APPROVAL OF LAW SCHOOL, *available at* http://www.americanbar.org/groups/legal_education/resources/standards.html. These outcomes should reflect knowledge of the substantive law, and the acquisition of skills and ethical judgment necessary to competently represent clients. *Id.* at Standard 302.

33. National Ass'n for Advancement of Multijurisdictional Practice v. Berch, 973 F. Supp. 2d 1082 (Ariz. 2013); *aff'd sub nom.* 773 F.2d 1037 (9th Cir. 2014).

applicant to show the requisite **good character and fitness** by a preponderance of the evidence.

Section 2 of the Restatement provides guidance in construing the "good moral character and fitness" requirement: "[t]he central inquiry concerns the present ability and disposition of the applicant to practice competently and honestly." United States Supreme Court Justice Felix Frankfurter believed good moral character involves "qualities of truth-speaking, of a high sense of honor, of granite discretion, [and] of the strictest observance of fiduciary responsibility."[34] Fitness also encompasses the principle that the bar candidate be free of chemical addiction or emotional stability problems that would prevent the lawyer from competently implementing the client's objectives.

Although the good moral character and fitness standard is broad and open to many interpretations, bar applicants must fully answer all the questions on the bar application, which requires an extensive personal history.[35] Applicants will be notified of any concerns based on the application or any other source, perhaps something regarding the applicant's criminal history or a record that lacks honesty, trustworthiness, or reliability. Possible factors affecting an applicant's character and fitness assessment include a violation of the honor code at the applicant's undergraduate or law school; a pattern of disregard for the law; failure to provide complete and accurate information concerning the applicant's past; evidence of psychological disorder that if left untreated would affect the person's ability to practice law; evidence of an existing and untreated chemical dependency; false statements; and acts involving dishonesty, fraud, deceit, misrepresentation, or neglect.[36]

In hope of promoting the integrity of the profession through a careful and thorough bar admission process, ABA Model Rule 8.1(a) prohibits the applicant, or a lawyer recommending the applicant, from knowingly making a false statement of a material fact in connection with a bar admission application. When the lawyer has knowledge of a falsehood and what constitutes a material fact is sometimes unclear, presenting difficult and debatable questions of fact.

Rule 8.1(b) imposes the affirmative duty on the applicant or a lawyer recommending the applicant to disclose facts necessary to correct any misapprehensions about the applicant to help provide admission authorities with a more complete picture of the applicant.[37] Rule 8.1(b) also directs applicants and lawyers to cooperate with a demand for information from admissions or disciplinary authorities, unless the information is protected by Rule 1.6. For example, if a lawyer represents the bar applicant in a matter separate from her application and learns unflattering information about the applicant, the lawyer would not have to volunteer that information to bar admission authorities under Rule 1.6.

---

34. Schware v. Board of Bar Examiners, 353 U.S. 232, 247 (1957).
35. *See* Konigsberg v. California, 366 U.S. 36 (1960) (upholding the denial of admission when the applicant failed to answer questions during a character investigation concerning his membership in the Communist party because it interfered with the character investigation).
36. Ohio Gov. Bar Rule I, §11(D)(3)(a)-(o).
37. *See* Mississippi Bar v. Johnson, No. 2017-BA-00955-SCT, 2019 Miss. LEXIS 188, at *9 (May 9, 2019) (suspending for three years a paralegal who had forged a judicial order while awaiting her successful bar examination results because she failed to supplement her bar application regarding the forgery as required under Rule 8.1(b) "to correct a misapprehension" about her character and fitness).

A local bar committee, commonly called the character and fitness or admissions committee, often meets with the applicant to further investigate any concerns that are flagged on the application. In some states, these committees will interview each candidate for the bar, irrespective of any red flags, to obtain additional information about a candidate's character.[38] If there is an adverse determination after the character and fitness committee's review, then the applicant generally may appeal to another administrative level of review and ultimately to the state's high court, which makes the final decision. Applicants must fully cooperate during the investigation and the entire process; the failure to cooperate can trigger adverse consequences. The United States Supreme Court held in Schware v. Board of Bar Examiners, 353 U.S. 232, 239 (1957), that states can require "high standards of qualifications, such as good moral character or proficiency in the law" for bar admission but such "qualifications must have a rational connection with the applicant's fitness or capacity to practice law." In *Schware*, the Court concluded the applicant's prior membership in the Communist party, several arrests without convictions that occurred many years ago, and his use of aliases to avoid anti-Semitism and to obtain work and be an effective labor activist did not show a lack of the requisite good character and fitness for bar admission. As a practical matter, relatively few applicants are denied admission for lack of good character and fitness, but a more substantial "number [are] deterred, delayed or harassed" in gaining admission.[39]

For example, in In re McKinney, 134 Ohio St. 3d 260 (2012), McKinney first wrote on the bar application that she left a former job because it conflicted with her school schedule. McKinney also wrote on the application that she was fired from the job for using the firm's email for personal reasons. In fact, she was fired for violating firm policy by using its email for personal reasons *and* creating fictitious letters on firm letterhead indicating McKinney was being transferred to another location for work. The work transfer scheme allowed McKinney to terminate her apartment lease without liability. McKinney also changed the voicemail on her sister's telephone to help the sister impersonate a fictitious human resource person at the firm in case the landlord called to verify McKinney's transfer.

Before conducting McKinney's character and fitness interview, the local admissions committee contacted the employer and learned of McKinney's scheme to defraud the landlord. The interviewers gave her open-ended questions to allow her to fully disclose the circumstances of her termination. Instead, she gave evasive answers, causing the committee to recommend disapproval of her application. McKinney appealed to a three-person panel of the Board of Commissioners on Character and Fitness, which noted her various volunteer work, including assistance at a domestic violence and sexual assault center and for a law student society. She also had five character reference letters, three of them from professors and one from a current lawyer-employer who testified he believed her to be honest and would retain her after bar admission. The panel also recommended disapproval of

---

38. *Id.* §11(C)(2) (also requiring the report of the National Conference of Bar Examiners that conducts a separate examination of the candidate's bar questionnaire).

39. ABA/BNA Man., *supra* note 6, at 21:705 (Aug. 31, 2010) (citing Deborah Rhode, *Moral Character as Professional Credential*, 94 Yale L.J. 491, 493-94 (1985)).

her application with an opportunity to reapply for the July 2014 bar exam. The full board adopted the panel's findings but decided McKinney could never establish her character and fitness to practice law, noting she was a 30-year-old law student at the time of her deceptive scheme and was evasive throughout the entire process.

The Ohio Supreme Court agreed McKinney had continued her deceitful scheme from her first year of law school through the admissions process and thus failed to show by clear and convincing evidence the requisite character and fitness to practice law. The court also noted that McKinney had applied herself in law school, had good references, including a lawyer who planned to hire her after the bar exam, and she appeared genuinely remorseful. The court rejected the full board's permanent ban on McKinney taking the exam, ruling McKinney could rehabilitate her character and reapply for the July 2014 bar examination subject to a full character and fitness investigation.

Other Character Examples — Immigration Status, Bigotry, Financial Neglect

As reflected in *McKinney*, an applicant's deceitful conduct generally prompts serious concerns about the applicant's character and fitness to practice law. In addition to the blatant deceit in *McKinney*, there are other forms of conduct that pose difficult questions for bar regulators in assessing an applicant's character. For example, what role, if any, do you think an applicant's immigration status should play in assessing whether the applicant has the requisite good character and fitness for bar admission?

In 2014, the California Supreme Court admitted an undocumented immigrant, Sergio C. Garcia, to the California bar following a newly enacted California law that authorized the court to admit "an applicant [to the bar] who is not lawfully present in the United States [but who] has fulfilled the requirements for admission to practice law."[40] The California Supreme Court held the new law complied with an exception in the federal law that prohibited states from granting professional licenses to undocumented immigrants, thus avoiding any conflict with federal law that would create a preemption issue under the Supremacy Clause. The state high court emphasized that although the Committee of Bar Examiners makes the initial determination on a case-by-case basis about whether the applicant has demonstrated the requisite good character, the California Supreme Court makes the final decision. It noted that "'[g]ood moral character' has been traditionally defined as the absence of conduct imbued with elements of 'moral turpitude.' It includes 'qualities of honesty, fairness, candor, and trustworthiness, observance of fiduciary responsibility, respect for and obedience to the laws of the state and the nation and respect for the rights of others and for the judicial process." The California Supreme Court decided an undocumented immigrant's unlawful presence in the United States does not itself demonstrate unfitness to be admitted to the bar. Reviewing Garcia's entire background, including "one or two problematical incidents" and the numerous strong references attesting to his good character, the court held Garcia

---

40. In re Garcia, 315 P.3d 117, 124 (Cal. 2014).

had demonstrated that "he possesses the requisite good character to qualify for a law license."

Sergio Garcia, the first undocumented lawyer to be granted a law license, began practicing law in California in 2014, after his successful legal battle to obtain his law license. After his acceptance into the California bar in June of 2015, Garcia received a green card, allowing him to live and work on a permanent basis in the United States. *Immigrant California Lawyer Finally Gets Green Card*, THE SAN MATEO DAILY J. (CAL.), June 5, 2015.

In another controversial case, Hale v. Committee on Character and Fitness to Practice for the State of Illinois, 335 F.3d 678 (7th Cir. 2003), the appeals court affirmed a dismissal of the applicant's §1983 claim that the state's Committee on Character and Fitness (Committee) had violated his First Amendment rights. Hale was denied admission to the Illinois bar because the committee found him unfit to practice law. Hale's life mission was to further the hegemony of the white race, to abolish equal protection, and to deport non-white Americans by nonviolent means. The committee believed that Hale was likely to engage in conduct inconsistent with bar membership and stated: "Hale's active commitment to bigotry . . . demonstrated a 'gross deficiency in moral character, particularly for lawyers who have a special responsibility to uphold the rule of law for all persons.'" A hearing panel affirmed this determination, and the Illinois Supreme Court refused to hear the appeal.

An applicant's financial situation is also a relevant factor in the character and fitness review. For example, in In re Anonymous, 889 N.Y.S.2d 713 (N.Y. App. Div. 2009), the applicant had passed the 2008 bar examination but was denied admission after reporting $430,000 in delinquent student loans covering a 20-year period without making any substantial payments. The applicant said the economic downturn and bad faith negotiations by some of the lenders caused the nonpayment. The court concluded: "His application demonstrates a course of action amounting to neglect of financial responsibilities" — the loans with interest now totaling $480,000. "His recalcitrance in dealing with lenders [was] incompatible with a lawyer's duties and responsibilities. . . ."

Case Preview

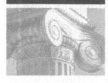

In re Glass

The *Glass* case was decided the same year as *In re Garcia*, discussed above. But in *Glass*, the California Supreme Court reached a result adverse to the applicant, denying Mr. Glass bar admission after he had passed the 2004 bar examination. The court did not believe Mr. Glass was sincere in contending he had rehabilitated his dishonest character.

In reading this case, consider the following:

1. As noted in *Glass*, applicants generally get the "benefit of the doubt" where there are "conflicting equally reasonable inferences" about one's fitness for the bar. Why did the court reject that approach here?

2. What facts led the court to conclude Glass's conduct was "reprehensible"?
3. What was the court's response to the witnesses who supported Glass's bar admission because they believed in his personal redemption?
4. Does the court suggest that its denial of Glass's admission was simply a case of an applicant seeking bar admission too soon after a serious infraction?

In re Glass
316 P.3d 1199 (Cal. 2014)

THE COURT:

Stephen Randall Glass made himself infamous as a dishonest journalist by fabricating material for more than 40 articles for The New Republic magazine and other publications. He also carefully fabricated supporting materials to delude The New Republic's fact checkers. The articles appeared between June 1996 and May 1998, and included falsehoods that reflected negatively on individuals, political groups, and ethnic minorities. During the same period, starting in September 1997, he was also an evening law student at Georgetown University's law school. Glass made every effort to avoid detection once suspicions were aroused, lobbied strenuously to keep his job at The New Republic, and, in the aftermath of his exposure, did not fully cooperate with the publications to identify his fabrications.

Glass applied to become a member of the New York bar in 2002, but withdrew his application after he was informally notified in 2004 that his moral character application would be rejected. In the New York bar application materials, he exaggerated his cooperation with the journals that had published his work and failed to supply a complete list of the fabricated articles that had injured others.

Glass passed the California Bar examination in 2006 and filed an application for determination of moral character in 2007. It was not until the California State Bar moral character proceedings that Glass reviewed all of his articles, as well as the editorials The New Republic and other journals published to identify his fabrications, and ultimately identified fabrications that he previously had denied or failed to disclose. In the California proceedings, Glass was not forthright in acknowledging the defects in his New York bar application.

I. FACTS

A. *Committee of Bar Examiners' Evidence*

In September 1995 Glass accepted a position at The New Republic magazine. In early June 1996 he began fabricating material for publication. The fabrications continued and became bolder and more comprehensive until he was exposed and fired in May 1998.

Glass testified at the State Bar Court hearing that he "wrote nasty, mean-spirited, horrible" things about people: "My articles hurt, and they were cruel. . . ." He testified that the fabrications gave him "A-plus" stories that afforded him status in staff meetings and also gave particular enjoyment to his colleagues. He said: "Overwhelmingly, what everyone remembers about my pieces are the fake things."

. . .

In [an] article, entitled *Deliverance*, published in November 1996, Glass recounted receiving unsatisfactory service from a named computer company, and claimed that his complaints to a telephone customer service representative were met with an anti-Semitic slur. In truth, no such slur ever was uttered. Glass also wrote a letter to the president of the company, repeating the accusation, and sent a copy to the Anti-Defamation League.

Glass also engaged in fabrications in freelance articles published by other magazines. [For example], Glass wrote an article entitled *The Vernon Question* for George magazine. The lengthy article, published in April 1998, concerned Vernon Jordan, an advisor to then President Clinton during the then emerging Monica Lewinsky scandal. In two paragraphs, Glass used nonexistent sources to describe Jordan's supposed reputation as a "boor" and attributed various fictitious statements to "political operatives," "socialites," "political hostesses" and officials. These persons assertedly stated that Jordan was well known for sexually explicit comments, unwanted sexual advances, and crude stares, and added that he was known in their circles as "Vern the Worm" or "Pussyman," and that young women needed protection against him. Another paragraph attributed to a fictional "watchdog" group contained certain claims about Jordan's asserted conflicts of interest and questionable corporate ethics. . . . These were all fabrications.

Charles Lane, who was the editor of The New Republic at the time of Glass's exposure, testified for the Committee of Bar Examiners (hereafter sometimes Committee) that he had received an early complaint about Glass concerning an article entitled *Boys on the Bus*, depicting the actor Alec Baldwin and his brother as silly celebrities whose efforts during a bus tour to campaign on the issue of campaign finance reform were based on ignorance. A representative of Baldwin's disputed the assertion in the article that the actor had been giving out autographs during the bus tour, but Glass repudiated the accusation in print in The New Republic.

Although at the time, the *Boys on the Bus* incident seemingly was resolved in Glass's favor, Lane's suspicions were aroused in May 1998 when a journalist employed by Forbes Digital Tool telephoned to warn him that factual assertions in Glass's recent article for George magazine, *Hack Heaven*, did not seem to be true. The article had described a teenager hacking a California software company and extorting money to stop the intrusion. The article described a convention in Bethesda, Maryland, where some of the events occurred, and when Lane challenged Glass, the latter journeyed with Lane to Bethesda, purporting to identify the building where the convention had been held. A person working in the building denied such a convention had occurred, and Lane became persuaded that Glass was lying. Lane pressed Glass about the factual basis for the article, and although Glass was evasive, he insisted the article was accurate. Glass spent the night at home fabricating what he would assert were his reporter's notes from interviews, fake business cards, a voicemail box, a Web site, and newsletters. He also induced his brother to impersonate a source.

[At one point while in the home office in Bethesda, Lane] . . . confronted Glass with evidence that Glass had used his brother as a false source in the *Hack Heaven* piece. Ultimately, during this exchange Glass admitted the article was fabricated, and Lane fired him.

Lane reviewed all of Glass's articles over the course of the following three or four weeks. He received a letter from Glass apologizing and saying he had instructed his lawyers to cooperate with The New Republic. Lane compiled a summary of the material in Glass's articles that he found suspicious and submitted the summary to Glass's counsel, who it was agreed would stipulate to those findings of Lane's that Glass believed to be correct. At the time, Lane concluded that 27 of the 42 articles Glass had written for the magazine contained fabrications, and Lane wrote two editorial articles informing the magazine's readership to this effect.

. . .

Glass graduated from law school in 2000, when he also took and passed the New York bar examination. He applied to become a member of the New York bar in 2002. After an evidentiary hearing before a subcommittee of a committee on character and fitness, and pursuant to apparent custom, in September 2004, a representative of that committee informed Glass informally that his application would be rejected, so he withdrew it. The record does not disclose the reason for the tentative decision.

In his application to the New York bar, Glass described his misconduct and firing. His application and supporting materials included only 20 articles containing fabrications. Glass wrote that he had apologized to the editor of The New Republic, saying, "I also worked with all three magazines [(referring to The New Republic, Harper's, and George magazines)] and other publications where I had written freelance articles to identify which facts were true and which were false in all of my stories, so they could publish clarifications for their readers."

At the hearing, Lane challenged the quoted statement as untrue. Lane believed that Glass had failed to come forward to actively assist The New Republic in identifying his fabrications, and instead had placed the entire burden of identifying his errors on Lane.

B. *Applicant's Evidence*

Once he was fired from The New Republic, Glass was distraught, suicidal, and unable to focus, almost immediately entering therapy. He nonetheless hired counsel whom he directed to "work with The New Republic." Glass testified that he believed that The New Republic wanted to conduct its own investigation because it did not trust him and testified that "I came to understand that they were going to provide me with a list of [fabricated] articles, and that I was to affirm whether or not the article was fabricated that they showed me or that they listed." He had fabricated more than The New Republic had discovered in its investigation, although he testified that due to his distress he did not realize this when he reviewed the list. . . . Glass testified that he had "no information" indicating that his lawyers had failed to convey information to The New Republic.

Members of Georgetown University's law school faculty testified on his behalf at the hearing, finding him to be bright, honest, trustworthy, and having learned from his wrongdoing. In addition, California attorney Paul Zuckerman testified that he decided to give Glass a chance as a law clerk. After initially assigning Glass minor projects and exercising close oversight, Zuckerman became convinced that Glass was one of the best employees in the firm, with a fine intellect, a good work ethic, and reliable commitment to honesty.

Also offered in support of Glass's application were affidavits that had been submitted in support of his New York bar application from the judges for whom Glass had worked during and immediately after completing law school. Both found him highly competent and honest at that time. Additional declarations from attorneys and friends that had been submitted with the New York bar application were offered in support.

. . .

II. DISCUSSION

A. Applicable Law

. . . "Persons of good character . . . do not commit acts or crimes involving moral turpitude — a concept that embraces a wide range of deceitful and depraved behavior." A lawyer's good moral character is essential for the protection of clients and for the proper functioning of the judicial system itself.

When the applicant has presented evidence that is sufficient to establish a prima facie case of his or her good moral character, the burden shifts to the State Bar to rebut that case with evidence of poor moral character. Once the State Bar has presented evidence of moral turpitude, the burden "falls squarely upon the applicant to demonstrate his [or her] rehabilitation."

Of particular significance for the present case is the principle that "the more serious the misconduct and the bad character evidence, the stronger the applicant's showing of rehabilitation must be." "Cases authorizing admission on the basis of rehabilitation commonly involve a substantial period of *exemplary* conduct following the applicant's misdeeds." (*Ibid.*, italics added.) Moreover, "truly exemplary" conduct ordinarily includes service to the community.

. . .

B. Analysis

Although an applicant ordinarily receives the benefit of the doubt as to "conflicting equally reasonable inferences" concerning moral fitness the State Bar Court majority failed to recognize that this rule does not materially assist applicants who have engaged in serious misconduct. This is because "[w]here serious or criminal misconduct is involved, positive inferences about the applicant's moral character are more difficult to draw, and negative character inferences are stronger and *more reasonable.*" When there have been very serious acts of moral turpitude, we must be convinced that the applicant "is no longer the same person who behaved so poorly in the past," and will find moral fitness "only if he [or she] has since behaved in exemplary fashion over a meaningful period of time."

. . .

Glass's conduct as a journalist exhibited moral turpitude sustained over an extended period. As the Review Department dissent emphasized, he engaged in "fraud of staggering proportions" and he "use[d] . . . his exceptional writing skills to publicly and falsely malign people and organizations for actions they did not do and faults they did not have." As the dissent further commented, for two years he "engaged in a multi-layered, complex, and harmful course of public dishonesty." Glass's journalistic dishonesty was not a single lapse of judgment, which we have sometimes excused, but involved significant deceit sustained unremittingly for a period of years. Glass's deceit also was motivated by professional ambition, betrayed a vicious, mean spirit and a complete lack of compassion for others, along with arrogance and prejudice against various ethnic groups. In all these respects, his misconduct bore directly on his character in matters that are critical to the practice of law.

Glass not only spent two years producing damaging articles containing or entirely made up of fabrications, thereby deluding the public, maligning individuals, and disparaging ethnic minorities, he also routinely expended considerable efforts to fabricate background materials to dupe the fact checkers assigned to vet his work. When exposure threatened, he redoubled his efforts to hide his misconduct, going so far as to create a phony Web site and business cards and to recruit his brother to pose as a source. In addition, to retain his position, he engaged in a spirited campaign among the leadership at The New Republic to characterize Lane's obviously well-founded concerns as unfair and to retain his position.

Glass's conduct during this two-year period violated ethical strictures governing his profession [of journalism]. [T]he Code of Ethics of the Society of Professional Journalists provides that "[t]he duty of the journalist is to further those ends by seeking truth and providing a fair and comprehensive account of events and issues. . . ." Glass's behavior fell so far short of this standard. . . .

Glass's misconduct was also reprehensible because it took place while he was pursuing a law degree and license to practice law, when the importance of honesty should have gained new meaning and significance for him.

. . .

The record also discloses instances of dishonesty and disingenuousness occurring after Glass's exposure, up to and including the State Bar evidentiary hearing in 2010. In the New York bar proceedings that ended in 2004, as even the State Bar Court majority acknowledged, he made misrepresentations concerning his cooperation with The New Republic and other publications and efforts to aid them identify all of his fabrications. He also submitted an incomplete list of articles that injured others. We have previously said about omissions on bar applications: "Whether it is caused by intentional concealment, reckless disregard for the truth, or an *unreasonable refusal to perceive the need for disclosure*, such an omission is itself strong evidence that the applicant lacks the 'integrity' and/or 'intellectual discernment' required to be an attorney."

Our review of the record indicates hypocrisy and evasiveness in Glass's testimony at the California State Bar hearing, as well. We find it particularly disturbing that at the hearing Glass persisted in claiming that he had made a good faith effort to work with the magazines that published his works. He went through many verbal twists and turns at the hearing to avoid acknowledging the obvious fact that in his

New York bar application he exaggerated his level of assistance to the magazines that had published his fabrications, and that he omitted from his New York bar list of fabrications some that actually could have injured real persons. . . . He has "not acted with the 'high degree of *frankness* and truthfulness' and the 'high standard of integrity' required by this process."

. . .

We also observe that instead of directing his efforts at serving others in the community, much of Glass's energy since the end of his journalistic career seems to have been directed at advancing his own career and financial and emotional well-being.

. . .

The Review Department majority relied heavily on the testimony of Glass's character witnesses, but the testimony of character witnesses will not suffice by itself to establish rehabilitation. Moreover, stressing that Glass's reputation as a journalist had been exploded and that so many years had passed, some of the character witnesses did not sufficiently focus on the seriousness of the misconduct, incorrectly viewing it as of little current significance despite its lingering impact on its victims and on public perceptions concerning issues of race and politics. They also did not take into account, as we do, that the misconduct reflected poorly on the particular commitment to honesty that Glass might have been expected to have had as a law student. For these reasons we believe the Review Department majority accorded too much probative value to the testimony of Glass's character witnesses.

Glass emphasized the remorse he expressed through his letters to victims, and characterized his novel and his appearance on *60 Minutes* as efforts to make amends. Remorse does not establish rehabilitation, however, and in any event, the weight of this evidence is diminished because the letters were not written near the time of his misconduct and exposure, when they might have been most meaningful to the victims, but rather seemed timed to coincide with his effort to become a member of the New York bar. The novel served Glass's own purposes, producing notoriety and a fee of $175,000, and the appearance on *60 Minutes* was timed to coincide with the release of the novel. . . .

The record of Glass's therapy does not represent "truly exemplary conduct in the sense of returning something to the community." To be sure, through therapy he seems to have gained a deep understanding of the psychological sources of his misconduct, as well as tools to help him avoid succumbing to the same pressures again. His treating psychiatrists are plainly highly competent and well regarded in their field, and they are convinced that he has no remaining psychological flaws tending to cause him to act dishonestly. Glass believed that he could best make amends by changing himself. But his 12 years of therapy primarily conferred a personal benefit on Glass himself. . . .

Glass points to the pro bono legal work he does for clients of his firm as evidence of sustained efforts on behalf of the community, but we observe that pro bono work is not truly *exemplary* for attorneys, but rather is expected of them.

Glass and the witnesses who supported his application stress his talent in the law and his commitment to the profession, and they argue that he has already paid a high enough price for his misdeeds to warrant admission to the bar. They emphasize his personal redemption, but we must recall that what is at stake is not compassion for Glass, who wishes to advance from being a supervised law clerk to enjoying a license to engage in the practice of law on an independent basis. Given our duty to protect the public and maintain the integrity and high standards of the profession, our focus is on the applicant's moral fitness to practice law. On this record, the applicant failed to carry his heavy burden of establishing his rehabilitation and current fitness.

III. CONCLUSION

For the foregoing reasons, we reject the State Bar Court majority's recommendation and decline to admit Glass to the practice of law.

Post-Case Follow-Up

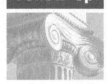

The *Glass* decision produced significant discussion about the bar admission process. Some critics believed that Glass had sufficiently demonstrated present fitness and good character to warrant admission to the bar or that the character review process is, at best, questionable when it comes to predicting how someone will act once admitted.[41] This may be related to the burden of proof. Should the courts apply a different standard of review for candidates seeking *admission* from those seeking *readmission*? For example, should first-time bar applicants be required to offer only "substantial," instead of "clear and convincing," evidence of their good character and fitness since they have not violated the profession's conduct code? What additional evidence could Glass have offered to meet his burden of showing by clear and convincing evidence that he possessed the requisite good character for admission?

Although the concept of rehabilitation is often discussed in the context of discipline and lawyers seeking readmission, *Glass* highlights the important role it plays in the admission process itself. The seriousness of some offenses appears to require a longer probationary period than others to reassure the courts that an applicant is truly rehabilitated and deserving of a license to practice law. Should there be some instances of misconduct, for example, the applicant murdering his wife and children,

In re Glass: After the Decision

In 2003, Stephen Glass wrote a self-serving novel entitled *The Fabulist* (Simon & Schuster 2003). This novel, an explanation piece, shows Glass's process through his turmoil and tribulations following the 1998 revelation of his scandalous behavior at *The New Republic* and how this led to his being denied bar admission in New York and California. Glass's story received even more attention when a made-for-TV movie, *Shattered Glass*, was released on the USA Network (Lions Gate Films, Inc. 2003). This movie portrayed Glass's rise to fame and dramatic fall. Shortly after Glass's last failed attempt to gain admission to the California bar, Hanna Rosin, a former colleague, conducted an interview with Glass in late 2013. Hanna Rosin, *Hello, My Name Is Stephen Glass, and I'm Sorry*, New Republic, Mar. 29, 2017, https://newrepublic.com/article/120145/stephen-glass-new-republic-scandal-still-haunts-his-law-career. During this interview,

---

41. *See* W. Bradley Wendel, *Stephen Glass, Situational Forces, and the Fundamental Attribution Error*, 4 J.L.: Periodical Laboratory of Legal Scholarship 99, 104-05 (2014) (raising questions about the basis for the decision).

Glass reflected on a variety of events in his life, including the challenges of obtaining a position as a paralegal. As of February 2017, Glass worked as the director of special projects at two firms, where he prepares the firms' clients for trial and helps them "discover their stories." Grant Rodgers, *Infamous Journalist Glass Works for Iowa Law Firm; Career Undone After Fabrications Found*, DES MOINES REGISTER, Feb. 6, 2017.

committing a series of rapes, failing to file income tax forms for seven years, or being a scofflaw driver (e.g., not paying 12 university parking tickets over a three-year period in law school), that should permanently disqualify one from admission to practice law?

In re Glass: Real Life Applications

1. Harold is 45 years old. In his mid-20s, he became involved in smuggling marijuana. Harold was indicted for his involvement and fled the country to escape prosecution. On return, Harold took responsibility for his actions and pleaded guilty to all charges. As part of his probation, Harold provided care for terminally ill AIDS patients. Harold attended the University of Maine law school, where he served on the law review and graduated summa cum laude. After graduation, he clerked for the Maine Supreme Court and recently applied for admission to the New Hampshire bar.

   As a member of the character and fitness committee, you have been asked to review Harold's application, which contains the information set out above. Do you feel comfortable recommending Harold as having the requisite character and fitness for bar admission? What additional questions might you ask Harold?

2. Petitioner M.C. filed an application for admission to the Florida bar. The Board of Bar Examiners investigated M.C. because of inconsistencies in his application and determined M.C. did not disclose on his application several financial debts and delinquent payments regarding outstanding student loans totaling $80,000. The board also found that M.C. owed roughly $17,000 in child support and that M.C. failed to file state and federal income tax returns for five years. During a board interview, M.C. expressed deep remorse for his past financial "issues" and promised to follow Florida's lawyer conduct rules. M.C. also submitted five letters in support of his good character, including two from college professors, two from employers, and one from a prominent local church pastor.

   Should the board recommend a denial of M.C.'s application for bar admission? Should the board recommend a permanent ban on his admission? Would you change your decision to deny M.C.'s application if he had satisfied all of his outstanding debts two months prior to taking the bar examination?

C. LAWYER DISCIPLINE

1. Misconduct Defined

Each state has a lawyer disciplinary system to protect clients, the public, the legal system, and the profession from lawyer misconduct. Given these important goals, there is no statute of limitations in most jurisdictions for filing lawyer discipline actions. As you continue reading this section, and at the risk of oversimplification, the following brief admonition might prove useful in avoiding the lawyer discipline system: "don't lie, steal, or cheat."

Under Rule 8.4 ("Misconduct"), lawyers commit professional misconduct and are subject to discipline when they violate or attempt to violate any Model Rule of Professional Conduct or knowingly induce or assist others to do so. The specific disciplinary rules that can result in sanctions are discussed in Chapters 3 through 10. But Rule 8.4 also contains several important "catchall" provisions that can result in lawyer discipline. Rule 8.4 defines misconduct to include criminal acts that adversely reflect on the lawyer's honesty, trustworthiness, or fitness to practice law, for example, income tax fraud, perjury, or money laundering. Misconduct also includes dishonesty, fraud, deceit, misrepresentation, or any conduct that is prejudicial to the administration of justice. For example, it is dishonest and unethical conduct for a lawyer to use web bugs to track email communications with opposing counsel to learn how much time they devoted to reviewing the bugged email and whether and to whom it was forwarded.[42] Finally, Rule 8.4 specifically prohibits lawyers from suggesting they are able to improperly influence a government agency or official and knowingly assisting a judge or judicial officer in violating judicial conduct rules.

In August 2016, the ABA added subsection (g) to Rule 8.4's list of misconduct. Under it, a lawyer shall not

> engage in conduct that the lawyer knows or reasonably should know is harassment or discrimination on the basis of race, sex, religion, national origin, ethnicity, disability, age, sexual orientation, gender identity, marital status or socioeconomic status in conduct related to the practice of law. This paragraph does not limit the ability of a lawyer to accept, decline or withdraw from a representation in accordance with Rule 1.16. This paragraph does not preclude legitimate advice or advocacy consistent with these Rules.

Rule 8.4(g) generated concern that its broad ban on conduct might deter constitutionally protected speech.[43] For example, the Texas Attorney General advised the state legislature that the adoption of Rule 8.4(g) "is unnecessary to protect against prohibited discrimination...and were it to be adopted, a court would likely invalidate it as unconstitutional" because it infringes on First Amendment free speech rights.[44] Other commentators believed that the ABA's new **antidiscrimination provision** in Rule 8.4(g) did not necessarily infringe on the First Amendment.[45]

---

42. ABA/BNA Man. *supra* note 6, at 638-39 (2016) (citing Alaska Bar Ass'n Ethics Comm. Op. 2016-1 as the second ethics opinion to ban web bugs for providing unfair advantage to the sender and stating that "[s]eeking to invade [the attorney-client relationship] through the use of tracking devices (whether disclosed or not) is dishonest and unethical").

43. Professor Margaret Tarkington wrote that Rule 8.4(g) poses a threat to a lawyer's First Amendment rights because it is exceedingly broad, prohibiting any verbal or physical conduct in any type of scenario that involves the practice of law, including social activities. She suggested modifying the rule so that it applies to "severe or pervasive" harassment or discrimination, as opposed to any type of harassment or discrimination. MARGARET TARKINGTON, VOICE OF JUSTICE: RECLAIMING THE FIRST AMENDMENT RIGHTS OF LAWYERS 244-78 (2018).

44. Texas Att'y Gen. Op. KP-0123 (2016), *available at* https://www.texasattorneygeneral.gov/sites/default/files/opinion-files/opinion/2016/kp0123.pdf. *See* TARKINGTON, *supra* note 43, at 244-45 (reporting that "Attorney Generals of Texas, South Carolina, Louisiana, and Tennessee have all written opinions that Rule 8.4(g) is unconstitutional, as violating attorneys' rights to freedom of speech, association and religion").

45. *See* Claudia E. Haupt, *Antidiscrimination in the Legal Profession and the First Amendment: A Partial Defense of Model Rule 8.4(g)*, 19 U. PA. J. CONST. L. ONLINE 1 (2017). *See generally* Veronica Root Martinez, *Combatting*

In 2020, the ABA Standing Committee on Ethics and Professional Responsibility addressed some of the concerns about Rule 8.4(g) in Formal Opinion 493. The committee stated that Rule 8.4(g) "does not prevent lawyers from freely expressing their opinions and ideas on matters of public concern, nor . . . limit . . . a lawyer's speech or conduct in settings unrelated to the practice of law." A "standard of objective reasonableness" would be used to assess whether a lawyer's conduct violates the rule, and then only "harmful [conduct] will be grounds for discipline." The committee further noted that violations of 8.4(g) will usually involve intentional conduct that is targeted at specific individuals or groups. The committee concluded that Rule 8.4(g) is constitutional and that its enforcement would play a critical role in "maintaining public confidence in the impartiality of the legal system and . . . trust in the legal profession. . . ."[46]

Rule 8.4's catchall provisions are broad and capture a wide variety of miscreant activity. The following subsections provide some common categories of misconduct that may result in discipline under Rule 8.4, with some representative cases.

Drug and Alcohol Abuse

Substance abuse affects a significant percentage of law students and lawyers and is reported to be higher than in other populations. Not surprisingly, substance abuse is a root cause for a significant amount of lawyer discipline. In Lawyer Disciplinary Board v. Sidiropolis, 828 S.E.2d 839 (W. Va. 2019), a lawyer suffered severe back pain because of an automobile accident and was prescribed vicodin and oxycodone. The lawyer, Sidiropolis, eventually became addicted to the drugs. After five to six years of drug use, he sought treatment for his addiction at a clinic, where he was given a drug called Suboxone. He continued to use the drug after he left treatment, buying it illegally along with heroin and other drugs, all to manage his pain. During this time, he began to wind down his practice, obtaining co-counsel for some of his cases as he readied to undergo more addiction treatment. Sidiropolis continued his drug use and was eventually pulled over with ten bricks of heroin in his car; he was arrested for driving under the influence and conspiracy to distribute heroin.

Sidiropolis self-reported that he was charged with one count to distribute heroin to the Office of Disciplinary Counsel (ODC). He also informed the ODC that he cooperated with federal and state drug task forces, participated in a twelve-step addiction recovery program, and was admitted into the Drug Court Program.

The court noted that Sidiropolis voluntarily stipulated that he had violated Rule 8.4(b), committing a criminal act adversely reflecting on his trustworthiness and fitness as a lawyer. The court found his efforts toward his recovery and his cooperation with the process to be mitigating factors. The court suspended his license for two years, with an automatic reinstatement of his license in 60 days, and the

---

Silence in the Profession, 105 U. Va. L. Rev. 805 (2019) (questioning, in part, Rule 8.4(g)'s effectiveness in achieving the ABA's goals of eliminating bias and promoting diversity in the profession and justice system, *id.* at 827; and noting that expansive comments to Rule 8.4(g) have engendered constitutional criticisms that create "noisy distractions" from the ABA's goals, *id.* at 831).
46. ABA Form Op. 493, at 14 (July 15, 2020).

remaining 22 months stayed with supervision by a licensed attorney in good standing. *See also* In re Minter, 367 P.3d 1238 (Kan. 2016) (holding indefinite suspension was appropriate because evidence established the attorney's possession of a controlled substance with intent to distribute warranted a severe sanction).

Financial Misconduct

Attending law school, starting and maintaining a practice, and additional personal obligations, such as purchasing a home or raising a family, demand substantial time and financial resources. Thus, another common cause of lawyer discipline involves financial misconduct. In Iowa Supreme Court Att'y Disciplinary Board v. Taylor, 2016 BL 375312, Iowa No. 16-0130 (Nov. 10, 2016), a lawyer was suspended for 6 months for failing to file income taxes for 11 years. The dissent sought a one-year suspension, writing that "[w]e would not hesitate to revoke the license of a lawyer who stole money from a client. Taylor, in effect stole money from all Iowans for many years." The Iowa Supreme Court Disciplinary Board recommended an 18-month suspension for violation of Rule 8.4(b) and (c) after the Iowa Grievance Commission had recommended a suspension for no more than 30 days. The court majority found that mitigating factors such as the lawyer's pro bono work, acceptance of responsibility, and efforts to pay back taxes warranted a lesser sanction. How do you explain the wide disparity in recommended sanctions? What sanction do you think is appropriate?

In In re Brost, 850 N.W.2d 699 (Minn. 2014), a lawyer was indefinitely suspended in 2009 for using the expired notary stamp of a deceased notary to fraudulently notarize the lawyer's own signature on a certificate of trust prepared for a client. The lawyer submitted the fraudulent document to a bank to steal funds. The court held Brost's theft of $43,000 from her client's annuity payments stemmed directly from Brost's fiduciary relationship with her client and constituted misconduct under Rule 8.4(b) and (c) warranting disbarment. In addition, Brost failed to cooperate in the investigation and had a prior disciplinary record, including being currently under indefinite suspension for similar dishonest and fraudulent misconduct.

Falsehoods and Other Deceptions

Another common category of misconduct under Rule 8.4 concerns lawyer deception. A New York appellate division case, In re Heffernan, 121 N.Y.S. 3d 144 (App. Div. 2020), provides an example. In this case, Heffernan, an assistant district attorney in the Narcotics Bureau, was asked to file an extension order to keep a pole camera operational for surveillance on a public street. The request came after the prior order had lapsed, so Heffernan backdated an extension order to keep the pole camera operational. Heffernan then had a detective sign the backdated order and presented the order, with backdated affidavits, to a trial judge who signed the order.

The court found that Heffernan violated Rules 8.4(c), engaging in conduct involving dishonesty and misrepresentation; 8.4(d), doing conduct prejudicial to the administration of justice; and 8.4(h), committing conduct that adversely reflects on his fitness as an attorney. The court noted that attorneys are officers of the court and that they must act "with the utmost honesty and candor when making submissions to the court"; this is especially so for public prosecutors who are duty bound to "seek[] justice." The court issued a public censure, however, having found "extraordinary mitigation," including no disciplinary history, Heffernan's tenure in public service as a prosecutor, his excellent reputation, tremendous family stress, and his resignation from the district attorney's office. *See* Neal v. Clinton, No. CIV 2000-5677 (Ark. 5th Div. 2001) (suspending President William Jefferson Clinton from the practice of law in Arkansas for five years for violating Rule 8.4(d) by engaging in conduct prejudicial to the administration of justice when he knowingly gave evasive and misleading answers concerning his relationship with Monica Lewinsky in the Paula Jones case), *available at* https://www.arcourts.gov/sites/default/files/opc_opinions/2000-013.pdf; *see generally*, Section 3 *infra* (discussing mitigation).

2. The Disciplinary Process

Clients may initiate the lawyer discipline process by complaining about their lawyer to statewide or local disciplinary counsel operating under the authority of that jurisdiction's highest court. A judge or opposing counsel may also initiate the process by alleging misconduct, and sometimes disciplinary counsel starts the process after learning of lawyer misconduct, perhaps through the media.

Although states' disciplinary processes differ, many share some common attributes. The following discussion in this subsection is based, in part, on the ABA Disciplinary Enforcement Processes that provides a useful model for better understanding the disciplinary process. MODEL RULES FOR LAWYER DISCIPLINARY ENFORCEMENT (AM. BAR ASS'N 2002). In general, the disciplinary authority or counsel evaluates the client's grievance at the intake stage of the disciplinary process to determine if sufficient facts are alleged, that if true, constitute a violation of a professional conduct rule.

Assuming the alleged facts, if true, would violate a professional conduct rule, the disciplinary counsel further investigates the matter. Counsel contacts the lawyer who is the subject of the grievance to obtain the lawyer's version of the facts and to obtain other possible evidence.

Lawyers who are the subject of investigations are well advised to spend time explaining their version of the facts and answering disciplinary counsel's questions in hope of having the grievance dismissed at intake. They may wish to confer with a lawyer specializing in professional responsibility matters even at this investigation phase of the process to help present their version of events concerning the client grievance in hope of facilitating a quick resolution.

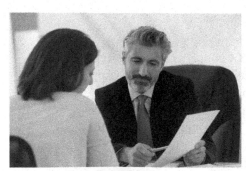

Lawyers need to maintain good communications with their clients to avoid misunderstandings that might lead to the filing of a disciplinary or malpractice action.
Shutterstock.com

Lawyers have an ethical duty under Rule 8.1 to cooperate with the disciplinary investigation, and their failure to cooperate is a separate chargeable disciplinary offense. For example, in In re Disciplinary Action Against Hansen, 868 N.W.2d 55 (Minn. 2015), the Minnesota Supreme Court ruled that an indefinite suspension with a 90-day minimum and a requirement that the respondent, Hansen, take the professional responsibility portion of the state bar exam before petitioning for reinstatement were appropriate sanctions given several acts of misconduct. This included improperly violating trust account requirements for almost a year and also a separate count for failing to cooperate with disciplinary counsel's investigations of the underlying trust problem and other matters.

Disciplinary counsel asked Hansen for a retainer agreement multiple times, but he never produced it, saying he was waiting for his client to sign a release. After months of delay, Hansen admitted there was no retainer; he then failed to respond to an ethics committee report and two follow-up letters. In the trust account matter, Hansen failed to respond to multiple requests for a written explanation of overdrafts. He sometimes said he would send all the documents but never did. Hansen finally admitted in a meeting several months later that he never kept any records. The court emphasized that failing to cooperate with an investigation "is serious misconduct and in itself generally warrants suspension." The cumulative effect of both the nature and the multiple instances of misconduct over a long period warranted a more severe sanction. Hansen's misconduct was also aggravated because he was already on disciplinary probation.

Lawyers or respondents are sometimes cleared of the underlying disciplinary charge but nevertheless disciplined for not cooperating during the investigation with disciplinary counsel or the relator.[47] Lawyers cannot be disbarred, however, for asserting their Fifth Amendment right not to testify in the discipline process, but the assertion can be considered "together with other evidence to substantiate a charge of other misconduct."[48]

After the investigation is completed, disciplinary counsel may dismiss the grievance; refer the respondent if involved in lesser misconduct to an **Alternative Discipline Program** (ADP); recommend probation or an admonition (i.e., a public or private reprimand depending on the jurisdiction's rules); file formal charges; or petition for a transfer to disability inactive status or for a stay. ADP occurs before disciplinary counsel files formal charges, and depending on the jurisdiction, might include arbitration, mediation, law office management assistance, lawyer assistance programs, psychological counseling, and continuing legal education.

---

47. *See* In re Disciplinary Action Against Cowan, 540 N.W.2d 825, 827 (Minn. 1995) (noting that the court has held that an "attorney's failure to cooperate can lead to indefinite suspension from the practice of law"); *see also* In re Sices, 289 So. 3d 1013 (La. 2020) (permanently disbarring a lawyer, in part, for not responding to any of disciplinary counsel's certified letters, such failure to cooperate under Rule 8.1(b) showed respondent intentionally harmed the legal profession).

48. WOLFRAM, *supra* note 9, at 104-05 (discussing Spevak v. Klein, 385 U.S. 511 (1967)). If a lawyer is granted immunity from future prosecution to testify in a case, any statements made under that immunity grant is admissible in a subsequent discipline proceeding because it is not a criminal prosecution. *Id.* (citing In re Daley, 549 F.2d 469 (7th Cir.), *cert. denied*, 434 U.S. 829 (1977)).

If disciplinary counsel files formal charges or a complaint against the lawyer with the disciplinary board, the respondent-lawyer gets a copy of the complaint and files a written answer. There is usually a board committee or panel that first hears the matter. The initial hearing panel consists of lawyers and sometimes non-lawyers; it is a formal trial process. The complainant gets to make a statement at the hearing, and the respondent can be represented by counsel at the hearing, cross-examine witnesses, and present evidence and arguments. The panel makes findings of fact and recommends a disposition in a report that is forwarded to the full board that approves, modifies, or disapproves the panel report.

The respondent or disciplinary counsel may file objections with the board concerning the panel's report. The full board conducts another hearing in which the parties can submit briefs and oral arguments, but it cannot consider any new evidence by the parties unless the opponent has an opportunity to respond. In this model, the panel is the trier of fact and the board provides the appellate review. The decision by the full board is then sent to the state's supreme court.

The state supreme court may review a matter on its own discretion or if the respondent or disciplinary counsel files objections to the board's report. If objections are filed, the parties may file briefs and present oral arguments in accordance with the rules governing civil appeals. Most state courts acting on bar disciplinary matters will apply a highly deferential standard of review to the board's finding of fact (clearly erroneous) but review *de novo* its application of law to facts, conclusions of law, and sanctions.

3. Sanctions — Aggravating and Mitigating Factors

What form of and how much discipline should be imposed? The ABA Standards for Imposing Lawyer Sanctions identify four factors that courts should consider in imposing appropriate discipline involving the following concerns: (1) the duty violated; (2) the lawyer's mental state (intentional or negligent); (3) the seriousness of the actual or potential injury; and (4) the existence of aggravating and mitigating factors.[49] Although the terms vary among jurisdictions, sanctions generally include **disbarment** (a permanent separation from the bar and with no chance of reinstatement in some jurisdictions); suspension (a removal from the bar for a set period, often ranging between 6 to 24 months, that permits the lawyer upon satisfactorily completing the suspension to automatically apply for reinstatement); public reprimand (a type of public censure with no removal from practice); and a private reprimand (a non-public admonition also without removal from practice). The court may also order the respondent to make full restitution to the complainant and attend and pay for a substance abuse or other treatment program.

Each disciplinary case involves unique circumstances and warrants consideration by the disciplinary authority of the particular misconduct and case precedent in hope of reaching a fair result. What qualifies as an aggravating or mitigating

---

49. *See II Theoretical Framework,* ABA STANDARDS FOR IMPOSING LAWYER SANCTIONS 48 (1986, amended in 1992).

factor may vary among jurisdictions, although some factors are well established and common in many jurisdictions. These factors can play a decisive role regarding the severity of the sanction following the establishment of misconduct. The following lists provide a good overview of both aggravating and mitigating factors and are based on factors adopted by Ohio.[50]

After the establishment of misconduct, **aggravating factors** calling for a more serious sanction include (1) prior disciplinary offenses; (2) a dishonest or selfish motive; (3) a pattern of misconduct; (4) multiple offenses; (5) a lack of cooperation; (6) the submission of false evidence, false statements, or other deceptive conduct during the disciplinary process; (7) a refusal to acknowledge wrongdoing; (8) the failure to make restitution; and (9) the vulnerability of and resulting harm to victims of the misconduct.

Some **mitigating factors** favoring a lesser sanction are (1) the lack of a prior disciplinary record; (2) the absence of a dishonest or selfish motive; (3) a timely, good faith effort to make restitution or rectify the consequences of misconduct; (4) full disclosure; (5) cooperation during the process; (6) imposition of other penalties (e.g., loss of employment); (7) good character or reputation; and (8) existence of a medical disorder. Another common mitigating factor is the lawyer's remorse for the misconduct.

> ### Insurance Policies and the Cost of Defense
>
> Lawyers should make sure their errors and omissions insurance policies, commonly referred to as malpractice insurance, cover the cost of defense in a disciplinary action. Some malpractice policies cover only the expenses of defense and civil judgment for actions in damages stemming from the lawyer's negligence or unintentional errors and omissions in delivering legal services. A discipline action is not a personal claim for damages resulting from the negligent delivery of legal services. It is instead an action by disciplinary counsel to protect the public's interest by seeking a sanction for a lawyer who violated professional conduct rules.

Many of these factors leave room for interpretation and application in any given disciplinary proceeding.[51] For example, should a recommendation for discipline that is before the state's high court but not yet decided count as a "prior offense"? How similar must the acts be and how close in time must they occur to constitute a "pattern"? Should all clients who are unsophisticated and are inexperienced with the court system be considered "vulnerable clients"? Should restitution or rectification of misconduct that is made reluctantly under the pressure of a disciplinary or criminal investigation or proceeding count as a "timely, good faith effort to make restitution or rectify consequences of misconduct"?

4. Disciplinary Authority; Choice of Law

One consequence of the increase in cross-border practice by lawyers is the potential risk of being less familiar with another jurisdiction's professional conduct rules

---

50. Ohio Gov. Bar Rule I, §13(A)-(C).
51. *See Evidence Required to Establish Aggravating and Mitigating Factors—Differing Views and Perspectives,* Miller-Becker Ctr. for Prof'l Responsibility Annual Disciplinary Program Panel (Oct. 21, 2016).

that differ from the lawyer's home jurisdiction or place of licensure. Rule 8.5 guides practitioners and disciplinary authorities concerning which jurisdiction's conduct rules will govern a lawyer's actions and possibly place the lawyer at risk of discipline. It states that any jurisdiction in which the lawyer is admitted retains authority to discipline the lawyer for misconduct occurring within or outside the jurisdiction.

For example, assume Roberta Gomez is a lawyer licensed in Maine who represents a Maine client in purchasing a home in Florida. Gomez negotiates the terms of the purchase contract in Florida, executes the contract there, and later returns to do the closing. During the closing, Gomez violates a Florida ethics rule. Maine retains authority to discipline its licensed lawyer, Gomez, even though the violation involves a Florida rule. Under Rule 8.5(a), Florida also can discipline Gomez because she is providing legal services within its jurisdiction even though Gomez is only licensed in Maine. Thus, both jurisdictions have authority to discipline Gomez.

If Maine elects to discipline Gomez for her work in Florida, Maine must decide whether it will apply its rules or Florida's in reviewing Gomez's conduct. Rule 8.5(b)(2) provides that the jurisdiction's rule where the conduct occurred or where the predominant effect of the conduct will occur determines which jurisdiction's rule applies to Gomez's conduct. Given the facts above, Maine should apply Florida's rule in the discipline proceeding since the terms of the purchase, the signing of the contract, and the closing occurred in Florida. Both the conduct and the predominant effect happened in Florida.

The "**predominant effects**" standard could change the result with different facts. For example, if the negotiation for the purchase, the financing, and the signing of the deal occur in Maine as well as the alleged misconduct, then arguably Maine should apply its rules because the conduct occurred in Maine. However, Gomez or Florida could also argue that Florida's rules should govern Gomez's conduct because the predominant effect of the conduct occurred in Florida where the closing took place and the property is located. In this scenario, Maine has to decide which rules, Maine's or Florida's, to apply in assessing Gomez's alleged misconduct. However, Rule 8.5(b)(2) provides a safe harbor for lawyers by not subjecting them to discipline for following the professional conduct rules of a state where the lawyer "reasonably believes" the predominant effects of his legal services occur.

The choice of law question in the disciplinary context is more straightforward when the lawyer is involved in litigation. In that context, the rules of the jurisdiction where the tribunal is located govern the disciplinary proceeding. To illustrate, if Gomez's work in Florida on behalf of a Maine client involved litigation before a Florida court or administrative agency, then Florida's rules would govern Gomez's conduct.

5. Reciprocal Discipline

Given the need for the lawyer discipline system to protect the public and the administration of justice from miscreant lawyers, courts commonly impose the same disciplinary sanction both in terms of length of time and severity as that which was issued by the other jurisdiction. After providing notice of the imposition of **reciprocal discipline**, the respondent bears the burden of showing that the predicate discipline was not appropriate, perhaps because of important procedural or substantive deficiencies, such as a lack of notice or proof. This is not an easy burden to meet. The following cases illustrate the concept of reciprocal discipline.

In Kentucky Bar Association v. Clifton, 504 S.W.3d 690 (Ky. 2016), the Ohio Supreme Court found Clifton knowingly made false statements of fact or law to a tribunal that warranted a public reprimand. Due to Clifton being a member of the Kentucky and Ohio bars, the Kentucky Bar Association initiated this proceeding against Clifton under Kentucky Supreme Court Rule 3.435(4), which states: "a lawyer shall be subject to identical discipline in the Commonwealth of Kentucky unless [he] proves by substantial evidence: (a) a lack of jurisdiction or fraud in the out-of-state disciplinary proceeding, or (b) that the misconduct established warrants substantially different discipline in this State." Because the Kentucky Bar Association found Clifton did violate Ohio's Rules of Professional Conduct, Kentucky also publicly reprimanded Clifton for the violations or imposed reciprocal discipline.

Midlen, the respondent in Attorney Grievance Commission of Maryland v. Midlen, 911 A.2d 852 (2008), represented the Jimmy Swaggart Ministries (JSM) in the royalty distribution process. Midlen would deduct his fees from JSM royalties and then remit the balance despite being asked numerous times by JSM to cease doing this. Further, Midlen failed to provide an accounting of the legal fees and deductions. The D.C. Court of Appeals found that Midlen violated the D.C. Rules of Professional Conduct and suspended him for 18 months for negligently misappropriating funds.

The Maryland Court of Appeals agreed that based on the findings of the D.C. court, Midlen's conduct also violated several Maryland Rules of Professional Conduct. The Maryland court rejected Midlen's claims that his due process rights were violated when the D.C. board did not adhere to the findings of the hearing panel because the board and the court were not strictly bound by its findings. Also, the Maryland court rejected Midlen's claims that the D.C. sanction was more severe than what Maryland normally imposed for similar conduct. The Maryland Court of Appeals disagreed and said it might have imposed a more severe sanction than D.C. but for the Maryland Bar Counsel's recommendation. The court also said that although the norm for reciprocal discipline is to have sanctions run concurrently, it was not doing so in this case because there was no evidence of when Midlen notified the bar counsel of the D.C. suspension or whether he continued to practice in Maryland after the D.C. suspension. *Compare* In re Peters, 2016 D.C. App. LEXIS 423 (D.C. 2016) (attorney's conduct warranted substantially different discipline in D.C. because reciprocal seven-year suspension was inappropriate as it exceeded D.C.'s disbarment rule that provided for five years with an opportunity to seek reinstatement, and is far longer than the three years that D.C. allows for suspensions under D.C. Bar R. XI, §§3(a)(2), 16(a)).

6. Lawyers' Duty to Report Misconduct

The legal profession has a strong tradition of self-regulation, although its effectiveness in protecting the public from incompetent and miscreant lawyers is subject to criticism. The Model Rules' Preamble recognizes that preserving self-regulation for the profession requires lawyers to ensure that other lawyers observe the Model Rules, including reporting lawyer misconduct.

Rule 8.3(a) requires a lawyer who knows about another lawyer's violation of a Model Rule to report it to the appropriate professional authority if the violations raise a "substantial question" about the lawyer's "honesty, trustworthiness or fitness to practice law." Rule 8.3(b) similarly obligates a lawyer who knows that a judge has violated the judicial ethics code in a way that raises a substantial question about the judge's honesty, trustworthiness, or fitness to serve as a judge. These obligations are sometimes derisively referred to as the "snitch" rules. When a lawyer "knows" that conduct violates a disciplinary rule and what kind of misconduct qualifies for reporting are fact-sensitive and often debatable questions.

A lawyer is not obliged to report every rule violation, only violations raising a "substantial question" about the lawyer's honesty and character fitness to practice law. Thus, according to Texas Ethics Opinion 632 (2013), a lawyer does not have to report another lawyer who impermissibly uses a trade name in Texas, without additional misconduct, because this does not raise a substantial question of honesty or trustworthiness under Rule 8.3. Other examples of misconduct that have not raised a substantial question of honesty or fitness involved dilatoriness, ineffective assistance, and "technical" violations.[52]

Some states, like Ohio, have a version of Rule 8.3(a) and (b) that imposes a greater duty of reporting. This version mandates the reporting of another lawyer's or judge's rule violation if it raises any "question," and not a "substantial question," about the lawyer's or judge's character and fitness. Thus, a lawyer might have to report a lawyer in Ohio for misconduct that raises a "question" about that lawyer's fitness to practice law while a lawyer would not have to report a lawyer for the same misconduct in another jurisdiction that requires reporting only if the misconduct raises a "substantial" question about the lawyer's fitness.

ABA Formal Opinion 94-383 prohibits a lawyer from threatening to file a disciplinary complaint against another lawyer under Rule 8.3 in order to gain an advantage in a matter, such as civil litigation. Rule 8.3 clearly requires the lawyer to report — not merely to *threaten* to report — conduct raising a substantial question about the lawyer's honesty and fitness to practice. Of course, it is not always clear when conduct constitutes a substantial question. The lawyer's failure to report under Rule 8.3(a) also constitutes a separate violation of Rule 8.4(a)'s duty not to violate, attempt to violate, or assist another to violate a rule. It is important to know what your jurisdiction's rules provide. Several states, including California, Texas, Illinois, Florida, Ohio, and the District of Columbia, have rules expressly banning threats to file disciplinary complaints.

Some state versions of Rule 8.3 identify the "appropriate professional authority" to receive reports of violations. The phrase likely includes statewide and local disciplinary counsel's offices or similar authorities that are better suited than the courts

---

52. *See* ABA/BNA Man., *supra* note 6, at 101:203.

to initiate the disciplinary investigation described in comment [1] of Rule 8.3. For example, in Ohio, a lawyer who needs to report another lawyer under Rule 8.3 can no longer discharge that obligation by informing the local court. Instead, the matter must be reported to the Office of Disciplinary Counsel or local certified grievance committee.[53]

Subsection (c) provides two exceptions to Rule 8.3's general reporting obligations. First, one does not have to report if knowledge of the violation is considered confidential and protected from disclosure under Rule 1.6. For example, if lawyer A seeks lawyer B's legal assistance concerning A's misconduct that raises a substantial question of A's honesty and fitness to practice law, B is not required under 8.3(c) to report A's misconduct to the appropriate disciplinary authorities. Second, the lawyer does not have to report misconduct learned in an approved lawyer assistance program. Thus, when a disabled lawyer joins a lawyer's assistance program and tells the program's lawyer that he has overcharged his clients, the program lawyer does not have to report the disabled lawyer's misconduct under 8.3(a). Another common scenario involves a lawyer representing a client who reveals the misconduct of his prior counsel. The lawyer would not have to report this misconduct because it is protected as confidential under Rule 1.6; but comment [2] to Rule 8.3 recommends the lawyer seek the client's permission to disclose the prior counsel's misconduct.

In In re Riehlmann, 891 So. 2d 1239 (La. 2005), the Louisiana Supreme Court addressed the question of when a lawyer has to report another lawyer's misconduct. It held Rule 8.3(a) requires a lawyer to promptly report another lawyer's misconduct whenever the evidence would permit "a reasonable lawyer under the circumstances" to form a firm belief that the conduct in question had "more likely than not occurred." Riehlmann and his friend, Deegan, were former prosecutors. While dying of cancer, Deegan told Riehlmann he had suppressed exculpatory blood evidence in an unnamed case; Deegan also rejected Riehlmann's suggestion to report his misconduct. Approximately five years after Deegan's passing, Riehlmann learned of a case where the crime lab found the perpetrator of the crime had a different blood type than the person on death row for the crime. Riehlmann spoke to the defendant's lawyer about his discussion with Deegan. Riehlmann then executed an affidavit to the Disciplinary Counsel's Office reporting his discussion with Deegan. Riehlmann was charged with a Rule 8.3(a) violation for failing to promptly report Deegan's misconduct. The Louisiana Supreme Court decided a lawyer must promptly report misconduct to facilitate a timely investigation of the matter and to protect the public and the profession from the lawyer's possible future misconduct. The court reprimanded Riehlmann and held a reasonable lawyer would have formed a firm belief at the time of Deegan's confession that the misconduct likely occurred.

---

53. Ohio Supreme Court Ethics Op. 2007-1.23 (concluding that a tribunal is not a "disciplinary authority" empowered to investigate or act upon misconduct under Ohio's Rule 8.3(a)).

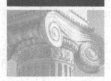

Case Preview

In re Himmel

In a disciplinary proceeding, Justice Stamos of the Illinois Supreme Court held that Attorney Himmel's failure to report the misconduct of another attorney who had formerly represented Himmel's client warranted a one-year suspension, not merely a private reprimand. The former attorney violated Illinois ethics rules when he converted the client's settlement funds from an insurance company. The client retained Himmel to help recover the stolen funds, and he managed to recover some of the funds. *In re Himmel* sent shock waves through the profession by underscoring the potentially significant consequences lawyers face when they breach their ethical duty to report other lawyers who violate the profession's ethics rules.

As you read *Himmel*, ask yourself the following questions:

1. What was the basis for the Illinois Supreme Court concluding that Himmel's information about the miscreant lawyer, Casey, was not protected from disclosure by the attorney-client privilege?
2. How does the court respond to Himmel's contention that he did not report Casey because his client told him not to report Casey?
3. At what point should Himmel have reported Casey?
4. What aggravating and mitigating factors did the court consider in determining the quantum of discipline to impose on Himmel?

In re Himmel
533 N.E.2d 790 (1988)

. . .

In October 1978, Tammy Forsberg was injured in a motorcycle accident. In June 1980, she retained John R. Casey to represent her in any personal injury or property damage claim resulting from the accident. Sometime in 1981, Casey negotiated a settlement of $35,000 on Forsberg's behalf. Pursuant to an agreement between Forsberg and Casey, one-third of any monies received would be paid to Casey as his attorney fee.

In March 1981, Casey received the $35,000 settlement check, endorsed it, and deposited the check into his client trust fund account. Subsequently, Casey converted the funds.

Between 1981 and 1983, Forsberg unsuccessfully attempted to collect her $23,233.34 share of the settlement proceeds. In March 1983, Forsberg retained respondent to collect her money and agreed to pay him one-third of any funds recovered above $23,233.34.

Respondent investigated the matter and discovered that Casey had misappropriated the settlement funds. In April 1983, respondent drafted an agreement in which

Casey would pay Forsberg $75,000 in settlement of any claim she might have against him for the misappropriated funds. By the terms of the agreement, Forsberg agreed not to initiate any criminal, civil, or attorney disciplinary action against Casey. This agreement was executed on April 11, 1983. Respondent stood to gain $17,000 or more if Casey honored the agreement. In February 1985, respondent filed suit against Casey for breaching the agreement, and a $100,000 judgment was entered against Casey. If Casey had satisfied the judgment, respondent's share would have been approximately $25,588.

The [Illinois Attorney Registration and Disciplinary Commission (Commission)] complaint stated that at no time did respondent inform the Commission of Casey's misconduct. According to the [Commission's] Administrator, respondent's first contact with the Commission was in response to the Commission's inquiry regarding the lawsuit against Casey.

A hearing on the complaint against the present respondent was held before the Hearing Board of the Commission on June 3, 1986 [and] . . . provided [the] additional facts.

Before retaining respondent, Forsberg collected $5,000 from Casey. . . . Forsberg told respondent that she simply wanted her money back and specifically instructed respondent to take no other action. Because of respondent's efforts, Forsberg collected another $10,400 from Casey. Respondent received no fee in this case.

The Hearing Board found that respondent received unprivileged information that Casey converted Forsberg's funds, and that respondent failed to relate the information to the Commission in violation of Rule 1-103(a) of the Code. The Hearing Board noted, however, that respondent had been practicing law for 11 years, had no prior record of any complaints, obtained as good a result as could be expected in the case, and requested no fee for recovering the $23,233.34. Accordingly, the Hearing Board recommended a private reprimand.

Upon the Administrator's exceptions to the Hearing Board's recommendation, the Review Board reviewed the matter. The Review Board's report stated that the client had contacted the Commission prior to retaining respondent and, therefore, the Commission did have knowledge of the alleged misconduct. Further, the Review Board noted that respondent respected the client's wishes regarding not pursuing a claim with the Commission. Accordingly, the Review Board recommended that the complaint be dismissed.

The Administrator now raises three issues for review: (1) whether the Review Board erred in concluding that respondent's client had informed the Commission of misconduct by her former attorney; (2) whether the Review Board erred in concluding that respondent had not violated Rule 1-103(a); and (3) whether the proven misconduct warrants at least a censure.

As to the first issue, the Administrator contends . . . that even if Forsberg had reported Casey's misconduct to the Commission, such an action would not have relieved respondent of his duty to report under Rule 1-103(a). Additionally, the Administrator argues that no evidence exists to prove that respondent failed to report because he assumed that Forsberg had already reported the matter.

Respondent argues . . . that the record is not clear that Forsberg failed to disclose Casey's name to the Commission. Respondent also argues that Forsberg directed respondent not to pursue the claim against Casey, a claim she had already begun to pursue.

We begin our analysis by examining whether a client's complaint of attorney misconduct to the Commission can be a defense to an attorney's failure to report the same misconduct. Respondent offers no authority for such a defense and our research has disclosed none. Common sense would dictate that if a lawyer has a duty under the Code, the actions of a client would not relieve the attorney of his own duty. Accordingly, while the parties dispute whether or not respondent's client informed the Commission, that question is irrelevant to our inquiry in this case. We have held that the canons of ethics in the Code constitute a safe guide for professional conduct, and attorneys may be disciplined for not observing them. The question is, then, whether or not respondent violated the Code, not whether Forsberg informed the Commission of Casey's misconduct.

As to respondent's argument that he did not report Casey's misconduct because his client directed him not to do so, we again note respondent's failure to suggest any legal support for such a defense. A lawyer, as an officer of the court, is duty-bound to uphold the rules in the Code. The title of Canon 1 reflects this obligation: "A lawyer should assist in maintaining the integrity and competence of the legal profession." A lawyer may not choose to circumvent the rules by simply asserting that his client asked him to do so.

As to the second issue, the Administrator argues that . . . respondent had unprivileged knowledge of Casey's conversion of client funds, and that respondent failed to disclose that information to the Commission. The Administrator states that respondent's knowledge of Casey's conversion of client funds was knowledge of illegal conduct involving moral turpitude [and] . . . that the information respondent received was not privileged under the definition of privileged information. Therefore, . . . respondent violated his ethical duty to report misconduct under Rule 1-103(a).

. . .

Our analysis of this issue begins with a reading of the applicable disciplinary rules. Rule 1-103(a) of the Code states:

(a) A lawyer possessing unprivileged knowledge of a violation of Rule 1-102(a)(3) or (4) shall report such knowledge to a tribunal or other authority empowered to investigate or act upon such violation."

Rule 1-102 of the Code states:

(a) A lawyer shall not
    (1) violate a disciplinary rule;
    (2) circumvent a disciplinary rule through actions of another;
    (3) engage in illegal conduct involving moral turpitude;
    (4) engage in conduct involving dishonesty, fraud, deceit, or misrepresentation; or
    (5) engage in conduct that is prejudicial to the administration of justice.

. . .

This court has also emphasized the importance of a lawyer's duty to report misconduct. We stated, "Under Disciplinary Rule 1-103 a lawyer has the duty to report the misconduct of other lawyers." Thus, if the present respondent's conduct did violate the rule on reporting misconduct, imposition of discipline for such a breach of duty is mandated.

The question whether the information that respondent possessed was protected by the attorney-client privilege, and thus exempt from the reporting rule, requires application of this court's definition of the privilege. We have stated that "'(1) [w]here legal advice of any kind is sought (2) from a professional legal adviser in his capacity as such, (3) the communications relating to that purpose, (4) made in confidence (5) by the client, (6) are at his instance permanently protected (7) from disclosure by himself or by the legal adviser, (8) except the protection be waived.'" . . . In this case, Forsberg discussed the matter with respondent at various times while her mother and her fiancé were present. Consequently, unless the mother and fiancé were agents of respondent's client, the information communicated was not privileged. Moreover, we have also stated that matters intended by a client for disclosure by the client's attorney to third parties, who are not agents of either the client or the attorney, are not privileged. The record shows that respondent, with Forsberg's consent, discussed Casey's conversion of her funds with the insurance company involved, . . . [and] with Casey himself. Thus, the information was not privileged.

Though respondent repeatedly asserts that his failure to report was motivated not by financial gain but by the request of his client, we do not deem such an argument relevant in this case. This court has stated that discipline may be appropriate even if no dishonest motive for the misconduct exists. In addition, we have held that client approval of an attorney's action does not immunize an attorney from disciplinary action. We have already dealt with, and dismissed, respondent's assertion that his conduct is acceptable because he was acting pursuant to his client's directions.

Respondent does not argue that Casey's conversion of Forsberg's funds was not illegal conduct involving moral turpitude under Rule 1-102(a)(3) or conduct involving dishonesty, fraud, deceit, or misrepresentation under Rule 1-102(a)(4). It is clear that conversion of client funds is, indeed, conduct involving moral turpitude. We conclude, then, that respondent possessed unprivileged knowledge of Casey's conversion of client funds, which is illegal conduct involving moral turpitude, and that respondent failed in his duty to report such misconduct to the Commission. Because no defense exists, we agree with the Hearing Board's finding that respondent has violated Rule 1-103(a) and must be disciplined.

The third issue concerns the appropriate quantum of discipline to be imposed in this case. The Administrator contends that respondent's misconduct warrants at least a censure, although the Hearing Board recommended a private reprimand and the Review Board recommended dismissal of the matter entirely. In support of the request for a greater quantum of discipline, the Administrator cites to the purposes of attorney discipline, which include maintaining the integrity of the legal profession and safeguarding the administration of justice. The Administrator argues that these purposes will not be served unless respondent is publicly disciplined so that the profession will be on notice that a violation of Rule 1-103(a) will not be tolerated. The Administrator argues that a more severe sanction is necessary because respondent deprived the Commission of evidence of another attorney's conversion and thereby interfered with the Commission's investigative function under Supreme Court Rule 752.

Citing to the Rule 774 petition filed against Casey, the Administrator notes that Casey converted many clients' funds after respondent's duty to report Casey arose. The Administrator also argues that both respondent and his client behaved in contravention of the Criminal Code's prohibition against compounding a crime by agreeing with Casey not to report him, in exchange for settlement funds.

In his defense, respondent reiterates his arguments that he was not motivated by desire for financial gain. He also states that Forsberg was pleased with his performance on her behalf. According to respondent, his failure to report was a "judgment call" which resulted positively in Forsberg's regaining some of her funds from Casey.

We have stated that while recommendations of the Boards are to be considered, this court ultimately bears responsibility for deciding an appropriate sanction. We reiterate our statement that "'[w]hen determining the nature and extent of discipline to be imposed, the respondent's actions must be viewed in relationship "to the underlying purposes of our disciplinary process, which purposes are to maintain the integrity of the legal profession, to protect the administration of justice from reproach, and to safeguard the public."'"

Bearing these principles in mind, we agree with the Administrator that public discipline is necessary in this case to carry out the purposes of attorney discipline. While we have considered the Board's recommendations in this matter, we cannot agree with the Review Board that respondent's conduct served to rectify a wrong and did not injure the bar, the public, or the administration of justice. Though we agree with the Hearing Board's assessment that respondent violated Rule 1-103 of the Code, we do not agree that the facts warrant only a private reprimand.

. . .

This failure to report resulted in interference with the Commission's investigation of Casey, and thus with the administration of justice. Perhaps some members of the public would have been spared from Casey's misconduct had respondent reported the information as soon as he knew of Casey's conversions of client funds. We are particularly disturbed by the fact that respondent chose to draft a settlement agreement with Casey rather than report his misconduct.

Both respondent and his client stood to gain financially by agreeing not to prosecute or report Casey for conversion. According to the settlement agreement, respondent would have received $17,000 or more as his fee. If Casey had satisfied the judgment entered against him for failure to honor the settlement agreement, respondent would have collected approximately $25,588.

We have held that fairness dictates consideration of mitigating factors in disciplinary cases, therefore, we do consider the fact that Forsberg recovered $10,400 through respondent's services, that respondent has practiced law for 11 years with no record of complaints, and that he requested no fee for minimum collection of Forsberg's funds. However, these considerations do not outweigh the serious nature of respondent's failure to report Casey, the resulting interference with the Commission's investigation of Casey, and respondent's ill-advised choice to settle with Casey rather than report his misconduct.

Accordingly, it is ordered that respondent be suspended from the practice of law for one year.

Post-Case Follow-Up

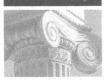

Himmel represents the uncommon case in which a lawyer is sanctioned for the sole violation of not reporting another lawyer's misconduct. Often the lawyer who fails to report is involved in additional misconduct. Following *Himmel*, lawyers became more sensitive about the potential costs of not reporting another lawyer's misconduct under Rule 8.3. For example, the rate of lawyer reporting jumped in Illinois during the period of 1992-1995 to 8.9 percent of all complaints received, with 18.2 percent of them resulting in formal disciplinary charges. *See* Laura Gaitland, *"Snitch Rule" Remains Controversial but Effective Especially in Illinois*, A.B.A. J. 24 (Apr. 1997).

It is important to note, however, that Rule 8.3(c) does not require the disclosure of information protected under Rule 1.6 (Confidentiality of Information). Rule 1.6(a) prohibits a lawyer from voluntarily disclosing information relating to the representation of a client, no matter the source of that information, unless the client gives informed consent, the revelation is impliedly authorized to carry out representation, or the disclosure falls within a few exceptions listed within the rule. Thus, when a lawyer learns from a client about the client's previous lawyer's misconduct, Rule 1.6 protects that information from disclosure. As you will learn in Chapter 5, *infra*, Rule 1.6 protects a broader range of information from disclosure than the attorney-client privilege standard used in *Himmel*.[54] Further, information a client told his lawyer in confidence under Rule 1.6 cannot be divulged to anyone without the client's permission, although the client may follow the lawyer's advice about whether to report or not. The lawyer should "encourage a client to consent to disclosure where prosecution would not substantially prejudice the client's interests."[55] Often times, when read together, Rules 8.3(c) and 1.6 trump the lawyer's duty to report lawyer misconduct.

In *Himmel*'s wake, there was a call for other states to sanction lawyers for nonreporting in the belief that lawyer reporting was particularly effective because of lawyers' familiarity with conduct rules and their contact with other lawyers. Lawyer reporting would help cleanse the profession of miscreant lawyers and support the profession's interest in self-regulation — both important goals. Whether imposing a mandatory lawyer reporting requirement is necessary to achieve these goals remains at least an open question. There is some evidence that lawyers will also report other lawyer misconduct even when such reporting is not mandatory. *See* Arthur F. Greenbaum, *The Attorney's Duty to Report Professional Misconduct: A Roadmap for Reform*, 16 GEO. J. LEGAL ETHICS 259 (2003). What do you think? Is it fair, or even efficient to expect lawyers to report the misconduct of fellow lawyers? Also, what should lawyers do when they suspect, but are not certain, that a fellow lawyer violated an ethics rule? Should the violation of any ethics rule trigger the lawyer's duty to report another lawyer?

---

54. *See* Chapter 5, *infra* (providing a detailed discussion of Rule 1.6 and other sources of lawyer-client secrecy, such as the attorney-client privilege and work product immunity doctrine).
55. *See* Rule 8.3 cmt. [2].

In re Himmel: Real Life Applications

An exotic dancer alleged that she was raped by three men at an early morning party hosted by members of the lacrosse team at a university in Vermont. Prosecutor Nitro oversaw the investigation and made several extrajudicial statements to the media. For example, he told CBS News that the "lacrosse team has not been fully cooperative," and implied that the men were uncooperative: "[i]f it's not the way it's been reported, then why are they so unwilling to tell us what, in their own words, did take place that night?" In fact, Nitro knew the three men were cooperative, including making voluntary statements and submitting DNA samples.

Nitro relied on Dr. Meehan, president of DNA Security Inc. (DSI), to conduct DNA tests. He informed Nitro that the DNA tests excluded the three defendants as possible contributors of the multiple male DNA from the rape kit. Nitro and Meehan orally agreed they would not include all of the DNA results in the DSI Report and instead would only include the positive results, effectively shielding potentially exculpatory evidence from the defendants. Nitro failed to memorialize his oral communications with Dr. Meehan as required by law. The DNA test from a vaginal swab also showed a sperm fraction from the victim's boyfriend.

Nitro did not tell the defendants that the statements from the other exotic dancer at the party that night were inconsistent with the victim's statements. Nitro also filed written documents with the court stating that "the State is not aware of any additional material or information which may be exculpatory in nature with respect to the defendants."

a. Assume a confidential source informs the lawyer for one of the three defendants about all of the above information related to the alleged rapes and Nitro's conduct. She would prefer not to report the information because the report may reveal the identity of the confidential source who is at risk of harm. Must the defense lawyer report this information to the disciplinary authorities?

b. Assume the defense lawyer contacts you, the Vermont statewide disciplinary counsel, and discloses all of the above information about the alleged rape and the related conduct of Nitro. What possible ethics standards did Nitro violate? What disciplinary sanctions, if any, would you recommend to the court? What aggravating factors might you argue support a more serious sanction?

D. LEGAL MALPRACTICE

1. Background

Lawyer self-regulation protects the public, the profession, and the courts from miscreant lawyers. The disciplinary system is not designed to compensate individuals for injuries caused by their lawyers' wrongful conduct, although clients may obtain some recompense by filing claims with state client protection funds that are supported by mandatory contributions from the bar. Instead, clients can file a civil action for damages, commonly known as a legal malpractice lawsuit, for injuries suffered because of their lawyers' wrongful conduct.

Legal malpractice cases generally involve claims of negligence, breach of fiduciary duty, or breach of contract against a lawyer and are often pled in the alternative. All three claims may be asserted in a single case. There is significant overlap in the application of these three claims as they all hinge on the lawyer breaching a standard of reasonable or ordinary care. The Restatement notes the similarities between legal malpractice actions based in negligence and breach of contract, stating the reasonable care element is viewed as an implied contract term. RESTATEMENT (THIRD) OF THE LAW GOVERNING LAWYERS §48 cmt. c, §55 cmt. c. That is why in legal malpractice cases involving a claim for breach of contract sometimes authorities note that "the contract claim sounds in tort." Thus, when the lawyer signs a written retention agreement to represent the plaintiff in an automobile collision case, an implied term of that agreement is the lawyer's duty to exercise reasonable or ordinary care in litigating the plaintiff's case. In this scenario, the lawyer arguably violates the duty of reasonable care when she fails to interview the only eyewitness to the accident and may find herself sued for legal malpractice.

In Volume 1, §1:2 of his treatise, LEGAL MALPRACTICE (2016), Ronald E. Mallen similarly recognizes the close relationship between negligence and breach of fiduciary duty:

> Often, the same conduct may be characterized as negligence and alternatively as a fiduciary breach. Although the terminology usually makes no substantive or procedural difference, the prevailing and better view is that legal malpractice encompasses any professional misconduct whether attributable to a breach of a standard of care or of the fiduciary obligations[, or of contract].

One practical difference concerning the three theories of legal malpractice is that the statute of limitations may vary for each claim, allowing the legal malpractice case to go forward based on one claim but not another. Some jurisdictions have one statute of limitation for the general category of legal malpractice lawsuits.[56]

2. Lawyer Negligence and Legal Malpractice

Traditional principles of negligence apply to **legal malpractice** actions.[57] Thus, in a negligence action for legal malpractice the plaintiff must prove the following elements by a preponderance of evidence: (1) the existence of an attorney-client relationship that establishes a duty on the part of the attorney; (2) a negligent act or omission constituting a breach of that duty; (3) the proximate cause (or legal cause) of the injury; and (4) the actual damages suffered by the plaintiff.

---

56. RESTATEMENT (THIRD) OF THE LAW GOVERNING LAWYERS §48 cmt. c.
57. *Id.* §§48 & 53.

The threshold for establishing the professional relationship is not a high one: it is the client's reasonable belief that the lawyer is the client's legal advisor. The client can form a reasonable belief in the lawyer's office as well as during a brief contact in an informal setting. Ideally, a retention agreement memorializes the creation of the professional relationship after an initial client interview in the office.

The lawyer owes a client a duty of reasonable care in rendering legal services following the creation of a professional relationship. Lawyers who hold themselves out as specialists are generally held to a stricter or higher standard of care; they are expected to practice with the care ordinarily used by lawyers in that specialty.[58]

Sometimes lawyers owe a duty of reasonable care to non-clients or third parties with whom they have no direct contact. Traditionally, the lawyer's duty and liability to third parties was limited by the doctrine of privity of contract. This restricted the lawyer's duty of care and liability to only persons with whom he had some contact. "The traditional privity defense has remained most effective in situations where the non-client is a clear adversary of the lawyer's client."[59]

Today, however, there are many exceptions to the privity defense to lawyer malpractice. Lawyers may owe a duty of reasonable care to third parties with whom the lawyer has never had any contact. This third-party duty of care and potential liability arises when the lawyer knows that his work is intended to benefit others or he is inviting others to rely on his opinion.[60] The classic example of third-party or non-client liability is when the client asks the lawyer to draft a trust for the benefit of a third party or to draft an opinion letter about the client's financial status to facilitate a bank loan for the client. The lawyer should know that these documents are benefitting the trust beneficiary or are inviting the bank's reliance. Restatement §51 identifies four circumstances in which a lawyer might be liable to a non-client: (1) where the non-client is a prospective client; (2) where the lawyer invites the non-client's reliance on the lawyer's work and the non-client is not too remote to be entitled to protection; (3) where the lawyer knows that his services are intended by the client to primarily benefit a non-client;[61] and (4) where the client acts as trustee, guardian, or fiduciary and the lawyer knowingly assists the client in breaching his obligations.[62]

After establishing a professional relationship or some other basis for the lawyer owing a duty of care, the parties usually offer expert testimony to define the

---

58. Ronald Mallen, with Allison Martin Rhodes, 2 LEGAL MALPRACTICE §20:4 (2016).

59. *See* ABA/BNA MAN., *supra* note 6, at 301:602.

60. *See id.* at 301: 608-09.

61. For example, in Bullis v. Downes, 612 N.W.2d 435 (Mich. Ct. App. 2000), the court held that the daughter of the decedent had standing to bring suit against the attorney who drafted the decedent's will and trust. The daughter was promised two specific real properties via the will; however, the properties were deeded to the trust, which contained no provision for the distribution of real property. As a result, she was deprived of one of the properties. The court of appeals concluded a third-party beneficiary has standing to sue for legal malpractice if the party was named as a beneficiary in the decedent's overall estate plan.

62. *See id.* at 608-09.

applicable standard of reasonable care. Sometimes courts reject the use of expert testimony as unnecessary for establishing the duty of care and the breach of it when both are readily apparent to the judge and jury. In many states, experts cite professional conduct rules as some evidence of what constitutes a reasonable standard of care. Restatement §52 reports that some authorities hold that professional conduct rules alone define the standard of care. Other authorities take a more limited view of the conduct rules in establishing the duty of care, as in Hizey v. Carpenter, 830 P.2d 646 (Wash. 1992), where the court prohibited the use of the language of the rule in a jury instruction. *See* Rios v. McDermott, Will & Emery, 613 So. 2d 544 (Fla. Dist. Ct. App. 1993) ("an alleged [ethics rule violation] does not state a cause of action for malpractice"). The Scope Section of the Model Rules notes that a rule violation "should not give rise to a cause of action against a lawyer nor should it create any presumption in such a case that a legal duty has been breached . . . nor warrant any other nondisciplinary remedy, such as disqualification of a lawyer in a pending proceeding. [The rules] are not designed to be a basis for civil liability." Even with the Scope Section's caveats, the rules often play a role in establishing the appropriate duty of care in legal malpractice cases. *See* Desimini v. Durkin, 2015 U.S. Dist. Lexis 68266 (D.N.H. May 27, 2015) (ethics rules are relevant in most jurisdictions for establishing standard of care in malpractice cases, and reporting *Hizey* is a minority view if it excludes opinions of ethics rule violations).

Once the plaintiff shows the lawyer owed a duty and breached it, the party must prove causation and damages. Where the defendant-lawyer's error or omission in a previous case caused an adverse judgment against the plaintiff in litigation, the plaintiff must show that he would have obtained a different result in the previous case but for the lawyer's negligence. This is commonly known as the "trial within a trial" or a "case within a case" requirement. For example, the plaintiff must show that he would have obtained a better damages award or settlement in the first case if the defendant-lawyer had exercised reasonable care in litigation. The same principle applies in the non-litigation context. The legal malpractice plaintiff has to show in the transactional setting that he would have obtained a different result but for the lawyer's negligence. For example, assume a former client retained a lawyer to negotiate a real estate lease that the client now claims is deficient. The former client must show that but for the lawyer's errors and omissions, the client would have obtained a different result, presumably a better lease.

In many jurisdictions, a criminal defendant may also sue for legal malpractice but only after the underlying conviction is set aside. The defendant must also show that, but for the lawyer's misconduct, the result in the previous criminal case would have been different. Other jurisdictions impose a stricter standard for relief. They require the criminal defendant to prove his actual innocence in addition to having the conviction set aside and showing that a different result would have occurred but for the lawyer's misconduct.

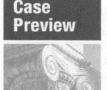

Case Preview

West Bend Mutual Insurance Co. v. Schumacher

In *West Bend Mutual Insurance Co. v. Schumacher*, the United States Court of Appeals for the Seventh Circuit ultimately affirmed the district court's dismissal of the plaintiff's legal malpractice case.

While reading the case, ask yourself the following questions:

1. What are the elements for legal malpractice under Illinois law?
2. Was Attorney Schumacher's conduct in representing West Bend consistent with the lawyer's duty to exercise reasonable care in providing professional services?
3. Why did the court find Schumacher's allegations concerning causation and damages to be deficient?
4. Finally, did the lawyer who represented West Bend in the instant legal malpractice case commit malpractice in not offering sufficient evidence to satisfy the "case within a case" requirement that is necessary for litigating a negligence claim in Illinois?

West Bend Mutual Insurance Co. v. Schumacher
844 F.3d 670 (7th Cir. 2016)

I. BACKGROUND

A

In December 2005, West Bend retained RLGZ to provide legal representation with respect to a workers' compensation claim filed by John Marzano against West Bend's insured, Nelson Insulation. Mr. Schumacher was the attorney with principal responsibility for defending against the Marzano claim.

. . .

According to the complaint, West Bend alleged that Mr. Schumacher breached duties to West Bend by virtue of "(a) his unauthorized stipulation concerning compensability; (b) his failure to adequately investigate the claim or claimant's pre-exi[s]ting medical condition; (c) his subsequent representations to [West Bend] regarding their litigation options[;] and (d) his failure to adequately advise [West Bend] of material facts and legal options prior to hearing." The specific allegations also concerned Mr. Schumacher's failure to depose Dr. Nelson [Marzano's independent medical expert whose testimony would be favorable to West Bend], his disclosure to Marzano's counsel of information beneficial to West Bend, and his failure to discover and remedy the unavailability of a relevant witness for the hearing.

All of these, West Bend alleged, resulted in its being "forced to accept a disadvantageous position which greatly compromised its ability to defend the claim." It also was "forced to pay additional sums and eventually chose to reach a disputed settlement in order to mitigate its exposure." . . .

B

The district court determined that, with respect to the bulk of West Bend's allegations about Mr. Schumacher's performance — including the failure to depose Dr. Nelson, the failure to contact witnesses prior to the hearing, and the disclosure of certain facts to Marzano's counsel — West Bend's complaint "does not . . . explain how any of these alleged acts and omissions harmed its defense." With respect to the allegation that Mr. Schumacher had represented that West Bend would accept liability, the district court stated:

> [P]laintiff admits that it could have contested the claim, despite the representation. In short, because plaintiff does not and cannot allege that defendants' representation was the cause of any damages it may have suffered, the representation cannot support a malpractice claim.

The court . . . concluded that West Bend had failed to state a claim in three successive complaints, [and] it terminated the case. West Bend now appeals.

II. DISCUSSION

A

2

The parties agree that Illinois law governs the elements of this legal malpractice action. The Supreme Court of Illinois has stated succinctly that a cause of action for legal malpractice includes the following elements: (1) the existence of an attorney-client relationship that establishes a duty on the part of the attorney, (2) a negligent act or omission constituting a breach of that duty, (3) proximate cause of injury, and (4) actual damages. Illinois courts have described the State's legal malpractice cause of action as following a case-within-a-case model:

> A legal malpractice suit is by its nature dependent upon a predicate lawsuit. Thus, a legal malpractice claim presents a case within a case. *[N]o* malpractice exists unless counsel's negligence has resulted in the loss of an underlying cause of action, or the loss of a meritorious defense if the attorney was defending in the underlying suit.

Therefore, in assessing the sufficiency of a complaint of legal malpractice we must focus on the underlying claim. The plaintiff must set forth a plausible statement not only that a breach of duty occurred but that the breach caused the plaintiff to lose a valid claim or defense in the underlying action and that, absent that loss, the underlying claim "would have been successful." "These elements effectively demand that the malpractice plaintiff present two cases, one showing that her attorney performed negligently, and a second or predicate 'case within a case' showing that she had a meritorious claim [or defense] that she lost due to her attorney's negligence." Mihailovich v. Laatsch, 359 F.3d 892, 904-05 (7th Cir. 2004).

B

There is no dispute that West Bend has described adequately the duty element in its malpractice claim. Nor is there any disagreement about the adequacy of

West Bend's narrative with respect to the alleged attorney conduct constituting a breach of that duty. In that respect, West Bend alleges that Mr. Schumacher, having assumed responsibility for the defense of the claim, failed to prepare adequately for the hearing, revealed inappropriately the defense theory of the case to Marzano's counsel, and then, without authorization, conceded liability for Marzano's workers' compensation claim.

The allegations with respect to causation and damages present, however, significant concerns. . . . While the complaint describes the conduct in some detail, it describes the underlying workers' compensation claim in rather summary fashion. Specifically, while the complaint identifies the injured party as John Marzano, it tells us nothing about his claimed injury or his claim against his employer. Instead, it summarily states that "[p]rior to August 2006, there existed *certain factual defenses and a medical causation defense* to the Marzano claim."

West Bend's brief on appeal invites our attention to paragraph 25 of the Second Amended Complaint as "set[ting] forth [its] factual allegations concerning defendants' breach of duty, proximate cause and damages." That paragraph of the complaint contains an abbreviated description of Mr. Schumacher's claimed errors, but, with respect to the crucial elements of causation and damages, says only that West Bend "was forced to accept *a disadvantageous position* which *greatly compromised* its ability to defend the claim." This same sort of general language appears in paragraph 28; there West Bend refers to a loss of "*valuable factual and legal defenses that* would have eliminated or substantially reduced any liability of [West Bend] to the claimant." These allegations are conclusory assertions and certainly do not set forth a plausible description of a lost defense that, absent Mr. Schumacher's alleged neglect, would have assured West Bend's success on the underlying claim.

West Bend has not invited our attention to any other factual allegations which detail the "valuable factual and legal defenses" lost because of Mr. Schumacher's litigation conduct.

With respect to the allegation that Mr. Schumacher had stipulated improperly to the compensability of the claim, West Bend at least makes the allegation that it was required to pay substantial amounts of money because of the stipulation. But it makes no concrete allegation that its final liability in this matter would have been any different if the stipulation had not occurred.

The . . . Complaint therefore leaves us to speculate as to whether and how West Bend would have prevailed on the underlying claim in the absence of the missteps of which it now accuses its former attorney. But, as our colleague in the district court recognized throughout West Bend's several attempts to improve the complaint, a plaintiff "must plead some facts that suggest a right to relief that is beyond the speculative level." The district court correctly concluded that the allegations that deal with the substance of the underlying compensation claim and defense fall short of that standard because they provide no plausible description as to how the attorney's negligence, if it occurred, was the cause of harm to West Bend. Even when evaluated as a whole, the complaint fails to describe, in even the most rudimentary of ways, "that but for [Mr. Schumacher's] negligence, the plaintiff would have been successful in th[e] underlying" workers' compensation action. . . .

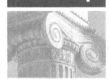

Post-Case Follow-Up

The *Schumacher* case highlights the need to be careful in pleading legal malpractice cases, especially in proving the lawyer's breach of a duty of reasonable care and that it caused the client's harm. Plaintiffs' lawyers may rely on multiple experts to establish these elements. For example, an ethics professor may testify about the defendant-lawyer's general duty of care under the jurisdiction's professional conduct rules, whether the defendant-lawyer's conduct breached that standard of care, and whether the breach caused the plaintiff's injury. A second expert who may be an experienced practitioner in the same or similar type of work giving rise to the instant legal malpractice claim may testify about how lawyers customarily act, whether the defendant-lawyer's conduct comported with the custom, and whether the breach caused the client's harm in the underlying case. Legal malpractice and the "trial within a trial" principle promise to remain a significant part of the litigation landscape. Based on West Bend's allegations of misconduct, what would you advise Schumacher to do differently in his next defense of a workers' compensation case? Would you hire Schumacher to represent you in light of his conduct in the *West Bend* case?

West Bend Mutual Insurance Co. v. Schumacher: Real Life Applications

1. After being eliminated from the Miss Universe beauty pageant, Monin took to social media and television to claim that the competition was rigged. The Miss Universe Organization filed an arbitration demand for $10 million, alleging breach of contract and defamation. Her attorney in the matter, Klineburger, advised Monin that the arbitration agreement did not apply because her copy of the agreement was unsigned. Klineburger notified the arbitrator that they were not obligated to participate in arbitration and refused to comply with discovery requests. Klineburger also demanded that the arbitrator communicate only with him as counsel for Monin, but he then did not relay information regarding the proceedings or hearing date to her. The arbitration proceeding that neither he nor Monin attended resulted in a $5 million award for the Miss Universe Organization as the arbitration clause was found applicable to Monin. The arbitrator noted that Monin's absence resulted in his drawing an adverse inference against her. It was at this time that Klineburger informed Monin of the proceedings and adverse judgment but stated that he could no longer represent her because he was not licensed in New York.

   Monin retains you to file a legal malpractice action against Klineburger to hopefully cover the $5 million judgment against her.

   a. What malpractice claims may you raise on her behalf?

   b. What ethics rules, if any, did Klineburger violate; and what is the significance of such violations in a legal malpractice action?

   c. Must you also report Klineburger to the statewide disciplinary counsel's office?

   d. Should you contact Klineburger before reporting him to the proper disciplinary authority?

   e. If Klineburger acted in good faith when he incorrectly advised Monin about the applicability of the arbitration clause, should the court in the discipline system be more forgiving of Klineburger's conduct?

2. A finance company sued attorney Ida Forti for legal malpractice for making a negligent misrepresentation in connection with loans made to Forti's brother-in-law, Dave King, a longtime and trusted client. King offered to secure the loan with farm machinery and asked Forti to prepare a letter stating there were no prior liens on the machinery. Relying on King's representation, Forti promptly prepared the letter without knowing that most of the farm machinery had already been pledged to other lenders. King obtained the loan, and a year later defaulted, then committed suicide.

   The finance company asks you, a local real estate lawyer who has done work for the company, if it can sue Forti for legal malpractice and what you think is its likelihood of success.

   a. Advise the company about any possible claims it might have against Forti for legal malpractice and the company's likelihood of success.

   b. In addition, the company believes Forti when she says she had no knowledge of the liens. The company's CEO feels sorry for her and does not want to jeopardize Forti's law license. The CEO asks you if there is any way to protect Forti's license.

   c. Should the fact that Forti relied on the representation of her "longtime and trusted" client insulate her from liability for either a legal malpractice claim or potential disciplinary action against her? Please discuss.

---

3. Legal Malpractice and Breach of Fiduciary Duty

The cornerstone of the fiduciary relationship is trust. This is reflected in traditional agency law, which is often used to characterize the lawyer-client professional relationship. The agent-lawyer owes a fiduciary duty to the principal-client to be trustworthy, including being loyal, competent, and protective of client confidences.

Case Preview

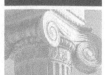

Burnett v. Sharp

Burnett identifies the core values of the fiduciary relationship as "integrity and fidelity." The case also demonstrates the close connection between the rules of professional conduct and the establishment of a fiduciary relationship. Plaintiffs often claim that a lawyer's violation of a duty contained in professional conduct rules is significant evidence that the lawyer breached his fiduciary responsibility to protect and promote the client's interests.

In reviewing *Burnett*, consider the following questions:

1. Did the court think there was a plausible justification for the lawyer believing he did not have to return the client's funds?
2. How does the court justify its holding that the lawyer's fiduciary duty to the client extends, even after the lawyer's discharge, until the lawyer returns funds belonging to the client?
3. What test does the court use to determine whether Burnett's claims have an arguable basis in the law?
4. Does the court provide for a change in its analysis if Burnett's decision to discharge his attorney was made in "bad faith"?

Burnett v. Sharp
328 S.W.3d 594 (Tex. App. 14th Dist. 2010)

[W]e construe the trial court's determination that Burnett "failed to state a cause of action as a matter of law" to be a determination that Burnett's claims have "no arguable basis in law." . . .

B. What Claims Did Burnett Plead?

. . .

Under a liberal construction of the petition, Burnett alleges the following:

- In June 2006, Burnett retained Sharp, a lawyer, to represent him in a criminal matter.
- Burnett gave Sharp a $3,000 retainer.
- Sharp had Burnett's case reset five times but did not provide any other legal services before Burnett replaced Sharp with another lawyer.
- Burnett called Sharp's office once, and Burnett's family called Sharp many times on behalf of Burnett, requesting a refund of the unearned portion of the retainer.
- Burnett served Sharp with a written demand for the return of the unearned portion of the retainer. Sharp did not respond to this demand, nor did Sharp return any part of the unearned retainer to Burnett.
- Sharp breached his fiduciary duty to Burnett by refusing to return the unearned part of Burnett's retainer.
- Sharp committed legal malpractice, negligence, and "deception."
- Burnett is seeking compensatory damages in the amount of $10,000.

Under a liberal construction of his petition, Burnett has pleaded claims for breach of fiduciary duty, money had and received, [and] conversion. . . . Avila v. Havana Painting Co. (Tex. App.-Houston [14th Dist.] 1988, writ denied) (holding that lawyer breached his fiduciary duty by refusing to return to former client funds in his possession which the former client was entitled to receive). The next question is whether the trial court erred in concluding that these claims have no arguable basis in law.

C. Do Burnett's Claims Have an Arguable Basis in Law?

Whether a claim has an arguable basis in law is a legal question to be reviewed de novo. A claim has no arguable basis in law only if it is based on (1) wholly incredible or irrational factual allegations; or (2) an indisputably meritless legal theory. An inmate's claim may not be dismissed merely because the court considers the allegations "unlikely." If Burnett's claims have an arguable basis in law, then the trial court erred in dismissing them as frivolous. Burnett's claims are not based on wholly incredible or irrational factual allegations. Therefore, the main issue on appeal is whether each of Burnett's claims is based on an indisputably meritless legal theory.

1. Breach-of-Fiduciary-Duty Claim

This court noted in *Avila* that, under a provision of the former Code of Professional Responsibility, a lawyer was required to promptly pay or deliver to the client all funds in the possession of the lawyer which the client was entitled to receive. The *Avila* court concluded that a lawyer's failure to promptly pay or deliver such funds constitutes a breach of fiduciary duty. In *Avila*, this court held that a lawyer breached his fiduciary duty by refusing to tender funds recovered for the client in a collection suit until after the client sued the lawyer for return of the funds. By the time the client sued the lawyer, the lawyer's representation must have been terminated. Therefore, the Avila court concluded that the lawyer had a fiduciary duty even after the lawyer's representation of the client in the collection suit had ended. A lawyer who refuses to pay or deliver funds belonging to his former client upon termination of the representation has breached a fiduciary duty owed to the former client.

The word fiduciary "'refers to integrity and fidelity.'" A breach of fiduciary duty occurs when a lawyer benefits improperly from his representation of the client by, among other things, a "failure to deliver funds belonging to the client." This court repeatedly has affirmed that a lawyer breaches his fiduciary duty if he refuses to give a client funds belonging to the client, and this court has never stated that this duty ceases if the client discharges the lawyer. Indeed, given that a client may be discharging his lawyer for good cause based on prior breaches by the lawyer of his fiduciary duty to the client, there are compelling reasons why this fiduciary duty should continue until the lawyer returns the client funds in his possession.

. . .

. . . Under Texas Disciplinary Rule of Professional Conduct 1.15(d), entitled "Declining or Terminating Representation," upon termination of a representation, the attorney shall, to the extent reasonably practical, surrender property that the client is entitled to receive to the client and shall refund any advance payment of attorney's fees that has not been earned. Given that, upon termination of the representation, a lawyer has a duty to return any unearned part of the retainer and any other client property to which the client is entitled, the return of such property to the client would appear to be one of the purposes of the representation and therefore would be part of the attorney-client relationship. . . .

For the reasons stated above, if, as alleged, Sharp refused to return uncarned retainer belonging to Burnett, then Sharp breached his fiduciary duty. Therefore, Burnett's breach-of-fiduciary duty claim is not based on an indisputably meritless legal theory, and the trial court erred in dismissing this claim as frivolous. . . .

. . .

III. CONCLUSION

Burnett's petition, liberally construed, contains claims for breach of fiduciary duty, money had and received, [and] conversion. . . . The first three claims are not based on (1) wholly incredible or irrational factual allegations; or (2) indisputably merit-less legal theories. Therefore, the trial court erred in dismissing these three claims as frivolous. . . . However, Burnett's negligence and intentionalmisrepresentation claims are based on indisputably meritless legal theories, and the trial court did not err in dismissing these claims as frivolous. Accordingly, . . . the judgment is . . . reversed, and remanded for further proceedings consistent with this opinion. . . .

Post-Case Follow-Up

Burnett highlights why plaintiffs allege more than one legal theory or claim when possible in a legal malpractice case. The *Burnett* court reversed the trial court's dismissal of the plaintiff's breach of fiduciary duty claim while affirming the dismissal of other claims, including the claim that Sharp was negligent. Burnett had not alleged a necessary element in his negligence claim, "that Sharp had exercised less care, skill or diligence than would be exercised by lawyers of ordinary skill and knowledge." Instead, Burnett's lawyer simply alleged in conclusory manner that Sharp was negligent. Lawyers must be careful to allege some factual basis to support each element of a negligence or fiduciary claim. In addition to the malpractice action, should Burnett's conduct also subject him to potential discipline? What sanction would you recommend? What strategies might you recommend to Burnett to help defend him in a discipline action?

Other courts have similarly held that the lawyer's failure to return client funds or property supports a breach of fiduciary duty claim. For example, in Hickey v. Scott, 738 F. Supp. 2d 55 (D.C. 2010), the parties signed a contract providing Scott would pay Hickey $225 per hour for legal services. In return, Hickey "will render [to Scott] a short summary statement of fees and disbursements for each month containing only the hours and fees spent on these matters along with a summary of disbursements spent during that month along with a reconciliation amount." After Scott won her Title VII action, a dispute arose concerning the amount owed to Hickey.

Hickey sued Scott for breach of contract, and she counterclaimed contending Hickey failed to provide competent legal services, violated D.C. Rule of Professional Conduct 1.5, and breached his fiduciary duty due to "a significant portion of hours which appear to have been excessive or inadequately documented." Both parties moved for summary judgment. The court held a jury could find on the record that Hickey violated the rules of professional conduct, and under the law such a finding would be sufficient to establish a breach of fiduciary duty, making summary judgment inappropriate.

Hickey highlights a common scenario. When a lawyer sues for legal fees, the client may respond by alleging the lawyer is not entitled to any fees because he committed malpractice and instead the lawyer owes the client damages. Professional conduct rules do not bar lawyers from suing clients for legal fees, but it should be a last resort strategy given the potential costs and adverse publicity associated with the effort.

Burnett v. Sharp: Real Life Applications

The Isley Brothers, a musical group, sued singer Coty Perez for copyright infringement, alleging Perez's 1991 hit "Love Is a Wonderful Thing" infringed on the Isley Brothers' copyright of their 1964 song with the same name. Mark Harris of Jones Night LLP jointly defended Perez; his record company, Sony Music Entertainment, Inc.; and Perez's music publishing company, Warner/Chappell, Inc. TIG, Warner/Chappell's insurance company, paid Jones Night for its joint representation. No one at Jones Night discussed the disadvantages of joint representation.

The Isley Brothers offered to settle the case for $700,000, but Harris never informed Perez of the offer. Nor did Harris inform Perez that an indemnification provision in his publishing contract would make him liable for damages if there was a final adverse judgment in the case. The case ended with a $5.4 million judgment against Perez and the other defendants. Perez believes there was a secret agenda between his lawyers and the publisher's insurance company to push the case to a final judgment instead of reaching a settlement, thereby triggering the indemnification provision in Perez's publishing contract and allowing TIG to recover from Perez.

He consults with you about suing Harris and his firm for $30 million for breach of fiduciary duty. Advise Perez.

---

4. Minimizing Liability for Legal Malpractice

Lawyers can minimize their exposure to legal malpractice claims by listening to their client's concerns and objectives, and establishing a good rapport to enhance client trust. This requires spending time with the client and promptly returning client calls and emails. Even if the lawyer cannot personally contact the client, someone in the lawyer's office should contact the client and provide an update, although non-lawyers have to be careful not to offer legal advice and commit the unauthorized practice of law. Also, lawyers can attend CLEs, periodically review office protocol, use a reliable calendaring and client intake process to safeguard against possible conflicts of interest, and conduct a peer review of firm forms or documents.

Another effective way for lawyers to minimize exposure to malpractice claims is to limit the scope of representation. Rule 1.2(c) permits this limitation "if the limitation is reasonable and the client gives informed consent." The rule assumes that the lawyer's legal services can be limited or compartmentalized without harming the client's overall legal objective. The lawyer is still obligated to provide competent representation even if the scope is limited. For example, a lawyer could agree to represent the author of a book for the limited purpose of only negotiating the publishing agreement once the author finds a publisher. This is unlike a situation where the lawyer undertakes the general representation of the author and is arguably responsible for a variety of related services, such as creating a corporation, tax planning, and marketing the book. The lawyer's obligation to negotiate the book can be neatly unbundled from the author's other related legal needs. Switch the matter to a contested divorce case and the result likely changes. A lawyer should not be permitted to agree to handle only the husband's property division in a contested divorce but not be responsible for the tax consequences of such a division or its effect on the custody battle over the children. These services are arguably inextricably bound together; it would be hard to competently negotiate a property division without taking into consideration its tax consequences and likely effect on custody.[63]

Another common method of limiting liability exposure among individual members in the firm is the creation of **limited liability partnerships** (LLPs) or **limited liability companies** (LLCs). General partnership doctrine holds partners jointly and individually liable for the misconduct of fellow partners. Following successful suits based on this doctrine, lawyers and other professional service providers advocated for these new limited liability structures. Under the structure, the firm still remains vicariously liable for a partner's, associate's, or part-time lawyer's malpractice, but individual partners' assets cannot be reached to satisfy a judgment beyond the LLP or firm insurance policy. In short, the LLP business form permits lawyers to be only personally liable for their own individual misfeasance should the firm's policy not cover a malpractice settlement or judgment.

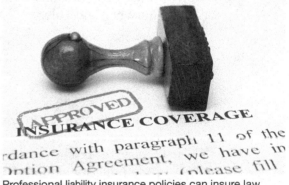

Professional liability insurance policies are technically labeled "errors and omissions" (E & O) policies, generally insuring the firm or individual lawyers for errors and omissions or negligent mistakes. E & O

Professional liability insurance policies can insure law firms and individual lawyers for errors and omissions or negligent mistakes.
Shutterstock.com

---

63. *See* Colo. Bar Ass'n, New Ethics Op. 101 (May 21, 2016), *available at* http://www.cobar.org/Portals/COBAR/ repository/ethicsOpinions/FormalEthicsOpinion_101.pdf; Stephanie L. Kimbro, *The Ethics of Unbundling*, 1 GPSolo eReport 3 (Oct. 2011), http://www.americanbar.org/publications/gpsolo_ereport/2011/october_2011/ ethics_ unbundling.html.

policies do not cover damages caused by a lawyer's intentional or criminal act, such as stealing client fees. Lawyers should also check their policy to see if it contains a "burning limit" provision that deducts the cost of defense from the policy coverage. Defense costs can be expensive, and this might expose the lawyer to financial risk if the damages exceed the policy cap. In addition, the lawyer needs to examine the policy's definition of legal services to ensure that the lawyer's work is covered. For example, will the policy cover advice to clients about where to invest the proceeds of a settlement?

Strong public policy reasons bar lawyers from contracting with clients to expressly limit their malpractice liability for professional work. It is unfair to force clients to waive future malpractice claims against their lawyers as the price for obtaining legal services and access to justice. The policy barring such contracts promotes public confidence in the profession because it precludes lawyers from contracting around liability for their misconduct, in effect discouraging shoddy services. Rule 1.8(h)(1) bars a lawyer from "mak[ing] an agreement prospectively limiting the lawyer's liability to a client for malpractice unless the client is independently represented in making the agreement." *See* Joann C. Rogers, *Mid-Representation Covered Future Malpractice*, 32 LAW. MAN. ON PROF. CONDUCT (ABA/BNA) 655 (2016) (discussing an Indiana case that permitted the firm to prospectively limit malpractice liability where client consulted independent counsel). In contrast, Restatement §54(4)(a) unconditionally prohibits a lawyer from prospectively limiting malpractice liability, a minority approach followed by a substantial number of states. Rule 1.8(h)(2) also bars lawyers from settling a claim or potential claim of malpractice without advising the client in writing of the desirability of seeking independent legal counsel in the matter. The lawyer must give the client adequate time to contact independent counsel. It is important to remember this rule as no one is perfect and the instinctive reaction for many lawyers is to reimburse the client as soon as possible for harm. Any ultimate settlement under this rule must be reasonable.

Chapter Summary

- Each state's high court has inherent authority to regulate the practice of law; federal courts and many government organizations (e.g., administrative agencies) also regulate the practice of law in their respective jurisdictions.
- Given the fiduciary nature of the lawyer-client relationship, courts generally require bar applicants to prove by clear and convincing evidence that they possess the requisite good character and fitness for bar admission.
- The legal profession is self-regulating, requiring lawyers to report misconduct that raises a substantial question about another lawyer's good character and fitness to practice law.
- Each state's high court normally disciplines lawyers for conduct code violations. Federal courts often adopt state disciplinary findings and sanctions.

■ Lawyer regulation is critical for protecting the public interest in access to justice, maintaining the integrity of the profession, and facilitating the administration of justice by the courts. The aim of the lawyer discipline system is to protect the public from miscreant lawyers through regulation; the purpose of legal malpractice lawsuits is to compensate clients and other private parties for harm caused by lawyers.

■ Lawyers may be civilly liable to clients and to some third parties for legal malpractice. Typical legal malpractice claims include breach of an express or implied contract, breach of fiduciary duty, and a breach of a duty of ordinary care or negligent representation.

Applying the Rules

1. John Burney applied for admission to the Massachusetts bar. In his application, Burney disclosed that he had been "wrongfully terminated" by two employers, and that he had brought multiple lawsuits involving separate incidents against former employers, attorneys, police officers, and a media outlet. These lawsuits alleged, in part, wrongful termination, violation of civil rights, defamation, breach of contract, malicious prosecution, and abuse of process.

   Due to inconsistencies with Burney's application, the board further investigated his litigation background and discovered information that Burney had failed to disclose in his application. During this investigation, it was determined that Burney represented himself *pro se*, and was reprimanded for various litigation misconduct, which resulted in Burney being sanctioned and held liable for costs and fees. Does Burney's personal history of litigation in his application alone suggest a lack of good character for bar admission? What, if any, effect do the board's investigation and findings have on your assessment of Burney's character and fitness for bar admission? If you were on the board, would you recommend that Burney reapply in a year?

2. Attorney Jupiter pled guilty in 2018 to one of four counts of making false, fictitious, or fraudulent claims to the IRS, arising out of his ill-advised scheme to claim $9.7 million in tax refunds. He served 18 months in prison. At his disciplinary hearing in 2018, Jupiter testified that he was at an "all time low" in his life when he committed the crime because of years of physical and emotional abuse by his wife, making him depressed and anxious. Jupiter was also going through a divorce and maintaining two households, and receiving counseling and taking antidepressant medication. Jupiter testified he never intended to obtain the tax refunds.

   According to his doctor, Jupiter suffered from a depressive disorder with psychotic features but because of subsequent treatment it was "highly unlikely that he would repeat the misconduct." His law partner for 25 years testified that Jupiter went "above and beyond the call of duty" to help his clients and that Jupiter appeared to be the victim of physical abuse on several occasions. Two of Jupiter's former clients also testified to his good character, with one being a friend who joined Jupiter on religious retreats.

In 2008, Jupiter was suspended for 6 months and again in 2014 for 18 months. The offenses included failing to communicate with a client and returning client files, neglecting a legal matter, failing to disburse settlement proceeds for more than a year, and maintaining an insufficient trust account balance. All but 30 days of the suspension time was stayed. You are part of the disciplinary board given the task of possibly disciplining Jupiter. What conduct rules has Jupiter violated? After considering possible aggravating and mitigating factors, what sanction would you recommend?

3. Attorney Rivera represented Jim Jones, the plaintiff in a medical malpractice case. Jones believed the surgeon committed malpractice during a routine "hip adjustment" at Mercy Hospital that left him unable to walk without a cane. Rivera had never handled a medical malpractice action, and before consulting anyone, including five other medical personnel in the operating room, Rivera sent a hasty demand letter to the surgeon and hospital seeking a $300,000 settlement. They both agreed to settle for that amount if Jones and Rivera kept the settlement confidential. Jones accepted the settlement based on Rivera's strong recommendation. Jones later learned from a nurse in the operating room that the surgeon was intoxicated during Jones's surgery and that the hospital had known about the surgeon's substance abuse problem for two years.

Jones contacts you to see if he has a potential malpractice claim against Rivera. Jones also tells you that Rivera reluctantly offered him $50,000 if Jones promised not to sue him for malpractice or file a disciplinary complaint. Advise Jones about the possibility of a legal malpractice lawsuit. Also, what, if any, ethics rules did Rivera violate?

Professional Responsibility in Practice

1. Should law schools play a greater gatekeeper role in screening graduates for good character and fitness for bar admission? How would schools assume a greater role? Outline your reasons why law schools should, or should not, assume a greater gatekeeper role and possible ways for law schools to implement such a role.

2. Explain the responsibility that individual lawyers have in the regulation of the profession. What are some of the practical problems associated with lawyers reporting the misconduct of other lawyers?

3. Research your state's law to learn if law firms, as well as individual lawyers, are subject to professional discipline. Is it a good idea to discipline law firms and not just individual lawyers? Articulate the reasons why law firms should, or should

not, be required to adopt proactive, management-based policies to ensure that their lawyers comply with ethics rules.

4. Should bar association websites post a lawyer's disciplinary history to protect the public? Should any posting include all grievances filed against a lawyer or only those resulting in discipline?

5. Identify the measures a lawyer can undertake in your state, consistent with professional conduct rules, to limit her exposure to a malpractice or disciplinary action.

6. There is literature discussing the benefits of doctors apologizing to their patients for their mistakes. Discuss the possible benefits and detriments of having lawyers or law firms apologize to their clients for their mistakes. Should an apology from a lawyer or law firm to a client for misconduct play any role in the lawyer disciplinary process?

The Attorney-Client Relationship

The Attorney-Client Relationship

The defining attribute of nearly all lawyering is the relationship between attorney and client. Lawyers work as agents for a client-principal — they work in a representative capacity, acting on behalf of other people or entities. This agency relationship entails fiduciary duties of the lawyer on behalf of the client. The lawyer owes the client core duties of loyalty, confidentiality, competence, communication, and conflict avoidance. The lawyer must protect the client's interests and must pursue the objectives of the client. The lawyer must fully disclose the nature of the engagement and any limitations on the lawyer's representation. The lawyer should undertake representation with the expectation that the lawyer will pursue it until completion. In addition, lawyers must not take advantage of their client-principal. They can only charge a reasonable fee and must safeguard client property. If the lawyer decides or is required to withdraw from a representation, the lawyer should work to mitigate any harm to the client flowing from that withdrawal. The lawyer is the client's loyal agent and must act as such in forming and dissolving the attorney-client relationship.

A. FORMING AN ATTORNEY-CLIENT RELATIONSHIP

As Susan Martyn summarizes, whenever an attorney-client relationship is created, either expressly or impliedly, "the law governing lawyers recognizes that the lawyer has assumed four core fiduciary obligations (the '4 C's'): Competence, Communication, Confidentiality, [and] Conflict of interest resolution."[1] The lawyer can be

Key Concepts

- Express and implied attorney-client relationships
- Duties owed to clients and prospective clients
- Allocation of authority between attorney and client
- Client identity: responsibilities to entity and government clients
- Charging and collecting attorneys' fees
- Handling client funds and property
- Terminating the attorney-client relationship

---

1. Susan R. Martyn, *Accidental Clients*, 33 HOFSTRA L. REV. 913, 914 (2005).

disqualified or subject to discipline or liability for breach of these core duties to her client. In a typical situation, the formation of the attorney-client relationship is done expressly—the attorney is formally hired by her client or appointed by a court and both the attorney and client are aware of the contours of the relationship and the obligations undertaken. Best and prudent practices commend an engagement letter or contract that clearly—in plain language that the client can understand—sets forth the terms of the relationship.

But best practices are not always possible. For example, on Friday, January 27, 2017, at 4:42 P.M. EST, President Donald Trump signed an executive order creating a three-month ban on entry into the United States by immigrants and non-immigrants from seven countries—Iraq, Syria, Sudan, Iran, Somalia, Libya, and Yemen. Federal officials from the Department of Homeland Security detained travelers—including those with valid green cards and visas—who arrived on flights beginning Friday evening and throughout Saturday and Sunday. Over that weekend, hundreds of lawyers throughout the United States went to international airports and offered to represent people who were being detained. Some lawyers had been recruited by the International Rescue Committee via email. Others were recruited through social media campaigns, and some lawyers saw news reports and just showed up at an airport. Lawyers held signs written in multiple languages offering free legal services and asked travelers who were disembarking if they knew of anyone who had been detained and then followed such leads.[2] Lawyers then filed petitions for writs of habeas corpus on behalf of these spur-of-the-moment clients, ultimately leading to several federal court preliminary injunctions as to certain classes of travelers.[3] Attorney Simon Sandoval-Moshenberg reported that he "reached out on Facebook trying to find potential plaintiffs and his inbox filled quickly. 'I was getting messages from people all over the world,' he said, 'including people who were writing in using the Wi-Fi from their planes. These are people who were lawfully boarding their flights, but as soon as the wheels hit the ground, they were covered by the executive order.'"[4] The exigency of the circumstances prescribed what would otherwise be very hastily made attorney-client relationships.

1. Implied Attorney-Client Relationships

An attorney-client relationship can also be implied—that is, the relationship is created without an express agreement. Courts have found an **implied attorney-client relationship** where attorneys received confidential information from a person and then provided legal advice. The relationships are found even though the attorney

---

2. *See, e.g.,* Jennifer Peltz & Frank Eltman, *Volunteer Lawyers Have Descended on Major Airports After Trump's Immigration Order,* AP NEWS, Jan. 31, 2017, *available at* https://apnews.com/article/5b0a350f937c4ee-0962a55221757c1f5; Jonah Engel Bromwich, *Lawyers Mobilize at Nation's Airports After Trump's Order,* N.Y. TIMES, Jan. 29, 2017, *available at* https://www.nytimes.com/2017/01/29/us/lawyers-trump-muslim-ban-immigration.html.
3. *See* Orin Kerr, *Four Federal Judges Issue Orders Blocking Parts of Trump's Executive Order on Immigration,* WASH. POST, Jan. 29, 2017, *available at* https://www.washingtonpost.com/news/volokh-conspiracy/wp/2017/01/29/four-federal-judges-issue-orders-blocking-parts-of-trumps-executive-order-on-immigration.
4. Dahlia Lithwick, *The Travelers Trapped in Horrific Limbo by Trump's Immigration Order,* SLATE, Jan. 29, 2017, *available at* https://slate.com/news-and-politics/2017/01/court-rulings-couldnt-protect-everyone-detained-because-of-trumps-immigration-order.html.

did not execute a formal contract or engagement agreement, did not receive a fee, and did not think that an attorney-client relationship had been formed. In certain situations, courts can and do infer — for purposes of malpractice, conflicts, confidentiality, and other duties — the existence of implied professional relationships between attorneys and clients.

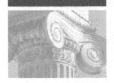

Case Preview

Togstad v. Vesely, Otto, Miller & Keefe

In *Togstad v. Vesely, Otto, Miller & Keefe*, attorney Jerre Miller was held liable for malpractice to the tune of $650,000 as to a client with whom Miller met for only 45 minutes and with whom he had no contract or engagement agreement. Indeed, Miller did not believe that he had undertaken an attorney-client relationship with the Togstads at all.

As you read *Togstad*, look for the following:

1. What actions did Miller undertake that led the court to find an implied professional relationship despite Miller's belief that no such relationship had been formed?
2. What are the two theories for finding an implied professional relationship set out by the court?
3. What could Miller have done to protect himself from malpractice in this case?

Togstad v. Vesely, Otto, Miller & Keefe
291 N.W.2d 686 (Minn. 1980)

This is an appeal by the defendants. . . . The jury found that the defendant attorney Jerre Miller was negligent and that, as a direct result of such negligence, plaintiff John Togstad sustained damages in the amount of $610,500 and his wife, plaintiff Joan Togstad, in the amount of $39,000. Defendants (Miller and his law firm) appeal to this court from the denial of their motion for judgment notwithstanding the verdict or, alternatively, for a new trial. We affirm.

In August 1971, John Togstad began to experience severe headaches and on August 16, 1971, was admitted to Methodist Hospital where tests disclosed that the headaches were caused by a large aneurism on the left internal carotid artery. The attending physician, Dr. Paul Blake, a neurological surgeon, treated the problem by applying a Selverstone clamp to the left common carotid artery. The clamp was surgically implanted on August 27, 1971, in Togstad's neck to allow the gradual closure of the artery over a period of days. . . . In the early morning hours of August 29, 1971, a nurse observed that Togstad was unable to speak or move. At the time, the clamp was one-half (50%) closed. Upon discovering Togstad's condition, the nurse called a resident physician, who did not adjust the clamp. Dr. Blake was also immediately informed of Togstad's condition and arrived about an hour later, at which time he opened the clamp. Togstad is now severely paralyzed in his right arm and leg, and is unable to speak.

Plaintiffs' expert, Dr. Ward Woods, testified that Togstad's paralysis and loss of speech was due to a lack of blood supply to his brain. Dr. Woods stated that the inadequate blood flow resulted from the clamp being 50% closed and that the negligence of Dr. Blake and the hospital precluded the clamp's being opened in time to avoid permanent brain damage. . . .

About 14 months after her husband's hospitalization began, plaintiff Joan Togstad met with attorney Jerre Miller regarding her husband's condition. . . .

Mrs. Togstad had become suspicious of the circumstances surrounding her husband's tragic condition due to the conduct and statements of the hospital nurses shortly after the paralysis occurred. . . .

Mrs. Togstad testified that she told Miller "everything that happened at the hospital," including the nurses' statements and conduct which had raised a question in her mind. She stated that she "believed" she had told Miller "about the procedure and what was undertaken, what was done, and what happened." She brought no records with her. Miller took notes and asked questions during the meeting, which lasted 45 minutes to an hour. At its conclusion, according to Mrs. Togstad, Miller said that "he did not think we had a legal case, however, he was going to discuss this with his partner." She understood that if Miller changed his mind after talking to his partner, he would call her. Mrs. Togstad "gave it" a few days and, since she did not hear from Miller, decided "that they had come to the conclusion that there wasn't a case." No fee arrangements were discussed, no medical authorizations were requested, nor was Mrs. Togstad billed for the interview.

Mrs. Togstad denied that Miller had told her his firm did not have expertise in the medical malpractice field, urged her to see another attorney, or related to her that the statute of limitations for medical malpractice actions was two years. She did not consult another attorney until one year after she talked to Miller. Mrs. Togstad indicated that she did not confer with another attorney earlier because of her reliance on Miller's "legal advice" that they "did not have a case." . . .

Miller's testimony was different in some respects from that of Mrs. Togstad. Like Mrs. Togstad, Miller testified that . . . the meeting [] lasted about 45 minutes. According to Miller, Mrs. Togstad described the hospital incident, including the conduct of the nurses. He asked her questions, to which she responded. Miller testified that "[t]he only thing I told her [Mrs. Tolgstad] after we had pretty much finished the conversation was that there was nothing related in her factual circumstances that told me that she had a case that our firm would be interested in undertaking."

Miller also claimed he related to Mrs. Togstad "that because of the grievous nature of the injuries sustained by her husband, that this was only my opinion and she was encouraged to ask another attorney if she wished for another opinion" and "she ought to do so promptly." He testified that he informed Mrs. Togstad that his firm "was not engaged as experts" in the area of medical malpractice, and that they associated with the Charles Hvass firm in cases of that nature. Miller stated that at the end of the conference he told Mrs. Togstad that he would consult with Charles Hvass and if Hvass's opinion differed from his, Miller would so inform her. Miller recollected that he called Hvass a "couple days" later and discussed the case with him. It was Miller's impression that Hvass thought there was no liability for malpractice in the case. Consequently, Miller did not communicate with Mrs. Togstad further.

. . .

Hvass stated that he had no recollection of Miller's calling him in October 1972 relative to the Togstad matter. He testified that: "when a person comes in to me about a medical malpractice action . . . I have to make a decision as to whether or not there probably is or probably is not . . . medical malpractice". . . . Hvass stated, however, that he would never render a "categorical" opinion. In addition, Hvass acknowledged that if he were consulted for a "legal opinion" regarding medical malpractice and 14 months had expired since the incident in question, "ordinary care and diligence" would require him to inform the party of the two-year statute of limitations applicable to that type of action.

. . . The jury found that Dr. Blake and the hospital were negligent and that Dr. Blake's negligence (but not the hospital's) was a direct cause of the injuries sustained by John Togstad; that there was an attorney-client contractual relationship between Mrs. Togstad and Miller; that Miller was negligent in rendering advice regarding the possible claims of Mr. and Mrs. Togstad; that, but for Miller's negligence, plaintiffs would have been successful in the prosecution of a legal action against Dr. Blake; and that neither Mr. nor Mrs. Togstad was negligent in pursuing their claims against Dr. Blake. The jury awarded damages to Mr. Togstad of $610,500 and to Mrs. Togstad of $39,000.

. . .

In a legal malpractice action of the type involved here, four elements must be shown: (1) that an attorney-client relationship existed; (2) that defendant acted negligently or in breach of contract; (3) that such acts were the proximate cause of the plaintiffs' damages; (4) that but for defendant's conduct the plaintiffs would have been successful in the prosecution of their medical malpractice claim.

This court first dealt with the element of lawyer-client relationship in the decision of Ryan v. Long, 35 Minn. 394, 29 N.W. 51 (1886). The *Ryan* case involved a claim of legal malpractice and on appeal it was argued that no attorney-client relation existed. This court, without stating whether its conclusion was based on contract principles or a tort theory, disagreed:

> [I]t sufficiently appears that plaintiff, for himself, called upon defendant, as an attorney at law, for "legal advice," and that defendant assumed to give him a professional opinion in reference to the matter as to which plaintiff consulted him. Upon this state of facts the defendant must be taken to have acted as plaintiff's legal adviser, at plaintiff's request, and so as to establish between them the relation of attorney and client.

Id. More recent opinions of this court, although not involving a detailed discussion, have analyzed the attorney-client consideration in contractual terms. . . . The trial court here . . . applied a contract analysis in ruling on the attorney-client relationship question. . . .

We believe it is unnecessary to decide whether a tort or contract theory is preferable for resolving the attorney-client relationship question raised by this appeal.

The tort and contract analyses are very similar in a case such as the instant one,[4] and we conclude that under either theory the evidence shows that a lawyer-client relationship is present here. The thrust of Mrs. Togstad's testimony is that she went to Miller for legal advice, was told there wasn't a case, and relied upon this advice in failing to pursue the claim for medical malpractice. In addition, according to Mrs. Togstad, Miller did not qualify his legal opinion by urging her to seek advice from another attorney, nor did Miller inform her that he lacked expertise in the medical malpractice area. Assuming this testimony is true, as this court must do, we believe a jury could properly find that Mrs. Togstad sought and received legal advice from Miller under circumstances which made it reasonably foreseeable to Miller that Mrs. Togstad would be injured if the advice were negligently given. Thus, under either a tort or contract analysis, there is sufficient evidence in the record to support the existence of an attorney-client relationship.

Defendants argue that even if an attorney-client relationship was established the evidence fails to show that Miller acted negligently in assessing the merits of the Togstads' case. They appear to contend that, at most, Miller was guilty of an error in judgment which does not give rise to legal malpractice. However, this case does not involve a mere error of judgment. The gist of plaintiffs' claim is that Miller failed to perform the minimal research that an ordinarily prudent attorney would do before rendering legal advice in a case of this nature. The record, through [expert testimony], contains sufficient evidence to support plaintiffs' position.

In a related contention, defendants assert that a new trial should be awarded on the ground that the trial court erred by refusing to instruct the jury that Miller's failure to inform Mrs. Togstad of the two-year statute of limitations for medical malpractice could not constitute negligence. . . .

The defect in defendants' reasoning is that there is adequate evidence supporting the claim that Miller was also negligent in failing to advise Mrs. Togstad of the two-year medical malpractice limitations period and thus the trial court acted properly in refusing to instruct the jury in the manner urged by defendants. One of defendants' expert witnesses, Charles Hvass, testified:

Q: Now, Mr. Hvass, . . . wouldn't ordinary care and diligence require that you inform them that there is a two-year statute of limitations within which they have to act or lose their rights?

A: Yes. I believe I would have advised someone of the two-year period of limitation, yes.

---

4. Under a negligence approach it must essentially be shown that defendant rendered legal advice (not necessarily at someone's request) under circumstances which made it reasonably foreseeable to the attorney that if such advice were rendered negligently, the individual receiving the advice might be injured thereby. *See, e.g.,* Palsgraf v. Long Island R. Co., 248 N.Y. 339 (1928). Or, stated another way, under a tort theory, "(a)n attorney-client relationship is created whenever an individual seeks and receives legal advice from an attorney in circumstances in which a reasonable person would rely on such advice." 63 MINN. L. REV. 751, 759 (1979). A contract analysis requires the rendering of legal advice pursuant to another's request and the reliance factor, in this case, where the advice was not paid for, need be shown in the form of promissory estoppel. *See,* 7 C.J.S., Attorney and Client, §65; *Restatement (Second) of Contracts,* § 90.

Consequently, . . . we must reject the defendants' contention, as it was reasonable for a jury to determine that Miller acted negligently in failing to inform Mrs. Togstad of the applicable limitations period.

. . .

Affirmed.

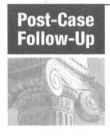

Post-Case Follow-Up

Mrs. Togstad and Miller report somewhat conflicting accounts of their meeting. When a client is under the impression that an attorney is representing her and testifies as much, is a jury likely to find more credible the testimony of the client or a conflicting account by the lawyer? Moreover, consider whether a judge is likely to place responsibility on the attorney to communicate clearly with a prospective client regarding whether or not the attorney is undertaking a representation.

In Westinghouse Elec. Corp. v. Kerr-McGee Corp., 580 F.2d 1311 (7th Cir. 1978), the United States Court of Appeals for the Seventh Circuit explained that an implied professional relationship arises "when the lay party submits confidential information to the [lawyer] with reasonable belief that the latter is acting as the former's attorney." Thus, in *Togstad*, the fact that Mrs. Togstad conveyed confidential information to Miller and reasonably believed he was acting as her attorney created an attorney-client relationship for purposes of malpractice. The onus is on the attorney to clarify the absence of a relationship whenever there is reasonable ambiguity. A common and prudent method to avoid such misunderstandings is by using a written declination letter memorializing that the attorney is not undertaking a representation or establishing an attorney-client relationship and advising the putative client of any statute of limitations or other deadlines and of the need to seek other legal counsel should she wish to pursue the matter.

Togstad v. Miller: Real Life Applications

1. Tamara is an attorney who is asked to speak at a local Chamber of Commerce event in her hometown about basic issues regarding small business operation and contracts. After the meeting, one of the attendees, Behzad, comes up and asks Tamara about the enforceability of a contract that he had entered into to perform contractor work, where the homeowner is obnoxious and has made it difficult for him to complete the work. He tells her he really wishes he didn't have to complete it. Tamara responds, "Don't we all wish that about our jobs! But it sounds to me like the owner maybe already breached the contract by making your work difficult — which would mean you wouldn't be obligated to finish." Assume that Behzad decides, based on this conversation, to stop working on the project and is successfully sued for $25,000 for breach of contract. Analyze whether Behzad had an attorney-client relationship with Tamara and whether he can sue her for legal malpractice.

2. Charles hired Joel to file a personal injury lawsuit on his behalf. Joel realized that the statute of limitations was running soon and that a complaint needed to be filed immediately. He was about to file the complaint when he realized that he had failed to pay his yearly bar dues and his license had lapsed for that failure. Joel called his friend, Thomas, and asked Thomas if he would just sign the complaint and file it for him, promising that Joel would then take care of serving the complaint, pay his dues and get his license reinstated, and take over the matter — Thomas need not do anything further. Thomas agreed, then affixed his name, signature, and attorney number on the complaint and had it filed. Unbeknownst to Thomas, Joel failed to timely serve the complaint. Charles's case was dismissed for failing to serve the complaint, and the statute of limitations had meanwhile run. Did Thomas have an attorney-client relationship with Charles, and can he be sued for malpractice or disciplined for incompetence in handling the case?

2. Prospective Clients

Model Rule 1.18 was added by the Ethics 2000 Commission and defines when someone is a **"prospective client"** and what duties are owed to those who fall within that category. The duties created by Rule 1.18 exist regardless of whether an express or implied attorney-client relationship is formed. Thus, even if an attorney makes it absolutely clear that he is not taking on a representation, the attorney will still owe the "prospective client" the duties set out in Rule 1.18. Yet the duties established in Rule 1.18 are watered down from the duties owed to a client under a normal express or implied attorney-client relationship. Under the rule, a prospective client is defined as "[a] person who consults with a lawyer about the possibility of forming a client-lawyer relationship with respect to a matter." The key term in this definition is "consult." If an attorney has consulted with a person, then that person is a prospective client.

How much communication is required for there to be a consultation triggering the application of Rule 1.18? Comment [2] to Rule 1.18 explains that it "depends on the circumstances," yet "a consultation is likely to have occurred if a lawyer, either in person or through the lawyer's advertising in any medium, specifically requests or invites the submission of information about a potential representation," and "a person provides information in response." On the other hand, the comment makes clear that where "a person communicates information unilaterally to a lawyer, without any reasonable expectation that the lawyer is willing to discuss the possibility of forming a client-lawyer relationship," the person is not a prospective client and the requirements of Rule 1.18 do not apply.

Could a prospective client seek a consultation with an attorney for the very purpose of creating a conflict so that the attorney cannot represent the opposing side? Indeed, couldn't a scheming person arrange to have initial consultations with all the best attorneys in a locality, purposefully disclose information, and then argue that the opposing side is conflicted out from using any of those attorneys?

Comment [2] to Model Rule 1.18 directly addresses this kind of **conflict shopping**, stating that "a person who communicates with a lawyer for the purpose of disqualifying the lawyer is not a 'prospective client'" under the rule and thus the duties imposed by Rule 1.18 do not apply. Nevertheless, it is not always easy to demonstrate that a party was engaged in conflict shopping rather than honestly seeking an excellent attorney.

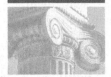

Case Preview

In re Marriage of Perry

In January 2008, Karen Perry called Gail Goheen's law office to discuss potentially filing for divorce from Karen's husband, Terance Perry. Karen spoke with Goheen's assistant and later with Goheen herself, but ultimately hired a different attorney. In 2009, Terance, himself an attorney, filed for divorce. He went through three different attorneys and even briefly represented himself. Then in February 2011 — three years after Karen had called Goheen's office and spoken with her — Terance hired Goheen to represent him in the divorce. Karen moved to disqualify Goheen, arguing both (1) that she had an implied professional relationship with Goheen; and (2) that she was Goheen's prospective client and thus Goheen was prohibited from representing Terance under Montana Rule 1.20 — which is nearly identical to Model Rule 1.18, although numbered differently.

As you read *Perry*, look for the following:

1. What is the standard for finding a disqualifying conflict of interest under Rule 1.18?
2. Did Goheen receive confidential information from Karen in the initial consultation? Was the information significantly harmful to Karen?
3. Did Goheen use or reveal confidential information she received from Karen? How does the court determine this issue?

In re Marriage of Perry
293 P.3d 170 (Mont. 2013)

On December 4, 2009, Terance filed for dissolution of his marriage to Karen in Missoula County. . . . [On February 25, 2011, Terance filed a substitution of counsel] naming Goheen as his counsel of record.

In January 2008, before any dissolution proceedings were filed, Karen contacted Goheen's office in Hamilton seeking legal advice concerning the potential filing of a dissolution action. Karen spoke with Goheen's assistant, Kailah Van Note (Van Note), and later Goheen herself.

Karen filed a motion to disqualify Goheen and an application for a preliminary injunction on March 1, 2011. Terance opposed the motion and filed two office memorandums and affidavits from Goheen and Van Note regarding their telephone conversations with Karen. A disqualification hearing was held on November 7, 2011. . . .

At the hearing, Karen testified that she provided personal information about herself and Terance during one telephone conversation with Van Note and two telephone conversations with Goheen. Karen said the conversations with Goheen lasted 45 minutes and 3 minutes, respectively. She said that she gave information about the marriage, including domestic abuse [which Terrance denied occurred] and finances, and that she asked for legal advice on her "position," which she described as: "[w]here I wanted to end up. If I could end up at a certain place. What would happen if I stayed here. What [would] happen if I left here. Goals of settlement. My weaknesses and fears." Karen testified that she identified individuals who were present during domestic disputes. She said Goheen quoted her a "ridiculously enormous" retainer, but conceded that she was never sent a retainer agreement and that Goheen had "denied representation." . . . Karen testified that she thought the information she gave to Goheen's office would be confidential. . . .

When asked "[h]ow does Gail Goheen's representation of your husband now, in this dissolution of marriage that he brought three years later, harm you," Karen responded:

[P]sychologically, it's like getting beat up again by him. It's like I can't trust anybody. There's nobody I can turn to. He took away everything and everybody I could trust. And now he's done it again with somebody who I confided in, who's now on the opposite side of the table. And it — I — I'm betrayed again. It's another form of abuse and control. . . .

[T]he District Court permitted Goheen to offer testimony about the length of the telephone conversations, her office procedures, and background information established in the court file. Goheen testified without another attorney questioning her. Goheen admitted to having one conversation with Karen in January 2008, which she said lasted less than 12 minutes because the time entry information on the record was left blank and it is her office policy that time information is left blank when a conversation lasts 12 minutes or less. Goheen denied having a second conversation with Karen. Explaining her office procedures for new clients, Goheen stated:

Whenever I meet with a client, Your Honor, I don't do it over the phone, in the sense of getting information. I sit down and I meet with the client for a half a day, usually, is my first meeting with a client on a divorce action. . . .

It's at that time that I go over everything I can think of . . . . All details.

I'm not interested in it, information, in terms of any details prior to that time. And my policy is that I never give anybody a retainer quote until I get all that information.

So I can state unequivocally [sic] that I would not have given a retainer quote to Karen Perry, or any other client under these circumstances.

Goheen said she was aware that Karen's husband was an attorney at Datsopoulos, MacDonald & Lind and that she does not represent someone against an attorney in Ravalli or Missoula County when the opposing attorney is from a firm that she regularly faces in divorce cases. Goheen said she did not remember the details of a conversation with Karen, relying on the office memorandums created from her and Van Note's conversations with Karen. Goheen said that a 45 minute telephone conversation did not occur, and that her telephone records indicate she made a two or three minute telephone call to refuse the case and refer Karen to someone else. Goheen said she was notified by Karen's current attorney that Karen had contacted Goheen's office in September 2009 and in January 2010 but that her telephone records revealed only two telephone conversations with Karen in January 2008. Van Note also testified about Goheen's office procedures.

[T]he District Court denied Karen's motion to disqualify and application for a preliminary injunction. . . .

DISCUSSION

1. Did the District Court err by denying Karen's motion to disqualify Goheen as counsel for Terance pursuant to Rule 1.20 of the Montana Rules of Professional Conduct?

Karen claims that the District Court erred by not disqualifying Goheen because an implied attorney-client relationship was formed between Karen and Goheen when Karen gave Goheen information that was "confidential" in nature. . . . Karen [argues] that she is "psychologically harmed" by the fact that Terance has hired Goheen and "[t]he district court did not properly address the correct standard or pertinent issue relative to Rule 1.20(c) with respect to the harm to Karen in determining Goheen's conflict of interest."

We have not yet addressed a lawyer's duty to prospective clients under the Montana Rules of Professional Conduct as amended in 2004. We considered this relationship under prior rules in *Pro-Hand Services*, stating:

> An implied attorney-client relationship may result when a prospective client divulges confidential information during a consultation with an attorney for the purpose of retaining the attorney, even if actual employment does not result. . . . In determining whether an implied attorney-client relationship exists, we will examine whether the alleged client reasonably believed that such relationship was formed.

. . . [At that time,] [i]f confidential information was not disclosed [by the client], then an attorney-client relationship did not exist. [Moreover,] "[i]f an attorney-client relationship was not formed, there is no conflict of interest," and an attorney could then represent a client in a matter that was adverse to the former prospective client.

In 2004, Rule 1.20 [the same as Model Rule 1.18], entitled "Duties to Prospective Clients" was adopted. Rule 1.20 defines and addresses a lawyer's relationship with a prospective client. It provides . . . :

> (a) A person who consults with or has had consultations with a lawyer about the possibility of forming a client-lawyer relationship with respect to a matter is a prospective client.
>
> (b) Even when no client-lawyer relationship ensues, a lawyer who has had consultations with a prospective client shall not use or reveal information learned in the consultation(s), except as Rule 1.9 would permit with respect to information of a former client.

(c) A lawyer subject to paragraph (b) shall not represent a client with interests materially adverse to those of a prospective client in the same or a substantially related matter if the lawyer received information from the prospective client that could be significantly harmful to that person in the matter, except as provided in paragraph (d). If a lawyer is disqualified from representation under this paragraph, no lawyer in a firm with which that lawyer is associated may knowingly undertake or continue representation in such a matter, except as provided in paragraph (d). . . .

Instead of determining whether an attorney-client relationship was created by disclosure of confidential information, Rule 1.20 creates duties to the prospective client "[e]ven when no client-lawyer relationship ensues." Mont. R. Pro. C. 1.20(b). Generally, and subject to exceptions discussed herein, a lawyer may not "use or reveal information learned in the consultation(s)" with a prospective client. Pertinent to the present issue, Rule 1.20 also prohibits a lawyer from representing a party with "interests materially adverse" to the prospective client in the same or substantially related proceeding "if the lawyer received information from the prospective client that could be significantly harmful to that person in the matter." Mont. R. Pro. C. 1.20(c). Thus, Rule 1.20 does not merely consider whether information was divulged by the prospective client but whether such information could be significantly harmful to that person in that or a related matter. Rule 1.18 of the American Bar Association's Model Rules of Professional Conduct (Model Rules) is nearly identical to Montana Rule 1.20. The Committee Comments to Model Rule 1.18 state "the lawyer is not prohibited from representing a client with interests adverse to those of the prospective client in the same or a substantially related matter unless the lawyer has received from the prospective client information that could be significantly harmful if used in the matter." Model R. Prof. Conduct 1.18 cmt. 6 (ABA 2012).

. . . Karen is a "prospective client" as defined by Rule 1.20(a) ("A person who consults with or has had consultations with a lawyer about the possibility of forming a client-lawyer relationship with respect to a matter is a prospective client."). Karen called Goheen's office more than once and spoke with Van Note and Goheen concerning representation. The question here does not depend on whether an attorney-client relationship was established or whether Karen reasonably believed such a relationship was formed, as in *Pro-Hand Services*. Rather, under Rule 1.20, the question [relevant to disqualification] is whether the information conveyed in Karen's conversations could be significantly harmful to Karen in this dissolution proceeding.

After hearing the testimony, the District Court found that the information conveyed by Karen to Goheen was not harmful to Karen. The court found that Goheen's office documentation of Karen's phone calls and the testimony of Goheen and Van Note were credible and that "there was nothing disclosed by Karen to Ms. Goheen or her staff 'that could be significantly harmful' to Karen in this matter." Karen claims a personal or psychological victimization by Goheen's representation of Terance. While we do not minimize the significance of such an effect, Rule 1.20 requires that the lawyer receive "information" that is "significantly harmful" to Karen in the proceeding. Karen did not establish that any information she divulged to Goheen in the telephone calls several years earlier could have any impact on the proceeding, particularly since, as discussed [], Goheen was not associated as counsel until three years into the proceeding, by which time substantially more information had been disclosed than the information Karen claims to have shared during those phone calls. We therefore conclude that the District Court did not abuse its discretion in denying Karen's motion to disqualify under Rule 1.20.

. . . Karen also argues that Goheen violated Rule 1.9 by using or disclosing information Karen had divulged to her. Because the provisions of Rule 1.9 regarding use of former client information are incorporated by Rule 1.20, governing the duties to prospective clients, we take up Karen's argument in that regard.

Rule 1.20(b) provides that "a lawyer who has had consultations with a prospective client shall not use or reveal information learned in the consultation(s), except as Rule 1.9 would permit with respect to information of a former client." Mont. R. Pro. C. 1.20(b). In turn, Rule 1.9 states, in pertinent part:

> (c) A lawyer who has formerly represented a client in a matter or whose present or former firm has formerly represented a client in a matter shall not thereafter: (1) use information relating to the representation to the disadvantage of the former client except as these Rules would permit or require with respect to a client, or when the information has become generally known; or (2) reveal information relating to the representation except as these Rules would permit or require with respect to a client.

Mont. R. Pro. C. 1.9(c).

. . . As established under Issue 1, Karen has not demonstrated that Goheen received information that could be significantly harmful to her in this proceeding. . . . The parties had previously filed information detailing Karen's and Terance's personal information, the parties' financial situations, and Karen's affidavits alleging spousal abuse. In its order, the District Court found that "any information regarding Terance's alleged abuse of Karen is now moot given what Karen herself subsequently disclosed early on in this case." The District Court permitted Goheen to testify concerning the background information in the court file, then permitted Goheen to testify as to the length of the telephone conversations with Karen, and Goheen's office procedures. It was permissible under the Rules for Goheen to use this information about her previous contact with Karen "to respond to allegations in any proceeding concerning the lawyer's representation of the client." Mont. R. Pro. C. 1.6(b)(3). The District Court properly limited Goheen's testimony to prevent disclosure of Karen's confidences, if any.

Karen's allegations against Goheen are generalized and vague. Goheen's limited use of Karen's information was permitted under Rules 1.6(b) and 1.9(c), and Goheen did not violate a duty to Karen.

Post-Case Follow-Up

In *Perry*, even though Karen had given Goheen confidential information, the court did not find a disqualifying conflict under Rule 1.18 because Goheen had not obtained "information from the prospective client that could be significantly harmful" to Karen. Karen argued that the information was "significantly harmful" because it was psychologically harmful to have someone she had confided in turn around and represent her husband. For Karen, it was the feeling of betrayal that was "significantly harmful" to her. What language from the rule did the court rely on in rejecting Karen's interpretation?

When is information "significantly harmful" to the prospective client such that a disqualification is appropriate? A Wisconsin ethics opinion surveys cases where information has been found to be significantly harmful within the meaning of Rule 1.18. The opinion synthesizes the cases to "fashion a loose definition of 'significantly harmful information.'" The opinion states:

> Information may be "significantly harmful" if it is sensitive or privileged information that the lawyer would not have received in the ordinary course of due diligence; or if it is information that has long-term significance or continuing relevance to the matter, such as motives, litigation strategies, or potential weaknesses. "Significantly harmful" may also be the premature possession of information that could have a substantial impact on settlement proposals and trial strategy; the personal thoughts and impressions about the facts of the case; or information that is extensive, critical, or of significant use.[5]

What happens when a consulting attorney receives information that is "significantly harmful" to the prospective client? Under Model Rule 1.18(c), the consulting attorney is prohibited from representing a client in the same or a substantially related matter adversely to the prospective client, and the disqualification is imputed to the entire firm. However, the lawyer and law firm can avoid imputation through a screening and notice procedure outlined in Model Rule 1.18(d). The screening and notice option is only available if the consulting lawyer "took reasonable measures to avoid exposure to more disqualifying information than was reasonably necessary to determine whether to represent the prospective client." If so, then the conflict is not imputed to the firm as long as the consulting lawyer is "timely screened" from the matter and "apportioned no part of the fee therefrom," and "written notice is promptly given to the prospective client."

In re Marriage of Perry: Real Life Applications

1. Kelly has just been injured in a car accident. She searches online for personal injury lawyers, opening the website of Jarret & Maine, a personal injury law firm. As soon as she opens the site, a chatbox pops up with the words, "Can we help you?" Kelly types in the facts of what happened in the lawsuit and submits it. She gets a response that Jarret & Maine will get back to her shortly. Kelly decides not to wait and closes the page. A couple months later, Kelly is sued by the other driver involved in the wreck, Jason. Jason is represented by Jarret & Maine. Consider whether Kelly is a prospective client of Jarret & Maine. Can the firm represent Jason against her?

---

5. Wisconsin State Bar Professional Ethics Committee, Wisconsin Ethics Op. EI-10-03: *Avoid Conflicts When Consulting with Prospective Clients. See also* ABA Formal Op. 492: *Obligations to Prospective Clients: Confidentiality, Conflicts and "Significantly Harmful" Information* (2020).

2. Attorney Carpenter has a friend, Thompson, who is an oil and gas landman. Thompson learns that a deceased person owned the mineral rights to a large portion of land. Thompson spent 300 hours researching the decedent's heirs. He discovers that part of the mineral rights were bequeathed to a local church. Thompson meets with Carpenter about potentially helping him lease the mineral rights from the church. Thompson shows Carpenter all of the documents that he has found pertaining to the mineral interests, including a prior notice from the surface owners that the mineral rights have lapsed. The next day Carpenter sends Thompson a letter stating that he cannot represent Thompson because he previously represented the church. Can someone else in Carpenter's firm represent Thompson? Can Carpenter represent the church? Can Carpenter notify the church of its rights and the potential lapse discovered by Thompson?

B. ALLOCATION OF ATTORNEY AND CLIENT AUTHORITY

Once an attorney-client relationship is formed, how should this agent-principal relationship work? Does the principal-client get to call the shots while the agent-lawyer simply takes orders? For example, imagine that a client comes to you and tells you about a situation where the client feels she has been wronged and wants to sue immediately on a whole panoply of claims. The area of law is one with which you are familiar and you know that some of the things for which your client wants to sue are not legally cognizable wrongs—although your client has one or two possible causes of action. Who makes the decision to sue or not? Who decides what claims and legal theories should be asserted? Who decides how much discovery should be done and how much should be spent on discovery? If the case goes to trial, who decides which witnesses to call? Who decides what the scope of cross-examination will be? Who decides whether to appeal an adverse judgment?

1. Basic Allocation of Authority

Model Rule 1.2 addresses the basic allocation of authority between the attorney and client. The rule explains that, in general, "a lawyer shall abide by a client's decisions concerning the objectives of the representation." In other words, it is the client who has the ultimate authority to decide the objectives, or as comment [1] puts it, "the purposes to be served," by the representation. Nevertheless, there are limits on the client's ability to determine the objectives of a representation—as indicated by Rule 1.2(d) and comment [1], the client's objectives must fall "within the limits imposed by law and the lawyer's professional obligations." Thus, a lawyer is prohibited under Rule 1.2(d) from counseling or assisting a client in knowingly criminal or fraudulent conduct—even (and perhaps especially) if that's what the client wants the lawyer to do.

While the client determines the objectives of the representation, the attorney is given more control over "the means by which [those objectives] are pursued."

Importantly, the attorney is required to "consult with the client" regarding those means as set forth in Rule 1.4. In addition, the attorney is permitted to "take such action on behalf of the client as is impliedly authorized to carry out the representation." *See* Model Rule 1.2(a). When there is a dispute between the attorney and client as to the means to be used, comment [2] provides a basic methodology for resolution:

> Clients normally defer to the special knowledge and skill of their lawyer with respect to the means to be used to accomplish their objectives, particularly with respect to technical legal and tactical matters. Conversely, lawyers usually defer to the client regarding such questions as the expense to be incurred and concern for third persons who might be adversely affected.

The comment explains that this basic dichotomy does not specify how all potential disputes should be resolved. If a lawyer and client disagree about whether to depose a certain person, for example, both interests are called into play — on the one hand, deposing someone is a tactical and technical matter for a case, yet it is also expensive and can adversely affect third persons (the person being deposed). Ultimately, comment [2] indicates that if a conflict cannot be resolved, the lawyer may withdraw on the basis of "a fundamental disagreement with the client" or the client can fire the attorney.

Attorneys should work with clients to resolve differences in an amicable and supportive manner. Badgering a client or being obnoxious or abusive will likely lead to being fired and may even lead to discipline. In *Sallee v. Tennessee Board of Professional Responsibility* (excerpted later in this chapter), attorney Yarboro Sallee wrote the following to her client when seeking additional fees:

> Your back seat driving will destroy [the case] . . . I will not brook [sic] anymore second guessing. . . . The cases need what they need Fran[,] and you don't know anything about it. . . . I will send you a proposal and you can agree to find someone else, but I will have the right to file against any funds recovered in the future by any other lawyer. . . . You are not the lawyer, I am. You don't know enough to know what I need. I do.

As we will see below, Sallee was charging her client a clearly excessive fee, and ultimately was fired and suspended from the practice of law.[6]

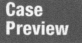
Case Preview

Red Dog v. Delaware

James Allen Red Dog, a Native American of the Lakota tribe of the Sioux, was sentenced to death for murder, kidnapping, and rape. He was executed by lethal injection on March 3, 1993.[7] A week before his execution, attorneys from the public defender's office representing him filed a motion for a stay of

---

6. Sallee v. Tennessee Board of Professional Responsibility, 469 S.W.3d 18, 24 (Tenn. 2015).
7. *See States Execute Two Murderers*, N.Y. Times, Mar. 4, 1993, *available at* http://www.nytimes.com/1993/03/04/us/states-execute-two-murderers.html.

execution. When the stay was denied, the attorneys filed an appeal. As the Supreme Court of Delaware explained, both the motion for the stay and the appeal were filed "without Red Dog's authorization and despite his express oral and written directions to the contrary."[8] Indeed, Red Dog had stated in a handwritten note: "I desire no appeals or any motions for stay of execution, scheduled for March 3, 1993 to be filed on my behalf." And when Red Dog learned about the motion for the stay of execution, "he personally advised the Superior Court in writing, on February 25, 1993, that the motion was 'against my wishes.'"[9] Red Dog asserted that disputing his death sentence "would violate his warrior's code."[10]

As you read *Red Dog*, consider the following:

1. Were the attorneys required to abide by Red Dog's desire to accept the death penalty and his instructions not to take any appeals?
2. What could the attorneys have done if they were strongly morally opposed to the death penalty?
3. Should a lawyer take actions (such as asserting a client's mental incompetence) that absolutely undermine the client's autonomy in order to pursue what the lawyer believes is in the client's "best interest" (here, the value of Red Dog's life)? Is it necessarily irrational for a client to prefer death over, say, life imprisonment?
4. If his attorneys truly believed that Red Dog was mentally incompetent to make decisions, what should they have done?

Red Dog v. Delaware
625 A.2d 245 (Del. 1993)

In Red Dog v. State, 620 A.2d 848 (1993), this Court affirmed a decision of the Superior Court which denied a stay of execution in a capital case. Therein, we held "that in the absence of a genuine issue of material fact as to Red Dog's present mental competency, the public defenders had no standing to file . . . a motion to stay his execution in derogation of his express directions to the contrary." *Id.* at 853. On independent and alternative grounds, we affirmed Red Dog's competency as well as the lack of standing of the Public Defender.

. . . Thereafter, Rules to Show Cause were directed to Lawrence M. Sullivan, the Public Defender of the State of Delaware, and Brian J. Bartley, Bernard J. O'Donnell, Edward C. Pankowski, and Nancy J. Perillo, all Assistant Public Defenders (collectively "Respondents"), directing responses as to why sanctions should not be imposed upon them for certain aspects of their representation of the defendant.

The Respondents filed written responses defending their actions as within the bounds of professional responsibility and required by the exigencies of representation of a defendant facing execution. . . .

---

8. *See* Red Dog v. State, 620 A.2d 848, 848 (Del. 1993).
9. *See id.* at 848-49.
10. *See States Execute Two Murderers, supra* note 7.

Respondents' efforts in pursuing an eleventh hour attempt to raise the question of the defendant's competency to forego further appeals or postconviction relief, despite the defendant's clearly expressed, longstanding and consistent desires to that effect, implicate conflicting ethical considerations. A defendant's wish to forego further appeals and accept the death penalty, like other decisions relating to the objectives of litigation, is essentially that of the client, whose decision the attorney must respect. Delaware Lawyers' Rules of Professional Conduct ("DLRPC") Rule 1.2(a). The means to be employed to achieve such objectives are "a matter on which the attorney is to consult with the client [and over which] the lawyer retains the ultimate prerogative to act." Modern Legal Ethics §4.3, p. 157. The deliberate decision of a defendant to accept the death penalty to avoid other penal alternatives is not, in itself, an irrational act. An attorney who is unable in good conscience to represent a client intent upon achieving such an objective, or to whom the death penalty is "repugnant," may seek leave to withdraw from the representation if the client's interests would not be prejudiced thereby. DLRPC Rule 1.16(b)(3).

If an attorney has a reasonable and objective basis to doubt a client's competency to make a decision foregoing further appeals, the attorney must, in a timely fashion, so inform the trial court and request the court to make a judicial determination of the defendant's competency. *See* DLRPC Rule 1.14(b). Where the lawyer's actions appear contrary to the client's stated decision, the lawyer who so moves, presumably in good faith, must, at a minimum, demonstrate an objective and reasonable basis for believing that the client cannot act in his own interest.

After full consideration of the circumstances surrounding the actions of Respondents in this matter, we find no basis for concluding that any of them acted in bad faith or were motivated by other than the best interests of their client. . . .

The Court recognizes the professional and personal demands which counsel experience in the defense of a capital case. A defendant facing execution is entitled to a vigorous and energetic defense, but a conscientious defense as well. A lawyer who renders such service is not free to fashion his or her own code of ethics. For members of the Bar of this Court those standards have already been established and they afford sufficient flexibility to accommodate proper zealous advocacy.

. . . Under such circumstances, we find no basis for the imposition of sanctions. . . .

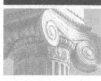

Post-Case Follow-Up

Red Dog illustrates that lawyers are required to abide by their client's lawful decisions regarding the objectives of the representation — even when the lawyer does not think that such a decision is in the best interest of the client or the decision conflicts with the lawyer's personal views. Rule 1.2 makes clear that a representation of a client "does not constitute an endorsement of the client's political, economic, social, or moral views or activities."

In May 2018, the Supreme Court decided McCoy v. Louisiana, 138 S. Ct. 1500 (2018). Robert McCoy was charged with murdering three members of his estranged wife's family. The evidence against McCoy was apparently overwhelming.

Nevertheless, McCoy maintained his innocence. His attorney, Larry English, determined that the best way to avoid a death sentence would be to concede that McCoy committed the murders. McCoy told English not to make the concession; instead, McCoy wanted English to "pursue acquittal." English understood McCoy's "complete opposition to English telling the jury that McCoy was guilty." Nevertheless, in his opening statement at trial, English told the jury that McCoy committed the three murders. McCoy objected and told the court that English was "selling him out." The trial court reiterated to McCoy that English was representing him, and that the court would not permit "any other outbursts" from McCoy. McCoy testified on his own behalf, "maintaining his innocence and pressing an alibi difficult to fathom." The jury returned a unanimous verdict of guilt and sentenced McCoy to death on each murder count. The Supreme Court reversed McCoy's conviction, holding that he was denied his Sixth Amendment right to effective assistance of counsel. The Court explained that the Sixth Amendment guarantees "assistance" of counsel, but that "an assistant, however expert, is still an assistant." The Court held:

> Counsel may reasonably assess a concession of guilt as best suited to avoiding the death penalty, as English did in this case. But the client may not share that objective. He may wish to avoid, above all else the opprobrium that comes with admitting he killed family members. Or he may hold life in prison not worth living and prefer to risk death for any hope, however small, of exoneration. . . . When a client expressly asserts that the objective of "*his* defence" is to maintain innocence of the charged criminal acts, his lawyer must abide by that objective and may not override it by conceding guilt. U.S. Const. Amdt. 6 (emphasis added); *see* ABA Model Rule of Professional Conduct 1.2(a) (2016) (a "lawyer shall abide by a client's decisions concerning the objectives of the representation").

Id. at 1508-09.

In addition to having the ultimate authority regarding the objectives of the representation, clients also have the ultimate authority in deciding whether to settle a case in a civil matter. In criminal matters, the client has the ultimate authority as to the "plea to be entered, whether to waive jury trial, and whether the client will testify." *See* Model Rule 1.2(a). Importantly, Rule 1.2 confers the authority to the criminal defendant to make these decisions "after consultation with the lawyer." The lawyer must first consult with the accused about the legal effects and consequences of those decisions. As discussed in Chapter 4, it may constitute a denial of the defendant's Sixth Amendment right to effective assistance of counsel for an attorney to fail to inform a client about significant consequences attendant to pleading guilty (such as deportation if the accused is not a citizen). Such consultation is also an integral part of the lawyer's duty to communicate with his client. Comment [2] to Rule 1.4 explains that if any of the rules require the client to make a particular decision, then Rule 1.4 in turn requires that the attorney "promptly consult" with the client about that decision and "secure the client's consent prior to taking action unless prior discussions with the client have resolved what action the client wants the lawyer to take."

Red Dog v. Delaware: Real Life Applications

1. You represent Kim in a medical malpractice case. You receive a phone call from opposing counsel, who makes a settlement offer of $25,000. You reasonably believe that a jury would give Kim at least $300,000. Further, you know that Kim needs at least $75,000 just to cover outstanding medical bills, so you are sure that Kim would not even consider — indeed, she would likely be insulted by — the offer. Can you decline the offer on her behalf?

2. Molly represents Joaquin in a criminal matter for transporting marijuana. Joaquin is a non-citizen, but has lived in the United States for 40 years and served in the U.S. armed forces. Molly tells Joaquin he does not need to worry about deportation because he has been in the United States so long. Relying on this advice, Joaquin accepts a deal and pleads guilty to a criminal charge that (unbeknownst to him at the time) mandates his deportation. Has Molly violated Rule 1.2? Does Joaquin have any recourse?

2. Counseling or Assisting the Client in Crime or Fraud

A very significant limit on the client's ultimate authority over the objectives of the representation is that a lawyer is prohibited from either counseling a client to engage or assisting clients "in conduct that the lawyer knows is criminal or fraudulent." Rule 1.2(d) refers to conduct that the lawyer "knows" is criminal or fraudulent, and the rules in turn define knowledge to require "actual knowledge," but such knowledge "may be inferred from the circumstances," as stated in Rule 1.0(f). As the ABA clarified in Formal Opinion 491:

> [A] lawyer who has knowledge of facts that create a high probability that a client is seeking the lawyer's services in a transaction to further criminal or fraudulent activity has a duty to inquire further to avoid assisting that activity under Rule 1.2(d). Failure to make a reasonable inquiry is willful blindness punishable under the actual knowledge standard of the Rule.[11]

Nevertheless, Rule 1.2 allows a lawyer to discuss with the client "the legal consequences of any proposed course of conduct" and to "counsel or assist a client to make a good faith effort to determine the validity, scope, meaning or application of the law."

For example, in People v. Chappell, 927 P.2d 829 (Colo. 1996), the Colorado Supreme Court disbarred attorney Lorraine Chappell for assisting her client in violating a child custody order. Chappell represented a mother who was pregnant with her second child in a child custody dispute. After learning from the court-ordered custody evaluator that she would recommend sole custody of both children to the father, Chappell told her client that "as an attorney" she would advise the client to stay in Colorado and comply with court orders, but "as a mother" she would advise her "to run." Chappell then undertook elaborate efforts to assist her client to evade

---

11. ABA Formal Op. 491, 2 (2020).

the court's orders and jurisdiction. Chappell "informed her client about a network of safehouses for people in her situation," "helped her to liquidate her assets and empty her bank accounts," arranged for a friend of the client to pack the belongings out of the marital home, and paid the friend moving and storage fees. Chappell kept the key to the storage unit where the belongings were kept. At the custody hearing, when the judge realized that Chappell's client likely had fled the jurisdiction with the children, the court ordered sole custody to the father. Ultimately, Chappell's client returned to Colorado, was convicted with a felony charge for violating a child custody order, and lost custody of her children — and Chappell was consequently disbarred.

A lawyer need not provide assistance to a client's crime or fraud to violate Rule 1.2(d). In In re Scionti, 630 N.E.2d 1358 (Ind. 1994), an attorney merely advised his client to violate a child custody order and not return his son to the mother (whom the client believed was abusive). The attorney was disciplined, and the client was convicted for contempt and incarcerated for 90 days. As a lawyer and an "officer of the court," advising or assisting a client to violate a court order will nearly always get you in serious trouble with the bar; it can also have substantial negative consequences for your client, as it did in *Chappell* and *Scionti*.

Transactional lawyers should take especial care to comply with Rule 1.2(d). A lawyer's knowing assistance in preparing for, closing, or otherwise effectuating a fraudulent transaction will violate Rule 1.2(d). Lawyers cannot issue bona fide, true sales, nonconsolidation, or other legal certifications if they know they are not true or are otherwise fraudulent. As explained in Chapter 1, the law requires that lawyers issue such legal opinions to effectuate legal transactions precisely because the lawyers — even as advocates — are supposed to maintain a level of gatekeeping for the rule of law.

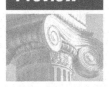

Case Preview

Iowa Supreme Court Attorney Disciplinary Board v. Engelmann

Marc Engelmann had practiced law, with a focus in real estate transactions, since 1976. As the Iowa Supreme Court summarized, prior to this case Engelmann "had practiced law for three decades with an unblemished record and had closed thousands of real estate transactions for his clients." Engelmann's legal career and exceptional reputation came to a tragic end after he closed nine real estate transactions for three swindlers. Engelmann was convicted of conspiracy, wire fraud, and bank fraud; he was sentenced to three years in prison and ordered to pay $392,937.73 in restitution to the defrauded lenders. Such charges, of course, also led to professional discipline.

As you read *Engelmann*, consider the following:

1. Did Engelmann profit financially from the ill-gotten gains obtained through the fraud?
2. What should Engelmann have done once he realized that his clients wanted him to create HUD forms that misrepresented the actual price paid for the homes?

Iowa Supreme Court Attorney Disciplinary Board v. Engelmann
840 N.W.2d 156 (Iowa 2013)

Engelmann was among the many casualties of the market crash in 2008, after purchasers of real estate sold by his clients defaulted on nine mortgage loans he helped obtain through fraud. On May 17, 2011, federal prosecutors filed a nine-count felony criminal indictment against him [for conspiracy, bank fraud, and wire fraud]. . . .

The transactions involved Laures as seller and Robert Herdrich (Herdrich) and Darryl Hanneken (Hanneken) as buyers. The parties agreed upon the purchase price for each property, but also agreed to list on the loan documents an inflated price of between $30,000 and $35,000 more than the actual purchase price for each property. The various lenders then loaned Herdrich and Hanneken money for the transaction based on the inflated price listed on the loan documents. Laures received the inflated price for each sale and then returned approximately $30,000 for each property to Herdrich and Hanneken after each closing as a "kickback."

Defendant admits he knew about the two different prices and that Laures returned money to the buyers. Defendant also knew that the inflated price was not being listed on the HUD-1 forms that were submitted to the lenders. Government witnesses testified that Defendant never disclosed the inflated price or the kickbacks to the lenders or the closing company, Excel Title. . . .

Engelmann charged a $350 fee for each of the nine closings, a volume discount from his standard $400 fee. There is no evidence or claim he otherwise personally benefited financially from these transactions. . . .

Rule 32:1.2(d) prohibits a lawyer from assisting a client "in conduct that the lawyer knows is criminal or fraudulent." Iowa R. Prof'l Conduct 32:1.2(d). Rule 32:1.16(a)(1) provides guidance to a lawyer confronted with a situation in which the lawyer's assistance will facilitate illegality. It states that "a lawyer shall not represent a client or, where representation has commenced, shall withdraw from the representation of a client if . . . the representation will result in violation of the Iowa Rules of Professional Conduct or other law."

Engelmann testified at trial that Laures had signed a contract to sell his properties to Herdrich and Hanneken before retaining Engelmann on the matter. This does not change the fact that Engelmann assisted the parties in executing their fraudulent contract by preparing the inaccurate forms and representing Laures at the closings. Comment 10 to rule 32:1.2(d) addresses this situation:

> When the client's course of action has already begun and is continuing, the lawyer's responsibility is especially delicate. The lawyer is required to avoid assisting the client, for example, by drafting or delivering documents that the lawyer knows are fraudulent or by suggesting how the wrongdoing might be concealed. A lawyer may not continue assisting a client in conduct that the lawyer originally supposed was legally proper but then discovers is criminal or fraudulent. The lawyer must, therefore, withdraw from the representation of the client in the matter.

Engelmann knew the true sales prices of the properties were less than stated on the HUD-1 forms. He also knew the buyers were receiving loans that exceeded the actual sales prices. As an experienced real estate lawyer, Engelmann knew or should have known that such a contract was not aboveboard. He helped the parties complete their fraudulent transaction by preparing documents that misrepresented the facts of the transaction, deceiving the lenders. The jury's finding that Engelmann was guilty of bank fraud and wire fraud establishes that he "knowingly did one or more overt acts for the purpose of carrying out" the fraud. We apply issue preclusion to find that Engelmann knowingly assisted his client in defrauding the buyers' lender, in violation of rule 32:1.2(d).

Engelmann should have declined to represent Laures in the transactions in the first instance. And, he should have withdrawn his representation before making misrepresentations. Engelmann had ample opportunity to withdraw. In fact, he had nine opportunities. But, instead of withdrawing, Engelmann continued to represent Laures in nine separate closings, misrepresenting the true price of the property in each transaction. We find Engelmann violated rule 32:1.16(a)(1).

. . .

For the reasons stated in this opinion, the license of the respondent, Marc R. Engelmann, is revoked. We assess costs to the respondent. . . .

Post-Case Follow-Up

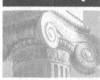

Engelmann charged a discounted rate of $350 per transaction to close these fraudulent deals. Thus, in total, Engelmann obtained $3,150 in fees for the nine closings. He paid dearly for those three thousand dollars — it cost him his license to practice law, three years in jail, and nearly $400,000 in restitution. It is certainly likely that some lawyers have closed deals containing fraudulent misrepresentations and were not caught. But it is absolutely never worth the risk. Assisting with client crime or fraud is not just a violation of Rule 1.2; it can easily lead to disbarment, civil liability, criminal indictment, and even imprisonment.

Iowa Supreme Court Attorney Disciplinary Board v. Engelmann: Real Life Applications

1. You work in a state that has legalized marijuana for medicinal and/or recreational use. Marijuana continues to be a Schedule I controlled substance under federal law, and thus it is a crime under federal law to use (for any purpose), manufacture, or distribute marijuana. A client comes to you and wants you to help him organize a business that distributes marijuana. Can you assist the client in organizing this business without violating Rule 1.2(d)?
2. Chen runs Sunrider, Inc., a business manufacturing health care products that Chen imports into the United States. Chen hires you to assist him in making

disclosures and paying tariffs to U.S. Customs. You begin examining Sunrider's documents and discover that Chen is reporting different prices to Customs than reported on his taxes to the IRS. Indeed, Chen has two sets of invoices for each product—a high one and a low one. Chen has been reporting the higher prices to the IRS (resulting in lower profits and thus lower taxes), while reporting lower prices to Customs (resulting in lower tariffs). You aren't sure which invoices are fake (the ones for taxes or the ones for tariffs), but you are confident one set of invoices is fraudulent. Can you assist in making the disclosures to U.S. Customs if you don't know whether the invoices you are using are fraudulent? If you determine that the invoices used for U.S. Customs are genuine, but the ones used for the IRS are fraudulent, can you continue assisting Chen as long as you don't assist with the taxes?

C. UNDERSTANDING THE IDENTITY OF THE CLIENT

When an attorney creates an attorney-client relationship with an individual person, there generally is no question as to the identity of the attorney's client. Thus, the attorney's duties of loyalty, confidentiality, competence, communication, and conflict avoidance clearly run to that individual client. But what happens when the client is an organization? To whom do the attorney's duties and loyalties run? For a corporate client, does the attorney represent just the corporation, or does she also represent the officers of the corporation with whom the attorney deals directly? What about attorneys for the government? Do they represent their immediate supervisor? Their branch of government? The entire body politic? What happens when an attorney works for an insurance company and represents an insured? Where an attorney's client has diminished mental capacity, should the attorney turn to others to make decisions for the client? In these and other situations, properly identifying the client and the duties owed to that client is critical.

1. Organizational Clients

When a lawyer represents an organization—be that a business association, a government entity, a union, or other association—the client is the organization itself and not any of the organization's individual constituents (such as officers, directors, employees, or shareholders). The rule holds even though the organization is a fictitious person—a creature of law—and can only operate through the actions of its human constituents. This **entity theory of organizational representation**, as Darian M. Ibrahim explains, "is based on two ideas: that an organization is a distinct legal entity; and that under the laws of agency, a lawyer, as agent of the entity-principal, owes her duties to the principal and not its other agents."[12] Although

---

12. Darian M. Ibrahim, *Solving the Everyday Problem of Client Identity in the Context of Closely Held Businesses*, 56 Ala. L. Rev. 181, 188 (2004).

other theories for organizational representation have been proffered,[13] the entity theory of representation dominates American law. Model Rule 1.13(a) adopts the "entity theory" — although using the term "organization" rather than "entity" — and addresses a lawyer's duties to an organizational client.[14]

Case Preview

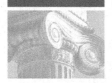

Yablonski v. United Mine Workers of America

Yablonski provides an example of attorneys whose loyalties were misplaced in favor of constituents and to the detriment of their actual organizational client. In 1969, Joseph Yablonski ran against incumbent Tony Boyle for the presidency of the union, United Mine Workers of America (UMWA). Boyle ended up winning the election, but Yablonski and other UMWA members filed several lawsuits contesting the election and the conduct of Boyle and the UMWA.[15] One of those lawsuits was a cause of action under §501 of the Labor Management Reporting and Disclosure Act brought against the UMWA, Boyle, and two other officers of the union. The §501 claim sought an accounting of UMWA funds and sought restitution for any misappropriated funds. Although the lawsuit was filed against both the UMWA and the individual officers, the cause of action was similar to a shareholder's derivative suit — the Yablonski group was arguing that the officers had violated their duties to the UMWA by misappropriating union funds. Any recovery of misappropriated funds from the individual officers in the lawsuit would go to the UMWA.

The UMWA was represented by its regular outside counsel, Williams and Connolly. When the case was initially filed, Williams and Connolly also represented Boyle and the individual officers. After six months of joint representation, Williams and Connolly withdrew from its representation of the individual defendants in the §501 case, but they continued to represent Boyle individually in the other related election cases. The Yablonski group moved to disqualify Williams and Connolly from representing the UMWA in the §501 case.

As you read *Yablonski*, consider the following:

1. Was it appropriate for Williams and Connolly to represent the UMWA and the individual defendants at the outset of the suit? Why? Were the interests of Boyle and the UMWA aligned?
2. What is the role of the entity's counsel in a §501 claim against a union or in a shareholder's derivative suit against a corporation?
3. Why did the UMWA need separate, independent counsel?

---

13. *See id.* at 181-218 (identifying and analyzing various theories and proffering a new theory for representation of closely held businesses).
14. *See id.* at 187 ("The entity theory—that the lawyer represents the entity itself and not its individual constituents — is the most widely accepted theory of entity representation . . . [and is] adopted by both the Model Rules and the Model Code. . . .").
15. *See* Yablonski v. UMWA, 466 F.2d 424 (D.C. Cir. 1972).

Yablonski v. United Mine Workers of America
448 F.2d 1175 (D.C. Cir. 1971)

This is an action under §501 of the Labor-Management Reporting and Disclosure Act brought by the late Joseph A. Yablonski and 48 other members of the United Mine Workers of America against the UMWA and three named officers — Boyle, President; Titler, Vice President; Owens, Secretary-Treasurer — asking for an accounting of UMWA funds disbursed by them and for restitution of funds allegedly misappropriated and misspent.

. . . At the outset of the lawsuit, [Williams and Connolly], the then counsel for all defendants set about with commendable diligence to delineate the real issues of the lawsuit, filing in behalf of the UMWA and the three individual defendants answers setting forth all customary general defenses, and filing 34 pages of interrogatories to develop more fully the scope of the case.

The appellants argue that this period of six months' prior representation in this same suit disqualifies the regular union outside counsel to continue its representation of the UMWA, even after its withdrawal as counsel for the three individual officer-defendants. With this we do not agree. It has been inferentially held that one lawyer can properly represent all defendants if a suit appears groundless, and that separate counsel is required only in a situation where there is a potential conflict between the interests of the union and those of its officers. We regard the actions of the regular UMWA counsel during its six-month representation of both the union and its officers as an effort to ascertain the exact nature of the lawsuit and protect the interests of all defendants, and by our ruling herein do not imply any censure of counsel's action during this period of joint representation. But there does exist in our judgment a more serious barrier to the continued representation of the UMWA by its regular outside counsel in this particular lawsuit.

. . . Of far more concern is the existence of other litigation in which the regular UMWA counsel is representing Boyle, sometimes in conjunction with representation of the union, at other times not. . . .

Each of these [other cases where Williams and Connolly represents Boyle individually] has been minutely examined by appellees' counsel to demonstrate that in no instance is the representation of Boyle individually in conflict with the good faith representation of the UMWA in this case; in effect, that the interests of the UMWA and of Boyle individually are the same. We are assured that if any conflict should arise appellees' counsel would be prompt to withdraw as counsel to the UMWA in this case.

While the issues involved in each of the individual cases, and the past or present existence or nonexistence of any conflict, are relevant to the propriety of the regular UMWA counsel continuing its representation of the union in the case at bar, yet we do not think that this analysis is determinative of the real problem here. It is undeniable that the regular UMWA counsel have undertaken the representation of Boyle individually in many facets of his activities as a UMWA official, as a Trustee of the Fund, as a Director of the Bank owned 74% by the union. With strict fidelity to this client, such counsel could not undertake action on behalf of another client which would undermine his position personally. Yet, in this particular litigation, counsel for the UMWA should be diligent in analyzing objectively the true interests of the UMWA as an institution without being hindered by allegiance to any individual concerned.[7]

We are not required to accept at this point the charge of the appellants that the "true interest" of the union is aligned with those of the individual appellants here; this may or may not turn out to be the fact. But in the exploration and the determination of the truth or falsity of the charges brought by these individual appellants against the incumbent officers of the union and the union itself as a defendant, the UMWA needs the most objective counsel obtainable. Even if we assume the accuracy of the appellee's position at the present time that there is no visible conflict of interest, yet we cannot be sure that such will not arise in the future.

. . . We think that the objectives of the Labor-Management Reporting and Disclosure Act[8] would be much better served by having an unquestionably independent new counsel in this particular case. The public interest requires that the validity of appellants' charges against the UMWA management of breach of its fiduciary responsibilities be determined in a context which is as free as possible from the appearance of any potential for conflict of interest in the representation of the union itself.

II. OBJECTIVE DETERMINATION OF THE UMWA'S INSTITUTIONAL INTEREST

Counsel for the appellees here have stressed the "institutional interest" of the UMWA in all of the issues raised, and particularly the institutional interest of the union in "repose." Counsel's interpretation of the "institutional interest" of the union appears to have been broad enough to authorize UMWA counsel to undertake practically everything worthwhile in the defense of this lawsuit. After the withdrawal of the regular union counsel from representation of Boyle individually in this case, the individual practitioner selected to represent Boyle has apparently contributed little to the defense.

By far the strongest laboring oar has been stroked by the regular UMWA counsel on behalf of the union. On oral argument appellees' counsel stated that it had

---

7. "Where, as here, union officials are charged with breach of fiduciary duty, the organization is entitled to an evaluation and representation of its institutional interests by independent counsel, unencumbered by potentially conflicting obligations to any defendant officer." Int'l Bhd. of Teamsters etc. v. Hoffa, 242 F. Supp. 246, 256 (D.D.C. 1965). . . .

8. 29 U.S.C. §401 (1964) sets forth the congressional declaration of findings, purposes and policy of the LMRDA, including inter alia the statement that "in order to accomplish the objective of a free flow of commerce it is essential that labor organizations, employers, and their officials adhere to the highest standards of responsibility and ethical conduct in administering the affairs of their organizations. . . ." The legislative history of the Act makes plain that a major congressional objective was to provide union members, as well as the Government in the public interest, with a variety of means to ensure that officials of labor organizations perform their duties in accordance with fiduciary standards. Both the Senate and House reports relating to the Act stressed the importance of such standards, the Senate Committee noting that:

Labor organizations are creations of their members; union funds belong to the members and should be expended only in furtherance of their common interest. A union treasury should not be managed as the private property of union officers, however well intentioned, but as a fund governed by fiduciary standards appropriate to this type of organization. The members who are the real owners of the money and property of the organization are entitled to a full accounting of all transactions involving their property. (S. Rep. No. 187, 86th Cong. 1st Sess. 8 (1959)). . . .

prepared 94 pages of answers to interrogatories, that the individual practitioner representing Boyle had agreed they should do this, as the UMWA had a definite interest that all questions as to the conduct of union affairs previously were accurately answered and that the accurate answers were to be found in the union records. We can see the UMWA interest in having such interrogatories answered accurately, but we would think that since it is the individual defendants who are charged with the misconduct, their counsel would be the one to initiate and to carry the burden. It appears that, since the division of work between the UMWA counsel and counsel for the individual defendants in July 1970, until 15 March 1971 approximately 250 pages of pleadings, motions, memoranda, exhibits, affidavits and papers relating to discovery were filed by the regular UMWA counsel, while the individual defendants' counsel contributed only about 50 pages of similar documents.

In the crucial area of discovery matters, clearly representing the vast bulk of the effort expended by the parties defendant at this stage of the litigation, UMWA counsel have prepared 174 pages of answers to plaintiffs' initial interrogatories which were directed to all defendants, while counsel for the individual defendants, until 2 April 1971, some 7 ½ months after the interrogatories were originally served, had contented himself with filing 2 pages of answers for each individual defendant, a total of 6 pages. On 2 April 1971 counsel finally filed additional answers on behalf of defendant Boyle; however, as of the date of argument of this appeal, answers on behalf of the other individual defendants had not been filed. . . .

This points up the difficulty of defining an "institutional interest" such as that of the union. In trying to achieve a valid definition of an institution's interest, it would seem that counsel charged with this responsibility should be as independent as possible. It appears that in 18 months of representation (6 months for both the UMWA and Boyle individually, and 12 months for the UMWA alone), the regular UMWA counsel has not brought forth a single issue on which the UMWA and the Boyle individual interest have diverged.

We think the analogy of the position of a corporation and its individual officers when confronted by a stockholder derivative suit is illuminating here. We believe it is well established that when one group of stockholders brings a derivative suit, with the corporation as the nominal defendant and the individual officers accused of malfeasance of one sort or another, the role of both the corporate house counsel and the regular outside counsel for the corporation becomes usually a passive one. Certainly no corporate counsel purports to represent the individual officers involved, neither in the particular derivative suit nor in other litigation by virtue of which counsel necessarily must create ties of loyalty and confidentiality to the individual officers, which might preclude counsel from the most effective representation of the corporation itself. The corporation has certain definite institutional interests to be protected, and the counsel charged with this responsibility should have ties on a personal basis with neither the dissident stockholders nor the incumbent officeholders.

Purportedly a stockholder derivative suit is for the benefit of the corporation, even though the corporation is a nominal defendant, just as the appellants here assert (yet to be proved) that their action is for the benefit of the UMWA and that the individual incumbent officers are liable to the union itself for their alleged misdeeds.

And, under established corporate law, if the individual officers are successful in the defense of a suit arising out of the performance of their duties as corporate officers, then they may justifiably seek reimbursement from the corporation for the costs of their successful defense.

In the ordinary case the action taken here by the regular UMWA counsel in the District Court might well have been the proper one, i.e., after establishing the nature of the lawsuit by interrogatories and filing answers on behalf of both the union and the individual officers in order fully to protect the position of all parties, then to step aside as counsel for the individual defendants and continue the representation of the union. But this particular case is a derivative action for the benefit of the union, and furthermore must be viewed in its relationship to this entire complex of numerous cases already pending or decided in this and the District Courts in which the regular UMWA counsel has already undertaken the representation of Boyle individually. Each and every one of these cases either directly arises out of or is directly connected with the struggle for power in the UMWA being waged by the Yablonski group on one side and the incumbent officers headed by President Boyle on the other. In this situation, the best interests of the UMWA and the purposes of the Labor-Management Reporting and Disclosure Act will be much better served by the disqualification of the regular union counsel in this particular suit and its continued representation of the individual Boyle in the other lawsuits.

We are cognizant that any counsel to represent the UMWA selected by President Boyle will be to some degree under his control. But such counsel will still only have one client — the UMWA — to represent in matters growing out of the union's affairs. Such counsel would never be professionally obligated to consider Boyle's personal interests, because they would not be representing him individually in related matters. And the extent of their labors would be gauged by the need to protect the UMWA position in this litigation.

Therefore, the Order of the District Court denying the appellants' motion to disqualify the regular UMWA outside counsel from representing the UMWA in this particular action is vacated. . . .

Post-Case Follow-Up

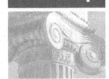

Consider whether Boyle's interests and the union's were the same. What indicators did Williams and Connolly have that their interests actually diverged dramatically? (As it turned out, Boyle was in fact misappropriating union funds and would ultimately be convicted of embezzlement.[16])

The *Yablonski* court indicated that it was proper for Williams and Connolly to initially represent both the UMWA and the individual defendants while determining whether or not the union needed separate counsel. Model Rule 1.13(g) seems to be in accord, stating: "A

---

16. *See* Wolfgang Saxon, *W.A. Boyle Dies*, N.Y. Times, June 1, 1985, *available at* http://www.nytimes.com/1985/06/01/us/wa-boyle-dies-led-miners-union.html.

Power Struggle in the UMWA: The Murder of the Yablonski Family

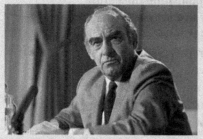

Joseph A. "Jock" Yablonski
AP Photo/Henry Burroughs

Joseph A. "Jock" Yablonski ran for president of the UMWA against decade-long incumbent William Anthony "Tony" Boyle in 1969. Boyle won by a 2-to-1 margin — results that Yablonski formally protested, giving rise to an investigation of the election by the Secretary of Labor. In addition, during the election and after his defeat, Yablonski filed several lawsuits against Boyle and the UMWA objecting to unlawful actions taken by the union against Yablonski during the election (including demoting Yablonski, using the union's official journal to promote Boyle's campaign, refusing to distribute Yablonski's campaign materials, and using unfair election processes).[19] In 1972, a federal court voided the 1969 election and ordered a new election. Arnold R. Miller defeated Boyle in the 1972 election. Tragically, Jock Yablonksi could not run against Boyle in 1972 because he, his wife Margaret, and his 25-year-old daughter Charlotte had been murdered on New Year's Eve 1969 — not long after Yablonski

lawyer representing an organization may also represent any of its directors, officers, employees, members, shareholders or other constituents, subject to the provisions of Rule 1.7." As you will see in Chapter 6, covering conflicts of interest, Rule 1.7 only allows a joint representation where the attorney reasonably believes that she can "provide competent and diligent representation to each affected client" and each affected client gives written informed consent — among other requirements. If an entity attorney does in fact represent both the entity and the individual officers, then pursuant to Rule 1.13(g) the necessary informed written consent must come from an entity official "*other than* the individual who is to be represented."

Comment [14] to Model Rule 1.13 goes even further by indicating that generally the entity attorney may represent the individual officers even in a shareholder's derivative suit — as such suits "are a normal incident of an organization's affairs, to be defended by the organization's lawyer like any other suit." The comment contains the caveat that such representation may produce a conflict prohibiting representation where "the claim involves serious charges of wrongdoing by those in control of the organization." Notably, the Model Rule's allowance of joint representation in derivative actions conflicts with the holding of several courts and the Restatement (Third) of the Law Governing Lawyers. As stated by the Third Circuit: "We have no hesitation in holding that — except in patently frivolous cases — allegations of directors' fraud, intentional misconduct, or self-dealing require separate counsel."[17] The Restatement asserts that in a derivative action, "[e]ven with informed consent of all affected clients, the lawyer for the organization ordinarily may not represent an individual defendant as well." Indeed, according to the Restatement, joint representation of the officers and the organization in a derivative suit is only allowed if "the *disinterested* directors conclude that *no basis exists* for the claim that the defending officers and directors have acted against the interests of the organization" and there is "effective consent of all clients."[18]

17. Bell Atlantic Corp. v. Bolger, 2 F.3d 1304, 1317 (3d Cir. 1998).
18. *See* Restatement (Third) of the Law Governing Lawyers §131(g) (emphasis added).
19. *See Yablonski*, 466 F.2d at 425-27 & n.2.

Yablonski v. United Mine Workers of America: Real Life Applications

1. Oliver is the attorney for the city of Springfield. He works very closely with the mayor, whom Oliver discovers has been taking municipal property for his personal use. The mayor comes to Oliver and asks for his assistance in the face of ethics charges being brought against him by the state. Whom does Oliver represent? Can he represent the mayor in this matter?

2. Newman represented 25 doctors who wanted to form a business entity for the limited purpose of buying a magnetic resonance imaging (MRI) machine. Newman meets with the individual doctors to discuss their goals and then organizes an appropriate entity, serving as the corporate counsel for that entity. Later, Dr. Danforth, one of the 25 physicians who met with Newman, is sued for medical malpractice, and Jacob, the attorney who represents the plaintiff in the med mal matter, is a partner at the same law firm as Newman. Dr. Danforth moves to disqualify Jacob on the theory that Danforth had a personal attorney-client relationship with Newman. Danforth argues that prior to the creation of the entity, Newman represented each of the doctors individually. Did Newman represent each of the individual doctors prior to the creation of the corporate entity?

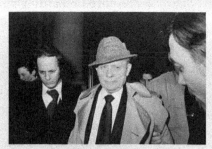

William Anthony "Tony" Boyle
AP Photo/Bill Ingraham

had objected to the election results. Yablonski and his family were shot and killed by three men — Paul Gilly, Claude Vealey, and Aubran Martin — who invaded the Yablonski farmhouse while the family slept. Ultimately, it was uncovered that these hitmen were hired by Boyle, who had paid them $20,000 in UMWA funds. In 1974, Boyle was convicted of three counts of first-degree murder and sentenced to life imprisonment. He died in 1985. Recall that the §501 lawsuit excerpted above alleged that Boyle was misappropriating union funds. Yet no one at that time realized that union funds had been used to finance the killing of Yablonski and his wife and daughter.[20]

"Mirandizing" the Organization's Constituents

An individual constituent (such as an officer, director, employee, shareholder, member) of an organization may not understand that the entity's lawyers do not represent the constituent. The constituent may believe, erroneously, that the attorney represents the constituent individually in addition to the organization. Consequently, Model Rule 1.13(f) requires the organization's attorney to clarify her role and "explain the identity of the client" to an organization's constituents "when the lawyer knows or reasonably should know that the organization's interests are adverse to those of the constituents with whom the lawyer is dealing." The Ninth Circuit has called this a "corporate *Miranda* warning."[21] Because the warning is

20. *See generally* Wolfgang Saxon, *W.A. Boyle Dies*, N.Y. TIMES, June 1, 1985, *available at* http://www.nytimes .com/1985/06/01/us/wa-boyle-dies-led-miners-union.html; *W.A. "Tony" Boyle, Ex-Union President Convicted of Murder*, United Press International, CHI. TRIB., June 1, 1985, *available at* http://articles.chicagotribune.com/1985-06-01/sports/8502040215_1_joseph-jock-yablonski-umw-district-mr-boyle.

21. *See* United States v. Ruehle, 583 F.3d 600, 604 n.3 (9th Cir. 2009). Chapter 5 examines Upjohn Co. v. United States, 449 U.S. 383 (1981), and covers the scope of an entity's attorney-client privilege.

required regarding representation of any entity or organization (not just corporations), we will call it the **entity warning**.

The requisite content of the entity warning is spelled out in Model Rule 1.13 and comment [10] thereto, which instruct attorneys to explain four basic points to constituents with interests potentially adverse to the organization: (1) that the lawyer represents the organization; (2) "that the lawyer cannot represent such constituent"; (3) "that such person may wish to obtain independent representation"; and (4) "that discussions between the lawyer for the organization and the individual may not be privileged." Despite the fact that comment [10] says that the "discussions . . . may not be privileged," in jurisdictions that follow the *Upjohn* rule (discussed in Chapter 5) most of the discussions between the attorney and organizational constituents will be covered by the attorney-client privilege — but it will be the *organization's* attorney-client privilege and not the constituent's. The comment is accurate in that there will not be an *individual* attorney-client privilege between the constituent and the attorney; thus, the individual constituent will not be able to invoke the privilege on her own behalf. Further, because the organization holds any privilege created by the communication, the organization can choose to waive the privilege and disclose the contents of the discussion to the detriment of the constituent. The Ninth Circuit presents an entity warning that explains this nuance:

> Such warnings [should] make clear that the corporate lawyers do not represent the individual employee; that anything said by the employee to the lawyers will be protected by the company's attorney-client privilege subject to waiver of the privilege in the sole discretion of the company; and that the individual may wish to consult with his own attorney if he has any concerns about his own potential legal exposure.[22]

In a similar vein, information shared by the constituent with the entity attorney is also covered by the attorney's duty of confidentiality — but again, the confidentiality is owed to the organization and not to the individual constituent. As the D.C. bar clarified in Ethics Opinion 269, "communications between the lawyer and the [constituent] being interviewed are protected by Rule 1.6 (Confidentiality of Information), but the protection accorded is for the benefit of the client corporation, not the interviewee."[23] The D.C. bar further explained that "the interviewee has no right to expect that disclosure or use of the information provided by him or her to the lawyer will be subject to his/her control under Rule 1.6, as the corporation will have the right to use the information to serve its purposes."[24]

If no entity warning or other clarification is provided to the individual constituent, can the constituent claim to have a personal attorney-client relationship with the entity attorney? In *Meehan v. Hopps*, 301 P.2d 10 (Cal. Ct. App. 1956), the California Court of Appeal held that Hopps, who had been a director and chairman of the board, could not claim an implied individual attorney-client relationship

---

22. *See Ruehle*, 583 F.3d at 604 n.3.
23. D.C. Bar Ethics Op. 269, *Obligation of Lawyer for Corporation to Clarify Role in Internal Corporate Investigation* (1997).
24. *Id.*

with corporate counsel. Hopps had given information to corporate counsel that implicated himself, and apparently he believed that corporate counsel would keep it confidential. The court held that because of Hopps's position in the company, Hopps had a fiduciary obligation to turn that information over to the entity attorneys. The court further explained:

> The attorney for a corporation represents it, its stockholders and its officers in their representative capacity. He in nowise represents the officers personally. It would be a sorry state of affairs if when a controversy arises between an attorney's corporate client and one of its officers he could not use on behalf of his client information which that officer was required by reason of his position with the corporation to give to the attorney.

In other words, the corporation was free to use against Hopps the information that Hopps provided to the corporation's attorneys.

However, some recent cases indicate that if no entity warning is given and the constituent reasonably believes that the entity attorney is acting on behalf of the constituent, then an implied attorney-client relationship may exist between the entity attorney and the individual constituent. But where adversity between the entity and the constituent exist, the finding of an implied individual attorney-client relationship with a constituent creates a conflict of interest with the attorney's representation of the organization, requiring the withdrawal or disqualification of the attorney from representing the entity.[25]

Individual constituents have been subjected to liability or even criminal prosecution based on statements made to the entity attorney. In *United States v. Ruehle*, the chief financial officer of Broadcom Corporation, William Ruehle, provided information in interviews with the entity attorneys regarding backdating company stock options. The backdating allegedly inflated the financial portfolio of the corporation by $2.2 billion. The information Ruehle conveyed to Broadcom's attorneys was initially provided to outside auditors and ultimately conveyed to the Securities and Exchange Commission (SEC) and the United States Attorney's Office. Ruehle was then indicted for securities and wire fraud. Ruehle argued that the information he had conveyed in interviews to Broadcom's attorneys was protected by an individual attorney-client privilege. While the district court agreed, the Ninth Circuit reversed and held that even if the Broadcom attorneys had failed to give an appropriate warning (the attorneys claimed they did warn him; Ruehle said they did not), Ruehle was not only aware that the information would be given to outside auditors, but provided the information for that very purpose. The court therefore held that Ruehle failed to show that the communications were intended to be confidential, and even if so, he waived any claim to privilege by the disclosure to the outside auditors. In a vein similar to *Meehan*, the court noted that Ruehle knew of

---

25. For example, in Home Care Industries Inc. v. Murray, 154 F. Supp. 2d 861 (D.N.J. 2001), the court found that the entity attorneys — who had not given an entity warning — had created an implied attorney-client relationship with the former chief executive officer (CEO) of the entity. Consequently, the court granted a motion to disqualify the entity attorneys from representing the entity against the CEO.

his corporate duty to disclose the information, and that the information had to be provided to outside auditors and the SEC.[26]

Reporting Up and Out

In the wake of Enron and other corporate scandals, Congress enacted the Sarbanes-Oxley Act, which required the SEC to create "minimum standards of professional conduct for attorneys appearing" before the SEC, and mandated that such standards include a requirement that attorneys report up to the chief legal officer any evidence the attorney received regarding a "material violation of securities law or breach of fiduciary duty" by the company or any constituent thereof. It further mandated that attorneys be required to report up to the board of directors, should the chief legal officer fail to appropriately respond (through remedial measures) to the violation. *See* 15 U.S.C. §7245 (2002). The SEC has promulgated such standards. *See* 17 C.F.R. §205.3.

The ABA followed suit and amended Model Rule 1.13(b) in 2003 to require attorneys to report up the corporate chain when the attorney knows that a constituent of an organizational client is violating or intends to violate "a legal obligation to the organization" or a violation of law that could be imputed to the organization and "is likely to result in substantial injury to the organization." Importantly, unlike the SEC regulations, a jurisdiction's version of Model Rule 1.13(b) does not just apply to attorneys practicing before the SEC, but to all attorneys in their representation of any kind of organizational client, including government clients.[27]

However, not all jurisdictions have adopted the 2003 amendments to Rule 1.13(b). As of March 2020, only 24 jurisdictions had adopted the 2003 amendments in toto, with other jurisdictions adopting part or a modified version thereof.[28] A number of jurisdictions still have in place the prior version of Rule 1.13(b) or a variation thereof, in which the attorney who knows of illegality by an

---

26. The Ninth Circuit stated:

> Ruehle was no ordinary Broadcom employee. He served as the public company's CFO — the senior corporate executive charged with primary responsibility for Broadcom's financial affairs. This was a sophisticated corporate enterprise with billions of dollars in sales worldwide, aided by accountants, lawyers, and advisors entrusted with meeting a multitude of regulatory obligations. The duties undertaken by Ruehle broadly encompassed not only accurately and completely reporting the company's historical and current stock option granting practices, but also Broadcom's strict compliance with reporting and record keeping requirements imposed through the Securities Exchange Act of 1934 and the Sarbanes-Oxley Act of 2002, among many other federal and state rules and regulations. As the head of finance, Ruehle cannot now credibly claim ignorance of the general disclosure requirements imposed on a publicly traded company with respect to its outside auditors or the need to truthfully report corporate information to the SEC.

Ruehle, 583 F.3d at 610. In an unusual twist, Ruehle was ultimately acquitted when the district court dismissed the charges rather than submitting the case to the jury because of prosecutorial misconduct involving intimidation of Ruehle's witnesses. *See generally* Peter J. Henning, *How the Broadcom Backdating Case Has Gone Awry*, N.Y. Times, Dec. 14, 2009; Associated Press, *Charges Dismissed Against 2 Broadcom Executives*, N.Y. Times, Dec. 15, 2009.

27. *See, e.g.*, In re Harding, 223 P.3d 303 (Kan. 2010) (city); In re DeMers, 901 N.Y.S.2d 858 (N.Y. App. Div. 2010) (zoning board).

28. *See* ABA, CPR Policy Implementation Committee, *Variations of the ABA Model Rules of Professional Conduct, Rule 1.13: Organization as Client* (March 10, 2020), *available at* https://www.americanbar.org/content/dam/aba/administrative/professional_responsibility/mrpc_1_13.pdf.

organizational constituent is required to "proceed as is reasonably necessary in the best interest of the organization" and then is given discretion as to what measures to take. The appropriate measures may (or may not) include reporting up the corporate ladder.[29]

Under the 2003 Model Rule approach, if an attorney has completed the mandatory report up to the highest authority that can act on behalf of an organization (usually the board of directors for corporate entities), and the highest authority has failed to fix or timely address the law violation, then the lawyer is permitted (but not required) to report outside the organization — regardless of whether an exception to confidentiality under Rule 1.6 would allow the disclosure. Notably, this *permissive* outside disclosure found in Rule 1.13(c) is allowed "only if and to the extent the lawyer reasonably believes necessary to prevent substantial injury to the organization." Further, Rule 1.13(c) does not apply to (and thus outside disclosure is not allowed by) attorneys who are hired by an organization to investigate or defend the organization as to allegations or claims of law violation. As comment [7] explains, this limitation on reporting out "is necessary in order to enable organizational clients to enjoy the full benefits of legal counsel in conducting an investigation or defending against a claim."

Not surprisingly, clients often are not particularly happy with attorneys who report their misdeeds. Lawyers should expect that taking such action may get them fired. If a lawyer is fired for disclosing information as required or permitted by Rule 1.13(b) and (c), the lawyer still owes duties to the organization. Of course, the lawyer owes duties of confidentiality and conflict of interest avoidance — the same as with all former clients. But Model Rule 1.13(e) additionally requires the attorney who is fired as a consequence of reporting information — or who withdraws under circumstances where the rule would require or permit reporting — to "proceed as the lawyer reasonably believes necessary to assure that the organization's highest authority is informed of the lawyer's discharge or withdrawal." For example, if an attorney for a corporation is fired by the CEO for reporting up illegalities, then the attorney needs to inform the board of directors of the situation and of the fact of being fired. This rule should preclude the ability of officers with firing authority from being able to fire the attorney to effectively stop the attorney's reporting up to the board of directors. It similarly eliminates the option for attorneys to withdraw as a method of avoiding their report up duties. If an attorney is obligated by Rule 1.13(b) to report up, the attorney cannot just withdraw from the representation

---

29. *See, e.g.,* Michigan Rule of Professional Conduct 1.13(b), which states:

> Any measures taken shall be designed to minimize disruption of the organization and the risk of revealing information relating to the representation to persons outside the organization. Such measures may include among others:
>
> (1) asking reconsideration of the matter;
> (2) advising that a separate legal opinion on the matter be sought for presentation to appropriate authority in the organization; and
> (3) referring the matter to higher authority in the organization, including, if warranted by the seriousness of the matter, referral to the highest authority that can act in behalf of the organization as determined by applicable law.

to avoid that obligation. Rule 1.13(e) requires the attorney to notify the highest authority for the organization of the withdrawal.

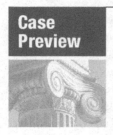

Case Preview

Pang v. International Document Services

If an attorney is fired for complying with Rule 1.13(b) or (c) by reporting up or out, can the attorney then sue the organization for wrongful discharge? In *Pang v. International Document Services*, the Utah Supreme Court addressed this issue.

As you read *Pang*, consider the following:

1. Should it be against public policy to allow organizations to freely fire attorneys for complying with the applicable rules of professional conduct?
2. Why might it be important to allow clients to freely fire their attorneys?
3. Do the report up requirements of Rule 1.13 protect public interests or only the private interests of the attorney and the client organization?
4. Will attorneys comply with duties to report up if the attorney cannot obtain any recourse in the event that the attorney is fired for that compliance?

Pang v. International Document Services
356 P.3d 1190 (Utah 2015)

This case requires us to determine whether rule 1.13(b) of the Utah Rules of Professional Conduct reflects a clear and substantial public policy of the kind sufficient to prevent companies from terminating in-house legal counsel for reporting illegal activity to management. David K. Pang, an attorney, filed a complaint against his employer alleging that he was terminated for refusing to ignore the company's violation of several states' usury laws. He asserted that the company had effectively asked him to violate the Utah Rules of Professional Conduct in order to keep his job. The district court dismissed his complaint, concluding that Mr. Pang was an at-will employee and that his firing did not violate a clear and substantial public policy of the State of Utah. We affirm the district court's decision. Rule 1.13(b) does not constitute a clear and substantial public policy that prevents the termination of an at-will employee. And even if it did, other rules of professional conduct evince strong policy choices that favor allowing clients to terminate the attorney-client relationship at any time, including firing an in-house lawyer with whom an organizational client disagrees.

. . .

Beginning in September 2011, Mr. Pang became concerned that the Company was violating "usury laws in numerous states by charging an interest rate above statutory limits and not registering as a loan institution." He warned the Company's owners "repeatedly" that these oversights "rendered their out of state practice illegal." Mr. Pang "made a final attempt to convince" the Company of its "illegal lending practices" in May 2012. He "printed, and took home, loan contracts from different states in order to develop a spreadsheet report to show the specific number of . . . usury violations." Two weeks later, the Company fired Mr. Pang "for taking home documents," citing a provision of the employee handbook that prohibited such conduct. "[A]t the time of his termination," Mr. Pang learned "for the first time" that "the owners were aware of the problems but did not plan to correct" them. And he "was told to ignore" the Company's "non-compliance."

According to Mr. Pang, the "real reason" for his termination was "the fear that [he] would expose [the Company's] illegal activities, and to punish and intimidate him into silence." He sued the Company for wrongful termination. . . .

. . . In Utah, all employment relationships are presumed to be at-will, meaning that the employer can terminate the relationship at any time for any reason, or no reason at all. There are several exceptions to the at-will employment doctrine. . . .

A. Mr. Pang's Complaint Does Not Implicate a State Public Policy of Sufficient Magnitude to Qualify as an Exception to At-Will Employment

On appeal, Mr. Pang has conceded that he was an at-will employee. But he argues that his firing falls within an exception to the at-will employment doctrine because he was terminated in "violation of a clear and substantial public policy." . . . [T]o support a wrongful discharge claim under the public policy exception, Mr. Pang's complaint must identify a public policy "so clear and weighty," and as to which "the public interest is so strong" that the policy should be "place[d] . . . beyond the reach of contract."

To make this determination, we consider a number of factors: (1) whether the policy at issue is reflected in authoritative sources of state public policy, (2) whether the policy affects the public generally as opposed to the private interests of the employee and employer, and (3) whether countervailing policies outweigh the policy at issue. Below, we discuss each factor and conclude that rule 1.13 does not reflect a public policy of sufficient magnitude to qualify as an exception to the at-will employment doctrine.

1. Mr. Pang has not raised a policy that is adequately reflected in the kind of sources we have recognized previously as authoritative expressions of Utah public policy

. . . [A] policy cannot be clear and substantial unless it is recognized by an authoritative source of Utah public policy. In other words, the policy must be "plainly defined" by authoritative sources of state law, such as "legislative enactments, constitutional standards, or judicial decisions." Rule 1.13 directs an in-house counsel to "refer" any "matter to higher authority in the organization" that "is a violation of a legal obligation to the organization, or a violation of law that reasonably might be imputed to the organization, and that is likely to result in substantial injury to the organization." . . .

We do not decide whether the rules of professional conduct qualify as "judicial decisions" that could independently establish an exception to at-will employment.

This is because even if some of the rules may reflect a public policy of sufficient magnitude to override at-will employment, rule 1.13, upon which Mr. Pang exclusively relies, clearly does not. . . .

2. Rule 1.13 regulates private attorney-client conduct, not matters of broad public importance

In addition to being defined by an authoritative source, clear and substantial public policies must be "of overarching importance to the public as opposed to the parties only." . . . Policies that "inure[] solely to the benefit of the employer and employee" are accordingly "insufficient to give rise to a substantial and important public policy." Mr. Pang has not shown that the policy he identifies in rule 1.13 meets this standard. . . . [W]hile rule 1.13, like many of the rules of professional conduct, indirectly benefits the public, its primary purpose is to regulate private conduct between a lawyer and his or her client. . . . Accordingly, rule 1.13 does not reflect a policy of sufficient public importance to qualify as an exception to at-will employment.

It is true that when in-house attorneys report illegal conduct to their superiors, the public reaps incidental benefits from corrective action the company might undertake to comply with the law. But rule 1.13 regulates conduct that is, at its core, a private matter between attorneys and their clients, not one of broad public concern. And in similar contexts, we have explicitly characterized an employee's duty to disclose information to an employer as "serv[ing] the private interest of the employer, not the public interest."

For instance, our caselaw has established that even though the public may reap incidental benefits when a company polices its own activity through hiring compliance officers, the principal benefits flow to the employer by minimizing its risk of liability. . . .

. . . [Mr. Pang] does not allege that he reported the Company's illegal activity to anyone outside the organization or that rule 1.13 required him to contact public authorities. And the fact that Mr. Pang had an ethical obligation as an attorney under rule 1.13 to take the action he did does not distinguish his case from [our prior cases where employees] acted on similar legal obligations to disclose information to their employers.

Moreover, rule 1.13's plain terms characterize the attorney's duty to "report up" as serving the employer's private interest, not an obligation to the public. The rule requires attorneys who suspect that their employer may be involved in illegal activity "that is likely to result in substantial injury to the organization" to "refer the matter to higher authority in the organization, including, if warranted by the circumstances, to the highest authority that can act on behalf of the organization." Other provisions in the rule allow disclosure of confidential information "to the extent the lawyer reasonably believes necessary to prevent substantial injury to the organization." And it instructs lawyers representing the employer to inform "directors, officers, [and] employees" within the organization that the lawyer represents the employer when its "interests are adverse to those of the constituents with whom the lawyer is dealing." Consequently, the duty to "report up" under the rule is like the regular duty an employee might have to "disclose information concerning the employer's business to [his or her] employer," a duty we characterized in [our prior cases] as distinctly private. Accordingly, we conclude that an in-house counsel's duty to "report up" illegal activity to his or her superiors is not the type of clear and substantial public policy that qualifies as an exception to the at-will employment doctrine.

This conclusion is buttressed by the significant weight and overarching importance of other clear and substantial public policies we have recognized previously, which contrast sharply with the private nature of the policy Mr. Pang has raised in this case. As we have already discussed, Utah public policy does not allow an employer to fire someone for refusing to commit a crime or for reporting illegal activity to law enforcement. This is because of the substantial benefits such policies confer on the public at large. . . . We have also held that an employer cannot terminate anyone for attempting to exercise his or her workers' compensation rights or for pressuring an employee to ignore state reporting requirements that "ensure [] the safety of financial institutions in the state."

These examples share a common feature — they involve overarching statutory frameworks designed by the legislature to protect the public from bodily injury and financial harm. Mr. Pang's claim, by contrast, involves an internal report he was required to make as in-house counsel to minimize the regulatory risks of his employer's out-of-state lending practices. It would be one thing if Mr. Pang's complaint invoked other rules of professional conduct — like rule 1.6 — that are designed to protect others from death, substantial bodily injury, and serious financial harm. That might be a different case. But here, the policy Mr. Pang asks us to recognize is a distinctly private matter of attorney-client relations, an issue that is qualitatively different than other public policies we have recognized previously.

3. Any policy reflected in rule 1.13 is outweighed by other countervailing interests

. . . [E]ven if an in-house counsel's duty to "report up" was clear and substantial, we are persuaded that other provisions of the ethical rules express countervailing policy interests that outweigh any Mr. Pang has raised in this case.

Two such policies are protecting a client's right to choose representation and deterring illegal conduct. And the rules strike a delicate balance between allowing clients to secure the representation of their choice and guarding against a client's use of an attorney's services to engage in criminal activity. For example, rule 1.2(a) provides that lawyers must "abide by a client's decisions concerning the objectives of representation" but cannot "assist a client[] in conduct that the lawyer knows is criminal or fraudulent." Other provisions give these directives some teeth — rule 1.16 requires an attorney to "withdraw from the representation of a client" if "the representation will result in violation of the rules of professional conduct or other law." And the lawyer must also withdraw if "the lawyer is discharged" by the client. Comment 4 to that rule further emphasizes that the client "has a right to discharge a lawyer at any time, with or without cause."

Accepting Mr. Pang's argument would upset this careful weighing of two important public policies — deterring crime and protecting a client's right to choose a lawyer. If organizational clients faced a potential wrongful termination suit every time they terminate an in-house lawyer with whom they disagreed, it would be more difficult for such clients to secure the representation of their choice—and there is no doubt that a client's right to choose a lawyer occupies a position of paramount importance throughout the rules of professional conduct. Accordingly, we conclude that countervailing policies outweigh the public policy Mr. Pang has raised in this case—that an in-house counsel who "reports up" illegal activity under rule 1.13 should be shielded from the consequences of the at-will employment doctrine.

In so concluding, we recognize that in-house attorneys are situated differently than those at law firms who can withdraw from a case without becoming unemployed. That may well cause attorneys who suspect their employer is engaged in harmful, illegal conduct trepidation. We emphasize, however, the narrow scope of our decision today—we do not hold that in-house attorneys may never raise a wrongful termination claim, nor do we foreclose the possibility that an attorney fired for complying with an ethical rule, such as reporting criminal activity to public authorities under rule 1.6, could ever make out such a claim. We hold only that an attorney's duty to "report up" illegal activity to an organizational client's highest authority is not founded in the type of clear and substantial public policy that qualifies as an exception to the at-will employment doctrine. We leave these broader issues to a future case that squarely presents them.

Post-Case Follow-Up

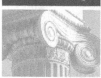

Some states have followed *Pang's* reasoning and similarly refused to provide a cause of action for wrongful discharge for attorneys — including in-house attorneys — who are fired because of compliance with rules that require an attorney to report up or report out. In Balla v. Gambro, Inc., 584 N.E.2d 104 (Ill. 1991), the Illinois Supreme Court held that former in-house counsel Roger Balla did not have an action for wrongful discharge against Gambro, Inc., for firing Balla when Balla disclosed to the U.S. Food and Drug Administration (FDA) that Gambro was selling defective kidney dialyzers, the use of which could cause serious injury or death. The FDA seized the dialyzers, prohibiting their distribution. Under the Illinois Rules of Professional Conduct, Balla was required to make this disclosure.[30] Nevertheless, citing the client's right to choose and fire counsel, the Illinois Supreme Court held that Balla could not sue for wrongful discharge. Balla argued that the lack of such a cause of action forces attorneys into a Scylla and Charybdis dilemma — either obey the rules but lose their job *or* keep their job but violate the rules and expose people to harm. The Illinois Supreme Court responded in strident terms:

> [I]n-house counsel plainly are not confronted with such a dilemma. In-house counsel do not have a choice of whether to follow their ethical obligations as attorneys licensed to practice law, or follow the illegal and unethical demands of their clients. In-house

---

30. Unlike Model Rule 1.6(b)(1), which only permits disclosure to prevent death or serious bodily injury, the Illinois Rules of Professional Conduct require attorneys to disclose confidential information in such situations. *See Balla*, 584 N.E.2d at 108 ("A lawyer *shall* reveal information about a client to the extent it appears necessary to prevent the client from committing an act that would result in death or serious bodily injury.").

counsel must abide by the Rules of Professional Conduct. Appellee had no choice but to report to the FDA Gambro's intention to sell or distribute these dialyzers. . . .[31]

Not all courts agree with the approach taken in *Pang* and *Balla*. For example, the Supreme Court of California in *General Dynamics Corp. v. Superior Court*, 876 P.2d 487 (1994), held that in-house counsel can sue for retaliatory discharge if "terminated for refusing to violate a mandatory ethical duty embodied in the Rules of Professional Conduct" or if discharged under circumstances where a non-attorney would have a claim for retaliatory discharge. Other states are in agreement with California.[32] In Van Asdale v. International Game Technology, 577 F.3d 989 (9th Cir. 2009), the Ninth Circuit held that in-house counsel who is fired for reporting up pursuant to obligations created by the Sarbanes-Oxley Act could bring claims under Nevada wrongful discharge laws and under Sarbanes-Oxley itself, which expressly provides a federal cause of action for retaliatory discharge. *See* 18 U.S.C. §1514A. Nevertheless, maintaining a successful cause of action for retaliatory discharge under Sarbanes-Oxley is quite difficult.[33]

Pang v. International Document Services: Real Life Applications

1. Lyle represents Ratchet, Inc. While working on a deal that requires certification of compliance with federal and state safety standards, Lyle discovers that Ratchet, Inc.'s tools do not comply with safety standards. Lyle meets with Ursula, who is in charge of safety and compliance. Ursula assures Lyle that while she has made mistakes in the past that have allowed noncompliant tools to be sold, that going forward Ratchet's products will be compliant with all safety standards. Under these circumstances, does Lyle need to report up regarding Ursula's past failures and noncompliance?
2. You are in-house counsel for Home Chefs, Inc., which makes high-quality kitchen utensils and appliances for home use. In preparing for a retail deal, you discover that the Home Chefs documents substantially misstate the financial status of the company. You decide to talk to the CFO about the problems. The CFO is evasive regarding your questions. You then go to the CEO who, upon hearing your concerns, fires you effective immediately. Are you really fired? What, if any, duties do you still owe to the company? How should you proceed? Can you sue for wrongful termination?

---

31. *See Balla*, 584 N.E.2d at 109.
32. *See, e.g.*, Crews v. Buckman Laboratories Int'l, Inc., 78 S.W.3d 852 (Tenn. 2002) (discussing split in authority); GTE Products Corp. v. Stewart, 653 N.E.2d 161, 167 (1995) (allowing narrow right to retaliatory discharge where attorney is fired for refusing to violate "(1) explicit and unequivocal statutory or ethical norms (2) which embody policies of importance to the public at large in the circumstances of the particular case, and (3) the claim can be proved without any violation of the attorney's obligation to respect client confidences and secrets").
33. *See* Megan E. Mowrey, L. Stephen Cash & Thomas L. Dickens, *Does Sarbanes-Oxley Protect Whistleblowers? The Recent Experience of Companies and Whistleblowing Workers Under SOX*, 1 Wm. & Mary Bus. L. Rev. 431 (2010).

2. Government Clients

Rule 1.13 applies to government clients as a specific type of organizational client. Thus, government lawyers are required to report up under Rule 1.13(b), to report to the highest authority regarding being fired for reporting up or out, and to provide entity warnings to their government client constituents whom the attorney does not represent. But who is the ultimate client of a government attorney and who is the "highest authority" that can act on behalf of the government client under Rule 1.13(b) and (c)?

Comment [9] explains that, although Rule 1.13 applies to government attorneys, "[d]efining precisely the identity of the client and prescribing the resulting obligations of such lawyers may be more difficult in the government context and is a matter beyond the scope of these Rules." Properly identifying the appropriate client is not only important for the obligations under Rule 1.13, but also for lawyers to fulfill their duties of competence, communication, confidentiality, and loyalty. For government attorneys, there is a wide range of possible ultimate clients. As Roger Cramton explains:

> The possibilities include: (1) the public (2) the government as a whole (3) the branch of government in which the lawyer is employed (4) the particular agency or department in which the lawyer works and (5) the responsible officers who make decisions for the agency. Although a scattering of support can be found for each possibility, the dispute has been primarily between a broader loyalty to "the public interest" or the government as a whole, on the one hand, and a more restricted vision of the government lawyer as the employee of a particular agency, on the other.[34]

Moreover, attorneys for the government perform nearly the whole range of legal activity — counseling, drafting, planning, negotiating, litigating — and they work in a manifold of legal specialties.[35] The vast range of government lawyer roles complicates defining a government client.

Kathleen Clark has argued that a universal definition of the government client is not attainable in light of the wide range of lawyer roles; rather, she argues that "one can determine a particular government lawyer's client by examining the particular context and the precise structure of governmental authority."[36] Thus, for example, Clark notes that some government attorneys, such as Judge Advocate General military defense lawyers, represent individual clients and have a typical individual attorney-client relationship with them. Similarly, she argues that most congressional lawyers represent individual legislators; however, some congressional lawyers represent a larger slice of the legislative branch, such as "the Senate Legal Counsel, [which] represents the Senate as an institution." As to the executive branch, Clark takes issue with the "unitary-executive view" that claims "that all executive-branch

---

34. Roger C. Cramton, *The Lawyer as Whistleblower: Confidentiality and Government Lawyer*, 5 Geo. J. Legal Ethics 291, 296 (1991).
35. *See id.* at 292.
36. Kathleen Clark, *Government Lawyers and Confidentiality Norms*, 85 Wash. U. L. Rev. 1033, 1056 (2007).

lawyers have as their client the entire executive branch, with the President ulti- mately responsible for defining client interests." She notes that some agencies are independent from the President. Thus, for example, lawyers for the SEC and the FCC should be seen as representing the agency rather than the executive branch as a whole. Nevertheless, Clark argues that the Justice Department and federal pros- ecutors represent the executive branch as a whole.[37] Significantly, Clark notes that while some government lawyers serve and answer to a specific government client or entity, others "serve both as the lawyer and essentially as a trustee, entrusted to make decisions that clients normally make."[38] For example, prosecutors make the decision whether to bring charges, appeal, or accept a plea deal — decisions usually allocated to the client in a traditional attorney-client relationship. Clark posits:

> While some have asserted that, for these lawyers, the "public interest" is their client, it makes more sense to conceive of these lawyers as trustees of the client (such as the state government) who can consider the public interest in making their decisions. . . .
>
> If a government lawyer has the authority to make client-like decisions (such as whether to bring or settle cases), then she also has the responsibility to act not just like any client, but in a way this particular client — a sovereign — should act. In our legal tradition, the sovereign is not free to act in the same way as any private litigant but is expected to act fairly and impartially.[39]

Because government lawyers ultimately represent a sovereign, "whose obli- gation to govern impartially is as compelling as its obligation to govern at all" — government lawyers may have a greater duty to ensure that their client is acting justly and in accordance with law.[40] Indeed, comment [9] to Rule 1.13 explains that "a government lawyer may have authority under applicable law to question" the conduct of government officials for whom the lawyer works "more extensively than that of a lawyer for a private organization in similar circumstances." This is so because where government is acting and is employing the weight and legitimacy of state power, "a different balance may be appropriate between maintaining confi- dentiality and assuring that the wrongful act is prevented or rectified."

3. Insureds

Insurance agreements generate another area with client identity complications. Insurers hire attorneys to represent an insured person in accordance with a policy between the insurer and the insured. In such a situation, does the attorney repre- sent the insurer (who is paying for the attorney) or the insured? The relationship

---

37. *Id.* at 1052-68. *See also* Kathleen Clark, *The Lawyers Who Mistook a President for Their Client*, 52 IND. L. REV. 271 (2019) (examining the DOJ's 150-year history of interpreting the Emoluments Clause as prohibiting accep- tance of any benefit from a foreign government until 2017, when the DOJ adopted the legal arguments of President Trump's personal lawyers "who were pushing for a narrow interpretation of the Clause in order to advance Trump's private financial interests").
38. Clark, *supra* note 36, at 1062.
39. *Id.* at 1069.
40. Berger v. United States, 295 U.S. 78, 88 (1935).

between the insured, the insurer, and the attorney hired by the insurer has been termed a **tripartite relationship**.[41] The Restatement (Third) of the Law Governing Lawyers maintains that the "lawyer designated to defend the insured has a client-lawyer relationship with the insured." Moreover, "[t]he insurer is not, simply by the fact that it designates the lawyer, a client of the lawyer."[42] The insurer may also have an attorney-client relationship with the attorney — in which case the attorney is representing the insured and the insurer as joint clients. Ellen Pryor and Charles Silver contend that the identity of the insurance defense lawyer depends entirely "on the agreement that actually is reached at the time the defense lawyer is engaged to handle the case."[43]

In many insurance contracts, the insured will have agreed to allow the insurer to control the defense, including whether or not to settle the claim. Given that the insured is either the sole or the joint client of the attorney, and that the decision to settle is given to the ultimate authority of the client, is such an arrangement permissible? Model Rule 1.2(c) generally allows an attorney to limit the scope of a representation with a client, as long as "the limitation is reasonable under the circumstances and the client gives informed consent." Read the following opinion, and consider what steps a lawyer has to take to successfully limit the scope of her relationship with an insured client to allow the insurer to control the defense and settlement of the claims.

Obligations of a Lawyer Representing an Insured Who Objects to a Proposed Settlement Within Policy Limits
ABA Formal Opinion 96-403 (1996)

. . . The Model Rules of Professional Conduct offer virtually no guidance as to whether a lawyer retained and paid by an insurer to defend its insured represents the insured, the insurer, or both. . . . The Model Rules assume a client-lawyer relationship established in accordance with state law, and prescribe the ethical obligations of the lawyer that flow from that relationship.

The insurer, the insured, and the lawyer may agree on the identity of the client or clients the lawyer is to represent at the outset. For example, the parties might agree that the lawyer will represent (1) the insured alone, (2) the insured and the insurer, or (3) the insured and the insurer for all purposes except settlement, and with respect to settlement the lawyer will represent the insurer alone. Provided there is appropriate disclosure, consultation, and consent, any of these arrangements would be permissible. Absent an express agreement specifying the identity of the lawyer's client or clients, however, a lawyer hired by an insurer to defend its insured may be held to

---

41. Charles Silver, *The Professional Responsibilities of Insurance Defense Lawyers*, 45 Duke L.J. 255, 264 (1995).
42. Restatement (Third) of the Law Governing Lawyers §134 cmt. f.
43. Ellen S. Pryor & Charles Silver, *Defense Lawyers' Professional Responsibilities: Part I — Excess Exposure Cases*, 78 Tex. L. Rev. 599, 607 (2000).

have a client-lawyer relationship with the insured alone or with both the insured and the insurer.

We have no reason to enter the debate as to whom the lawyer represents in this context absent an express agreement as to the identity of the client. For purposes of this opinion, nothing fundamental turns on whether the lawyer represents the insured alone or both the insurer and the insured. If a lawyer hired and paid by an insurer to defend a claim against an insured represents the insured — whether alone or jointly with the insurer, whether by virtue of a provision in an engagement letter or otherwise — the Rules of Professional Conduct govern the lawyer's obligations to the insured, and "[t]he essential point of ethics involved is that the lawyer so employed shall represent the insured as his client with undivided fidelity. . . ." ABA Committee on Professional Ethics, Formal Opinion 282 (1950) (construing the 1908 Canons of Professional Ethics). Whatever the rights and duties of the insurer and the insured under the insurance contract, that contract does not define the ethical responsibilities of the lawyer to his client.

If the lawyer is to proceed with the representation of the insured at the direction of the insurer, the lawyer must make appropriate disclosure sufficient to apprise the insured of the limited nature of his representation as well as the insurer's right to control the defense in accordance with the terms of the insurance contract. Generally a lawyer must abide [by] his client's decisions as to the objectives of the litigation and specifically as to whether to accept a settlement. . . .

Rule 1.2(c) provides that a "lawyer may limit the objectives of the representation," but only if "the client consents after consultation" with the lawyer. "Consultation" "denotes communication of information reasonably sufficient to permit the client to appreciate the significance of the matter in question." Model Rules of Professional Conduct, Terminology. . . .

We presume that in the vast majority of cases the insured will have no objection to proceeding in accordance with the terms of his insurance contract. Nonetheless, communication between the lawyer and the insured is required. Rule 1.2 explicitly requires the lawyer to communicate with the client, and convey information "sufficient to permit the client to appreciate the significance of the matter in question." We cannot assume that the insured understands or remembers, if he ever read, the insurance policy, or that the insured understands that his lawyer will be acting on his behalf, but at the direction of the insurer without further consultation with the insured.

A short letter clearly stating that the lawyer intends to proceed at the direction of the insurer in accordance with the terms of the insurance contract and what this means to the insured is sufficient to satisfy the requirements of Rule 1.2 in this context. We do not believe extended discussion is required or, indeed, that any oral communication is necessary. As long as the insured is clearly apprised of the limitations on the representation being offered by the insurer and that the lawyer intends to proceed in accordance with the directions of the insurer, the insured has sufficient information to decide whether to accept the defense offered by the insurer or to assume responsibility for his own defense at his own expense. No formal acceptance or written consent is necessary. The insured manifests consent to the limited representation by accepting the defense offered by the insurer after being advised of the terms of the representation being offered.

4. Clients with Diminished Capacity

Lawyers may represent clients who have diminished mental capacity. This diminished capacity may exist because of the client's age (whether due to youth or old age) or other mental impairments. For example, if a lawyer represents a 13-year-old boy in a juvenile proceeding, should the lawyer follow the instructions of the 13-year-old, even when the lawyer believes such action is not in her client's interest? Jurisdictions differ on the precise answer to that question.[44] For example, in some states the attorney is to consider the juvenile client's wishes, yet the lawyer is not required to follow the juvenile's instructions if it does not appear to be in the client's best interests.[45] In stark contrast, other jurisdictions maintain that the attorney must comply with the juvenile's instructions — even when it does not appear to be in the client's best interests.[46] Attorneys representing juvenile clients, or other clients with potential diminished capacities, should take care to examine the approach of the pertinent jurisdiction.

Model Rule 1.14 sets out the basic principle that the attorney should — whenever possible — treat the client as a normal client in an attorney-client relationship, with the client making decisions for the representation. Only in exigent circumstances — situations where the client "is at risk of substantial physical, financial or other harm unless action is taken" and "cannot adequately act in the client's own interest" — should the lawyer take "reasonably necessary protective action." *See* Model Rule 1.14(b). Moreover, attorneys should undertake protective measures that are the least intrusive to client autonomy as possible given the circumstances. Again, comment [5] counsels that in taking protective measures:

> the lawyer should be guided by such factors as [1] the wishes and values of the client . . . , [2] the client's best interests . . . , [3] the goals of intruding into the client's decision-making autonomy to the least extent feasible, [4] maximizing client capacities and [5] respecting the client's family and social connections.

Guardianship should be sought only when absolutely necessary, as a guardianship eviscerates the decision-making autonomy of the client. Often, even with a diminished capacity, a client will have "the ability to understand, deliberate upon, and reach conclusions about matters affecting the client's own well-being." *See* Model Rule 1.14 cmt. [1]. And even when protective measures are appropriate, there are many options far less intrusive to the client than guardianship. As comment [5] points out, "[s]uch measures could include consulting with family members, using a reconsideration period to permit clarification or improvement of circumstances, using voluntary surrogate decisionmaking tools such as durable powers of attorney or consulting with support groups, professional services, adult-protective agencies" and the like. Importantly, wherever possible, the attorney must keep in mind the identity of his client, to whom the attorney owes duties

---

44. *See* ANNOTATED MODEL RULES OF PROF'L CONDUCT, Rule 1.14, Representation of a Minor.
45. *See id.; see, e.g.,* In re Christina W., 639 S.E.2d 770 (W. Va. 2006).
46. *See, e.g.,* Mass. Ethics Op. 93-6 (1993).

of communication, confidentiality, and loyalty. Thus, for example, when the client needs the assistance of family to communicate with the attorney or make decisions, the lawyer must do his best to ensure that the client's family is not interfering with the attorney's duties to his actual client.

D. ATTORNEY AS FIDUCIARY

Attorneys are supposed to be the champion of their client's interests (within the bounds of the law), yet there are aspects of the attorney-client relationship where the lawyer's interest and the client's interest inevitably diverge — most notably in the charging and payment of attorneys' fees. In such situations where the lawyer's and client's interests actually or potentially diverge, lawyers cannot take advantage of their clients. The lawyer owes the client the duties of a fiduciary — the client trusts the lawyer to safeguard the client's interests in charging a fee, handling client funds and property, and withdrawing from the case.

1. Fees

Fees create an inherent adversity of interest between the attorney and client. It is in the client's financial interest to pay a lower fee, while it is in the lawyer's financial interest to charge a higher one. Further, when a fee must be collected, the lawyer and client enter into an adverse relationship as creditor and debtor. Yet the lawyer is still the fiduciary of the client — even in the charging or collecting of a fee; the client trusts and the rules require that the lawyer will protect the client's interests.

Communicating the Fee to the Client

Clients, especially those who are unfamiliar with legal services, may not appreciate (or have the slightest concept of) the cost of legal representation in a matter. Thus, the first obstacle in the charging of a fee is effectively communicating to the client what the basis or rate of the fee will be. The Model Rules require attorneys to "communicate[] to the client" the basis or rate of both the fee and the expenses that the client will be responsible to pay. The lawyer is also required to communicate "the scope of the representation" to the client, meaning that the lawyer must communicate what legal actions the lawyer is agreeing to undertake and/or any limitations on the scope of the lawyer's services. *See* Model Rule 1.5(b). This requirement goes hand in hand with communicating the fee so that the client understands what it is she is (and is not) purchasing when hiring the attorney. Notably, Model Rule 1.2 allows an attorney to limit the scope of a representation, as long as the "limitation is reasonable under the circumstances and the client gives informed consent."

The Model Rules themselves do not require that non-contingent fee agreements be in writing; rather, Rule 1.5 only requires communication to the client, while stating that a writing is preferable. However, any marginally prudent lawyer will put the fee agreement in writing. Moreover, a number of jurisdictions require a written communication outlining the basis and rate whenever a fee is charged.

Contingent Fees

The Model Rules generally allow an attorney to charge a contingent fee, with a couple of important exceptions. Under Rule 1.5, attorneys cannot charge a contingent fee in a criminal matter or if the contingent fee is prohibited by other law. In addition, attorneys are prohibited in domestic relations cases from charging a fee that "is contingent upon the securing of a divorce or upon the amount of alimony or support or property settlement in lieu thereof."

Further, Model Rule 1.5(c) requires that two writings accompany any contingent fee agreement with a client. First, at the outset of the representation, the contingent fee agreement must be made in writing and be signed by the client. This first writing must contain several components: (1) "the method by which the fee is to be determined," which itself must include "the percentages that shall accrue to the lawyer in the event of settlement, trial or appeal"; (2) "litigation and other expenses to be deducted from the recovery"; (3) "whether such expenses are to be deducted before or after the contingent fee is calculated"; and (4) a statement of any expenses that the client must pay whether or not the client prevails. The second required writing comes at the conclusion of the contingency case. The lawyer is required to prepare "a written statement" that informs the client both of the final disposition of the action and of the "remittance to the client and the method of its determination" as to any recovery.

A Reasonable Fee

Model Rule 1.5(a) expressly prohibits a lawyer from agreeing to, charging, or collecting "an unreasonable fee or an unreasonable amount for expenses." The requirement of reasonableness applies whether the fee is calculated on an hourly or a contingent basis. The rule sets out a list of eight factors to consider in determining the reasonableness of a fee, which will be discussed in the *Sallee* case below. Importantly, there is not a safe harbor where a fee will be deemed reasonable if the fee is calculated by multiplying the hours actually and honestly worked by the agreed-upon hourly rate.[47] In Board of Professional Responsibility, Wyoming State Bar v. Casper, 318 P.3d 790 (2014), the Wyoming Supreme Court held that a lodestar determination ("reasonable hours times a reasonable rate") is only a first step to examining reasonableness. The second step requires considering other factors to "adjust the fee either upward or downward." The Wyoming Supreme Court explained:

> The second step requires the application of "billing judgment," which usually is demonstrated by the attorney writing off unproductive, excessive, or redundant hours. Billing

---

47. In re Fordham, 668 N.E.2d 816, 821, 824 (Mass. 1996) (rejecting "safe harbor" that a fee is reasonable "as long as an agreement existed between a client and an attorney to bill a reasonable rate multiplied by the number of hours actually worked").

for legal services . . . should not be a merely mechanical exercise. . . . A reasonable fee can only be fixed by the exercise of judgment, using the mechanical computations simply as a starting point. . . .[48]

Thus, in In re Fordham, 668 N.E.2d 816 (Mass. 1996), the Massachusetts Supreme Judicial Court held that a $50,000 fee for defending an accused for operating a motor vehicle under the influence of alcohol (OUI) was unreasonable where the standard fee in the locality was between $1,500 and $5,000. One of the most significant factors set out in Rule 1.5 for measuring the reasonableness of a fee is "the fee customarily charged in the locality for similar legal services." Fordham's fee was ten times the customary fee for the location. Thus, the fee was unreasonable even though the attorney honestly and diligently worked each of the hours billed, secured an excellent result (acquittal), and the client agreed to the hourly rate. The court noted that Fordham, who had not previously performed criminal work, had charged for the time spent to educate himself regarding criminal defense. The court explained that Fordham could not charge for his education, stating: "It cannot be that an inexperienced lawyer is entitled to charge three or four times as much as an experienced lawyer for the same service."[49] Importantly, the first factor for determining reasonableness in Model Rule 1.5(a) is not the time actually *spent* by the attorney, but "the time and labor *required*" — that is, the time that would be taken by a reasonably proficient attorney.

In a similar vein, the Utah Supreme Court held that an attorney could not charge fees that were generated by the attorney's own incompetence and attempts to fix that incompetence. In Dahl v. Dahl, 2015 UT 79, excerpted in Chapter 4, Christensen sought an award of attorneys' fees for his representation in a divorce. Christensen made numerous procedural errors that led to nearly all of his exhibits being excluded at trial, the exclusion of expert witness testimony on behalf of his client, and the exclusion of evidence regarding his client's financial need. Consequently, his client was not awarded either temporary or permanent alimony and the client's ex-husband was awarded sole custody of their children. Nevertheless, Christensen sought an award of fees and expenses of over $2.1 million, including $327,000 related to experts that were largely excluded from trial (because Christensen did not prepare proper expert reports). The court noted that many of the hours billed were for review of the file with "huge, almost impossible hours recorded during the trial months" that were billed "to gain an understanding of evidence and facts that should have been mastered months earlier."[50] In addition, many of the hours billed were for motions to reconsider rulings that resulted from Christensen's poor handling of the case. In sum, the court held that Christensen's fee was "unreasonable as a matter of law" and that "most of the fees and expenses seem to have been driven by Mr. Christensen's inability to effectively manage basic discovery and pretrial disclosure procedures."[51] The court admonished:

---

48. *Casper,* 318 P.3d at 796 (internal citations omitted).
49. *Fordham,* 668 N.E.2d at 822-23.
50. *Dahl,* 2015 UT 79, ¶179.
51. *Id.* ¶211, ¶205.

When an attorney proceeds competently, but nonetheless is unsuccessful for his client, we ascribe no error. But when an attorney consistently fails to perform basic skills in a competent manner, and the client is harmed as a result, we will not allow that attorney to collect [what has become] patently unreasonable fees.[52]

Just as in *Fordham*, where an inexperienced attorney cannot charge more than an experienced attorney, so too an incompetent attorney cannot charge more than a competent attorney despite actually spending significant time engaged in or seeking to undo wasteful or even counterproductive measures.

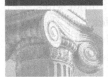

Case Preview

Sallee v. Tennessee Board of Professional Responsibility

Attorney Yarboro Sallee was suspended from the practice of law for one year for charging an unreasonable fee in a wrongful death case, failing to communicate the rate and basis of the fee to the client, and failing to protect her client's interests once her client fired her.

As you read *Sallee*, consider the following:

1. What made Sallee's fees unreasonable? Which of the factors outlined in Rule 1.5(a) indicated an unreasonable fee? What types of activities did Sallee charge for that the court found inappropriate?
2. Was Sallee's failure to communicate her rate and basis of fee the primary problem? If Sallee had employed the "preferable" path of a written fee agreement fully explaining her rate and basis of fee (including the charges for time and a half) and provided clear billing statements, would Sallee's fee have been reasonable?

Sallee v. Tennessee Board of Professional Responsibility
469 S.W.3d 18 (Tenn. 2015)

The case that prompted this disciplinary complaint arose from a tragic occurrence. On October 15, 2009, Lori Noll fell down steps in her home. She died five days later. Ms. Noll was a wife, mother of two children, and the daughter of the claimants in this

---

52. *Id.* ¶206. The court was also concerned that Christensen devoted so much of his presentation to the court to secure his own fees rather than to protect his client's interests. The court noted:

> Ms. Dahl's counsel devoted nearly seventeen pages of her appellate brief to her request for attorney fees while devoting less than two pages to Ms. Dahl's request for joint custody of her children. While counsel is certainly entitled to pursue an award of fees on his client's behalf, the focus on the attorney fees issue to the exclusion of issues such as custody raises serious concerns.

See id. ¶210.

case, Frances Rodgers and Vearl Bible (collectively, the "Claimants"). Despite a medical examiner's finding that the death was accidental, the Claimants suspected that their daughter's husband, Adam Noll, was responsible for her death, motivated by a one-million dollar insurance policy on Ms. Noll's life. A close friend of the Claimants recommended Attorney Sallee to advise them on their legal options.

On September 18, 2010, the Claimants had an initial meeting with Attorney Sallee, to discuss the feasibility of a wrongful death action on behalf of their deceased daughter. . . . At this initial meeting, Attorney Sallee did not discuss her compensation with the Claimants. . . .

A few days later, on September 21, 2010, Attorney Sallee met with the Claimants to discuss the 911 call Mr. Noll made regarding their daughter's death. In the 911 call, Mr. Noll gave the dispatcher a questionable explanation for Ms. Noll's fall and his subsequent actions. After Attorney Sallee conveyed her preliminary thoughts, the Claimants agreed to retain Attorney Sallee and wrote her a check for $5,000. In this meeting, the Claimants orally agreed to pay Attorney Sallee $250 per hour for her services.

. . . Even though she had only an oral representation agreement, in light of the looming expiration of the limitations period, Attorney Sallee launched into intensive work on the case. . . . [O]n October 13, 2010, Attorney Sallee told the Claimants that, in order to continue representing them, she would need a $20,000 retainer. Despite the absence of a written representation agreement, Ms. Rodgers wrote Attorney Sallee a check for an additional $15,000. . . . During this time, Attorney Sallee did not provide the Claimants with any sort of billing statement.

On October 15, 2010, Attorney Sallee filed a timely wrongful death complaint against Mr. Noll in the Circuit Court of Knox County, Tennessee. Attorney Sallee's agreement was to represent only the Claimants. Despite this, the complaint drafted by Attorney Sallee was filed on behalf of not only the Claimants, but also on behalf of Ms. Noll's children and the estate of Ms. Noll. The complaint did not plead the claim by the grandparents as "next friend" of the grandchildren.

On October 19, 2010, Attorney Sallee sent another email to Ms. Rodgers. . . . That same day, Ms. Rodgers received a visit at her home from the friend who had initially recommended Attorney Sallee to the Claimants. The friend admonished Ms. Rodgers that the Claimants had not given Attorney Sallee enough money for her retainer. This prompted Ms. Rodgers to immediately write Attorney Sallee an additional check, in the amount of $10,000. The friend then delivered Ms. Rodgers' check to Attorney Sallee.

. . . Finally, in early December 2010, the Claimants asked Attorney Sallee for a written contract addressing her representation of them. In response, Attorney Sallee gave the Claimants several confusing draft agreements that included "a conglomeration of hourly charges, plus contingency [fees]." The inclusion of contingency fees in the draft agreements came as a surprise to the Claimants; they had been under the impression that Attorney Sallee was to receive only hourly fees, not contingency fees. In view of this discrepancy, the Claimants declined to sign the proposed agreements. . . .

In an apparent attempt to pressure the Claimants into executing her proposed fee agreement, in early January 2011, Attorney Sallee threatened to "drop [the

Claimants] from the case." Finally fed up, the Claimants instead "decided it was time to drop her." The Claimants sent Attorney Sallee a formal letter terminating her representation of them in all matters.

. . . When the Claimants requested their file, Attorney Sallee refused to provide them the entire file. As justification, Attorney Sallee asserted that the Claimants owed her "eighty-plus thousand dollars, in addition to what [they had] already paid her." She mailed the Claimants a letter to this effect on January 5, 2011.

In mid-January 2011, Mr. Bible and Ms. Rodgers each sent a complaint letter to the Tennessee Board of Professional Responsibility ("BPR" or "the Board"), outlining some of the difficulties with Attorney Sallee's representation of them. . . .

In early February 2011, Attorney Sallee sent the BPR her initial response to the Claimants' complaints: a 21-page letter, single-spaced. Although she had never given the Claimants an itemization of her time spent on their cases, Attorney Sallee attached to her BPR response an itemized "billing statement" with detailed time entries on the work she claimed to have done for the Claimants.[4]

Despite the Claimants' complaint to the BPR, Attorney Sallee continued to refuse to turn over to the Claimants items from their files. This forced the Claimants to hire another attorney, Larry Vaughan, to obtain the withheld items. To that end, in early March 2011, Attorney Vaughan filed an action on behalf of the Claimants against Attorney Sallee in the Knox County Chancery Court. The lawsuit specifically sought medical records on Ms. Noll that Attorney Sallee had retrieved from the hospital, as well as brain tissue slides from Ms. Noll's autopsy that were in Attorney Sallee's possession.

The filing of the chancery court complaint did not persuade Attorney Sallee to turn over the disputed items to the Claimants. . . . In early April 2011, the chancellor ordered Attorney Sallee to turn over the remaining items to the Claimants. . . .

. . .

Attorney Sallee contends that the record does not contain substantial and material evidence to support the Panel's finding that the fee she charged to the Claimants was excessive. She argues strenuously that her fee was "on average per hour less tha[n] the average hourly fee of attorney[s] in Knoxville" and that "the record is replete with hundreds of e-mails and proof of calls every day" demonstrating her constant communication with the Claimants.

. . . Rule 1.5 of the Tennessee Rules of Professional Conduct at [the time of the misconduct] required that "[a] lawyer's fee and charges for expenses shall be reasonable" and mandated that "the basis or rate of the fee shall be communicated to the client, preferably in writing, before or within a reasonable time after commencing the representation." Tenn. Sup. Ct. R. 8, RPC 1.5(a) and (b) (2010). In determining whether an attorney fee is reasonable, courts examine the following factors:

---

4. . . . The "billing statement" has time entries for the time period of September 16, 2010 (the date of the initial meeting) to December 3, 2010, totaling 493.5 hours. Of this total, 135 hours were shown at a rate of $375 per hour, and the remaining 358.5 hours were shown at the agreed rate of $250 per hour. According to Attorney Sallee's "billing statement," in a time span of less than three months, the accrued hourly charges on the Claimants' legal matters came to over $140,000. Subtracting the $54,000 the Claimants had already paid, Attorney Sallee maintained that the Claimants still owed her over $86,000. The "billing statement" provided to the BPR did not include the contingency fees Attorney Sallee sought in addition to the hourly charges.

(1)   The time and labor required, the novelty and difficulty of the questions involved, and the skill requisite to perform the legal service properly;

(2)   The likelihood, if apparent to the client, that the acceptance of the particular employment will preclude other employment by the lawyer;

(3)   The fee customarily charged in the locality for similar legal services;

(4)   The amount involved and the results obtained;

(5)   The time limitations imposed by the client or by the circumstances;

(6)   The nature and length of the professional relationship with the client;

(7)   The experience, reputation, and ability of the lawyer or lawyers performing the services;

(8)   **Whether the fee is fixed or contingent;**

(9)   **Prior advertisements or statements by the lawyer with respect to the fees the lawyer charges; and**

(10) **Whether the fee agreement is in writing.**

Tenn. Sup. Ct. R. 8, RPC 1.5(a) (2010). The Panel's written decision demonstrates that it properly considered these factors in reaching its decision. . . . We consider them as well.

Initially, we confess a certain amount of skepticism about Attorney Sallee's claim that she in fact worked well over 493.5 hours on the Claimants' matters in a span of three months, while also continuing to service the 28 to 30 other clients she claimed she had during that time period.[24] Nevertheless, we assume, for purposes of this appeal, that she actually worked those hours. Attorney Sallee's arguments are considered in light of this assumption.

. . .

The record indicates that Attorney Sallee initially represented to the Claimants that she had considerable experience relevant to their legal concerns. She told the Claimants that her legal qualifications were such that she normally commanded $500 per hour for her time but, in this instance, she was willing to give them a "discounted" rate of $250 per hour. She estimated that the contemplated wrongful death lawsuit would cost the Claimants no more than $100,000. A mere three months later, Attorney Sallee claims, she had amassed charges totaling over $140,000.[25] For this fee, in the wrongful death case, she had accomplished only the filing of a basic wrongful death complaint — which was pled incorrectly — and the gathering of the recording of the 911 call and a few pertinent documents and medical records. She had taken no witness statements, prepared no expert statements, taken no depositions, propounded no discovery requests. She had, however, engaged in a prodigious amount of wheel-spinning, spending countless hours, charged at a lawyer

24. Asked about time entries on the "billing statement" indicating that she worked up to 19 or even 23 hours in a single day, Attorney Sallee insisted that she actually worked those hours, but added vaguely that certain columns on the so-called "billing statement" may not have lined up correctly.

25. This total comes from the so-called "billing statement" that Attorney Sallee gave to the BPR. The entries on the document are confusing and disorganized, with time spent on each of the Claimants' matters combined. The entries are generally billed at a minimum increment of 0.5 hours. While the document has been referred to in these proceedings as a "billing statement," it is in fact no such thing, since it was never given to the Claimants until they filed complaints with the Board. We consider it instead to be an exhibit created by Attorney Sallee for the purpose of defending the BPR complaint.

rate, in activities such as watching *48 Hours* television episodes, waiting in hospitals for medical records, and doing internet research on strangulation. Her communications with the Claimants referred to the hours she had worked only in general terms, and only in the context of badgering them for more money. At no point did she tell them that her original estimate had quickly proven unrealistic, that she was charging them a "time-and-a-half" $375 per hour rate for tasks performed after business hours, or that she intended to charge them lawyer rates for administrative tasks and watching television. At no point did she give them an itemized statement of her charges. As the final straw, toward the end of the three-month period, she insisted that the Claimants sign a representation agreement that would entitle her to charge contingency fees in addition to the high hourly rates she was already charging them.

The Rules governing lawyers require transparency and candor with clients. Many a lawyer has been asked by a prospective client to estimate how much a contemplated legal matter will cost. If the lawyer has sufficient experience, such an estimate can be given. However, under most circumstances, once it becomes reasonably clear to the lawyer that the estimate is inaccurate, this fact should be communicated to the client, so the client can make an informed decision about going forward with the case. In this case, if Attorney Sallee's "billing statement" is to be believed, her fees reached the $100,000 level of her original estimate for the entire wrongful death litigation only two months after her engagement, at a time when the litigation was just getting started. Yet, she said nothing to the Claimants about the inaccuracy of her estimate. Thus, the Panel did not err in considering the fact that Attorney Sallee did not tell the Claimants that her original estimate of $100,000 for the entire wrongful death action had proven inaccurate.

Clients who are being charged hourly rates should be kept reasonably informed about the amount of work being done by the lawyer, the type of work being done, and the rates being charged for the hours worked. Here, the Claimants had no way to know the enormous number of total hours Attorney Sallee was claiming to have worked. They were not told that Attorney Sallee sought to change the oral representation agreement to charge them "time and a half" for time spent working after regular business hours, or that she intended to charge them contingency fees in addition to hourly fees. They were not told that she intended to charge them lawyer rates, either $250 per hour or $375 per hour depending on the time of day, for tasks such as sitting at a hospital to wait for medical records. . . .

Assuming *arguendo* that the hourly rate of $250 per hour is reasonable for Attorney Sallee's experience and ability,[26] it is important under the Rules that the lawyer ensure that the work for which he or she seeks to charge the client is "reasonable." For example, a lawyer who represents criminal clients may be interested in watching *Perry Mason* or *Breaking Bad* on television, and may even pick up a useful tidbit or two from doing so. The lawyer may not, however, equate that to research for which

---

26. Our review of the time entries on the "billing statement" Attorney Sallee furnished to the BPR shows she spent many hours on activities for which an attorney with sufficient experience in wrongful death actions to command $250 per hour would not have spent his or her billable time. This indicates that the rate Attorney Sallee sought to charge the Claimants was not commensurate with her experience and ability.

he or she may charge a client. In this case, the Panel did not err in considering the many hours Attorney Sallee sought to charge the Claimants for watching television shows such as *48 Hours*. In addition, the Panel considered the explanations offered by Attorney Sallee for charging the Claimants a lawyer's rate for many, many hours spent on essentially administrative tasks, and it found that she did not have adequate justification under the facts of this case for such charges. The Panel did not err in considering either of these factors in reaching the conclusion that Attorney Sallee sought to charge the Claimants for work that was not reasonable. RPC 1.5 cmt. 5 (2010) ("A lawyer should not exploit a fee arrangement based primarily on hourly charges by using wasteful procedures.").

In assessing the reasonableness of the charges, the lawyer must also take into account the "results obtained." At the time her representation of the Claimants was terminated, the legal matters for which Attorney Sallee was hired were far from resolved, so the ultimate result was not yet known. However, as outlined above, after three months' work, she had achieved little more than filing the wrongful death complaint and gathering obvious documents and records. Attorney Sallee was obliged to recognize that the $140,000 she sought to charge the Claimants at that juncture was outlandish in light of how little had been accomplished, and reduce her fee to a level commensurate with the very modest results she had obtained for the Claimants at that point. The Panel did not err in concluding that the fee Attorney Sallee sought to charge the Claimants was not reasonable in light of the minimal results accomplished for the Claimants at the time of the termination.

Based on our careful review of the record, and considering all of Attorney's Sallee's conduct with regard to the fees she sought to charge the Claimants, we find material and substantial evidence to support the Panel's determination that Attorney Sallee violated Rules 1.4 [Communication] and 1.5 [Fees] of the Tennessee Rules of Professional Conduct. . . .

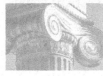

Post-Case Follow-Up

Notice that Tennessee's Rule 1.5 contains two additional factors beyond the eight found in Model Rule 1.5(a). Several other jurisdictions have either added factors or modified the eight standard factors listed in Rule 1.5(a). Although the court gave Sallee the benefit of the doubt, the court expressed skepticism as to whether Sallee in fact worked all of the hours she billed. As noted below, if Sallee did not work those hours, she is charging a fraudulent fee and is engaged in theft.

The court noted in footnote 25 that the smallest increment in Sallee's bills was 0.5 hours. Would that alone render the fee unreasonable? In Board of Professional Responsibility, Wyoming State Bar v. Casper, 318 P.3d 790 (Wyo. 2014), the attorney, Stacy Casper, billed her client in increments of 15 minutes (.25 hours). The court noted that of the 106 entries in the billing record, "few if any of those tasks would reasonably require a quarter hour of her time." Indeed, Casper "routinely billed .25 hours each to sign such documents as subpoenas, stipulated orders and pleadings." The court ultimately found Casper had charged an unreasonable fee and expounded:

> Use of billing with minimum time increments does not necessarily result in an unreasonable fee. The Court recognizes that use of minimum billing increments is a useful tool which is not, in and of itself, unethical. The Task Force on Lawyer Business Ethics has explained:
>
>> For convenience, lawyers generally keep track of the time spent using standard increments of time, commonly six minutes (0.1 hour), ten minutes (1/6 hour) or fifteen minutes (1/4 hour). This approach is essential and should not be objectionable unless the increments are unreasonably large or are used in an abusive manner. It would not be practical to keep track of time in constantly varying measurements, and minimum increments serve the practical needs of both lawyers and clients. On the other hand, the practice should not be abused. Legitimate use of a minimum time increment may depend on how the lawyer records the balance of the increment. Two fifteen-minute charges for two five-minute calls within the same fifteen-minute period seem inappropriate; some balancing should be used.

Sallee v. Tennessee Board of Professional Responsibility: Real Life Applications

1. Josh is an attorney who has consistently had low billable hours compared with others in his firm. He decides to perform extra work to make up the difference. For example, he makes his own copies of motions and briefs for filing, rather than having his secretary do it. He also personally delivers discovery requests to the office of opposing counsel and files documents rather than having the courier perform those tasks. Making these changes in his habits has allowed Josh to work an extra 30 hours a month. Are there any problems with Josh billing this time to his clients?

2. Michelle practices law at a New York City law firm, where she charges, as a new partner, $780 an hour. She decides to move her practice to Boise, Idaho, where she grew up. The going rate in Boise is $250 an hour for partners. Michelle believes that she should be able to charge for her "big city" experience, and decides to charge a middle-ground rate of $450 an hour. Under Rule 1.5, what hourly rate can Michelle charge in Boise?

Fraudulent Fees

The charging of a fraudulent fee is *per se* unreasonable under Rule 1.5 — it additionally can lead to criminal charges or civil liability for the lawyer. Many lawyers have gone to prison for fraudulent billing.[53]

---

53. *See, e.g.*, Lisa G. Lerman, *Blue-Chip Bilking: Regulation of Billing and Expense Fraud by Lawyers*, 12 GEO. J. LEGAL ETHICS 205 (1999). Lerman examines the cases of 16 lawyers who were indicted for fraudulent billing — some of them sentenced to multiple years in prison. *See id.* at 211-15.

Observance of a few basic principles will protect a lawyer from the pitfall of fraudulent billing. First, only charge your client for time you actually work. As noted in ABA Formal Opinion 93-379, "a lawyer who has undertaken to bill on an hourly basis is never justified in charging a client for hours not actually expended." Padding a bill by adding or increasing time that was not actually spent working is not only unethical, it is theft. While it is generally permissible to bill clients in agreed-upon increments of time (typically tenths of an hour), lawyers cannot fraudulently inflate the bill with time they did not work. Lisa Lerman provides a few examples of fraudulent billing:

- Some lawyers are just sloppy about keeping time records.
- Some systematically "pad" timesheets, or bill one client for work done for another.
- Some create entirely fictitious timesheets.
- Some record hours based on work done by other lawyers, paralegals or secretaries, representing that they did the work. This may result in nonbillable time being billed, or in work being billed at a rate higher than that of the person who actually did the work.
- Some lawyers bill for time that their clients might not regard as legitimately billable — for schmoozing with other lawyers, chatting with clients about sports or families, for doing administrative work that could be done by a non-lawyer, or for thinking about a case while mowing the lawn or watching television.[54]

Second, do not bill an impossible number of hours. Many lawyers have gotten into serious trouble when they have billed for hours that they could not possibly have worked. An Ohio attorney, Kristen Stahlbush, received a two-year suspension for billing "more than 24 hours per day on at least three occasions" with numerous other days billed at "14 to 24 hours." Indeed, "[i]n one 96-hour period [she] billed 90.3 hours, and in a separate 144-hour period, she billed 139.5 hours."[55] Similarly, Jerome Berg was disbarred for repeatedly billing an insurance company more than 24 hours per day — and on some days he billed 100 hours.[56]

Third, do not **double bill** or otherwise charge for the same hour of work more than once. If you work for one hour, you can only charge for one hour — even if you are representing multiple clients, acting in multiple capacities (such as trustee and attorney), or want to use the same work product in another case. Double billing occurs when a lawyer charges multiple clients each for the same block of time spent. Billing recycled work product means billing a subsequent client for the time spent for (and already billed to) a prior client for reusing the work product. In Formal Opinion 93-379, the ABA condemned these practices as unethical:

A lawyer who spends four hours of time on behalf of three clients has not earned twelve billable hours. A lawyer, who flies for six hours for one client, while working for five hours

---

54. *See id.* at 208.
55. Toledo Bar Association v. Stahlbush, 933 N.E.2d 1091 (Ohio 2010).
56. In re Berg, 3 Cal. State Bar Ct. Rptr. 725 (1997).

on behalf of another, has not earned eleven billable hours. A lawyer who is able to reuse old work product has not re-earned the hours previously billed and compensated when the work product was first generated. Rather than looking to profit . . . , the lawyer who has agreed to bill solely on the basis of time spent is obliged to pass the benefits of these economies on to the client. The practice of billing several clients for the same time or work product, since it results in the earning of an unreasonable fee, therefore is contrary to the mandate of the Model Rules.

Thus, for example, if you travel for one client and work for another client while on the airplane, you are going to have to reasonably apportion the travel hours between the two.

Fourth, do not churn the bill. **Churning** — unnecessarily overstaffing a case or performing duplicative or unnecessary work to drive up a bill — is a form of fraudulent billing. David Segal relates the story of Sporicidin Co., which wanted to hire a couple of high-end lawyers, and ended up with "53 attorneys and paralegals" working on the case, billing $830,000 in less than a year and a half.[57] Adam Victor hired DLA Piper to assist with a bankruptcy, but then objected to the bill as being excessive. DLA Piper sued Victor for the $675,000 bill. During the lawsuit, emails were uncovered from firm lawyers, one reading, "I hear we are already 200k over our estimate — that's Team DLA Piper!" and another noting that "random people" were being added to work "full time on random research projects in standard 'churn that bill, baby!' mode."[58] DLA Piper released a statement that "the emails were in fact an offensive and inexcusable effort at humor, but in no way reflect actual excessive billing"[59] — yet, whether made in jest or for other purposes, the statements were revelatory.[60] Victor amended his counterclaim in light of these emails, adding a claim for fraud and seeking $22.5 million in punitive damages — a claim that DLA Piper settled in 2013.[61] The pressure to produce billable hours may result in churning. While some of these examples are extreme, any time a lawyer performs duplicative or unnecessary work — such as unnecessarily rereading or reviewing a document or filing — in order to drive up one's billable hours, that constitutes a violation of Rule 1.5.

There are other problematic billing practices — such as charging for firm overhead or having an attorney perform and charge for work that should be done by a

---

57. David Segal, *In the Business of Billing? The Ethics Squeeze*, WASH. POST, Mar. 22, 1998, *available at* http://www .washingtonpost.com/wp-srv/business/longterm/ethics/ethics2.htm.

58. *See* Martha Neil, *"Churn That Bill, Baby!" Email Surfaces in Fee Dispute with DLA Piper*, A.B.A. J., Mar. 25, 2013, *available at* http://www.abajournal.com/news/article/sued_by_dla_piper_for_675k_ex-client_discovers _lighthearted_churn_that_bill.

59. *Id.*

60. In 2016, one of the lawyers involved in the emails, Erich Eisenegger, sued the firm that represented DLA Piper in the fee dispute for turning over the emails. Eisenegger said he lost his job (he had left DLA Piper prior to the publicizing of the email) and suffered reputational damage because of the publicity surrounding the emails. He also contended that the email statements were taken out of context and were "part of a much more thoughtful and serious discussion amongst associates and a DLA partner about DLA's billing habits." *See* Martha Neil, *Ex-DLA Piper Partner Caught in "Churn That Bill, Baby!" Crossfire Sues Firm's Counsel*, A.B.A. J., Mar. 24, 2016, *available at* http://www.abajournal.com/news/article/ex_dla_piper_partner_caught_in_churn_that_bill_baby_crossfire_sues _law_firm.

61. *See* Neil, *Churn That Bill, Baby!, supra* note 58. The lawsuit was settled in April 2013. *See DLA Piper Settles $22.5M Suit over "Churn That Bill" Emails*, LAW360, Apr. 17, 2013, *available at* https://www.law360.com/articles/ 433837/dla-piper-settles-22-5m-suit-over-churn-that-bill-emails.

less-expensive worker, such as a paralegal, secretary, or courier. Always remember that the lawyer is the client's fiduciary. Any billing practices that take advantage of or otherwise defraud the client will violate the lawyer's duties.

2. Safeguarding Client Funds and Property

An attorney, as the fiduciary of the client, holds client funds and property in sacred trust. As an attorney, you will be responsible to hold client funds and property. If you cannot be trusted (whether due to malfeasance or negligence) to safeguard client money and property, then you cannot be an attorney. The seriousness of mishandling client funds cannot be overstated. The presumptive sanction in most jurisdictions for misappropriating client funds is disbarment. In the words of the Colorado Supreme Court, "lawyers are almost invariably disbarred for knowing misappropriation of client funds."[62]

Despite the extreme potential sanction, many lawyers steal or misappropriate client funds. States take measures to prevent misappropriation and partially reimburse victimized clients. Nearly all states have adopted laws requiring banks to notify the bar of overdrafts in any client trust account.[63] Further, all states administer client protection fund programs whereby monies collected from licensed attorneys through state bar fees are used to partially reimburse clients whose lawyers misappropriate funds. A survey performed from 2014 to 2016 of client protection funds found that on average, each state received requests for reimbursements of approximately $4 to $7.5 million per year (that's about $200 to $375 million per year nationwide).[64] Most states reimburse victimized clients at a fraction of what they lost through attorney malfeasance.[65]

Attorneys have five basic fiduciary duties relating to handling client funds and property: (1) **segregation**; (2) **record keeping**; (3) **notification**; (4) **delivery**; and (5) **accounting**. The first two are set out in Model Rule 1.15(a) to (c), while the last three are described in 1.15(d).

Segregation

As noted in Rule 1.15(a), a lawyer is required to keep a client's funds or property "separate from the lawyer's own property." Client money must be placed in a client trust account. The lawyer is absolutely forbidden from commingling her own funds

---

62. People v. Rhodes, 107 P.3d 1177, 1185 (2005).

63. *See* ABA, Standing Committee on Client Protection, *State by State Adoption of ABA Client Protection Programs* (December 2015), *available at* http://www.americanbar.org/content/dam/aba/administrative/professional _responsibility/state_by_state_cp_programs.authcheckdam.pdf.

64. *See* ABA, Standing Committee on Client Protection, *2014-2016 Survey of Lawyers' Funds for Client Protection*, Part III: Fund Claim Experiences at 6, *available at* https://www.americanbar.org/content/dam/aba/administrative/ professional_responsibility/2014_16_survey_of_lawyers_funds_for_client_protection_final.pdf.

65. *See id.* (noting that in the same years where per state reimbursement requests were approximately 4 to 7.5 million dollars on average, the average total of awards approved during each year was approximately 1 million dollars). *See also* Harriet L. Turney & John A. Holtaway, *Client Protection Funds — Lawyers Put Their Money Where Their Mouths Are*, 9 No. 2 Prof. Law. 18 (1998) (noting that because of the number and size of claims, most client protection funds cap the reimbursement an aggrieved client can receive).

with those of the client. Thus, a lawyer cannot put her own money in the client trust account. Rule 1.15(b) allows a limited exception in that an attorney can deposit the attorney's own money in a client trust account "for the sole purpose of paying bank service charges on that account." But even for this exception, the attorney is allowed to deposit only the requisite amount to cover bank service charges.

If a lawyer is holding funds for several clients, the lawyer generally is permitted to deposit the funds of multiple clients into the same client trust account. If an attorney is holding a substantial amount for a specific client for an extended time, or is holding estate or trust monies, then the attorney should place the funds in their own interest-bearing account, which interest belongs to the client. *See* Model Rule 1.15 cmt. [1]. Because attorneys often hold the funds of multiple clients in one pooled client trust account, with each client's funds only being held for short periods of time, individual clients do not recover interest on their funds. Before the 1980s, lawyers simply held such funds in a non-interest-bearing trust account (as it was unethical for the lawyer to profit from handling client funds by collecting the interest from the pooled client monies).[66] Today, states instead require attorneys to participate in the state's IOLTA program. **IOLTA (Interest on Lawyers' Trust Accounts)** is a program through which the interest earned on the pooled client funds in attorneys' general client trust accounts escheats to the state to pay for charitable programs, primarily the state's legal aid services for people with low incomes. The U.S. Supreme Court upheld the constitutionality of IOLTA programs against a challenge that they constituted an unconstitutional taking of property. The Court noted that the client's pecuniary loss under IOLTA is zero[67] — because without IOLTA, clients received no interest from funds placed in lawyer trust accounts. All states have IOLTA programs, and attorney participation is mandatory in all but four states.[68]

Non-monetary property of the client that is given to the attorney during a representation must be "identified" as client property and "appropriately safeguarded."[69] Comment [1] to Rule 1.15 directs lawyers to keep securities in a safe deposit box absent "special circumstances" that warrant different arrangements.

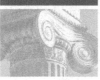

Case Preview

In re Sather

What happens when a client pays a retainer or flat fee to an attorney at the outset of a representation? Does the money belong to the client until it is earned (in which case it should be placed in the client trust account) or does the money belong to the attorney? In *Sather*, Frank Perez hired attorney

---

66. *See* ABA, Commission on Interest on Lawyer Trust Accounts, *Overview*, *available at* http://www.americanbar.org/groups/interest_lawyers_trust_accounts/overview.html.
67. *See* Brown v. Legal Found. of Wash, 538 U.S. 216, 240 (2003).
68. Four states allow lawyers to opt out of IOLTA (Alaska, Kansas, Nebraska, Virginia). *See* ABA, Commission on Interest on Lawyer Trust Accounts, *Status of IOLTA Programs*, *available at* http://www.americanbar.org/groups/interest_lawyers_trust_accounts/resources/status_of_iolta_programs.html.
69. Model Rule 1.15(a).

Larry D. Sather to represent Perez in a civil rights lawsuit. Sather charged Perez a "non-refundable" flat fee of $20,000 for the representation, and Sather filed the lawsuit. A few months later, Sather was suspended from the practice of law due to a separate disciplinary proceeding, and, consequently, Perez fired him. Perez asked for a refund of any unearned fees. Sather agreed that he had not earned approximately $13,000 of the fee but could not immediately make a refund because he had spent the entire $20,000.

As you read *In re Sather*, consider the following:

1. According to the court, what are the underlying interests served by requiring attorneys to keep client funds separated from an attorney's personal funds?
2. What should Sather have done with the $20,000 when he received it? Had he earned any of the fee at that time? According to the court, when has an attorney "earned" a fee?
3. The court divides retainers into two basic categories. What are those categories?
4. When, if ever, can an attorney charge a retainer at the outset of a case that is earned upon receipt and can immediately be placed in the attorney's account as property of the attorney? Even then, is the fee completely nonrefundable?

In re Sather
3 P.3d 403 (Colo. 2000)

Sather agreed to represent Franklin Perez in a lawsuit against the Colorado State Patrol and certain individual troopers [for allegedly] violat[ing] his civil rights during a traffic stop. . . . [O]n November 15, 1996, Sather and Perez entered into a written agreement for legal services, captioned "Minimum Fee Contract." Sather drafted the agreement, the terms of which required Perez to pay Sather $20,000 plus costs to represent Perez in the case against the State Patrol. . . .

The contract stated that Perez understood his obligation to pay this fee "regardless of the number of hours attorneys devote to [his] legal matter" and that no portion of the fee would be refunded "regardless of the time or effort involved or the result obtained." The contract acknowledged Perez's right to discharge Sather as his attorney, but the contract informed Perez that in no circumstance would any of the funds paid be refunded:

> IN ALL EVENTS, NO REFUND SHALL BE MADE OF ANY PORTION OF THE MINIMUM FEE PAID, REGARDLESS OF THE AMOUNT OF TIME EXPENDED BY THE FIRM. . . .

Perez paid Sather $5,000 of the minimum fee on November 17, 1996. He paid the remaining $15,000 on December 16th. Sather spent the $5,000 soon after receiving the money. Sather kept the second payment of $15,000 for approximately one month before spending these funds. Sather did not place any of these funds in his trust account before spending them . . . because he believed he earned the fees upon receipt. . . .

. . . [O]n December 6, 1996, Sather filed suit in Denver District Court on behalf of Perez against the State Patrol and three troopers. . . .

On April 21, 1997, in a matter unrelated to the Perez case, this court suspended Sather from the practice of law for thirty days, effective May 21, 1997. As required, Sather notified Perez of his suspension and Perez responded on May 23, requesting an accounting of the hours Sather worked on his case. . . . [O]n June 4, 1997, Perez faxed Sather notice discharging him from his case because of the suspension. . . . [Perez, acting *pro se*, settled the lawsuit for $6,000.]

Sather provided the accounting requested by Perez on June 27, 1997. Sather claimed that his fees, his paralegal assistant's fees, costs and expenses in Perez's case as of the date of discharge totaled $6,923.64. . . .

Despite acknowledging his duty to return the unearned $13,076.36 to Perez, Sather did not refund any money to Perez because at the time of discharge he had spent Perez's funds. On September 3, 1997 — three months after Perez discharged him — Sather paid Perez $3,000. Sather paid the remaining $10,076.36 on November 2, 1997. The hearing board found that this delay prejudiced Perez because he did not have access to his funds for almost five months. . . .

III. DISCUSSION

Sather contends that under Colorado law it is unclear whether an attorney must deposit all advance fees — including flat fees — into a trust account until the fees are earned. Sather further argues that an attorney earns flat fees upon receipt and the fees are thus the attorney's property and not subject to the trust requirements of Colo. RPC 1.15. Sather's fee agreement also raises the issue of "non-refundable" fees.

In order to address the issues raised in this case, we examine first Colo. RPC 1.15's requirement that attorneys segregate their property and funds from their clients'. Second, we discuss when and under what circumstances a client's property or funds are earned by an attorney and may therefore be treated as the attorney's property. Thirdly, we address whether an attorney may charge a "non-refundable" fee.

A. Colo. RPC 1.15 Requires Segregation of Attorney and Client Property

Initially, we address Colo. RPC 1.15(a), which requires that an attorney keep client funds separate from the attorney's own property:

In connection with representation, *an attorney shall hold property of clients or third persons that is in an attorney's possession separate from the attorney's own property. Funds shall be kept in a separate account* maintained in the state where the attorney's office is situated, or elsewhere with the consent of the client or third person. . . . Complete records of such account funds and other property shall be kept by the attorney and shall be preserved for a period of seven years after termination of representation.

(Emphasis added.) In addition to this subsection of the rule, Colo. RPC 1.15(f)(1)[9] requires that an attorney maintain client funds submitted to the attorney as advance fees in a separate trust account until the attorney earns the fees. . . .

. . . Thus, Colo. RPC 1.15(a) and (f) indicate that an attorney has an obligation to keep clients' funds separate from his own, and that advance fees remain the property of the client until such time as the fees are "earned." . . .

The rule requiring that an attorney segregate funds advanced by the client from the attorney's own funds serves important interests. As a fiduciary to the client, one of an attorney's primary responsibilities is to safeguard the interests and property of the client over which the attorney has control. Requiring the attorney to segregate all client funds — including advance fees — from the attorney's own accounts unless and until the funds become the attorney's property protects the client's property from the attorney's creditors and from misuse by the attorney. Thus, Colo. RPC 1.15(a) and (f) further the attorney's fiduciary obligation to protect client property.

In addition to protecting client property, requiring an attorney to keep advance fees in trust until they are earned protects the client's right to discharge an attorney. . . . Upon discharge, the attorney must return all unearned fees in a timely manner, even though the attorney may be entitled to quantum meruit recovery for the services that the attorney rendered and for costs incurred on behalf of the client.

If an attorney suggests to a client that any pre-paid or advance funds are "non-refundable" or constitute the attorney's property regardless of how much or how little work the attorney performs for the client, then the client may fear loss of the funds and may refrain from exercising his right to discharge the attorney. Because the unearned portion of the advance fees must be kept in trust and cannot be treated as the attorney's property until earned, the client will not risk forfeiting fees for work to be performed in the future if the client chooses to discharge his attorney. Thus, the requirement that the attorney place advance fees in trust protects the client's right to discharge his attorney.

B. An Attorney Earns Fees by Conferring a Benefit on or Providing a Service for the Client

As we discussed, rule 1.15's requirement that an attorney hold in trust all unearned fees furthers important interests central to the attorney-client relationship. When a client pays an attorney before the attorney provides legal services, the crucial issue becomes whether funds are "earned on receipt" and may be treated as the attorney's property, or whether the fees are unearned, in which case the funds must be segregated in a trust account under Colo. RPC 1.15. As one publication aptly framed this dilemma:

> The basic question is, Whose money is it? If it's the client's money in whole or in part, it is subject to the trust account requirements. If it is the lawyer's money, placing it into a trust account would violate the anti-commingling rule.

---

9. We note that Colo. RPC 1.15(f)(1) became effective July 1, 1999, after Sather's conduct in this case. However, we include Colo. RPC 1.15(f)(1) in our discussion because it helps clarify the current state of the rules.

ABA/BNA Lawyers' Manual on Professional Conduct 45:109 (1993). We hold that an attorney earns fees only by conferring a benefit on or performing a legal service for the client. Unless the attorney provides some benefit or service in exchange for the fee, the attorney has not earned any fees and, with a possible exception in very limited circumstances, the attorney cannot treat advance fees as her property.

Funds given by clients to attorneys as advance fees or retainers benefit attorneys and clients. Some forms of advance fees or retainers appropriately compensate an attorney when the fee is paid because the attorney makes commitments to the client that benefit the client immediately. Such an arrangement is termed a "general retainer" or "engagement retainer," and these retainers typically compensate an attorney for agreeing to take a case, which requires the attorney to commit his time to the client's case and causes the attorney to forego other potential employment opportunities as a result of time commitments or conflicts. Although an attorney usually earns an engagement retainer by agreeing to take the client's case, an attorney can also earn a fee charged as an engagement retainer by placing the client's work at the top of the attorney's priority list. Or the client may pay an engagement retainer merely to prevent the attorney from being available to represent an opposing party. In all of these instances, the attorney is providing some benefit to the client in exchange for the engagement retainer fee.

In contrast to engagement retainers, a client may advance funds — often referred to as "advance fees," "special retainers," "lump sum fees," or "flat fees" — to pay for specified legal services to be performed by the attorney and to cover future costs. We note that unless the fee agreement expressly states that a fee is an engagement retainer and explains how the fee is earned upon receipt, we will presume that any advance fee is a deposit from which an attorney will be paid for specified legal services. *See* Draft Restatement §50 cmt. (g) ("A fee payment that does not cover services already rendered and that is not otherwise identified is presumed to be a deposit against future services.").

Advance fees present an attractive option for both the client and the attorney. Like engagement retainers, advance fees allow clients to secure their choice of counsel. Additionally, some forms of advance fees, e.g., "lump sums" or "flat fees," benefit the client by establishing before representation the maximum amount of fees that the client must pay. In these instances, the client knows how much the total cost for legal fees will be in advance, permitting the client to budget based on a fixed sum rather than face potentially escalating hourly fees that may exceed the client's ability to pay. So long as the fees are reasonable, such arrangements do not violate ethical rules governing attorney fees.

Advance fees benefit the attorney because the attorney can secure payment for future legal services, eliminating the risk of non-payment after the attorney does the work. Often, attorneys collect a certain amount from the client in advance of any work and deduct from that amount according to the hours worked or mutually agreed-upon "milestones" reached during representation (e.g., investigation, pretrial work and motions, negotiations, filings, handling a company's initial public offering, etc.). Attorneys often deduct costs from advance payments as they incur the costs, similar to the manner in which they deduct their fees as they are earned. Advance fees represent an alternative method of obtaining legal assistance that accommodates legitimate needs of both clients and attorneys, and by this opinion we do not intend to discourage these fee arrangements provided the fee agreements comply with the ethical principles discussed in this case.

In the case of both advance fees and engagement retainers, the attorney performs a service or provides a benefit to the client in exchange for the fee. We recognize that we have not previously explained the ethical principle that determines when an attorney may treat funds paid as engagement retainers or advance fees as property of the attorney. Because this principle is a crucial element of the attorney-client relationship, we make our interpretation of the underlying ethical principle explicit: an attorney earns a fee only when the attorney provides a benefit or service to the client. Under Colo. RPC 1.15(a) and (f), all client funds — including engagement retainers, advance fees, flat fees, lump sum fees, etc. — must be held in trust until there is a basis on which to conclude that the attorney "earned" the fee; otherwise, the funds must remain in the client's trust account because they are not the attorney's property.

With respect to fees mutually agreed to be "earned on receipt," an attorney must describe in writing the nature of the benefit being provided to a specific client in order to claim some portion or all of an engagement retainer as earned when paid. . . . That is, an attorney cannot treat a fee as "earned" simply by labeling the fee "earned on receipt" or referring to the fee as an "engagement retainer." Rather, the attorney must explain in detail the nature of the benefit being conferred on the client, whether it is the attorney's guarantee of availability, prioritization of the client's work, or some other appropriate consideration.

. . .

C. "Non-refundable" Fees

. . . [W]e [now] address Sather's characterization of his fee as "non-refundable." Because fees are always subject to refund under certain conditions, labeling a fee "non-refundable" misleads the client and may deter a client from exercising their rights to refunds of unearned fees under Colo. 1.16(d). Thus, we hold that attorneys cannot enter into "non-refundable" retainer or fee agreements. . . .

A fee labeled "non-refundable" misinforms the client about the nature of the fee and interferes with the client's basic rights in the attorney-client relationship. Attorney fees are always subject to refund if they are excessive or unearned. A fee agreement that suggests that advance fees are "non-refundable" undermines the client's understanding of her rights and may discourage a client from seeking refunds to which the client may be entitled.

In addition to misinforming the client, "non-refundable fees" may discourage the client from discharging his attorney for fear that the client will not be able to recover advance fees for which the attorney has yet to perform any work. Because the label is inaccurate and misleading, and discourages a client from exercising the right to discharge an attorney, we hold that attorneys may not enter into "non-refundable fee" agreements or otherwise communicate to their clients that the fees are "non-refundable."

We acknowledge that in some instances a client may agree with an attorney to allow the attorney to treat funds paid in advance of legal services or other consideration as property of the attorney and thus not subject to the trust account requirements. Although we do not address the exact contours of such an arrangement in this opinion and recognize that narrow exceptions to this rule may exist, we caution that at minimum such arrangements will be construed against the attorney and in favor of the client. Furthermore, the attorney must expressly communicate to the client verbally and in writing that the attorney will treat the advance fee as the attorney's property upon receipt; that the client must understand the attorney can keep the fee only by providing a benefit or providing a service for which the client has contracted; that the fee agreement must spell out the terms of the benefit to be conferred upon the client; and that the client must be aware of the attorney's obligation to refund any amount of advance funds to the extent they are unreasonable or unearned if the representation is terminated by the client. Further, any arrangement that allows the attorney to treat unearned advance fees as his own property must protect the client's property interests in the funds and the client's right to discharge the attorney at any time without being penalized by "non-refundable" fees or retainers.

In the limited circumstances in which an attorney earns fees before performing any legal services (i.e., engagement retainers) or where an attorney and client agree that the attorney can treat advance fees as the attorney's property before the attorney earns the fees by supplying a benefit or performing a service, the fee agreement must clearly explain the basis for this arrangement and explain how the client's rights are protected by the arrangement. In either of these situations, however, an attorney's fees are always subject to refund if excessive or unearned, and an attorney cannot communicate otherwise to a client.

. . .

Because we have not previously made clear an attorney's obligation to deposit all forms of advance fees into trust accounts or explained the prohibition against "non-refundable" fees, we do not sanction Sather for violating these rules. . . . Because Sather knowingly failed to return unearned fees and knowingly misrepresented the nature of the fees paid by a client, and in light of his disciplinary history, we hold that Sather be suspended for six months.

Post-Case Follow-Up

Retainers are typically split into two overarching categories: the general retainer and the special retainer. The court in *Sather* adopted this dichotomy but tried to clarify the types by calling general retainers "engagement retainers" and calling special retainers "advance fees." Using the *Sather* court's terminology, a general or an engagement retainer is a fee that is earned upon receipt. But notice the very limited circumstances under which the court will allow an engagement retainer — the attorney must provide some benefit to the client in return for that retainer and must explain as much in writing to the client. Further, the engagement retainer cannot be truly nonrefundable despite being the attorney's property upon receipt because, according to the court, all fees are subject to refund if found to be unreasonably excessive or unearned. What possible benefits to the client does the court list as potentially justifying an engagement retainer?

The other type of retainer is the special retainer or advance fee. This type of retainer is the standard type of retainer used by attorneys — and if there is any question as to which type of retainer is created, it will be presumed to be an advance fee. An advance fee or special retainer is the client's upon receipt by the attorney. Thus, the attorney must place the advance fee in a client trust account. The attorney can withdraw funds from the advance fee only as she earns them. As the *Sather* court noted, even flat fees paid upfront are still advance fees or special retainers. Thus, the attorney must put the flat fee in a client trust account and can only make withdrawals as they are earned. Model Rule 1.15(c) endorses this view, requiring attorneys to deposit "legal fees and expenses that have been paid in advance" into a client trust account and allowing the lawyer to make withdrawals "only as fees are earned or expenses incurred."

In re Sather: Real Life Applications

1. New Alliance Bank is reorganizing and is selling stock to patrons in priority of those who hold certain amounts of money in their accounts. Larry has a client trust account with New Alliance Bank. He would like to purchase stock, but to obtain priority, he needs the client trust account to maintain a higher balance. Larry deposits some of his own money in the client trust account in order to obtain the priority to buy the stock. Larry decides that he will "forgo" ownership of any money that he placed into the client trust account in order to avoid commingling. Has Larry violated the rules?
2. Mason handles complex business disputes and wants to start charging an engagement retainer of $2,500 that is his upon receipt. What must Mason do to successfully charge an engagement retainer?

Record Keeping

Rule 1.15(a) requires that attorneys keep "[c]omplete records of such account funds and other property." As noted in comment [1], such records must be kept current and must be kept in accordance with generally accepted accounting practices (GAAP) in addition to "any recordkeeping rules established by law or court order." The rule further requires that such records be preserved by the attorney for a period of years following the end of the representation. The Model Rule recommends a record preservation period of five years, but many states have selected a longer preservation period, ranging from six to eight years.[70]

---

70. *See* ABA, CPR Policy Implementation Committee, *Variations of the ABA Model Rules of Professional Conduct, Rule 1.15: Safekeeping Property* (Feb. 25, 2020), *available at* https://www.americanbar.org/content/dam/aba/administrative/professional_responsibility/mrpc_1_15.pdf.

Notification, Delivery, and Accounting

Rule 1.15(d) covers three fiduciary duties owed as to client property and funds. First, if the lawyer receives funds or other property (commonly a settlement check) as to which the client or another person has an interest, the lawyer must "promptly notify the client or third person." Second, the attorney is then required to "promptly deliver" the funds or property to the client or third person with the ownership interest. Finally, if a client or a third person claiming an interest in property or funds held by the attorney makes a request for an accounting, the lawyer is required to "promptly render a full accounting regarding such property."

Disputes over Property Held by the Attorney

Model Rule 1.15(e) sets out how an attorney is to handle disputes over ownership of property, especially money. Third parties, including creditors of the client, may have enforceable claims against client funds held by the attorney.[71] Yet, not too surprisingly, the most common situation in which there is a dispute over ownership of money held by the attorney involves disputes between the attorney and client. For example, the attorney will deposit an advance fee into the client trust account. The attorney then bills the client, who objects to the attorney's bill as being excessive. Or, the attorney receives a settlement check for the client, but the attorney is owed fees or expenses — and then the client objects to the attorney taking as much as the attorney asserts he is owed under a contingent or other fee agreement. So how much, if anything, can an attorney withdraw in such cases (and in other cases where a third party may assert an interest in client funds)?

Model Rule 1.15(e) states that "the property shall be kept separate by the lawyer until the dispute is resolved," but also that "the lawyer shall promptly distribute all portions of the property as to which the interests are not in dispute." Thus, the attorney is required to distribute any undisputed portions, but must keep any disputed portions in the client trust account. So if an attorney bills a client for $2,000, and the client thinks the attorney has only earned $1,000, then the attorney must withdraw the $1,000 that both agree the attorney has earned — but the attorney must also keep the disputed $1,000 in the client trust account until the dispute is resolved.

There is a split in authority as to whether an attorney must return funds to the client trust account if the attorney makes a disbursement prior to learning of a dispute, but thereafter becomes aware that the disbursement is disputed. In *In re Martin*, the D.C. Court of Appeals held that where an attorney disbursed settlement funds to himself from the trust account but learned shortly thereafter that the client disputed the disbursement, the attorney was required to return the disputed portion to the client trust account. However, the court noted the existence of conflicting authority, citing both courts that agreed with its holding and courts

---

71. For example, comment [4] to Rule 1.15(a) notes that a creditor of the client may have "a lien on funds recovered in a personal injury action."

that held that once an attorney has disbursed funds, she need not return disputed portions to the client trust account.[72]

3. Terminating the Representation

An attorney should undertake a representation only if it appears that he can carry it through to completion. *See* Model Rule 1.16 cmt. [1]. Completion occurs when the attorney has performed the assistance for which the client hired him. *See id.* Certainly, as long as the limitation is reasonable, an attorney and client can agree at the outset to narrow the scope of the representation so that an attorney is hired only to undertake limited or preliminary tasks as to a legal matter.[73] But as fiduciaries of their clients, attorneys cannot willy-nilly abandon a client's matter. As noted in the *Pang* and *Sather* cases above, clients have a right to discharge their lawyer at any time with or without cause,[74] but an attorney lacks a similar right and cannot always withdraw from a representation with which the attorney is dissatisfied. At the same time, the rules require attorneys to withdraw under certain circumstances. But even then, the attorney's withdrawal may require permission from a tribunal. The bottom line is that attorneys cannot count on being able to easily withdraw from a matter — especially if withdrawing will prejudice the client or interfere with a court's adjudication of a case.

Model Rule 1.16 divides attorney withdrawal into two basic categories: mandatory withdrawal and permissive withdrawal. Model Rule 1.16(a) covers mandatory withdrawal — situations in which the attorney is required to withdraw; while 1.16(b) covers permissive withdrawal — situations in which an attorney is allowed to withdraw. If an attorney wishes to withdraw and cannot fit the withdrawal into one of the categories outlined in Rule 1.16(a) and (b), the attorney cannot withdraw. Moreover, under Rule 1.16(c), a lawyer will have to obtain permission from the tribunal, in accordance with local law, in order to effectuate withdrawal in a case involving an adjudicative proceeding. If the court denies the attorney's petition to withdraw, the attorney must continue with the representation even if Rule 1.16(a) or (b) would have permitted or required the attorney to withdraw.[75]

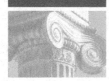

Case Preview

In re Kiley

Michael McGibbon hired Thomas M. Kiley and Associates to assert a medical malpractice claim on his behalf. McGibbon entered a contingency fee contract with the firm, and Pamela Swift, an attorney for the firm, filed suit and entered an

---

72. *See In re Martin*, 67 A.3d 1032, 1045-46 & n.14 (D.C. Ct. App. 2013) (collecting conflicting authority).
73. Model Rule 1.2(c) allows an attorney, with client informed consent, to undertake representations that are limited in scope, as long as "the limitation is reasonable under the circumstances."
74. *See also* Model Rule 1.16 cmt. [4].
75. *See* Model Rule 1.16(c) (explaining that when a court so orders, "a lawyer shall continue representation notwithstanding good cause for terminating the representation").

appearance on McGibbon's behalf. Swift decided to take a "sabbatical from the practice of law." She notified McGibbon that he needed to seek successor counsel. McGibbon's search for successor counsel was unsuccessful. Nevertheless, Swift moved to withdraw from the case, which motion the court denied because no successor counsel had appeared. Swift moved to reconsider, and after a hearing, the court allowed Swift to withdraw, but ordered that Kiley, the named partner of the Kiley firm, represent McGibbon. The court explained that McGibbon had a valid contract to have the Kiley firm represent him and that the case was "falling behind" the court-ordered schedule for its disposition. Nevertheless, Kiley informed McGibbon by letter that their contingency contract had been terminated; however, the judge would not let Kiley out of the case. Kiley filed an interlocutory appeal, which is excerpted here.

As you read *In re Kiley*, consider the following:

1. Under the Massachusetts rules, which follow the Model Rules, when is an attorney required to withdraw? When is an attorney permitted to withdraw?
2. When an attorney seeks court permission to withdraw, what factors do the Massachusetts courts consider in deciding whether to allow the attorney to withdraw?
3. When an attorney who practices with a law firm enters an appearance, is the law firm also bound to continue that appearance if the individual attorney is unable to complete the representation?
4. If a lawyer undertakes a case on contingency, but comes to realize after filing the case that it will not be profitable for the lawyer, is the lawyer free to withdraw on that basis?

In re Kiley
459 Mass. 645 (2011)

An attorney who has entered an appearance in a case filed in court may not withdraw from the representation of the client without complying with two rules: Mass. R. Prof. C. 1.16, which identifies the limited circumstances under which an attorney must or may withdraw; and Mass. R. Civ. P. 11(c), which identifies the limited circumstances where withdrawal may be done without leave of court and otherwise requires leave of court.

Under rule 1.16(a), an attorney "shall" withdraw from representation where the client discharges the lawyer, where continued representation will result in violation of the rules of professional conduct or other law, or where the lawyer's physical or mental condition materially impairs the lawyer's ability to represent the client. Under rule 1.16(b), a lawyer "may" withdraw from representation where the withdrawal can be accomplished "without material adverse effect on the interests of the client." Where withdrawal will have a material adverse effect on the client's interests, a lawyer may withdraw only if at least one of the following circumstances is present:

(1) the client persists in a course of action involving the lawyer's services that the lawyer reasonably believes is criminal or fraudulent;

(2) the client has used the lawyer's services to perpetrate a crime or fraud;

(3) a client insists upon pursuing an objective that the lawyer considers repugnant or imprudent;

(4) the client fails substantially to fulfil an obligation to the lawyer regarding the lawyer's services and has been given reasonable warning that the lawyer will withdraw unless the obligation is fulfilled;

(5) the representation will result in an unreasonable financial burden on the lawyer or has been rendered unreasonably difficult by the client; or

(6) other good cause for withdrawal exists.

Mass. R. Prof. C. 1.16(b). Regardless whether a lawyer must or may withdraw in these circumstances, where the lawyer has entered an appearance on behalf of the client and "the rules of a tribunal" require approval of the withdrawal by the tribunal, the lawyer shall not withdraw the appearance without the tribunal's permission. Mass. R. Prof. C. 1.16(c).

Where an attorney has entered an appearance in a civil proceeding in a Massachusetts court, the "rules of [the] tribunal" require the attorney to obtain leave of court before withdrawing from a case unless three conditions are met: the notice of withdrawal is accompanied by the entry of appearance of successor counsel, no motions are pending, and no trial date has been set. Mass. R. Civ. P. 11(c). Where at least one of these conditions is not met, the decision whether to allow an attorney's withdrawal is left to the sound discretion of the judge and will be reversed only for an abuse of discretion.

As reflected in these two rules, an attorney may not terminate an agreement to represent a client simply because the attorney no longer wishes to continue the representation. *See* Rusinow v. Kamara, 920 F. Supp. 69, 72 (D.N.J. 1996) ("Sudden disenchantment with a client or a cause is no basis for withdrawal. Those who cannot live with risk, doubt and ingratitude should not be trial lawyers"). Even if an attorney has not entered an appearance on behalf of the client, the attorney may withdraw in accordance with rule 1.16 only if the withdrawal will not have a material adverse effect on the client's interests or if at least one of the circumstances requiring or permitting withdrawal is present. . . .

Where, as here, the client enters into a representation agreement with a law firm rather than a sole practitioner, the law firm may not terminate the agreement simply because the attorney who had been handling the case has died, left the practice of law, or moved to a different firm. While the departure of the responsible attorney may cause the client to leave the firm, it may not cause the firm to leave the client if withdrawal will have a material adverse effect on the client's interests and none of the circumstances requiring [or] permitting withdrawal is present.

Because McGibbon was unable to retain successor counsel to prosecute his medical malpractice case, the Kiley firm's withdrawal would have had a material adverse effect on the client's interest in prevailing at trial or obtaining a reasonable settlement. Apart from conclusory assertions of "irreconcilable differences" with the client, neither Swift nor Kiley had identified any justification under rule

1.16(b) or (c) to terminate representation. . . . While McGibbon was willing to discharge Swift in light of her intention to leave the practice of law, he wanted the Kiley firm to continue to represent him in the case. Kiley's letter to the client on June 21, 2010, in which he declared that his law firm was "unilaterally terminating" the agreement to represent the client in the medical malpractice case, effective immediately, demonstrates his apparent disregard of the dictates of rule 1.16 and rule 11(c), as well as the judge's order, because it suggests that an attorney has the authority unilaterally to terminate an agreement to represent a client even where the attorney has filed a complaint on behalf of the client and entered an appearance in the case.

Even if there had been a permissible basis under rule 1.16 for the Kiley firm to move to withdraw from the case, the judge did not abuse his discretion by allowing Swift's motion to withdraw but requiring the Kiley firm to continue the representation and file an appearance. "[An] attorney who agrees to represent a client in a court proceeding assumes a responsibility to the court as well as to the client." V.H. v. J.P.H., *supra.* In deciding whether to allow the withdrawal of an attorney or the attorney's law firm, a judge may consider the impact of a withdrawal on the timely and fair adjudication of the case and the "reasonable expectation of the opposing party to have a case efficiently adjudicated." Zabin v. Picciotto, 73 Mass. App. Ct. 141, 165 (2008). The judge noted in his findings that he had been informed by defense counsel that the dispute over McGibbon's representation had "severely retarded discovery progress" in the case, and that the case was already three years old and was "falling behind" in its compliance with time standards. In view of all these circumstances, we conclude that the judge did not abuse his discretion in denying what was, in effect, the Kiley firm's motion to withdraw. . . .

The judge also did not abuse his discretion in refusing to allow withdrawal of the Kiley firm after Kiley, in his motion to vacate or reconsider the June 16 findings and order, provided the judge with documents that McGibbon had sent to opposing counsel. . . .

Kiley contends that, as a result of the production of these documents to opposing counsel, continued representation "has been rendered unreasonably difficult by the client" and justified termination of the representation under rule 1.16(b)(5). The judge did not address this issue in denying the motion for reconsideration, but the record provides ample basis for us to conclude that the denial of the motion was within his discretion. There is nothing in the record to suggest that McGibbon provided these documents to opposing counsel to sabotage his own case or otherwise acted in bad faith. Kiley cannot improperly abandon his client and then, when the client injures his position during settlement negotiations because the Kiley firm was no longer advising him, argue that the client's error now justifies his firm's withdrawal from the case. Moreover, even if McGibbon's conduct provided a ground for the Kiley firm to withdraw from the representation under rule 1.16(b)(5), the judge did not abuse his discretion in refusing to release the Kiley firm from the representation where the case was already three years old, discovery was delayed, and no successor counsel could be found.

The judge erred however, in requiring Kiley himself to file an appearance. . . . The language of the agreement is clear that the agreement is between McGibbon and Kiley's law firm, not Kiley individually.

When an attorney who is a partner, shareholder, or employee of a law firm enters an appearance in a civil case, the appearance binds both the individual attorney and that law firm to appear on behalf of the client. . . . Where an attorney leaves a law firm and moves to withdraw, and where successor counsel from another law firm does not file an appearance, a judge is entitled to expect that another attorney from the law firm will enter an appearance and continue to represent the client. In such circumstances, unless specified in the order, the allowance by a judge of a departing attorney's motion to withdraw does not also permit the law firm to withdraw its representation in the case. A judge may allow the attorney's motion but require the law firm to select another attorney to enter an appearance and continue the representation. A judge may not, however, select the attorney in the law firm who will enter the appearance; the law firm may select the appropriate attorney.

On remand, the single justice is to affirm the judge's order only to the extent that it denies the Kiley law firm's motion to withdraw from the representation and requires another attorney affiliated with the Kiley firm to file an appearance on behalf of McGibbon. . . .

We address briefly the argument raised in one of the amicus briefs that motions to withdraw filed by attorneys who are retained on a contingency fee should be more generously allowed to prevent claims that are meritless from being brought to trial, "at no cost to the client, but at great cost to all others involved." Nothing in the record suggests that McGibbon's claim is without merit. . . .

A law firm, after agreeing to represent a client for a contingent fee and filing a complaint that presumably complies with the requirement of a good faith basis under Mass. R. Civ. P. 11(a) may not withdraw from a case simply because it recognizes belatedly that the case will not be profitable for the law firm. A lawyer's miscalculation of the time or resources necessary to represent a client, the likelihood of success, or the amount of damages "is usually a dubious ground" for withdrawal, because lawyers are better able than clients to forecast these matters. . . . Attorneys who agree to represent clients on a contingent fee basis must choose their cases carefully, because the law does not allow them easily to jettison their mistakes, especially after the complaint has been filed.

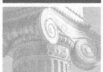

Post-Case Follow-Up

In re Kiley illustrates the reality that attorneys cannot abandon their clients should the representation prove less profitable than initially thought — the lawyer's circumstance must fall within one of the provisions of Rule 1.16 to allow appropriate withdrawal. Further, where attorneys are associated in a firm, the fact that one lawyer must withdraw due to personal reasons does not give license to the entire firm to withdraw from the client.

In re Kiley: Real Life Applications

1. Peter works for the law firm Price and French. Peter personally represents Mike in a civil rights lawsuit that's been filed in federal district court. Peter is diagnosed with cancer and is required to take a leave of absence. He tells Mike that he is going to have to withdraw because his physical condition completely impairs his ability to continue the representation. Assume no one else at Price and French wants to take on Mike's case. What should Peter do? What should Price and French do?

2. Heather, an attorney, learns that opposing counsel previously represented her client in a different matter years before the case. Heather's client is not interested in a quick resolution of the case because the client will likely be held liable. The client recommends that Heather move to disqualify opposing counsel, but wants to wait until close to trial in order to delay the proceedings. Is this a good idea? Is such a plan likely to be successful?

Mandatory Withdrawal

As noted in *Kiley* and Model Rule 1.16(a), a lawyer is required to withdraw under three circumstances. First, the lawyer must withdraw when "the representation *will result* in violation" of the jurisdiction's professional conduct rules or other law. Often this occurs when a lawyer is faced with an unconsented to or nonconsentable conflict of interest. But it may also include other situations where continued representation will result in a violation of the rules, for example, the prohibition in Rule 1.2(d) from assisting a client in crime or fraud. Withdrawal is also required when the lawyer is too sick to handle a case. Be it a physical or mental impairment, the lawyer is required to withdraw if the ailment "materially impairs the lawyer's ability to represent the client." *See* Model Rule 1.16(a)(2). Finally, a lawyer must withdraw when the client fires the lawyer. The client has the right to fire the lawyer "at any time, with or without cause." *See* Model Rule 1.16 cmt. [4]. However, if the situation involves appointed counsel of a criminal defendant — particularly if this is not the first time that a defendant has fired an appointed attorney in the matter — negative consequences may follow the defendant's firing and the attorney should inform the defendant of such. Specifically, the appointing authority may determine "that appointment of successor counsel is unjustified, thus requiring self-representation by the client." *See* Model Rule 1.16 cmt. [5]. Again, even with mandatory withdrawal, the lawyer will have to obtain permission to withdraw if a proceeding has been filed. While courts are likely to grant permission in such situations, the court may deny permission if withdrawal is unduly prejudicial. Courts have denied petitions for mandatory withdrawal, for example, where the withdrawal is sought on the eve of trial.[76]

---

76. *See, e.g.,* Georgia Baptist Health Care System, Inc. v. Hanafi, 559 S.E.2d 746, 747-49 (Ga. Ct. App. 2002) (denying motion to disqualify made at conclusion of discovery and initially raised 17 months after learning of the conflict); Velazquez-Velez v. Molina-Rodriguez, 2017 WL 395105, at *2 (D.P.R. 2017) (noting that the "great majority of cases where motions to disqualify were denied as untimely involved motions filed on the eve of trial").

Permissive Withdrawal

Permissive withdrawal can also be categorized into three basic types: (1) lack of harm to the client; (2) the client's bad or otherwise repugnant acts; and (3) the client's failure to pay or otherwise fulfill an obligation to the attorney. In addition, Rule 1.16(b)(7) is a catchall provision allowing for withdrawal when "other good cause for withdrawal exists."

As the *Kiley* court explained, an attorney is permitted to withdraw under Rule 1.16(b)(1) whenever withdrawal can be accomplished "without material adverse effect on the interests of the client." The attorney needs no other reason to withdraw if it will not harm his client. This basis for withdrawal indicates that in the other forms of permissive withdrawal, the withdrawal may adversely affect the client's interests.

Several of the bases for permissive withdrawal center around a client's bad or otherwise repugnant actions. Thus, under Rule 1.16(b)(2) and (b)(3), a lawyer is permitted to withdraw (1) if the client is using the lawyer's services to engage in conduct that the lawyer "reasonably believes is criminal or fraudulent" or (2) if the client has previously "used the lawyer's services to perpetrate a crime or fraud." In both of these situations, the client is not currently using the lawyer's services to perpetrate a known crime or fraud, which would trigger mandatory withdrawal. Nevertheless, the lawyer is not required to maintain a relationship with a client who is using or has used the lawyer's services in potentially criminal or fraudulent ways that are just shy of triggering mandatory withdrawal. Similarly, Rule 1.16(b)(4) allows an attorney to withdraw from representing a client who "insists upon taking action that the lawyer considers repugnant" or fundamentally disagrees with. Notably, if an attorney decides to continue a representation, despite personally disagreeing with the client's views or ends, the attorney is not thereby endorsing the client's views.[77]

The final bases under which a lawyer can permissively withdraw revolve around a client's failure to pay fees or comply with other obligations to the attorney, or a representation that will create an unreasonable financial burden on the attorney. As noted in ABA Formal Opinion 476, courts have generally held under Rule 16(b)(5) and (b)(6) that "if a client fails over time to pay a lawyer's fees, and that failure continues after a lawyer provides a reasonable warning to the client, the lawyer may be permitted to withdraw."

Comment [3] to Rule 1.16 instructs lawyers to carefully guard their duty of confidentiality (covered in Chapter 5) in moving to withdraw from a court proceeding. The comment explains that if a court seeks an explanation, the lawyer may be prohibited by the duty of confidentiality from disclosing facts constituting the explanation. However, in such instances, the attorney is to provide the court with the following explanation as the reason for withdrawal: "professional considerations

---

77. *See* Model Rule 1.2(b) (maintaining that the representation of a client does not constitute an endorsement of the client's views or claims).

require termination of the representation." Comment [3] indicates that normally this explanation should suffice.[78]

Duties Owed to the Client After Termination

The lawyer continues to owe duties to the client even after termination. Rule 1.16(d) requires a withdrawing attorney to take reasonable measures "to protect a client's interests." The rule lists four such measures: (1) providing the client with reasonable notice of the withdrawal; (2) giving the client time to hire another attorney; (3) returning papers and property to the client; and (4) refunding advance payments of fees and expenses.

Protecting the client's interests as a fiduciary requires that the client be notified of the intent to withdraw with sufficient time to obtain successor counsel who can continue the representation. Further, the client will need the file and other documents and evidence held by the attorney to successfully proceed with the matter. Recall from *Sallee* above that the attorney was additionally disciplined for refusing to return the entire file, including medical records and brain-tissue slides from the client's daughter's autopsy, which the attorney withheld, claiming that she had no obligation to turn them over until her clients paid her over $80,000 in fees. Most jurisdictions maintain that the entire file presumptively belongs to the client. However, a minority view adopts the "end product" approach whereby the client has a right to the lawyer's end product documents, but "is not entitled to preliminary documents . . . such as internal legal memoranda, preliminary drafts of pleadings, and other preliminary documents."[79]

Whether an attorney can withhold parts of the file as a security for payment of fees — a "retaining lien" — depends on the law of the particular jurisdiction, as indicated in Rule 1.16(d).[80] A number of jurisdictions expressly prohibit retaining liens,[81] while others only allow them if the retention of the papers will not prejudice

---

78. Nevertheless, in ABA Formal Opinion 476, the ABA noted that many courts require further factual enhancement and offered the following guidance on how an attorney should proceed in safeguarding the duty of confidentiality when moving to withdraw on the basis of nonpayment of fees. The attorney could

> (1) initially submit a motion providing no confidential client information apart from a reference to "professional considerations" or the like; (2) upon being informed by the court that further information is necessary, respond, when practicable, by seeking to persuade the court to rule on the motion without requiring the disclosure of confidential client information, asserting all non-frivolous claims of confidentiality and privilege; and if that fails; (3) thereupon under Rule 1.6(b)(5) submit only such information as is reasonably necessary to satisfy the needs of the court and preferably by whatever restricted means of submission, such as *in camera* review under seal, or such other procedures designated to minimize disclosure as the court determines is appropriate. If the court expressly orders the lawyer to make further disclosure, the exception in Rule 1.6(b)(6) for disclosures required to comply with a court order will apply. . . .

ABA Formal Op. 476 (2016).
79. SEC v. McNaul, 277 F.R.D. 439, 444-45 (2011).
80. *See* Model Rule 1.16(d) (allowing a lawyer to retain papers after withdrawal "to the extent permitted by other law").
81. *See, e.g.,* MINN. R. PROF'L CONDUCT 1.16(g) ("A lawyer shall not condition the return of client papers and property on payment of the lawyer's fee or the cost of copying the files or papers.").

the client.[82] It is essential that attorneys contemplating a retaining lien carefully consult the applicable law in their jurisdiction.

Further, as noted in *Sather*, attorneys who have obtained an advance fee — even if a flat fee — must refund any unearned portions upon withdrawal from a case. Client receipt of such funds is not solely a matter of obtaining an entitled refund — it also can provide the means for the client to obtain successor counsel and appropriately proceed with the representation.

Chapter Summary

- Attorney-client relationships can be created either expressly or impliedly; whenever such a relationship exists, attorneys owe the client core duties of loyalty, communication, competence, confidentiality, and conflict avoidance.
- Attorneys owe specific but more limited duties to prospective clients.
- The client has the ultimate authority to determine the objectives of the representation (within the bounds of the law), while the attorney has more control regarding the means by which such objectives are pursued.
- In a civil matter, the client has the ultimate authority as to whether to settle a case; in a criminal matter, the client has the ultimate authority as to the plea to enter, whether to testify, and whether to waive jury trial.
- The attorney for an organization represents the organization and not its constituents, and so the attorney must provide a clarifying entity warning to constituents with interests potentially adverse to the entity. The attorney must protect the entity's interest, including by reporting up when required under the rules.
- Attorneys act as fiduciaries of their clients even when the lawyer's interest and the client's interest diverge; the lawyer must safeguard the client's interests in charging a fee, handling client funds and property, and withdrawing from the case.
- Attorneys must communicate the basis and rate of their fee to the client and are forbidden from charging an unreasonable or fraudulent fee.
- Attorneys have five basic fiduciary duties relating to handling client funds and property: (1) segregation; (2) record keeping; (3) notification; (4) delivery; and (5) accounting.
- Attorneys can only withdraw when required or allowed by the rules and, if a case is before a tribunal, permitted by the court; moreover, the attorney must take measures to protect the client's interests upon withdrawal.

---

82. *See, e.g.*, Iowa State Bar Association, Ethics Op. 07-08 (2007) ("An Attorney may not assert a statutory retaining lien against a client's original documents if, by doing so the client would be otherwise prejudiced.").

Applying the Rules

1. Matt lives in a small community and is suing a contractor who substantially damaged his home. There are only three attorneys in the community that could competently handle the matter. Otherwise, a person would have to hire an attorney at a substantially higher price from a metropolitan area 50 miles to the west. Matt meets with each of the three attorneys in the community and tells them about his case in detail. Matt believes this will not only help him determine who to hire, but it will preclude those attorneys (having heard Matt's side of the story) from being able to represent the contractor he plans to sue. Under the rules, has Matt succeeded in conflicting out the competent local counsel from representing the contractor?

2. You represent Dave, who is a "high maintenance" client with a short temper and unrealistic expectations. Opposing counsel calls and asks you for a 15-day extension to respond to a motion for summary judgment because his out-of-state daughter had an emergency C-section with a premature baby. Opposing counsel has previously asked for extensions for discovery and pleading, to which you objected at Dave's behest. Both extensions of time were then granted as a matter of course by the judge, who was annoyed to have to rule on motions for modest extensions of time. Dave knows the summary judgment response is due and is anxiously awaiting it. You tell him of opposing counsel's request and he demands that you deny it, threatening to fire you if you do not. How should you proceed?

3. Ella wants to sell off her family farm for commercial or residential development. She asks John to represent her in the transaction. Ella tells John she cannot afford to pay him a cash fee, but she will give him ten acres of the land in payment. John asks Ella what the land is worth, and she tells him she thinks it is worth $3,000 an acre. John agrees to undertake the representation and to accept the ten acres as payment. John writes up an agreement that simply states that John agrees to represent Ella in the development of her land and that Ella agrees to transfer to him ownership of ten acres of the land. Assume that unbeknownst to Ella or John the land is actually worth $50,000 an acre. Has John charged an unreasonable fee? Are there any other Model Rules he needs to consider regarding collecting such a fee?

4. Melody hired Karl to represent her in a personal injury action, from which she recovered $50,000. Karl set up a special needs trust for Melody, with himself as trustee, to ensure that the assets were not depleted quickly and to preserve Melody's ability to remain on public assistance. Melody decided she wanted to obtain access to the trust principal. She talked to an attorney, Mindy. Mindy said she would represent Melody on a contingency fee basis whereby Mindy would get "one-third of whatever is in the trust." Melody agreed and signed a contingency fee agreement to that effect. Mindy called Karl, informed Karl of

Melody's desires, and asked him to step aside as trustee. Karl agreed to do so. Mindy created a short document naming herself as the successor trustee. She then prepared documents terminating the trust. Mindy and Melody then went to the bank together and depleted the trust assets, with Mindy receiving the full fee of $16,667 for a couple hours of work. Has Mindy violated the rules?

5. You represent Star Corp and are preparing to close a major deal. The CFO sends you an email asking you to come speak with him. When you arrive, the CFO begins telling you that he is concerned because his malfeasance has resulted in some financial setbacks that have not yet been reflected on Star Corp's financial statements. He is concerned that if these setbacks are accurately reported, it will mess up the deal. What do you tell the CFO? How do you proceed?

Professional Responsibility in Practice

1. Eli comes to you asking you to represent him in a slip and fall case against his neighbor, Cyrus, for an incident that occurred ten months ago. You meet with him for a half hour, but decide you do not want to take his case. Draft an appropriate declination letter to Eli.

2. Same facts as above, only this time you decide to take Eli's case and want to charge a one-third contingency fee. Draft a contingency fee agreement that complies with Rule 1.5.

3. Research whether an in-house attorney has a cause of action for wrongful discharge when fired for complying with mandatory rules of professional conduct in the state where you plan to practice or are attending law school.

4. Select a state that has decided to legalize marijuana. Research the ethics opinions in that state to see how that state approaches the problem of compliance with Rule 1.2(d) where state law expressly allows marijuana use but federal law criminalizes it.

4

Competence — The Lawyer's Indispensable Duty

Competence is the lawyer's indispensable duty. Clients come to attorneys to protect client life, liberty, and property interests, yet attorneys who act incompetently can cripple those rights. The very person whom clients pay and trust to vindicate their rights and interests becomes the instrument through which those rights and interests are impaired and perhaps lost entirely. Attorneys have a duty to act with competence — to have or obtain the requisite skill, legal knowledge, and expertise to handle the client's matter, to undertake thorough preparation and perform necessary investigation to obtain the requisite factual knowledge about the case, to act with diligence to advance the client's interests, and to communicate with and counsel the client. Competence, diligence, and communication are core duties essential to protecting client rights and avoiding discipline. Moreover, in criminal cases, the Sixth Amendment guarantees that the accused shall have "the assistance of counsel for his defence." Thus, an attorney who violates duties of competence also undermines her client's constitutional right to effective assistance of counsel.

Attorneys who fulfill the duties of competence, diligence, and communication can literally save their clients' lives, families, and fortunes. Yet, as examples in this chapter will illustrate, an attorney's incompetence can cause irreparable harm to clients: clients have lost custody of children, have gone to prison or have even been executed, have been deported, have had adoptions nullified, and have been evicted from their homes — all due to the incompetence of their own attorneys. In

Key Concepts

- Competence requires legal knowledge, skill, thoroughness, and preparation
- The consequences to clients of attorney incompetence
- The lawyer's duty to act with diligence and promptness
- Attorney-client communication as essential to successful representation
- The criminal defendant's right to effective assistance of counsel
- Substance abuse, mental health, and competence

addition, incompetent attorneys completely undermine their own role in the justice system when their actions divest rather than protect the liberty and property — and in some cases even the life — of their client, the very person who has entrusted those rights to their care.

A. THE COMPETENT ATTORNEY

Clients come to attorneys because clients lack the requisite knowledge, skill, and ability to protect their own legal interests and rights. Attorneys who are incompetent violate their first and basic duty to their clients: to protect their clients' interests. Indeed, incompetent attorneys not only fail to protect client interests, but often impair and destroy client rights.

The whole theory underlying the licensure of attorneys and accompanying unauthorized practice of law rules is that it is essential to the protection of clients and their legal interests to allow only those who have the *specialized knowledge and training* to practice law. If those who are licensed are not willing to become and remain competent in the practice of law, what is the justification for restricting practice to licensed attorneys? As discussed in Chapter 1, attorneys have a social contract with the public, whereby in exchange for an exclusive license they agree to maintain high standards of minimum conduct in order to protect the public and safeguard justice, the profession's public good. The profession must insist on minimum standards of competence to properly protect these interests.

Importantly, the Supreme Court has held that it is not unjust for a client to be bound by his attorney's incompetence: "[The client] voluntarily chose this attorney as his representative in the action, and he cannot now avoid the consequences of the acts or omissions of this freely selected agent. Any other notion would be wholly inconsistent with our system of representative litigation, in which each party is deemed bound by the acts of his lawyer-agent."[1] Thus, the rights of clients can be nullified by their own lawyer's incompetence without full recourse to undo the legal consequences created by that incompetence. Often, and for individual clients generally, the client has no way of measuring or appreciating the incompetence of her counsel precisely because the client lacks the requisite training and skill to protect her own legal rights — which is why the client hired an attorney in the first place. An action for attorney malpractice can sometimes provide monetary compensation to clients harmed by attorney incompetence. But often when legal rights are at stake, money damages cannot provide full compensation for what was lost through attorney incompetence, as will be illustrated repeatedly in this chapter.

Competence — along with the cognate duties of diligence and communication — are placed first in the Model Rules — a reminder of their preeminent importance to protecting your client's rights. Model Rule 1.1 requires attorneys to "provide competent representation to a client," which the rule then explains consists of four basic components: "legal knowledge, skill, thoroughness and preparation."

---

1. Link v. Wabash Railroad Co., 370 U.S. 626, 633-34 (1962).

1. Legal Knowledge and Skill

Attorneys must obtain the requisite legal knowledge and skill to handle their cases. Comment [1] to Rule 1.1 explains that while expertise in a particular field may be required in some cases, nevertheless, in "many instances, the required proficiency is that of a general practitioner." The comment goes on to explain that generalized legal skills are of primary importance in many types of cases. These skills include "analysis of precedent, the evaluation of evidence, and legal drafting." The comment posits that "[p]erhaps the most fundamental legal skill consists of determining what kind of legal problems a situation may involve"—commonly known to lawyers and law students as "issue-spotting."

Legal knowledge includes not only knowledge of substantive law, but also knowledge of procedural rules and requirements to successfully handle a case. The importance of attorney competence in procedure can hardly be overstated. An attorney who understands procedure can use it skillfully to vindicate client rights, while the attorney who makes procedural missteps can easily forfeit a client's meritorious claims and rights. Notably, an attorney's failure to read, understand, or follow procedural rules does not constitute a basis for obtaining relief from a judgment under Federal Rule of Civil Procedure 60(b).[2] Thus, failure to comply with procedural requirements may lead to a client forfeiting rights and being unable to recover them.

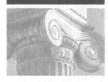

Case Preview

Dahl v. Dahl

Dahl v. Dahl is an appeal from a divorce proceeding where the husband, a cardiologist, divorced his wife, who had been the primary caretaker of their two children and had not worked outside of the home during their 18 years of marriage. Counsel for Ms. Dahl made several major procedural errors. Notably, he failed to file proper expert witness reports as to experts that he had designated to testify in favor of Ms. Dahl relating to child custody. He also failed to make proper pretrial disclosures and provide an exhibit list, and he failed to file or designate for trial the requisite financial declaration to obtain temporary or permanent alimony. Consequently, at trial, the trial court refused to allow Ms. Dahl's experts to testify beyond what was disclosed in their meager reports and excluded from evidence nearly all of Ms. Dahl's trial exhibits. Full custody of the children was awarded to Mr. Dahl, and Ms. Dahl was denied any award of alimony. Ms. Dahl appealed, arguing that a trial in which she was not allowed to introduce most of her exhibits and was not allowed to have child custody experts testify on her behalf was an abuse of the trial court's discretion.

---

2. Pioneer Inv. Services Co. v. Brunswick Associates Ltd., 507 U.S. 380, 392 (1993) ("[I]nadvertence, ignorance of the rules, or mistakes concerning construing the rules do not usually constitute 'excusable' neglect," under Rule 60(b) allowing for relief from judgment.).

As you read *Dahl v. Dahl*, consider the following:

1. Why is competence so important? What did attorney incompetence cost Ms. Dahl?
2. The Utah Supreme Court indicated that Ms. Dahl could alleviate her losses by suing her attorney for malpractice. Would malpractice fully compensate a client like Ms. Dahl?
3. Is it really fair to bind clients to the mistakes of their "freely selected agent attorney" when an attorney makes egregious procedural missteps?

Dahl v. Dahl
2015 UT 79

Dr. Charles Dahl and Ms. Kim Dahl were married for nearly eighteen years.... The divorce proceedings were extremely contentious. The parties fiercely disputed custody of their children, Ms. Dahl's right to temporary and permanent alimony, and the proper distribution of the marital estate. The discovery process was rife with abuses on both sides, which delayed trial. The pretrial disclosure process was similarly fraught and ultimately resulted in the exclusion of most of Ms. Dahl's trial exhibits and expert witnesses. The district court aptly described the pretrial proceedings as a "train wreck."

. . .

B. THE DISTRICT COURT DID NOT ABUSE ITS DISCRETION IN ITS PRETRIAL EVIDENTIARY RULINGS

Ms. Dahl [] argues that the district court abused its discretion [in its evidentiary rulings].... We find no abuse of discretion. Rather, the rulings were appropriate because Ms. Dahl's counsel failed to comply with basic rules of procedure....

2. *The District Court Did Not Abuse Its Discretion When It Limited the Number of Exhibits Ms. Dahl Was Allowed to Introduce at Trial*

At a June 17, 2009 pretrial conference, the district court ordered the parties to exchange "an actual schedule of the people [they planned] to call and the exhibits [they planned] to use" no later than two weeks before the first day of trial....

The exhibit list submitted by Ms. Dahl's counsel failed to comply with the court's order. Nor did it comport with any reasonable standards of pretrial disclosure. The exhibit list encompassed the entire universe of potential exhibits and was accompanied by a CD containing digital copies of over 8,000 documents. For example, the first exhibit listed was "[a]ny and all documents exchanged by the parties as potential exhibits in this matter on August 31, 2009, to the extent that they are admissible." Other listed exhibits included "[a]ny and all documents maintained in the Court's file"; "[a]ll affidavits filed in this matter"; "[a]ll email communications and other written communications between the parties"; "[a]ny and all admissible information, received pursuant to Subpoena Duces Tecum or other discovery method in the above-entitled matter"; and "[a]ny rebuttal exhibits." The list was so broad and overinclusive as to be meaningless. It failed to identify any particular exhibit by an identifying number or a particularized description and made no effort to link the general categories of documents to the electronic documents contained on the CD. In short, the exhibit list failed to identify any single document with enough particularity to allow the court or opposing counsel to identify it as one Ms. Dahl planned to introduce at trial.

At the final pretrial motion hearing on September 15, 2009, the court . . . noted the problems with the exhibit list, stating:

> I thought my direction to you was clear. It's the same direction I give to every litigant who prepares for trial. I tell them to prepare a list of the actual exhibits, one by one that they intend to introduce and you've given me a list that says all the documents maintained, all the affidavits, all the records relied upon, all the marital communications. That's completely unworkable. I'm not going to allow you to simply dump all your discovery on my desk and tell me to sort it out.

The court thereafter struck the exhibit list and ordered counsel to resubmit a list that would identify particular documents that he would use with particular witnesses. In response, Ms. Dahl's counsel filed an amended exhibit list on September 22, 2009, the first day of trial. The amended list, though improved, continued to include designations such as "[a]ny and all documents exchanged by the parties as potential exhibits in this matter on August 31, 2009, to the extent they are admissible." The court again expressed its displeasure at counsel's failure to specifically identify which exhibits he planned to use at trial, citing the need to give all parties fair notice. . . .

On the next trial date, the court noted that counsel for Ms. Dahl had yet to submit an acceptable witness or exhibit list. By October 7, the fifth day of trial, counsel continued to attempt to introduce exhibits that had not previously been disclosed to the court or opposing counsel. The district court properly refused to allow these exhibits. On October 23 and November 4, counsel for Ms. Dahl filed supplemental exhibit lists, which identified particular documents, but did not identify which witness would be used to introduce the documents. Because Ms. Dahl's counsel failed to submit a proper exhibit list, the district court was confronted with the daunting task of determining, on a document-by-document basis during the course of trial, which exhibits had been previously produced. If a document had been previously produced to opposing counsel, the trial court admitted it. If not, the court excluded it.

Ms. Dahl argues that the district court abused its discretion when it excluded *most of her exhibits* based on counsel's failure to submit a proper exhibit list. . . . We disagree. The district court's order clearly directed the parties to designate particular documents to be used with particular witnesses and to exchange those documents with opposing counsel. And even if the district court's order were unclear, counsel was given numerous opportunities to rectify the situation and failed to do so. The district court would have been justified in excluding all of Ms. Dahl's exhibits based on her failure to submit a proper exhibit list prior to the start of trial. And it appropriately exercised its discretion when it excluded all documents except those that the parties stipulated had been previously disclosed during discovery.

3. *The District Court Did Not Abuse Its Discretion When It Limited the Testimony of Ms. Dahl's Expert Witnesses*

Ms. Dahl argues that the district court abused its discretion when it limited the testimony of two of her expert witnesses, Dr. Barden and Dr. Mejia. Ms. Dahl timely designated Drs. Barden and Mejia as experts prior to trial. Although the district court allowed these two experts to testify, it limited the scope of their testimony to the reports and affidavits the experts had filed earlier in the litigation. Ms. Dahl asserts that this limitation was an abuse of discretion. We disagree. . . .

. . . Though counsel for Ms. Dahl filed what were styled as expert witness reports for Drs. Barden and Mejia, neither report complied with the requirements of [Utah Civil Procedure] rule 26.

The expert report for Dr. Barden consisted of a mere four pages, contained no summary of Dr. Barden's qualifications or list of his publications, and identified the proposed subject matter of his testimony only in the most cursory way. . . .

The expert report for Dr. Mejia was similarly deficient. The report was less than two pages and contained only vague descriptions of Dr. Mejia's proposed testimony. The report failed to include a list of Dr. Mejia's publications or of previous cases in which he had testified.

Despite these shortcomings, the district court allowed Drs. Mejia and Barden to testify, but limited their testimony to that consistent with reports they had filed previously in the litigation. Given Ms. Dahl's failure to provide the kind of proper notice of expert testimony contemplated by rule 26, the district court did not abuse its discretion in limiting these experts' testimony in this way.

Pretrial discovery and disclosure are basic skills that we expect all attorneys to possess. Our already overworked district court judges should not be required to provide remedial instructions to counsel on how to properly conduct discovery, designate trial exhibits, or prepare expert reports. Our courts rely heavily on the competence and diligence of counsel. The evidentiary rulings Ms. Dahl complains of were largely the result of her counsel's inability to follow basic rules of procedure and properly manage discovery. Accordingly, we conclude that the district court did not abuse its discretion in its pretrial evidentiary rulings.

. . .

C. THE DISTRICT COURT DID NOT ABUSE ITS DISCRETION IN DENYING MS. DAHL'S REQUESTS FOR BOTH TEMPORARY AND PERMANENT ALIMONY

Ms. Dahl next challenges the district court's denial of her requests for temporary and permanent alimony. . . . We conclude that although Ms. Dahl may have qualified for an award of both temporary and permanent alimony, the district court did not abuse its discretion in refusing to make such an award because Ms. Dahl's counsel repeatedly failed to provide the credible financial documentation necessary for the district court to make an adequate finding as to Ms. Dahl's financial need.

. . . At the hearing on Ms. Dahl's first request for temporary alimony, the commissioner determined that Ms. Dahl's declaration was not sufficiently detailed and did not have enough evidentiary support for him to comply with the rules, statutes, and case law governing alimony awards. . . . Two months later, Ms. Dahl filed an affidavit in support of her request for temporary alimony. The affidavit, however, did not include any verification of the expenses she claimed, nor did it include any verification of her current financial condition or need. Instead, Ms. Dahl attached a 2005 tax return and an appraisal of the marital home in which she was no longer living. The commissioner again found the evidence insufficient to support an alimony award and ordered Ms. Dahl to file a financial declaration that complied with rule 101(d) of the Utah Rules of Civil Procedure.

A third hearing on this issue was held, but Ms. Dahl had not yet complied with the court's prior order that she provide a financial declaration. The commissioner again, relying on the Rules of Civil Procedure, the Utah Code, and relevant case law, declined to award temporary alimony. The matter was then raised in the district court at a hearing just four days later. The district court ordered Ms. Dahl to comply with the commissioner's order for a financial declaration.

Ms. Dahl made a third attempt at documenting her financial need a month and a half later when she filed a "Verified Financial Declaration." In contrast to her first declaration, where she testified to just over $11,000 in monthly expenses, she testified to over $40,000 in monthly expenses. . . . But Ms. Dahl again failed to provide verification of any of these expenses. She provided no proof of income, no bills, no checks, no lease agreement, no bank statements. In short, she provided absolutely no evidence to support the claimed expenses. The commissioner again ruled that Ms. Dahl had failed to provide sufficient evidence to support an alimony award under Utah law. . . . When the district court reviewed and ruled on the commissioner's recommendation, Ms. Dahl had still not complied with the commissioner's order for a financial declaration, and the district court therefore adopted the commissioner's findings. . . .

Nearly a year after the divorce petition had been filed, Ms. Dahl filed another motion for temporary alimony, accompanied by a new affidavit. . . . Again, there was no supporting documentation for this amount. One day prior to the hearing on the motion, Ms. Dahl submitted a notice of errata to her affidavit, which finally, after a year of litigation, included a copy of a rent check, other checks written for unknown purposes, utility bills, and past-due medical bills. These bills totaled $2,651.78.

At the hearing the next day, the commissioner treated this second motion for temporary alimony as a motion to reconsider the court's prior rulings that no temporary alimony was warranted. . . . The district court ultimately adopted the commissioner's recommendation [and] found that "[Ms. Dahl's] [c]ounsel was previously permitted to re-file this Motion several times" but each time had failed to include the necessary supporting documents.

. . . In this case, although Dr. Dahl submitted sufficient evidence to the court to demonstrate his ability to pay alimony, Ms. Dahl's counsel repeatedly failed to comply with the district court's order to supply the court with documentation. . . . Instead of supplying the court with the requested documentation, Ms. Dahl submitted a new declaration, requesting over $40,000 in monthly alimony. . . . And because Ms. Dahl's counsel again provided no evidence to substantiate Ms. Dahl's alleged monthly expenses or earning ability, the district court appropriately denied her request for temporary alimony. . . .

2. *The District Court Did Not Abuse Its Discretion in Denying Ms. Dahl's Request for Permanent Alimony*

Ms. Dahl next . . . asserts that the district court abused its discretion when it denied her request for permanent alimony. We disagree. . . .

As the party seeking an award of permanent alimony, Ms. Dahl bore the burden of providing the district court with sufficient credible evidence of each factor listed in the Alimony Statute. . . . She provided no financial declaration, no supporting financial documentation, and no expert testimony. . . . We therefore conclude that Ms. Dahl failed to meet her burden of showing her financial need — a necessary prerequisite to an award of permanent alimony.

. . . Any harm Ms. Dahl may have suffered by receiving no permanent alimony was not a result of error on the part of the district court, but instead was due to her counsel's failure to present the evidence necessary to support an award of permanent alimony.[23]

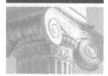

Post-Case Follow-Up

The Utah Supreme Court emphasized that understanding and complying with procedural rules and requirements, including pretrial disclosure of evidence, "are basic skills that we expect all attorneys to possess." Yet, as *Dahl v. Dahl* exemplifies, not all attorneys in fact possess such skills and their clients suffer from such incompetence. Reading, double-checking, and staying current on revisions to and interpretations of procedural rules are all essential to a competent practice. Comment [1] to Rule 1.1 advises lawyers to "maintain the requisite knowledge and skill" for their practice, "to keep abreast of changes in the law and its practice," and to "engage in continuing legal education requirements to which the lawyer is subject."

Dahl v. Dahl: Real Life Applications

1. What, if anything, could Ms. Dahl have done to protect her interests in this case? Could she have fired her attorney during trial once it was clear he had not properly prepared the expert reports or the pretrial disclosures?

2. Madison is an attorney who is filing a claim on behalf of George against the estate of Samuel Zuckerman. Letters testamentary were issued on October 25, 2019. Madison files the claims against the estate on October 15, 2020. Under state law, all claims against the estate are subject to a one-year statute of limitations from the date the letters testamentary are issued. Madison has the executrix served

---

23. To the extent these deficiencies are due to the negligence of Ms. Dahl's counsel, her remedy lies in a civil action for malpractice. But attorney negligence does not provide a basis for us to sidestep the legal standard that our statutes and case law prescribe for alimony determinations.

on November 5, 2020. Assume that the law of the state requires that service on the executrix must take place to satisfy the statute of limitations. Can Madison obtain relief from the statute by arguing that she misread or misunderstood the statute of limitations and honestly believed that all she had to do was file the complaint within the year? Can George, Madison's client, argue that the statute of limitations should not bar his claim because George relied on his attorney to understand and follow the rules?

2. Inexperienced Lawyers

According to comment [2] to Rule 1.1, "[a] newly admitted lawyer can be as competent as a practitioner with long experience." This is so because, as noted, many legal problems require the same basic legal skills. In deciding whether an attorney can competently undertake a representation, comment [1] identifies several factors for consideration: "the relative complexity and specialized nature of the matter, the lawyer's general experience, the lawyer's training and experience in the field in question, the preparation and study the lawyer is able to give the matter and whether it is feasible to refer the matter to, or associate or consult with, a lawyer of established competence in the field in question." Comment [2] further indicates that for an inexperienced attorney—one undertaking a case in a wholly novel field—the requisite competence can be obtained in one of two ways: (1) through necessary study and preparation; and/or (2) through association with an attorney of established competence.

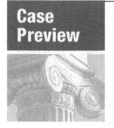

Case Preview

Attorney Grievance Commission of Maryland v. Kendrick

Karin Kendrick was a close personal friend of Judith Kerr and was appointed a co-personal representative of Kerr's estate, along with Kerr's brother. Although Kendrick apparently sincerely believed that her legal assistance would benefit her friend's estate, Kendrick was not experienced in probate matters. She committed numerous missteps causing the small estate to be open from 1999 until 2007.

As you read through *Kendrick*, consider the following:

1. What could and should Kendrick have done once it became clear that she lacked the knowledge and skill to handle the estate?
2. How important is it for an attorney to engage in candid self-evaluation to recognize and admit her own lack of knowledge or skill? At what point in a case should an attorney stop stubbornly insisting that she can handle a matter when she actually lacks the competence to do so?

Attorney Grievance Commission of Maryland v. Kendrick

943 A.2d 1173 (Md. 2008)

. . .

Respondent [] excepts to the hearing judge's conclusion that she violated Rule 1.1 (Competence). Respondent claims that her "alleged failure to file [the] Third and Final Administration Account . . . is due to the fact that Respondent . . . has been continually harassed by the Orphans' Court [and its] failure to give Respondent . . . notice and due process." . . .

Respondent's exception does not address the underlying reasoning for the hearing judge's conclusion that she violated Rule 1.1 (Competence), except to complain about her treatment by the Orphans' Court. The hearing judge concluded that Respondent's handling of the Estate violated Rule 1.1 because "despite the eight years of problems that she ha[d] been experiencing with several courts in administering this Estate, [] Respondent refuse[d] to admit her ignorance of the probate procedures involved or to seek and accept help from qualified legal professionals in getting her problems solved." The hearing judge found that "[h]er stubbornness over the past eight years to find the guidance necessary to close the Estate amounts to incompetence." The record clearly supports the hearing judge's conclusion. The record shows that Judith Nina Kerr died on February 27, 1999. According to the records of the Register of Wills of Baltimore County, the Estate, valued at approximately $60,000, was not closed until December 20, 2007. Those findings indicate 8 years, 9 months and 23 days had lapsed from the date of Ms. Kerr's death until the closing of her Estate. . . .

Moreover, the record shows that Respondent failed to timely file many of the documents necessary to administer the Estate, leading to her removal as Co-Personal Representative. Pursuant to §7-201, Respondent and/or Mr. Kerr had the duty to file an Inventory with the Register of Wills within three months after their appointments as Co-Personal Representatives. On June 11, 1999, the Orphans' Court issued a Delinquent Notice to Mr. Kerr and Respondent for their failure to file an Inventory and Information Report. Thereafter, a summons and a request for show cause order was issued to the Sheriff of Baltimore County to "cite and summons" Respondent to appear before the Orphans' Court to explain why the Inventory had not been filed as of July 13, 1999. On July 26, 1999, Respondent filed the required Inventory.

On December 10, 1999, the Orphans' Court issued a Delinquent Notice to Mr. Kerr and Respondent for their failure to render and file a First Administration Account for the Estate. Pursuant to §7-305(a)(1), Respondent and Mr. Kerr were required to render an account of the Estate within 9 months of their appointment, on or before December 4, 1999. In response to the notice, Respondent requested two extensions, which were granted; however, a second Delinquent Notice was then issued on February 18, 2000, when Respondent did not comply with the extended deadline. A hearing on the delinquency was then scheduled for March 8, 2000; neither Respondent nor Mr. Kerr appeared for that hearing. On March 9, 2000, the Orphans' Court issued a summons and a request for show cause order was issued to the Sheriff of Baltimore County to "cite and summons" Respondent and Mr. Kerr to appear before the Orphans' Court to explain why the First Administration Account had not been filed as of February 11, 2000. Respondent and Mr. Kerr did not file the "First, Not Final Administration Account" with the Register of Wills until April 10, 2000.

The Orphans' Court's issuance of Delinquent Notices and Summonses continued throughout the administration of the Estate. [The court lists several instances through the issuance of a *sixth* Delinquent Notice for failing to make requisite filings.] . . .

Despite repeated interactions with the Register of Wills and the Orphans' Court regarding Respondent's and Mr. Kerr's tardiness in filing the documents, Respondent and Mr. Kerr did not seek assistance in the administration of the Estate. Consequently, on May 3, 2002, a petition to remove Respondent and Mr. Kerr as Co-Personal Representatives was initiated by the Orphans' Court because of Respondent's and Mr. Kerr's failure to file a Supplemental Inventory, a Supplemental Information Report, and a Third Administration Account. The petition was granted and the Court removed Respondent and Mr. Kerr as Co-Personal Representatives of the Estate on August 28, 2002. The Order mandated that Respondent and Mr. Kerr file the "Third and Final Administration Account" and turn over all assets and financial records in their possession within thirty days of the date of the Order. Despite this significant action, Respondent failed to file the Third and Final Administration Account within the 30 day time-limit prescribed by the order of the Orphans' Court, leading to additional court interactions including the imposition of Civil Contempt by the Orphans' Court on June 2, 2005.

It is clear from the record that Respondent's failure to properly comply with probate law in the administration of the Estate was due to her inexperience and her unwillingness to obtain the help she needed to properly administer the estate. As the hearing judge stated in his analysis, "inexperience does not necessarily amount to a violation of this Rule." We have said, however, that attorneys who undertake legal work in areas unfamiliar to them "must take careful thought as to their competence to practice in 'specialty' areas," like the administration of estates. If an attorney "plunges into a field in which he or she is not competent, and as a consequence makes mistakes that demonstrate incompetence, the Code [of Professional Responsibility] demands that discipline be imposed; that one is simply a general practitioner who knew no better is no defense." *Brown*, 308 Md. at 234-35. . . .

It is clear that Respondent did not employ the requisite knowledge and skill to administer the Estate or to comply with the Orphans' Court's orders. . . .

Post-Case Follow-Up

As indicated in *Kendrick* and Model Rule 1.1 comment [2], "[a] lawyer can provide adequate representation in a wholly novel field through necessary study" or "through association of a lawyer of established competence in the field." Importantly, though, the lawyer cannot charge her client for the extra time taken to educate herself to become competent.

For example, in In re Fordham, 668 N.E.2d 816 (Mass. 1996), the Massachusetts Supreme Judicial Court explained:

> It cannot be that an inexperienced lawyer is entitled to charge three or four times as much as an experienced lawyer for the same service. A client should not be expected to pay for the education of a lawyer when he spends excessive amounts of time on tasks which, with reasonable experience, become matters of routine.

Attorney Grievance Commission of Maryland v. Kendrick: Real Life Applications

1. Maria is a brand-new attorney who decides to start her own practice. A potential client, JaNeal, calls Maria and says that she's been sued in a case. After consulting briefly, JaNeal tells Maria she wants to hire her and to please appear on her behalf in the case. Maria has no idea how to make an appearance. She researches appearances for a few hours, and then drafts an appearance and files it. The appearance she files is compliant with all laws and local rules; however, an experienced attorney normally spends less than five minutes preparing an appearance. Can Maria competently continue with the representation? If so, can she charge JaNeal for the time she actually spent on making an appearance in the case?

2. Robert is a criminal defense attorney who is asked by Eugene to represent him in a civil contract dispute. Robert has not done any civil litigation in the 15 years that he's been practicing law. Eugene does not have much money to spend and does not want Robert to spend too much time on the case. Robert thinks that he remembers civil procedure from law school pretty well. The opposing party files a lengthy motion for summary judgment. Robert decides that since Eugene has denied the allegations in his Answer, summary judgment is not appropriate and — just as when his criminal clients plead not guilty — Eugene will be entitled to a trial based on Eugene's pleading. The court grants summary judgment for the opposing party and against Eugene on all claims, explaining that in civil litigation, the non-movant cannot rest on the allegations of his pleadings but must produce evidence showing there is a genuine issue for trial. What should Robert have done differently? What two basic options did he have?

3. Thoroughness and Preparation

Under Model Rule 1.1, competence requires "thoroughness and preparation." Lawyers have a duty to undertake preparations reasonable to the case, including obtaining the requisite factual information regarding a case. As Monroe Freedman and Abbe Smith expound: "Competent representation requires that a lawyer be 'fully informed of all the facts of the matter he is handling.'"[3] Thus, lawyers must

---

3. Monroe H. Freedman & Abbe Smith, Understanding Lawyers' Ethics 128 (4th ed. 2010) (quoting UpJohn Co. v. United States, 449 U.S. 383, 391 (1981)).

thoroughly investigate the facts of a case and make sufficient preparation for legal proceedings and transactions. Numerous disciplinary proceedings have been brought against lawyers who proverbially dropped the ball and "failed to discover and present readily available evidence supporting" their client's case or "failed to prepare" necessary documentation, briefing, or other materials for court proceedings or transactions.[4]

In some situations, lawyers agree to limit the scope of their representation pursuant to Rule 1.2. Nevertheless, the duty of competence still applies. Thus, in In re Seare, 493 B.R. 198 (Bankr. D. Nev. 2013), the court explained:

> Whether a lawyer fulfilled the duty of competence depends on the client's objectives. The lawyer's duty is to competently attain the client's goals of representation. In the absence of a valid limitation on services, a lawyer *must provide the bundle of services that are reasonably necessary to achieve the client's reasonably anticipated result*, unless and until grounds exist for the lawyer's withdrawal. . . . [T]he duty of competence both informs and survives any and all limitations on the scope of services. The *baseline obligation to inquire into the facts and circumstances of a case and analyze the possible legal issues* is not changed when the scope of services is limited.

A lawyer's failure to thoroughly prepare a matter can have disastrous consequences for the client. Consider what the lack of preparation of pretrial disclosures and expert reports cost Ms. Dahl. Another example occurred in Albrechtsen v. Board of Regents of the University of Wisconsin, 309 F.3d 433 (7th Cir. 2002). Professor Albrechtsen prevailed in a jury trial on a Title VII claim against his employer, the University of Wisconsin. The university filed an appeal to the Seventh Circuit, arguing that there was insufficient evidence to support the jury verdict. Notably, the university had a very difficult hurdle to overcome in order to prevail on its appeal — as it was trying to vacate a jury verdict as a matter of law. Conversely, Albrechtsen's lawyer had a very easy burden on appeal — all he had to do was marshal enough evidence introduced at trial to show that there was a sufficient basis in evidence to support the jury's verdict. Nevertheless, Albrechtsen's lawyer failed to include a statement of facts with citations to the trial transcript in his brief. Instead, "the half-page portion of the brief captioned 'Statement of Facts'" simply referred the Seventh Circuit to examine "the district court's opinion denying the University's motion for summary judgment." The Seventh Circuit explained that this was entirely unacceptable because the summary judgment order (entered before a trial was held) contained no cites to the record at trial or summation of the evidence admitted at trial. Instead, the order simply summarized pretrial discovery showing that there were genuine issues of fact necessitating a trial. The Seventh Circuit concluded, "Albrechtsen has effectively provided no statement of facts at all." Consequently, in ruling on the appeal, the Seventh Circuit said that it would treat Albrechtsen's "silence as assent to the [university's] presentation" of the facts. At oral argument, the appellate court gave Albrechtsen's counsel another opportunity,

---

4. People v. Boyle, 942 P.2d 1199 (Colo. 1997).

asking him to identify the evidence admitted at trial that would support the jury verdict. Albrechtsen's lawyer's response was disheartening and betrayed his lack of preparation: "The entire record." The Seventh Circuit explained: "That will not do. . . . Courts are entitled to assistance from counsel, and an invitation to search without guidance is no more useful than a litigant's request to a district court at the summary judgment stage to paw through the assembled discovery material. Judges are not like pigs, hunting for truffles buried in the record." The Seventh Circuit ruled in favor of the university and overturned Albrechtsen's jury verdict.

Albrechtsen's lawyer did not prepare for the appeal. He should have taken the time to prepare a thorough statement of facts with citations to the trial transcript and other evidence admitted at trial. He did not know the trial record at all — at oral argument he could not pinpoint a single piece of evidence or testimony from trial that would support the verdict and thereby preserve his client's jury victory. Thoroughness indicates that lawyers should not take unwarranted shortcuts. The decision of Albrechtsen's counsel to incorporate the trial court's summary judgment order rather than take the time to read the trial transcript, examine the admitted evidence, and then marshal and present that evidence in a statement of facts (with citations) was a devastating shortcut for Albrechtsen. It cost him a jury verdict and award of nearly $150,000, handing his victory to the opposing party.

4. Competence and Technology

Technological advances have made significant changes to the ways in which lawyers practice law — including in how they communicate with clients and maintain client files. What level of technological competence is required of attorneys? Comment [8] to Model Rule 1.1 explains: "To maintain the requisite knowledge and skill, a lawyer should keep abreast of changes in the law and its practice, including the benefits and risks associated with relevant technology."

A number of jurisdictions have examined whether attorneys should use cloud computing and storage and, correspondingly, what steps attorneys should take to remain competent in the use of such technologies to protect client communications and confidences. The use of cloud computing has become nearly ubiquitous. As the Pennsylvania Bar Association summarized, "[i]f an attorney uses a Smartphone or an iPhone, or uses web-based electronic mail (e-mail) such as Gmail, Yahoo!, Hotmail or AOL Mail, or uses products such as Google Docs, Microsoft Office 365 or Dropbox, the attorney is using 'cloud computing.'"[5] What are the obligations of attorneys who use these now common technologies in their practice? The California bar has opined:

---

5. Pennsylvania Bar Association Committee on Legal Ethics and Professional Responsibility, Formal Op. 2011-200, *Ethical Obligations for Attorneys Using Cloud Computing/Software as a Service While Fulfilling the Duties of Confidentiality and Preservation of Client Property,* available at https://www.pabar.org/members/catalogs/Ethics%20Opinions/formal/F2011-200.pdf.

Many attorneys, as with a large contingent of the general public, do not possess much, if any, technological savvy. Although the Committee does not believe that attorneys must develop a mastery of the security features and deficiencies of each technology available, the duties of confidentiality and competence that attorneys owe to their clients do require a basic understanding of the electronic protections afforded by the technology they use in their practice. If the attorney lacks the necessary competence to assess the security of the technology, he or she *must seek additional information or consult with someone who possesses the necessary knowledge*, such as an information technology consultant.[6]

This approach is entirely consistent with Rule 1.1's basic tenet that attorneys must obtain competence either through necessary study or through association with one who is competent.

Use of Cloud Computing Services
Ohio State Bar Association Informal Advisory Opinion 2013-03

The "cloud" is "merely 'a fancy way of saying stuff's not on your [own] computer.'" More formally, cloud storage is the use of "internet-based computing in which large groups of remote servers are networked so as to allow . . . centralized data storage."

Due to "recent advances in . . . technology, the ways attorneys are able to perform and deliver legal services have drastically changed." The applicable Ohio Rules of Professional Conduct, however, are adaptable to address new technologies. Regarding cloud storage, the key rules are those relating to competent representation, communicating with the client, preserving client confidentiality, safeguarding the client's property and supervising nonlawyers that provide support services. The obligations expressed in these rules operate as they traditionally have for older data storage methods. . . .

This approach — applying existing principles to new technological advances while refraining from mandating specific practices — is a practical one. Because technology changes so quickly, overly-specific rules would become obsolete as soon as they were issued. For example, rules about exactly what security measures are required in order to protect client data stored in the cloud would be superseded quickly by technological advances.

Against that background, there are four main issues to consider in applying the Ohio Rules of Professional Conduct to cloud storage of client data: competently selecting an appropriate vendor; preserving confidentiality and safeguarding the client's data; supervising cloud storage vendors; and communicating with the client.

---

6. State Bar of California Standing Committee on Professional Responsibility and Conduct, Formal Op. No. 2010-179, *available at* http://www.calbar.ca.gov/Portals/0/documents/ethics/Opinions/2010-179-Interim-No-08-0002-PAW.pdf (emphasis added).

1. COMPETENTLY SELECTING AN APPROPRIATE VENDOR FOR CLOUD STORAGE

The duty of competence under ORPC 1.1 requires a lawyer to exercise the "legal knowledge, skill, thoroughness, and preparation reasonably necessary for the representation." In Ohio Advisory Opinion 2009-6 (Aug. 14, 2009), the Ohio Board of Commissioners on Grievances and Discipline ("Board") opined that a lawyer who selects a vendor for any type of support services that are provided outside the lawyer's firm must exercise "due diligence as to the qualifications and reputation of those to whom services are outsourced," and also as to whether the outside vendor will itself provide the requested services competently and diligently.

Knowing the qualifications, reputation and longevity of your cloud storage vendor is necessary. But in addition, just as you would review and assess the terms of a contract for off-site storage of your clients' paper files in a brick-and-mortar facility, so you must read and understand the agreement you enter into with an online data storage service—sometimes called a "Service Level Agreement." Some commonly-occurring issues include:

- What safeguards does the vendor have to prevent confidentiality breaches?
- Does the agreement create a legally enforceable obligation on the vendor's part to safeguard the confidentiality of the data?
- Do the terms of the agreement purport to give "ownership" of the data to the vendor, or is the data merely subject to the vendor's license?
- How may the vendor respond to government or judicial attempts to obtain disclosure of your client data?
- What is the vendor's policy regarding returning your client data at the termination of its relationship with your firm?
- What plans and procedures does the vendor have in case of natural disaster, electric power interruption or other catastrophic events?
- Where is the server located (particularly if the vendor itself does not actually host the data, and uses a data center located elsewhere)? Is the relationship subject to international law?

2. PRESERVING CONFIDENTIALITY AND SAFEGUARDING CLIENT PROPERTY

Under ORPC 1.6(a), a lawyer "shall not reveal information relating to the representation of a client," with only limited exceptions. . . . [T]he ABA House of Delegates added Model Rule 1.6(c) in August 2012, requiring a lawyer to make "reasonable efforts to prevent the inadvertent or unauthorized disclosure of, or unauthorized access to, information relating to the representation of a client." . . .

[And] in Advisory Opinion 99-2 . . . the Board said that communicating with clients by e-mail was covered by the confidentiality rule. . . . "The duty extends to communications by electronic methods just as it extends to other forms of communication used by an attorney." . . .

. . . [S]toring client data in the cloud involves yielding exclusive control over the information and puts it in the hands of a third party, just as storing a client's paper files off-site does. And similar to storing a client's paper files off-site, cloud storage raises the risk that "a third party could illegally gain access to . . . confidential client data." . . . Therefore, a lawyer's duty under the ORPC to preserve the confidentiality of cloud-stored client data is to exercise competence (1) in selecting an appropriate vendor, (2) in staying abreast of technology issues that have an impact on client data storage and (3) in considering whether any special circumstances call for extra protection for particularly sensitive client information or for refraining from using the cloud to store such particularly sensitive data. . . .

3. SUPERVISING CLOUD VENDORS

. . . [U]nder Rule 5.3(a)-(b), lawyers who contract with a cloud-storage vendor must make reasonable efforts to ensure that the vendor's conduct is compatible with the lawyer's own professional obligations.

While the extent of supervision needed is a matter of professional judgment for the lawyer, the lawyer must exercise due diligence in ascertaining whether the vendor will be capable of conduct consistent with the lawyer's own obligations.

4. COMMUNICATING WITH THE CLIENT

Rule 1.4(a)(2) requires a lawyer to "reasonably consult with the client" about how the client's objectives are to be accomplished. We do not conclude that storing client data in "the cloud" always requires prior client consultation, because we interpret the language "reasonably consult" as indicating that the lawyer must use judgment in order to determine if the circumstances call for consultation. . . . In exercising judgment about whether to consult with the client about storing client data in "the cloud," the lawyer should consider, among other things, the sensitivity of the client's data.

5. ETHICS OPINIONS FROM OTHER JURISDICTIONS REGARDING CLOUD STORAGE

Our conclusion that cloud storage is permissible under the ORPC is echoed by ethics authorities in other jurisdictions. To date, at least 14 states have issued ethics opinions regarding or related to cloud data storage. All have concluded that their respective lawyer conduct rules permit lawyers to store client data in the cloud, with due regard for their state ethics rules, usually their states' versions of ORPC 1.1, 1.6, 1.15 and 5.3. . . .

5. Diligence

Model Rule 1.3 requires lawyers to "act with reasonable diligence and promptness in representing a client." Diligence requires that the lawyer pursue a client's case "despite opposition, obstruction or personal inconvenience to the lawyer, and take whatever lawful and ethical measures are required to vindicate a client's cause or endeavor." *See* Model Rule 1.1 cmt. [1]. The very nature of our adversarial system of justice creates a likelihood of unfairness when only one side in a controversy has counsel or only one side has competent and diligent counsel. Attorneys can improve the quality of justice both by representing people regardless of any opposition or personal inconvenience (including taking unpopular cases and performing pro bono representation) and also by fully and diligently pursuing their own client's interests, thus ensuring that their clients are not put at a disadvantage.

As noted in comment [2], in order to be diligent, lawyers must control their workload so that they are able to competently handle each and every case. When an attorney is an associate or other employee whose caseload is assigned by another, this requirement may be more difficult. Subordinate lawyers must communicate with senior and assigning lawyers if their caseload is more than they can realistically handle competently. Similarly, public defenders and other public employee lawyers may have less ability to control their caseload, but they still can take actions to protect their clients' interests, as will be addressed later in this chapter.

As comment [3] cautions, "Perhaps no professional shortcoming is more widely resented than procrastination." Why is this so? The comment explains: "A client's interests often can be adversely affected by the passage of time or the change of conditions; in extreme instances, as when a lawyer overlooks a statute of limitations, the client's legal position may be destroyed." Even where procrastination doesn't directly impact a client's rights, "unreasonable delay can cause a client needless anxiety." *See* Model Rule 1.3 cmt. [3]. In Shakespeare's famous "To be or not to be" soliloquy, Hamlet lists reasons that would make a person want to commit suicide ("not to be"), and among them is "the law's delay."[7] Legal processes generally take far more time than clients expect even where an attorney acts promptly, with diligence and competence. When attorneys do not act diligently, cases will languish — along with the client.

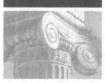

Case Preview

In re Disciplinary Action Against Howe

Sometimes clients actually want to delay a proceeding. For example, a client may wish to delay proceedings that could lead to time in jail, deportation, or other serious personal consequences. A client may want evidence that is adverse to him to become stale. In the following case, attorney Henry Howe represented the Camachos, a couple who were undocumented immigrants faced with deportation even though they had lived in the United States for over 20 years and had four children who were United States citizens. Howe claimed to have engaged in a dilatory strategy to keep the Camachos in the United States for as long as possible.

---

7. WILLIAM SHAKESPEARE, HAMLET, act 3, sc. 1 ("For who would bear the whips and scorns of time, The oppressor's wrong, the proud man's contumely, The pangs of despised love, the law's delay, The insolence of office and the spurns That patient merit of the unworthy takes, When he himself might his quietus make With a bare bodkin?").

As you read *Howe*, consider the following:

1. Was Howe's alleged strategy of delay helpful to his clients?
2. Even if a client wants to delay proceedings, should the lawyer engage in tactics solely for the purpose of delay?

In re Disciplinary Action Against Howe
843 N.W.2d 325 (N.D. 2014)

Attorney Henry H. Howe objected to a report of a hearing panel of the Disciplinary Board.... We order that Howe be suspended from the practice of law for six months and one day, [and] that he pay $8,871.34 in costs of the disciplinary proceedings....

This proceeding arises from Howe's representation of Elias Angel Camacho-Banda and Margarita Maya-Morales (collectively "Camachos"). The Camachos, undocumented Mexican nationals, have lived in the United States for over twenty years. The Camachos have four United States citizen children and one Mexican citizen child. Subsequent to a February 2007 traffic incident, authorities discovered the Camacho adults and one child did not have legal immigration status. The Camachos were placed in removal proceedings before the Executive Office for Immigration Review, Immigration Court, in Bloomington, Minnesota. The Camachos retained Howe to represent them in the removal proceedings.

During the immigration court's May 16, 2007, master calendar hearing, Howe conceded the Camachos were removable for staying in the United States past the time permitted and stated he would file their applications for cancellation of removal and adjustment of status. To prevail in canceling removal, the Camachos needed to establish removal would result in "exceptional and extremely unusual hardship to the alien's . . . child, who is a citizen of the United States" under 8 U.S.C. §1229b(b)(1)(D). The immigration judge informed Howe he needed significant documentation of hardship, including documentation of one child's alleged learning disability. On May 16, 2007, Howe received an information sheet for gathering "biometrics," which explained the process for collecting fingerprints and personal information as required at immigration proceedings before final status decisions are made. Howe did not file the applications for cancellation of removal until November 21, 2008.

A merits hearing was held on December 1, 2008. Howe had not completed the biometrics process, including failing to obtain the Camachos' fingerprints. When asked why he did not complete the biometrics process, Howe blamed a calendaring error by his paralegal. Howe did not provide the hardship documentation requested by the judge, instead supplying only the children's school records. Further, the Camachos were the only witnesses called. The immigration judge chastised Howe for being unprepared, but allowed him thirty days to augment the Camachos' application for cancellation of removal. In addition to the clarification Howe already received on May 16, 2007, regarding supplemental materials the judge sought, the judge directed Howe to augment the file concerning the

Camachos' son's learning disability, including letters from teachers and doctors and information regarding the special educational prospects in Mexico for a child with a learning disability.

The merits hearing was rescheduled for January 13, 2009. The Camachos were not present at the hearing because Howe failed to notify them of the rescheduled hearing. . . . The judge agreed to reschedule the merits hearing from January 13, 2009, to October 21, 2009, warning Howe that if the Camachos again failed to appear, he would issue a removal order in their absence. . . .

Before the rescheduled merits hearing, Howe resubmitted duplicate documents, including country conditions and school records. Howe's submission was rejected for failing to comply with filing requirements. Howe attempted to fix the issues by resending his submission. The court noted that all the documents still were improperly submitted, but that it would nonetheless accept them. On April 23, 2010, Howe submitted additional articles about violence in Mexico, offered to demonstrate hardship. The Camachos' merits hearing was rescheduled to April 8, 2011. Howe obtained letters from the Camacho children's teachers, including a letter from the special education teacher and case manager for the child with the learning disability. Howe argues that while he possessed the letters, in his opinion the letters would not have helped meet the exceptional and extremely unusual hardship standard and possibly could have made things worse.

On April 8, 2011, Howe and the Camachos appeared at the rescheduled merits hearing, but because an interpreter was not available, the judge reserved the case for written submissions and closing arguments to be submitted within two weeks. Howe did not provide additional materials or submit written closing arguments. On November 15, 2011, the judge ordered the Camachos deported to Mexico. Howe was discharged, and the Camachos retained new counsel.

. . .

Rule 1.3, N.D.R. Prof. Conduct, provides that "[a] lawyer shall act with reasonable diligence and promptness in representing a client." Reasonable diligence is defined as: "A fair degree of diligence expected from someone of ordinary prudence under circumstances like those at issue." Black's Law Dictionary 468 (7th ed. 1999). Prompt is defined as: "quick to act or to do what is required[.]" Webster's New World Dictionary 1137 (2nd ed. 1980). "Perhaps no professional shortcoming is more widely resented than procrastination." N.D.R. Prof. Conduct 1.3 cmt. 3.

Howe failed to diligently represent the Camachos in several ways. While Howe paid the biometrics fee and filed the biometrics forms, he did not obtain the Camachos' fingerprints and, therefore, did not complete the biometrics process before the merits hearing. The judge cannot make a decision regarding the Camachos' legal status in the United States until their updated criminal background information is obtained. . . . Even after the judge admonished Howe at the December 1, 2008 hearing to complete biometrics, Howe did not make an appointment for the Camachos to be fingerprinted before the January 13, 2009 merits hearing. Howe blamed a calendaring error to excuse his unpreparedness regarding the biometrics information, but he had more than a month to obtain the fingerprints, or at least make an appointment, before the January 13, 2009 hearing. Howe also failed to timely submit the applications for cancellation of removal. Howe stated on May 16, 2007 that he would file the

Camachos' applications for cancellation of removal, yet he waited until November 21, 2008 to file the applications. The result was that the applications were filed just days before the merits hearing on December 1, 2008.

Howe also failed to communicate with his clients concerning important hearing dates, causing them to miss their January 13, 2009 merits hearing. Howe first blamed the communication failure on a change in office personnel. He later testified he spoke with the Camachos concerning the hearing date, but that a miscommunication occurred because the Camachos' daughter who usually translated was not present. Howe's arguments blaming his paralegal and changes in office personnel are to no avail because he is responsible for ensuring his nonlawyer staff's conduct comports with his professional obligations as an attorney under Rule 5.3(b), N.D.R. Prof. Conduct.

We conclude clear and convincing evidence establishes that Howe did not meet the diligence requirements for the Camachos' case and that he violated Rule 1.3, N.D.R. Prof. Conduct.

. . .

Howe argues in his objection to the hearing panel's recommendations and in his briefing to this Court that his three-part strategy was disregarded, ignored or not understood. Howe's three-part strategy for the Camachos included petitioning for cancellation of removal by showing exceptional and extremely unusual hardship, taking necessary steps to protect the status and assets of the Camacho family and keeping the Camachos in the United States for as long as possible.

Although Rule 3.2, N.D.R. Prof. Conduct, was not included by the disciplinary counsel in its petition for discipline, Howe's arguments implicate Rule 3.2, providing: "A lawyer shall make reasonable efforts to expedite litigation consistent with the interests of the client." "The question is whether a competent lawyer acting in good faith would regard the course of action as having some substantial purpose other than delay." N.D.R. Prof. Conduct 3.2 cmt. 2. Howe's argument that he sought delay at any cost for his clients is legally untenable under Rule 3.2 because a competent and diligent immigration lawyer would not seek delay by purposely failing to timely file documents requested by the judge, and would not refrain from telling clients about hearing dates in the hopes trial would be postponed. A competent and diligent lawyer would not do these things because the judge is not required to show lenience for failure to follow requirements, and lawyers can never predict how a judge will react to such failures. Despite noting Howe's unpreparedness at the December 1, 2008 hearing, the immigration judge allowed thirty extra days to augment the file. Despite Howe failing to tell the Camachos of the rescheduled merits hearing, the immigration judge showed lenience and rescheduled the merits hearing rather than immediately issuing a removal order in their absence. Further, the immigration court showed lenience with Howe's inability or unwillingness to follow document submission requirements. The Camachos are still in the United States and in the appeal process for nothing but the grace of the immigration court judge, rather than due to Howe's alleged strategy.

Howe's arguments on review fail. . . . The numerous egregious risks Howe took during his representation of the Camachos are dispositive. Clear and convincing evidence establishes he violated Rules 1.1, 1.3 and 1.4, N.D.R. Prof. Conduct.

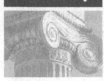

Post-Case Follow-Up

In disciplining Howe under Rule 1.3, the court also invoked Rule 3.2, requiring "reasonable efforts to expedite litigation consistent with the interests of the client." As comment [1] to that rule explains, acting solely to delay proceedings is not permissible under the rule: "Nor will a failure to expedite be reasonable if done for the purpose of frustrating an opposing party's attempt to obtain rightful redress or repose." As the court in *Howe* noted, "[t]he question is whether a competent lawyer acting in good faith would regard the course of action as having some substantial purpose other than delay." Notably, the comment clarifies that such client interests cannot be the realization of "financial or other benefit *from* otherwise improper delay."

In re Disciplinary Action Against Howe: Real Life Applications

1. Janet is representing Devon as a defendant in a personal injury lawsuit. The discovery deadline is March 31. Janet does not know if she will want to do discovery yet or not, but neither she nor her client wants to proceed to trial. Her client, Devon, is hoping to sell some real estate before a potential judgment is entered adverse to him. Thus, Janet files a motion with the court to obtain a 60-day extension of time for the discovery deadline, arguing that she needs more time to conduct discovery, including specific depositions. Over the plaintiff's objection, the court grants the 60-day extension. Janet does not conduct any discovery during the 60 days, but her client is able to sell his real estate and is very pleased with the delay. Has Janet violated the rules?

2. Suppose that you represent Sara in a divorce proceeding from her husband, Ray. Sara indicates to you that she is actually thinking of reconciling and asks you to proceed as slowly as possible while she considers reconciliation. Consequently, you ask the court for several extensions of time on various motions (which are granted), with the primary purpose of delaying the proceedings. Ultimately, however, Sara decides to go through with the divorce. Have you violated the rules?

6. Communication

In the animated sitcom "King of the Hill," Peggy Hill, the wife of the protagonist, Hank Hill, asks a neighbor how to improve her marriage, but adds the caveat, "And don't say 'communicate,' because there are some things Hank just will not do." Of course, the joke is that communication is essential to maintaining good relationships with people. And communication is particularly important for successful attorney-client relationships. As Eli Wald has observed:

> Communications between clients and attorneys are the cornerstone of the attorney-client relationship. Because the vast majority of civil and criminal trials settle and

plea-bargain, respectively, many clients never actually enter the courtroom, interact with a judge or a jury, or meet the opposing party or its attorney. Consequently, for a good number of Americans, communicating with their own lawyers will constitute most, if not all, of their exposure to law and the legal system. Communications between clients and their own attorneys thus become the main arena in which clients gain any experience with lawyers and the law.[8]

A lawyer's communication with a client is the method whereby a client knows what is going on in her lawsuit — and for many clients a lawsuit implicates intimately important personal interests that weigh heavily and constantly on the client's mind (think of criminal charges, housing, child custody, employment, medical benefits, disability, social security, probate, etc.). Melvin Hirshman, as Bar Counsel for the Maryland Attorney Grievance Commission, urged lawyers to "'step into your client's shoes' and realize how important their legal matter is to them." Hirshman contends that "[e]ven the delivery of bad news is better than no news if that be the case"; rather, "[i]t is the unknown that causes anxiety [] for many clients." Thus, he concludes: "It is not too much to require an attorney to communicate with a client, truthfully and promptly."[9]

In addition to the client's need to hear from the attorney about her case, it is critically important for the attorney to hear from and communicate with the client in order for the attorney to ascertain the client's objectives. Again, Wald observes:

> [T]he attorney-client relationship is an agency relationship in which a lawyer-agent serves the interests of a client-principal. Communications are the mechanism by which the client controls the agency relationship, informs the attorney about his goals and objectives, and provides the lawyer with necessary and relevant information about the representation. Successful representation requires effective communications, without which the attorney-agent cannot know, understand, or represent the client's goals.[10]

The client is also the primary source for obtaining the facts of a case. Lawyers simply must communicate with clients to effectively represent the client and appropriately pursue the client's actual interests and goals. Thus, Model Rule 1.4(b) requires lawyers to "explain a matter to the extent reasonably necessary to permit the client to make informed decisions regarding the representation." How much information does the client need? Comment [5] provides a guideline: the client needs "sufficient information to participate intelligently" in making decisions regarding the representation. Notably, a good attorney-client relationship will likely include far more communication than what is required at a minimum by the rules.

Model Rule 1.4 sets out basic categories of required communication. First, the rule requires that the lawyer "promptly inform the client of any decision or circumstance with respect to which the client's informed consent . . . is required by these Rules." When is the client's informed consent required — thus triggering the

---

8. Eli Wald, *Taking Attorney-Client Communications (and Therefore Clients) Seriously*, 42 U.S.F. L. Rev. 747, 747-48 (2008).
9. Melvin Hirshman, *Communication*, 43-Feb. Md. B.J. 61 (2010).
10. Wald, *supra* note 8, at 747, 748.

communication requirement? Remember that under Rule 1.2(a), there are certain actions that the client has the ultimate authority to decide. In civil cases, the client has ultimate authority to decide whether to settle a matter, and in criminal cases, the client has the ultimate authority regarding entering a plea, waiving a jury trial, and testifying on her own behalf. Thus, in these matters, Rule 1.4 plainly requires the attorney to communicate with the client — and to do so *promptly*. Comment [2] explains that "a lawyer who receives from opposing counsel an offer of settlement in a civil controversy or a proffered plea bargain in a criminal case must promptly inform the client of its substance." A lawyer may only forgo telling a client of a plea or settlement offer if "the client has previously indicated that the proposal will be acceptable or unacceptable or has authorized the lawyer to accept or reject the offer." *See* Model Rule 1.4 cmt. [2].

Communicating with the client about matters that are the client's to decide does not mean merely informing the client of his choice without discussing the issue thoroughly. Indeed, the attorney must counsel with the client so that the client can make a truly informed decision. Thus, in communicating settlement and plea offers to a client, the lawyer should consult with the client about the pros, cons, and material consequences of accepting or rejecting such an offer. For example, and as discussed later in this chapter, in the plea bargaining context attorneys should explain to the client material consequences of pleading guilty — including deportation consequences for non-citizen defendants. Similarly, in counseling with a criminal defendant regarding whether to testify on his own behalf, the attorney should explain to the criminal defendant that testifying may allow the prosecution to introduce the prior criminal record of the accused to impeach his credibility. In making these decisions, the client should not act blindly, but should act knowingly, which she can only do with proper counseling from the attorney.

Recognize that if a rule requires informed consent, that triggers the attorney's obligation under Rule 1.4 to promptly communicate the circumstance to the client. The Model Rules require client informed consent in several other instances, notably in waiving conflicts of interest or permitting disclosure of confidential information.

The Model Rules themselves do not define the term "promptly," but as indicated in the *Howe* and *Helmedach* cases in this chapter, jurisdictions take a common parlance approach, construing prompt to mean "quick to act" or "without delay." As *Helmedach* indicates, where a lawyer has ample opportunity to communicate something to a client and fails to do so, the lawyer has not acted promptly.

Rule 1.4 also requires that a lawyer "reasonably consult with the client about the means by which the client's objectives are to be accomplished" and "keep the client reasonably informed about the status of the matter." As comment [3] elucidates, there are times when a lawyer is required to consult with the client prior to acting, but that depends "on both the importance of the action under consideration and the feasibility of consulting with the client." Further, whenever there are material developments in the status of a client's case, the lawyer needs to communicate such developments to the client.

Unfortunately, material developments that a lawyer must communicate to the client can include the lawyer's own mistakes that negatively affect a representation. Some attorneys have gone to extraordinary lengths to hide their own incompetence from their clients. For example, in In re Mays, 495 S.E.2d 30 (Ga. 1998), the attorney allowed the statute of limitations to run, and instead of so informing his client, the attorney lied to his client, telling him about a non-existent settlement offer, and then used his own money to pay a fake settlement. Obviously, such deceit of one's client will only make matters worse—much worse—for the attorney. Malpractice—or even incompetence under the rules—may warrant slight if any sanction from the bar and perhaps an increase in one's malpractice insurance premiums, but actively defrauding and deceiving one's own client about those same mistakes will likely result in a suspension if not disbarment. So when must an attorney disclose her own mistakes in a representation to her client? The following North Carolina Ethics Opinion discusses that issue.

Disclosing Potential Malpractice to a Client
North Carolina State Bar Ethics Opinion (2015)

INTRODUCTION

Lawyers will, inevitably, make errors, mistakes, and omissions (referred to herein as an "error" or "errors") when representing clients. Such errors may constitute professional malpractice, but are not necessarily professional misconduct. [As] explained in comment [9] to Rule 1.1, Competence:

> An error by a lawyer may constitute professional malpractice under the applicable standard of care and subject the lawyer to civil liability. However, conduct that constitutes a breach of the civil standard of care owed to a client giving rise to liability for professional malpractice does not necessarily constitute a violation of the ethical duty to represent a client competently. A lawyer who makes a good-faith effort to be prepared and to be thorough will not generally be subject to professional discipline, although he or she may be subject to a claim for malpractice....

Although an error during the representation of a client may not constitute professional misconduct, the actions that the lawyer takes following the realization that she has committed an error should be guided by the requirements of the Rules of Professional Conduct. This opinion explains a lawyer's professional responsibilities when the lawyer has committed what she believes may be legal malpractice....

INQUIRY #1

When the lawyer determines that an error that may constitute legal malpractice has occurred, is the lawyer required to disclose the error to the client?

OPINION #1

Disclosure of an error to a client falls within the duty of communication. Rule 1.4(a)(3) requires a lawyer to "keep the client reasonably informed about the status of the matter," while paragraph (b) of the rule requires a lawyer to "explain a matter to the extent reasonably necessary to permit the client to make informed decisions regarding the representation." Comment [3] to the rule explains that paragraph (a)(3) requires that the lawyer keep the client reasonably informed about "significant developments affecting the timing or the substance of the representation." Comment [7] to Rule 1.4 adds that "[a] lawyer may not withhold information to serve the lawyer's own interest or convenience or the interests or convenience of another person."

In the spectrum of possible errors, material errors that prejudice the client's rights or claims are at one end. These include errors that effectively undermine the achievement of the client's primary objective for the representation, such as failing to file the complaint before the statute of limitations runs. At the other end of the spectrum are minor, harmless errors that do not prejudice the client's rights or interests. These include nonsubstantive typographical errors in a pleading or a contract or missing a deadline that causes nothing more than delay. Between the two ends of the spectrum are a range of errors that may or may not materially prejudice the client's interests.

Whether the lawyer must disclose an error to a client depends upon where the error falls on the spectrum and the circumstances at the time that the error is discovered. The New York State Bar Association, in a formal opinion, described the duty as follows:

> [W]hether an attorney has an obligation to disclose a mistake to a client will depend on the nature of the lawyer's possible error or omission, whether it is possible to correct it in the present proceeding, the extent of the harm resulting from the possible error or omission, and the likelihood that the lawyer's conduct would be deemed unreasonable and therefore give rise to a colorable malpractice claim.

N.Y. State Bar Ass'n Comm. Prof'l Ethics, Op. 734 (2000). Under this analysis, it is clear that material errors that prejudice the client's rights or interests as well as errors that clearly give rise to a malpractice claim must always be reported to the client. Conversely, if the error is easily corrected or negligible and will not materially prejudice the client's rights or interests, the error does not have to be disclosed to the client.

Errors that fall between the two extremes of the spectrum must be analyzed under the duty to keep the client reasonably informed about his legal matter. If the error will result in financial loss to the client, substantial delay in achieving the client's objectives for the representation, or material disadvantage to the client's legal position, the error must be disclosed to the client. Similarly, if disclosure of the error is necessary for the client to make an informed decision about the representation or for the lawyer to advise the client of significant changes in strategy, timing, or direction of the representation, the lawyer may not withhold information about the error. Rule 1.4. When a lawyer does not know whether disclosure is required, the lawyer should err on the side of disclosure or should seek the advice of outside counsel, the State Bar's ethics counsel, or the lawyer's malpractice carrier.

Perhaps the most obvious duty to communicate is also the most frequent basis for client complaints — the duty to respond to client requests for information. Model Rule 1.4 states that the lawyer shall "promptly comply with reasonable requests for information." Failure to return phone calls or emails is one of the most common client complaints made to the bar. Martin Cole, who acted as the Director of the Office of Lawyers Professional Responsibility of the Minnesota Bar, called noncommunication and neglect the "hardiest perennials."[11] Noncommunication is a hardy perennial because complaints against attorneys for failing to return calls and emails—like poison ivy or other noxious weeds—come in year after year and seem resilient against warnings and measures undertaken by the bar to improve lawyer communication.

Martin Cole, The Hardiest Perennials
64 Bench & B. Minn. 12 (2007)

In the October 1971 issue of Bench & Bar of Minnesota, Richey Reavill, the first director of the Office of Lawyers Professional Responsibility, wrote in this column, "As of July 31, the new procedures have been in effect for six months. During that period, almost 45 percent of the complaints which crossed our desk involved neglect of clients' business and the failure to keep the client and others entitled thereto advised as to the status quo. Neglect and failure to communicate seem to go hand in hand, probably because the only response the neglectful lawyer can make to an inquiry is that he has done nothing." . . .

In November 1985, William Wernz, in his first column as director . . . described neglect and noncommunication as a "hardy perennial." He added that "[f]ormer directors Richey Reavill, Paul Sharood, Walt Bachman and Mike Hoover all lamented the number of complaints of attorney neglect and noncommunication with clients. In 1984, as in 1971, 40-45 percent of all complaints alleged such failures."

The Office of Lawyers Professional Responsibility has been in existence for 36 years now, and while some things have changed immensely, others clearly have not. By a wide margin, neglect and noncommunication remain the most common source of client unhappiness and thus of client complaints. A few months ago, in the March 2007 Bench & Bar "Summary of Admonitions," I wrote that, "As in most years, the majority of admonitions last year involved a lack of diligence and/or communication by the attorney." Surely, neglect and noncommunication must be considered the hardiest perennials after so many years without change.

LEARNING FROM HISTORY

After all these years, why is this so? Aren't we supposed to learn from the lessons of history? By now shouldn't we recognize procrastination, lack of diligence, neglect (whatever we call it), when we see it? Do we know it only when we see it in others, while failing to recognize it in ourselves? The applicable Rules of Professional Conduct don't seem especially difficult to understand. . . .

---

11. Perennials are plants that come up year after year without needing to be replanted—and "hardy" perennials will come up despite efforts to kill them.

Noncommunication can be . . . tricky to pin down, depending on the circumstances. Not returning one or two phone calls, while a poor business practice, is often forgiven by the client if an apology is proffered. Routinely failing to return phone calls or not replying to correspondence from clients or opposing counsel eventually *will* lead to disciplinary problems. . . .

MINIMIZING THE RISK

Since there isn't a clear line of demarcation announcing when an attorney's conduct goes from "that can happen" to "that simply shouldn't happen," the easiest and best solution is not to put yourself so close to the line that you need to be worried about it. Proper office management skills are attainable even for a busy solo practitioner. An office calendar and "tickler system" for court appearances, meetings and the like are essential. An assistant who may handle some routine inquiries or return some phone calls on the attorney's behalf is certainly permissible and can help eliminate much client frustration (that said, systematically making it impossible for clients to get beyond support staff or ever talk directly with the lawyer may violate the lawyer's duty to communicate). . . .

As noted, admonitions issued for neglect and/or noncommunication remain common. The annual summary of admonitions published in this column rarely provides details of these admonitions, however. This past year, attorneys were admonished for taking almost one year to complete a QDRO [Qualified Domestic Relations Order] in a marital dissolution matter, taking over two years to complete a generally uncomplicated estate matter, and putting research on an issue concerning the sale of a client's motor home "on the back burner" (the attorney's words) for many months. Attorneys who failed to communicate with their clients for several months at a time, usually despite several calls or letters from the client requesting (eventually begging) for a response, also received admonitions. Admonitions are generally appropriate when the matter is the lawyer's first valid complaint and the ultimate financial harm to the client was minimal. Frustration is a given. . . .

So, one last exhortation: "Don't procrastinate and do communicate!" Do those two things and odds are we'll never meet because of a complaint.

In a similar vein, comment [4] to Rule 1.4 provides a simple rule for complying with client requests for information: promptly respond or acknowledge the communication. The comment says that "when a client makes a reasonable request for information . . . [the rule] requires prompt compliance with the request, or if a prompt response is not feasible, that the lawyer, or a member of the lawyer's staff, acknowledge receipt of the request and advise the client when a response may be expected." Thus, where a lawyer doesn't yet have the requested information or is in the middle of a trial or other time-consuming matter and cannot fully respond to the client request promptly, the lawyer should still acknowledge the client communication and give the client an idea of when the attorney will be able to respond more fully. Respond or acknowledge promptly — it's really that simple.

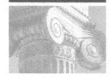

Case Preview

Utah Bar Journal, Discipline Corner

The following is an excerpt from the *Utah Bar Journal's* Discipline Corner, which provides a summary of disciplinary proceedings. The excerpt regards attorney Karen Thomas, who failed to communicate (and act diligently and competently) on behalf of her client in securing an adoption.

As you read this excerpt, consider the following:

1. Where did Thomas go wrong? What could and should she have done differently?
2. What impact, including emotional distress, did Thomas cause her client?

Discipline Corner
Utah Bar Journal (Jan/Feb 2007)

On October 30, 2006, the Honorable Sandra N. Peuler, Third Judicial District Court, entered Findings of Fact and Conclusions of Law, and Order of Discipline: Suspension suspending Karen Thomas for six months from the practice of law for violations of Rules 1.1 (Competence), 1.3 (Diligence), 1.4(a) (Communication), 1.5(a) (Fees), 1.16(d) (Declining or Terminating Representation), 3.2 (Expediting Litigation), 8.1(b) (Bar Admission and Disciplinary Matters), and 8.4(a) (Misconduct) of the Rules of Professional Conduct. Ms. Thomas's suspension was effective thirty days from the date of its entry.

Ms. Thomas was hired to finalize an adoption, in which the natural mother had agreed to relinquish her parental rights. The client paid Ms. Thomas for the drafting of the adoption agreement, the finalization of the adoption and the filing fee. The client notified Ms. Thomas of the birth of the baby. The client took the baby home from the hospital. Five weeks after the baby's birth, Ms. Thomas had not arranged for the natural mother to sign the required relinquishment papers in front of a signing judge. The client left numerous messages for Ms. Thomas concerning the status of the relinquishment. Ms. Thomas failed to keep the client informed of the status and failed to promptly comply with the client's requests for information. Ms. Thomas informed her client that the delay was due in part because the signing judge was out of town. The natural mother became frustrated with Ms. Thomas and the delay. The client arranged, on her own, for the natural mother to appear before the judge to sign the relinquishment papers. At the hearing, the natural mother demanded that the baby be returned. The court ordered that the client return the baby within an hour's time. Ms. Thomas informed the client that she would help the client try to get the baby back without charge to the client. Ms. Thomas did not earn the fees she collected from the client. Ms. Thomas collected an excessive fee given the work performed in the adoption.[12]

---

12. *Discipline Corner*, UTAH BAR J., Jan.-Feb. 2007, at 52, *available at* https://www.utahbar.org/wp-content/uploads/2017/11/2007_jan_feb.pdf.

Post-Case Follow-Up

The Karen Thomas disciplinary matter underscores the importance of these basic core duties that generally go hand in hand: competence, diligence, and communication. Imagine the distress felt by Ms. Thomas's client when she was forced to return a baby she had brought home from the hospital, taken care of and nurtured for over five weeks, and considered her own child. Competently protecting a client's interests is the attorney's indispensable duty.

Thomas Disciplinary Summary: Real Life Applications

1. Shaniqua is representing James in defending against an action to collect a debt James owes. James sells his only major asset — a small commercial building — and obtains $70,000 cash on October 30. The plaintiff in the action checks the title records in mid-November and learns that James sold the building. The plaintiff moves the court for a temporary restraining order (TRO) prohibiting James from disbursing any of the proceeds of the sale and requiring James to make an accounting of the funds at a hearing ten days later, which the court grants the same day. At the hearing, James fails to provide an accounting, and says that all but $15,000 of the sale proceeds have already been spent, transferred, or given away. Further, he indicates that Shaniqua, who was served with the signed TRO ten days previously, had only told him about the TRO the day before the hearing so he had not had adequate time to prepare an accounting and had continued to use the proceeds up until that time. Under the rules, when did Shaniqua need to tell James about the TRO?

2. Larry is an attorney, representing Karen in a contentious divorce. Karen is very worried about how child custody will play out, and so she contacts Larry frequently. Larry is tired of responding to Karen's phone calls. Do the rules require him to do so?

B. INEFFECTIVE ASSISTANCE OF CRIMINAL DEFENSE COUNSEL

When a criminal defense attorney performs poorly, more than the duty of competence is at stake. Incompetent criminal defense attorneys also deprive their clients of their constitutional right to effective assistance of counsel. The Sixth Amendment to the Constitution declares that "[i]n all criminal prosecutions, the accused shall . . . have the Assistance of Counsel for his defence." The Sixth Amendment guarantee was a break from eighteenth-century criminal procedure in England, where a defendant accused of a felony was *prohibited* from having or employing counsel to assist in her defense, and instead was required to "speak for yourself."[13] Yet in the American colonies, the English rule had been rejected even before the federal Constitution's creation. Nearly every colony had provided by law that an accused had a right to have counsel for his defense—and thus that right was an integral part of American conceptions of justice at the time of the creation of the Bill of Rights.

This history underlying the Sixth Amendment was recited by the Supreme Court in Powell v. Alabama, 287 U.S. 45 (1932), wherein the Supreme Court held that states were required by the Due Process Clause of the Fourteenth Amendment to provide effective assistance of counsel to an accused in certain cases. In *Powell*, nine Black teenagers (commonly referred to as the "Scottsboro boys") had been convicted of gang-raping two Caucasian women on a slow-moving train. The defendants were tried within days of the alleged incident. Immediately before their trials were to begin, the defendants were appointed counsel—characterized by the Supreme Court as being "pro forma [rather] than zealous and active." The trials were completed quickly with all defendants convicted and all but one sentenced to death.[14] The Supreme Court reversed the convictions noting that the appointment of counsel and trials had gone forward not in the "spirit of regulated justice but . . . with the haste of the mob":

> The defendants, young, ignorant, illiterate, surrounded by hostile sentiment, haled back and forth under guard of soldiers, charged with an atrocious crime regarded with especial horror in the community where they were to be tried, were thus put in peril of their lives within a few moments after counsel for the first time charged with any degree of responsibility began to represent them.

According to the State, the appointed counsel "thought there was no defense" and thus "exercised their best judgment in proceeding to trial without preparation." The Court rejected this argument, stating: "Neither [appointed counsel] nor the court could say what a prompt and thorough-going investigation might disclose as to the facts. No attempt was made to investigate. No opportunity to do so was given. Defendants were immediately hurried to trial." Moreover, the Court noted that defendants had not been provided with any counsel "during perhaps the most critical period of the proceedings against these defendants, that is to say, from the time of their arraignment until the beginning of their trial, when consultation, thorough-going investigation and preparation were vitally important"—indeed, the Court emphasized, "they were as much entitled to such aid during that period as at the trial itself." Ultimately, the Court concluded that "in a capital case, where the defendant is unable to employ counsel, and is incapable adequately of making his own defense . . . it is the duty of the court, whether requested or not, to assign

---

13. *See* John H. Langbein, *Shaping the Eighteenth-Century Criminal Trial: A View from the Ryder Sources*, 50 U. CHI. L. REV. 1, 123-30 & nn.515-16 (1983). In the first half of the eighteenth century, the accused could not have any assistance of counsel, although later in the century, the accused could employ counsel to cross-examine witnesses and address points of law. Nevertheless, defense counsel could only speak as to issues of law (and not fact), and defense "counsel was forbidden to 'address the jury,' that is, to make opening and closing statements." Thus, the accused could not use an attorney "for his 'defense'"—instead the accused had to speak for himself. *See id.*

14. The jury was hung as to life imprisonment or death as the appropriate sentence for Roy Wright, who was 13 years old.

The Scottsboro Boys and the Moral Courage of Judge James E. Horton, Jr.

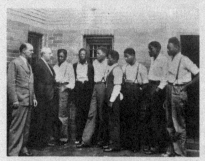

Attorney Samuel Leibowitz and his clients, the "Scottsboro boys."
AP Photo

On remand after *Powell*, the Scottsboro boys were represented for no fee[15] by Samuel Leibowitz — a renowned Jewish criminal defense attorney from New York, who had obtained 77 acquittals in the course of 78 criminal trials. Haywood Patterson was the first to be retried. The venue was moved from Scottsboro, and Judge James E. Horton, Jr. was assigned to preside. Judge Horton addressed the jury venire: "So far as the law is concerned, it knows neither native nor alien, Jew or Gentile, black or white. This case is no different than any other. We have only our duty to do without fear or favor."[16] Leibowitz masterfully undermined the prosecution's case. He had the Lionel Corporation build a 32-foot replica of the train to show the implausibility of the accusations, including that a gang rape had taken place in a gondola

counsel for him as a necessary requisite of due process of law; and that duty is not discharged by an assignment at such a time or under such circumstances as to preclude the giving of effective aid in the preparation and trial of the case." The Supreme Court thus indicated the need for *effective* assistance of counsel, which had not been satisfied in *Powell* by a pro forma appointment without real substance. In making its determination, the Court eloquently explained:

> The right to be heard would be, in many cases, of little avail if it did not comprehend the right to be heard by counsel. Even the intelligent and educated layman has small and sometimes no skill in the science of law. If charged with crime, he is incapable, generally, of determining for himself whether the indictment is good or bad. He is unfamiliar with the rules of evidence. Left without the aid of counsel he may be put on trial without a proper charge, and convicted upon incompetent evidence, or evidence irrelevant to the issue or otherwise inadmissible. He lacks both the skill and knowledge adequately to prepare his defense, even though he have a perfect one. He requires the guiding hand of counsel at every step in the proceedings against him. Without it, though he be not guilty, he faces the danger of conviction because he does not know how to establish his innocence. If that be true of men of intelligence, how much more true is it of the ignorant and illiterate, or those of feeble intellect?

In Gideon v. Wainwright, 372 U.S. 335 (1963), the Supreme Court expressly incorporated the Sixth Amendment's guarantee of assistance of counsel as applying to the states through the Fourteenth Amendment, and in Argersinger v. Hamlin, 407 U.S. 25 (1972), the Court extended that right to less serious offenses, holding that "absent a knowing and intelligent waiver, no person may be imprisoned for any offense, whether classified as petty, misdemeanor, or felony, unless he was represented by counsel at his trial."

15. J.Y. Smith, *Samuel Leibowitz, Noted Judge Dies*, Wash. Post, Jan. 12, 1978, *available at* https://www.washingtonpost.com/archive/local/1978/01/12/samuel-leibowitz-noted-judge-dies/30cc052b-afa3-4b7c-9326-6838070eb364/?utm_term=.22685be8581f.

16. Regarding the information in this paragraph, see generally Douglas O. Linder, *Without Fear or Favor: Judge James Edwin Horton and the Trial of the "Scottsboro Boys,"* 68 UMKC L. Rev. 549 (2000).

1. The Constitutional Test for Ineffective Assistance of Counsel

The Supreme Court's recognition and incorporation of the Sixth Amendment's guarantee of assistance of counsel to state prosecutions, as well as federal, did not directly address the problem of incompetent counsel. What should happen if an attorney is appointed, but proceeds incompetently? When, if ever, is an attorney's incompetence so severe that it constitutes a denial of the Sixth Amendment's right to the provision of counsel? Lower courts approached this problem in differing manners until the Supreme Court in *Strickland v. Washington* established a test for determining whether a defendant had been denied his Sixth Amendment right to effective assistance of counsel.

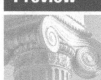

Case Preview

Strickland v. Washington

The facts of *Strickland* are quite unsympathetic. David Leroy Washington was convicted of committing "three groups of crimes, which included three brutal stabbing murders, torture, kidnapping, severe assaults, attempted murders, attempted extortion, and theft." Washington repeatedly went against his attorney's advice by confessing to the murders, pleading guilty to all charges, and waiving his right to a jury trial. Washington's attorney advised Washington to invoke a right to an advisory jury for the sentencing phase, and again, Washington ignored his attorney's advice and waived that right. The attorney then performed a very limited investigation for the sentencing hearing—he talked to Washington's wife and mother over the phone. He also successfully moved to exclude Washington's rap sheet. But defense counsel didn't do further

car that was filled with chert (small jagged rocks) to within a foot and a half of the roof. He elicited medical testimony that the sperm found vaginally less than two hours after the alleged rape was old and "non-motile" and that the women had no scrapes or bruises (despite the chert). Leibowitz's final witness was Ruby Bates, one of the two women allegedly raped, who recanted her prior accusations and said they had invented the story to avoid vagrancy charges. Nevertheless, the jury convicted Patterson and sentenced him to death. The prosecution had stated in closing argument, "Show them that Alabama justice can't be bought and sold with Jew money from New York." After the verdict, Judge Horton received numerous letters of praise regarding his handling of the case and the result. But then Horton surprised his native Alabama constituency. On June 22, 1933, Judge Horton opened court by granting the defense's motion for a new trial on the basis of insufficiency of the evidence. Horton reviewed all the improbabilities and inconsistencies in the prosecution's case and set aside the verdict and the sentence of death. "Deliberate injustice," he said, "is more fatal to the one who imposes it than to the one on whom it is imposed." Horton lost his judicial seat in the 1934 election.[17]

---

17. *See id.* Patterson and Clarence Norris were retried by a different judge, convicted, and sentenced to death. The U.S. Supreme Court reversed the convictions again, this time based on Alabama's total exclusion of Black persons on juries—an argument Leibowitz had been making and preserving since the first day of jury selection in Patterson's case before Judge Horton. Charges against four of the boys were then dropped, but the others were retried and convicted yet again—each ultimately serving a lengthy prison sentence. *See The Scottsboro Boys: A Chronology, available at* http://law2.umkc.edu/faculty/projects/ftrials/scottsboro/SB_chron.html.

investigation or preparation because of a "sense of hopelessness about overcoming the evidentiary effect of respondent's confessions to the gruesome crimes." The trial court sentenced Washington to death on each of the murders, which convictions and sentences were upheld on direct appeal. Washington then sought state collateral relief and ultimately federal habeas corpus relief, arguing that he was denied effective assistance of counsel at the sentencing hearing based on his attorney's failure to investigate and present mitigating evidence, such as psychiatric, character, and medical evidence.

As you read through *Strickland*, consider the following:

1. What is the Court's two-prong test for determining ineffective assistance of counsel?
2. Under the Court's test, how competent must a defense attorney be to satisfy the Sixth Amendment guarantee? How much deference is given to the attorney?
3. In applying the two-prong test, does it matter which prong a court examines first — and why does that matter?
4. When, if ever, is prejudice presumed? How is the test different where the attorney proceeds with a criminal representation under a conflict of interest?
5. Why does Justice Marshall object to the prejudice prong? Is the Sixth Amendment only for the protection of the innocent, or is it also a guarantee for the guilty?

Strickland v. Washington
466 U.S. 668 (1984)

. . .

III

A convicted defendant's claim that counsel's assistance was so defective as to require reversal of a conviction or death sentence has two components. First, the defendant must show that counsel's performance was deficient. This requires showing that counsel made errors so serious that counsel was not functioning as the "counsel" guaranteed the defendant by the Sixth Amendment. Second, the defendant must show that the deficient performance prejudiced the defense. This requires showing that counsel's errors were so serious as to deprive the defendant of a fair trial, a trial whose result is reliable. Unless a defendant makes both showings, it cannot be said that the conviction or death sentence resulted from a breakdown in the adversary process that renders the result unreliable.

A

As all the Federal Courts of Appeals have now held, the proper standard for attorney performance is that of reasonably effective assistance. . . . When a convicted defendant complains of the ineffectiveness of counsel's assistance, the defendant must show that counsel's representation fell below an objective standard of reasonableness.

More specific guidelines are not appropriate. The Sixth Amendment refers simply to "counsel," not specifying particular requirements of effective assistance. It relies instead on the legal profession's maintenance of standards sufficient to justify the law's presumption that counsel will fulfill the role in the adversary process that the Amendment envisions. The proper measure of attorney performance remains simply reasonableness under prevailing professional norms.

Representation of a criminal defendant entails certain basic duties. Counsel's function is to assist the defendant, and hence counsel owes the client a duty of loyalty, a duty to avoid conflicts of interest. From counsel's function as assistant to the defendant derive the overarching duty to advocate the defendant's cause and the more particular duties to consult with the defendant on important decisions and to keep the defendant informed of important developments in the course of the prosecution. Counsel also has a duty to bring to bear such skill and knowledge as will render the trial a reliable adversarial testing process. *See* Powell v. Alabama, 287 U.S., at 68-69.

These basic duties neither exhaustively define the obligations of counsel nor form a checklist for judicial evaluation of attorney performance. In any case presenting an ineffectiveness claim, the performance inquiry must be whether counsel's assistance was reasonable considering all the circumstances. Prevailing norms of practice as reflected in American Bar Association standards and the like, e.g., ABA Standards for Criminal Justice 4-1.1 to 4-8.6 (2d ed. 1980) ("The Defense Function"), are guides to determining what is reasonable, but they are only guides. No particular set of detailed rules for counsel's conduct can satisfactorily take account of the variety of circumstances faced by defense counsel or the range of legitimate decisions regarding how best to represent a criminal defendant. Any such set of rules would interfere with the constitutionally protected independence of counsel and restrict the wide latitude counsel must have in making tactical decisions. Indeed, the existence of detailed guidelines for representation could distract counsel from the overriding mission of vigorous advocacy of the defendant's cause. Moreover, the purpose of the effective assistance guarantee of the Sixth Amendment is not to improve the quality of legal representation, although that is a goal of considerable importance to the legal system. The purpose is simply to ensure that criminal defendants receive a fair trial.

Judicial scrutiny of counsel's performance must be highly deferential. It is all too tempting for a defendant to second-guess counsel's assistance after conviction or adverse sentence, and it is all too easy for a court, examining counsel's defense after it has proved unsuccessful, to conclude that a particular act or omission of counsel was unreasonable. A fair assessment of attorney performance requires that every effort be made to eliminate the distorting effects of hindsight, to reconstruct the circumstances of counsel's challenged conduct, and to evaluate the conduct from counsel's perspective at the time. Because of the difficulties inherent in making the evaluation, a court must indulge a strong presumption that counsel's conduct falls within the wide range of reasonable professional assistance; that is, the defendant must overcome the presumption that, under the circumstances, the challenged action "might be considered sound trial strategy." There are countless ways to provide effective assistance in any given case. Even the best criminal defense attorneys would not defend a particular client in the same way. . . .

Thus, a court deciding an actual ineffectiveness claim must judge the reasonableness of counsel's challenged conduct on the facts of the particular case, viewed as of the time of counsel's conduct. A convicted defendant making a claim of ineffective assistance must identify the acts or omissions of counsel that are alleged not to have been the result of reasonable professional judgment. The court must then determine whether, in light of all the circumstances, the identified acts or omissions were outside the wide range of professionally competent assistance. In making that determination, the court should keep in mind that counsel's function, as elaborated in prevailing professional norms, is to make the adversarial testing process work in the particular case. At the same time, the court should recognize that counsel is strongly presumed to have rendered adequate assistance and made all significant decisions in the exercise of reasonable professional judgment.

These standards require no special amplification in order to define counsel's duty to investigate, the duty at issue in this case. As the Court of Appeals concluded, strategic choices made after thorough investigation of law and facts relevant to plausible options are virtually unchallengeable; and strategic choices made after less than complete investigation are reasonable precisely to the extent that reasonable professional judgments support the limitations on investigation. In other words, counsel has a duty to make reasonable investigations or to make a reasonable decision that makes particular investigations unnecessary. In any ineffectiveness case, a particular decision not to investigate must be directly assessed for reasonableness in all the circumstances, applying a heavy measure of deference to counsel's judgments.

The reasonableness of counsel's actions may be determined or substantially influenced by the defendant's own statements or actions. Counsel's actions are usually based, quite properly, on informed strategic choices made by the defendant and on information supplied by the defendant. In particular, what investigation decisions are reasonable depends critically on such information. For example, when the facts that support a certain potential line of defense are generally known to counsel because of what the defendant has said, the need for further investigation may be considerably diminished or eliminated altogether. And when a defendant has given counsel reason to believe that pursuing certain investigations would be fruitless or even harmful, counsel's failure to pursue those investigations may not later be challenged as unreasonable. In short, inquiry into counsel's conversations with the defendant may be critical to a proper assessment of counsel's investigation decisions, just as it may be critical to a proper assessment of counsel's other litigation decisions.

B

An error by counsel, even if professionally unreasonable, does not warrant setting aside the judgment of a criminal proceeding if the error had no effect on the judgment. The purpose of the Sixth Amendment guarantee of counsel is to ensure that a defendant has the assistance necessary to justify reliance on the outcome of the proceeding. Accordingly, any deficiencies in counsel's performance must be prejudicial to the defense in order to constitute ineffective assistance under the Constitution.

In certain Sixth Amendment contexts, prejudice is presumed. Actual or constructive denial of the assistance of counsel altogether is legally presumed to result in prejudice. So are various kinds of state interference with counsel's assistance. *See United States v. Cronic*, 466 U.S., at 659, and n. 25. Prejudice in these circumstances is so likely that case-by-case inquiry into prejudice is not worth the cost. Moreover, such circumstances involve impairments of the Sixth Amendment right that are easy to identify and, for that reason and because the prosecution is directly responsible, easy for the government to prevent.

One type of actual ineffectiveness claim warrants a similar, though more limited, presumption of prejudice. In Cuyler v. Sullivan, 446 U.S., at 345-350, the Court held that prejudice is presumed when counsel is burdened by an actual conflict of interest. In those circumstances, counsel breaches the duty of loyalty, perhaps the most basic of counsel's duties. Moreover, it is difficult to measure the precise effect on the defense of representation corrupted by conflicting interests. Given the obligation of counsel to avoid conflicts of interest and the ability of trial courts to make early inquiry in certain situations likely to give rise to conflicts, it is reasonable for the criminal justice system to maintain a fairly rigid rule of presumed prejudice for conflicts of interest. Even so, the rule is not quite the per se rule of prejudice that exists for the Sixth Amendment claims mentioned above. Prejudice is presumed only if the defendant demonstrates that counsel "actively represented conflicting interests" and that "an actual conflict of interest adversely affected his lawyer's performance." Cuyler v. Sullivan, *supra*.

Conflict of interest claims aside, actual ineffectiveness claims alleging a deficiency in attorney performance are subject to a general requirement that the defendant affirmatively prove prejudice. The government is not responsible for, and hence not able to prevent, attorney errors that will result in reversal of a conviction or sentence. Attorney errors come in an infinite variety and are as likely to be utterly harmless in a particular case as they are to be prejudicial. . . . Representation is an art, and an act or omission that is unprofessional in one case may be sound or even brilliant in another. Even if a defendant shows that particular errors of counsel were unreasonable, therefore, the defendant must show that they actually had an adverse effect on the defense.

It is not enough for the defendant to show that the errors had some conceivable effect on the outcome of the proceeding. Virtually every act or omission of counsel would meet that test, and not every error that conceivably could have influenced the outcome undermines the reliability of the result of the proceeding. . . .

On the other hand, we believe that a defendant need not show that counsel's deficient conduct more likely than not altered the outcome in the case. . . . [Where there is ineffective assistance of counsel], [t]he result of a proceeding can be rendered unreliable, and hence the proceeding itself unfair, even if the errors of counsel cannot be shown by a preponderance of the evidence to have determined the outcome.

Accordingly, the appropriate test for prejudice [is:] . . . The defendant must show that there is a reasonable probability that, but for counsel's unprofessional errors, the result of the proceeding would have been different. A reasonable probability is a probability sufficient to undermine confidence in the outcome.

. . .

The governing legal standard plays a critical role in defining the question to be asked in assessing the prejudice from counsel's errors. When a defendant challenges a conviction, the question is whether there is a reasonable probability that, absent the errors, the factfinder would have had a reasonable doubt respecting guilt. When a defendant challenges a death sentence such as the one at issue in this case, the question is whether there is a reasonable probability that, absent the errors, the sentencer — including an appellate court, to the extent it independently reweighs the evidence — would have concluded that the balance of aggravating and mitigating circumstances did not warrant death. . . .

IV

A number of practical considerations are important for the application of the standards we have outlined. . . . Although we have discussed the performance component of an ineffectiveness claim prior to the prejudice component, there is no reason for a court deciding an ineffective assistance claim to approach the inquiry in the same order or even to address both components of the inquiry if the defendant makes an insufficient showing on one. In particular, a court need not determine whether counsel's performance was deficient before examining the prejudice suffered by the defendant as a result of the alleged deficiencies. The object of an ineffectiveness claim is not to grade counsel's performance. If it is easier to dispose of an ineffectiveness claim on the ground of lack of sufficient prejudice, which we expect will often be so, that course should be followed. Courts should strive to ensure that ineffectiveness claims not become so burdensome to defense counsel that the entire criminal justice system suffers as a result. . . .

V

. . . Application of the governing principles is not difficult in this case. The facts as described above, make clear that the conduct of respondent's counsel at and before respondent's sentencing proceeding cannot be found unreasonable. They also make clear that, even assuming the challenged conduct of counsel was unreasonable, respondent suffered insufficient prejudice to warrant setting aside his death sentence. . . .

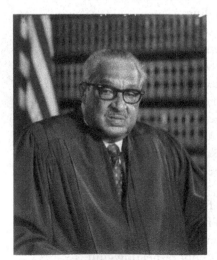

Thurgood Marshall
Library of Congress Prints and
Photographs Division, Washington, D.C.

Justice MARSHALL, dissenting.

The Sixth and Fourteenth Amendments guarantee a person accused of a crime the right to the aid of a lawyer in preparing and presenting his defense. It has long been settled that "the right to counsel is the right to the effective assistance of counsel." The state and lower federal courts have developed standards for distinguishing effective from inadequate assistance. Today, for the first time, this Court attempts to synthesize and clarify those standards. For the most part, the majority's efforts are unhelpful. Neither of its two principal holdings seems to me likely to improve the adjudication of Sixth Amendment claims. . . .

I

The opinion of the Court revolves around two holdings. First, the majority ties the constitutional minima of attorney performance to a simple "standard of reasonableness."

Second, the majority holds that only an error of counsel that has sufficient impact on a trial to "undermine confidence in the outcome" is grounds for overturning a conviction. I disagree with both of these rulings.

A

My objection to the performance standard adopted by the Court is that it is so malleable that, in practice, it will either have no grip at all or will yield excessive variation in the manner in which the Sixth Amendment is interpreted and applied by different courts. To tell lawyers and the lower courts that counsel for a criminal defendant must behave "reasonably" and must act like "a reasonably competent attorney," is to tell them almost nothing. In essence, the majority has instructed judges called upon to assess claims of ineffective assistance of counsel to advert to their own intuitions regarding what constitutes "professional" representation, and has discouraged them from trying to develop more detailed standards governing the performance of defense counsel. In my view, the Court has thereby not only abdicated its own responsibility to interpret the Constitution, but also impaired the ability of the lower courts to exercise theirs.

. . .

The majority defends its refusal to adopt more specific standards primarily on the ground that "[n]o particular set of detailed rules for counsel's conduct can satisfactorily take account of the variety of circumstances faced by defense counsel or the range of legitimate decisions regarding how best to represent a criminal defendant." I agree that counsel must be afforded "wide latitude" when making "tactical decisions" regarding trial strategy, but many aspects of the job of a criminal defense attorney are more amenable to judicial oversight. For example, much of the work involved in preparing for a trial, applying for bail, conferring with one's client, making timely objections to significant, arguably erroneous rulings of the trial judge, and filing a notice of appeal if there are colorable grounds therefor could profitably be made the subject of uniform standards.

The opinion of the Court of Appeals in this case represents one sound attempt to develop particularized standards designed to ensure that all defendants receive effective legal assistance. By refusing to address the merits of these proposals, and indeed suggesting that no such effort is worthwhile, the opinion of the Court, I fear, will stunt the development of constitutional doctrine in this area.

B

I object to the prejudice standard adopted by the Court for two independent reasons. First, it is often very difficult to tell whether a defendant convicted after a trial in which he was ineffectively represented would have fared better if his lawyer had been competent. Seemingly impregnable cases can sometimes be dismantled by good defense counsel. On the basis of a cold record, it may be impossible for a reviewing court confidently to ascertain how the government's evidence and arguments would have stood up against rebuttal and cross-examination by a shrewd, well-prepared lawyer. The difficulties of estimating prejudice after the fact are exacerbated by the possibility that evidence of injury to the defendant may be missing from the record precisely because of the incompetence of defense counsel. In view of all these impediments to a fair evaluation of the probability that the outcome of a trial was affected by ineffectiveness of counsel, it seems to me senseless to impose on a defendant whose lawyer has been shown to have been incompetent the burden of demonstrating prejudice.

Second and more fundamentally, the assumption on which the Court's holding rests is that the only purpose of the constitutional guarantee of effective assistance of counsel is to reduce the chance that innocent persons will be convicted. In my view, the guarantee also functions to ensure that convictions are obtained only through fundamentally fair procedures. The majority contends that the Sixth Amendment is not violated when a manifestly guilty defendant is convicted after a trial in which he was represented by a manifestly ineffective attorney. I cannot agree. Every defendant is entitled to a trial in which his interests are vigorously and conscientiously advocated by an able lawyer. A proceeding in which the defendant does not receive meaningful assistance in meeting the forces of the State does not, in my opinion, constitute due process.

In Chapman v. California, 386 U.S. 18, 23 (1967), we acknowledged that certain constitutional rights are "so basic to a fair trial that their infraction can never be treated as harmless error." Among these rights is the right to the assistance of counsel at trial. In my view, the right to effective assistance of counsel is entailed by the right to counsel, and abridgment of the former is equivalent to abridgment of the latter. I would thus hold that a showing that the performance of a defendant's lawyer departed from constitutionally prescribed standards requires a new trial regardless of whether the defendant suffered demonstrable prejudice thereby.

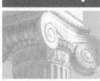

Post-Case Follow-Up

Strickland continues to state the test for determining when an accused has received ineffective assistance of counsel in contravention of the Sixth Amendment. The two-pronged approach requires a defendant to prove (1) deficient performance of counsel and (2) prejudice. As to the first prong, deficient performance of counsel, *Strickland* continues to state the basic standard: "reasonableness under prevailing professional norms." Further, reviewing courts are to engage in a "strong presumption that counsel's conduct falls within the wide range of reasonable professional assistance." *Strickland* also continues to state the basic standard for determining prejudice: "The defendant must show that there is a reasonable probability that, but for counsel's unprofessional errors, the result of the proceeding would have been different."

Strickland v. Washington: Real Life Applications

1. Melinda is charged with shoplifting, a misdemeanor, but a high-level one that carries a potential sentence of incarceration. She is appointed a public defender, Yvonne, to defend her. Yvonne and Melinda meet briefly before the arraignment,

where Melinda declares her innocence. She pleads not guilty. Yvonne receives and conveys to Melinda several plea deals, but Melinda refuses all of them, and wants to proceed to trial. Yvonne does very little preparation for trial and decides not to cross-examine the state's primary witness, Don, an employee at the shop Melinda allegedly stole from who called the police. Melinda is convicted. Is Melinda likely to succeed on an ineffective assistance of counsel claim? What if there is not much evidence of guilt? What if there is substantial evidence of guilt, such as a store security tape clearly showing Melinda taking items and hiding them in her clothes?

2. Sullivan, Carchidi, and DiPasquale are all indicted for the first-degree murders of two individuals. DiBona, an attorney, represents all three of them, who are to be tried separately. Sullivan's trial is first. DiBona is concerned that exposing defense witnesses to examination in the first trial could harm the trials of Carchidi and DiPasquale. Consequently, he decides not to use any defense witnesses in Sullivan's case. Sullivan is convicted. In their subsequent trials, where DiBona puts on a full defense with witnesses, Carchidi and DiPasquale are acquitted. Can Sullivan prevail on an ineffective assistance of counsel claim to undo the conviction? What if there is substantial evidence of guilt?

2. *Strickland*'s First Prong: Deficient Performance

Why should prevailing professional norms define the constitutional standard for effective assistance of counsel? Aren't there some essential components of competent criminal representation that should be constitutionally required, regardless of common practice? In a different context, Judge Learned Hand maintained:

> [I]n most cases reasonable prudence is in fact common prudence; but strictly it is never its measure; a whole calling may have unduly lagged in the adoption of new and available devices. It never may set its own tests, however persuasive be its usages. Courts must in the end say what is required; there are precautions so imperative that even their universal disregard will not excuse their omission.[18]

Are there actions that are "so imperative" in the practice of law that "even their universal disregard will not excuse their omission"? A study of homicide cases in New York City indicated that in over 70 percent of cases, the defense attorneys did not turn in receipts for investigation and did not file any legal motions.[19] If no investigation and no legal motions is a prevailing professional norm, does and should that render such representation compliant with the Constitution? Consider whether it would be a good idea to have the prevailing professional norms found

---

18. The T.J. Hooper v. Northern Barge Corp., 60 F.2d 737, 740 (2d Cir. 1932).
19. Michael McConville & Chester L. Mirsky, *Criminal Defense of the Poor in New York City*, 15 N.Y.U. Rev. L. & Soc. Change 581 (1987), *cited in* Hazard et al., The Law and Ethics of Lawyering 900 (5th ed. 2010).

among law enforcement set the standard for the constitutionality of searches and seizures or excessive force under the Fourth Amendment.

Failure to Investigate

In *Strickland*, Washington's defense attorney did not investigate in preparation for the sentencing hearing; yet the Court held that his actions did not constitute deficient performance under the first prong of its test. The Court indicated that the attorney's failure to investigate could be sound strategy. But when can failure to investigate a criminal case be a sound strategy? With a possible exception for physical incriminating evidence (e.g., a murder weapon),[20] criminal defense attorneys generally are not required to disclose inculpatory evidence that they find as part of their investigation of a client's case. Thus, if an investigation reveals evidence that is helpful to the client, the criminal defense attorney can use it. If the investigation reveals evidence that is harmful to the client, the criminal defense attorney has no obligation to use it at trial or to disclose it to the prosecution. As criminal defense lawyer William Genego said of the *Strickland* Court:

> The Court was wrong. Having a client examined by a psychiatrist in preparation for a capital sentencing proceeding does not mean that an attorney must introduce the report or the psychiatrist's testimony at the hearing. If a report had been done on Washington and it had been unfavorable, the attorney could have chosen not to introduce the report at the sentencing proceeding. . . . The critical point is that Washington's attorney could not make a reasonable strategic decision about the utility of relying on psychiatric testimony without having his own doctor examine Washington. . . . The Court was similarly misguided about the failure of Washington's attorney to interview character witnesses. In his collateral challenge, Washington introduced fourteen affidavits from friends, neighbors and relatives who said that, had they been asked, they would have testified on his behalf. . . . [Washington's] attorney, however, could not have intelligently speculated about the utility of such evidence . . . [because] the attorney had no idea what the fourteen character witnesses could have said about Washington's request that he be allowed to live.[21]

In more recent cases, however, the Supreme Court has more readily recognized that a failure to investigate can constitute deficient performance of counsel under *Strickland*'s first prong. In Kimmelman v. Morrison, 477 U.S. 365 (1986), the Court held that "a total failure to conduct pre-trial discovery" constituted deficient performance. In addition, in Andrus v. Texas, 140 S. Ct. 1875 (2020), the Court declared it "unquestioned" that "under prevailing professional norms," defense "counsel had an obligation to conduct a thorough investigation of the defendant's background" for the penalty phase. The Court elaborated: "In any ineffectiveness case, a particular decision not to investigate must be directly assessed for reasonableness in all

---

20. Whether a criminal defense lawyer must turn over physical incriminating evidence to the prosecution or law enforcement is discussed in Chapter 8.
21. William J. Genego, *The Future of Effective Assistance of Counsel: Performance Standards and Competent Representation*, 22 AM. CRIM. L. REV. 181 (1984).

the circumstances, applying a heavy measure of deference to counsel's judgment." Nevertheless, the Court concluded that in *Andrus,* the "failure to investigate thoroughly resulted from inattention, not reasoned strategic judgment."[22]

Failure to Communicate

As noted in the first part of this chapter, attorneys have duties to communicate with their clients and are required to communicate certain matters over which the client must give informed consent or that fall within the absolute authority of the client to decide. When does an attorney's failure to communicate with her client constitute ineffective assistance of counsel?

In Missouri v. Frye, 566 U.S. 134 (2012), the United States Supreme Court held "as a general rule," that "defense counsel has the duty to communicate formal offers from the prosecution to accept a plea on terms and conditions that may be favorable to the accused." Thus, Frye's attorney acted deficiently under *Strickland*'s first prong by failing to communicate a formal plea offer to the accused and allowing the plea offer to expire. The Court relied in part on the ABA rules and standards requiring communication of such offers to criminal defendants.

Case Preview

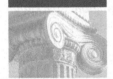

Helmedach v. Commissioner of Correction

Helmedach deals with a specific application of *Frye* and an interpretation of the duty to communicate found in Rule 1.4. Richard Reeve represented Jennifer Helmedach, who was being tried for felony murder, first degree burglary, and related offenses. During the trial, on the morning that the defense was to begin presenting its case, the prosecution told Reeve that it was offering Helmedach a plea with a ten-year sentence. Reeve did not communicate the plea offer to Helmedach until after she had finished testifying at trial—two and a half days later. When Helmedach learned of the plea offer, she wanted to take it, but the prosecution had withdrawn the plea offer. Helmedach was found guilty at trial and sentenced to 35 years in prison.

As you read *Helmedach,* consider the following:

1. How promptly must defense counsel inform a client of plea offers? What if there is not an express time for expiration of the offer?
2. Did attorney Reeve have a justified trial strategy in delaying communication of the plea offer to Helmedach?
3. Are there other communication obligations found in Rule 1.4, the non-compliance with which might constitute ineffective assistance of counsel in criminal cases?

---

22. *Andrus,* 140 S. Ct. at 1881-83.

Helmedach v. Commissioner of Correction
148 A.3d 1105 (Conn. 2016)

. . . [T]he petitioner filed an amended petition for a writ of habeas corpus, alleging ineffective assistance of trial counsel. . . . [T]he habeas court granted the petition . . . and concluded that Reeve's failure to relay the favorable offer to the petitioner in a timely manner before it was withdrawn fell below the objective standard of reasonableness required by attorneys under the state and federal constitutions. . . .

The respondent . . . contends that the habeas court improperly relied on *Missouri v. Frye* in finding that Reeve's performance was deficient, because [*Frye* doesn't address] whether it is reasonable trial strategy for a defense attorney to delay informing the client of a plea offer if valid strategic reasons exist for that decision. . . .

In response, the petitioner argues that Reeve's conduct could not be reasonable trial strategy because, as a matter of law, the decision made by Reeve to delay informing the petitioner of a favorable plea offer is not one that counsel constitutionally is allowed to make because it undermined the petitioner's ability to meaningfully exercise a right that belongs solely to her. Thus, in the petitioner's view, Reeve's conduct cannot be characterized as a matter of trial strategy. . . . We agree with the petitioner that Reeve's decision to delay informing the petitioner about a plea offer was not within the realm of strategic decisions that an attorney is allowed to make.

. . .

"To succeed on a claim of ineffective assistance of counsel, a habeas petitioner must satisfy the two-pronged test articulated in *Strickland v. Washington. Strickland* requires that a petitioner satisfy both a performance prong and a prejudice prong. . . .

"The Sixth Amendment guarantees a defendant the right to have counsel present at all critical stages of the criminal proceedings." *Missouri v. Frye, supra.* "[P]lea bargains have become so central to the administration of the criminal justice system that defense counsel have responsibilities in the plea bargain process, responsibilities that must be met to render the adequate assistance of counsel that the Sixth Amendment requires in the criminal process at critical stages. Because ours is for the most part a system of pleas, not a system of trials . . . it is insufficient simply to point to the guarantee of a fair trial as a backstop that inoculates any errors in the pretrial process. . . . In today's criminal justice system, therefore, the negotiation of a plea bargain, rather than the unfolding of a trial, is almost always the critical point for a defendant." . . .

In the present case, the respondent concedes that if indeed Reeve performed deficiently, the habeas court properly determined that the petitioner suffered prejudice on the basis of a reasonable probability that (1) the petitioner would have accepted the ten year plea offer had it been conveyed to her immediately, and (2) the trial court would have accepted the plea agreement and sentenced the petitioner accordingly. Our review and analysis, therefore, is confined to the first prong of *Strickland*, the performance prong. . . .

"Judicial scrutiny of counsel's performance must be highly deferential." *Strickland.* . . . At the same time, however, if the choice at issue implicates a fundamental right of constitutional magnitude, such a choice is "distinguishable from [a] tactical trial [right] that [is] not personal to the defendant and that counsel may choose to [make] as part of trial strategy." . . . But certain decisions regarding the exercise or waiver of basic trial rights are of such moment that they cannot be made for the defendant by a surrogate. A defendant has the ultimate authority to determine whether to plead guilty, waive a jury, testify in his or her own behalf, or take an appeal. Concerning those decisions, an attorney must both consult with the defendant and obtain consent to the recommended course of action.

"A guilty plea . . . is an event of signal significance in a criminal proceeding. By entering a guilty plea, a defendant waives constitutional rights that inhere in a criminal trial, including the right to trial by jury, the protection against self-incrimination, and the right to confront one's accusers. . . . While a guilty plea may be tactically advantageous for the defendant . . . the plea is not simply a strategic choice; it is itself a conviction . . . and the high stakes for the defendant require the utmost solicitude. . . ." Florida v. Nixon, 543 U.S. 175 (2004). . . .

We agree with the petitioner that this court need not consider whether, under the circumstances, Reeve's challenged action might be considered sound trial strategy, because the challenged action does not fall under the umbrella of trial strategy at all. The habeas court found that although Reeve "believed that ten years was a very favorable offer, he was concerned about relaying it to the petitioner immediately prior to her testimony because she was young and flustered, and he believed that this unexpected news would negatively impact her testimony." Such paternalistic decision-making on the part of defense counsel infringed upon the petitioner's basic trial right to plead guilty, which she, alone, had the ultimate authority to determine whether to exercise.[7]

Moreover, defense counsel's decision was not a matter of trial strategy, let alone a reasonable strategic decision, because, pursuant to *Frye*, if defense counsel violates his duty to communicate timely to the accused formal plea offers from the prosecution, he fails to render the effective assistance that the United States constitution requires. The basis for this rule is grounded largely in professional performance standards that govern the practice of law.

In *Frye*, the defendant was charged with a felony arising from driving with a revoked license. The prosecution sent a letter to his defense counsel that offered a choice between two plea bargains, with the offers set to expire on a fixed date. Defense counsel did not inform the defendant of the offers, and after they lapsed, the defendant pleaded guilty but on more severe terms. The court held that, "as a general rule, defense counsel has the duty to communicate formal offers from the prosecution to accept a plea on terms and conditions that may be favorable to the accused. . . . When defense counsel allowed the offer to expire without advising the defendant or allowing him to consider it, defense counsel did not render the effective assistance the Constitution requires. Though the standard for counsel's performance is not determined solely by reference to codified standards of professional practice, these standards can be important guides.

---

7. By not timely informing the petitioner of the ten year plea offer, defense counsel not only deprived the petitioner of critical information that might have resulted in her foregoing the remainder of the trial in favor of pleading guilty, but, by virtue of the point in the trial during which the plea offer was made, deprived her of critical information that may well have factored into how she internally weighed the risks and benefits of testifying in her own defense. The decision made by the petitioner to testify was thus arguably based upon an incomplete calculus. Ultimately, the petitioner was entitled to make both decisions — whether to plead guilty and whether to testify in her own defense — fully informed of the state's very favorable plea offer.

The American Bar Association recommends defense counsel 'promptly communicate and explain to the defendant all plea offers made by the prosecuting attorney,' ABA Standards for Criminal Justice, Pleas of Guilty 14-3.2(a) (3d ed. 1999). . . . The standard for prompt communication and consultation is also set out in state bar professional standards for attorneys." *Id.*

The respondent argues that the holding in *Frye* does not apply to the facts of the present appeal because this is not a "lapsed plea" case, i.e., Reeve did not allow the state's ten year plea offer to expire without first advising the petitioner of it. . . .

We agree with the respondent that *Frye* does not necessarily control this case. We decline, however, to read *Frye* as narrowly as urged by the respondent because the respondent's assertion essentially ignores the thorough reasoning that the court provided for the general rule in *Frye*. . . . As previously discussed, the court repeatedly emphasized the requirement for prompt communication between defense counsel and client as set forth in both American Bar Association and state bar professional standards for attorneys. *Id.* Indeed, rule 1.4 of this state's Rules of Professional Conduct provides in relevant part: "(a) A lawyer shall: (1) promptly inform the client of any decision or circumstance with respect to which the client's informed consent . . . is required by these Rules . . . [and] (3) keep the client reasonably informed about the status of the matter. . . . (b) A lawyer shall explain a matter to the extent reasonably necessary to permit the client to make informed decisions regarding the representation." One such circumstance in which an attorney is required to promptly relay information to the client is set forth in rule 1.2(a) of the Rules of Professional Conduct, which provides in relevant part: "In a criminal case, the lawyer shall abide by the client's decision, after consultation with the lawyer, as to a plea to be entered, whether to waive jury trial and whether the client will testify. . . ."

In determining whether Reeve acted promptly, within the confines of *Frye*, when he delayed informing the petitioner of the ten year plea offer until after her trial testimony had concluded, it is necessary to define the meaning of "promptly" as it is used in rule 1.4(a)(1) of our Rules of Professional Conduct. When pressed at oral argument, the respondent conceded that defense attorneys have a duty to communicate plea offers promptly to their clients, but contended that *Frye* does not stand for the proposition that defense attorneys are required to communicate plea offers immediately to their clients. . . . [W]e employ our well established tools of statutory construction to determine the term's meaning. . . .

We first note that rule 1.0 of the Rules of Professional Conduct, entitled "Terminology," does not define "promptly." Absent this definition, in order to assign "promptly" its ordinary definition, "[w]e look to the dictionary definition of the [term] to ascertain [its] commonly approved meaning." The eleventh edition of *Merriam-Webster's Collegiate Dictionary* defines "prompt" as "being ready and quick to act as occasion demands . . . performed readily or immediately." In addition, *Random House Webster's Unabridged Dictionary* defines "prompt" as "done, performed, delivered, etc., at once or without delay." Similarly, although *Black's Law Dictionary* does not offer a definition for the word "prompt" used in the form of an adjective or adverb, it defines the verb form of "prompt" as "[t]o incite, esp. to immediate action." In turn, *Black's Law Dictionary* defines "immediate" as "[o]ccurring without delay; instant...."

On the basis of these "commonly approved" definitions, an interpretation of the term "promptly" that would allow an attorney to delay informing his client about a plea offer well after counsel had an opportunity to do so, would be unreasonable. Each of these dictionary definitions references either immediacy or a lack of delay, concepts which the petitioner advanced in her construction of the term "promptly."...

In applying the common meaning of "promptly" to the facts of the present case, it is clear that Reeve did not act promptly in informing the petitioner of the plea offer. Once Reeve received the extremely advantageous ten year offer from Nicholson on the morning of October 9, he decided to wait to tell the petitioner about the offer until after she had taken the stand in her own defense and gone through her entire trial testimony, which ultimately took two and one-half days to complete. Significantly, the respondent does not claim on appeal that Reeve was prevented by circumstances outside of his control from communicating the plea offer to his client for several days. Because the trial proceeded on October 9, the very same day Reeve received the offer from Nicholson, Reeve obviously was interacting with his client throughout each of the following days and had ample time to communicate the offer and to discuss the risks and benefits of accepting or rejecting it. In making the conscious decision to delay delivering this information to his client, Reeve did not act immediately or without delay within the definition of "promptly." Nicholson's agreement to keep the offer open did not obviate Reeve's duty to promptly inform his client of the offer. Therefore, Reeve failed to comply with our Rules of Professional Conduct and, by extension, failed to fulfill his duty to timely communicate offers from the state in derogation of *Frye*.

Because defense counsel's actions prevented the petitioner from properly exercising her constitutional right to plead guilty and to make a fully informed decision as to whether to testify on her own behalf, we agree with the petitioner that Reeve's decision may not properly be viewed as trial strategy at all, much less a reasonable trial strategy. Nevertheless, even if we were to consider counsel's decision to delay communicating the plea offer as falling within the penumbra of trial strategy, we would find that Reeve's decision was not reasonable under the circumstances.

Post-Case Follow-Up

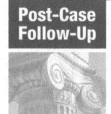

Helmedach underscores the necessity of prompt communication of plea offers as a constitutional duty and under the Model Rules. Communicating promptly means to do so "without delay"—and even immediately in situations such as in *Helmedach* where the attorney is actively associating with the pertinent client throughout the day and has ample opportunities to communicate the plea.

Helmedach v. Commissioner of Correction: Real Life Applications

1. Beth is charged with residential burglary. She hires a defense attorney, Keith. Keith initially keeps in close contact with Beth and conveys several plea offers to her, which she rejects. As the date for trial becomes imminent, Beth sends Keith numerous letters and leaves him short phone messages (she can make free one-minute phone calls twice a week). Keith fails to respond to Beth's messages and meets her again at a pretrial conference set the week of trial. Beth tells Keith that she needed to talk to him about trial strategy and potential witnesses on her behalf. She tells Keith the names of a couple of friends whom she believes would be willing to act as witnesses. Keith is unable to get ahold of the witnesses prior to trial that week. The state presents overwhelming evidence that Beth committed the burglaries and Beth is convicted. Did Keith violate the Model Rules? Does Beth have a valid claim for ineffective assistance of counsel?

2. Robin represents Wayne in a criminal prosecution for allegedly murdering Lance. Wayne explains to Robin that he shot Lance because he believed that Lance had a gun under his pillow and was about to pull it out and kill him. The police did not find a gun in Lance's apartment in the investigation of the crime. On the eve of trial, Wayne tells Robin that he is planning on testifying in his own behalf and is going to say that he saw Lance pull out a metallic object from under his pillow, which is why he shot him. Robin reminds Wayne that he must testify truthfully, but Wayne insists that it is necessary to his claim of self-defense to say he actually saw a weapon. Robin tells Wayne that he will not let Wayne testify falsely, and thus he will not allow Wayne to testify at all in light of Wayne's proposed testimony. At trial, Wayne tells Robin that he will testify truthfully if Robin will allow him to testify on his own behalf. Robin agrees, and Wayne testifies truthfully and is convicted. Did Robin violate the Model Rules? Does Wayne have a valid claim for ineffective assistance of counsel?

Deportation Consequences of a Plea

As in *Frye*, the Court has indicated that certain practices will typically constitute deficient performance of counsel under the first prong of the *Strickland* test. Notably, in Padilla v. Kentucky, 559 U.S. 356 (2010), the Supreme Court held that it was constitutionally deficient performance of counsel for an attorney to fail to inform a non-citizen criminal defendant of the potential deportation consequences of a guilty plea. Jose Padilla had been a lawful permanent resident of the United States for more than 40 years and had served in the Vietnam War as a member of the U.S. armed forces. He was charged with transporting a large amount of marijuana. His counsel told him that he did not need to worry about deportation because Padilla had been in the United States so long. Relying on this advice, Padilla accepted a deal and pled guilty to a criminal charge that (unbeknownst to him at the time) mandated his deportation. Padilla sought post-conviction relief, arguing that he would have insisted on going to trial rather than pleading guilty had he known that he would be deported as a direct result of his plea. The Supreme Court held as to the first *Strickland* prong that "[t]he weight of prevailing professional norms supports the view that counsel must advise her client regarding the risk of deportation." The Court remanded as to the prejudice prong. The Court also explained that where immigration laws are complex or make deportation consequences unclear or uncertain, "a criminal defense attorney need do no more than advise a noncitizen client that pending criminal charges may carry a risk of adverse immigration consequences."[23]

3. *Strickland*'s Second Prong: Prejudice

Strickland's prejudice prong is a serious roadblock to a successful assertion of ineffective assistance of counsel. In cases where there is substantial evidence of guilt, it is nearly impossible to overcome the prejudice prong and show that there is a reasonable probability that but for the errors of counsel the outcome would be different—because in light of the substantial evidence, it appears that the defendant would have been convicted anyway. This hurdle effectively blocks claims despite even substantial errors and incompetence of counsel.

In cases dealing with guilty pleas, the prejudice prong must be considered differently depending on whether the defendant did not accept a favorable plea due to counsel's incompetence (as in *Frye*) or accepted an unfavorable plea due to counsel's incompetence (as in *Padilla*). The Court in *Frye* explained how to determine prejudice in these situations:

> To show prejudice from ineffective assistance of counsel where a plea offer has lapsed or been rejected because of counsel's deficient performance, defendants must demonstrate a reasonable probability they would have accepted the earlier plea offer had they been afforded effective assistance of counsel. Defendants must also demonstrate a reasonable probability the plea would have been entered without the prosecution canceling it or the trial court refusing to accept it, if they had the authority to exercise that discretion under state law. . . .
>
> . . . In cases where a defendant complains that ineffective assistance led him to accept a plea offer as opposed to proceeding to trial, the defendant will have to show a reasonable probability that, but for counsel's errors, he would not have pleaded guilty and would have insisted on going to trial.[24]

Thus, in situations like *Padilla* where the accused accepted an unfavorable plea, the defendant has to show that she would not have pled guilty absent her attorney's incompetence but would have proceeded to trial instead; and in situations like *Frye* where the accused failed to accept a favorable plea, the defendant must show both "a reasonable probability [defendant] would have accepted the earlier plea offer"

---

23. *Padilla*, 559 U.S. at 369.
24. *Frye*, 566 U.S. at 147-48 (internal citations omitted).

and "that, if the prosecution had the discretion to cancel it or if the trial court had the discretion to refuse to accept it, there is a reasonable probability neither the prosecution nor the trial court would have prevented the offer from being accepted or implemented."[25]

There are also situations in which prejudice is presumed and the defendant is relieved of the obligation to prove it to succeed on a claim of ineffective assistance of counsel. As the Supreme Court recognized in United States v. Cronic, 466 U.S. 648 (1984), decided the same day as *Strickland*, there are "circumstances that are so likely to prejudice the accused that the cost of litigating their effect in a particular case is unjustified." Such a presumption was appropriate where it was shown "that [defense] counsel failed to function in any meaningful sense as the Government's adversary." Citing *Powell v. Alabama* as an example, the Court said that it had "uniformly found constitutional error without any showing of prejudice when counsel was either totally absent, or prevented from assisting the accused during a critical stage of the proceeding" or where defense counsel "entirely fail[ed] to subject the prosecution's case to meaningful adversarial testing."[26] In United States v. Ragin, 820 F.3d 609 (4th Cir. 2016), the United States Court of Appeals for the Fourth Circuit found that *Cronic*'s presumption of prejudice was warranted where defense attorney Nikita Mackey slept through a "substantial portion" of the trial and had to be punched awake by his client when called on.[27]

In McCoy v. Louisiana, 138 S. Ct. 1500 (2018), the United States Supreme Court explained that the normal *Strickland* analysis would not apply where counsel had conceded guilt over the client's objection. Accordingly, the defendant need not show prejudice to obtain a new trial for denial of the defendant's Sixth Amendment right to counsel. The Court explained:

> Because a client's autonomy, not counsel's competence, is in issue, we do not apply our ineffective-assistance-of-counsel jurisprudence. To gain redress for attorney error, a defendant ordinarily must show prejudice. Here, however, the violation of [defendant] McCoy's protected autonomy right was complete when the court allowed counsel to usurp control of an issue within McCoy's sole prerogative. Violation of a defendant's Sixth Amendment-secured autonomy ranks as error of the kind our decisions have called "structural." . . . The trial court's allowance of [the attorney's] English's admission of McCoy's guilt despite McCoy's insistent objections was incompatible with the Sixth Amendment. Because the error was structural, a new trial is the required corrective.[28]

---

25. *Id.*

26. Nevertheless, the Court held that a presumption of prejudice was unwarranted under the facts of *Cronic* itself—even though a young real estate attorney, who had never previously conducted a jury trial, was appointed to represent a defendant charged with mail fraud just 25 days before trial (the government had taken four and a half years for its own investigation and preparation for the trial).

27. *Ragin*, 820 F.3d 609, 615, 619 (4th Cir. 2016) ("We . . . hold that a defendant's Sixth Amendment right to counsel is violated when that defendant's counsel is asleep during a *substantial* portion of the defendant's trial"). The Fourth Circuit elaborated in a footnote: "Whether a lawyer slept for a substantial portion of the trial should be determined on a case-by-case basis, considering, but not limited to, the length of time counsel slept, the proportion of the trial missed, and the significance of the portion counsel slept through." *See id.* at 622 n.11.

28. *McCoy*, 138 S. Ct. at 1510-12.

Additionally, where a criminal defense counsel's performance is affected by a conflict of interest, the Supreme Court has not required a showing of prejudice. In Cuyler v. Sullivan, 446 U.S. 335 (1980), the Supreme Court held that where a criminal defendant suffers from a conflict of interest (in that case, counsel represented three co-defendants), the defendant need only show (1) the existence of an actual conflict of interest; and (2) that the conflict adversely affected counsel's performance.

C. WHEN INCOMPETENCE IS NOT YOUR FAULT

What should an attorney do when incompetence is seemingly forced upon him either through being assigned an unmanageable caseload or being appointed to a representation with insufficient time to prepare? This situation has been a continuous problem, particularly, for many public defenders. In Formal Opinion 06-441, the ABA addressed the problem of unmanageable caseloads for public defenders, reiterating that the duty of competence belongs to all attorneys.

Ethical Obligations of Lawyers Who Represent Indigent Criminal Defendants When Excessive Caseloads Interfere with Competent and Diligent Representation
ABA Formal Opinion 06-441 (2006)

In this opinion, we consider the ethical responsibilities of lawyers, whether employed in the capacity of public defenders or otherwise, who represent indigent persons charged with criminal offenses, when the lawyers' workloads prevent them from providing competent and diligent representation to all their clients. Excessive workloads present issues for both those who represent indigent defendants and the lawyers who supervise them.

ETHICAL RESPONSIBILITIES OF A PUBLIC DEFENDER IN REGARD TO INDIVIDUAL WORKLOAD

Persons charged with crimes have a constitutional right to the effective assistance of counsel. Generally, if a person charged with a crime is unable to afford a lawyer, he is constitutionally entitled to have a lawyer appointed to represent him. The states have attempted to satisfy this constitutional mandate through various methods, such as establishment of public defender, court appointment, and contract systems. Because these systems have been created to provide representation for a virtually unlimited number of indigent criminal defendants, the lawyers employed to provide representation generally are limited in their ability to control the number of clients they are assigned. Measures have been adopted in some jurisdictions in attempts to control workloads, including the establishment of procedures for assigning cases to lawyers outside public defenders' offices when the cases could not properly be directed to a public defender, either because of a conflict of interest or for other reasons.

Model Rules of Professional Conduct 1.1, 1.2(a), 1.3, and 1.4 require lawyers to provide competent representation, abide by certain client decisions, exercise diligence, and communicate with the client concerning the subject of representation. These obligations include, but are not limited to, the responsibilities to keep abreast of changes in the law; adequately investigate, analyze, and prepare cases; act promptly on behalf of clients; communicate effectively on behalf of and with clients; control workload so each matter can be handled competently; and, if a lawyer is not experienced with or knowledgeable about a specific area of the law, either associate with counsel who is knowledgeable in the area or educate herself about the area. The Rules provide no exception for lawyers who represent indigent persons charged with crimes.

Comment 2 to Rule 1.3 states that a lawyer's workload "must be controlled so that each matter may be handled competently." The Rules do not prescribe a formula to be used in determining whether a particular workload is excessive. National standards as to numerical caseload limits have been cited by the American Bar Association. Although such standards may be considered, they are not the sole factor in determining if a workload is excessive. Such a determination depends not only on the number of cases, but also on such factors as case complexity, the availability of support services, the lawyer's experience and ability, and the lawyer's nonrepresentational duties. If a lawyer believes that her workload is such that she is unable to meet the basic ethical obligations required of her in the representation of a client, she must not continue the representation of that client or, if representation has not yet begun, she must decline the representation.

A lawyer's primary ethical duty is owed to existing clients. Therefore, a lawyer must decline to accept new cases, rather than withdraw from existing cases, if the acceptance of a new case will result in her workload becoming excessive. When an existing workload does become excessive, the lawyer must reduce it to the extent that what remains to be done can be handled in full compliance with the Rules.

When a lawyer receives appointments directly from the court rather than as a member of a public defender's office or law firm that receives the appointment, she should take appropriate action if she believes that her workload will become, or already is, excessive. Such action may include the following:

- requesting that the court refrain from assigning the lawyer any new cases until such time as the lawyer's existing caseload has been reduced to a level that she is able to accept new cases and provide competent legal representation; and
- if the excessive workload cannot be resolved simply through the court's not assigning new cases, the lawyer should file a motion with the trial court requesting permission to withdraw from a sufficient number of cases to allow the provision of competent and diligent representation to the remaining clients.

If the lawyer has sought court permission to withdraw from the representation and that permission has been denied, the lawyer must take all feasible steps to assure that the client receives competent representation.

When a lawyer receives appointments as a member of a public defender's office or law firm, the appropriate action to be taken by the lawyer to reduce an excessive workload might include, with approval of the lawyer's supervisor:

- transferring non-representational responsibilities within the office, including managerial responsibilities, to others;
- refusing new cases; and
- transferring current case(s) to another lawyer whose workload will allow for the transfer of the case(s).

If the supervisor fails to provide appropriate assistance or relief, the lawyer should continue to advance up the chain of command within the office until either relief is obtained or the lawyer has reached and requested assistance or relief from the head of the public defender's office. . . .

In State v. Miller, 76 A.3d 1250 (N.J. 2013), the New Jersey Supreme Court held that there had not been ineffective assistance when the defendant, Terrence Miller, was represented at trial and convicted of drug-related offenses under the following circumstances:

On Thursday, December 6, 2007, defendant's new attorney was informed by his supervisors at the Mercer County OPD that he would be transferred from his current assignment in the Mercer County OPD's juvenile unit to a trial team responsible for cases overseen by the trial judge in this case. The attorney was told that day that he would serve as defendant's trial counsel and that defendant's trial was expected to begin on the following Monday, December 10, 2007. It would be his first adult criminal trial in seven years. Defendant's attorney, concerned that he was being assigned a case with an imminent trial date, immediately went to the trial judge's chambers, explained the reassignment and informally requested that the trial date be adjourned. The trial judge denied his request and advised him that the case would proceed to trial as scheduled.

The attorney spent several hours before Monday preparing, but "[h]e had no contact with defendant in the days leading up to trial." Indeed, the attorney met Miller for the first time on December 10, 2007, when the court held a suppression hearing, with trial proper starting on December 11. After being introduced, "counsel and defendant conferred for approximately twenty-five minutes in a window area of an empty stairwell between two floors of the courthouse." Again, counsel moved for an adjournment, which the court denied despite no opposition from the prosecution. Miller was convicted. On appeal, Miller argued that he had been denied effective assistance of counsel; he also noted that under the circumstances of his representation Miller had not been able to locate and call witnesses that could corroborate Miller's version of the facts, which was essential in both the suppression hearing and the trial. Nevertheless, the New Jersey Supreme Court upheld his conviction, holding that Miller had failed to show that he suffered prejudice under *Strickland*.

Case
Preview

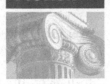

Ohio v. Jones

In upholding the conviction in *Miller*, the New Jersey Supreme Court relied in part on the fact that Miller's attorney stated on the record at the beginning of trial that he was prepared to proceed. What if the defense lawyer had stated on the record that he was *not* prepared and couldn't competently go forward? Might the appeal have gone differently? In *Ohio v. Jones*, a criminal defense attorney took that different path.

As you read *Ohio v. Jones*, consider the following:

1. What efforts should a defense attorney take to preserve the right of the criminal defendant to have a fair trial when the state has the burden to prove guilt beyond reasonable doubt (and the defendant has the presumption of innocence on her side)? Is the opportunity to argue ineffective assistance of counsel on appeal an adequate substitute for having competent counsel at trial?

2. What are the costs to the criminal defendant to proceed with a representation when an attorney is simply unprepared and has not been given sufficient time or resources to prepare?

Ohio v. Jones
2008-Ohio-6994 (Ohio Ct. App. 2008)

Appellant, Brian Jones, appeals from the January 7, 2008, judgment entry of the Portage County Municipal Court, Kent Division, in which he was sentenced for contempt.

Appellant, an attorney with the Portage County Public Defender's Office, was appointed on August 15, 2007, to represent Jordan Scott ("defendant Scott") on a charge of misdemeanor assault in State v. Scott. The case was set for trial the following day.

According to appellant's affidavit, on the morning of the trial, he met with six other clients before receiving the Scott file. Appellant then met with defendant Scott for twenty minutes. When the case was called, appellant informed Portage County Municipal Court Judge John J. Plough ("Judge Plough") that he would be filing a jury demand. After Judge Plough stated that the matter was set for trial, appellant indicated that he had been appointed to the case the day before. Appellant voiced concerns that he would not be effective as defendant Scott's counsel and would not feel comfortable representing him. Appellant said that he would need more time to talk to the witnesses. Judge Plough replied that three witnesses were present and the trial would proceed after lunch. Appellant indicated that he needed to speak with other witnesses whom the state had not subpoenaed.

Following the break, the trial court reconvened and proceeded with the Scott case. As appellant attempted to raise a pretrial matter, Judge Plough asked him whether he was ready to start the trial. Appellant replied that he was not and that he did not have an opportunity to interview the witnesses. Judge Plough warned appellant that he would be held in contempt of court if he did not proceed with the trial. Over objection by defense counsel, Judge Plough ordered the trial to commence. Appellee, the state of Ohio, waived its opening statement and appellant informed the trial court that he was not able to participate in the case. Judge Plough threatened appellant that if he did not proceed, he would be taken to jail immediately. . . . Judge Plough wanted appellant to proceed with the trial, and if a conviction resulted, the defendant could file an appeal on the basis of ineffective assistance of counsel. Appellant did not comply. The trial court found appellant in direct criminal contempt and ordered him to be taken into custody.

. . .

In the instant matter, the record reveals that appellant was appointed to represent defendant Scott the day before the case was set for trial. Appellant orally requested a continuance, which was denied by Judge Plough. . . . Here, the facts demonstrate that a continuance was warranted. . . . In addition, the continuance requested by appellant was for legitimate reasons and his conduct did not give rise to the need for one. Again, appellant was permitted merely two hours to familiarize himself with the facts, the witnesses, and his client, before preparing and constructing a defense based upon his findings. The mere fact that defendant Scott was charged with misdemeanor assault does not render the matter simple or inconsequential. Based on the information available to appellant, there may have been any number of potential witnesses and defenses pertinent to the assault charge and it was his obligation to conduct a complete investigation.

Under these circumstances, effective assistance and ethical compliance were impossible as appellant was not permitted sufficient time to conduct a satisfactory investigation as required by Rule 1.1 of the Ohio Rules of Professional Conduct, and the Sixth Amendment of the United States Constitution. It would have been unethical for appellant to proceed with trial as any attempt at rendering effective assistance would have been futile. Appellant properly refused to put his client's constitutional rights at risk by proceeding to trial unprepared.

"The rights of indigent defendants to appointment and effective assistance of counsel are neither lofty philosophical ideals nor rights that only function to give us all faith in the criminal justice system. . . . The rights to appointment of counsel and to effective assistance ultimately impact not only whether people are convicted of crimes based on fair processes but moreover, whether innocent people are convicted of crimes they did not commit. These are both outcomes whose probabilities should be reduced whenever and however feasible." . . .

The rights guaranteed to citizens under the Constitution are clearly defined and include the right to effective and competent assistance of counsel, the right to subpoena witnesses, the right to confront one's accusers and above all a right to a fair trial. Counsel must be given ample opportunity to prepare, investigate and discover the facts of the accusation. Furthermore, counsel must have time to investigate witness testimony, the nature of the allegations, and develop possible defenses in order to properly represent his or her client and provide effective assistance. The right to a speedy trial is a right both constitutional and statutory which inures to the defendant not the court.

By denying appellant's motion for a continuance, Judge Plough improperly placed an administrative objective of controlling the court's docket above its supervisory imperative of facilitating effective, prepared representation and a fair trial. . . .

In his third assignment of error, appellant alleges that [an appellate] court was not the proper forum for curing the types of defects in this matter. [This argument is in response to Judge Plough's suggestion to Jones that any incompetence could be fixed on appeal through a claim of ineffective assistance of counsel.]

Strickland v. Washington (1984), 466 U.S. 668, 687, states:

> . . . "When a convicted defendant complains of the ineffectiveness of counsel's assistance, the defendant must show that counsel's representation fell below an objective standard of reasonableness." *Id*. . . . [Additionally,] "[t]o warrant reversal, '(t)he defendant must show that there is a reasonable probability that, but for counsel's unprofessional errors, the result of the proceeding would have been different. A reasonable probability is a probability sufficient to undermine confidence in the outcome.'"

In the case sub judice, had defendant Scott been convicted, his right to the presumption of innocence would have been unfairly replaced by a burden on appeal to demonstrate a "reasonable probability" that the result of the proceeding would have been different if appellant had been prepared. In denying a continuance, Judge Plough improperly relied on the appellate process to correct the likely deprivation of defendant Scott's constitutional right to effective assistance of counsel. Direct appeal is not a reliable remedy to fix an obvious error, which could have been prevented at inception. The judicial system, the state, the defendant, and the public are always best served when the proceedings and the trial are performed with a "best practices" approach to adhere to constitutional and statutory requirements, especially when the trial record is limited. Also, by the time an appeal would have been perfected, defendant Scott's sentence would have likely been expired. Appellate courts should not be used to correct errors, especially those involving constitutional rights that a trial court has anticipated and which could have been prevented.

. . .

For the foregoing reasons, . . . [t]he judgment of the Portage County Municipal Court, Kent Division, is reversed with respect to holding appellant in contempt.

Post-Case Follow-Up

Consider what would have happened had Jones proceeded with the trial unprepared and his client had been convicted. What remedy would the client have? Of course, the client could seek to overturn the conviction, claiming ineffective assistance of counsel — but in that situation, the client would have the burden of proof to overcome the "strong presumption" that his attorney acted with reasonable proficiency. Further, the client would have had to prove prejudice — that but for the lack of preparation, there was a reasonable probability that he would not have been convicted. Compare this immense uphill burden for the defendant with what the criminal defendant should have been given: his constitutional right to have competent counsel prepare his case adequately with the presumption of innocence on his side and the burden on the state to prove guilt beyond a reasonable doubt. Jones's contempt preserved these essential constitutional rights of his client, including his right to effective assistance of counsel.

Ohio v. Jones: Real Life Applications

1. A junior public defender is assigned nearly twice as many cases as she can handle. According to ABA Formal Opinion 06-441, what can and should the public defender do?

2. Sandra is an attorney who has just opened her own solo practice. She wants to bring in clientele, so she participates in a Groupon deal of the day. Under the deal, Sandra sells for $50 the first ten hours of legal work on any family law matter. She pledges to complete the work within a month of the purchase of the deal. One hundred people buy the deal on the day it is promoted, meaning that Sandra has to complete 1,000 hours of legal work within the month (there are only 744 hours in the month). What should Sandra do? What should she have done to avoid this problem if she wanted to participate in the Groupon deal of the day?

D. COMPETENCE, MENTAL HEALTH, AND SUBSTANCE ABUSE

In a 2007 article published in *The Professional Lawyer*, J. Nick Badgerow identified an "apocalypse at law," arguing that "four horsemen" are destroying the lives of a sizable contingent of our profession — along with their ability to competently care for their clients' matters. The "four horsemen of the modern bar" Badgerow identified are "drugs, alcohol, gambling, and depression."[29]

Is Badgerow's apocalyptic diagnosis overstated? Probably not. Alcoholism, drug use, depression, and other mental health issues plague the legal profession and lead to incompetent handling of cases and professional discipline.[30] Badgerow reviews case after case where attorneys suffering with these issues have, for example, failed to communicate with clients; failed to perform the requisite legal services for a matter; failed to maintain client files, records, and appropriate accounts; failed to notify clients of receipt of funds; failed to return prepaid unearned fees; misappropriated client funds; and failed to respond to the bar's investigation of their conduct.

---

29. J. Nick Badgerow, *Apocalypse at Law: The Four Horsemen of the Modern Bar*, 18(3) Prof. Law. 2 (2007).
30. As noted in Badgerow's article, gambling is also a significant and problematic addiction among attorneys — in part because attorneys have access to client funds and often addicted gamblers convince themselves to "borrow" them, sure that their luck will turn and they can repay the money with ease. *See id.*

Patrick Krill has summarized:

As it turns out, attorneys who struggle with alcohol dependence — who struggle with the disease of addiction — are substantially more likely to underserve their clients, commit malpractice, face disciplinary action and disbarment, fall victim to mental health problems, and even take their own lives. Notably, at least 25 percent of attorneys who face formal disciplinary charges from their state bar are identified as suffering from addiction or other mental illness, with substance abuse playing at least some role in 60 percent of all disciplinary cases. Furthermore, approximately 60 percent of all malpractice claims and 85 percent of all trust fund violation cases involve substance abuse.[31]

It thus appears that alcoholism and substance abuse create a fairly sure path to the problems with attorney incompetence delineated throughout this chapter (and the resultant harms to clients). Krill subsequently co-authored a study conducted jointly by the ABA Commission on Lawyer Assistance Programs and the Hazelden Betty Ford Foundation, which was published in 2016 in the *Journal of Addiction Medicine*.[32] As summarized by James Podgers, the study revealed two main trends:

First, the levels of problem drinking and mental health issues in the legal profession appear to be higher than indicated by previous studies. And second, younger lawyers are the segment of the profession most at risk of substance abuse and mental health problems. Previous studies indicated that older lawyers were more at risk for developing problems in both areas.[33]

Indeed, the 2016 study showed that "20.6 percent of the lawyers and judges surveyed reported problematic alcohol use," but "using a variation of the questionnaire that focuses solely on the frequency of alcohol consumption, [] 36.4 percent of the respondents qualified as problem drinkers."[34] (Keep in mind that for the general adult population, 6.4 percent have an alcohol use disorder.[35]) Further, the study found that "being in the early stages of one's legal career is strongly correlated with a high risk of developing an alcohol use disorder."[36]

Why would substance abuse and mental health problems be more prevalent among younger lawyers? Linda Albert and Patrick Krill surmise:

Many lawyers find themselves working long hours; getting minimal sleep; not eating well; and distancing themselves from family, friends, and colleagues as they attempt to

---

31. Patrick Krill, *If There Is One Bar a Lawyer Cannot Seem to Pass: Alcoholism in the Legal Profession*, 44(1) THE BRIEF, (2014).
32. *See* Patrick R. Krill, Ryan Johnson & Linda Albert, *The Prevalence of Substance Use and Other Mental Health Concerns Among American Attorneys*, 10 J. ADDICT. MED. 46 (2016).
33. *Younger Lawyers Are Most at Risk for Substance Abuse, and Mental Health Problems, a New Study Reports*, A.B.A. J., Feb. 7, 2016, *available at* http://www.abajournal.com/news/article/younger_lawyers_are_most_at_risk_for_substance_abuse_and_mental_health_prob.
34. *See id.*
35. *See* Linda Albert & Patrick Krill, *Wellness and the Legal Profession: Implications of the 2016 Landmark Study on the Prevalence of Substance Use and Mental Health Concerns Among U.S. Attorneys*, B. EXAM'R 50, 54 (2016). The 6.4 percent correlates with the 21 percent of lawyers with problematic drinking. But even as to the questionnaire producing the 36 percent number for problematic drinking by lawyers, the same questionnaire was used to survey problematic drinking among physicians in 2012, with a resultant 15 percent. *See id.* at 52.
36. *See* Krill, Johnson & Albert, *supra* note 32, at 51.

keep up with the demands of the profession. These patterns are reinforced by organizations that impose heavy workloads on their employees without consideration for the impact upon those employees. Young lawyers are having difficulties finding jobs and paying off student loans and often struggle to maintain adequate social support, while also postponing life events such as marriage and starting a family. It is possible, if not probable, that these circumstances contribute to the higher level of distress symptoms we see among lawyers during their first 15 years of practice.[37]

Do the addictive behaviors destructive of the careers (and lives) of attorneys and the legal rights of their clients begin (or blossom) in law school? The 2016 Survey of Law Student Well-Being (SLSWB) gathered information from law students at 15 U.S. law schools, which resulted in the following statistics as to the law students surveyed:

- 53 percent drank enough to become drunk at least once in the prior 30 days
- 43 percent binge drank at least one time in the prior two weeks
- 22 percent binge drank two or more times in the prior two weeks
- 25 percent used marijuana in the prior year
- 14 percent used marijuana in the prior 30 days
- 6 percent used cocaine in the prior year
- 2 percent used cocaine in the prior 30 days
- 14 percent used prescription drugs without a prescription in the prior year
- 17 percent screened positive for depression (using Patient Health Questionnaire-2)
- 37 percent screened positive for anxiety (using Kessler (K6) questionnaire)[38]

Despite these numbers, only 4 percent of surveyed students had actually sought help for drug or alcohol problems. Around 23 percent had sought help for mental illness problems. Why didn't more seek help? The survey asked about deterrents to seeking help, and over 60 percent of respondents indicated a concern of a potential threat to bar admission or finding a job (hence the title of the findings from the survey, "Suffering in Silence").[39]

So what can be done? Albert and Krill contend that wellness needs to be taught and emphasized in law school and to legal professionals. They explain: "Wellness concepts include teaching law students and legal professionals about stress management as well as building hardiness and resiliency skills; the importance of physical exercise, good sleep, and quality nutrition; minimizing alcohol use; and incorporating interpersonal connectedness into their lives."[40] Learning to deal with stress in ways other than alcohol and substance abuse is key—and that learning needs to start and be encouraged during law school. Certainly law school is stressful—but law practice is also stressful—thus students who find themselves turning

---

37. *See* Albert & Krill, *supra* note 35, at 54-55.
38. Jerome M. Organ, David B. Jaffe & Katherine M. Bender, *Suffering in Silence: The Survey of Law Student Well-Being and the Reluctance of Law Students to Seek Help for Substance Use and Mental Health Concerns*, 66 J. LEGAL EDUC. No. 1 (2016).
39. *See id.*
40. Albert & Krill, *supra* note 35, at 55.

to alcohol and substance abuse or who have mental health issues in law school need to recognize that graduating and moving on to law practice will not solve problems. Each student should engage in serious self-reflection on whether she is at risk and take appropriate actions, including where appropriate seeking help from health professionals, Lawyer Assistance Programs, or university or law school counselors. Every jurisdiction in the United States has a Lawyers Assistance Program, which offers assistance to both lawyers and law students struggling with substance abuse or other mental or emotional health problems.[41] In many jurisdictions, obtaining help from a Lawyer Assistance Program is confidential. The 2017 Report of the National Task Force on Lawyer Well-Being recommended that law schools, state bars, legal employers, and other stakeholders reduce any stigma or adverse consequences associated with seeking help and, instead, encourage "help-seeking behaviors" while taking other active steps to instill and improve wellness in the legal profession.[42]

The Struggle
Above the Law (Aug. 22, 2016)[43]

Hi, my name is [redacted], and I am in recovery from alcoholism and depression. Less than a year ago, I would have never imagined uttering those words. Depression was not even on my radar, and how could I possibly have a drinking problem? At 25 years old, I was in my third year of law school, and successfully interning at two different legal organizations. On the outside, I had my life together. However, on the inside, I was really struggling.

In order to better explain "my law school struggle," I need to briefly explain my past. I grew up in a loving family but also in a family who buried emotions — the "pull yourself up by your own bootstraps" mentality. Growing up, my idea of strength was suffering in silence. It wasn't until a family tragedy occurred right before law school that I even contemplated seeking outside help. However, I quickly dismissed the idea of mental health therapy, as I was afraid of how that could negatively affect my future legal career. Therefore, I continued to suffer in silence and began law school with unresolved grief and trauma issues. Moreover, while I was a social drinker before law school, my drinking greatly increased during law school, as I was now turning to alcohol as a way to cope with my emotions and the increased stress and pressure I was faced with on a daily basis as a law student.

---

41. The ABA keeps a directory of Lawyer Assistance Programs for each jurisdiction on its website at http://www.americanbar.org/groups/lawyer_assistance/resources/lap_programs_by_state.html.

42. National Task Force on Lawyer Well-Being, *The Path to Lawyer Well-Being: Practical Recommendations for Positive Change*, at 13 (2017), *available at* https://www.americanbar.org/content/dam/aba/images/abanews/thepathtolawyerwellbeingreportrevfinal.pdf.

43. Anonymous law student story excerpted from Staci Zaretsky, *The Struggle: Will Alcoholism Treatment Affect Your Character and Fitness Review?*, Above the Law, Aug. 22, 2016, *available at* http://abovethelaw.com/2016/08/the-struggle-will-alcoholism-treatment-affect-your-character-and-fitness-review/.

By my second year of law school, I was suffering from depression and I began abusing alcohol in an attempt to "get happy." However, self-medicating with alcohol only increased my depression and by my third year in law school, I became suicidal and developed signs of alcoholism. While I functioned during the day, my evenings and weekends were spent binge drinking alone in my apartment. I no longer saw the point of living and drank myself into a stupor on multiple occasions. At this point, I knew I needed help but I was too afraid and ashamed to admit it.

Finally, I confided in a mentor who urged me to seek help and I listened. While I was fearful that mental health and addiction treatment could negatively impact my admission to the bar, I knew I had to address these issues before I started my legal career—my life was at risk. Therefore, right before my law school graduation, and to the surprise of my friends and family, I electively entered a thirty-day inpatient treatment program for mental health and alcohol addiction.

Today, I am over nine months sober and I can honestly say my life is now worth living. For the first time in a long time, I am happy and healthy. Unfortunately, I cannot say my journey to health, happiness, and sobriety has been an easy one. It has taken a lot of self-care, mental health therapy, and recovery support to get to this point.

Chapter Summary

- Clients hire attorneys because clients lack the requisite knowledge, skill, and ability to protect their own legal interests and rights; thus, attorneys who are incompetent violate their first and basic duty to their clients: to protect their clients' interests.
- Competence requires that an attorney act with the requisite legal knowledge and skill to handle a case; attorneys can obtain competence in a new area of law through necessary study or by associating with an attorney of established competence.
- Competence requires lawyers to thoroughly investigate the facts of a case and make sufficient preparation, including the preparation of appropriate documents and filings, for legal proceedings and transactions.
- Attorneys have a duty to act with reasonable diligence and promptness in representing a client, which requires lawyers to manage their workload and avoid procrastination.
- Communication is essential to a successful attorney-client relationship: the attorney and client must communicate both (1) for the attorney to properly pursue the client's actual objectives and to determine the factual bases for the claims; and (2) for the client to meaningfully participate in the matter and be informed regarding the status of the case.
- Attorneys must communicate any circumstance regarding which the client must give informed consent, which includes those matters within the sole authority of the client to decide, such as whether to settle a civil matter and, in criminal cases, the plea to be entered, waiver of jury trial, and whether the defendant will testify in her own behalf.

- Attorneys must promptly respond to a client's reasonable request for information, which means the attorney must respond to or at least acknowledge receipt of the communication.
- Criminal defendants have a constitutional right to the effective assistance of counsel. In order to prevail on such a claim, the defendant must show both (1) deficient performance — counsel's conduct fell measurably below that expected of a reasonable attorney gauged by prevailing professional norms; and (2) prejudice — there is a reasonable probability that but for counsel's errors, the result of the proceeding would have been different.
- Alcohol and other substance abuse and mental health problems are particularly prevalent among lawyers and often lead to incompetence, failure to communicate or act with diligence, and other disciplinary problems — all of which inure to the detriment of the client.

Applying the Rules

1. Joel is a solo practitioner who has primarily done criminal defense representation, but wants to change his area of practice. A wealthy neighbor, Sally, asks Joel to draft a will for her. Joel is excited about the opportunity to do something different. However, he knows absolutely nothing about wills or estate planning. Joel wants to have a friend of his, Ralph, assist with the will because Ralph is an established attorney with his own estate planning practice. Does Joel need to tell Sally about his desire to have Ralph assist with the representation? Does Sally need to consent to bringing Ralph into the matter? (Consult comment [6] to Rule 1.1, as well as Rule 1.4.)

2. Mattie is an attorney who has practiced entirely in state court. Mattie decides to file a lawsuit in federal court on behalf of a new client, Landblast, Inc. She reads Rule 8(a) of the Federal Rules of Civil Procedure (FRCP) and sees that it is identical in language to the state civil procedure rule 8(a). In the state where she lives, civil procedure rule 8(a) is construed to only require notice pleading. However, in federal court, and unbeknownst to Mattie, the Supreme Court in the *Twombly* and *Iqbal* cases reinterpreted FRCP 8(a) to require that an attorney plead sufficient facts to plausibly state a claim and held that legal conclusions are not entitled to an assumption of truth. Mattie files a complaint in federal court that contains almost no factual assertions but is just a recital of legal conclusions. The federal trial court grants the opposing party's FRCP 12(b)(6) motion to dismiss for failure to state a claim upon which relief can be granted, and orders Mattie to file a new amended complaint that complies with federal pleading standards within ten days or the complaint will be dismissed with prejudice. The court's order also directly chastises Mattie for her obvious failure to stay abreast of the Supreme Court's interpretation of Rule 8(a). Has Mattie violated the Model Rules? Must Mattie disclose the court's

order to her client or can she just quietly fix it by filing an amended complaint? What does she need to do to ensure that she proceeds in a competent manner?

3. Taylor was in an automobile wreck with Simon. Taylor sued Simon, and Jane undertook the representation of Simon. After lengthy pretrial proceedings, the court ordered that the case be transferred to mandatory arbitration. Jane was aware of this order. Jane did not ever receive notice about the case being scheduled on the arbitration calendar, but four months later, she learned that she had missed the mandatory hearing and the arbitration court had entered a $10,000 default arbitration award against Simon for failure to appear. Jane moved to vacate the award, arguing that she had received no notice of the hearing. The court responded that a postcard notice had been mailed to her, and even if she had not received it she should have checked the mandatory arbitration calendar herself in the intervening four months from the initial order to determine the date of the arbitration hearing. Did Jane have a duty to inquire into the dates if she really did not see the notice (regardless of the reason for her not receiving the notice)?

4. Henry is a bankruptcy attorney who handles a high volume of relatively simple bankruptcy petitions for individuals. Henry delegates most of the work in drafting and handling the bankruptcy petitions to his paralegals. The bankruptcy court determines that the debts of Henry's client, George, are nondischargeable, and the court issues an order stating that the bankruptcy was neither filed nor handled in a competent manner. George files a grievance with the bar. Can Henry be disciplined for the incompetence of his paralegals' work? What should Henry have done?

5. Tanya is a criminal defense lawyer who has a very heavy caseload and is worn out. She is appointed to represent Trevor in a prosecution for felony murder. At trial, she repeatedly falls asleep during the State's presentation of evidence — and even a few times during the State's cross-examination of her own witnesses. The State presents substantial evidence of guilt, and Trevor is convicted. Does Trevor have a meritorious claim for ineffective assistance of counsel?

Professional Responsibility in Practice

1. You are an associate at the law firm Moore & Less. Three different partners email you an assignment on Monday morning: one needs you to write a summary judgment motion in a large case, one needs you to draft discovery requests and respond to the opposition's discovery requests, and one needs you to prepare pretrial disclosures for an upcoming trial. All three assignments must be completed by the end of the week. You work diligently for a couple days and realize

you cannot complete all three assignments by the end of the week, and perhaps cannot complete any one of them. How should you proceed and how soon should you do so? Plan out what you would actually say to a partner under these circumstances.

2. You have a client, Darrin, who calls or emails you daily to discuss the progress of his case. You have taken the case on contingency, so you are not charging Darrin an hourly rate for the time it takes to answer and respond to his inquiries. Darrin's case does not need constant attention — indeed, you have just sent out discovery requests, and it will be 30 days before you receive responses and have any new information to disclose to Darrin. In addition, you have several other matters that need your full attention. Draft an email to your client that will not strain your relationship with him, will fulfill your communication duties to him, and will also allow you to devote your time to your other matters.

3. A number of jurisdictions have adopted ethics opinions about the risks and competent use of cloud computing and other new or emerging technologies. Research whether there are any such opinions in the state in which you now live or intend to practice and write a brief summary of any such opinion.

Confidentiality, the Attorney-Client Privilege, and Work-Product Immunity

The attorney-client relationship is a **fiduciary** one that creates obligations of loyalty and secrecy on the part of the lawyer. The attorney must keep her client's information secret, and may not disclose confidences learned during the relationship to the disadvantage of the client. This **confidentiality** obligation is imposed for two primary reasons. First, it furthers the normative goal of protecting the autonomy of the client and her authority to control the purposes and direction of the representation. Second, it serves the utilitarian function of encouraging clients to communicate fully and frankly with their lawyers, even on embarrassing or sensitive topics. The premise here is that lawyers need full and accurate information from their clients in order to render sound legal advice.

There are three sources of the attorney's secrecy obligations—the ethical duty of confidentiality under Model Rules 1.6 and 1.9, the **attorney-client privilege** under the Rules of Evidence, and the common law **work-product immunity** in litigation. You can think of these three secrecy obligations as partially over-lapping circles, with the ethical duty of confidentiality being the largest circle, the attorney-client privilege being the second largest circle, and the work-product protection being the smallest circle. *See* Figure 5.1, Three Circles of Lawyer "Secrets," *infra* at page 303.

Key Concepts

- The ethical obligation to keep client information confidential
- Exceptions to the duty of confidentiality: to defend a claim against the lawyer, or to prevent certain future harms
- Protecting the confidentiality of client communications under the attorney-client evidentiary privilege
- The attorney-client privilege is subject to waivers and exceptions
- Work-product immunity protects from discovery a lawyer's preparations in anticipation of litigation

The three doctrines can be and often are confused by laymen and by law students; nevertheless, they derive from distinct sources, impose different rights and responsibilities upon attorneys, and carry different exceptions. We will examine each doctrine in turn, and then compare them in the Chapter Summary.

A. THE DUTY OF CONFIDENTIALITY

Confidentiality is part of the professional duty of loyalty (fiduciary duty) that agents owe to their principals. The basic duty of confidentiality is set forth in Model Rule 1.6(a) with exceptions in 1.6(b). The duty of confidentiality prohibits lawyers from voluntarily disclosing information that they learn in the course of representing a client to others (third parties, the media, opposing counsel) unless they have the express or implied permission of their client, or unless an exception applies. Put simply, you cannot blab about non-public aspects of your client's case to other people. Lawyers who breach this confidentiality obligation may be subject to professional discipline and may be sued by their clients in tort for breach of fiduciary duty.

Students often confuse the duty of confidentiality under Rule 1.6 with the attorney-client privilege. But there are important differences. The first is the source of the information. In this regard, the ethical rule of confidentiality is much broader than the rule of privilege.

As you will see below, the privilege protects only information communicated in secret between the client and the attorney. The confidentiality rule, by contrast, protects not only information communicated from the client himself, but also information that the lawyer learns from talking to third-party witnesses, from consulting with experts and consultants, and from preexisting documents that the client provides to the lawyers. Rule 1.6 defines **confidential material** as any "information relating to the representation of a client." Given this very broad definition, even *the fact* of representation may be confidential if the client has not expressly or impliedly authorized it to be revealed. For example, if a famous professional athlete is thinking about getting a divorce and approaches a small law firm that is renowned for litigating high-profile probate matters to discuss his options, that firm could not reveal its representation of the athlete before he makes a final decision to pursue a divorce because this may disadvantage the client.

Given this very broad definition of confidential information, lawyers need to understand that even casual conversations with friends or loved ones about their work on behalf of a client (over dinner or at the gym) may violate the disciplinary rules. Talking about a case in terms of a generalized hypothetical is permissible so long as the listener is not able to ascertain the identity of the client or the particulars of the client's situation. *See* Model Rule 1.6 cmt. [4].

A second important difference between the duty of confidentiality and the rule of privilege is that the privilege is a shield that protects against judicially compelled disclosure (that is, the lawyer or client may refuse to answer or produce documents in response to a subpoena). The ethical rule of confidentiality, by contrast, prohibits at any time the *voluntary* disclosure of client information to third parties (casual friends or acquaintances, opposing counsel, other parties contemplating lawsuits, the media, etc.). The rule of confidentiality cannot be asserted to block disclosure of information that is compelled by a court-sanctioned request for information (subpoena, deposition question, interrogatory); for that you would need to rely on the privilege, which is a rule of evidence, not a rule of professional ethics. In other words, a subpoena can reach information that is confidential, but it cannot reach information that is privileged.

A third respect in which the rules of confidentiality are broader than the rules of privilege is that under the rules of confidentiality a lawyer may not *use* confidential information to the disadvantage of the client, even if that information is never revealed to anyone. *See* Model Rule 1.8(b). Because confidential information is provided to the lawyer in a fiduciary capacity, it is impermissible for the lawyer to use that information to the disadvantage of the principal. For example, if an attorney learns of a business client's intention to relocate its manufacturing facility in the future to a remote part of the state, it would be impermissible for the lawyer to buy a piece of property in that area with the hope of increasing its value in the time period prior to the company's relocation. *See* Model Rule 1.8(b). An exception to this prohibition of "use" of client information is for information that is generally known in the community. *See* Restatement (Third) of the Law Governing Lawyers §59 and Model Rule 1.9(c). If the same business client had publicly announced its future plans to move the manufacturing plant and this announcement was the subject of newspaper articles in local business journals, it would not be impermissible for the lawyer to speculate on real property in the area of future relocation.

Both the rule of confidentiality and the rule of privilege apply to a lawyer's dealings with **prospective clients**. *See* Model Rules 1.18(b) and 1.9(c). A lawyer who is interviewing a prospective client has a duty not to disclose confidential client information, and not to use it to the prospective client's disadvantage. Both sources of confidentiality survive the death of the client or the termination of the lawyer-client relationship. *See* Rule 1.6 cmt. [20]. So if a client is deceased, the lawyer must obtain any required permissions to waive confidentiality from the client's estate.

Lawyers have a duty to *protect* confidential client information as well as a duty not to disclose it or use it to the client's disadvantage. The duty of confidentiality under Rule 1.6(c) requires lawyers to take "reasonable efforts to prevent the inadvertent or unauthorized disclosure" of client information. So a lawyer cannot carelessly leave her client's file at a coffee shop, cannot talk about the matter with another firm attorney in an audible voice while seated in a crowded subway car, and cannot dispose of client documents in the trash without shredding them. In an era of hacking and surreptitious electronic surveillance, what security protocols will constitute "reasonable efforts" to protect client information is a constantly evolving question.

The exceptions to a lawyer's duty of confidentiality under Rule 1.6 are both numerous and controversial. We will start with the exceptions that are fairly standard from state to state. A lawyer may reveal confidential client information if that disclosure is explicitly or impliedly authorized by the client. *See* Rule 1.6(a). Explicit authorization requires **informed consent** — defined as express agreement after the client has been advised about the risks and available alternatives. *See* Rule 1.0(c).

So a politician who is being criticized by his opponent for failing to release his tax returns may authorize his tax lawyer to release those returns and discuss them with the media. But in the absence of such informed consent, the tax attorney would be acting unethically by revealing the politician's tax returns to the media unilaterally, even if he thought it was in the best interests of his client.

Disclosure of confidential client information is "**impliedly authorized**" if it is necessary in order to carry out the purposes of the representation. For example, if a motor vehicle accident victim engages an attorney to sue the driver allegedly responsible for the crash, the attorney may include as factual allegations in the complaint information that the attorney learns from interviewing the client, reviewing her medical records, and consulting her physician. Implicit authorization may be inferred from the circumstances—such as where it is consistent with the goals of the representation. An attorney may write a demand letter to opposing counsel revealing factual information learned from his intake interview with his client and documents provided by the client, if such a demand letter would facilitate a settlement that is desired by the client.

There are four other fairly standard exceptions to client confidentiality that are reflected in Model Rule 1.6(b). A lawyer may reveal confidential client information to the extent the lawyer reasonably believes necessary to secure ethical advice about the lawyer's own responsibilities. *See* Model Rule 1.6(b)(4). For example, a lawyer might consult another lawyer, a retired judge, or a bar ethics committee for advice about complying with the disciplinary rules in the context of a particular legal engagement; in that context, the limited disclosure of client information is permissible to the extent necessary to accurately convey the factual issues involved. Second, a lawyer may reveal client information if reasonably necessary to establish a claim or defense in a controversy between the lawyer and the client, or in a criminal, civil, or disciplinary complaint against the lawyer brought by someone else alleging misconduct by the lawyer in his representation of that client. *See* Model Rule 1.6(b)(5). This is known as the "self-defense" exception. If a lawyer is sued for malpractice, subjected to discipline for alleged ethical misconduct, or has to sue the client for unpaid legal fees, the revelation of confidences is allowed because the lawyer would not be able to assert his claim or defense without revealing client information.

Third, a lawyer may reveal client information for the limited purpose of complying with conflict checks when the lawyer changes jobs and moves to a new law firm or when a group of lawyers create a new firm or merge with another firm. *See* Model Rule 1.6(b)(7). In these situations, a lawyer may reveal the names of his clients and the general nature of the matters involved in the representation for the purpose of being "screened" for any potential conflicts at a new firm, so long as that limited revelation does not disclose privileged material or in any way disadvantage the prior client.

Fourth, a lawyer may reveal confidential client information if necessary to "comply with other law or a court order." Rule 1.6(b)(6). As noted above, confidentiality may be trumped by a judicial subpoena, unless the material is also privileged. Other professional conduct rules may also require revelation of otherwise confidential material held by attorneys under Rule 1.6. As we will see when we study the lawyer's duty with respect to client perjury in Chapter 7, Rule 3.3(b) requires a lawyer to rectify any fraud that the client has perpetrated on an adjudicative tribunal, and this legal obligation trumps the duty of confidentiality under Rule 1.6. *See* Model Rule 3.3(c).

Finally, most states allow exceptions to their confidentiality rules for disclosures that are necessary to prevent certain **future harms**. These exceptions are complex and vary considerably from state to state. In fact, there is more variation in these future harm exceptions than in any other area of legal ethics, so students need to be attentive to their local rules. We suggest that students compare Model Rule 1.6(b) with the correlative rule in the state in which they intend to practice.

With respect to future harms, bar committees and state supreme courts drafting the exceptions to Rule 1.6 typically are trying to balance four objectives: encouraging frank communications between lawyers and clients; respecting a client's autonomy and his right to control the principal-agent relationship; protecting members of the public from harm; and protecting the integrity of the profession by not allowing legal services to be used for criminal or fraudulent purposes. Proponents of broad exceptions for future harms argue that client candor is not as important as countervailing societal interests in avoiding injury; and anyway, much of what is considered "confidential" under Rule 1.6 comes from non-clients, so disclosure will not impede future candor by clients. Proponents of narrow exceptions for future harms argue that respect for client autonomy and control should outweigh a lawyer's obligations to third parties in all but the most extreme instances.

In order to understand the disagreement among state rulemakers on the issue of future harms, it may be helpful to think of confidentiality exceptions for future harms as running along four possible tracks or axes: (1) is disclosure mandatory, or is it permissive?; (2) is disclosure required/allowed when it is necessary to prevent certain *crimes*, or is it also required/allowed when it is necessary to prevent certain *crimes or frauds*?; (3) is disclosure required/allowed when it is necessary to prevent only serious bodily injury or death to another, or is it also allowed when it is necessary to prevent substantial financial injury to another?; and (4) is disclosure required/allowed only when the *client* is expected to engage in future injurious behavior, or is it also required/allowed when the future harm is likely to be committed by a *third party*?

It is impossible to catalogue here all the state variations with respect to future harm exceptions. In some jurisdictions, revelation may be required; in others it may be permissive; and in still others it may be forbidden. For example, California has a really narrow future harms exception, permitting disclosure only when necessary to prevent a crime involving death or substantial bodily harm. *See* CAL. R. PROF'L CONDUCT, R. 1.6(b). New Jersey has an extremely broad exception, *requiring* disclosure when either a client or a third party threatens to commit a crime or a fraud that will result in death, substantial bodily harm, substantial financial injury, or fraud on a tribunal. *See* N.J. R. PROF'L CONDUCT 1.6(b).

The ABA Model Rules, as you might expect, take an intermediate approach. Disclosure is permissive, but is not mandatory. While disclosure is allowed to prevent anyone (including a third party) from causing death or serious bodily injury to another person, it is only permitted to prevent a *client* from committing a crime or fraud that is likely to result in substantial financial injury, and even then, only if the client has *used the lawyer's services* in furtherance of that crime or fraud. *See* Model Rule 1.6(b)(2). ABA Model Rule 1.6 was amended to add this financial injury component in 2003 in response to the Enron corporate fraud scandal. Thus, an attorney can disclose client confidences to prevent substantial financial injury to others, but only if the client is the perpetrator and only when the client has used the lawyer's services in an attempt to perpetrate that financial fraud.[1]

Imagine a lawyer for a wealthy businessman who is in the process of purchasing a piece of commercial real estate. The lawyer learns in the course of the representation that the client has inflated his assets on a multi-million-dollar loan application that is pending with a bank. If the client used the lawyer's services in completing that loan application, the lawyer may reveal the client confidence to the bank in order to prevent substantial financial harm. But if the client completed the bank loan application without the lawyer's assistance, such revelation would not be permitted under ABA Model Rule 1.6(b)(2). However, before the loan closes and the funds are disbursed for the purchase of real estate, the lawyer might have to withdraw from representation in order to avoid assisting a crime or fraud. *See* ABA Model Rule 1.2(d). Many lawyers would resolve this dilemma by informing the client that they are ethically required to **withdraw** before the bank closing and purchase, unless the client either remedies his false statements to the bank (by updating or amending his loan application) or gives permission to the lawyer to do so under Rule 1.6(a).

This hypothetical bank fraud scenario is further complicated by Rule 4.1(b). Rules 1.6(b)(2) and (3) permit but do not require disclosure of client confidences when the lawyer's services were used to further a substantial financial injury. Rule 4.1(b) provides that in the course of representing a client, a lawyer shall not knowingly "fail to disclose a material fact when disclosure is necessary to avoid assisting a criminal or fraudulent act by a client, unless disclosure is *prohibited* by Rule 1.6" (emphasis supplied). Rule 4.1 requires disclosure, while Rule 1.6(b) allows disclosure. Because Rule 4.1(b) is mandatory regarding disclosure, unless it is prohibited by Rule 1.6, the expansion of permissive disclosures under Rule 1.6(b) may arguably lead to more mandatory disclosures to third persons under Rule 4.1(b) with respect to financial crimes likely to cause substantial injury where the lawyer's services were used in the fraud.

The intersection between Rule 1.6(b)(2) and (3) and Rule 4.1(b), which were enacted at different times and using different language, is imprecise and undertheorized by courts and commentators. As Professors Mark Cady and Gregory Sisk have explained:

> [W]hen the stringent requisites for both Rule 1.6(b)(2) or (3) and Rule 4.1(b) are present in a case, the lawyer is required, and not merely authorized, to make the disclosure. Somewhere in the combined operation of subparagraphs (b) (2) and (3) of Rule 1.6

---

1. Lawyers for organizational clients have wider latitude in revealing client confidences to prevent future financial harms than lawyers for individual clients. As we saw in Chapter 3, ABA Model Rule 1.13(c) allows a lawyer for an organization who knows that an officer, employee, or other person associated with the organization has engaged in a violation of law that might be imputed to the organization and is likely to result in substantial injury to the organization to report that violation out of the organization after unsuccessfully reporting it up the ladder, irrespective of whether the lawyer's services were used in furtherance of the fraud. *See* Rule 1.13(c) and cmt. [6]. Securities and Exchange Commission regulations mirror Rule 1.13(c) in this regard. *See* 17 C.F.R. §205.3(d)(2).

and of Rule 4.1(b) is to be found a newly vitalized and mandatory duty to disclose information about client fraud or crime, although this remains an area of professional responsibility that is still evolving and the parameters of that duty consequently remain uncertain.[2]

The rules are incongruent, however, in that Rules 1.6(b)(2) and (3) refer to substantial financial injury caused by a client's crime or fraud in furtherance of which the client has "*used*" the lawyer's assistance, whereas Rule 4.1(b) does not have the substantiality requirement, is not limited to financial injury, and requires disclosure where necessary to avoid "*assisting*" with a crime or fraud. That is, Rule 1.6(b) *permits* but does not require disclosure when the client is using the lawyer's past work in committing a crime of fraud, even when the lawyer is not now actively assisting. Rule 4.1(b) *requires* disclosure where the client is actively and currently using the lawyer's help in committing the crime or fraud, in the sense that the lawyer would be liable as an accomplice.

Let's return to the hypothetical bank fraud scenario discussed above. If the loan application was filled out by the client without the lawyer's assistance, the lawyer may not reveal the falsity of the information to the bank under Rule 1.6(b). He may, however, withdraw from representation or threaten to do so if the client does not reveal the false statements, because the falsity "involves" the lawyer's services. *See* Rule 1.16 (b)(2). If the loan application was filled out or filed by the lawyer based on information provided by the client and the lawyer *subsequently* learns of the falsity of the information, the lawyer may disclose under Rule 1.6(b)(2) because his legal assistance is being "used" by the client to commit a crime or fraud. However, a lawyer would be "assisting" with a crime or fraud within the meaning of Rule 4.1(b) only if the attorney helps the client fill out the bank application with knowledge of its falsity, or subsequently learns of the falsity of the information while somehow continuing to affirm or warranty the accuracy of the application to the bank. The difference between a permissive disclosure under Rule 1.6(b)(2) and a mandatory disclosure under Rule 4.1(b) thus appears to turn on the mental state of the lawyer.[3]

---

2. Mark S. Cady & Gregory C. Sisk, 16 Lawyer and Judicial Ethics §5:6(h)(3), Iowa Practice Series (2019).

3. Lawrence J. Fox illustrated this complicated and somewhat contested interplay between Rules 1.6(b) and 4.1(b) in Chapter 4 of his book, Legal Tender (ABA Section of Litigation, 1995). Fox posits a case where a lawyer helps a large maintenance company secure lending from a bank. In the course of the multi-million-dollar banking transaction, the lawyer writes an opinion letter to the bank detailing and explaining the maintenance company's biggest assets, over 200 five-year contracts with area municipalities to replace their street lights and traffic controls, and the enforceability of those contracts. Based on that opinion letter, the bank loans the client $5 million to purchase new trucking equipment, to be distributed in quarterly installments of $300,000 over a four-year period. After one year of loan distributions, the maintenance company learns that its lead salesman fabricated some of the municipal contracts by reporting them to the company as five-year service agreements when actually they were two- or three-year service agreements, in order to inflate his commissions. The lawyer's opinion letter written one year previously is thus false. The company fires its first lawyer and replaces him with another attorney in an attempt tactically to prevent the first attorney from revealing the fraud to the bank. If the lawyer no longer represents the company and had no knowledge of the falsity of the opinion letter when it was written, he has no mandatory duty to disclose under Rule 4.1(b), because arguably he is not "assisting" a crime or fraud. But does he have an *option* to disclose under Rule 1.6(b)(2)? If the client (through the new lawyer) lets the original opinion letter remain at the bank uncorrected before the next $300,000 distribution, is the client "using" the lawyer's services to commit a crime or fraud?

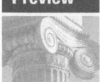

Case Preview

Purcell v. District Attorney for the Suffolk District

After receiving an order to vacate his apartment, Joseph Tyree sought legal advice from a legal services attorney, Jeffrey Purcell. Tyree had recently been discharged from his employment as a maintenance man at the apartment building where he resided. During their consultation, Purcell became suspicious that Tyree intended to burn down the apartment building. Purcell informed the Boston Police Department of his suspicions. The police then searched Tyree's apartment pursuant to a warrant and found incendiary materials, gasoline, and several bottles with wicks attached. The smoke detectors had been disconnected and gasoline had been poured on the floor. Tyree was arrested and charged with attempted arson. Purcell was later subpoenaed to testify at Tyree's trial, but he asserted the attorney-client privilege. The trial judge found that the statements Tyree made to Purcell were not protected by the attorney-client privilege, and denied Purcell's motion to quash the subpoena. Purcell sought extraordinary relief in a petition before the state supreme court.

As you read *Purcell*, ask yourself the following:

1. Was there a way that Attorney Purcell could reasonably have protected the inhabitants of the apartment building without revealing his client's statement and identity?
2. Suppose that Purcell believed he could talk his client out of the attempted arson and assure that incendiary materials were removed from the premises. Would the lawyer still be allowed to reveal the client confidence to authorities?
3. What social value is advanced by making the disclosure for future deadly harms permissive rather than mandatory under Rule 1.6? That is, don't the lives of innocents *always* outweigh the autonomy of clients?

Purcell v. District Attorney for the Suffolk District
676 N.E.2d 436 (Mass. 1997)

. . .

There is no question before this court, directly or indirectly, concerning the ethical propriety of Purcell's disclosure to the police that Tyree might engage in conduct that would be harmful to others. As bar counsel agreed in a memorandum submitted to the single justice, this court's disciplinary rules regulating the practice of law authorized Purcell to reveal to the police "[t]he intention of his client to commit a crime and the information necessary to prevent the crime." S.J.C. Rule 3:07, Canon 4, DR 4-101(C)(3), as appearing in 382 Mass. 778 (1981). The fact that the disciplinary code permitted Purcell to make the disclosure tells us nothing about the admissibility of the information that Purcell disclosed.

. . .

The attorney-client privilege is founded on the necessity that a client be free to reveal information to an attorney, without fear of its disclosure, in order to obtain informed legal advice. It is a principle of long standing. The debate here is whether Tyree is entitled to the protection of the attorney-client privilege in the circumstances.

The district attorney announces the issue in his brief to be whether a crime-fraud exception to the testimonial privilege applies in this case. He asserts that, even if Tyree's communication with Purcell was made as part of his consultation concerning the eviction proceeding, Tyree's communication concerning his contemplated criminal conduct is not protected by the privilege. We shall first consider the case on the assumption that Tyree's statements to Purcell are protected by the attorney-client privilege unless the crime-fraud exception applies.

"It is the purpose of the crime-fraud exception to the attorney-client privilege to assure that the 'seal of secrecy,' . . . between lawyer and client does not extend to communications 'made for the purpose of getting advice for the commission of a fraud' or crime." There is no public interest in the preservation of the secrecy of that kind of communication.

Our cases have not defined a crime-fraud exception to the attorney-client privilege with any precision. In *Matter of John Doe Grand Jury Investigation*, the court stated that there was "no legitimate interest of a client and no public interest would be served by a rule that would preserve the secrecy of" a conversation between attorney and client in a conference related to the possible future defrauding of an insurance company. We cited *Commonwealth v. Dyer*, in which we said that "[t]here is no privilege between attorney and client where the conferences concern the proposed commission of a crime by the client." The cases cited in our *Dyer* opinion and the facts of that case — the attorney was alleged to be part of the conspiracy — demonstrate that the exception asserted concerned conferences in which the attorney's advice was sought in furtherance of a crime or to obtain advice or assistance with respect to criminal activity.

We, therefore, accept the general principle of a crime-fraud exception. The Proposed Massachusetts Rules of Evidence adequately define the crime-fraud exception to the lawyer-client privilege set forth in rule 502(d)(1) as follows: "If the services of the lawyer were sought or obtained to enable or aid anyone to commit or plan to commit what the client knew or reasonably should have known to be a crime or fraud." We need not at this time consider seemingly minor variations of the exception expressed in various sources. The applicability of the exception, like the existence of the privilege, is a question of fact for the judge.

The district attorney rightly grants that he, as the opponent of the application of the testimonial privilege, has the burden of showing that the exception applies. In its *Zolin* opinion, the Supreme Court did not have to decide what level of showing the opponent of the privilege must make to establish that the exception applies. We conclude that facts supporting the applicability of the crime-fraud exception must be proved by a preponderance of the evidence. However, on a showing of a factual basis adequate to support a reasonable belief that an in camera review of the evidence may establish that the exception applies, the judge has discretion to conduct such an in camera review. Once the judge sees the confidential information, the burden of proof normally will be unimportant.

In this case, in deciding whether to conduct a discretionary in camera review of the substance of the conversation concerning arson between Tyree and Purcell, the judge would have evidence tending to show that Tyree discussed a future crime with Purcell and that thereafter Tyree actively prepared to commit that crime. Without this evidence, the crime of arson would appear to have no apparent connection with Tyree's eviction proceeding and Purcell's representation of Tyree. With this evidence, however, a request that a judge inquire in camera into the circumstances of Tyree's apparent threat to burn the apartment building would not be a call for a "fishing expedition," and a judge might be justified in conducting such an inquiry. The evidence in this case, however, was not sufficient to warrant the judge's finding that Tyree consulted Purcell for the purpose of obtaining advice in furtherance of a crime. Therefore, the order denying the motion to quash because the crime-fraud exception applied cannot be upheld.

There is a consideration in this case that does not appear in other cases that we have seen concerning the attorney-client privilege. The testimony that the prosecution seeks from Purcell is available only because Purcell reflectively made a disclosure, relying on this court's disciplinary rule which permitted him to do so. Purcell was under no ethical duty to disclose Tyree's intention to commit a crime. He did so to protect the lives and property of others, a purpose that underlies a lawyer's discretionary right stated in the disciplinary rule. The limited facts in the record strongly suggest that Purcell's disclosures to the police served the beneficial public purpose on which the disciplinary rule was based.

We must be cautious in permitting the use of client communications that a lawyer has revealed only because of a threat to others. Lawyers will be reluctant to come forward if they know that the information that they disclose may lead to adverse consequences to their clients. A practice of the use of such disclosures might prompt a lawyer to warn a client in advance that the disclosure of certain information may not be held confidential, thereby chilling free discourse between lawyer and client and reducing the prospect that the lawyer will learn of a serious threat to the well-being of others. To best promote the purposes of the attorney-client privilege, the crime-fraud exception should apply only if the communication seeks assistance in or furtherance of future criminal conduct. When the opponent of the privilege argues that the communication itself may show that the exception applies and seeks its disclosure in camera, the judge, in the exercise of discretion on the question whether to have an in camera proceeding, should consider if the public interest is served by disclosure, even in camera, of a communication whose existence is known only because the lawyer acted against his client's interests under the authority of a disciplinary rule. The facts of each situation must be considered.

It might seem that this opinion is in a posture to conclude by stating that the order denying the motion to quash any subpoena to testify is vacated and the matter is to be remanded for further proceedings concerning the application of the crime-fraud exception.

However, the district attorney's brief appears to abandon its earlier concession that all communications between Tyree and Purcell should be treated as protected by the attorney-client privilege unless the crime-fraud exception applies. The question whether the attorney-client privilege is involved at all will be open on remand. We, therefore, discuss the issue.

The attorney-client privilege applies only when the client's communication was for the purpose of facilitating the rendition of legal services. See Rule 502(b) of the Proposed Massachusetts Rules of Evidence. The burden of proving that the attorney-client privilege applies to a communication rests on the party asserting the privilege. The motion judge did not pass on the question whether the attorney-client privilege applied to the communication at all but rather went directly to the issue of the crime-fraud exception, although not using that phrase.

A statement of an intention to commit a crime made in the course of seeking legal advice is protected by the privilege, unless the crime-fraud exception applies. That exception applies only if the client or prospective client seeks advice or assistance in furtherance of criminal conduct. It is agreed that Tyree consulted Purcell concerning his impending eviction. Purcell is a member of the bar, and Tyree either was or sought to become Purcell's client. The serious question concerning the application of the privilege is whether Tyree informed Purcell of the fact of his intention to commit arson for the purpose of receiving legal advice or assistance in furtherance of criminal conduct. Purcell's presentation of the circumstances in which Tyree's statements were made is likely to be the only evidence presented.

This is not a case in which our traditional view that testimonial privileges should be construed strictly should be applied. A strict construction of the privilege that would leave a gap between the circumstances in which the crime-fraud exception applies and the circumstances in which a communication is protected by the attorney-client privilege would make no sense. The attorney-client privilege "is founded upon the necessity, in the interest and administration of justice, of the aid of persons having knowledge of the law and skilled in its practice, which assistance can only be safely and readily availed of when free from the consequences or the apprehension of disclosure." Unless the crime-fraud exception applies, the attorney-client privilege should apply to communications concerning possible future, as well as past, criminal conduct, because an informed lawyer may be able to dissuade the client from improper future conduct and, if not, under the ethical rules may elect in the public interest to make a limited disclosure of the client's threatened conduct.

A judgment should be entered in the county court ordering that the order denying the motion to quash any subpoena issued to Purcell to testify at Tyree's trial is vacated and that the matter is remanded for further proceedings consistent with this opinion.

So ordered.

Post-Case Follow-Up

The Massachusetts disciplinary rule was amended in 2015 to create a permissive exception to the duty of confidentiality "to prevent reasonably certain death or substantial bodily harm, or to prevent the wrongful execution or incarceration of another." MASS. R. PROF'L CONDUCT 1.6(b)(1). Note how this future harms exception in Massachusetts is now both *narrower* and *broader* than the future harms exception in

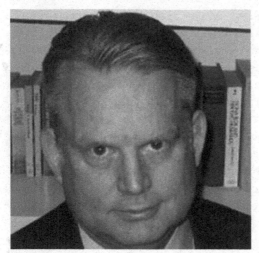

Jeffrey W. Purcell

effect in Massachusetts at the time of the *Purcell* decision: it is narrower because only certain highly dangerous future acts are included, but it is broader because the attorney may reveal client confidences to the extent reasonably necessary to prevent someone *other than the client* from committing those acts.

Why were Tyree's threats to burn down the apartment building protected *at all* under the attorney-client privilege in the *Purcell* case? Is it clear that the client's statements to Purcell were part and parcel of a communication made for the purposes of obtaining legal advice? The Supreme Judicial Court ruled that they were, because a construction of the privilege "that would leave a gap between the circumstances in which the crime-fraud exception applies and the circumstances in which a communication is protected by the attorney-client privilege would make no sense." Is that so obvious? We will return to this question after you read Section B, below.

Purcell v. District Attorney for the Suffolk District: Real Life Applications

1. Suppose that Purcell had represented a client in an employment action against a manufacturing company that had terminated the client from his job as a maintenance man. Imagine further that the client confessed to Purcell that he had unlawfully discharged toxic chemicals into the river behind the company in retribution for his discharge. The river flows into a reservoir that supplies drinking water to the public. May Purcell reveal *that* confidence to authorities? In other words, does the deadly bodily harm have to be imminent under either the 2015 Massachusetts rule or the ABA Model Rule in order for the exception to the confidentiality rule to apply? Although neither rule uses the word "imminent" in its text, the immediacy of the harm may be taken into account by the lawyer in determining whether disclosure "is reasonably necessary to prevent *reasonably certain*" death or substantial bodily harm. *See* Model Rule 1.6 cmt. [6]. Is the harm reasonably certain in the above situation?

Ordinarily, when a client comes to a lawyer and admits that he has done something wrong in the past (robbed a bank, cheated on his taxes, stolen from an employer), the lawyer's role is to help the client avoid or minimize liability for that past misconduct. No matter how bad the conduct is or how high the stakes are, the lawyer may not favor society's interests over his client's, and must protect the client's confidences. We will return to this issue in Chapter 8, where we discuss the so-called "Buried Bodies Case," New York State Bar Association, Formal Opinion 479 (1978).

With respect to financial harms, however, section (b)(3) of Rule 1.6 goes one step further than section (b)(2) and permits a lawyer to reveal a client confidence if reasonably necessary "to mitigate or rectify" a past crime or fraud that is reasonably certain to result in substantial financial injury to another and in furtherance of which the client has used the lawyer's services. This allows a lawyer to reveal information needed to rectify certain limited *past* misconduct, not just future misconduct. If the act causing substantial financial injury is past and the client used the lawyer's services to perpetrate that financial fraud, the lawyer may reveal confidences to the extent reasonably necessary to rectify the fraud. Here the rulemakers have valued the integrity of the profession over the client's autonomy because the client has inappropriately used legal services to assist with financial misdealing. The drafters refused to distinguish between past financial frauds and threats of future financial frauds because with financial injury — unlike with purely physical injury — that temporal line is much more difficult to draw; the manager of a company might tell a lie about the financial status of the company in a prospectus or annual report and stakeholders might rely on this fraudulent misstatement days, weeks, or months later. If the lawyer's services were used to assist with that misrepresentation in the prospectus or annual report, Rule 1.6(b)(3) would allow the lawyer to reveal client confidences if necessary to rectify the fraud. This confidentiality exception for limited past crimes or frauds is controversial; over a dozen states have declined to adopt the Model Rule formulation.

Where **confidentiality exceptions** are permissive (as they are in Model Rule 1.6(b)(1) through (7)), the exceptions allow a lawyer to reveal confidential information "to the extent the lawyer reasonably believes necessary" to meet one of the enumerated objectives. So the lawyer cannot disclose client confidences when some other course of conduct would reasonably be expected to meet the same objective; moreover, when the lawyer does reveal client information, the disclosure may be no greater than reasonably necessary to accomplish that objective. In other words, the lawyer cannot use a sledgehammer when a scalpel will suffice. With respect to disclosures reasonably believed necessary to prevent future harms, the lawyer, where feasible, must first make a good faith effort to persuade the client to prevent the harmful conduct, including advising the client of the lawyer's ability to reveal information if the client chooses not to do so. *See* Model Rule 1.6, cmt. [16]. If that fails, the lawyer may disclose only as much information as necessary to prevent the future harm.

Now that you have learned these complex — and in places ambiguous — exceptions to the rule of client confidentiality, how would you advise a new client about your professional obligation of secrecy? Many lawyers begin their discussions with new clients by saying something like "What you share with me is confidential, and I am ethically obliged to keep it secret." While this short introduction may have the advantage of simplicity (and of putting the client at ease), you now know that it is both incomplete and inaccurate. Would it be better to say nothing? We will return to this subject after addressing the attorney-client privilege.

B. THE ATTORNEY-CLIENT PRIVILEGE

1. Introduction

The attorney-client privilege is one of the oldest and broadest evidentiary privileges at common law. A cornerstone of the legal profession, the privilege permits clients to resist being compelled by legal process from disclosing confidential communications with their lawyer for legal services. Thus, a client may refuse a formal request in an interrogatory or a question on cross-examination for his or her confidential communications with counsel.

Evidentiary privileges permit the non-disclosure of otherwise relevant evidence to further important social policies unrelated to the relevancy or significance of the evidence. The attorney-client privilege promotes society's interest in the free flow of communications from the client to the lawyer and generally from the lawyer to the client; a sort of two-way communications street. Clients will hopefully communicate more candidly with their lawyers because the privilege protects their communications. Armed with a better understanding of their client's problem, lawyers can provide more informed representation and better advise their clients to observe the law.

Attorney-Client Privilege Elements Defined

Professor Wigmore's treatise on evidence provides a classic definition of the attorney-client privilege:

> (1) Where legal advice of any kind is sought (2) from a professional legal advisor in his capacity as such, (3) the communications relating to that purpose, (4) made in confidence (5) by the client,[4] (6) are at his instance permanently protected (7) from disclosure by himself or by the legal adviser, (8) except the protection be waived.

Section 68 of the Restatement (Third) of the Law Governing Lawyers (Restatement) similarly provides that the attorney-client privilege protects "(1) a communication (2) made between privileged persons (3) in confidence (4) for the purpose of obtaining or providing legal assistance for the client." The Restatement's more concise formula of the attorney-client privilege is widely accepted by state and federal courts.

---

4. Although not expressly stated in the Wigmore formulation, EVIDENCE IN TRIALS AT COMMON LAW §2292 (McNaughton ed. 1961), the attorney-client privilege also protects lawyer communications to the client providing legal advice. *See* RESTATEMENT (THIRD) OF THE LAW GOVERNING LAWYERS §70, at 537 [hereinafter Restatement].

Although many states have codified the attorney-client privilege in varying forms, there is no similar codification on the federal level. Instead, Congress enacted the current Rule 501, which broadly states that federal "common law . . . [generally] governs a claim of privilege," underscoring that the attorney-client privilege is a common law rule in federal courts. Federal courts will apply state attorney-client privilege rules, however, when state law provides the rule of decision in a civil action or proceeding, such as in federal cases where jurisdiction is based on diversity of citizenship or a federal cause of action that contains a pendant state law claim.[5]

2. Scope of the Privilege

The Confidential and Privileged Relationship

Privileges do not automatically preclude the disclosure of evidence; the **privilege holder** must make a timely refusal to disclose the evidence. The client is the holder of the attorney-client privilege and ultimately decides whether to assert or waive it. Given their **agency relationship**, the lawyer may sometimes assert or waive the privilege to protect the client's interests.[6] The privilege claimant bears the burden of proving its applicability. The lawyer should ideally advise the client about the scope of the privilege, including possible exceptions and risks of waiver, during the initial interview or soon thereafter. *See* Rules 1.2 and 1.3.

Communications for the Purpose of Legal Advice

The attorney-client privilege protects the client's oral and written confidential communications to the lawyer in his or her professional capacity for the purpose of obtaining legal services. The client needs only a **reasonable belief** that he is consulting with a licensed lawyer to have otherwise qualified communications protected by the privilege. Once the privilege applies, its protection against compelled disclosure continues even after the client's death.[7]

The privilege also protects the lawyer's oral and written communications to the client providing legal advice or services. For example, a lawyer's email to a client describing the legal strategy for representing him in an automobile accident is a privileged communication. Under the privilege, both the lawyer and the client may refuse to disclose the contents of the lawyer's strategy email and any client response to that email.

---

5. Gray v. Bicknell, 86 F.3d 1472 (8th Cir. 1996). STEVEN I. FRIEDLAND & JACK P. SAHL, EVIDENCE PROBLEMS AND MATERIALS 479 (6th ed. 2020) [hereinafter EVIDENCE PROBLEMS].
6. Drimmer v. Appleton, 628 F. Supp. 1249 (S.D.N.Y. 1986).
7. Swidler & Berlin v. United States, 524 U.S. 399, 410 (1998). *See* Rebecca Blair, *A Novel View of Cravath*, AM. LAW. 15 (Sept. 2016) (reporting that the author of a novel about business giant George Westinghouse's battle with Thomas Edison in the 1880s over the patent for the lightbulb was denied access by Cravath, Swain & Moore to a box of letters from Westinghouse to his lawyer, Paul Cravath, because they are protected by the attorney-client privilege).

Observations are not communications. Evidence that anyone could observe about the client's mental state or appearance during lawyer-client communications is not privileged. Thus, a lawyer's observations that the client looked sad or had a black eye are not privileged and are subject to disclosure.

The privilege protects only client communications with his lawyer that the client intends to be confidential. A client who discloses confidential communications with his lawyer to a friend at dinner, to a third party during an investigation, or in answers to an interrogatory has no reasonable claim that he intended the communications to be confidential. *See* Nguyen v. Excel Corp., 197 F.3d 200 (5th Cir. 1999). In general, the identity of the client, the fact of consultation, the amount of the fee, the general subject matter of consultation, and the client's location are not protected under the evidentiary privilege because this information does not disclose the content of the client's confidential communications.[8] Some courts in criminal cases have used what is referred to as the "**last link doctrine**" to hold that a client's identity is protected by the attorney-client privilege when it connects the client to the offense.[9]

The presence of third parties during client-lawyer communications generally defeats a claim that the communications were intended to be confidential. The privilege is not lost, however, by the presence of representatives assisting the lawyer in the delivery of legal services. Representatives may include a secretary, accountant, paralegal, or junior partner who are present during confidential client communications.[10]

The test for determining when the privilege covers a lawyer's representative is whether: (1) the lawyer is directing the representative's assistance, and (2) the lawyer is rendering legal advice.[11] Thus, there is no privilege when the client contacts the firm's paralegal to seek her opinion about legal strategy. However, the privilege would apply when the lawyer advises the client about legal strategy in the presence of the paralegal while directing the paralegal to take notes of the meeting.

Sometimes third parties accompanying the client during communications will not defeat the client's claim that he intended the communications to be confidential. For instance, a client who brings an interpreter to facilitate communications will not lose the privilege if the client believes the interpreter will not reveal the communications. Nor will the privilege be lost if the client is a family caretaker who brings a young child or an aged relative to a legal consultation. *See* Stroh v. Gen. Motors Corp., 623 N.Y.S.2d 873 (N.Y. App. Div. 1995).

---

8. The attorney-client privilege does prohibit such disclosure to the extent it reveals the content of the client's communications. *See* J. Media Grp. Inc. v. N.J. Dep't of Law & Pub. Safety, No. A-5833-13T4, 2016 BL 259485 (N.J. Super. Ct. App. Div. Aug. 11, 2016) (finding the identities of state employees and their requests for representation and/or indemnification, and any written denial of such requests, are entitled to non-disclosure under state lawyer ethics rules *if not the attorney-client privilege* in the infamous 2013 Bridgegate matter — the linking of the George Washington Bridge lane closures to New Jersey governor Chris Christie's administration) (emphasis added); Ralls v. United States, 52 F.3d 223, 226 (9th Cir. 1995) (involving fee-payer who sought lawyer's advice about fee-payer's involvement in a crime for which the defendant was arrested and holding that fee-payer's identity and fee arrangement were privileged because they were intertwined with confidential communications).

9. Baird v. Koerner, 279 F.2d 623 (9th Cir. 1960). *Cf.* Restatement §69 cmt. g, at 527-28 (reporting the privilege does not prohibit disclosure merely because it might incriminate the client).

10. United States v. Evans, 113 F.3d 1457 (7th Cir. 1997).

11. Bloomingburg Jewish Educ. Ctr. v. Village of Bloomingburg, 171 F. Supp. 3d 136, 140 (S.D.N.Y. 2016).

The privilege does not cover communications between the client and lawyer that do not involve the rendition of legal services. A client who asks his lawyer about whether a private or public high school offers his child the best opportunity to play sports is not a communication seeking legal advice. Similarly, a client request seeking the lawyer's recommendation about whether to invest client funds with one stock broker over another is a request for financial advice. The attorney-client privilege does not cover requests for pure financial or business advice.

Mixed Communications

Client-lawyer communications sometimes involve a mix of legal and non-legal advice, such as business, financial, or personal advice. Whether the privilege protects **mixed communications** from disclosure is a fact-dependent question for the courts. As with all testimonial privileges, courts narrowly construe the attorney-client privilege because it "contravene[s] the fundamental principle that the public has a right to every man's evidence" for a fair and efficient search for the truth.[12] While some courts will protect a communication from disclosure if it has a "legal component," others require a greater degree of legal advice.[13] Most courts hold that if the primary purpose for the communications was to seek legal advice, then the confidential communications are privileged.[14] The privilege claimant must show that the nature of the particular communication involved the lawyer acting in a professional legal capacity, providing advice, and that the client subjectively believed the communication was confidential.[15]

The District of Columbia Circuit Court of Appeals recognized in In re Kellogg Brown & Root, 756 F.3d 754 (D.C. Cir. 2014), that determining the primary purpose for a communication can be a difficult, if not "inherently impossible task" when the primary purpose is motivated by two overlapping purposes, for example, one business and one legal. In *Kellogg*, an employee claimed that KBR had defrauded the U.S. government while administering military contracts in wartime Iraq. The *Kellogg* court held that the primary purpose test is met and the privilege applies if just "one of the significant purposes" of the communication was to obtain or provide legal advice, as was the case here. The appeals court concluded that KBR conducted the internal investigation to comply with regulatory requirements, its own corporate policy, and to obtain or provide legal advice, making the internal investigation documents privileged.

The privilege protects only communications made during the attorney-client relationship or by a prospective client during an initial interview whether or not the lawyer represents the prospective client and whether or not there has been an exchange or an agreement for compensation. The communications can be in electronic form.

---

12. In re Pacific Pictures Corp., 679 F.3d 1121, 1126 (9th Cir. 2012) (quoting Trammel v. United States, 445 U.S. 40, 50 (1980)).
13. *Compare* U.S. Postal Service v. Phelps Dodge Refinance Corp., 852 F. Supp. 156 (E.D.N.Y. 1994), *with* United States v. Mejia, 655 F.3d 126, 132 (2d Cir. 2011) (communications must be solely for obtaining or providing legal advice).
14. FTC v. Boehringer Ingelheim Pharm., Inc., 892 F.3d 1264, 1267 (D.C. Cir. 2018).
15. *See* United States v. Chen, 99 F.3d 1495, 1502 (9th Cir. 1996); Restatement §71 cmt. b.

No Privilege for Preexisting Client Documents and Underlying Facts

The privilege does not cover a client's statements or documents that were made before the client conferred with or retained the lawyer. For instance, the privilege would not protect a box of letters and tax documents that the client prepared two years before hiring counsel. Depositing this box of preexisting written materials with the lawyer does not alter the fact that these materials were not communications made to the client's lawyer. The client would have to disclose the preexisting materials upon a discovery request but the client's "act of deposit" to the lawyer is a communicative act that would not have to be revealed.

The privilege protects communications, not the underlying facts. For example, the attorney-client privilege protects from disclosure the defendant-client's confidential statement to his lawyer that he was looking at his children in the rear of his car when he struck the plaintiff's vehicle. Although the privilege protects the defendant-client's communication from disclosure, the plaintiff may prove the same fact through non-privileged means. Thus, the plaintiff may offer a bystander's eyewitness testimony that he saw the defendant-client look toward the rear of his car at the time of the collision even if that same fact was independently communicated to a lawyer. The plaintiff may also ask the defendant at trial about whether he was looking in the rear of the car at the time of the accident and the defendant would be required to answer the underlying fact question. The defendant cannot be asked, however, about what he told his attorney as that communication is privileged.

Entity Clients and the Privilege

Although corporations do not have a Fifth Amendment right to refuse to testify, corporations and other legal entities can claim the attorney-client privilege as a basis for refusing to disclose confidential communications between them and their lawyers. *See* Nguyen v. Excel Corp., 197 F.3d 200 (5th Cir. 1999). A common challenge for lawyers in representing entities is determining who is the client or who speaks on behalf of the legal entity. In general, the lawyer is taking direction from the CEO or president concerning the assertion of, or waiver of, the privilege. The leading case on the attorney-client privilege as it applies to corporations is Upjohn Co. v. United States, 449 U.S. 383 (1981).

Case Preview

Upjohn Co. v. United States

Since mid- and lower-level employees may embroil their corporations in legal difficulties, entity lawyers may need to confer with these employees to gather facts to adequately advise their entity-clients. In *Upjohn*, the corporation's general counsel directed all of Upjohn's foreign general and area managers to provide him and outside counsel with information about possible questionable payments to obtain government business. The general counsel also described the investigation as "highly confidential" and directed the managers to discuss the investigation only with Upjohn employees who might be helpful in providing the requested information.

As you read *Upjohn*, consider the following questions:

1. How does the Court describe the underlying policy for the attorney-client privilege?
2. What particular facts concerning the nature of Upjohn general counsel's request for information prompted the Court to note that Upjohn employees knew their responses would be confidential and for the purpose of legal assistance?
3. Why did the appellate court reject the argument that extending the privilege beyond the "control group" was unnecessary?
4. How does the Court address the appellate court's concern that extending the privilege to non–control group employees will place a burden on discovery?

Upjohn Co. v. United States
449 U.S. 383 (1981)

We granted certiorari in this case to address important questions concerning the scope of the attorney-client privilege in the corporate context and the applicability of the work-product doctrine in proceedings to enforce tax summonses. With respect to the privilege question the parties and various *amici* have described our task as one of choosing between two "tests" which have gained adherents in the courts of appeals. We are acutely aware, however, that we sit to decide concrete cases and not abstract propositions of law. We decline to lay down a broad rule or series of rules to govern all conceivable future questions in this area, even were we able to do so. We can and do, however, conclude that the attorney-client privilege protects the communications involved in this case from compelled disclosure and that the work-product doctrine does apply in tax summons enforcement proceedings.

Petitioner Upjohn Co. manufactures and sells pharmaceuticals here and abroad. In January 1976 independent accountants conducting an audit of one of Upjohn's foreign subsidiaries discovered that the subsidiary made payments to or for the benefit of foreign government officials in order to secure government business. The accountants, so informed petitioner, Mr. Gerard Thomas, Upjohn's Vice President, Secretary, and General Counsel. . . . It was decided that the company would conduct an internal investigation of what were termed "questionable payments." As part of this investigation the attorneys prepared a letter containing a questionnaire which was sent to "All Foreign General and Area Managers" over the Chairman's signature. . . . Managers were instructed to treat the investigation as "highly confidential" and not to discuss it with anyone other than Upjohn employees who might be helpful in providing the requested information. Responses were to be sent directly to Thomas. Thomas and outside counsel also interviewed the recipients of the questionnaire and some 33 other Upjohn officers or employees as part of the investigation.

. . .

... On November 23, 1976, the Service issued a summons pursuant to 26 U.S.C. §7602 demanding production of:

> All files relative to the investigation conducted under the supervision of Gerard Thomas to identify payments to employees of foreign governments and any political contributions made by the Upjohn Company or any of its affiliates since January 1, 1971 and to determine whether any funds of the Upjohn Company had been improperly accounted for on the corporate books during the same period.
>
> The records should include but not be limited to written questionnaires sent to managers of the Upjohn Company's foreign affiliates, and memorandums or notes of the interviews conducted in the United States and abroad with officers and employees of the Upjohn Company and its subsidiaries.

The company declined to produce the documents specified in the second paragraph on the grounds that they were protected from disclosure by the attorney-client privilege. . . . Federal Rule of Evidence 501 provides that "the privilege of a witness . . . shall be governed by the principles of the common law as they may be interpreted by the courts of the United States in light of reason and experience." The attorney-client privilege is the oldest of the privileges for confidential communications known to the common law. Its purpose is to encourage full and frank communication between attorneys and their clients and thereby promote broader public interests in the observance of law and administration of justice. The privilege recognizes that sound legal advice or advocacy serves public ends and that such advice or advocacy depends upon the lawyer's being fully informed by the client. As we stated last Term: . . . "The lawyer-client privilege rests on the need for the advocate and counselor to know all that relates to the client's reasons for seeking representation if the professional mission is to be carried out." [W]e recognized the purpose of the privilege to be "to encourage clients to make full disclosure to their attorneys." . . . Admittedly complications in the application of the privilege arise when the client is a corporation, which in theory is an artificial creature of the law, and not an individual; but this Court has assumed that the privilege applies when the client is a corporation. . . .

The Court of Appeals, however, considered the application of the privilege in the corporate context to present a "different problem," since the client was an inanimate entity and "only the senior management, guiding and integrating the several operations, . . . can be said to possess an identity analogous to the corporation as a whole." The first case to articulate the so-called "control group test" adopted by the court below, reflected a similar conceptual approach:

> [T]he most satisfactory solution, I think, is that if the employee making the communication, of whatever rank he may be, is in a position to control or even to take a substantial part in a decision about any action which the corporation may take upon the advice of the attorney, . . . then, in effect, *he is (or personifies) the corporation* when he makes his disclosure to the lawyer and the privilege would apply." (Emphasis supplied.)

Such a view, we think, overlooks the fact that the privilege exists to protect not only the giving of professional advice to those who can act on it but also the giving of information to the lawyer to enable him to give sound and informed advice. . . .

Middle-level — and indeed lower-level — employees can, by actions within the scope of their employment, embroil the corporation in serious legal difficulties, and it is only natural that these employees would have the relevant information needed by corporate counsel if he is adequately to advise the client with respect to such actual or potential difficulties.

The control group test adopted by the court below thus frustrates the very purpose of the privilege by discouraging the communication of relevant information by employees of the client to attorneys seeking to render legal advice to the client corporation. The attorney's advice will also frequently be more significant to noncontrol group members than to those who officially sanction the advice, and the control group test makes it more difficult to convey full and frank legal advice to the employees who will put into effect the client corporation's policy.

The narrow scope given the attorney-client privilege by the court below not only makes it difficult for corporate attorneys to formulate sound advice when their client is faced with a specific legal problem but also threatens to limit the valuable efforts of corporate counsel to ensure their client's compliance with the law. In light of the vast and complicated array of regulatory legislation confronting the modern corporation, corporations, unlike most individuals, "constantly go to lawyers to find out how to obey the law," particularly since compliance with the law in this area is hardly an instinctive matter. The test adopted by the court below is difficult to apply in practice, though no abstractly formulated and unvarying "test" will necessarily enable courts to decide questions such as this with mathematical precision. But if the purpose of the attorney-client privilege is to be served, the attorney and client must be able to predict with some degree of certainty whether particular discussions will be protected. An uncertain privilege, or one which purports to be certain but results in widely varying applications by the courts, is little better than no privilege at all. The very terms of the test adopted by the court below suggest the unpredictability of its application. The test restricts the availability of the privilege to those officers who play a "substantial role" in deciding and directing a corporation's legal response.

The communications at issue were made by Upjohn employees to counsel for Upjohn acting as such, at the direction of corporate superiors in order to secure legal advice from counsel. . . . The communications concerned matters within the scope of the employees' corporate duties, and the employees themselves were sufficiently aware that they were being questioned in order that the corporation could obtain legal advice. . . . Pursuant to explicit instructions from the Chairman of the Board, the communications were considered "highly confidential" when made and have been kept confidential by the company. Consistent with the underlying purposes of the attorney-client privilege, these communications must be protected against compelled disclosure.

The Court of Appeals declined to extend the attorney-client privilege beyond the limits of the control group test for fear that doing so would entail severe burdens on discovery and create a broad "zone of silence" over corporate affairs. Application of the attorney-client privilege to communications such as those involved here, however, puts the adversary in no worse position than if the communications had never taken place.

[W]e conclude that the narrow "control group test" . . . sanctioned by the Court of Appeals, in this case cannot, consistent with "the principles of the common law as . . . interpreted . . . in the light of reason and experience," Fed. Rule Evid. 501, govern the development of the law in this area.

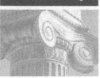

Post-Case Follow-Up

The *Upjohn* decision and its rationale have become firmly rooted in federal common law for determining the application and scope of the attorney-client privilege. Many states have also adopted the *Upjohn* decision, recognizing that lawyers need as much information as possible from their entity-clients, which may involve casting a large net to capture facts from a wide range of entity constituents to promote corporate compliance with the law. Some questions about the privilege in the corporate setting remain. For example, when must the lawyer for the corporate entity who is interviewing an entity employee disclose that the employee's interest conflicts with the client-entity's interest and that the employee should retain separate counsel?

Upjohn Co. v. United States: Real Life Applications

1. Imagine the CEO of a local construction company contacts you and your firm to conduct an investigation of the company possibly paying kickbacks to government officials for public contracts. What steps would you take to ensure that communications with company employees are protected by the attorney-client privilege? In the course of your investigation, you find it necessary to interview a former company employee. He asks whether you are representing him too and, if so, whether his communications to you are protected by the attorney-client privilege. Discuss the former employee's situation with him.

2. Jane Hankins manages a 40-person law firm. She suspects a firm partner, Tom Jones, of mishandling a client's funds. Hankins asks two associates to conduct an internal factual investigation of the matter. The grand jury subpoenas the two associates to learn about their discussions with Hankins. The two associates claim that as lawyers their discussions with Hankins are protected by the attorney-client privilege. The government contends, however, that the privilege is inapplicable because the two associates are merely employees on a fact-finding mission. Hankins asks you, a professional responsibility expert, whether the firm will be successful in claiming the privilege protects her communications with the two associates. Discuss the firm's chances of success.

3. Attorney Irving represents a company and its CEO concerning his executive assistant's recent allegation that she was wrongfully terminated. She alleges that the CEO began sexually harassing her after she confronted the CEO about his financial misrepresentations about the company to lenders. She claims her termination is really a case of sexual discrimination. The executive assistant's lawyers have not yet filed an action in court but are threatening one unless a suitable settlement is offered. Attorney Irving asks for all of the executive assistant's emails on her company laptop for the period of the alleged sexual harassment up to her termination, including emails to the lawyers representing her in this wrongful termination matter. The executive assistant refuses to turn over

the laptop and her emails to her lawyers, claiming they are protected by the attorney-client privilege. Attorney Irving has concluded based on preliminary investigation that the employee's allegations may have some merit but that there is also evidence supporting the CEO's claim that the executive assistant's work was unsatisfactory.

Are the former executive assistant's emails privileged? How does the fact that her lawyers have not filed a complaint affect Attorney Irving's strategy in resolving this matter? What other possible ethics issues loom in Attorney Irving's decision to represent the company and the CEO?

Government Lawyers and the Privilege

The attorney-client privilege generally protects communications between government agencies or members of the executive branch and their agency's in-house counsel or the U.S. Department of Justice when the purpose is for legal advice in a civil case. *See* In re County of Erie, 473 F.3d 413 (2d Cir. 2007). Courts differ on whether the privilege protects similar communications in criminal cases.

In In re Grand Jury Investigation, 399 F.3d 527 (2d Cir. 2005), the government sought private communications of Connecticut governor John Rowland and his staff with his office's former chief legal counsel for advice concerning federal grand jury proceedings about possible criminal conduct for the receipt of gifts from persons doing business with the state. The Second Circuit held that it was "crucial" for a government official who faces criminal prosecution to be able to fully consult with counsel to observe the law while working for the public. "Upholding the privilege [in this case promotes the public interest by furthering] a culture in which consultation with government lawyers is accepted . . . [as an] indispensable part of conducting public business."

Other circuit courts considering the same question in grand jury proceedings take a contrary view. For example, the court in In re Grand Jury Subpoena Duces Tecum, 112 F.3d 910, 920 (8th Cir. 1997), concluded that "the general duty of public service calls upon government employees and agencies to favor disclosure over concealment." That same court noted that the "difference between the public and the private interest is perhaps, by itself, reason enough to find *Upjohn* unpersuasive." Unlike private corporations, government entities cannot be held criminally liable. The Eighth Circuit Court also noted a "strong public interest in honest government" and in the revelation of wrongdoing by public officials.[16] Finally, government officials faced with criminal liability can hire their own private lawyers.

The attorney-client privilege covers "communications between the attorney and all agents or employees who are authorized to act or speak" for the government entity concerning the subject matter of the communication.[17] As in the corporate

---

16. In re Grand Jury Subpoena Duces Tecum, 112 F.3d 910, 921 (8th Cir. 1997). *See also* In re Lindsey, 148 F.3d 1100, 1109 (D.C. Cir. 1998) (noting the public interest in honest government and exposing government officials' wrongdoing).

17. Scott Paper Co. v. United States, 943 F. Supp. 489, 499 (E.D. Pa. 1996), *aff'd*, 943 F. Supp. 501 (E.D. Pa. 1996).

context, the dissemination of legal advice is limited to employees who "need to know" given the scope of their responsibilities, and the privilege belongs to the government client-entity, not to a particular government employee.[18] This means the government entity can waive the privilege over an employee's objection. The government bears the burden of demonstrating all of the requisite elements of the privilege.

Common Interest Doctrine

Sometimes parties need to share or pool confidential information and coordinate strategies in a matter of common legal interest. The **common interest doctrine** involves multiple parties and multiple lawyers — each party having separate counsel — and is distinguishable from the "**joint client**" situation where multiple clients share a lawyer (see the Joint-Clients Exception subsection, *infra* at page 296).

The common interest doctrine treats all lawyers and clients pursuing a common legal interest as a single attorney-client unit where the pooling of information remains privileged or confidential.[19] The common interest doctrine protects attorney-client communications even when common interest members disagree on some matters but still agree to pursue one common legal interest.[20]

For communications to be privileged under the common interest doctrine, all of the usual requirements for the attorney-client privilege must be met. For example, the client's communication must be confidential, and made to a lawyer for the purpose of obtaining legal advice. However, the common interest doctrine provides a safe harbor from the general rules that the privilege does not encompass communications to a third party or communications between the lawyer for one party and the lawyer for another.

Although not uniformly followed, the Restatement notes that the common interest doctrine applies to both litigation and non-litigation situations.[21] The doctrine is sometimes referred to as the "joint defense" or "pooled information" rule.[22] The common interest doctrine promotes the policies of the attorney-client privilege by encouraging full client disclosure for effective representation. The doctrine also promotes cost-efficient representation as common interest members can share information and expenses, such as the cost of empirical studies, experts, or investigators, in pursuit of their common legal matter.

The common interest doctrine protects attorney-client communications when the privilege holder discloses them to another lawyer who represents a person

---

18. In re Cty. of Erie, 473 F.3d 413 (2d Cir. 2007).
19. Stephen A. Saltzburg, Michael M. Martin & Daniel J. Capra, 2 Federal Rules of Evidence §501.02[5][e] (11th ed. 2015) [hereinafter Evidence Manual].
20. Eisenberg v. Gagnon, 766 F.2d 770, 787-88 (3d Cir. 1985).
21. Restatement §76, at 584. *But see* Ambac Assurance Corp. v. Countrywide Home Loans, Inc., 57 N.E.3d 30 (N.Y. 2016) (common interest privilege in New York only applies to communications related to pending or anticipated litigation).
22. United States v. Gonzalez, 669 F.3d 974 (9th Cir. 2012).

in a matter of common legal interest.[23] Although the common interest doctrine should theoretically apply to (1) communications among group member clients and (2) client communications with another group member's lawyer, the safest policy is for a client's lawyer to communicate with another member's lawyer so there is no question that the communication is advancing the agreed-upon common legal interest.[24] Communications among group member clients with no lawyer present are generally not privileged.[25] One court has also rejected a common interest privilege when one common interest member spoke with another group member's lawyer without ever consulting his own lawyer before or after speaking with the other group member's lawyer.[26] The common interest privilege will not protect the confidentiality of member communications in joint strategy meetings when one member in the meeting decides to use any communication in the meeting against another member in adverse litigation.[27] Nor can one member of a common interest agreement prevent another party to the agreement from revealing work-product materials because that would enlarge work-product protection and be contrary to public policy.[28]

The common interest privilege claimant must show (1) that all clients and attorneys with access to the communication had in fact agreed upon a joint approach to the matter communicated; and (2) that the information was imparted with the intent to further the common purpose.[29] The failure to meet the requirements of the "common legal interest" doctrine may result in a court finding that the client waived the attorney-client privilege concerning the subject matter of the communication to the third lawyer. In federal courts, a party cannot seek an immediate interlocutory appeal of a court's rejection of the attorney-client privilege because disclosure is unlikely to deter clients and lawyers from seeking the benefits of full communication in their professional relationship.[30]

EXHIBIT 5.1   **Sample Joint Defense and Common Interest Agreement***

THIS JOINT DEFENSE AND COMMON INTEREST AGREEMENT (the "Agreement") is entered into by and among the undersigned Counsel, as of _____, 2010, acting for and on behalf of their respective clients ("the Parties"), each of whom is a defendant in litigation filed by _____ asserting claims of, among other things, _____. The Parties share an interest in the defense of the claims or potential claims of patent infringement concerning the _____ Patent (the "Infringement Claims"), including, without limitation, demonstrating that the _____ Patent is invalid and unenforceable and that

---

23. United States v. McPartlin, 595 F.2d 1321 (7th Cir. 1979) (noting common interest doctrine applies even when co-defendants have conflicting defenses but share a common interest in discrediting diary).
24. EVIDENCE MANUAL, *supra* note 19, §501.02[5][e].
25. United States v. Gotti, 771 F. Supp. 535, 545 (E.D.N.Y. 1991).
26. United States v. Bay State Ambulance & Hosp. Rent. Serv., 874 F.2d 20, 29 (1st Cir. 1989).
27. United States v. Almeida, 341 F.3d 1318, 1326-27 (11th Cir. 2003).
28. In re Grand Jury, 274 F.3d 563, 574-75 (1st Cir. 2001).
29. In re Teleglobe Communications Corp., 493 F.3d 345 (3d Cir. 2007).
30. Mohawk Indus. v. Carpenter, 558 U.S. 100 (2009).

the Parties do not infringe any claim of the _____ Patent. Because the undersigned wish to continue to pursue their separate but common interests and to avoid any suggestion of waiver of the confidentiality of privileged communications or documents, they hereby agree as follows:

1. **Definition of Counsel**—For purposes of this Agreement, the term "Counsel" means and includes both outside and in-house Counsel for any Party, and execution of this Agreement by either outside or in-house counsel for a Party binds that Party and all in-house and outside Counsel retained to provide legal services in connection with the Infringement Claims at any time.

2. **Defense Materials**—The Parties and their counsel have concluded that it is in each of their individual and mutual best interests in the defense of the Infringement Claims to share certain information related to that defense with some or all of Counsel and/or the Parties in writing and/or orally. These communications may include but are not limited to written communications, the disclosure of documents, factual and legal analyses, summaries, and memoranda, opinions, legal strategies, interview reports and reports of experts, consultants or investigators, joint meetings between defense counsel, the parties, their representatives and employees, and any meetings with prospective witnesses or consulting experts or litigation support service providers in connection with the litigation in person, by telephone or in any other form, and records or reports of such communications, all of which are included within the term "Defense Materials" used herein. However, nothing in this Agreement shall be construed to affect the separate and independent representation of each client by its respective Counsel.

3. **Common Interest**—The Parties and their counsel agree that all sharing and pooling of information pursuant to this Agreement will be done within the context of and in furtherance of the Parties' common goal and effort in defending against the Infringement Claims.

4. **Privileged Communications**—Some or all of the Defense Materials may be protected from disclosure to adverse or other Parties as a result of the attorney-client privilege, the work-product doctrine, or other applicable privileges, protections or immunities. It is the desire, intention, and mutual understanding of the Parties hereto (a) that the sharing of Defense Materials among one another is not intended to, and shall not, waive or diminish in any way the confidentiality of such materials or their continued protection under the attorney-client privilege, the work-product doctrine or other applicable privileges, protections or immunities; and (b) that all Defense Materials provided by a Party pursuant to this Agreement that are entitled to protection under the attorney-client privilege, the work-product doctrine or other applicable privileges, protections or immunities, shall remain entitled to such protection under the common interest doctrine, and may not be disclosed to persons other than those described in Paragraph 5 without the consent of the providing party. The Parties also intend and understand that any disclosure of Defense Materials pursuant to this Agreement will not constitute a waiver of any available privilege, protection or immunity.

5. **Disclosure of Defense Materials**—Each of the undersigned Counsel has further agreed that he or she will not disclose any exchanged Defense Materials received by him or her from another Party to this Agreement or Counsel for another Party to this Agreement to anyone except (a) in-house counsel, employees or officers of each Party who are responsible for the defense of the Infringement Claims on behalf of their employer; (b) outside Counsel of record for any Party to this Agreement; and (c) paralegals, support staff, or experts who are directly employed by or retained by and assisting

outside Counsel in the defense of the Infringement Claims. All persons permitted access to Defense Materials (collectively, "Authorized Persons") shall be specifically advised that the Defense Materials are privileged and subject to the terms of this Agreement.

6. **Limited Use of Defense Materials**—Any shared Defense Materials, and the information contained therein, are to be used by each person or Party receiving them solely in connection with the defense of the Infringement Claims. Neither the Defense Materials nor the information contained therein may be used by any person or Party receiving them for any other purpose whatsoever.

7. **Previously Exchanged Defense Materials**—All Defense Materials exchanged between and among any of the undersigned counsel pursuant to prior oral agreements or any previous joint defense agreement are now subject to this Agreement. This Agreement specifically preserves the protections afforded to those materials shared between the parties from the time that the commonality of interest came into being until execution of this Agreement under the same terms as contained in this Agreement.

8. **Privilege Not Waived**—The privileges and protections for the Defense Materials to which this Agreement is applicable may not be waived by any Party to this Agreement without the prior written consent of the Party that provided the Defense Materials. Any inadvertent or purposeful disclosure of Defense Materials exchanged pursuant to this Agreement that is made by a Party contrary to the terms of this Agreement shall not constitute a waiver of any privilege or protection. If any Party is required by court order or rule of law to produce or reveal any confidential information, documents or privileged materials which are part of the Parties' efforts pursuant to this Agreement, reasonable notice shall be given to each Party who has executed this Agreement before responding to, or complying with, such requests so that any Party may, at its own cost, have the opportunity to resist the production of such information by timely and appropriate process. In the event the Party from whom disclosure is sought has no objection to the disclosure, such Party shall nevertheless invoke this Agreement during the pendency of any action taken by the objecting Party and shall otherwise make reasonable efforts to prevent disclosure until the final resolution of the objection of the objecting Party.

9. **Withdrawal**—In the event that a Party determines that it no longer has a commonality of interest in the defense of the Infringement Claims, such Party shall withdraw from this Agreement. Each undersigned Counsel has a duty to withdraw from the Agreement when, in good faith, he or she reasonably believes that a commonality of interest no longer exists and to give prompt written notice of such withdrawal to each of the undersigned. Notwithstanding a Party's withdrawal, this Agreement shall remain operative as to: (a) all other remaining Parties to this Agreement; and (b) all previously furnished Defense Materials. Any Party may withdraw from this Agreement on written notice to all of the undersigned Counsel. Any such withdrawal will be solely on a prospective basis and any Defense Materials provided pursuant to this Agreement prior to such withdrawal shall continue to be governed by the terms of this Agreement.

10. **Settlement or Dismissal**—A party who is dismissed or settles all pending claims will be deemed to have withdrawn from the Agreement in accordance with terms of paragraph 9 as of the date of the dismissal or settlement.

11. **Modification**—The provisions of this Agreement may be modified only by written agreement of all affected Parties, and it shall be binding upon all successors and assigns of the Parties.

12. **Additional parties**—The parties recognize that other counsel and their clients may be permitted to join this Agreement at a future time by signing a copy of this Agreement. Any such additions shall be made only with the permission of all then-current signatories to this Agreement.

13. **No endorsement or authorization**—While the undersigned believe that their clients are well served by the sharing of information under this Agreement, they also understand that participation in this Agreement represents neither an endorsement of, nor an authorization to control, the defense strategy or decisions of other participating counsels' clients.

14. **Protective Order obligations**—Nothing in this Agreement shall relieve the Parties or their counsel from any obligation or obligations pursuant to the terms of any protective order or similar order entered by any court regarding the disclosure of dissemination of information pertaining to any Infringement Claims.

15. **Independent work product**—Nothing in this Agreement shall limit the right of any Party to use or disclose any documents or information or work product that have been independently obtained or generated by such Party (i.e. they were not obtained or generated as part of the common defense efforts made pursuant to this Agreement), whether or not such documents, information or work product have been provided to any other Party pursuant to this Agreement.

16. **Effect on Other Agreements**—Nothing in this Agreement shall prevent the Parties from entering into common interest agreements with other parties or among themselves, and this Agreement shall not be deemed to supersede or nullify, in whole or in part, any common interest agreement any Party has entered into prior to the date of its execution of this Agreement.

17. **Scope of Protection**—This Agreement shall be interpreted so as to afford the broadest and greatest protection possible of Defense Materials from disclosure to third parties.

18. **No Attorney-Client Relationship**—Nothing in this Agreement is intended to create any attorney-client relationship for the purposes of conflicts or otherwise. Each undersigned counsel understands that it is his or her sole responsibility to represent his or her or their respective client and that none of the other signatories to this Agreement have in any way assumed any such responsibility. Moreover, the participation in, execution or receipt of any information pursuant to this Agreement shall not disqualify any representative of a signatory (including a law firm) from accepting any other future engagement.

19. **No Admission of Liability**—Nothing in this Agreement is intended as, nor shall be construed or deemed to be, an admission of liability by any Party, or of the existence of facts upon which liability could be based.

20. **Continuing Obligation**—This Agreement shall continue in full force and effect notwithstanding any conclusion or resolution as to any Party of the Infringement Claims.

21. **Confidentiality of Terms**—The contents of this Agreement are confidential and shall not be released to any person or entity not a Party to this Agreement or as necessary to enforce the terms of this Agreement.

22. **Counterparts**—This Agreement may be signed in counterparts. All executed counterparts shall comprise the entire Agreement. This Agreement may be executed by counsel for a Party. Each counsel signing this Agreement represents that

he or she has been authorized by his or her client to execute this Agreement on behalf of the client.

IN WITNESS WHEREOF, the Parties have executed this Agreement on the dates indicated below.

By: _____   By: _____

Counsel for _____   Counsel for _____

Dated: _____   Dated: _____

---

*This agreement was originally presented as part of a panel titled "Best Practices in Multi-Defendant Litigation," at the Intellectual Property Owners Association (IPO) 2010 Annual Meeting. The following panelists who created the document have granted permission to reprint it: Moderator: "Betty" Ann Morgan, The Morgan Law Firm P.C., Atlanta, GA; William Bergmann, Baker & Hostetler, LLP, Washington, DC; Julianne Hartzell, Marshall, Gerstein & Borun LLP, Chicago, IL; and Preston K. Ratliff, Paul, Hastings, Janofsky & Walker LLP, New York, NY.

Common legal interest agreements should be memorialized in writing. Written agreements provide evidence of the nature and scope of the common legal interest, facilitate the determination of which communications relate to that nature and scope, and permit signatories to waive the use of their common interest communications in future litigation against another common interest member.[31]

Case Preview

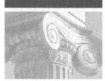

Schaeffler v. United States

The appellant, Georg F.W. Schaeffler, is the majority owner of the Schaeffler Group that sought to acquire a minority interest in a German company, Continental AG. The Schaeffler Group found a consortium (Consortium) of banks to loan it 11 billion euros for the acquisition. On July 30, 2008, the Schaeffler Group offered Continental AG shareholders a fixed price for their stock with the offer set to expire on September 16, 2008. The 2008 economic crisis caused a loss of market value for Continental AG. German law governed the acquisition and prevented Schaeffler from retracting its offer, which was oversubscribed. The oversubscription threatened the Schaeffler Group's solvency. The Schaeffler Group and the Consortium refinanced the acquisition debt and restructured the Group, which affected Schaeffler's personal tax liability to the IRS. The Group anticipated IRS scrutiny and hired a tax law firm and Ernst & Young (EY) to advise Schaeffler on federal tax implications and possible future litigation. The Group was unsuccessful in moving to quash an IRS summons for numerous documents created by EY and provided to "outside parties," including the Consortium.

---

31. EVIDENCE MANUAL, *supra* note 19, §501.02[5][e].

The Second Circuit held that the appellant, Schaeffler Group, had not waived the attorney-client privilege when it provided documents to the Consortium because they shared a "common legal interest" in the tax treatment of the refinancing and corporate restructuring caused by the acquisition.

In reading *Schaeffler*, consider the following:

1. What, if any, additional action could the appellant have taken to clarify that it was sharing communications with the Consortium not only for economic and business reasons but also to pursue a common legal strategy?
2. What weight should the court attach to a written agreement titled "Common Legal Interest" between Schaeffler and the Consortium in deciding whether the common interest privilege applies?
3. Given that financial matters often involve tax consequences, does *Schaeffler* open the door to additional common interest privilege claims in financial or corporate litigation?

Schaeffler v. United States
806 F.3d 34 (2d Cir. 2015)

BACKGROUND

A. *The Acquisition*

. . .

To finance the offer [to purchase an interest in the company, Continental AG], the Schaeffler Group executed an eleven-billion Euro loan agreement with a consortium of banks. The offer made July 30, 2008 expired on September 16, 2008. The timing of the offer was unlucky, to say the least. On September 14, 2008, two days before the offer expiration date, Lehman Brothers Holding Inc. announced its bankruptcy, the stock market collapsed, and the economic crisis worsened. The market price of Continental AG shares, already declining, fell accordingly. Because German law prohibited the Schaeffler Group from withdrawing its tender offer, far more shareholders than expected or desired accepted the offer, leaving the Schaeffler Group the owner of nearly 89.9% of outstanding Continental AG shares.

These circumstances combined to threaten the Schaeffler Group's solvency and ability to meet its payment obligations to the Consortium. As a result, appellants and the Consortium perceived an urgent need to refinance the acquisition debt and to restructure the Schaeffler Group. Because Mr. Schaeffler is an 80% owner of the ultimate parent of the Schaeffler Group, the tax consequences of his companies' debt refinancing and restructuring substantially affected his personal tax liability to the IRS. Given the complex and novel refinancing and restructuring that ensued, appellants anticipated scrutiny by the IRS. Therefore, they retained Ernst & Young ("EY") and Dentons U.S. LLP ("Dentons") to advise on the federal tax implications of the transactions and possible future litigation with the IRS.

As anticipated, the IRS began an audit of appellants that led to the issuance of the summons at issue in this appeal. The summons sought documents that were

(a) created by Ernst & Young and (b) "provided to parties outside" appellants; the summons did not therefore seek documents that were prepared by Dentons, appellant's law firm, or that were prepared by EY and shared only with appellants' counsel. The IRS specifically demanded "all documents . . . including but not limited to legal opinions, analysis and appraisals . . . that relate to [the restructuring]." Appellants produced several thousand documents in response to the information document request from the IRS but sought to quash the demand for legal opinions. For example, appellants sought to withhold memoranda, such as an EY memorandum ("EY Tax Memo") that identified potential U.S. tax consequences of the refinancing and restructuring, identified and analyzed possible IRS challenges to the Schaeffler Group's tax treatment of the transactions, and discussed in detail the relevant statutory provisions, U.S. Treasury regulations, judicial decisions, and IRS rulings.

B. The District Court's Ruling

In denying the petition to quash, the district court held that appellants had waived their attorney-client privilege by sharing the withheld documents with the Consortium. The court noted that "[b]y all accounts, the Schaeffler Group, Ernst & Young, and Dentons worked closely with the Bank Consortium not only in effectuating the refinancing and restructuring but also in analyzing the tax consequences of the [Continental AG] acquisition." The court held that the "common legal interest" or "joint defense privilege" exception to the waiver by third-party disclosure rule did not apply. In the court's view, the Consortium "lack[ed] . . . any common legal stake in Schaeffler's putative litigation with the IRS," because it would not be named as a co-defendant in the anticipated litigation and "only the Consortium's economic interests," as opposed to its legal interests, "were in jeopardy." Therefore, appellants and the Consortium did not have a common legal interest and were not "formulating a common legal strategy." Accordingly, appellants' attorney-client privilege had been waived.

. . .

DISCUSSION

A. Waiver of the Attorney-Client Privilege

We review the district court's finding of waiver of the attorney-client privilege for abuse of discretion. An abuse of discretion occurs when a district court: (i) bases a decision on an error of law or a clearly erroneous factual finding, or (ii) reaches a decision that is outside the range of permissible decisions.

The IRS summons seeks only those documents prepared by EY "that were provided to parties outside the Schaeffler Group." Because there is no evidence indicating disclosure of some or all of the documents beyond the Consortium, we need only determine the effect of disclosure to the Consortium. As noted, the district court held that appellants waived attorney-client privilege by sharing the contested documents with the Consortium because the Consortium's interest was commercial rather than legal.

The purpose of the attorney-client privilege is to enable attorneys to give informed legal advice to clients, which would be undermined if an attorney had to caution a client about revealing relevant circumstances lest the attorney later be compelled to disclose those circumstances. The privilege, and by extension the tax practitioner privilege, protects communications between a client and its attorney that are intended to be, and in fact were, kept confidential. A party that shares otherwise privileged communications with an outsider is deemed to waive the privilege by disabling itself from claiming that the communications were intended to be confidential. Moreover, the purpose of the communications must be solely for the obtaining or providing of legal advice. Communications that are made for purposes of evaluating the commercial wisdom of various options as well as in getting or giving legal advice are not protected.

While the privilege is generally waived by voluntary disclosure of the communication to another party, the privilege is not waived by disclosure of communications to a party that is engaged in a "common legal enterprise" with the holder of the privilege. Under United States v. Schwimmer, 892 F.2d 237 (2d Cir. 1989), such disclosures remain privileged "where a joint defense effort or strategy has been decided upon and undertaken by the parties and their respective counsel . . . in the course of an ongoing common enterprise . . . [and] multiple clients share a common interest about a legal matter." "The need to protect the free flow of information from client to attorney logically exists whenever multiple clients share a common interest about a legal matter."

Parties may share a "common legal interest" even if they are not parties in ongoing litigation. The common-interest-rule serves to "protect the confidentiality of communications passing from one party to the attorney for another party where a joint defense effort or strategy has been decided upon and undertaken by the parties and their respective counsel." "[I]t is therefore unnecessary that there be actual litigation in progress for the common interest rule of the attorney-client privilege to apply[.]" However, "[o]nly those communications made in the course of an ongoing common enterprise and intended to further the enterprise are protected." The dispositive issue is, therefore, whether the Consortium's common interest with appellants was of a sufficient legal character to prevent a waiver by the sharing of those communications. We hold that it was.

The original relationship between the Schaeffler Group and the Consortium arose before the economic crisis and the resultant oversubscription to the Schaeffler Group's tender offer that necessitated the refinancing and restructuring. . . . As a result of the oversubscription, the Schaeffler Group faced a threat of insolvency that would in turn cause a default on the Consortium's eleven-billion Euros loan. The Group and the Consortium could avoid this mutual financial disaster by cooperating in securing a particular tax treatment of a refinancing and restructuring. Securing that treatment would likely involve a legal encounter with the IRS. Both appellants and the Consortium, therefore, had a strong common interest in the outcome of that legal encounter.

On this record, the nature and viability of the refinancing and restructuring had a commercial component and tax law component. . . . [T]he nature and viability of the transaction was driven by U.S. tax law, and both appellants and the Consortium had a common interest in seeing that law applied in a particular way. The documents in question were all directed to the tax issues, a legal problem albeit with commercial consequences, namely the possible insolvency of the Schaeffler Group and its default on the Consortium loan. Appellants' interest was in securing a refinancing. The Consortium's interest was in funding a refinancing that would protect its earlier investment and would itself be repaid, goals dependent on the resolution of legal tax issues. The fact that eleven-billion Euros of sunken investment and any additional sums advanced in the refinancing were at stake does not render those legal issues "commercial," and sharing communications relating to those legal issues is not a waiver of the privilege.

For example, when the possibility of default loomed, the Consortium's counsel became familiar with the Schaeffler Group's organizational structure and advised it during negotiations to restructure the Group and refinance its acquisition. The Consortium needed "access to confidential tax information and analyses" to "assess its credit exposure for potential tax liabilities of Mr. Schaeffler." Together, appellants and the Consortium agreed that Appellants should request an IRS private letter ruling. With regard to issues not resolved by the letter ruling, they agreed to share "certain core tax advice prepared by the U.S. tax advisors." This information was exchanged pursuant to the confidentiality agreement.

The mutual obligations that appellants and the Consortium undertook under the agreement, reflect a common legal strategy. The Consortium agreed, subject to limitations not pertinent here, to permit Mr. Schaeffler to pay up to 885 million Euros in personal tax liabilities before repaying the Schaeffler Group's debt. It further agreed to extend him an additional line of credit to pay tax liabilities up to 250 million Euros. In return, Mr. Schaeffler's right to act unilaterally was restricted. He was required to give notice to the Consortium of any material audit or investigation. The Consortium also retained a right of refusal limiting Mr. Schaeffler's freedom of action with regard to the IRS, *e.g.* paying taxes, suing for a refund, or settling. The communications regarding tax opinions were, therefore, "made in the course of an ongoing common enterprise" and "intended to further the enterprise."

. . . It is true that cases involving criminal prosecutions usually describe the definition of a common defense strategy according to the contours of a particular charging instrument. In the context of civil proceedings, however, these cases emphasized the need of the parties to identify a common legal interest or strategy in obtaining a particular legal goal whether or not litigation is ongoing. . . .

No caselaw in this or another circuit compels us to hold that the Consortium's interest in appellants' obtaining favorable tax treatment for the refinancing and restructuring transaction is not a sufficient common legal interest. In our view, the fact that the Consortium stood to lose a lot of money (along with appellants) if appellants' tax arguments failed is not support for the position that no common legal interest existed. To the contrary, it was the interest in avoiding the losses that established a common legal interest. A financial interest of a party, no matter how large, does not preclude a court from finding a legal interest shared with another party where the legal aspects materially affect the financial interests.

For example, the Consortium's legal interest is underlined by the extent to which the Consortium essentially insured appellants, by extending credit and subordinating its debt, and retained control over Mr. Schaeffler's legal decisions to settle, pay, or sue. . . . See Travelers Cas. & Sur. Co. v. Excess Ins. Co., 197 F.R.D. 601, 607 (S.D. Ohio

2000) (holding that members of a reinsurance group facing similar environmental pollution claims by United States insurance and reinsurance companies "shared [legal] interests sufficiently common or joint to create a need for full and frank communication between and among counsel and their clients").

We, therefore, conclude that appellants did not waive their attorney-client privilege.

. . .

CONCLUSION

[Judgment vacated and remanded] "to determine [consistent with this opinion] whether any remaining documents are protected by the attorney-client privilege or work-product doctrine."

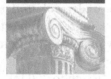

Post-Case Follow-Up

Soon after *Schaeffler*, the New York Court of Appeals issued a significant opinion clarifying the state's approach to the common legal interest doctrine in Ambac Assurance Corp. v. Countrywide Home Loans, Inc., 57 N.E.3d 30 (N.Y. 2016). The *Ambac* court noted that the Restatement and some federal appellate courts had "eliminated the common law requirement that shared communications [had to] relate to pending or anticipated litigation" to remain privileged from disclosure. The court reported nevertheless that a number of jurisdictions have not followed this expansion of the doctrine, including 11 that statutorily restrict the doctrine to communications shared in the context of ongoing litigation. *Id.* at 36 n.2. The *Ambac* court decided to take a "narrow approach" to the common legal interest doctrine by restricting it to only cases where there is pending or anticipated ligation. The *Ambac* court held that a broad construction of the common legal interest doctrine is inconsistent with the trend of liberal discovery rules and would create an obstacle to the truth-finding process by excluding pertinent information. The dissent in *Ambac* was willing to extend the common legal interest doctrine to the instant transactional setting where parties exchanged confidential information for the purpose of obtaining legal and regulatory advice to complete the merger even though there was no anticipated litigation. Ultimately, lawyers must know their jurisdiction's approach to the common legal interest doctrine because jurisdictions differ concerning the doctrine's standards and application.

Schaeffler v. United States: Real Life Applications

1. The Acme Company and Boxcar Company were engaged in merger negotiations. The two firms exchanged documents created by each company's lawyers for their respective CEOs concerning information about their patents, tax issues, and other internal corporate affairs based on a detailed confidentiality

agreement. You represent the Hercules Company in a lawsuit against the Boxcar Company. You seek some of the Boxcar documents exchanged with Acme claiming that Boxcar waived the attorney-client privilege. Advise Hercules about the likelihood of the court finding a waiver of the privilege.

2. Nordbank is the administrative agent for five lenders who agreed to loan Hickory Hill, Ltd. up to $200 million to build a condominium complex in Florida. Under the loan agreement, Nordbank is a co-lender and solely responsible for enforcing any rights or remedies in the agreement to protect all of the lenders' interests. The principals of Hickory Hill, Cohen and Smith, executed a Guaranty of Payment, which jointly and severally guaranteed full payment of any unpaid loan balance. The Florida real estate market deteriorated and Nordbank claimed that Hickory Hill defaulted on the loan. Nordbank sued Cohen and Smith for breach of contract and sought immediate repayment of the outstanding loan balance. During the course of discovery, the plaintiff withheld nine documents claiming they are privileged. In these nine documents, Nordbank's lawyer communicated directly with the CEOs of the five non-party co-lenders about the best legal strategy for obtaining relief against Cohen and Smith. The defendants filed a motion to compel the disclosure of the nine documents asserting that they are not privileged under the common legal interest doctrine because the only common interest is a business one. The defendants further asserted that even if the documents involved common legal interests, the communications from Nordbank's lawyer to the non-party lender CEOs waived the privilege because the Nordbank lawyer could only communicate with the other co-lenders' lawyers. Nordbank consults you for your opinion about whether the nine documents are privileged. Discuss your opinion.

3. Waivers

A client can waive the protection of the attorney-client privilege in several ways. The client can consent to waive the privilege or authorize agents to relinquish the privilege. For example, the client's lawyer, an agent, generally has implied authority both to waive and to assert the privilege.[32]

The client also permanently waives the privilege by voluntarily disclosing confidential communications to a third party, such as a reporter or a close friend. The client's voluntary disclosure of the communication undermines any claim that the client intended the communications to be confidential.[33]

The client's voluntary disclosure of a *fact* contained in a privileged communication does not necessarily waive the privilege, but it may be used as evidence that the client never intended the communication to be confidential.[34] For example, in

---

32. In re Pacific Pictures Corp., 679 F.3d 1121, 1126 (9th Cir. 2012); Restatement §79 cmt. b.
33. In re Pacific Pictures Corp., 679 F.3d at 1121, 1126-27; Restatement §78, at 596.
34. *See* Restatement §79, at 597-98 (reporting that the public disclosure of facts communicated in confidence to a lawyer does not waive the attorney-client privilege unless the disclosure also reveals that the facts were communicated to the lawyer).

a personal injury case a defendant made a privileged communication to his law-yer about the circumstances of an automobile accident, including a statement that "the light was red." At the subsequent trial, opposing counsel asked the client, "Did you see the light was red?"[35] The client replied, "The light was red," but disclosed no other details of his earlier privileged communication. The client's factual reply about the light being red does not constitute a waiver of his privileged communi-cation.[36] Contrast this question with a different one: "Did you tell your lawyer the light was red?" If the client replies: "Yes, I told my lawyer, 'the light was red,'" then the client will be deemed to have waived the privilege for that communication with his lawyer.[37]

Protecting the Privilege in Adversarial Proceedings and During Representation

Parties must take effective steps to protect the confidentiality of their communica-tions. For example, the failure to timely object to another party's use of privileged information in a proceeding constitutes a waiver of the attorney-client privilege.[38] Similarly, parties must object to discovery requests for documents containing priv-ileged communications to successfully assert the privilege and prevent disclosure. The lawyer's failure to take steps to protect the confidentiality of client communi-cations exposes the lawyer to malpractice and disciplinary actions for incompetent representation.

Malpractice and disciplinary claims typically result in a general waiver of privilege to all related privileged communications between the claimant and lawyer.[39] It would be unfair to allow the party to pursue claims against the lawyer for inadequate legal assistance while prohibiting the lawyer from using privileged communications necessary to defend his work. However, lawyers should never view allegations of inadequate representation as an unlimited license for them to retaliate against their clients by revealing confidences unrelated to the claims of inadequacy. For example, a lawyer who represented a client in a real estate trans-action and is then sued for malpractice related to alleged incompetence in that matter is not permitted, in retaliation, to disclose privileged communications about the client's extramarital affairs arising out of the lawyer's representation of the client in an earlier child custody dispute.

Selective Waiver

Most courts, including every federal circuit court that has considered the ques-tion except the Eighth Circuit, reject the idea of a "selective" or "limited waiver"

---

35. *See* Restatement §69 cmt. d, at 526; §79 cmt. e, at 598.
36. *See id.*
37. *See id.*
38. *Id.* §78(3), at 593.
39. In re Lott, 424 F.3d 446, 452-53 (6th Cir. 2005).

where a party voluntarily waives the privilege for communications in one case but later asserts the privilege over the same communications in a different case.[40] For example, a corporate defendant in a lawsuit brought by a government agency might selectively waive the attorney-client privilege regarding a particular communication and then claim it in a different lawsuit brought by a private litigant. Courts believe that "selective waiver" might be used abusively as a tactical maneuver and that permitting selective waivers is not necessary to accomplish the purpose of the privilege, which is to encourage full and candid communications by clients with their lawyers.[41]

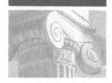

Case Preview

In re Pacific Pictures Corp.

DC Comics, a comic book publisher, sued the following parties: the heirs of the creators of Superman, an attorney who was involved in a joint venture with the heirs, and three entities in which that same attorney held a controlling interest (collectively, the "Petitioners"). DC Comics claimed that the attorney had interfered with the publisher's contractual relationships with the heirs. After the instant suit was filed, the U.S. Attorney's Office in another matter issued a grand jury subpoena for documents of the Petitioners. The government promised not to disclose the documents to non-government third parties and the Petitioners complied with the subpoena. DC Comics then sought disclosure of those same documents in the instant

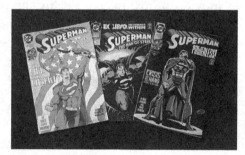

DC Comics/Superman
AP Photo/Ed Bailey

suit. The magistrate judge found the Petitioners waived the attorney-client privilege when they disclosed the documents to the government in the other matter. Thus, the magistrate ordered the Petitioners to turn over the documents to DC Comics. The Petitioners requested a writ of mandamus, seeking to overturn the district court's order. This case provided the Ninth Circuit Court of Appeals with an opportunity to consider the theory of selective waiver.

In reviewing *In re Pacific Pictures Corp.*, consider the following:

1. What facts does the court discuss concerning the lawyer's decision to voluntarily disclose otherwise privileged materials to the government?

---

40. In re Pacific Pictures Corp., 679 F.3d 1121 (9th Cir. 2012) (noting the ruling in Diversified Industries, Inc. v. Meredith, 572 F.2d 596 (8th Cir. 1978) (en banc)). DAVID M. GREENWALD, ROBERT R. STAUFFER & ERIN R. SCHRANTZ, 1 TESTIMONIAL PRIVILEGES §1:102 (3d ed. 2015).
41. In re Pacific Pictures Corp., 679 F.3d at 1121, 1127.

2. What is this court's rationale for holding that a client's voluntary disclosure of otherwise privileged materials to selected recipients constitutes a general waiver of the privilege?

3. Why does the court find that selective waiver does not serve the purpose of the attorney-client privilege?

4. Why does the court reject the Petitioners' argument that waiver should not apply to these disclosures because they were made pursuant to a government subpoena?

In re Pacific Pictures Corp.
679 F.3d 1121 (9th Cir. 2012)

We must decide whether a party waives attorney-client privilege forever by voluntarily disclosing privileged documents to the federal government. . . .

Marc Toberoff, a Hollywood producer and a licensed attorney, stepped into the fray around the turn of the millennium. As one of his many businesses, Toberoff pairs intellectual property rights with talent and markets these packages to movie studios. Having set his sights on Superman, Toberoff approached the Heirs with an offer to manage preexisting litigation over the rights Siegel and Shuster had ceded to D.C. Comics. He also claimed that he would arrange for a new Superman film to be produced. To pursue these goals, Toberoff created a joint venture between the Heirs and an entity he owned. Toberoff served as both a business advisor and an attorney for that venture. The ethical and professional concerns raised by Toberoff's actions will likely occur to many readers, but they are not before this court.

While the preexisting litigation was pending, Toberoff hired a new lawyer to work for one of his companies. This attorney remained in Toberoff's employ for only about three months before allegedly absconding with copies of several documents from the Siegel and Shuster files. Unsuccessful in his alleged attempt to use the documents to solicit business from the Heirs, this attorney sent the documents to executives at D.C. Comics. While he did not include his name with the package, he did append a cover letter, written in the form of a timeline, outlining in detail Toberoff's alleged master plan to capture Superman for himself.

. . .

In 2010, D.C. Comics filed this lawsuit against Toberoff, the Heirs, and three entities in which Toberoff owned a controlling interest (collectively, the "Petitioners"), claiming that Toberoff interfered with its contractual relationships with the Heirs. The attorney's cover letter formed the basis of the lawsuit and was incorporated into the complaint. Toberoff has continued to resist the use of any of the documents taken from his offices, including those already disclosed to D.C. Comics and especially the cover letter.

About a month after the suit was filed, Toberoff asked the Office of the United States Attorney for the Central District of California to investigate the theft [of documents from his office]. In response to a request from Toberoff, the U.S. Attorney's Office issued a grand jury subpoena for the documents as well as a letter stating that if Toberoff voluntarily complied with the subpoena the Government would "not provide the . . . documents . . . to non-governmental third parties except as may be required by law or court order." The letter also confirmed that disclosure would indicate that "Toberoff has obtained all relevant permissions and consents needed (if any) to provide the . . . documents . . . to the government." Armed with this letter, Toberoff readily complied with the subpoena, making no attempt to redact anything from the documents.

D.C. Comics immediately requested all documents disclosed to the U.S. Attorney, claiming that the disclosure of these unredacted copies waived any remaining privilege. Examining the weight of authority from other circuits, the magistrate judge agreed that a party may not selectively waive attorney-client privilege. The magistrate judge reasoned that, because a voluntary disclosure of privileged materials breaches confidentiality and is inconsistent with the theory behind the privilege, such disclosure waives that privilege regardless of whether the third party is the government or a civil litigant. Having delivered the documents to the government, the magistrate judge concluded, Petitioners could not rely on the attorney-client privilege to shield them from D.C. Comics.

. . .

III

Under certain circumstances, the attorney-client privilege will protect communications between clients and their attorneys from compelled disclosure in a court of law. . . .

Nonetheless, because, like any other testimonial privilege, this rule "contravene[s] the fundamental principle that the public has a right to every man's evidence," we construe it narrowly to serve its purposes. In particular, we recognize several ways by which parties may waive the privilege. Most pertinent here is that voluntarily disclosing privileged documents to third parties will generally destroy the privilege. The reason behind this rule is that, "'[i]f clients themselves divulge such information to third parties, chances are that they would also have divulged it to their attorneys, even without the protection of the privilege.'" Under such circumstances, there simply is no justification to shut off judicial inquiry into these communications. Petitioners concede that this is the general rule, but they assert a number of reasons why it should not apply to them.

A

Petitioners' primary contention is that because Toberoff disclosed these documents to the government, as opposed to a civil litigant, his actions did not waive the privilege as to the world at large. That is, they urge that we adopt the theory of "selective waiver" initially accepted by the Eight Circuit, Diversified Industries, Inc. v. Meredith, 572 F.2d 596 (8th Cir. 1978) (en banc), but rejected by every other circuit to consider the issue since.

As the magistrate judge noted, we have twice deferred judgment on whether we will accept a theory of selective waiver. But we share the concerns expressed by many of our sister circuits about the cursory analysis behind the *Diversified* rule. The Eighth Circuit — the first court of appeals to consider the issue — adopted what has become a highly controversial rule only because it concluded that "[t]o hold otherwise may have the effect of thwarting the developing procedure of corporations to employ independent outside counsel to investigate and advise them in order to protect stockholders." This apprehension has proven unjustified. Officers of public corporations, it seems, do not require a rule of selective waiver to employ outside consultants or voluntarily to cooperate with the government. More importantly, such reasoning does little, if anything, to serve the public good underpinning the attorney-client privilege. That is, "selective waiver does not serve the purpose of encouraging full disclosure to one's attorney in order to obtain informed legal assistance; it merely encourages voluntary disclosure to government agencies, thereby extending the privilege beyond its intended purpose."

. . .

It is not beyond our power to create such a privilege. But as doing so requires balancing competing societal interests in access to evidence and in promoting certain types of communication, the Supreme Court has warned us not to "exercise this authority expansively." Put simply, "[t]he balancing of conflicting interests of this type is particularly a legislative function."

Since *Diversified*, there have been multiple legislative attempts to adopt a theory of selective waiver. Most have failed. Given that Congress has declined broadly to adopt a new privilege to protect disclosures of attorney-client privileged materials to the government, we will not do so here. *Univ. of Pa.*, 493 U.S. at 189 (requiring federal courts to be particularly cautious when legislators have "considered the relevant competing concerns but [have] not provided the privilege").

. . .

D

Petitioners also argue that they should be treated differently because Toberoff produced these documents subject to a subpoena. Involuntary disclosures do not automatically waive the attorney-client privilege. But without the threat of contempt, the mere existence of a subpoena does not render testimony or the production of documents involuntary. Instead, whether the subpoenaed party "chose not to assert the privilege when it was appropriate to do so is [also] relevant to the waiver analysis."

Toberoff both solicited the subpoena and "chose not to assert the privilege when it was appropriate to do so. . . ." That is, even though the subpoena specifically contemplated that Toberoff may choose to redact privileged materials, he did not. Petitioners assert that the U.S. Attorney would not have been satisfied with redacted documents, but we will never know because Toberoff never tried. As such, we conclude that the district court properly treated the disclosure of these documents as voluntary. . . .

IV

Because Petitioners have not established error, we need not discuss the other . . . factors. The petition for mandamus is DENIED.

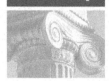

Post-Case Follow-Up

A number of federal and state cases after *In re Pacific Pictures Corp.* have rejected the concept of selective waiver. *E.g.*, Gruss v. Zwirn, 09 Civ. 6441 (PGG) (MHD), 2013 U.S. Dist. LEXIS 100012 (S.D.N.Y. July 10, 2013); Feinstein v. Keenan, No. FSTCV106007235S, 2012 Conn. Super. LEXIS 1456 (June 6, 2012). Their reasons for rejection generally track those in *In re Pacific Pictures Corp.*, for example, their concern that selective waiver "has little, if any, relation to fostering frank communication between a client and her attorney" — the public good underlying the privilege. There is also the belief that clients should not be allowed to use selective waiver for their own tactical or strategic benefit to pick and choose among opponents. Finally, there is an appreciation for the general concept that courts should construe privileges narrowly because they exclude information that might assist in the truth-finding process. Thus, these courts hold that when one voluntarily discloses privileged information to third parties, it destroys the privilege.

In one case, the court noted that the attorney-client privilege is not always waived when a party makes an involuntary disclosure. In In re Western States Wholesale Natural Gas Antitrust Litigation, 2016 U.S. Dist. LEXIS 61371 (D. Nev. May 5, 2016), the court cited *In re Pacific Pictures Corp.* for the principle that the mere issuance of a subpoena is insufficient to make a disclosure coerced or involuntary; there must also be the threat of contempt. *Western States* acknowledged, however, a contrary California evidence rule that was inapplicable but provides that a subpoena is sufficient to constitute coercion, making the disclosure involuntary and thus not waiving the privilege. It is important to check state evidence rules and cases to see what constitutes a voluntary disclosure and a waiver of the privilege in that jurisdiction.

In re Pacific Pictures Corp.: After the Case

Following the Ninth Circuit's *In re Pacific Pictures Corp.* decision rejecting selective waiver, a court granted summary judgment in favor of Toberoff finding that DC Comics' claims of tortious interference with contractual relations were barred by the statute of limitations. DC Comics v. Pacific Pictures Corp., 938 F. Supp. 2d 941 (C.D. Cal. 2013). (This ruling was appealed to the Ninth Circuit by DC Comics, but the parties settled and the case was dismissed.)

The heirs of Joe Shuster, one of the Superman creators, did not fare as well. The district court granted DC Comics' motion for summary judgment regarding the validity of the heirs' copyright termination notice. DC Comics v. Pacific Pictures Corp., No. CV 10-3633 ODW RZ, 2012 U.S. Dist. LEXIS 149532, at *9 (C.D. Cal. Oct. 17, 2012), *aff'd*, 545 F. App'x 678 (9th Cir. 2013). The United States Supreme Court refused to hear an appeal of the decision against the heirs. In 1976, Congress changed the copyright law to allow authors and their heirs to terminate previous copyright grants made prior to January 1, 1978. The purpose of the termination provision was to safeguard against unfair copyright transfers made early in an artist's career when the parties had unequal bargaining power. Such was the case with the teenage Superman creators, Jerome Siegel and Joe Shuster, who sold the rights to Superman to DC Comics in 1938 for $130. Due to public pressure, DC Comics provided pensions to the impoverished Siegel and Shuster in 1975. In 1992, Shuster's heirs entered into an agreement with DC Comics to increase the amount of the pension to $25,000 a year. The court held that the 1992 agreement superseded the 1938 copyright transfer, and regranted the copyrights to DC Comics. Thus, the heirs could not avail themselves of the Copyright Act termination provisions, because the transfer occurred after 1978.

In re Pacific Pictures Corp.: Real Life Applications

1. The defendants produced documents, including Exhibits 3, 8, 22, 25, and 34, that they wished to claw back under the court's blanket protective order concerning discovery and protection of possible privileged information. The defendants raised a generalized objection that these exhibits were protected by the attorney-client privilege. The plaintiffs filed a motion to compel re-production. Exhibits 3, 8, and 25 were entered as exhibits, formed the basis of questions, and were partially read into the record. The defendants did not object to introduction of Exhibits 22 and 34 and permitted the plaintiffs' counsel to use the exhibits to ask a witness questions. Did the defendants' conduct constitute an inadvertent waiver of the privilege?

2. During discovery, the defendant disclosed two letters written to him by his attorney. The plaintiff argued that this disclosure constituted a voluntary waiver of the defendant's attorney-client privilege and, as a result, the plaintiff asked to review all of the files and records of the defendant's attorney. The defendant maintains the letters were inadvertently disclosed by his paralegals during a large document request. The defendant argues that the privilege is only waived, if at all, regarding these two letters, and not as to other, related documents. Did the production of the two letters during discovery act as a waiver of the attorney-client privilege?

Partial Disclosures and Subject Matter Waivers

A party who voluntarily discloses a privileged communication before a factfinder, for example, in a complaint, in a pretrial proceeding or hearing, or in settlement negotiations, is deemed to have intentionally and completely waived the privilege concerning the subject matter of that particular disclosure.[42] The voluntary disclosure, however, may be misleading because it represents only a fraction of a more extensive communication on the subject matter. A party may seek all portions of a single communication and related privileged communications to prevent the opposing party from unfairly distorting the context or meaning of its partial disclosure.[43] In this situation, courts will find a general waiver of the entire subject matter of the communication or related privileged communications "that are reasonably necessary to provide a complete and balanced presentation."[44] The concern

---

42. Restatement §79 cmt. f.
43. *Id.* at 598-99.
44. *Id.* at 598. SEC v. Brady, 238 F.R.D. 429, 441 (N.D. Tex. 2006).

regarding fairness and subject matter waiver highlights a familiar refrain: that the "privilege is a shield not a sword," meaning that it is unfair to allow a party to selectively offer only a portion of a privileged communication while withholding less favorable portions.

Courts draw a distinction between testimonial and non-testimonial settings in deciding whether to find **subject matter waiver**. In a testimonial setting, there is a concern that a partial disclosure will mislead the factfinder and cause an unfair result. In a non-testimonial setting, such as pretrial discovery, there is no factfinder present to be misled and thus no need for the court to find subject matter waiver following a partial disclosure.[45] Nevertheless, a majority of courts will also find broad subject matter waiver of the privilege when a partial disclosure, even one not intended to mislead others, occurs in a non-testimonial setting or in pretrial discovery because courts expect parties who want to assert the privilege to take effective steps to prevent partial disclosure.[46] The prominent case of In re von Bulow, 828 F.2d 94 (2d Cir. 1987), suggests, however, that not all courts automatically find a broad waiver of the privilege in the non-testimonial setting, at least where the client's lawyer makes the partial disclosure.

Claus von Bülow was convicted of assault with intent to murder his wife. The Rhode Island Supreme Court reversed the conviction and he was acquitted upon retrial. Harvard Law professor Alan Dershowitz represented him on appeal. With von Bülow's consent and encouragement, in 1986, Dershowitz published his book, *Reversal of Fortune: Inside the von Bulow Case*, chronicling the case and disclosing some confidential client communications.

The decedent-wife's children from a prior marriage sued von Bülow on behalf of their mother in a civil action, alleging, in part, common law assault, negligence, and fraud. They "moved to compel discovery of certain discussions between [Claus] and his attorneys based on the alleged waiver of the attorney-client privilege with respect to those communications in the book." The Second Circuit held that von Bülow had waived the

In re von Bulow

Claus von Bülow, a Danish-German aristocrat living in London, met Sunny (née Martha Crawford), an American heiress, in the 1960s. The couple got married in 1966, soon after Sunny's divorce from the Austrian prince Alfred von Ausperg, with whom she had two children, Annie Laurie and Alexander. The von Bülows had a daughter, Cosima, in 1967, and in 1968, Claus left his position with J. Paul Getty and moved to America, to reside in Newport, Rhode Island with his family. In December 1979, Sunny slipped into a coma induced by low blood sugar, but was revived. About a year later, she suffered a brain injury that left her in a persistent vegetative state for nearly 28 years. In the meantime, the von Bülows' marriage experienced difficulties. Based *inter alia* on Annie Laurie and Alexander's suspicions, Claus was investigated as a suspect and later charged with and convicted of two counts of assault with intent to murder Sunny von Bülow by insulin injection. These convictions were reversed on appeal and Claus was acquitted upon retrial. After the acquittal, Alexander and Annie Laurie filed a civil action in federal court against Claus on behalf of their mother alleging common law assault, negligence, fraud, and RICO violations and seeking $56 million in damages. The suit was based upon the same facts as the Rhode Island criminal proceedings and ended in an out-of-court settlement in 1988. Claus agreed to divorce

---

45. Restatement §79 cmt. f, at 599.
46. *Id.*

Sunny, to renounce all claims to her fortune, to leave the country, and to relinquish all rights to write books or earn money from the case. He returned to England where he worked as an art and theater critic.

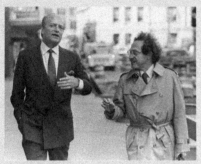

Claus von Bülow with Alan Dershowitz, who represented von Bülow on appeal.
AP Photo/Charles Krupa

privilege "as to the particular matters *actually disclosed* in the book" but that it was an abuse of discretion to broaden the waiver to include those portions of conversations that remained *undisclosed* in the book and any communications on the same or related matters. The court noted that the "fairness doctrine" would warrant a general waiver of the privilege "requir[ing] the production of the remainder" of the communications concerning the book disclosures if they were offered in litigation. The fairness doctrine does not apply, however, "when the privilege-holder or his attorney has made extrajudicial disclosures, and those disclosures have not subsequently been placed at issue during litigation."

Inadvertent Disclosures: Limiting Attorney-Client Privilege and Work-Product Waivers

Litigators fear that the disclosure of confidential communications — no matter how minimal or inadvertent — will constitute a general waiver of all communications or information concerning the subject matter of the disclosure. This fear causes additional litigation expense as lawyers carefully review discovery requests for documents and other information. The fear of subject matter waiver and related costs has exponentially increased with the advent of the electronic age and digital data.[47]

An **inadvertent disclosure** is one where the "disclosing person took precautions reasonable in the circumstances to guard against [the] disclosure" but nevertheless the communication or information was accidently disclosed.[48] The accidental disclosure may not constitute a waiver of the privilege if the client took reasonable precautions to protect the confidential nature of the communications and promptly seeks to "**claw back**" the communication and reestablish its confidentiality.[49] Determining whether reasonable precautions were taken involves looking at the importance of the content of the disclosure; the efficacy of and the availability of additional precautions; externally imposed time pressures or the volume of the required disclosure; whether the disclosure was by the client, the lawyer, or some third person; and the degree of disclosure to non-privileged persons.[50]

Federal Rule of Evidence (FRE) 502 recognizes the significant concern that lawyers have in the digital age about complying with discovery requests for large

---

47. Zubulake v. UBS Warburg LLC, 220 F.R.D. 212 (S.D.N.Y. 2003). Judge Scheindlin opined that lawyers are ethically obligated to fully and accurately comply with reasonable discovery requests for electronic communications no matter how onerous, although courts may order the requesting party to pay some of the discovery expense.
48. FRE 502; *see* Restatement §79 cmt. h, at 600.
49. *See* Gray v. Bicknell, 86 F.3d 1472, 1483-84 (8th Cir. 1996) (discussing Hydraflow, Inc. v. Enidine, Inc., 145 F.R.D. 626 (W.D.N.Y. 1993), and its five-step analysis for determining whether inadvertent disclosure constituted waiver and whether the waiver covers related documents).
50. Restatement §79 cmt. h, at 600.

amounts of information while at the same time avoiding any inadvertent disclosure that might waive the attorney-client privilege for a particular subject. FRE 502 provides, in part, that an inadvertent disclosure in federal court will not operate as a waiver in any federal or state court if the privilege holder took reasonable steps to prevent the disclosure and then also to promptly rectify the error.[51] A party's use of advanced analytical software applications and linguistic tools in screening for privilege and work-product immunity in some instances may constitute reasonable steps to prevent disclosure.[52]

A party who learns of an inadvertent disclosure should immediately request the document's return and possibly seek a protective order from the court to prevent its further use.[53] FRE 502 also permits federal judges to issue orders that preclude a waiver of the privilege or work-product immunity to assist with discovery as litigants will no longer fear losing protection for confidential information.[54] Litigants can create their own private agreements under FRE 502(e) to limit the waiver of the privilege or work-product immunity, which may be incorporated in the court order.[55]

Ardon v. City of Los Angeles

Ardon v. City of Los Angeles, 366 P.3d 996 (Cal. 2016) illustrates the concern courts have about whether inadvertent disclosures of privileged communications constitute a waiver of the attorney-client privilege or work-product immunity (*see* Section C, *infra*, discussing work-product immunity). *Ardon* involved a class action lawsuit filed against the City of Los Angeles, challenging the validity of a certain tax and seeking a refund of taxes already paid. During discovery, a city entity was served a business records subpoena pursuant to the California Public Records Act (PRA). The PRA required the release of all requested public records, unless a specified exemption applied, such as the attorney-client or work-product privileges. Further, the PRA provided that the disclosure of a public record waived such privileges, but it was unclear whether the PRA waiver provision included inadvertent disclosures.

The city informed the plaintiff that, pursuant to its production request, the city had inadvertently released three documents protected by the attorney-client and work-product privileges. The plaintiff's attorney refused to return the documents, contending that the city's release of them had waived any privilege claim.

---

51. FRE Advisory Committee Note.
52. Id. *See* Orthopaedic Hosp. v. DJO Global, Inc., No. 3:19-cv-00970-JLS-AHG, 2020 U.S. Dist. LEXIS (S.D. Cal. Sept. 8, 2020) (holding the attorney-client privilege was waived where an attorney allowed four minutes of questioning about a privileged document without objecting and then promptly seeking to claw back the disclosure as required by FRE 502; also rejecting a broader claim of subject matter waiver as to all related documents because that is reserved for unusual situations where fairness requires broader disclosure of protected information to prevent the selective and misleading presentation of evidence).
53. EVIDENCE PROBLEMS, *supra* note 5, at 490.
54. FRE 502(d). FRE 502(d) does not authorize "selective waiver" — where a litigant waives the privilege against one party but claims it against the rest of the world. CHRISTOPHER B. MUELLER & LAIRD C. KIRKPATRICK, 2 FEDERAL EVIDENCE §5.35 (4th ed. 2013). FRE 502(d) also applies to both intentional and inadvertent disclosures. *Id.*
55. FRE 502(e) (permitting parties to craft their own agreements to facilitate discovery); EVIDENCE PROBLEMS, *supra* note 5, at 490.

The city filed a motion to compel Ardon to return the documents and to disqualify the plaintiff's lawyer. The trial court determined that the city's inadvertent release of the documents waived any claim of privilege under the PRA. The Court of Appeals affirmed the trial court's decision and found that the PRA's legislative history showed it was intended to prevent selective waiver, which would occur if the city were permitted to reclaim the privilege after having already disclosed the documents to the plaintiffs.

The California Supreme Court reversed the appellate court, holding that the PRA waiver provision applied to intentional, not inadvertent, disclosures; therefore, a government entity's inadvertent release of privileged documents did not waive the privilege. The court rejected the appellate court's concern about possible selective disclosure; when there is an inadvertent release there is "no 'selection' because [the City] has not exercised choice in making the release [;][i]t was an accident." *Id.* at 1001 (internal citations omitted).

The California Supreme Court noted that construing the PRA waiver provision as excluding inadvertent disclosures of attorney-client or work-product material was consistent with the way in which the attorney-client and work-product privileges have been construed. "Both privileges serve important purposes. The former safeguards 'the confidential relationship between clients and their attorneys so as to promote full and open discussion of the facts and tactics surrounding individual legal matters.' The latter enables 'a lawyer [to] work with a certain degree of privacy, free from unnecessary intrusion by opposing parties and their counsel.'" *Id.* at 1001 (internal citations omitted).

The *Ardon* court recognized that both of these privileges can be waived under Evidence Code §912 (a), which "generally provides the attorney-client privilege 'is waived with respect to a communication protected by the privilege if any holder of the privilege, without coercion, has disclosed a significant part of the communication or has consented to disclosure made by anyone.'" However, the court also recognized that case law has construed §912 restrictively. For example, in State Compensation Ins. Fund v. WPS, Inc., 70 Cal. App. 4th 644 (1999), the court held "that 'waiver' does not include accidental, inadvertent disclosure of privileged information by the attorney." The *State Compensation Fund* court also quoted from another case in which the court found no waiver of the attorney-client privilege: "'[plaintiff] invites us to adopt a "gotcha" theory of waiver, in which an underling's slip-up in a document production becomes the equivalent of actual consent. We decline. The substance of an inadvertent disclosure under such circumstances demonstrates that there was no voluntary release.'"

As cited in *Ardon*, the *State Compensation Fund* court explained that its conclusion was "fundamentally based on the importance which the attorney-client privilege holds in the [state's] jurisprudence. . . . Without it, full disclosure by clients to their counsel would not occur, with the result that the ends of justice would not be properly served. We believe a client should not enter the attorney-client relationship fearful that an inadvertent error by its counsel could result in the waiver of privileged information or the retention of the privileged information by an adversary who might abuse and disseminate the information with impunity." *Ardon*, 366 P.3d at 1002.

The *Ardon* court also noted the practical consequences of adopting a contrary position to the rule announced in *State Compensation Fund*, given that, today

> document production may involve massive numbers of documents. A contrary holding could severely disrupt the discovery process . . . "[T]he party responding to a request for mass production must engage in a laborious, time consuming process. If the document producer is confronted with the additional prospect that any privileged documents inadvertently produced will become fair game for the opposition, the minute screening and re-screening that inevitably would follow not only would add enormously to that burden but would slow the pace of discovery to a degree sharply at odds with the general goal of expediting litigation." *Id.* at 1002-03.

4. Exceptions

There are several exceptions to the attorney-client privilege. For example, the privilege does not apply to a communication that is relevant to an issue among competing parties claiming inheritance through the same deceased client, or to a communication concerning the attestation of a document when the lawyer was the attesting witness.[56]

Exceptions are distinguishable from waivers because exceptions involve situations that preclude a finding that the privilege ever arose or existed to protect the communications from disclosure. In contrast, with waivers the elements for a valid privilege arose or existed but the client's subsequent conduct rendered the privilege lost or ineffective.[57] There are three noteworthy exceptions: the crime-fraud exception, the exception for joint clients, and the exception for self-defense.

Crime-Fraud Exception

The **crime-fraud exception** to the attorney-client privilege provides that a client's confidential communications with counsel are not protected from disclosure when made for the purpose of furthering a crime or fraud. The purpose of the privilege is to promote the client's full disclosure and observance of the law, not to allow clients to use lawyers for unlawful purposes.

It is the client's, not the lawyer's, intention to commit the crime or fraud, now or in the future, which ultimately determines whether the client's communications are privileged.[58] Even if the intended crime or fraud never takes place, the client's intent alone triggers the crime-fraud exception and requires disclosure; it does not matter whether the lawyer unwittingly participated in the client's scheme.[59] Discerning client intent is a fact-based and sometimes difficult inquiry.

---

56. *See* Proposed FRE 503(d)(2) & (4); Restatement §81, at 612-13.
57. Squire, Sanders & Dempsey, L.L.P. v. Givaudan Flavors Corp., 937 N.E.2d 533 (Ohio 2010); *see* In re Lott, 424 F.3d 446 (6th Cir. 2005).
58. EVIDENCE MANUAL, *supra* note 19, §501.02[5][l][iii], at 501-64-66; Restatement §82(a), at 613-14. The Restatement also provides that the "crime-fraud exception applies even if the client's purpose was benign at the time of consultation, but later the client used the consultation to commit a crime or fraud." Restatement §82(b) cmt. c. & Reporter's Note at 613-14.
59. EVIDENCE MANUAL, *supra* note 19, §501.02[5][l][iii].

The crime-fraud exception does not apply to client communications concerning the criminal propriety of a proposed course of conduct.[60] The privilege is designed to encourage clients to consult with lawyers about their future conduct to promote compliance with the law. The exception is triggered, however, when the client approaches the lawyer with a preconceived plan that he knows is criminal or fraudulent and uses the lawyer to implement it.[61]

Client disclosure of a past crime or fraud does not trigger the crime-fraud exception.[62] Client communications intended to help the lawyer defend the client's past or current conduct are also privileged. But communications aimed at covering up past or ongoing criminal conduct are not privileged.[63]

The party challenging the applicability of the attorney-client privilege bears the burden of establishing a prima facie case that the client intended his communications to further a crime or fraud. In United States v. Zolin, 491 U.S. 554 (1989), the Supreme Court did not decide the quantum of proof necessary to make the "threshold" or prima facie showing, but it noted "many blatant abuses of privilege which cannot be substantiated by extrinsic [or independent] evidence." Accordingly, the Court held that judges may examine the allegedly privileged statements *in camera* and outside the presence of the party asserting the crime-fraud exception to determine the exception's applicability. The Court also held that "before a district court may engage *in camera* review, . . . the party opposing the privilege . . . must present evidence to support a reasonable belief that *in camera* review may yield evidence that establishes the exception's applicability." Although the Court rejected the view that only evidence independent of the alleged privileged communications could be used in making a prima facie showing for the crime-fraud exception, independent evidence remains important. Examples of independent evidence include a prosecutor's statements or good faith affidavit about testimony already presented to the grand jury or a corporate employee's self-serving testimony that corporate counsel asked him to commit perjury.[64]

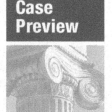

Case Preview

In re Grand Jury Investigation

In *In re Grand Jury Investigation*, the appellant corporation operated a call center that marketed surgical devices to medical centers. The FDA believed that the corporation's advertising violated the Food, Drug, and Cosmetics Act by not providing relevant risk information about the devices. The government believed that the corporation's lawyers' responses to FDA letters contained false statements designed to distract the investigators. Under the crime-fraud exception, the grand jury issued subpoenas to three lawyers

---

60. *See* In re Grand Jury Proceedings (Corporation), 87 F.3d 377, 381 (9th Cir. 1996).
61. EVIDENCE MANUAL, *supra* note 19, §501.02[5][l][iii].
62. *See* In re Grand Jury Proceedings (Corporation), 87 F.3d at 377, 381.
63. *See* In re Sealed Case, 754 F.2d 395, 403 (D.C. Cir. 1985); EVIDENCE MANUAL, *supra* note 19, §501.02(5)(l)(iii).
64. In re Grand Jury Investigation of Schroeder, 842 F.2d 1223 (11th Cir. 1987); White v. American Airlines, 915 F.2d 1414 (10th Cir. 1983).

to produce, among other items, all communications, including documents, notes, and the sources of the information, relating to their FDA correspondence. The lawyers did not fully comply with the subpoena. In a matter of first impression in the circuit, the court held that the district court had committed an error when it ordered the defendants to produce all attorney-client documents without *in camera* review to determine whether they were made in furtherance of a contemplated or ongoing crime or fraud.

In reading *In re Grand Jury Investigation*, consider the following questions:

1. What two-part test did the court use to determine the applicability of the crime-fraud exception?
2. Does the court require an *in camera* review of communications to establish the first part of the crime-fraud exception test?
3. What requirement does the court impose on district courts to comply with the second part of the crime-fraud exception test?

In re Grand Jury Investigation
810 F.3d 1110 (9th Cir. 2016)

I

Appellant Corporation was a call center that marketed a surgical device for medical facilities. In December 2010, the director and health officer for Los Angeles County Public Health sent a letter to the FDA raising concerns that the Corporation's advertisements (large billboards, bus placards, and direct mail) were "inadequately inform[ing] consumers of potential risks" of the surgical device. After the Corporation received this letter from a local columnist, the company — through counsel — sent its own letter to the FDA disputing many of the letter's assertions and attempting in various ways to dissuade the FDA from investigating.

Despite the attorney's letter, the FDA opened an investigation and sent warning letters to the Corporation and a few medical centers in California. The letters stated that the FDA believed the Corporation's advertising violated the Food, Drug, and Cosmetic Act (FDCA) by not providing "relevant risk information regarding the use of the [device], age and other qualifying requirements for the [surgical] procedure, and the need for ongoing modification of [lifestyle] habits." New counsel for the Corporation responded by letter to the FDA warning letter. A third attorney responded on behalf of the medical centers.

The government alleged that these responses contained false statements designed to obstruct the FDA investigation. Under the crime-fraud exception to attorney-client privilege, grand jury subpoenas were issued to the three lawyers to produce "(1) all communications relating to their correspondence to the FDA, including documents and notes showing the information received and identifying the sources of information for the statements and representations made and (2) retainer agreements and billing records identifying the client(s) who retained and paid for their services in communicating with the FDA on the subject matter of the correspondence."

The attorneys provided some information, but they did not fully comply with the subpoenas.

The government filed a motion to compel compliance with the subpoenas. Without reviewing any documents in camera, the district court determined from independent, non-privileged evidence that the government had established a prima facie case that the lawyers' services were obtained "in furtherance of and . . . sufficiently related to ongoing" crimes, i.e., false statements to and obstruction of the FDA. The district court rejected the argument that in camera review of the privileged documents was necessary to determine whether the government established a prima facie case of crime-fraud. The district court granted the government's motion to compel production of all "matters identified in the subpoenas."

II

While the attorney-client privilege is "arguably most fundamental of the common law privileges recognized under Federal Rule of Evidence 501," it is "not absolute." In re Napster, Inc. Copyright Litig., 479 F.3d 1078, 1090 (9th Cir. 2007). Under the crime-fraud exception, communications are not privileged when the client "consults an attorney for advice that will serve him in the commission of a fraud" or crime. *Id.* To invoke the crime-fraud exception, a party must "satisfy a two-part test":

> First, the party must show that "the client was engaged in or planning a criminal or fraudulent scheme when it sought the advice of counsel to further the scheme." Second, it must demonstrate that the attorney-client communications for which production is sought are "sufficiently related to" and were made "*in furtherance of* [the] intended, or present, continuing illegality."

Id.

Appellants first contend that the district court could not find a prima facie case of crime-fraud without examining the privileged documents in camera. The district court correctly rejected this contention. District courts may find a prima facie case of crime-fraud either by examining privileged material in camera or by examining independent, non-privileged evidence.

As *In re Napster* stated, however, the existence of a prima facie case is only step one of the inquiry. In this case, the government relied on independent, non-privileged evidence to establish reasonable cause that the attorneys were enlisted to make false statements to the FDA. No evidence has been presented regarding the second step in the analysis: whether "the attorney-client communications for which production is sought are 'sufficiently related to' and were made 'in furtherance of [the] intended, or present, continuing illegality.'" In re Napster, 479 F.3d at 1090. Thus far, the litigation has not focused on any individual documents. Instead, the district court broadly ordered the attorneys to produce everything identified in the government's subpoenas, without first examining any specific documents in camera to determine whether they contained communications in furtherance of the asserted crime-fraud.

. . .

[W]e agree with the Sixth Circuit. While in camera review is not necessary during step one to establish a prima facie case that "the client was engaged in or planning a criminal or fraudulent scheme when it sought the advice of counsel to further the scheme," a district court must examine the individual documents themselves to determine that the specific attorney-client communications for which production is sought are "sufficiently related to" and were made "in furtherance of the intended, or present, continuing illegality."

For these reasons, we VACATE and REMAND the order compelling production of all subpoenaed documents so the district court may examine the documents in camera to determine the proper scope of the production order, i.e., which documents contained communications in furtherance of the crime-fraud.

Post-Case Follow-Up

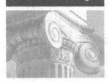

In re Grand Jury Investigation followed the U.S. Supreme Court's well-established approach in United States v. Zolin, 491 U.S. 554 (1989), that requires courts to conduct an *in camera* review of specific privileged documents to determine whether they further a crime or fraud and thus are excepted from the attorney-client privilege. *In re Grand Jury Investigation* also represents one approach to an issue left unresolved in *Zolin*: whether a court also has to conduct an *in camera* review of privileged documents to establish the prerequisite finding of a crime or fraud for the application of the crime-fraud exception. The *In re Grand Jury Investigation* approach of not requiring the court to conduct an *in camera* review to establish a crime or fraud seems to strike a reasonable balance between competing interests. It conserves the court's and litigants' time and resources while also protecting the attorney-client privilege by requiring the court, after a prerequisite finding of a crime or fraud, to conduct an *in camera* review of specific communications before ordering their disclosure.

In re Grand Jury Investigation: Real Life Applications

1. Over a year ago, a high-ranking political figure from a poor nation met with Attorney Fonseca in his New York City law office. The politician asked Fonseca how he could "discreetly" bring large sums of money into the United States for the purchase of valuable real estate and manufacturing businesses. The client wanted to avoid publicity and insisted that Fonseca handle everything. The client preferred to transact business on a cash-only basis. Fonseca helped the client with several transactions. The U.S. Attorney has charged Fonseca with money laundering and has asked him for all of his documents regarding this client as well as disclosure of the nature of their communications. The government told Fonseca that if he cooperates, he will not be charged with a crime. Fonseca believes that the documents and communications are protected by the attorney-client privilege, but he wants to know whether he can make the disclosures to avoid criminal charges. He contacts you, a professional responsibility and criminal defense lawyer, for advice. Advise Fonseca.

2. Imagine that the CEO of a small local bank recently retired from his position. The new CEO is a friend of yours and consults you about possible financial improprieties by the former CEO. When you contact the former CEO, he says that he relied on the advice of the bank's lawyer at the time. The former CEO and that lawyer refuse to disclose their communications about the legal propriety of the former CEO's financial dealings, claiming that the dealings are protected by the attorney-client privilege. Are the former CEO and the lawyer correct?

Joint-Clients Exception

The **joint-clients exception** recognizes that sometimes multiple clients with a common legal interest may want the same lawyer to represent them. Joint representation offers the clients and the lawyer potential savings in time and expense. Joint representation also offers the strategic benefit of a unified defense, making it less likely that the opposing party can succeed with a "divide and conquer" approach.

The joint-clients exception provides that a communication to a lawyer that is relevant to a matter of common interest between the joint clients is not privileged when one joint client proceeds against another joint client. To illustrate, clients A and B retain Attorney Jones to defend them in a common matter involving defamation. A's and B's communications to Jones, whether communicated separately or in a joint conference, are privileged from any third-party disclosure request. However, the privilege will not prevent client A from offering her or client B's confidential communications to their joint attorney in a subsequent action by client A against client B.

Self-Defense Exception

The attorney-client privilege does not protect confidential communications related to a client's action against his counsel concerning the quality of his representation.[65] Fairness requires that the lawyer be able to use these communications to defend herself against client allegations of lawyer malpractice, ineffective assistance of counsel, and other misconduct.[66] The lawyer is permitted to disclose only privileged client communications necessary to defend herself against the client's claims of misconduct. The lawyer should not use the **self-defense exception** as an excuse to retaliate against the client by disclosing communications unrelated to the client's claims of misconduct. Some courts permit the lawyer under this exception to use confidential communications to establish a claim for compensation against the client.[67]

---

65. EVIDENCE MANUAL, *supra* note 19, §501.02[5][l][i].
66. *Id.*
67. *Id.*

C. WORK-PRODUCT IMMUNITY

Work-product immunity prevents the discovery of mental impressions, conclusions, opinions, or legal theories of attorneys or their representatives involved in or preparing for litigation.[68] Work-product immunity at the federal level is found both in **Rule 26(b)(3) of the Federal Rules of Civil Procedure** and in federal common law.[69] Most states have codified the immunity doctrine in statutes or court rules.[70]

Work-product immunity reflects, in part, the belief that even with liberal discovery rules, the truth-seeking process is best advanced by a competitive and confidential development of facts and legal information by opposing parties.[71] The immunity promotes client interests in diligent legal assistance because lawyers know that their work is beyond the reach of opposing parties who may appropriate or "free ride" on their diligent preparations for litigation.[72]

The Restatement (Third) of the Law Governing Lawyers notes that immunity applies when there is a reasonable *anticipation* of litigation, which requires an objective examination of the facts surrounding the preparation and nature of the materials and the role of the lawyer.[73] The *actual* commencement of litigation is not a prerequisite for successfully asserting work-product protection. Litigation includes any adversarial proceeding in which parties contest factual issues or present competing legal arguments, such as criminal and civil trials, proceedings before administrative agencies, claims commissions, and arbitration panels and mediations.[74]

Work-product immunity covers the lawyer's preparation, collection, and assembly of tangible evidence or its intangible equivalents.[75] For example, tangible work product would include the lawyer's photographs of an accident, photographs of the accident that the lawyer collected from a bystander, or pictures the lawyer assembled from a magazine that covered the accident. Other tangible work product can include written notes, for example of witness interviews; financial and other analyses; computer databases; electronic recordings; tapes; surveys; and diagrams.[76] Intangible equivalents of the same work in unwritten, oral, or remembered form are also entitled to work-product protection.[77] For example, the lawyer's unrecorded recollection of a witness's description of an automobile accident would be protected from discovery under work-product immunity.[78]

---

68. Evidence Problems, *supra* note 5, at 488.
69. Hickman v. Taylor, 329 U.S. 495 (1947).
70. Restatement §87, at 640.
71. *Id.* at 638.
72. *Id.*
73. *Id.* at 642; Schaeffler v. United States, 806 F.3d 34, 43-45 (9th Cir. 2015).
74. Restatement §87, at 641.
75. In re Cendant Corp. Sec. Litig., 343 F.3d 658 (3d Cir. 2003).
76. *Id.*
77. *Id.*
78. Restatement §87, at 640-41.

1. Two Types of Work Product: Ordinary and Opinion

Work product falls into two general categories: ordinary and opinion. **Ordinary work product,** for example, a witness's statement to the lawyer, written or oral, would generally be immune from discovery. The immunity is not absolute, however. The court can compel the lawyer's disclosure of the witness's statement if the inquiring party can show (1) a substantial need for the material in order to prepare for trial, and (2) that the party is unable without undue hardship to obtain the substantial equivalent of the material by other means.[79] For example, a lawyer's notes of the only eyewitness statements about an accident probably warrant disclosure under the "**substantial need–undue hardship**" exception to work-product immunity if the witness died recently. There is a substantial need for the eyewitness's testimony since she saw the accident and any other way of obtaining the information would impose an undue hardship since the eyewitness is dead. The party seeking disclosure should be able to show that she will likely be prejudiced by the absence of discovery of the eyewitness's statements.[80]

Opinion work product includes the lawyer's mental impressions, opinions, and strategy in litigation — often referred to as the "core" work product. For example, the lawyer retains an undisclosed trial consultant to develop a psychological plan for winning the case and attacking the credibility of the opposing party's key witnesses. The consultant will not testify but meets with witnesses and sends the lawyer a document containing a psychological roadmap for winning the case. The lawyer adds some notes reflecting his mental impressions of the roadmap and his thoughts about how to implement the roadmap. The consultant's document, the contents of his discussion with witnesses, and the lawyer's additional notes are considered opinion work product.[81] Opinion work product is extremely difficult to obtain. The inquiring party must show extraordinary circumstances to justify disclosure — a standard that the Restatement notes has never been intelligibly defined.[82]

2. Waivers and Exceptions to Work-Product Immunity

Parties or their agents can agree to waive work-product immunity.[83] A party who fails to object in a tribunal to another person attempting to offer work-product evidence waives the immunity.[84] Waiver also occurs when the holder of the immunity discloses the work product to third parties and there is a "significant likelihood that

---

79. Baker v. Gen. Motors Corp., 209 F.3d 1051 (8th Cir. 2000).
80. Restatement §88 cmt. b, at 651.
81. In re Cendant Corp. Sec. Litig., 343 F.3d at 658 (holding that it was opinion work product when a trial consultant, here Dr. Phil McGraw who now hosts a television show, prepares a trial plan and talks with witnesses; an attorney's tactical planning is considered opinion work product).
82. Restatement §89 cmt. b, at 656.
83. *Id.* §91, at 661-62.
84. *Id.*

an adversary or potential adversary in anticipated litigation will obtain it."[85] A party waives immunity if the material is used to aid or impeach a witness or when the party alleges in a proceeding that the lawyer was ineffective or negligent, or otherwise committed misconduct. Work-product immunity does not protect material if the client uses the work product in furtherance of a crime or fraud that is later accomplished.[86]

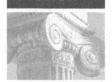

Case Preview

Schaeffler v. United States

Recall our discussion of the corporate acquisition in *Schaeffler*, *supra* at page 273. In that case, the Schaeffler Group was unsuccessful in moving to quash an IRS summons for numerous documents created by EY and provided to "outside parties," including the Consortium. In reviewing *Schaeffler v. United States*, consider the kinds of evidence the appellant offered to show that the documents were prepared in anticipation of litigation.

Further, consider the following:

1. What additional kinds of evidence might support such a finding in other cases?
2. Did this case involve ordinary or opinion work product?
3. What is the significance of designating work product as ordinary or opinion?
4. What are the potential costs or disadvantages to the IRS in pursuing its case against Schaeffler given the court's ruling that the EY Tax Memo and other documents are protected by the work-product immunity?

Schaeffler v. United States
806 F.3d 34 (2d Cir. 2015)

BACKGROUND

A.

[The full statement of facts in *Schaeffler v. United States* is provided in this chapter at pages 274-278.]

---

85. *Id. See* United States v. Sanmina Corp., 968 F.3d 1107 (9th Cir. 2020) (holding, in part, that a party's disclosure of its in-house corporate counsel memoranda to a firm helping that party with an IRS matter was not an express waiver of the work-product rule because it was not a disclosure to an adversary nor "conduct inconsistent with maintaining secrecy against an adversary" (here, the IRS) (*id.* at 1125); also holding that when the party used the firm's report containing a footnote to the memoranda during the investigation, the court concluded that while "the fairness principle does not require the categorical disclosure" of the memoranda, the party implicitly waived work-product protection to the factual portions of the memoranda but not to any opinion work product — i.e., the in-house attorneys' "mental impressions, conclusions, opinions, or legal theories" (*id.* at 1126)).
86. Restatement §93, at 673.

B. District Court's Ruling

. . .

[T]he district court held that the EY Tax Memo and, presumably, other similar documents were not entitled to work-product protection. After conducting an *in camera* review of the EY Tax Memo, the district court described it as containing: (i) "detailed legal analysis of the federal tax issues implicated," (ii) "assert[ions] that there is no law clearly on point," (iii) "language such as 'although not free from doubt,' 'the better view is that,' 'it may be argued,' and 'it is not inconceivable that the IRS could assert'"; and (iv) "arguments and counter-arguments that could be made by Schaeffler and the IRS with regard to the appropriate tax treatment of [the refinancing and restructuring]."

The district court noted that the EY Tax Memo "does not specifically refer to litigation . . . by discussing what actions peculiar to the litigation process [the parties] might take or what settlement strategies might be considered." The court concluded that appellants would have engaged in the "detailed and complex process of resolving" the unusual tax issues even if they did not anticipate any litigation. It reasoned that "Schaeffler is a rational businessperson" who "would have sought out the type of tax advice provided by Ernst & Young about the transaction had he not been concerned about an audit or litigation with the IRS." Because "any sophisticated businessperson engaging in a complex financial transaction will naturally wish to obtain advice on the relevant tax laws so that the transaction can be structured in such a way as to receive the most favorable tax treatment possible," the court ruled that, "given our assumption that Schaeffler is a rational businessperson who routinely makes efforts to comply with the law, we find that, even had he not anticipated an audit or litigation with the IRS, he still would have had to obtain the type of legal assistance provided by Ernst & Young to carry out the refinancing and restructuring transactions in an appropriate manner."

The court further stated that "petitioners have presented no facts suggesting that Ernst & Young would have acted any differently" or given advice "different in content or form had it known that no audit or litigation would ensue." . . . The court also relied on its view that the language of the EY Tax Memo did not "indicate that the authors are describing any particular anticipated litigation," notwithstanding the document's detailed discussion of legal strategies. Accordingly, the court ruled that the EY Tax Memo and related documents were not protected from disclosure under the work-product doctrine.

. . .

C. Application of Work-Product Doctrine

[W]e address only the district court's view that the EY Tax Memo and related documents were not entitled to work-product protection.

Attorney work product is of course protected from discovery. *See* Hickman v. Taylor, 329 U.S. 495 (1947); *see also* Fed. R. Civ. P. 26(b)(3). The doctrine "is intended to preserve a zone of privacy in which a lawyer can prepare and develop legal theories and strategy with an eye toward litigation, free from unnecessary intrusion by his adversaries." Documents prepared in anticipation of litigation are work product, even when they are also intended to assist in business dealings. We review the district court's ruling on a work-product claim for abuse of discretion.

The district court acknowledged that the EY Tax Memo was prepared at a time when appellants believed litigation was highly probable and contained analyses of the strengths, weaknesses, and likely outcomes of potential legal arguments. Nevertheless, the court found that appellants would have sought and received advice "created in essentially similar form" even if they had not anticipated litigation. On this ground, the court denied work-product protection.

Adlman is the governing precedent. It established a test to determine whether documents should be deemed prepared "in anticipation of litigation" and therefore subject to work-product protection. A document will be protected if, "in light of the nature of the document and the factual situation in the particular case, the document can fairly be said to have been prepared or obtained *because of* the prospect of litigation." Conversely, protection will be withheld from "documents that are prepared in the ordinary course of business or that would have been created in essentially similar form irrespective of the litigation." The district court's application of the "ordinary course of business" or "essentially similar form" example to the documents at issue in this appeal appears to us to virtually swallow the work-product protection *Adlman* extended to documents "prepared or obtained because of the prospect of litigation."

Adlman held that work-product protection would be withheld only from documents that were prepared in the ordinary course of business in a form that would not vary regardless of whether litigation was expected. In the present case, such records would include the supporting records and papers that appellants' external tax return preparers collected and created in the ordinary course of annually completing appellants' federal tax returns.

The tax advice in the EY Tax Memo was quite different. It was specifically aimed at addressing the urgent circumstances arising from the need for a refinancing and restructuring and was necessarily geared to an anticipated audit and subsequent litigation, which was on this record highly likely. *See Adlman*, 134 F.3d at 1195 (predicted litigation was virtually inevitable because of size of transaction and losses).

We also disagree with the district court's characterization of the form of the advice EY would be ethically and legally required to give appellants even in the absence of anticipated litigation. Neither professional standards, tax laws, nor IRS regulations required that appellants' tax advisors provide the kind of highly detailed, litigation-focused analysis and advice included in the EY Tax Memo. The standards relied upon by the district court all target concerns over the "audit lottery," in which aggressive tax advisors might recommend risky tax positions solely because the particular clients were statistically unlikely ever to be audited. That policy concern is simply not implicated here where appellants would not have sought the same level of detail if merely preparing an annual routine tax return with no particular prospect of litigation.

Finally, we address the district court's construct of a hypothetical scenario in which appellants faced exactly the same business and tax issues but did not anticipate litigation. This scenario appears to us to ignore reality. The size of a transaction and the complexity and ambiguity of the appropriate tax treatment are important variables that govern the probability of the IRS's heightened scrutiny and, therefore, the likelihood of litigation. To hypothesize the same size of the transaction and the same complexity and ambiguity of the tax issues but also a lack of any anticipation of litigation posits a factual situation at odds with reality. . . .

Finally, we note that the district court's holding appears to imply that tax analyses and opinions created to assist in large, complex transactions with uncertain tax consequences can never have work-product protection from IRS subpoenas. This is contrary to *Adlman*, which explicitly embraces the dual-purpose doctrine that a document is eligible for work-product protection "if 'in light of the nature of the document and the factual situation in the particular case, the document can fairly be said to have been prepared or obtained *because of* the prospect of litigation.'"

In our view, the EY Tax Memo contains "legal analysis that falls squarely within [Hickman v. Taylor, 329 U.S. 495 (1947)]'s area of primary concern — analysis that candidly discusses the attorney's litigation strategies [and] appraisal of likelihood of success." They are therefore, protected under the work-product doctrine.

CONCLUSION

[Judgment vacated and remanded] "to determine [consistent with this opinion] whether any remaining documents are protected by the attorney-client privilege or work-product doctrine."

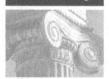

Post-Case Follow-Up

The question in *Schaeffler* about whether the documents were prepared in anticipation of litigation and therefore entitled to work-product immunity is a common one. The standard that is widely cited by courts for answering this question is "whether in light of the nature of the document, and the factual situation in the particular case, the document can fairly be said to have been prepared or obtained because of the prospect of litigation."[87] The *Schaeffler* court focused on the detailed legal advice in the challenged document, including possible legal strategies, and the likelihood of an IRS proceeding. These facts played a key role in the court's finding that the documents were prepared in anticipation of litigation. The *Schaeffler* formula of legal advice, including possible legal strategies and the likelihood of an adversarial proceeding, are important considerations for litigators as they attempt to protect their work and efforts in preparation for litigation. Litigators need to create and preserve evidence to demonstrate compliance with the *Schaeffler* formula. The requirement that work product be in anticipation of litigation is highly fact specific and promises to consume the attention of both litigators and the courts.

---

87. *Id.* §87 cmt. i, at 649 (citing 8 C. WRIGHT, A. MILLER & R. MARCUS, FEDERAL PRACTICE AND PROCEDURE 343 (2d ed. 1994)).

Schaeffler v. United States: Real Life Applications

1. An elementary school teacher is accused of sexually molesting students over several years. Criminal charges are filed against the teacher and several victims sue the principal and school district, claiming that the defendants knew about the alleged abuse but took no action. The school district hired the Smith law firm to investigate the incident. The district's lawyers interviewed 100 people and took only written notes of each interview. The firm summarized its findings in memoranda sent to the district. The Smith firm does not represent the defendants in this litigation. The plaintiffs issue a subpoena for the firm's notes and other internal legal memoranda in its possession concerning its investigation. The Smith firm refuses to produce the documents, relying on the attorney-client privilege and the work-product doctrine. The plaintiffs argue that the law firm was hired to provide only investigative services and not legal advice. How should the judge rule on the Smith claim that (a) the attorney-client privilege protects the documents and (b) that work-product immunity protects the documents?

2. Using the facts above, assume that the district's new litigation firm, Jones and Dower, retains a school-security expert who will testify that the defendant-district's conduct was appropriate in the above sexual molestation case. The security expert submits an expert report. The plaintiffs request the expert's three preliminary drafts of his final expert report. Jones and Dower refuses to comply and claims the preliminary drafts are protected by work-product immunity. How should the court rule on the Jones and Dower claim?

Chapter Summary

FIGURE 5.1   Three Circles of Lawyer "Secrets"

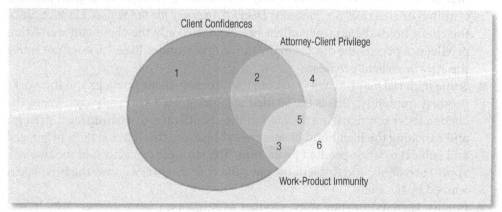

- It may be helpful to think of the three sources of client secrecy as interlocking but not coterminous circles. Look at the diagram above and review the material in this chapter by reference to the number in each section of the circle.

■ The largest circle, designated #1, is the protection for client confidences under Model Rule 1.6. This is the largest of the three circles because all information that the lawyer learns while representing a client on any type of matter, regardless of its source, is confidential, unless the client has given express or implied authorization for its disclosure.

■ The next circle, #2, is the attorney-client privilege, a creature of evidence law. The attorney-client privilege furthers the policy of encouraging clients to make full and candid disclosures to their lawyers and of encouraging lawyers to provide solid and effective advice to their clients. This circle is smaller than the protection for client confidences circle because the privilege applies only to information communicated directly between the client and the lawyer for the purposes of legal advice — not to preexisting documents, and not to information gathered by the lawyer from third parties. The client holds the attorney-client privilege and ultimately must decide whether to assert it or waive it. There are exceptions to the privilege — most notably for litigation between the client and the attorney (the "self-defense" exception) and the crime-fraud release. Corporations and other legal entities may claim the attorney-client privilege, but the privilege belongs to the corporation and not to its constituents.

■ The third circle, #3, is the work-product immunity. This provides qualified protection from discovery for documents that contain the mental impressions, opinions, and conclusions of lawyers during litigation. This is the smallest of the three circles because work-product immunity applies only to attorneys and agents involved in *litigation or anticipated litigation*; to documents or tangible things (photographs, charts) prepared by the lawyer or his agents (not documents prepared by the client); and to documents or tangible things that somehow contain or memorialize the mental impressions of the lawyer. There is both "ordinary" and "opinion" work product.

■ The section of attorney-client circle privilege that extends beyond the rule of confidentiality (shaded area #4) reflects the fact that a lawyer may engage in a permissive disclosure of confidential information under Rule 1.6, but the information obtained from the client will still remain privileged if subpoenaed in a criminal or civil case. *See Purcell v. District Attorney for the Suffolk District.* Since the client holds the attorney-client privilege and only the client can waive that privilege, a permissive disclosure by the attorney under Rule 1.6 does not waive the attorney-client privilege.

■ Some material may be subject to both the attorney-client privilege and the work-product immunity. This is the shaded area designated #5. If a lawyer writes the client a letter summarizing the facts of the client's case, discussing legal strategy, and assessing the likelihood of success in litigation, this letter is both privileged and subject to work-product protection. The stronger protection of the two will apply (privilege), and this letter is not subject to discovery unless the privilege is waived by the client.

■ Finally, there is attorney work product in litigation that is neither confidential under Rule 1.6 nor privileged under the rules of evidence (shaded area #6). If a lawyer handling a products liability case asks his associate to read and summarize every products liability decision from the state supreme court in the past 20 years, the associate's memo — if it contains pure legal research and no facts communicated from the client or gathered from third parties — is neither confidential under Rule 1.6 nor privileged under the rules of evidence. Nonetheless, it is the work product of the law firm and it would be protected in discovery during litigation as "opinion" rather than "ordinary" work product.

Applying the Rules

1. Imagine that you work for a law firm that represents one of the nation's largest sports equipment and apparel companies. You have just been asked to work on an endorsement contract under which a major recording artist has tentatively agreed to appear in radio and television commercials endorsing your client's products. The corporation has also agreed to manufacture and market a new sports clothing line bearing the trade name of the recording artist. You are working on all the licensing and trademark agreements. The deal has not yet been made public. You are very excited about this new assignment and confident that it will be challenging and rewarding. Assume that you are out to dinner with your best friend from law school. She asks, "What's new at work?" What can you tell her about your new assignment, if anything?

2. Art Gorski, a non-veteran, represented to federal agencies from 2016 until 2020 that Legion was a Service-Disabled Veteran Owned Small Business Entity (SDVOSB) to obtain government contracts. To be eligible for such contracts, the entity must be at least 51 percent owned by one or more service-disabled veterans and they must control it, making long-term decisions and managing the entity's daily operations. From 2016 until early 2020, veteran A, who is service disabled, owned 55 percent of Legion and Gorski owned 45 percent but controlled the company's daily operations.

   Gorski retained the Gomez law firm on March 1, 2020 to restructure Legion in order to comply with new regulations that became effective on February 8, 2020. The regulations did not change any of the ownership and control requirements pertaining to SDVOSBs. Although the restructuring took place on March 23, 2020, the documents were dated February 1, 2020 by Gomez. It was important that the restructuring occur prior to the new regulations coming into force if Legion was to remain eligible for government contracts as an SDVOSB. The restructuring, however, did not change the fact that veteran A retained majority ownership and that Gorski maintained control of the entity's daily operations. A competitor challenged Legion's status, prompting an agency inquiry. The Gomez firm crafted a response on April 1, 2020, purporting to show that Legion was restructured on February 1, 2020, and still eligible to obtain SDVOSB contracts.

Gorski is indicted for conspiracy to defraud the United States. The U.S. Attorney issues subpoenas to Legion and Gomez for documents from November 2019 to December 2020 concerning Legion's ownership and SDVOSB eligibility and documents concerning their response to the agency inquiry. Legion and Gomez refuse to comply with the subpoena claiming that the items are protected by the attorney-client privilege. The U.S. Attorney consults you and asks several questions.

a. Are there any exceptions to the privilege that might permit disclosure by Gomez?

b. What is the significance, if any, of the fact that the Gomez firm never intended to help Legion evade the law?

c. What standards and processes will the court use to determine whether the crime-fraud exception applies?

3. Plaintiff-surgeon resigned from practice at the Defendant-Benton Hospital (BH). He alleges that the BH participated in race and ethnicity discrimination by entertaining charges of professional misconduct that BH knew were false and harmful to his reputation. The surgeon seeks two chains of emails. The first chain (Jan. 29-30, 2020) was between several hospital employees, including doctors, nurses, the human resources department (HR), and the CEO. This chain discussed the surgeon's alleged misconduct and certain emails in the chain were carbon copied (CC) to BH's in-house counsel.

The second email chain (Mar. 26-28, 2020), between BH's custodian of hospital records and the chief medical officer, concerned the surgeon's request for his personnel record. Assume that BH does not assert work-product immunity for the second email chain but does claim it is protected by the attorney-client privilege. Are either of the email chains protected by the attorney-client privilege? Explain your reasoning.

4. Two investors, Dayton and Smith, jointly retain Attorney Barton to create a partnership to purchase real estate. Following the partnership's first real estate purchase, Smith alleges that the attorney made several mistakes concerning the purchase and the creation of the partnership. Barton has not returned Smith's calls and Smith sues Barton for legal malpractice. Barton hires you to defend him in the malpractice action and asks the following questions:

a. In his defense, can he disclose confidential communications with Dayton and Smith concerning the partnership and real estate purchase?

b. Barton is angry about the malpractice suit. He once represented Smith in a contested divorce in which Smith confidentially informed him of an extramarital affair with a prominent official. Can Barton use this information to help defend himself in Smith's malpractice action?

Professional Responsibility in Practice

1. Imagine that you represent a defendant in a child rape prosecution. The defendant allegedly lured a child into the woods where he sexually assaulted her at knifepoint. The perpetrator allegedly abandoned the attack and ran off when a jogger approached. In the course of your representation, the defendant suddenly and unexpectedly reveals to you that he is responsible for a kidnapping, rape, and murder of another child five years earlier in the same park. You research that event and discover that another defendant was charged and convicted of that crime, and is now serving life in prison. Check the law in the state where you intend to practice. Are you authorized to reveal your client's confession to that crime in order to prevent the continued wrongful incarceration of an innocent man? If so, when and to whom?

2. The state has asked your firm to draft two model statutes, one defining the attorney-client privilege and the other work-product immunity. Draft such statutes.

3. Imagine a husband and wife visit your law office and ask you to draft individual wills for them containing similar provisions, essentially leaving everything to the surviving spouse. Their adult daughter has driven them to the appointment and wishes to sit in on the counseling session. What action would you take to ensure that the attorney-client privilege protects the confidentiality of their communications with you? How would you describe the scope of the attorney-client privilege to the husband and wife?

4. Research the law in your jurisdiction to determine if the common interest privilege protects the confidentiality of group member communications in both litigation and non-litigation matters (e.g., contract negotiations). What is the scope of the common interest doctrine in your jurisdiction? For example, will communications among group members at a joint strategy session without a lawyer present be privileged? Would the common interest doctrine protect a group member's communication with another group member's lawyer?

5. Research and compare (a) a case in your jurisdiction that found material protected by ordinary work-product immunity with (b) a case that found material protected by opinion work-product immunity.

6

Conflicts of Interest

Loyalty and the preservation of client confidences are two fundamental values of the legal profession. As noted in Chapter 3, lawyers are fiduciaries for clients, owing them duties of independent judgment, competence, undivided loyalty, and the protection of client confidences from unauthorized disclosure or misuse.

Sometimes conflicts of interest arise that impair the ability of lawyers to faithfully execute their fiduciary duties. According to §121 of the Restatement (Third) of the Law Governing Lawyers, a conflict of interest exists when there is a substantial risk that the lawyer's ability to perform her fiduciary duties is materially and adversely affected by the lawyer's own competing interests or the lawyer's duties to others. Absent a **conflict of interest waiver**, professional conduct codes and court decisions prohibit lawyers from entering into or continuing with representation that potentially involves a conflict of interest. Lawyers are subject to disqualification, fee disgorgement, professional discipline, and civil liability for violating this "conflict" prohibition.

Conflicts of interest fall into four general categories: current client (where the lawyer's responsibilities to multiple current clients clash); former client (where the lawyer's duties to a current client compromise the lawyer's ongoing duties to a former client); third party (where another party's interests collide with the lawyer's duty to a current client); and the lawyer's

Key Concepts

- Conflicts of interest rules promote fiduciary values
- Four conflict categories—concurrent, former, third-party, and a lawyer's personal interest
- Concurrent conflicts—directly adverse or a significant risk of material limitation
- Waivable and nonwaivable conflicts
- "Substantial relationship" test applies to former client conflicts
- Imputing a lawyer's conflicts to other firm members
- "Personal and substantial participation" test governs government lawyer-employee conflicts
- Screening to avoid imputation
- Conflict violations—disqualification and other consequences

**Client Intake:
A Practical Tip**

It is important for lawyers, during
the client intake process and
thereafter, to learn as much as
possible about the client and the
client's matter to avoid potential
conflicts of interest. Lawyers should
pay attention at the intake stage
to any personal reactions they
develop about the client that might
forewarn of a potential personal
or other conflict involving the
client or client matter. Sometimes
one's moral compass for avoiding
disloyalty and conflicts of interest
is a good, albeit limited, first step
in assessing the ethical propriety of
providing legal services.

personal interest (where the lawyer's and the client's
interests are at odds). ABA Model Rules 1.7 through
1.12 govern these four conflict categories.

Today's marketplace for the delivery of legal
services is undergoing significant change, providing a
fertile landscape for conflicts of interest. The changing landscape includes the increasing consolidation
of economic enterprises with their network of allied
businesses and interlocking boards of directors, the
globalization of legal services, and the growth of
new technologies that facilitate the easy and rapid
development of professional and personal relationships. These developments enhance the potential
to enmesh lawyers and clients in conflicts of interest. Given these developments and the significant
costs associated with conflicts of interest for clients
and lawyers, conflicts of interest promise to continue to attract substantial attention in case law and
literature.

A. CURRENT-CLIENT CONFLICTS AND CLIENT WAIVERS

1. Directly Adverse and Material Limitation Conflicts

The starting block for understanding conflict analysis is Rule 1.7, *Conflicts of
Interest: Current Clients*. Rule 1.7(a) establishes a baseline for lawyers to assess the
nature of current-client (i.e., **concurrent client**) conflicts, distinguishing "**directly
adverse**" conflicts from those less obvious conflicts that involve "**a significant risk
that the conflict will materially limit**" the lawyer's representation. These two conflict designations arise in both litigation and non-litigation or transactional settings.

Rule 1.7(b) provides lawyers with a roadmap for obtaining a current-client
waiver of a Rule 1.7(a) conflict. Rule 1.7(b)'s waiver provision applies to both
"directly adverse" conflicts and to "significant risk of . . . material limit[ation]"
conflicts. Rule 1.7(b)'s waiver provision also generally applies to the other conflicts of interest situations (e.g., former client) covered in Rules 1.8 through 1.12.[1]
The following four requirements are necessary to constitute a valid waiver under
Rule 1.7(b).

First, the lawyer must reasonably believe at the outset of representing a client in
a matter that she can independently represent the client in a competent and diligent

---

1. Some rules impose additional requirements for a valid conflict of interest waiver beyond those outlined in Rule
1.7(b). For example, Rule 1.8(a) addresses business transactions between a client and lawyer and imposes additional waiver requirements. It requires the client's written consent to the conflict and that the consent be signed by
the client after the client has been advised in writing of the desirability of having independent counsel review the
client's business transaction with another lawyer.

manner. It is incumbent for lawyers to deliberate on this point. Disciplinary authorities and the courts in a civil matter will review or "Monday morning quarterback" the lawyer's "reasonableness determination." They will ask whether an objectively reasonable lawyer would have concluded that she could competently and diligently represent a client given her duties to other clients. Second, the representation cannot be prohibited by law; and third, "the representation [must] not involve the assertion of a claim by one client against another client represented by the lawyer in the same litigation or proceeding before a tribunal." Rule 1.7(b)'s fourth waiver requirement, perhaps the most important, mandates that "each affected client give[] informed consent, confirmed in writing." Whether the client gave informed consent and the lawyer was reasonable at the outset in believing she could provide competent and diligent representation are fact-dependent questions that have spawned much debate and litigation.

The following excerpt from Professor W. Bradley Wendel's article, *Conflicts of Interest Under the Revised Model Rules*, discusses Rule 1.7's significance and application to current-client conflict situations. It also highlights the prominent role of informed consent in Rule 1.7(b)'s conflict-waiver process and the rule's parameters.

W. Bradley Wendel, Conflicts of Interest Under the Revised Model Rules
81 Neb. L. Rev. 1363 (2003)

[Concurrent representation conflicts, s]ometimes called "current-client" conflicts, [are] cases [that] involve a lawyer simultaneously representing two or more clients whose interests may be somehow at odds. . . . The key to the analysis here is the concept of independent professional judgment. Under agency law as well as the more specific law governing lawyers, a lawyer is required to be an effective, diligent, loyal representative of the client. The lawyer must be able to give advice about all of the client's options, without holding anything back for fear of interfering with another client's interests. When a lawyer takes on a new client, she must ask whether the duties she is assuming with respect to the new client — competence, diligence, confidentiality, loyalty, and so on — will require her to do something for the new client that will impair her ability to discharge those same duties to existing clients. The essence of a concurrent conflict of interest is therefore the inability of a lawyer to fulfill her professional obligations to one client because of the need to fulfill professional obligations to another client.

. . . A concurrent conflict of interest is defined as the representation of one client *directly adverse* to another client, or a case in which there is a significant risk that the representation of one client will be *materially limited* by the lawyer's obligations to another client. The clearest case of direct adversity is easy to imagine — one client suing another, with the lawyer representing both in the same litigation. As the comments to Rule 1.7 make clear, however, direct adversity conflicts can arise in transactional matters, as where the same lawyer represents both the buyer and seller, or in litigation where the lawyer must cross-examine one client, who appears as a witness, while representing another client at trial. Material limitation conflicts are simply those conflicts that are less severe than direct adversity conflicts, but which nevertheless interfere with the lawyer's ability to exercise independent professional judgment on behalf of all affected clients.

It is important to understand direct adversity and material limitation not as conceptually distinct, but as points along a continuum. Consider, as an example, a well-known case that appears in many professional responsibility textbooks. The case involved civil rights litigation against the State of New Hampshire by two classes of plaintiffs, mentally handicapped children who lived in a state institution, and female prison inmates. Both classes were represented by the same legal aid office, but a conflict arose when the State offered to settle the prisoner litigation by constructing a better facility for the female inmates — on the grounds of the school for the handicapped kids! The court handled the conflict for the legal aid lawyers as one of material limitation, but it would not have been wrong to analyze it as a direct adversity conflict. In any event, nothing in the remainder of the analysis turns on whether the conflict is one of direct adversity or material limitation. For this reason, the Ethics 2000 revision of the *Model Rules* rewrote the current-client conflicts rule so that the question is posed as whether a concurrent conflict of interest exists; this term is further defined as either direct adversity or material limitation, and it is clear from the rule that the subsequent analysis of consentability is not affected by what kind of concurrent conflict of interest is present. . . .

The Ethics 2000 version of the *Model Rules* provides a much clearer analysis of the issue of consentability. Under Rule 1.7(b), most concurrent representation is permissible provided that each affected client gives informed consent, confirmed in writing. "Informed consent" is a term of art in the *Model Rules*, drawn from the law of medical malpractice. It means consent by the client after the lawyer has communicated adequate information about the risks of simultaneous representation and the reasonably available alternatives. This information must include "possible effects on loyalty, confidentiality and the attorney-client privilege and the advantages and risks involved." Lawyers often err by disclosing too little, perhaps trying to "finesse" the clients into consenting. In one Nebraska disciplinary proceeding, a lawyer represented a husband and wife jointly in a personal-injury action. A few months later, the wife approached the lawyer to request that he represent her in divorce proceedings. The lawyer requested that the husband (still his client in the personal-injury litigation) consent to him representing the wife in the divorce case, and had him sign a handwritten note, but did not advise the husband of the consequences of his consent. This was a serious error by the lawyer, because without full disclosure of the possible risks to the husband, his consent to the lawyer representing his wife in the divorce proceedings would be ineffective. For example, it is unlikely that the husband, an individual inexperienced in litigation, would have appreciated the potential effect on confidentiality of the multiple representation. In the course of the injury litigation, the lawyer would have access to a great deal of confidential information about the husband, some of which might be useful to the wife in the divorce. Perhaps the lawyer would have to cross-examine the husband at trial if the divorce proceedings went that far, and the lawyer would be in the position of having to attack the credibility of his own client. The husband would likely feel betrayed by this development, because he may assume that his own lawyer would never turn on him in any way. Although in sanctioning the lawyer the court focused on the sexual relationship that later developed between the wife and the lawyer, the lawyer could just as readily have been disciplined for representing the wife in the divorce case without first obtaining informed consent, after full disclosure, from the husband.

Some conflicts are not consentable, even with the most complete disclosure. The *Model Rules* list three categories of non-consentable conflicts:

1. *Representations prohibited by law,* which include cases of former government lawyers who are barred by federal or state statutes from undertaking the representation of particular clients for a given length of time, and representatives of government entities that are prohibited from consenting to conflicts of interest.
2. *Asserting a claim on behalf of one client in litigation in which the same lawyer represents the opponent.* The traditional view, still followed in many jurisdictions, is that a lawyer may never assert a claim against another current client, even if the matters are unrelated and the client is represented by other counsel in the litigation in question. An emerging trend, by contrast, is to permit a lawyer to represent a client in a lawsuit against another client, provided that the lawyer is representing the second client on an unrelated matter. The cases I am aware of that approve of a lawyer suing her own client on behalf of another client all involve large, sophisticated entity clients with diverse operations. It is almost inconceivable that a lawyer could proceed in this kind of case where the clients are individuals.
3. *Other cases in which the lawyer does not reasonably believe that she can provide competent and diligent representation to each affected client.* The key here is to focus on the lawyer's professional duties, and ask whether it is possible for the lawyer to be an effective, vigorous, loyal representative of all clients simultaneously. I sometimes refer to these cases as "zero-sum" conflicts, to capture the idea that there is no way one client can get the best possible result if their lawyer is also trying to get the best possible result for the other client. These cases can arise in business transactions, where there are risks and benefits that have to be allocated among the parties, and there is no win-win solution under which all of the parties come out ahead.

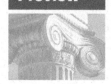

Case Preview

Cinema 5, Ltd. v. Cinerama, Inc.

In *Cinema 5*, the Second Circuit was asked to consider whether the trial judge abused his discretion in disqualifying a plaintiff's lawyer who was suing a defendant who was represented by the plaintiff-lawyer's partner in another law firm in litigation unrelated to the subject matter of the plaintiff's lawsuit. The individual plaintiff-lawyer's conflict of interest was imputed to other members of his firm (see *infra* Section D) warranting their disqualification. In reviewing *Cinema 5*, consider the impact of the decision for large law firms with satellite offices and large corporate clients. The size of these firms and their clients may increase the chance of having a request to represent a client in adverse litigation against another current client in an unrelated matter.

As you read *Cinema 5*, also consider the following:

1. Do you think the appellate court reached the right result? What do you think of the appellant's unsuccessful argument that the lawyer's representation of both clients should be permissible because the representation involved issues not "substantially related"?

2. Did this case involve representation that was a "directly adverse" conflict or instead pose a "significant risk of a material limitation" conflict for the firm? Does the conflict designation matter?

3. What did you think of the firm offering to drop one of the two adverse clients? Should law firms be permitted to draft around the *Cinema 5* prohibition by having clients agree in advance to let their lawyers sue them on unrelated matters?

Cinema 5, Ltd. v. Cinerama, Inc.
528 F.2d 1384 (2d Cir. 1976)

Attorney Manly Fleischmann is a partner in Jaeckle, Fleischmann and Mugel of Buffalo and in Webster, Sheffield, Fleischmann, Hitchcock and Brookfield of New York City. He divides his time between the two offices. Cinerama is a distributor of motion pictures and the operator of several large theater chains. In January 1972 the Jaeckle firm was retained to represent Cinerama and several other defendants in an action brought in the United States District Court for the Western District of New York. Plaintiffs in that suit are local upstate theater operators who allege anti-trust violations resulting from discriminatory and monopolistic licensing and distribution of motion pictures in the Rochester area. A similar action involving allegedly illegal distribution in the Buffalo area was commenced in March 1974, and the Jaeckle office represents the interests of Cinerama in this action also. Both suits are presently pending in the Western District.

The instant action, brought in the Southern District of New York in August 1974, alleges a conspiracy among the defendants to acquire control of plaintiff corporation through stock acquisitions, with the intention of creating a monopoly and restraining competition in New York City's first-run motion picture theater market. Judge Brieant found that there was sufficient relationship between the two law firms and the two controversies to inhibit future confidential communications between Cinerama and its attorneys and that disqualification was required to avoid even the appearance of professional impropriety. . . .

Appellant's counsel strongly dispute these findings. They say that they should not be disqualified unless the relationship between the controversies is substantial, and they contend there is nothing substantial in the relationship between an upstate New York conspiracy to deprive local theater operators of access to films and an attempted corporate take-over in New York City.

The "substantial relationship" test is indeed the one that we have customarily applied in determining whether a lawyer may accept employment against a former client. However, in this case, suit is not against a former client, but an existing one. One firm in which attorney Fleischmann is a partner is suing an actively represented client of another firm in which attorney Fleischmann is a partner. The propriety of this conduct must be measured not so much against the similarities in litigation, as against the duty of undivided loyalty which an attorney owes to each of his clients.

A lawyer's duty to his client is that of a fiduciary or trustee. Hafter v. Farkas, 498 F.2d 587, 589 (2d Cir. 1974); Wise, *Legal Ethics* 256 (2d ed.). When Cinerama retained Mr. Fleischmann as its attorney in the Western District litigation, it was entitled to feel that at least until that litigation was at an end, it had his undivided loyalty as its advocate and champion, Grievance Committee v. Rottner, 152 Conn. 59, 65, 203 A.2d 82 (1964), and could rely upon his "undivided allegiance and faithful, devoted service." Because "no man can serve two masters," Matthew 6:24; Woods v. City Nat'l Bank and Trust Co., 312 U.S. 262, 268 (1941) it had the right to expect also that he would "accept no retainer to do anything that might be adverse to his client's interests." Needless to say, when Mr. Fleischmann and his New York City partners undertook to represent Cinema 5, Ltd., they owed it the same fiduciary duty of undivided loyalty and allegiance.

Ethical Considerations 5-1 and 5-14 of the American Bar Association's Code of Professional Responsibility [principles reflected today in Model Rule 1.7] provide that the professional judgment of a lawyer must be exercised solely for the benefit of his client, free of compromising influences and loyalties, and this precludes his acceptance of employment that will adversely affect his judgment or dilute his loyalty. The Code has been adopted by the New York State Bar Association, and its canons are recognized by both Federal and State Courts as appropriate guidelines for the professional conduct of New York lawyers.

Under the Code, the lawyer who would sue his own client, asserting in justification the lack of "substantial relationship" between the litigation and the work he has undertaken to perform for that client, is leaning on a slender reed indeed. Putting it as mildly as we can, we think it would be questionable conduct for an attorney to participate in any lawsuit against his own client without the knowledge and consent of all concerned. This appears to be the opinion of the foremost writers in the field, *see* Wise, *supra*, at 272; Drinker, *Legal Ethics* 112, 116, and it is the holding of the New York courts. In Matter of Kelly, 23 N.Y.2d 368, 376, 296 N.Y.S.2d 937 (1968), New York's highest court said that "with rare and conditional exceptions, the lawyer may not place himself in a position where a conflicting interest may, even inadvertently, affect, or give the appearance of affecting, the obligations of the professional relationship." Nor is New York alone in this view. In Grievance Committee v. Rottner, *supra*, 152 Conn. at 65, Connecticut's highest court held that the maintenance of public confidence in the bar requires an attorney to decline employment adverse to his client, even though the nature of such employment is wholly unrelated to that of his existing representation.

Whether such adverse representation, without more, requires disqualification in every case, is a matter we need not now decide. We do hold, however, that the "substantial relationship" test does not set a sufficiently high standard by which the necessity for disqualification should be determined. That test may properly be applied only where the representation of a former client has been terminated and the parameters of such relationship have been fixed. Where the relationship is a continuing one, adverse representation is prima facie improper, Matter of Kelly, *supra*, 23 N.Y.2d at 376, and the attorney must be prepared to show, at the very least, that there will be no actual or *apparent* conflict in loyalties or diminution in the vigor of his representation. We think that appellants have failed to meet this heavy burden and that, so long as Mr. Fleischmann and his Buffalo partners continue to represent Cinerama, he and his New York City partners should not represent Cinema 5, Ltd. in this litigation.

Because he is a partner in the Jaeckle firm, Mr. Fleischmann owes the duty of undivided loyalty to that firm's client, Cinerama. Because he is a partner in the Webster firm, he owes the same duty to Cinema 5, Ltd. It can hardly be disputed that there is at least the appearance of impropriety where half his time is spent with partners who are defending Cinerama in multi-million dollar litigation, while the other half is spent with partners who are suing Cinerama in a lawsuit of equal substance.

Because "an attorney must avoid not only the fact, but even the appearance, of representing conflicting interests," Edelman v. Levy, 42 App. Div. 2d 758, 346 N.Y.S.2d 347 (2d Dept. 1973) (mem.), this requires his disqualification. Moreover, because of the peculiarly close relationship existing among legal partners, if Mr. Fleischmann is disqualified, his partners at the Webster firm are disqualified as well. Laskey Bros., Inc. v. Warner Bros. Pictures, Inc., 224 F.2d 824, 826 (2d Cir. 1955) cert. denied, 350 U.S. 932 (1956).

Nothing that we have heretofore said is intended as criticism of the character and professional integrity of Mr. Fleischmann and his partners. We are convinced that the dual representation came about inadvertently and unknowingly, and we are in complete accord with Judge Brieant's finding that there has been no actual wrongdoing. Furthermore, the record shows that after learning of the conflict which had developed, the Jaeckle firm, through Mr. Fleischmann, offered to withdraw its representation of Cinerama in the Western District actions. However, that offer was not accepted, and Mr. Fleischmann continued, albeit reluctantly, to have one foot in each camp.

Under the circumstances, Judge Brieant's order of disqualification cannot be construed as an abuse of his discretion. We therefore affirm.

Post-Case Follow-Up

The *Cinema 5* decision and its prohibition against a lawyer simultaneously representing current clients who are adverse parties in the same or unrelated litigation is widely cited and followed in federal and state courts. The lawyer's loyalty to a client is necessarily called into question when the lawyer simultaneously represents one client suing another current client, or as the court aptly stated: "'No man can serve two masters.' Where the relationship is a continuing one, adverse representation is prima facie improper, and the attorney must be prepared to show, at the very least, that there will be no actual or *apparent* conflict in loyalties or diminution in the vigor of his representation."

Professor Wendel noted in his article earlier in this chapter "an emerging trend" whereby some courts permit a lawyer on behalf of a current client to sue another current client on an unrelated matter. Thus, a lawyer on behalf of current client #1 could sue current client #2 provided the lawyer's representation of client #2 involves a matter unrelated to client #1's lawsuit. Given the lawyer's division of loyalty in such a scenario, one or both of the clients may question whether the lawyer is pulling punches in favor of the other client. Not surprisingly, the Restatement §128 cmt. c requires the lawyer to obtain the informed consent of both client #1 and client #2 to file the lawsuit.[2] When a lawyer is in doubt about the existence of a potential conflict of interest involving current clients or any other situation, a prudent lawyer should seek the informed consent from each affected client. Of course, as Wendel emphasized, some conflicts are not consentable; thus following Rule 1.7(b)'s waiver roadmap is not a guarantee that a firm will not be subject to a successful disqualification motion or a related malpractice or discipline action.

Cinema 5, Ltd. v. Cinerama, Inc.: Real Life Applications

1. The Tarton Company is a wholly owned subsidiary of CLI. Tarton and CLI share a unity of personnel and are located in the same building in Cleveland, Ohio. Both companies share the same legal department and George Hawk acts as general counsel and statutory agent for both companies. Mr. Hawk currently supervises Tarton's antitrust defense in *Amway v. Tarton* in federal district court.

   Mr. Hawk also supervised Gomez & Baker LLP in its defense of CLI in an antitrust matter in *Moore v. CLI*, in the Sixth Circuit Court of Appeals. The Sixth Circuit case was still pending when Gomez & Baker entered an appearance for Amway. The two cases overlapped for two months. Gomez & Baker's conflicts check revealed that the firm had never represented Tarton, although it had represented Tarton's parent, CLI, in the antitrust case of *Moore v. CLI*. Gomez & Baker never divulged the potential conflict to either party in *Amway v. Tarton*, or to CLI. Hawk consults you about seeking the disqualification of Gomez & Baker in *Amway*. Advise Hawk.

2. Arthur Goldberg meets Stefanie Stark in 2017. They become romantically involved and at Goldberg's request, she gives up her businesses and moves to New Jersey to care for him. Goldberg is a wealthy, longtime client of the Jaffe & Asher (J & A) law firm. At his request, the firm continually represented Stark on a variety of matters. Goldberg died on October 1, 2019, and his will did not leave anything to Stark. The estate's directors retained J & A that same day to deal with any forthcoming litigation.

---

2. Restatement (Third) of the Law Governing Lawyers §128 cmt. c(ii) [hereinafter Restatement].

Stark retained attorney Rosen on December 1, 2019 to file a palimony suit. On December 2, Rosen provided a draft of the complaint to the estate's directors and agreed not to file it while settlement negotiations were pending. The directors shared Rosen's letter with J & A. On December 22, 2019, the firm sent Stark a letter stating, in part:

> [S]ince you have commenced an action against the Goldberg estate, a conflict of interest has arisen in our representation of you and we must withdraw immediately as your lawyers. We ask that you pay in full your current outstanding legal bills in arrears, including for the last two service dates of December 17 and 20, 2019.

Stark consults you, exclaiming: "I've never consented to being dropped like a 'hot potato.' They say 'too bad, you're now a former client.'" Stark plans to file her palimony complaint and wants you to move to disqualify J & A from representing the estate based on Rule 1.7(a). Discuss with Stark what the chances are for winning the disqualification motion.

Joint Clients and the Attorney-Client Privilege: A Practical Tip

When representing joint clients, it is important to remind them that what each client communicates to her lawyer is protected by the attorney-client privilege. However, the privilege will not prevent a joint client from revealing an otherwise privileged communication; a joint client is free to disclose her communication or her fellow joint clients' communications to their lawyer. Also, lawyers for joint clients will want to inform them that the lawyer will not keep one joint client's communication secret from another joint client.

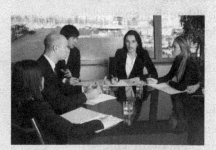

Lawyers sometimes represent multiple clients in a matter. This is called multiple, dual, or joint representation. *Shutterstock.com*

Multiple/Joint Representation Conflicts

Lawyers occasionally represent multiple clients in a matter; this is sometimes called multiple, dual, or **joint representation**. These terms all mean that the lawyer is simultaneously representing more than one client on the same matter. When lawyers undertake joint or multiple representation in civil and criminal matters there is often a risk for a potential conflict of interest. Client matters in all kinds of settings, whether a litigation or a transactional setting, have a life of their own. Even when multiple clients' interests appear aligned at the outset of representation, client needs and other developments may change and affect their objectives. For example, clients may revise settlement claims or liabilities, and there is always the prospect that the discovery of new evidence may create differing interests among multiple or joint clients. Also, it is important to note that when multiple representation fails, the lawyer ordinarily must withdraw from representing all of the multiple clients.[3]

---

3. Restatement §121 cmt. e(i); Model Rule 1.7 cmt. [29].

EXHIBIT 6.1 **Joint Representation Checklist**

1. Identify with precision your clients and the matter in which you will be representing them.
2. Identify anyone in the vicinity who is not a client (but who might somehow think they are), and tell them you are not their lawyer, preferably in writing.
3. Evaluate whether any conflict of interest exists in jointly representing these clients in this matter.
4. If there is a conflict, evaluate whether the clients may ethically waive it, watching out for any prohibited joint representations.
   a. If the conflict is one that may be waived, consider whether, under all the circumstances, a waiver is prudent, both for you as the lawyer and for the clients.
   b. If so, work through the consent process to obtain a waiver from the clients.
   c. Memorialize the waiver in writing.
5. Even if there is no conflict of interest, seriously consider discussing with the clients the possibility that a conflict may arise down the road.
6. Regardless of whether there is a conflict of interest, consider whether, under all the circumstances, joint representation is prudent, both for you as the lawyer and for the clients.
7. Discuss with the clients how confidentiality works in a joint representation; obtain their agreement to your sharing confidential and privileged information between or among them; and consider memorializing the agreement in writing.
8. Establish clearly with all clients who is obligated to pay your fees and expenses, including the specifics of any shared obligation, and seriously consider putting [that] in writing.
9. If someone other than the clients is obligated to pay your fees and expenses, confirm with all the clients and this third person that this third person is not your client; that this third person cannot direct or control your work, unless the clients agree; and that you cannot share information about the matter with this third person, unless the clients consent. Consider putting all this in writing.
10. If the ethics rules require that the fee agreement be in writing, put it in a form that complies with the rules.
11. Consider whether you should discuss and reach agreement with the clients on a plan for your continued representation of fewer than all the clients if a conflict of interest does arise later. If this is a good idea under the circumstances, discuss and memorialize the discussion and agreement.
12. Before, during, and after the representation, treat all of the clients equally in all respects, including loyalty, confidentiality, communication, and decision making. . . .
13. Throughout the joint representation, be aware of the possibility of conflicts of interest arising, and carefully monitor developments that may lead to conflicts, including changes in the facts and procedural posture of the matter, the positions of the clients concerning the matter, and relationships among the clients.
14. If a conflict of interest arises in the midst of the representation, evaluate and address it promptly before continuing in the representation.

Reprinted with permission from Lucian T. Pera. Lucian T. Pera, *The Ethics of Joint Representation*, 40(1) Litig. 45 (2013).

Criminal Cases

Lawyers undertaking joint representation in criminal cases need to be familiar with Rule 44 of the Federal Rules of Criminal Procedure. It recognizes that a defendant who is unable to obtain counsel is entitled to have one appointed at every stage of the proceeding unless the defendant waives the right. The rule is designed to protect defendants from unknowingly waiving their right to separate representation. Rule 44(c) directs the courts to inquire about the propriety of joint representation to safeguard the defendant's constitutional right to effective representation.

> **(c) Inquiry into Joint Representation.**
> **(1) Joint Representation.** Joint representation occurs when:
> **(A)** two or more defendants have been charged jointly under Rule 8(b) or have been joined for trial under Rule 13; and
> **(B)** the defendants are represented by the same counsel, or counsel who are associated in law practice.
> **(2) Court's Responsibilities in Cases of Joint Representation.** The court must promptly inquire about the propriety of joint representation and must personally advise each defendant of the right to the effective assistance of counsel, including separate representation. Unless there is good cause to believe that no conflict of interest is likely to arise, the court must take appropriate measures to protect each defendant's right to counsel.

The Supreme Court addressed joint representation in criminal cases in the prominent case of Holloway v. Arkansas, 435 U.S. 475 (1978). There, the Court reversed a conviction in which a trial judge ignored a defendant's objections to the judge's order of joint representation. The Court stated that a lawyer should "ordinarily decline" multiple representation of clients in a criminal matter given the potential for conflicts of interest and the important interests at stake for defendants. The Court specifically noted that the conflict in *Holloway* may have precluded counsel from pursuing plea negotiations and perhaps having the client testify for the government in return for a lesser sentence.[4] Depending on the criminal matter, other potential conflicts of interest involved in joint representation may include each co-defendant having different levels of criminal responsibility, criminal and family history records, financial support obligations to family and others, and financial ability to pay for representation and damages. In addition, differing interests may arise when one co-defendant asserts the Fifth Amendment and refuses to testify or alternatively when one co-defendant insists on testifying. All of these factors pose a potential conflict of interest. Quoting the ABA, the *Holloway* Court noted that multiple representation should occur only in "unusual situations when,

---

4. For another case illustrating the concern about multiple representation and its effect on plea negotiations, *see* State ex rel. Yurish v. Faircloth, No. 19-1160, 2020 W. Va. LEXIS 330 (May 28, 2020) (affirming the disqualification of a lawyer jointly representing three co-defendants because the state offered cooperation plea agreements to each of them which created "an actual conflict of interest . . . because [the attorney] could not advise one [defendant about taking such a plea] without violating his professional obligations to the other[s] . . . regardless of [the co-defendants'] waivers." *Id.* at 19-20).

after careful investigation, it is clear no conflict is likely to develop and when the co-defendants give informed consent to the multiple representation." The concerns expressed in *Holloway* about joint representation in criminal litigation represent the prevailing view.[5]

In Cuyler v. Sullivan, 446 U.S. 335 (1980), the Court examined an issue left unresolved in *Holloway* about whether the mere *possibility* of a conflict of interest is enough to conclude that the defendant was deprived of his Sixth Amendment right to effective assistance of counsel and thus calling into question the defendant's conviction. The Court found that it is not; the defendant must establish the existence of an *actual* conflict of interest that had an adverse effect on his lawyer's representation. However, the Court added that once it is established that an actual conflict affected the adequacy of representation, the defendant does not have to show prejudice in order to obtain relief. On this basis, the Court vacated the decision of the court of appeals and remanded the case to afford Sullivan an opportunity to demonstrate that an actual conflict of interest existed.[6]

Although one should approach joint representation in a criminal case as if handling a porcupine, the Supreme Court has recognized the important right of criminal defendants to choose their counsel, and thus trial courts must carefully review motions to disqualify a defendant's choice of joint counsel.[7] For example, in United States v. Turner, 594 F.3d 946 (7th Cir. 2010), the district court disqualified Roosevelt Turner's counsel from representing him in a cocaine-conspiracy case because the attorney was also representing an alleged co-conspirator in sentencing proceedings. Though both defendants waived any conflict of interest, the district court judge found that because the defendants may turn on each other, the conflicts were "absolute," "specific," and that "[t]here's no way that any waiver can overcome these conflicts." The appellate court disagreed, finding the district court's decision to disqualify the attorney was based on the mere possibility that either defendant may turn on the other. Citing Rule 1.7 comment [8], the appellate court considered "the likelihood that a difference in interests will eventuate and, if it does, whether it will materially interfere with the lawyer's independent professional judgment in considering alternatives or foreclose courses of action that reasonably should be pursued on behalf of the client." The court found nothing in the record to suggest that the potential conflict of interest identified by the district court had a serious likelihood of maturing into an actual conflict. Nor was there anything to support a conclusion that the conflict was sufficiently severe to jeopardize Turner's right to

---

5. Similarly, Rule 1.7's comment [23] provides: "The potential for conflict of interest in representing multiple defendants in a criminal case is so grave that ordinarily a lawyer should decline to represent more than one codefendant."

6. *See* Harvey v. United States, 798 F. App'x 879, 884 (6th Cir. 2020) (stating that the Supreme Court "left open the question [of] whether the *Sullivan* presumption of prejudice [concerning the simultaneous representation of defendants] applies to claims of ineffective counsel based on conflicts arising from successive representation" and declining to extend such a presumption; also rejecting Harvey's ineffective counsel claims because he did not show "an actual conflict adversely affect[ing his lawyer's] representation").

7. *See* RICHARD E. FLAMM, CONFLICTS OF INTEREST IN THE PRACTICE OF LAW 689-90 (noting that " 'an element of [the Sixth Amendment guarantee is that the defendant has a right] to choose who will defend him,' " and adding this is especially true when the client is paying for counsel (citing United States v. Gonzalez-Lopez, 548 U.S. 140, 144 (2006))) [hereinafter FLAMM]. *See also* Wheat v. United States, 486 U.S. 153, 159 (1988) (stating that "the right to select and be represented by one's preferred attorney is comprehended by the Sixth Amendment . . . ," although the case goes on to discuss the limitations of this right).

effective counsel. The court held that as a general matter, an attorney may represent multiple clients notwithstanding a conflict of interest, if the client gives informed consent.

Civil Cases

Lawyers generally have more leeway to represent persons having similar interests in civil litigation than in criminal cases. Simultaneous representation of parties in civil litigation whose interests may differ is generally permissible if the lawyer complies with the waiver provisions in Rule 1.7(b)(1)-(4), in particular, obtaining the informed consent of each party involved in the common representation.[8] "The mere possibility of subsequent harm does not itself require disclosure and consent." Rather, the critical questions are (1) what is the likelihood a conflict will eventuate; and (2) will it materially interfere with the lawyer's ability to provide independent advice or "foreclose courses of action that reasonably should be" undertaken for the client.[9] The effectiveness of any waiver depends on the client's ability to understand the material risks involved in proceeding with the conflicted representation. The more sophisticated the client, the greater the likelihood that the waiver will be upheld, and the waiver is presumptively valid if the client consults independent counsel about the waiver. However, lawyers need to remember that clients can revoke consent at any time. Waivers may need to be updated to reflect new developments in cases or matters that might render the earlier waiver invalid. In general, advance waivers of conflicts of interest are more likely to be upheld when they are more comprehensive in explaining the conflict risks and are more recent in time.

In the non-litigation or transactional setting, a lawyer may also ordinarily represent multiple clients provided their interests are generally aligned or only marginally different. A lawyer may not engage in common or joint representation if the clients' interests are fundamentally antagonistic to each other.[10]

For example, assume four neighbors jointly hired a lawyer to help them limit the size of a home being remodeled on a parcel of land adjacent to each landowner's property. All four joint clients want the size of the remodeled house to be as small as possible, ideally not over 2,500 square feet in living area nor over 35 feet high. They informed the lawyer at a group meeting that limiting the house size is their primary goal. They noted several zoning regulations that permit them to object to the proposed remodeling but are willing to let the project proceed if the new owner limits the house size. One neighbor-client also informed the lawyer that he prefers the remodeled garage to be limited to two bays and three of the four clients prefer the new home to retain its unpaved driveway to fit in with the neighborhood's ambience. The lawyer's joint representation here is permissible because the four clients' interests align on the central purpose for the representation, limiting the house size. The other client preferences about the number of garage bays and an

---

8. Model Rule 1.7 cmt. [23].
9. Model Rule 1.7 cmt. [8].
10. Model Rule 1.7 cmt. [28].

unpaved driveway represent marginal differences of preference. These preferences are not fundamentally antagonistic to the position of another client; for example, no client is saying that another key purpose for retaining the lawyer is to have the driveway paved, while another fundamentally disagrees and insists that it remain unpaved. If the positions are generally aligned and only marginally inconsistent as in this example, then the lawyer may assert the inconsistent marginal positions along with his primary position of limiting the house size, although it may be wise to acknowledge the inconsistent positions in the engagement letter and obtain the four clients' informed consent to the representation.

The case of Van Kirk v. Miller, 869 N.E.2d 534 (Ind. Ct. App. 2007), applied the "general alignment of interests" doctrine to the sale of a business. Although some states, like New Jersey, bar lawyers from representing both the buyer and seller in some real estate closings, Indiana took a different approach at least where the parties negotiated the terms of the sale.[11] In *Van Kirk*, Attorney Miller represented Summers who gave Miller permission to contact potential buyers for his B&T Sports Bar. Miller contacted Van Kirk, his client in unrelated matters, and gave Van Kirk Summers's contact information after Van Kirk expressed an interest in the B&T sale. After independently negotiating with Summers and deciding to purchase B&T, Van Kirk decided Miller should represent both him and Summers in the transaction because it would "save money." As Van Kirk admitted in his deposition, he knew that after negotiating with Summers "there would have to be a closing and Mr. Miller . . . [would] handle the written agreements and whatever legal documents needed to be done." Since Miller would be representing both parties, he prepared a conflict of interest waiver that both parties signed.

When Summers called off the closing and sold B&T to someone else, Van Kirk sued Miller for malpractice. Van Kirk also claimed the conflict waiver was invalid because Miller's joint representation of both the seller and buyer constituted a non-consentable conflict of interest. The appellate court disagreed and ruled the waiver valid. It found the parties' interests were generally aligned; they had a common goal — the finalization of the B&T transaction. Comment [28] to Rule 1.7 provides that dual representation is permissible where the clients' interests are "generally aligned . . . even though there [are] some difference[s]." Further, Summers and Van Kirk independently negotiated the terms of the transaction and contacted Miller

---

11. The New Jersey Supreme Court has issued a "bright-line rule" prohibiting dual representation of the buyer and seller "in commercial real estate transactions where large sums of money are at stake, where contracts contain complex contingencies, or where options are numerous." Boswell v. Price Meese Shulman & D'Arminio, P.C., No. A-4531-13T2, 2016 N.J. Super. Unpub. LEXIS 1924, at *29 (Super. Ct. App. Div. Aug. 18, 2016). The New Jersey Supreme Court has not issued a blanket prohibition against dual representation of a buyer and seller outside of complex commercial real estate transactions, but its Advisory Committee on numerous occasions has condemned the practice. 13A N.J. Prac., Real Estate Law and Practice §26:9 Conflicts of interest (3d ed. 2013 & 2019 Update). Some case law deems it inherently improper for a lawyer to represent both buyer and seller — e.g., Iowa Supreme Court Attorney Disciplinary Bd. v. Qualley, 2013 BL 34482, 828 N.W.2d 282 (Iowa 2013) — but ethics committees are divided on this issue. *Compare* North Carolina Ethics Op. 99-8 (1999) (approving dual representation), *with* Florida Ethics Op. 97-2 (1997) (advising against dual representation). According to Restatement §122, cmt. g(iv), a lawyer may not represent both a buyer and seller in negotiating and documenting a complex real estate transaction where the parties are in "sharp disagreement" on several key issues or where the parties should receive extensive counseling concerning their rights and possible alternative arrangements.

to draft an agreement that would finalize the deal. Miller did not sit on both sides of the table during the negotiations. Instead, Miller was simply employed to draft the agreement memorializing the terms that Summers and Van Kirk had independently negotiated.

Sometimes a lawyer may take a position on behalf of one client that is adverse to another client in unrelated matters. This is commonly referred to as a "positional" or an "issue" conflict, which may occur in litigation, transactional, and rule-making settings. In the litigation context, taking inconsistent positions on issues for different clients may or may not constitute a conflict of interest under Rule 1.7. Comment [24] to Rule 1.7 provides that the "mere fact that advocating a legal position on a legal matter [for one client] might create precedent adverse to the interests of a client represented by the lawyer in an unrelated matter does not create a conflict of interest." However, a conflict does exist if advocating for one client's interests presents a significant risk of materially limiting the lawyer's effectiveness in advocating another client's interests in a different matter. Comment [24] identifies factors for deciding whether a significant risk of a material limitation exists, including "where the cases are pending, whether the issue is substantive or procedural, the temporal relationship between the matters, the significance of the issue to the immediate and long-term interests of the clients involved and the clients' reasonable expectation in retaining the lawyer." If these or other factors show a significant risk of a material limitation on the lawyer's effectiveness, then absent informed consent from all of the affected parties, the lawyer needs to refuse one of the representations or withdraw from one or both representations.

Courts have a heightened concern about positional conflicts in criminal litigation given what is at stake: the possible deprivation of life, liberty, and property. In this situation, a conflict of interest exists if the lawyer takes a position for client A that creates precedent that seriously undermines the lawyer's different position for client B. *See* Model Rule 1.7 cmt. [24].

Williams v. State, 805 A.2d 880 (Del. 2002), provides a striking example in a criminal case of the danger of creating adverse precedent. There, the defense lawyer appealed Williams's capital murder case to the Delaware Supreme Court. The lawyer contended on appeal that Williams could argue that the trial court erred in concluding it *had to give great weight* to the jury's 10-2 vote in favor of imposing the death penalty. The lawyer also believed, however, that he may have a conflict in raising this argument for Williams because of another capital murder case that he argued and was still pending on appeal before the Delaware Supreme Court. In the pending case, the lawyer took the exact opposite position and argued that the trial court erred when it *failed to give great weight* to the jury's 2-10 vote rejecting the death penalty.

The lawyer filed a motion to withdraw as counsel for Williams due to a conflict of interest. The Delaware Supreme Court granted the motion to withdraw, finding that the lawyer identified a disqualifying positional conflict of interest. The state supreme court further held that the lawyer could not "effectively argue both sides of the same legal question without compromising the interests of one client or the other."

B. LAWYER PERSONAL-INTEREST CONFLICTS WITH CLIENTS

At the beginning of this chapter we noted four general categories of conflicts of interests. Section A addressed concurrent client conflicts. Section B examines another category of conflicts where the lawyer's personal interests interfere with the lawyer's fiduciary duties to be loyal and competent, and to preserve client confidences. In general, the lawyer's superior training and experience places the lawyer in a unique position to take advantage of the client for the lawyer's own personal interest or aggrandizement. The profession has developed specific rules for certain recurring personal-interest conflict situations. Although not an exclusive list, Rule 1.8(a)-(i) governs lawyer conduct in some very common **personal-interest conflict** situations.

1. Business Transactions and Using Client Information

When a lawyer becomes involved in a business transaction with a client or acquires a pecuniary interest potentially adverse to the client while serving as the client's counsel, there is a risk that the lawyer's self-interest will undermine his duty of loyalty to the client. Examples of such business transactions include the lawyer who while representing the client on a related matter also sells the client title insurance or financial services, provides a loan to the client, or purchases assets of a client's estate.[12] When the lawyer provides legal services as part of her contribution to a business venture, there is a heightened concern about the client's vulnerability to lawyer overreaching and a potential personal-interest conflict.[13] For example, assume a lawyer's longstanding client wishes to develop her farmland and she has already retained an engineer to help with the project. They both seek the lawyer's help because they lack the money to develop the land and to pay for legal services. The lawyer incorporates the proposed business and convinces the client to convey her land to the corporation. In return for his present and future legal services, the lawyer receives a 20 percent ownership share in the development company with the others each getting 40 percent.[14] Rule 1.8(a) governs the lawyer's conduct in this example and in any other situation where the lawyer "knowing[ly] acquire[s] an ownership, possessory, security or other pecuniary interest adverse to a client." Ultimately, the ethical propriety of the lawyer's conduct here requires his full compliance with all of Rule 1.8(a)'s provisions.

---

12. Model Rule 1.8(a) cmt. [1].

13. *See* Model Rule 1.8(a) cmt. [2] (warning that risk of harm to the client is greatest where the lawyer is expected to represent the client in the transaction or "when the lawyer's financial interest . . . poses a significant risk that the lawyer's representation will be materially limited by the lawyer's financial interest in the transaction").

14. For a case involving somewhat similar facts, see Committee on Professional Ethics v. Mershon, 316 N.W.2d 895 (Iowa 1982) (although the court found that the lawyer had been "forthright and honest" it nevertheless reprimanded the lawyer for violating professional conduct standards that today are in Rule 1.8(a); holding that as a fiduciary the lawyer must ensure that the "client either has independent advice in the matter" or the equivalent from the lawyer, which means more than simply making the client "fully aware of the nature and terms of the transaction").

Rule 1.8(a)(1)-(3) provides an important prophylactic process for protecting the client from any overreaching while allowing the lawyer and client to enter into a business transaction. First, the lawyer shall explain the transaction in an understandable manner in writing for the client and the terms must be "fair and reasonable to the client." Second, the lawyer shall advise the client to have independent counsel review the terms of the transaction and give the client an opportunity to obtain such review. Finally, the lawyer shall obtain the informed consent of the client in a writing signed by the client. The lawyer's compliance with these three steps does not guarantee court approval of the lawyer's involvement with a client in a business transaction if the client subsequently challenges the propriety of the business transaction. However, the failure to strictly follow the Rule 1.8(a)(1)-(3) provisions almost certainly guarantees judicial disapproval of the transaction, even if the terms are fair and reasonable. The court may invalidate the transaction and order the lawyer to disgorge any proceeds.

Rule 1.8(a) does not apply to standard commercial business transactions between the lawyer and client. In those transactions, there is less concern for potential overreaching by the lawyer. The lawyer is not providing legal services and is less likely to exploit her fiduciary role as the client's advisor to benefit the lawyer's self-interest. Thus, the lawyer's purchase of a car from the client's auto dealership would not trigger the application of Rule 1.8(a), nor would the creation of a cleaning company by the lawyer and client where each contributes $10,000 startup capital and the lawyer is not providing legal services.

Another potential personal-interest conflict involves a lawyer having the opportunity to use client confidential information for the lawyer's own benefit. Consistent with the lawyer's fiduciary duties and absent client consent, Rule 1.8(b) bars lawyers from using confidential information to the client's disadvantage.

Rule 1.8(b) does not prohibit the lawyer from using client confidential information for the lawyer's own personal benefit. But one should check the applicable jurisdiction's agency law to ensure that such use of client information is permitted. Traditional agency principles proscribe agents, in this case lawyers, from personally benefitting from the use of the principal's, here the client's, confidential information, at least without the principal's permission.[15] The lawyer may have to disgorge any personal benefit gained from the use of the client's information under traditional agency law. Thus, if a lawyer obtains confidential information that his client is developing a mall on Whiteacre and the value of the adjacent parcel, Blackacre, is likely to increase, the lawyer may purchase it under professional conduct rules if it will not disadvantage the client. Of course, the lawyer is well advised to ask the client if he has any objections to the lawyer purchasing the adjacent Blackacre, and, although not required, memorializing the client's approval in a follow-up communication. For example, the lawyer may send an email stating: "Thanks for meeting with me today to get your thoughts on the proposed mall development and your approval for my purchase of Blackacre. . . ."

---

15. RESTATEMENT (THIRD) OF AGENCY §8.05 *Use of Principal's Property; Use of Confidential Information* (2006). "An agent has a duty . . . (2) not to use or communicate confidential information of the principal for the agent's own purposes or those of a third party."

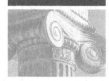

Case Preview

In re Disciplinary Proceedings Against Creedy

In re Disciplinary Proceedings Against Creedy illustrates the ease with which lawyers may find themselves involved in a business transaction with clients. The informality surrounding Creedy's business arrangement with his client is striking — there was no written agreement.

As you review *Creedy*, ask yourself:

1. Would more formality have helped Creedy to appreciate that the business venture with his client was the type of matter covered by Rule 1.8(a)?
2. Would an absolute bar to all lawyer-client business transactions be a better approach for protecting clients from possible lawyer overreaching than Rule 1.8(a)'s current approach?
3. Do you think Creedy's conduct warranted more than a public reprimand? Remember the bar had asked for a four-month suspension.
4. Also, is it fair to punish Creedy for violating Rule 1.8(b)'s ban on using client confidential information when he assisted the government in prosecuting Murphy?
5. Should the lawyer's purpose for violating Rule 1.8(b) matter? Should Creedy's purpose be a mitigating factor concerning possible discipline?

In re Disciplinary Proceedings Against Creedy
854 N.W.2d 676 (Wis. 2014)

Attorney Creedy was admitted to the practice of law in Wisconsin in 1980. . . . He has no previous disciplinary history.

Most of the allegations in the OLR's [Office of Lawyer Regulation's] complaint involve Attorney Creedy's business relationship with a client named Joseph Murphy. Murphy, who is not an attorney, created a company called American Disability Entitlements LLC, intended to represent claimants in Social Security disability matters. Social Security laws and procedures permit nonlawyers to represent such claimants. Murphy learned that if an attorney provides similar services, the attorney can have fees paid directly to the attorney by the Social Security Administration out of any award. Murphy approached Attorney Creedy to see if they could work together representing disability claimants in order to ensure receipt of any fees.

Murphy and Attorney Creedy both represented claimants before the Social Security Administration. They would discuss and mutually agree upon a fair division of fees. They did not have a written agreement.

Murphy was routinely accepting unlawful fee advances, a practice prohibited by applicable Social Security rules and procedures. The parties disputed whether Attorney Creedy knew that Murphy was routinely accepting unlawful fee advances.

Attorney Creedy maintained that he first learned this was occurring in March of 2010, when an attorney representing a claimant advised Attorney Creedy that the claimant had been improperly assessed two fees: one paid by the claimant directly to Murphy, and another later paid to Attorney Creedy by the Social Security Administration. Upon receiving and confirming this information, Attorney Creedy promptly refunded one set of fees to the claimant. He then began dissolving the business arrangement with Murphy.

Meanwhile, law enforcement was investigating Murphy in connection with a variety of matters. Attorney Creedy voluntarily met and provided law enforcement with some information about Murphy.

On June 27, 2013, the OLR filed an eight-count complaint against Attorney Creedy seeking a four-month suspension of his license to practice law. Attorney Creedy filed an answer and the court appointed the referee, who conducted an evidentiary hearing in February 2014.

After the hearing, the parties executed a stipulation whereby the OLR voluntarily dismissed [several] Counts. . . . Attorney Creedy withdrew his answer and pled no contest to the remaining allegations of misconduct. . . .

As relevant to this matter, the referee explicitly stated that he found Attorney Creedy to be both credible and professional. He believed that Attorney Creedy was unaware that Murphy was improperly accepting advance fees until confronted by a claimant's lawyer in March 2010. He deemed Murphy to be a less than credible witness, noting that Murphy is currently serving time for felony convictions related to a variety of fraud-related transactions. Moreover, the referee observed that "it was clear that [Murphy] had personal animosity toward [Attorney] Creedy and went out of his way to express that animosity."

. . .

Count Two of the complaint relates to Attorney Creedy's failure to comply with supreme court rules, specifically in violation of SCR 20:1.8(a), in the manner in which he entered the business arrangement with Murphy to represent Social Security claimants. It is undisputed that Attorney Creedy never disclosed, in writing, the terms upon which the business relationship was based, never advised Murphy in writing of the desirability of seeking the advice of independent legal counsel on the transaction, and never obtained written, informed consent from Murphy to the essential terms of the transaction and to Attorney Creedy's role in the transaction.

The referee noted that it was apparent that Murphy was a sophisticated business person, but this does not excuse failure to comport with the requirements of the rule. Accordingly, the OLR alleged, Attorney Creedy stipulated, and the referee agreed that the record evidence supported a conclusion that Attorney Creedy violated SCR 20:1.8(a).

. . .

In Count Eight, the OLR alleged that Attorney Creedy violated SCR 20:1.8(b) by providing information obtained in the course of his representation of Murphy to the disadvantage of Murphy, without Murphy's consent. It is undisputed that the Green County District Attorney's Office and the Monroe Police Department investigated Murphy. Attorney Creedy met with these entities and provided certain information that was adverse to Murphy, without obtaining Murphy's informed consent. The investigation into Murphy's conduct ultimately led to felony charges and convictions of Murphy. Accordingly, the OLR alleged, Attorney Creedy stipulated, and the referee concluded that by providing information obtained in the course of his representation of Murphy to the Green County District Attorney's Office and the Monroe Police Department to the disadvantage of Murphy, without obtaining Murphy's informed consent, Attorney Creedy violated SCR 20:1.8(b).

Initially the OLR sought a four-month suspension but, following the evidentiary hearing, the parties submitted a joint stipulation agreeing that a public reprimand was sufficient. The referee observed that there was no evidence that any member of the public, other than perhaps Murphy, was harmed by Attorney Creedy's conduct, and characterized any harm to Murphy as de minimus and the proven ethical violations as technical. Indeed, the referee commented that a private reprimand might have been a sufficient sanction. However, he accepted the parties' stipulation and recommends that this court impose a public reprimand.

The only remaining dispute involves whether the court should impose the full costs of this proceeding on Attorney Creedy. The OLR seeks imposition of all costs, which total $17,801.64 as of May 21, 2014. Attorney Creedy filed a timely objection, arguing that no costs should be imposed.

The court's general policy is that upon a finding of misconduct it is appropriate to impose all costs, including the expenses of counsel for the office of lawyer regulation, upon the respondent. In some cases the court may, in the exercise of its discretion, reduce the amount of costs imposed upon a respondent. . . .

The referee carefully considered each of these criteria and recommended, both before and after the filing of Attorney Creedy's objection, that Attorney Creedy should pay one-half of the costs of the proceedings. . . . His statements regarding imposition of costs are telling:

> . . . I have to confess that I find the requested imposition of almost $18,000 in costs to be extraordinarily large. As I wrote in my original Decision, I felt Respondent was "both professional and credible" in his appearance and testimony before me. I thought he acted properly in promptly returning one set of fees to a client as soon as he learned of it and verified it (*Ibid.*, p. 9, 10). I found no evidence that his other two violations harmed either a client or the public.

The referee reminds the court ". . . [t]he violations of the Supreme Court Rules were by no means flagrant." He notes further that Attorney Creedy cooperated fully with the disciplinary process. We agree with the referee's assessment. . . .

IT IS ORDERED that Attorney Carl H. Creedy is publicly reprimanded for professional misconduct [and that he] . . . pay to the Office of Lawyer Regulation one-half the costs of this proceeding.

Post-Case Follow-Up

Creedy underscores the importance of respondent-lawyers having credibility during the disciplinary process. The referee found that Creedy was "'both professional and credible' in his appearance and testimony. . . ." The court also valued Creedy's quick repayment of the fee owed to a client-claimant who was improperly assessed two fees and Creedy's quick dissolution of his business with his client, Murphy. One important take-away from *Creedy* is that when a lawyer has any question about whether he is involved in a business transaction with a client, the lawyer should follow the guidelines of Rule 1.8(a)(1)-(3). Some law firms require a lawyer who is becoming involved in a business transaction with a client to have the arrangement approved by other members in the law firm and to have another firm lawyer draft any agreements or other documents related to the lawyer-client business transaction. This protocol minimizes the risk of any overreaching by the lawyer directly involved in a business transaction with the client.

In re Disciplinary Proceedings Against Creedy: Real Life Applications

1. Gerry Wysocki works in a Midwestern law firm, where he frequently represents farmers in various matters relating to their agricultural businesses. Tom Takala consults with Gerry because he fears that the government will take a substantial part of his land through eminent domain. In explaining his situation, Tom also reveals that his farming business is struggling and that he was thinking of selling other parts of his land to investors willing to take a chance with his business. Because Gerry knows the region's economy rather well, he sees this as a great opportunity to invest some inheritance money. Besides, Gerry thinks that he would be able to build a successful truck stop on Tom's land if Tom's farm fails. Gerry advises Tom on Tom's eminent domain question and then proposes to draft a contract to buy Tom's land that would contain certain clauses regarding Gerry's future participation in Tom's business. How should Gerry proceed to acquire Tom's land?

2. Attorney helped his client obtain a $200,000 settlement for his client after she was involved in an automobile accident. Following the settlement, the client, who stated she had an alcohol problem, asked the attorney to hold the money on her behalf. He later advised her that she should invest her settlement, with him as an equal partner, in purchasing Coca-Cola collectibles (and other business ventures) to later resell for a profit. Their business was ultimately a bust and she lost a significant portion of her settlement. The attorney argues that upon receiving the settlement, he was no longer acting as her attorney, that he was merely trying to help her financially as a friend. The client contacts you, a local lawyer, and contends that her lawyer acted unethically and seeks your help in recovering her lost money. Discuss her options.

---

2. No Gift Solicitations (or Writing Testimonial Bequests to Yourself)

Lawyers are prohibited from soliciting any substantial gift from a client, unless the gift is from a relative. The rationale for this rule is that given the lawyer's fiduciary and personal relationship with a client, there is a real risk of overreaching and manipulation. The lawyer is free to accept token gifts, for example, a holiday gift basket. If a client insists, however, on giving the lawyer a substantial gift, the lawyer can accept it provided he does not solicit it or prepare an instrument giving him the gift unless it is from a relative. *See* Model Rule 1.8(c). Substantial gifts to lawyers are voidable under the doctrine of undue influence.[16]

In In re Disciplinary Matter Involving Stepovich, 386 P.3d 1205 (Alaska 2016), the lawyer, Michael Stepovich, and a client had been friends for several decades. When the client was diagnosed with cancer, he asked Stepovich to draft his will. Although probate was outside Stepovich's normal practice areas, he had helped other friends with "very simple" wills, and agreed to help the client because of their friendship. The will named the client's "good friend, Michael Stepovich," as the sole contingent beneficiary. The client died about six weeks after signing his will, leaving a considerable estate. Because his wife survived, Stepovich received nothing as the contingent beneficiary.

The Alaska Supreme Court emphasized that "[n]aming one[self] as a contingent devisee in a client's will is an obvious conflict of interest that should have been recognized as a problem even absent specific knowledge of Rule 1.8(c)." The court suspended Stepovich for one year and required him to retake and pass the MPRE before reinstatement for failing to follow Rule 1.8(c) and because he had prior history of misconduct.

3. Literary Rights and Financial Assistance

Every state but California has an ethics rule that prohibits lawyers from making or negotiating an agreement for media rights concerning information related to representing a client.[17] The fear is that the lawyer's interest in the media rights will take priority over the client's interests in an efficient, fair, and favorable outcome. The client's desired outcome may not be the best course of conduct for a lawyer interested in maximizing the value of publicity.

One case addressing the impropriety of lawyers acquiring media rights is Harrison v. Mississippi Bar, 637 So. 2d 204 (Miss. 1994). There, the lawyer, Garnett Harrison, faced several allegations of professional misconduct concerning her representation of two clients, including Dorrie Singley. These two cases involved highly charged child custody disputes with allegations of child sexual abuse by the fathers. While still representing the estate of Dorrie Singley, Harrison signed an option contract for $10,000 with a movie production company for the rights to her life story, "The Garnett Harrison Story." The life story was to include a section on her

---

16. Model Rule 1.8(c) cmt. [6]. *See* Attorney Grievance Comm'n of Maryland v. Lanocha, 896 A.2d 996, 997 n.1 (Md. 2006).

17. Model Rule 1.8(d). *See* ABA/BNA Law. Man. on Prof'l Conduct §51:701 (stating the rule does not bar a lawyer from obtaining media rights related to a completed case if the former client provides informed consent) [hereinafter ABA/BNA Man.]. *See also* Burt v. Titlow, 571 U.S. 12 (2013) (although a lawyer probably engaged in unethical conduct by having the client sign over the publication rights to her prosecution as part of his fees, Justice Alito held that a violation of the rules of professional conduct, in and of itself, did not constitute a violation of the Sixth Amendment because it did not make the lawyer *per se* ineffective).

representation of Singley and the founding of Mothers Against Raping Children (MARC). Based on the option contract, Harrison sought and obtained a "permission and release" from Singley's estate. Harrison claimed that she did not intend to violate Mississippi Rule of Professional Conduct 1.8(d) (which mirrored ABA Model Rule 1.8(d)). Harrison also argued that the Singley story was only a small part of her story and did not harm the client. Nevertheless, the Supreme Court of Mississippi held that "the potential serious injury to the profession is manifest. Realization of personal profit from representation of a client creates an appearance of impropriety which the profession can ill afford. Therefore, disbarment is proper under this Rule."

In general, Rule 1.8(e) prohibits lawyers from providing financial assistance to a client for anticipated or pending litigation. The underlying concern is that if lawyers were permitted to provide such assistance, it may encourage clients to bring lawsuits that otherwise would not be brought, and may give the lawyer too great of a financial stake in the outcome.[18] The lawyer's creditor interest in repayment of his financial assistance or loan may interfere with the lawyer's duty of loyalty and independent judgment to promote the client's best interests.

There are three exceptions to Rule 1.8(e)'s general ban on lawyers providing financial assistance to clients. First, Rule 1.8(e)(1) provides a lawyer "may advance court costs and expenses of litigation" if the repayment is "contingent on the outcome of the matter." The rationale for this exception is that advanced court costs "are virtually indistinguishable from contingent fees," which are permissible, and permitting these advances would help indigent clients access the courts.[19] Under this exception, if lawyers lose, they do not get reimbursed for their expense advances. Second, Rule 1.8(e)(2) authorizes lawyers to simply pay an indigent client's court costs with no expectation of repayment, again to facilitate access to the courts. In essence, the lawyer gifts the litigation expenses, such as filing fees and the cost of medical examinations and expert testimony. Third, Rule 1.8(e)(3) allows lawyers representing indigent clients pro bono to "provide modest gifts" to them for their basic living expenses, including food, rent, transportation, and medicine, with no expectation of repayment.[20] This narrow exception is "intended to increase access to justice for [the] most vulnerable citizens."[21]

An example of a violation of Rule 1.8(e) was found in Rubio v. BNSF Ry. Co., 548 F. Supp. 2d 1220 (D.N.M. 2008). Before the client's lawsuit was filed in *Rubio*, the client and his attorneys jointly borrowed $86,400 from a bank to subsidize the

---

18. Model Rule 1.8(e) cmt. [10]. *See* The Philadelphia Bar Ass'n Prof'l Guidance Comm. Op. 2013-8 (2014) (recognizing the ban on living expense advances given Pennsylvania State Bar Opinion 2005-100).

19. Model Rule 1.8(e) cmt. [10].

20. MODEL RULES OF PROF'L CONDUCT, Rule 1.8(e) (reporting Rule 1.8(e)(3)'s adoption by the ABA on August 4, 2020), *available at* https://www.americanbar.org/groups/professional_responsibility/committees_commissions/ethicsandprofessionalresponsibility/.

21. The narrow scope of this exception is reflected, in part, in Model Rule 1.8(e)(3)(i)-(iii) (barring lawyers from: promising or implying such gifts prior to retention or as an inducement to continuing a client relationship; "seek[ing] reimbursement from the client or anyone affiliated with the client; and publiciz[ing] . . . a willingness to provide such gifts to prospective clients"), *available at* https://www.americanbar.org/groups/professional_responsibility/publications/model_rules_of_professional_conduct/rule_1_8_current_clients_specific_rules/.

client's living expenses, in violation of N.M. R. Ann. 16-108(E), which was modeled on ABA Model Rule 1.8(e). The court noted that the purpose for the rule is to prevent a lawyer from acquiring "too great a financial stake in the litigation" as the relationship between a creditor and a debtor is inherently adversarial. The court determined that the attorneys' violation of the rule warranted their disqualification because the loan was not necessary to allow the client access to the courts, there was "no evidence that [the attorneys] co-signed the loan for humanitarian or charitable reasons, 'disqualification' would serve the purposes behind [the rule]," and the loan created a conflict of interest. The court rejected the argument that advances of living expenses should be considered in the same light as contingency fees and indigent expense advances that facilitate access to courts. Some commentators similarly argue that such advances should be permissible because "clients gain financial assistance and more meaningful access to the courts, lawyers can engage in humanitarian acts, and the public learns that the legal profession seeks to assist all citizens in obtaining justice."[22] In addition to the ABA, at least 11 jurisdictions (two of those because of judicial decisions) permit lawyers to advance some form of living expenses for humanitarian purposes. Nevertheless, many states continue to bar lawyers from providing such assistance for **humanitarian expenses**. What do you think?

4. Aggregate Settlements

Lawyers need to be mindful that it is the *client's* and not the lawyer's cause of action or legal matter when providing legal representation in a group setting. The client is the principal in the lawyer-client relationship and "owns" the legal action or matter irrespective of how invested the lawyer-agent becomes in the client's matter. Model Rule 1.8(g) recognizes this fundamental principle and the fact that multiple clients are likely to differ in making or accepting a settlement or in accepting a plea. Thus, Rule 1.8(g) bars lawyers from participating in an aggregate settlement of the claims for or against multiple clients and making an aggregate guilty or nolo contendere agreement unless each client provides informed consent in writing.[23] This rule is consistent with Rule 1.2(a) that similarly recognizes that only a client is authorized to accept a settlement or plea.

In Arce v. Burrow, 958 S.W.2d 239 (Tex. App. 1997) *aff'd and rev'd in part*, 997 S.W.2d 229 (Tex. 1999), Arce and others hired Burrow and others as their attorneys to file individual suits against Phillips 66 in relation to an explosion at a chemical plant that left numerous people dead or injured. The clients agreed to pay the attorneys on a contingency fee basis. The attorneys reached an aggregate settlement with Phillips 66 for the entire lawsuit, allegedly without discussion or

---

22. *See* Jack P. Sahl, *The Cost of Humanitarian Assistance: Ethical Rules and the First Amendment*, 34 ST. MARY'S L.J. 795, 827 (2003) (arguing that lawyers should be permitted to provide and advertise humanitarian assistance). *See also* Philip G. Schrag, *The Unethical Ethics Rule: Nine Ways to Fix Model Rule of Professional Conduct 1.8(e)*, 28 GEO. J. LEGAL ETHICS 39, 72 (2014) (criticizing the text of Rule 1.8(e) prior to the adoption of 1.8(e)(3) as contributing "to homelessness, inadequate medical care, starvation, and in some cases, a denial of access to justice because clients are forced by their poverty to accept inadequate settlements").

23. Model Rule 1.8(g).

individual authority from the clients, save for a 20-minute meeting to discuss settlement arrangements. The clients sued the attorneys for a breach of fiduciary duty and sought fee forfeiture. The court examined the issue of whether the attorneys breached their fiduciary duties to the clients by entering into an aggregate settlement. The attorneys argued that there was no aggregate settlement. The court defined the term "aggregate settlement" as relating to the situation where "an attorney, who represents two or more clients, settles the entire case on behalf of those clients without individual negotiations on behalf of any one client." The court noted that unless there is informed consent, attorneys representing multiple clients have an ethical responsibility, based on their duty of loyalty and good faith to each client, to obtain an individual settlement for each client. Otherwise, mass settlements are unfair to clients and may "result in a benefit to the attorney (speedy resolution and payment of fees) to the detriment of the clients (decreased recovery)." Because of this unfairness, the court concluded the attorneys breached their fiduciary duties to their clients when they entered into aggregate settlements without client consent and that the aggregate settlements violated the Texas Disciplinary Rules of Professional Conduct. The court remanded the case to the lower court for a determination of the amount of forfeiture.

Unlike the aggregate settlement scenario, in class action representation where a lawyer represents a class of plaintiffs or defendants, the lawyer may not have a full attorney-client relationship with each class member.[24] Upon class certification, the lawyer needs to comply with applicable rules concerning notice and other procedural requirements to protect the entire class.[25]

5. No Prospective Malpractice Limitations

All states have an ethics rule that prohibits lawyers from entering into an agreement to prospectively limit their liability for malpractice.[26] There is one exception to the prohibition in those "rare circumstances" when, under Rule 1.8(h)(1), the client retains independent counsel in making the agreement and, even then, not every state recognizes this exception.[27] Indeed, the potential for overreaching with these malpractice agreements is significant. Lawyers act as trusted fiduciaries for their clients and asking clients to forgo possible malpractice claims against their lawyers is unfair when many clients may not fully appreciate the significance of signing such an agreement. This is especially true at the formation of the professional relationship when there is likely a dearth of information available to the client, for example, information about the risks involved in representation. Also, the malpractice limitation may serve as a disincentive for the lawyer to diligently and competently advance the client's interest. Courts generally frown on any attempt by a lawyer to limit liability. Rule 1.8(h) does not prohibit agreements with clients

---

24. Model Rule 1.8(g) cmt. [13].
25. *Id.*
26. ABA/BNA Man. §51:1101.
27. *Id.* (reporting the exception as occurring in "rare circumstances").

to arbitrate legal malpractice claims in jurisdictions where such agreements are enforceable and clients appreciate the significance of the agreement.

Rule 1.8(h)(2) prohibits a lawyer from settling a claim or potential claim for malpractice with an unrepresented client or former client unless the client is advised in writing of the benefit of having independent counsel and the client is given an opportunity to seek such independent advice. By way of an example, in In re Carson, 991 P.2d 896 (Kan. 1999), an attorney had a fee dispute with his former client. Carson submitted an agreement to his client without advising her to seek independent counsel concerning a provision that waived malpractice claims against the lawyer. The former client signed the agreement without the benefit of independent counsel. The attorney was charged with a violation of Kansas Rule of Professional Conduct 1.8(h). Carson argued that Rule 1.8(h) could not have applied to him as the agreement was signed by a former client who had not at that time asserted a claim for malpractice against him. The court was unconvinced by the attorney's "technical arguments" and found him in violation of the second part of Rule 1.8(h). It did not matter that no actual claim existed at that time.

6. No Proprietary Interest in Client Matter

Lawyers are prohibited from acquiring a proprietary interest in the subject matter of the client's litigation or other matter under Model Rule 1.8(i). The rule is designed to prevent lawyers from unfairly using their knowledge and fiduciary position to take such an interest. There is also the concern that once the lawyer acquires a proprietary interest, the lawyer's self-interest in protecting that interest may interfere with the lawyer's duty of loyalty to advance the client's interests. There are two exceptions to the Rule 1.8(i) prohibition. First, lawyers can acquire a lien, for example a charging lien[28] or retaining lien,[29] authorized by law to secure his fees or expenses. Second, lawyers are permitted to contract for a contingency fee in a civil case.

In In re Fisher, 202 P.3d 1186 (Colo. 2009), the attorney represented the wife in a marital dissolution case and was charged with several professional conduct rule violations, including what is now Colorado Rule of Professional Conduct 1.8(i), a rule identical to the ABA Model Rule. Fisher was concerned that his client would not pay his professional fees and asked her to sign a promissory note in the amount of $3,102, secured by a deed of trust in her marital residence. He explained that it was necessary to ensure payment of his fees. The marital residence

---

28. A charging lien is a lien for services rendered by an attorney "in procuring a judgment, decree, or award for the client" and attaching "to the client's cause of action, verdict and judgment, and the proceeds thereof." R.L. ROSSI, 2 ATTORNEYS' FEES §12.13 (3d ed. 2016). Rossi notes that a charging lien is "only applicable to charges rendered for the particular action involved," but does not require possession. *Id.*
29. Atty. Grievance Comm'n of Md. v. Rand, 128 A.3d 107 (Md. 2015) ("A retaining lien permits the attorney to 'secure' his claim for unpaid fees through retention of client property [or funds] in his possession." (citing CHARLES W. WOLFRAM, MODERN LEGAL ETHICS §9.6.3 Attorney Liens, at 558-59 (1986))). The attorney "holds the property until the client pays the balance of the fees owed or possibly provides some other security." *See* ROSSI, *supra* note 28 (adding that the retaining lien may be used to "compel payment of any or all professional charges, whether connected with the action or not").

was subsequently sold and Fisher attempted to have the title company pay all proceeds to him. Fisher argued that this was permissible under Colorado Rule 1.8(i) as his interest in the marital residence constituted a "lien authorized by law" within the meaning of the rule.

The Colorado Supreme Court examined the comments to Colorado Rule 1.8(i) to determine which liens are authorized by law. The comments provided liens "may include liens granted by statute, liens originating in common law, and liens acquired by contract with the client," but ultimately it is "the law of each jurisdiction" that determines which liens are excluded from Rule 1.8(i)'s prohibition. The court concluded that "[a]ttorney's charging liens . . . specifically provided for by statute are excepted" from Rule 1.8(i)'s ban on lawyers obtaining a proprietary interest in the subject matter of the representation. In contrast to charging liens that give lawyers an interest in their clients' judgment for legal services rendered, deeds of trust are not authorized by law but rather granted by an individual. Thus, the court held that Fisher violated Rule 1.8(i) by acquiring an interest in the marital residence.

7. Sexual Relations with Clients

Another example of lawyers seeking personal aggrandizement is when they get involved in sexual relations with a client after the commencement of representation. Professional conduct standards prohibit a lawyer from having sexual relations with a client unless the relations existed before the formation of the lawyer-client relationship.[30] There is concern that the lawyer will take advantage of his or her fiduciary position with a client to have such relations, especially with vulnerable clients, and that it will affect the independent judgment of both parties.

In In re Stanton, 376 P.3d 693 (Alaska 2016), the attorney began a sexual relationship with a young woman after he agreed to represent her in a child custody case. Although "sexual relationship" is not defined under Alaska's Professional Conduct Rules, the parties agreed that sexting and physical contact between the lawyer and client constituted a sexual relationship prohibited by Rule 1.8(j). The Alaska Supreme Court noted that "Stanton's pursuit of sexual gratification — either by initiating or answering the client's sexual overtures with genital photos and sexually provocative texts — advanced his personal interests to the detriment of his client." The court further concluded that the "[d]isclosure of the sexual relationship reinforced allegations that his client was a mixed up, troubled young woman who might not be the best parent for a young child. [Stanton's] conflict required him

---

30. Model Rule 1.8(j). Nearly every state has adopted disciplinary rules regarding sexual relations either under Rule 1.7 or Rule 1.8(j). RONALD J. MALLEN, 2 LEGAL MALPRACTICE §16 (2017). *See* ABA CPR Policy Implementation Committee, *Variations on the ABA Model Rules of Prof'l Conduct: Rule 1.8: Conflict of Interest: Current Clients: Specific Rules* (March 2020), *available at* https://www.americanbar.org/content/dam/aba/administrative/professional_responsibility/mrpc_1_8.pdf. *See also* Lawyer Disciplinary Bd. v. Campbell, 807 S.E.2d 817 (W. Va. 2017) (where a lawyer had sex with her client, a prior boyfriend, after commencement of representation, the court held that a "longstanding and continuous, albeit intermittent sexual relationship, though dormant at the commencement of the attorney-client relationship, constitutes a preexisting relationship" covered by Rule 1.8(j)'s exception. *Id.* at 825-26).

to withdraw and left his client without legal counsel in a contested custody proceeding." The court suspended Stanton from the practice of law in Alaska for three years.[31]

8. Prospective-Client Conflicts and Advance Waivers

Chapter 3 provided a discussion of prospective clients. It is important to understand that such clients pose a risk to lawyers in the conflicts of interest area. The general rule prohibits a lawyer from representing a client with "interests materially adverse to those of a prospective client in the same or substantially related matter if the lawyer received information that might be significantly harmful to the prospective client."[32] Sometimes clients interview several lawyers or law firms before selecting representation that is best suited in terms of expertise and expense to handle their legal needs. This search process is occasionally referred to as a "beauty contest." Lawyers must be concerned about prospective clients laying the groundwork for a subsequent motion to disqualify them by disclosing certain information during the initial interview and before the formation of the lawyer-client relationship.

Some law firms provide prospective clients with written statements warning clients about the risk of disclosing confidential information at the initial consultation. The prospective client may also waive confidentiality for information he provides to the attorney during the initial interview.[33] If the lawyer discovers during the interview a potential conflict of interest, she should inform the prospective client of the conflict and decline to represent the client.[34]

However, a firm may also ask prospective clients to waive their right to file a disqualification motion against the firm should it represent a party in the same or substantially related matter against the prospective clients. The validity of such future conflict of interest waivers ("**advance conflict waivers**") depends on the facts and the extent to which a client meaningfully understood the material risks involved in the waiver. In general, the more detailed the explanation about potential conflicts of interest, the more sophisticated the client, and the more recent the waiver, the more likely a court will find a valid advance waiver. In contrast, vague and broad statements about the firm being permitted to represent adverse interests in anything substantially related to the client's disclosures is generally less likely to be upheld as a valid waiver.[35] The enforceability of advance conflict waivers is greater when a prospective or current client has independent counsel, for example, in-house counsel, reviewing the advance waiver and explaining its material risks to

---

31. For another example of a Rule 1.8(j) violation, see In re Albrecht, 845 N.W.2d 184, 192 (Minn. 2014) (disbarring an attorney who had sexual relations with a client over an extended period of time and pressured her for sex whenever she sought legal advice; rejecting the claim there was no client harm because the sex began as consensual and stating the lawyer-client relationship is "'almost always unequal' and can be 'unfairly exploited' in a sexual relationship regardless of how the relationship began" as here when Albrecht sought sex despite the client's objections).
32. Model Rule 1.18(c). *See* Model Rule 1.9(a).
33. Restatement §122 cmt. d.
34. Restatement §122(1).
35. Marian C. Rice, *A Perspective on Prospective Waivers*, A.B.A. L. Prac. Mag., May/June 2014, at 6.

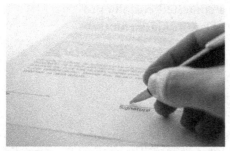

A firm may ask a client to sign a future conflict of interest waiver.
Shutterstock.com

the client. In summary, absent a waiver, lawyers should be careful to limit any discussion with a prospective client that might constitute a basis for disqualifying the firm from representing a current or future client. Of course, advance waivers, like other types of consent to conflicts, may be revoked at any time by the client.

In addition, lawyers must be mindful that certain future conflicts of interest are not consentable under Rule 1.7(b) and an advance waiver would not make them consentable. Therefore, advance waivers are only valid for future conflicts to which a client may consent in accordance with Rule 1.7.[36]

9. Advocate-Witness Conflict

Lawyers are prohibited from serving as an advocate in a case in which they are likely to be called as a necessary witness. The concern is that combining the roles of advocate and witness may prejudice the tribunal and the opposing party.[37] The factfinder may be confused about whether the lawyer is testifying to facts from personal knowledge or, as is the case with advocates, commenting and explaining the testimony of others.[38] The jury may overvalue the lawyer's testimony, or poor or weak testimony by an advocate-witness may harm his client's interests.

The dual role as advocate and witness may also create a conflict of interest under Rule 1.7 (current-client conflicts) or Rule 1.9 (former-client conflicts) if the advocate's testimony may reflect adversely on his client.[39] For example, a substantial conflict between the advocate's and his client's testimony would create a Rule 1.7 conflict requiring client consent to continue with representation. The advocate's inability to testify about facts because of his duty to preserve a former client's confidential information would create a Rule 1.9 conflict.[40]

Fognani v. Young, 115 P.3d 1268, 1272 (Colo. 2005), illustrates some of these concerns and discusses Colorado's Rule of Professional Conduct (CRPC) 3.7, its **advocate-witness rule**, which was modeled largely on ABA Model Rule 3.7. The rule states that an attorney "cannot maintain dual roles as advocate and witness in the same matter before the same tribunal." Attorney John D. Fognani, a partner at Fognani Guibord & Homsy, LLP (FGH), was representing his parents in a medical malpractice suit against Dr. Young. Attorney Fognani was named in pretrial disclosures as a fact witness, including with regard to his father's medical condition, the care and treatment he received from Dr. Young, and Dr. Young's alleged apology and admission of fault — "that he was not completely abreast of modern treatment

---

36. See *supra* at pages 310-13 for a discussion of Rule 1.7 and waiver.
37. Model Rule 3.7 cmt. [1].
38. Model Rule 3.7 cmt. [2].
39. Model Rule 3.7 cmt. [6].
40. *Id.*

measures that would have averted the injuries." Defendants moved to disqualify Attorney Fognani pursuant to CRPC 3.7.

In examining CRPC 3.7, the Colorado Supreme Court acknowledged the wide discretion that trial courts have to order disqualification. It also noted that motions to disqualify opposing counsel are abused sometimes for dilatory or tactical reasons; thus opposing counsel cannot be disqualified on mere "speculation or conjecture" but only upon facts that show a potential violation of CRPC 3.7.[41]

The court considered the rationales behind the rule, including avoiding jury confusion, and quoted one of its earlier decisions. "[A] lawyer who intermingles the functions of advocate and witness diminishes the effectiveness of both. . . . The client's case is subject to criticism that it is being presented through the testimony of an obviously interested witness who on that account is subject to impeachment, and, of equal importance, placed in the unseemly position of arguing his own credibility to the jury."[42]

CRPC 3.7's prohibition applies when the lawyer is "likely to be a necessary witness." The court stated that if the advocate's testimony is merely cumulative of other testimony, then it is not necessary. The court held that "'likely to be a necessary witness' involves a consideration of the nature of the case, with emphasis on the subject of the lawyer's testimony, the weight the testimony might have in resolving disputed issues, and the availability of other witnesses or documentary evidence which might independently establish the relevant issues." The court opined that Fognani's testimony about Dr. Young's declarations of not keeping abreast of modern treatment measures, if proven true, could subject him to liability and thus made Fognani a necessary witness.[43]

The Colorado Supreme Court next considered the three exceptions to the CRPC 3.7 prohibition. The first two exceptions allow a lawyer to testify to an uncontested matter or about the nature and value of legal services rendered in the case. These exceptions are not relevant in the instant case. The third exception allows a lawyer to serve as an advocate and witness if disqualifying the lawyer would work a "substantial hardship on the client." This rule is designed to protect the client; substantial hardship means something more than that the lawyer has invested significant time and expense in the case. The trial court must consider all relevant factors imposing a substantial hardship on the client, for example, "the nature of the case, financial hardship, giving weight to the stage in the proceedings, and the time at which the attorney became aware of the likelihood of his testimony." Weighing these factors, the Colorado Supreme Court concluded that Fognani's disqualification would not impose a substantial hardship on the client.[44]

---

41. Fognani v. Young, 115 P.3d 1268, 1272 (Colo. 2005). The advocate-witness rule's requirements that an advocate be a "necessary witness" with testimony relating to a contested issue help to limit the possible tactical abuse by lawyers who seek to disqualify opposing counsel by calling her as a witness. *See* Model Rule 3.7(a).
42. *Fognani*, 115 P.3d at 1272 (quoting Williams v. Dist. Court, 700 P.2d 549, 553 (Colo. 1985)).
43. *See also* Brooks v. S.C. Comm'n on Indigent Def., 797 S.E.2d 402, 406 (S.C. App. 2017) (disqualifying under Rule 3.7's "necessary witness" standard a lawyer-wife from representing her lawyer-husband in his alleged overbilling of a commission because she "was an active participant in [her husband's] overbilling" and her information would be material, relevant, and unobtainable elsewhere, regarding the "full extent of her involvement" with the overbilling).
44. *See also id.* (rejecting appellant's argument that disqualifying his lawyer-wife as his counsel falls within Rule 3.7's substantial hardship exception because she "had only been involved in the case for two months and 'the expense of hiring new counsel [did] not outweigh the prejudice that would occur to [the Commission]' should they not be allowed to call [her] as [a] witness").

The court concluded that disqualification pursuant to Rule 3.7 did not necessarily preclude participation in pretrial matters. On this basis, the court limited the scope of Fognani's disqualification to the trial, but allowed the trial court on remand to extend the disqualification to pretrial activity if Fognani's participation would be disclosed to the jury, thereby undermining Rule 3.7.

The Colorado Supreme Court also found that CRPC 3.7(b) did not impose an automatic vicarious disqualification of Fognani's firm, FGH. It remanded the case, however, for a further determination of whether the requirements of CRPC 1.7 had been met and, in particular, whether the plaintiffs consented to be continuously represented by FGH given their son's disqualification.

C. FORMER-CLIENT CONFLICTS OF INTEREST

In an era of increasing lawyer and client mobility and other economic developments, such as the merger of businesses, lawyers may find themselves being asked to represent a current client against a former client. This could create a potential conflict of interest if the lawyer is in a position to use the former client's confidences for the current client's benefit. In former-client conflict cases, courts are primarily concerned about protecting the former client's confidences from lawyer misuse. Lawyers are fiduciaries for their clients and have an ongoing duty, even after the conclusion of client representation, to preserve client confidences from intentional and inadvertent disclosure or misuse. If there was no ongoing duty, clients would not be able to trust their lawyers with their confidences.

There is also a concern about loyalty when considering former clients and conflicts of interest. Former clients expect their lawyers not to represent parties with material adverse interests that involve the same or a substantially similar matter that the lawyer worked on for them. Permitting lawyers to represent adverse parties against former clients on substantially similar matters would betray former clients' trust in the loyalty of their lawyers and have a corrosive effect on the public's perception of the profession.

"According to Rule 1.9(a), lawyers may proceed against former clients when either the current client's interests are not *materially adverse* to the former client's interests *or* the current client's matter is not *substantially related* to the work the lawyer did for the former client."[45] When the matter is substantially related, courts will presume the lawyer had access to confidential information that can be used to the former client's disadvantage, and may disqualify the lawyer from the case.[46]

A lawyer who sues a former client on a matter that is not substantially related to prior work the lawyer did for the former client is not required to consult the former client. However, if the former client is not already represented, the lawyer may

---

45. *See* T.C. Theatre Corp. v. Warner Bros. Pictures, Inc., 113 F. Supp. 265 (S.D.N.Y. 1953) (Judge Weinfeld is generally credited with establishing the "substantial relationship" test in this landmark case).

46. *See* Model Rule 1.9(c) (barring the use or revelation of former client information). One way to view Rule 1.9(c) is that the "lawyer's lips are sealed" forever, regarding confidential client information, absent a few exceptions such as where the client consents to disclosure or one of the permissive disclosure provisions under Rule 1.6(b)(1)-(7) is applicable.

consider communicating with the former client for the purpose of reassuring her that the lawyer cannot reveal any of her confidential information.

Sometimes, a question arises about whether a client is a current client or a former client for purposes of Rule 1.9. This question is important, because, as discussed earlier in this chapter, when considering *Cinema 5*, a lawyer is generally prohibited from suing a current client on behalf of another current client, even on unrelated matters.[47]

The court in IBM Corp. v. Levin, 579 F.2d 271, 281 (3d Cir. 1978), addressed this question. There, IBM moved to disqualify Carpenter, Bennett & Morrissey (CBM), Levin's counsel in a private antitrust action against IBM, on the ground that CBM represented both IBM and Levin while the case was pending. While CBM did not represent IBM in the antitrust action, CBM had provided occasional legal work for IBM in labor matters prior to the commencement of that action. The Third Circuit Court of Appeals examined, among other issues, whether IBM was a current client of CBM or whether it was a former client.

The trial court found that CBM "had an on-going attorney-client relationship with both IBM and the plaintiffs." The appellate court agreed with this assessment: "Although CBM had no specific assignment . . . from IBM on hand on the day the antitrust complaint was filed and even though CBM performed services for IBM on a fee for service basis rather than pursuant to a retainer arrangement, the pattern of repeated retainers, both before and after the filing of the complaint, supports the finding of a continuous relationship." Thus, IBM was a current client and not a former client for purposes of conflict analysis and this warranted disqualification of CBM.[48]

The following two cases, *Gillette Co. v. Provost* and *Damron v. Herzog*, demonstrate how courts apply the substantial relationship test with differing results. Note the fact-intensive inquiry and the courts' concern for both enforcing the lawyers' duty of loyalty and for protecting the confidential information of the former clients.

In Gillette Co. v. Provost, 33 Mass. L. Rptr. 327 (Mass. Super. Ct. 2016), Cekala worked as a patent lawyer for Gillette from 1987 to 1990 and again from 1992 through May 2006. During that period, Cekala "had access to privileged communications and information" concerning Gillette's patents and technologies and developed "detailed knowledge" about Gillette's patents and related licensing agreements.

In 2012, Cekala started working for ShaveLogic on patent matters, and became its general counsel in 2013. ShaveLogic informed investors and prospective business partners that Cekala's "intimate knowledge of Gillette's intellectual property portfolio and patent strategy" gave ShaveLogic "a competitive edge in the market." ShaveLogic hired Cekala "to provide freedom to operate opinions respecting Gillette patents, including patents whose prosecution he oversaw, and to identify potential

---

47. *See* FLAMM, *supra* note 7, at 141 (2015) (noting "[i]t is generally considered . . . improper for an attorney to act in manner . . . adverse to the interests of a current client, even in a matter wholly unrelated to any counsel [the lawyer] is handling on that client's behalf, and both state and federal courts have so held").

48. An "end of engagement" letter is a good practice for firms to follow in memorializing the conclusion of their professional relationships with clients. After such letters, those clients should be treated as former clients for purposes of a conflict of interest review.

voids in Gillette's patent portfolio." While employed by ShaveLogic, Cekala also provided similar assistance to other companies competing with Gillette. Gillette complained that Cekala had represented ShaveLogic in matters that were substantially related to those in which he previously represented Gillette, that he had done so without Gillette's consent, and that as a result Cekala had breached his continuing fiduciary duty to Gillette.

The court granted the defendant's motion to dismiss Gillette's claim and held that Cekala owes a continuing fiduciary duty to Gillette but that the scope of his duty to Gillette today is narrower than the broad duty of undivided loyalty that he owed while employed by Gillette. The court added: "[T]he facts . . . do not plausibly suggest that Cekala has breached any fiduciary duty owed to Gillette under Mass. R. Prof. Conduct 1.9, because they do not suggest that Cekala's current representation of ShaveLogic and alleged assistance to other companies is 'materially adverse' to Gillette's legal interests or that it is 'substantially related' to any work Cekala did [for] Gillette."

The court in Damron v. Herzog, 67 F.3d 211 (9th Cir. 1995), reached a different result than in *Gillette*. The appellate court in *Damron* reversed and remanded for a new trial a former client's malpractice action against Attorney Herzog, who represented Damron in the 1982 sale of his cemetery business. As part of the sale, he drafted a stock purchase agreement that called for payments through 1997. Herzog never represented Damron again but he did represent the purchasers following the sale in various matters, including advising them in 1991 to cease making payments under the stock purchase agreement. Damron sued Herzog for malpractice, although he did not claim that Herzog used confidential information from his former representation of Damron. The appellate court concluded nevertheless that because the lawsuit involved the same matter that Herzog worked on for Damron, Herzog was presumed to have had access to confidential information when he advised the purchasers who had material and adverse interests to Damron. The court emphasized that it is not the actual misuse but the potential misuse of confidential information that is required for a conflict of interest. Thus, Damron had a potential cause of action against Herzog for breaching his duty to protect his former client's confidences. Also, the court held that Herzog's duty of loyalty to his former client "re-attached" once Herzog became involved in advising the purchasers about the same matter he worked on for Damron. This required him not to betray his former client's trust.

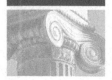

Case Preview

Western Sugar Coop. v. Archer-Daniels-Midland Co.

In the high-profile case of *Western Sugar Coop. v. Archer-Daniels-Midland Co.* (*Western Sugar*), the federal trial court considered the possible disqualification of a large law firm, Squire, Patton & Boggs (SPB), on conflict of interest grounds. The SPB firm was the result of a recent mega-merger of two longstanding and nationally prominent law firms: Squire, Sanders and Dempsey and Patton Boggs.

SPB's failure to identify potential conflicts of interests stemming from the merger proved costly to both the firm and its former and current clients.

As you examine *Western Sugar*, consider the following:

1. How does Patton Boggs's Attorney Smitha Stansbury's post-merger departure affect the outcome of this case? Should it have any effect?
2. What facts in the case support the court's ruling that the Patton Boggs former representation of Ingredion is "substantially related" to its successor firm's, SPB's, representation of Western Sugar?
3. Do you think the court gave sufficient weight to the Patton Boggs lawyers who worked on Ingredion matters before the merger and who declared that they never shared any information post-merger with the Squire Sanders lawyers representing the Western Sugar plaintiffs?
4. What is the significance of the July 2014 meeting when a Patton Boggs lawyer consulted with the plaintiff's expert witness, David Kessler, and the former Squire Sanders attorney, John Burlingame, who is the co-lead attorney for the Western Sugar plaintiffs?
5. Why does the court find a conclusive presumption that SPB possessed confidential information? Is it a fair presumption?
6. Do you agree with the court's view that "[i]t is the possibility of the breach of confidence, not the fact of the breach that triggers disqualification"?

Western Sugar Coop. v. Archer-Daniels-Midland Co.
98 F. Supp. 3d 1074 (C.D. Cal. 2015)

II. PROCEDURAL AND FACTUAL BACKGROUND

The underlying case arises from false advertising claims relating to the marketing of high-fructose corn syrup ("HFCS"), pitting the sugar industry against the corn-refining industry. Plaintiffs are sugar industry manufacturers, trade groups, and associations: Western Sugar Cooperative . . . and the Sugar Association, Inc. (collectively the "Sugar Plaintiffs"). Defendants are manufacturers and trade groups and associations active in the corn and HFCS industry: Archer-Daniels-Midland Company ("ADM"); Ingredion Inc. ("Ingredion"); Tate & Lyle Ingredients Americas, Inc. ("Tate & Lyle"); and The Corn Refiners Association ("CRA") (collectively "Defendants").

Plaintiffs, represented by the legacy law firm of Squire Sanders & Dempsey, LLP ("Squire Sanders"), filed the instant lawsuit on April 22, 2011, and the SAC [Second Amended Complaint] on November 21, 2011. The SAC asserts one cause of action for false advertising under the Lanham Act, alleging that Defendants misled consumers by use of the term "corn sugar."

On September 4, 2012, Defendants ADM, Cargill, Ingredion, and Tate & Lyle each filed a counterclaim against Plaintiff the Sugar Association. Defendants' counterclaim asserts one cause of action for false advertising in violation of the Lanham Act, alleging that the Sugar Association misrepresented HFCS as unhealthy.

A. *The Patton Boggs and Squire Sanders Merger*

On June 1, 2014, the law firms of Patton Boggs LLP ("Patton Boggs") and Squire Sanders combined to form Squire Patton Boggs ("SPB"). SPB remains the Sugar Plaintiffs' counsel of record. Ingredion and Tate & Lyle each filed motions to disqualify SPB from representing the Sugar Plaintiffs in this action because SPB is now adverse to both Ingredion and Tate & Lyle — long-standing clients of the legacy firm Patton Boggs.

B. *Patton Boggs' and SPB's Representation of Tate & Lyle*

. . . Tate & Lyle entered into an attorney-client relationship with Patton Boggs in or about February 1998, as documented in a letter dated February 11, 1998, signed by Stuart Pape of Patton Boggs (the "1998 Engagement Letter").

Tate & Lyle has relied on multiple lawyers at Patton Boggs for legal advice on a wide range of matters since 1998 and through the merger in June 2014. . . . Tate & Lyle's counsel declares that Patton Boggs' lawyers advised Tate & Lyle on matters that required a thorough understanding of its business operations, including its operations and processing of ingredients such as HFCS.

1. Tate & Lyle Bring the Conflict to SPB's Attention

In late July 2014, Tate & Lyle's counsel, Heidi Balsley, contacted SPB attorney, who was formerly a Patton Boggs attorney, Dan Waltz, inquiring whether he knew of the pending lawsuit, which he did not. . . . They explained that a paralegal at Patton Boggs had prepared a list of clients with conflicts for considerations as part of the pre-merger conflicts diligence, and Tate & Lyle had been inexplicably omitted from the list. During that call, they asked Tate & Lyle for a conflict waiver.

. . .

2. Tate & Lyle Does Not Agree to Waive the Conflict

[On August 4, 2014], Tate & Lyle [told SPB it] would not waive the conflict [and] requested that SPB withdraw from its representation of the Sugar Plaintiffs.

Thereafter on August 10, 2014, SPB's counsel sent a letter to Tate & Lyle's counsel, enclosing a copy of the 1998 Engagement Letter. The letter states, "the terms of Tate & Lyle's engagement of Patton Boggs . . . provided us with Tate & Lyle's advance consent that we would represent other clients on matters adverse to Tate & Lyle so long as those matters were unrelated to our work for Tate & Lyle." . . .

3. SPB Withdraws from Its Representation of Tate & Lyle

On August 18, 2014, SPB sent a letter to Tate & Lyle's counsel terminating its relationship with Tate & Lyle. [L]awyers at SPB were actively providing services to Tate & Lyle up until SPB's termination on August 18, 2014.

C. *Patton Boggs' Representation of Ingredion*

Defendant Ingredion provides ingredients to food and beverage companies and refines corn to produce HFCS. Ingredion first retained Patton Boggs in May

2004, and Patton Boggs continued to perform work for Ingredion over the years and last performed work for Ingredion in September 2013. Patton Boggs has provided legal services to Ingredion on at least fifty-six different occasions, and since 2004, Ingredion has paid Patton Boggs over $230,000 in legal fees.

Shortly after Tate & Lyle's counsel raised the conflict, SPB sent Ingredion's counsel a letter dated July 31, 2014, advising it of the merger and that Squire Sanders had been representing the Sugar Plaintiffs and SPB would continue to do so going forward. The letter stated that if Ingredion wanted to have its lawyers from Patton Boggs do any new work, it would be necessary to obtain a waiver from Ingredion due to the conflict presented by SPB's role in the present case.

Ingredion and Tate & Lyle each move to disqualify SPB from representing the Sugar Plaintiffs in this action, contending that the merger resulted in SPB simultaneously representing adverse clients.

III. LEGAL STANDARD

Motions to disqualify counsel are governed by state law. . . . The decision to disqualify counsel is within the trial court's discretion limited by applicable legal principles. Because of the potential for abuse, disqualification motions are subject to strict judicial scrutiny. A court should examine the implications of disqualification, including "a client's right to chosen counsel, an attorney's interest in representing a client, the financial burden on a client to replace disqualified counsel, and the possibility that tactical abuse underlies the disqualification motion."

Motions to disqualify generally arise in one of two contexts: (1) in cases of successive representation, where an attorney seeks to represent a client with interests that are potentially adverse to a former client; and (2) in cases of simultaneous representation, where an attorney seeks to represent in a single action multiple parties with potentially adverse interests. The primary fiduciary duty at stake in each of these contexts differs, and the applicable disqualification standards vary accordingly.

A. Successive Representation of Adverse Clients

The rules regarding successive representation of clients with adverse interests focus on an attorney's duty of confidentiality. If an attorney undertakes to represent a client adverse to a former client without obtaining informed consent, the former client may disqualify the attorney by showing a "substantial relationship" between the subjects of the prior and current representations. This protects the enduring duty to preserve client confidences that survives the termination of the attorney's representation. When a substantial relationship between the representations is established, the attorney is automatically disqualified from representing the second client.

In determining whether there is a "substantial relationship," a court should first analyze whether there was a direct relationship with the former client and whether the relationship touched on issues related to the present litigation. The substantial relationship test requires evidence supporting a rational conclusion that "information material to the evaluation, prosecution, settlement or accomplishment of the former representation given its factual and legal issues is material to the evaluation, prosecution, settlement or accomplishment of the current representation given its factual and legal issues."

If the former representation involved a direct relationship with the client and the matters are substantially related, the former client need not prove that the attorney possesses actual confidential information; instead, the attorney is presumed to possess confidential information. The presumption that an attorney has access to confidential information relevant to the subsequent representation and resulting disqualification extends vicariously to the entire firm. . . .

. . .

IV. DISCUSSION

. . .

B. SPB Is Subject to Disqualification Due to Its Prior Representation of Ingredion in Matters Substantially Related to the Present Action

1. Ingredion Was a Former Client of SPB

Ingredion first retained Patton Boggs in May 2004, and Patton Boggs has continued to perform work for Ingredion over the years and last performed work for Ingredion in September 2013.

Ingredion contends that it was an existing client at the time of the merger because during the firm's decade-long representation, Ingredion reached out to Patton Boggs on an as-needed basis, but time gaps never resulted in a termination of the attorney-client relationship. Ingredion contends that it was treated as an existing client and was not asked to enter into a new fee agreement when it approached Patton Boggs in February 2009, May 2013, or on other occasions following time gaps. All work was billed to Ingredion's existing account with Patton Boggs.

An engagement letter dated December 14, 2005 (the "2005 Engagement Letter") from Patton Boggs' attorney, Stuart Pape, enclosed Patton Boggs' Standard Terms of Engagement. The Standard Terms of Engagement provides, "[i]t is our policy that the attorney-client relationship will terminate upon our completion of any service that you have retained us to perform." Patton Boggs completed services for Ingredion in September 2013, eight months prior to the merger in June 2014, and under the terms of the 2005 Engagement Letter, its attorney-client relationship with Ingredion ended.

Ingredion contends that it was not rendered a former client by the statements in Patton Boggs' Standard Terms of Engagement because (1) it did not expressly agree to those terms; and (2) the 2005 Engagement Letter that accompanied the Standard Terms of Engagement shows that Ingredion retained Patton Boggs not for a discrete issue or litigation, but to provide ongoing representation in connection with FDA regulation of Ingredion's products.

Ingredion was not required to take any action to show its assent to the Standard Terms of Engagement. The 2005 Engagement Letter from Mr. Pape provides, "[t]his letter supplements and modifies the enclosed terms of engagement. . . . If you agree with these terms and conditions, including those set forth in the [Standard Terms of Engagement], no further action is required. . . ."

The 2005 Engagement Letter also provides that Patton Boggs was retained to "represent [Ingredion] in connection with FDA regulation of the Company's

Products." It does not specify that Patton Boggs' representation is ongoing, continuing or open-ended. The Standard Terms of Engagement provides that the attorney client relationship would end upon completion of Patton Boggs' services and states that should Ingredion continue to retain Patton Boggs, the attorney-client relationship would be re-established at that time. Once Patton Boggs completed its representation of Ingredion in September 2013, the attorney-client relationship terminated.

Accordingly, Ingredion was a former client of Patton Boggs at the time of the June 2014 merger. Whether SPB can represent the Sugar Plaintiffs in this action after previously representing Ingredion depends on whether SPB can do so while maintaining its duty of confidentiality it owes to Ingredion. That, in turn, depends on whether the former and current matters are "substantially related."

2. The Prior and Current Representations Are "Substantially Related"

a. Patton Boggs' Prior Work for Ingredion vs. Its Work in the Present Action

Patton Boggs' attorneys advised Ingredion regarding permissible, common or unusual names for HFCS. Evidence filed *in camera* shows lawyers billed time in 2006 for researching regulations on advertising products with HFCS; reviewing FDA and Department of Agriculture rules and regulations on HFCS, and discussing research and common or unusual names for HFCS with each other and Ingredion.

Patton Boggs' attorneys also advised Ingredion regarding FDA statements and enforcement actions following a letter issued from the FDA dated July 3, 2008, signed by Geraldine June (the "Geraldine June Letter"). The Geraldine June Letter describes aspects of manufacturing HFCS and whether a resulting product could be considered "natural." Ingredion received advice from Patton Boggs regarding interpretation of the Geraldine June Letter, including advice concerning a key aspect of the HFCS manufacturing process and how that might affect whether the resulting HFCS product could be described as "natural." Patton Boggs' lawyers billed time in 2009 for researching and discussing FDA statements and natural claims internally and with Ingredion.

Ingredion contends that in the Geraldine June Letter, the FDA concluded that HFCS qualifies as "natural." Counsel for Ingredion declares that it and other Defendants are relying on the Geraldine June Letter in this action in support of their position that it is not a misrepresentation to claim that HFCS is "natural."

SPB represents Plaintiffs in this lawsuit against Defendants, alleging that they engaged in false advertising of HFCS. Plaintiffs allege that this lawsuit is a response to an educational campaign initiated by Defendant CRA in 2008 that sought to educate the public about HFCS and to address the Sugar Plaintiffs' purported vilification and myths about HFCS with facts and scientific studies. Sugar Plaintiffs allege that Defendant CRA's campaign constitutes false advertising under the Lanham Act, identifying two categories of false and/or misleading representations: the first category is Defendants' use of the term "corn sugar," and the second category is Defendants' statements that HFCS is a "natural" product.

Defendants, including Ingredion, defend that the term "corn sugar" accurately depicts HFCS and that the FDA has confirmed methods of producing HFCS that qualifies as "natural." Ingredion's defense relies, in part, on the Geraldine June Letter. The Geraldine June Letter has been explored in multiple depositions, it is expected to be discussed in motions for summary judgment, and it will likely be addressed at trial.

b. Legal and Factual Similarities

The evaluation of whether the two representations are substantially related centers upon the factual and legal similarities of the representations.

SPB contends that none of the four billing entries from August 2006 relating to HFCS concern the use of the word "sugar" or any other term at issue in this litigation. SPB further argues that there was no question related to whether the word "sugar" could be used for HFCS in labeling, or any question regarding the relative benefits of sugar versus HFCS, and the inquiry did not relate to advertising.

SPB contends that the Geraldine June Letter is only at issue in this litigation regarding whether Defendants can rely on it as an FDA endorsement of marketing HFCS as "natural." SPB further contends that work performed in August 2009, was performed by attorneys Paul Rubin, who left Patton Boggs in August 2012 (two years before the merger) and Smitha Stansbury, who left SPB in July 2014 (almost two months *after* the merger).

A "substantial relationship" does not necessarily mean an exact match between the facts and issues involved in the two representations. The work Patton Boggs performed for Ingredion in 2006 and 2009 relates to the propriety of characterizing HFCS as "natural" under FDA policy — advice that is germane to issues concerning marketing and advertising HFCS as natural and whether such claims could be false or misleading. Accordingly, the similarities of the legal and factual issues of Patton Boggs' prior representation of Ingredion put Patton Boggs, now SPB, in a position where confidential information material to its current representation of the Sugar Plaintiffs was likely imparted to counsel. Moreover, the fact that former Patton Boggs attorneys Smitha Stansbury and Paul Rubin are no longer at SPB does not change the outcome, particularly since Ms. Stansbury left SPB *after* the merger.

Ingredion has established that there is a "substantial relationship" between the prior and current representations, and the attorneys at Patton Boggs, now SPB, are presumed to possess confidential information. SPB is thus subject to automatic disqualification from this action.

3. SPB's Evidence Does Not Overcome the Presumption

SPB provides declarations from attorneys [who] have worked on the instant lawsuit on behalf of the Sugar Plaintiffs. These attorneys declare that they have never received any information from any lawyer who was with Patton Boggs about either Ingredion or Tate & Lyle, and they have not performed work on any matter for Tate & Lyle after the merger. SPB's counsel declares that the only lawyers who remain at SPB who have worked on Ingredion matters after 2010 are Stuart Pape, Carey Nuttall, and Ann Spiggle. These lawyers declare that they have never provided any information to any lawyer who was at Squire Sanders about Ingredion, and after the firms merged, they did not work on any matter for the Sugar Plaintiffs.

Shortly after the merger in July 2014, Stuart Pape — the Patton Boggs attorney who signed the engagement letters for both Ingredion and Tate & Lyle — consulted with the Sugar Plaintiffs' expert witness, David Kessler, and the former Squire Sanders attorney, John Burlingame, who is co-lead attorney for the Sugar Plaintiffs in this action. This consultation occurred prior to any formal ethical walls being in place. There is a real risk that confidential information was in fact compromised.

In any event, whether the attorneys actually possessed or conveyed confidential information is not the test. Rather, because Ingredion has met its burden showing that a "substantial relationship" exists between the two representations, SPB is *conclusively presumed* to possess confidential information material to the present action. . . . The "substantial relationship" test ensures that clients are not forced to reveal the confidences the rule is intended to protect. *Trone*, 621 F.2d at 999 ("It is the possibility of the breach of confidence, not the fact of the breach, that triggers disqualification").

The Court finds that SPB is subject to automatic disqualification because it previously represented Ingredion in matters substantially related to the present action, and SPB is thus presumed to possess client confidences revealed in the prior representations. Evidence showing that the Patton Boggs attorney who signed the engagement letters for Ingredion and Tate & Lyle actually consulted with Sugar Plaintiffs' counsel and expert witness following the merger reinforces the Court's finding.

D. Other Alternatives to Disqualification

A disqualification motion may involve considerations such as a client's right to chosen counsel and the possibility that tactical abuse underlies the disqualification motions. The Court balances the need to maintain ethical standards of professional responsibility, preservation of public trust in the scrupulous administration of justice, and the integrity of the bar against a client's right to chosen counsel, and the burden on the client if its counsel were disqualified.

SPB and Plaintiff Sugar Association contend that Ingredion and Tate & Lyle filed their Motions to obtain an improper tactical advantage in this litigation. The merger was highly publicized, and counsel for Sugar Plaintiffs, Mr. Burlingame, opines that the Motions have been filed by Defendants to "gain a tactical advantage both by delaying this [a]ction and by removing The Sugar Association's chosen and experienced counsel." At various depositions, Defendants' counsel never raised the prospect that the merger would create any conflict. Similarly, on June 2, 2014, SPB filed and served a notice, reflecting the firm's name change, and no one called the legacy Squire Sanders lawyers to raise any issue upon the filing. It was not until July 23, 2014 that Tate & Lyle's counsel first raised the conflict.

The Court does not conclude from the evidence provided that the Motions were brought for tactical reasons. The Motions were filed days after Tate & Lyle's counsel met and conferred with SPB's counsel and after it became clear that Tate & Lyle would not consent to the existing conflict. SPB cannot minimize its breach of ethical duties owed to its clients by placing the burden on them to identify and raise the conflicts sooner.

In UMG Recordings v. MySpace, [526 F. Supp. 2d 1046 (C.D. Cal. 2007),] the district court fashioned an alternative remedy to disqualification. . . . Unlike in *UMG Recordings*, . . . SPB's representation of Ingredion regarding the characterization of HFCS as "natural" is an issue that goes to the heart of this lawsuit.

. . . Also unlike in *UMG Recordings*, where the law firm implemented an ethical wall some seven months *before* the events that led plaintiff to complain of the conflict, here, SPB implemented a formal ethical wall *after* the motions to disqualify were filed, and *after* counsel for the Sugar Plaintiffs met with Mr. Pape, the attorney who engaged both Tate & Lyle and Ingredion.

Additionally, in *UMG Recordings*, the law firm made "crystal clear" that it would not agree to represent the plaintiff UMG unless it agreed to waive any conflict that would prevent the law firm from representing an adverse party in cases concerning infringement of intellectual property rights on the internet. Plaintiff UMG signed the waiver that put it on notice that its law firm might represent a specific party (like the defendant), even if UMG were still an active client of the law firm. Here, the advanced waivers contained in Patton Boggs' Standard Terms of Engagement is a generalized advanced waiver with no specificity and could not have put Ingredion or Tate & Lyle on notice of the conflicts it was agreeing to waive.

The Sugar Plaintiffs have a right to their counsel of choice, and declare that they have relied on SPB as their trusted counsel, who have become "case experts" on "extraordinarily complex issues" central to this litigation. Indeed, disqualification at this late stage would undoubtedly impose hardship on Plaintiffs. The parties have engaged in extensive discovery and motion practice, and Plaintiffs have incurred over $12 million in fees from Squire Sanders/SPB in this matter, reflecting over 20,000 hours of professional time, demonstrating the depth of the firm's involvement. The Sugar Plaintiffs contend that no replacement firm could master these issues without near-identical effort.

Having considered the competing interests of Plaintiffs' right to chosen counsel and the prejudice they would face if SPB were disqualified against the paramount concern of preserving public trust in the scrupulous administration of justice and the integrity of the bar, the Court finds that no alternative short of disqualification will suffice. While the Court is mindful that this outcome imposes hardship on the Sugar Plaintiffs, "the important right to counsel of one's choice must yield to ethical considerations that affect the fundamental principles of our judicial process."

V. CONCLUSION

The Court hereby GRANTS Tate & Lyle's and Ingredion's Motion to Disqualify Squire Patton Boggs LLP.

Post-Case Follow-Up

The situation presented in *Western Sugar Coop. v. Archer-Daniels-Midland Co.* is certainly not unique. Law firms continue to consider ways to increase market share for the delivery of legal services, for example, through law firm mergers and acquisitions. *Western Sugar* highlights the costly risks involved for clients and lawyers involved in a merger or acquisition where a conflict of interest was not identified. Law firms must remain mindful of how these mergers and acquisitions occur and how they are carried out in order to limit to the greatest extent the possibility of conflicts of interest.

Western Sugar Coop. v. Archer-Daniels-Midland Co.: Real Life Applications

1. Sue Ortiz was terminated by Zena Liu, her employer. Ortiz alleges her termination was in retaliation for filing a workers' compensation action. Ortiz hired attorney Nakisha Williams, who filed an action against Liu seeking damages for Ortiz's wrongful termination. In response, Liu's attorney filed a motion to disqualify both Williams and her law firm because Williams had served as Liu's in-house counsel for 14 years. Liu's counsel alleges that during Williams's 14 years of employment with Liu, Williams had obtained confidential information about Liu's company and that Williams was now directly involved in similar actions. Should Williams be disqualified?

2. Ms. Rodriguez contacted the Justice Project ("JP") seeking legal assistance in her dispute with Mr. Petrof and various collateral matters related to her rental property. Upon visiting JP, Rodriguez spoke to paralegal Keyda Montalban. In her initial conversation, Rodriguez gave Montalban basic information pertaining to her legal problems concerning accessibility to Rodriguez's apartment. Rodriguez also conveyed relevant financial and background information to determine her eligibility for legal assistance. While employed at JP, Attorney Phillips was responsible for reviewing Montalban's intake file, but the parties dispute the extent of that review function.

   With Rodriguez's consent, JP subsequently referred her case to the Legal Assistance Corporation of Central (LACC) for legal assistance, which filed an action against Petrof eight weeks later. Petrof hired the law firm of Kemp and Kemp as defense counsel and it assigned the case to a newly hired lawyer, Attorney Phillips.

   Rodriguez filed a motion to disqualify Phillips as the defendant's counsel on conflict of interest grounds because Phillips worked at JP, which had advised Rodriguez about her dispute with Petrof. The judge asks you to draft a memorandum discussing how you would rule on the case. Should Phillips be disqualified? Should the entire firm of Kemp and Kemp be disqualified?

D. IMPUTATION OF CLIENT CONFLICTS

Rule 1.10(a) recognizes a longstanding rule that when one lawyer in a firm is prohibited from representing a client because of a conflict of interest under Rules 1.7 and 1.9, then all other firm members are generally prohibited from undertaking the representation. In short, the individual lawyer's conflict is imputed to each lawyer associated with the "conflicted lawyer's" firm. The rationale for the imputation or vicarious disqualification rule is based on the two fundamental concepts that lawyers owe clients loyalty and that lawyers must protect clients' information.

These principles become at risk when lawyers practice in law firms or any other association where they presumably have access to sensitive client information and files. Firm lawyers also share mutual financial interests, which creates a heightened risk that any confidential information that a firm or firm member has may be accessible to others in the firm and used to a client's disadvantage. Consequently, if one lawyer is disqualified because of a conflict of interest due to his having confidential information, then all firm members must be vicariously disqualified to safeguard the confidential information from misuse. The **imputation doctrine** has generated much debate, with some arguing that it is unfair to think that a firm lawyer with a conflict of interest would not protect client confidences from others in the firm who might use it to the client's disadvantage if there were no imputation rule.

The imputation rule does not apply to "personal" conflict situations where a lawyer's duty of loyalty or protection of client confidential information is not at risk.[49] For example, a lawyer's firmly held political or religious convictions should not generally be imputed to others in the firm. Thus, lawyers in a firm could represent an abortion clinic even though a leading partner in the firm is a "right to life" advocate and refuses to assist in the representation of the clinic. However, if the "right to life" partner's interest would materially limit the representation by others in the firm, then that partner's interest would be imputed to them.[50]

The question sometimes arises as to who is a firm member for purposes of the imputation rule. Rule 1.0(c) defines a firm to be "a lawyer or lawyers in a law partnership, professional corporation, sole proprietorship, or other association, authorized to practice law; or lawyers employed in a legal services organization or the legal department of a corporation or other organization." It does not include lawyers who are acting as co-counsel in a case but who are not in the same firm.[51] In general, a conflict may be imputed to the entire firm from an individual partner, associate, or lawyer serving as "of counsel," and occasionally others, for example, a temporary lawyer,[52] paralegal,[53] or summer intern. The key concern in all of these

---

49. Model Rule 1.10(a)(1) & cmt. [3].

50. Model Rule 1.10 cmt. [3]. Also, Rule 1.8(j)'s prohibition on a lawyer having sexual relations with a client after the commencement of the lawyer-client relationship is not a conflict that is imputed to other firm members. *See* Model Rule 1.8(k).

51. ABA/BNA Man. §51:2025.

52. ABA Comm. on Prof'l Ethics & Grievances, Formal Op. 88-356 (1988) considered whether temporary lawyers are "associated" with a firm for purposes of imputing conflicts of interest. "Ultimately, whether a temporary lawyer is treated as being 'associated with a firm' while working on a matter for the firm depends on whether the nature of the relationship is such that the temporary lawyer has access to information relating to the representation of firm clients other than the client on whose matters the lawyer is working and the consequent risk of improper disclosure or misuse of information relating to representation of other clients of the firm."

53. *See, e.g.*, Hodge v. URFA-Sexton, LP, 758 S.E.2d 314 (Ga. 2014). In *Hodge*, the appellant had retained an attorney in a law firm to pursue claims associated with the death of the appellant's sister. A paralegal at the law firm knew the appellant for approximately ten years. Subsequently, the paralegal went to work for the firm that represented appellees. Appellant filed a motion to disqualify appellees' law firm because of the migrating paralegal. The court held that a non-lawyer's conflict of interest can be remedied as in this case by implementing proper screening measures so as to avoid disqualification of an entire law firm.

situations is the risk that a lawyer may have acquired client confidential information and is now in a position to misuse it.

In general, the imputation rule does not apply to office sharing arrangements, but it could. Whether conflicts are imputed among lawyers who share office space depends on the facts and the degree of risk that client confidential information may be improperly shared by them. Important questions to consider in investigating an office sharing arrangement include the following: Are client files and confidential information accessible by others in the office? Do the lawyers sharing space have a protocol in place to protect against inadvertent sharing of client confidences? Do they market themselves as a group and resemble a law firm, thus warranting similar treatment and the application of the imputation rule?[54] The more an office sharing arrangement resembles a classic law firm, the greater the risk of the misuse of client confidences and the more likely the court will impute conflicts to others in the office.

Sometimes law firms are affiliated with other firms even in different jurisdictions, often for cross-referrals of work and other marketing purposes. Firms claiming to be affiliated are generally treated as one firm for purposes of conflict of interest analysis and imputation.[55]

Imputation may apply to legal aid societies, depending on the facts, namely whether there is physical or organizational separation of the attorneys.[56] In general, if multiple clients seek representation from a non-profit legal services agency and their interests conflict, a private lawyer or a lawyer from an autonomous agency must provide the representation.[57] Authority is split concerning the imputation of conflicts of interest in public defender's offices and legal aid offices. Some courts will not automatically disqualify an entire public defender's office based on the disqualification of a single attorney. These courts contend the financial incentives in the organization are absent for lawyers to use confidential information to the disadvantage of another client or to lessen advocacy provided for a client.[58] There is also the concern that automatic disqualification would diminish the pool of defenders.[59] But other courts find a public defender's office is like all other law firms and must be treated as such.[60]

Some jurisdictions had adopted **screening** as an exception to the imputation rule in recognition of the increased mobility of lawyers changing firms. In 2009,

---

54. *See* Restatement §123 cmt. e. *See also* Terminology, Annotated Model Rules of Prof'l Conduct §1.0 cmt. [2] (acknowledging that whether two or more lawyers constitute a firm depends on the facts); Imputation of Conflicts of Interest: General Rule, Annotated Model Rules of Prof'l Conduct §1.10 (citing Monroe v. City of Topeka, 988 P.2d 228 (Kan. 1999), and noting "indicia of lawyers presenting themselves to public as a firm for purposes of imputed disqualification include sharing office space, telephone, facsimile number, and mailing address").

55. *See* ABA/BNA Practice Guide 51-2022. *See also* ABA Comm. on Prof'l Ethics & Grievances, Formal Op. 94-388 (1994) ("As the two firms become more inextricably linked, the need to consider the conflict potential becomes more pronounced." "[W]here two law firms have a relationship in which they have shared profits, it is highly unlikely one could represent a client whose interests are adverse to clients of the other firm without following the procedure proscribed by 1.7(b). . . .").

56. Restatement §123 cmt. d(v).

57. *Id.*

58. ABA/BNA Practice Guide 51-2024.

59. *See* People v. Shari, 204 P.3d 453 (Colo. 2009).

60. *See* Scott v. State, 991 So. 2d 971 (Fla. Dist. Ct. App. 2008); Restatement §123 cmt. d(iv).

the ABA adopted Rule 1.10(a)(2) that similarly permits screening as an exception to the imputation of conflicts under Rules 1.7 and 1.9 in the private law firm market (the ABA already permitted screening in the government sector, as is discussed later in Section E of this chapter). Rule 1.10's screening applies only to lawyers moving between private law firms. It is important when law firms hire lawyers from other firms, called lateral hires, that the hiring firm have a reliable conflicts of interest check system in place to identify potential conflicts of interest. The following examples illustrate how screening under Rule 1.10 applies.

The XYZ law firm laterally hires lawyer A from the Peterson firm, where he and several Peterson colleagues represent client #1. Assume lawyer B is already at the XYZ firm and represents a longtime XYZ client, client #2, who is suing client #1. Lawyer A can make the lateral move or switch sides and move to the XYZ firm, but he will need to be "screened." Lawyer A is presumed to possess confidential information pertaining to client #1's lawsuit with XYZ's client #2 and is thus disqualified under Rule 1.9 (former-client conflict of interest rule) from participating in the suit against his former client #1. Lawyer A's disqualification will be imputed to everyone in the XYZ firm unless that firm institutes a timely screen to ensure that the migrating lawyer A cannot share any of his former client #1 confidences with his new XYZ firm.

It is worth noting several variations of the above migrating lawyer example to better understand the scope of the imputation rule and how it may be applied in other scenarios, appreciating that courts may differ on the application of the imputation rule.

I

First, in the original scenario, the Peterson law firm can continue representing client #1 after lawyer A leaves Peterson for XYZ as lawyer A's departure for XYZ does not disqualify Peterson with regard to client #1. (See *Goldberg v. Warner/Chappell Music, Inc., infra.*)

II

Let us vary the original scenario as follows. Suppose that CW, a large law firm based in New York City, is representing client #3 in proceedings against client #1 and retains XYZ's help as local counsel in matters relating to the case. If XYZ is conflicted out (i.e., disqualified) because of its lawyer A's former involvement with client #1, XYZ's conflict of interest is generally not imputed up to CW unless lawyer A actually shared client #1 confidential information with someone at CW. Thus, CW could continue representing client #3 against client #1 provided the CW and XYZ firms are not deemed to be affiliated with each other. In deciding whether firms are affiliated or not, ABA Formal Opinion 94-388 (Dec. 5, 1994) indicated that important considerations including whether the law firms' relationship is "close and regular, continuing and semi-permanent" would be relevant to addressing the issue. However, here it appears that CW retained XYZ as local counsel to handle routine matters, such as serving papers, and would not be affiliated.

III

What if lawyer A in the original scenario had only attended one or two meetings with client #1 as a junior associate and had otherwise not participated in the representation of client #1? The general presumption is that lawyer A acquired confidential information pertaining to client #1 while he worked at Peterson, but he will be allowed to rebut this presumption by showing that he did not in fact acquire any such confidential information. (Silver Chrysler Plymouth, Inc. v. Chrysler Motors Corp., 518 F.2d 751 (2d Cir. 1975); Adams v. Aerojet-General Corp., 104 Cal. Rptr. 2d 116 (Ct. App. 2001).)

Screening under Rule 1.10 does not apply where lawyers A and B already both work in the XYZ law firm and lawyer A wishes to represent a new client, client #3, whose interest conflicts with the interest of a current XYZ firm client represented by lawyer B. Screening lawyer A from lawyer B to allow lawyer A to represent the new client is not permitted here since both lawyers, A and B, already work in the XYZ firm. There is no migrating lawyer in this scenario so screening will not work to allow lawyer A to represent the new client. It is possible, although unlikely, that lawyer A could represent the new client who has a conflict of interest with lawyer B's current client if each affected client consents to the conflicted representation under Rule 1.7(b).[61]

Rule 1.0(k) defines a screen as a complete "isolation of a lawyer from any participation in a matter . . ." in a timely manner "to protect information that the isolated lawyer is obligated to protect under these Rules or other law." The failure to have a timely screen in place, ideally before the lawyer joins his new firm, often results in the disqualification of the migrating lawyer's new firm. An effective screen must be opaque. Ideally, this usually means that the new or migrating lawyer who is presumed to have confidential information that might harm his old firm's former client is physically separated from his new firm's colleagues handling the matter in conflict with his or his old firm's client. The new firm should clearly communicate to its lawyers not to communicate with the migrating lawyer about the case, for example, by denying the lawyer access to email communications among the lawyers and anyone else involved in the case matter against the lawyer's former client. The migrating lawyer should not have any opportunity to share his old client's information with his new firm's lawyers opposing his old client. Remember, under Rule 1.9(c) the migrating lawyer should never use his former client's information to the client's disadvantage by sharing it with his new firm.

In addition, Rule 1.10(a)(2)(i) requires that the disqualified migrating lawyer be apportioned no fee from his new firm's case against his former client. Rule 1.10(a)(2)(ii) further requires that the migrating lawyer promptly provide written notice to any affected former client to enable that client to ascertain whether the lawyer is in compliance with the rule, including a description of the screening

---

61. The provisions of Rule 1.9(a) will apply instead if lawyer B's client becomes a former client of XYZ at some point. Lawyer A thus will not be allowed to represent his new client in the same or a substantially related matter in which his client's interests are materially adverse to the interests of lawyer B's former client unless lawyer B's former client gives written informed consent.

procedures, a statement by the screened lawyer and the firm of its compliance with the screening rules, and an indication of the ability of the former client to seek review of the procedures. Finally, the firm must also agree to promptly respond to any written questions or concerns about the screening procedures and provide certifications of compliance with the rule at reasonable intervals upon the former client's written request.

Finally, Rule 1.10(d) makes clear that when a lawyer joins a private firm after representing the government, questions about imputation are governed not by Rule 1.10 but by Rule 1.11(b) and (c) (*see* Section E, *infra*).

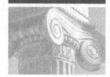

Case Preview

Goldberg v. Warner/Chappell Music, Inc.

Goldberg is a prominent case in which the court refused to find and impute a conflict of interest to other lawyers in the firm of Mitchell Silberberg & Knupp LLP (MSK). It highlights the fact-intensive nature of conflict of interest analysis in disqualification cases and the importance of preserving client confidences as a predicate for granting (or not granting) disqualification.

In reading *Goldberg*, consider the following questions:

1. Did Goldberg have a valid reason for feeling that MSK betrayed its duty of loyalty to her?
2. Is there an appearance of impropriety in allowing the firm to represent Goldberg's former employer?
3. What are the benefits and risks of disqualifying lawyers on an "appearance of impropriety" basis?
4. Is the public and profession best served by such a broad and general standard?
5. Finally, would the result in this case be different if Salomon were still at the Mitchell firm? If he were still there, should Salomon's conflict be imputed to all MSK lawyers under Rule 1.10?

Goldberg v. Warner/Chappell Music, Inc.
125 Cal. App. 4th 752 (2005)

[Ilene Goldberg sued the respondents, Warner/Chappell Music, Inc. (Warner), her former employer, and her former supervisor, Edward Pierson, for wrongful termination. She claimed that she was terminated as retaliation for complaining about gender-based discrimination and] "blowing the whistle" on Pierson's illegal conduct, including practicing law without a license.

FACTUAL AND PROCEDURAL BACKGROUND

. . .

Motion to Disqualify

Goldberg formally moved to disqualify [Mitchell Silberberg & Knupp LLP] (MS&K) on December 10, 2003. In her moving papers, she presented evidence that in 1997, while still employed at Warner, she was given a written employment agreement to sign. She asked Salomon, then a partner with MS&K, to advise her with respect to the agreement. She met with Salomon for an hour and a half on May 9, 1997, to go over the terms of the agreement. She purportedly "disclosed confidential information to him including the nature and term of [her] employment agreement, [her] compensation and benefits, disability, termination by [Warner], [her] ability to retain, disclose, and use confidential/privileged information concerning [her] employment relationship with [Warner], scripts and other literary works created by [her], the effect of a change in control of [Warner], expiration of the employment agreement, and [Warner's] obligations under state and federal law." She also had "other conversations and correspondence with [Salomon] relating to his advice about the terms and conditions of [her] employment agreement." On July 29, 1997, she sent him a letter and draft of a proposed employment agreement, and promised to send the final agreement "for [his] files." She asked him to send her a bill for his advice, but he refused to do so.

Subsequently, Goldberg retained MS&K to work on various matters for Warner, and she "did not have an objection to [MS&K's] representation of [Warner] in matters that did not conflict with [MS&K's] prior representation of [her]."

Opposition

Respondents presented evidence in their opposition that in April 1997, one month prior to Goldberg's purported consultation with Salomon, MS&K began legal work on a copyright matter for Warner. A formal retention letter between MS&K and Warner was signed on May 2, 1997.

The executive director of MS&K stated in a declaration that there was no record in any of MS&K's files of Goldberg ever having been a client of the firm, and that the policy of the firm was to execute a formal, written engagement letter before taking on legal representation.

. . .

Salomon stated in a declaration that he practiced law at MS&K from October 1987 through October 2000, when he moved to another firm. He denied that he had been retained by Goldberg to represent her in her contract negotiations with Warner. Instead, Goldberg "told [Salomon] she was going to represent herself in negotiations over the contract, but asked if [Salomon] would talk to her about these agreements generally to get a sense of how [Warner] lawyers dealt with the contract's various provisions." He told Goldberg he "would be glad to talk to her about what she could expect in the course of her negotiations." They primarily discussed "what she might expect with respect to the boilerplate issues." Salomon "never discussed with any other lawyer at [MS&K] what was said in [his] conversation with Ms. Goldberg."

. . .

Trial Court's Ruling

The court denied the motion to disqualify. At the hearing, the court stated that the only potential basis for disqualification was Goldberg's contact with Salomon, not her personal and professional relationships with other MS&K attorneys. The court concluded that there was an attorney-client relationship between Goldberg and Salomon even though Salomon appeared to be helping her "as a friend." The court agreed that if Salomon were still with MS&K, the firm would be disqualified. However, because Salomon had left the firm, there was no need for vicarious disqualification.

In its order, the court specifically found: "The evidence is undisputed that [MS&K] and Salomon never opened a file for Ms. Goldberg. They never billed her. There are no notes or records in their files about the meeting and no documents were prepared. No telephone calls were made. It was simply a meeting late one afternoon where Ms. Goldberg and Mr. Salomon sat down and discussed the meaning of the employment contract she was being offered and what provisions she might request. . . . There is no evidence that Mr. Salomon talked to anyone about this matter when he was with [MS&K]. And more importantly, he had left the firm approximately three years before this matter began. There is no fear of him talking about the case in the lunch room, or having his files seen by other members of the firm, as he is no longer there."

Goldberg filed a petition for writ of mandate for review of the order. By order dated March 24, 2004, the petition was denied, with one dissent. Goldberg noticed an appeal. . . .

DISCUSSION

(2) Rule 3-310(E) of the [California] Rules of Professional Conduct provides that an attorney "shall not, without the informed written consent of the client or former client, accept employment adverse to the client, or former client where, by reason of the representation of the client or former client, the member has obtained confidential information material to the employment." There is no question that an attorney can and should be disqualified for representing a party adverse to a former client where the attorney possesses confidential information that could be helpful to the new client and hurtful to the old. . . .

(3) The courts do not generally inquire into whether the attorney actually possesses confidential information. Instead, the substantial relationship test is applied. "'*When a substantial relationship has been shown to exist between the former representation and the current representation*, and when it appears by virtue of the nature of the former representation or the relationship of the attorney to his former client confidential information material to the current dispute would normally have been imparted to the attorney or to subordinates for whose legal work he

was responsible, *the attorney's knowledge of confidential information is presumed.*'" (Rosenfeld Construction Co. v. Superior Court (1991) 235 Cal. App. 3d 566, 574 [286 Cal. Rptr. 609], italics added.)

(4) In addition, "[i]t is now firmly established that where the attorney is disqualified from representation due to an ethical conflict, the disqualification extends to the entire firm." (Adams v. Aerojet-General Corp., *supra*, 86 Cal. App. 4th at p. 1333.) "[W]here an attorney is disqualified because he formerly represented and therefore possesses [either actually or presumptively] confidential information regarding the adverse party in the current litigation, vicarious disqualification of the entire firm is compelled as a matter of law." . . .

(5) There is, however, a recognized "limited exception to this conclusive presumption in the rare instance where the lawyer can show that there was no *opportunity* for confidential information to be divulged."

. . .

The court explained why it distinguished the situation before it from the situation where the attorney who sought to undertake adverse representation was still working with the attorneys who had acquired the former client's confidential information: "'No amount of assurances or screening procedures, no "cone of silence," could ever convince the opposing party that the confidences would not be used to its disadvantage. . . . No one could have confidence in the integrity of a legal process in which this is permitted to occur without the parties' consent.' Once an attorney departs the firm, however, a blanket rule to prevent future breaches of confidentiality is not necessary because the departed attorney no longer has presumptive access to the secrets possessed by the former firm. The court need no longer rely on the fiction of imputed knowledge to safeguard client confidentiality. Instead, the court may undertake a dispassionate assessment of whether and to what extent the attorney, during his tenure with the former firm, was reasonably likely to have obtained confidential information material to the current lawsuit."

The court [in *Adams v. Aerojet-General Corp.*] found further support for its decision in the realities of modern law firm practice: "Disqualification based on a conclusive presumption of imputed knowledge derived from a lawyer's past association with a law firm is out of touch with the present day practice of law. Gone are the days when attorneys (like star athletes) typically stay with one organization throughout their entire careers. . . . We have seen the dawn of the era of the 'mega-firm.' Large law firms (like banks) are becoming ever larger, opening branch offices nationwide or internationally, and merging with other large firms. Individual attorneys today can work for a law firm and not even know, let alone have contact with, members of the same firm working in a different department of the same firm across the hall or a different branch across the globe." [*Id.* at 1336.]

From this, the court concluded that "a rule which disqualifies an attorney based on imputed knowledge derived solely from his membership in the former firm and without inquiry into his actual exposure to the former client's secrets sweeps with too broad a brush, is inconsistent with the language and core purpose of rule 3-310(E), and unnecessarily restricts both the client's right to chosen counsel and the attorney's freedom of association. It also clashes with the principle that applying the remedy of disqualification '"when there is no realistic chance that confidences were disclosed [to counsel] would go far beyond the purpose" of the substantial relationship test.'"

We agree with the court in Adams v. Aerojet-General Corp., *supra*, 86 Cal. App. 4th 1324, that at some point, it ceases to make sense to apply a presumption of imputed knowledge as a lawyer moves from firm to firm. Salomon, while at MS&K, gave advice to Goldberg concerning the terms of her contract with Warner. We agree with the trial court that, despite the informality, an attorney-client relationship existed between them. Moreover, if Salomon were still practicing at MS&K, MS&K would likely have to be disqualified from the current litigation because there would be no practical way of ensuring that, despite his best intentions, Salomon would not let slip some confidential information he may not even be aware that he possesses. But Salomon is no longer with MS&K. We need not be concerned that he will inadvertently pass on confidential information to his colleagues in the future because he is no longer there "in the lunch room" as the trial court said. It was appropriate under the circumstances for the trial court to make an assessment of whether Salomon actually passed on confidential information. Since the court found he had not, there was no basis for disqualification.

. . .

(6) If an attorney worked on a matter "substantially related" to the matter in which he or she seeks to represent a party adverse to a former client, the presumption is conclusive that the *attorney* is possessed of confidential information that would impact the present matter. Where tainted attorneys and nontainted attorneys are working together at the same firm, there is not so much a conclusive presumption that confidential information has passed as a pragmatic recognition that the confidential information will work its way to the nontainted attorneys at some point. When, however, the relationship between the tainted attorneys and nontainted attorneys is in the past, there is no need to "rely on the fiction of imputed knowledge to safeguard client confidentiality" and opportunity exists for a "dispassionate assessment" of whether confidential information was actually exchanged. This is precisely what the trial court did here.

(7) Our conclusion that the trial court analyzed the matter correctly is also in line with the ABA Model Rules of Professional Conduct, which California courts may consult when a matter is not addressed by the California Rules. . . . Model Rule 1.10(b) provides: "When a lawyer has terminated an association with a firm, the firm is not prohibited from thereafter representing a person with interests materially adverse to those of a client represented by the formerly associated lawyer and not currently represented by the firm, unless (1) the matter is the same or substantially related to that in which the formerly associated lawyer represented the client; and (2) any lawyer remaining in the firm has [protected] information . . . that is material to the matter." Courts from other jurisdictions have followed the ABA Model Rule in situations analogous to the present one: where an attorney who presumptively acquired confidential information from a former client leaves the firm, the firm is not automatically disqualified if it chooses to represent a party adverse to the former client. . . . This is further basis to uphold the trial court's determination.

. . .

The order is affirmed.

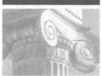

Post-Case Follow-Up

Goldberg highlights, in part, the risk and relative ease of establishing an attorney-client relationship. MSK and Salomon never opened a client file for Goldberg, made documents for her, telephoned her, created meeting notes for a file, and never billed her, although she requested a bill. "Despite the informality[,]" the appellate court nevertheless agreed with the trial court that an attorney-client relationship existed between Goldberg and Salomon. *Goldberg* is also well known for recognizing an important limitation on the imputation doctrine reflected in ABA Model Rule 1.10(b). It provides that once a tainted lawyer with a potential conflict of interest leaves the firm (Salomon in this case), the risk of his divulging confidential information to others remaining in the firm is reduced. In *Goldberg*, the concern that Salomon may accidently slip and divulge information no longer existed following his departure from the firm. Thus, absent Salomon actually sharing Goldberg's confidential information with another MSK lawyer who may then slip and divulge it to others, there is little need to vicariously disqualify the entire MSK firm.

Goldberg v. Warner/Chappell Music, Inc.: Real Life Applications

1. Plaintiffs, Celebrity Chefs, are suing Kmart for breach of contract, conversion, and trademark infringement. Alleging a conflict of interest, plaintiffs filed a motion to disqualify Kmart's counsel and his firm. The law firm representing Kmart, Seltzer Caplan, had previously represented the plaintiffs in two cases to recover sponsorship and advertising fees. Plaintiffs allege that during the course of these two representations, Seltzer Caplan learned confidential information about their business and litigation strategies. They argue that because Seltzer Caplan possesses this knowledge, counsel and Seltzer Caplan as a whole must be disqualified.

   However, Seltzer Caplan argue that not only is the current case not related to its prior representation of the plaintiffs, but also, the attorneys who worked on those cases did not disclose the confidential information to anyone else in the firm, and they are no longer with Seltzer Caplan. How should the motion be decided?

2. Former employees are suing the defendant, Boston Scientific, for unlawfully firing them when they reported fraudulent billing within the company. Attorney Hasan was employed as in-house counsel for the defendant corporation prior to the initiation of this suit. During her time as in-house counsel, her duties included investigating matters directly related to those at issue here. Two years after leaving the defendant-corporation, Hasan became associated with the plaintiff's law firm, Tank & Blank. Upon learning of her new employment, Boston Scientific moved to disqualify Hasan and to impute her conflict of interest under Rules 1.9 and 1.10 to her new firm, Tank & Blank.

Tank & Blank argues that even though there was not a proper screen in place, Hasan was de facto screened because she was not in the office very often nor did she disclose any confidential information. Should Hasan be disqualified? Should Hasan's conflict of interest be imputed to Tank & Blank?

3. As an associate at his law firm, Attorney Johnson performed work for Thompson Property Corp., which was in active litigation with Korner Tech over several patents. The lawsuit was still pending between the parties when Johnson left his firm and began working at the ABC law firm, which represented Korner. Though Johnson worked in ABC's Chicago office and the lawyers representing Korner worked in ABC's Tampa office, the law firm nevertheless used a screening protocol to prevent Johnson from disclosing any information he might have about Thompson Corp. Johnson also sent a written notice to Thompson advising the company of his ABC employment and the screening measures taken by ABC. In response, Thompson filed a disqualification motion alleging that because Johnson had performed significant work on the case, screening could not be used to rebut the presumption that he had shared confidential information with the defendant's lawyers (i.e., his colleagues) working on this case or that he will do so in the future. Advise how the court would rule on Johnson's disqualification. Is it likely that the law firm will also be imputed?

E. CONFLICTS OF INTERESTS FOR CURRENT AND FORMER LAWYERS IN GOVERNMENT SERVICE

The conflicts rules governing lawyers who have left private practice to enter government service or have left government service for private practice diverge slightly from the rules governing all other lawyers because they serve some different purposes. Like the rules governing conflicts of interest for lawyers in private practice, protection of former clients' confidential information is paramount. Thus, under Rule 1.11, government lawyers and former government lawyers are subject to the prohibition in Rule 1.9(c) that they shall not reveal their former client's confidential information or use that information to the disadvantage of their former clients.

In the situation of former government lawyers, however, other policy considerations are present. First, government lawyers should not be able to take advantage of their status as government lawyers to improve their opportunities in private practice. At the same time, government agencies need to be able to recruit good lawyers, and overly strict rules would discourage lawyers from entering government service if they could not take advantage of that governmental experience to some degree when they move into private practice. Finally, the public benefits from having lawyers in private practice who served in the government and understand government practice and policy. In theory, these former government lawyers may encourage greater compliance with the law.

As a result, the conflicts rules governing former government lawyers are narrower in some respects and broader in others. Rule 1.11(a) is narrower than

Rule 1.9 in that it only limits a former government lawyer from representing a private client "in connection with a matter in which the lawyer *participated personally and substantially*" as a government lawyer, unless the government agency gives informed consent in writing. Thus, a former prosecutor may not turn around and defend a client that he personally prosecuted, but he may defend a client who was prosecuted by the office that he worked in if he did not personally participate in the prosecution.

Further, Rule 1.11(b) contains a special imputation rule that permits nonconsensual screening: the conflict is not imputed to the firm if the "disqualified lawyer is timely screened" and "written notice is promptly given to the appropriate government agency." Thus, a former prosecutor can join a law firm and the firm can continue to defend clients who are being prosecuted by that office, even a client who the new lawyer personally prosecuted, provided that the former prosecutor is timely screened and the firm provides notice to the prosecutor's office. This imputation rule ensures that a private law firm will not be discouraged from hiring a former government lawyer.

Rule 1.11(c) is broader than Rule 1.9, however, in that the prohibition extends to *any* representation related to the lawyer's government work even if it is not adverse. Thus, a Securities and Exchange Commission lawyer who personally prosecuted a defendant for securities fraud cannot leave government service and represent plaintiffs in a civil suit against the same defendant. In that way, the former government lawyer is not able to take special advantage of his former role as a government lawyer to benefit other clients.

As for current government lawyers, under Rule 1.11(d)(1) they are subject to both Rules 1.7 and 1.9. Thus, consistent with Rule 1.9, a government lawyer may not represent the government adverse to a former client in a matter that is substantially related to the former representation unless the former client gives informed consent in writing. Rule 1.11(d)(2) also contains an additional limitation for government lawyers: they may not participate in any matter in which they personally and substantially participated while in private practice, *whether or not the current matter is adverse* to their former client, unless the government agency gives its informed consent in writing. Finally, a government lawyer's personal conflicts are not imputed to the government agency, but Rule 1.11 comment [2] suggests that it would be "prudent" to screen conflicted lawyers.

F. SPECIFIC CONFLICT RULES: JUDGES, ARBITRATORS, AND OTHERS

Rule 1.12 parallels Rule 1.11 and addresses potential conflicts of interest involving lawyers who are former judges, adjudicative officers, clerks, arbitrators, mediators, and other third-party neutrals. "Adjudicative officers" includes referees, masters, hearing officers, and other officials who play a role in deciding or resolving disputes between parties. Just like Rule 1.11, Rule 1.12 forbids such persons, without written informed consent from all parties, from representing anyone in connection with a matter in which they participated personally and substantially as a judge or other adjudicative officer or law clerk or as an arbitrator, mediator, or other third-party neutral. It also imputes the conflict to the lawyer's law firm, unless the lawyer is screened and apportioned no fee pertaining to the matter and proper written notice is given to the parties and the tribunal. The rule finds its basis in the duty of confidentiality and its keystone is therefore whether the lawyer participated "personally and substantially" in the related matter. A former judge who exercised administrative responsibility in a court does not prevent the former judge from acting as a lawyer in a matter where the judge had previously exercised remote administrative responsibility that did not affect the merits.

In James v. Miss. Bar, 962 So. 2d 528 (Miss. 2007), a former judge sought to represent a party in a divorce case related to a domestic abuse case over which she had previously presided. Similar to ABA Model Rule 1.12(a), Mississippi Rule of Professional Conduct 1.12(a) prohibited a lawyer from representing anyone in connection with a matter in which the lawyer participated personally and substantially as a judge. The court examined whether the former judge had "substantially participated" in the matter, reviewing her interaction with the case and the litigants in her capacity as judge. The court found that she had substantially participated in the domestic abuse case because she had read motions, conducted hearings, heard testimony, and entered orders. Furthermore, the court found that the divorce case in which she was currently involved was connected to the earlier domestic abuse. Although the two cases did not share the same docket numbers, both cases involved the same parties, the same issues, and the same concerns. As a result, the court held that the former judge was precluded from representing either party from the domestic abuse case in the subsequent divorce matter without informed consent in writing from all of the parties.

Chapter Summary

- A lawyer has a fiduciary relationship with a client and owes the client loyalty, competence, and confidentiality. These duties extend to some degree to former clients and prospective clients.
- A conflict of interest exists when there is a significant risk of a material limitation on the ability of the lawyer to exercise independent judgment on behalf of the client or preserve the client's confidential information. When confronted with a conflict of interest, the lawyer should decline or discontinue representation.
- A concurrent conflict of interest exists when the lawyer's independent professional judgment may be compromised because the lawyer represents multiple current clients with potentially differing interests. If the lawyer's independent judgment is compromised, the lawyer must withdraw from representation while preserving the client's confidential information.
- Some concurrent conflicts of interest are waivable when the lawyer reasonably believes that she can provide competent and diligent representation to each

client. The lawyer must obtain each client's informed consent in writing, assuming the conflict is waivable, for example, not prohibited by law.

■ When lawyers represent a current client against a former client there is a concern about protecting the former client's confidences. Absent both the current and former clients' consent, lawyers are barred from representing a client against a former client in a matter that is substantially related to the lawyer's work for the former client.

■ If a lawyer undertakes to represent a client with interests adverse to a former client, without first obtaining the informed consent of both the former and current client, the lawyer risks disqualification if there is a showing of a "substantial relationship" between the subjects of the prior and current representation.

■ In general, if a lawyer has a conflict of interest, the conflict will be imputed to all members of the firm. The conflict of interest of a lawyer who moves from one firm to a new firm will not be imputed to a new firm if the lawyer is timely screened from any involvement in the matter and notice is provided to the former firm.

■ Where there is no concern about loyalty or protecting confidential information, a conflict of interest based on a lawyer's personal, political, or moral feelings will not be imputed to the entire firm unless the representation by others in the firm would be materially limited. Nor will a lawyer's violation of Rule 1.8(j) involving a sexual relationship with a client be imputed to others in a firm.

■ The general rule of imputation also affects non-lawyers of law firms, i.e., paralegals, law clerks, secretaries, and the like.

Applying the Rules

1. Michael Newman retained Jim Jones of the Jones Firm to represent his interests in the formation of the N&F law partnership with John Ferraro, who was separately represented by Rafferty LLP. Attorneys at the Jones Firm drafted the partnership, financing, and security agreements, and other legal documents relating to the N&F partnership formation. Over the next nine years, Jim Jones and the Jones Firm represented both Michael Newman, his wife Lynn Newman, and Michael Newman's interest in the N&F partnership on a wide variety of legal, business, and personal matters.

   Michael and Ferraro decided to renegotiate their partnership. During this process, Michael passed away. Notwithstanding Michael and his wife's relationship with Jim Jones and his firm, Ferraro retained the Jones Firm to represent his interests in an anticipated dispute with the estate of Michael Newman shortly after Michael's death.

   The dispute concerned the partnership agreement that the Jones Firm drafted to protect Michael Newman's interests. It provided that upon dissolution of the partnership for any reason, including the death of Michael Newman, Ferraro was obligated to pay 40 percent of the law firm's gross revenues to Lynn

Newman. Lynn Newman is upset about the Jones Firm representing Ferraro and consults you for legal advice. Discuss your advice for Lynn.

2. Natalie and David Parrott are brother and sister. David and Natalie were charged separately with several criminal violations concerning marijuana and weapons found in their apartment.

   The state offered a joint plea deal to the Parrotts of ten years' imprisonment with the possibility of probation if they successfully completed a program of shock incarceration. In response, defense counsel wrote a joint letter, advising them both not to take the offer. Defense counsel also acknowledged that the state's case against Natalie was much weaker than its case against David, stating: "I really don't see how the Prosecutor thinks he has any case against Natalie for cultivation. Even the charge of possession against Natalie may be rather weak."

   After the initial plea deal was withdrawn, the prosecution offered Natalie a better deal if she would testify against her brother. The prosecution noted that this new plea deal created a conflict of interest concerning defense counsel's joint representation of David and Natalie. The state said it might move to disqualify defense counsel because "[y]ou would not be able to successfully represent Natalie's interest and her brother's." This plea deal involving Natalie's testimony was also rejected.

   After more negotiations, the prosecution offered 15 years contingent on both Natalie and David entering a plea of guilty but without requiring Natalie's testimony against her brother. The Parrotts' attorney was able to convince his clients to accept the plea deal. David and Natalie are now unhappy with the case outcome and seek your help as a local defense expert. They ask, "What can be done — if anything — to get the plea deal thrown out?" Natalie states, "Due to a conflict of interest, he didn't protect me!" Advise the Parrotts.

3. Company A had a meeting with a large law firm regarding a potential lawsuit against company B and requests information about the firm's services. Expecting to receive an engagement letter from the firm, company A was surprised when the firm decided to represent company B in a lawsuit against company A in a similar, but separate matter. The firm claims it screened the attorneys that met with company A, but company A still moved to disqualify the firm under Rule 1.18 for failing to maintain confidences and sharing privileged information received during their meeting. Company A has provided no concrete evidence on what information was shared and has not shown proof that the firm's representation of company B caused significant harm. Advise how the court should decide the disqualification motion. Does the fact that the firm screened the attorneys that attended the meeting with company A make a difference?

Professional Responsibility in Practice

1. Think of a conflict of interest matter (e.g., involving a politician, businessperson, or public servant) that you have recently heard of or read about in the media. What issues did that conflict matter present? How, if at all, were the values of loyalty, independent judgment, and confidentiality involved in the matter? How was the conflict resolved (or not)?

2. Now, find a recent conflict of interest matter in the news that involves a lawyer. How were the lawyer's fiduciary values of loyalty, independent judgment, confidentiality, and competence placed in issue in the matter? Comparing the conflict of interest matters you considered in question 1 above with conflicts of interest problems involving lawyers, what similarities and dissimilarities, if any, do you find in how the conflicts were addressed and resolved? Would you have withdrawn from representation if you were in that lawyer's position? How would you feel if you were the client?

3. Imagine you own a law practice, and a prospective client schedules an initial consultation with you regarding her recent termination from employment. What strategies and protocols might you implement in the initial interview and thereafter to uncover any potential conflicts of interest? What are some of the questions you might ask in the initial interview to identify potential conflicts of interest? Prepare a list of five questions to help you identify any potential conflicts of interest issues in handling the unjust dismissal claim.

4. Assume three clients asked you to jointly represent them in the unjust dismissal claim in question 3, above. How would this change your initial interview discussion and questions concerning possible conflicts of interest? For example, would your explanation about the preservation of their confidences be any different than in question 3? What additional follow-up action might you institute to avoid any future conflicts of interest given your representation of multiple clients?

Lawyer as Advocate

Fairness in Adjudication

An attorney's obligation of loyalty to his client and obligation of candor to the tribunal may collide in the context of litigation. When they do, an attorney's obligations as an officer of the court[1] typically trump her obligations of zealous representation.[2] Lying to the court, assisting or permitting a client or witness to perjure, and counseling a client to destroy documents after they have been subpoenaed are perhaps the most obvious examples of behavior that offends a lawyer's obligation to preserve the integrity of judicial proceedings. But there are many others.

A. MERITORIOUS CLAIMS AND EXPEDITING LITIGATION

Model Rule 3.1 prohibits filing claims, defending lawsuits, or advancing issues within litigation that are "frivolous." Whether a claim is **frivolous** is assessed from an objective standard of what a reasonable attorney would have known in the actor's situation, rather than a subjective standard of malice or motive to harass.

A lawyer is permitted to file a civil complaint or answer with a lesser factual foundation than subsequent pleadings, if she believes in good faith that facts will be developed during litigation to support her initial claim or defense. Comment (2) to Rule 3.1 states that "[t]he filing of an action or defense or similar action taken for a client is not frivolous merely because the facts have not first been fully substantiated or because the lawyer expects to develop vital evidence only by discovery."

Key Concepts

- The attorney's obligation to be honest with the court
- The attorney's responsibility to prevent and remedy perjury
- Why the concealment or destruction of evidence is unlawful
- An attorney's duty to act fairly in dealing with opposing counsel

---

1. Preamble to the Model Rules of Professional Conduct, [1].
2. As will be discussed *infra*, with respect to frivolous factual and legal contentions, Rule 3.1 partially exempts criminal defense lawyers by providing that "[a] lawyer for the defendant in a criminal proceeding . . . may nevertheless so defend the proceeding as to require that every element of the case be established."

Courts tend to be in a better position than bar disciplinary committees to assess the merits of factual claims. Understanding a legal and factual record well enough to assess whether a complaint, answer, motion, or discovery response is well grounded would impose tremendous information costs on bar counsel. Moreover, litigants have little to gain from referring these cases to bar disciplinary agencies, because even if fines are imposed, they will not end up compensating complainants. For both of these reasons Rule 3.1 is infrequently invoked to discipline lawyers. But courts have their own tools to police frivolous pleadings. Rule 11(c) of the Federal Rules of Civil Procedure and its analogue in many states allows a court to sanction a party who signs a written complaint, motion, or other pleading that is not supported by existing law or a good faith argument for an extension of the law, or which is based on factual contentions that have no evidentiary support or are unlikely to derive evidentiary support after reasonable inquiry.[3] Like Rule 3.1, Rule 11 determines the issue of frivolousness by assessing whether an attorney conducted an *objectively reasonable* investigation into the factual and legal predicate for a filing.[4] But unlike Rule 3.1, Rule 11 requires that any factual contentions in a pleading that have not been substantiated be specifically identified as being filed "on information or belief." In order to invoke the sanctions machinery of Rule 11, opposing counsel must serve a separate motion on the offending party requesting sanctions but not file this motion with the court. The attorney accused of misconduct then has a 21-day "safe harbor" to withdraw or correct the challenged pleading before the court is authorized to hold a sanctions hearing.[5]

Case Preview

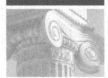

In re Olsen

The following case excerpt stems from a federal employment claim Olsen filed on behalf of his client, Melissa Mellott, against her former employer, MSN Communications. Olsen sought back pay, equal pay, front pay, and benefits for his client. Maintaining that the suit was frivolous, MSN presented documentary evidence (including W-2s) showing that Mellott

---

3. Federal Rule of Civil Procedure 11(b) provides:

> By presenting to the court a pleading, written motion, or other paper—whether by signing, filing, submitting, or later advocating it—an attorney or unrepresented party certifies that to the best of the person's knowledge, information, and belief, formed after an inquiry reasonable under the circumstances:
>   (1) it is not being presented for any improper purpose, such as to harass, cause unnecessary delay, or needlessly increase the cost of litigation;
>   (2) the claims, defenses, and other legal contentions are warranted by existing law or by a nonfrivolous argument for extending, modifying, or reversing existing law or for establishing new law;
>   (3) the factual contentions have evidentiary support or, if specifically so identified, will likely have evidentiary support after a reasonable opportunity for further investigation or discovery; and
>   (4) the denials of factual contentions are warranted on the evidence or, if specifically so identified, are reasonably based on belief or a lack of information.

4. Business Guides v. Chromatic Communications, 498 U.S. 533, 541 (1991).
5. Fed. R. Civ. P. 11(c)(2); Star Mark Management, Inc. v. Koon Chun Hing Kee Soy & Sauce Factory, Ltd., 682 F.3d 170, 175 (2d Cir. 2012).

had been employed for substantial compensation since her termination, that she was fraudulently using someone else's social security number to hide income while collecting unemployment, and that she lied to the district court when she asserted that she had moved to Germany. Olsen filed a memorandum opposing MSN's motion to dismiss the lawsuit as being frivolous, without conducting his own investigation. The Office of Attorney Regulation subsequently filed a suit against Olsen alleging he violated several of Colorado's Rules of Professional Conduct.

As you read *Olsen*, ask yourself the following questions:

1. Was Olsen's professional misstep the filing of the complaint, or the filing of the opposition to the motion to dismiss?
2. Was Olsen guilty of lying in this pleading, or of deliberate indifference to the truth?
3. How could Olsen have prepared his case differently to avoid this sanction?

In re Olsen
326 P.3d 1004 (Colo. 2004)

. . .

II

We affirm the Hearing Board's conclusions that Olsen violated Rules of Professional Conduct 3.1 and 8.4(d), but we reverse its imposition of a six-month suspension with the requirement of reinstatement and instead order that Olsen be, and hereby is, publicly censured for his misconduct. . . .

B. *Hearing Board Findings on Rule Violations*

. . . [T]he Board concluded that Olsen violated two rules of Professional Conduct. It concluded that he violated Rule 3.1 by advancing three frivolous arguments on behalf of his client in the underlying federal litigation: (i) Mellott's claim for lost wages; (ii) Mellott's theories for why she used multiple SSNs; and (iii) that Mellott had moved to Europe and was unavailable to appear in person for several hearings before the federal magistrate and district court judges. The Board also concluded that Olsen violated Rule 8.4(d) by engaging in protracted and unnecessary litigation that wasted considerable judicial resources and prejudiced the administration of justice. We agree with the Board's conclusions that Olsen violated Rules 3.1 and 8.4(d).

Rule 3.1 states, in pertinent part: "A lawyer shall not bring or defend a proceeding, or assert or controvert an issue therein, unless there is a basis in law and fact for doing so that is not frivolous, which includes a good faith argument for an extension, modification or reversal of existing law." We interpret Rule 3.1 broadly to include all proceedings in which factual and legal contentions are made, including post-trial and disciplinary proceedings. An objective standard is used to determine whether an attorney's claim is frivolous. See Colo. RPC Preamble cmt. 20 ("[The] Rules . . . establish standards of conduct by lawyers . . . a lawyer's violation of a Rule may be evidence of [a] breach of the applicable standard of conduct."). While an attorney is permitted to rely on factual accounts given by a client, it may not be objectively reasonable to continue to rely exclusively on a client's statement of facts when the attorney is presented with credible contradictory evidence. See Colo. RPC 3.1 cmt. 2 ("What is required of lawyers . . . is that they inform themselves about the facts of their clients' cases . . . and determine that they can make good faith arguments in support of their clients' positions.").

The Board found that Olsen advanced his client's frivolous arguments first in the underlying federal lawsuit, and again in the post-trial proceedings concerning attorney fees and other sanctions. The Board reasoned that "it should have been obvious to [Olsen] that [his client's] shifting narratives were completely contradicted by credible evidence" and also that there was a "dearth of credible evidence indicating that [Olsen] conducted a reasonable investigation of his client's implausible factual assertions."

We agree that Olsen had an ongoing professional duty to independently assess the factual and legal bases for Mellott's claims. At the same time, we recognize that an attorney's role is to advocate for the client. The dissenting Hearing Board member correctly observes that an attorney has a duty of loyalty to the client, along with a duty of candor to the court, and attorneys should generally resolve doubts about the factual underpinnings of a claim in favor of their clients.

Nevertheless, Rule 8.4(d) states, in pertinent part: "It is professional misconduct for a lawyer to . . . engage in conduct that is prejudicial to the administration of justice." The record before us contains ample evidence that Olsen's conduct prejudiced the administration of justice in the underlying federal lawsuit. His unprofessional demeanor in dealing with opposing counsel, Judge Brimmer, and Magistrate Judge Watanabe exceeded the bounds of acceptable litigation strategy and evidenced a disregard for his professional responsibility to the tribunals. As a result of Olsen's pursuit of his client's frivolous arguments, Judge Brimmer and Magistrate Judge Watanabe were each required to expend significant judicial resources scheduling, preparing for, and continuing hearings, and ruling on Olsen's repetitive and often unsupported motions. For these reasons, there is adequate evidence in the record to uphold the Board's conclusion that Olsen violated Rule 8.4(d).

. . .

III

We affirm the Hearing Board's conclusions that Olsen violated Rules of Professional Conduct 3.1 and 8.4(d), but we reverse its imposition of a six-month suspension with the requirement of reinstatement. We hereby censure John R. Olsen for his misconduct.

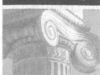

Post-Case Follow-Up

In the underlying federal litigation in *Olsen*, the district court awarded the defendant $25,000 in attorneys' fees under 28 U.S.C. §1927 (a predecessor to FRCP 11) as a sanction for Olsen's misconduct. Do you think that this case-based sanction influenced the Colorado Supreme Court's decision to reduce the lawyer's discipline from suspension to public censure? Why or why not?

Is public censure of an attorney an effective sanction for ethical misconduct, or is it a mere "slap on the wrist"? Does this depend on how informed and cohesive the legal community is in the particular jurisdiction?

In re Olsen: Real Life Applications

1. Both Rule 3.1 and FRCP 11 allow an attorney to file a factual claim with a tribunal if he reasonably believes that the claim will have evidentiary support after discovery. Does this mean that an attorney may rely solely on his client's factual allegations in drafting and filing a civil complaint, without *any* factual inquiry whatsoever? Suppose that you are a workers' compensation attorney and a new client approaches you claiming to have been injured on the job site. The client has no visible signs of injury. May you file a workers' compensation claim on his behalf without seeking and analyzing documents substantiating both his employment and his injury? Should you?

2. You are an insurance defense attorney. Your client, Providential Insurance Co., represents a chain of "big box" stores. A large percentage of your practice is defending "slip and fall" cases that allegedly occur on store property. May you routinely include a defense of contributory negligence in your answers to complaints without conducting any interviews or analyzing video security footage to determine whether the plaintiff may have been partially responsible for the accident?

As we have just seen, there must be non-frivolous support for an attorney's *factual* claims. But an attorney's *legal* argument may be based on a creative or novel theory that presses for changes in the law. A legal claim or argument is not frivolous within the meaning of Rule 3.1 if it is supported by "a good faith argument for an extension, modification, or reversal of existing law." The comment to this rule recognizes that an action or defense is not frivolous "even though the lawyer believes that the client's position ultimately will not prevail."[6]

Rule 3.4(d) imposes obligations on an attorney with respect to discovery requests and responses that parallel Rule 3.1's obligations with respect to pleadings. Again, the emphasis is on candor to the tribunal and avoiding frivolous tactics that abuse the litigation process. Rule 3.4(d) provides that a party shall not "make a frivolous discovery request or fail to make reasonably diligent effort to comply with a legally proper discovery request by an opposing party." Examples of discovery conduct that may violate Rule 3.4(d) include overusing depositions or interrogatories, engaging in questioning techniques that seek embarrassing but irrelevant information, unreasonably delaying document production, and instructing deposition

---

6. Model Rule 3.1 cmt. [2].

witnesses not to answer clearly pertinent inquiries that call for non-privileged information.

B. OBLIGATION TO BE TRUTHFUL

The attorney's obligation of **candor to the tribunal** may arise in a variety of contexts: for example, when the lawyer makes statements of law to the court during oral argument; when the lawyer cites or fails to cite legal authority in written memoranda or briefs; and when the lawyer calls a witness who makes false statements during testimony. The attorney's ethical obligations are slightly different in each instance. The attorney clearly cannot directly make false statements of her own to the court, nor can she assist her client to make false statements. The attorney's responsibility with respect to a witness who makes false statements is significantly more complex.

With regard to false statements to a tribunal, the responsibilities of an attorney require a delicate balance of three professional obligations: (1) the lawyer must learn as much about the client's case as possible in order to be able to represent the client competently (Rule 1.1); (2) the lawyer must keep confidential any private information divulged by the client, with certain exceptions (Rule 1.6); and (3) the lawyer must not knowingly participate in a fraud on the tribunal (Rule 3.3). This three-way tension is often referred to as the lawyer's "trilemma." Where these tensions collide in the context of litigation, the Model Rules emphasize the attorney's third obligation of candor to the tribunal over the first two, requiring a lawyer to take remedial action to prevent or rectify any fraud on the court.[7] Some states may rank these duties differently, particularly with respect to client perjury where the witness is a criminal defendant, which is discussed later in Chapter 8.

1. Candor to the Court

Rule 3.3(a) provides that a lawyer shall not "knowingly make a false statement of law or fact to a tribunal" or "fail to correct a false statement of material fact or law previously made to the tribunal by the lawyer." If the judge or magistrate[8] asks a lawyer at a criminal bail hearing "does your client have a job," the lawyer must answer truthfully, and is subject to discipline if she fails to do so. An attorney preparing a brief for appeal may not misstate or overstate testimony from the record below in order to render a legal argument more persuasive.

A lawyer violates Rule 3.3(a) when he makes a statement to the court knowing that it is false; mere suspicion of falsity or recklessness toward the truth will not suffice. Nonetheless, the comment to the rule recognizes that "knowledge that

---

7. *See* ABA Formal Op. 87-353 (1987).
8. The use of the word "tribunal" in Rule 3.3 means that the obligation of candor applies to all types of adjudicative proceedings, including administrative hearings and arbitrations. *See* Model Rule 1.0(m). For the purposes of discussion in this chapter the authors will use the words tribunal and court interchangeably.

evidence is false . . . can be inferred from the circumstances."[9] While an attorney may resolve doubts or suspicions regarding the truth of statement in favor of the client, a lawyer cannot ignore an obvious falsehood by putting his head in the sand to avoid actual knowledge.

Note that a lawyer's obligations with regard to truthful statements to a tribunal differ depending on their timing. If the lawyer knows that the statement is false at the time he makes it, he may not make the statement to the court, regardless of how significant or trivial the subject. But if a lawyer makes a statement and *subsequently* learns of its falsehood, the attorney has a duty to correct the falsity only if the statement is "**material**." *See* Rule 3.3(a)(3). For example, if a lawyer advises the court at a hearing on a motion for a preliminary injunction in a case involving the sale of real property that his client's ownership of real estate is limited to the client's primary residence, he has a duty to correct that statement at a subsequent court hearing with respect to that same litigation if he subsequently learns that his client owns a vacation home.[10] But if a lawyer argues to the court at the same motion hearing that his client is 52 years of age when actually he is 53, the lawyer has no duty to subsequently correct that misstatement.

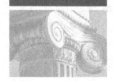

Case Preview

In re Richards

The underlying litigation that lead to this disciplinary action against attorney Robert Richards stems from a case he brought *pro se* against Arthur Adair, represented by George Scarborough. Richards sought to depose a nonparty, Rodeo Nites, but it did not show up for the deposition. Adair and his attorney successfully moved for lost wages and attorneys' fees for their wasted day. Richards filed a motion for a new hearing, believing that Scarborough should not have been able to argue the attorneys' fees and lost wages issue on the same day as his show cause hearing. In his appeal from the district court order, Richards alleged that he objected to Scarborough's motion on that day. He presented the transcript from the hearing as evidence, but omitted crucial aspects of the transcript in order to bolster his argument.

As you read *In re Richards*, ask yourself the following:

1. Why are appellate courts especially vulnerable to misrepresentation or deception by counsel of record?
2. Could Richards have made a non-frivolous argument that his objection was preserved below without using ellipses to redact the lower court transcript?

---

9. Model Rule 3.3 cmt. [8].
10. The duty to take remedial measures may require the lawyer to reveal information that otherwise would be protected by the lawyer's duty of confidentiality under Rule 1.6. *See* Model Rule 3.3 cmt. [10].

In re Richards
943 P.2d 1032 (N.M. 1997)

. . .

This matter came before the Court on the recommendation of the disciplinary board that Robert Richards be publicly censured for knowingly making a false statement of material fact in a brief filed in the New Mexico Court of Appeals for the purpose of deceiving the appellate court. This Court, having considered the recommendation and being sufficiently advised, adopts the recommendation and orders that respondent be publicly censured for violation of his duty of candor to the court.

. . .

We agree completely with the Court of Appeals' concluding remarks, that it "expect[s] candor in the memoranda submitted . . ." and that respondent's "memorandum failed to meet that standard."

In his defense, respondent has maintained that the deletion of a portion of the quote did not change the meaning, because he intended to object on two grounds: that Scarborough was representing adverse interests in Adair and Rodeo Nites, and that he had not received notice that Adair's motion would be heard at that hearing. Respondent contended that the trial court cut him off before he could articulate the second basis for his objection. This was not, he argued, fatal to his objection, because Rule 1-046 of the Rules of Civil Procedure for the District Courts provides that, to preserve a question for appeal, it is only necessary that the party makes known to the court the objection to the ruling. From this, respondent argues that his redacted quotation showed that the district court knew that he was objecting to Adair's motion being heard, because she referenced Scarborough's request to have Adair's motion heard and stated she was going to hear it.

Respondent is the only person in the world who knows whether he did intend to object on the additional basis that he had not received proper notice that Adair's motion would be heard. What respondent apparently does not understand is that this point is not determinative of whether he made a material misrepresentation to the Court of Appeals. If respondent had recited the entire discussion he had with Judge Maes, he could have argued to the Court of Appeals (1) that he would have objected on the notice basis had he not been interrupted or (2) that under Rule 1-046, an objection is preserved if the record shows the court understood the basis for the objection, even if it was not articulated by the objecting party. The Court of Appeals, with all relevant information before it, could have decided whether the record supported respondent's version of what objection he was making and whether respondent's interpretation of the requirements for preserving error was correct.

Instead, respondent engaged in a form of advocacy that was deceitful and dishonest. The Court of Appeals was not told that the record failed to reflect an objection on the notice issue, but rather reflected an objection on another topic altogether. Moreover, not only did respondent omit material language, but he also made the affirmative statement that the trial court understood his objection to address the issue of hearing Mr. Adair's motion. As the Court of Appeals noted, respondent achieved this impression by omitting language that showed the objection he actually made.

Certainly a lawyer is expected to make the best argument he or she can to enhance the chance of success. The lawyer's arguments must, however, be based upon the actual state of events, not a distorted version of what occurred. Contrary to respondent's contention, the portion he omitted did change the meaning of the text. If included, there was a very real possibility that the Court of Appeals would find that he had not objected to the motion being heard, but rather had only raised an objection concerning who Scarborough represented. By omitting that portion of the dialogue, respondent attempted to increase the chance that the court would believe he had actually objected to Adair's motion being heard. That is not advocacy; it is deceit.

. . .

We therefore adopt the recommendation of the disciplinary board and find that respondent violated Rule 16-303(A)(1), by knowingly making a false statement of material fact to the Court of Appeals. . . .

Post-Case Follow-Up

Would Richards's conduct have been any less egregious or violative of Rule 3.3 if he had been represented by private counsel in the underlying litigation, and then represented himself *pro se* on appeal?

We tend to think that professional and strategic considerations are distinct, but are they? Where an attorney gains a reputation among judges for playing fast and loose with the facts, could that make her less effective as an advocate?

In re Richards: Real Life Applications

1. You are scheduled to try a motor vehicle accident case, and your primary witness (the plaintiff) inexplicably fails to show up to court. The case is marked "no further continuances," and you know that the judge will be reluctant to grant you an extension. May you tell the judge that your client has had a medical emergency and request a continuance on that basis?

2. You are representing one party to a divorce action in probate court. Your client is seeking alimony from her longtime husband. At the preliminary hearing after the divorce complaint is filed, you lodge an affidavit of financial condition stating that your client is an unemployed homemaker. After oral argument, the judge orders the husband to make a temporary payment of $1,000 per week to your client pending a final decree of divorce. Following this preliminary hearing, your client obtains a part-time job earning $750 per week. Although your statement to the court was accurate when made, it no longer reflects the financial condition of the client. Do you have an *ethical* duty to inform the court of your client's recent employment, or does that duty, if any, rest on the procedural rules of the probate court?

2. Failure to Disclose Adverse Facts in *Ex Parte* Proceedings

Attorneys typically are not required to disclose adverse facts to the court during a trial, because in an adversarial system, litigants are expected to present their cases in the best possible light. Adverse facts generally will be disclosed by opposing counsel if it is his tactical advantage to do so. But this presumption breaks down in *ex parte* (one-sided) proceedings, where opposing counsel is not present. Applications for a search warrant or wiretap authorization in criminal cases, and motions for a *lis pendens* or temporary restraining order in civil cases, are examples of *ex parte* **proceedings**. Model Rule 3.3(d) provides that in an *ex parte* proceeding a lawyer must inform the tribunal of "all material facts known to the lawyer that will enable the tribunal to make an informed decision, whether or not the facts are adverse." The principle behind the rule is that hiding material adverse facts from the judge or magistrate in an *ex parte* proceeding would disable the court from making an informed decision.[11]

Suppose that a litigator files a complaint for breach of a real estate contract, and at the time of the filing of the complaint brings a motion for a temporary restraining order asking the court to prevent the defendant and owner of the property from conveying the property to another during the pendency of the proceeding. The plaintiff's theory of breach of contract is that the defendant signed a purchase and sale agreement but then reneged on the sale when he got a higher offer. If the purchase and sale agreement required the plaintiff to secure financing by a specified date and the plaintiff missed that contractual deadline by 24 hours, this would be a "material" adverse fact that the plaintiff's lawyer would be required to bring to the court's attention at the hearing.

A lawyer's duty to reveal material adverse facts at an *ex parte* hearing *includes* facts that are protected by client confidences. Rule 1.6 creates an exception to the obligation of confidentiality for those disclosures that are necessary to comply with law.[12] However, lawyers are not required by Rule 3.3(d) to reveal at *ex parte* hearings information that is protected by the attorney-client privilege.[13]

3. Failure to Disclose Controlling Legal Authority

The duties with respect to factual representations pertain to affirmative misstatements to the tribunal. The *omission* of facts or the failure to reveal facts to the tribunal are not explicitly covered by Rule 3.3(a). Except at an *ex parte* proceeding,[14] a lawyer typically has no affirmative duty to reveal contrary facts to the court unless specifically asked about them, because contrary facts are ordinarily expected to be revealed by opposing counsel to their advantage. However, where the attorney is aware of undisclosed facts that make her factual presentation to the

---

11. Model Rule 3.3(d) cmt. [14].
12. Model Rule 1.6(b)(6) and cmt. [12]. *See* People v. Ritland, 327 P.3d 914 (Colo. 2014) (in *ex parte* petition for adoption of child, lawyer impermissibly misrepresented biological father of child).
13. Restatement (Third) of the Law Governing Lawyers §112 cmt. [b] [hereinafter Restatement].
14. *See* Section B.2, *supra*.

court *fundamentally misleading*, the omission of those facts may rise to the level of "dishonesty, fraud, deceit, or misrepresentation" within the meaning of a separate section of the rules. *See* Model Rule 8.4(c).[15]

With respect to legal argument, however, an attorney has both a duty not to knowingly *misstate* the law and a duty to *reveal* controlling legal authority. Rule 3.3(a)(2) provides that a lawyer has the duty to disclose "legal authority in the controlling jurisdiction known to the lawyer to be directly adverse to the position of the client and not disclosed by opposing counsel." The premise here is that, as an officer of the court, a lawyer has an obligation to assist the court in determining the legal authority properly applicable to the case. Of course, dealing with negative authority is also good lawyering, because usually the opposing counsel or judge is going to uncover it themselves, so it is better tactically to address — and if possible distinguish — negative precedent "up front."

Case Preview

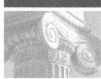

In re Thonert

The following is an excerpt from an Indiana Supreme Court decision upholding discipline on attorney, Richard Thonert. Thonert represented a client charged with operating a motor vehicle while intoxicated. The defendant sought to withdraw his guilty plea and retained Thonert. Thonert failed to inform his client of a directly relevant similar matter in which he represented the defendant and had not prevailed, *Fletcher v. State*. The holding in *Fletcher* was binding precedent on his client's case, but Thonert did not argue for changing or extending the *Fletcher* holding. Instead, both Thonert and the opposing counsel failed to disclose the case to the court on appeal.

As you read *In re Thonert*, ask yourself the following:

1. Why was it so clear that Thonert had actual knowledge of the adverse legal authority within the meaning of Rule 3.3?
2. How does the obligation to disclose adverse legal authority coincide with the right of an attorney under Rule 3.3 to press for changes in the law or the overruling of controlling precedent?

In re Thonert
733 N.E.2d 932 (Ind. 2000)

The respondent in this attorney disciplinary matter is charged with failing to disclose to an appellate tribunal controlling authority known to him, not disclosed by opposing counsel, that was directly adverse to his client's position. He also failed to

---

15. *See* In re Cardwell, 50 P.3d 897 (Colo. 2002). *See also* Model Rule 3.3 cmt. [3] ("there are circumstances where failure to make a [factual] disclosure is the equivalent of an affirmative misrepresentation").

advise his client of the adverse legal authority when his client was contemplating his legal options.

. . .

The respondent represented the defendant in Fletcher v. State, 649 N.E.2d 1022 (Ind. 1995). In that case, this Court addressed the questions that the respondent raised in his client's case. The ruling in *Fletcher* was adverse to the arguments that the respondent offered on appeal of his client's case. The respondent had served as counsel of record for defendant Fletcher in the appeal before this Court. This Court's ruling in *Fletcher* was issued on May 1, 1995, over one year before the respondent filed his appeal on behalf of the client. In his appellate brief filed on behalf of the client, the respondent failed to cite to *Fletcher* or argue that its holding was not controlling authority in the client's case. The respondent also failed to argue that the holding in *Fletcher* should be changed or extended. . . .

Indiana Professional Conduct Rule 3.3(a)(3) provides that a lawyer shall not knowingly fail to disclose to a tribunal legal authority in the controlling jurisdiction known to the lawyer to be directly adverse to the position of the client and not disclosed by opposing counsel. The concept underlying this requirement of disclosure is that legal argument is a discussion seeking to determine the legal premises properly applicable to the case. *Comment* to Ind. Professional Conduct Rule 3.3. The respondent's intimate familiarity with *Fletcher* is established by his having served as counsel to the defendant. Accordingly, we find that the respondent violated the rule by failing to disclose *Fletcher* to the Court of Appeals in his legal arguments on behalf of the client.

. . .

It is, therefore, ordered that the respondent, Richard J. Thonert, is hereby reprimanded and admonished for his violations of Prof. Cond. R. 3.3(a)(3). . . .

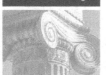

Post-Case Follow-Up

Rule 3.3 allows for discipline of the lawyer only where the adverse legal authority is both known by the attorney and non-disclosed by the opposition. So the provision of this rule does not often present a dilemma for lawyers, because normally an opposing party will disclose authority favorable to her case.

Note how Rule 1.1 and Rule 3.3 work together here. If a lawyer does not conduct adequate research to reveal the controlling legal authority, he may not have actual "knowledge" within the meaning of Rule 3.3 (although knowledge may be inferred from the circumstances under Rule 1.0). But by pleading *negligence*, the attorney may be opening himself up to a charge of incompetence under Rule 1.1.

In re Thonert: Real Life Applications

1. Is *dicta* in an appellate opinion suggesting how a court would likely come out in a factual setting not immediately before the court ever "authority" within

the meaning of Rule 3.3(a)(2)? Even if it is "authority," can it ever be "directly" adverse to the position of a client?

2. Suppose that you are an assistant district attorney representing the state on appeal from an assault and battery conviction. The defendant unsuccessfully raised a claim of self-defense at trial. The trial judge refused to allow the defendant to admit evidence of prior violent conduct on the part of the victim that was unknown to the defendant at the time of the fight. Your case is on direct appeal before the state supreme court. You are aware of an opinion from a three-judge panel of the state appeals court in another case holding that prior acts of violence of the victim should be admitted in a case involving self-defense, even if those acts were not known to the defendant. Defense counsel does not cite this opinion in his brief. Do you have an obligation to cite it in your brief, even if you go on to argue that it was erroneously decided? That is, does the word "controlling" in Rule 3.3(a) refer to the word "authority" or to the word "jurisdiction"?

4. Client or Other Witness Giving False Testimony in Civil Litigation

Paragraph (a)(3) of Rule 3.3 sets forth an attorney's duties with respect to a client or a witness called by the attorney who gives materially false testimony at an adjudicative proceeding (which includes a deposition, pretrial hearing, trial, or arbitration). In the next chapter, we deal with the responsibilities of defense lawyers in criminal cases. Here we discuss the obligation of lawyers in civil cases when they know that their client or a witness they have called has lied under oath on a material matter. In these situations, the attorney's obligation of candor to the tribunal takes priority over her obligation of confidentiality under Rule 1.6. Even when the witness is the attorney's client, the lawyer who knows that a witness has testified falsely as to a material matter, either on direct or cross-examination, must "take reasonable remedial measures, including, if necessary, disclosure to the tribunal."[16] The comment to the rule suggests that **reasonable remedial measures** include remonstrating with the witness and encouraging the witness to withdraw such testimony, withdrawal from representation upon approval of the court if it will undo the effects of the false testimony, or disclosure to the tribunal of the falsity.[17]

The obligations of an attorney under Model Rule 3.3 differ depending on when the attorney learns of the falsity. If a witness reveals to an attorney his *intention* to commit perjury before testifying, the lawyer is obliged to remonstrate with the witness, attempt to convince him of the dangers and consequences of testifying falsely, and, where the witness is a client, threaten to withdraw from representation if the witness persists in his intention. Usually that will work. But what if it doesn't work, or if the witness surprises the attorney by testifying falsely notwithstanding

---

16. Model Rule 3.3(a)(3).
17. *Id.* cmt. [10].

contrary indications? In those circumstances, the obligation of the attorney to take "remedial measures" depends on the materiality of the evidence. Where the testimony relates to a trivial or inconsequential matter, the attorney may do nothing. Where the testimony relates to a material matter, the attorney must ask the witness to correct his testimony, and if that remonstration fails, disclose the false testimony to the court.[18]

An attorney's duty with respect to false testimony applies in both the trial and pretrial contexts. Nevertheless, the ABA has recognized that the "remedial measures" available to a lawyer may be broader when a witness or client gives false answers in the discovery context — such as with interrogatories or depositions — than when he gives false testimony at trial. In the former situation, it may be sufficient for the attorney to disaffirm the work product, supplement the discovery provided, or notify opposing counsel where the witness persists in giving false evidence.[19]

The requirements of Rule 3.3(a)(3) that we have been discussing apply only if the attorney actually *knows* that her witness's or client's testimony is false. The attorney may suspect or believe that the witness's testimony is false, but in the absence of affirmative knowledge, the lawyer does not need to remonstrate with the witness or inform the court. However, knowledge may be inferred from the circumstances. Comment [8] to Rule 3.3 provides that "although a lawyer should resolve doubts about the veracity of testimony or other evidence in favor of the client, the lawyer cannot ignore an obvious falsehood."[20]

If the attorney suspects but does not know that a witness's testimony will be false before presenting it, the attorney has discretion to refuse to offer the testimony. The attorney may simply refuse to call the person as a witness if he thinks the person is going to lie. But the attorney is not required to do so; the discretion in such instance rests with the attorney. We will soon see that there is an important exception to this rule for criminal cases where the witness is the attorney's client.

Case Preview

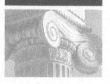

Committee on Professional Ethics v. Crary

Unbeknownst to Sue Evans Curtis and William Crary, Sue's husband hired a private investigator to follow them around and document their love affair. During this period, Mrs. Curtis repeatedly lied to her husband about her whereabouts — occasionally for weeks at a time. When Mrs. Curtis filed for divorce, she employed her paramour as one of the attorneys to represent her in the divorce proceedings. During her deposition, her husband's attorney, armed with all the knowledge of the private investigator, asked Sue Evans Curtis about her alleged trips out of town. Rather than reveal the relationship, she

---

18. *See* ABA Formal Op. 87-353 (1987).
19. *See* ABA Formal Op. 93-376 (1993).
20. Model Rule 3.3(a)(3) cmt. [9].

lied under oath while Crary sat idly by allowing her to perjure herself for two days. After the divorce, Curtis and Crary married and a custody battle ensued for her children in which he helped her circumvent the court order awarding custody to her husband. The Iowa State Bar Association filed a complaint with the Grievance Commission of the Iowa Supreme Court against Crary for his unethical conduct with regards to both the perjury incident and the frustration of the custody decree.

As you read this opinion, ask yourself the following:

1. At what point in the proceedings could and should Crary have made different decisions?
2. How does the court dispose of Crary's self-incrimination argument? Is it convincing?

Committee on Professional Ethics v. Crary
245 N.W.2d 298 (Iowa 1976)

II. THE DEPOSITION PERJURY

The charge involving perjury . . . presents two subsidiary problems.

A. *The First Problem Is Procedural*

[The court first addressed the interplay between an Iowa statute prohibiting a lawyer from misleading a judge by any artifice or false statement and the Model Code of Professional Responsibility.]

B. *The Second Problem Involves the Merits of the Charge Relating to the Perjury*

What are the *facts* of the matter? Mr. and Mrs. Curtis were husband and wife, lived together, and had three children. Respondent began to see Mrs. Curtis and stayed with her at various places and slept with her—both before and after Mrs. Curtis commenced her divorce suit against Mr. Curtis.

. . .

Respondent contends . . . that the record contains no express testimony by him or Mrs. Curtis that he put her up to the false stories she related in the deposition. Yet those stories did not come out of thin air; they took some contriving. We doubt that Mrs. Curtis simply developed those stories about Mrs. Needham as the deposition progressed or that she developed them alone.

We think respondent was involved in the whole shameful episode, but we will accept arguendo his contention that he did not contrive the perjury with Mrs. Curtis. Then we have a situation in which respondent as an attorney at a deposition listened, his client started to lie under oath, he knew she was lying, and he just "sat there" and let her lie. More than that, the deposition recessed over Thursday, and respondent did nothing to stop Mrs. Curtis from lying some more. She resumed her lying on Friday and respondent still just sat there.

What is the *law* of this matter? We are not disposed to read §§610.14(3) and 610.24(3) of the Iowa Code in a narrow, technical, or legalistic manner. Assuming respondent did not know in advance that Mrs. Curtis was going to lie, his guilt was in failing to stop her or otherwise to call a halt when she started to lie.

Central to the administration of justice is the fact-finding process. Legislatures and courts can devise the finest rules of law, but if those rules are applied to false "facts," justice miscarries.

The attorney functions at the heart of the fact-finding process, both in trial and in pre- and post-trial proceedings. If he knowingly suffers a witness to lie, he undermines the integrity of the fact-finding system of which he himself is an integral part. Thus the fundamental rule is unquestioned that *an attorney must not knowingly permit a witness to lie.* . . .

But respondent contends he was not required to volunteer to opposing counsel or the court that Mrs. Curtis' testimony was false, since this could have provided evidence for building an adultery case against him. He cites authority that an attorney like others is privileged not to produce evidence which will incriminate him. . . .

Respondent does not seem to grasp the point here. We do not place the decision on respondent's failure to inform opposing counsel or the court of the truth. In the present case no need really existed for this. Opposing counsel was not misled. His subsequent questions revealed he knew the facts; he made Mrs. Curtis' perjury patent. The vice of respondent's conduct was not in failing to reveal the truth but in participating in the corruption of the fact-finding system by knowingly permitting Mrs. Curtis to lie. Indeed if Mr. Curtis had not had private investigators, the falsity of this testimony might never have come to light; Mrs. Curtis' perjury, countenanced by respondent, might have subsequently carried the day in court. Contrast with respondent's conduct the acts of Mr. Gray. When that attorney suspected on Friday that Mrs. Curtis was lying he confronted respondent and upon learning the truth said, "She can't sit there and tell this story." He thereupon recessed the deposition.

Apart from self-incrimination, respondent contends that his duty to protect his client, Mrs. Curtis, conflicted with his duty to the justice system to divulge the falsity, and that he properly placed his duty to his client first. He bases this contention on the attorney-client privilege.

Respondent confuses the duty to divulge the truth after perjury is committed with the duty not to permit a witness to give false testimony in the first place. We will proceed on this contention, however, on respondent's basis, as though respondent's breach was in not divulging the truth to opposing counsel or the court after the false testimony was given. We address respondent's contention as he does under the attorney-client privilege and without reference to any other privilege.

The difficulty with respondent's contention is that it proceeds from a false premise. He cites the article entitled Perjury, The Lawyer's Trilemma, in *Litigation* (Winter 1975 Journ. of A.B.A. Litigation Section). From this article, he concludes that a conflict between two duties exists: one to the client, the other to the justice system.

The flaw in respondent's reasoning is that no duty exists to the client when the client perjures himself to the knowledge of the attorney. Such conduct by the client falls outside the attorney-client relationship. When a prospective client approaches an attorney, he may expect that the attorney will assist him to the best of the attorney's ability. He may not expect, however, that the attorney will tolerate lying or any other species of fraud in the process. . . .

The office of attorney does not permit, much less does it demand of him for any client, violation of law or any manner of fraud or chicane. He must obey his own conscience and not that of his client. Canons of Professional Ethics (A.B.A. 1957).

Correspondingly, the present rules state that "A lawyer shall not . . . engage in conduct involving dishonesty, fraud, deceit, or misrepresentation," "engage in conduct that is prejudicial to the administration of justice," "participate in the creation or preservation of evidence when he knows or it is obvious that the evidence is false," or "counsel or assist his client in conduct that the lawyer knows to be illegal or fraudulent." Iowa Code of Professional Responsibility for Lawyers (1971) DR1-102(A)(4) and (5), DR7-102(A)(6) and (7).

We hold that respondent acted unethically in knowingly permitting Mrs. Curtis to commit perjury on the first day of the deposition and to resume the perjury two days later, and that in so doing he violated §§610.14(3) and 610.24(3) of the Iowa Code.

. . .

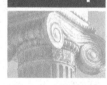

Post-Case Follow-Up

Was Crary prohibited by any other ethical rule from agreeing to represent in a divorce proceeding a client with whom he was having a sexual relationship? What about the conflict of interest rules? The attorney-witness rule?

Mr. Crary's client lied in two days of deposition testimony. One typical and acceptable response to client perjury is to remonstrate privately with the client and attempt to convince her to correct the misstatement. Suppose that Crary intended to remonstrate with his client after the first day of deposition was concluded, but before he could do so, opposing counsel approached him with a settlement offer. Would settling the case without correcting the record violate Rule 3.3 or any other rule?

Committee on Professional Ethics v. Crary: Real Life Applications

1. Suppose that you represent a defendant in a motor vehicle tort case. You have examined your client's phone records and compared them to the police report. You know to a substantial degree of certainty that your client was on her cell phone to her boyfriend at the time of the accident. At her deposition in response to questions from opposing counsel, your client denies that she was "using" her cell phone at the time of the crash. What are your options under comment [10] to Rule 3.3?

2. Imagine a similar case as in hypothetical #1, but the client's testimony occurs at trial. Your client has testified in a way that contradicts not only her cell phone

records (produced by the plaintiff in discovery) but also her prior statements to you during private meetings. What are your options at trial? Would a motion to withdraw from representation (a so-called noisy withdrawal) be an adequate substitute for affirmatively disclosing the adverse fact to the court? Can such a motion "undo the effect" of the false evidence within the meaning of comment [10]?

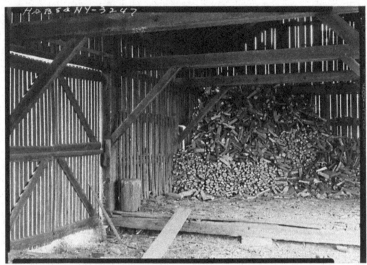

When does "woodshedding" a witness cross the line?
Library of Congress Prints and Photographs Division, Washington, D.C.

Rule 3.4(b) prohibits an attorney from counseling or assisting a witness to testify falsely. This prohibition applies regardless of the materiality of the testimony, consistent with the prohibition in Rule 3.3(a)(3) of knowingly presenting false testimony. An attorney may help prepare a witness to present her testimony in the light most favorable to the attorney's client, by suggesting convincing manners of expression or emphasis. But an attorney may not suggest that a witness knows facts that she does not know, or pressure the witness to testify in a way that is inconsistent with the witness's actual memory or belief.

Exactly when does rehearsing or **"woodshedding"** a witness cross the line between helping to shape the most accurate and powerful testimony and helping to fashion false or misleading testimony? This question was the subject of the following Ethics Opinion from the District of Columbia Bar.

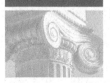

Case Preview

D.C. Bar Legal Ethics Committee Formal Opinion 79

This opinion issued by the D.C. Legal Ethics Committee addresses three questions raised regarding a lawyer's role in preparing a witness's testimony. The committee, in interpreting the D.C. Code of Professional Responsibility—replaced in 1991 by the D.C. Rules of Professional Conduct—determined that lawyers are allowed to prepare or assist in preparing a witness's testimony so long as he or she did not know or should not have reasonably known that the testimony was false or misleading.

As you read this opinion, ask yourself whether the required mental state for a violation of Rule 3.4(b) hinders or promotes perjured testimony.

Limitations on a Lawyer's Participation in the Preparation of a Witness's Testimony
D.C. Bar Legal Ethics Committee Formal Opinion 79 (1979)

The particular questions put by the inquirer are whether it is ethically proper for a lawyer actually to write the testimony the witness will adopt under oath; whether, if so, the lawyer may engage in "practice cross-examination exercises" intended to prepare the witness for questions that may be asked at the hearing.

In order to present those issues in a more inclusive setting, the questions may usefully be rephrased as follows:

(1) What are the ethical limitations on a lawyer's suggesting the actual language in which a witness's testimony is to be presented, whether in written form or otherwise?

(2) What are the ethical limitations on a lawyer's suggesting that a witness's testimony include information that was not initially furnished to the lawyer by the witness?

(3) What are the ethical limitations on a lawyer's preparing a witness for the presentation of testimony under live examination, whether direct or cross, and whether by practice questioning or otherwise?

A single prohibitory principle governs the answer to all three of these questions: it is, simply, that a lawyer may not prepare, or assist in preparing, testimony that he or she knows, or ought to know, is false or misleading. So long as this prohibition is not transgressed, a lawyer may properly suggest language as well as substance of testimony, and may — indeed should — do whatever is feasible to prepare his or her witnesses for examination.

It follows, therefore — to address the first question here raised — that the fact that the particular words in which testimony, whether written or oral, is cast originated with a lawyer rather than the witness whose testimony it is has no significance so long as the substance of that testimony is not, so far as the lawyer knows or ought to know, false or misleading. If the particular words suggested by the lawyer, even though not literally false, are calculated to convey a misleading impression, this would be equally impermissible from the ethical point of view.

The second question raised by the inquiry — as to the propriety of a lawyer's suggesting the inclusion in a witness's testimony of information not initially secured from the witness — may, again, arise not only with respect to written testimony but with oral testimony as well. In either case, it appears to us that the governing consideration for ethical purposes is whether the substance of the testimony is something the witness can truthfully and properly testify to. If he or she is willing and (as respects his or her state of knowledge) able honestly so to testify, the fact that the inclusion of a particular point of substance was initially suggested by the lawyer rather than the witness seems to us wholly without significance. There are two principal hazards here. One hazard is the possibility of undue suggestion: that is, the risk that the witness may thoughtlessly adopt testimony offered by the lawyer simply because it is so offered, without considering whether it is testimony that he or she may appropriately give under oath. The other hazard is the possibility of a suggestion or implication in the witness's resulting testimony that the witness is testifying on a particular matter of his own knowledge when this is not the fact the cases. . . . [H]owever, there should be no difficulty, for a reasonably skilled and scrupulous lawyer, in avoiding the hazards in question.

We turn, finally, to the extent of a lawyer's proper participation in preparing a witness for giving live testimony—whether the testimony is only to be under cross-examination, as in the particular circumstances giving rise to the present inquiry, or, as more usually the case, direct examination as well. Here again it appears to us that the only touchstones are the truth and genuineness of the testimony to be given. The mere fact of a lawyer's having prepared the witness for the presentation of testimony is simply irrelevant: indeed, a lawyer who did not prepare his or her witness for testimony, having had an opportunity to do so, would not be doing his or her professional job properly.

It matters not at all that the preparation of such testimony takes the form of "practice" examination or cross-examination. What does matter is that whatever the mode of witness preparation chosen, the lawyer does not engage in suppressing, distorting or falsifying the testimony that the witness will give.

D.C. Bar Legal Ethics Committee Formal Opinion 79: Real Life Applications

1. The D.C. Ethics Committee opined that it would not violate the jurisdiction's disciplinary rules for a lawyer to "script" testimony of a witness before her appearance at a tribunal, so long as the attorney was not putting words into the witness's mouth that the attorney knows or should know to be false. But is such formal scripting *wise* as a tactical matter? Imagine what impression such rigid adherence to a script might leave on the finder of fact, and how it might be exposed on cross-examination. Federal Rule of Evidence 612 allows a court to order opposing counsel to inspect any writing used by a witness to refresh the witness's recollection, either *before* or during testimony.

The Restatement (Third) of the Law Governing Lawyers suggests that the following methods of **witness preparation** are ethically appropriate: explaining the law that applies to the case; telling the witness about likely testimony from others and documents that will be admitted in evidence; suggesting words or phrases that will help make the witness's meaning clearer; and preparing for possibly hostile cross-examination.[21]

C. FAIRNESS TO OPPOSING PARTY AND COUNSEL

1. Obstruction, Alteration, or Destruction of Evidence

Destroying or altering documents after they have been designated by a subpoena or civil discovery request is behavior antithetical to a lawyer's duty of candor and

---

21. Restatement §116 cmt. b.

to his obligation as an officer of the court. Model Rule 3.4(a) provides that a lawyer may not "unlawfully obstruct another party's access to evidence or unlawfully alter, destroy, or conceal a document or other material having potential evidentiary value." Because the rule states that a lawyer may not "unlawfully" perform these acts, this is an area of legal ethics in which the attorney must be cognizant of substantive law — including criminal, tort, and procedural law. Whether handling of physical evidence or documents[22] is "unlawful" will depend on the substantive law in your jurisdiction, including the crime of obstruction of justice.

Typically, **obstruction** statutes prohibit destruction or concealment of evidence only if the individual knows or reasonably believes that an official proceeding has been commenced or is about to be instituted. An attorney's professional responsibilities will thus depend on the timing of destruction, whether proceedings are pending or likely to be filed, and the state of mind of the lawyer. In civil cases, if documents are destroyed or altered when a legal proceeding is clearly foreseeable, not only may the attorney face bar disciplinary charges, but the judge also may allow the finder of fact to find an adverse inference against the client in litigation. A lawyer who counsels or assists his client to dispose of potential evidence may end up undermining the client's case if the court gives a **spoliation of evidence**[23] instruction to the jury.

Sometimes lawyers are provided or shown physical evidence by their clients in conjunction with an ongoing proceeding. Imagine that you represent one spouse in a contested divorce and child custody matter. During one of your initial interviews you ask your client if she uses Facebook. If she answers "yes," may you advise your client to "clean up" her Facebook page by deleting any photographs or messages that might reflect poorly on her as a mother? In Opinion 2014-5, the Philadelphia Bar Association Professional Guidance Committee answered this question in the context of a lawyer representing a client in pending litigation. The committee opined that it was permissible for a lawyer to advise a client to change her privacy settings on Facebook, since that simply restricts permissive access to information rather than conceals it. But a lawyer may only counsel the client to delete material from Facebook if that instruction is accompanied by "appropriate action to preserve" electronic or hard copies of the deleted information in the event that this material is later subject to a subpoena or request for production of documents.

Counseling a client to discard documents does not always run afoul of Rule 3.4(a). The rule speaks to the "potential evidentiary value" of evidence. This language requires the lawyer to assess the probability of future litigation. For example, if a commercial lawyer discovers documents several years old that suggest that a client may be liable to a third party for contract non-performance or breach, but the lawyer does not know whether that party will ever file suit, arguably such documents need not be preserved. Particularly when an attorney is representing an organizational client, it would be impracticable to require retention of all documents against the mere possibility that an adversary proceeding may be commenced at some future date. One crucial counseling function of a lawyer is to help his clients establish appropriate document retention policies. Document retention policies must both

---

22. Rule 3.4(a) applies to both documents and physical evidence.
23. *See, e.g.,* Vodusek v. Bayliner Marine Corp., 71 F.3d 148, 155 (4th Cir. 1995).

assure compliance with applicable laws while avoiding impracticable accumulation of paper and unnecessary storage costs. It is presumptively lawful to act pursuant to a bona fide document retention program if it is consistently followed.[24]

Much of the legal authority concerning concealment and alteration of physical evidence arises in the context of criminal investigations. We return to this subject in the next chapter.

2. Discovery Obligations

Evasive or incomplete responses to discovery requests appear to be a pervasive problem in the United States.[25] It seems that many litigators adhere to the standard conception of zealous advocacy by exploiting advantages in resources through excessive discovery, narrowly construing discovery demands, and purposefully delaying depositions and production of documents for strategic advantage. Students should appreciate that such discovery abuse can be counterproductive, especially where it provokes a motion for sanctions or equally abusive conduct by opposing counsel. It may also tend to undermine constructive settlement efforts.

Intentional or even reckless failure to comply with discovery requests may violate Model Rule 3.4(d), which provides that "a lawyer shall not . . . fail to make a reasonably diligent effort to comply with a legally proper discovery request by an opposing party." If opposing counsel makes a discovery request in litigation that is overbroad, burdensome, or seeks protected information, the proper response is to assert these objections affirmatively, rather than merely failing to reply or only partially responding to the request. A lawyer may not knowingly withhold a document that has been requested in discovery unless he does so in a procedurally proper form.[26] In addition, a lawyer responding to discovery requests may not mix together both responsive and non-responsive documents in order to obscure the responsive document's evidentiary value, for such conduct would involve "deceit" within the meaning of Model Rule 8.4(c).

In addition to bar discipline, discovery abuse in civil litigation may lead to imposition of attorneys' fees and punitive damages.[27] Indeed, **discovery abuse** is far more likely to be sanctioned by the courts in the context of ongoing litigation than by bar disciplinary authorities,[28] because judges presiding over the case are thought to be more likely to have a grasp of the complex factual and legal issues involved.

Model Rule 3.2 requires lawyers to make "reasonable efforts to expedite litigation consistent with the interests of the client." That last clause in this sentence is an important limitation on the principle that may swallow the general rule. It recognizes that sometimes the client may *wish* to delay litigation — such as where the client is anticipating persuasive appellate authority in a pending case, is expecting a global settlement of a related matter, or thinks that damages may be impacted by

---

24. *See* Restatement §118 cmt. c.
25. Douglas N. Frenkel, Robert L. Nelson & Austin Sarat, *Ethics: Beyond the Rules*, 67 Fordham L. Rev. 697, 706 (1998) (discussing research by ABA Section on Litigation).
26. Restatement §110 cmt. e.
27. Fed. R. Civ. P. 37.
28. Restatement §110 cmt. b.

further factual developments. According to the ABA, "[t]he question is whether a competent lawyer acting in good faith would regard the course of action as having some substantial purpose other than delay." Protracting discovery for the sole purposes of running up the attorney's bill would clearly violate the rule. But what about exhausting the resources of your opponent and forcing him into settlement? If that is what the client wishes to do and can afford to pay for it, is it permitted by Rule 3.2? The ABA seems to have punted on this difficult question.

Finally, Model Rule 4.4(b) contains an important provision about a lawyer's responsibility pertaining to **inadvertent discovery**. The rule provides that an attorney who receives a document or electronically stored information relating to the representation of a client and knows or reasonably should know that the document was sent to him inadvertently must promptly notify the sender so that he or she can take protective measures. For example, if opposing counsel attaches the wrong document to an email or includes information in a discovery packet that he obviously did not intend to convey (e.g., a legal memorandum prepared by an associate that is clearly work product), the receiving attorney must notify the sending attorney. The rule does not address the receiving attorney's responsibility with respect to the document (e.g., destruction or return) but rather leaves that issue to the Rules of Civil Procedure, the Rules of Evidence, and the inherent powers of the court.

D. TRIAL TACTICS

Several types of obstreperous or disruptive trial tactics may violate attorney disciplinary rules. Here the attorney must be concerned not only with her obligations as a fair adversary, but also with her obligations as an officer of the court.

1. Disruption

While an advocate must be persuasive and should be passionate in representing a client's interests before the court, he must also refrain from "abusive" or "obstreperous" conduct.[29] The Model Rules prohibit conduct during the course of litigation that is "intended to disrupt a tribunal."[30] Examples of **disruptive conduct** may include impugning the integrity of the court;[31] refusing to comply with the court's directives;[32] shouting or using profanity;[33] and assaulting or threatening to assault witnesses, parties, opposing counsel, or court personnel.[34]

---

29. Model Rule 3.5(d).
30. Model Rule 3.5(d), cmt. [4].
31. In re Romious, 240 P.3d 945 (Kan. 2010) (lawyer called court "kangaroo court" during public proceedings); In re Larvadain, 664 So. 2d 395 (La. 1995) (lawyer attacked integrity of judge by accusing him of being racist).
32. In re Disciplinary Action Against Kirschner, 793 N.W.2d 196, 201 (N.D. 2011) (attorney ignored denial of continuance and did not appear at trial).
33. *See* In re Romious, 240 P.3d at 948 (attorney shouted profanities at court house security officials when he triggered the metal detector).
34. *See* Fla. Bar v. Martocci, 791 So. 2d 1074 (Fla. 2001) (attorney threatened to "beat up" father of party in open court, discipline imposed under "conduct prejudicial to administration of justice" rule).

A certain amount of contentiousness may be inevitable in the adversarial setting of a courtroom. Lawyers have a professional obligation to protect their client's interests by raising evidentiary objections, and by preserving grounds for appeal where they believe that the court's evidentiary or legal rulings are erroneous. Nevertheless, a court has inherent power to hold a lawyer in contempt where the lawyer persists in a line of inquiry notwithstanding clear instructions from the judge, or exposes the jury to evidence that definitively has been ruled inadmissible.[35] Both the attorney disciplinary rule and a court's inherent contempt power are limited to attorney conduct that actually disrupts the proceedings; as one commentator has argued, tribunals should not confuse an "offense to their sensibilities" with actual obstruction of the judicial process.[36]

2. Civility

While the Model Code expressed a professional norm of "zealous" representation,[37] in the Model Rules this standard conception of a lawyer's role was relegated to the Preamble[38] and to a comment to Rule 1.3.[39] This change in emphasis signaled recognition by the ABA that the traits of zealousness and civility may sometimes be in tension. In fact, comment [1] to Model Rule 1.3 provides that "[t]he lawyer's duty to act with reasonable diligence does not require the use of offensive tactics or preclude treating all persons involved in the legal process with courtesy and respect." Although there is no express provision in the ABA Model Rules dealing with **civility**, profoundly discourteous or rude behavior in the context of legal practice could be disciplined under the catchall provisions of Rule 8.4(d).[40]

In In re Snyder, 472 U.S. 634 (1985), Chief Justice Burger cautioned lawyers to fulfill their responsibilities toward clients with civility:

> All persons involved in the judicial process — judges, litigants, witnesses, and court officers — owe a duty of courtesy to all other participants. The necessity for civility in the inherently contentious setting of the adversary process suggests that members of the bar cast criticisms of the system in a professional and civil tone.[41]

---

35. In re Levine, 27 F.3d 594, 595-96 (D.C. Cir. 1994) (lawyer repeatedly asked witness about evidence the court ruled inadmissible).
36. *See* Louis Raveson, *Advocacy and Contempt: Constitutional Limitations on the Judicial Contempt Power*, 65 WASH. L. REV. 477, 514 (1990).
37. MODEL CODE OF PROF'L RESPONSIBILITY EC 7-1 ("A lawyer shall represent a client zealously within the bounds of the law.").
38. Model Rules Preamble cmt. [2] ("As an advocate, a lawyer zealously asserts the client's position under the rules of the advocacy system").
39. Model Rule 1.3 cmt. [1] ("A lawyer must also act with commitment and dedication to the interests of the client and with zeal in advocacy upon the client's behalf.").
40. Model Rule 8.4(d) prohibits conduct "prejudicial to the administration of justice." *Cf.* Carroll v. Jacques Admiralty Law Firm, 110 F.3d 290 (5th Cir. 1997) (recognizing inherent authority of federal court to sanction lawyer for profanity and abusiveness toward opposing counsel during deposition).
41. *Id.* at 647.

Notwithstanding that admonition, however, the Court reversed the Eighth Circuit's suspension of a criminal defense attorney for writing an allegedly rude letter to a district court judge's secretary setting forth his decision not to take any more Criminal Justice Act appointments, or to submit any more documentation in support of prior appointments. The Court held that "even assuming that the letter exhibited an unlawyerlike rudeness, a single incident of rudeness or lack of professional courtesy — in this context — does not support a finding of contemptuous or contumacious conduct, or a finding that a lawyer is 'not presently fit to practice law in the federal courts.' "[42]

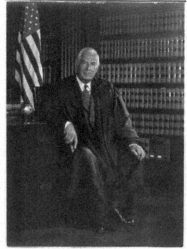

Chief Justice Warren Burger, proponent of civility
Library of Congress Prints and Photographs Division, Washington, D.C.

In response to abusive litigation tactics and what some observers see as the inherent limitations of bar discipline, many states have adopted voluntary and nonbinding "civility" codes.[43] Although the contents of these codes differ, many contain exhortations such as "cooperate in scheduling" and "avoid excessive zeal."[44] A few states also require lawyers to take "civility" oaths upon admission to practice.[45] To date there is little evidence that such oaths or codes have had a substantial influence on lawyer behavior. But even if such empirical evidence is lacking, do you think that the profession may benefit collectively from being perceived as willing and able to reach consensus around civility norms?

E. MAINTAINING THE IMPARTIALITY OF THE TRIBUNAL

Lawyers have a responsibility as officers of the court to avoid conduct that will compromise the fairness and impartiality of the judicial proceedings. This responsibility carries with it an obligation to avoid *ex parte* contact with judges or jurors, to refrain from (and report) any attempts to destroy evidence or improperly influence or intimidate witnesses, and to avoid acting as advocate in cases where the attorney is also likely to be called as a witness.

Under Model Rule 3.5(b), attorneys are prohibited from engaging in ***ex parte communications*** with judges or jurors on the subject of the litigation unless authorized by law. Fairness in adversary proceedings requires that the opposing counsel (or opposing party if self-represented) be present whenever an attorney addresses

---

42. *Id.*

43. Katherine Sylvester, *I'm Rubber, You're Sued: Should Uncivil Lawyers Receive Ethical Sanctions?*, 26 Geo. J. Legal Ethics 1015, 1016 (2013) (distinguishing civility from ethics and discussing the role of voluntary civility codes in regulating attorney conduct).

44. *See, e.g.*, Colorado Bar Association, Principles of Professionalism (2011), http://www.cobar.org/For-Members/Committees/Professionalism-Coordinating-Council/Principles-of-Professionalism (last visited July 11, 2017). For a list of states with civility codes, see http://www.americanbar.org/groups/professional_responsibility/resources/professionalism/professionalism_codes.html.

45. S.C. App. Ct. Rules 402(h), 402(k); Tex. Gov't Code Ann. §82.037 (West 2015).

the court, seated jurors, or prospective jurors. Lawyers and judges often interact socially at bar association events and other professional gatherings. They may also meet each other in the hallways or other common areas of the courthouse. Rule 3.5(d) does not prohibit attorneys from talking to judges or magistrates about matters unrelated to the pending case (e.g., the news, sports, or weather) because those topics are not considered *ex parte* communications; nevertheless, an attorney must scrupulously avoid talking about the matter being litigated, because that could potentially compromise the judge's impartiality.

Paying a bribe or offering a monetary reward to a judge, juror, or fact witness[46] obviously compromises the **impartiality of a tribunal**, and in many instances will constitute a crime under state and federal law. Rule 3.5(a) prohibits a lawyer from "seek[ing] to influence a judge, juror, prospective juror or other official by means prohibited by law." A lawyer has a duty not only to refrain from engaging in such conduct, but also to *report* such conduct if he learns that it has been done by another. Rule 3.3(b) provides that a lawyer representing a client in an adjudicative proceeding "who knows that a person intends to engage, is engaging, or has engaged in criminal or fraudulent conduct relating to the proceeding" must take reasonable remedial measures, including disclosure to the court if necessary. For example, if a relative or friend of the client informs the lawyer that they have offered a bribe to a potential witness or juror, or that they destroyed or altered evidence, the attorney has an obligation to notify the court, even if that notice requires revealing a client confidence under Rule 1.6. If the same person discloses his intent to offer a bribe to a juror or a witness, the lawyer has a duty to do everything in his power to talk the person out of doing so.

Model Rule 3.5 also limits the situations where an attorney may contact jurors *after* a verdict has been rendered in a case. A lawyer may desire post-verdict contact with jurors because the initial case resulted in a mistrial and the lawyer wants to learn from the first case about what strategies were effective or ineffective before retrying the case in front of another jury. Or, the attorney may seek to contact individual jurors after a verdict because he believes that there might have been impermissible and extraneous matters injected in juror deliberations that could give cause for a motion for new trial. These legitimate objectives, however, are in tension with common law presumptions that jury deliberations are privileged and that verdicts are final. For these reasons, attorneys may not communicate with jurors after a verdict if (1) the communication is prohibited by law or court order; (2) the juror has made known a desire not to be contacted; or (3) the communication involves misrepresentation, coercion, duress, or harassment. Lawyers must be familiar with particular attorney discipline rules and court decisions in the jurisdictions in which they practice, because states differ widely in their allowance of post-verdict contact with jurors. For example, some states prohibit any lawyer-initiated contact with jurors unless authorized by the court,[47] and some states require notice to opposing counsel and a waiting period before contact may be made.[48]

---

46. Expert witnesses may be compensated for their testimony under both state and federal law.
47. *See, e.g.*, Del. Lawyers' R. Prof'l Conduct 3.5(c).
48. Commonwealth v. Moore, 474 Mass. 541 (2016).

Except in narrow situations, under Model Rule 3.7 an attorney may not serve as both an advocate and a witness in the same proceeding. This is known as the **advocate-witness rule**. There are several purported justifications for the rule, none of which are entirely persuasive. The rule may prevent prejudice to the client where the attorney gives factual testimony that differs from that offered by the client or other witnesses. Second, even if an attorney testifies favorably to his client, allowing an attorney to serve as a witness may in some situations prejudice the opposing party, because an attorney may be perceived as having added credibility compared to a lay witness. The jury may be confused as to how to evaluate an attorney's testimony (are they testifying as a fact witness or an expert witness?) and thereby give it inordinate weight. Both of these concerns have led to a presumption that proceedings cannot be fair and impartial where an attorney plays a dual role in the same litigation. But Rule 3.7 contains three notable exceptions: the advocate may serve as a witness in the same proceeding if (1) the testimony relates to an uncontested issue; (2) the testimony relates only to the nature and value of legal services; or (3) disqualification would impose a substantial hardship on the client.

F. PUBLIC COMMENT ON PENDING CIVIL LITIGATION

Disciplinary proceedings against lawyers in civil cases for talking to the media are rare. The likelihood of a lawyer materially prejudicing a civil proceeding by talking to the press is relatively low, because civil cases are less sensational than criminal cases, and because nobody's liberty is at stake. We discuss restrictions on talking to the press in criminal cases in the next chapter, including the Supreme Court's seminal decision in *Gentile v. State Bar of Nevada*.

Rule 3.6(a) prohibits a lawyer participating in the litigation of an ongoing matter from making an "extrajudicial statement" that the lawyer "knows or reasonably should know will be disseminated by means of public communication" and that will have "a substantial likelihood of materially prejudicing an adjudicative proceeding in the matter."[49] Because one of the primary dangers of statements to the press is tainting the jury pool, the likelihood of prejudice from **media statements** is highest in cases that will be tried to a jury, and higher still the closer the matter gets to time of trial. Civil cases that are tried to a judge or arbitrator present the lowest possible risk of prejudice by comments to the media.[50] In addition to complying with Rule 3.6, once a civil trial has started the attorney must also comply with any **gag order** or restriction on media contact that is imposed by the court.[51]

Model Rule 3.6 (b) contains a "safe harbor" provision that allows an attorney to comment on specific subjects, irrespective of how likely they are to prejudice the proceedings. This section provides that "[n]otwithstanding" the prohibitions of Rule 3.6(a), a lawyer may permissibly comment on (1) the claim, offense, or defense

---

49. Model Rule 3.6(a).
50. Model Rule 3.6(a) cmt. [6].
51. *See* Sheppard v. Maxwell, 384 U.S. 333, 363 (1966) ("The courts must take such steps by rule and regulation that will protect their [trial] processes from prejudicial outside interferences.").

involved; (2) information contained in a public record; (3) the fact that an investigation of a matter is in progress; (4) the scheduling or result of any step in litigation; (5) a request for assistance in obtaining evidence; and (6) a warning to the public of any dangers. Lawyers facing media inquiries regarding pending litigation should be mindful of the protection afforded by these six categories of information.

The broadest of these so-called safe harbor provisions is the public records exception. If a lawyer has already made a statement in court or in a written court submission, unless the matter is under seal the information may be repeated to the press. The attorney may also discuss with the press the content of any documents that have been marked in evidence or are otherwise made part of the public record in the case. Rule 3.6 also contains a "**fighting fire with fire**" provision, which allows an attorney to make a public statement that a reasonable lawyer "would believe is required to protect a client from the substantial undue prejudicial effect of recent publicity not initiated by the lawyer or the lawyer's client."

Lawyers may not use spokespeople to undertake conduct that would be impermissible if engaged in by the attorney. Model Rule 5.3(c) states that a lawyer shall be responsible for conduct of another if the lawyer "order[s]" or "ratif[ies]" that conduct, or if the lawyer has direct supervisory authority over a non-lawyer in a law firm and knows about that person's conduct in time to avoid its consequences but fails to do so. *See also* Rule 8.4(a) (which prohibits violating the rules "through the acts of another"). Thus, an attorney violates Rule 3.6 with respect to pretrial publicity if she asks a communications or public relations specialist either within the firm or outside of the firm to make a statement to the media that is prejudicial, or if the attorney assists the spokesperson with making such a statement.

| **Case Preview** | ***Maldonado v. Ford Motor Co.*** |

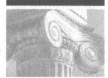

Justine Maldonado filed suit against Ford Motor Co., alleging that her supervisor, Daniel Bennett, sexually harassed her. Maldonado and her attorney repeatedly publicized Bennett's prior indecent exposure conviction that was subsequently expunged and denied admission as evidence in the harassment suit. Their actions included issuing a press release, meeting with the media to generate news coverage of the expunged conviction, and handing out leaflets containing information about the conviction at "Justice for Justine" rallies. Maldonado's attorney participated in the demonstrations, spoke to a local news station, and accused the judge of being under the influence of Ford Motor Co. This opinion of the Michigan Supreme Court highlights the interaction between Rule 3.6 and the First Amendment.

As you read *Maldonado*, consider the following:

1. Was Maldonado's attorney at fault for violating Rule 3.6 directly, or by doing so through the actions of another (his client) under Rule 8.4(a)?

2. If the trial judge had not entered an order expressly prohibiting public comment on the indecent exposure conviction, would dismissal of a civil complaint be an available remedy for violation of an attorney disciplinary rule?

Maldonado v. Ford Motor Co.
719 N.W.2d 809 (Mich. 2006)

. . .

III. ANALYSIS

. . .

B. *The Trial Court's Authority to Dismiss This Case*

. . .

Not only did plaintiff and her counsel disregard Judge Macdonald's order and Judge Giovan's explicit warning to respect the order, counsel violated numerous rules of professional conduct. Plaintiff's counsel's public references to Bennett's excluded conviction violated MRPC 3.6, which was the basis for Judge Giovan's dismissal. Plaintiff's counsel reasonably knew or should have known that their comments would have a substantial likelihood of materially prejudicing the proceedings by improperly influencing prospective jurors regarding Bennett's propensities to commit sexual harassment, especially since trial was approximately two weeks away.

Plaintiff argues that Judge Giovan improperly relied on MRPC 3.6 in dismissing plaintiff's case. She contends that Judge Giovan's dismissal was solely based on plaintiff's comments, and that MRPC 3.6 does not apply to nonlawyers. Plaintiff correctly argues that the Michigan Rules of Professional Conduct do not apply to nonlawyers, but mistakenly contends that Judge Giovan relied only on her behavior in ordering a dismissal. Plaintiff also erroneously contends that she is free to engage in improper pretrial publicity designed to taint the potential jury pool. The Michigan Court Rules do apply to plaintiff. They authorize the trial court to impose sanctions such as dismissal for party misconduct. MCR 2.504(B)(1). Judge Giovan expressly warned plaintiff that if she continued to disseminate information regarding Bennett's excluded conviction in violation of Judge Macdonald's order, he would dismiss her case. Plaintiff failed to obey this warning and, thus, Judge Giovan properly dismissed her case. In any event, even if plaintiff is not bound by MRPC 3.6, plaintiff's counsel's repeated public references to Bennett's excluded conviction, coupled with Ms. Massie's statement five days before trial that "Metro Detroit" judges were biased in favor of the Ford Motor Company, were substantially likely to materially prejudice the proceedings and improperly influence prospective jurors.

. . .

C. The First Amendment and a Trial Court's Ability to Restrict Speech

. . .

We agree with the majority of the States that the "substantial likelihood of material prejudice" standard [of Rule 3.6] constitutes a constitutionally permissible balance between the First Amendment rights of attorneys in pending cases and the State's interest in fair trials.

When a state regulation implicates First Amendment rights, the Court must balance those interests against the State's legitimate interest in regulating the activity in question. The "substantial likelihood" test . . . is constitutional . . . for it is designed to protect the integrity and fairness of a state's judicial system and it imposes only narrow and necessary limitations on lawyers' speech. The limitations are aimed at two principal evils: (1) comments that are likely to influence the actual outcome of the trial, and (2) *comments that are likely to prejudice the jury venire, even if an untainted panel can ultimately be found.* [*Gentile*, 501 U.S at 1075 (emphasis added).]

The Court noted that "[l]awyers representing clients in pending cases are key participants in the criminal justice system, and the State may demand some adherence to the precepts of that system in regulating their speech as well as their conduct." Id. at 1074. . . . The Court further observed that "[f]ew, if any, interests under the Constitution are more fundamental than the right to a fair trial by 'impartial' jurors, and an outcome affected by extrajudicial statements would violate that fundamental right." Id. at 1075. . . .

. . .

More important, however, is that the plaintiff should not be heard to make her argument, which goes like this: "We deny that our behavior was intended to have a substantial likelihood of prejudice. But even if you establish that it was, you cannot dismiss the plaintiff's case until you establish that it has achieved its intended effect."

We believe otherwise. That is not an acceptable standard for preserving the integrity of a court system. The behavior in question has been intentional, premeditated, and intransigent. It was designed to reach the farthest boundaries of the public consciousness. It should be presumed to have had its intended effect.

The Court of Appeals acknowledged that the applicable test under *Gentile* is whether the conduct generated a "substantial likelihood" of prejudice, yet remanded for an evidentiary hearing to determine whether "actual" prejudice occurred.

We hereby affirm the trial court's understanding of *Gentile*. Plaintiff's and her counsel's numerous public references to Bennett's inadmissible, expunged indecent exposure conviction, despite a court order excluding such evidence, were obviously intended to prejudice potential jurors. The trial court thus warned the parties and counsel that all public references to the expunged conviction in violation of the ethical rules would result in dismissal. This limitation on plaintiff's and her counsel's speech only applied to speech that was substantially likely to have a materially prejudicial effect and that, therefore, violated the rules of ethics. It did not prohibit plaintiff and her counsel from speaking about sexual harassment or the general nature of plaintiff's case.

. . .

The Court of Appeals requirement that actual prejudice be shown conflicts not only with the "substantial likelihood" test set forth in *Gentile*, but also with the plain language of MRPC 3.6. Moreover, the Court of Appeals standard has no practical workability. It would be impossible to determine "actual prejudice" to a potential jury pool three years after the incident in question. We decline to order an evidentiary hearing that is no more than a fool's errand.

. . .

V. CONCLUSION

We hold that the trial court's explicit warning prohibiting any references to Bennett's excluded conviction did not violate the First Amendment. Accordingly, we reverse the judgment of the Court of Appeals and reinstate the trial court's order dismissing plaintiff's case.

Post-Case Follow-Up

Rule 3.6 focuses on *pretrial* comments that have potential to prejudice an adversarial proceeding. In addition, disciplinary rules in effect in many jurisdictions prohibit an attorney from knowingly or recklessly making false comments about the qualifications or integrity of a judge — either before or after the proceeding. *See* Model Rule 8.2(a). Under Rule 8.2 it is improper for an attorney participating in litigation to make untruthful comments that call into question the competence of the court. But since criticism of the government is a very core protection of the First Amendment,[52] this method of preserving public confidence in the integrity of the judiciary bumps squarely up against constitutional protections. Because Rule 8.2 prohibits comments that the lawyer knows or should know are untruthful, it puts the risk on lawyers to carefully evaluate the truthfulness of their speech before publicly making any statements that impugn the reputation of judges before whom they appear.[53]

Maldonado v. Ford Motor Co.: Real Life Applications

Imagine a lawyer who makes a statement to the media following a trial that "this was one of the most poorly conducted trials that I have ever participated in; I am confident that the trial judge's ill-conceived and biased evidentiary rulings will be overturned on appeal." Does this statement violate either Rule 3.6 or Rule 8.2? If the trial is over, is there any "substantial likelihood" that this public statement could prejudice the proceeding within the meaning of Rule 3.6? Is the statement about the way the judge conducted the trial a statement of opinion or fact? If the former, is that something that can either be true or false within the meaning of Rule 8.2? If the latter, is it a statement about the judge's "qualifications" or "integrity"?

52. Gentile v. State Bar of Nevada, 501 U.S. 1030, 1055 (1991).
53. In re Wilkins, 777 N.E.2d 714, 716-17 (Ind. 2002), *modified*, 782 N.E.2d 985 (Ind. 2003) (disciplining lawyer who called the Indiana Court of Appeals' decision "disturbing," accused the judges of making affirmative misstatements of fact, and suggested that they were biased in favor of other party).

G. COMMUNICATING WITH REPRESENTED PERSONS

Model Rule 4.2, often called the **"no-contact" rule**, prohibits an attorney from communicating with a person represented by counsel on the subject of that representation without permission of the client's attorney. In substance, when a person is known to be represented in a matter, an attorney must first go through that person's counsel for permission to speak with the client. The purposes of the "no-contact" rule are threefold: (1) to encourage professional courtesy by requiring permission before one lawyer speaks with another lawyer's client; (2) to prevent a lawyer, through overreaching or superior bargaining power, from tricking a represented witness or party into making damaging admissions or concessions; and (3) to discourage uncounseled waivers of the attorney-client privilege.

All 50 states contain a "no-contact" provision in their attorney disciplinary rules, although state rules vary considerably in their terminology and exceptions. The Model Rules provision was amended in 1995 to apply to represented "persons" rather than "parties." Some states still apply their "no-contact" rule only to represented "parties."[54] This is perhaps the most common deviation among states. The potential significance of this distinction will be discussed below.

Where the "no-contact" rule applies to represented parties, an attorney would be subject to discipline if he contacts an opposing party directly to discuss a potential settlement of the case without receiving permission from opposing counsel. Even "cc'ing" the client on a letter to counsel proposing a settlement without the lawyer's permission would violate the rule, because the attorney is "communicating" with the party on the subject of the representation. Note that the rule is not waivable by the client, but only by the attorney. Thus, a prosecutor who is approached by a represented defendant[55] outside of the courtroom must decline to speak to that opposing party without his attorney's permission, or risk being found in violation of the rule.

Even in jurisdictions that apply their "no-contact" rule to represented "parties," the protections of the rule apply outside of the litigation context. Courts and bar disciplinary authorities have declined to limit the rule's application to opposing parties after litigation has been commenced, and have construed the term "party" to apply to clients in a business setting who stand on the opposite side of a transaction.[56] For example, where an attorney is negotiating a commercial lease on behalf of a business tenant and the owner of the premises is known to be represented by counsel, the lawyer may not have communication directly with the owner without that attorney's permission.

Where the jurisdiction applies its "no-contact" rule to a represented "person" an attorney must also be careful not to communicate directly with any *witness* who is represented by counsel. For example, a plaintiff in an employment discrimination suit might seek to take the statement of a former co-worker about the conditions of their employment. If that former co-worker has also retained counsel for purposes of conducting negotiations with the company, the attorney for the plaintiff must seek permission of that lawyer before speaking with the co-worker, even

---

54. *See* Ariz. R. Prof'l Conduct 4.2; Conn. R. Prof'l Conduct 4.2.
55. Where the party is self-represented, communication is permissible.
56. N.Y. R. Prof'l Conduct. 4.2; *see* United States v. Galanis, 685 F. Supp. 901, 902 (S.D.N.Y. 1988).

if that former co-worker is not yet a party to any formal litigation and is ostensibly on the "same side." In the same vein, a prosecutor may normally speak to the victim of a crime unencumbered by any proscriptions about obtaining advance permission, but if that victim has retained a lawyer (for example, in order to advise the victim on potential civil recoveries for the same injury), the prosecutor must first go through counsel.

The term "person" in Rule 4.2 includes artificial persons — business entities such as corporations, partnerships, and trusts that are represented by counsel. Those business entities can only act through natural persons, but the question is which of those natural persons — from top management to lower-level employees — are considered "represented" by corporate counsel and thereby shielded from contact under the rule. Here we see that a balance is necessary between protecting attorney-client relationships and providing the public and putative litigants with the ability to gather evidence to investigate wrongdoing. Taking the position that "all employees" are represented by corporate counsel would curtail the informal discovery process and force litigants to conduct expensive depositions. Taking the position that only the senior management of a company is represented by counsel for the purposes of the rule would handicap corporate lawyers from shielding their clients from damaging admissions or revelations of privileged information by lower-level employees. Pay careful attention to how the Massachusetts Supreme Judicial Court resolved these competing tensions in a sex discrimination suit against Harvard University.

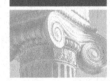

| **Case Preview** | ***Messing, Rudavsky & Weliky, P.C. v. President and Fellows of Harvard College*** |

Kathleen Stanford was a sergeant with the Harvard University Police Department who claimed that Harvard and its chief of police discriminated against her because of her gender. During the course of the litigation, a partner with the law firm of Messing, Rudavsky & Weliky (MR&W) contacted five employees of the Harvard Police Department — none of whom were involved in the alleged discrimination — without first seeking permission from Harvard's attorneys. The trial court sanctioned MR&W under Massachusetts Rule of Professional Conduct 4.2, which prohibits a lawyer from communicating directly with any person known to be represented by a lawyer.

As you read *Messing*, ask yourself:

1. How does the "**control group**" test for deciding who is a represented person under Rule 4.2 insufficiently protect organizations from damaging admissions by employees?
2. How does an interpretation of Rule 4.2 that synchronizes the "no-contact" standard with the test for admissions under the Rules of Evidence impede informal discovery? What are the financial consequences of erecting such a barrier in litigation?

Messing, Rudavsky & Weliky, P.C. v. President and Fellows of Harvard College
764 N.E.2d 825 (Mass. 2002)

. . . This appeal raises the issue whether, and to what extent, the rule prohibits an attorney from speaking ex parte to the employees of an organization represented by counsel. . . .

On appeal, MR & W contends that the judge's construction of the rule is overly broad and results from an incorrect interpretation of the rule's commentary.

. . .

The rule has been justified generally as "preserv[ing] the mediating role of counsel on behalf of their clients . . . protect[ing] clients from overreaching by counsel for adverse interests," and "protecting the attorney-client relationship." . . .

When the represented person is an individual, there is no difficulty determining when an attorney has violated the rule; the represented person is easily identifiable. In the case of an organization, however, identifying the protected class is more complicated.

Because an organization acts only through its employees, the rule must extend to some of these employees. However, most courts have rejected the position that the rule automatically prevents an attorney from speaking with all employees of a represented organization.

. . .

According to comment [4] to rule 4.2, an attorney may not speak ex parte to three categories of employees: (1) "persons having managerial responsibility on behalf of the organization with regard to the subject of the representation"; (2) persons "whose act or omission in connection with that matter may be imputed to the organization for purposes of civil or criminal liability"; and (3) persons "whose statement may constitute an admission on the part of the organization." Mass. R. Prof. C. 4.2 comment [4], 426 Mass. 1403 (1998).

. . .

Some jurisdictions have adopted the broad reading of the rule endorsed by the judge in this case. . . . Courts reaching this result do so because, like the Superior Court, they read the word "admission" in the third category of the comment as a reference to Fed. R. Evid. 801(d)(2)(D) and any corresponding State rule of evidence. Id. This rule forbids contact with practically all employees because "virtually every employee may conceivably make admissions binding on his or her employer". . . .

At the other end of the spectrum, a small number of jurisdictions has interpreted the rule narrowly so as to allow an attorney for the opposing party to contact most employees of a represented organization. These courts construe the rule to restrict contact with only those employees in the organization's "control group," defined as those employees in the uppermost echelon of the organization's management. . . .

Other jurisdictions have adopted yet a third test that, while allowing for some ex parte contacts with a represented organization's employees, still maintains some protection of the organization. The Court of Appeals of New York articulated such a rule in Niesig v. Team I, 76 N.Y.2d 363, 559 N.Y.S.2d 493, 558 N.E.2d 1030 (1990), rejecting an approach that ties the rule to Fed. R. Evid. 801(d)(2)(D). Instead, the court defined a represented person to include "employees whose acts or omissions in the matter under inquiry are binding on the corporation . . . or imputed to the corporation for purposes of its liability, or employees implementing the advice of counsel." Id. at 374, 559 N.Y.S.2d 493, 558 N.E.2d 1030.

. . .

We instead interpret the rule to ban contact only with those employees who have the authority to "commit the organization to a position regarding the subject matter of representation." . . . The employees with whom contact is prohibited are those with "speaking authority" for the corporation who "have managing authority sufficient to give them the right to speak for, and bind, the corporation". . . . Employees who can commit the organization are those with authority to make decisions about the course of the litigation, such as when to initiate suit, and when to settle a pending case. . . . We recognize that this test is a retrenchment from the broad prohibition on employee contact endorsed by the comment.

This interpretation, when read in conjunction with the other two categories of the comment, would prohibit ex parte contact only with those employees who exercise managerial responsibility in the matter, who are alleged to have committed the wrongful acts at issue in the litigation, or who have authority on behalf of the corporation to make decisions about the course of the litigation. This result is substantially the same as the *Niesig* test because it "prohibit[s] direct communication . . . 'with those officials . . . who have the legal power to bind the corporation in the matter or who are responsible for implementing the advice of the corporation's lawyer . . . or whose own interests are directly at stake in a representation.'" Niesig v. Team I, *supra* at 374, 559 N.Y.S.2d 493, 558 N.E.2d 1030. . . .

Our test is consistent with the purposes of the rule, which are not to "protect a corporate party from the revelation of prejudicial facts" . . . but to protect the attorney-client relationship and prevent clients from making ill-advised statements without the counsel of their attorney. Prohibiting contact with all employees of a represented organization restricts informal contacts far more than is necessary to achieve these purposes. See Niesig v. Team I, supra at 372-373, 559 N.Y.S.2d 493, 558 N.E.2d 1030. The purposes of the rule are best served when it prohibits communication with those employees closely identified with the organization in the dispute. The interests of the organization are adequately protected by preventing contact with those employees empowered to make litigation decisions, and those employees whose actions or omissions are at issue in the case. We reject the "control group" test, which includes only the most senior management, as insufficient to protect the "principles motivating [Rule 4.2]." See id. at 373, 559 N.Y.S.2d 493, 558 N.E.2d 1030. The test we adopt protects an organizational party against improper advances and influence by an attorney, while still promoting access to relevant facts. See id. at 373-374, 559 N.Y.S.2d 493, 558 N.E.2d 1030. The Superior Court's interpretation of the rule would grant an advantage to corporate litigants over nonorganizational parties. It grants an unwarranted benefit to organizations to require that a party always seek prior judicial approval to conduct informal interviews with witnesses to an event when the opposing party happens to be an organization and the events at issue occurred at the workplace.

. . .

Applying rule 4.2 to the employees interviewed by MR & W. The five Harvard employees interviewed by MR & W do not fall within the third category of the comment as we have construed it. As employees of the HUPD, they are not involved in directing the litigation at bar or authorizing the organization to make binding admissions. In fact, Harvard does not argue that any of the five employees fit within our definition of this category.

The Harvard employees are also not employees "whose act or omission in connection with that matter may be imputed to the organization for purposes of civil or criminal liability." Mass. R. Prof. C. 4.2 comment [4]. Stanford's complaint does not name any of these employees as involved in the alleged discrimination. In fact, in an affidavit she states that the two lieutenants "had no role in making any of the decisions that are the subject of my complaint of discrimination and retaliation," and Harvard does not refute this averment. All five employees were mere witnesses to the events that occurred, not active participants.

We must still determine, however, whether any of the interviewed employees have "managerial responsibility on behalf of the organization with regard to the subject of the representation." Mass. R. Prof. C. 4.2 comment [4]. Although the two patrol officers and the dispatcher were subordinate to Stanford and had no managerial authority, the two lieutenants exercised some supervisory authority over Stanford. However, not all employees with some supervisory power over their coworkers are deemed to have "managerial" responsibility in the sense intended by the comment. . . . "[S]upervision of a small group of workers would not constitute a managerial position within a corporation." . . . Even if the two lieutenants are deemed to have managerial responsibility, the Massachusetts version of the comment adds the requirement that the managerial responsibility be in "regard to the subject of the representation." Mass. R. Prof. C. 4.2 comment [4]. Thus, the comment includes only those employees who have supervisory authority over the events at issue in the litigation. There is no evidence in the record that the lieutenants' managerial decisions were a subject of the litigation. The affidavits of the two lieutenants indicate that they did not complete any evaluations or offer any opinions of Stanford that Chief Riley considered in reaching his decisions.

5. Conclusion. Because we conclude that rule 4.2 did not prohibit MR & W from contacting and interviewing the five HUPD employees, we vacate the order of the Superior Court judge and remand the case for the entry of an order denying the defendant's motion for sanctions.

Post-Case Follow-Up

The comment to Model Rule 4.2 was amended in 2002 to adopt the *Messing* refinement,[57] limiting the implied representation of corporate employees by corporate counsel to three classes of employees. However, not all states agree with this middle-ground approach to classifying who is represented by corporate counsel for purposes of the "no-contact" rule.

---

57. Model Rule 4.2 cmt. [7].

As the discussion by the Massachusetts Supreme Judicial Court in *Messing* indicates, some states limit the rule's prohibition to those in the corporate control group (which has the effect of permitting more informal fact investigation) while other states broaden the rule to prevent communication with any employee whose statements might constitute an "admission" at trial — which under the Federal Rules of Evidence constitutes any employee speaking about a subject matter within the scope of her employment — thus preventing informal discovery and requiring resort to depositions.

Messing, Rudavsky & Weliky, P.C. v. President and Fellows of Harvard College: Real Life Applications

1. With little knowledge of a company's business, how is a lawyer supposed to know which employees are considered "represented" by corporate counsel for purposes of the *Messing* test? Suppose that you represent a golfer who was injured when he tripped over an unmarked sprinkler head at a private country club. After filing suit, you wish to conduct informal interviews with the president of the club, the head greenskeeper, an employee of the club who was mowing the grass nearby the accident at the time your client tripped, and your client's caddy. Which individuals may you interview without getting permission from counsel for the country club?

2. You represent one spouse in an increasingly bitter divorce. After a contentious pretrial hearing, your client informs you, "I just want to talk to my husband personally and see if we can work out some of these issues between ourselves." May you counsel your *client* to talk to a represented opposing party without running afoul of Rules 4.2 and 8.4? What values behind the "no-contact" rule are at risk and what values are not at risk in a situation involving party-to-party contact?

3. Suppose that you want to investigate an opposing party in litigation. May you ask a paralegal to send the party a "friend request" on Facebook so that the two of you can peruse the party's personal information, without running afoul of Rule 4.2?

Where corporate employees are concerned, lawyers would be well advised to consult precedent of their individual jurisdiction for an interpretation of Rule 4.2. Most states agree that *former* employees of the corporation are not automatically represented by counsel for the corporation unless they have been expressly retained, because they are no longer part of the relationship sought to be fostered and protected by the rule.[58]

Note that Model Rule 8.4(a) makes it professional misconduct for an attorney to violate a disciplinary rule "through the acts of another." Where an attorney is

---

58. *Id. See also* ABA Formal Op. 91-359 (1991); Restatement §100 cmt. g.

prevented from contacting a represented person or party under Rule 4.2, the attorney is also prohibited from instructing a paralegal or private investigator to engage in that same contact.

The "no-contact" rule allows an attorney to conduct communications with a represented person without permission of counsel if he is "authorized to do so by law or a court order."[59] What types of *ex parte* communications might be authorized by law? Service of a subpoena to testify at trial or deposition is clearly authorized, because most jurisdictions' rules of procedure allow for in-person service. What else might this include? The "authorized by law" exception has generated heated debate among the criminal justice community about what investigatory steps are allowed by prosecutors with regard to represented targets prior to bringing an indictment. Some of these issues are discussed in the next chapter.

H. COMMUNICATING WITH UNREPRESENTED PERSONS

In representing a client an attorney often comes into contact with persons whose legal rights and obligations may be at issue in the case, but who have not retained their own lawyer. For example, in a motor vehicle accident case involving a multiple car pileup, an attorney for one plaintiff may interview witnesses who also have potential causes of action against the defendant, but who have not contemplated or commenced litigation. A real estate attorney may negotiate a commercial lease of a business premises directly with an owner who is not represented by counsel. In order to avoid misleading unrepresented persons in these situations, Model Rule 4.3 prohibits a lawyer from stating or implying that a lawyer is disinterested when he is dealing with an unrepresented party. Often times lay witnesses are confused about whom the lawyer represents and what the lawyer's goals are in conducting an interview. Where it is clear to the lawyer that an unrepresented person is confused about the lawyer's role in the matter, the lawyer has an affirmative obligation under Rule 4.3 to correct the misunderstanding. For example, the lawyer representing the plaintiff in our hypothetical motor vehicle accident who is interviewing the driver of another car struck by the defendant, if asked "how much money will I get if you win your case" must explain that the pending proceeding is not a class action, that he represents only one alleged tort victim, and that if the witness seeks to recover on his own he must file his own civil action or speak directly to the defendant's insurance company.

A lawyer must also avoid the conflict of interest that would arise in giving legal advice to someone whose interests are adverse to those of the lawyer's client. Rule 4.3 prohibits the provision of legal advice, other than the "advice to secure counsel," to someone whose interests have a reasonable possibility of being adverse to the interests of the lawyer's client. For example, in the commercial lease example cited above, the owner of the building and the future tenant have interests that may be in conflict. If the building owner does not understand a term of the draft lease and

---

59. Model Rule 4.2.

asks the lawyer for the tenant what a particular legal term means and what his legal rights are under that clause of the draft contract, the attorney must explain to the owner that he is not allowed to give him legal advice and that if he wants a legal explanation he needs to engage his own lawyer. In this scenario, the rule recognizes that determining precisely where the lawyer crosses the line between explaining factual terms in a contract and providing "legal advice" to an unrepresented person will depend on "the experience and sophistication of the unrepresented person, as well as the setting in which the behavior and comments occur."[60]

I. TRUTHFULNESS IN STATEMENTS TO OTHERS

Model Rule 4.1 prohibits a lawyer from making a false statement of material fact to a third person during the course of his representation of a client. The rule also requires disclosure of a material fact where necessary to prevent a crime or fraud, *unless* such disclosure is prohibited by Rule 1.6. With respect to omissions and third parties, the duty of confidentiality thus trumps the duty of candor. Compare this to a lawyer's duty of candor to a tribunal in *ex parte* proceedings (Section B.2, *supra*) and with respect to witness perjury (Section B.4, *supra*), where a lawyer's duty as an officer of the court trumps his duty to protect client confidences.

Note the difference between commissions and omissions in Rule 4.1(a) and (b). A lawyer may not make a false statement of material fact to a third party, period. However, a lawyer's duty to affirmatively correct a false statement made by his client or another is considerably more complicated.

The *commission* component of Rule 4.1(a) would prohibit a personal injury lawyer from advising a prospective witness to a motor vehicle accident that his client lost his job as a result of the accident, if in fact his client was unemployed at the time of the crash. This misstatement is material because it might engender sympathy in the client, increase the witness's view of damages, and cause the witness to be willing to cooperate when otherwise he might not be inclined to do so. On the other hand, Rule 4.1(a) would *not* be violated if that same lawyer misrepresented himself as a relative of the witness in order to get through to the witness on the office switchboard. Such a statement, while false, is irrelevant to the car accident and therefore not material.

Now consider the *omission* component of Rule 4.1(b). A lawyer must disclose a material fact to a third person only if such disclosure (1) is necessary to avoid assisting a criminal or fraudulent act by the client, *and* (2) such disclosure does not violate the rule of client confidences. Here, the protection for client confidences under Rule 1.6 trumps the obligation of truthfulness. For example, a lawyer may discover during his representation of a client in the purchase of real property that his client has substantially misstated his assets on a loan application to a bank. If rectifying this misstatement would require the lawyer to reveal a client confidence (for example, if the lawyer knows this information only as a result of his representation

---

60. Model Rule 4.3 cmt. [2].

of the client), the lawyer generally may not reveal the information and has not violated Rule 4.1(b). However, if the lawyer assists the client in purchasing the real property *based* on this false mortgage application, he may be assisting in a crime or fraud in violation of Rule 1.2(d). If that is the case, the lawyer must correct the material misstatement if he intends to continue the representation, unless the revelation would violate Rule 1.6. Since the "exceptions" to client confidences in Rule 1.6(b)(1)-(7) are phrased in terms of **permissive disclosures**, exercising discretion to reveal a confidence in one of those enumerated instances would not be "prohibited" by the rule. Thus, with respect to material omissions, the permissive disclosures under Rule 1.6(b) become mandatory disclosures if necessary to avoid assisting in a criminal or fraudulent act by your client. In the case of our supposed bank fraud, the lawyer's options in that situation are either to withdraw from representation; to urge the client to correct the misrepresentation to the bank; to seek the client's permission to breach the client confidence and inform the bank himself; or — and only if the lawyer reasonably believes it is necessary to prevent substantial injury to the financial interests or property of another — to reveal the misstatement to the bank himself. *See* Model Rule 1.6(b)(3).

The Model Rule's prohibition of material misstatements by a lawyer to a third party contains a "puffing" exception. During legal representation a lawyer may engage in negotiations with a third party as to price or value. For example, in the real estate transaction cited above, the client may engage the lawyer to make an offer on his behalf for the purchase of residential real estate. The lawyer may offer $500,000. After a counteroffer of $550,000, the lawyer may meet in the middle and offer $525,000, stating that "this is as high as my client has authorized me to go." If the client has in fact authorized him to purchase the property for as much as $600,000, this is a material misstatement of fact. Nevertheless, it is unlikely to result in bar discipline in most jurisdictions. Comment [2] to Model Rule 4.1 provides that under "generally accepted conventions in negotiations," statements regarding price, value, or settlement intentions are generally considered statements of opinion rather than fact for the purposes of the rule. This "puffing" exception for misstatements to third parties seems to be a pragmatic concession to the limits of attorney regulation with regard to a lawyer's role in negotiations.

With regard to misstatements to others, attorneys must be aware that Model Rule 8.4(c) is broader than Model Rule 4.1 and constrains conduct that would not violate the former rule. Rule 8.4(c) provides that an attorney may not "engage in conduct involving dishonesty, fraud, deceit or misrepresentation." Rule 8.4 is broader than Rule 4.1 because the false statement or misrepresentation does not have to be material and the statement does not have to be in the course of representation of a client. Rule 8.4(c) is thus a broader, potential "catchall" provision that could arguably apply even to an attorney's private affairs. For example, Rule 8.4(c) could be invoked to sanction a lawyer for dishonesty in his personal business dealings or political pursuits.[61]

---

61. Finely v. Kentucky Bar Ass'n, 378 S.W.3d 313, 314 (Ky. 2012) (lawyer used his office's Westlaw account to conduct research for personal profit).

Should either Rule 4.1 or Rule 8.4 contain an exception allowing attorneys to misrepresent their identity or purpose in order to investigate conduct they believe to be unlawful? Some commentators believe that civil attorneys should be able to engage in or direct "testing" (i.e., undercover investigations) in order to expose unlawful activities. One prominent attorney in Massachusetts thought so, and proceeded to conduct an undercover investigation of alleged judicial misconduct that got him disbarred.

Case Preview

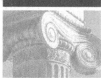

In re Crossen

Attorney Crossen represented one of the family members in a multi-million-dollar shareholder derivative suit involving control of the Demoulas supermarket empire. In an effort to have a Massachusetts superior court judge recused from the case, Crossen took part in an intricate plot designed to uncover evidence of the trial judge's bias. Crossen set up and recorded sham job interviews with the judge's former law clerk in order to coax the clerk into unveiling facts about the judge's deliberative process and alleged bias. Crossen also placed the law clerk under surveillance and threatened to interfere with his state bar application if he did not cooperate. The disciplinary board recommended Crossen be disbarred, and this appeal followed.

Although *In re Crossen* involved a Massachusetts disciplinary rule that predated the state's adoption of the Model Rules, it is instructive as to the limits of a private attorney's authority to engage in misrepresentation.

As you read *In re Crossen*, consider the following:

1. Do you think Crossen's investigatory tactics were influenced by his prior experiences as a prosecutor and Assistant U.S. Attorney? Should they have been?
2. In handing out its sanction of disbarment, the Supreme Judicial Court was influenced by the "unusual scope" of the respondent's misconduct. Do you think the court was motivated by a unique desire to protect the deliberative processes of judges and their law clerks? Would a lawyer's fraud and deceit have warranted such severe discipline if the "victim" had not been the court system itself?

In re Crossen
880 N.E.2d 352 (Mass. 2008)

(ii) Use of a sham interview. The board properly determined that Crossen's participation in the New York interview, including the surreptitious tape recording, violated Canon 1, DR 1-102(A)(2) and (4)-(6), and Canon 7, DR 7-102(A)(5) and (7). That the New York interview involved "dishonesty, fraud, deceit, or misrepresentation," Canon 1, DR 1-102(A)(4), and "false" statements and "fraudulent" conduct, Canon 7, DR 7-102(A)(5) and (7), cannot seriously be doubted.

. . .

The board also correctly concluded that the surreptitious tape recording of the New York interview violated DR 1-102(A)(4) and DR 7-102(A)(5). Crossen is correct that no legal barrier prevented him from secretly tape recording the law clerk's conversation in New York. However, when Crossen orchestrated the surreptitious tape recording in 1997, there was long-standing authority that lawyers violate the ethical rules when they tape record a person without his consent, even if the recording is legal. ABA Formal Op. 337 (1974). In any event, we will not detach the legal act of one-party tape recording in New York from the web of knowing and deliberate misstatements and falsehoods in which it was integrally embedded in this case. . . . The legality of the tape recording does not mask its improper purpose. Where the surreptitious tape recording of the law clerk was in furtherance of an effort to coerce or even manufacture sworn testimony against a judge in a pending matter, Crossen's tape recording of the sham interview not only violated his obligations to eschew misstatement, deceit, and falsehood in his professional dealings, but also manifestly worked to the prejudice of the administration of justice and impugned his own bona fides as an attorney.

. . .

(iii) Threats and surveillance. The board concluded that Crossen violated Canon 1, DR 1-102(A)(4)-(6), and Canon 7, DR 7-102(A)(5) and (7), when he threatened that, unless the law clerk stated under oath that Judge Lopez was biased against the Telemachus Demoulas family in the shareholder derivative suit, he, Crossen, would disclose the "embarrassing or compromising" statements the law clerk made during the sham job interviews, including the information that the law clerk, in connection with his bar application, had submitted a letter of recommendation from a person whom he did not know. The board also concluded that Crossen violated the same disciplinary rules, with the exception of DR 1-102(A)(5), when he deliberately misrepresented to the law clerk that there existed a tape recording of the Halifax meeting. These conclusions find ample support in the record.

. . .

Again, we consider Crossen's available choices. When the New York interview did not yield the results Crossen sought, Crossen did not lay the matter to rest. He did not confront Curry[62] — whom he was advised by at least three highly regarded cocounsel to view with caution — with exaggerating what the law clerk said in Halifax. Rather, Crossen sought to obtain the results his client wanted by offering the law clerk a stark quid pro quo: an implicit bargain not to make public the law clerk's bar application if the law clerk offered sworn testimony that Judge Lopez had prejudged the Demoulas defendants' case. To further pressure the law clerk, the quid pro quo was presented under a deadline that did not exist. This conduct goes far beyond what a reasonable attorney zealously representing his client would consider either proper investigation of the facts or permissible hard-nosed bargaining. Crossen's most coercive actions occurred *after* the sham interview yielded equivocal results and *after* he was warned about Curry's credibility. . . .

---

62. Kevin Curry was another attorney representing the Demoulas family who had originally interviewed the law clerk and informed Crossen that the law clerk had heard the judge make prejudicial statements about his client. — Eds.

With regard to surveillance, there was substantial evidence for the board to conclude that Crossen intentionally lied to the law clerk when he denied any involvement in or awareness of surveillance of the law clerk in late August. We agree with the board that this misrepresentation is of a piece with his other misstatements and falsehoods in violating DR 1-102(A)(4) and (6).

. . .

b. Investigative techniques. Crossen argues that he had a good faith belief that his conduct was proper, and that his "subjective belief was objectively reasonable, as illustrated by contemporaneous scholarly commentary." He leans particularly on an article coauthored by a former chair of the American Bar Association's Standing Committee on Professional Responsibility. . . . Crossen does not claim that he took guidance from, or even read, the ethics article in the course of the relevant events in this case. More importantly, the ethics article does not discuss, much less endorse, the kind of ruse at issue here. The ethics article's thrust, as Crossen says, is that public and private attorneys who act as investigators and testers conducting undercover investigations or undertaking discrimination testing to gather evidence they otherwise would be unlikely to obtain voluntarily, or who supervise others in such conduct, do not violate rules 4.1(a) and 8.4(c) of the ABA Model Rules of Professional Conduct, which forbid making false statements or material misrepresentations. . . . However, Crossen omits the important caveat of the ethics article's thesis, namely, that it applies only to "elementary, and essential, misrepresentations as to identity and purpose made by discrimination undercover investigators and testers". . . . ("Rule 8.4[c], which prohibits conduct involving dishonesty, fraud, deceit or misrepresentation, would not apply to misrepresentations of the *mild sort necessarily* made by discrimination testers and undercover investigators" [emphasis added]). The article makes clear that where the "misrepresentations are of a graver kind, or when a tester/ investigator is used by the lawyer specifically for something the lawyer is forbidden to do, or when the lawyer directs a tester/investigator to engage in activities that violate the rights of others," the Model Rules of Professional Conduct are implicated, regardless whether the attorney is private or public counsel. . . . According to the authors of the ethics article, specific conduct that violates Model Rules 4.1(a) and 8.4(c) includes a lawyer acting in his or her capacity as a lawyer who makes "misrepresentations of material fact" . . . as well as a lawyer engaging in conduct or supervising conduct that employs "excessively intrusive investigative techniques," "entrapment," or involves "an actionable invasion of privacy". . . . It is clear from what we have said to this point that Crossen's conduct fails even the ethics article's test.

. . .

We conclude as well that, acting with reason, Crossen should have known that his efforts to intimidate the law clerk with threats of disclosure unless the law clerk produced sworn statements damaging to Judge Lopez was prejudicial to the administration of justice: it was intended or was likely to produce from the law clerk testimony more critical of Judge Lopez than the law clerk otherwise would or could have given.

. . .

6. Sanction

. . .

In considering whether the sanction of disbarment is markedly disparate from sanctions in comparable cases, we are immediately struck, as was the special hearing officer, by the sui generis nature of the law clerk episode, ultimately orchestrated and driven by Crossen. Countless bar disciplinary cases concern relatively discrete events of misconduct involving one attorney, and one or a few transactions or clients. We have found none that involves such a large number of attorneys and their agents, or deceit so exquisitely choreographed as to include in one bundle surreptitious tape recording, traveling out of State to avoid the laws of Massachusetts, the masking of multiple identities, the procurement of sham business cards and sham business information, multiple sham interviews, covert surveillance, and multiple threats and attempts at coercion, among other things.

. . .

That there is no blueprint in our prior cases for the facts of this proceeding should come as no surprise, reflecting the unusual scope of the misconduct. The sanction of disbarment we impose is appropriate to ensure that the law clerk episode (or anything like it) remains sui generis.

. . .

7. Conclusion. For the reasons stated above, we adopt the recommendation of the board and remand to the county court where a judgment of disbarment shall enter.

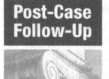

Post-Case Follow-Up

If Crossen had truly believed that the judge before whom he appeared was corrupt and unethical, how could he have substantiated that claim in a way that did not violate Rule 8.4? Exactly where and how did he go too far?

Sometimes it is not the conduct that gets you into trouble, but the cover-up. How many lies did Crossen tell after perpetrating the initial ruse?

Food Fight: Inside the Battle for the Market Basket

The *Demoulas v. DeMoulas* case, which was the inter-family dispute undergirding the *Crossen* disciplinary matter, was the subject of an award-winning documentary entitled "Food Fight."

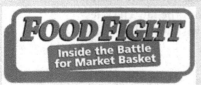

A documentary by Food Fight Films, LLC

http://www.foodfightfilm.com/

In re Crossen: Real Life Applications

1. Suppose that the heirs of a recently deceased widow bring a civil action in state court alleging fraud by the widow's next-door neighbor, who happens to be a lawyer. According to the heirs, the lawyer defrauded the elderly and confused woman out of a strip of property between their houses by falsely claiming that she was conveying an easement and not a fee simple. The lawyer subsequently enlarged his estate using the strip of land, to the disadvantage of the neighbor who was deprived of access to a nearby beach. At the time they file the civil fraud suit, the heirs also report the lawyer to the state bar disciplinary authority. If proven, is this conduct a violation of Rule 8.4(c)?

Even if it is, is this the type of conduct that you think bar disciplinary agencies should regulate? Why or why not?

2. Imagine that you represent a client who alleges that he was not hired for a position of salesperson at a retail clothing store because of his race. In order to develop evidence of discrimination before filing a lawsuit on his behalf, may you ask paralegals or investigators in your office to go "undercover" to the clothing store and apply for the same job? If your state does not have an "investigatory" exception to Rule 8.4, either expressly in the rule or by judicial construction, would you be comfortable putting your license on the line by engaging in such deception?

Many lawyers use, or direct their subordinates to use, covert investigative techniques designed to gather evidence of wrongdoing. Prosecutors supervise the undercover operations of police officers, which often involve shams. Civil rights lawyers send their agents in to pose as "testers" to ascertain whether a business may be discriminating unlawfully. Do these acts of misidentification in order to gather evidence violate Rule 8.4(c)? This remains an unsettled area of the law. Note that the Supreme Judicial Court in *In re Crossen* refused to address whether there should be an investigatory exception to the Massachusetts predecessor to Rule 8.4(c), because the court ruled that Crossen's deceit with respect to the law clerk was not the sole basis for discipline, and that Crossen's entire course of conduct was highly prejudicial to the administration of justice. Some courts have ruled that misidentifying yourself and your purpose in order to gather evidence of wrongdoing is not a violation of the rule prohibiting dishonesty and deceit,[63] while others have concluded that it is.[64] Some states have amended their disciplinary codes to expressly allow for an investigatory exception to Rule 8.4, but even those states disagree on whether such an exception should apply only to criminal lawyers working for the government,[65] or also to civil lawyers engaged in covert activity to investigate violations of civil or constitutional rights.[66]

Chapter Summary

■ A lawyer may not knowingly make false statements to the court. If a lawyer makes a materially false statement to the court and comes to know of its falsity after the statement is made but before the conclusion of the proceedings, the lawyer must correct the false statement.

---

63. Apple Corps Ltd. v. International Collectors Society, 15 F. Supp. 2d 456, 475 (D.N.J. 1998) (lawyers hired private investigators to pose as members of the general public wishing to buy exclusive Beatles stamps from the defendant).

64. In re Gatti, 8 P.3d 966, 974 (Or. 2000) (lawyer claimed to be a chiropractor for the purpose of obtaining information from insurance claims reviewer as to how it was conducting medical screening); In re Pautler, 47 P.3d 1175, 1180 (Colo. 2002) (lawyer presented himself to at-large murder suspect as a public defender for the purpose of apprehending him).

65. Fla. St. Bar Rule 4-8.4(c).

66. Or. R. Prof'l Conduct 8.4(b); Iowa R. Prof'l Conduct 32:8.4(c), cmt. [6].

- A lawyer must disclose adverse legal authority in the controlling jurisdiction to the court, if not disclosed by opposing counsel.

- A lawyer may not counsel or assist a witness to commit perjury, and may not put a witness on the stand in a civil case who he knows will commit perjury. If a witness called by the lawyer surprises the lawyer by testifying falsely on a material matter, the lawyer must take remedial measures.

- During pendency of the litigation, a lawyer may not have any *ex parte* contact with the presiding judge or a juror unless authorized by law.

- A lawyer may not communicate with a person represented by counsel on the subject of that representation without first obtaining permission of the person's lawyer.

- A lawyer may not engage in conduct involving fraud, deceit, or misrepresentation, even in his private dealings.

Applying the Rules

1. You represent a UPS driver who claims that he suffered a back injury on the job. In litigation against the company, the plaintiff testified during his deposition that he now walks with a cane and that he is unable to carry on normal day-to-day activities like carrying groceries, picking up his small children, and bending over to tie his shoes. Prior to trial, opposing counsel presents you with photographs allegedly taken by his private investigator showing your client jogging, skiing, and playing golf since the time of the alleged accident. What should you do?

2. You represent one spouse in a divorce contest. You have made a generous settlement offer to opposing counsel, but she has not responded, and she has failed to return several of your phone calls. May you send opposing counsel a registered letter reiterating the offer, and this time copy her client on the letter so that you can be sure the opposing party has been informed?

3. One of your clients is a small automobile repair shop with fewer than ten employees. The owner comes to your office one day and states that she is being investigated by the state attorney general for failing to pay mechanics overtime in violation of the state prevailing wage law. The client delivers to you her laptop computer, which she claims contains all of her payroll records for the past three years. What should you do with the computer?

4. You represent a defendant corporation in a shareholder derivative action. The federal district judge granted summary judgment in favor of your client. Plaintiffs have filed a brief on appeal to the Circuit Court. They have neglected to cite a case from another Circuit that directly supports their position in the litigation. Do you have an obligation to cite this case in your brief, even if it is to distinguish the case or argue that its reasoning is unpersuasive?

Professional Responsibility in Practice

1. Research the law in the jurisdiction in which you intend to practice. Is there any case law or commentary that recognizes an investigative exception to Rule 8.4(c)?

2. Suppose that you represented a plaintiff in an employment discrimination matter. After a two-week jury trial, the jury returned a verdict in favor of the defendant corporation. The day after the verdict, you receive an email from a juror informing you that she was very distraught by the deliberations process and feels like several members of the jury made improper racial comments during deliberations harmful to your client. Research the law of your jurisdiction to determine how, if at all, you may respond to the juror's email or otherwise communicate with the juror.

8

Special Ethical Issues in Criminal Practice

The ethical restraints in litigation we discussed in the previous chapter apply to both civil and criminal practitioners. However, there are certain attorney discipline rules that apply only to prosecutors, and others that are more relevant and acute in the context of criminal defense.

A. THE PROSECUTOR

Because she represents the entire community rather than any single client or entity, the prosecutor has unique professional obligations. The source and meaning of such obligations will be discussed below.

1. Who Do You Represent?

Unlike a traditional advocate, a prosecutor does not represent an individual or organizational client, but rather the sovereign at large. This puts the prosecutor in the position of being at the same time both a principal and agent. Unlike a traditional advocate, whose job is to provide his client with informed advice and then to pursue the client's objectives zealously within the bounds of the law, the prosecutor must first make decisions about what is in the best interests of society before ascertaining a course of action to pursue

Key Concepts

- Sources of a prosecutor's duty to "seek justice"
- The prosecutor's duty to turn over exculpatory evidence
- The "no-contact" rule and limits on the government's investigation of represented suspects
- The prosecutor and the press—obligations that exceed Rule 3.6
- Dangers for the criminal defense attorney in taking possession of physical evidence
- The criminal defense attorney's "trilemma," and how to handle client perjury

those goals. Because a prosecutor represents the collective "sovereign," she has no personal client to direct her course of action. She has constituents — the police, the victim(s) of crime, the probation department, members of the public, and even the defendant himself — but none of these constituents can be treated as traditional clients entitled to control the objectives of litigation. As the Supreme Court has recognized, "[the prosecutor] is the representative not of an ordinary party to a controversy, but of a sovereignty whose obligation to govern impartially is as compelling as its obligation to govern at all; and whose interest, therefore, in a criminal prosecution is not that it shall win a case, but that justice shall be done."[1]

The uniqueness of the prosecutor's role — whether it stems from the distinctive nature of the prosecutor's client or the awesome power wielded by the government — has important consequences for a prosecutor's conduct in investigating and prosecuting criminal cases. The ABA has enacted a specific rule of professional conduct applicable only to prosecutors — Model Rule 3.8 — detailing these special responsibilities. Comment [1] to Rule 3.8 is particularly instructive because it describes the prosecutor's role in the following general terms: "A prosecutor has the responsibility of a **minister of justice** and not simply that of an advocate. This responsibility carries with it a specific obligation to see that the defendant is accorded procedural justice [and] that guilt is decided upon the basis of sufficient evidence. . . ." (Emphasis supplied.)

How does a prosecutor go about assessing what constitutes "justice" in any particular case? Professor Fred Zacharias attempts to unpack this "minister of justice" obligation in the following law review article. He suggests that it has both substantive and procedural components. What are they?

Fred Zacharias, Structuring the Ethics of Trial Advocacy
44 Vand. L. Rev. 45 (1991)

II. THE MEANING OF JUSTICE IN THE CONTEXT OF ADVERSARIAL TRIALS

One obvious concern underlying the prosecutor's special ethical duty is to prevent punishment of innocent defendants. At the charging, plea bargaining, and sentencing stages, the heart of the codes' mandate to do justice seems clear: the prosecutor should exercise discretion so as to prosecute only persons she truly considers guilty, and then only in a manner that fits the crime. Many codes reinforce the prosecutor's general obligation with specific rules limiting pretrial conduct along these lines.

Once a case reaches trial, this duty is no longer very meaningful. The prosecutor already has made her good faith determination that the defendant is guilty. Unless some unexpected development makes her reconsider her conclusion, she may pursue a conviction. Thus, in extending the prosecutor's justice obligation to the trial

---

1. Berger v. United States, 295 U.S. 78, 88 (1935).

stage, the codes almost by definition intend a higher obligation than simply avoiding unjustified prosecutions. The American Bar Association (ABA) proposed specific standards for trial conduct in the 1970s, but these standards were not adopted in the later Model Rules. All modern codes are silent on the meaning of justice at trial.

Reputable scholars have advanced the proposition that the adversary system is ineffective in producing accurate verdicts. Interpreting the codes from that perspective, one might assume that "doing justice" requires prosecutors to temper their zeal. One can hypothesize open-minded prosecutors who present facts neutrally and encourage courts and jurors to emphasize defendants' procedural rights. These idealized government attorneys constantly would reevaluate the strength of their case. They would adjust the content and force of each evidentiary presentation to further the outcome that they believe the jury should reach on the current state of the evidence.

It is beyond the scope of this Article to discuss whether adversarial theory is essentially flawed, whether the image of prosecutorial nonpartisanship is realistic, or whether prosecutors and all other lawyers have uncodified obligations to bring about socially beneficial results. For our purposes, it suffices to recognize that the noncompetitive approach to prosecutorial ethics is inconsistent with the professional codes' underlying theory. The codes are concerned specifically with structuring adversarial practice. They do not exempt prosecutors from the requirements of zealous advocacy. Reading the cursory "do justice" language as a denunciation of competitive fact-finding therefore would create an internal contradiction.

. . .

The Adversary System's General Approach to Lawyer Ethics

. . .

Nevertheless, as David Luban and other commentators have pointed out, law's version of adversary process may not be an effective method for achieving accurate verdicts. The view that a process of contradiction alone exposes truth is counterintuitive and, at least in some circumstances, simply wrong. Proponents of adversaries therefore have looked to alternative justifications to support the system.

One rationale is that adversary process assures procedural fairness, including assertion of all the parties' rights. Aligning attorneys solely with their clients' interests creates an incentive for lawyers to be active and to take full advantage of the law's protections. Ensuring that the parties' views are presented — even if extreme — may make the parties feel as if the legal system has treated them evenhandedly. Not only is that sense of fairness an independent "good," but ultimately, it helps some litigants accept even unfavorable results.

Proponents also argue that the system is an efficient mechanism for resolving disputes. Adversarial process causes lawyers to frame and narrow the issues for the fact finder and creates a system of checks and balances. The attorneys keep an eye on one another and on the judge to make sure that they all perform their assigned roles in proper and ethical fashion.

When the various justifications for the adversary system are considered as a whole, one can see that the "justice" it strives for has several elements. Ascertaining the true facts is not the only or paramount goal. Fairness and respect for client

individuality play an equal part, even though full assertion of client rights may interfere with truth-seeking. Efficient fact-finding also is an important objective.

B. How Prosecutors Fit Within the Adversarial Scheme

To the extent that the adversary system works according to theory, government
lawyers promote justice by playing the same role at trial as private advocates. They
contribute to truth by defending their own factual hypotheses and contesting those
of their opponents. Prosecutors help courts assess defendants' rights; the claims of
defendants' champions must be contested to determine their validity. Prosecutors
also enhance the efficiency aspects of the process by acting adversarially. By challenging defense counsels' positions at every step, prosecutors force defenders to remain
vigilant and to frame the issues clearly for proper adjudication.

At one level, the prosecutor thus helps achieve the appropriate systemic
results — does adversarial justice — simply by performing as an aggressive advocate. In the context of an adversarial model of adjudication, even prosecutors who
develop "conviction psychology" seem justified; ordinarily it is not up to a lawyer
to act contrary to her side's interests. Having proceeded to trial, the prosecutor
represents the community's interest in conviction. Court-enforced constitutional
safeguards (such as the beyond-a-reasonable-doubt standard) arguably suffice to
protect the innocent.

The notion that a prosecutor sometimes should refrain from acting as a pure
advocate stems from the fact that she has no single client. The prosecutor is simultaneously responsible for the community's protection, victims' desire for vengeance,
defendants' entitlement to a fair opportunity for vindication, and the state's need for
a criminal justice system that is efficient and appears fair. Described accurately, the
prosecutor represents "constituencies" — and several of them at one time.

This multirepresentation is significant for the structure of prosecutorial ethics.
Private lawyers confronting ethical dilemmas usually find themselves torn between
promoting a single client's goals and safeguarding their own professional or moral
self-interest. The disciplinary rules resolve these conflicts largely by casting trial lawyers as agents who must champion client interests, subject only to narrow limits on
extreme behavior.

Prosecutors, in contrast, face conflicts among their constituents' interests as
well as between constituent and personal interests. Code drafters could have used
an agency analysis to shape prosecutorial ethics. The rules simply could state which
constituent's interests take precedence in particular situations. The decision not to
codify priorities reflects the drafters' sense that prosecutors' multirepresentational
role requires an independent framework for governing prosecutorial conduct.

The framework that the drafters have chosen consists primarily of the "do justice" rule. The prosecutor's relative independence provides a theoretical justification
for the rule's departure from adversarial norms. As discussed above, drafters committed to the adversary system would not expect the advocate for the prosecution
routinely to disavow zeal. But because a prosecutor need not focus exclusively on a
single client's interests, her role in promoting the system's goals of procedural fairness and efficient fact-finding becomes more dominant. The code envisions limited

circumstances in which she can temper her competitive spirit, yet still contribute to results that the adversary system deems appropriate.

. . .

Moreover, the prosecutor benefits from unique prestige and symbolic power. Because she represents the community, she commonly carries more influence with juries than attorneys allied solely with individual clients. The prosecutor can rely on jurors' natural instincts to be protected against crime. She can draw upon jurors' tendencies to believe that persons a grand jury singles out for prosecution probably are guilty.

Finally, a prosecutor enjoys practical advantages over her adversaries. She benefits from the state's hefty investigative and litigation resources. Through the police and grand jury, she monopolizes the ability to coerce testimony and obtain cooperation in the investigation of crimes. The literature is replete with discussions of ways in which a prosecutor can misuse her singular tools.

The fear of prosecutorial abuses thus explains why code drafters have chosen to adopt a "do justice" obligation. The drafters reasonably expect that, as the symbol of fair criminal justice, prosecutors should not take undue advantage of their built-in resources. Prosecutors who overreach undermine "confidence, not only in [their] profession, but in government and the very ideal of justice itself."

The nature of the prosecutor's unique power also suggests that the duty takes on special meaning at the trial stage. Aspects of prosecutorial power — such as the unusual influence over jurors — come into play solely at trial. Confining the codes' requirements to instituting and maintaining prosecutions in good faith thus would understate the drafters' concerns. The "do justice" rule may not contemplate half-hearted advocacy, but it clearly addresses the use of techniques that tilt trials toward convictions in an unfair way.

To fix the scope of the "do justice" rule, one must consider its theoretical justification and underlying practical concerns in tandem. It would be reading too much into two words — "do justice" — to conclude that the rule embodies a counter-traditional theoretical conception of prosecutors as nonadversarial lawyers. The paradigm of the prosecutor as an unaligned "minister of the system" makes sense in the trial context only if it targets situations in which competitive fact-finding will not produce results that are "acceptable" within the meaning of the adversary system. Yet we have seen that when the adversary system operates in its intended fashion, competition by definition produces appropriate results. The "do justice" rule, therefore, must focus on cases in which the system itself is defective — in which defendants are not tried in accordance with the system's basic, structural elements.

Interpreting prosecutors' obligation to do justice with reference to "adequate adversarial process" rather than "accurate outcomes" helps identify when prosecutors should depart from an advocate's stance: prosecutors must strive for adversarially valid results rather than factually correct results. This systemic approach also defines limits to prosecutors' ethical duty. The codes assign prosecutors a special role within the system because prosecutors are unencumbered by client ties. It follows that the codes accord prosecutors leeway to repair flaws in the process, but impose no general duty to help defendants win.

C. Defining the Prosecutor's Duty to Do Justice at Trial

The key to understanding this adversarial interpretation of justice is to identify the essential elements of adversarial process and isolate ways in which they may fail. When the system breaks down in a significant respect, the codes can no longer expect competition to achieve adversarially appropriate results. If the evidence is in conflict, an ethical prosecutor cannot rationalize a conviction simply on the ground that the trial is fair.

. . .

Consider a case in which a judge deprives one party of an opportunity to present the facts by cowing defense counsel into avoiding relevant lines of questioning. Arguably, the trial does not satisfy the adversary system's design. The premises of a passive tribunal and an equal opportunity to put forth a case may be lacking. The litigant's capacity to obtain a systemically appropriate result is at risk.

. . .

The prosecutor's unique prestige helps justify holding her to a higher ethical responsibility. In the hypothetical scenario, practical considerations might prevent a private attorney from taking advantage of the court's one-sided attitude. The attorney reasonably may fear that the jury will perceive him to be bullying the opponent. In contrast, because a prosecutor starts out with an aura of respectability, she can get away with more. Practical limitations do not restrain her conduct to the same extent.

The prosecutor's resource advantages also weigh in favor of making her rectify the system's failure. By virtue of her access to the grand jury and her relationship with law enforcement agencies, the prosecutor has an institutional identity that helps her deal with the hypothetical judge's conduct. The judge can do without a private attorney's affection and, consequently, may retaliate for the attorney's attempt to challenge him. In contrast, the judge needs the prosecutor's goodwill almost as much as the prosecutor needs his. The court must have the cooperation of the prosecutor's office to manage the criminal justice system; offending one prosecutor may offend them all. Within limits, the nature of the prosecutor's office as the institution in charge of law enforcement resources thus enables individual prosecutors to serve as checks on failures elsewhere in the system.

Hence, viewed from the code drafters' adversarial perspective, "justice" does take on special meaning for government attorneys. The codes impose a different duty to role differentiate than they impose on private lawyers. Once a prosecutor determines the prosecution should proceed, her function is to advocate the defendant's guilt. But when the system breaks down, she at least temporarily must set aside her view that the defendant should be convicted. Her role is not to help him win, yet neither may she passively accept systemically faulty outcomes. As a "minister" of the system, the codes require her to help restore adversarial balance.

. . .

2. Quantum of Proof Necessary for Charging

The invocation of the state's charging power has immeasurable reputational and economic consequences for a defendant, even if he is subsequently acquitted at trial. Zacharias suggests that in making pretrial decisions (e.g., charging, plea bargaining) prosecutors should prosecute only individuals that they truly believe are guilty, and then only in a manner and to a degree that fits the crime.

What quantum of evidence must a prosecutor possess before commencing charges? The non-binding ABA Standards for Criminal Justice suggest that as a "minister of justice" a prosecutor should not commence criminal proceedings unless the state possesses sufficient admissible evidence to prove its case beyond a reasonable doubt (essentially the directed verdict standard).[2] Note, however, that Rule 3.8(a) of the Model Rules of Professional Conduct suggests a lower threshold, that of "**probable cause**." While the probable cause standard is concededly higher than the standard for filing a civil complaint (i.e., Rule 3.1 prohibits only "frivolous" complaints), it is still remarkably low. It allows for the consideration of hearsay, and it allows a prosecutor to leave questions about the constitutional and legal admissibility of evidence for resolution by the court.

Why do Zacharias and the Criminal Justice Committee of the ABA recommend a higher charging threshold than the attorney discipline rules in effect in most jurisdictions? Or, to phrase the question in the negative, when would it ever be a legitimate exercise of state power for a prosecutor to charge a crime that meets the probable cause threshold, but not the sufficient admissible evidence of guilt threshold?

At the other end of the spectrum, how should a prosecutor conduct himself when objectively there is sufficient admissible evidence to support a finding of guilt, but the prosecutor *personally* believes that the defendant is innocent? ABA Standard 3-4.3 states as an aspirational matter that "[a] prosecutor's office should not file or maintain charges if *it* believes the defendant is innocent, no matter what the state of the evidence." (Emphasis supplied.) But how helpful is this non-binding ABA guideline? "Offices" cannot "believe"; only "individuals" can "believe." As a representative of the sovereign, may a prosecutor decline to commence charges when there is sufficient admissible evidence to support a conviction, but the prosecutor herself has lingering personal doubts about the defendant's guilt?

The following story of Daniel Bibb from the Manhattan District Attorney's Office may test the limits of the "do justice" mandate.

Benjamin Weiser, Doubting Case, a Prosecutor Helped the Defense
N.Y. Times, June 23, 2008

The Manhattan district attorney, Robert M. Morgenthau, had a problem. The murder convictions of two men in one of his office's big cases — the 1990 shooting of a bouncer outside the Palladium nightclub — had been called into question by a stream of new evidence.

---

2. ABA STANDARDS FOR CRIMINAL JUSTICE: PROSECUTION FUNCTION, Standard 3-4.3(a) (4th ed. 2015).

So the office decided on a re-examination, led by a 21-year veteran assistant, Daniel L. Bibb.

Mr. Bibb spent nearly two years reinvestigating the killing and reported back: He believed that the two imprisoned men were not guilty, and that their convictions should be dropped. Yet top officials told him, he said, to go into a court hearing and defend the case anyway. He did, and in 2005 he lost.

But in a recent interview, Mr. Bibb made a startling admission: He threw the case. Unwilling to do what his bosses ordered, he said, he deliberately helped the other side win.

He tracked down hard-to-find or reluctant witnesses who pointed to other suspects and prepared them to testify for the defense. He talked strategy with defense lawyers. And when they veered from his coaching, he cornered them in the hallway and corrected them.

"I did the best I could," he said. "To lose."

Today, the two men are free. At the end of the hearing, which stretched over six weeks, his superiors agreed to ask a judge to drop the conviction of one, Olmedo Hidalgo. The judge granted a new trial to the other, David Lemus, who was acquitted in December.

Mr. Bibb, 53, who said it was painful to remain in the office, resigned in 2006 and is trying to build a new career as a defense lawyer in Manhattan — with some difficulty, friends say, in a profession where success can hang on the ability to cut deals with prosecutors.

Mr. Morgenthau's office would not comment on Mr. Bibb's claims. Daniel J. Castleman, chief assistant district attorney, would say only: "Nobody in this office is ever required to prosecute someone they believe is innocent. That was true then, as it is now. That being the case, no useful purpose would be served in engaging in a debate with a former staff member." The office has said it had good reason to believe that the two men were guilty.

Yet whatever the facts of the murder, the dispute offers an unusual glimpse of a prosecutor weighing the demands of conscience against his obligation to his office, and the extraordinary measures he took to settle that conflict in his own mind.

"I was angry," Mr. Bibb said, "that I was being put in a position to defend convictions that I didn't believe in."

The case also reveals a rare public challenge to one of the nation's most powerful district attorneys from within his office. As the hearing unfolded in 2005, Mr. Morgenthau, running for re-election, was sharply criticized by an opponent who said he had prosecuted the wrong men.

By then, the Palladium case had become one of the most troubled in the city's recent history, stirred up every few years by fresh evidence, heralded in newspaper and television reports, that pointed to other suspects.

It is not as if Mr. Morgenthau has refused to admit mistakes. In 2002, in spectacular fashion, his office recommended dismissing the convictions of five men in the attack on a jogger in Central Park, after its reinvestigation showed that another man had acted alone. "It's my decision," Mr. Morgenthau said then. "The buck stops here."

In fact, the prosecutor who led that inquiry, Nancy E. Ryan, was Mr. Bibb's supervisor in the Palladium case — though Mr. Bibb would not detail his conversations with her or other superiors, saying they were privileged.

Defense lawyers confirmed that Mr. Bibb helped them, though he never explicitly stated his intentions. Some praised his efforts to see that justice was done. Others involved in the case suggested he did a disservice to both sides — shirking his duty as an assistant district attorney, and prolonging an injustice by not quitting the case, or the office.

And some blame Mr. Bibb's superiors. Steven M. Cohen, a former federal prosecutor who pushed Mr. Morgenthau's office to reinvestigate, said that while Mr. Bibb should have refused to present the case, his bosses should not have pressed him.

"If Bibb is to be believed, he was essentially asked to choose between his conscience and his job," Mr. Cohen said. "Whether he made the right choice is irrelevant; that he was asked to make that choice is chilling."

At 6-foot-6, Mr. Bibb looks every inch the lawman, with a square jaw, a gravelly voice and a negotiating style that lawyers describe as brutally honest. He joined the district attorney's office right out of Seton Hall Law School in 1982 and went on to handle some of its major murder cases and cold-case investigations.

The Palladium case certainly looked open and shut in 1992, when Mr. Lemus and Mr. Hidalgo were sentenced to 25 years to life. Several bouncers identified them as the men they scuffled with outside the East Village nightclub. Mr. Lemus's ex-girlfriend said he claimed to have shot a bouncer there.

But the next decade brought a string of nagging contradictions. A former member of a Bronx drug gang confessed that he and a friend had done the shooting. That spurred new examinations by the district attorney's office, federal prosecutors, defense lawyers, the police and the press.

When Mr. Morgenthau's office was asked to take another look, Mr. Bibb said, his supervisors gave him carte blanche. "It really was, leave no stone unturned," he said.

Over 21 months, starting in 2003, he and two detectives conducted more than 50 interviews in more than a dozen states, ferreting out witnesses the police had somehow missed or ignored.

Mr. Bibb said he shared his growing doubts with his superiors. And at a meeting in early 2005, he recalled, after defense lawyers won court approval for a hearing into the new evidence, he urged that the convictions be set aside. "I made what I considered to be my strongest pitch," he said.

Instead, he said, he was ordered to go to the hearing, present the government's case and let a judge decide — a strategy that violated his sense of a prosecutor's duty.

"I had always been taught that we made the decisions, that we made the tough calls, that we didn't take things and throw them up against the wall" for a judge or jury to sort out, he said. "If the evidence doesn't convince me, then I'm never going to be able to convince a jury."

Still, Mr. Bibb said, he worried that if he did not take the case, another prosecutor would — and possibly win.

Defense lawyers said he plunged in. In long phone conversations, he helped them sort through the new evidence he had gathered.

"If I make a mistake in my interpretation of what he said, he'll correct me," said Gordon Mehler, who represented Mr. Lemus. "If there's a piece of evidence that bears on another piece of evidence I'm talking about, he'll remind me of it. That's not something that a prosecutor typically does."

As the defense decided which witnesses to call, he again hunted them down — sometimes in prison or witness protection — and, when necessary, persuaded them to testify in State Supreme Court in Manhattan.

"I made sure all of their witnesses were going to testify in a manner that would have the greatest impact, certainly consistent with the truth," Mr. Bibb said. "I wasn't telling anybody to make anything up."

He told them what questions to expect, both from the defense and his own cross-examination — which he admitted felt "a little bit weird." Defense lawyers say they first met some of their witnesses on the day of testimony, outside the courtroom.

During breaks, Mr. Bibb confronted the lawyers when he felt they were not asking the right questions. "Don't you understand?" one lawyer recalled him saying. "I'm your best friend in that courtroom."

Cross-examining the witnesses, Mr. Bibb took pains not to damage their credibility. Facing a former gang member who had pleaded guilty to six murders, he asked only a few perfunctory questions about the man's record.

Daniel J. Horwitz, the other defense lawyer, said the help was invaluable. "Did Dan play a useful role in making sure that justice prevailed in that courtroom? The answer is unequivocally yes."

When the testimony was over, Mr. Bibb said he made one last appeal to his superiors to drop the convictions. They agreed to do so for Mr. Hidalgo, but not for Mr. Lemus — who was still implicated by "strong evidence," the office said at the time.

"I said, 'I'm done,'" Mr. Bibb recalled. "I wanted nothing to do with it."

Another prosecutor made final written arguments, and in October 2005, Justice Roger S. Hayes ordered the new trial for Mr. Lemus. Demoralized by the case, Mr. Bibb resigned a few months later.

A close friend, Robert Mooney, a New York City police detective, said that if not for the Palladium case, Mr. Bibb "would have spent his entire professional life at the prosecutor's office.

"He's brokenhearted that he's not doing this anymore."

In a brief interview after he quit, Mr. Bibb defended Mr. Morgenthau against criticism that the case had been mishandled. "There was never any evil intent on the part of the D.A.'s office," Mr. Bibb said then.

But around the same time, he distanced himself from the office's decisions in remarks to "Dateline NBC." He said that during the hearing, he already believed the two men were not guilty, but proceeded because he had a client to represent: Mr. Morgenthau.

"He was aware of what was going on," Mr. Bibb told the interviewer. "The decision to go to a hearing was not made in my presence."

As for Mr. Bibb's new revelation that he helped the defense, lawyers and others are divided.

Stephen Gillers, a legal ethics professor at the New York University School of Law, said he believed that Mr. Bibb had violated his obligation to his client, and could conceivably face action by a disciplinary panel. "He's entitled to his conscience, but his conscience does not entitle him to subvert his client's case," Mr. Gillers said. "It entitles him to withdraw from the case, or quit if he can't."

On the other hand, he added, Mr. Morgenthau could have defused any conflict by assigning another prosecutor.

John Schwartz, a former detective who worked to exonerate the convicted men, said Mr. Bibb did them no favor by continuing in the case. "He effectively took part in keeping two innocent men in prison an additional year at least, for not going with what he felt was the truth," Mr. Schwartz said.

But Mr. Mehler, the defense lawyer, said Mr. Bibb acted honorably. While lawyers on both sides must advocate for their clients, he said, "a prosecutor has an additional duty to search out the truth.

"I say that he lived up to that."

Today, Mr. Bibb says he does not believe he crossed any line.

"I didn't work for the other side," he said. "I worked for what I thought was the right thing."

After this news story ran, the New York Bar Disciplinary Committee investigated Bibb and concluded that there was "no basis" for any discipline of Bibb pertaining to the Palladium nightclub prosecution.[3] Do you agree?

Professor Stephen Gillers from New York University, quoted in the *Times* story above, argues that Bibb violated a duty of loyalty to his client by actively aiding the defense. Is he correct? The state is not a corporeal client, but it is a client nonetheless. Did Bibb subvert his client's interests? Note that in aiding the defense before and during the hearing on defendants' motion for new trial, Bibb drew the line at refusing to disclose confidential communications between himself and his superiors in the Manhattan District Attorney's Office. Bibb thus appears to have implicitly recognized that the state is a client who can have confidences under Rule 1.6. Why isn't the state also a client who can control the objectives of litigation (Rule 1.2) and demand competent representation toward those objectives (Rule 1.1)? What were Bibb's other alternatives if he doubted the defendants' guilt?

3. Disclosure of Exculpatory Evidence

Failure to disclose **exculpatory evidence** is one of the most frequent contributors to wrongful convictions, along with flawed witness identifications and ineffective assistance of defense counsel. Several high-profile cases in recent years have highlighted prosecutorial failures with respect to this disclosure obligation. The conviction of former Senator Ted Stevens from Alaska was reversed after it was revealed that federal prosecutors withheld notes of an interview with a key government witness that undercut that witness's trial testimony. In Texas, Michael Morton was freed from jail after serving 25 years for murdering his wife after it was revealed that the prosecutor failed to disclose notes of an interview with the defendant's child indicating that someone else was in the house at the time of the brutal act. Former Durham County North Carolina District Attorney Mike Nifong was disbarred for failing to disclose to the defense exculpatory DNA evidence that showed

---

3. Benjamin Weiser, *Lawyer Who Threw a City Case Is Vindicated, Not Punished*, N.Y. TIMES, Mar. 4, 2009, *available at* http://www.nytimes.com/2009/03/05/nyregion/05da.html.

the presence of multiple unidentified males on a rape kit specimen extracted from an erotic dancer who falsely accused members of the Duke lacrosse team of rape. These stories and others have made the public and the judiciary more highly attuned than ever to prosecutorial misconduct with respect to discovery.

Rules of Criminal Procedure in effect in most jurisdictions require prosecutors after arraignment to disclose police reports, grand jury transcripts, witness statements, and forensic reports, and to make available for inspection by defense counsel any physical exhibits that the government intends to introduce as evidence at trial. *See, e.g.*, FED. R. CRIM. P. 16. Normally, these items — known as "inculpatory" evidence — will link the defendant to the crime in some important respect. Disclosure is required so that the defendant has a fair preview of the government's case.

However, prosecutors also have a duty to disclose to defense counsel any "exculpatory" evidence in their possession — that is, evidence that is helpful to the defendant because it could be used to prove that the defendant did *not* commit the alleged offense, or committed a lesser offense. In other words, prior to the trial a prosecutor must reveal not only the government's case, but must also reveal any evidence that would be helpful to the defendant in building its own case.

This prosecutorial duty to disclose exculpatory evidence dates back at least to the Supreme Court's 1963 decision in *Brady v. Maryland*, excerpted below. It is traditionally justified on two grounds: the imbalance in investigatory resources between the government and the defendant, and the prosecutor's obligation as "minister of justice" to seek the truth rather than to pursue partisan victory. In this regard, the prosecutor's duty of helpful disclosures is one-sided; the defense has no corresponding duty to reveal to the prosecutor evidence in its possession that could help prove the defendant's guilt, and indeed may be committing malpractice if it did so.

Case Preview

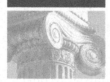

Brady v. Maryland

The petitioner in this case, Brady, and his companion, Boblit, were separately convicted of first degree murder and sentenced to death. At his trial, Brady did not deny playing a role in the murder but, seeking to avoid the death penalty, testified that Boblit did the actual killing. While on death row, Brady moved for a new trial after discovering statements made by Boblit — in which Boblit admitted to doing the actual killing — that had previously been withheld by the prosecutor.

As you read the *Brady* decision, ask yourself:

1. Is the withholding of exculpatory evidence really analogous to the knowing presentation of perjured testimony?
2. If so, why does the Court conclude that the Due Process Clause is violated "irrespective of the good faith or bad faith of the prosecution"?
3. What use could Brady have made of Boblit's statement at his sentencing hearing?

Brady v. Maryland
373 U.S. 83 (1963)

We agree with the Court of Appeals that suppression of [Boblit's] confession was a violation of the Due Process Clause of the Fourteenth Amendment. . . .

This ruling is an extension of Mooney v. Holohan, 294 U.S. 103, where the Court ruled on what nondisclosure by a prosecutor violates due process:

> It is a requirement that cannot be deemed to be satisfied by mere notice and hearing if a state has contrived a conviction through the pretense of a trial which in truth is but used as a means of depriving a defendant of liberty through a deliberate deception of court and jury by the presentation of testimony known to be perjured. Such a contrivance by a state to procure the conviction and imprisonment of a defendant is as inconsistent with the rudimentary demands of justice as is the obtaining of a like result by intimidation.

In Pyle v. Kansas, 317 U.S. 213, 215, we phrased the rule in broader terms:

> Petitioner's papers are inexpertly drawn, but they do set forth allegations that his imprisonment resulted from perjured testimony, knowingly used by the State authorities to obtain his conviction, and from the deliberate suppression by those same authorities of evidence favorable to him. These allegations sufficiently charge a deprivation of rights guaranteed by the Federal Constitution, and, if proven, would entitle petitioner to release from his present custody. Mooney v. Holohan, 294 U.S. 103.

. . .

We now hold that the suppression by the prosecution of evidence favorable to an accused upon request violates due process where the evidence is material either to guilt or to punishment, irrespective of the good faith or bad faith of the prosecution.

The principle of *Mooney v. Holohan* is not punishment of society for misdeeds of a prosecutor but avoidance of an unfair trial to the accused. Society wins not only when the guilty are convicted but when criminal trials are fair; our system of the administration of justice suffers when any accused is treated unfairly. An inscription on the walls of the Department of Justice states the proposition candidly for the federal domain: "The United States wins its point whenever justice is done its citizens in the courts." A prosecution that withholds evidence on demand of an accused which, if made available, would tend to exculpate him or reduce the penalty helps shape a trial that bears heavily on the defendant. That casts the prosecutor in the role of an architect of a proceeding that does not comport with standards of justice, even though, as in the present case, his action is not "the result of guile," to use the words of the Court of Appeals. 226 Md. at 427.

Affirmed.

Post-Case Follow-Up

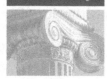

Although the Court's decision in *Brady* referenced the prosecutor's constitutional duty to turn over exculpatory evidence "on demand" of defense counsel, subsequent decisions have clarified that this duty is self-executing; that is, it applies whether or not the defendant specifically requested the withheld material. *See, e.g.,* United States v. Agurs, 427 U.S. 97, 107 (1976).

Nine years after the *Brady* decision, the Court expanded the definition of "exculpatory" evidence to include evidence that could be used by the defendant on cross-examination of a government witness to demonstrate bias. *Giglio v. United States*, 405 U.S. 150, 154-55 (1972). Under *Giglio*, the government must disclose to the defendant any promises, rewards, or inducements made to a government witness in exchange for his testimony.

In *Brady*, the Court ruled that the good faith or bad faith of the prosecutor is irrelevant to the constitutional violation. Three decades later, the Court clarified in *Kyles v. Whitley* that even if the prosecutor does not know about the existence of the exculpatory evidence, so long as that evidence is in possession of a government agent (*e.g.*, police officer, investigator) and material, its nondisclosure offends due process protections for the accused. 514 U.S. 418 (1995). Thus, prosecutors have an affirmative duty to ferret out and turn over exculpatory evidence possessed by anyone "acting on the government's behalf" in the case. *Id.* at 437.

Note that evidence is only exculpatory for due process purposes under *Brady* if it is "material." *Brady*, 373 U.S. at 87. Withheld evidence that would have provided only trivial or cumulative assistance to the accused will not lead to a reversal of the defendant's conviction. In *United States v. Bagley*, the Court defined materiality as "a reasonable probability that, had the evidence been disclosed to the defense, the result of the proceeding would have been different." 473 U.S. 667, 682 (1985). Material evidence is thus evidence that has the capacity to undermine confidence in the outcome of the trial. Scholars have critiqued this materiality standard as unworkable, because it is a retrospective test for a prospective disclosure obligation; that is, in order to determine whether the disclosure of a particular piece of evidence is constitutionally required, the prosecutor must look ahead and forecast its likely impact on a trial that has not yet occurred.[4]

Brady v. Maryland: Real Life Applications

1. Three eye witnesses to the armed robbery of a liquor store are shown a photo array of potential suspects following the incident. Two of the witnesses pick out the accused, but one witness states that he does not see the perpetrator in the photo array. Must the third witness's statement be disclosed to the defense?

2. An alleged get-away driver at a bank robbery is offered a deal by the government. If he testifies against his co-defendant and tells the truth at trial, the charges against him will be reduced to conspiracy and the prosecutor will recommend a suspended sentence on that charge. Must this arrangement be disclosed to the defense prior to trial? Does it matter whether the agreement is reduced to writing?

3. The victim of an alleged sexual assault is taken by ambulance to a nearby hospital. A police officer accompanies her in the ambulance. Dazed and partially incoherent, the victim describes her assailant as a light-skinned Black male wearing a dark sweatshirt. The police officer follows up with the victim the

---

4. *See, e.g.*, Daniel S. Medwed, *Brady's Bunch of Flaws*, 67 Wash. & Lee L. Rev. 1522, 1542 (2010).

following morning in the hospital and the victim gives a more detailed statement of the attack. In this second statement, which is written down and signed, the victim describes her assailant as "Black or Hispanic" and wearing a "dark green hoodie." The prosecutor does not know about the first statement in the ambulance and thus does not disclose it to the defense. Has there been a *Brady* violation?

Like the Due Process Clause, Model Rule 3.8(d) requires a prosecutor to disclose exculpatory evidence; the disciplinary rule provides in part that a prosecutor must "make timely disclosure to the defense of all evidence or information known to the prosecutor that tends to negate the guilt of the accused or mitigates the offense. . . ." Most states have adopted language in their attorney conduct rules that closely tracks this "tends to negate guilt" standard. Prosecutors thus have both a constitutional and an ethical duty to disclose so-called exculpatory evidence to the defense in criminal cases. As the following advisory opinion from the ABA suggests, however, the disclosure obligations of Model Rule 3.8(d) and *Brady* may differ in several important respects.

Prosecutor's Duty to Disclose Evidence and Information Favorable to the Defense
ABA Formal Opinion 09-454 (2009)

THE SCOPE OF THE PRETRIAL DISCLOSURE OBLIGATION

A threshold question is whether the disclosure obligation under Rule 3.8(d) is more extensive than the constitutional obligation of disclosure. A prosecutor's constitutional obligation extends only to favorable information that is "material," *i.e.*, evidence and information likely to lead to an acquittal. . . . The following review of the rule's background and history indicates that Rule 3.8(d) does not implicitly include the materiality limitation recognized in the constitutional case law. The rule requires prosecutors to disclose favorable evidence so that the defense can decide on its utility.

Courts recognize that lawyers who serve as public prosecutors have special obligations as representatives "not of an ordinary party to a controversy, but of a sovereignty whose obligation to govern impartially is as compelling as its obligation to govern at all; and whose interest, therefore, in a criminal prosecution is not that it shall win a case, but that justice shall be done." Similarly, Comment [1] to Model Rule 3.8 states that: "A prosecutor has the responsibility of a minister of justice and not simply that of an advocate. This responsibility carries with it specific obligations to see that the defendant is accorded procedural justice, that guilt is decided upon the basis of sufficient evidence, and that special precautions are taken to prevent and to rectify the conviction of innocent persons."

. . .

Unlike Model Rules that expressly incorporate a legal standard, Rule 3.8(d) establishes an independent one. Courts as well as commentators have recognized that the ethical obligation is more demanding than the constitutional obligation. The ABA Standards for Criminal Justice likewise acknowledge that prosecutors' ethical duty of disclosure extends beyond the constitutional obligation.

In particular, Rule 3.8(d) is more demanding than the constitutional case law, in that it requires the disclosure of evidence or information favorable to the defense without regard to the anticipated impact of the evidence or information on a trial's outcome. The rule thereby requires prosecutors to steer clear of the constitutional line, erring on the side of caution.

Under Rule 3.8(d), evidence or information ordinarily will tend to negate the guilt of the accused if it would be relevant or useful to establishing a defense or negating the prosecution's proof. Evidence and information subject to the rule includes both that which tends to exculpate the accused when viewed independently and that which tends to be exculpatory when viewed in light of other evidence or information known to the prosecutor.

Further, this ethical duty of disclosure is not limited to admissible "evidence," such as physical and documentary evidence, and transcripts of favorable testimony; it also requires disclosure of favorable "information." Though possibly inadmissible itself, favorable information may lead a defendant's lawyer to admissible testimony or other evidence or assist him in other ways, such as in plea negotiations. In determining whether evidence and information will tend to negate the guilt of the accused, the prosecutor must consider not only defenses to the charges that the defendant or defense counsel has expressed an intention to raise but also any other legally cognizable defenses. Nothing in the rule suggests a de minimis exception to the prosecutor's disclosure duty where, for example, the prosecutor believes that the information has only a minimal tendency to negate the defendant's guilt, or that the favorable evidence is highly unreliable.

. . .

THE KNOWLEDGE REQUIREMENT

Rule 3.8(d) requires disclosure only of evidence and information "known to the prosecutor." Knowledge means "actual knowledge," which "may be inferred from [the] circumstances." Although "a lawyer cannot ignore the obvious," Rule 3.8(d) does not establish a duty to undertake an investigation in search of exculpatory evidence.

The knowledge requirement thus limits what might otherwise appear to be an obligation substantially more onerous than prosecutors' legal obligations under other law. Although the rule requires prosecutors to disclose *known* evidence and information that is favorable to the accused, it does not require prosecutors to conduct searches or investigations for favorable evidence that may possibly exist but of which they are unaware. For example, prior to a guilty plea, to enable the defendant to make a well-advised plea at the time of arraignment, a prosecutor must disclose known evidence and information that would be relevant or useful to establishing a defense or negating the prosecution's proof. If the prosecutor has not yet reviewed voluminous files or obtained all police files, however, Rule 3.8 does not require the prosecutor to review or request such files unless the prosecutor actually knows or infers from the circumstances, or it is obvious, that the files contain favorable evidence or information. In the hypothetical, for example, the prosecutor would have to disclose that two eyewitnesses failed to identify the defendant as the assailant and that an informant attributed the assault to someone else, because the prosecutor knew that information from communications with the police. Rule 3.8(d) ordinarily would not require the prosecutor to conduct further inquiry or investigation to discover other evidence or information favorable to the defense unless he was closing his eyes to the existence of such evidence or information.

THE REQUIREMENT OF TIMELY DISCLOSURE

In general, for the disclosure of information to be timely, it must be made early enough that the information can be used effectively. Because the defense can use favorable evidence and information most fully and effectively the sooner it is received, such evidence or information, once known to the prosecutor, must be disclosed under Rule 3.8(d) as soon as reasonably practical.

Evidence and information disclosed under Rule 3.8(d) may be used for various purposes prior to trial, for example, conducting a defense investigation, deciding whether to raise an affirmative defense, or determining defense strategy in general. The obligation of timely disclosure of favorable evidence and information requires disclosure to be made sufficiently in advance of these and similar actions and decisions that the defense can effectively use the evidence and information. Among the most significant purposes for which disclosure must be made under Rule 3.8(d) is to enable defense counsel to advise the defendant regarding whether to plead guilty. Because the defendant's decision may be strongly influenced by defense counsel's evaluation of the strength of the prosecution's case, timely disclosure requires the prosecutor to disclose evidence and information covered by Rule 3.8(d) prior to a guilty plea proceeding, which may occur concurrently with the defendant's arraignment. Defendants first decide whether to plead guilty when they are arraigned on criminal charges, and if they plead not guilty initially, they may enter a guilty plea later. Where early disclosure, or disclosure of too much information, may undermine an ongoing investigation or jeopardize a witness, as may be the case when an informant's identity would be revealed, the prosecutor may seek a protective order.

. . .

THE OBLIGATIONS OF SUPERVISORS AND OTHER PROSECUTORS WHO ARE NOT PERSONALLY RESPONSIBLE FOR A CRIMINAL PROSECUTION

Any supervisory lawyer in the prosecutor's office and those lawyers with managerial responsibility are obligated to ensure that subordinate lawyers comply with all their legal and ethical obligations. Thus, supervisors who directly oversee trial prosecutors must make reasonable efforts to ensure that those under their direct supervision meet their ethical obligations of disclosure, and are subject to discipline for ordering, ratifying or knowingly failing to correct discovery violations. To promote compliance with Rule 3.8(d) in particular, supervisory lawyers must ensure that subordinate prosecutors are adequately trained regarding this obligation. Internal office procedures must facilitate such compliance.

For example, when responsibility for a single criminal case is distributed among a number of different lawyers with different lawyers having responsibility for investigating the matter, presenting the indictment, and trying the case, supervisory lawyers must establish procedures to ensure that the prosecutor responsible for making disclosure obtains evidence and information that must be disclosed. Internal policy might be designed to ensure that files containing documents favorable to the defense are conveyed to the prosecutor providing discovery to the defense, and that favorable information conveyed orally to a prosecutor is memorialized. Otherwise, the risk would be too high that information learned by the prosecutor conducting the investigation or the grand jury presentation would not be conveyed to the prosecutor in subsequent proceedings, eliminating the possibility of its being disclosed. Similarly, procedures must ensure that if a prosecutor obtains evidence in one case that would negate the defendant's guilt in another case, that prosecutor provides it to the colleague responsible for the other case.

In Formal Opinion 09-454, the ABA Standing Committee on Ethics and Professional Responsibility concluded that Rule 3.8(d) imposes obligations broader than the Due Process Clause in two critical respects: it rejects any consideration of materiality, and it requires prosecutors to disclose exculpatory evidence in advance of a guilty plea.[5] However, in one other critical respect the committee believed that Model Rule 3.8(d) is *narrower* than its constitutional counterpart, because a prosecutor can be subject to bar discipline only if he *knows* of the existence of the exculpatory evidence and fails to disclose it. Under Supreme Court precedent, due process is violated even in the absence of actual knowledge, where the police possess exculpatory information that is never turned over to the prosecutor. This essentially equates to a "knew or should have known" standard.[6]

Not all states agree with the ABA that their state's version of Rule 3.8(d) imposes greater disclosure responsibilities on a prosecutor than the due process requirements of *Brady*. For example, Ohio, Colorado, and Wisconsin[7] have rejected constructions of their attorney disciplinary rules that dispense with a materiality requirement. In Massachusetts and Virginia,[8] however, the pertinent state ethical rule has been interpreted to impose obligations that exceed *Brady*. This difference may be largely a matter of semantics. It is still fairly uncommon for state bar disciplinary committees to discipline prosecutors who violate their *Brady* obligations, perhaps because they believe reversal of the criminal conviction will impose a

---

5. In United State v. Ruiz, 536 U.S. 622 (2002), the Supreme Court concluded that the primary purpose of the *Brady* doctrine was to protect the defendant's right to a fair trial, and that due process was not violated where the government conditioned a fast-track plea agreement on the defendant's waiver of certain discovery.
6. Kyles v. Whitley, 514 U.S. 418, 437 (1995) (prosecutor has affirmative duty to learn of and turn over exculpatory evidence possessed by anyone "acting on the government's behalf" in the case).
7. In re Riek, 834 N.W.2d 384, 390-91 (Wis. 2013); Disciplinary Counsel v. Kellogg Martin, 923 N.E.2d 125, 130 (Ohio 2010); In re Attorney C, 47 P.3d 1167, 1173 (Colo. 2002).
8. Mass. R. Prof'l Conduct. 3.8, cmt. [3A]; Va. State Bar Legal Ethics Op. 1862 (2012).

sufficient deterrent effect on the government, or perhaps due to separation of powers or institutional competence concerns.[9] If states are not disciplining attorneys for failing to turn over material exculpatory evidence before trial and conviction, they are not likely to discipline prosecutors for failing to turn over less important evidence, or material exculpatory information prior to a guilty plea.

4. Contact with Represented Suspects

Recall that in Chapter 7, we explored the contours of Rule 4.2 (the "no-contact" rule), which prohibits an attorney from communicating with a represented party/person without permission of that person's lawyer. This rule has two important implications for criminal prosecutors because it may inhibit criminal investigations that would otherwise comply with constitutional protections.

In states that prohibit *ex parte* communications with represented "persons," prosecutors must be mindful of police undercover contact with suspects who have "lawyered up" prior to their arrest or indictment. Often times suspects secure counsel as soon as they learn that they are being investigated for a crime. Imagine a murder investigation where the police have focused their suspicions on the victim's former boyfriend. Does the suspect's act of securing counsel prohibit the government from continuing with routine undercover investigations directed toward that individual, such as sending a willing (and perhaps "wired") informant in to discuss the crime, or purchase contraband such as weapons? Rule 4.2 applies only to attorneys, but Rule 5.3 states that an attorney who has direct supervisory authority over a non-lawyer is responsible for the conduct of that non-lawyer if the attorney orders the conduct or ratifies the conduct having knowledge of it. Rule 8.4(a) also makes it professional misconduct for a lawyer to violate the Rules of Professional Conduct "through the acts of another." In the pre-indictment context, police investigatory conduct that might not violate the Fourth Amendment's prohibition of unreasonable searches and seizures or the Fifth Amendment protection against compelled self-incrimination could arguably violate the "no-contact" rule where the suspect has lawyered up and the prosecutor participates in planning or ratifying an undercover operation. In a Formal Opinion, the ABA Committee on Ethics and Professional Responsibility has taken the position that pre-charging undercover contacts with represented persons are not prohibited by Rule 4.2 because these contacts are "authorized by law" within the meaning of the rule, at least where they comport with Fourth and Fifth Amendment guarantees and any applicable statutory constraints on searches and electronic surveillance.[10] Most courts agree. One of the few federal courts that has prohibited pre-charging undercover contact with a represented person did so on the ground that the prosecutor engaged

---

9. R. Michael Cassidy, Prosecutorial Ethics 64 (2d ed. 2013).
10. ABA Formal Op. 95-396 (1995) (reasoning that undercover investigations by police were accepted practice at time of adoption of Rule 4.2, and that there is a strong public interest in continuing to investigate crime that may outweigh interests served by the "no contact" rule in pre-indictment context, at least where prosecutor does not participate directly in the undercover ruse).

in misconduct during the undercover investigation by issuing a fake grand jury subpoena to encourage the target to have a conversation with an undercover informant, and therefore the contact was not deemed "authorized by law."[11]

A second difficult application of the "no-contact" rule pertains to **post-indictment contact** with a represented party who wishes to cooperate with the government without his counsel knowing about it. Cooperating defendants may fear for their safety if persons close to a criminal enterprise were to learn of their informant status. This problem can arise in a jurisdiction that applies its "no-contact" rule to either represented persons or parties. The Sixth Amendment guarantees a criminally accused the right to the assistance of counsel — intentional interference with this right after it has attached (arraignment) may lead to suppression of evidence gained during the communication.[12] But the Sixth Amendment right to counsel is a right that may be *waived by the client*; if the client wishes to talk to the government without his counsel being present, he may voluntarily choose to do so. However, the "no-contact" rule is not a right of the client, it is an ethical rule that requires the *attorney's* permission prior to contact. What should a prosecutor do when a defendant awaiting trial sends a message through the police that he would like to meet with the government to discuss cooperation, but without his attorney's knowledge? This was the dilemma facing the Assistant U.S. Attorney in *Lopez*, below.

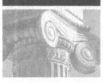

Case Preview

United States v. Lopez

Lopez, represented by Tarlow, and Escobedo, represented by Twitty, were both indicted for distribution of cocaine and heroin. Tarlow informed Lopez that it was his general policy not to negotiate pleas with the government in exchange for cooperation. When Twitty began negotiating a plea for Escobedo, Lopez asked to be included in the negotiations. He did not want Tarlow to find out for fear that he would not represent him if the case went to trial. During the course of negotiations, the prosecutor, Lyons, met with Lopez multiple times and did not inform Tarlow. When Tarlow found out from a mutual acquaintance of Lyons, he withdrew from representing Lopez. Represented by new counsel, Lopez successfully moved to dismiss the indictments against him due to prosecutorial misconduct. The district court concluded that Lyons had violated California Rule 2-100, the state equivalent of the Model Rule's "no-contact" provision. This appeal followed.

---

11. United States v. Hammad, 858 F.2d 834, 840 (2d Cir. 1988). *Cf.* United States v. Carona, 660 F.3d 360 (2d Cir. 2011) (although court will take case-by-case approach in assessing the propriety of pre-indictment contacts, normally undercover operations by police or informants do not violate the "no contact" rule). Such undercover operations have been ruled unethical where, as in *Hammad*, the prosecutor herself engages in fraud or deceit. *See* In re Pautler, 47 P.3d 1175 (Colo. 2002) (prosecutor subject to discipline for impersonating a public defender and engaging in telephone conversation with murder suspect to talk him into surrendering). *See also* Model Rule 8.4(c) (prohibiting conduct by a lawyer that involves "dishonesty, fraud, deceit or misrepresentation").
12. Massiah v. United States, 377 U.S. 201, 206 (1964).

As you read *Lopez*, ask yourself:

1. Why was the prosecutor's conversation with the defendant not "authorized by law," given that the judge had approved the communication beforehand following an *ex parte* hearing?
2. What are some of the reasons that a criminal defendant may not want his counsel to know that he is considering cooperating with the government? Are these legitimate concerns that the judiciary should accommodate?

United States v. Lopez
4 F.3d 1455 (9th Cir. 1993)

. . .

Having retained substitute counsel, Lopez filed a motion to dismiss the indictment on September 27, 1990. Lopez alleged that the government infringed upon his Sixth Amendment rights as well as Rules of Professional Conduct of the State Bar of California Rule 2-100 (1988). Binding pursuant to Local Rule 110-3 in the Northern District of California, Rule 2-100 generally prohibits a lawyer from communicating with another party in the case without the consent of that party's lawyer.

. . .

Rule 2-100 of the Rules of Professional Conduct of the State Bar of California governs communications with a represented party:

(A) While representing a client, a member shall not communicate directly or indirectly about the subject of the representation with a party the member knows to be represented by another lawyer in the matter, unless the member has the consent of the other lawyer.

. . .

(C) This rule shall not prohibit:
   (1) Communications with a public officer, board, committee, or body;
   (2) Communications initiated by a party seeking advice or representation from an independent lawyer of the party's choice; or
   (3) Communications otherwise authorized by law.

Rule 2-100's prohibition against communicating with represented parties without the consent of their counsel is both widely accepted and of venerable heritage. The California rule tracks the language of Rule 4.2 of the American Bar Association's Model Rules of Professional Conduct, which in turn is nearly identical to its predecessor in the Model Code of Professional Responsibility, Disciplinary Rule 7-104(A)(1). . . .

The rule against communicating with a represented party without the consent of that party's counsel shields a party's substantive interests against encroachment by opposing counsel and safeguards the relationship between the party and her attorney. As Tarlow's withdrawal upon discovering the secret communication between Lopez and the government exemplifies all too well, the trust necessary for a successful attorney-client relationship is eviscerated when the client is lured into clandestine meetings with the lawyer for the opposition. As a result, uncurbed communications with represented parties could have deleterious effects well beyond the context of the individual case, for our adversary system is premised upon functional lawyer-client relationships.

A

The government argues, however, that Rule 2-100 was not intended to apply to prosecutors pursuing criminal investigations. . . . In People v. Sharp, 197 Cal. Rptr. 436 (1983), decided under the predecessor of Rule 2-100, the court noted that:

> [b]ecause the prosecutor's position is unique — he represents authority and the discretion to make decisions affecting the defendant's pending case — his contact carries an implication of leniency for cooperative defendants or harsher treatment for the uncooperative. Such contact intrudes upon the function of defense counsel and impedes his or her ability to negotiate a settlement and properly represent the client, whose interests the rule is designed to protect.

Id. 197 Cal. Rptr. at 439-40. . . .

The cases advanced by the government in support of its position are largely irrelative. [Citations omitted.] In addition, they have noted that during investigation of the case and prior to indictment,

> the contours of the "subject matter of the representation" by [the suspect's] attorneys, concerning which the code bars "communication," [are] less certain and thus even less susceptible to the damage of "artful" legal questions the Code provisions appear designed in part to avoid.

Lemonakis, 485 F.2d at 956; compare Rule 2-100 (barring communication "about the subject of the representation").

The government's insistence that there are no salient differences between the pre- and post-indictment contexts for purposes of Rule 2-100 is puzzling. The prosecutor's ethical duty to refrain from contacting represented defendants entifies upon indictment for the same reasons that the Sixth Amendment right to counsel attaches:

> The initiation of judicial criminal proceedings is far from a mere formalism. It is the starting point of our whole system of adversary criminal justice. For it is only then that the government has committed itself to prosecute, and only then that the adverse positions of government and defendant have solidified.

. . .

B

The government next adopts the position that Lyons' conduct falls within the "communications otherwise authorized by law" exception to the rule against attorney communication with represented parties. See Rule 2-100(C)(3). The government argues that Lyons' contact with Lopez was authorized by statutes enabling prosecutors to conduct criminal investigations, and that the meetings were authorized by the magistrate judge's approval.

1

The government reasons that federal prosecutors operate pursuant to a "statutory scheme" that permits them to communicate with represented parties in order to detect and prosecute federal offenses. Citing 28 U.S.C. §§509, 515(a) and (c), 516, 533 and 547, the government argues that Justice Department attorneys fall within the "authorized by law" exception to California Rule 2-100 and its counterparts.

The comment to California Rule 2-100 notes that:

> Rule 2-100 is intended to control communications between a member [of the bar] and persons the member knows to be represented by counsel unless a statutory scheme or case law will override the rule. There are a number of express statutory schemes which authorize communications between a member and person who would otherwise be subject to this rule. . . . Other applicable law also includes the authority of government prosecutors and investigators to conduct criminal investigations, as limited by the relevant decisional law.

(Emphasis supplied.) Thus, the "authorized by law" exception to Rule 2-100 requires that a statutory scheme expressly permit contact between an attorney and a represented party. While recognizing the statutory authority of prosecutors to investigate crime, however, Rule 2-100 is intended to allow no more contact between prosecutors and represented defendants than the case law permits. We agree with the district court that the statutes cited by the government are nothing more than general enabling statutes. Nothing in these provisions expressly or impliedly authorizes contact with represented individuals beyond that permitted by case law. As discussed above, "the authority of government prosecutors and investigators to conduct criminal investigations" is "limited by the relevant decisional law" to contacts conducted prior to indictment in a non-custodial setting. Lyons' discussions with Lopez were not so authorized.

2

The government also maintains that by obtaining the prior approval of a magistrate judge, Lyons brought his conversations with Lopez within the realm of the "authorized by law" exception to California Rule 2-100. We agree that in an appropriate case, contact with a represented party could be excepted from the prohibition of Rule 2-100 by court order. See Rule 2-100 cmt. (Rule 2-100 forbids communication with represented persons "unless . . . case law will override the rule."). But, as in other areas of the law, judicial approval cannot absolve the government from responsibility for wrongful acts when the government has misled the court in obtaining its sanction. [Citations omitted.] When seeking the authorization of the district court, the prosecutor had an affirmative duty to avoid misleading the court. Rules of Professional Conduct of the State Bar of California Rule 5-200(B) (1988) ("In presenting a matter to a tribunal, a member . . . [s]hall not seek to mislead the judge, judicial officer or jury by an artifice or false statement of fact or law.").

The district court concluded that the magistrate judge approved the meeting between Lyons and Lopez in the mistaken belief, fostered by Lyons, that:

> Tarlow[ ] was being paid by a third party with interests inimical to those of Lopez and that Lopez feared that if Tarlow became aware of his client's interest in cooperating with the government, he would pass the information on to others who would harm Lopez and/or his family.

765 F. Supp. at 1452. The district court thus concluded that the magistrate judge's approval could not legally authorize Lyons to meet with Lopez.

The district court found that Lyons materially misled the magistrate judge regarding the facts surrounding Lopez's request to speak directly with the prosecutor. We agree that the magistrate judge apparently did not have a full understanding of the facts surrounding Lopez's request. Without that understanding, she could not have made an informed decision to authorize the communications.

Although it is not necessary to our determination in this case to decide whether the district court erred in its finding that Lyons materially misled the magistrate judge, we suggest that the finding is not sustainable without resolving certain conflicts in the testimony of Twitty, Lyons, and Lopez as to what Lyons knew and when he knew it (the district court, for whatever reason, said it was not necessary to resolve these conflicts). On remand, were the district court to consider lesser sanctions than dismissal of the indictment, resolution of these conflicts would be essential.

C

The government makes several related arguments regarding the effect of Lopez's waiver on its ethical obligations. We note initially that it would be a mistake to speak in terms of a party "waiving" her "rights" under Rule 2-100. The rule against communicating with represented parties is fundamentally concerned with the duties of attorneys, not with the rights of parties. Lyons' duties as an attorney practicing in the Northern District of California extended beyond his obligation to respect Lopez's rights. Consequently, as the government concedes, ethical obligations are personal, and may not be vicariously waived.

The government also argues, however, that Lopez created a form of "hybrid representation" by waiving his right to counsel for the limited purpose of negotiating with the government, while retaining Tarlow as his counsel for all other purposes. Since Lopez would be unrepresented for purposes of discussions with the government, it would presumably not be a violation of Rule 2-100 for the government to communicate with him directly. We have in the past held, however, that "[i]f the defendant assumes any of the 'core functions' of the lawyer, . . . the hybrid scheme is acceptable only if the defendant has voluntarily waived counsel." United States v. Turnbull, 888 F.2d 636, 638 (9th Cir. 1989) (quoting United States v. Kimmel, 672 F.2d 720, 721 (9th Cir. 1982)), cert. denied, 498 U.S. 825 (1990). Representing a client in negotiations with the government is certainly one of the core functions of defense counsel, and there is no question that Lopez did not waive his right to counsel. In fact, the magistrate judge, following the hearing with Lopez, clearly communicated to Lyons that while Lopez was waiving his right to have counsel present while inquiring about the possibility of cooperating with the government, he was not waiving his right to counsel. The district court found Lopez did not wish to waive his right to have an attorney present. In Kimmel, we explained that:

> [w]hen the accused assumes functions that are at the core of the lawyer's traditional role . . . he will often undermine his own defense. Because he has a constitutional right to have his lawyer perform core functions, he must knowingly and intelligently waive that right.

672 F.2d at 721. While we are not immediately concerned with the constitutional dimensions of Lopez's communications with the government, it is clear that the magistrate judge's intervention could not, as a matter of law, have created a form of "hybrid representation." To the contrary, Lyons was notified by the court that Lopez was still represented by Tarlow, and consequently he could not evade his duty under Rule 2-100 on this basis.

For the same reason, we reject the government's claim that enforcing the ethical prohibition against communication with represented parties would interfere, under these circumstances, with the party's constitutional rights. The government relies on the doctrine established in Faretta v. California, 422 U.S. 806 (1975), that it is unconstitutional to require a criminal defendant to be represented by an attorney. We see no conflict between Faretta and Rule 2-100. Of course, Rule 2-100 does not bar communications with persons who have waived their right to counsel, for by its express terms the rule only applies to "communications with a represented party." (Emphasis supplied.) Because Lopez did not waive his right to counsel, Faretta is immaterial.

D

We therefore conclude that the district court was correct in holding that Lyons had an ethical duty to avoid communicating directly with Lopez regarding the criminal prosecution so long as Lopez was represented by Tarlow.

. . .

Post-Case Follow-Up

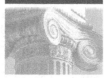

In an excerpted portion of this opinion, the Ninth Circuit concluded that even if Assistant U.S. Attorney Lyons violated California Disciplinary Rule 2-100 by talking to Lopez without permission of his lawyer, Tarlow, the district court erred in imposing the drastic sanction of dismissal of the indictment. What would have been an appropriate "remedy" for such an ethical violation?

Why was the Ninth Circuit unwilling to conclude that Lopez had waived his right to counsel at the negotiations, and therefore was not "represented" within the meaning of Rule 2-100?

United States v. Lopez: Real Life Applications

1. Sally Smith is arrested for shoplifting. At arraignment she waives her right to an attorney and agrees to proceed *pro se*. After the arraignment Smith approaches the prosecutor in the hallway of the courthouse and wishes to discuss a plea agreement. May the prosecutor speak to Smith outside of court?

2. Joe Jones is arrested for possession with intent to distribute cocaine. He is assigned a public defender at arraignment. While Jones is out on bail, the government receives information that Jones is now selling handguns out of his apartment in addition to cocaine. An informant approaches the police and states that he is willing and able to go undercover to purchase a handgun from Jones. Pursuant to common practice in the jurisdiction, the police seek the prosecutor's permission to "wire" the informant. Is there any advice or direction the prosecutor may give to the police regarding the new operation without violating Rule 4.2?

3. Three suspects are arrested for bank robbery. They are represented by separate defense counsel. One of the defendants sends word to the police through the jail that he would be interested in cooperating and testifying against his confederates, but for security reasons he does not want his attorney to know about his cooperation until a deal is in place. What should the prosecutor do?

Controversy over the "no-contact" rule's application to federal prosecutors and the ways in which it may impose limitations on criminal investigations beyond constitutional protections led to several directives from the Department of Justice in the 1990s trying to limit its reach. For an excellent history of this controversy, see Bruce A. Green, *Whose Rules of Professional Conduct Should Govern Lawyers in Federal Court and How Should the Rules Be Created?*, 64 GEO. WASH. L. REV. 460, 470-79 (1996). This matter was settled in 1998 when Congress enacted the **McDade Amendment**,[13] making it clear that Justice Department prosecutors must abide by the attorney discipline rules in the states in which they practice.

5. Statements to the Media

Prosecutors are in a vital and perhaps unequaled position to keep the public informed about issues of public safety in their communities. Explaining the reasons for prosecutorial decisions is also essential to fulfill the deterrent aims of the criminal law. Yet because prosecutors are in possession of reams of sensitive information about the character and background of the defendant — some of which may not be admissible at trial — the prosecutor is also in a position to potentially taint the jury pool and undermine the presumption of innocence by making pretrial statements that cast the defendant in a highly negative light.

---

13. Pub. L. No. 105-277, §801(a), 112 Stat. 2681, codified as amended at 28 U.S.C. §530B.

As we saw in Chapter 7, all lawyers participating in adjudication are prohibited under Rule 3.6 from making **public statements** that have a "substantial risk of materially prejudicing an adjudicative proceeding." This standard was upheld against a First Amendment attack by the Supreme Court's plurality opinion in *Gentile v. State Bar of Nevada*, 501 U.S. 1030 (1991).[14] Comment [5] to Rule 3.6 sets forth a list of certain subject matters that "are more likely than not" to have a material prejudicial effect on proceedings, in effect creating a presumption that public discussion of those identified topics will violate the rule. Several of those "off-limits" topics are particularly relevant to prosecutors: the defendant's criminal record, any confessions made by the defendant, the results of any scientific tests performed in the case, and information that the lawyer knows is not likely to be admissible in evidence. The theory behind comment [5] is that these facts will likely be the subject of pretrial litigation and ultimately may not be admitted in evidence at trial; once the public (and potential jury pool) hears such damaging information, they may be unable to "unhear" it.

Rule 3.8(f) imposes two additional responsibilities on prosecutors with respect to media comments about pending cases. First, the rule mandates that a prosecutor refrain from making extrajudicial comments that serve no "legitimate law enforcement purpose" and serve only to "heighten[] public condemnation of the accused." Whereas Rule 3.6 looks to the likelihood of *prejudicing the proceeding*, Rule 3.8(f) looks to the likelihood of *disparaging the accused* and holding him up to public opprobrium. Examples may include making a graphic or gory description of a heinous crime scene, displaying shocking or disturbing physical evidence to the media, disclosing criminal associations or uncharged crimes of the defendant, or arranging a "perp walk" for the sole purpose of giving the media footage of the defendant being transported in shackles. Mike Nifong, the prosecutor in the infamous Duke Lacrosse case, was censured by the North Carolina Bar Disciplinary Committee under Rule 3.8(f) for analogizing the alleged gang rape to a "cross burning," and for criticizing the suspects before the media for "refus[ing] to speak to investigators" upon "advice of counsel."[15]

Model Rule 3.8(f) also places an affirmative duty on prosecutors to try to rein in public comments by the police. Police departments often hold press conferences detailing the nature of an arrest and the attendant crime. Normally, an attorney is only responsible for conduct of non-lawyers if the attorney directs, supervises, or ratifies that conduct. But recognizing the synergistic relationship between the prosecutor and the police, Rule 3.8(f) requires prosecutors to "exercise reasonable care" to prevent investigators and other persons assisting or associated with the criminal case from making extrajudicial statements that the prosecutor would be prohibited from making under either Rule 3.6 or Rule 3.8.

---

14. For a criticism of *Gentile* and its premise that the "substantial risk" standard of Rule 3.6 can be applied equally to prosecutors and defense counsel without offending First Amendment principles, see Margaret Tarkington, *Lost in the Compromise: Free Speech, Criminal Justice, and Attorney Pre-Trial Publicity*, 66 FLA. L. REV. 1873, 1879 (2014).

15. For a more fulsome discussion of the flaws in the Duke Lacrosse prosecution, see Robert P. Mosteller, *The Duke Lacrosse Case: Innocence, False Identifications, and a Fundamental Failure to "Do Justice,"* 76 FORDHAM L. REV. 1337 (2007).

B. THE CRIMINAL DEFENSE LAWYER

The common perception of the criminal defense lawyer is the zealous advocate on steroids. If all lawyers are bound to advocate strenuously and competently on behalf of their clients, many believe that the criminal defense lawyer's mission is even more one-sided, because these lawyers are upholding the presumption of innocence and protecting their clients from the coercive power of the state. Where and exactly how a criminal defense lawyer's mission may be different from advocates in civil cases will be explored in the following three sections.

1. Taking Possession of Physical Evidence

Sometimes a defense lawyer will discover or be given a piece of real evidence that has evidentiary value — stolen property, a weapon used in a crime, documents that reveal the client's plan or intentions, or a laptop containing incriminating material. This **real evidence** is not itself a communication between the attorney and the client, but the act of giving it to the attorney (if given for the purposes of providing legal advice and intended to be confidential) may be privileged.

Such real evidence may be damaging to the client if revealed to authorities. So the attorney in this situation is faced with a choice between client loyalty and obligation to the justice system. When should the attorney refuse to accept the real evidence? If he does take possession of it, when does the lawyer have a duty to reveal it to the authorities? Ethicists have grappled with these complex questions for centuries. The answer to them, to the extent that there are clear answers, lies at the intersection of criminal law, criminal procedure, and legal ethics.

We saw in Chapter 7 that Model Rule 3.4 prohibits an attorney from "unlawfully" obstructing another party's access to evidence or "unlawfully" altering, destroying, or concealing evidence. So the rule prohibits only what the law prohibits — and that law may come from various sources: court orders, discovery obligations under the rules of criminal procedure, and the substantive criminal law. "Concealment" of real evidence is impermissible if the lawyer has some legal obligation to disclose the evidence independent of the ethical rule. "Destruction" of the evidence is unlawful if the conduct would violate an **obstruction of justice** statute.

The federal obstruction of justice statutes are particularly broad — they punish alteration, concealment, or destruction of real evidence and inducement of others to do so, where the person's intent is to keep the item from use in an official proceeding (civil, criminal, or agency administrative action).[16] The proceeding does not have to be already initiated so long as it is *foreseeable*.[17]

---

16. The two most commonly invoked federal statutes are the general obstruction of justice prohibition, 18 U.S.C. §1503 (penalizing one who corruptly interferes, obstructs, or impedes the due administration of justice) and the anti-shredding provisions of the Sarbanes-Oxley law, 18 U.S.C. §1519 (penalizing whoever knowingly "alters, destroys, mutilates, conceals, covers up, falsifies, or makes a false entry" in any record, document, or tangible object with the intent to impede a federal investigation). Although there are several differences between the elements of these two crimes, for present purposes the most notable is that the former applies both to the destruction of documents and physical objects, while the Supreme Court has interpreted the latter to apply only to documents and electronic records that are capable of storing information. Yates v. United States, 574 U.S. 528 (2015) (fisherman who directed crew to throw undersize fish overboard before inspector boarded ship could not be convicted under §1519).

17. *See, e.g.*, 18 U.S.C. §1512(c).

A lawyer who is offered physical evidence by a client in a criminal case should not become the repository of the evidence permanently if he knows or should know that the police will be looking for it, for that may constitute "concealment."[18] An attorney may return the evidence to its source unless there is an applicable state or federal statute that requires citizens to turn over to authorities the fruits or instrumentalities of a crime.[19] But an attorney clearly may not return physical evidence to its source with suggestions to destroy or conceal the evidence, because

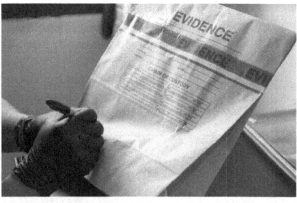

Should an attorney ever refuse to accept real evidence?
Shutterstock.com

that conduct would constitute "counsel(ing) or assist(ing)" another to obstruct access to evidence in violation of Rule 3.4 (a).

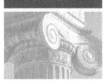

Case Preview

The Buried Bodies Case

The following opinion from the New York State Bar Association, commonly referred to as the "Buried Bodies Case," answers four main questions that arose from actions taken by an attorney in the course of representing a client charged with murder. The client confessed to his attorneys to having committed two prior murders and disclosed the location of those bodies. The client also drew a diagram of their location. One of the attorneys traveled to the location of one of the bodies and, upon discovering the corpse, began to photograph it. While taking pictures, the attorney moved the body slightly to bring it within the range of his camera. At a later date, the attorney destroyed the photographs as well as all record of his conversation with his client concerning the previous murders, including the diagram. Later, while discussing with the prosecutor a possible plea disposition, the lawyer suggested that in exchange for favorable consideration for his client the lawyer might be in position to provide information concerning several unsolved murders. The government refused the plea proposal, trial ensued, and in the context of raising an insanity defense, the client actually testified to having committed the other murders. Public outrage over the lawyer's

---

18. In re Ryder, 263 F. Supp. 360, 361 (E.D Va.), *aff'd*, 381 F.2d 713 (4th Cir. 1967) (lawyer who transferred stolen money and gun from client's safety deposit box to his own safety deposit box violated predecessor to Rule 3.4(a) by assisting his client to conceal evidence, and by unlawfully possessing sawed-off shotgun).

19. Professor Gillers has argued that state laws requiring citizens to turn over fruits or instrumentalities of a crime may be unconstitutional as applied to criminal defense attorneys who receive such evidence from their clients, because they could deprive the defendant of his right to the effective assistance of counsel under the Sixth Amendment. Stephen A. Gillers, *Guns, Fruits, Drugs and Documents: A Criminal Defense Lawyer's Responsibility for Real Evidence*, 63 STAN. L. REV. 813, 827 (2011).

secret conduct then led the New York Bar Association to take up the controversial subject in a formal ethics opinion.

As you read Formal Opinion 479, ask yourself:

1. When and how could the lawyers possibly have made different decisions, given their obligations of client confidentiality under Rule 1.6?
2. Why was the public so outraged by their conduct when it came to light?

Client's Confidences and Secrets; Past Crimes Disclosed to Lawyer; Plea Bargaining
New York State Bar Association Formal Opinion 479 (1978)

QUESTIONS

1. Under the circumstances alleged, would a lawyer be acting improperly in failing to disclose to the authorities his knowledge of the two prior murders and the location of the bodies?

2. Under the circumstances alleged, would a lawyer be acting improperly in withholding and destroying (a) the records of his conversation with the client, (b) the photographs taken by him of the bodies of the victims and (c) the diagram showing the physical location of the bodies?

3. Under the circumstances alleged, would a lawyer be acting improperly in moving parts of one of the bodies prior to taking photographs?

4. Under the circumstances alleged, would a lawyer be acting improperly, in his attempt to negotiate a plea disposition, in suggesting to the District Attorney that he had information concerning two unsolved murders?

OPINION

The questions raised are complex and difficult. Legal issues, upon which we do not pass, may be inextricably interwoven with ethical considerations. Illegal conduct involving moral turpitude is per se unethical. DR1-102(A)(3).

1. The lawyer's failure to disclose his knowledge of the two unrelated homicides was not improper, assuming, as the facts given us indicate, that the information came to the lawyer during the course of his employment. Furthermore, the requirements of Canon 4 that "a lawyer should preserve the confidences and secrets of a client," and of EC 4-1 and DR 4-101(B), would have been violated if such disclosure had been made. . . .

Proper representation of a client calls for full disclosure by the client to his lawyer of all possibly relevant facts, even though such facts may reveal the client's commission of prior crimes. To encourage full disclosure, the client must be assured of confidentiality, a requirement embodied by law in the attorney-client privilege and broadly incorporated into Canon 4 of the Code and the EC's and DR's thereunder.

Frequently clients have a disposition to withhold information from lawyers. If the client suspects that his confidences will not be adequately protected or may in some way be used against him, he will be far more likely to withhold information which he believes may be to his detriment or which he does not want generally known. The client who withholds information from his lawyer runs a substantial risk of not being accorded his full legal rights. At the same time, the lawyer from whom such information is withheld may well be required to assert, in complete good faith and with no violation of EC 7-26 or DR 7-102(A), totally meritless or frivolous claims or defenses to which his client has no legal right. Thus, the interests served by the strict rule of confidentiality are far broader than merely those of the client, but include the interests of the public generally and of effective judicial administration.

Narrow and limited exceptions to the rule of confidentiality have been incorporated in DR 4-101(C) and DR 7-102(B)(1), the most important of which relate to information involving the intention of the client to commit a crime in the future or the perpetration of a fraud during the course of the lawyer's representation of the client, or where the client consents following full disclosure. The future crime exception recognizes both the possible preventability of the crime, as well as the total absence of any societal need to encourage criminal clients to make such disclosures to their lawyers. . . .

Thus, the lawyer was under an injunction not to disclose to the authorities his knowledge of the two prior murders, and was duty bound not to reveal to the authorities the location of the bodies. The lawyer's knowledge with respect to the location of the bodies was obtained solely from the client in confidence and in secret. Without the client's revelation in secret and in confidence, he would not have been in a position to assist the authorities in this regard. Thus, his personal knowledge is a link solidly welded to the chain of privileged communications and, without the client's express permission, must not be disclosed. The relationship between lawyer and client is in many respects like that between priest and penitent. Both lawyer and priest are bound by the bond of silence. . . .

2. A lawyer's obligation to hold a client's confidences and secrets inviolate extends beyond information imparted orally and embraces written material from the client "coming into existence merely as a communication to the attorney." See 8 Wigmore, Evidence §2307 (McNaughton Rev. 1961).

The memorialization by a lawyer of statements, information and documents received from a client, whether by shorthand or longhand notes, dictated and typed memoranda, speedwriting, electronic or magnetic recording, Xerox, Photostat, photograph or other form of recordation or reproduction does not alter the fact that the communication from the client is privileged. Such memorialization may be useful in facilitating the handling of a matter by the lawyer and is part of the lawyer's work product. When the lawyer's purpose is served, the work product may be destroyed without violation of ethical standards.

Similarly, written material prepared by the client for his lawyer is a form of written communication and falls within the attorney-client privilege. Such documents are not instruments or fruits of the crime, which under certain circumstances the lawyer might be obliged to turn over to authorities. See *State v. Olwell*, supra. Accordingly, neither the lawyer nor his client was obliged to reveal an incriminating diagram, whether prepared by the client for his lawyer or by the lawyer on the basis of information gained by him during the course of the client's representation, under EC 7-27 and DR 7-102. Provided it was not contrary to his client's wishes for him to do so, there was no ethical inhibition against its destruction by the lawyer.

3. This Committee does not pass upon the legality of alleged conduct, but if such conduct is illegal, it would of course be unethical, with rare exceptions of inadvertent violations involving no moral turpitude. Thus, any tampering, concealment or destruction of physical evidence in violation of N.Y. Penal Law §215.40 would also be violative of the Code. Even in the absence of any violation of law and in the absence of an intention on the part of the lawyer to tamper, conceal or destroy evidence, there could be an appearance of impropriety in violation of Canon 9 in moving a part of one of the bodies. Such conduct should be avoided to prevent even the appearance that there might have been an intent to tamper with or suppress evidence.

4. There is no ethical impropriety in the lawyer's discussing with the District Attorney the possibility of an appropriate plea disposition, provided that the lawyer had the express consent of his client before making such disclosure. Plea bargaining is an accepted part of our criminal procedures today. A lawyer engaged or attempting to engage in it with his client's consent would be properly serving his client. Thus, the lawyer's suggestion to the District Attorney that he might be in a position to assist the authorities in resolving open cases during such a discussion would appear to involve no violation of proper professional standards. One can conceive of a variety of circumstances in which such a disclosure might be helpful to a client. For example, the disclosure of the client's commission of prior crimes of violence might very well establish the client's need for confinement for medical treatment rather than imprisonment.

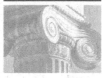

Post-Case Follow-Up

Attorney Francis Belge, the attorney who was the subject of this formal opinion, was also criminally charged under two sections of the New York Public Health statute making it a misdemeanor to fail to report the death of someone who died without medical assistance. Although Belge was subsequently exonerated by the trial judge in that criminal matter, the public outcry over the choices he made in the Buried Bodies case undercut his standing in the small-town community and ultimately his law practice. His life was ruined in many ways for "stepping up" to take on a difficult case, and then making a very courageous and unpopular decision within the context of that case.

Defendant Garrow in the Buried Bodies case was actually represented by two attorneys — Francis Belge and Frank Armani. Armani was not present when Belge observed and photographed one of the bodies, so he escaped indictment. In interviews after the Garrow prosecution, both attorneys explained that one of their motivations for checking to see if the bodies were located where the client said they would be was that they thought their client had mental health issues and might be fabricating the other crimes. Is this the sort of "preparation" contemplated by Rule 1.1?

As the New York State Bar Committee acknowledged, where a client informs his attorney of the location of physical evidence but does *not* deliver that evidence to the attorney, the communication is privileged if intended to be confidential. However, that privilege may be lost if the attorney thereafter acts on this information by moving the evidence, altering it, or destroying it. Because the attorney has compromised the ability of the state to make use of the evidence, some courts have ruled that this form of unethical conduct defeats the privilege.[20]

> ## More on the Buried Bodies Case
>
> For a fascinating discussion of the Belge matter, including interviews with the participants, listen to the 2016 RadioLab podcast *The Buried Bodies Case, available at* http://www.radiolab.org/story/the_buried_bodies_case.

Compare the Buried Bodies case with *People v. Meredith*, discussed in footnote 20. In the former case, the lawyer left the bodies where he found them and escaped any discipline. In the latter case, the lawyer's investigator moved the victim's discarded wallet but later turned it over to authorities; nonetheless, the defense team was forced to make the government "whole" by testifying at trial as to where the wallet was found. Why should the client — who had not waived the privilege in either instance — be in any worse position in the *Meredith* case than in the Buried Bodies case?

The Buried Bodies Case: Real Life Applications

1. Suppose that you represent a local parish. The rector for the parish comes to your office and tells you that the parish recently fired its youth minister after discovering child pornography on the employee's work laptop. The client delivers the laptop to you and asks that you take whatever steps necessary to protect the client from adverse publicity and potential liability with respect to the matter. Although possession of child pornography is a crime, to your knowledge the FBI has not opened an investigation into the youth minister. What should you do with the computer?

2. Imagine that a prominent local businessman comes to you with a problem. He thinks he may have been involved in a hit and run accident the previous night. He didn't stop his car because he was drunk, disoriented, and scared. But this morning he noticed a large dent in his front right fender. He also saw a news report on a local television station saying that a pedestrian was "clinging to life" in a local hospital after being hit by a car matching the general description of his car. Your visitor asks you what should be done with the car. How do you advise him? May it be repaired? May you engage a chemist to test the fender for fibers, blood, or hair? Does that depend on whether such testing would destroy the evidentiary value of the site of impact?

---

20. People v. Meredith, 631 P.2d 46, 53 (Cal. 1981) (where the attorney or his agent removes or alters evidence as a result of confidential communication with client, there exists an exception to the attorney-client privilege and the defense lawyer's investigator may be called to testify as to where he found it).

3. Your client is under investigation for murder and conspiracy to commit murder with respect to a drive-by shooting. The client suspects that one of his former friends and associates may be cooperating with the government. He comes to you for advice. During your discussions you ask the client if and when he ever had any communications with the cooperating witness. He tells you that they have texted each other regularly for the past two months, and hands you his cell phone. Should you take possession of the cell phone? If so, what can and should you do with it?

The attorney-client privilege further complicates the attorney's responsibility with respect to real evidence. While a preexisting document or physical object is not subject to the privilege, the fact that a client gives or attempts to give that evidence to his attorney will likely *itself* be considered a communicative act subject to the attorney-client privilege.[21] If the lawyer is forced to deliver the physical evidence to the authorities pursuant to some legal obligation, search warrant, or subpoena, the lawyer may thereafter argue that the state may not use this "act of production" against the client because to do so would whipsaw the attorney between a privileged communication and a legal obligation.[22]

It is thus relatively clear what a lawyer cannot do — destroy likely evidence or counsel his client to do so, or keep the evidence and alter its evidentiary value (e.g., by wiping a gun for fingerprints or deleting the hard drive of a computer). Further, some criminal statutes make it unlawful to even possess certain types of evidence altogether — narcotics, stolen property, firearms — and in those jurisdictions a criminal defense lawyer should not take even temporary possession of such items because then the lawyer would be committing a crime.

Short of those two extremes are actions with respect to physical evidence that pose extremely complex and challenging ethical problems for a criminal defense lawyer. To avoid some of those ambiguities, many lawyers simply refuse to take possession of physical evidence offered to them by a criminal suspect. But there may be cases in which an attorney thinks it is in the best interests of his client to take possession of an item temporarily to have it examined or tested. One state has provided explicit guidance on this question, ruling that it is permissible for an attorney to inspect and test an object of physical evidence and then deliver it to authorities so long as the attorney does not tell the government where he obtained it.[23] Yet another jurisdiction has adopted a third-party intermediary strategy. In the District of Columbia, an attorney who receives incriminating physical evidence may return it to its rightful owner if it is not yet under subpoena and if such return would not compromise client confidences or violate state law. But if returning the evidence to its owner would prejudice the client by implicitly revealing

---

21. State v. Olwell, 394 P.2d 681 (Wash. 1964) (attorney given knife by client could turn it over to government with assurances that prosecution must refrain from telling jury where it came from).
22. *Id. See* Fisher v. United States, 425 U.S. 391, 407 (1976).
23. *Olwell*, 394 P.2d at 684. Professor Gregory Sisk posits that a lawyer may retain the physical evidence long enough to conduct a physical test on it, and then return it to its source, without running afoul of Rule 3.4(a). Gregory Sisk, *The Legal Ethics of Real Evidence*, 89 WASH. L. REV. 819, 881 (2014).

client confidences, or if substantive criminal law requires delivery of the evidence to authorities, the attorney may give the physical evidence to the D.C. Bar Counsel and ask that bar counsel turn it over. *See* D.C. R. Prof'l Conduct 3.4(a) cmt. [5].

2. Putting Your Client on the Stand

In Chapter 7, we discussed a lawyer's duty of candor to the tribunal and responsibility for remedying perjury. The obligations of a criminal defense lawyer in this regard are more nuanced, because a defendant has a constitutional right to present a defense and to the effective assistance of counsel under the Sixth Amendment. This has sometimes been referred to as the "**lawyer's trilemma**." A lawyer must guard the client's secrets, must act diligently in gathering as much information as will enable him to counsel the accused and competently mount a defense, and must be candid to the court. How can a criminal defense lawyer do all three at the same time, if in gathering information from the accused the lawyer learns that he intends to testify falsely? With regards to civil cases, we saw that when there is a tension between these duties the obligation of candor takes precedence. Should the same be true of a criminal defense attorney? One important difference is that the criminal defendant's Sixth Amendment right to present a defense has been interpreted by the Supreme Court to include the right to take the stand in one's own defense, even against the advice of counsel.[24] In a criminal context where we expect lawyers to take an adversarial stance against the government's attempt to deprive the defendant of liberty and to prefer the client's interests at almost all costs over that of the society, does that justify a different result?

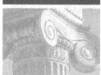

Case Preview

Nix v. Whiteside

Nix v. Whiteside arose from a drug deal gone horribly wrong in which Emanuel Whiteside showed up at Calvin Love's apartment late one night hoping to procure marijuana. An argument broke out between the two and Whiteside, fearing that Love was reaching for a gun, fatally stabbed Love. Whiteside repeatedly told his attorney, Gary L. Robinson, that he had not actually seen the gun, but was convinced Love had one. However, a week before the trial, Whiteside told Robinson for the first time that he had seen something metallic in Love's hand. Robinson immediately saw through Whiteside's attempt to strengthen his self-defense claim, and warned Whiteside that if he insisted on committing perjury, he would withdraw from representation. Whiteside elected not to commit perjury and was convicted of second degree murder. The Supreme

---

24. Rock v. Arkansas, 483 U.S. 44 (1987); Harris v. New York, 401 U.S. 222 (1971).

Court granted certiorari to decide whether the trial attorney's conduct deprived Whiteside of his Sixth Amendment right to counsel.

As you read *Whiteside*, ask yourself:

1. How did Attorney Robinson "know" that Whiteside intended to commit perjury within the meaning of Rule 3.3?
2. What does the Court identify as the "range of reasonable professional conduct" in response to a criminal defendant's intent to commit perjury?

Nix v. Whiteside
475 U.S. 157 (1986) (citations omitted)

I

A

Whiteside gave him a statement that he had stabbed Love as the latter "was pulling a pistol from underneath the pillow on the bed." Upon questioning by Robinson, however, Whiteside indicated that he had not actually seen a gun, but that he was convinced that Love had a gun. No pistol was found on the premises; shortly after the police search following the stabbing, which had revealed no weapon, the victim's family had removed all of the victim's possessions from the apartment. Robinson interviewed Whiteside's companions who were present during the stabbing, and none had seen a gun during the incident. Robinson advised Whiteside that the existence of a gun was not necessary to establish the claim of self-defense, and that only a reasonable belief that the victim had a gun nearby was necessary even though no gun was actually present.

Until shortly before trial, Whiteside consistently stated to Robinson that he had not actually seen a gun, but that he was convinced that Love had a gun in his hand. About a week before trial, during preparation for direct examination, Whiteside for the first time told Robinson and his associate Donna Paulsen that he had seen something "metallic" in Love's hand. When asked about this, Whiteside responded:

"[I]n Howard Cook's case there was a gun. If I don't say I saw a gun, I'm dead."

Robinson told Whiteside that such testimony would be perjury and repeated that it was not necessary to prove that a gun was available but only that Whiteside reasonably believed that he was in danger. On Whiteside's insisting that he would testify that he saw "something metallic" Robinson told him, according to Robinson's testimony:

[W]e could not allow him to [testify falsely] because that would be perjury, and as officers of the court we would be suborning perjury if we allowed him to do it; . . . I advised him that if he did do that it would be my duty to advise the Court of what he was doing and that I felt he was committing perjury; also, that I probably would be allowed to attempt to impeach that particular testimony. [App. to Pet. for Cert. A-85.]

Robinson also indicated he would seek to withdraw from the representation if Whiteside insisted on committing perjury.

Whiteside testified in his own defense at trial and stated that he "knew" that Love had a gun and that he believed Love was reaching for a gun and he had acted swiftly in self-defense. On cross-examination, he admitted that he had not actually seen a gun in Love's hand. Robinson presented evidence that Love had been seen with a sawed-off shotgun on other occasions, that the police search of the apartment may have been careless, and that the victim's family had removed everything from the apartment shortly after the crime. Robinson presented this evidence to show a basis for Whiteside's asserted fear that Love had a gun.

The jury returned a verdict of second-degree murder, and Whiteside moved for a new trial, claiming that he had been deprived of a fair trial by Robinson's admonitions not to state that he saw a gun or "something metallic." . . .

. . .

B

In *Strickland v. Washington*, we held that to obtain relief by way of federal habeas corpus on a claim of a deprivation of effective assistance of counsel under the Sixth Amendment, the movant must establish both serious attorney error and prejudice. To show such error, it must be established that the assistance rendered by counsel was constitutionally deficient in that "counsel made errors so serious that counsel was not functioning as 'counsel' guaranteed the defendant by the Sixth Amendment." *Strickland*, 466 U.S. at 687. To show prejudice, it must be established that the claimed lapses in counsel's performance rendered the trial unfair so as to "undermine confidence in the outcome" of the trial. Id. at 694. In *Strickland*, we acknowledged that the Sixth Amendment does not require any particular response by counsel to a problem that may arise. Rather, the Sixth Amendment inquiry is into whether the attorney's conduct was "reasonably effective." To counteract the natural tendency to fault an unsuccessful defense, a court reviewing a claim of ineffective assistance must "indulge a strong presumption that counsel's conduct falls within the wide range of reasonable professional assistance." Id. at 689. In giving shape to the perimeters of this range of reasonable professional assistance, *Strickland* mandates that "[p]revailing norms of practice as reflected in American Bar Association Standards and the like, . . . are guides to determining what is reasonable, but they are only guides." Id. at 688.

Under the *Strickland* standard, breach of an ethical standard does not necessarily make out a denial of the Sixth Amendment guarantee of assistance of counsel. When examining attorney conduct, a court must be careful not to narrow the wide range of conduct acceptable under the Sixth Amendment so restrictively as to constitutionalize particular standards of professional conduct and thereby intrude into the state's proper authority to define and apply the standards of professional conduct applicable to those it admits to practice in its courts. In some future case challenging attorney conduct in the course of a state-court trial, we may need to define with greater precision the weight to be given to recognized canons of ethics, the standards established by the state in statutes or professional codes, and the Sixth Amendment, in defining the proper scope and limits on that conduct. Here we need not face that question, since virtually all of the sources speak with one voice.

C

We turn next to the question presented: the definition of the range of "reasonable professional" responses to a criminal defendant client who informs counsel that he will perjure himself on the stand. We must determine whether, in this setting, Robinson's conduct fell within the wide range of professional responses to threatened client perjury acceptable under the Sixth Amendment.

In *Strickland*, we recognized counsel's duty of loyalty and his "overarching duty to advocate the defendant's cause." Ibid. Plainly, that duty is limited to legitimate, lawful conduct compatible with the very nature of a trial as a search for truth. Although counsel must take all reasonable lawful means to attain the objectives of the client, counsel is precluded from taking steps or in any way assisting the client in presenting false evidence or otherwise violating the law. This principle has consistently been recognized in most unequivocal terms by expositors of the norms of professional conduct since the first Canons of Professional Ethics were adopted by the American Bar Association in 1908. . . .

. . .

These principles have been carried through to contemporary codifications of an attorney's professional responsibility. Disciplinary Rule 7-102 of the Model Code of Professional Responsibility (1980), entitled "Representing a Client Within the Bounds of the Law," provides:

> (A) In his representation of a client, a lawyer shall not:
> (4) Knowingly use perjured testimony or false evidence.
> (7) Counsel or assist his client in conduct that the lawyer knows to be illegal or fraudulent.

This provision has been adopted by Iowa, and is binding on all lawyers who appear in its courts. See Iowa Code of Professional Responsibility for Lawyers (1985). The more recent Model Rules of Professional Conduct (1983) similarly admonish attorneys to obey all laws in the course of representing a client:

> *RULE 1.2* SCOPE OF REPRESENTATION
> (d) A lawyer shall not counsel a client to engage, or assist a client, in conduct that the lawyer knows is criminal or fraudulent. . . .

Both the Model Code of Professional Responsibility and the Model Rules of Professional Conduct also adopt the specific exception from the attorney-client privilege for disclosure of perjury that his client intends to commit or has committed. DR 4-101(C)(3) (intention of client to commit a crime); Rule 3.3 (lawyer has duty to disclose falsity of evidence even if disclosure compromises client confidences). Indeed, both the Model Code and the Model Rules do not merely *authorize* disclosure by counsel of client perjury; they *require* such disclosure. See Rule 3.3(a)(4); DR 7-102(B)(1).

These standards confirm that the legal profession has accepted that an attorney's ethical duty to advance the interests of his client is limited by an equally solemn duty to comply with the law and standards of professional conduct; it specifically ensures that the client may not use false evidence. This special duty of an attorney to prevent and disclose frauds upon the court derives from the recognition that perjury is as much a crime as tampering with witnesses or jurors by way of promises and threats, and undermines the administration of justice. See 1 W. Burdick, Law of Crime §§293, 300, 318-336 (1946).

. . .

It is universally agreed that at a minimum the attorney's first duty when confronted with a proposal for perjurious testimony is to attempt to dissuade the client from the unlawful course of conduct. Model Rules of Professional Conduct, Rule 3.3, Comment; Wolfram, Client Perjury, 50 S. Cal. L. Rev. 809, 846 (1977). A statement directly in point is found in the commentary to the Model Rules of Professional Conduct under the heading "False Evidence":

> When false evidence is offered by the client, however, a conflict may arise between the lawyer's duty to keep the client's revelations confidential and the duty of candor to the court. Upon ascertaining that material evidence is false, the lawyer *should seek to persuade the client that the evidence should not be offered* or, if it has been offered, that its false character should immediately be disclosed. [Model Rules of Professional Conduct, Rule 3.3, Comment (1983) (emphasis added).]

The commentary thus also suggests that an attorney's revelation of his client's perjury to the court is a professionally responsible and acceptable response to the conduct of a client who has actually given perjured testimony. Similarly, the Model Rules and the commentary, as well as the Code of Professional Responsibility adopted in Iowa, expressly permit withdrawal from representation as an appropriate response of an attorney when the client threatens to commit perjury. Model Rules of Professional Conduct, Rule 1.16(a)(1), Rule 1.6, Comment (1983); Code of Professional Responsibility, DR 2-110(B), (C) (1980). Withdrawal of counsel when this situation arises at trial gives rise to many difficult questions including possible mistrial and claims of double jeopardy.

The essence of the brief *amicus* of the American Bar Association reviewing practices long accepted by ethical lawyers is that under no circumstance may a lawyer either advocate or passively tolerate a client's giving false testimony. This, of course, is consistent with the governance of trial conduct in what we have long called "a search for truth." The suggestion sometimes made that "a lawyer must believe his client, not judge him" in no sense means a lawyer can honorably be a party to or in any way give aid to presenting known perjury.

D

Considering Robinson's representation of respondent in light of these accepted norms of professional conduct, we discern no failure to adhere to reasonable professional standards that would in any sense make out a deprivation of the Sixth Amendment right to counsel. Whether Robinson's conduct is seen as a successful attempt to dissuade his client from committing the crime of perjury, or whether seen as a "threat" to withdraw from representation and disclose the illegal scheme, Robinson's representation of Whiteside falls well within accepted standards of professional conduct and the range of reasonable professional conduct acceptable under *Strickland*.

. . .

The Court of Appeals' holding that Robinson's "action deprived [Whiteside] of due process and effective assistance of counsel" is not supported by the record since Robinson's action, at most, deprived Whiteside of his contemplated perjury. Nothing counsel did in any way undermined Whiteside's claim that he believed the victim was reaching for a gun. Similarly, the record gives no support for holding that Robinson's action "also impermissibly compromised [Whiteside's] right to testify in his own defense by conditioning continued representation . . . and confidentiality upon [Whiteside's] *restricted* testimony." The record in fact shows the contrary: (a) that Whiteside did testify, and (b) he was "restricted" or restrained only from testifying falsely and was aided by Robinson in developing the basis for the fear that Love was reaching for a gun. Robinson divulged no client communications until he was compelled to do so in response to Whiteside's post-trial challenge to the quality of his performance. We see this as a case in which the attorney successfully dissuaded the client from committing the crime of perjury.

Paradoxically, even while accepting the conclusion of the Iowa trial court that Whiteside's proposed testimony would have been a criminal act, the Court of Appeals held that Robinson's efforts to persuade Whiteside not to commit that crime were improper, *first*, as forcing an impermissible choice between the right to counsel and the right to testify; and, *second*, as compromising client confidences because of Robinson's threat to disclose the contemplated perjury.

Whatever the scope of a constitutional right to testify, it is elementary that such a right does not extend to testifying *falsely*. In *Harris v. New York*, we assumed the right of an accused to testify "in his own defense, or to refuse to do so" and went on to hold:

"[T]hat privilege cannot be construed to include the right to commit perjury. . . ."

. . . *Harris* and other cases make it crystal clear that there is no right whatever — constitutional or otherwise — for a defendant to use false evidence.

The paucity of authority on the subject of any such "right" may be explained by the fact that such a notion has never been responsibly advanced; the right to counsel includes no right to have a lawyer who will cooperate with planned perjury. A lawyer who would so cooperate would be at risk of prosecution for suborning perjury, and disciplinary proceedings, including suspension or disbarment.

Robinson's admonitions to his client can in no sense be said to have forced respondent into an *impermissible* choice between his right to counsel and his right to testify as he proposed for there was no permissible choice to testify falsely. For defense counsel to take steps to persuade a criminal defendant to testify truthfully, or to withdraw, deprives the defendant of neither his right to counsel nor the right to testify truthfully. In *United States v. Havens, supra*, we made clear that "when defendants testify, they must testify truthfully or suffer the consequences." *Id.*, 446 U.S. at 626. When an accused proposes to resort to perjury or to produce false evidence, one consequence is the risk of withdrawal of counsel.

On this record, the accused enjoyed continued representation within the bounds of reasonable professional conduct and did in fact exercise his right to testify; at most he was denied the right to have the assistance of counsel in the presentation of false testimony. Similarly, we can discern no breach of professional duty in Robinson's admonition to respondent that he would disclose respondent's perjury to the court. The crime of perjury in this setting is indistinguishable in substance from the crime of threatening or tampering with a witness or a juror. A defendant who informed his counsel that he was arranging to bribe or threaten witnesses or members of the jury would have no "right" to insist on counsel's assistance or silence. Counsel would not be limited to advising against that conduct. An attorney's duty of confidentiality, which totally covers the client's admission of guilt, does not extend to a client's announced plans to engage in future criminal conduct. In short, the responsibility of an ethical lawyer, as an officer of the court and a key component of a system of justice, dedicated to a search for truth, is essentially the same whether the client announces an intention to bribe or threaten witnesses or jurors or to commit or procure perjury. No system of justice worthy of the name can tolerate a lesser standard.

The rule adopted by the Court of Appeals, which seemingly would require an attorney to remain silent while his client committed perjury, is wholly incompatible with the established standards of ethical conduct and the laws of Iowa and contrary to professional standards promulgated by that State. The position advocated by petitioner, on the contrary, is wholly consistent with the Iowa standards of professional conduct and law, with the overwhelming majority of courts, and with codes of professional ethics. Since there has been no breach of any recognized professional duty, it follows that there can be no deprivation of the right to assistance of counsel under the *Strickland* standard.

E

. . .

Whether he was persuaded or compelled to desist from perjury, Whiteside has no valid claim that confidence in the result of his trial has been diminished by his desisting from the contemplated perjury. Even if we were to assume that the jury might have believed his perjury, it does not follow that Whiteside was prejudiced.

In his attempt to evade the prejudice requirement of *Strickland*, Whiteside relies on cases involving conflicting loyalties of counsel. In Cuyler v. Sullivan, 446 U.S. 335 (1980), we held that a defendant could obtain relief without pointing to a specific prejudicial default on the part of his counsel, provided it is established that the attorney was "actively represent[ing] conflicting interests." *Id.* at 350.

Here, there was indeed a "conflict," but of a quite different kind; it was one imposed on the attorney by the client's proposal to commit the crime of fabricating testimony without which, as he put it, "I'm dead." This is not remotely the kind of conflict of interests dealt with in *Cuyler v. Sullivan.* Even in that case we did not suggest that all multiple representations necessarily resulted in an active conflict rendering the representation constitutionally infirm. If a "conflict" between a client's proposal and counsel's ethical obligation gives rise to a presumption that counsel's assistance was prejudicially ineffective, every guilty criminal's conviction would be suspect if the defendant had sought to obtain an acquittal by illegal means. Can anyone doubt what practices and problems would be spawned by such a rule and what volumes of litigation it would generate?

Whiteside's attorney treated Whiteside's proposed perjury in accord with professional standards, and since Whiteside's truthful testimony could not have prejudiced the result of his trial, the Court of Appeals was in error to direct the issuance of a writ of habeas corpus and must be reversed.

Reversed.

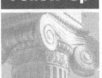

Post-Case Follow-Up

In *Whiteside*, the Court ruled that Model Rule 3.3 is constitutional where a criminal defense attorney *threatens* to withdraw or reveal the perjury, and the client does not testify. The Court did not say that this is the *only* course of conduct that would satisfy Sixth Amendment protections. This leaves states free to adopt ethical rules that pose other solutions to the problem of client perjury. Justice Blackmun emphasized this very narrow ground of the Court's ruling in his concurrence: "The only federal issue in this case is whether Robinson's behavior deprived Whiteside of the effective assistance of counsel; it is not whether Robinson's behavior conformed to any particular code of legal ethics. . . . It is for the States to decide how attorneys should conduct themselves in state criminal proceedings, and this Court's responsibility extends only to ensuring that the restrictions a State enacts do not infringe a defendant's federal constitutional rights." *Id.* at 189-90.

Whiteside did not testify at trial that he had seen a gun. Suppose that he had? If his attorney had then revealed the perjury to the court (consistent with Rule 3.3) and Whiteside was convicted, would Whiteside have a stronger claim that his Sixth Amendment right to counsel was violated? Presumably, if threatening to do something is permissible, actually doing the same thing should also be permissible. But the Supreme Court has never directly confronted and answered that question.

The Model Rule's solution to client perjury in Rule 3.3(a)(3) represented a major policy change from prior attorney discipline standards. By contrast, the 1969 Model Code of Professional Responsibility, DR 7-102(A)(4), provided that an attorney "shall not knowingly *use* perjured testimony or false evidence." Unlike the rules, the Code did not require revelation of attorney-client confidences to remedy client perjury; if a client lied on the witness stand notwithstanding the lawyer's remonstrations to the contrary, the attorney would satisfy his ethical obligations if he refrained from *using* that evidence in closing argument. Would the client feel any less betrayed by this approach? Does it not have the same effect of making clear to the judge (and perhaps the jury) that the client lied?

Nix v. Whiteside: Real Life Applications

1. Your client is accused of rape. The alleged attack was committed in a public park between strangers at night. The defendant tells you that he met the victim while strolling through the park, they struck up a conversation, and it led to hand holding, kissing, and then consensual intercourse in a secluded area. You doubt your client's version of events, and you think that a mistaken identification defense is more likely to succeed. The perpetrator used a condom and no male DNA samples were recovered from the victim. What do you do?

2. Your client is accused of armed robbery while masked. He insists he did not commit the crime and offers an alibi for the date and time of the offense. You interview the two alibi witnesses. In your view, they are not credible. Their stories are full of holes and they have criminal convictions that could be used to impeach them at trial. May you refuse to put these two witnesses on the stand?

3. You are a public defender who is assigned to represent a defendant charged with assault and battery after a barroom brawl. You interview your client on the morning of his arraignment and he tells you that he was drunk and that he punched the victim in the face after the victim insulted his girlfriend. After you receive in discovery the police report and witness statements, you determine that the case against your client is very strong. Your client will not agree to a plea bargain because a criminal conviction will jeopardize his job. Prior to trial, your client tells you for the first time that the victim pushed him, before he struck back in self-defense. What advice do you give to your client, and how do you proceed if he insists on testifying?

There are two significant differences with regard to the ethical obligation of a criminal defense lawyer faced with **perjury by a client** compared to other lawyers. First, lawyers for any other type of client or witness (including a criminal prosecutor) may refuse to put the witness on the stand if they reasonably believe the witness will lie. Under Rule 3.3(a)(3), however, out of respect for a criminal defendant's constitutional right to testify in his own defense, a criminal defense lawyer may not refuse to put the defendant on the witness stand unless she actually *knows* the client will lie. Actual knowledge may be rare as an epistemological matter. In *Nix* the lawyer had actual knowledge, because Whiteside stated that he did not see a gun or any other object on one occasion, and then modified his story to describe seeing something "metallic" because he insisted that if he did not do so he would be "dead." The circumstances would have been different if Whiteside had simply embellished his version of the events over time with new details that had not been disclosed earlier. Although a criminal defense lawyer has an important counseling role to play as a strategic matter in advising his client when implausible testimony will hurt the case, there is nothing wrong with giving the client the benefit of the doubt with respect to the truth of proposed testimony.[25] For this reason, some criminal defense lawyers avoid asking their clients directly if they committed the crime, because full knowledge of the facts may turn out to hamstring the lawyer's options ethically in deciding how to structure a defense. By contrast, civil lawyers typically like to learn as much about factual circumstances of the client's case as possible in order to enable them to mount a case.

Second, with respect to prospective perjury of a criminal defendant, some states require a different solution to the "trilemma" than Model Rule 3.3(a). Massachusetts, Wisconsin, and the District of Columbia,[26] for example, require the criminal defense lawyer who is unable to dissuade his client from committing perjury and unable to withdraw from representation to follow a "narrative" approach: allow the defendant to take the stand, and then ask the defendant to tell the jury what happened in an open-ended, narrative fashion. The attorney may not assist the perjury by structuring the testimony in the form of "question and answer." Nor may the attorney argue the facts gleaned from the narrative in closing argument (which would amount to lack of candor to the tribunal). Chief Justice Burger seemed to reject the wisdom of the narrative approach in footnote 6 of the *Nix* opinion,[27] but as Justice Blackmun's concurring opinion reminds us, states are free to craft their own rules of professional conduct. Comment [7] to Model Rule 3.3 recognizes that some jurisdictions favor the narrative solution, and concedes that this may be an appropriate "remedial measure" in jurisdictions that do so. The benefits of the narrative approach are that the attorney's role in advancing the perjury are minimized, it avoids the instances where the client is deprived of the right to testify because the attorney mistakenly believed that the client would lie, and the attorney is not directly involved in revealing any client confidences. Advocates of the narrative approach also argue that it avoids kicking the problem of client perjury over to the judge: what is a judge supposed to do in a criminal case when an attorney goes to sidebar or chambers and reveals the falsity of the defendant's testimony? Strike the testimony? Declare a mistrial? Even in the rare situation where withdrawal of counsel would not prejudice the client, what would withdrawal accomplish from a systemic point of view — defendant presumably would get a new lawyer and the process would start all over again, although this time the client

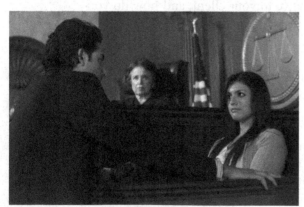

The attorney may not assist the perjury of a criminal defendant by structuring the testimony in the form of "question and answer."
Shutterstock.com

---

25. In *United States v. Midgett*, the Fourth Circuit ruled that the defendant was denied his constitutional right to testify when his lawyer refused to put him on the stand and threatened to withdraw upon a mere belief, "albeit a strong one," that the testimony would be false. 342 F.3d 321, 327 (4th Cir. 2003).

26. Mass. R. Prof'l Conduct 3.3(e); Wis. Stat. §20:3.3(a); D.C. R. Prof'l Conduct 3.3(b). For a list of jurisdictions that follow the narrative approach, see State v. Chambers, 994 A.2d 1248, 1258 n.12 (Conn. 2010).

27. 475 U.S. at 170 n.6.

would likely be slightly less forthcoming with new counsel. In real life, most judges who are informed of a criminal defendant's perjury in states that follow Model Rule 3.3(a)(3) do *nothing* and leave it to the jury to sort out the truth of the evidence after cross-examination. If that is the most likely factual outcome, what has been accomplished by Rule 3.3(a)'s requirement of revelation, other than insulating the lawyer from any possible suggestion of complicity in the lie?

3. Cross-Examining a Truthful Witness

A lawyer's duty of candor to the tribunal precludes him from offering evidence that he knows to be false. Is a criminal defense attorney "offering" evidence when he attempts to impeach a witness on cross-examination who he knows to be telling the truth (such as with prior convictions, bias, inconsistent statements, problems in perception, etc.)? **Discrediting truthful testimony** may not be the same thing as offering a false fact, but it certainly has a similar effect.

In 1987, Harry Subin and John Mitchell engaged in a vigorous debate on this very issue in the *Georgetown Journal of Legal Ethics*. Subin criticized the arbitrary lines between "presenting" false evidence through your own witnesses (which violates Rule 3.3) and (1) cross-examining a truthful witness to suggest she is fabricating her testimony, or (2) arguing a false inference to the jury from known truthful testimony.[28] Using the example of a rape victim who the defense attorney learns is telling the truth, Subin argues that there is no socially redeeming value in permitting the attorney to discredit her testimony or arguing in closing that the sex was consensual. According to Subin, the criminal defense attorney's sole legitimate role in defending a case where he knows that the victim is telling the truth is to assert all available procedural defenses on behalf of his client, and thereafter act as "monitor" to ensure that the government has satisfied its burden of proof beyond a reasonable doubt. Mitchell's response follows.

John Mitchell, Reasonable Doubts Are Where You Find Them: A Response to Professor Subin's Position on the Criminal Lawyer's "Different Mission"
1 Geo. J. Legal Ethics 339 (1987)

I. INTRODUCTION

In *A Criminal Lawyer's "Different Mission": Reflections on the "Right" to Present a False Case*, Professor Harry L. Subin attempts to draw what he considers to be the line between attorney as advocate, and attorney as officer of the court. Specifically,

---

28. Harry I. Subin, *The Criminal Defense Lawyer's "Different Mission": Reflections on a "Right" to Present a False Case*, 1 Geo. J. Legal Ethics 125 (1987).

he "attempts to define the limits on the methods a lawyer should be willing to use when his client's goals are inconsistent with truth." This is no peripheral theme in professional responsibility. Quite the contrary, Professor Subin has chosen a difficult issue which touches upon the very nature of our criminal justice system, the role of the attorney in that system, the relationship of the individual to the state, and the Constitution. Further, Professor Subin takes a tough and controversial stand on this issue and, although I disagree with him, I respect his position.

. . .

. . . While Professor Subin directs his attack on the notion that a criminal defense attorney has a "different mission" than uncovering truth, in my view it is the criminal justice system itself which has a "different mission."

II. PROFESSOR SUBIN'S ASSUMPTIONS

Professor Subin rests his entire analysis on two basic premises: (1) the principle goal of the criminal justice system is "truth"; and (2) it is contrary to the goal of "truth" to permit a criminal defense attorney to put on a "false defense." In Subin's terms, a false defense is an attempt to "convince the judge or jury that facts established by the state and known to the attorney to be true are not true, or that facts known to the attorney to be false are true." Such a defense is put on by: ". . . (1) cross-examination of truthful government witnesses to undermine their testimony or their credibility; (2) direct presentation of testimony, not in itself false, but used to discredit the truthful evidence adduced by the government, or to accredit a false theory; and, (3) argument to the jury based on any of these acts." I take exception to both of these premises, as set out below.

The Principal Concern of the Criminal Justice System Is Not "Truth"

The idea that the focus of the criminal justice system is not "truth" may initially sound shocking. I have valued truth throughout my life and do not condone lying in our legal system. But the job of our criminal justice system is simply other than determining "truth." Professor Subin himself recognizes that there are rules within the criminal justice system which are barriers to truth, but which are nevertheless supported by strong policy (e.g., privilege, suppression of illegally obtained evidence). Nevertheless, he states early in his article that he "shall argue" that the criminal justice system has the determination of truth as its principle goal. Apparently he means that he shall adopt this fundamental premise by fiat, for nowhere does he articulate an argument for this proposition. I believe there is a good reason for this omission. It is emotionally easy (and perhaps even rhetorically convincing) to proclaim the virtue of "truth" in the abstract; it is more difficult to extol "truth's" virtues when analyzing the American criminal justice system. An analysis of the American criminal justice system in actual operation is appropriate at this point.

A system focused on truth would first collect all information relevant to the inquiry. In our system, the defendant is generally the best source of information in the dispute, but he is not available unless he so chooses. The police may not question him. He may not be called to the stand with his own lawyer beside him and with a judge controlling questioning under the rules of evidence. The prosecutor may not even comment to the jury about the defendant's failure to testify, even though fair inferences may be drawn from the refusal to respond to serious accusations.

A system focused on truth would have the factfinder look at all the information and then decide what it believed had occurred. In our system, the inquiry is dramatically skewed against finding guilt. "Beyond a reasonable doubt" expresses the deep cultural value that "it is better to let ten guilty men go than convict one innocent man." It is a system where, after rendering a verdict of not guilty, jurors routinely approach defense counsel and say, "I thought your guy was guilty, but that prosecutor did not prove it to me beyond a reasonable doubt." What I have just described is not a "truth system" in any sense in which one could reasonably understand that term. Truth may play a role, but it is not a dominant role; there is something else afoot. The criminal defense attorney does not have a "different mission"; the system itself has a "different mission."

Embodying this "different mission" is the concept of "legal guilt" and its distinction from "factual guilt." The latter refers to "did he do it?"; the former to "did the prosecution prove he did it beyond a reasonable doubt?" The criminal justice system focuses exclusively upon "legal guilt." . . .

[T]he criminal justice system protects the individual from the police power of the executive branch of government. Between the individual citizen and the enormous governmental power residing in the executive stands a panel of that individual's peers — a jury. Through them, the executive must pass. Only if it proves its case "beyond a reasonable doubt," thereby establishing legal guilt, may the executive then legitimately intrude into the individual citizen's life. Thus, "factual" guilt or innocence, or what Professor Subin would call "truth," is not the principle issue in the system. Our concern is with the legitimate use of the prosecutor's power as embodied in the concept of "legal guilt."

. . .

A. Defense Attorney Acting in a Manner Meeting with Subin's Disapproval Is Not Putting on a "False Defense"

When placed in the "reasonable doubt" context, Professor Subin's implicit distinction between "true" and "false" defenses misportrays both how a defense attorney may actually function in a case, and the very nature of evidence in that case. His categories are too imprecise to capture the subtle middle ground of a pure reasonable doubt defense, in which counsel presents the jury with alternative possibilities that counsel knows are false, without asserting the truth of those alternatives.

For example, imagine I am defending a young woman accused of shoplifting a star one places on top of Christmas trees. I interview the store manager and find that he stopped my client when he saw her walk straight through the store, star in hand, and out the door. When he stopped her and asked why she had taken the star without paying, she made no reply and burst into tears. He was then about to take her inside to the security office when an employee called out, "There's a fire!" The manager rushed inside and dealt with a small blaze in the camera section. Five minutes later he came out to find my client sitting where he had left her. He then took her back to the security room and asked if she would be willing to empty her pockets so that he could see if she had taken anything else. Without a word, she complied. She had a few items not belonging to the store and a ten-dollar bill. The star was priced at $1.79.

In an interview with my client, she admitted trying to steal the star: "It was so pretty, and would have looked so nice on the tree. I would have bought it, but I also wanted to make a special Christmas dinner for Mama and didn't have enough money to do both. I've been saving for that dinner and I know it will make her so happy. But that star. . . . I could just see the look in Mama's eyes if she saw that lovely thing on our tree."

At trial, the manager tells the same story he told me, except he leaves out the part about her waiting during the fire and having a ten-dollar bill. If I bring out these two facts on cross-examination and argue for an acquittal based upon my client "accidentally" walking out of the store with the star, surely Professor Subin will accuse me of raising a "false defense." I have brought out testimony, not itself false, to accredit a false theory and have argued to the jury based on this act. But I am not really arguing a false theory in Professor Subin's sense.

My defense is not that the defendant accidentally walked out, but rather that the prosecution cannot prove the element of intent to permanently deprive beyond a reasonable doubt. Through this theory, I am raising "doubt" in the prosecution's case, and therefore questioning the legitimacy of the government's lawsuit for control over the defendant. In my effort to carry out this legal theory, I will *not assert* that facts known by me to be true are false or those known to be false are true. As a defense attorney, I do not have to prove what *in fact* happened. That is an advantage in the process I would not willingly give up. Under our constitutional system, I do not need to try to convince the factfinder about the truth of any factual propositions. I need only try to convince the factfinder that the prosecution has not met its burden. . . .

. . .

In our shoplifting example, the prosecution will elicit that the defendant burst into tears when stopped by the manager. From this information will run a chain of inferences: defendant burst into tears; people without a guilty conscience would explain their innocence, not cry; defendant has a guilty conscience; her guilty conscience is likely motivated by having committed a theft. Conversely, if the defense brings out that the manager was shaking a lead pipe in his hand when he stopped the defendant, defense counsel is *not asserting* that defendant did not have a guilty conscience when stopped. Counsel is merely *weakening* the persuasiveness of the prosecution's inference by raising the "possibility" that she was crying not from guilt, but from fear. By raising such "possibilities," the defense is making arguments against the ability of the prosecution's inferences to meet their burden of "beyond a reasonable doubt." The defense is not arguing what are true or false facts (i.e., that the tears were from fear as opposed to guilt). Whatever Professor Subin cares to call it, this commentary on the prosecution's case, complete with raising possibilities which weaken the persuasiveness of central inferences in that case, is in no ethical sense a "false case." "False case" is plainly a misnomer. In a system where factual guilt is not at issue, Professor Subin's "falsehoods" are, in fact, "reasonable doubts."

. . .

To illustrate, imagine I am representing a defendant accused of robbery. I have seen the victim at a preliminary hearing, and based upon the circumstances of the identification and my overall impression of the witness, I am certain that he is truthful and accurate. My client has confessed his factual guilt. And therefore I "know" (in Professor Subin's sense) beyond a reasonable doubt that my client has been accurately identified.

In his direct examination, the victim states, "The defendant had this big, silvery automatic pistol right up near my face the whole time he was asking for money." In accordance with Professor Subin's view that defense counsel can "persuade the jury that there are legitimate reasons to doubt the state's evidence," may I raise the general vagaries of eyewitness identification? . . . Perhaps Subin would say I cannot make the misidentification argument. He might argue that the "legitimacy" of reasons to doubt the state's evidence is not to be judged from the perspective of a reasonable juror hearing the prosecution's evidence but from my subjective knowledge. Since I "know" that there was no difficulty with the identification, I cannot put forward a "legitimate" reason to doubt. If this is Professor Subin's meaning, I, as monitor, am left with the following closing argument: "Ladies and gentlemen, thank you for your attention to this case. Remember, the prosecution must prove each element beyond a reasonable doubt. Thank you." . . .

"Legitimate reason" to doubt must refer to a reasonable juror's perception of the state's evidence, not to the defense attorney's private knowledge. Bringing out reasonable doubts in the state's evidence concerning the identification therefore must be legitimate, and yet this would seem to raise a "false defense" (i.e., mistaken identification). Presumably, Subin would permit this defense because of a greater policy than "truth," i.e., the right to have the state prove guilt beyond a reasonable doubt. If this is permissible in Subin's view, it is difficult to understand why it would not be permissible to call an expert on eyewitness identification to testify.

. . .

Another indication that Subin would not adhere to the "stark" definition of lawyer as monitor is that he would allow the defense to demonstrate the inaccuracy of information that may be harmful to its case. Imagine that the robbery victim in my hypothetical testifies that Bloogan's Department Store, directly across the street from where the nighttime robbery occurred, had all of its lights on at the time of the robbery. In fact, I find out in investigation that Bloogan's was closed for remodeling that evening. Subin would undoubtedly allow me to bring this out. What, after all, would a "truth" theory be if I were not permitted to confront "lies" and "misperceptions." If Professor Subin permits me to bring out this "inaccuracy" on cross-examination and/or through other witnesses, he must also allow me to use it in closing or my initial access to this information would be meaningless. In closing, my only real use for this information would be in support of my "false defense" of mistaken identification. The line between advocate and monitor is again blurred.

. . .

B. Bigger Problems: Constitutional Concerns and Jeopardizing an Independent Defense Bar

If Professor Subin's approach is more than a statement of his own private ethics, the vagueness and uncertainty of the line which divides the advocate from the monitor presents a serious problem. First, constitutional concerns additional to those already expressed may arise. Criminal defense representation touches significant interests: 1) protection of the individual from the state; 2) the freedom of the defendant in a nation which values liberty; and 3) significant constitutional rights (fourth, fifth, sixth, eighth, and fourteenth amendments). It is within these areas that the impreciseness in Professor Subin's categories comes to the fore. To the extent defense attorneys are guided by ethical rules which are vague about what conduct is proper, the representation of clients is hampered. Counsel, uncertain as to appropriate behavior, may fall into a "conflict" between pushing the client's interests as far as is legitimate and protecting himself against charges of unethical conduct. Attorneys' decisions may then tend to fall on the self-protective side, raising constitutional concerns regarding zealous representation.

Second, if Subin's approach were enforced as a rule of professional conduct, the independent defense bar would be seriously jeopardized. Professor Subin may or may not be correct that the public and the bar have a low view of the criminal defense bar. Nonetheless, the independence of that bar has provided all citizens with significant protection against governmental oppression. With Professor Subin's approach, however, if an acquittal were gained by a defense attorney who was a thorn in the government's side, the prosecutor's office might be tempted to file an ethical complaint stating that defense counsel should have known he put on a "false defense." Subin's position now becomes a weapon of repression in the hands of the government. Even if vindication follows upon a disciplinary hearing, time, expense, and public humiliation might ensue. This will deliver a powerful message to defense attorneys. Don't risk fighting, plead your clients guilty.

Mitchell seems to have won this debate with Subin among most practitioners, scholars, and judges. Commentators now agree that it is ethically appropriate — if not required — for a criminal defense attorney to impeach a witness who he knows to be testifying truthfully. Some rest their arguments on the presumption of innocence and the advocate's obligation to hold the government to its extraordinarily high burden of proof in criminal cases.[29] Monroe Freedman has argued that this license stems from the defense lawyer's access to confidential information from the client — which often is the source of the attorney's knowledge of the witness's truthfulness; if a defense lawyer declines to cross-examine a witness based upon what his client has told him, it will dissuade clients in the future from being forthcoming with information.[30] Still others have argued that zealous advocacy on behalf of a client needs to be at its apex in the criminal defense context because we want to curtail the power of the state to punish its citizens.[31] Is Mitchell's position an amalgamation of these arguments, or something distinct? Does it resonate with you?

---

29. David G. Bress, *Professional Ethics in Criminal Trials: A View of Defense Counsel's Responsibility*, 64 MICH. L. REV. 1493, 1494 (1966); Warren E. Burger, *Standards of Conduct for Prosecution and Defense Personnel: A Judge's Viewpoint*, 5 AM. CRIM. L.Q. 11, 14-15 (1966). This position has come to be known as the "Burger-Bress" argument in support of a criminal defense attorney's right to impeach a truthful witness.

30. Monroe H. Freedman, *Professional Responsibility of the Criminal Defense Lawyer: The Three Hardest Questions*, 64 MICH. L. REV. 1469, 1474-75 (1966).

31. *See* David Luban, *The Adversary System Excuse*, in THE GOOD LAWYER 83, 92 (David Luban ed., 1984).

Clearly siding with Mitchell, Section 4-7.7(b) of the aspirational and non-binding ABA Standards for the Administration of Criminal Justice: Defense Function states that "[d]efense counsel's belief or knowledge that a witness is telling the truth does not preclude vigorous cross-examination, even though defense counsel's cross-examination may cast doubt on the testimony." As ministers of justice, should prosecutors be given the same or less leeway in cross-examining defense witnesses who they believe to be telling the truth?[32]

Chapter Summary

- The prosecutor has a responsibility as "minister of justice" to make sure that criminal charges are supported by probable cause, that they fairly reflect the gravity of the offense, and that adversarial proceedings are conducted fairly.
- The "no-contact" rule prohibits prosecutors from contacting represented defendants without their lawyer's permission, and thus imposes obligations that exceed Fifth and Sixth Amendment guarantees.
- A prosecutor must disclose to defense counsel all exculpatory evidence in possession of the government, unless relieved of this obligation by an order of the tribunal.
- The prosecutor must avoid media comments about pending cases that heighten public condemnation of the accused and that serve no legitimate law enforcement purpose.
- A criminal defense attorney, unlike a prosecutor, acts properly when she cross-examines a witness who she knows to be telling the truth in order to undermine that witness's credibility.
- A criminal defense attorney who knows that his client intends to commit perjury may not counsel or assist that perjury, and may withdraw from representation if allowed by the court.

Applying the Rules

1. Suppose that you serve as a prosecutor in a local district court, and you are preparing for trial in a domestic assault and battery case. The defendant was arrested after police were called to his marital home to break up a fight. The police took a statement from the victim and took photographs of her injuries. In preparing the case for trial, you call the victim in to your office for an interview. The victim says she does not want to go forward with the case. She says that she lied to the police officers because she was mad at her husband and

---

32. For a discussion of that question, see R. Michael Cassidy, *Character and Context: What Virtue Theory Can Teach Us About a Prosecutor's Ethical Duty to "Seek Justice,"* 82 NOTRE DAME L. REV. 635, 667 (2006).

wanted to get back at him. She denies that the defendant hit her, and instead insists that she received her injuries by falling down the stairs. What do you do with this information? How do you decide whether to proceed with the case?

2. Imagine that you represent the state in a rape prosecution. The defendant is a star professional athlete accused of sexual assaulting a female after escorting her home from a nightclub. The victim has hired a lawyer to commence a civil tort suit against the athlete. May you speak with the alleged rape victim in order to prepare her for the criminal trial without obtaining permission from her counsel in the civil case?

3. Imagine that you are a criminal defense attorney for the same athlete charged with rape in hypothetical #2 above. In interviewing the defendant after his arraignment, the defendant claims that he was "set up" and that the sex was purely consensual. The athlete tells you that he has security cameras throughout his home and that the video will corroborate his account of the consensual encounter. Should you take any steps to obtain and watch this video?

4. Suppose that you are a public defender assigned to represent a defendant accused of robbing an elderly victim of her purse at knifepoint. When you meet with your client, he confesses to the crime and tells you that he committed the robbery in order to support a drug habit. If you are unsuccessful in obtaining a plea bargain and the case proceeds to trial, should you call your client as a witness? If you decide not to put your client on the witness stand and instead assert a reasonable doubt defense, may you cross-examine the victim to call into question her ability to perceive the perpetrator due to the poor lighting conditions and her fright upon feeling a knife against her back?

Professional Responsibility in Practice

1. Research the law in the jurisdiction in which you intend to practice and determine whether any appellate courts or the state bar have recognized an undercover investigatory exception to Rule 4.2.

2. Imagine that you represent a defendant accused of rape. The government's allegations are that your client forced himself on the victim in his bedroom during a fraternity party. Both the defendant and the victim agree to having consumed large quantities of alcohol during the party. But defendant insists that the sex was consensual. Right before the case is scheduled to go to trial, the defendant tells you for the first time that the victim insisted he use a condom and that she actually unwrapped the condom and put it on the defendant. This is the first time the defendant has revealed this "fact" to you. He did not discuss it with police officers when he was interviewed during the investigation, nor did he reveal it to you during any prior interviews. Play the role of the defense counsel and have a conversation with your client about whether he will testify about the condom.

Delivery of Legal Services and Access to Justice

Practicing Law: Issues in Group Lawyering and the Unauthorized Practice of Law

This chapter addresses several issues related to the business and organization of law practice. It begins by examining the ethical responsibilities of lawyers who work in group settings. What are the responsibilities of lawyers with managerial and supervisory authority with respect to those lawyers that they oversee? What are the responsibilities of junior lawyers who are ordered to do something that they believe might violate the Rules of Professional Conduct?

The remainder of the chapter covers several other regulations on law practice including the traditional prohibition on lawyers going into business with non-lawyers and non-lawyers engaging in the practice of law. These rules reflect longstanding concerns about lawyer independence and protecting the public from incompetent services, but they have come under increasing scrutiny as the nature of law practice has changed due to technology and globalization, and countries around the world have liberalized their rules on these issues.

Key Concepts

- The responsibility of lawyers with managerial authority to ensure compliance with ethical obligations
- The independent responsibility of subordinate lawyers to act in compliance with their ethical obligations
- Professional independence of lawyers
- Prohibitions on practicing with non-lawyers
- Agreements restricting lawyer practice
- Prohibitions on practicing law without a license

A. LAW FIRMS AND ASSOCIATIONS

Most lawyers work in a group setting, such as law firms (large and small), non-profit organizations, the corporate counsel division of for-profit businesses, or government law offices. The hierarchical structure of these practices complicates ethical decision making, because lawyers may face institutional pressures or incentives that conflict with their own personal values and professional responsibilities. In the next sections of this chapter, we explore two questions: when supervisory lawyers are responsible for the conduct of junior lawyers within a law practice, and when subordinate lawyers may reasonably rely on ethical judgments made by their superiors.

1. Responsibility of Supervisors

Partners in law firms and other senior lawyers with comparable managerial authority in non–law firm settings are required to make "reasonable efforts" to create procedures and structures to ensure compliance with the applicable disciplinary rules by all lawyers working within that organization. *See* Model Rule 5.1(a). This rule recognizes that the environment in which one practices can have a huge impact on ethical decision making, and it calls upon lawyers with managerial responsibility to take adequate steps to foster a workplace where attention is paid to professionalism. According to comment [2], such steps will include establishing a firm procedure for detecting and resolving conflicts of interest, accounting for client funds and trust property, creating reasonable filing and case tracking systems, and ensuring that inexperienced lawyers are adequately trained and supervised.

Supervisory lawyers may be found to have vicarious responsibility for the actual professional misconduct of junior lawyers in the organization in two instances: when they order or ratify the junior lawyer's conduct, or when they have either general managerial authority over the lawyer or "direct supervisory authority" over the specific legal matter and they learn of the junior lawyer's conduct at a time when its consequences can be avoided and they fail to take reasonable remedial measures. *See* Model Rule 5.1(c). The power to impose vicarious responsibility on senior lawyers under the rules is thus fairly broad — it can sweep in lawyers who have no formal supervisory role or title if they order or ratify the conduct (such as a more senior associate working on the case — *see* Model Rule 5.1(c)(1)), and it can sweep in partners or department heads who are not actively working on the matter in question, but who come to know about the professional misconduct of a junior lawyer in time to prevent or remedy it and fail to do so.

Partners in law firms and managing attorneys in non-partnership settings (government, legal aid, in-house counsel) also have a responsibility to create an environment of professionalism for non-legal staff. Rule 5.3 recognizes that lawyers often rely on non-lawyers to complete their work — such as accountants, investigators, paralegals, and messengers. Rule 5.3 parallels Rule 5.2 in that it requires lawyers with supervisory authority to take efforts to ensure the conduct of non-lawyer assistants is compatible with the professional obligations of the lawyer.

A messenger who is sent to deliver privileged and confidential material to a client must have some training on the requirements of confidentiality so he does not leave the file open in a coffee shop. A bookkeeper must be properly trained not to commingle client assets with assets of the firm.[1]

Just like with Rule 5.2, a lawyer can have vicarious responsibility for the actual actions of a non-lawyer assistant if she either directs or ratifies the conduct, or is a supervisory lawyer and comes to learn of the conduct in time to avoid or mitigate the consequences but fails to do so. *See* Model Rule 5.3(c). For example, where a lawyer is prohibited from talking to an opposing party without her counsel's permission under the "no contact" rule, *see* Model Rule 4.2, the lawyer violates the rule when he directs an investigator or paralegal to make that very same contact.

2. Responsibility of Junior Lawyers

There is no "Nuremberg" or "following orders" defense to charges of professional misconduct. Model Rule 5.2(a) quite clearly states that "[a] lawyer is bound by the Rules of Professional Conduct notwithstanding that the lawyer acted at the direction of another person." That is, an associate or junior lawyer cannot escape responsibility for violation of the disciplinary rules by arguing that a senior lawyer "made me do it." All lawyers take an oath to uphold the canons of the legal profession, and a junior lawyer cannot escape liability for her own personal actions by relying on a chain of hierarchy within an organization. If a junior lawyer is asked to do something that she knows clearly violates the disciplinary rules, the only acceptable answer is "no."

Rule 5.2(a) creates a limited safe harbor for subordinate lawyers who act "in accordance with a supervisory lawyer's reasonable resolution of an arguable question of professional duty." The comment to the rule recognizes that where a question of professional ethics is a close one, someone has to decide on a course of action, and placing the responsibility on the senior lawyer is consistent with the typical disparity in experience and judgment between the relevant players. But note the limitations of this limited safe harbor—in order for a subordinate lawyer to avoid professional discipline for conduct he is instructed to take by a supervisor, the subordinate lawyer must do *at least enough* factual and legal research to ascertain whether the supervisor's direction is a "reasonable resolution" of an "arguable question." If the ethical question is clear cut, or if it is a gray area and the supervisor's resolution is not "reasonable," the subordinate lawyer cannot rely on the safe harbor of Rule 5.2(a).

Usually, we think of vicarious responsibility as flowing upward: that is, bosses can have responsibility for acts of their subordinates, but usually subordinates do not have responsibility for actions of their bosses (unless they are complicit in those actions). We just saw how this doctrine works with respect to Rule 5.1. Thus, a

---

1. *See* In re Bailey, 821 A.2d 851 (Del. 2003) (managing partner of law firm disciplined under Rule 5.3 for failing to exercise "even a modicum of diligence" to make sure that the firm's bookkeeper paid relevant taxes and did not invade client trust accounts to pay debts of the firm).

junior lawyer will not normally have responsibility for professional misconduct committed by a partner or senior lawyer in the organization, unless he *participated* in the misconduct. This comports with our sense of moral as well as ethical responsibility — someone who is in a position to alleviate or prevent the misconduct has broader responsibilities than a subordinate who does not have the power to control the conduct of others. However, the Model Rules recognize one important exception to this traditional construction of principal/agency relationships. Model Rule 3.3(b) governs a lawyer's obligations of candor to the tribunal, and provides that "[a] lawyer who represents a client in an adjudicative proceeding and who knows that *a person* intends to engage, is engaging, or has engaged in criminal or fraudulent conduct related to the proceeding shall take reasonable remedial measures. . . ." (Emphasis supplied.) The use of the generic term "person" applies to both witnesses, clients, and *lawyers* involved in the case. In the context of litigation, therefore, there may be instances where a junior lawyer needs to speak up or risk being punished for the conduct of a senior lawyer with whom he is litigating the case. For example, if the senior lawyer makes a false statement of material fact to the court and the junior associate knows of its falsity, the associate has violated Rule 3.3(b) by remaining silent.[2]

Case Preview	### Davis v. Alabama State Bar

Attorneys Davis and Goldberg were suspended from the practice of law for 60 days for, among other infractions, failing to ensure that lawyers in their firm complied with the Rules of Professional Conduct (Rule 5.1) and failing to ensure that activities of non-lawyer assistants were compatible with professional standards (Rule 5.3). The partners in the firm essentially "churned" civil complaints by taking on an extremely large volume of cases (particularly bankruptcy and social security disability claims) and thereafter neglecting client files. Several of the witnesses against Davis and Goldberg were former associates or secretarial assistants of the firm.

As you read the *Davis* decision, ask yourself:

1. What economic incentives might have led these two small-firm lawyers to establish the following practices at their firm?
   a. Having non-lawyer assistants complete and serve bankruptcy filings;
   b. Requiring associates to open a certain quota of cases per month;
   c. Forbidding associates from returning client phone calls; and
   d. Forbidding associates from interviewing clients before the first scheduled court appearance.

---

2. For a powerful discussion of the responsibilities of principal and subordinate lawyers in the context of the Berkey-Kodak antitrust litigation, see David Luban, *The Ethics of Wrongful Obedience*, *in* Ethics in Practice: Lawyers' Roles, Responsibilities and Regulation (Deborah L. Rhode ed., 2003).

Davis v. Alabama State Bar
676 So. 2d 306 (Ala. 1996)

. . .

Two attorneys appeal from Alabama State Bar disciplinary proceedings. They challenge the sufficiency of the evidence presented at their disciplinary hearing, claiming that the disciplinary proceeding was nothing more than a "witch-hunt" that they say the Bar conducted because it did not approve of the attorneys' advertising practices. They further challenge the penalties imposed as being too severe.

The Alabama State Bar Disciplinary Board found William Dowsing Davis III and Dan Arthur Goldberg to be violating Rule 1.1, Alabama Rules of Professional Conduct (failure to provide competent representation); Rule 1.4(a) and (b) (failure to keep clients reasonably informed and failure to reasonably explain a matter so as to permit a client to make an informed decision); Rule 5.1 (failure to make reasonable efforts to ensure that the lawyers in their firm conformed to the Rules of Professional Conduct); Rule 5.3(b) (failure to ensure that the activities of a nonlawyer under an attorney's supervision are compatible with professional standards); Rule 5.5(b) (providing assistance to a person engaging in the unauthorized practice of law); Rule 8.4(a) (violation of the Rules of Professional Conduct through the acts of another); Rule 8.4(d) (engaging in conduct prejudicial to the administration of justice); and Rule 8.4(g) (engaging in conduct that adversely reflects on a lawyer's fitness to practice law). Both of the attorneys were suspended from the practice of law for 60 days.

The record before this Court is voluminous. Several former and present attorneys and secretaries of these attorneys' firm testified at the disciplinary hearing. Several clients of the firm also testified.

These two attorneys were the sole partners in the law firm of Davis & Goldberg. The firm spent approximately $500,000 annually on advertising, primarily television advertising, and the advertising attracted a large number of clients. As a result of this large expenditure and the volume of clients produced by the advertising, the attorneys implemented several policies, described below, designed to minimize expenses and maximize profits.

The Bar presented evidence, for example, that Davis and Goldberg allowed nonlawyer secretaries to provide legal services. It was also shown to be common practice at the firm for secretaries to interview clients and prepare legal filings, especially bankruptcy petitions. Evidence also indicated that nonlawyer staff members gave clients legal advice, such as "informing" clients of the differences between Chapter 7 and Chapter 13 bankruptcy. One former associate attorney testified that it was the firm's practice that attorneys would not interview or have any contact with the client before the first scheduled court appearance.

There was further testimony that these two attorneys imposed unmanageable caseloads on associate attorneys, many of whom were inexperienced. Some associate attorneys, for example, maintained caseloads of nearly 600 active cases. Former associates testified that because of the sheer volume of cases, the amount of time that could be spent on each case was so limited as to make it impossible for them to adequately represent their clients. At the hearing before the Disciplinary Board, the attorneys' own expert witness on Social Security law, Charles Tyler Clark, testified that the Social Security caseload, as described by a former associate of the firm, could not have been adequately handled by the one attorney assigned to it.

There was testimony that the firm had an inadequate supply of filing cabinets for case files and that files were simply stacked in various parts of the office, including the employees' break room and the hallway near the bathrooms. The evidence further tended to show that associate attorneys were given the barest of support staffs and that this fact, coupled with the huge volume of cases imposed upon the associates, created a situation in which files were mishandled, resulting in harm to the interests of clients.

The harm resulting from what could be described as a practice of the firm is best illustrated in the testimony of a former client, Brenda Marie Wood. Her husband, Douglas Wayne Wood, suffers from acute peripheral neuropathy and is dying. He was awarded Social Security disability benefits, but did not begin receiving his payments until eight months after he was supposed to. Mr. and Mrs. Wood saw a Davis & Goldberg television commercial that promised that the firm would "cut through the Social Security red tape" and get its clients' Social Security benefits fast. Because of the statement made in the advertisement, Mr. Wood hired the firm of Davis & Goldberg in October 1991 to represent him in his claim for past-due benefits. The firm lost Wood's file three times, and each time Wood was required to fill out a new set of forms. Wood was continuously assured by the firm's staff that his claim had been filed, when in fact it had not been. In February 1992, Wood received a letter from the firm informing him that the deadline for filing the claim had passed, and that it was too late to file his appeal.

The associates employed by Davis & Goldberg were also subjected to policies that interfered with their adequate and professional representation of their clients. These policies included the imposition of time limits or restrictions on the amount of time that they could spend with clients and on cases; the imposition of a quota system that required associates to open a specified number of files in a certain time period; and the imposition of a policy requiring associates not to return the phone calls of existing clients, so that the attorneys could free more time to sign new clients.

The appellants contend that the Bar did not meet its burden of proof as to the allegations against them. The standard of review applicable to an appeal from an order of the Disciplinary Board is "that the order will be affirmed unless it is not supported by clear and convincing evidence or misapplies the law to the facts." . . . We disagree with the attorneys' claims that the evidence was insufficient. In fact, the evidence presented amply showed that the two attorneys, in an effort to turn over a huge volume of cases, neglected their clients and imposed policies on associate attorneys that prevented the attorneys from providing quality and competent legal services. The evidence more than met the clear and convincing standard, and the Board's findings that these lawyers had violated the Rules of Professional Conduct are due to be affirmed.

Even though we affirm the findings that these lawyers had violated the Rules of Professional Conduct, we elect to address their argument that the disciplinary proceeding amounted to a "witch-hunt" conducted because the Bar does not approve of the firm's advertising practices. We reject this contention. Instead, we find that the Disciplinary Board properly fulfilled its role of being a guardian of the image of the legal profession, and, thus, acted as a guardian of the profession itself. We cannot find, as the attorneys ask us to find, that the Bar was conducting a "witch-hunt." In fact, there was evidence that the Bar examined the attorneys' advertising practices; it could have found that their advertisements were misleading, specifically in that the attorneys did not provide the quality legal service advertised. The Disciplinary Board heard evidence that one specific advertisement was misleading as it related to a United States Supreme Court ruling on the availability of Social Security benefits. Even the appellants' expert witness testified that the advertisement could have been misleading under certain circumstances.

This Court recognizes that attorneys have a First Amendment right to engage in various forms of commercial speech. We uphold the discipline imposed upon these attorneys, but we are not upholding it because they advertised; rather, we uphold it because the advertising was misleading in that the attorneys did not provide what they said they would provide. False and misleading advertising by attorneys can, and probably has, greatly harmed the public's perception of the legal profession, at a time when the public's confidence in attorneys has diminished. Indeed, the vast majority of those in the legal profession think advertising is harmful to the image of attorneys.

Justice O'Connor warned in her dissent in *Shapero v. Kentucky Bar Ass'n*, that the advertising practices of some attorneys, similar to those practices followed by these two attorneys, will "undermine professional standards" by giving an attorney "incentives to ignore (or avoid discovering) the complexities that would lead a conscientious attorney to treat some clients' cases as anything but routine." 486 U.S. at 486. . . .

Evidence was presented that these two attorneys placed advertisements that were false and misleading. There can be no constitutional right to advertise in a false and misleading way. The evidence tends to show that these two attorneys' ethical violations were caused by their advertising practices and desire to turn over a huge volume of cases. The harm caused by this practice seems apparent.

Additionally, this Court finds no error or abuse in regard to the sanction the Board imposed, a 60-day suspension of the licenses of Davis and Goldberg. The violations were serious, and we cannot hold that the Board acted improperly in imposing the punishment. Consequently, the orders of the Disciplinary Board are affirmed.

In their application for rehearing, the attorneys argue that in its opinion of December 15, 1995, the Court erred in upholding the disciplinary sanctions based solely on allegations of misleading or false advertising. They are apparently referring to the Board's acquittal as to the charge of violating Rule 7.1, Alabama Rules of Professional Conduct. The Court affirmed the Disciplinary Board's numerous findings of violations of ethical rules, but did not address the Board's acquittal of the alleged violation of Rule 7.1. Instead, the Court addressed the attorneys' contention that the Disciplinary Board had conducted a "witch-hunt" against them because the Board did not approve of their advertising policies.

However, the Disciplinary Board found the attorneys in violation of Rule 8.4(g), which states:

It is professional misconduct for a lawyer to:

> . . .

> (g) Engage in any other conduct that adversely reflects on his fitness to practice law.

As we have stated earlier, much evidence was presented at the disciplinary hearing that proved that the attorneys' advertising practices and the procedures and policies adopted by Davis & Goldberg adversely affected the attorneys' ability to practice law in the manner required by the Rules of Professional Conduct. Further, Rule 8.4(g) is broad enough to require that attorney advertisements be honest and accurate and that an attorney's practice of law centered around such heavy advertisement be professional and competent as generally required by the Rules of Profession Conduct.

The evidence presented to the Disciplinary Board showed that Davis & Goldberg advertised that the firm provided legal services of a very high standard, but that the firm's representation of its clients failed to meet the high standard presented in its advertising. This evidence of a failure on the part of Davis & Goldberg to do what was promised in its advertisements, taken with the evidence regarding harmful policies and practices adopted by the firm in response to the fact that a large number of clients were attracted to the firm by its advertising practices, is more than sufficient to support the Board's finding that the attorneys violated Rule 8.4(g).

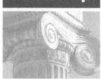

Post-Case Follow-Up

Many associates of the Davis & Goldberg firm became so dissatisfied with the working conditions that they quit. Thus, the firm was not only churning cases, it was also churning associates.

1. Before they quit, could the associates have insulated themselves from ethical responsibility by following office policies and the demands of the partners? That is, Davis and Goldberg were disciplined for failing adequately to supervise associates in the office. Couldn't the associates also have been disciplined for failure to provide competent representation under Rule 1.1? *See* Model Rule 5.2(a). Why weren't they? Is this a reasonable exercise of the bar disciplinary committee's discretion? Didn't the associates *know* that failure to return client phone calls and failure to interview clients impeded their ability to provide competent representation in individual cases? This wasn't an "arguable question of professional duty," was it? *See* Model Rule 5.2(b).

2. One of the reasons that Davis & Goldberg needed to churn cases was that it spent $500,000 per year on advertising. Keeping labor costs low and minimizing non-advertising expenses was important to maximize the firm's profits. Bar counsel originally charged Davis and Goldberg with false or misleading advertising in violation of Rule 7.1. Does a lawyer who advertises that he will get clients "social security benefits *fast*" engage in false or misleading conduct by his *subsequent* failure to do so? As you see from the opinion above, the hearing officer found that the state had not met its burden of proof on the misleading advertising charge by clear and convincing evidence. We discuss the constitutional limits on regulating lawyer advertising in Chapter 10. The court in *Davis* ruled that the close connection between mass advertising and an unsustainable volume of cases constituted "conduct prejudicial to the administration of justice." Did the Alabama Supreme Court essentially find a Rule 7.1 violation through the back door of Rule 8.4(c)?

3. Is resignation the appropriate step for a lawyer to take when confronted with unprofessional office policies and working conditions? If so, had the associates at Davis & Goldberg been working in a state that recognized the so-called snitch rule,

Model Rule 8.3(a), would they also have had to inform the state bar on their way out the door? Is that a realistic expectation?

Davis v. Alabama State Bar: Real Life Applications

1. You serve as an associate at a large law firm. You are coordinating discovery in a complex commercial antitrust dispute. You uncover a letter in your client's files that is arguably responsive to the request for production of documents, but it is also highly damaging. The letter is from an expert retained by the company to analyze the potential market for one of its new products. The partner who is supervising you on the case brusquely asks you to "withhold it" because the document is a "letter" and not a memorandum or report. How do you engage the partner in a discussion of this discovery issue to assure yourself that you are complying with your professional obligations?

2. You are an associate specializing in patent litigation at a large law firm. The partner for whom you do most of your work calls you late one night to tell you that the son of an important client was arrested for disorderly conduct, being a minor in possession of alcohol, and assault and battery on a police officer. The partner asks you to go to court the following morning and represent the 20-year-old young man at his arraignment — even though you do not have one iota of criminal experience. The partner assures you that "the arraignment will be short and sweet — it's just a formality. Tell the client to plead not guilty and get a new date. We will refer the matter out to a criminal lawyer by the time of the pretrial conference." Can you cover the arraignment without violating Rule 1.1? If so, how do you prepare yourself?

3. You are a partner in a mid-size law firm specializing in commercial real estate matters. Your firm has not historically conducted a formal training program for new associates — relying instead on a "train as you go" model. In working closely with one particular new associate, you notice that the young lawyer does not maintain orderly files, and does not regularly document his communications with clients. None of the clients have yet complained, but you know that the associate's sloppy procedures will eventually reflect poorly on the firm. How do you address these deficiencies in a way that satisfies your obligations under Rule 5.1? Can you wait until the associate's annual performance review?

B. THE LAWYER'S INDEPENDENCE

Since the founding of the United States, an important ideal of lawyer professionalism has been a lawyer's independence.[3] Model Rule 2.1 requires lawyers to "exercise independent professional judgment and render candid advice."

---

3. Rebecca Roiphe traces this ideal of independence to Alexander Hamilton's statements in *The Federalist Papers*. *See* Rebecca Roiphe, *Redefining Professionalism*, 26 U. FLA. J.L. & PUB. POL'Y 193, 203 (2015).

What does **lawyer independence** mean? There are multiple potential facets to lawyer independence. As Bruce Green states, "[t]he term turns out to be elusive, in part because the various meanings seem to be inconsistent with each other or internally contradictory."[4] Nevertheless, certain meanings of lawyer independence are significant, and as Rebecca Roiphe contends, have "played an important role in American democracy."[5]

First, as noted in Chapters 1 and 2, United States lawyers have largely engaged in "self-regulation," which, as the Preamble to the Model Rules notes, "helps maintain the legal profession's independence from government domination." Indeed, a primary meaning of lawyer independence is independence from government control. This aspect of independence is essential to the lawyer's role in the United States justice system. Lawyers help ensure that government does not overstep its bounds or trample on clients' constitutional and other legal rights. By bringing suits on behalf of aggrieved individuals, lawyers are constantly challenging the legitimacy of government actions — from local and state government action (ranging from the police to governor), to Congress, to federal agencies and officials, including the President. Moreover, every appeal filed by an attorney is also a check on judicial power. Lawyer independence from and probing of government power has been an essential part of the success of our democratic experiment.

Even when government pays for lawyers, the lawyers must retain their independent professional judgment. For example, when Congress created the Legal Services Corporation, there was deep concern that lawyers hired by or accepting LSC funds would not be independent from their government employer in taking on cases for low-income clients. But such fears were unfounded. Lawyers hired by the LSC and accepting LSC funding understood their independence from the government and their loyalty to their clients.[6] In fact, Congress attempted to restrict the ability of LSC lawyers representing welfare recipients from making any arguments challenging the validity of existing welfare law. In Legal Services Corporation v. Velazquez, 531 U.S. 533 (2001), the Supreme Court struck down such restrictions, explaining that the lawyer, even though funded by the government, "is not the government's speaker" but "speaks on behalf of the client in a claim against the government." Further, the Court indicated that a congressional restriction that forbade lawyers from challenging the validity of congressional laws also threatened the judiciary — the "primary mission" of which is to interpret the law and Constitution, "to say what the law is" — but which can only perform that mission when lawyers bring clients' claims or controversies to court. Congress could not "insulate" its laws from judicial review by restricting lawyer advocacy — even when Congress paid for those lawyers.[7] The Court touted the importance of lawyer independence: "An informed, independent judiciary presumes an informed, independent bar." *See id.* at 542-46.

---

4. Bruce Green, *Lawyers' Professional Independence: Overrated or Undervalued*, 46 AKRON L. REV. 599, 601 (2013).
5. *See* Roiphe, *supra* note 3, at 230.
6. *See id.* at 216-21 (describing the history of the LSC, the concerns about its independence, and that ultimately the LSC lawyers showed "fierce and combative independence" from the government).
7. *Velazquez*, 531 U.S. at 546 ("The restriction imposed by the statute here threatens severe impairment of the judicial function . . . [by] sift[ing] out cases presenting constitutional challenges in order to insulate the Government's laws from judicial inquiry.").

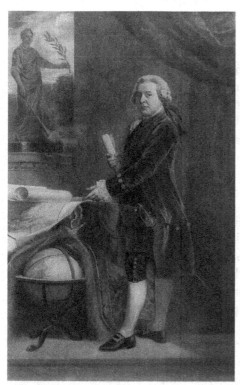 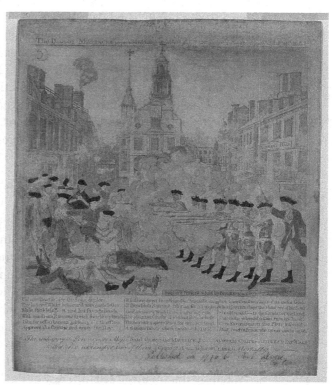

John Adams represented British soldiers involved in the Boston Massacre, ensuring a fair process despite his personal alignment with the revolutionary cause.
Library of Congress Prints and Photographs Division, Washington, D.C.

Going hand in hand with independence from government control is the idea of independence from popular opinion or prejudice. Lawyers recognize an obligation to undertake the representation of unpopular clients and causes[8] — to help in the protection of minority interests from majoritarian tyranny inherent in democracy[9] and to assist in the struggles of the poor and underserved against the wealthy and well-represented. Part of lawyer independence is a recognition that representing a client does not constitute an endorsement of the client's views or actions — it instead provides access to law despite popular suspicions. *See* Model Rule 1.2(b). As noted in Chapter 1, this tradition in the United States dates back to John Adams's representation of British soldiers who were tried for their role in the Boston Massacre.

Lawyer independence from popular opinion and prejudice is a type of individual lawyer independence from pressure by third parties. Model Rule 5.4(c) expresses another aspect of independence from third parties — namely loyalty to the client when a lawyer is paid, recommended, or employed by a third party. According to Rule 5.4(c), lawyers must not allow that third person to "direct or regulate the lawyer's professional judgment in rendering such legal services."

Finally, independence also denotes the lawyer's independence from her own client. A lawyer is an officer of the court, who has sworn to uphold state and federal constitutions and has independent obligations to the rule of law, to the profession,

---

8. *See* Model Rule 6.2 cmt. [1] (noting lawyer responsibility to accept "a fair share of unpopular matters or indigent or unpopular clients").

9. *See* THE FEDERALIST No. 10 (James Madison) (expressing concern that "measures are too often decided, not according to the rules of justice and the rights of the minor party, but by the superior force of an interested and overbearing majority").

and to the public good. While representing a client is not an endorsement of that client's views, nevertheless, the lawyer must resist pressure from the client to disregard the lawyer's legal and ethical obligations. Each lawyer is independently obligated to follow the Rules of Professional Conduct and uphold the law. Just as junior lawyers cannot rely on unethical instructions of supervising lawyers, a lawyer cannot advise or assist a client in conduct that is criminal or fraudulent or a violation of the rules — despite a client's wishes for the lawyer to do so. Even as the advocate of the client, the lawyer retains her own essential independence.

1. Independence from Non-Lawyers in Practicing Law

In addition to the conceptions of independence outlined above, the ABA has maintained as an enforceable part of lawyer independence a requirement that, in practicing law, lawyers cannot go into business with non-lawyers. This restriction is reiterated in three basic prohibitions found in Model Rule 5.4: (1) a prohibition on multidisciplinary practice; (2) a prohibition on sharing fees with non-lawyers; and (3) a prohibition on non-lawyer ownership or direction of law firms. Many commentators have decried the ABA's and state bars' insistence on this type of independence, which Green argues "equat[es] professional independence with professional isolation."[10] Historically, the creation of these restrictions was "transparently motivated by the financial self-interest of the bar's leadership" — specifically, to squelch "competition from corporations and, at least implicitly, to protect the profession's native-born, middle- and upper-class elite against competition."[11]

Indeed, Thomas Morgan contends that the prohibitions are outdated, as the practice of law has changed in the past 50 years from being almost exclusively individual lawyer provision of services to "institutional law practice" involving "the multi-person provision of legal services through organizations."[12] He argues that these prohibitions in Rule 5.4 should be liberalized in light of clients' modern needs for lower-cost bundled services and the fact that international firms in the United Kingdom and Australia are allowed to practice with non-lawyers and are competing with U.S. firms. Rather than prohibiting practice with non-lawyers, Morgan argues "the only sensible question is how to embrace it and make it better serve the public interest," including by regulating such businesses "to require competent service, protection of privileged information, and avoidance of conflicts of interest."[13]

As Green quips, the alleged fear driving these prohibitions is that, if allowed, "lawyers are likely to succumb to the improper influence of their nonlawyer[] allies, sell out their clients, divulge client confidences, represent clients ineptly, violate solicitation rules, and disregard their public obligations."[14] Green argues that the prohibitions on non-lawyer alliances trivialize the important meanings of lawyer independence outlined above:

> In much of the bar's rhetoric in other contexts, the threats to the bar's independence come from the executive and legislative branches of government or the general public.

---

10. Bruce A. Green, *The Disciplinary Restrictions on Multidisciplinary Practice, Their Derivation, Their Development, and Some Implications for the Core Values Debate*, 84 Minn. L. Rev. 1115 (2000).
11. *See id.* at 1145, 1157.
12. Thomas D. Morgan, *The Rise of Institutional Law Practice*, 40 Hofstra L. Rev. 1005, 1008 (2012).
13. *See id.* at 1020, 1026.
14. *See* Green, *supra* note 10, at 1117.

In the one ethics rule with "independence" in its title, these threats are not identified; nor are lawyers encouraged to stare them down. Rather, the enemy at the gate of independence is envisioned as . . . accountants! The rule trivializes the ideal of professional independence as it diminishes legal professionals. Surely, the bar could project a loftier ideal of independence and express greater confidence in lawyers' fortitude.[15]

Despite such critics, in all U.S. jurisdictions except Washington, D.C., the prohibitions remain on multidisciplinary practice, fee-sharing with non-lawyers, and non-lawyer investment or management of law firms.

Multidisciplinary Practice

Model Rule 5.4(b) prohibits lawyers from "form[ing] a partnership with a non-lawyer if any of the activities of the partnership consist of the practice of law." This rule prohibits **multidisciplinary practices (MDPs)** — that is, businesses that offer bundled services that include the practice of law in addition to other professional services, such as accounting, banking, insurance, public relations, securities dealing, financial planning, etc. Under Model Rule 5.4, lawyers are prohibited from forming MDPs with non-lawyer professionals offering related services. The ABA has considered proposals to change this rule twice since 2000 and rejected it both times, relying on the importance of lawyer independence.[16]

Sharing Fees with Non-Lawyers

With a few narrow exceptions, Rule 5.4(a) prohibits the sharing of legal fees with non-lawyers. The exceptions are limited to (1) paying to the estate or heirs of a deceased lawyer fees owed to that lawyer or money obtained from the sale of that lawyer's law practice; (2) including "nonlawyer employees in a compensation or retirement plan"; and (3) sharing "court-awarded legal fees with a nonprofit organization" that "employed, retained or recommended" the lawyer. The narrowness of these exceptions is blatant. Lawyers generally cannot share fees with non-lawyers — even if the non-lawyer recommended the lawyer or greatly assisted the lawyer in the representation. Non-lawyers include paralegals; secretaries; attorneys who have been suspended or disbarred; attorneys on inactive status; and expert consultants or investigators who assist with the representation.

Model Rule 5.4(a)'s restriction on sharing fees with non-lawyers for *recommending* the lawyer mirrors the restriction in Rule 7.2(b) that prohibits a lawyer from giving "anything of value to a person [lawyer or non-lawyer] for recommending the lawyer's services."[17] Rule 7.2(b) makes an exception, allowing lawyers to participate in a non-profit lawyer referral service that has been approved by the state bar or other regulatory agency.[18] Importantly, Rule 7.2(b) also allows lawyers to enter into a **reciprocal referral agreement** with non-lawyer professionals (or

---

15. Green, *supra* note 4, at 619.
16. *See* Morgan, *supra* note 12, at 1019.
17. Note, however, that Model Rule 7.2(b)(5) allows a lawyer "to give nominal gifts as an expression of appreciation that are neither intended nor reasonably expected to be a form of compensation for recommending a lawyer's services."
18. Model Rule 7.2 cmt. [6] ("A qualified lawyer referral service is one that is approved by an appropriate regulatory authority as affording adequate protections for the public.").

other lawyers), whereby the lawyer and the non-lawyer professional refer clients to each other — without paying each other for such referrals. Such a reciprocal referral agreement cannot be exclusive, and the referred client has to be informed "of the existence and nature of the agreement." *See* Model Rule 7.2(b)(4). Thus, despite Rule 5.4, a lawyer can enter into a reciprocal referral agreement with a non-lawyer professional (such as an accountant) as long as no one is being paid for the referral and the other conditions of Rule 7.2(b) are met.

In 2016, Avvo Legal Services, a for-profit corporation with non-lawyer officers and directors,[19] unrolled its online legal services program in 25 states.[20] The program matched lawyers with clients for limited services and charged a "marketing fee." Several bar associations responded by issuing ethics opinions concluding that lawyer participation in such a program violated the rules.[21] In 2018, Avvo was purchased by Internet Brands, which discontinued "Avvo Legal Services" as of July 31, 2018 — specifically shutting down Avvo's online fixed-fee legal services program in light of the pressure from state bars.[22]

Read the following opinion from the Pennsylvania Bar Association from 2016, and examine the several ways in which the bar association considered Avvo Legal Services — and any future company wishing to offer similar flat-fee limited-scope services online — to be a threat to a lawyer's exercise of independent professional judgment. Is allowing attorneys to practice with non-lawyers more difficult and a greater threat to independent professional judgment than indicated above by the critiques of Green and Morgan? Could the problems identified by the Pennsylvania Bar Association be alleviated through appropriate amendment of the rules to accommodate non-lawyer involvement and still enforce lawyer obligations regarding confidentiality, handling client property, limiting the scope of representation, etc.?

Ethical Considerations Relating to Participation in Fixed Fee Limited Scope Legal Services Referral Programs

Pennsylvania Bar Association Legal Ethics and Professional Responsibility Formal Opinion 2016-200 (2016)

I. SUMMARY

The Pennsylvania Bar Association Legal Ethics and Professional Responsibility Committee (the "Committee") has reviewed the potential ethics issues arising from lawyers participating in legal services referral programs meeting the following description:

---

19. *See* Avvo, *Leadership Team* (visited Mar. 9, 2017), *available at* https://www.avvo.com/about_avvo/leadership.
20. *See* Samson Habte, *Third Ethics Panel Dings Avvo Flat-Fee Referral Service*, Oct. 5, 2016, ABA/BNA LAW. MAN. ON PROF'L CONDUCT, Current Reports.
21. The opinions do not name Avvo Legal Services, but Josh King, Avvo's chief legal officer, said that it was clear that the opinions were about Avvo Legal Services. *See id; see also* Jason Tashea, *Avvo's Fixed-Cost Service to Be Discontinued by Internet Brands*, A.B.A. J., July 6, 2018, *available at* https://www.abajournal.com/news/article/accordingly_we_have_decided_to_discontinue_avvo_legal_services (noting that "Indiana, New Jersey, New York, Ohio, Pennsylvania, South Carolina and Utah have all ruled that lawyers participating in for-profit referral services, like Avvo Legal Services, violate state professional rules").
22. *See* Tashea, *supra* note 21.

A for-profit business (the "Business"), which is not a law firm or lawyer-owned, assists in pairing up potential clients seeking certain so-called "limited scope" or "unbundled" legal services with lawyers who are willing to provide such services for a flat fee, with the amount of the fee established by the Business. The client remits the full fee, in advance, to the Business. The Business then forwards the fee to the lawyer after confirming, according to its own procedures and standards, that the requested services were performed. The lawyer then separately pays the Business what is described as a "marketing fee" for each assignment completed. The so-called "marketing fee" charged regarding one type of service may represent a different percentage of the legal fee than the marketing fee charged for another type of service; but, in any event, the amount of the "marketing fee" varies directly with the amount of the flat fee for the legal services. In other words, the greater the amount of the flat fee, the greater the amount of the marketing fee, with the marketing fee typically ranging between 20% to 30% of the legal fee.

Based on this description, the Committee concludes that a Pennsylvania lawyer's participation in such a program (. . . a "Flat Fee Limited Scope" or "FFLS" program) would violate the following provisions of the Pennsylvania Rules of Professional Conduct ("RPCs"):

1. RPC 5.4(a), which generally prohibits sharing legal fees with non-lawyers; and
2. RPC 1.15(i), which requires legal fees paid in advance to be deposited in the lawyer's Trust Account.

Participation in such a program also poses a substantial risk that the lawyer could violate the following RPCs:

1. RPC 2.1, which requires a lawyer to exercise independent professional judgment;
2. RPC 5.4(c), which, in pertinent part, prohibits a lawyer from allowing a person who recommends a lawyer to direct or regulate the lawyer's professional judgment;

   [The opinion also lists RPC 5.3(c)(1) (lawyer responsible for conduct of non-lawyer); RPC 8.4(a) (lawyer cannot violate RPCs through the acts of another); RPC 1.16(d) (lawyer must refund unearned advance payment on termination); RPC 1.2(c) (lawyer can limit scope of representation only if reasonable and client provides informed consent); RPC 1.6(a) (confidentiality of information relating to the representation); RPC 7.7(a) (limiting lawyer referrals); RPC 5.5(a) (assisting unauthorized practice of law).]

II. ETHICAL CONSIDERATIONS RELATING TO FEE SHARING WITH NONLAWYERS AND PAYING FOR RECOMMENDING A LAWYER'S SERVICES

An obvious concern presented by the FFLS programs described above is whether they involve the sharing of legal fees with non-lawyers, which is prohibited under RPC 5.4(a). The Businesses which operate such programs, presumably in recognition of this concern, typically structure payment in such a way that the actual payment of funds by the client is not directly "shared" between the lawyer and the non-lawyer

Business. Instead, as described previously, the client pays a flat fee to the Business and, upon the Business supposedly verifying that the lawyer has earned the fee, the Business remits the full amount of the flat fee to the lawyer, typically by electronic bank transfer to the lawyer's operating account. Then, in an ostensibly separate transaction, the Business collects its marketing fee related to the completed assignment from the lawyer, typically through a pre-authorized, monthly direct debit from the same operating account into which the fees are deposited.

The manner in which the payments are structured is not dispositive of whether the lawyer's payment to the Business constitutes fee sharing. Rather, the manner in which the amount of the "marketing fee" is established, taken in conjunction with what the lawyer is supposedly paying for, leads to the conclusion that the lawyer's payment of such "marketing fees" constitutes impermissible fee sharing with a non-lawyer.

Outright payment of referral fees to a non-lawyer would violate RPC 7.2(c), which prohibits a lawyer from giving "anything of value for recommending the lawyer's services." Comment [6] to RPC 7.2 explains that a "communication contains a recommendation if it endorses or vouches for a lawyer's credentials, abilities, competence, character, or other professional qualities." One FFLS program website lauds all participating lawyers with such terms and descriptions as "highly rated," "top reviewed," "qualified," "experienced," and "licensed to practice anywhere in your state." The individual lawyer profiles prominently feature "star" ratings, on a scale of one to five stars, based on client reviews, as well as the lawyer's score under the program operator's proprietary, "1 to 10" numerical rating system. The profiles also include excerpts from client reviews. Such communications fit the definition of "recommendations" in the Comment to RPC 7.2. . . .

[In any event], payments to a lawyer referral service remain subject to RPC 5.4(a)'s prohibition against sharing fees with non-lawyers. Ethics opinions that have considered similar compensation arrangements have concluded that marketing, advertising, or referral fees paid to for-profit enterprises that are based upon whether a lawyer received any matters, or how many matters were received, or how much revenue was generated by the matters, constitute impermissible fee sharing under RPC 5.4(a). For example, Ohio Opinion 2016-3, which addresses the same types of FFLS programs discussed in this Opinion, states that "a fee-splitting arrangement that is dependent upon the number of clients obtained or the legal fee earned does not comport with the Rules of Professional Conduct." S.C. Opinion 16-06, which also addressed a FFLS program, reached the same conclusion. . . .

. . . The proponents of FFLS programs have also claimed that the lawyer's payment of marketing fees which vary based upon (1) the number of matters received, and (2) on the amount of legal fees generated by those matters, is not impermissible fee sharing, because such payments supposedly do not interfere with the lawyer's professional independence. Even if this were accurate, it would not be dispositive of the issue. Moreover, while the premise that the primary policy underlying RPC 5.4(a) is the preservation of the lawyer's professional independence is valid, the assumption that the lawyer's payment to a non-lawyer of marketing fees amounting to 20% to 30% of legal fees earned does not interfere with the lawyer's professional independence is, at a minimum, of questionable validity. As discussed elsewhere in this Opinion, there are a number of aspects of the FFLS programs that pose a substantial risk of interfering with a lawyer's professional independence.

. . .

III. ETHICAL CONSIDERATIONS RELATING TO HANDLING OF CLIENT FUNDS

As discussed above, the non-lawyer Business collects the client's advance fee payment prior to commencement of the lawyer-client relationship and then retains the advance fee until the Business concludes, to its satisfaction, that the fees have been earned by, and should be remitted to, the lawyer. This poses several ethical issues. Such an arrangement effectively, and exclusively, delegates to a non-lawyer several critical decisions and functions that fall within the exclusive domain of the practice of law. This includes, for example, the decision whether the professional services the client requested of the lawyer have been satisfactorily completed, such that the advance fee has been earned by and is payable to the lawyer. Such delegation violates RPC 2.1, which requires a lawyer to exercise independent professional judgment, and RPC 5.4(c), which prohibits a lawyer from allowing a person who recommends, employs or pays the lawyer to render legal services for another to direct or regulate the lawyer's professional judgment in rendering such legal services.

In at least some circumstances, the Business [] consider[s] the completion of a telephone call between the lawyer and the client on the Business's phone system (which apparently does not monitor content) as alone sufficient to establish that the advance fee has been "earned" and can be remitted to the lawyer's operating account. Clearly, a lawyer would not be permitted to make this determination in such a mechanistic fashion. . . .

These problems highlight a broader issue with the FFLS programs: The delegation of the possession and distribution of advance fee payments to a non-lawyer violates RPC 1.15(i), which provides:

> A lawyer shall deposit into a Trust Account legal fees and expenses that have been paid in advance, to be withdrawn by the lawyer only as fees are earned or expenses incurred, unless the client gives informed consent, confirmed in writing, to the handling of fees and expenses in a different manner.

The only way to rectify the issues discussed above would be for the Business to immediately remit advance fee payments to the lawyer, for deposit in the lawyer's Trust Account, as defined in RPC 1.15(a)(11), as soon as a lawyer-client relationship is established. This would not only comply with RPC 1.15(i), but would also allow the lawyer to independently fulfill his or her non-delegable obligations with respect to the disposition of the funds, as required under RPCs 2.1, 5.4(c), and 1.16(d). However, as presently constituted, the FFLS programs do not accommodate this requirement.

IV. ETHICAL CONSIDERATIONS RELATING TO "LIMITED SCOPE" REPRESENTATION

"Limited scope" representation is authorized under RPC 1.2(c). . . . The two operative requirements for limited scope representation are that (1) the limitation be "reasonable," and (2) "the client gives informed consent." When a prospective client contacts a Business operating a FFLS program seeking legal assistance, the Business, as a non-lawyer, cannot properly assess whether the limited scope legal services the prospective client seeks are appropriate for the client, or that the limitations on the scope of the representation offered through the FFLS program would be "reasonable" within the meaning of RPC 1.2(c), given the prospective client's particular circumstances. The Business cannot secure the prospective client's informed consent to the limitations to the representation, because this is also a nondelegable responsibility of the lawyer who ultimately undertakes the representation.

. . .

In theory, at least, it would be possible for a lawyer who decides to accept a FFLS program referral to fulfill these obligations. . . . [H]owever, given the time and financial constraints imposed by of [*sic*] the FFLS programs, it will be challenging, if not impossible, for a lawyer to make the necessary assessment of the appropriateness and reasonableness of the limited scope assignment, to secure the client's informed consent to such limitations, and to then provide the requested professional services. . . .

The burden on the lawyer to verify the appropriateness of the "limited scope" services to meet the client's needs, as well as the reasonableness of the limitation on the scope of services to be provided, is further heightened by the broad and vague descriptions of limited scope services that are offered on a flat fee basis through a typical FFLS program operator, such as: Document Review; Create a Termination Letter; Create a Business Contract; Create an Operating Agreement; Create a Business Partnership; Create an Asset Purchase Agreement; Create an Estate Plan Bundle; Create a Living Trust Bundle (Couple); Create a Parenting Plan; and Create a Commercial Lease Agreement. Even if the prospective client selects the correct general category of service, the prospective client's perception of what is needed may differ from what is actually required, and the lawyer would have no way of ascertaining the scope and magnitude of the effort required to meet the prospective client's true needs until after speaking with the client, possibly at great length.

This is not to mention that the lawyer must also conduct a proper conflict check which, in most cases, cannot be completed until the lawyer is in direct communication with the prospective client.

. . .

VI. ETHICAL CONSIDERATIONS RELATING TO CONFIDENTIALITY

The structure of the FFLS programs exposes the Business to significant information that would ordinarily be considered confidential under RPC 1.6(a). . . . RPC 1.6(a) prohibits a lawyer from "revealing" confidential information, subject to various exceptions. Under the FFLS program, it is the prospective client who chooses to reveal the information described above to the Business, and that choice is made before the lawyer-client relationship has even been established. Therefore, the client's disclosure of information to the Business prior to formation of a lawyer-client relationship does not directly implicate the lawyer's duty of confidentiality under RPC

1.6(a). The program does, however, place information at risk of disclosure in future litigation, since the communications between the client and the Business would not be protected by the lawyer-client privilege.

With one exception, the FFLS program does not require, or anticipate, further disclosure of potentially confidential information to the Business once the lawyer-client relationship has been established. The one exception is that the Business must be informed, or at least reach the conclusion, that the assignment has been completed, in order to release the advance fee payment to the lawyer. The completion of the assignment, as well as the nature of the work performed is itself "information relating to representation of the client" subject to RPC 1.6(a). No exception to the prohibition against disclosure applies. Disclosure is not "impliedly authorized in order to carry out the representation." Rather, disclosure to the Business is merely the Business's externally-imposed condition to the lawyer's receipt of the client's advance fee payment, which has nothing to do with "carrying out the representation." . . . The lawyer could request the client's informed consent to the disclosure. . . .

. . .

IX. ACCESS TO LEGAL SERVICES

Operators of FFLS programs argue that "unbundling" legal services reduces the cost to clients, thereby making legal services more accessible. Expanding access to legal services is, of course, an important goal that all lawyers, and the organized Bar, should support. However, the manner in which these FFLS programs currently operate raises concerns about whether they advance the goal of expanding access to legal services. Further, compliance with the RPCs should not be considered inconsistent with the goal of facilitating greater access to legal services.

Any lawyer can offer "unbundled" or "limited scope" legal services at, or even below, the rates prescribed by an FFLS program, provided the lawyer can do so in a manner that complies with his or her professional and ethical obligations, including the obligation of competence (see RPC 1.1) and full disclosure of and informed consent to any limitations on the scope of the legal services rendered. If a lawyer cannot fulfill those obligations working outside the scope of an FFLS program, he or she almost certainly would not be able to do so working within such a program. If anything, services offered through FFLS programs would be expected to be even more costly than they otherwise would have to be, because of the burden of substantial "marketing fees" that vary in direct relation to the revenue derived from such legal services and that bear no relationship to the actual cost of any marketing services provided. . . .

Non-Lawyer Ownership or Direction of Law Firms

Rule 5.4(d) also prohibits lawyers from practicing law "for profit" in a business organization in which "a nonlawyer owns any interest therein," or a non-lawyer is an officer, director, or someone with similar managerial responsibility, or "a non-lawyer has the right to direct or control the professional judgment of a lawyer." For example, if Avvo had directly hired lawyers to provide the limited legal services it offered, those lawyers would be prohibited from engaging in the practice of law because Avvo had non-lawyer officers and directors.

Washington, D.C. has liberalized its version of Rule 5.4 to allow lawyers to practice in a business organization "in which a financial interest is held or managerial authority is exercised by an individual nonlawyer who performs professional services which assist the organization in providing legal services to clients." The D.C. rule requires, among other things, that non-lawyers "having such managerial authority or holding a financial interest undertake to abide by these Rules of Professional Conduct."[23]

In a similar vein, as part of Ethics 20/20, the ABA considered, but ultimately rejected, a proposal to amend the Model Rules to allow **Alternative Business Structures (ABSs)** with non-lawyer ownership and management. However, the percentage of non-lawyer ownership would be limited, with a recommended 25 percent maximum, so that any ABS would be controlled by lawyers owning a majority interest.[24] Thomas Morgan argues that the current rule, which absolutely prohibits non-lawyer investment in law firms, has negative effects — it "both denies law firms the ability to raise a potentially important form of capital and reduces the incentive a firm can give its members to help build the firm as an effective, ethical institution that would be attractive to outside investors."[25]

The state of Arizona is forging ahead to allow such innovations and non-lawyer investments. In rule amendments that will take effect January 2021, Arizona recently eliminated Rule 5.4, thus allowing fee-sharing between lawyers and non-lawyers. The rules also expressly authorize the creation and licensing of ABSs, specifically "recogniz[ing] that lawyers may provide legal services through firms that include nonlawyers as economic interest holders, owners, managers, shareholders, officers, or other nonlawyers who hold decision-making authority."[26] The Arizona rules nonetheless require that, in any licensed ABS, "legal services are *only* provided by persons authorized to do so and in compliance with the Rules of Supreme Court."[27]

2. Restrictions on Lawyer's Practice

Another area where state bars have asserted lawyer independence is in protecting the ability of individual lawyers to freely compete with other lawyers and change

---

23. *See* D.C. RULE OF PROF'L CONDUCT 5.4(b). The D.C. rule allows non-lawyer ownership or managerial authority but only if the following circumstances are met: (1) the sole purpose of the organization has to be the provision of "legal services to clients"; (2) the non-lawyer managers or interest-holders must "undertake to abide by these Rules of Professional Conduct"; (3) the lawyers with managerial or financial interest in the organization "undertake to be responsible for the nonlawyer participants to the same extent as if nonlawyer participants were lawyers under Rule 5.1"; and (4) these "conditions are set forth in writing." *See id.*

24. *See* Morgan, *supra* note 12, at 1020 and nn.100-08.

25. *See id.* at 1022.

26. *See* ARIZ. R. PROF'L CONDUCT, ER 5.3, cmt. 2021 Amendment, *available at* https://www.azcourts.gov/Portals/215/Documents/082720FOrderR-20-0034LPABS.pdf.

27. *See* ARIZ. R. SUP. CT. 31.1(c) (2021) (emphasis added), *available at* https://www.azcourts.gov/Portals/215/Documents/082720FOrderR-20-0034LPABS.pdf.

their practice or employment. Thus, Model Rule 5.6 prohibits **covenants not to compete** and other restrictions on an attorney's ability to practice law or compete after terminating employment with a firm or company as a lawyer.

Case Preview	## *In re Truman* If an associate decides to leave a law firm, can the associate take firm clients with her? Can the law firm restrict the ability of the associate to do so? In *In re Truman*, a law firm attempted to do exactly that. As you read *In re Truman*, consider the following:

1. What is the court's rationale underlying the rule prohibiting restrictions on practice?
2. Did the associate's position in a law firm help him obtain these clients? If so, should the firm be able to restrict the ability of the associate to then take the clients with him?
3. How would it affect client choice of counsel if law firms could restrict the ability of departing lawyers from taking clients?

In re Truman
7 N.E.3d 260 (Ind. 2014)

We find that Respondent, Karl N. Truman, engaged in attorney misconduct by making an employment agreement that restricted the rights of a lawyer to practice after termination of the employment relationship. For this misconduct, we conclude that Respondent should receive a public reprimand. . . .

BACKGROUND

In October 2006, Respondent hired an associate ("Associate") to work in his law firm. As a condition of employment, Associate signed a Confidentiality/Non-Disclosure/Separation Agreement ("the Separation Agreement"). If Associate left the firm, the Separation Agreement provided that only Respondent could notify clients that Associate was leaving, prohibited Associate from soliciting and notifying clients that he was leaving, and prohibited Associate from soliciting and contacting clients after he left. The Separation Agreement also included provisions for dividing fees if Associate left the firm that were structured to create a strong financial disincentive to prevent Associate from continuing to represent clients he had represented while employed by the firm.

In October 2012, Associate informed Respondent that he was leaving the firm. At the time, Associate had substantial responsibility in representing more than a dozen clients ("Associate's Clients"). Respondent insisted on enforcing the terms of the Separation Agreement regarding these clients. Respondent sent notices to Associate's Clients announcing Associate's departure. Not all of the notices explained that these clients could continue to be represented by Associate if they so chose, and the notices did not provide clients with Associate's contact information. The Separation Agreement provided that Respondent would provide Associate's Clients with his contact information only if they requested it, and Respondent provided the information to any such clients who specifically requested it.

Despite the provisions of the Separation Agreement, Associate sent out notices to Associate's Clients that explained that the client could choose to be represented by Respondent or by Associate, and that included Associate's contact information. In response, Respondent filed a complaint against Associate seeking to enforce the Separation Agreement. A settlement was reached through mediation.

Immediately after the Commission began its investigation in this matter, Respondent discontinued his use of the Separation Agreement, and he has not enforced any similar provisions against any other former associates.

. . .

DISCUSSION

Indiana Professional Conduct Rule 5.6(a) is for the protection of both lawyers and clients. Comment [1] to this rule states: "An agreement restricting the right of lawyers to practice after leaving a firm not only limits their professional autonomy but also limits the freedom of clients to choose a lawyer." The Separation Agreement hampered both Associate's right to practice law and Associate's Clients' freedom to choose a lawyer by restricting Associate's ability to communicate with the clients and creating an unwarranted financial disincentive for Associate to continue representing them.

The Ohio Supreme Court recently addressed a similar situation. In that case, an attorney's employment agreement with his associates restrained them from taking clients with them when the associates left the attorney's firm by requiring a departing associate to remit to the attorney 95% of the fees generated in a case involving a former firm client, regardless of the proportion of the work that the attorney and the associate performed on the client's case. The Ohio Supreme Court found that the attorney violated Ohio's Professional Conduct Rules 5.6 and 1.5 (prohibiting excess fees) and approved an agreed public reprimand. *See* Cincinnati Bar Assn. v. Hackett, 950 N.E.2d 969 (2011). A client's "absolute right to discharge an attorney or law firm at any time, with or without cause, subject to the obligation to compensate the attorney or firm for services rendered prior to the discharge[,] . . . would be hollow if the discharged attorney could prevent other attorneys from assuming the client's representation." *Id.* at 970. . . .

The Court concludes that Respondent violated Indiana Professional Conduct Rule 5.6(a) by making an employment agreement that restricted the rights of a lawyer to practice after termination of the employment relationship. For Respondent's professional misconduct, the Court imposes a public reprimand.

Post-Case Follow-Up

Truman represents the majority approach to restrictions on lawyer practice. Nevertheless, a number of jurisdictions do allow a law firm to enter into employment and partnership agreements that impose "reasonable" financial disincentives for terminating employment and taking firm clients. A leading case is Howard v. Babcock, 863 P.2d 150, 156 (Cal. 1993), in which the Supreme Court of California asserted that "a revolution in the practice of law has occurred requiring economic interests of the law firm to be protected as they are in other business enterprises." The court argued:

> It seems to us unreasonable to distinguish lawyers from other professionals such as doctors or accountants, who also owe a high degree of skill and loyalty to their patients and clients. The interest of a patient in a doctor of his or her choice is obviously as significant as the interest of a litigant in a lawyer of his or her choosing. Yet for doctors, reasonable noncompetition agreements binding upon withdrawing partners are permitted.[28]

Quoting Justice Rehnquist, the court noted that "[i]nstitutional loyalty appears to be in decline." Thus, one of the "changes rocking the legal profession is the propensity of withdrawing partners in law firms to 'grab' clients of the firm and set up a competing practice." Seeking "to achieve a balance between the interest of clients in having the attorney of choice, and the interest of law firms in a stable business environment," the court held that "an agreement among partners imposing a reasonable cost on departing partners who compete with the law firm in a limited geographical area is not inconsistent with [the rules] and is not void on its face as against public policy." The court held that its "recognition of a new reality in the practice of law" would not have a "deleterious effect on the current ability of clients to retain loyal, competent counsel of their choice." *See id.* at 157-61.

In re Truman: Real Life Applications

1. Jason is hired as in-house counsel for We Care, Inc. We Care has Jason sign an employment contract that contains the following clause: "During employment and for one year after termination of employment, employee agrees to not accept employment or provide any services to a competitor of We Care, Inc." Two years later, Jason receives a more lucrative job offer from The Caring Corp., a competitor of We Care. Can Jason accept the job at The Caring Corp.? If the agreement violates the rules, does that make it unenforceable?

2. Maria is a 61-year-old partner at the law firm of Morgan & Taylor, where she has practiced for 32 years. Maria is asked by the other partners to resign. Maria resigns and begins to receive monthly retirement benefits from Morgan & Taylor.

---

28. *Howard*, 863 P.2d at 160.

Maria would like to continue practicing law and considers taking a position at another firm, Harris & Martinez. Maria is aware that under her partnership agreement with Morgan & Taylor, a person is only eligible for retirement benefits if a person is (1) over 60 years of age; (2) has been associated with Morgan & Taylor for more than 30 years; and (3) has ceased practicing law. Indeed, the agreement states that if a person receiving retirement benefits resumes practicing law, then she must refund any retirement benefits received. Is Morgan & Taylor's restriction on receiving retirement benefits in violation of Rule 5.6?

3. Sale of a Law Practice

Traditionally, the sale of a law practice was viewed as unethical — because law was perceived to be a profession involving lawyer loyalty to individual clients rather than a business. In 1990, Model Rule 1.17 was adopted to allow an attorney who is leaving the practice of law (or a certain practice area) to sell his practice. Nevertheless, Rule 1.17 places rigid restrictions on such a sale, only allowing sales under limited and specific conditions. Indeed, comment [1] reiterates the rationale for the traditional prohibition: "The practice of law is a profession, not merely a business" and "[c]lients are not commodities that can be purchased and sold at will."

Under Rule 1.7, a lawyer can only sell a law practice (or an area of practice) — and a lawyer can only buy one — if all of the following conditions are met: (1) the seller must cease practicing law or practicing the specific area of law in that jurisdiction; (2) the seller must be selling the entire law practice or entire area of practice; (3) the seller has to provide a specified notice to clients; and (4) the fees charged to clients cannot be increased because of the sale.

Notably, the first condition is a significant limitation on the right to sell a law practice. Only if a lawyer is planning to stop entirely practicing law or a given area of law can the lawyer sell her practice. There are several situations where this could happen beyond retirement. For example, a lawyer could become a judge or take another public office requiring him to forgo law practice. In addition, a lawyer may move to a different jurisdiction, and the rule allows a lawyer to sell her law practice in the jurisdiction from which she is moving. Further, even in the same jurisdiction, comment [2] clarifies that a lawyer who sells his practice can accept subsequent employment "as a lawyer on the staff of a public agency or a legal services entity that provides legal services to the poor, or as in-house counsel to a business." Further, a lawyer is permitted to sell off just one area of her practice, but the lawyer "must cease accepting any matters in the area of practice that has been sold."[29] The rationale for requiring attorneys to sell the entire practice or area of practice (rather than specific matters separately) is to protect "clients whose matters are less lucrative."[30]

Clients must be given written notice of the sale and be informed of their right "to retain other counsel or take possession of the file" rather than have their matter

---

29. Model Rule 1.17 cmt. [5].
30. Model Rule 1.17 cmt. [6].

undertaken by the purchasing attorney. Further, the notice must tell the client that the client's matter will be undertaken by the purchasing attorney if the client does not take other action within 90 days. If a client cannot be located, the transfer of the case to the purchasing attorney must be done by court order. *See* Model Rule 1.17(c).

C. UNAUTHORIZED PRACTICE OF LAW (UPL)

State law defines the "practice of law" and prohibits individuals who are not licensed from practicing law or holding themselves out as being able to practice law.[31] **UPL** is a crime in many states subjecting the violator to imprisonment and a fine. Depending on the jurisdiction, the prosecutor's office or the state attorney general's office may enforce UPL laws while state and local disciplinary counsel or bar committees may enforce court regulations barring UPL. UPL enforcement is a persistent concern for the profession; state and local bar associations have created committees to promote investigation and litigation of UPL. State supreme courts have established UPL boards to review UPL charges brought by bar counsel and to recommend sanctions for the courts' adoption. The level of UPL enforcement among states varies and depends upon a jurisdiction's resources and other pressing prosecutorial needs. In addition to civil and criminal penalties for UPL violations, a lawyer engaging or assisting another in UPL may face possible disciplinary sanctions. UPL is a concern not just for those who are not licensed to practice law in any jurisdiction but also for those lawyers who practice law in a jurisdiction where they are not licensed.

1. Justifications for the Professional Monopoly

The prohibition on the practice of law by non-lawyers is intended to "protect[] the public against rendition of legal services by unqualified persons."[32] Indeed, incompetent services performed by untrained lay people can and do cause great harm to the public. Immigrants, for example, have frequently been victimized by non-lawyer immigration consultants (sometimes known as "notarios") who charge large fees to process fraudulent or frivolous applications for them.

But many commentators have criticized UPL restrictions as being intended to protect lawyers from competition rather than the public from incompetent services. A broad prohibition on the unauthorized practice of law protects the profession's monopoly on the delivery of legal services by limiting competition and allowing lawyers to charge higher prices to the potential detriment of the public who might benefit from less expensive services offered by alternative service providers.[33] The Federal Trade Commission (FTC) has long advocated that "non-attorneys should

---

31. Model Rule 5.5(a) & cmt. [1]-[2].
32. Model Rule 5.5(a) cmt. [2]; RESTATEMENT (THIRD) OF THE LAW GOVERNING LAWYERS §2 [hereinafter Restatement].
33. Jack P. Sahl, *Cracks in the Profession's Monopoly Armor*, 82 FORDHAM L. REV. 2635, 2636, nn.4-5 (2014) (also citing Thomas D. Morgan, *The Evolving Concept of Professional Responsibility*, 90 HARV. L. REV. 702, 207 (1977), who asserts lawyers draft rules to promote their own interests in a self-regulatory context).

be permitted to compete with attorneys," particularly in areas "where no specialized legal knowledge and training is demonstrably necessary to protect the interests of consumers."[34] One area of focus for the FTC has been real estate closings: in some states, non-lawyers (real estate brokers and title agents, for example) may perform the critical tasks at real estate closings; in other states, however, only a lawyer may perform those functions even though no empirical evidence exists suggesting that the use of lawyers in real estate closings protects the public.[35] As Professor Deborah Rhode has argued, in the absence of "evidence of significant injuries resulting from lay assistance, individuals should be entitled to determine the cost and quality of legal services that best meet their needs."[36]

2. Defining the Practice of Law

What constitutes the practice of law is controversial. In 2002, the ABA chartered a task force on the subject, which proposed the following definition: "The practice of law is the application of legal principles and judgment with regard to the circumstances or objectives of a person that requires the knowledge and skill of a person trained in the law."[37] Under this broad standard, a real estate broker consulting with a client about which terms to include in a lease or a sales agreement and a coach advising a player about the terms and benefits of signing a specific agency or endorsement agreement all might constitute the practice of law. The following scenarios also are arguably covered by the ABA's broad standard: a non-lawyer neighbor advising a landowner about the legal meaning of a variance and assisting him in developing evidence and a strategy to obtain the variance; a mailman advising a friend about how to devise his estate and legally challenge an IRS audit; and a legal secretary or second-year law student informing a firm's client who plans to file for a divorce about the consequences of moving out of the marital residence.

The ABA Task Force ultimately abandoned its task of drafting a model definition of the practice of law and recommended that states develop their own definitions. Those definitions have provided little clarity beyond a few basic areas of agreement:

- In most jurisdictions, only lawyers may represent clients in court, draft certain legal documents, and hold themselves out as lawyers.
- All jurisdictions recognize the right of an individual to represent himself in litigation and in other non-litigation matters, such as negotiating and preparing

---

34. *See* Letter from the Fed. Trade Comm'n Office of Policy Planning to the Rules Comm. of the Superior Court 2 (May 17, 2007), *available at* https://www.ftc.gov/sites/default/files/documents/advocacy_documents/ftc-staff -comment-mr.carl-e.testo-counsel-rules-committee-superior-court-concerning-proposed-rules-definition -practice-law/v070006.pdf.

35. In a closely followed case, the Rhode Island Supreme Court upheld the right of non-lawyer title company employees to conduct residential real estate closings and prepare routine documents, such as residency affidavits and limited durable powers of attorney. The court held, however, that only a licensed attorney can conduct the examination of title for marketability and draft a deed. In reaching this conclusion, the court surveyed the various approaches taken by jurisdictions across the country. In re Paplauskas, 228 A.3d 43 (R.I. 2020).

36. Deborah L. Rhode, *Policing the Professional Monopoly: A Constitutional and Empirical Analysis of Unauthorized Practice Prohibitions*, 34 STAN. L. REV. 1, 98-99 (1981).

37. ABA Task Force on the Model Definition of the Practice of Law, Draft Report (Sept. 18, 2002), *available at* https://www.americanbar.org/groups/professional_responsibility/task_force_model_definition_practice_law/ model_definition_definition/.

a lease or a contract for the sale of personal property, or drafting a will.[38] This personal right, however, does not entitle the individual to assist others with their legal needs. In addition, in most states, a business association cannot proceed *pro se* but instead must be represented by counsel in court proceedings.

■ By custom or explicit rule, states generally do not enforce unauthorized practice of law prohibitions against other professionals. For example, Texas specifically excludes licensed real estate agents from its unauthorized practice of law statute.[39]

■ Some jurisdictions permit limited practice by non-lawyers in particular contexts. For example, federal regulations permit non-lawyers to represent individuals before certain federal administrative agencies. Patent agents, for example, do not need to be lawyers. In Sperry v. Florida Bar, 373 U.S. 379 (1963), the Supreme Court prohibited Florida from enjoining a non-lawyer agent from preparing and prosecuting patents before the U.S. patent office when both a federal statute and USPTO rules authorized non-lawyers to perform this work. Even though the agents' work constituted the practice of law in Florida, the Supremacy Clause prohibited the state from interfering with the "accomplishment of the federal objectives."

■ Several states permit non-lawyers to perform various tasks in order to assist unrepresented litigants in navigating the court system. *See* Chapter 11.

■ In August 2020, the Utah Supreme Court announced that it was establishing a "pilot legal regulatory sandbox." The sandbox, to be overseen by a newly created Office of Legal Services Innovation, would "allow individuals and entities to explore creative ways to safely allow lawyers and non-lawyers to practice law."[40] Other states, including Arizona and California, are considering similar innovations.

Beyond that, however, what constitutes the practice of law is a gray area, and most states' definitions sweep just as broadly as the ABA's proposed definition. State definitions of the practice of law are also notoriously circular and vague. For example, the District of Columbia defines the practice of law, in part, to include

> ## Formalities of the Practice of Law
>
> In *Florida Bar v. Brumbaugh*, discussed on page 500, the Florida bar sued for an injunction against Marilyn Brumbaugh to prevent her from engaging in the unauthorized practice of law. Fla. Bar v. Brumbaugh, 355 So. 2d 1186 (Fla. 1978). In the late 1970s, Brumbaugh provided typing services for "do-it-yourself" uncontested divorces. *Id.* at 1190. For $50(!), Brumbaugh would prepare "all papers deemed by her to be needed for the pleading, filing, and securing of a dissolution of marriage, as well as detailed instructions as to how the suit should be filed, notice served, hearings set, trial conducted, and the final decree secured." *Id.*
>
> Brumbaugh never held herself out as a lawyer, and her ads were clearly directed to people seeking to obtain a divorce *pro se. Id.* In the course of the case, Brumbaugh was jailed for pleading the Fifth Amendment when she refused to answer the referee's questions. *Id.* Brumbaugh made sure to fly under the radar after the Florida Supreme Court ruled on her case, although she still provided forms, just without any advice. Kevin Spear, *Typist's Trade Is Divorce*, ORLANDO SENTINEL, Mar. 26, 1988, *available at* http://articles.orlandosentinel.com/1988-03-26/news/0030020242_1_divorce-papers-do-it-yourself-divorce-divorce-kits. She stated, "I'm paranoid and I think I always will be. I think I have been a threat to the legal system. All they would have to do is catch me giving legal advice, and I'd go back to jail." *Id.*

---

38. Restatement §4 cmt. d.
39. Tex. Bus. & Com. Code §83.001.
40. Utah Supreme Court Standing Order No. 15 (Aug. 14, 2020), *available at* http://www.utcourts.gov/utc/rules-approved/wp-content/uploads/sites/4/2020/08/final-utah-supreme-court-standing-order-no.-15.pdf.

the "provision of professional legal advice. . . ."[41] The Mississippi Supreme Court has said that "any exercise of intelligent choice in advising another of his legal rights and duties brings the activity within the practice of the legal profession."[42]

A current area of controversy is how UPL regulation applies to LegalZoom, Avvo, and other companies that deliver legal information, legal services, and other products on the Internet. To the extent that these companies provide legal information and legal forms to consumers without advising a particular consumer about his or her problem, they are in the clear. In New York County Lawyers' Ass'n v. Dacey, 234 N.E.2d 459 (N.Y. 1967), the New York Court of Appeals held that a non-lawyer had the right to publish his book *How to Avoid Probate!* because he was providing information about the law and not practicing law. Similarly, in Florida Bar v. Brumbaugh, 355 So. 2d 1186 (Fla. 1978), the Florida Supreme Court held that a non-lawyer "may sell printed material purporting to explain legal practice and procedure to the public in general . . . and sample legal forms." The court further held that she could type out those forms for her clients, though she could "not make inquiries nor answer questions from her clients as to the particular forms which might be necessary, how best to fill out such forms, where to properly file such forms, and how to present necessary evidence at the court hearings."

These modern businesses go far beyond merely providing legal information, however. LegalZoom, for example, uses interactive branching technology to help consumers complete wills, trademarks applications, incorporation papers, and many other legal documents. The company has been operating since 2001 and has served

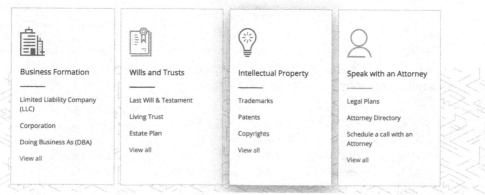

A current area of controversy is how UPL regulation applies to LegalZoom, Avvo, and other companies that deliver legal information, legal services, and other products on the Internet.
avvo.com

---

41. D.C. App. R. 49.
42. Darby v. Miss. State Board of Bar Admissions, 185 So. 2d 684 (Miss. 1966).

millions of customers notwithstanding a number of UPL lawsuits across the country. In one case, *Janson v. LegalZoom*, 82 F. Supp. 2d 1053 (W.D. Mo. 2011), a federal district court held that LegalZoom was engaged in the unauthorized practice of law. The court seemed to be particularly troubled by the fact that non-lawyer employees were reviewing the legal documents for completeness, spelling, grammatical errors, consistency, and formatting. But the parties subsequently settled that litigation with LegalZoom making some changes to its business model. Similarly, in Opinion 2016-200 (excerpted above) regarding Avvo's legal services program, the Pennsylvania Bar Association opined that lawyers who participated in the program would possibly violate Rule 5.5 by assisting non-lawyers in the unauthorized practice of law, inasmuch as the non-lawyer operators of the program make initial "judgments and decisions which are only appropriately made by lawyers."

In 2015, LegalZoom also settled a dispute with the North Carolina bar in which the bar had said that LegalZoom was engaged in the unauthorized practice of law, and LegalZoom had countered with antitrust claims. Under the settlement, LegalZoom agreed to submit its documents for review by a North Carolina lawyer and inform its customers that their use of LegalZoom's templates is not a substitute for the advice of an attorney. In return, the state bar agreed to support legislation to clarify the definition of "unauthorized practice of law." The parties also agreed to support legislation permitting interactive legal-help websites.[43] On the heels of these settlements, the tide of litigation against LegalZoom seems to have slowed. And in Utah's new "legal regulatory sandbox," companies that deliver legal services can be specifically approved to provide those services by the new Office of Legal Services Innovation.

D. MULTIJURISDICTIONAL PRACTICE (MJP)

For several decades, lawyers have increasingly practiced in multiple jurisdictions as they try to meet clients' needs across state and national borders. Advances in technology help facilitate MJP as lawyers can more easily communicate and deliver services across territorial boundaries. Is it a problem for a lawyer who is a member of the Pennsylvania Bar to help a client in Florida? Lawyers generally did not worry about this issue until the California Supreme Court gave them a wakeup call.

Case Preview

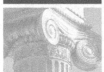

Birbrower, Montalbano, Condon & Frank v. Superior Court

In 1992 and 1993, two lawyers at Birbrower, a New York law firm, represented ESQ, a California client with its principal place of business in California. No Birbrower lawyer was licensed in California at that time. In 1992, the law firm and ESQ signed a retention agreement in New York obligating the

---

43. Terry Carter, *LegalZoom Resolves $10.5M Antitrust Suit Against North Carolina State Bar*, A.B.A. J., Oct. 23, 2015, *available at* http://www.abajournal.com/news/article/legalzoom_resolves_10.5m_antitrust_suit_against_north_carolina_state_bar. In October 2019, LegalZoom settled yet another lawsuit — this time the case was brought by a

firm to provide legal services, including representing ESQ in the investigation and pursuit of all claims against Tandem Computers Incorporated, a Delaware corporation with its principal place of business in Santa Clara. The dispute involved a software development and marketing contract between ESQ and Tandem. The contract provided that California law would govern the validity of the agreement and related claims. After ESQ settled the case, it sued Birbrower for malpractice and related claims, and the firm filed a counterclaim for unpaid fees. ESQ argued that the fee agreement was unenforceable because Birbrower engaged in the unauthorized practice of law in California.

As you read the *Birbrower* decision, ask yourself:

1. What constitutes the practice of law in California?
2. What actions by the Birbrower lawyers constituted the practice of law in California?
3. What purpose does the enforcement of California's UPL statute against the Birbrower lawyers serve?

Birbrower, Montalbano, Condon & Frank v. Superior Court
949 P.2d 1 (Cal. 1998)

CHIN, J.

. . .

The facts with respect to the unauthorized practice of law question are essentially undisputed. Birbrower is a professional law corporation incorporated in New York, with its principal place of business in New York. During 1992 and 1993, Birbrower attorneys, defendants Kevin F. Hobbs and Thomas A. Condon (Hobbs and Condon), performed substantial work in California relating to the law firm's representation of ESQ. Neither Hobbs nor Condon has ever been licensed to practice law in California. None of Birbrower's attorneys were licensed to practice law in California during Birbrower's ESQ representation.

ESQ is a California corporation with its principal place of business in Santa Clara County. In July 1992, the parties negotiated and executed the fee agreement in New York, providing that Birbrower would perform legal services for ESQ, including "All matters pertaining to the investigation of and prosecution of all claims and causes of action against Tandem Computers Incorporated [Tandem]." The "claims and causes of action" against Tandem, a Delaware corporation with its principal place of business in Santa Clara County, California, related to a software development and marketing contract between Tandem and ESQ dated March 16, 1990 (Tandem

---

business rival—that asserted, among other things, that LegalZoom engages in the unauthorized practice of law. *See* Blake Brittain, *LegalZoom, LegalForce Settle 'Trademarkia' Trademark Dispute*, Oct. 7, 2019, *available at* https://news .bloomberglaw.com/ip-law/legalzoom-legalforce-settle-trademarkia-trademark-dispute.

Agreement). The Tandem Agreement stated that "The internal laws of the State of California (irrespective of its choice of law principles) shall govern the validity of this Agreement, the construction of its terms, and the interpretation and enforcement of the rights and duties of the parties hereto." Birbrower asserts, and ESQ disputes, that ESQ knew Birbrower was not licensed to practice law in California.

While representing ESQ, Hobbs and Condon traveled to California on several occasions. In August 1992, they met in California with ESQ and its accountants. During these meetings, Hobbs and Condon discussed various matters related to ESQ's dispute with Tandem and strategy for resolving the dispute. They made recommendations and gave advice. During this California trip, Hobbs and Condon also met with Tandem representatives on four or five occasions during a two-day period. At the meetings, Hobbs and Condon spoke on ESQ's behalf. Hobbs demanded that Tandem pay ESQ $15 million. Condon told Tandem he believed that damages would exceed $15 million if the parties litigated the dispute.

Around March or April 1993, Hobbs, Condon, and another Birbrower attorney visited California to interview potential arbitrators and to meet again with ESQ and its accountants. Birbrower had previously filed a demand for arbitration against Tandem with the San Francisco offices of the American Arbitration Association (AAA). In August 1993, Hobbs returned to California to assist ESQ in settling the Tandem matter. While in California, Hobbs met with ESQ and its accountants to discuss a proposed settlement agreement Tandem authored. Hobbs also met with Tandem representatives to discuss possible changes in the proposed agreement. Hobbs gave ESQ legal advice during this trip, including his opinion that ESQ should not settle with Tandem on the terms proposed.

ESQ eventually settled the Tandem dispute, and the matter never went to arbitration. But before the settlement, ESQ and Birbrower modified the contingency fee agreement. The modification changed the fee arrangement from contingency to fixed fee, providing that ESQ would pay Birbrower over $1 million. The original contingency fee arrangement had called for Birbrower to receive "one-third (1/3) of all sums received for the benefit of the Clients ... whether obtained through settlement, motion practice, hearing, arbitration, or trial by way of judgment, award, settlement, or otherwise. ..."

In January 1994, ESQ sued Birbrower for legal malpractice and related claims in Santa Clara County Superior Court. Birbrower ... filed a counterclaim, which included a claim for attorney fees for the work it performed in both California and New York. ... ESQ moved for summary judgment ... argu[ing] that by practicing law without a license in California and by failing to associate legal counsel while doing so, Birbrower violated section 6125, rendering the fee agreement unenforceable. Based on these undisputed facts, the Santa Clara Superior Court granted ESQ's motion. ... The court concluded that: (1) Birbrower was "not admitted to the practice of law in California"; (2) Birbrower "did not associate California counsel"; (3) Birbrower "provided legal services in this state"; and (4) "The law is clear that no one may recover compensation for services as an attorney in this state unless he or she was a member of the state bar at the time those services were performed."

Although the trial court's order stated that the fee agreements were unenforceable, at the hearing on the summary adjudication motion, the trial court also observed: "It seems to me that ... if they aren't allowed to collect their attorney's fees here, I don't think that puts the attorneys in a position from being precluded from collecting all of their attorney's fees, only those fees probably that were generated by virtue of work that they performed in California and not that work that was performed in New York."

. . .

We granted review to determine whether Birbrower's actions and services performed while representing ESQ in California constituted the unauthorized practice of law under section 6125 and, if so, whether a section 6125 violation rendered the fee agreement wholly unenforceable.

II. DISCUSSION

A. *The Unauthorized Practice of Law*

The California Legislature enacted section 6125 in 1927 as part of the State Bar Act (the Act), a comprehensive scheme regulating the practice of law in the state. Since the Act's passage, the general rule has been that, although persons may represent themselves and their own interests regardless of State Bar membership, no one but an active member of the State Bar may practice law for another person in California. The prohibition against unauthorized law practice is . . . designed to ensure that those performing legal services do so competently.

. . .

Although the Act did not define the term "practice law," case law explained it as "'the doing and performing services in a court of justice in any matter depending therein throughout its various stages and in conformity with the adopted rules of procedure.'" [This court] included in its definition legal advice and legal instrument and contract preparation, whether or not these subjects were rendered in the course of litigation. [This court] later determined that the Legislature "accepted both the definition already judicially supplied for the term and the declaration of the Supreme Court that it had a sufficiently definite meaning to need no further definition. The definition . . . must be regarded as definitely establishing, for the jurisprudence of this state, the meaning of the term 'practice law.'"

In addition to not defining the term "practice law," the Act also did not define the meaning of "in California." In today's legal practice, questions often arise concerning whether the phrase refers to the nature of the legal services, or restricts the Act's application to those out-of-state attorneys who are physically present in the state.

Section 6125 has generated numerous opinions on the meaning of "practice law" but none on the meaning of "in California." In our view, the practice of law "in California" entails sufficient contact with the California client to render the nature of the legal service a clear legal representation. In addition to a quantitative analysis, we must consider the nature of the unlicensed lawyer's activities in the state. Mere fortuitous or attenuated contacts will not sustain a finding that the unlicensed lawyer practiced law "in California." The primary inquiry is whether the unlicensed lawyer engaged in sufficient activities in the state, or created a continuing relationship with the California client that included legal duties and obligations.

Our definition does not necessarily depend on or require the unlicensed lawyer's physical presence in the state. Physical presence here is one factor we may consider in deciding whether the unlicensed lawyer has violated section 6125, but it is by no means exclusive. For example, one may practice law in the state in violation of section 6125 although not physically present here by advising a California client on California law in connection with a California legal dispute by telephone, fax, computer, or other modern technological means. Conversely, although we decline to provide a comprehensive list of what activities constitute sufficient contact with the state, we do reject the notion that a person *automatically* practices law "in California" whenever that person practices California law anywhere, or "virtually" enters the state by telephone, fax, e-mail, or satellite. . . .

This interpretation acknowledges the tension that exists between interjurisdictional practice and the need to have a state-regulated bar. As stated in the American Bar Association Model Code of Professional Responsibility, Ethical Consideration EC 3-9, "Regulation of the practice of law is accomplished principally by the respective states. Authority to engage in the practice of law conferred in any jurisdiction is not per se a grant of the right to practice elsewhere, and it is improper for a lawyer to engage in practice where he is not permitted by law or by court order to do so. However, the demands of business and the mobility of our society pose distinct problems in the regulation of the practice of law by the states. In furtherance of the public interest, the legal profession should discourage regulation that unreasonably imposes territorial limitations upon the right of a lawyer to handle the legal affairs of his client or upon the opportunity of a client to obtain the services of a lawyer of his choice in all matters including the presentation of a contested matter in a tribunal before which the lawyer is not permanently admitted to practice."

. . .

Exceptions to section 6125 do exist, but are generally limited to allowing out-of-state attorneys to make brief appearances before a state court or tribunal. They are narrowly drawn and strictly interpreted. . . .

In addition, with the permission of the California court in which a particular cause is pending, out-of-state counsel may appear before a court as counsel pro hac vice. A court will approve a pro hac vice application only if the out-of-state attorney is a member in good standing of another state bar and is eligible to practice in any United States court or the highest court in another jurisdiction. The out-of-state attorney must also associate an active member of the California Bar as attorney of record and is subject to the Rules of Professional Conduct of the State Bar.

. . .

B. *The Present Case*

. . . As the Court of Appeal observed, Birbrower engaged in unauthorized law practice *in California* on more than a limited basis, and no firm attorney engaged in that practice was an active member of the California State Bar. As noted, in 1992 and 1993, Birbrower attorneys traveled to California to discuss with ESQ and others various matters pertaining to the dispute between ESQ and Tandem. Hobbs and Condon discussed strategy for resolving the dispute and advised ESQ on this strategy. Furthermore, during California meetings with Tandem representatives in August 1992, Hobbs demanded Tandem pay $15 million, and Condon told Tandem he believed damages in the matter would exceed that amount if the parties proceeded to litigation. Also in California, Hobbs met with ESQ for the stated purpose of helping to reach a settlement agreement and to discuss the agreement that was eventually proposed. Birbrower attorneys also traveled to California to initiate arbitration proceedings before the matter was settled. As the Court of Appeal concluded, ". . . the Birbrower firm's in-state activities clearly constituted the [unauthorized] practice of law" *in California.*

Birbrower contends, however, that section 6125 is not meant to apply to *any* out-of-state *attorneys.* Instead, it argues that the statute is intended solely to prevent nonattorneys from practicing law. This contention is without merit because it contravenes the plain language of the statute. Section 6125 clearly states that *no person* shall practice law in California unless that person is a member of the State Bar. The statute does not differentiate between attorneys or nonattorneys, nor does it excuse a person who is a member of another state bar. . . .

Birbrower next argues that we do not further the statute's intent and purpose — to protect California citizens from incompetent attorneys — by enforcing it against out-of-state attorneys. Birbrower argues that because out-of-state attorneys have been licensed to practice in other jurisdictions, they have already demonstrated sufficient competence to protect California clients. But Birbrower's argument overlooks the obvious fact that other states' laws may differ substantially from California law. Competence in one jurisdiction does not necessarily guarantee competence in another. By applying section 6125 to out-of-state attorneys who engage in the extensive practice of law in California without becoming licensed in our state, we serve the statute's goal of assuring the competence of all attorneys practicing law in this state.

. . .

Assuming that section 6125 does apply to out-of-state attorneys not licensed here, Birbrower alternatively asks us to create an exception to section 6125 for work incidental to private arbitration or other alternative dispute resolution proceedings. Birbrower points to fundamental differences between private arbitration and legal proceedings, including procedural differences relating to discovery, rules of evidence, compulsory process, cross-examination of witnesses, and other areas. As Birbrower observes, in light of these differences, at least one court has decided that an out-of-state attorney could recover fees for services rendered in an arbitration proceeding.

. . .

We decline Birbrower's invitation to craft an arbitration exception to section 6125's prohibition of the unlicensed practice of law in this state. Any exception for arbitration is best left to the Legislature, which has the authority to determine qualifications for admission to the State Bar and to decide what constitutes the practice of law. . . . In the face of the Legislature's silence, we will not create an arbitration exception under the facts presented.

Finally, Birbrower urges us to adopt an exception to section 6125 based on the unique circumstances of this case. Birbrower notes that "Multistate relationships are a common part of today's society and are to be dealt with in commonsense fashion." In many situations, strict adherence to rules prohibiting the unauthorized practice of law by out-of-state attorneys would be " 'grossly impractical and inefficient.' "

Although . . . we recognize the need to acknowledge and, in certain cases, to accommodate the multistate nature of law practice, the facts here show that Birbrower's extensive activities within California amounted to considerably more than any of our state's recognized exceptions to section 6125 would allow. Accordingly, we reject Birbrower's suggestion that we except the firm from section 6125's rule under the circumstances here.

C. Compensation for Legal Services

Because Birbrower violated section 6125 when it engaged in the unlawful practice of law in California, the Court of Appeal found its fee agreement with ESQ unenforceable in its entirety. Without crediting Birbrower for some services performed in New York, for which fees were generated under the fee agreement, the court reasoned that the agreement was void and unenforceable because it included payment for services rendered to a California client in the state by an unlicensed out-of-state lawyer. . . . We agree with the Court of Appeal to the extent it barred Birbrower from recovering fees generated under the fee agreement for the unauthorized legal services it performed in California. We disagree with the same court to the extent it implicitly barred Birbrower from recovering fees generated under the fee agreement for the limited legal services the firm performed in New York.

It is a general rule that an attorney is barred from recovering compensation for services rendered in another state where the attorney was not admitted to the bar. The general rule, however, has some recognized exceptions.

[The court found that none of the recognized exceptions applied to Birbrower.]

Birbrower asserts that even if we agree with the Court of Appeal and find that none of the above exceptions allowing fees for unauthorized California services apply to the firm, it should be permitted to recover fees for those limited services it performed exclusively in *New York* under the agreement. In short, Birbrower seeks to recover under its contract for those services it performed for ESQ in New York that did not involve the practice of law in California, including fee contract negotiations and some corporate case research. Birbrower thus alternatively seeks reversal of the Court of Appeal's judgment to the extent it implicitly precluded the firm from seeking fees generated in New York under the fee agreement.

We agree with Birbrower that it may be able to recover fees under the fee agreement for the limited legal services it performed for ESQ in New York to the extent they did not constitute practicing law in California, even though those services were performed for a California client. Because section 6125 applies to the practice of law in California, it does not, in general, regulate law practice in other states. Thus, although the general rule against compensation to out-of-state attorneys precludes Birbrower's recovery under the fee agreement for its actions in California, the severability doctrine may allow it to receive its New York fees generated under the fee agreement, if we conclude the illegal portions of the agreement pertaining to the practice of law in California may be severed from those parts regarding services Birbrower performed in New York.

. . .

In this case, the parties entered into a contingency fee agreement followed by a fixed fee agreement. ESQ was to pay money to Birbrower in exchange for Birbrower's legal services. The object of their agreement may not have been entirely illegal, assuming ESQ was to pay Birbrower compensation based in part on work Birbrower performed in New York that did not amount to the practice of law in California. The illegality arises, instead, out of the amount to be paid to Birbrower, which, if paid fully, would include payment for services rendered in California in violation of section 6125.

Therefore, we conclude the Court of Appeal erred in determining that the fee agreement between the parties was entirely unenforceable because Birbrower violated section 6125's prohibition against the unauthorized practice of law in California. Birbrower's statutory violation may require exclusion of the portion of the fee attributable to the substantial illegal services, but that violation does not necessarily entirely preclude its recovery under the fee agreement for the limited services it performed outside California.

Thus, the portion of the fee agreement between Birbrower and ESQ that includes payment for services rendered in New York may be enforceable to the extent that the illegal compensation can be severed from the rest of the agreement. . . .

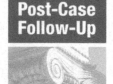

Post-Case Follow-Up

The *Birbrower* decision unsettled many lawyers who were already engaged in national and international cross-border practice, particularly given the court's expansive definition of practicing law *in California*. In the wake of the *Birbrower* decision, the ABA appointed the Multijurisdictional Practice (MJP) Commission in 2000 to study and report on the application of ABA ethics rules to multijurisdictional practice. Based on the MJP Commission's recommendations, in 2002 the ABA adopted amendments to Rule 5.5 that most states have adopted in some form.[44]

Rule 5.5(a) reiterates the fundamental principle that lawyers shall not practice law in a jurisdiction or assist another without being admitted to that jurisdiction's bar. Rule 5.5(b) prohibits lawyers from holding themselves out to others as being admitted to practice law or having an office or systemic presence in the jurisdiction for the practice of law. Rule 5.5(c) provides lawyers with four safe harbors to provide legal services on a temporary basis in jurisdictions where they are not admitted if (1) the non-admitted lawyer associates local counsel who actively participates in the matter; (2) the non-admitted lawyer's services are related to a pending or potential proceeding before a tribunal in which the lawyer is authorized or reasonably expects to be authorized to appear; (3) the services are reasonably related to a pending or potential arbitration, mediation, or other alternative dispute resolution proceeding and they arise out of or are reasonably related to the lawyer's practice in the jurisdiction in which he is admitted and do not require pro hac vice admission; and (4) the

---

44. Preface ABA MODEL RULES OF PROFESSIONAL CONDUCT, ABA COMPENDIUM OF PROFESSIONAL RESPONSIBILITY RULES AND STANDARDS 7 (2015) (reporting the ABA also amended Rule 8.5). Most jurisdictions have either adopted a rule identical to Model Rule 5.5 or a similar rule. STATE IMPLEMENTATION OF ABA MODEL RULE 5.5. *See* ABA, CPR Policy Implementation Committee, *Variations of the ABA Model Rules of Professional Conduct, Rule 5.5: Unauthorized Practice of Law; Multijurisdictional Practice of Law* (Feb. 20, 2020), *available at* http://www.americanbar.org/content/dam/aba/administrative/professional_responsibility/mrpc_5_5 .authcheckdam.pdf.

services are not covered by (c)(3) and (c)(4) but arise out of or are reasonably related to the lawyer's practice in the jurisdiction in which the lawyer is admitted.

Even after the changes to Rule 5.5, the extent to which a lawyer may practice law outside of her home state remains a gray area. Some situations are clear. First, a lawyer admitted in one state may not open an office in another state or engage in regular practice in that state without being admitted to practice law in that state. Second, lawyers in litigation matters can avoid a UPL claim by applying to a tribunal for pro hac vice status, a request to the court for authorization to represent a client in only the instant litigation before it. Once approved, the lawyer may engage in any activity a regularly admitted lawyer to the bar can undertake, for example, deposing witnesses and negotiating and drafting a contract or settlement related to the litigation.

There is no comparable procedure in transactional matters, however, and lawyers in non-litigation matters face uncertainty when they engage in practice across state lines. Under Model Rule 5.5(c)(4), these services are permissible if they are "reasonably related" to the lawyer's practice in his state of admission. The Restatement explains that several factors are relevant in determining that issue, including

> whether the lawyer's client is a regular client of the lawyer or, if a new client, is from the lawyer's home state, has extensive contacts with that state, or contacted the lawyer there; whether a multistate transaction has other significant connections with the lawyer's home state; whether significant aspects of the lawyer's activities are conducted in the lawyer's home state; whether a significant aspect of the matter involves the law of the lawyer's home state; and whether either the activities of the client involve multiple jurisdictions or the legal issues involved are primarily either multistate or federal in nature. Because lawyers in a firm often practice collectively, the activities of all lawyers in the representation of a client are relevant. The customary practices of lawyers who engage in interstate law practice is one appropriate measure of the reasonableness of a lawyer's activities out of state.[45]

Enforcement in multijurisdictional cases is erratic, but lawyers need to proceed with caution even when they are just doing favors for friends or family members. In In re Charges of Unprofessional Conduct in Panel File No. 39302, 884 N.W.2d 661 (Minn. 2016), the Minnesota Supreme Court issued a private reprimand to a Colorado lawyer who assisted his Minnesota in-laws when their condominium association attempted to collect a $2,368.13 judgment against them. The court found that by sending multiple emails "over several months, advis[ing] Minnesota clients on Minnesota law in connection with a Minnesota legal dispute and attempt[ing] to negotiate a resolution of that dispute with a Minnesota attorney," the Colorado lawyer had engaged in the practice of law in Minnesota even though he was not physically present in Minnesota. The court further concluded that the legal services provided were not related to the Colorado lawyer's environmental and personal injury practice in Colorado; therefore, he could not take advantage of the safe-harbor provision of Rule 5.5(c)(4).

---

45. Restatement §3 cmt. e. *See also* Model Rule 5.5 cmt. [14] (listing similar factors).

Birbrower, Montalbano, Condon & Frank v. Superior Court: *Real Life Applications*

1. A Pennsylvania-licensed lawyer has an office in Philadelphia. New Jersey is right across the river from Philadelphia, and the lawyer periodically gets inquiries from New Jersey clients. May the lawyer see clients from New Jersey in his Philadelphia office and advise them on issues of New Jersey law? May the lawyer open an office in New Jersey to better serve these clients?

2. A lawyer is admitted to practice and has an office in New York and practices in the area of trusts and estates. One of the lawyer's clients retires to Florida and calls the lawyer to request that she revise his will. The client also recommends his lawyer to his new neighbor in Florida, and the lawyer agrees to perform estate planning for the new client. Has the lawyer engaged in the unauthorized practice of law?

Chapter Summary

- Lawyers with managerial authority in a legal organization have a responsibility to create procedures, training programs, and reporting structures that promote compliance with ethical obligations by members of the organization.
- Supervisory lawyers will have vicarious responsibility for ethical missteps of subordinate lawyers if they order or ratify their conduct, or if they become aware of the conduct in time to prevent it and fail to do so.
- Professional independence of lawyers has manifold meanings, including independence from government control, independence from public opinion and prejudice, independence from third-party interference with the attorney-client relationship, and independence from one's own client.
- The Model Rules enforce professional independence from non-lawyers by prohibiting lawyers from going into business with non-lawyers, including prohibiting each of the following: multidisciplinary practice, fee-sharing with non-lawyers, and non-lawyer financial investments or direction of law firms.
- The Model Rules prohibit employment agreements that restrict a lawyer's ability to practice law; however, some jurisdictions allow reasonable restrictions on competition.
- A lawyer who is ceasing to practice law or to practice a particular area of law can sell that entire law practice or area of practice as long as certain conditions are met, including notice to affected clients.
- State law and the Model Rules generally prohibit non-lawyers from practicing law, though state definitions of the practice of law vary widely and are notoriously vague.

Applying the Rules

1. Shana works as a litigation associate at a boutique criminal defense firm. She is tasked with writing an appellate brief for a client convicted of first degree murder. In her draft brief, Shana cites and attempts to distinguish a prior decision of the state supreme court on an issue of law critical to the case. She provides the draft brief to the partner supervising the case. The partner provides her written feedback, suggesting that she delete the paragraph discussing the allegedly controlling precedent and stating that "we will distinguish that case at oral argument if the prosecutor relies on it in her brief." Shana disagrees with this recommendation by the partner. May she sign the brief?

2. You represent a claimant seeking social security benefits. The claimant was previously represented by an authorized non-attorney advocate. Upon completion of the representation, you are paid your fee, but are aware that the non-attorney advocate was not paid. You would like to give the non-attorney advocate the portion of the fee paid to you representing an appropriate amount for the non-attorney's initial work in the matter. Can you give the non-attorney advocate part of the fee? If not, do you have any other options to help the non-attorney receive her appropriate share?

3. Kyle is an attorney who is confused about a difficult area of procedural law. He asks Professor Robertson, his former Civil Procedure and Complex Litigation professor, for some guidance in handling the case. Professor Robertson — whose license is on inactive status in the jurisdiction — gives Kyle some very helpful suggestions for how to properly move forward. Kyle recovers a substantial fee in the case. Can Kyle give part of it to Professor Robertson? Should Professor Robertson have helped out with the case? What if Kyle had hired Professor Robertson as a consulting expert rather than asking for assistance as a lawyer?

4. Assume that a business, Arrow Legal Services (Arrow), offers a Flat Fee Limited Scope (FFLS) program, like that discussed in Pennsylvania Bar Association Opinion 2016-200. Arrow reviews the Pennsylvania opinion and decides to alter its program. The fee charged to the client is still held by Arrow until completion of the services by the lawyer, but rather than depositing the money into the attorney's own operating account, Arrow deposits the fee into the lawyer's client trust account. Then Arrow deducts the marketing fee from the operating account. The business leaves it up to the lawyer to withdraw the "earned" fee from the client trust account. Has Arrow avoided violating the rules by making this change?

5. A Texas-licensed lawyer moved to Wisconsin and opened a Michigan office but was denied admission to the Wisconsin and Michigan bars. The attorney subsequently was admitted to practice in the U.S. District Court for the Western

District of Michigan, where the local rule provides that "[a] person who is duly admitted to practice in a court of record of a state, and who is in active status and in good standing, may apply for admission to the bar of this Court. . . ." The lawyer limited his services to practicing law in federal court. Is he engaged in the unauthorized practice of law?

Professional Responsibility in Practice

1. Research whether the law in the state where you are planning to practice or are attending law school interprets Rule 5.6 to permit reasonable restrictions on lawyer practice and competition.

2. You are an associate in a law firm representing a corporation that is accused of fraud. You are responding to discovery and find a non-privileged document within the scope of the request that strongly indicates that your client is liable. You show the document to a partner who says, "Make that document go away." Consider how you should handle the situation. Draft an appropriate response to the partner.

3. Research the definition of "practice of law" and what activities constitute "unauthorized practice of law" in the jurisdiction where you plan to practice or are attending law school.

Marketing Legal Services

Lawyers need clients. Although lawyer marketing is often thought of as limited to personal injury lawyers making flashy television commercials, big firm lawyers also market their services through firm websites, blogs, and golf games with high-ranking corporate officers. In today's competitive legal market, moreover, lawyers in all areas of practice are taking advantage of new methods to market their services; in addition to websites and blogs, many lawyers use LinkedIn, Facebook, Twitter, and some are even creating apps or podcasts to attract clients.

The state bars have traditionally shown hostility to marketing, and, in the first half of the twentieth century, lawyer marketing was essentially prohibited. In a series of decisions beginning with *Bates v. State Bar of Arizona*,[1] however, the United States Supreme Court recognized that attorney advertising deserves protection as commercial speech and struck down overly restrictive advertising rules under the First Amendment.

The Rules of Professional Conduct today largely reflect the balance struck by the Court: lawyers have the right to market themselves in a truthful, non-deceptive manner, but, in the interest of protecting the public and the reputation of lawyers, states can continue to regulate (and, in some cases, prohibit) marketing that presents a danger of "fraud, undue influence, intimidation, overreaching, and other forms of vexatious conduct."[2] This chapter considers the constitutional doctrine that creates the backdrop for the rules of professional conduct governing lawyer marketing as well as the rules themselves.

Key Concepts

- Rules governing lawyer marketing and their constitutional limits
- **Communications/advertising** (marketing directed to a broad audience) treated differently than **solicitation** (targeted communication directed to a specific person)
- The application of the rules of professional conduct to modern forms of marketing

---

1. 433 U.S. 350 (1977).
2. Ohralik v. Ohio State Bar Ass'n, 436 U.S. 447, 462 (1978).

A. COMMUNICATIONS VS. SOLICITATION

Outside of the legal world, solicitation is generally understood as a form of advertising, but the Rules of Professional Conduct distinguish "solicitation" from all other communications about a lawyer's services and regulate them differently. The rules define "solicitation" as "communication initiated by or on behalf of a lawyer or law firm that is directed to a specific person the lawyer knows or reasonably should know needs legal services in a particular matter and that offers to provide . . . legal services for that matter."[3] While Rule 7.3 (Solicitation of Clients) prohibits lawyers (with some limited exceptions) from soliciting clients by "live person-to-person contact," lawyers may generally market their services subject to a number of conditions; principally, that the communications cannot be "false or misleading." In considering situations involving lawyer marketing, a lawyer must first decide whether the conduct is prohibited solicitation under Rule 7.3. If it is not, then the lawyer must consider whether the marketing is permissible under Rules 7.1 and 7.2, which govern all other communications about the lawyer's services.

B. REGULATION OF LAWYER ADVERTISING

In deciding how to market their services, lawyers must consult the Model Rules of Professional Conduct. These rules are shaped by four decades of Supreme Court decisions concerning the constitutionality of regulations governing lawyer marketing. This section considers that constitutional doctrine before turning to the rules governing lawyer advertising.

1. Constitutional Limits on the Bar's Power to Restrict Advertising

The 1908 ABA Canons reflected the organized bar's traditional attitude toward lawyer marketing: "It is unprofessional to solicit professional employment by circulars, advertisements, through touters or by personal communications or interviews not warranted by personal relations. Indirect advertisements for professional employment . . . and all other like self-laudation, offend the traditions and lower the tone of our profession and are reprehensible. . . ."[4] Proponents of restricting lawyer advertising typically argue that law is a "learned profession," not a trade or business, and that marketing demeans the reputation of the profession. In the first-half of the twentieth century, lawyer advertising was prohibited.

   In Bates v. State Bar of Arizona, 433 U.S. 350 (1977), however, the United States Supreme Court held for the first time that lawyer advertising is constitutionally protected commercial speech. The lawyers in *Bates* operated a low-cost legal clinic that offered routine legal services, such as uncontested divorces, uncontested adoptions, and simple personal bankruptcies. To support their practice, they

---

3. Model Rule 7.3(a).
4. MODEL CODE OF PROF'L RESPONSIBILITY Canon 27 (AM. BAR ASS'N 1908) (repealed 1963).

DO YOU NEED
A LAWYER?

LEGAL SERVICES
AT VERY REASONABLE FEES

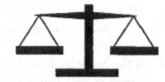

- **Divorce or legal separation--uncontested
  (both spouses sign papers)**

  $175.00 plus $20.00 court filing fee

- **Preparation of all court papers and instructions on
  how to do your own simple uncontested divorce**

  $100.00

- **Adoption--uncontested severance proceeding**

  $225.00 plus approximately $10.00 publication cost

- **Bankruptcy--non-business, no contested proceedings**

  Individual
  $250.00 plus $55.00 court filing fee

  Wife and Husband
  $300.00 plus $110.00 court filing fee

- **Change of Name**

  $95.00 plus $20.00 court filing fee

  **Information regarding other types of cases
  furnished on request**

Legal Clinic of Bates & O'Steen
**617 North 3rd Street
Phoenix, Arizona 85004
Telephone (502) 252-8838**

This is the advertisement that led to the U.S. Supreme Court's seminal decision in
Bates v. State Bar of Arizona, 433 U.S. 350 (1977).

placed an advertisement in a Phoenix newspaper stating that they offered "legal services at very reasonable fees," and listed their fees for certain services. At that time, Arizona prohibited all lawyer advertising.[5] In a 5-4 decision, the Court struck down Arizona's ban as it applied to the lawyers' "truthful advertis[ing] concerning the availability and terms of routine legal services."[6]

In a series of cases following *Bates*, the Court offered further constitutional protection to lawyers using truthful, non-deceptive marketing to promote their qualifications. In each of these cases, the Court held that states' attempts to discipline lawyers for such advertising was unconstitutional under the First Amendment. In *In re RMJ*, the Court held that a lawyer may advertise his areas of practice and where he is admitted to practice.[7] In *Peel v. Attorney Registration & Disciplinary Commission*, the Court found that a lawyer's letterhead could state that he was a "Certified Civil Trial Specialist" by the National Board of Trial Advocacy.[8] And in *Ibanez v. Florida Department of Business and Professional Regulation*, the Court held that the lawyer could promote her practice by stating in her marketing materials that she was a CPA and certified financial planner.[9]

In two other cases, the Supreme Court protected a lawyer's right to target her marketing to a particular group of clients with an identifiable legal problem. In *Zauderer v. Office of Disciplinary Counsel*, the Court upheld the constitutional right of a lawyer to run a newspaper ad announcing his willingness to represent women who had suffered injuries resulting from their use of a contraceptive known as the Dalkon Shield Intrauterine Device.[10] The advertisement featured a drawing of the device and stated that the Dalkon Shield had generated a large amount of lawsuits and that women should not assume that their claims were time-barred.[11] In *Shapero v. Kentucky Bar Ass'n*, the Court went even further in protecting lawyer marketing when it upheld the right of a lawyer to send direct mailings to potential clients who had foreclosure suits filed against them.[12] The letter advised potential clients that: "you may be about to lose your home"; "[f]ederal law may allow you to . . . ORDE[R] your creditor to STOP"; "you may call my office . . . for FREE information"; and "[i]t may surprise you what I may be able to do for you."[13] Since the letter did not constitute "face-to-face" communication, the Court treated it as advertising rather than solicitation and applied its commercial speech jurisprudence.[14] (As we will discuss later in this chapter, the Court has held that states may ban in-person solicitation by lawyers.) The Court held that the state could not categorically prohibit lawyers from soliciting business for pecuniary gain by sending truthful and non-deceptive letters to potential clients known to face particular legal problems.

The Supreme Court's latest opportunity to analyze the constitutionality of restrictions on lawyer marketing came in the 1995 case of *Florida Bar v. Went For It, Inc.*

---

5. *Bates*, 433 U.S. at 354-55.
6. *Id.* at 384.
7. 455 U.S. 191, 205-07 (1982).
8. 496 U.S. 91, 96, 110-11 (1990).
9. 512 U.S. 136, 143-49 (1994).
10. 471 U.S. 626, 630-31, 639-47 (1985).
11. *Id.* at 630-31.
12. 486 U.S. 466, 477-78 (1988).
13. *Id.* at 469.
14. *Id.* at 472-78.

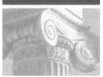

Case Preview

Florida Bar v. Went For It, Inc.

State advertising rules vary widely. In 1990, the Florida bar, which has been one of the most aggressive regulators of lawyer marketing, issued two novel rules that, in combination, prohibited plaintiffs' lawyers from contacting accident victims or their families for 30 days following the accident. In March 1992, lawyer G. Stewart McHenry, owner of a lawyer referral service called Went For It, Inc., brought suit to challenge the constitutionality of the regulation under the First Amendment.

The case is significant for at least three reasons. First, it serves as an example of the wide variety of ways in which states attempt to regulate lawyer advertising. Second, it illustrates the Court's most recent application of the commercial speech doctrine to lawyer advertising. Third, the majority opinion and dissent lay out some of the core policy arguments advanced on both sides of the lawyer advertising issue.

As you read the case, consider the following:

1. Is the direct mail at issue in this case "communication" or "solicitation" within the meaning of the Rules of Professional Conduct?
2. What test does the Court apply to the advertising rule at issue, and how does the Court apply that test in this case?
3. What were the state interests that the Florida bar was trying to protect?
4. How does the dissent differ from the majority concerning the policy behind this restriction on lawyer speech?

Florida Bar v. Went For It, Inc.
515 U.S. 618 (1995)

Justice O'CONNOR delivered the opinion of the Court.

Rules of the Florida Bar prohibit personal injury lawyers from sending targeted direct-mail solicitations to victims and their relatives for 30 days following an accident or disaster. This case asks us to consider whether such Rules violate the First and Fourteenth Amendments of the Constitution. We hold that in the circumstances presented here, they do not.

I

In 1989, the Florida Bar (Bar) completed a 2-year study of the effects of lawyer advertising on public opinion. After conducting hearings, commissioning surveys, and reviewing extensive public commentary, the Bar determined that several changes to its advertising rules were in order. In late 1990, the Florida Supreme Court adopted the Bar's proposed amendments with some modifications. . . . Two of these amendments are at issue in this case. Rule 4-7.4(b)(1) provides that "[a] lawyer shall not send, or knowingly permit to be sent, . . . a written communication to a prospective client for the purpose of obtaining professional employment if: (A) the written communication concerns an action for personal injury or wrongful death or otherwise relates to an accident or disaster involving the person to whom the communication is addressed or a relative of that person, unless the accident or disaster occurred more than 30 days prior to the mailing of the communication." Rule 4-7.8(a) states that "[a] lawyer shall not accept referrals from a lawyer referral service unless the service: (1) engages in no communication with the public and in no direct contact with prospective clients in a manner that would violate the Rules of Professional Conduct if the communication or contact were made by the lawyer." Together, these Rules create a brief 30-day blackout period after an accident during which lawyers may not, directly or indirectly, single out accident victims or their relatives in order to solicit their business.

In March 1992, G. Stewart McHenry and his wholly owned lawyer referral service, Went For It, Inc., filed this action for declaratory and injunctive relief in the United States District Court for the Middle District of Florida challenging Rules 4-7.4(b)(1) and 4-7.8(a) as violative of the First and Fourteenth Amendments to the Constitution. . . .

The District Court . . . entered summary judgment for the plaintiffs. . . . The Eleventh Circuit affirmed. . . . We granted certiorari . . . and now reverse.

II

A

Constitutional protection for attorney advertising, and for commercial speech generally, is of recent vintage. Until the mid-1970's, we adhered to the broad rule . . . that, while the First Amendment guards against government restriction of speech in most contexts, "the Constitution imposes no such restraint on government as respects purely commercial advertising." In 1976, the Court changed course. In Virginia Bd. of Pharmacy v. Virginia Citizens Consumer Council, Inc. . . . we invalidated a state statute barring pharmacists from advertising prescription drug prices. At issue was speech that involved the idea that " 'I will sell you the X prescription drug at the Y price.' " Striking the ban as unconstitutional, we rejected the argument that such speech "is so removed from 'any exposition of ideas,' and from 'truth, science, morality, and arts in general, in its diffusion of liberal sentiments on the administration of Government,' that it lacks all protection."

In Bates v. State Bar of Arizona, the Court struck a ban on price advertising for what it deemed "routine" legal services. . . . Expressing confidence that legal advertising would only be practicable for such simple, standardized services, the Court rejected the State's proffered justifications for regulation.

Nearly two decades of cases have built upon the foundation laid by Bates. It is now well established that lawyer advertising is commercial speech and, as such, is accorded a measure of First Amendment protection. . . . Such First Amendment protection, of course, is not absolute. We have always been careful to distinguish commercial speech from speech at the First Amendment's core. " '[C]ommercial speech [enjoys] a limited measure of protection, commensurate with its subordinate position in the scale of First Amendment values,' and is subject to 'modes of regulation that might be impermissible in the realm of noncommercial expression.' "

Mindful of these concerns, we engage in "intermediate" scrutiny of restrictions on commercial speech, analyzing them under the framework set forth in Central Hudson Gas & Elec. Corp. v. Public Serv. Comm'n of N.Y. Under Central Hudson, the government may freely regulate commercial speech that concerns unlawful activity or is misleading. Commercial speech that falls into neither of those categories, like the advertising at issue here, may be regulated if the government satisfies a test consisting of three related prongs: First, the government must assert a substantial interest in support of its regulation; second, the government must demonstrate that the restriction on commercial speech directly and materially advances that interest; and third, the regulation must be "'narrowly drawn.'"

B

The Bar asserts that it has a substantial interest in protecting the privacy and tranquility of personal injury victims and their loved ones against intrusive, unsolicited contact by lawyers.... Because direct-mail solicitations in the wake of accidents are perceived by the public as intrusive, the Bar argues, the reputation of the legal profession in the eyes of Floridians has suffered commensurately. The regulation, then, is an effort to protect the flagging reputations of Florida lawyers by preventing them from engaging in conduct that, the Bar maintains, "'is universally regarded as deplorable and beneath common decency because of its intrusion upon the special vulnerability and private grief of victims or their families.'"

We have little trouble crediting the Bar's interest as substantial....

Under Central Hudson's second prong, the State must demonstrate that the challenged regulation "advances the Government's interest 'in a direct and material way.'" ... That burden, we have explained, "'is not satisfied by mere speculation or conjecture; rather, a governmental body seeking to sustain a restriction on commercial speech must demonstrate that the harms it recites are real and that its restriction will in fact alleviate them to a material degree.'" In Edenfield, the Court invalidated a Florida ban on in-person solicitation by certified public accountants (CPA's). We observed that the State Board of Accountancy had "present[ed] no studies that suggest personal solicitation of prospective business clients by CPA's creates the dangers of fraud, overreaching, or compromised independence that the Board claims to fear." Moreover, "[t]he record [did] not disclose any anecdotal evidence, either from Florida or another State, that validate[d] the Board's suppositions...." Finding nothing in the record to substantiate the State's allegations of harm, we invalidated the regulation.

The direct-mail solicitation regulation before us does not suffer from such infirmities. The Bar submitted a 106-page summary of its 2-year study of lawyer advertising and solicitation to the District Court. That summary contains data — both statistical and anecdotal — supporting the Bar's contentions that the Florida public views direct-mail solicitations in the immediate wake of accidents as an intrusion on privacy that reflects poorly upon the profession. As of June 1989, lawyers mailed 700,000 direct solicitations in Florida annually, 40% of which were aimed at accident victims or their survivors. A survey of Florida adults commissioned by the Bar indicated that Floridians "have negative feelings about those attorneys who use direct mail advertising." Fifty-four percent of the general population surveyed said that contacting persons concerning accidents or similar events is a violation of privacy. A random sampling of persons who received direct-mail advertising from lawyers in 1987 revealed that 45% believed that direct-mail solicitation is "designed to take advantage of gullible or unstable people"; 34% found such tactics "annoying or irritating"; 26% found it "an invasion of your privacy"; and 24% reported that it "made you angry." Significantly, 27% of direct-mail recipients reported that their regard for the legal profession and for the judicial process as a whole was "lower" as a result of receiving the direct mail. . . .

In light of this showing . . . we conclude that the Bar has satisfied the second prong of the Central Hudson test.

In reaching a contrary conclusion, the Court of Appeals determined that this case was governed squarely by Shapero v. Kentucky Bar Assn. Making no mention of the Bar's study, the court concluded that " 'a targeted letter [does not] invade the recipient's privacy any more than does a substantively identical letter mailed at large. The invasion, if any, occurs when the lawyer discovers the recipient's legal affairs, not when he confronts the recipient with the discovery.' " In many cases, the Court of Appeals explained, "this invasion of privacy will involve no more than reading the newspaper."

While some of Shapero's language might be read to support the Court of Appeals' interpretation, Shapero differs in several fundamental respects from the case before us. First and foremost, Shapero's treatment of privacy was casual. . . . Second, in contrast to this case, Shapero dealt with a broad ban on all direct-mail solicitations, whatever the time frame and whoever the recipient. Finally, the State in Shapero assembled no evidence attempting to demonstrate any actual harm caused by targeted direct mail. The Court rejected the State's effort to justify a prophylactic ban on the basis of blanket, untested assertions of undue influence and overreaching. Because the State did not make a privacy-based argument at all, its empirical showing on that issue was similarly infirm. . . .

Here . . . the harm targeted by the Bar cannot be eliminated by a brief journey to the trash can. The purpose of the 30-day targeted direct-mail ban is to forestall the outrage and irritation with the state-licensed legal profession that the practice of direct solicitation only days after accidents has engendered. The Bar is concerned not with citizens' "offense" in the abstract, but with the demonstrable detrimental effects that such "offense" has on the profession it regulates. Moreover, the harm posited by the Bar is as much a function of simple receipt of targeted solicitations within days of accidents as it is a function of the letters' contents. Throwing the letter away shortly after opening it may minimize the latter intrusion, but it does little to combat the former. . . .

Passing to Central Hudson's third prong, we examine the relationship between the Bar's interests and the means chosen to serve them. With respect to this prong, the differences between commercial speech and noncommercial speech are manifest. [T]he "least restrictive means" test has no role in the commercial speech context. "What our decisions require," instead, "is a 'fit' between the legislature's ends and the means chosen to accomplish those ends," a fit that is not necessarily perfect, but reasonable; that represents not necessarily the single best disposition but one whose scope is 'in proportion to the interest served;' that employs not necessarily the least restrictive means but . . . a means narrowly tailored to achieve the desired objective. . . ."

We are not persuaded by respondents' allegations of constitutional infirmity. . . . Rather than drawing difficult lines on the basis that some injuries are "severe" and some situations appropriate (and others, presumably, inappropriate) for grief, anger, or emotion, the Bar has crafted a ban applicable to all postaccident or disaster solicitations for a brief 30-day period. Unlike respondents, we do not see "numerous and obvious less-burdensome alternatives" to Florida's short temporal ban. The Bar's rule is reasonably well tailored to its stated objective of eliminating targeted mailings whose type and timing are a source of distress to Floridians, distress that has caused many of them to lose respect for the legal profession.

III

Speech by professionals obviously has many dimensions. There are circumstances in which we will accord speech by attorneys on public issues and matters of legal representation the strongest protection our Constitution has to offer. This case, however, concerns pure commercial advertising, for which we have always reserved a lesser degree of protection under the First Amendment. Particularly because the standards and conduct of state-licensed lawyers have traditionally been subject to extensive regulation by the States, it is all the more appropriate that we limit our scrutiny of state regulations to a level commensurate with the " 'subordinate position' " of commercial speech in the scale of First Amendment values.

We believe that the Bar's 30-day restriction on targeted direct-mail solicitation of accident victims and their relatives withstands scrutiny under the three-pronged Central Hudson test that we have devised for this context. The Bar has substantial interest both in protecting injured Floridians from invasive conduct by lawyers and in preventing the erosion of confidence in the profession that such repeated invasions have engendered. The Bar's proffered study, unrebutted by respondents below, provides evidence indicating that the harms it targets are far from illusory. The palliative devised by the Bar to address these harms is narrow both in scope and in duration. The Constitution, in our view, requires nothing more.

The judgment of the Court of Appeals, accordingly, is Reversed.

Justice KENNEDY, with whom Justice STEVENS, Justice SOUTER, and Justice GINSBURG join, dissenting.

Attorneys who communicate their willingness to assist potential clients are engaged in speech protected by the First and Fourteenth Amendments. That principle has been understood since Bates. The Court today undercuts this guarantee in an important class of cases and unsettles leading First Amendment precedents, at the expense of those victims most in need of legal assistance. With all respect for the Court, in my view its solicitude for the privacy of victims and its concern for our profession are misplaced and self-defeating, even upon the Court's own premises.

I take it to be uncontroverted that when an accident results in death or injury, it is often urgent at once to investigate the occurrence, identify witnesses, and preserve evidence. Vital interests in speech and expression are, therefore, at stake when by law an attorney cannot direct a letter to the victim or the family explaining this simple fact and offering competent legal assistance. Meanwhile, represented and better informed parties, or parties who have been solicited in ways more sophisticated and indirect, may be at work. Indeed, these parties, either themselves or by their attorneys, investigators, and adjusters, are free to contact the unrepresented persons to gather evidence or offer settlement. This scheme makes little sense. As is often true when the law makes little sense, it is not first principles but their interpretation and application that have gone awry.

Although I agree with the Court that the case can be resolved by following the three-part inquiry we have identified to assess restrictions on commercial speech, a preliminary observation is in order. Speech has the capacity to convey complex substance, yielding various insights and interpretations depending upon the identity of the listener or the reader and the context of its transmission. It would oversimplify to say that what we consider here is commercial speech and nothing more, for in many instances the banned communications may be vital to the recipients' right to petition the courts for redress of grievances. The complex nature of expression is one reason why even so-called commercial speech has become an essential part of the public discourse the First Amendment secures. If our commercial speech rules are to control this case, then, it is imperative to apply them with exacting care and fidelity to our precedents, for what is at stake is the suppression of information and knowledge that transcends the financial self-interests of the speaker. . . .

[T]he State and the opinion of the Court [emphasize the importance of] protecting the reputation and dignity of the legal profession. The argument is, it seems fair to say, that all are demeaned by the crass behavior of a few. . . . While disrespect will arise from an unethical or improper practice, the majority begs a most critical question by assuming that direct-mail solicitations constitute such a practice. The fact is, however, that direct solicitation may serve vital purposes and promote the administration of justice, and to the extent the bar seeks to protect lawyers' reputations by preventing them from engaging in speech some deem offensive, the State is doing nothing more . . . than manipulating the public's opinion by suppressing speech that informs us how the legal system works. The disrespect argument thus proceeds from the very assumption it tries to prove, which is to say that solicitations within 30 days serve no legitimate purpose. This, of course, is censorship pure and simple; and censorship is antithetical to the first principles of free expression. . . .

Even were the interests asserted substantial, the regulation here fails the second part of the Central Hudson test, which requires that the dangers the State seeks to eliminate be real and that a speech restriction or ban advance that asserted state interest in a direct and material way. . . .

It is telling that the essential thrust of all the material adduced to justify the State's interest is devoted to the reputational concerns of the Bar. It is not at all clear that this regulation advances the interest of protecting persons who are suffering trauma and grief, and we are cited to no material in the record for that claim. . . .

Were it appropriate to reach the third part of the Central Hudson test, it would be clear that the relationship between the Bar's interests and the means chosen to serve them is not a reasonable fit. The Bar's rule creates a flat ban that prohibits far more speech than necessary to serve the purported state interest. . . .

The accident victims who are prejudiced to vindicate the State's purported desire for more dignity in the legal profession will be the very persons who most need legal advice, for they are the victims who, because they lack education, linguistic ability, or familiarity with the legal system, are unable to seek out legal services. . . .

The reasonableness of the State's chosen methods for redressing perceived evils can be evaluated, in part, by a commonsense consideration of other possible means of regulation that have not been tried. Here, the Court neglects the fact that this problem is largely self-policing: Potential clients will not hire lawyers who offend them. And even if a person enters into a contract with an attorney and later regrets it, Florida, like some other States, allows clients to rescind certain contracts with attorneys within a stated time after they are executed. . . . The State's restriction deprives accident victims of information which may be critical to their right to make a claim for compensation for injuries. The telephone book and general advertisements may serve this purpose in part; but the direct solicitation ban will fall on those who most need legal representation: for those with minor injuries, the victims too ill informed to know an attorney may be interested in their cases; for those with serious injuries, the victims too ill informed to know that time is of the essence if counsel is to assemble evidence and warn them not to enter into settlement negotiations or evidentiary discussions with investigators for opposing parties. . . . The very fact that some 280,000 direct-mail solicitations are sent to accident victims and their survivors in Florida each year is some indication of the efficacy of this device. . . .

It is most ironic that, for the first time since Bates, the Court now orders a major retreat from the constitutional guarantees for commercial speech in order to shield its own profession from public criticism. Obscuring the financial aspect of the legal profession from public discussion through direct-mail solicitation, at the expense of the least sophisticated members of society, is not a laudable constitutional goal. There is no authority for the proposition that the Constitution permits the State to promote the public image of the legal profession by suppressing information about the profession's business aspects. If public respect for the profession erodes because solicitation distorts the idea of the law as most lawyers see it, it must be remembered that real progress begins with more rational speech, not less. . . .

Post-Case Follow-Up

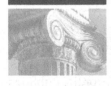

In *Went For It*, the Court held that Florida's 30-day blackout period on direct mail solicitation by plaintiffs' attorneys does not violate the First Amendment. Applying its commercial speech doctrine, the Court recognized the Florida bar's substantial interest in protecting the privacy of personal injury victims and the reputation of Florida lawyers. Moreover, the Court found that the 30-day blackout period "advances the Government's interest in a direct and material way" relying primarily on evidence that the Florida bar accumulated during a two-year study of lawyer marketing. Finally, the Court held that there is a "fit" between the bar's goals and the means chosen to accomplish its goals. Although the Model Rules do not contain a 30-day blackout period, a few other states — including Alabama, Connecticut, Kentucky, Louisiana, Maryland, New York, and Texas — have adopted similar rules either in their professional codes or through legislation.

Did *Went For It* Go Too Far With It?

Do you think the Court gave undue weight to the report submitted by the Florida bar? Consider this: less than one-third of the pages in the report mentioned targeted, direct-mail solicitations. Further, the report contained few quotes that supported lawyer advertising or direct-mail solicitations, and the ones it did include were not flattering, for example: "The issue is, don't we all — even attorneys — have the constitutional right to make ourselves look trashy . . . ?" and "The Supreme Court said lawyers can advertise. There's no reason to treat our ads differently than those of the lottery or race tracks or banks." Douglas W. Swalina, Note, *The Florida Bar Went For It, But It Went Too Far,* 26 Stetson L. Rev. 437, 461 n.142 (1996).

The dissent took issue with the report, calling it "noteworthy for its incompetence" and stating that *Central Hudson* required "more than a few pages of self-serving and unsupported statements by the State." Fla. Bar v. Went For It, Inc., 515 U.S. 618, 640-41 (1995) (Kennedy, J., dissenting).

Finally, look again at Justice O'Connor's description of the report and the statistics that she quotes—do they really support the majority's conclusion?

The Supreme Court has not revisited the topic of lawyer marketing since *Went For It*, and the Court's decision leaves some significant unanswered questions. In particular, what other types of limited restrictions on lawyer advertising might the Court find constitutional?

Florida Bar v. Went For It, Inc.: Real Life Applications

1. A state bar association is considering a new rule that would prohibit lawyers from sending "written or electronic solicitations to accident victims and their relatives for 60 days following an accident or disaster." You serve on the state's ethics committee. What would you advise the state bar?

2. A state rule provides: "All advertisements shall be predominantly informational. No drawings, animations, dramatizations, music, or lyrics shall be used in connection with televised advertising. No advertisement shall rely in any way on techniques to obtain attention that depend upon absurdity and that demonstrate a clear and intentional lack of relevance to the selection of counsel; included in this category are all advertisements that contain any extreme portrayal of counsel exhibiting characteristics clearly unrelated to legal competence."[15] Is this provision constitutional?

2. Rules Governing Communications Concerning a Lawyer's Services

The restrictions contained in the Model Rules of Professional Conduct reflect the balance struck by the Supreme Court: lawyers have the right to market themselves in a truthful, non-deceptive manner, even if those advertisements strike other lawyers or the public as crass or distasteful.[16] This section discusses the most common pitfalls lawyers face in marketing themselves.

---

15. N.J. Rules of Prof'l Conduct r. 7.2(a) (2018).
16. A comment to an earlier version of the rules stated that "questions of effectiveness and taste in advertising are matters of speculation and subjective judgment." *See* Model Rule 7.2 cmt. [3] (repealed 2018).

False or Misleading Communications

The primary rule of thumb is that lawyer marketing may not be "false or mislead ing." *See* Model Rules of Professional Conduct, Rule 7.1. Thus, lawyers can be dis ciplined for false advertising but also for communications about their services that are truthful but nevertheless misleading.

The prohibition on false advertising is straightforward, but understanding the prohibition on "misleading" communications is more difficult. The comments to Rule 7.1 shed some light on this standard: a truthful statement is misleading "if it omits a fact necessary to make the lawyer's communication considered as a whole not materially misleading." Similarly, a truthful statement is "misleading if a sub stantial likelihood exists that it will lead a reasonable person to formulate a specific conclusion about the lawyer or the lawyer's services for which there is no reason able factual foundation."

Deciding whether a particular advertisement is misleading must be done on a case-by-case basis, but there are several recurring situations in which lawyers have run into trouble. First, lawyers who compare themselves to other lawyers need to be very careful. Model Rule 7.1, comment [3], states that "an unsubstantiated comparison of the lawyer's or law firm's services or fees with those of other lawyers or law firms, may be misleading if presented with such specificity as would lead a reasonable person to conclude that the comparison or claim can be substantiated." Thus, a lawyer probably cannot claim that he is "the best trial lawyer in town."[17]

Second, lawyers may not promise future results. Some states have even enacted specific prohibitions against this kind of marketing. In *Public Citizen, Inc. v. Louisiana Attorney Disciplinary Board*, the Fifth Circuit upheld Louisiana's rule barring communications that "promise results" because "[a] promise that a party will prevail in a future case is necessarily false and deceptive. No attorney can guar antee future results."[18]

A third potential way in which lawyers can violate the prohibition on mislead ing advertising is by marketing past successes. Although the Model Rules do not specifically ban such advertising, Rule 7.1, comment [3], states: "A communication that truthfully reports a lawyer's achievements on behalf of clients or former cli ents may be misleading if presented so as to lead a reasonable person to form an unjustified expectation that the same results could be obtained for other clients in similar matters without reference to the specific factual and legal circumstances of each client's case." Again, some states have enacted specific bans on such marketing. First Amendment challenges to such bans have led to mixed results. In *In re Frank*, for example, the lawyer obtained the names of individuals who had been charged with drunk driving but had no attorney and sent them letters in which he described "his successful experience in plea bargaining such cases." The Court held that his conduct "serves to unduly influence the legally unsophisticated persons into believ ing that [they] could and would get a favorable resolution of their case."[19] More

---

17. *See* Medina Cty. Bar Ass'n v. Grieselhuber, 678 N.E.2d 535, 537 (1997) (disciplining a lawyer for advertising "We Do It Well" because it was an unverifiable and misleading claim).
18. 632 F.3d 212, 218 (5th Cir. 2011).
19. 440 N.E.2d 676, 676-77 (Ind. 1982).

recently, however, in *Rubenstein v. Florida Bar*, a Florida district court struck down a Florida advertising rule that banned lawyers from advertising their past success in indoor or outdoor displays, television, and radio commercials. Although the court recognized that the state has substantial interests in regulating lawyer advertising (including protection of the public), the court found that completely banning lawyers from sharing truthful information did not advance those interests.[20] The Fifth Circuit reached the same conclusion concerning a Louisiana rule that "prohibit[ed] communications that contain a reference or testimonial to past successes or results obtained except" when provided in response to a client request.[21]

Fourth, lawyers need to be careful about using nicknames, which states have tried to limit with a number of different justifications. In *Florida Bar v. Pape*, the Florida Supreme Court held that a lawyer's use of a pit bull logo and the telephone number 1-800-PIT-BULL violated Florida's prohibition on depictions that are "deceptive, misleading, or manipulative." The Court said that these "advertising devices would suggest to many persons not only that the lawyers can achieve results but also that they can engage in a combative style of advocacy. The suggestion is inherently deceptive because there is no way to measure whether the attorneys in fact conduct themselves like pit bulls so as to ascertain whether this logo and phone number convey accurate information." Accordingly, the court concluded that the nickname is misleading because it is not objectively verifiable. The Court rejected the lawyer's First Amendment challenge to these prohibitions.[22]

The Louisiana bar has also taken a dim view of nicknames. In its *Handbook on Lawyer Advertising and Solicitation*,[23] the bar has created examples of complying and noncomplying advertisements. As the following ad demonstrates, the Louisiana bar believes that the nickname "The Golden Retriever" "implies an ability to obtain results" in violation of Louisiana's version of Rule 7.1.[24]

The Fifth Circuit has upheld Louisiana's ban on communications that "utilize[] a nickname, moniker, motto or trade name that states or implies an ability to obtain results in a matter."[25]

On the other hand, several courts and ethics opinions have concluded that lawyers may tout their selection by ratings services such as Super Lawyers, Best Lawyers in America, and Martindale Hubbell. For example, Super Lawyers are nominated and voted on by other lawyers. The company also does independent research. In the end, only 5 percent of lawyers are selected to be Super Lawyers.[26] The title "Super Lawyer" (like Pit Bull or Golden Retriever) may be misleading in the sense that the lawyer does not actually wear a cape and fly around. Calling oneself a "Super Lawyer" also might tend to imply an ability to obtain results, but

---

20. Rubenstein v. Fla. Bar, 72 F. Supp. 3d 1298, 1315-17 (S.D. Fla. 2014). Florida was the only state to ban such advertising.

21. Public Citizen, Inc. v. La. Att'y Disciplinary Bd., 632 F.3d 212, 217, 221-23 (5th Cir. 2011).

22. 918 So. 2d 240, 244, 247-49 (2005).

23. Louisiana State Bar Ass'n Rules of Prof'l Conduct Comm., Handbook on Lawyer Advertising and Solicitation (2008), *available at* https://www.lsba.org/documents/lawyeradvertising/lawyeradhandbook.pdf.

24. *Id.* at 42.

25. *Public Citizen, Inc.*, 632 F.3d at 224-27. In contrast, the Second Circuit struck down New York's similar rule. *See* Alexander v. Cahill, 598 F.3d 79, 94-95 (2d Cir. 2010).

26. *Selection Process*, Super Lawyers, http://www.superlawyers.com/about/selection_process.html (last visited July 28, 2020).

This fake advertisement appears in the Louisiana bar's *Handbook on Lawyer Advertising and Solicitation* to show lawyers examples of complying and noncomplying advertisements.

authorities considering the title have concluded that it is permissible provided that lawyers who tout this achievement provide sufficient context — "the lawyer's advertising must state accurately the publication by which he or she was ranked, the year of the ranking, and the field of the ranking, if one was specified."[27] In that sense, it is distinguishable from Florida's "Pit Bull" and Louisiana's "Golden Retriever."

Fifth, consistent with *Peel*, *R.M.J.*, and *Ibanez*, in which the Supreme Court recognized lawyers' constitutional rights to market themselves in truthful, non-deceptive ways, comment [9] to Rule 7.2 permits a lawyer to "communicate that

27. Alaska Bar Ass'n, Op. 2009-2 (2009).

the lawyer does or does not practice in particular areas of law" and to state that she "'concentrates in' or is a 'specialist,' practices a 'specialty,' or 'specializes in' particular fields based on the lawyer's experience, specialized training or education," provided that such a statement is not "false or misleading." Lawyers need to be careful about claims of certification, however. Concerned that the public will misunderstand the basis for such claims, Rule 7.2(c) states that a "lawyer shall not state or imply that a lawyer is certified as a specialist in a particular field of law, unless: (1) the lawyer has been certified as a specialist by an organization that has been approved by an appropriate authority of the state, the District of Columbia, or a U.S. Territory, or that has been accredited by the American Bar Association; and (2) the name of the certifying organization is clearly identified in the communication."

Sixth, Rule 7.1 generally proscribes law firm names that are misleading. Comment [5] to this rule specifically prohibits a law firm from using a trade name or other designation if it "implies a connection with a government agency, with a deceased lawyer who was not a former member of the firm, with a lawyer not associated with the firm or a predecessor firm, with a nonlawyer or with a public or charitable legal services organization." For example, a law firm located across from a university may not call itself "University Law Firm" if it has no connection with the university.

Required Disclosures

Finally, the Supreme Court has said that states may require lawyers to provide some additional information in their advertisements "as long as disclosure requirements are reasonably related to the State's interest in preventing deception of consumers."[28] Given this leeway by the Court, states impose a wide variety of requirements. The Model Rules only impose one: any communication must "include the name of, and contact information for, the lawyer or law firm."[29]

3. Social Media and Other Forms of Electronic Advertising

In this competitive market, lawyers are increasingly turning to social media and other electronic forms of marketing. In the 2019 ABA Legal Technology Survey Report, 80 percent of lawyers reported that their firms maintain a social media presence.[30] Lawyers use websites, blogs, and social media sites, such as LinkedIn, Facebook, Martindale, Avvo, and Twitter, to market themselves and their practices.

In some cases, applying the advertising rules to online marketing is simple: just like traditional advertising, online advertising cannot be false or misleading, and it must also follow the other rules outlined in the previous section. But social media marketing also raises some novel issues, and relatively little authority addresses those issues.

---

28. Zauderer v. Office of Disciplinary Counsel of Supreme Court of Ohio, 471 U.S. 626, 651 (1985).
29. Model Rule 7.2 cmt. [12].
30. Allison Shields, *Social Media, in* ABA Techreport 2019 (2019), *available at* https://www.americanbar.org/groups/law_practice/publications/techreport/abatechreport2019/websitesmarketing2019.

Do the Advertising Rules Apply to Social Media?

A threshold issue is whether the rules that govern a lawyer's professional conduct apply to a lawyer's posts on social media. In its recent amendment to Rule 7.2(a), the ABA made clear that they do cover a lawyer's communications "regarding the lawyer's services through *any media*," including social media. This is consistent with a 2010 ABA Ethics Opinion, concluding that standard lawyer websites that provide biographical information about lawyers constitute "communication about the lawyer or the lawyer's services" within the meaning of the rules.[31]

Nevertheless, social media remains a gray area. Whenever a lawyer communicates about the services she provides on social media, she is subject to the rules. It may not always be clear, however, whether the lawyer is communicating about her services (covered by the rules) or just updating her Twitter followers on what she is doing tonight (not covered by the rules). A 2012 California Ethics Opinion is one of the only authorities to analyze this precise issue.

The State Bar of California Standing Committee on Professional Responsibility and Conduct Formal Opinion No. 2012-186[32]

Consider the following examples of Attorney's use of personal social media sites for status postings which are visible to all of her "friends," "connections," or "followers" (although not to the public at large):

Example Number 1: "Case finally over. Unanimous verdict! Celebrating tonight."

In the Committee's opinion, this statement, standing alone, is not [subject to the advertising rules] because it is not a message or offer "concerning the availability for professional employment," whatever Attorney's subjective motive for sending it. Attorney status postings that simply announce recent victories without an accompanying offer about the availability for professional employment generally will not qualify as a communication.

Example Number 2: "Another great victory in court today! My client is delighted. Who wants to be next?"

Similarly, the statement "Another great victory in court today!" standing alone is not a communication [subject to the advertising rules] because it is not a message or offer "concerning the availability for professional employment." However, the addition of the text, "[w]ho wants to be next?" [does constitute advertising] because it suggests availability for professional employment. . . .

---

31. ABA Comm. on Ethics & Prof'l Responsibility, Formal Op. 10-457 (2010) (emphasis added).
32. Cal. Bar Comm. on Prof'l Responsibility & Conduct, Formal Op. 2012-186 (2012), *available at* https://www .calbar.ca.gov/Portals/0/documents/ethics/Opinions/CAL%202012-186%20%2812-21-12%29.pdf. The California rules define "communications" subject to the advertising rules as "any message or offer made by or on behalf of a member concerning the availability for professional employment of a member or a law firm directed to any former, present, or prospective client. . . ." CAL. R. PROF'L CONDUCT r. 7.2 (2018).

Example Number 3: "Won a million dollar verdict. Tell your friends to check out my website."

In the Committee's opinion, this language also qualifies as [an advertisement subject to the rules] because the words "tell your friends to check out my website," in this context, convey a message or offer "concerning the availability for professional employment." It appears that Attorney is asking the reader to tell others to look at her website so that they may consider hiring her. . . .

Example Number 4: "Won another personal injury case. Call me for a free consultation."

Again, the Committee concludes that this posting is [advertising] due primarily to the second sentence.

[An advertisement] has to include an offer about availability for professional employment so the "free" consultation language at first might indicate the posting is not [an advertisement]. Yet the rule does not limit "communications" to messages seeking financial compensation for services. To the contrary, a communication includes any "message or offer made by or on behalf of a member concerning the availability for professional employment of a member or a law firm." . . . An offer of a free consultation is a step toward securing potential employment, and the offer of a free consultation indicates that the lawyer is available to be hired. On balance, this example in the Committee's opinion constitutes [advertising].

Example Number 5: "Just published an article on wage and hour breaks. Let me know if you would like a copy."

In this instance, we believe the statement does not concern "availability for professional employment." The attorney is merely relaying information regarding an article that she has published, and is offering to provide copies. . . .

In its opinion, the California bar's determination of whether a social media item constitutes advertising within the meaning of the rules turns on whether the post includes an offer from the lawyer concerning her availability for professional employment. The Florida bar has come to the same conclusion: "Pages appearing on networking sites that are used to promote the lawyer or law firm's practice are subject to the lawyer advertising rules."[33]

Unique Dangers of Social Media and Other Forms of Electronic Advertising

If the Internet content is subject to the marketing rules, then the lawyer must, of course, ensure that the content complies with all of the rules that would apply to traditional marketing. But social media and other forms of electronic marketing, such as websites and blogs, also pose some unique dangers.

---

33. FLA. BAR COMM. ON ADVERTISING, THE FLORIDA BAR STANDING COMM. ON ADVERTISING GUIDELINES FOR NETWORKING SITES 1 (May 9, 2016), *available at* https://www-media.floridabar.org/uploads/2019/11/guidelines-social-networking-sites-2019.pdf.

A central concern is that social media and other forms of electronic advertising often enable third parties to post content on the lawyer's website (or blog or social media posting). Are lawyers responsible for content created by others? In other words, if a third party posts content on a lawyer's Avvo page and that content would violate the Rules of Professional Conduct if the lawyer posted it herself, is the lawyer subject to discipline? In a 2010 ethics opinion, the South Carolina Ethics Advisory Committee concluded that once a lawyer "claims" his website listing, he is "responsible for conforming all information in the . . . listing to the Rules of Professional Conduct. . . . [A] lawyer should monitor a 'claimed' listing to keep all comments in conformity with the Rules. If any part of the listing cannot be conformed to the Rules (e.g., if an improper comment cannot be removed), the lawyer should remove his or her entire listing and discontinue participation in the service."[34] The New York State Bar Association's Social Media Committee reached the same conclusion:

> A lawyer is responsible for all content that the lawyer posts on her social media website or profile. A lawyer also has a duty to periodically monitor her social media profile(s) or blog(s) for comments, endorsements and recommendations to ensure that such third-party posts do not violate ethics rules. If a person who is not an agent of the lawyer unilaterally posts content to the lawyer's social media, profile or blog that violates the ethics rules, the lawyer must remove or hide such content if such removal is within the lawyer's control and, if not within the lawyer's control, she must ask that person to remove it. . . .
>
> A lawyer must ensure the accuracy of third-party legal endorsements, recommendations, or online reviews posted to the lawyer's social media profile. To that end, a lawyer must periodically monitor and review such posts for accuracy and must correct misleading or incorrect information posted by clients or other third-parties.[35]

In addition, electronic advertising poses other risk management concerns:

- First, lawyers need to be careful about forming inadvertent attorney-client relationships. Although a lawyer may provide legal information on a website, if a lawyer "provide[s] specific legal advice on a social media network . . . a lawyer's responsive communications may be found to have created an attorney-client relationship."[36]
- Second, lawyers who invite website visitors to contact them may create a prospective client relationship within the meaning of Rule 1.18.[37]

---

34. S.C. Bar Ethics Advisory Comm., Op. 09-10 (2009), *available at* https://www.scbar.org/lawyers/legal-resources-info/ethics-advisory-opinions/eao/ethics-advisory-opinion-09-10/. *But see* Conn. Bar Ass'n Prof'l Ethics Comm., Informal Op. 2012-03 (2012), *available at* https://www.ctbar.org/docs/default-source/publications/ethics-opinions-informal-opinions/2012/informal_opinion_2012-03.pdf (concluding that lawyers are not responsible for Martindale.com ratings because they "cannot control the content of client reviews" that appear on the website).
35. N.Y. Bar Ass'n Com. & Fed. Lit. Section, Social Media Ethics Guidelines, Guidelines No. 2.C, 2.D (Jun. 9, 2015) [hereinafter N.Y. Social Media Guidelines], *available at* https://nysba.org/app/uploads/2020/02/NYSBA-Social-Media-Ethics-Guidelines-Final-6-20-19.pdf.
36. *Id.* at Guideline No. 3.A. *See supra* Chapter 3.
37. *See supra* Chapter 3.

C. REGULATION OF SOLICITATION

Although the Supreme Court recognized in *Bates* that lawyer advertising is constitutionally protected commercial speech, the *Bates* decision did not address the constitutionality of in-person solicitation. The Supreme Court took up that issue the next year in *Ohralik v. Ohio State Bar Association.* This section considers that constitutional doctrine before turning to the rules governing lawyer solicitation.

1. Constitutional Limits on the Bar's Power to Limit Solicitation

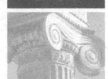

Case Preview

Ohralik v. Ohio State Bar Association

Like most states, the Ohio bar prohibited solicitation with some limited exceptions. In February 1974, attorney Albert Ohralik solicited two clients who had been involved in an automobile accident, one in the hospital and one at home after she was released from the hospital. The Ohio bar subsequently brought disciplinary proceedings against Ohralik and suspended him indefinitely. Relying on *Bates,* Ohralik argued that the application of the solicitation ban against him violated his First Amendment rights. The Supreme Court disagreed and upheld Ohralik's suspension.

As you read the case, consider the following:

1. How does the lawyer's conduct at issue in *Bates* and *Went For It* differ from the lawyer's conduct in this case?
2. What are the Ohio bar's interests in banning solicitation? How does that state interest justify the outcome in this case?
3. How should the holding and rationale of *Ohralik* apply to solicitation using social media and other electronic means?

Ohralik v. Ohio State Bar Association
436 U.S. 447 (1978)

Mr. Justice POWELL delivered the opinion of the Court.

In *Bates v. State Bar of Arizona*, this Court held that truthful advertising of "routine" legal services is protected by the First and Fourteenth Amendments against blanket prohibition by a State. The Court expressly reserved the question of the permissible scope of regulation of "in-person solicitation of clients-at the hospital room or the accident site, or in any other situation that breeds undue influence-by attorneys or their agents or 'runners.'" Today we answer part of the question so reserved, and hold that the State-or the Bar acting with state authorization-constitutionally may discipline a lawyer for soliciting clients in person, for pecuniary gain, under circumstances likely to pose dangers that the State has a right to prevent.

I

Appellant, a member of the Ohio Bar, lives in Montville, Ohio. . . . On February 13, 1974 . . . appellant learned . . . about an automobile accident that had taken place on February 2 in which Carol McClintock, a young woman with whom appellant was casually acquainted, had been injured. Appellant [visited] Ms. McClintock's parents, who . . . explained that their daughter had been driving the family automobile on a local road when she was hit by an uninsured motorist. Both Carol and her passenger, Wanda Lou Holbert, were injured and hospitalized. In response to the McClintocks' expression of apprehension that they might be sued by Holbert, appellant explained that Ohio's guest statute would preclude such a suit. When appellant suggested to the McClintocks that they hire a lawyer, Mrs. McClintock retorted that such a decision would be up to Carol, who was 18 years old and would be the beneficiary of a successful claim.

Appellant proceeded to the hospital, where he found Carol lying in traction in her room. After a brief conversation about her condition, appellant told Carol he would represent her and asked her to sign an agreement. Carol said she would have to discuss the matter with her parents. She did not sign the agreement, but asked appellant to have her parents come to see her. Appellant also attempted to see Wanda Lou Holbert, but learned that she had just been released from the hospital. He then departed for another visit with the McClintocks.

On his way appellant detoured to the scene of the accident, where he took a set of photographs. He also picked up a tape recorder, which he concealed under his raincoat before arriving at the McClintocks' residence. Once there, he . . . discovered that the McClintocks' insurance policy would provide benefits of up to $12,500 each for Carol and Wanda Lou under an uninsured-motorist clause. . . . The McClintocks . . . told appellant that Carol had phoned to say that appellant could "go ahead" with her representation. Two days later appellant returned to Carol's hospital room to have her sign a contract, which provided that he would receive one-third of her recovery.

[Appellant subsequently] visited Wanda Lou at her home, without having been invited. He again concealed his tape recorder and recorded most of the conversation with Wanda Lou. . . . [A]ppellant told Wanda Lou that he was representing Carol and that he had a "little tip" for Wanda Lou: the McClintocks' insurance policy contained an uninsured-motorist clause which might provide her with a recovery of up to $12,500. The young woman, who was 18 years of age and not a high school graduate at the time, replied to appellant's query about whether she was going to file a claim by stating that she really did not understand what was going on. Appellant offered to represent her, also, for a contingent fee of one-third of any recovery, and Wanda Lou stated "O. K."

Wanda's mother attempted to repudiate her daughter's oral assent the following day, when appellant called on the telephone to speak to Wanda. . . . Appellant insisted that Wanda had entered into a binding agreement. A month later Wanda confirmed in writing that she wanted neither to sue nor to be represented by appellant. She requested that appellant notify the insurance company that he was not her lawyer, as the company would not release a check to her until he did so. Carol also eventually discharged appellant. Although another lawyer represented her in concluding a settlement with the insurance company, she paid appellant one-third of her recovery in settlement of his lawsuit against her for breach of contract.

Both Carol McClintock and Wanda Lou Holbert filed complaints against appellant with the Grievance Committee of the Geauga County Bar Association. [After a disciplinary hearing, the Board of Commissioners on Grievances and Discipline of the Supreme Court of Ohio found that appellant had violated Disciplinary Rules (DR) 2-103(A) and 2-104(A) of the Ohio Code of Professional Responsibility.[38] The Supreme Court of Ohio adopted the findings of the Board and suspended him indefinitely.]

The decision in *Bates* was handed down after the conclusion of proceedings in the Ohio Supreme Court. We noted probable jurisdiction in this case to consider the scope of protection of a form of commercial speech, and an aspect of the State's authority to regulate and discipline members of the bar, not considered in *Bates*. We now affirm the judgment of the Supreme Court of Ohio.

II

. . .

A

Appellant contends that his solicitation of the two young women as clients is indistinguishable, for purposes of constitutional analysis, from the advertisement in *Bates*. Like that advertisement, his meetings with the prospective clients apprised them of their legal rights and of the availability of a lawyer to pursue their claims. According to appellant, such conduct is "presumptively an exercise of his free speech rights" which cannot be curtailed in the absence of proof that it actually caused a specific harm that the State has a compelling interest in preventing. But in-person solicitation of professional employment by a lawyer does not stand on a par with truthful advertising about the availability and terms of routine legal services, let alone with forms of speech more traditionally within the concern of the First Amendment.

. . .

B

The state interests implicated in this case are particularly strong. In addition to its general interest in protecting consumers and regulating commercial transactions,

---

38. DR 2-103(A) of the Ohio Code (1970), which was in force at that time, provided: "A lawyer shall not recommend employment, as a private practitioner, of himself, his partner, or associate to a non-lawyer who has not sought his advice regarding employment of a lawyer." DR 2-104(A) (1970) provided: "A lawyer who has given unsolicited advice to a layman that he should obtain counsel or take legal action shall not accept employment resulting from that advice, except that: (1) A lawyer may accept employment by a close friend, relative, former client (if the advice is germane to the former employment), or one whom the lawyer reasonably believes to be a client."

the State bears a special responsibility for maintaining standards among members of the licensed professions. "The interest of the States in regulating lawyers is especially great since lawyers are essential to the primary governmental function of administering justice, and have historically been 'officers of the courts.'" While lawyers act in part as "self-employed businessmen," they also act "as trusted agents of their clients, and as assistants to the court in search of a just solution to disputes."

. . .

The substantive evils of solicitation have been stated over the years in sweeping terms: stirring up litigation, assertion of fraudulent claims, debasing the legal profession, and potential harm to the solicited client in the form of overreaching, overcharging, underrepresentation, and misrepresentation. The American Bar Association, as amicus curiae, defends the rule against solicitation primarily on three broad grounds: It is said that the prohibitions embodied in DR2-103(A) and 2-104(A) serve to reduce the likelihood of overreaching and the exertion of undue influence on lay persons, to protect the privacy of individuals, and to avoid situations where the lawyer's exercise of judgment on behalf of the client will be clouded by his own pecuniary self-interest.

We need not discuss or evaluate each of these interests in detail as appellant has conceded that the State has a legitimate and indeed "compelling" interest in preventing those aspects of solicitation that involve fraud, undue influence, intimidation, overreaching, and other forms of "vexatious conduct. . . ."

III

Appellant's concession that strong state interests justify regulation to prevent the evils he enumerates would end this case but for his insistence that none of those evils was found to be present in his acts of solicitation. He challenges what he characterizes as the "indiscriminate application" of the Rules to him and thus attacks the validity of DR 2-103(A) and DR 2-104(A) not facially, but as applied to his acts of solicitation. And because no allegations or findings were made of the specific wrongs appellant concedes would justify disciplinary action, appellant terms his solicitation "pure," meaning "soliciting and obtaining agreements from Carol McClintock and Wanda Lou Holbert to represent each of them," without more. Appellant therefore argues that we must decide whether a State may discipline him for solicitation per se without offending the First and Fourteenth Amendments.

We agree that the appropriate focus is on appellant's conduct. . . . [But] Appellant's argument misconceives the nature of the State's interest. The Rules prohibiting solicitation are prophylactic measures whose objective is the prevention of harm before it occurs. The Rules were applied in this case to discipline a lawyer for soliciting employment for pecuniary gain under circumstances likely to result in the adverse consequences the State seeks to avert. In such a situation, which is inherently conducive to overreaching and other forms of misconduct, the State has a strong interest in adopting and enforcing rules of conduct designed to protect the public from harmful solicitation by lawyers whom it has licensed.

The State's perception of the potential for harm in circumstances such as those presented in this case is well founded. The detrimental aspects of face-to-face selling even of ordinary consumer products have been recognized and addressed by the Federal Trade Commission, and it hardly need be said that the potential for over-reaching is significantly greater when a lawyer, a professional trained in the art of persuasion, personally solicits an unsophisticated, injured, or distressed lay person. Such an individual may place his trust in a lawyer, regardless of the latter's qualifications or the individual's actual need for legal representation, simply in response to persuasion under circumstances conducive to uninformed acquiescence. Although it is argued that personal solicitation is valuable because it may apprise a victim of misfortune of his legal rights, the very plight of that person not only makes him more vulnerable to influence but also may make advice all the more intrusive. Thus, under these adverse conditions the overtures of an uninvited lawyer may distress the solicited individual simply because of their obtrusiveness and the invasion of the individual's privacy, even when no other harm materializes. Under such circumstances, it is not unreasonable for the State to presume that in-person solicitation by lawyers more often than not will be injurious to the person solicited.

The efficacy of the State's effort to prevent such harm to prospective clients would be substantially diminished if, having proved a solicitation in circumstances like those of this case, the State were required in addition to prove actual injury. Unlike the advertising in *Bates*, in-person solicitation is not visible or otherwise open to public scrutiny. Often there is no witness other than the lawyer and the lay person whom he has solicited, rendering it difficult or impossible to obtain reliable proof of what actually took place. This would be especially true if the lay person were so distressed at the time of the solicitation that he could not recall specific details at a later date. If appellant's view were sustained, in-person solicitation would be virtually immune to effective oversight and regulation by the State or by the legal profession, in contravention of the State's strong interest in regulating members of the Bar in an effective, objective, and self-enforcing manner. It therefore is not unreasonable, or violative of the Constitution, for a State to respond with what in effect is a prophylactic rule. . . .

Accordingly, the judgment of the Supreme Court of Ohio is affirmed.

Post-Case Follow-Up

In *Ohralik*, the Court held that Ohio's ban on solicitation was constitutional as applied to Ohralik's in-person solicitation. The Court recognized that the state has a strong interest in protecting consumers from "fraud, undue influence, intimidation, overreaching and other forms of 'vexatious conduct'" and that the state's absolute ban on in-person solicitation was a necessary "prophylactic measure[]" intended to prevent harm before it occurs.

Ohralik is the only case in which the Court has upheld a categorical ban on lawyer marketing. The question that remains after *Ohralik* is whether the state may ban any other forms of solicitation. As noted earlier, the Supreme Court subsequently found that states may not ban a lawyer's targeted marketing by other means to a particular group of clients with an identifiable legal problem. In Zauderer v. Office of Disciplinary Counsel, 471 U.S. 626 (1985), the Court upheld the constitutional right of a lawyer to run a newspaper advertisement announcing his willingness to represent women who had suffered injuries resulting from their use of a contraceptive known as the Dalkon Shield Intrauterine Device, and in Shapero v. Kentucky Bar Association, 486 U.S. 466 (1988), the Court upheld the right of a lawyer to send direct mailings to potential clients who had foreclosure suits filed against them. Since the letter did not constitute "face-to-face" communication, the Court treated it as advertising rather than solicitation and applied its commercial speech jurisprudence.

On the same day that it handed down *Ohralik*, the Supreme Court also placed another limit on *Ohralik*'s reach when it decided In re Primus, 436 U.S. 412 (1978), in which the Court offered constitutional protection to solicitation in pro bono cases. Edna Smith Primus was a lawyer in Columbia, South Carolina and a cooperating lawyer with the Columbia branch of the American Civil Liberties Union (ACLU).[39] The ACLU learned that pregnant mothers in Aiken County, South Carolina were being sterilized or threatened with sterilization if they wanted to continue receiving Medicaid benefits, and Ms. Primus sent a letter to a prospective litigant communicating the ACLU's offer to represent her for free.[40] The South Carolina Supreme Court publicly reprimanded Ms. Primus for soliciting a client in violation of South Carolina's Canon of Ethics.[41] The U.S. Supreme Court reversed, holding that Primus' letter was a form of protected political association under the First Amendment and that she may not be subject to discipline without proof of actual wrongdoing.[42] The Court said that her motivation was to "express personal political beliefs and to advance the civil-liberties objectives of the ACLU."[43] Unlike *Ohralik*, "[t]his was not in-person solicitation for pecuniary gain. [Ms. Primus] was communicating an offer of free assistance by attorneys associated with the ACLU, not an offer predicated on entitlement to a share of any monetary recovery. And her actions were undertaken to express personal political beliefs and to advance the civil liberties objectives of the ACLU, rather than to derive financial gain."[44]

Ohralik v. Ohio State Bar Association: Real Life Applications

1. A state bar association is considering bringing a disciplinary case against two different lawyers. Based on *Ohralik* and *Primus*, what would you advise the state bar concerning the constitutionality of bringing these cases?
   a. One lawyer tweeted at an accident victim that he was available to represent her.
   b. The other lawyer went to the hospital of a Black female patient who was assaulted by the police and asked her if she wanted to bring a civil rights suit against the police.

---

39. In Re Primus, 436 U.S. at 414.
40. *Id.* at 415-16.
41. *Id.* at 421.
42. *Id.* at 434.
43. *Id.* at 422.
44. *Id.*

2. After a gas line exploded in an apartment complex resulting in massive property loss (but no injuries), a law firm set up a Recreational Vehicle with the firm's name on it 100 feet from the emergency shelter where the accident victims were staying. What would you advise the state bar about the constitutionality of trying to discipline the firm's lawyers?

2. Rules Governing Solicitation

Following *Ohralik,* Model Rule 7.3 defines solicitation as "a communication initiated by or on behalf of a lawyer or law firm that is directed to a specific person the lawyer knows or reasonably should know needs legal services in a particular matter and that offers to provide, or reasonably can be understood as offering to provide, legal services for that matter." The rule states that a "lawyer shall not solicit professional employment by live person-to-person contact when a significant motive for the lawyer's doing so is the lawyer's or law firm's pecuniary gain." Comment [2] to the rule states that solicitation is dangerous because of the "private importuning of the trained advocate in a direct interpersonal encounter. . . . The situation is fraught with the possibility of undue influence, intimidation, and over-reaching."

The rule does have some narrow exceptions: lawyers may solicit other lawyers, those who have a "family, close personal, or prior business or professional relationship with the lawyer or law firm," and those "who routinely use[] for business purposes the type of legal services offered by the lawyer." A lawyer may not solicit even this group, however, if the "target of the solicitation has made known to the lawyer a desire not to be solicited," or "the solicitation involves coercion, duress or harassment."

Remember that even if a lawyer's communication with a prospective client does not constitute solicitation, that communication still must satisfy the marketing rules discussed above.

In a 2018 amendment to Rule 7.3, the ABA clarified an ambiguity by defining impermissible "live person-to-person contact" as "face-to-face, live telephone and other real-time visual or auditory person-to-person communications where the person is subject to a direct personal encounter without time for reflection."[45] The rule now explicitly permits communication through "chat rooms, text messages or other written communications that receipients may easily disregard," which was not clear under the prior rule. The new rule makes sense since the rationale for banning solicitation is the "possibility of undue influence, intimidation, and over-reaching."[46] These dangers are not present when a consumer receives an email, text message, or Tweet from a lawyer soliciting business because the consumer can simply ignore those communications. Thus, these communications are permissible so long as they are not "false or misleading" and otherwise comply with Rules 7.1 and 7.2.

---

45. Model Rule 7.3 cmt. [2].
46. *Id.*

Indeed, a state almost certainly could not constitutionally ban solicitations made through email, text message, Twitter, or other methods that could be easily disregarded by the receipient. Recall that in *Shapero*, the Supreme Court held that a state could not categorically ban lawyers from sending direct mailings to potential clients who had foreclosure suits filed against them. The *Shapero* Court emphasized that the Court's decision in *Ohralik* turned on the fact that, unlike direct mail, face-to-face solicitation is "a practice rife with possibilities for overreaching, invasion of privacy, the exercise of undue influence, and outright fraud" and distinguished it from direct mail.

> Unlike the potential client with a badgering advocate breathing down his neck, the recipient of a letter and the "reader of an advertisement . . . can 'effectively avoid further bombardment of [his] sensibilities simply by averting [his] eyes,'" A letter, like a printed advertisement (but unlike a lawyer), can readily be put in a drawer to be considered later, ignored, or discarded. In short, both types of written solicitation "conve[y] information about legal services [by means] that [are] more conducive to reflection and the exercise of choice on the part of the consumer than is personal solicitation by an attorney."[47]

Chapter Summary

- Advertising generally refers to marketing that is directed to a broad audience, whereas solicitation is a targeted communication initiated by the lawyer that is directed to a specific person.
- In a series of cases, the Supreme Court has recognized that lawyer marketing is protected under the commercial speech doctrine and that lawyers therefore have a constitutional right to advertise in a truthful, non-deceptive manner.
- As *Went For It* demonstrates, however, states may impose limits on lawyer marketing to serve a variety of government interests including protecting the public and the reputation of lawyers.
- Under the Model Rules, the primary limit on lawyer marketing is that it may not be false or misleading.
- In *Ohralik*, the Supreme Court upheld a categorical ban on in-person, face-to-face solicitation for pecuniary gain, finding that such conduct is necessary to protect consumers from "fraud, undue influence, intimidation, overreaching and other forms of vexatious conduct."
- The Model Rules ban solicitation, defined as "live person-to-person contact when a significant motive for the lawyer's doing so is the lawyer's or law firm's pecuniary gain."

---

47. Shapero v. Ky. Bar Ass'n, 486 U.S. 466, 475-76 (1988) (citations omitted) (alterations in original).

Applying the Rules

1. In its opinion above, the California bar determined that examples 2, 3, and 4 constitute advertising within the meaning of the Rules of Professional Conduct. Do those statements violate the rules?

2. Your law firm has been hired to represent two personal injury lawyers.

   a. The first created a television commercial in which he called himself "The Hammer" and stated that he would "hammer the insurance company."
   b. The second lawyer referred to herself and her partners in the firm's marketing as "The Heavy Hitters."

   The bar has opened an investigation into the propriety of these ads and ordered a hearing. Are the ads permissible under the Model Rules of Professional Conduct? Would it be constitutional for the bar to discipline the lawyers in these ads?

3. You are a third-year associate in the commercial litigation department at a large law firm and have decided to join LinkedIn to help build your reputation and attract clients. Can you list "Legal Research" under the "Skills and Expertise" section of your LinkedIn page? Can you accept an endorsement for "Legal Research" from a law school classmate? If your law school classmate endorses you for "Tax Advice," what should you do?

4. A lawyer sponsored a poster on the public bus that showed his firm's name and stated: "ACCIDENT VICTIM AWARDED $1,000,000 VERDICT." This statement was true. Is the attorney subject to discipline?

5. A tax lawyer offered an educational seminar on new provisions of the IRS Code that affect small businesses. Fifty small business owners attended. At the end of the seminar, the lawyer announces that the attendees can hire him to help them ensure that their businesses are in compliance with the new provisions. Is the lawyer subject to discipline?

6. A woman tweeted that her car was hit while she was unloading groceries and said "Is it smart to post photographs of car accidents online? Can insurance companies use this against you?" An attorney tweeted back: "If you are interested in suing the other driver, I would be happy to represent you." Is the lawyer subject to discipline?

Professional Responsibility in Practice

1. Advertising rules vary greatly from state to state. Look up your state's rules and compare them to the Model Rules.

2. Pick an area of law in which you might engage in private practice. Develop a marketing plan for your practice.

3. Find some examples of advertisements created by local attorneys. Do they follow your state's rules? If not, how would you alter them to make them comply?

Access to Justice and Pro Bono Services

We often think about the United States as having the world's greatest justice system; although our system has its flaws, it is, by many measures, a model for the rest of the world. But when it comes to access to justice, we fall far short. The World Justice Project scores the United States 30th out of the 37 countries in our income group under the factor "Civil Justice," and that poor rating is largely due to the United States' woeful score on "accessibility and affordability," where the United States ranks 103d out of the 126 countries surveyed.[1]

Most lawyers charge hundreds of dollars per hour for their services, which prices them far above what most low- and moderate-income Americans can afford. Moreover, the Supreme Court has refused to recognize any right to a lawyer in civil cases. Nor is funding anywhere close to sufficient to meet the public's needs: "Providing even one hour of attorney time to everyone in the United States with a legal problem would cost around $40 billion, but total expenditures on legal aid (both public and private) are just 3.5% of that amount."[2]

Key Concepts

- Parties in civil cases have no right to counsel under federal law, though some states provide lawyers in limited categories of cases
- With no legal right to counsel, low- and moderate-income Americans lack adequate access to representation
- Lawyers, courts, innovators, commentators, and others have proposed a wide range of potential solutions to address the **access-to-justice gap**[3]

---

1. World Justice Project, World Justice Project Rule of Law Index 2020, at 154 (2020), *available at* https://worldjusticeproject.org/sites/default/files/documents/WJP-ROLI-2020-Online_0.pdf.
2. Solomon, Rhode & Wanless, *How Reforming Rule 5.4 Would Benefit Lawyers and Consumers, Promote Innovation, and Increase Access to Justice*, Stanford Center on the Legal Profession, Stanford Law School, https://www-cdn.law.stanford.edu/wp-content/uploads/2020/04/Rule_5.4_Whitepaper_-_Final.pdf (citing Gillian Hadfield & Deborah Rhode, *How to Regulate Legal Services to Promote Access, Innovation, and the Quality of Lawyering*, 67 Hastings L.J. 1191, 1193 (2016)).
3. Although serious problems exist in our criminal justice system, criminal defendants are guaranteed the right to counsel under the Sixth Amendment, while parties in civil matters enjoy no such protection. This chapter focuses on access to justice for parties in civil matters.

More than 40 years ago, President Jimmy Carter observed, "Ninety percent of our lawyers serve 10 percent of our people."[4] If anything, the situation has grown worse. Every year, millions of Americans face legal crises — mortgage foreclosure proceedings, child custody disputes, debt collection actions, and other serious legal issues — without the help of a lawyer. The economic upheaval caused by the COVID-19 pandemic is exacerbating the situation.

Do lawyers bear some responsibility for improving this state of affairs? Professor Deborah Rhode, who has long been a leading voice on access-to-justice issues, articulates two primary reasons why they do:

> [First,] the legal profession has a monopoly on the provision of essential services. Lawyers have special privileges that entail special obligations. In the United States, attorneys have a much more extensive and exclusive right to provide legal assistance than attorneys in other countries. The American bar has closely guarded those prerogatives and its success in restricting lay competition has helped to price services out of the reach of many consumers. . . .
>
> An alternative justification for imposing special obligations on lawyers stems from their special role in our governance structure. As [a New York Committee Report on access to justice] explained, much of what lawyers do
>
> > is about providing justice, [which is] . . . nearer to the heart of our way of life . . . than services provided by other professionals. The legal profession serves as indispensable guardians of our lives, liberties and governing principles. . . . Like no other professionals, lawyers are charged with the responsibility for systemic improvement of not only their own profession, but of the law and society itself.[5]

One way to improve access to justice would be to guarantee individuals the right to a lawyer in at least some category of civil cases, but the courts and legislatures have largely refused to do so. This chapter begins by describing the very limited rights of civil litigants to the assistance of a lawyer. Without a right to counsel, the vast majority of individuals are left to face legal problems on their own. The chapter then turns to the access-to-justice gap before discussing some potential solutions.

A. "CIVIL GIDEON"

In the famous case of Gideon v. Wainwright, 372 U.S. 335 (1963), the Supreme Court held that indigent defendants in criminal cases have a right to court-appointed counsel under the Sixth Amendment.[6] The Supreme Court has also held that indigent defendants have the right to court-appointed counsel in criminal contempt proceedings (other than summary proceedings).[7] The Court has made clear,

---

4. *Remarks at the 100th Anniversary Luncheon of the Los Angeles Bar Association*, 1 PUB. PAPERS 834, 836 (May 4, 1978); *see* Deborah Rhode, *Access to Justice: Connecting Principles to Practice*, 17 GEO. J. LEGAL ETHICS 369, 371 (2004).
5. Deborah L. Rhode, *Cultures of Commitment: Pro Bono for Lawyers and Law Students*, 67 FORDHAM L. REV. 2415, 2419 (1999) (footnote omitted).
6. Gideon v. Wainwright, 372 U.S. at 339-40.
7. United States v. Dixon, 509 U.S. 688, 696 (1993).

however, that the Sixth Amendment does not apply in civil cases. In recent years, advocates of what is commonly referred to as the "Civil Gideon" movement, have argued in courts and legislatures for recognition of an expanded right to counsel in civil cases. In the federal courts, the Civil Gideon movement has achieved little success. Although the U.S. Supreme Court recognized a right to counsel for juveniles in delinquency proceedings in the 1967 case of In re Gault, 387 U.S. 1, 41 (1967), the Court has not expanded that right beyond *Gault*. The latest setback came in *Turner v. Rogers*.[8]

Case Preview

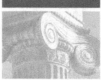

Turner v. Rogers

Michael Turner was a father who allegedly owed child support. South Carolina enforces its child support orders by threatening incarceration for civil contempt for those who are able to comply with a child support order but fail to do so. Turner had previously been held in contempt several times and, in some cases, had served time in jail before he paid the amount due. In January 2008, Turner appeared again pro se before the South Carolina family court, this time owing $5,728.76 in back child support to his wife, who was also unrepresented. After a very brief hearing, the court sentenced him to 12 months in jail. On appeal, Turner argued that as an indigent person facing potential incarceration, he was entitled to counsel under the Due Process Clause of the Fourteenth Amendment.

As you read *Turner*, consider the following:

1. What do you think about the proceeding at which Turner was found in contempt? How does it compare to your idea of what courtroom proceedings are like? How does it compare to the depiction of legal proceedings in popular media?
2. Why does the Court conclude that Turner was not entitled to counsel?
3. Are the "alternative procedures" required by the Court an adequate replacement for a lawyer?

Turner v. Rogers
564 U.S. 431 (2011)

Justice BREYER delivered the opinion of the Court.

South Carolina's Family Court enforces its child support orders by threatening with incarceration for civil contempt those who are (1) subject to a child support order, (2) able to comply with that order, but (3) fail to do so. We must decide whether

---

8. 564 U.S. 431 (2011).

the Fourteenth Amendment's Due Process Clause requires the State to provide counsel (at a civil contempt hearing) to an *indigent* person potentially faced with such incarceration. We conclude that where as here the custodial parent (entitled to receive the support) is unrepresented by counsel, the State need not provide counsel to the noncustodial parent (required to provide the support). But we attach an important caveat, namely, that the State must nonetheless have in place alternative procedures that assure a fundamentally fair determination of the critical incarceration-related question, whether the supporting parent is able to comply with the support order.

I

A

South Carolina family courts enforce their child support orders in part through civil contempt proceedings. Each month the family court clerk reviews outstanding child support orders, identifies those in which the supporting parent has fallen more than five days behind, and sends that parent an order to "show cause" why he should not be held in contempt. The "show cause" order and attached affidavit refer to the relevant child support order, identify the amount of the arrearage, and set a date for a court hearing. At the hearing that parent may demonstrate that he is not in contempt, say, by showing that he is not able to make the required payments. If he fails to make the required showing, the court may hold him in civil contempt. And it may require that he be imprisoned unless and until he purges himself of contempt by making the required child support payments (but not for more than one year regardless).

B

In June 2003 a South Carolina family court entered an order, which (as amended) required petitioner, Michael Turner, to pay $51.73 per week to respondent, Rebecca Rogers, to help support their child. . . . Over the next three years, Turner repeatedly failed to pay the amount due and was held in contempt on five occasions. The first four times he was sentenced to 90 days' imprisonment, but he ultimately paid the amount due (twice without being jailed, twice after spending two or three days in custody). The fifth time he did not pay but completed a 6–month sentence.

After his release in 2006 Turner remained in arrears. On March 27, 2006, the clerk issued a new "show cause" order. And after an initial postponement due to Turner's failure to appear, Turner's civil contempt hearing took place on January 3, 2008. Turner and Rogers were present, each without representation by counsel.

The hearing was brief. The court clerk said that Turner was $5,728.76 behind in his payments. The judge asked Turner if there was "anything you want to say." Turner replied,

> Well, when I first got out, I got back on dope. I done meth, smoked pot and everything else, and I paid a little bit here and there. And, when I finally did get to working, I broke my back, back in September. I filed for disability and SSI. And, I didn't get straightened out off the dope until I broke my back and laid up for two months. And, now I'm off the dope and everything. I just hope that you give me a chance. I don't know what else to say. I mean, I know I done wrong, and I should have been paying and helping her, and I'm sorry. I mean, dope had a hold to me.

The judge then said, "[o]kay," and asked Rogers if she had anything to say. After a brief discussion of federal benefits, the judge stated,

> If there's nothing else, this will be the Order of the Court. I find the Defendant in willful contempt. I'm [going to] sentence him to twelve months in the Oconee County Detention Center. He may purge himself of the contempt and avoid the sentence by having a zero balance on or before his release. I've also placed a lien on any SSI or other benefits.

The judge added that Turner would not receive good-time or work credits, but "[i]f you've got a job, I'll make you eligible for work release." When Turner asked why he could not receive good-time or work credits, the judge said, "[b]ecause that's my ruling." *Ibid.*

The court made no express finding concerning Turner's ability to pay his arrearage (though Turner's wife had voluntarily submitted a copy of Turner's application for disability benefits . . .). Nor did the judge ask any followup questions or otherwise address the ability-to-pay issue. After the hearing, the judge filled out a prewritten form titled "Order for Contempt of Court," which included the statement: "Defendant (was) (was not) gainfully employed and/or (had) (did not have) the ability to make these support payments when due." But the judge left this statement as is without indicating whether Turner was able to make support payments.

C

While serving his 12–month sentence, Turner, with the help of *pro bono* counsel, appealed. He claimed that the Federal Constitution entitled him to counsel at his contempt hearing. The South Carolina Supreme Court decided Turner's appeal after he had completed his sentence. And it rejected his "right to counsel" claim. . . .

Turner sought certiorari [and the Supreme Court granted the writ].

. . .

II

[The Court held that the case was not moot even though Turner is no longer incarcerated.]

III

We must decide whether the Due Process Clause grants an indigent defendant, such as Turner, a right to state-appointed counsel at a civil contempt proceeding, which may lead to his incarceration. This Court's precedents provide no definitive answer to that question. This Court has long held that the Sixth Amendment grants an indigent defendant the right to state-appointed counsel in a *criminal* case. Gideon v. Wainwright, 372 U.S. 335 (1963). And we have held that this same rule applies to *criminal contempt* proceedings (other than summary proceedings).

But the Sixth Amendment does not govern civil cases. Civil contempt differs from criminal contempt in that it seeks only to "coerc[e] the defendant to do" what a court had previously ordered him to do. A court may not impose punishment "in a civil contempt proceeding when it is clearly established that the alleged contemnor is unable to comply with the terms of the order." And once a civil contemnor complies with the underlying order, he is purged of the contempt and is free.

Consequently, the Court has made clear (in a case not involving the right to counsel) that, where civil contempt is at issue, the Fourteenth Amendment's Due Process Clause allows a State to provide fewer procedural protections than in a criminal case.

This Court has decided only a handful of cases that more directly concern a right to counsel in civil matters. And the application of those decisions to the present case is not clear. On the one hand, the Court has held that the Fourteenth Amendment requires the State to pay for representation by counsel in a *civil* "juvenile delinquency" proceeding (which could lead to incarceration). In re Gault, 387 U.S. 1 (1967). Moreover, in Vitek v. Jones, 445 U.S. 480 (1980), a plurality of four Members of this Court would have held that the Fourteenth Amendment requires representation by counsel in a proceeding to transfer a prison inmate to a state hospital for the mentally ill. Further, in Lassiter v. Department of Social Servs. of Durham Cty., 452 U.S. 18 (1981), a case that focused upon civil proceedings leading to loss of parental rights, the Court wrote that the "pre-eminent generalization that emerges from this Court's precedents on an indigent's right to appointed counsel is that such a right has been recognized to exist only where the litigant may lose his physical liberty if he loses the litigation." And the Court then drew from these precedents "the presumption that an indigent litigant has a right to appointed counsel only when, if he loses, he may be deprived of his physical liberty."

On the other hand, the Court has held that a criminal offender facing revocation of probation and imprisonment does *not* ordinarily have a right to counsel at a probation revocation hearing. And, at the same time, *Gault, Vitek,* and *Lassiter* are readily distinguishable. The civil juvenile delinquency proceeding at issue in *Gault* was "little different" from, and "comparable in seriousness" to, a criminal prosecution. In *Vitek,* the controlling opinion found *no* right to counsel. And the Court's statements in *Lassiter* constitute part of its rationale for *denying* a right to counsel in that case. We believe those statements are best read as pointing out that the Court previously had found a right to counsel "*only*" in cases involving incarceration, not that a right to counsel exists in *all* such cases. . . .

B

Civil contempt proceedings in child support cases constitute one part of a highly complex system designed to assure a noncustodial parent's regular payment of funds typically necessary for the support of his children. Often the family receives welfare support from a state-administered federal program, and the State then seeks reimbursement from the noncustodial parent. Other times the custodial parent (often the mother, but sometimes the father, a grandparent, or another person with custody) does not receive government benefits and is entitled to receive the support payments herself.

The Federal Government has created an elaborate procedural mechanism designed to help both the government and custodial parents to secure the payments to which they are entitled. These systems often rely upon wage withholding, expedited procedures for modifying and enforcing child support orders, and automated data processing. But sometimes States will use contempt orders to ensure that the custodial parent receives support payments or the government receives reimburse-ment. Although some experts have criticized this last-mentioned procedure, and the Federal Government believes that "the routine use of contempt for non-payment of child support is likely to be an ineffective strategy," the Government also tells us that "coercive enforcement remedies, such as contempt, have a role to play." South Carolina, which relies heavily on contempt proceedings, agrees that they are an important tool.

We here consider an indigent's right to paid counsel at such a contempt proceed-ing. It is a civil proceeding. And we consequently determine the "specific dictates of due process" by examining the "distinct factors" that this Court has previously found useful in deciding what specific safeguards the Constitution's Due Process Clause requires in order to make a civil proceeding fundamentally fair. As relevant here those factors include (1) the nature of "the private interest that will be affected," (2) the comparative "risk" of an "erroneous deprivation" of that interest with and without "additional or substitute procedural safeguards," and (3) the nature and magnitude of any countervailing interest in not providing "additional or substitute procedural requirement [s]."

The "private interest that will be affected" argues strongly for the right to coun-sel that Turner advocates. That interest consists of an indigent defendant's loss of personal liberty through imprisonment. The interest in securing that freedom, the freedom "from bodily restraint," lies "at the core of the liberty protected by the Due Process Clause." And we have made clear that its threatened loss through legal pro-ceedings demands "due process protection."

Given the importance of the interest at stake, it is obviously important to assure accurate decisionmaking in respect to the key "ability to pay" question. Moreover, the fact that ability to comply marks a dividing line between civil and criminal contempt, reinforces the need for accuracy. That is because an incorrect decision (wrongly clas-sifying the contempt proceeding as civil) can increase the risk of wrongful incarcer-ation by depriving the defendant of the procedural protections (including counsel) that the Constitution would demand in a criminal proceeding. And since 70% of child support arrears nationwide are owed by parents with either no reported income or income of $10,000 per year or less, the issue of ability to pay may arise fairly often.

On the other hand, the Due Process Clause does not always require the provision of counsel in civil proceedings where incarceration is threatened. And in determin-ing whether the Clause requires a right to counsel here, we must take account of opposing interests, as well as consider the probable value of "additional or substitute procedural safeguards."

Doing so, we find three related considerations that, when taken together, argue strongly against the Due Process Clause requiring the State to provide indigents with counsel in every proceeding of the kind before us. First, the critical question likely at issue in these cases concerns, as we have said, the defendant's ability to pay. That question is often closely related to the question of the defendant's indigence. But when the right procedures are in place, indigence can be a question that in many—but not all—cases is sufficiently straightforward to warrant determination *prior* to providing a defendant with counsel, even in a criminal case. Federal law, for example, requires a criminal defendant to provide information showing that he is indigent, and therefore entitled to state-funded counsel, *before* he can receive that assistance.

Second, sometimes, as here, the person opposing the defendant at the hearing is not the government represented by counsel but the custodial parent *un*represented by counsel. The custodial parent, perhaps a woman with custody of one or more children, may be relatively poor, unemployed, and unable to afford counsel. Yet she may have encouraged the court to enforce its order through contempt. She may be able to provide the court with significant information. A requirement that the State provide counsel to the noncustodial parent in these cases could create an asymmetry of representation that would "alter significantly the nature of the proceeding." Doing so could mean a degree of formality or delay that would unduly slow payment to those immediately in need. And, perhaps more important for present purposes, doing so could make the proceedings *less* fair overall, increasing the risk of a decision that would erroneously deprive a family of the support it is entitled to receive. The needs of such families play an important role in our analysis.

Third, as the Solicitor General points out, there is available a set of "substitute procedural safeguards," which, if employed together, can significantly reduce the risk of an erroneous deprivation of liberty. They can do so, moreover, without incurring some of the drawbacks inherent in recognizing an automatic right to counsel. Those safeguards include (1) notice to the defendant that his "ability to pay" is a critical issue in the contempt proceeding; (2) the use of a form (or the equivalent) to elicit relevant financial information; (3) an opportunity at the hearing for the defendant to respond to statements and questions about his financial status, (*e.g.*, those triggered by his responses on the form); and (4) an express finding by the court that the defendant has the ability to pay. In presenting these alternatives, the Government draws upon considerable experience in helping to manage statutorily mandated federal-state efforts to enforce child support orders. It does not claim that they are the only possible alternatives, and this Court's cases suggest, for example, that sometimes assistance other than purely legal assistance (here, say, that of a neutral social worker) can prove constitutionally sufficient. But the Government does claim that these alternatives can assure the "fundamental fairness" of the proceeding even where the State does not pay for counsel for an indigent defendant.

While recognizing the strength of Turner's arguments, we ultimately believe that the three considerations we have just discussed must carry the day. In our view, a categorical right to counsel in proceedings of the kind before us would carry with it disadvantages (in the form of unfairness and delay) that, in terms of ultimate fairness, would deprive it of significant superiority over the alternatives that we have mentioned. We consequently hold that the Due Process Clause does not *automatically* require the provision of counsel at civil contempt proceedings to an indigent individual who is subject to a child support order, even if that individual faces incarceration (for up to a year). In particular, that Clause does not require the provision of counsel where the opposing parent or other custodian (to whom support funds are owed) is not represented by counsel and the State provides alternative procedural safeguards equivalent to those we have mentioned (adequate notice of the importance of ability to pay, fair opportunity to present, and to dispute, relevant information, and court findings).

We do not address civil contempt proceedings where the underlying child support payment is owed to the State, for example, for reimbursement of welfare funds paid to the parent with custody. Those proceedings more closely resemble debt-collection proceedings. The government is likely to have counsel or some other competent representative. And this kind of proceeding is not before us. Neither do we address what due process requires in an unusually complex case where a defendant "can fairly be represented only by a trained advocate."

IV

The record indicates that Turner received neither counsel nor the benefit of alternative procedures like those we have described. He did not receive clear notice that his ability to pay would constitute the critical question in his civil contempt proceeding. No one provided him with a form (or the equivalent) designed to elicit information about his financial circumstances. The court did not find that Turner was able to pay his arrearage, but instead left the relevant "finding" section of the contempt order blank. The court nonetheless found Turner in contempt and ordered him incarcerated. Under these circumstances Turner's incarceration violated the Due Process Clause.

We vacate the judgment of the South Carolina Supreme Court and remand the case for further proceedings not inconsistent with this opinion.

Justice THOMAS, with whom Justice SCALIA joins, and with whom THE CHIEF JUSTICE and Justice ALITO join as to Parts I–B and II, dissenting.

The Due Process Clause of the Fourteenth Amendment does not provide a right to appointed counsel for indigent defendants facing incarceration in civil contempt proceedings. Therefore, I would affirm. Although the Court agrees that appointed counsel was not required in this case, it nevertheless vacates the judgment of the South Carolina Supreme Court on a different ground, which the parties have never raised. Solely at the invitation of the United States as *amicus curiae,* the majority decides that Turner's contempt proceeding violated due process because it did not include "alternative procedural safeguards." Consistent with this Court's longstanding practice, I would not reach that question. . . .

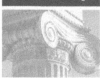

Post-Case Follow-Up

Although the U.S. Supreme Court has declined to recognize a civil right to counsel under federal law, many states mandate or authorize (at the court's discretion) a right to counsel in certain limited circumstances. The most common situations in which states guarantee a right to counsel are: proceedings in which parents are accused of abuse or neglect, state-initiated termination of parental rights cases, involuntary commitment proceedings, litigation concerning medical treatment, and guardianship proceedings.[9] In many cases, these rights are provided by statute, though in some cases they are established by court opinions. Again, however, the reach of these laws is quite limited, and most people in most states are not guaranteed counsel in most civil cases.

---

9. For a comprehensive list of state resources, see the directory at ABA COMM. ON LEGAL AID & INDIGENT DEFENSE, *available at* https://www.americanbar.org/groups/legal_aid_indigent_defense/civil_right_to_counsel1/ (last visited July 21, 2020); *see also* National Coalition for a Civil Right to Counsel, Status Map, *available at* http://www.civilrighttocounsel.org/map (last visited July 21, 2020).

Turner v. Rogers: Real Life Applications

1. Under a divorce decree, Father was awarded visitation every other weekend. Over several years, Mother denied Father regular visitation, stating that the children were afraid of their father although she could not give any specific reason why. The court held several contempt hearings. Father filed yet another application for contempt after being denied visitation. At the hearing, Father appeared without a lawyer. The court asked Mother if she was prepared to proceed without counsel, even though the hearing could result in jail time, and she agreed. The hearing took about an hour and 20 minutes. Mother offered her own testimony and letters from the minor children detailing how they felt about Father and their visitations with him, as the court would not allow them to testify. The court found that Mother failed to purge her contempt and sentenced her to 30 days in jail. Did the Court err in jailing Mother without first providing her with counsel?

2. In her divorce, Mother was ordered to pay child support. Eight years later, the county child support enforcement agency filed a motion for contempt against Mother for failing to pay. Mother appeared at the hearing without counsel. The magistrate said to Mother, "I'm going to deny your request for counsel at this time. There [was] a recent U.S. Supreme Court decision that came down on contempt citations regarding child support, [holding] that obligors that are facing jail time in civil contempts are not entitled to court-appointed counsel." Agency counsel presented evidence that Mother owed over $16,000 in child support. Mother testified that she was not aware of the obligation and that she could not afford the payments since her income consisted of $200 per month in food stamps, and she had a medical condition that prevented her from working. The magistrate found Mother in contempt and sentenced her to 30 days in jail. Should Mother appeal?

B. THE JUSTICE GAP

A woman living in poverty receives a notice from her landlord that she is being evicted from her apartment. She cannot afford a lawyer; what should she do? The best option for low-income Americans is to try to obtain the services of a legal services lawyer, funded by the Legal Services Corporation (LSC). LSC, a non-profit organization established by Congress in 1974, is the single largest funder of civil legal aid for low-income Americans.[10] LSC does not deliver legal services itself but rather funds legal service providers in every state in the country. Only individuals who live in households with annual incomes below 125 percent of the federal poverty guidelines — $15,950 in household income for a single person and $32,750 for a family of four — are eligible for LSC-funded services.[11]

---

10. *About LSC*, LEGAL SERVS. CORP., http://www.lsc.gov/about-lsc (last visited July 21, 2020).
11. Income Level for Individuals Eligible for Assistance, 85 Fed. Reg. 8190 (Feb. 13, 2020) (to be codified at 45 C.F.R. pt. 1611 app. A), *available at* https://www.federalregister.gov/documents/2020/02/13/2020-01824/income-level-for-individuals-eligible-for-assistance.

Legal services offices also fund their budgets with resources derived from some combination of state funding, private fundraising, and grants from Interest On Lawyer Trust Accounts (IOLTA). The availability of funding varies dramatically from state to state, prompting an ABA report to observe that when it comes to the availability of legal services "geography is destiny."[12] As a general matter, state government funding and grants from IOLTA have declined dramatically. The National Association of IOLTA Programs (NAIP), which administers state-based sources of funding, including IOLTA, state court filing fees, and legislative appropriations, projected a $157.4 million loss of revenue available for civil legal aid in 2020 because of economic disruptions caused by the COVID-19 pandemic.[13]

Given the overwhelming demand for legal services and the drop in state funding, even the record-level of federal funding[14] that LSC received for fiscal year 2020 is insufficient to meet the demand for LSC lawyers. As a result, LSC-funded offices simply do not have sufficient staffing to meet the needs of individuals with legal problems and have to turn away more than half of those who approach them.[15]

Where else can our tenant facing eviction go? A variety of public interest organizations provide free legal services in specific locations for particular client groups. In addition to low-income persons, public interest organizations provide services to the elderly, people with disabilities, members of Native American populations, people with HIV/AIDS, people who are homeless, and veterans. They also provide services on particular legal issues, for example, housing, immigration, or civil rights. Again, the services available to the public vary greatly from state to state and within individual states.

Law school clinics also provide legal assistance to the poor, but the impact that these clinics can make is limited. To ensure a high-quality educational experience for and careful supervision of law students, the ABA requires clinics to maintain a small faculty-student ratio thereby limiting the number of cases that law

IOLTA Funding and the Fifth Amendment

IOLTA funding has survived several constitutional attacks. In 1998, the Supreme Court held that the interest earned from clients' money in a lawyer's trust account is private property subject to the Fifth Amendment. Phillips v. Wash. Legal Found., 524 U.S. 156 (1998). The Court remanded the case to determine whether that property had been taken for public use without just compensation.

Without a definite answer, litigation continued. Finally, in 2003, the Court settled the issue in Brown v. Legal Found. of Wash., 538 U.S. 216 (2003). The Court found that the use of the interest to benefit those who could not afford lawyers was a public use and a *per se* taking. Nevertheless, it upheld IOLTA funding as constitutional. Since the Fifth Amendment is only violated when there is a taking without just compensation, which is measured by the property owner's loss, the court concluded that the Fifth Amendment was not violated as the client has lost nothing. Lawyers only deposit client funds into IOLTA accounts when those funds could not earn net interest because the funds are too small and/or they are being held for such a short time that the administrative costs of a separated interest-bearing account would exceed the interest earned by the individual client.

---

12. *Report on the Future of Legal Services in the United States (2016)*, ABA COMM'N ON THE FUTURE OF LEGAL SERVS., *available at* https://www.americanbar.org/content/dam/aba/images/abanews/2016FLSReport_FNL_WEB.pdf (last visited July 25, 2020).
13. *$157.4 Million Projected Loss in Critical Sources of State Funding for Civil Legal Aid*, NAIP Press Release, 2020, *available at* https://www.iolta.org/images/NAIP-Press-Release-5-29-20.pdf.
14. Marilyn Odendahl, *"Boost in LSC Funding Likely to Bring More Dollars to Indiana,"* THE INDIANA LAWYER, 2019, *available at* https://www.theindianalawyer.com/articles/boost-in-lsc-funding-likely-to-bring-more-dollars-to-indiana.
15. *2017 Annual Report Justice Gap*, LEGAL SERVICES CORP., *available at* https://www.lsc.gov/media-center/publications/2017-annual-report-justice-gap.

school clinics can take. Although many law school clinics deliver outstanding legal services to their low-income clients, the principle purpose of clinics remains education, not service.

If our tenant were lucky, she might be able to find a lawyer willing to offer her services pro bono. Pro bono work by lawyers in private practice is another significant resource for low-income persons, but the good work done by many lawyers does not come anywhere close to solving the problem: "providing one hour of pro bono per justice problem would require over 200 hours of pro bono work per attorney per year, but the average pro bono hours worked per attorney is only 42.8."[16]

Although we have assumed so far that our tenant lives in poverty, a middle-income American served with an eviction notice might have almost as much difficulty finding a lawyer. These individuals do not meet the income qualifications for LSC-funded lawyers or most other legal aid providers, yet they often still cannot afford to hire attorneys. The Economic Policy Institute provides a calculator to measure the income that a family needs to attain a "modest yet adequate standard of living."[17] In Memphis, Tennessee, one of the least expensive cities in the country, that amount is $71,800 per year, which is higher than the median family income in the city's metropolitan area. As this example illustrates, most middle-income families do not have money in their budget to hire lawyers when the need arises.

The resulting situation is bleak. A leading researcher concluded that "well over 100 million Americans [are] living with civil justice problems, many involving what the American Bar Association has termed 'basic human needs'" relating to shelter, sustenance, safety, health, and child custody.[18] Yet most of these individuals must deal with these problems without the help of a lawyer or other legal service provider: "[o]ver four-fifths of the legal needs of the poor and a majority of the needs of middle-income Americans remain unmet."[19]

One significant consequence of this justice gap is that our court system is witnessing an enormous and growing number of unrepresented litigants. One study concluded that more than 80 percent of low-income litigants are unrepresented in cases involving basic life needs (debt collection cases, mortgage foreclosures, child support and custody cases, etc.).[20] Depending on the type of case and particular jurisdiction, the numbers are even worse. According to a recent study between 2010 and 2019, less than 10 percent of defendants in debt collection cases were represented by legal counsel.[21] The large numbers of unrepresented litigants impact the entire justice system.

---

16. Solmon, Rhode & Wanless, *How Reforming Rule 5.4 Would Benefit Lawyers and Consumers, Promote Innovation, and Increase Access to Justice*, Stanford Center on the Legal Profession, Stanford Law School, 2020, *available at* https://www-cdn.law.stanford.edu/wp-content/uploads/2020/04/rule_5.4_whitepaper_-_final.pdf.

17. *Family Budget Calculator*, Economic Policy Institute, https://www.epi.org/resources/budget/ (last visited July 23, 2020).

18. Rebecca L Sandefur, *What We Know and Need to Know About the Legal Needs of the Public*, 67 S.C. L. Rev. 433, 446 (2016).

19. Deborah L. Rhode, *What We Know and Need to Know About the Delivery of Legal Services by Nonlawyers*, 67 S.C. L. Rev. 429, 429 (2016).

20. *Documenting the Justice Gap in America*, Legal Services Corporation (2009), *available at* https://www.lsc .gov/sites/default/files/LSC/pdfs/documenting_the_justice_gap_in_america_2009.pdf.

21. *How Debt Collectors are Transforming the Business of State Courts*, The PEW Charitable Trusts, May 6, 2020, *available at* https://www.pewtrusts.org/en/research-and-analysis/reports/2020/05/how-debt-collectors -are-transforming-the-business-of-state-courts.

Beyond affordable legal services, groundbreaking research by Professor Rebecca Sandefur has uncovered another reason for the justice gap: many people do not know that their problems are *legal* problems; they just know that they are problems. And partly as a result of this dynamic, people seldom go to lawyers for help in solving their legal problems. Instead, they may seek assistance from churches, housing counselors, social workers, city agencies, the Better Business Bureau, and their elected representatives. The most common course of action, however, is self-help.[22] Interestingly, although most people do not identify their legal problems as such, when asked what they want in terms of assistance, those same people are seeking what we would define as legal advice: an understanding of their rights, advice on the situation, and help with filling out forms or writing letters.[23]

C. POSSIBLE SOLUTIONS

1. Simplifying Court Procedures

Our court system is complex and intimidating to those who seek to represent themselves. As one judge testified:

> Most individuals would not attempt to play a sport, play a game, take an exam, or fill out an important application without knowing the rules and instructions. Indeed, we give people clear rules or instructions on how to complete these tasks. But, we . . . do not always provide unrepresented litigants the rules, instructions and necessary tools when they are attempting to navigate the courts. In our adversarial system, the information, rules and forms unrepresented litigants need to be successful on their case are often not available or accessible. We often hide the ball necessary to play the game. It is time to stop hiding the ball, so the game is fair. . . .
>
> In order to achieve a major step forward in access to justice, standardization and simplification of forms and procedures is an effort we must embrace and get done. . . . [J]ustice should not be stymied by obstacles we can remove.[24]

To help unrepresented litigants, our courts need to develop what one commentator has called "The Self-Help Friendly Court."[25] Courts could help unrepresented litigants by simplifying courtroom and other procedures to make them more readily accessible to everybody and by providing standardized and uniform

---

22. Rebecca L. Sandefur & American Bar Found., Accessing Justice in the Contemporary USA: Findings from the Community Needs and Services Study 3-4, 7 (2014) (Only 9 percent of those experiencing a civil justice situation described their problem as "legal."), *available at* http://www.americanbarfoundation.org/uploads/cms/documents/sandefur_accessing_justice_in_the_contemporary_usa._aug._2014.pdf.

23. Rebecca L. Sandefur, *Legal Advice from Nonlawyers: Consumer Demand, Provider Quality, and Public Harms*, 16 Stan. J. C.R. & C.L. 283, 291 (2020).

24. *The Chief Judge's 2011 Hearings on Civil Legal Services, First Dep't (Sept. 26, 2011)* 2, 3-4 (written statement of Hon. Fern Fisher, Deputy Chief Administrative Judge for New York City Courts and Director of the New York State Courts Access to Justice Program), *available at* http://ww2.nycourts.gov/sites/default/files/document/files/2018-04/2011_1stDeptTestifying_0.pdf.

25. Richard Zorza, The Self-Help Friendly Court: Designed from the Ground Up to Work for People Without Lawyers (2002).

forms that are written in plain language. Judges and court personnel could also be trained in assisting self-represented litigants. Some jurisdictions are developing these resources,[26] but significant work remains to be done.

2. Mandatory Pro Bono

The Model Rules do not require that lawyers engage in pro bono work; rather, Rule 6.1 states that a lawyer "***should*** aspire to render at least (50) hours of pro bono" service per year.[27] For several decades, states have discussed requiring lawyers to perform pro bono work. In 1977, the State Bar of California proposed that practicing lawyers be required to perform 40 hours per year, but the proposal was ultimately rejected. In 2010, the Mississippi Supreme Court proposed mandatory pro bono rules but withdrew the proposal after receiving negative feedback from lawyers. Nine states require mandatory *reporting* of pro bono work in the hope of promoting such work, but do not require the actual performance of pro bono.[28]

In 2013, New York became the first state to mandate pro bono work, but only for *applicants* to the bar, not members of the bar. To become a member of the bar in New York, applicants must perform 50 hours of pro bono work in law school or some other time before they are admitted.[29] Other states are considering a similar requirement. Supporters argue that a mandatory pro bono rule for bar applicants will provide at least some help to indigent parties while also allowing future lawyers the opportunity for some practical experience. Critics, on the other hand, argue that it is unfair to impose this requirement on applicants but not on lawyers and, moreover, that compelled assistance from inexperienced lawyers is worse than nothing at all.

3. Technology

Through its adoption of comment [8] to Rule 1.1, the ABA has made clear that a lawyer's duty of competence includes understanding and using technology to benefit clients. Technology also holds great promise for improving access to justice.

Technology is being employed in a variety of ways to improve the delivery of legal services. For example, many legal aid offices and public interest law firms (in addition to private law firms and companies) are using document assembly software to assist clients. These tools are similar to TurboTax: the user is asked a series of questions and the software uses sophisticated branching technology to generate legal

---

26. ABA Groups, Standing Committee on the Delivery of Legal Services, Unbundling Resource Center, *Self-Help Centers*, ABA, *available at* https://www.americanbar.org/groups/delivery_legal_services/resources/pro_se_unbundling_resource_center/self_service_centers/.
27. Model Rule 6.1 (emphasis added).
28. ABA Groups, Standing Committee on Pro Bono & Public Service, Policy, *Pro Bono Reporting*, ABA, March 19, 2020, *available at* https://www.americanbar.org/groups/probono_public_service/policy/arguments/.
29. *Bar Admission Requirements, The Legal Profession – Pro Bono*, NYCourts.gov, http://ww2.nycourts.gov/attorneys/probono/baradmissionreqs.shtml (last visited July 23, 2020).

documents — for example, wills, leases, or other contracts — based on the user's responses. A lawyer can then review the document and make any necessary changes, but the software saves significant time allowing the lawyer to operate more efficiently and serve more clients.

In some cases, these resources are available online as part of a unified legal portal that can direct individuals who need legal assistance to the most appropriate form of assistance, whether it be document assembly software, other self-help resources, or the names of attorneys with relevant expertise. An excellent example of such a portal is Illinois Legal Aid Online (www.illinoislegalaid.org), where consumers can find articles, videos, and forms.

Many other technological innovations hold the promise of making the delivery of legal services faster, better, and cheaper. For example, companies have developed artificial intelligence tools that can perform legal research, draft legal documents, review contracts as part of due diligence, predict the outcome of pending cases, and perform many other tasks.[30]

Courts are also using technology to improve access to the justice system. For example, some courts are using technology to make services available remotely, such as document filing, document preparation, record searches, and similar services. A particularly powerful example of this is in Arizona where some individuals who live north of the Grand Canyon have to travel up to seven hours to reach their local courthouse on the south side of the Grand Canyon. In order to make the court system more accessible to those residents, the County placed a kiosk in a motor vehicles division building on the north side of the Grand Canyon so that residents who live there can access the courts without having to make that long drive. Residents can use the kiosk for a variety of purposes: for example, they can make appearances in cases that do not involve mandatory jail time. They can also talk with the clerk of the court, ask questions about civil filings, and print court forms. The cost of the kiosk was approximately $7,000, and the only ongoing expense is $75/month for the Internet connection.[32]

A Robot Lawyer Helps Overturn Parking Tickets

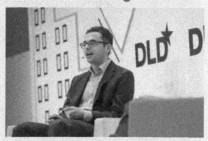

Joshua Browder, creator of the Robot Lawyer app
AP Images

Joshua Browder, a 20-year-old Stanford student, has developed an artificial intelligence app that helps people in New York and Chicago overturn parking tickets. The robot asks the user a series of questions to determine the factual background behind the ticket and then looks for loopholes to overturn the ticket. The bot then generates a letter to send to the city and guides the user through the appeal process. The success rate is 60 percent, higher than other apps using actual lawyers. Browder has said that his goal is to "level the playing field so anyone can have the same legal access under the law."[31]

Browder's app has been expanded beyond parking, helping with landlord/tenant disputes, unexplained banking charges, and a variety of tasks. *See* https://donotpay.com.

30. Daniel Fagella, *AI in Law and Legal Practice — A Comprehensive View of 35 Current Applications*, EMERJ, The AI Research and Advisory Company (March 14, 2020), *available at* https://emerj.com/ai-sector-overviews/ai-in-law-legal-practice-current-applications/.
31. Arezou Rezvani, *"Robot Lawyer" Makes the Case Against Parking Tickets*, NPR (Jan. 16, 2017), *available at* https://www.npr.org/2017/01/16/510096767/robot-lawyer-makes-the-case-against-parking-tickets.
32. Stephanie Francis Ward, *Kyle Rimel: Using Technology to Bring Court Services to Remote Areas,* Legal Rebels Profile, A.B.A. J., (Sept. 16, 2015), *available at* http://www.abajournal.com/legalrebels/article/kyle_rimel_profile.

Self-help centers are another technological innovation offered at more than 500 courthouses across the country. These self-help centers provide a variety of services including live and/or telephone assistance, referrals, web-based information, and document support.[33]

There are many other examples of technological innovations from across the country and the world. The expansion of these programs and the development of new technological innovations hold great promise in improving access to justice.

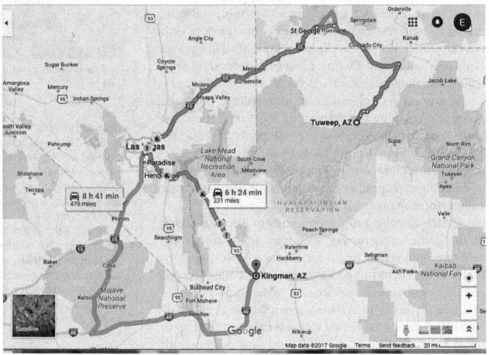

Residents of Tuweep, Arizona have to travel over six hours to the courthouse in Kingman. The self-pay kiosk improves their access to the legal system.
Google Maps

4. Unbundled Legal Services

In the traditional attorney-client relationship, the lawyer endeavors to help the client with her legal problem until the issues are fully resolved no matter what is involved or how long the assistance takes. In some cases, however, taking on a complicated and time-consuming pro bono case might seem daunting to a lawyer who otherwise might be interested in helping a client for low or no fee. Similarly, clients might not be able to afford full-service representation but might have sufficient funds to pay a lawyer to do certain discrete tasks. One answer to these situations is to allow lawyers to provide unbundled legal services — i.e., services limited

---

33. ABA Groups, Standing Committee on the Delivery of Legal Services, Unbundling Resource Center, *Self-Help Centers*, ABA, https://www.americanbar.org/groups/delivery_legal_services/resources/pro_se_unbundling _resource_center/self_service_centers/ (last visited July 23, 2020).

in their scope. Rule 1.2 permits lawyers to limit the scope of their representation if that representation is reasonable under the circumstances, and the client provides informed consent. Lawyers may offer a range of activities as unbundled services: advice, research, document drafting, or court appearances. The lawyer and client could also agree to limit the representation to certain issues: for example, a lawyer could help a client in a landlord-tenant matter with maintaining possession of her apartment but not represent the client on other issues.

5. Regulatory Changes

The legal market is heavily regulated. Among the most significant regulations are (1) the requirement that only lawyers can deliver legal services and (2) the prohibitions on non-lawyer ownership of law firms, non-lawyer management of law firms, and sharing fees with non-lawyers (except under very limited circumstances). The debate over whether to change these rules is among the most controversial in the legal profession. The ABA recently took a significant step by passing a resolution that encourages states to explore regulatory innovations that could improve access to justice and to collect data on those programs.[34] Following in the spirit of this resolution, in August 2020, the Utah Supreme Court announced that it was establishing a "pilot legal regulatory sandbox" and an Office of Legal Services Innovation with the explicit goal of improving access to justice. Subject to oversight by the Utah Supreme Court, the Innovation Office will oversee and regulate "the practice of law by nontraditional legal service providers or by traditional providers offering nontraditional legal services."[35] Other states, including Arizona and California, are considering similar innovations. Could these regulatory changes improve access to justice?

Non-Lawyers Delivering Legal Services

When you get sick, a doctor is not the only one who can help you. In the health care field, nurse practitioners, physician's assistants, and other professionals are able to supplement the work that doctors do by providing certain basic medical services at a lower price. Similarly, some legal problems may not require a lawyer, and some U.S. jurisdictions have authorized legal service providers other than lawyers to assist individuals in addressing their legal needs.

Federal legislation has long authorized the use of non-lawyers under limited circumstances. For instance:

■ Bankruptcy petition preparers who are not lawyers may assist debtors in filling out the paperwork necessary to file for bankruptcy in United States Bankruptcy Court.

---

34. Brenda Sapino Jeffreys, *ABA Approves Innovation Resolution, with Revisions to Limit Regulatory Changes*, The American Lawyer, Law.com (February 17, 2020), *available at* https://www.law.com/americanlawyer/2020/02/17/aba-approves-innovation-resolution-with-revisions-to-limit-regulatory-changes/?slreturn=20200404214026.
35. Utah Supreme Court Standing Order No. 15 (Aug. 14, 2020), *available at* http://www.utcourts.gov/utc/rules-approved/wp-content/uploads/sites/4/2020/08/FINAL-Utah-Supreme-Court-Standing-Order-No.-15.pdf.

- Qualified non-lawyers can represent individuals in immigration proceedings before the Executive Office for Immigration Review.
- The Social Security Administration permits non-lawyers to represent claimants seeking benefits.
- A variety of different professionals, including certified public accountants, are authorized to practice before the IRS.
- Patent agents who are not lawyers may prepare and file patent applications with the Patent and Trademark Office.[36]

Many states are experimenting with new forms of legal service providers:

- New York and Arizona permit specially trained and lawyer-supervised college students to be "Court Navigators." Under New York's program, launched in 2014, Court Navigators assist unrepresented litigants in nonpayment proceedings in housing court or consumer debt cases by researching information about the law, collecting necessary documents, and responding to a judge's questions about the case. Under Arizona's program, which began in 2015, Court Navigators help guide self-represented litigants through the court process in family law cases.
- In California and Washington State, non-lawyer "Courthouse Facilitators" provide unrepresented individuals in family law cases with information about court procedures and legal forms.
- Arizona, California, and Nevada authorize specially trained non-lawyer "Document Preparers" to prepare legal documents on specific legal matters.[37]
- The Arizona Supreme Court recently announced a "licensure process that will allow nonlawyers, called 'Legal Paraprofessionals' (LPs) to provide limited legal services to the public, including being able to go into court with their client."[38]

Up until the summer of 2020, Washington State was at the forefront of this movement. In 2012, the Washington Supreme Court approved the role of Limited License Legal Technician (LLLT), "the first independent legal paraprofessional in the United States that is licensed to give legal advice"[39] and a precursor to Arizona's Legal Paraprofessionals. In order to practice, the court required that LLLTs have an associate's degree or higher; complete 45 credit hours of a core curriculum through a program approved by the ABA or the LLLT Board; pass family law courses offered at the University of Washington School of Law; take part in 3,000 hours of paralegal work; and pass practice area and professional responsibility exams. Once admitted to practice, LLLTs were permitted to do most of the work that lawyers can do, except that they could not represent clients in court nor negotiate on behalf of

---

36. *Report on the Future of Legal Services in the United States (2016)*, ABA COMM'N ON THE FUTURE OF LEGAL SERVS., at 20-27 (2016), https://www.americanbar.org/content/dam/aba/images/abanews/2016FLSReport_FNL _WEB.pdf (last visited July 25, 2020).

37. *Id.* at 19-24.

38. Arizona Supreme Court, News Release, "Arizona Supreme Court Makes Generational Advance in Access to Justice" (Aug. 27, 2020), *available at* https://www.azcourts.gov/portals/201/pressreleases/2020releases/ 082720rulesagenda.pdf.

39. Paula C. Littlewood, *The Practice of Law in Transition*, NW LAW, July-Aug. 2015, at 13, *available at* https:// wabarnews.wsba.org/wabarnews/july-august_2015/MobilePagedReplica.action?pm=2&folio=12#pg14.

clients, and they could only prepare legal documents approved by the LLLT Board. The Board also passed the LLLT Rules of Professional Conduct, similar to those for lawyers, which sought to ensure ethical behavior. LLLTs were authorized to practice family law, but new practice areas were under consideration.

The Washington Supreme Court adopted the LLLT rule after a lengthy and, at times, heated discussion among the bench and bar.[40] The primary argument that the court made in favor of the rule was the need for it in light of the "ever-growing gap in necessary legal and law related services for low and moderate income persons." The Court explained: "[m]any individuals will need far more help than the limited scope of law related activities that a limited license legal technician will be able to offer. These people must still seek help from an attorney. But there are people who need only limited levels of assistance that can be provided by non-lawyers trained and overseen within the framework of the regulatory system developed by the Practice of Law Board. This assistance should be available and affordable. Our system of justice requires it."[41]

On June 5, 2020, however, the Washington Supreme Court, abruptly voted 7-2 to "sunset" the program, prohibiting anybody not already in the pipeline from pursuing the license.[42] The court cited the "overall costs of sustaining the program and the small number of interested individuals." Indeed, fewer than 40 individuals have become LLLTs throughout the duration of the program. Despite the end of Washington's program, several other states in addition to Arizona are exploring similar programs.

Alternative Business Structures (ABS)

The Model Rules of Professional Conduct prohibit non-lawyer ownership of law firms, non-lawyer management of law firms, and sharing fees with non-lawyers (except under very limited circumstances). The term Alternative Business Structure (ABS) generally refers to a business model that deviates from this rule in some way. For some time, the District of Columbia has permitted non-lawyers to have a financial interest and hold managerial authority in a law firm,[43] though very few firms have taken advantage of this provision. In August 2020, Arizona became the first state to completely eliminate Rule 5.4.[44] The Arizona Supreme Court described this move as a "generational advance in access to justice."[45]

---

40. *See* Brooks Holland, *The Washington State Limited License Legal Technician Practice Rule: A National First in Access to Justice*, 82 Miss. L.J. 75 (2013), *available at* https://papers.ssrn.com/sol3/papers.cfm?abstract_id=2196607.

41. *In the Matter of the Adoption of New APR 28 — Limited Practice Rule for Limited License Legal Technicians*, Order No. 25700-A-1005 (Wash. June 15, 2012)

42. Lyle Moran, *Washington Supreme Court Sunsets Limited License Program for Nonlawyers*, A.B.A. J., (June 8, 2020), *available at* https://www.abajournal.com/news/article/washington-supreme-court-decides-to-sunset-pioneering-limited-license-program.

43. D.C. R. PROF'L CONDUCT 5.4, *available at* https://www.dcbar.org/for-lawyers/legal-ethics/rules-of-professional-conduct/law-firms-and-associations/professional-independence-of-a-lawyer.

44. Order Amending the Arizona Rules of the Supreme Court and the Arizona Rules of Evidence (Aug. 27, 2020), *available at* https://www.azcourts.gov/portals/215/documents/082720forderr-20-0034l pabs.pdf.

45. Arizona Supreme Court, News Release, "Arizona Supreme Court Makes Generational Advance in Access to Justice" (Aug. 27, 2020), *available at* https://www.azcourts.gov/portals/201/pressreleases/2020releases/082720rulesagenda.pdf.

Outside of the United States, many jurisdictions, including Australia, England and Wales, Singapore, Scotland, Italy, Spain, Denmark, Germany, Netherlands, Poland, Spain, Belgium, New Zealand, and some Canadian provinces permit various forms of ABS.[46] What each jurisdiction allows varies. There are a wide variety of arguments for and against liberalizing the rules concerning ABS, but one relates to the topic of access to justice. Proponents of ABS believe that it will increase access to affordable legal services. As one commentator explained:

> First, [limits on non-lawyer funding] constrain the supply of capital for law firms, thereby increasing the cost which the firms must pay for it. To the extent that this cost of doing business is passed along to consumers, it will increase the price of legal services. Second, bigger firms might be better for access to justice, due to risk-spreading opportunities and economies of scale and scope. Individual clients . . . must currently rely on small partnerships and solo practitioners, and allowing non-lawyer capital and management into the market might facilitate the emergence of large consumer law firms. Large firms would plausibly find it easier than small ones to expand access through flat rate billing, reputational branding, and investment in technology. Finally, insulating lawyers from non-lawyers precludes potentially innovative inter-professional collaborations, which might bring the benefits of legal services to more people even if firms stay small.[47]

To date, however, there is limited empirical data about whether the liberal regulatory schemes in jurisdictions that permit ABS actually increase access to justice.

Chapter Summary

- Parties in civil litigation generally have no right to counsel. In its most recent pronouncement on this issue, the Supreme Court ruled in *Turner v. Rogers* that the Due Process Clause does not require the state to provide counsel to an indigent defendant who faces incarceration for civil contempt where the custodial parent was also unrepresented. The majority did hold, however, that the state must provide some basic procedural protections. Some states guarantee lawyers in limited categories of cases by statute or court decision.
- With no legal right to counsel, low- and moderate-income Americans lack adequate access to representation. More than 80 percent of the legal needs of the poor and a majority of the needs of moderate-income Americans go unmet.

---

46. *Report on the Future of Legal Services in the United States,* ABA Comm'n on the Future of Legal Services in the United States (2016), *available at* https://www.americanbar.org/content/dam/aba/images/abanews/2016FLSReport_FNL_WEB.pdf (last visited July 25, 2020).

47. Noel Semple, Legal Services Regulation at the Crossroads: Justitia's Legions 158 (2015) (emphasis omitted); *see* Gillian K. Hadfield, *The Cost of Law: Promoting Access to Justice through the (Un)Corporate Practice of Law,* 38 Int'l Rev. L. & Econ. 43 (2014).

■ Lawyers, courts, innovators, commentators, and others have proposed a wide range of potential solutions to address the access-to-justice gap. These include simplifying court procedures, allowing greater use of non-lawyers to deliver legal services, technological innovations, loosening of regulatory restrictions, and mandatory pro bono services.

Applying the Rules

1. To demonstrate the power of a good legal website, let's pretend that you are a handyman living in Waukegan in Lake County, Illinois. You performed extensive work for a local business that now refuses to pay you the $4,600 they owe you. Go to www.illinoislegalaid.org to find out information about your legal rights and what steps you might take to try to collect what you are owed.

2. Figure out if you or those in your family can afford legal services. Go to the Economic Policy Institute's Family Budget Calculator (www.epi.org/resources/budget/) to calculate how much money you need to earn to attain a "modest yet adequate standard of living." If you suddenly face an unexpected legal issue, do you have several hundred (or thousand) dollars left over to hire a lawyer?

Professional Responsibility in Practice

1. As noted earlier, when it comes to access to legal services, "geography is destiny." Find out what resources are available in your state/city/community.

2. Imagine that you have a legal problem: you have received an eviction notice, you plan to get divorced, you have received a complaint in a debt collection action, or some other issue. You plan to solve that problem without a lawyer. How would you proceed? What resources are available in your jurisdiction to help? Would you consider hiring a licensed non-lawyer (the equivalent of an LLLT)?

3. Visit a local courthouse that hears cases involving low- and moderate-income litigants (small claims court, housing court, etc.). Document what you see. Do the parties have lawyers? How does the judge treat those who do not? How do unrepresented litigants fare?

4. Innovators from all over the world have devised innovations that employ technology to improve the delivery of legal services. Get on the Internet and find one.

5. Beginning with Washington State in 1994, most states launched Access to Justice Commissions to study the justice gap and possible solutions. The final reports of these commissions are a good way to learn about some of the specific barriers to justice in those states. To find your state's Access to Justice Commission and to see what you can learn about the unique issues facing your state, follow this link: https://public.tableau.com/views/AccesstoJusticeCommissions/Dashboard1.

The Judiciary

Judicial Ethics

Lawyers need to know the laws and rules governing judges for at least three reasons. First, Rule 8.4(f) of the Rules of Professional Conduct provides that a lawyer shall not "knowingly assist a judge or judicial officer in conduct that is a violation of applicable rules of judicial conduct or other law." Thus, lawyers must know the rules governing judges in order to avoid getting in trouble themselves. Second, some lawyers will run for judicial office. Rule 8.2(b) provides that "[a] lawyer who is a candidate for judicial office shall comply with the applicable provisions of the Code of Judicial Conduct." Third, lawyers need to know the circumstances under which they should move to disqualify a judge.

The regulatory structure for lawyers is similar to the regulatory structure for judges. The ABA has issued a Model Code of Judicial Conduct, which states are free to accept, modify, or reject. The Code applies to all individuals who perform "judicial functions" even if they are not full-time judges, and it follows a format similar to the Model Rules of Professional Conduct. The Model Code, which has been largely adopted by the states, was substantially amended in 2007. In contrast to its predecessors, the 2007 Code is similar to a piece of legislation, providing black letter rules for judges to follow that are organized around four canons, or overarching principles. As with the Model Rules, a judge who violates a rule is subject to discipline, and most states have commissions comprised of judges and lawyers to enforce their state codes, though in a recent investigative series, Reuters documented significant

Key Concepts

- The requirement that judges perform their **judicial duties** "impartially, competently, and diligently"
- The requirement that judges' **extrajudicial activities** not interfere with the performance of their judicial duties
- The standards for disqualification under the Rules of Professional Conduct and the United States Constitution
- Understanding and applying the limits on **political activity by judicial candidates** and the First Amendment implications of those limits

underenforcement of judicial misconduct.[1] The Model Code also sets forth the circumstances in which judges should be disqualified.[2]

With its emphasis on judicial independence and integrity, Canon 1 sets the tone for the entire Code: "[a] judge shall uphold and promote the independence, integrity, and impartiality of the judiciary, and shall avoid impropriety and the appearance of impropriety." Among the specific edicts under Canon 1: judges shall "comply with the law";[3] "act at all times in a manner that promotes public confidence in the independence, integrity, and impartiality of the judiciary";[4] "avoid impropriety and the appearance of impropriety";[5] and "not abuse the prestige of judicial office to advance the personal or economic interests of the judge or others."[6]

This chapter explores the specific applications of these concepts in four distinct areas: (A) judges' performance of their judicial duties, (B) judges' involvement in extrajudicial activities, (C) judicial disqualification, and (D) judicial campaigns and other political activity.

A. PERFORMANCE OF JUDICIAL DUTIES

Canon 2 governs a judge's conduct in performing her judicial duties and requires a judge to "perform the duties of judicial office impartially, competently, and diligently."[7] These judicial duties "take precedence over all of a judge's personal and extrajudicial activities."[8] The rules under Canon 2 serve to ensure the critical principles of fidelity to the law, independence, and impartiality in several ways.

First, Rule 2.2 states the obvious[9]: judges must "uphold and apply the law"; yet on occasion, judges are sanctioned for violating this rule. In *In re Hague*, a Michigan trial judge was suspended for repeatedly refusing to follow the rulings of the Michigan Appellate Court.[10] More recently, the Alabama Court of the Judiciary suspended then-Alabama Supreme Court Chief Justice Roy Moore for violating several provisions of the Alabama Code of Judicial Conduct, including Alabama's equivalent to Rule 2.2.[11] After the U.S. Supreme Court had issued its decision in *Obergefell v. Hodges*, holding that "same-sex couples may exercise the fundamental right to marry" in all states,[12] Chief Justice Moore issued an administrative order to Alabama's 68 probate judges that they should continue to follow Alabama state

---

1. *The Teflon Robe*, Reuters Investigates, Reuters.com (2020), *available at* https://www.reuters.com/investigates/section/usa-judges/.
2. MODEL CODE OF JUDICIAL CONDUCT r. 2.11. Judges are also subject to other federal and state laws regarding disqualification. For example, 28 U.S.C. 455 (2012), which contains essentially the same disqualification standard as Rule 2.11 of the Model Code of Judicial Conduct, governs federal judges. In addition, as discussed below, the Due Process Clause of the United States Constitution requires judges to recuse themselves in some extreme cases.
3. MODEL CODE OF JUDICIAL CONDUCT r. 1.1 (AM. BAR. ASS'N 2011).
4. *Id.* r. 1.2.
5. *Id.*
6. *Id.* r. 1.3.
7. *Id.* Canon 2.
8. *Id.* r. 2.1.
9. Rule references in this chapter are to the Model Code of Judicial Conduct, unless otherwise noted.
10. 315 N.W.2d 524 (1982) (suspending the judge for 60 days without pay).
11. Moore v. Alabama Judicial Inquiry Commission, 234 So. 3d 458 (Ala. 2017).
12. 574 U.S. 644, 675 (2015).

law forbidding same-sex marriage and therefore not issue any marriage licenses to same-sex couples.[13] The Alabama Court of the Judiciary concluded that Moore should be disciplined because "'the undeniable consequence of [Chief Justice Moore's administrative order] was to order and direct the probate judges to deny marriage licenses in direct defiance of the decision of the United States Supreme Court in *Obergefell*.'"[14] The Alabama Supreme Court affirmed the decision.

Second, judges must perform their duties competently and diligently,[15] which requires, among other things, "prompt disposition of the court's business."[16] Judges who fail to complete their work in a timely manner are subject to discipline.[17]

Third, related to the duty to uphold the law is the judge's duty to report misconduct by lawyers and other judges. This duty is similar to the lawyer's duty to report misconduct, found in Model Rule of Professional Conduct 8.3, but broader. As with lawyers, a judge who *knows* about a rules violation by a lawyer or a code violation by a judge that raises a "substantial question" regarding the lawyer or judge's "honesty, trustworthiness or fitness," must inform "the appropriate authority."[18] But the judge's duty goes further: if a judge "receives information indicating a substantial likelihood" that a judge has committed a violation of the Code, or that a lawyer has committed a violation of the Rules of Professional Conduct, then she must "take appropriate action." "Appropriate action" includes "communicating directly" with the lawyer or judge or "reporting the suspected violation to the appropriate authority."[19]

Fourth, to ensure that judges are impartial and independent, the rules constrain the judge in her decision-making process in several ways. First, judges must perform their duties "without bias or prejudice"[20] and free from "external influences."[21] Second, a judge may not engage in *ex parte* communications with a lawyer, except under limited circumstances.[22] Third, judges may not engage in independent investigation (including social media research) concerning the facts of a case.[23] This is a surprisingly easy prohibition to violate in the digital age: a North Carolina judge was publicly reprimanded for Googling one of the parties.[24] With respect to the law, a judge may hire an independent expert, but she must let both the parties know.[25]

---

13. *Moore*, No. 46, 9-13.

14. *Id.* at 32.

15. MODEL CODE OF JUDICIAL CONDUCT r. 2.5 (AM. BAR. ASS'N 2011).

16. *Id.* cmt. [3].

17. *See In re Astrowski*, Disposition of Complaints 19-362 and 19-363, May 19, 2020, *available at* https://www .azcourts.gov/portals/137/reports/2019/19-362.pdf; *see also In re Corretore*, Determination, State of N.Y. Commission on Judicial Conduct, June 22, 2020, (judge failed to issue decisions in small claims matters, where the judge must render judgment within 30 days from the time the case is submitted, for between five and 47 months), *available at* http://www.cjc.ny.gov/determinations/c/corretore.david.t.2020.06.22.det.pdf.

18. MODEL CODE OF JUDICIAL CONDUCT r. 2.15 (AM. BAR. ASS'N 2011).

19. *Id.* cmt. [2].

20. MODEL CODE OF JUDICIAL CONDUCT r. 2.3 (AM. BAR. ASS'N 2011).

21. *Id.* r. 2.4.

22. *Id.* r. 2.9.

23. *Id.* r. 2.9(c); r. 2.9 cmt. [6].

24. Public Reprimand of B. Carlton Terry, Jr., No. 08-234 (N.C. Jud. Standards Comm'n Apr. 1, 2009), *available at* https://www.nccourts.gov/assets/inline-files/Public-Reprimand-08-234-Terry.pdf.

25. Model Code r. 2.9(a)(2).

Finally, the rules also limit what a judge can say about a case. Rule 2.10 provides that a judge "shall not make any public statement that might reasonably be expected to affect the outcome or impair the fairness of a matter pending or impending."[26] Similarly, judges may not make "pledges, promises or commitments" in connection with a case.[27] The constitutionality of the "pledges and promises" ban, which also applies to judicial candidates, is discussed below.

B. EXTRAJUDICIAL ACTIVITIES

Off the bench, judges must conduct their activities "to minimize the risk of conflict" with their judicial obligations.[28] Again, the principal guiding factors are the maintenance and appearance of judicial independence and impartiality. Accordingly, Rule 3.1 states rather broad principles: a judge shall not participate in activities that "will interfere with the proper performance of the judge's judicial duties," "will lead to frequent disqualification of the judge," or "would appear to a reasonable person to undermine the judge's independence, integrity, or impartiality."[29]

Subject to the limitations of Rule 3.1, judges may engage in a variety of activities off the bench, including "activities sponsored by organizations or governmental entities concerned with the law, the legal system or the administration of justice, and those sponsored by or on behalf of educational, religious, charitable, fraternal, or civic organizations not conducted for profit. . . ."[30] In response to an inquiry, a New York ethics opinion recently concluded that a full-time judge may volunteer as a disc jockey for a not-for-profit college radio station.[31] Judges can also accept compensation and reimbursement of expenses in connection with such extrajudicial activities, "unless such acceptance would appear to a reasonable person to undermine the judge's independence, integrity or impartiality."[32]

But the limitations of Rule 3.1 are significant and severely curtail judges' ability to participate in civic activities. For example, judges cannot solicit contributions for such organizations (except from family members); can only solicit membership for the organization if the "entity is concerned with the law, the legal system, or the administration of justice"; and can only participate in a fundraising event for that organization if the "event concerns the law, the legal system, or the administration of justice."[33] Ethics committees have been strict in instructing judges that they cannot participate in extrajudicial activities that interfere with their judicial duties. The Connecticut Committee on Judicial Ethics recently issued an Informal Opinion, concluding that judges should not participate in "A Silent March of Black Female

---

26. *Id.* r. 2.10(a).
27. *Id.* r. 2.10(b).
28. *Id.* Canon 3.
29. *Id.* r. 3.1.
30. Model Code r 3.7.
31. N.Y. Advisory Comm. on Judicial Ethics, Op. 20-49, (March 19, 2020), *available at* https://www.nycourts.gov/legacyhtm/ip/judicialethics/opinions/20-49.htm.
32. Model Code r. 3.12, 3.14.
33. Model Code r. 3.7.

Attorneys of Connecticut" protesting George Floyd's death and similar instances of police abuse because, among other things, "the Judicial Official may be called upon to rule in cases that involve claims of police brutality or police abuse, [and the judge's] participation in this extrajudicial activity may appear to a reasonable person to undermine the judge's independence and impartiality in violation of Rule 3.1."[34] Similarly, the Judicial Council of the Seventh Circuit reprimanded a federal judge for a law review article he wrote entitled "The Roberts Court's Assault on Democracy." The Council recognized that "most of the article is an example of . . . permissible judicial writing on law-related subjects," but concluded that the judge crossed the line with his opening two sentences, in which the author described Chief Justice Roberts' confirmation testimony equating a Supreme Court Justice's role to an umpire calling balls and strikes as a "masterpiece of disingenuousness" and "misleading." The Council said that this criticism "could be seen as inconsistent with a judge's duty to promote public confidence in the integrity and impartiality of the judiciary and as reflecting adversely on the judge's impartiality."[35]

The rules go on to offer several more specific prohibitions. First, judges cannot use the prestige of their office to advance their own or others' interests. Thus, a judge cannot appear before governmental bodies (with some limited exceptions)[36] or testify as a character witness (unless subpoenaed).[37] This is another rule that is easily broken in the digital age with a simple "like" on Facebook. The California Supreme Court recently added a comment to its Code of Judicial Ethics to clarify this point: "[i]f a judge posts on social networking sites such as Facebook or crowd-sourced sites such as Yelp or TripAdvisor, the judge may not lend the prestige of judicial office to advance the pecuniary or personal interests of the judge or others. For example, a judge may not comment on, recommend, or criticize businesses, products, or services on such sites if it is reasonably likely that the judge can be identified as a judge."[38]

Further, because it is important for judges to maintain the public's confidence in the integrity and impartiality of the judiciary, judges "shall not hold membership in any organization that practices invidious discrimination on the basis of race, sex, gender, religion, national origin, ethnicity, or sexual orientation."[39]

Finally, judges may not accept "any gifts, loans, bequests, benefits, or other things of value, if acceptance is prohibited by law or would appear to a reasonable person to undermine the judge's independence, integrity or impartiality."[40] The rule goes on to list a number of items that judges may accept, including "items with little intrinsic value."[41]

---

34. Conn. Comm. on Judicial Ethics, Informal Op. No. 2020-03 (June 5, 2020), *available at* https://jud.ct.gov/Committees/ethics/sum/2020-03.pdf.

35. *Resolution of the Judicial Misconduct Complaints about District Judge Lynn Adelman,* Judicial Council of the Seventh Jud. Dist., Nos. 07-20-90044, 07-20-90045, 07-20-90046 (June 22, 2020), *available at* http://www.ca7.uscourts.gov/judicial-conduct/judicial-conduct_2020/07-20-90046_90044.pdf.

36. Model Code r. 3.2.

37. *Id.* r. 3.3.

38. Cal. Code of Judicial Ethics Canon 2, Advisory Comm. Commentary: Canon 2B (Cal. 2020).

39. Model Code r. 3.6(a).

40. *Id.* r. 3.13.

41. *Id.* r. 3.31(b)(1).

C. JUDICIAL DISQUALIFICATION

Disqualification is perhaps the most difficult doctrinal issue in the field of judicial ethics. This section considers the issue of when judges should be disqualified under the Code of Judicial Conduct, including the possibility that judges' social media use could lead to disqualification, before turning to the exceptional circumstances under which the Due Process Clause of the United States Constitution requires disqualification.

1. Disqualification Under the Code

Rule 2.11 and the federal statute (28 U.S.C. 455) that applies to federal judges both require that judges disqualify themselves "in any proceeding in which the judge's impartiality might reasonably be questioned,"[42] even in the absence of a motion.[43] Most states have similar statutory provisions for their state judges.[44] This standard goes beyond cases of actual bias and also prohibits judges from sitting in cases involving the appearance of impropriety. A comment to the Code provides: "The test for appearance of impropriety is whether the conduct would create in reasonable minds a perception that the judge violated this Code or engaged in other conduct that reflects adversely on the judge's honesty, impartiality, temperament, or fitness to serve as a judge."[45] The words "reasonably" in the Code provision and "reasonable" in the comments indicate that this is an objective standard.

Judges also have an affirmative obligation to disclose on the record information that the parties or their lawyers "might reasonably consider relevant" to the disqualification issue, even if the judge believes that disqualification is not warranted.[46] In most circumstances, judges may also ask the parties to waive disqualification.[47]

The Rule provides a *non-exclusive* list of circumstances requiring disqualification, which includes:

(1) the judge has a "personal bias or prejudice concerning a party or a party's lawyer" or "personal knowledge" of the facts in dispute;
(2) the judge or a family member is a party, lawyer or material witness in the proceeding;
(3) the judge or a close family member has an economic interest in the proceeding;
(4) the judge previously served as a lawyer in the matter.

---

42. *Id.* r. 2.11(a). The statute applicable to federal judges, 28 U.S.C. §455 contains an almost identical standard: "Any justice, judge, or magistrate judge of the United States shall disqualify himself in any proceeding in which his impartiality might reasonably be questioned." 28 U.S.C. §455(a) (2012).
43. Model Code r. 2.11 cmt. [2].
44. Richard E. Flamm, Judicial Disqualification: Recusal and Disqualification of Judges §5.2 (2d ed. 2007 & Supp. 2016).
45. Model Code r. 1.2 cmt. [5].
46. *Id.* r. 2.11 cmt. [5].
47. *Id.* r. 2.11(c).

The more difficult question is what circumstances, outside of these enumerated in the rule, require disqualification. Judges' social relationships with litigants, lawyers, or witnesses in pending matters present a particularly knotty issue. Courts have recognized that such a friendship certainly can create an "appearance of partiality."[48] The specific concern is that the personal relationship will cause "a reasonable person knowing all the circumstances [to] believe that the judge will accord different credibility to the testimony or statements of the person known to the judge."[49]

Distinguishing which social relationships are impermissible under the "appearance of impropriety" standard is a challenge, particularly in the context of friendship. For that reason, some commentators have justifiably criticized the standard.[50] The Code does not define the level of friendship with the parties or lawyers that would require a judge to recuse himself. Moreover, judges are certainly permitted — if not encouraged — to maintain a social life and certainly do not have to, as one court put it, "withdraw from society and live an ascetic, antiseptic and socially sterile life."[51] The Code accepts that judges may have a social life by recognizing that judges who accept "ordinary social hospitality" do not run afoul of the prohibition on receiving gifts.[52]

Because of their shared interests and backgrounds, judges are quite likely to have social relationships with lawyers. There is obviously nothing wrong with such a relationship *per se*, but at some point that relationship becomes disqualifying, perhaps because the relationship is so close or because the judge is interacting with the lawyer while the case is pending. The courts and ethics authorities have struggled to determine what constitutes permissible "ordinary social hospitality," versus an impermissible "appearance of impropriety." Further complicating the matter is Rule 2.7, which imposes on judges a "duty to sit." This rule requires judges to "hear and decide matters assigned to the judge, except when disqualification is required."[53] In other words, judges should not recuse themselves for frivolous reasons, nor should they necessarily err on the side of disqualification in close cases. In 2019, the ABA released a Formal Opinion on the issue that nicely summarized these policy considerations but ultimately reiterated that every situation must be reviewed on a case-by-case basis: "Whether judges must disqualify themselves when a party or lawyer is a friend or shares a close personal relationship with the judge or should instead take the lesser step of disclosing the friendship or close personal relationship to the other lawyers and parties, depends on the circumstances."[54]

---

48. *See, e.g.*, United States v. Kelly, 888 F.2d 732, 745 (11th Cir. 1989) (holding that trial judge, who was close friends with a key defense witness, improperly failed to disqualify himself under the federal disqualification statute).
49. Leslie W. Abramson, *Appearance of Impropriety: Deciding When a Judge's Impartiality "Might Reasonably Be Questioned,"* 14 Geo. J. Legal Ethics 55, 96 (2000).
50. Jeremy M. Miller, *Judicial Recusal and Disqualification: The Need for a* Per Se *Rule on Friendship (Not Acquaintance)*, 33 Pepp. L. Rev. 575, 577 (2006) (criticizing the "glaring gap in the law on the issue of when a judge must recuse himself or herself because a party or advocate in the case is a friend").
51. United Farm Workers of Am. v. Superior Court, 170 Cal. App. 3d 97, 100 (Cal. Ct. App. 1985).
52. Model Code r. 3.13(b)(3).
53. *Id.* r. 2.7.
54. ABA, Standing Comm. on Ethics and Prof'l Responsibility, Formal Op. 488 (2019), *Judges' Social or Close Personal Relationships with Lawyers or Parties as Grounds for Disqualification or Disclosure*, available at https://www.americanbar.org/content/dam/aba/administrative/professional_responsibility/aba_formal_opinion_488.pdf.

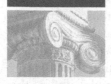

Case Preview

Cheney v. United States District Court for the District of Columbia

During President George W. Bush's first term (2000-2004), he appointed Vice President Dick Cheney to chair the National Energy Policy Development Group, the administration's energy task force. As part of this work, Cheney and the other government officials on the task force allegedly met behind closed doors with energy industry officials and lobbyists.[55] Two public interest groups with very different political leanings — The Sierra Club and Judicial Watch — filed suit against Cheney seeking records from the task force, arguing that the secretive meetings violated an open government law entitled the Federal Advisory Committee Act (FACA), 5 U.S.C. app'x §§1-16 (2012). The administration maintained that the meetings were not subject to FACA. These meetings were politically significant, particularly during President Bush's 2004 reelection campaign against John Kerry, when Kerry and other critics of the Bush administration argued that these meetings demonstrated that the administration was letting big energy corporations dictate the nation's energy policy.

On December 15, 2003 (less than a year before the Presidential election), the U.S. Supreme Court agreed to hear Vice President Cheney's appeal from a lower court ruling ordering him and other senior officials to produce information about the work of the task force. Three weeks later, in mid-January 2004, Vice President Cheney and Justice Antonin Scalia, who were longtime friends, went duck hunting together at a private camp in southern Louisiana. On February 23, 2004, the Sierra Club moved to disqualify Justice Scalia from hearing the FACA case. Consistent with its historic practice, the motion was referred to Justice Scalia.

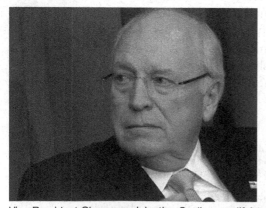 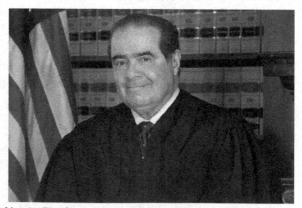

Vice President Cheney and Justice Scalia were lifelong friends. The Sierra Club moved to disqualify Justice Scalia from hearing the FACA case.
Albert H. Telch / Shutterstock.com; Collection of the Supreme Court of the United States

---

55. Bill Mears, *High Court Hears Arguments on Cheney Task Force*, CNN, June 24, 2004, *available at* http://www.cnn.com/2004/LAW/04/27/scotus.cheney/.

As you read Justice Scalia's decision and Lawrence Fox's commentary that follows, consider the following:

1. What are Justice Scalia's most convincing arguments in support of his conclusion that he should not recuse himself? What are Professor Fox's most convincing counter-arguments? Who do you think is right?
2. After reading Justice Scalia's opinion, are you more or less likely to question his impartiality in this case?
3. What is the procedure for handling disqualification motions at the Supreme Court? Can you think of ways to improve the procedure? How is a motion to disqualify a Supreme Court Justice different than a motion to disqualify a trial judge?

Cheney v. United States District Court for the District of Columbia
541 U.S. 913 (2004)

Memorandum of Justice SCALIA.

. . .

I

The decision whether a judge's impartiality can "'reasonably be questioned'" is to be made in light of the facts as they existed, and not as they were surmised or reported. The facts here were as follows:

For five years or so, I have been going to Louisiana during the Court's long December-January recess, to the duck-hunting camp of a friend whom I met through two hunting companions from Baton Rouge, one a dentist and the other a worker in the field of handicapped rehabilitation. The last three years, I have been accompanied on this trip by a son-in-law who lives near me. Our friend and host, Wallace Carline, has never, as far as I know, had business before this Court. He is not, as some reports have described him, an "energy industry executive" in the sense that summons up boardrooms of ExxonMobil or Con Edison. He runs his own company that provides services and equipment rental to oil rigs in the Gulf of Mexico.

During my December 2002 visit, I learned that Mr. Carline was an admirer of Vice President Cheney. Knowing that the Vice President, with whom I am well acquainted (from our years serving together in the Ford administration), is an enthusiastic duck hunter, I asked whether Mr. Carline would like to invite him to our next year's hunt. The answer was yes; I conveyed the invitation (with my own warm recommendation) in the spring of 2003 and received an acceptance (subject, of course, to any superseding demands on the Vice President's time) in the summer. The Vice President said that if he did go, I would be welcome to fly down to Louisiana with him. (Because of national security requirements, of course, he must fly in a Government plane.)

That invitation was later extended — if space was available — to my son-in-law and to a son who was joining the hunt for the first time; they accepted. The trip was set long before the Court granted certiorari in the present case, and indeed before the petition for certiorari had even been filed.

We departed from Andrews Air Force Base at about 10 a.m. on Monday, January 5, flying in a Gulfstream jet owned by the Government. We landed in Patterson, Louisiana, and went by car to a dock where Mr. Carline met us, to take us on the 20-minute boat trip to his hunting camp. We arrived at about 2 p.m., the 5 of us joining about 8 other hunters, making about 13 hunters in all; also present during our time there were about 3 members of Mr. Carline's staff, and, of course, the Vice President's staff and security detail. It was not an intimate setting. The group hunted that afternoon and Tuesday and Wednesday mornings; it fished (in two boats) Tuesday afternoon. All meals were in common. Sleeping was in rooms of two or three, except for the Vice President, who had his own quarters. Hunting was in two- or three-man blinds. As it turned out, I never hunted in the same blind with the Vice President. Nor was I alone with him at any time during the trip, except, perhaps, for instances so brief and unintentional that I would not recall them-walking to or from a boat, perhaps, or going to or from dinner. Of course we said not a word about the present case. The Vice President left the camp Wednesday afternoon, about two days after our arrival. I stayed on to hunt (with my son and son-in-law) until late Friday morning, when the three of us returned to Washington on a commercial flight from New Orleans.

II

Let me respond, at the outset, to Sierra Club's suggestion that I should "resolve any doubts in favor of recusal." That might be sound advice if I were sitting on a Court of Appeals. There, my place would be taken by another judge, and the case would proceed normally. On the Supreme Court, however, the consequence is different: The Court proceeds with eight Justices, raising the possibility that, by reason of a tie vote, it will find itself unable to resolve the significant legal issue presented by the case. Thus, as Justices stated in their 1993 Statement of Recusal Policy: "We do not think it would serve the public interest to go beyond the requirements of the statute, and to recuse ourselves, out of an excess of caution, whenever a relative is a partner in the firm before us or acted as a lawyer at an earlier stage. Even one unnecessary recusal impairs the functioning of the Court." Moreover, granting the motion is (insofar as the outcome of the particular case is concerned) effectively the same as casting a vote against the petitioner. The petitioner needs five votes to overturn the judgment below, and it makes no difference whether the needed fifth vote is missing because it has been cast for the other side, or because it has not been cast at all.

Even so, recusal is the course I must take-and will take-when, on the basis of established principles and practices, I have said or done something which requires that course. I have recused for such a reason this very Term. I believe, however, that established principles and practices do not require (and thus do not permit) recusal in the present case.

A

My recusal is required if, by reason of the actions described above, my "impartiality might reasonably be questioned." 28 U.S.C. §455(a). Why would that result follow from my being in a sizable group of persons, in a hunting camp with the Vice President, where I never hunted with him in the same blind or had other opportunity for private conversation? The only possibility is that it would suggest I am a friend of his. But while friendship is a ground for recusal of a Justice where the personal fortune or the personal freedom of the friend is at issue, it has traditionally *not* been a ground for recusal where *official action* is at issue, no matter how important the official action was to the ambitions or the reputation of the Government officer.

A rule that required Members of this Court to remove themselves from cases in which the official actions of friends were at issue would be utterly disabling. Many Justices have reached this Court precisely because they were friends of the incumbent President or other senior officials — and from the earliest days down to modern times Justices have had close personal relationships with the President and other officers of the Executive. John Quincy Adams hosted dinner parties featuring such luminaries as Chief Justice Marshall, Justices Johnson, Story, and Todd, Attorney General Wirt, and Daniel Webster. Justice Harlan and his wife often "'stopped in'" at the White House to see the Hayes family and pass a Sunday evening in a small group, visiting and singing hymns. Justice Stone tossed around a medicine ball with members of the Hoover administration mornings outside the White House. Justice Douglas was a regular at President Franklin Roosevelt's poker parties; Chief Justice Vinson played poker with President Truman. A no-friends rule would have disqualified much of the Court in *Youngstown Sheet & Tube Co. v. Sawyer,* the case that challenged President Truman's seizure of the steel mills. Most of the Justices knew Truman well, and four had been appointed by him. A no-friends rule would surely have required Justice Holmes's recusal in *Northern Securities Co. v. United States*, the case that challenged President Theodore Roosevelt's trust-busting initiative.

It is said, however, that this case is different because the federal officer (Vice President Cheney) is actually a *named party*. That is by no means a rarity. At the beginning of the current Term, there were before the Court (excluding habeas actions) no fewer than 83 cases in which high-level federal Executive officers were named in their official capacity — more than 1 in every 10 federal civil cases then pending. That an officer is named has traditionally made no difference to the proposition that friendship is not considered to affect impartiality in official-action suits. Regardless of whom they name, such suits, when the officer is the plaintiff, seek relief not for him personally but for the Government; and, when the officer is the defendant, seek relief not against him personally, but against the Government. That is why federal law provides for *automatic substitution* of the new officer when the originally named officer has been replaced. . . .

Richard Cheney's name appears in this suit only because he was the head of a Government committee that allegedly did not comply with the Federal Advisory Committee Act (FACA), and because he may, by reason of his office, have custody of some or all of the Government documents that the plaintiffs seek. If some other person were to become head of that committee or to obtain custody of those documents, the plaintiffs would name that person and Cheney would be dismissed. Unlike the defendant in *United States v. Nixon* or *Clinton v. Jones*, Cheney is represented here, not by his personal attorney, but by the United States Department of Justice in the person of the Solicitor General. And the courts at all levels have referred to his arguments as (what they are) the arguments of "the government."

The recusal motion, however, asserts the following:

> Critical to the issue of Justice Scalia's recusal is understanding that this is not a run-of-the-mill legal dispute about an administrative decision. . . . Because his own conduct is central to this case, the Vice President's "reputation and his integrity are on the line." (*Chicago Tribune.*)

I think not. Certainly as far as the legal issues immediately presented to me are concerned, this *is* "a run-of-the-mill legal dispute about an administrative decision." I am asked to determine what powers the District Court possessed under FACA, and whether the Court of Appeals should have asserted mandamus or appellate jurisdiction over the District Court. Nothing this Court says on those subjects will have any bearing upon the reputation and integrity of Richard Cheney. Moreover, even if this Court affirms the decision below and allows discovery to proceed in the District Court, the issue that would ultimately present itself *still* would have no bearing upon the reputation and integrity of Richard Cheney. That issue would be, quite simply, whether some private individuals were *de facto* members of the National Energy Policy Development Group (NEPDG). It matters not whether they were caused to be so by Cheney or someone else, or whether Cheney was even aware of their *de facto* status; if they *were de facto* members, then (according to D.C. Circuit law) the records and minutes of NEPDG must be made public.

The recusal motion asserts, however, that Richard Cheney's " 'reputation and his integrity are on the line' " because "respondents have alleged, *inter alia*, that the Vice President, as the head of the Task Force and its subgroups, was responsible for the involvement of energy industry executives in the operations of the Task Force, as a result of which the Task Force and its subgroups became subject to FACA."

As far as Sierra Club's *complaint* is concerned, it simply is not true that Vice President Cheney is singled out as having caused the involvement of energy executives. But even if the allegation had been made, it would be irrelevant to the case. FACA assertedly requires disclosure if there were private members of the task force, *no matter who* they were — "energy industry executives" or Ralph Nader; and *no matter who* was responsible for their membership — the Vice President or no one in particular. I do not see how the Vice President's " 'reputation and . . . integrity are on the line' " any more than the agency head's reputation and integrity are on the line in virtually all official-action suits, which accuse his agency of acting (to quote the Administrative Procedure Act) "arbitrar[ily], capricious[ly], [with] an abuse of discretion, or otherwise not in accordance with law." Beyond that always-present accusation, there is nothing illegal or immoral about making "energy industry executives" members of a task force on energy; some people probably think it would be a good idea. If, in doing so, or in allowing it to happen, the Vice President went beyond his assigned powers, that is no worse than what every agency head has done when his action is judicially set aside.

To be sure, there could be political consequences from disclosure of the fact (if it be so) that the Vice President favored business interests, and especially a sector of business with which he was formerly connected. But political consequences are not my concern, and the possibility of them does not convert an official suit into a private one. That possibility exists to a greater or lesser degree in virtually all suits involving agency action. To expect judges to take account of political consequences — and to assess the high or low degree of them — is to ask judges to do precisely what they should not do. It seems to me quite wrong (and quite impossible) to make recusal depend upon what degree of political damage a particular case can be expected to inflict.

In sum, I see nothing about this case which takes it out of the category of normal official-action litigation, where my friendship, or the appearance of my friendship, with one of the named officers does not require recusal.

B

The recusal motion claims that "the fact that Justice Scalia and his daughter [sic] were the Vice President's guest on Air Force Two on the flight down to Louisiana" means that I "accepted a sizable gift from a party in a pending case," a gift "measured in the thousands of dollars." Let me speak first to the value, though that is not the principal point. Our flight down cost the Government nothing, since space-available was the condition of our invitation. And, though our flight down on the Vice President's plane was indeed free, since we were not returning with him we purchased (because they were least expensive) round-trip tickets that cost precisely what we would have paid if we had gone both down and back on commercial flights. In other words, none of us saved a cent by flying on the Vice President's plane. The purpose of going with him was not saving money, but avoiding some inconvenience to ourselves (being taken by car from New Orleans to Morgan City) and considerable inconvenience to our friends, who would have had to meet our plane in New Orleans, and schedule separate boat trips to the hunting camp, for us and for the Vice President's party. . . .

The principal point, however, is that social courtesies, provided at Government expense by officials whose only business before the Court is business in their official capacity, have not hitherto been thought prohibited. Members of Congress and others are frequently invited to accompany Executive Branch officials on Government planes, where space is available. That this is not the sort of gift thought likely to affect a judge's impartiality is suggested by the fact that the Ethics in Government Act of 1978, which requires annual reporting of transportation provided or reimbursed, excludes from this requirement transportation provided by the United States. I daresay that, at a hypothetical charity auction, much more would be bid for dinner for two at the White House than for a one-way flight to Louisiana on the Vice President's jet. Justices accept the former with regularity. While this matter was pending, Justices and their spouses were invited (*all* of them, I believe) to a December 11, 2003, Christmas reception at the residence of the Vice President — which included an opportunity for a photograph with the Vice President and Mrs. Cheney. Several of the Justices attended, and in doing so they were fully in accord with the proprieties.

III

When I learned that Sierra Club had filed a recusal motion in this case, I assumed that the motion would be replete with citations of legal authority, and would provide some instances of cases in which, because of activity similar to what occurred here, Justices have recused themselves or at least have been asked to do so. In fact, however, the motion cites only two Supreme Court cases assertedly relevant to the issue here discussed, and nine Court of Appeals cases. Not a single one of these even involves an official-action suit. And the motion gives not a single instance in which, under even remotely similar circumstances, a Justice has recused or been asked to recuse. Instead, the argument section of the motion consists almost entirely of references to, and quotations from, newspaper editorials. The core of Sierra Club's argument is as follows:

> "Sierra Club makes this motion because . . . damage [to the integrity of the system] is being done right now. As of today, 8 of the 10 newspapers with the largest circulation in the United States, 14 of the largest 20, and 20 of the 30 largest have called on Justice Scalia to step aside. . . . Of equal import, there is no counterbalance or controversy: not a single newspaper has argued against recusal. Because the American public, as reflected in the nation's newspaper editorials, has unanimously concluded that there is an appearance of favoritism, any objective observer would be compelled to conclude that Justice Scalia's impartiality has been questioned. These facts more than satisfy Section 455(a), which mandates recusal merely when a Justice's impartiality 'might reasonably be questioned.'"

The implications of this argument are staggering. I must recuse because a significant portion of the press, which is deemed to be the American public, demands it.

The motion attaches as exhibits the press editorials on which it relies. Many of them do not even have the facts right. The length of our hunting trip together was said to be several days (San Francisco Chronicle), four days (Boston Globe), or nine days (San Antonio Express-News). We spent about 48 hours together at the hunting camp. It was asserted that the Vice President and I "spent time alone in the rushes," "huddled together in a Louisiana marsh," where we had "plenty of time . . . to talk privately" (Los Angeles Times); that we "spent . . . quality time bonding [together] in a duck blind" (Atlanta Journal-Constitution); and that "[t]here is simply no reason to think these two did not discuss the pending case" (Buffalo News). As I have described, the Vice President and I were never in the same blind, and never discussed the case. (Washington officials know the rules, and know that discussing with judges pending cases — their own or anyone else's — is forbidden.) The Palm Beach Post stated that our "transportation [was] provided, appropriately, by an oil services company," and Newsday that a "private jet . . . whisked Scalia to Louisiana." The Vice President and I flew in a Government plane. The Cincinnati Enquirer said that "Scalia was Cheney's guest at a private duck-hunting camp in Louisiana." Cheney and I were Wallace Carline's guests. Various newspapers described Mr. Carline as "an energy company official" (Atlanta Journal-Constitution), an "oil industrialist" (Cincinnati Enquirer), an "oil company executive" (Contra Costa Times), an "oil-man" (Minneapolis Star Tribune), and an "energy industry executive" (Washington Post). All of these descriptions are misleading. . . .

Such a blast of largely inaccurate and uninformed opinion cannot determine the recusal question. It is well established that the recusal inquiry must be "made from the perspective of a *reasonable* observer who is *informed of all the surrounding facts and circumstances.*"

IV

While Sierra Club was apparently unable to summon forth a single example of a Justice's recusal (or even motion for a Justice's recusal) under circumstances similar to those here, I have been able to accomplish the seemingly more difficult task of finding a couple of examples establishing the negative: that recusal or motion for recusal did *not* occur under circumstances similar to those here.

Justice White and Robert Kennedy

The first example pertains to a Justice with whom I have sat, and who retired from the Court only 11 years ago, Byron R. White. Justice White was close friends with Attorney General Robert Kennedy from the days when White had served as Kennedy's Deputy Attorney General. In January 1963, the Justice went on a skiing vacation in Colorado with Robert Kennedy and his family, Secretary of Defense Robert McNamara and his family, and other members of the Kennedy family. . . . At the time of this skiing vacation there were pending before the Court at least two cases in which Robert Kennedy, in his official capacity as Attorney General, was a party. In the first of these, moreover, the press might have said, as plausibly as it has said here, that the reputation and integrity of the Attorney General were at issue. There the Department of Justice had decreed deportation of a resident alien on grounds that he had been a member of the Communist Party. (The Court found that the evidence adduced by the Department was inadequate.)

Besides these cases naming Kennedy, another case pending at the time of the skiing vacation was argued to the Court *by Kennedy* about two weeks later. That case was important to the Kennedy administration. . . . When the decision was announced, it was front-page news. Attorney General Kennedy argued for affirmance of a three-judge District Court's ruling that the Georgia Democratic Party's county-unit voting system violated the one-person, one-vote principle. This was Kennedy's only argument before the Court, and it certainly put "on the line" his reputation as a lawyer, as well as an important policy of his brother's administration.

Justice Jackson and Franklin Roosevelt

The second example pertains to a Justice who was one of the most distinguished occupants of the seat to which I was appointed, Robert Jackson. Justice Jackson took the recusal obligation particularly seriously. Nonetheless, he saw nothing wrong with maintaining a close personal relationship, and engaging in " 'quite frequen[t]' " socializing with the President whose administration's acts came before him regularly.

In April 1942, the two "spent a weekend on a very delightful house party down at General Watson's in Charlottesville, Virginia. I had been invited to ride down with the President and to ride back with him." Pending at the time, and argued the next month, was one of the most important cases concerning the scope of permissible federal action under the Commerce Clause, *Wickard v. Filburn,* 317 U.S. 111 (1942). Justice Jackson wrote the opinion for the Court. Roosevelt's Secretary of Agriculture, rather than Roosevelt himself, was the named federal officer in the case, but there is no doubt that it was important to the President.

I see nothing wrong about Justice White's and Justice Jackson's socializing — including vacationing and accepting rides — with their friends. Nor, seemingly, did anyone else at the time. (The Denver Post, which has been critical of me, reported the White-Kennedy-McNamara skiing vacation with nothing but enthusiasm.) If friendship is basis for recusal (as it assuredly is when friends are sued personally) then activity which suggests close friendship must be avoided. But if friendship is *no* basis for recusal (as it is not in official-capacity suits) social contacts that do no more than evidence that friendship suggest no impropriety whatever. . . .

V

Since I do not believe my impartiality can reasonably be questioned, I do not think it would be proper for me to recuse. That alone is conclusive; but another consideration moves me in the same direction: Recusal would in my judgment harm the Court. If I were to withdraw from this case, it would be because some of the press has argued that the Vice President would suffer political damage *if* he should lose this appeal, and *if,* on remand, discovery should establish that energy industry representatives were *de facto* members of NEPDG — and because some of the press has elevated that possible political damage to the status of an impending stain on the reputation and integrity of the Vice President. But since political damage often comes from the Government's losing official-action suits; and since political damage can readily be characterized as a stain on reputation and integrity; recusing in the face of such charges would give elements of the press a veto over participation of any Justices who had social contacts with, or were even known to be friends of, a named official. That is intolerable.

My recusal would also encourage so-called investigative journalists to suggest improprieties, and demand recusals, for other inappropriate (and increasingly silly) reasons. The Los Angeles Times has already suggested that it was improper for me to sit on a case argued by a law school dean whose school I had visited several weeks before-visited not at his invitation, but at his predecessor's. The same paper has asserted that it was improper for me to speak at a dinner honoring Cardinal Bevilacqua given by the Urban Family Council of Philadelphia because (according to the Times's false report) that organization was engaged in litigation seeking to prevent same-sex civil unions, and I had before me a case presenting the question (whether same-sex civil unions were lawful? — no) whether homosexual sodomy could constitutionally be *criminalized.* While the political branches can perhaps survive the constant baseless allegations of impropriety that have become the staple of Washington reportage, this Court cannot. The people must have confidence in the integrity of the Justices, and that cannot exist in a system that assumes them to be corruptible by the slightest friendship or favor, and in an atmosphere where the press will be eager to find foot-faults.

. . .

As I noted at the outset, one of the private respondents in this case has not called for my recusal, and has expressed confidence that I will rule impartially, as indeed I will. Counsel for the other private respondent seek to impose, it seems to me, a standard regarding friendship, the appearance of friendship, and the acceptance of social favors, that is more stringent than what they themselves observe. Two days before the brief in opposition to the petition in this case was filed, lead counsel for Sierra Club, a friend, wrote me a warm note inviting me to come to Stanford Law School to speak to one of his classes. (Judges teaching classes at law schools normally have their transportation and expenses paid.) I saw nothing amiss in that friendly letter and invitation. I surely would have thought otherwise if I had applied the standards urged in the present motion.

There are, I am sure, those who believe that my friendship with persons in the current administration might cause me to favor the Government in cases brought against it. That is not the issue here. Nor is the issue whether personal friendship with the Vice President might cause me to favor the Government in cases in which *he* is named. None of those suspicions regarding my impartiality (erroneous suspicions, I hasten to protest) bears upon recusal here. The question, simply put, is whether someone who thought I could decide this case impartially despite my friendship with the Vice President would reasonably believe that I *cannot* decide it impartially because I went hunting with that friend and accepted an invitation to fly there with him on a Government plane. If it is reasonable to think that a Supreme Court Justice can be bought so cheap, the Nation is in deeper trouble than I had imagined.

As the newspaper editorials appended to the motion make clear, I have received a good deal of embarrassing criticism and adverse publicity in connection with the matters at issue here — even to the point of becoming (as the motion cruelly but accurately states) "fodder for late-night comedians." If I could have done so in good conscience, I would have been pleased to demonstrate my integrity, and immediately silence the criticism, by getting off the case. Since I believe there is no basis for recusal, I cannot. The motion is *Denied*.

Lawrence J. Fox, I Did Not Sleep with That Vice President
15 No. 2 Prof. Law. 1 (2004)

. . . Why is the Scalia memorandum extraordinary? First, there is the question of its length. . . . Me thinks the gentleman doth protest too much.

The tone of the memorandum does not help. Justice Scalia is known for his rapier pen. He often demonstrates how clever he is in terms that must leave the litigants with whom he doesn't agree and his fellow Justices in similar circumstances quivering at the poverty of their own cognitive powers. But with his own integrity on the line, one would have hoped — as it turns out, against hope — that Justice Scalia would have adopted a less belligerent, cynical and dismissive voice in defending his willingness to sit on this important case. Instead we get a strident brief, dripping with annoyed sarcasm that anyone would question his rectitude and, as it turns out, one that raises far more questions than it answers, one that highlights the infirmities of the good Justice's self-assured stance.

Make no mistake about it. Justice Scalia thinks he is a trial lawyer. Right from the beginning he goes for our sympathy vote. How else can one explain Justice Scalia's remarkable narrative, which begins by telling us the totally irrelevant fact that the Justice was introduced to the man who hosted this exclusive soirée by a dentist and, drum roll please, a worker in handicapped rehabilitation? With that as a starting point, one cannot help but feeling all warm and fuzzy about the down to earth altruistic folk who brought the Justice and the veep together.

Next, Justice Scalia addresses the issue of his host, Wallace Carline, a magnanimous gentleman, who has been inviting Justice Scalia to Louisiana for years. On this occasion Mr. Carline agreed, at Justice Scalia's request, to invite the Vice-President, an avid duck hunter, as well, an invitation the host permitted Justice Scalia to extend personally.

Justice Scalia tells us a lot more about what the host is not, than what he is. But this must be very important because twice in the memorandum Justice Scalia addresses the issue of how his host makes his less than modest living.

The host is not:

"an energy industry executive,"
"an oil company executive,"
"an oil man,"
"an energy company official," or
"an oil industrialist. . . ."

In fact his host, far from being an oil industrialist — drum roll please — "runs his own company that provides services and equipment rental to" — pause — "*oil rigs.*" (Emphasis added). Certainly doesn't sound like an "oil industrialist" to me. In fact — how could anyone make such a mistake? He was in point of fact an "oil rig and oil equipment industrialist." The gauze is lifted from our eyes.

What Justice Scalia apparently wanted to make clear was that his host was not an "ExxonMobil" or "Con Ed" executive; he apparently was not a Halliburton executive either, though the host's wholly-owned company does sound an awful lot like a competitor of Halliburton. I guess Justice Scalia is asserting that these oil field supply folks, unlike the BP Unocal gang, are totally indifferent to the administration's energy policy, not caring one way or the other whether the Bush-Cheney administration allows offshore or North Slope drilling for petroleum.

Justice Scalia then tells us — a real confidence builder here — that the trip was set even before certiorari was granted, and was completed long before the case is to be argued. Justice Scalia does not, however, cite any authority for the remarkable proposition that it would be okay to preside over a case involving a litigant with whom you spent the weekend before oral argument, but not okay to arrange for same thing after certiorari is granted.

Only then does Justice Scalia address the trip on Air Force Two, the Vice President's personal jet that whisked Scalia and party to Louisiana. One of the most interesting aspects of this disquisition is what Scalia does not address. While later we learn who was with whom during the duck hunt, in the section of the opinion dealing with the sumptuous air travel arrangements, that subject is studiously not discussed. From the opinion, all one learns is that the complement included the Vice President and his staff and security detail, Justice Scalia and his son and son-in-law, quite a cozy group for a multiple-hour plane ride on a Gulfstream jet. Perhaps the cabin was too noisy for any conversation, unlike a duck blind. We will never know, though somehow we doubt it. In any event, we receive no assurance that the justice was sequestered from the litigant.

But if we were concerned about this omission our fears are quickly put to rest by Justice Scalia's assertion that, when he rode on Air Force Two, the trip cost the tax-payers nothing; the plane was flying there anyway and Justice Scalia received nothing of value when his son, son-in-law and he were offered these otherwise vacant seats on Air Force Two. This is because — damnit — they were only able to hitch a one-way ride with the Vice President. This meant — groan — the Scalia party had to buy one-way tickets back. But since one-way tickets, in addition to being a clear sign that the flyers are terrorists, are so much more expensive than round-trip tickets, the Scalia group bought round-trip tickets and, in violation of the airline's rules, tore up the other half. So the out-of-pocket expense for the Scalia party was the same as it would have been if the Vice President had never offered this little perquisite. In Justice Scalia's flamboyant rhetoric, "none of us saved a cent." End of discussion.

Well, not quite. Not many have flown on private jets. The author was lucky enough to do it once. And let me tell you there is real value to flying in the rarefied world of the dedicated private Gulfstream. The plane leaves when you want. It makes no stops. There is no racing through a hub to change planes. The space is luxurious. The food custom prepared. I can still taste the smoked salmon sandwiches served on monogrammed china aboard the Merrill Lynch Gulfstream. And you land not in New Orleans — how inconvenient — but at a private airport in Morgan City right next to your duck-hunting destination.

Justice Scalia grudgingly recognizes that even if he did not save any money, there was some very small value in what he received. But he wants us to put that value into perspective. He observes that at a charity auction one would bid far more for a dinner at the White House — something typically provided to Supreme Court justices — than for a trip on Air Force Two.

Does Justice Scalia think for one minute that this astonishing assertion proves that a trip on Air Force Two is not valuable? I have no idea what people would bid for seats at a Christmas dinner at the White House, but it would certainly be in the thousands. That certainly leaves lots of room to value the Air Force Two trip at a very high number as well — even if it could be snared at a lower dollar figure than dinner at the White House. . . .

Finally, Justice Scalia addresses the duck hunting itself. We are told there were 13 hunters in all, a group Justice Scalia characterizes as "not intimate," even "siz-able," perhaps because he found the flight down so much more *intime*. We learn they took meals together. One day they went fishing — in two boats. And though Justice Scalia studiously fails to tell us whether he was in the Vice President's fishing boat, we know in our hearts that is where he fished because when it came to the duck hunting, Justice Scalia makes it quite clear that Mr. Cheney and he never shared a duck blind, as it sadly turns out. Finally, lest you were worried about the Vice President having a Clinton problem, we are told that, although virtually everyone shared sleeping rooms, this sharing did not include the Vice President, who was not forced to sleep with Justice Scalia, his son or his son-in-law.

I make light of Justice Scalia's exegesis of the facts. I might even be accused of adopting a Scalia-like tone. But the fact that Justice Scalia spends all this time arguing the facts is really quite informative. Taking the time to share them with us, Justice Scalia must feel that they are critical, if not dispositive to dismissing any allegations that he should recuse himself. But what is he really saying?

If I had been introduced to my host by an oil man, not someone—tears now—who works with the handicapped, then I would have been forced to recuse.

If the host was an oil man and not an oil rig man, then I would have been forced to recuse.

If certiorari had been granted before the trip was set, then I would have been forced to recuse.

If I took a round trip on Air Force Two—and saved the cost of a round-trip ticket—then I would have been forced to recuse.

If I had been in the same duck blind—like he was in the same small plane and same small fishing boat—I would have been forced to recuse.

If I had shared a room with the Vice President, I would have been forced to recuse.

Why *is* Justice Scalia telling us all this? In my view, it demonstrates the weakness of his position. Should any motion to recuse turn on the facts to which Justice Scalia so tenaciously clings? The fact is Justice Scalia spent this huge amount of time with a litigant with a present matter before the court. No amount of tap dancing about who introduced who to whom, whether the host was an oil man or an oil rig man, or whether they were in the same duck blind changes the substance of what occurred. Justice Scalia engaged in conduct vis-à-vis the Vice President that required him to recuse himself. From the point of view of the adverse litigants this situation is intolerable. . . .

It is true that different standards might apply in personal versus official capacity lawsuits. The Social Security Administrator might well be indifferent to the fact that he or she is sued hundreds of times a month. And the idea that a judge played golf with that administrator while hearing some poor soul's social security appeal might not raise serious questions of judicial ethics. But to analogize such an unremarkable prosaic circumstance to *this* lawsuit against *this* vice president is surely to exalt form above substance.

It is also certainly true, as Justice Scalia repeatedly observes, that the Vice President has been sued in his official capacity. But the concept of official capacity-private capacity cannot be an on-off switch for deciding when a justice must recuse himself. Some official capacity lawsuits are far more personal than lawsuits that are classified as personal. Despite Justice Scalia's naked assertion to the contrary, this lawsuit raises an issue that has garnered significant attention for years—the highly charged question of who was sitting down in secret with the former CEO of Halliburton to decide our country's energy policy. Who were these oil industrialists? Oil men? Energy industry executives? It is an issue on which the Vice President has literally staked his reputation, one that might even affect the Vice President's re-nomination or re-election. And to assert that the Vice President does not have a deep, abiding and personal interest in whether he is going to be forced to share this information with an inquisitive world is to ignore the dozens of editorials that have been written on the topic.

And that is something we know Justice Scalia did not do. Indeed, he proclaims that the unanimous view of these editorial writers, whose facts he so carefully has checked, is not going to persuade him to recuse himself. That lesson is one conclusion of the Justice with which I agree. Just because 20 newspapers say a judge should recuse himself is no reason to do it. But that 20 newspapers thought this case was so important that they commented on the recusal issue demonstrates in a dramatic way that Justice Scalia's attempts to assure his participation in this case on the basis that this case is just like any garden variety run-of-the-mill Social Security appeal does not pass the straight face test.

But I have spent too much time addressing Justice Scalia on his own terms (this is all about the Vice President and me) and not nearly enough confronting the very serious ethical lapse his failure to recuse creates. Imagine you are a lawyer. You are handling a major case for a distraught client. The case will be tried next month to a judge. Your client, on your advice, takes a weekend of rest and relaxation at the Homestead. The client enters the elegant dining room with his wife and, as they are escorted to their table, they notice the judge, the adversary and the adversary's wife hoisting martini glasses filled with a silver liquid, laughing boisterously. As your client passes their way, there is an embarrassed silence followed by the judge's halting comment, "Great to see you, Mr. Jones. Just down here for some trout fishing. Of course, we haven't discussed that little matter."

How does that client feel? How do you feel? What has this done to the system of justice? Can the client ever be convinced that the judge will still be impartial? Should there be a need to convince the client of that fact? Even if you know the judge will be impartial, the appearance of bias is both profound and destructive. There is no place for judges fraternizing with litigants who have matters before them. And that is precisely what Justice Scalia brazenly and insensitively did and yet, when called on it, instead of curing the problem by graciously acknowledging the conflict of interest, he launches a rhetorical broadside that only fans the flames.

This Homestead scenario also highlights how useless is Justice Scalia's reliance on the matter being one in which Cheney is sued in his official capacity. If at our dining room scene our dismayed client had also been told, "Don't worry. The case I'm deciding next week is against my olive-loving friend in his official capacity," do you suppose the client would feel relieved, any lingering concerns evaporating once those words were uttered by the convivial judge? You see the problems with the personal-official distinction, are that (a) the offended party, a layman, will not understand the distinction and (b) even if he did, in the eyes of the offended party the betrayal looks identical. While the judge may think it is perfectly alright to go duck hunting with a litigant whose case is pending before him (so long as he does not occupy the same duck blind) because the matter involves the litigant in the litigant's official capacity, that fact is of no consequence to the litigant who was not invited to join the hunting party.

What does all of this teach us? I think there are two lessons here. First, Supreme Court practice apparently provides that the Justice who is the subject of a recusal motion decides whether the motion should be granted. Thus, we are the recipients of Justice Scalia's twenty-page pronuncimento. How much better would it be if every justice but the justice who is the object of attention were to decide this matter? These other justices are fully cognizant of the special considerations that must inform a Supreme Court motion to recuse, given the fact if one Justice steps down there is no one to take her place. Moreover, they are objective in a way that any judge who is the subject of such a motion cannot be. You can be sure that if the present eight Justices, without Scalia participating, had decided this motion, the world would have been treated, in the best sense of that word, to a far shorter and more persuasive opinion — even if the Court decided to deny the motion — than the one Scalia handed down. And the world would also have far more confidence that the result that was reached was a fair one.

Second, we could not find a better poster child than Justice Scalia's conduct and his defense for the importance of maintaining an appearance standard, if not the current appearance of impropriety standard, in our canons of judicial conduct. Since Justice Scalia may be completely unaffected by his sojourn with Dick Cheney, some of us might agree with Justice Scalia's assertion that if a Justice of the Supreme Court could be corrupted by this little fishing adventure then the nation is in real trouble. On the other hand, the appearance that Justice Scalia would be biased as a result of his Louisiana sojourn is something our canons of judicial ethics cannot condone or ignore. . . .

In the world of judging, appearances count and anyone who thinks that a requirement that judges be unfettered, honest and erudite in all things is enough, if what the judges appear to be doing goes unregulated, is failing to recognize how fragile is the trust the American public is currently willing to repose in our judiciary. . . .

What is it then that we don't want our judges to appear to be doing, even if they are not in fact doing it? We don't want them to engage in conduct that might lead the public to question their impartiality. We don't want them to engage in conduct that might lead the public to question their independence. We don't want them to engage in conduct that might lead the public to question their honesty. And we don't want them to engage in conduct that might lead the public to question their competence. . . .

Justice Scalia's adventure with Vice President Cheney not only reflected an appearance of impropriety, but also reflected an appearance that Justice Scalia was not impartial. . . .

For so many of us, the Supreme Court is the most important symbol of both the separation of powers and the rule of law. Maintaining the Court's dignity is critical to both of its symbolic roles. Gentle reader, please read Justice Scalia's 21-page tirade again. Has Justice Scalia enhanced the dignity of the Court by providing us with this? Do we feel better about the Court knowing that this Justice did not recuse himself because he did not sleep with Vice President Cheney? I don't think so and I'll bet you don't either.

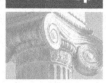

Post-Case Follow-Up

Justice Scalia declined to recuse himself because he did not believe that his duck hunting trip with the vice president created a situation where his "impartiality might be reasonably questioned."

In its subsequent decision on the merits, the Supreme Court, with Justice Scalia joining the seven-justice majority, declined to force Vice President Cheney to disclose the requested information under FACA and sent the case back to the D.C. Circuit.[56] The D.C. Circuit subsequently dismissed the case.[57] The Bush administration's allegedly cozy relationship with big corporations and special interests continued to be a major issue in the 2004 presidential campaign, which ultimately saw President Bush win reelection for a second term.

The entire incident brought renewed attention to the issue of judicial recusal. First, Justice Scalia's opinion provided little in the way of clarity concerning the recusal standard. It remains difficult to distinguish which social relationships are impermissible under the "appearance of impropriety" standard.

Second, the case brought scrutiny to the procedures the Supreme Court and other courts use for deciding recusal motions. For example, at the Supreme Court level, some like Professor Fox have called for recusal motions to be referred to the entire court rather than to the justice who is the subject of the motion while others have called for allowing retired justices or court of appeals judges to sit in place of disqualified justices.

Cheney v. United States District Court: Real Life Applications

1. Arizona trial judge Mary H. Murguia was presiding over a highly controversial case. Plaintiffs had filed suit against infamous Maricopa County Sheriff Joseph M. Arpaio and the County, alleging that Defendants were engaging in racial profiling and unlawful detention of persons of Hispanic appearance and descent. Judge Murguia's identical twin sister was the President and CEO of the National Council of La Raza, the largest Latino civil rights organization in the United States. Defendants moved to recuse Judge Murguia based on this relationship. How should she rule?

2. Given the important political cases that come before the Supreme Court, it is not surprising that calls for justices to recuse themselves remain a hot topic, particularly in politically charged cases. No formal motions were made in any of the following cases. Do you think any of these justices should have recused themselves? What are the best arguments for and against recusal?

56. Cheney v. United States Dist. Ct., 542 U.S. 367 (2004).
57. In re Cheney, 406 F.3d 723 (D.C. Cir. 2005).

a. When the constitutionality of the Affordable Care Act was pending before the Supreme Court, activists on both sides of the issue argued that justices who were likely to vote against their position should recuse themselves.

   i. Opponents of the ACA said that Justice Elena Kagan should recuse herself because she had been solicitor general in President Barack Obama's administration when the health care law was moving through Congress.

   ii. Those who supported the ACA said that Justice Thomas should recuse himself because of the political advocacy work that his wife had done to fight the law. Virginia Thomas was the founder and head of a non-profit group named Liberty Central, which described itself as opposed to the leftist "tyranny" of President Obama and dedicated to "protecting the [nation's] core founding principles." Mrs. Thomas was a vocal critic of the ACA and gave public speeches describing "Obamacare" as a "disaster" for small businesses and arguing that it was unconstitutional.[58]

b. After the Supreme Court decided Citizens United v. FEC, 558 U.S. 310 (2010), in which the Court struck down limits on political expenditures by non-profit organizations, Common Cause, a liberal advocacy group, asked the Justice Department to investigate whether Justices Scalia and Thomas should have recused themselves in that case because they had allegedly attended political retreats organized by the conservative businessman Charles Koch, who opposed limits on campaign spending.

c. Opponents of gay marriage said that Justices Elena Kagan and Ruth Bader Ginsburg should recuse themselves in Obergefell v. Hodges, 574 U.S. 644 (2015), in which the Supreme Court considered (and ultimately struck down) state laws banning same-sex marriage because both justices had previously officiated same-sex marriages.

d. During the 2016 presidential campaign, Justice Ginsburg criticized then-candidate Donald Trump as a "faker," saying "[h]e has no consistency about him. He says whatever comes into his head at the moment. He really has an ego. . . . How has he gotten away with not turning over his tax returns? The press seems to be very gentle with him on that."[59] Justice Ginsburg subsequently apologized; but after he was elected, President Trump publicly called on her to recuse herself on "anything having to do with Trump or Trump-related."[60]

2. Judges' Use of Social Media

While Justice Scalia's duck hunting involved traditional, in-person friendship, social media poses a new challenge for judges. Should judges participate in social

---

58. George Zornick, *The Nation: Clarence Thomas v. Legal Ethics,* National Public Radio, Nov. 15, 2011, *available at* http://www.npr.org/2011/11/15/142339329/the-nation-clarence-thomas-vs-legal-ethics.

59. Joan Biskupic, *Justice Ruth Bader Ginsburg Calls Trump a "Faker," He Says She Should Resign,* CNN, July 13, 2016, *available at* https://www.cnn.com/2016/07/12/politics/justice-ruth-bader-ginsburg-donald-trump-faker/index.html.

60. Devan Cole et al., *Trump Calls for Sotomayor, Ginsburg to Recuse Themselves from "Trump-Related" Cases as He Has a Lot at Stake Before the Court,* CNN, Feb. 25, 2020, *available at* https://www.cnn.com/2020/02/25/politics/donald-trump-ruth-bader-ginsburg-sonia-sotomayor-recusal/index.html.

media at all? When judges do participate in social media, under what circumstances should their social media "friendships" disqualify them?

The American Bar Association and several jurisdictions have issued ethics opinions addressing these issues. All of the ethics opinions endorse judges using social media, albeit in a "judicious" way. As the opinion from the ABA concluded, such use "can benefit judges in both their personal and professional lives" and also keep them from being "thought of as isolated or out of touch."[61]

The more difficult question is whether judges' social media connections with lawyers and litigants who may appear before them create an "appearance of impropriety" requiring disqualification; on this issue, the ethics opinions are divided.

Some states, such as Florida, adhere to a restrictive view, and forbid a judge from Facebook "friending" lawyers who may appear before the judge. The Florida Committee reasoned that when a judge "friends" a lawyer, he is selecting a special class of accepted individuals while rejecting others. That preference is then publicly communicated through social networking, which conveys the impression that the lawyer is in a special position to influence the judge. The Florida Committee reached the same conclusion concerning LinkedIn connections.[62] On the other hand, states in the more permissive camp generally allow judges to be "friends" with lawyers who may appear before them. For example, the Kentucky Ethics Committee concluded that a judge does not violate the Judicial Code simply by connecting with a lawyer on social media.[63] Similarly, the New York Committee concluded that social network connections are allowed, but judges must consider whether the circumstances of each case would indicate a "close social relationship" and require disclosure, recusal, or both.[64] The ABA's Opinion strikes somewhat of a middle ground declining to offer any *per se* rule. Instead, the ABA mentioned that state committees "have expressed a wide range of views" on the issue and noted that "designation as [a social media] connection does not, in and of itself, indicate the degree or intensity of a judge's relationship with a person." The opinion concluded that "context is significant."[65]

3. Constitutional Dimensions of Disqualification

Although "most matters relating to judicial disqualification [do] not rise to a constitutional level,"[66] in extreme cases, the Supreme Court has held that the Due Process Clause requires a judge to recuse herself.[67] The standard is whether there is a "serious risk of actual bias."

---

61. ABA Comm. on Ethics & Prof'l Responsibility, Formal Op. 462 at 1, 4 (2013).
62. *See, e.g.,* Fla. Judicial Ethics Advisory Comm., Op. 2009-20 (2009), *available at* http://www.jud6.org/ LegalCommunity/LegalPractice/opinions/jeacopinions/2009/2009-20.html. In a 2018 opinion, the Florida Supreme Court disagreed with this conclusion and found that a Facebook "friendship" with an attorney appearing before a judge did not, standing alone, constitute a basis for disqualification. Law Offices of Herssein & Herssein v. United Servs. Auto. Ass'n, 271 So. 3d 889 (Fla. 2018).
63. Ethics Comm. of Ky. Judiciary, Formal Op. JE-119 at 2 (2010).
64. N.Y. Advisory Comm. on Judicial Ethics, Op. 08-176 (2009).
65. ABA Comm'n on Ethics & Prof'l Responsibility, Formal Op. 462 at 2, 3 (2013).
66. FTC v. Cement Inst., 333 U.S. 683, 702 (1948).
67. Caperton v. A.T. Massey Coal Co., 556 U.S. 868, 884 (2009).

In three older cases, the Court found constitutional violations where the judge had a direct pecuniary stake in the outcome of the case. First, in *Tumey v. Ohio,* the Court struck down an Ohio statute that permitted local mayors to sit as judges and be paid out of the fines collected from those convicted of violating Ohio's Prohibition Act. The mayors only received compensation if they convicted the defendants. The Court said the scheme was impermissible under the Fourteenth Amendment because it gave the mayor "a direct, personal, pecuniary interest in convicting the defendant who came before him for trial."[68] Forty-five years later, in *Ward v. Village of Monroeville,* the Court considered another Ohio statute that incentivized the presiding mayor to convict defendants. In *Ward,* the fines did not go to the mayor personally, but went instead into his town's coffers and made up a "substantial portion" of the municipality's budget. The Court said that this scheme was impermissible because it created a "possible temptation" for the mayor to "maintain the high level of contribution from the mayor's court."[69] Finally, in *Aetna Life Insurance Co. v. Lavoie,* the Court found that it was impermissible for an Alabama Supreme Court justice to hear a case involving allegations of bad faith against an insurance company, where he was a plaintiff in a lawsuit involving a "very similar bad-faith-refusal-to-pay" in another Alabama court. As in *Tumey* and *Ward,* the Court held that the judge had a "direct, personal, substantial and pecuniary" interest in the case and that his participation therefore violated due process.[70]

More recently, in *Caperton v. A.T. Massey Coal Co.,* the Supreme Court addressed for the first time the circumstances under which the Due Process Clause requires a judge to recuse himself as a result of campaign contributions received from one of the parties. The facts of *Caperton* are so compelling that they inspired John Grisham to write a novel. (*See* sidebar, *infra.*) The *Caperton* plaintiffs, who operated a coal company, sued the much larger Massey Coal Company for anti-competitive behavior and won a $50 million verdict at trial, which Massey appealed to the Supreme Court of Appeals of West Virginia. While the appeal was pending, Don Blankenship, Massey's chairman, decided to support a conservative candidate, Brent Benjamin, in an effort to unseat one of the Court's more liberal members Justice Warren McGraw, in the belief that Benjamin would be more likely to overturn the verdict than McGraw. He contributed the statutory maximum $1,000 to Benjamin's campaign committee, donated almost $2.5 million to his political action committee, and made more than $500,000 in individual expenditures for direct mailings soliciting donations and for television and newspaper advertisements. The $3,000,000 that Blankenship spent was more than the total amount spent by all other Benjamin supporters and three times the amount spent by Benjamin's own campaign committee. Benjamin won the seat.

When the appeal came before the West Virginia Supreme Court, Caperton moved on three separate occasions to disqualify Justice Benjamin because of Blankenship's support for his campaign, but Justice Benjamin denied each motion, concluding that he had no direct pecuniary interest in the case: he did not stand to

---

68. 273 U.S. 510, 523-24 (1927).
69. 409 U.S. 57, 58-60 (1972).
70. 475 U.S. 813, 822-25 (1986).

gain anything from the outcome. The court reversed the jury verdict in a 3-2 decision (with Justice Benjamin in the majority), and Caperton filed a petition for certiorari in the U.S. Supreme Court.

The Supreme Court agreed to hear the case and reversed in a controversial 5-4 decision. Writing for the majority, Justice Kennedy concluded:

> Not every campaign contribution by a litigant or attorney creates a probability of bias that requires a judge's recusal, but this is an exceptional case. We conclude that there is a serious risk of actual bias — based on objective and reasonable perceptions — when a person with a personal stake in a particular case had a significant and disproportionate influence in placing the judge on the case by raising funds or directing the judge's election campaign when the case was pending or imminent. The inquiry centers on the contribution's relative size in comparison to the total amount of money contributed to the campaign, the total amount spent in the election, and the apparent effect such contribution had on the outcome of the election.

In reaching this conclusion, the Court stressed the size of Blankenship's campaign contributions, particularly "in comparison to the total amount contributed to the campaign . . . [and] spent in the election." The Court also emphasized that this case was unusual, repeatedly describing it as "extraordinary," "extreme," and "rare."[71] In his dissent, Chief Justice Roberts criticized the Court for providing "no guidance to judges and litigants about when recusal will be constitutionally required" and listed 40 "fundamental questions" that the Court's decision failed to address. He also predicted that the uncertainty of the standard would "inevitably lead to an increase in allegations that judges are biased."[72]

The Supreme Court's most recent decision addressing the application of the Due Process Clause to recusal issues is *Williams v. Pennsylvania*. This case concerned the role of Ronald Castille in Terrance Williams' prosecution and subsequent appeal. Castille had been the District Attorney of Philadelphia when the decision was made to seek the death penalty against Williams. As the head of the office, Castille reviewed the trial prosecutor's memorandum in support of seeking the death penalty and wrote a note

Straight Out of (or Into?) a Grisham Novel?

If you think that the facts of the *Caperton* case seem fantastic enough to be the subject of a legal thriller, you would be right. The events surrounding the case inspired bestselling author John Grisham to write *The Appeal*. In *The Appeal,* the plaintiff sues a chemical company for allowing pollutants to seep into the town's water supply, killing her husband and son. The jury awards $41 million in damages. The billionaire majority stockholder of the defendant company then vows to do "whatever it takes" to preserve his company, appealing the judgment to the Mississippi Supreme Court. He then recruits an inexperienced, naïve candidate for the Mississippi Supreme Court to unseat a justice up for re-election who is known to be plaintiff-friendly, and pumps millions of dollars into the campaign. The billionaire's candidate wins and immediately starts overturning judgments on appeal. We won't spoil the end for you—you'll have to read *The Appeal* yourself to find out whether the candidate overturns the judgment against the corporation that helped him get elected.

One other note: Grisham, a notoriously fast writer, was able to write his book and get it published before the U.S. Supreme Court managed to issue its decision in *Caperton.*

---

71. 556 U.S. 868, 872-75, 884-87, 890 (2009).
72. *Id.* at 890-91, 893-98 (Roberts, J. dissenting).

at the bottom of the document, "Approved to proceed on the death penalty." Thirty years later, Castille sat as Chief Justice of the Pennsylvania Supreme Court when the Commonwealth's appeal of Williams' habeas petition came before the Court. Williams moved to recuse Castille based on a provision in the Pennsylvania Code of Judicial Conduct (similar to the Model Code) that disqualifies judges from any proceeding in which "they served as a lawyer in the matter in controversy." Chief Justice Castille declined to recuse himself without any explanation. The Pennsylvania Supreme Court, with Chief Justice Castille joining the majority opinion, vacated the trial court's order staying Williams' execution and ordering a new sentencing hearing.

The U.S. Supreme Court reversed, finding that Chief Justice Castille's participation in the appeal violated due process. The Court held: "[w]here a judge has had an earlier significant, personal involvement as a prosecutor in a critical decision in the defendant's case, the risk of actual bias in the judicial proceeding rises to an unconstitutional level." Writing for the 5-3 majority, Justice Kennedy stated:

> When a judge has served as an advocate for the State in the very case the court is now asked to adjudicate, a serious question arises as to whether the judge, even with the most diligent effort, could set aside any personal interest in the outcome. There is, furthermore, a risk that the judge "would be so psychologically wedded" to his or her previous position as a prosecutor that the judge "would consciously or unconsciously avoid the appearance of having erred or changed position." In addition, the judge's "own personal knowledge and impression" of the case, acquired through his or her role in the prosecution, may carry far more weight with the judge than the parties' arguments to the court.[73]

D. JUDICIAL CAMPAIGNS AND OTHER POLITICAL ACTIVITY

Although federal judges are appointed, judges in many states are elected. Thirty-eight states have some form of judicial election for their highest state court; 32 of the 41 states that have intermediate appellate courts elect those judges; and 39 states hold elections for their trial courts.[74] The form of election varies — some are partisan, some are nonpartisan, and in some cases, judges face uncontested retention elections after their initial appointment. If judges in these states hope to get elected, they must raise funds and campaign for office. Their actions on the campaign trail raise a number of ethical issues.

1. Fundraising

Judges have to raise money for their campaigns, and those campaigns have become expensive — a 2019 study concluded that $39.7 million was spent on campaigns for

---

73. 136 S. Ct. 1899, 1903-10 (2016) (citations omitted).
74. For an interactive map showing judicial selection methods by court level and phase of selection (first full term, interim selection, and additional terms), see *Judicial Selection: An Interactive Map*, BRENNAN CTR. FOR JUSTICE, http://judicialselectionmap.brennancenter.org/?court=Supreme (last visited July 28, 2020).

state supreme court seats between 2017 and 2018.[75] Moreover, the amount of money spent on campaigns correlates to success at the ballot box. In one study, 90 percent of the contested seats were won by the candidate who spent the most money.[76]

The existence of money in judicial elections poses a threat to the public's confidence in the independence and impartiality of the judiciary. Is it reasonable for citizens to infer that judges will favor litigants and/or lawyers who contributed money to them? Even if judges are not actually biased by contributions, will the public perceive that a problem exists? In public opinion surveys, the large majority of citizens (87 percent in one survey) express concern that money in judicial elections is impacting the judges' decision making.[77]

The Model Code of Judicial Conduct provides that a judge should recuse herself where: "The judge knows or learns by means of a timely motion that a party, a party's lawyer, or the law firm of a party's lawyer has within the previous [insert number] year[s] made aggregate contributions to the judge's campaign in an amount that [is greater than $[insert amount] for an individual or $[insert amount] for an entity] [is reasonable and appropriate for an individual or an entity]."[78] Thus, the Model Code leaves it up to each state to decide whether to select an express dollar limit or instead use a "reasonable and appropriate" standard. In addition to the Code of Judicial Conduct, as we saw in *Caperton*, in extreme cases, the Due Process Clause requires judges who receive substantial donations from parties to recuse themselves.

Rule 4.1 also prohibits candidates from personally soliciting campaign contributions as opposed to through a committee. In its most recent decision addressing speech by judicial candidates, the Supreme Court upheld this restriction. *See* Williams-Yulee v. Florida Bar, 575 U.S. 433 (2015). In that case, Lanell Williams-Yulee sent a letter to local voters announcing her candidacy for county court judge in Hillsborough County, Florida and asking for a contribution. The Florida bar filed a complaint against her for violating Florida's ban on personal solicitation of funds, a restriction that Williams-Yulee claimed was a violation of her First Amendment rights. The Supreme Court held that this was a "rare case" in which the restriction was narrowly tailored to serve the state's interest in protecting the integrity of the judiciary and maintaining the public's confidence in an impartial judiciary: "[s]imply put, Florida and most other States have concluded that the public may lack confidence in a judge's ability to administer justice without fear or favor if he comes to office by asking for favors."[79]

---

75. Douglas Keith et al., *New Report Finds $39.7 Million Spent on Campaigns for State Supreme Court Judgeships in 2017-2018, $10.8 Million of It by Special Interest Groups*, Brennan Ctr. for Justice (Dec. 11, 2019), *available at* https://www.brennancenter.org/our-work/analysis-opinion/new-report-finds-397-million-spent-campaigns -state-supreme-court.

76. Scott Greytak et al., *Bankrolling the Bench: The New Politics of Judicial Elections 2013-14*, Brennan Ctr. for Justice at 1 (Oct. 2015), *available at* https://www.brennancenter.org/sites/default/files/publications/The_ New_Politics_of_Judicial_Election_2013_2014.pdf. *But see* Ronald D. Rotunda, *Judicial Elections, Campaign Financing, and Free Speech*, 2 Election L.J. 79 (2003); Ronald D. Rotunda, *A Preliminary Empirical Inquiry into the Connection Between Judicial Decision Making and Campaign Contributions to Judicial Candidates*, Prof. Law. at 16 (Winter 2003), in which Professor Rotunda concluded that there was no such correlation.

77. *Justice at Stake*, Brennan Center National Poll (Oct. 22-24, 2013), https://www.brennancenter.org/sites/default/ files/toplines337_B2D51323DC5D0.pdf.

78. Model Code of Judicial Conduct r. 2.11(a)(4) (Am. Bar Ass'n 2011).

79. 575 U.S. 444-45 (2015).

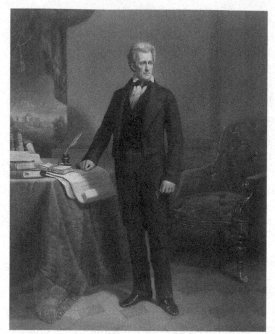 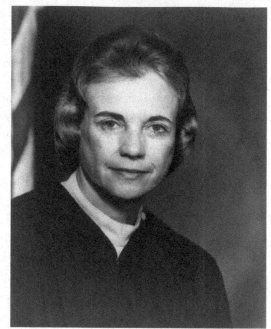

President Andrew Jackson championed electing judges to give ordinary people more power over the justice system. Since she retired from the bench, Justice Sandra Day O'Connor has been a strong advocate of depoliticizing the selection of judges. Her judicial selection plan can be found here: https://iaals.du.edu/sites/default/files/documents/ publications/oconnor_plan.pdf.
Library of Congress Prints and Photographs Division, Washington, D.C.

2. Other Political Activity

Even without the need to raise money, when judges and judicial candidates engage in political activity, that conduct poses a significant threat to judges' impartiality, or at least the appearance of impartiality. The public expects judges to make decisions based upon the facts and law in particular cases and not for political reasons. When judges engage in political activity, it could cause them to base their decisions on the political impact of those decisions, or at least give the public that impression. For that reason, Canon 4 provides that "[a] judge or candidate for judicial office shall not engage in political or campaign activity that is inconsistent with the independence, integrity, or impartiality of the judiciary." To that end, Rule 4.1 imposes broad restrictions on political activity by judges and judicial candidates. For example, judges and judicial candidates cannot act as leaders for a political organization,[80] make speeches for a political organization, publicly endorse political

---

80. The Terminology section of the Code defines "political organization" as "a political party or other group sponsored by or affiliated with a political party or candidate, the principal purpose of which is to further the election or appointment of candidates for political office."

candidates for any office, or solicit funds or make contributions to a political organization or political candidate.

Judicial campaigns pose yet another quandary: judicial candidates need to be able to communicate their views to the public so that voters can make an informed decision about how to vote. At the same time, it is important that judges have an open mind once they reach the bench and actually hear cases, and it is equally important that the public perceives them to have an open mind. Statements that judges made on the campaign trail could lead litigants and the public to believe that the judge has already made up her mind about an issue. Thus, states have an interest in limiting judicial campaign speech, but any restrictions on judicial candidates' political speech pose significant First Amendment concerns.

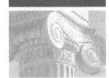

Case Preview

Republican Party of Minnesota v. White

For more than 30 years, Minnesota, like most states, followed an ABA Model Code provision, known as the "announce clause" that stated that a "candidate for a judicial office, including an incumbent judge," shall not "announce his or her views on disputed legal or political issues."[81] In 1996, Gregory Wersal ran for associate justice of the Minnesota Supreme Court, and, during his campaign, criticized several Minnesota Supreme Court decisions on crime, welfare, and abortion. The Office of Lawyers Professional Responsibility brought disciplinary proceedings against him for violating the announce clause. Those charges were subsequently dismissed, but Wersal nevertheless withdrew from the election. In 1998, Wersal ran again and sought an advisory opinion from the Lawyers Board about whether it planned to enforce the announce clause. After the Lawyers Board stated that it could not answer his question because he had not submitted a list of the announcements he wished to make, he filed suit arguing that the announce clause violated his First Amendment rights.

As you read the case, consider the following:

1. What is the Minnesota Office of Lawyer Professional Responsibility's interest in enforcing the announce clause?
2. How is Minnesota's "announce" clause different than the "promises and pledges" clause? Is this difference significant?
3. How does Justice Scalia's majority opinion define "impartiality" and what is the significance of that understanding for the Court's conclusion?

---

81. Model Code Canon 7(b)(1)(c) (1972) (repealed 1990).

Republican Party of Minnesota v. White
536 U.S. 765 (2002)

Justice SCALIA delivered the opinion of the Court.

The question presented in this case is whether the First Amendment permits the Minnesota Supreme Court to prohibit candidates for judicial election in that State from announcing their views on disputed legal and political issues.

I

Since Minnesota's admission to the Union in 1858, the State's Constitution has provided for the selection of all state judges by popular election. . . . Since 1974, they have been subject to a legal restriction which states that a "candidate for a judicial office, including an incumbent judge," shall not "announce his or her views on disputed legal or political issues." Minn. Code of Judicial Conduct, Canon 5(A)(3)(d)(i) (2000). This prohibition . . . is known as the "announce clause. . . ."

In 1996, one of the petitioners, Gregory Wersal, ran for associate justice of the Minnesota Supreme Court. In the course of the campaign, he distributed literature criticizing several Minnesota Supreme Court decisions on issues such as crime, welfare, and abortion. A complaint against Wersal challenging, among other things, the propriety of this literature was filed with the Office of Lawyers Professional Responsibility. . . . The Lawyers Board dismissed the complaint; with regard to the charges that his campaign materials violated the announce clause, it expressed doubt whether the clause could constitutionally be enforced. Nonetheless, fearing that further ethical complaints would jeopardize his ability to practice law, Wersal withdrew from the election. In 1998, Wersal ran again for the same office. Early in that race, he sought an advisory opinion from the Lawyers Board with regard to whether it planned to enforce the announce clause. The Lawyers Board responded equivocally, stating that, although it had significant doubts about the constitutionality of the provision, it was unable to answer his question because he had not submitted a list of the announcements he wished to make.

Shortly thereafter, Wersal filed this lawsuit in Federal District Court against respondents, seeking, *inter alia,* a declaration that the announce clause violates the First Amendment and an injunction against its enforcement. . . .

Other plaintiffs in the suit, including the Minnesota Republican Party, alleged that, because the clause kept Wersal from announcing his views, they were unable to learn those views and support or oppose his candidacy accordingly. . . .

II

Before considering the constitutionality of the announce clause, we must be clear about its meaning. Its text says that a candidate for judicial office shall not "announce his or her views on disputed legal or political issues."

We know that "announc[ing] . . . views" on an issue covers much more than *promising* to decide an issue a particular way. The prohibition extends to the candidate's mere statement of his current position, even if he does not bind himself to maintain that position after election. All the parties agree this is the case, because the Minnesota Code contains a so-called "pledges or promises" clause, which *separately* prohibits judicial candidates from making "pledges or promises of conduct in office other than the faithful and impartial performance of the duties of the office," — a prohibition that is not challenged here and on which we express no view.

There are, however, some limitations that the Minnesota Supreme Court has placed upon the scope of the announce clause that are not (to put it politely) immediately apparent from its text. The statements that formed the basis of the complaint against Wersal in 1996 included criticism of past decisions of the Minnesota Supreme Court. One piece of campaign literature stated that "[t]he Minnesota Supreme Court has issued decisions which are marked by their disregard for the Legislature and a lack of common sense." It went on to criticize a decision excluding from evidence confessions by criminal defendants that were not tape-recorded, asking "[s]hould we conclude that because the Supreme Court does not trust police, it allows confessed criminals to go free?" It criticized a decision striking down a state law restricting welfare benefits, asserting that "[i]t's the Legislature which should set our spending policies." And it criticized a decision requiring public financing of abortions for poor women as "unprecedented" and a "pro-abortion stance." Although one would think that all of these statements touched on disputed legal or political issues, they did not (or at least do not now) fall within the scope of the announce clause. The Judicial Board issued an opinion stating that judicial candidates may criticize past decisions, and the Lawyers Board refused to discipline Wersal for the foregoing statements because, in part, it thought they did not violate the announce clause. . . .

There are yet further limitations upon the apparent plain meaning of the announce clause: In light of the constitutional concerns, the District Court construed the clause to reach only disputed issues that are likely to come before the candidate if he is elected judge. The Eighth Circuit accepted this limiting interpretation by the District Court, and in addition construed the clause to allow general discussions of case law and judicial philosophy. The Supreme Court of Minnesota adopted these interpretations as well when it ordered enforcement of the announce clause in accordance with the Eighth Circuit's opinion.

It seems to us, however, that — like the text of the announce clause itself — these limitations upon the text of the announce clause are not all that they appear to be. First, respondents acknowledged at oral argument that statements critical of past judicial decisions are *not* permissible if the candidate also states that he is against *stare decisis*. Thus, candidates must choose between stating their views critical of past decisions and stating their views in opposition to *stare decisis*. Or, to look at it more concretely, they may state their view that prior decisions were erroneous only if they do not assert that they, if elected, have any power to eliminate erroneous decisions. Second, limiting the scope of the clause to issues likely to come before a court is not much of a limitation at all. One would hardly expect the "disputed legal or political issues" raised in the course of a state judicial election to include such matters as whether the Federal Government should end the embargo of Cuba. Quite obviously, they will be those legal or political disputes that are the proper (or by past decisions have been made the improper) business of the state courts. And within that relevant category, "[t]here is almost no legal or political issue that is unlikely to come before a judge of an American court, state or federal, of general jurisdiction." Third, construing the clause to allow "general" discussions of case law and judicial philosophy turns out to be of little help in an election campaign. At oral argument, respondents gave, as an example of this exception, that a candidate is free to assert that he is a "'strict constructionist.'" But that, like most other philosophical generalities, has little meaningful content for the electorate unless it is exemplified by application to a particular issue of construction likely to come before a court — for example, whether a particular statute runs afoul of any provision of the Constitution. Respondents conceded that the announce clause would prohibit the candidate from exemplifying his philosophy in this fashion. Without such application to real-life issues, all candidates can claim to be "strict constructionists" with equal (and unhelpful) plausibility.

In any event, it is clear that the announce clause prohibits a judicial candidate from stating his views on any specific nonfanciful legal question within the province of the court for which he is running, except in the context of discussing past decisions — and in the latter context as well, if he expresses the view that he is not bound by *stare decisis*.

Respondents contend that this still leaves plenty of topics for discussion on the campaign trail. These include a candidate's "character," "education," "work habits," and "how [he] would handle administrative duties if elected." Indeed, the Judicial Board has printed a list of preapproved questions which judicial candidates are allowed to answer. These include how the candidate feels about cameras in the courtroom, how he would go about reducing the caseload, how the costs of judicial administration can be reduced, and how he proposes to ensure that minorities and women are treated more fairly by the court system. Whether this list of preapproved subjects, and other topics not prohibited by the announce clause, adequately fulfill the First Amendment's guarantee of freedom of speech is the question to which we now turn.

III

. . .

The Court of Appeals concluded that respondents had established two interests as sufficiently compelling to justify the announce clause: preserving the impartiality of the state judiciary and preserving the appearance of the impartiality of the state judiciary. Respondents reassert these two interests before us, arguing that the first is compelling because it protects the due process rights of litigants, and that the second is compelling because it preserves public confidence in the judiciary. Respondents are rather vague, however, about what they mean by "impartiality. . . ."

A

One meaning of "impartiality" in the judicial context — and of course its root meaning — is the lack of bias for or against either *party* to the proceeding. Impartiality in this sense assures equal application of the law. That is, it guarantees a party that the judge who hears his case will apply the law to him in the same way he applies it to any other party. This is the traditional sense in which the term is used. . . .

We think it plain that the announce clause is not narrowly tailored to serve impartiality (or the appearance of impartiality) in this sense. Indeed, the clause is barely tailored to serve that interest *at all,* inasmuch as it does not restrict speech for or against particular *parties,* but rather speech for or against particular *issues.* To be sure, when a case arises that turns on a legal issue on which the judge (as a candidate) had taken a particular stand, the party taking the opposite stand is likely to lose.

But not because of any bias against that party, or favoritism toward the other party. *Any* party taking that position is just as likely to lose. The judge is applying the law (as he sees it) evenhandedly.

B

It is perhaps possible to use the term "impartiality" in the judicial context (though this is certainly not a common usage) to mean lack of preconception in favor of or against a particular *legal view.* This sort of impartiality would be concerned, not with guaranteeing litigants equal application of the law, but rather with guaranteeing them an equal chance to persuade the court on the legal points in their case. Impartiality in this sense may well be an interest served by the announce clause, but it is not a *compelling* state interest, as strict scrutiny requires. A judge's lack of predisposition regarding the relevant legal issues in a case has never been thought a necessary component of equal justice, and with good reason. For one thing, it is virtually impossible to find a judge who does not have preconceptions about the law. . . . Indeed, even if it were possible to select judges who did not have preconceived views on legal issues, it would hardly be desirable to do so. "Proof that a Justice's mind at the time he joined the Court was a complete *tabula rasa* in the area of constitutional adjudication would be evidence of lack of qualification, not lack of bias." The Minnesota Constitution positively forbids the selection to courts of general jurisdiction of judges who are impartial in the sense of having no views on the law. Minn. Const., Art. VI, §5 ("Judges of the supreme court, the court of appeals and the district court shall be learned in the law"). And since avoiding judicial preconceptions on legal issues is neither possible nor desirable, pretending otherwise by attempting to preserve the "appearance" of that type of impartiality can hardly be a compelling state interest either.

C

A third possible meaning of "impartiality" (again not a common one) might be described as open-mindedness. This quality in a judge demands, not that he have no preconceptions on legal issues, but that he be willing to consider views that oppose his preconceptions, and remain open to persuasion, when the issues arise in a pending case. This sort of impartiality seeks to guarantee each litigant, not an *equal* chance to win the legal points in the case, but at least *some* chance of doing so. It may well be that impartiality in this sense, and the appearance of it, are desirable in the judiciary, but we need not pursue that inquiry, since we do not believe the Minnesota Supreme Court adopted the announce clause for that purpose.

Respondents argue that the announce clause serves the interest in openmindedness, or at least in the appearance of openmindedness, because it relieves a judge from pressure to rule a certain way in order to maintain consistency with statements the judge has previously made. The problem is, however, that statements in election campaigns are such an infinitesimal portion of the public commitments to legal positions that judges (or judges-to-be) undertake, that this object of the prohibition is implausible. Before they arrive on the bench (whether by election or otherwise) judges have often committed themselves on legal issues that they must later rule upon. More common still is a judge's confronting a legal issue on which he has expressed an opinion while on the bench. Most frequently, of course, that prior expression will have occurred in ruling on an earlier case. But judges often state their views on disputed legal issues outside the context of adjudication—in classes that they conduct, and in books and speeches. Like the ABA Codes of Judicial Conduct, the Minnesota Code not only permits but encourages this. See Minn. Code of Judicial Conduct, Canon 4(B) (2002) ("A judge may write, lecture, teach, speak and participate in other extra-judicial activities concerning the law . . ."); Minn. Code of Judicial Conduct, Canon 4(B), Comment. (2002) ("To the extent that time permits, a judge is encouraged to do so . . ."). That is quite incompatible with the notion that the need for open-mindedness (or for the appearance of open-mindedness) lies behind the prohibition at issue here.

The short of the matter is this: In Minnesota, a candidate for judicial office may not say "I think it is constitutional for the legislature to prohibit same-sex marriages." He may say the very same thing, however, up until the very day before he declares himself a candidate, and may say it repeatedly (until litigation is pending) after he is elected. As a means of pursuing the objective of openmindedness that respondents now articulate, the announce clause is so woefully underinclusive as to render belief in that purpose a challenge to the credulous. . . .

IV

To sustain the announce clause, the Eighth Circuit relied heavily on the fact that a pervasive practice of prohibiting judicial candidates from discussing disputed legal and political issues developed during the last half of the 20th century. It is true that a "universal and long-established" tradition of prohibiting certain conduct creates "a strong presumption" that the prohibition is constitutional. . . . The practice of prohibiting speech by judicial candidates on disputed issues, however, is neither long nor universal.

. . .

The first code regulating judicial conduct was adopted by the ABA in 1924. It contained a provision akin to the announce clause: "A candidate for judicial position . . . should not announce in advance his conclusions of law on disputed issues to secure class support. . . ." ABA Canon of Judicial Ethics 30 (1924). The States were slow to adopt the canons, however. "By the end of World War II, the canons . . . were binding by the bar associations or supreme courts of only eleven states." Even today, although a majority of States have adopted either the announce clause or its 1990 ABA successor, adoption is not unanimous. Of the 31 States that select some or all of their appellate and general-jurisdiction judges by election, 4 have adopted no candidate-speech restriction comparable to the announce clause, and 1 prohibits only the discussion of "pending litigation." This practice, relatively new to judicial elections and still not universally adopted, does not compare well with the traditions deemed worthy of our attention in prior cases.

. . .

There is an obvious tension between the article of Minnesota's popularly approved Constitution which provides that judges shall be elected, and the Minnesota Supreme Court's announce clause which places most subjects of interest to the voters off limits. (The candidate-speech restrictions of all the other States that have them are also the product of judicial fiat.) The disparity is perhaps unsurprising, since the ABA, which originated the announce clause, has long been an opponent of judicial elections. That opposition may be well taken (it certainly had the support of the Founders of the Federal Government), but the First Amendment does not permit it to achieve its goal by leaving the principle of elections in place while preventing candidates from discussing what the elections are about. "[T]he greater power to dispense with elections altogether does not include the lesser power to conduct elections under conditions of state-imposed voter ignorance. If the State chooses to tap the energy and the legitimizing power of the democratic process, it must accord the participants in that process . . . the First Amendment rights that attach to their roles."

The Minnesota Supreme Court's canon of judicial conduct prohibiting candidates for judicial election from announcing their views on disputed legal and political issues violates the First Amendment. Accordingly, we reverse the grant of summary judgment to respondents and remand the case for proceedings consistent with this opinion.

[Justice O'Connor, concurred with the majority opinion to emphasize the following point: "Minnesota has chosen to select its judges through contested popular elections instead of through an appointment system or a combined appointment and retention election system along the lines of the Missouri Plan. In doing so the State has voluntarily taken on the risks to judicial bias described above. As a result, the State's claim that it needs to significantly restrict judges' speech in order to protect judicial impartiality is particularly troubling. If the State has a problem with judicial impartiality, it is largely one the State brought upon itself by continuing the practice of popularly electing judges."]

. . .

[In his dissenting opinion, joined by three other Justices, Justice Stevens reasoned as follows: "By recognizing a conflict between the demands of electoral politics and the distinct characteristics of the judiciary, we do not have to put States to an all or nothing choice of abandoning judicial elections or having elections in which anything goes. As a practical matter, we cannot know for sure whether an elected judge's decisions are based on his interpretation of the law or political expediency. . . . But we do know that a judicial candidate, who announces his views in the context of a campaign, is effectively telling the electorate: 'Vote for me because I believe X, and I will judge cases accordingly.' Once elected, he may feel free to disregard his campaign statements, but that does not change the fact that the judge announced his position on an issue likely to come before him *as a reason to vote for him*. Minnesota has a compelling interest in sanctioning such statements.]

[In her dissenting opinion, Justice Ginsburg emphasized the interrelationship between the "Pledges and Promises" clause and the "Announce" clause: "Uncoupled from the Announce Clause, the ban on pledges or promises is easily circumvented. By prefacing a campaign commitment with the caveat, 'although I cannot promise anything,' or by simply avoiding the language of promises or pledges altogether, a candidate could declare with impunity how she would decide specific issues. . . . By targeting statements that do not technically constitute pledges or promises but nevertheless 'publicly mak[e] known how [the candidate] would decide' legal issues, the Announce Clause prevents this end run around the letter and spirit of its companion provision. No less than the pledges or promises clause itself, the Announce Clause is an indispensable part of Minnesota's effort to maintain the health of its judiciary, and is therefore constitutional for the same reasons."]

Post-Case Follow-Up

In *White*, the Court held that Minnesota's "announce clause" (which mirrored the ABA Model Code's language) was unconstitutional. The court found that the ban on judicial candidates announcing their views on disputed legal or political issues was not narrowly tailored to serve the state's stated goal of ensuring the judiciary's impartiality.

The *White* decision had a real impact on judicial elections. At a minimum, it enabled judicial candidates to speak more freely about contested political issues. Some have argued that the *White* decision marked a significant shift in the tone and intensity of judicial elections since it allows judicial candidates to engage in aggressive campaigning on issues, though the research on *White*'s impact is mixed.[82]

Following *White*, the drafters of the Model Code of Judicial Conduct removed the announce clause, but retained the ban on pledges and promises. Thus, a judicial candidate shall not "in connection with cases, controversies, or issues that are likely to come before the court, make pledges, promises, or commitments that are inconsistent with the impartial performance of the adjudicative duties of judicial office."[83] As a result, it is permissible for a judicial candidate to announce that he disagrees with *Roe v. Wade* and favors laws restricting a woman's ability to get an abortion, but it is unlawful for a candidate to state that if he is elected, he promises to uphold any restriction on abortions. Comment [13] to Rule 4.1 states that whether a statement is a "pledge, promise, or commitment is not dependent upon, or limited to, the use of any specific words or phrases; instead, the totality of the statement must be examined to determine if a reasonable person would believe that the candidate for judicial office has specifically undertaken to reach a particular result."

Republican Party v. White: Real Life Applications

1. The *White* majority did not address the constitutionality of the "pledges and promises" clause of the Minnesota rules (which is substantially similar to Rule 4.1 of the current Model Code). What are the arguments for and against the constitutionality of this provision?

---

82. *See* David M. O'Brien, *State Court Elections and Judicial Independence*, 31 J.L. & POL. 417 (2016).
83. Model Code r. 4.1(a)(13).

2. Willie Singletary was a candidate for traffic court judge in Philadelphia. While campaigning for the primary election, he spoke to a gathering of a motorcycle club. During the meeting, he asked attendees to donate to his campaign and stated, "You're going to need me in traffic court, am I right about that? . . . Now you all want me to get there, you're all going to want my hook-up, right?" Is Judge Singletary subject to discipline?

3. As noted earlier, Model Rule 4.1 prohibits judges from "act[ing] as a leader in, or hold[ing] an office in, a political organization," "mak[ing] speeches on behalf of a political organization," "mak[ing] a contribution to a political organization or a candidate," and "publicly endors[ing] . . . a candidate for any public office." Are these restrictions on political activity a good idea? Are they constitutional?

4. Some states hold nonpartisan elections. Are these restrictions a good idea? Are they constitutional?

5. Other states impose restrictions on judicial candidates' ability to associate themselves with political parties. For example:

    a. Kentucky used to prohibit judicial candidates from disclosing their party affiliation "in any form of advertising, or when speaking to a gathering" except in answer to a question by a voter one-on-one or in "very small private informal" settings.
    b. Ohio permits judicial candidates to run in partisan primaries but does not allow them to list their party affiliation on the general election ballot.[84]

Are these restrictions a good idea? Are they constitutional?

Chapter Summary

- The guiding principle behind the Model Code of Judicial Conduct is ensuring that judges act with independence, integrity, and impartiality, and promoting the appearance of the same.
- On the bench, judges must perform their duties impartially, competently, and diligently. For example, judges must "uphold and apply the law" and avoid bias, prejudice, and other external influences in their decision making. Judges must also limit their public statements about pending cases.
- Off the bench, judges must minimize activities that conflict with their judicial obligations. For example, judges may not use the prestige of their office to advance their own or others' interests or hold membership in discriminatory organizations.
- Judges should be disqualified "in any proceeding in which the judge's impartiality might reasonably be questioned." This standard is vague and can be difficult

---

84. OHIO REV. CODE ANN. §3505.04 (LexisNexis 2013 & Supp. 2016).

to apply, particularly with respect to judges' social relationships with lawyers and parties who appear before the judge. Justice Scalia declined to recuse himself after he went duck hunting with Vice President Cheney while a case in which Cheney was a named defendant was pending before the Supreme Court.

■ The Model Code and the states impose a wide variety of restrictions on political activity by judges and judicial candidates. In *White*, the Supreme Court held that Minnesota's "announce clause" (which mirrored the ABA Model Code's language) was unconstitutional. The Court did not address the "pledges and promises" clause or a host of other restrictions on political activity by judicial candidates.

Applying the Rules

1. What does the duty of impartiality mean, and how should it be applied?

   a. Is a judge subject to discipline if she steps down from the bench before a criminal trial starts and shakes the defendant's hand in front of potential jurors to emphasize the defendant's presumption of innocence?

   b. Is a judge subject to discipline for wearing rainbow-flag pins on his judicial robes or posting safe place placards on courtroom doors to convey his acceptance of LGBTQ youth?

2. In 1978, Judge George C. Paine II, Chief Judge of the United States Bankruptcy Court for the Middle District of Tennessee became a member of the Belle Meade Country Club, which has no female or Black members. In 1990, Judge Paine wrote a strong letter to the Club's Board of Directors stating that he thought it "long overdue that the Club have Jewish and black associate and resident members" and that it was "patently preposterous that there are not persons in these racial and religious groups who would not be excellent participating members of the Club." Despite Judge Paine's letter, the club continued to lack female and minority members. Is Judge Paine subject to discipline?

3. James Singleton is a candidate for trial court judge in a state election. To support his campaign, he creates a Facebook page. Can he link his personal page to the campaign page? Can the campaign page include a place where the public could contribute? Can James send a digital invitation to his campaign launch to all of his Facebook friends? James's college roommate and best friend Michael Schwartz is running for Congress and has set up a Facebook page to support his congressional campaign. Can James "like" Michael's page?

4. After President George W. Bush nominated Harriet Miers to the U.S. Supreme Court, Texas Supreme Court Justice Nathan Hecht, a longtime friend, gave over 100 interviews about her:

   ■ He shared information about Miers' background and experience.
   ■ He described Miers' views on religion and abortion.

- He shared his positive view of her nomination, describing the appointment as "great," "solid," and "strong."
- He described her in various interviews as being "remarkable," "charming," "gracious," "solid," "strong," "sterling," and "stellar."
- He said that after the American public had a chance to review her record, they were "going to herald this nomination as a good one" and that her detractors were "going to be happy as clams" after they learned more about her.
- He predicted that during the confirmation process, Senators would be "convinced that this is the right person for the job." . . .
- He described their close personal relationship acknowledging his "admiration" for her.

Is Justice Hecht subject to discipline for these comments?

5. Attorney Sandra Perlman represented defendant Lawrence Braynen in a criminal case. Perlman was one of 34 members serving on the steering committee for a judicial candidate that opposed circuit judge Cheryl Aleman in the recent election. Perlman moved to recuse Judge Aleman. Should Judge Aleman grant the motion?

Professional Responsibility in Practice

1. The Code of Judicial Conduct varies greatly from state to state. Look up your state's Code and compare it to the Model Code.

2. The 1972 Code of Judicial Conduct effectively prohibited broadcast media in the courtroom, but since 1982, the Code has not contained such a prohibition, and it is up to each court to consider the issue. In Chandler v. Florida, 449 U.S. 560 (1981), the Supreme Court held that there was no constitutional prohibition on a state permitting radio, television, or photographic coverage of a criminal trial. Some courts now permit video cameras in the courtroom while others, including the U.S. Supreme Court, do not (though the U.S. Supreme Court did permit audio streaming at the outset of the COVID-19 pandemic). Should courts permit live coverage of court proceedings?

3. Research how judges are selected in your state. How does it compare to other states? What do you think are the pros and cons of your state's process?

4. Justice Sandra Day O'Connor has long championed changes to how states select judges. Evaluate the pros and cons of Justice O'Connor's plan, which can be found here: https://iaals.du.edu/sites/default/files/documents/publications/oconnor_plan.pdf.

Glossary

access-to-justice gap The gap between the legal needs of low- and moderate-income Americans and the resources available to meet those needs. (Ch. Eleven)

accounting Lawyer's fiduciary duty to provide a full accounting of any funds or property, if a client or a third person claiming an interest in property or funds held by the attorney makes a request. (Ch. Three)

advance conflict waivers Document that asks prospective clients to waive their right to file a disqualification motion against the firm should it represent a party in the same or substantially related matter against the prospective clients. (Ch. Six)

advertising/communications Marketing that is directed to a broad audience. (Ch. Ten)

advocate-witness rule An attorney cannot maintain dual roles as advocate and witness in the same matter before the same tribunal. (Chs. Six, Seven)

agency relationship Relationship between parties whereby one agrees to act on behalf of another. (Ch. Five)

aggravating factors After the establishment of misconduct, these factors establish the severity of sanctions needed. (Ch. Two)

alternative business structures (ABS) Proposed structures that allow for non-lawyer ownership and/or management of a business or firm. Also known as alternative legal practice structures. (Chs. Nine, Eleven)

alternative discipline program (ADP) Occurs before disciplinary counsel files formal charges, and depending on the jurisdiction, might include arbitration, mediation, law office management assistance, lawyer assistance programs, psychological counseling and continuing legal education. (Ch. Two)

antidiscrimination provision Bars conduct and speech related to the practice of law that a lawyer should reasonably know is harassment or discrimination on the basis of 11 grounds, including race, sex, religion, and age. (*See* Model Rule 8.4(g).) (Ch. Two)

attorney-client privilege Client's privilege to refuse disclosure of confidential communications between the client and the attorney. (Ch. Five)

autonomous self-interest Ideology that views clients as individualistic and atomistic entities whose goal is to pursue and maximize their self-interest without regard to others. (Ch. One)

candor to the tribunal The attorney's obligation to be truthful to the court. (Ch. Seven)

churning Unnecessarily overstaffing a case or performing duplicative or unnecessary work to drive up a bill. A form of fraudulent billing. (Ch. Three)

Civil Gideon   A movement to recognize an individual's right to counsel in civil cases. (Ch. Eleven)

civility   Obligation to act with courtesy and respect. (Ch. Seven)

clawback   To get something back. (Ch. Five)

common interest doctrine   When multiple parties and multiple lawyers share or pool confidential information and coordinate strategies in a matter of common legal interest. (Ch. Five)

communication   The method of conveying information so that the attorney accurately ascertains the client's objectives, and the client thereafter is kept apprised of what is going on in the matter or transaction. (Ch. Four)

competence   For attorneys, consists of four components: legal knowledge, skill, thoroughness, and preparation. (Ch. Four)

concurrent client   Another term for current client. (Ch. Six)

confidential material   Any information relating to the representation of a client. (Ch. Five)

confidentiality   The state of keeping or being kept secret or private. (Ch. Five)

confidentiality exceptions   Exceptions that allow a lawyer to reveal confidential information to the extent the lawyer reasonably believes necessary for particular purposes. (Ch. Five)

conflict of interest   Exists when there is a substantial risk that the lawyer's ability to perform her fiduciary duties is affected by the lawyer's own competing interests or the lawyer's duties to others. (Ch. Six)

conflict of interest waiver   Legal document stating that a conflict of interest may be present in a situation, all parties are aware, and steps are being taken to keep things fair and reasonable. (Ch. Six)

conflict shopping   When someone arranges to have initial consultations with several attorneys with the purpose of disclosing information and subsequently arguing that the opposing side is conflicted out from using any of those attorneys. (Ch. Three)

continuing legal education   Professional education for attorneys that takes place after their initial admission to the bar. (Ch. Two)

control group test   One possible test used to determine whether the attorney-client privilege protects communications made by corporate employees to the company's lawyer. (*See* Model Rule 4.2) (Chs. Five, Seven)

covenants not to compete   An agreement in which one party agrees not to work for the other party's direct competition in a specified area for a certain amount of time. (Ch. Nine)

crime-fraud exception   Provides that a client's confidential communications with counsel are not protected by the attorney-client privilege from compelled disclosure when made for the purpose of furthering a crime or fraud. (Ch. Five)

deficient performance   Defined by *Strickland* as "unreasonableness" under prevailing professional norms. Reviewing courts engage in a "strong presumption that counsel's conduct falls within the wide range of reasonable professional assistance." (Ch. Four)

delivery   Lawyer's fiduciary duty to promptly deliver any funds or property to the client (or third person with the ownership interest.) (Ch. Three)

diligence   Requires that the lawyer pursue a client's case "despite opposition, obstruction or personal inconvenience to the lawyer, and take whatever lawful and ethical measures are required to vindicate a client's cause or endeavor." (*See* Model Rule 1.1, Comment [1]) (Ch. Four)

disbarment   A permanent separation from the bar, with no chance of reinstatement in some jurisdictions. (Ch. Two)

discovery abuse   The misuse of the discovery process by making unnecessary requests for information, by responding to opponent's discovery requests in an improper manner, or by conducting discovery for an improper purpose. (Ch. Seven)

double bill   Charging for the same hour of work more than once. (Ch. Three)

entity theory of organizational representation   When a lawyer represents an organization, the client is the organization itself and not any of the organization's individual constituents (such as officers, directors, employees or shareholders). (Ch. Three)

entity warning   Requirement under Model Rule 1.13(f) that an organization's attorney should clarify her role and "explain the identity of the client" to an organization's constituents "when the lawyer knows or reasonably should know that the organization's interests are adverse to those of the constituents with whom the lawyer is dealing." (Ch. Three)

ex parte communications   Any communication between a judge or juror and a party to a legal proceeding or his counsel outside of the presence of the opposing party or the opposing party's attorney. (Ch. Seven)

ex parte proceedings   One-sided proceedings, where opposing counsel is not present. (Ch. Seven)

exculpatory evidence   Evidence that is favorable to the defendant in a criminal case in that it tends to negate guilt. (Ch. Eight)

extrajudicial duties   Activities of a judge off of the bench. Should be conducted in such a manner that minimizes the risk of conflict with their judicial obligations. (Ch. Twelve)

fiduciary   A relationship of trust that creates obligations of loyalty, care, and secrecy on the part of the lawyer. (Ch. Five)

frivolous   Groundless. In the context of litigation, whether a pleading is frivolous will be assessed from an objective standard of what a reasonable attorney would have known in the actor's situation, rather than a subjective standard of malice or motive to harass. (Ch. Seven)

future harms   Potential harms. In the context of professional responsibility, most states also contain exceptions to their confidentiality rules for disclosures that are necessary to prevent these. (Ch. Five)

gag order   Restriction on media contact that is imposed by the court. (Ch. Seven)

good character and fitness   Requirement for admission to the bar. Concerned with the present ability and disposition of the applicant to practice competently and honestly. (Ch. Two)

humanitarian expenses   In limited situations, a lawyer may provide a modest gift to cover such client expenses as food, rent, transportation, medicine, and other basic living expenses. (*See* Model Rule 1.8(e)(i)-(iii).) (Ch. Six)

implied attorney-client relationship   When an attorney-client relationship is created without an express agreement. (Ch. Three)

impliedly authorized   Authorization for a lawyer to do what is reasonably necessary in order to effectively perform his explicit duties. (Ch. Five)

imputation doctrine   Where one lawyer is disqualified because of a conflict of interest due to his having confidential information, then all firm members must be vicariously disqualified to safeguard the confidential information from misuse. (Ch. Six)

***in camera* review**   A legal proceeding where a judge privately examines documents or a witness in chambers. (Ch. Five)

inadvertent disclosure   Occurs when the disclosing person took precautions reasonable in the circumstances to guard against a disclosure but the communication or information was still accidently revealed. (Ch. Five)

ineffective assistance of counsel   Denial of an accused's Sixth Amendment right to counsel. The two-pronged approach to determine ineffective assistance is defined by *Strickland v. Washington*, requiring a defendant to prove (1) deficient performance of counsel and (2) prejudice. (Ch. Four)

informed consent   Express agreement after the client has been advised about the risks and available alternatives. (Ch. Five)

interest on lawyer trust accounts (IOLTA)   Interest received on client funds held in trust accounts in situations when it is impractical for the attorney to establish a separate account for each client. (Ch. Eleven)

integrated state bar association   State bar association where the high court requires bar membership to practice law. (Ch. Two)

joint client   A situation where multiple clients share a lawyer. (Ch. Five)

joint representation   When a lawyer represents more than one client in the same matter. (Ch. Six)

joint-clients exception   Provides that a communication to a lawyer that is relevant to a matter of common interest between joint clients is not privileged when one joint client proceeds against another joint client. (Ch. Five)

judicial duties   Duties of judicial office that must be performed impartially, competently, and diligently. (Ch. Twelve)

last link doctrine   Holding of courts that a client's identity is protected by the attorney-client privilege when it connects the client to the offense. (Ch. Five)

lawyer independence   Requirement of Model Rule 2.1. Multiple facets include independence from government control, need for independent professional judgment, independence from popular opinion and prejudice, and independence from clients. (Ch. Nine)

lawyer's trilemma   Situation where lawyer considers whether to put his client on the witness stand. A lawyer must simultaneously act diligently in gathering as much information as will enable him to counsel the client, guard the client's secrets, and be candid to the court. (Ch. Eight)

legal malpractice   Negligence, breach of fiduciary duty, or breach of contract by an attorney that causes harm to his or her client. To establish legal malpractice, the following must be shown: (1) the existence of an attorney-client relationship that establishes a duty on the part of the attorney, (2) a negligent act or omission constituting a breach of that duty, (3) the proximate cause (or legal cause) of the injury, and (4) the actual damages suffered by the plaintiff. (Ch. Two)

Legal Services Corporation (LSC)   A non-profit organization established by Congress in 1974, which is the single largest funder of civil legal aid for low-income Americans. (Ch. Eleven)

limited liability companies (LLC)   Form of business enterprise, recognized in all states, offering the pass-through tax status of a partnership and the limited liability of a corporation. (Ch. Two)

limited liability partnership (LLP)   Form of partnership in which a partner has no personal liability for the misconduct of another partner (and, in 49 jurisdictions, no personal liability for contractual obligations of the partnership). (Ch. Two)

Limited License Legal Technicians (LLLTs)   Independent legal paraprofessionals licensed to give legal advice in Washington State. (Ch. Eleven)

material   Important; affecting the merits of a case. (Ch. Seven)

McDade Amendment   Federal law that makes it clear that Justice Department prosecutors must abide by the attorney discipline rules in the states in which they practice. (Ch. Eight)

minister of justice   Designation of the special role of a prosecutor, as described in Model Rule 3.8. (Ch. Eight)

mitigating factors   After the establishment of misconduct, these factors help determine whether a lesser sanction is appropriate. (Ch. Two)

mixed communications   Mix of legal and non-legal advice, such as business, financial, or personal advice. (Ch. Five)

moral dialogue   Discussion with the client to determine the client's actual desires and moral ends. (Ch. One)

multidisciplinary practices (MDPs)   Businesses that offer "bundled services" that include the practice of law in addition to other professional services. Under Model Rule 5.4, lawyers are prohibited from forming MDPs with nonlawyer professionals offering related services. (Ch. Nine)

no contact rule   Prohibits an attorney from communicating with a person represented by counsel on the subject of that representation without permission of the client's attorney. (*See* Model Rule 4.2) (Ch. Seven)

non-integrated state bar association   State bar association where bar membership is voluntary. (Ch. Two)

notification   Lawyer's fiduciary duty to promptly notify a client (or third party with an ownership interest) when funds or other property in which the client has an interest are received. (Ch. Three)

obstruction   Any attempt to hinder or interfere with the administration of justice. (Chs. Seven, Eight)

opinion work product   Work product that includes the lawyer's mental impressions, opinions, and strategy in litigation, also referred to as the "core" workproduct. The inquiring party must show extraordinary circumstances to justify disclosure. (Ch. Five)

ordinary work product   Work product that is the result of gathering basic facts or conducting interviews with witnesses. This is generally immune from discovery except upon establishment of a substantial need for the material and the inability to obtain the substantial equivalent of the material without substantial hardship. (Ch. Five)

perjury   The offense of willfully telling an untruth in a court after having taken an oath or affirmation. (Ch. Eight)

permissive disclosures   The "exceptions" to client confidences in Rule 1.6(b) 1-7 where attorneys may exercise discretion to reveal a confidence in one of those enumerated instances. (Ch. Seven)

personal-interest conflict   Where the lawyer's personal interests interfere with the lawyer's fiduciary duties to be loyal and competent, and to preserve client confidences. (Ch. Six)

political activity by judicial candidates   Fundraising, campaigning, and other political activity by judges and candidates who seek judicial office. (Ch. Twelve)

post-indictment contact   Pertains to a prosecutor's communication with a represented party after arraignment. (Ch. Eight)

predominant effects   Standard that the jurisdiction where the predominant effect of the conduct will occur determines which jurisdiction's rule applies to conduct. (Ch. Two)

prejudice   The second prong of the test for showing ineffective assistance of counsel, as defined by *Strickland*, that "the defendant must show that there is a reasonable probability that, but for counsel's unprofessional errors, the result of the proceeding would have been different." (Ch. Four)

privilege holder   The one with the ability to assert a privilege. The client is the holder of the attorney-client privilege and ultimately decides whether to assert or waive it. (Ch. Five)

pro bono   Legal work performed voluntarily and without payment. (Ch. Eleven)

pro hac vice admission   Practice where a lawyer who has not been admitted to practice in a certain jurisdiction is allowed to participate in a case in that jurisdiction. (Ch. Two)

probable cause   Sufficient reason based upon known facts to believe a crime has been committed. (Ch. Eight)

professional liability insurance   Insures the firm or individual lawyers for errors and omissions or negligent mistakes. Also called "errors and omissions" ("E & O") policies. (Ch. Two)

prospective clients   Rule 1.18 defines prospective clients as "a person who consults with a lawyer about the possibility of forming a client-lawyer relationship." Lawyers owe specific limited duties to prospective clients. (Chs Three, Five)

real evidence   Physical evidence. (Ch. Eight)

reasonable belief   What an ordinary person of average intelligence and sound mind would believe. (Ch. Five)

reciprocal discipline   Practice of courts of commonly imposing the same disciplinary sanction both in terms of length of time and severity as to that which was issued by another jurisdiction. A lawyer disciplined for misconduct in one state is subject to reciprocal discipline in every other jurisdiction in which he or she is admitted to practice. (Ch. Two)

reciprocal referral agreement   Agreement whereby a lawyer and nonlawyer professional refer clients to each other—without paying each other for such referrals. (Ch. Nine)

record keeping   Requirement that attorneys keep complete records of trust account funds and other property. (Ch. Three)

relational self-interest   Ideology that understands clients as attempting to pursue and maximize their self-interest in relation to others. (Ch. One)

role morality   Occurs when a lawyer acts as an agent for the client's purposes. (Ch. One)

sanctions   Penalties or other means of enforcement used to provide incentives for obedience. For lawyers, can include disbarment, suspension, public reprimand, private reprimand, and financial restitution. (Ch. Two)

screening   Segregating lawyers or administrative staff who may have a conflict of interest in regards to current clients of the law firm or former clients of the lawyer or administrative staff. (Ch. Six)

segregation   Requirement that client money must be placed in a client trust account, separate from lawyer's funds. The lawyer is absolutely forbidden from commingling her own funds with those of the client. (Ch. Three)

self-defense exception   The lawyer is permitted to disclose only privileged client communications necessary to defend herself against the client's claims of misconduct. (Ch. Five)

solicitation   Targeted marketing communication initiated by a lawyer that is directed to a specific person. (Ch. Ten)

spoliation of evidence Intentional or reckless destruction of, or tampering with, evidence that is relevant to a legal proceeding. (Ch. Seven)

subject matter waiver A party may seek all portions of a single communication and related privileged communications to prevent the opposing party from unfairly distorting the context or meaning of its partial disclosure. (Ch. Five)

substantial need–undue hardship When demonstrated, provides limited circumstances when an opposing party may discover or compel disclosure of work product. (Ch. Five)

tripartite relationship The relationship between the insured, the insurer, and the attorney hired by the insurer. (Ch. Three)

unauthorized practice of law Engaging in the practice of law by persons or entities not authorized to practice law. (Ch. Nine)

withdraw To cease representing a client. (Ch. Five)

woodshedding Rehearsing a witness in advance of their testimony by telling them exactly how to answer questions. (Ch. Seven)

work-product immunity A rule that an opposing party generally may not discover or compel disclosure of written or oral materials prepared by or for an attorney in the course of litigation. (Ch. Five)

Table of Cases

Principal cases are indicated by italics.

A

ABA Formal Op. 06-441 (2006), 231
ABA Formal Op. 09-454 (2009), 433
ABA Formal Op. 96-403 (1996), 144
Adams v. Aerojet-General Corp, 355, 359-360
Adoption of New APR 28 — Limited Practice
   Rule for Limited License Legal Technicians,
   Matter of, 561
Aetna Life Ins. Co. v. Lavoie, 592
Agurs; United States v., 431
Albrecht, In re, 337
Albrechtsen v. Board of Regents of Univ. of
   Wis., 193
Alexander v. Cahill, 526
Almeida; United States v., 269
Ambac Assurance Corp. v. Countrywide Home
   Loans, Inc., 268, 278
Amway v. Tarton, 317
Andrus v. Texas, 222-223
Anonymous, In re, 54
Apple Corps Ltd. v. International Collectors
   Soc'y, 415
Arce v. Burrow, 333
Ardon v. City of L.A., 289, 290-291
Argersinger v. Hamlin, 212
Astrowski, In re, 569
Attorney C, In re, 436
Attorney Grievance Comm'n of Md. v. Kendrick,
   189, *190*, 191
Attorney Grievance Comm'n of Md. v.
   Lanocha, 331
Attorney Grievance Comm'n of Md. v.
   Midlen, 71
Attorney Grievance Comm'n of Md. v.
   Rand, 335
Avila v. Havana Painting Co., 89, 90

B

Bagley; United States v., 432
Bailey, In re, 475
Baird v. Koerner, 260
Baker v. General Motors Corp., 298
Balla v. Gambro, Inc., 140-141

Bates v. State Bar of Ariz., 513-516, 518, 532,
   534, 536
Bay State Ambulance & Hosp. Rental Serv.;
   United States v., 269
Bell Atlantic Corp. v. Bolger, 130
Berg, In re, 157
Berger v. United States, 143, 420
Birbrower, Montalbano, Condon & Frank v.
   Superior Court, 501, *502*, 508
Bloomingburg Jewish Educ. Ctr. v. Village of
   Bloomingburg, 260
Board of Prof'l Responsibility, Wyo. State Bar v.
   Casper, 148, 149, 155
Boehringer Ingelheim Pharm., Inc.; FTC v., 261
Boswell v. Price Meese Shulman & D'Arminio,
   P.C., 323
Boyle; People v., 193
Brady v. Maryland, 430, *431*, 432, 433, 436
Brady; SEC v., 286
Brooks v. South Carolina Comm'n on Indigent
   Def., 339
Brost, In re, 65
Brown v. Legal Found. of Wash., 160, 553
Bullis v. Downes, 82
Burnett v. Sharp, 88, *89*, 91
Burt v. Titlow, 331
Business Guides v. Chromatic Commc'ns, 372

C

Caperton v. A.T. Massey Coal Co., 591, 592,
   593, 595
Cardwell, In re, 381
Carona; United States v., 438
Carroll v. Jacques Admiralty Law Firm, 394
Carson, In re, 335
Case of Attorney Karen Thomas, 209
Cement Inst.; FTC v., 591
Cendant Corp. Sec. Litig., In re, 297, 298
Central Hudson Gas & Elec. Corp. v. Public
   Serv. Comm'n of N.Y. Under Cent.
   Hudson, 519
Chambers; State v., 462
Chandler v. Florida, 607

Chapman v. California, 220
Chappell; People v., 120
Charges of Unprofessional Conduct in Panel
    File No. 39302, In re, 509
Chen; United States v., 261
Cheney, In re, 589
Cheney v. United States Dist. Court for D.C.,
    574, *575*
Christina W., In re, 146
Cincinnati Bar Ass'n v. Hackett, 494
Cinema 5, Ltd. v. Cinerama, Inc., 313, *314*, 316
Citizens United v. FEC, 590
Clinton v. Jones, 578
Committee on Prof'l Ethics v. Crary, 384, *385*
Committee on Prof'l Ethics v. Mershon, 325
Commonwealth v. *See name of opposing party*
Connick v. Thompson, 4, 5
Corretore, In re, 569
County of. *See name of county*
Cowan, In re Disciplinary Action Against, 67
Creedy, In re Disciplinary Proceedings Against,
    327, 329-330
Crews v. Buckman Labs. Int'l, Inc., 141
Cronic; United States v., 5, 216, 230
Crossen, In re, 411
Cuyler v. Sullivan, 217, 231, 321, 459

D

Dahl v. Dahl, 149, 183, *184*, 188
Daley, In re, 67
Damron v. Herzog, 341, 342
Darby v. Mississippi State Bd. of Bar
    Admissions, 500
Davis v. Alabama State Bar, 476, *477*, 480
DC Comics v. Pacific Pictures Corp., 285
DeMers, In re, 134
Demoulas v. DeMoulas, 414
Desimini v. Durkin, 83
Disciplinary Actions Against. *See name
    of party*
Disciplinary Counsel v. Kellogg Martin, 436
*District of Columbia Bar Legal Ethics Comm.
    Formal Op. 79 (1979)*, 389
Diversified Indus., Inc. v. Meredith, 281,
    283-284
Dixon; United States v., 544
Drimmer v. Appleton, 259
Dyer; Commonwealth v., 253

E

Edelman v. Levy, 316
Eisenberg v. Gagnon, 268
Erie, County of, In re, 267, 268
Evans; United States v., 260

F

Faretta v. California, 443
Feinstein v. Keenan, 285
Finely v. Kentucky Bar Ass'n, 410
Fisher, In re, 335
Fisher v. United States, 452
Fletcher v. State, 381, 382
Florida v. Nixon, 225
Florida Bar v. Brumbaugh, 499, 500
Florida Bar v. Martocci, 393
Florida Bar v. Pape, 526
Florida Bar v. Went For It, Inc., 516, *517*,
    523-524, 532, 539
Fognani v. Young, 338, 339
Fordham, In re, 148-150, 192
Frank, In re, 525
FTC v. *See name of opposing party*

G

Galanis; United States v., 402
Garcia, In re, 44, 53, 54
Gatti, In re, 415
Gault, In re, 545, 548
General Dynamics Corp. v. Superior Court, 141
Gentile v. State Bar of Nev., 397, 400, 401, 445
Georgia Baptist Health Care Sys., Inc. v.
    Hanafi, 174
Gideon v. Wainwright, 212, 544, 547
Giglio v. United States, 432
Gillette Co. v. Provost, 341
Glass, In re, 54, *55*, 61
Goldberg v. Warner/Chappell Music, Inc., 354,
    356, 361
Gonzalez; United States v., 268
Gonzalez-Lopez; United States v., 321
Gotti; United States v., 269
Grand Jury, In re, 269
Grand Jury Investigation, In re, 267, 292,
    293, 295
Grand Jury Investigation of Schroeder, In
    re, 292
Grand Jury Proceedings, In re, 292
Grand Jury Subpoena Duces Tecum, In re, 267
Gray v. Bicknell, 259, 288
Grievance Comm. v. Rottner, 315
Gruss v. Zwirn, 285
GTE Prods. Corp. v. Stewart, 141

H

Hafter v. Farkas, 315
Hague, In re, 568
Hale v. Committee on Character & Fitness to
    Practice for the State of Ill., 54
Hammad; United States v., 438

Hansen, In re Disciplinary Action Against, 67
Harding, In re, 134
Harris v. New York, 453, 458
Harrison v. Mississippi Bar, 331
Harvey v. United States, 321
Havens; United States v., 458
Heffernan, In re, 65
Helmedach v. Commissioner of Corr., 204, 223, 224, 227
Hickey v. Scott, 91-92
Hickman v. Taylor, 297, 300, 302
Himmel, In re, 74, 79
Hizey v. Carpenter, 83
Hodge v. URFA-Sexton, LP, 352
Holloway v. Arkansas, 320-321
Home Care Indus. Inc. v. Murray, 133
Howard v. Babcock, 495
Howe, In re Disciplinary Action Against, 198, 199, 204
Hydraflow, Inc. v. Enidine, Inc., 288

I

Ibanez v. Florida Dep't of Bus. & Prof'l Regulation, 516, 527
IBM Corp. v. Levin, 341
In re. *See name of party*
International Bhd. of Teamsters v. Hoffa, 127
Iowa Supreme Court Attorney Disciplinary Bd. v. Engelmann, 121, *122*
Iowa Supreme Court Attorney Disciplinary Bd. v. Qualley, 323
Iowa Supreme Court Attorney Disciplinary Bd. v. Taylor, 65

J

James v. Mississippi Bar, 364
Janson v. LegalZoom, 501
J. Media Group Inc. v. New Jersey Dep't of Law & Pub. Safety, 260
John Doe Grand Jury Investigation, Matter of, 253

K

Keller v. State Bar of Cal., 45
Kellogg Brown & Root, In re, 261
Kelly, Matter of, 315, 316
Kelly; United States v., 573
Kentucky Bar Ass'n v. Clifton, 71
Kiley, In re, 169, *170*, 173-175
Kimmel; United States v., 442
Kimmelman v. Morrison, 222
Kirschner, In re Disciplinary Action Against, 393
Konigsberg v. California, 51
Kyles v. Whitley, 432, 436

L

Larvadain, In re, 393
Laskey Bros., Inc. v. Warner Bros. Pictures, Inc., 316
Lassiter v. Department of Soc. Servs. of Durham Cty., 548
Lathrop v. Donohue, 45
Law Offices of Herssein & Herssein v. United Servs. Auto. Ass'n, 591
Lawyer Disciplinary Bd. v. Campbell, 336
Lawyer Disciplinary Bd. v. Sidiropolis, 64
Legal Servs. Corp. v. Velazquez, 482
Levine, In re, 394
Lindsey, In re, 267
Link v. Wabash R.R. Co., 182
Lopez; *United States v.*, 438, *439*
Lott, In re, 280, 291

M

Maldonado v. Ford Motor Co., 398, *399*
Marbury v. Madison, 37
Marriage of. *See name of party*
Martin, In re, 168, 169
Massiah v. United States, 438
Matter of. *See name of party*
Mays, In re, 205
McCoy v. Louisiana, 118, 230
McKinney, In re, 52, 53
McNaul; SEC v., 176
McPartlin; United States v., 269
Medina Cty. Bar Ass'n v. Grieselhuber, 525
Meehan v. Hopps, 132
Mejia; United States v., 261
Meredith; People v., 451
Messing, Rudavsky & Weliky, P.C. v. President & Fellows of Harvard Coll., 403, *404*, 406-407
Midgett; United States v., 462
Mihailovich v. Laatsch, 85
Milavetz, Gallop & Milavetz v. United States, 6
Miller; State v., 233, 234
Minter, In re, 65
Mississippi Bar v. Johnson, 51
Missouri v. Frye, 223-229
Mohawk Indus. v. Carpenter, 269
Monroe v. City of Topeka, 353
Mooney v. Holohan, 431
Moore v. Alabama Judicial Inquiry Comm'n, 568
Moore v. CLI, 317
Moore; Commonwealth v., 396

N

Napster, Inc. Copyright Litig., In re, 294
National Ass'n for Advancement of
  Multijurisdictional Practice v. Berch, 50
Neal v. Clinton, 66
New York Cty. Lawyers' Ass'n v.
  Dacey, 500
*New York State Bar Ass'n Formal Op. 479
  (1978), 448*
Nguyen v. Excel Corp., 260, 262
Niesig v. Team I, 404-405
Nix v. Whiteside, 453, *454*, 460, 462
Nixon; United States v., 578
Northern Sec. Co. v. United States, 577

O

Obergefell v. Hodges, 568-569, 590
Ohio v. Jones, 234
*Ohio State Bar Ass'n Informal Advisory Op.
  2013-03, 195*
Ohralik v. Ohio State Bar Ass'n, 513, *532*,
  536-539
Olsen, In re, 372, *373*, 375
Olwell; State v., 449, 452
Orthopaedic Hosp. v. DJO Global,
  Inc., 289

P

Pacific Pictures Corp., In re, 261, 279, 281,
  282, 285
Padilla v. Kentucky, 228, 229
Palsgraf v. Long Island R.R. Co., 106
Pang v. International Document Servs., 136,
  140-141, 169
Paplauskas, In re, 498
Pautler, In re, 415, 438
Peel v. Attorney Registration & Disciplinary
  Comm'n, 516, 527
*Pennsylvania Bar Ass'n Legal Ethics & Prof'l
  Responsibility Formal Op. 2016-200
  (2016), 486*
People v. *See name of opposing party*
Perry, In re Marriage of, 109, 113
Peters, In re, 71
Phillips v. Washington Legal
  Found., 553
Pioneer Inv. Servs. Co. v. Brunswick Assocs.
  Ltd., 183
Powell v. Alabama, 211-212, 215, 230
Primus, In re, 537
Public Citizen, Inc. v. Louisiana Attorney
  Disciplinary Bd., 525, 526
Purcell v. District Attorney for Suffolk Dist., 252,
  256, 304
Pyle v. Kansas, 431

R

Ragin; United States v., 230
Ralls v. United States, 260
Red Dog v. Delaware, 625 A.2d 245 (Del. 1993),
  116, *117*, 118
Red Dog v. State, 620 A.2d 848 (Del. 1993), 117
Republican Party of Minn. v. White, 597, *598*,
  604, 606
Rhodes; People v., 159
Richards, In re, 377, *378*
Riehlmann, In re, 73
Riek, In re, 436
Rios v. McDermott, Will & Emery, 83
Ritland; People v., 380
RMJ, In re, 516, 527
Rock v. Arkansas, 453
Roe v. Wade, 604
Romious, In re, 393
Rosenfeld Constr. Co. v. Superior Court, 359
Rubenstein v. Florida Bar, 526
Rubio v. BNSF Ry. Co., 332
Ruehle; United States v., 131-134
Ruiz; United States v., 436
Rusinow v. Kamara, 171
Ryan v. Long, 105
Ryder, In re, 447

S

Sallee v. Tennessee Bd. of Prof'l Responsibility,
  116, 148, *150*, 176
Sanmina Corp.; United States v., 299
Sather, In re, 160, *161*, 166-167, 169, 177
Schaeffler v. United States, 273, *274*, 278, 297,
  299, 302
Schware v. Board of Bar Exam'rs, 51, 52
Schwimmer; United States v., 276
Scionti, In re, 121
Scott v. State, 353
Scott; State v., 234
Scott Paper Co. v. United States, 267
Sealed Case, In re, 292
Seare, In re, 193
SEC v. *See name of opposing party*
Shapero v. Kentucky Bar Ass'n, 479, 516, 520,
  537, 539
Shari; People v., 353
Sharp; People v., 440
Sheppard v. Maxwell, 397
Sices, In re, 67
Silver Chrysler Plymouth, Inc. v. Chrysler
  Motors Corp., 355
Snyder, In re, 394
Spaulding v. Zimmerman, 17, *18*, 22-24
Sperry v. Florida Bar, 499
Spevak v. Klein, 67

Squire, Sanders & Dempsey, LLP v. Givaudan Flavors Corp., 291
Stanton, In re, 336
Star Mark Mgmt., Inc. v. Koon Chun Hing Kee Soy & Sauce Factory, Ltd., 372
State v. *See name of opposing party*
State Bar of Cal. Standing Comm. on Prof'l Responsibility & Conduct Formal Op. No. 2012-186, 529
State Comp. Ins. Fund v. WPS, Inc., 290-291
State ex rel. *See name of party*
Stepovich, In re Disciplinary Matter Involving, 331
Strickland v. Washington, 213, *214*, 220, 222, 224, 228-230, 233, 236, 455-456, 458, 459
Stroh v. General Motors Corp., 260
Supreme Court of N.H. v. Piper, 49
Supreme Court of Va. v. Friedman, 49
Swidler & Berlin v. United States, 259

T

T.C. Theatre Corp. v. Warner Bros. Pictures, Inc., 340
Teleglobe Commc'ns Corp., In re, 269
Thonert, In re, 381
T.J. Hooper v. Northern Barge Corp., 221
Togstad v. Vesely, Otto, Miller & Keefe, 103, 107
Toledo Bar Ass'n v. Stahlbush, 157
Trammel v. United States, 261
Travelers Cas. & Sur. Co. v. Excess Ins. Co., 277
Truman, In re, 493, 495
Tumey v. Ohio, 592
Turnbull; United States v., 442
Turner v. Rogers, 545, 562
Turner; United States v., 321

U

UMG Recordings v. MySpace, 350
United Farm Workers of Am. v. Superior Court, 573
United States v. *See name of opposing party*
Upjohn Co. v. United States, 131, 132, 192, 262, *263*, 266, 267
U.S. Postal Serv. v. Phelps Dodge Refinance Corp., 261

V

Van Asdale v. International Game Tech., 141
Van Kirk v. Miller, 323
Velazquez-Velez v. Molina-Rodriguez, 174
V.H. v. J.P.H., 172
Virginia Bd. of Pharmacy v. Virginia Citizens Consumer Council, Inc., 518
Vitek v. Jones, 548
Vodusek v. Bayliner Marine Corp., 391
von Bulow, In re, 287

W

Ward v. Village of Monroeville, 592
West Bend Mut. Ins. Co. v. Schumacher, 84, 87
Western States Wholesale Natural Gas Antitrust Litig., In re, 285
Western Sugar Coop. v. Archer-Daniels-Midland Co., 342, 343, 350
Westinghouse Elec. Corp. v. Kerr-McGee Corp., 107
Wheat v. United States, 321
White v. American Airlines, 292
Wickard v. Filburn, 582
Wiesmueller v. Kosobucki, 49
Wilkins, In re, 401
Williams v. District Court, 339
Williams v. Pennsylvania, 593
Williams v. State, 324
Williams-Yulee v. Florida Bar, 595
Woods v. City Nat'l Bank & Trust Co., 315

Y

Yablonski v. United Mine Workers of Am., 125, 126, 129, 130
Yates v. United States, 446
Youngstown Sheet & Tube Co. v. Sawyer, 577
Yurish, State ex rel. v. Faircloth, 320

Z

Zabin v. Picciotto, 172
Zauderer v. Office of Disciplinary Counsel, 516, 528, 536
Zolin; United States v., 253, 292, 295
Zubulake v. UBS Warburg LLC, 288

Table of Rules

ABA FORMAL OPINIONS

Opinion	Page(s)
06-441	231-233, 237
09-454	433-436
10-457	529 n.31
87-353	376 n.7, 384 n.18
88-356	352 n.52
91-359	407 n.58
93-376	384 n.19
93-379	157
94-383	72
94-388	353 n.55, 354
95-396	437 n.10
96-403	144-145
337 (1974)	412
462 (2013)	591 n.61, 591 n.65
476 (2016)	175, 176 n.78
488 (2019)	573 n.54
491 (2020)	120, 120 n.11
492 (2020)	114 n.5
493 (2020)	64, 64 n.46

ABA MODEL CODE OF JUDICIAL CONDUCT

Rule	Page(s)
1.1	568 n.3
1.2	568 n.4
1.2 cmt. [5]	572 n.45
1.3	568 n.6
2.1	568 n.8
2.2	568
2.3	569 n.20
2.4	569 n.21
2.5	569 n.15
2.5 cmt. [3]	569 n.16
2.7	573, 573 n.53
2.9	569 n.22
2.9(a)(2)	569 n.25
2.9(c)	569 n.23
2.9 cmt. [6]	569 n.23
2.10	570
2.10(a)	570 n.26
2.10(b)	570 n.27
2.11	568 n.2, 572
2.11(a)	572 n.42
2.11(a)(4)	595 n.78
2.11(c)	572 n.47
2.11 cmt. [2]	572 n.43
2.11 cmt. [5]	572 n.46
2.15	569 n.18
2.15 cmt. [2]	569 n.19
3.1	570, 570 n.29, 571
3.2	571 n.36
3.3	571 n.37
3.6(a)	571 n.39
3.7	570 n.30, 570 n.33
3.12	570 n.32
3.13	571 n.40
3.13(b)(3)	573 n.52
3.14	570 n.32
3.31(b)(1)	571 n.41
4.1	595, 596, 604, 605
4.1(a)(13)	604 n.83
4.1 cmt. [13]	604
Canon 1	568
Canon 2	568, 568 n.7
Canon 3	570 n.28
Canon 4	596

ABA MODEL CODE OF PROFESSIONAL RESPONSIBILITY

Disciplinary Rule 2-110(B)	457
Disciplinary Rule 2-110(C)	457
Disciplinary Rule 4-101(C)(3)	456
Disciplinary Rule 6-101	46
Disciplinary Rule 7-102	439
Disciplinary Rule 7-102(A)(4)	457
Disciplinary Rule 7-102(B)(1)	456
Disciplinary Rule 7-104(A)(1)	439
Canon 6	46

ABA MODEL RULES OF PROFESSIONAL CONDUCT

Rule	Page(s)
PREAMBLE	29, 30, 72, 371 n.1, 394, 482
PREAMBLE cmt. [1]	371 n.1
PREAMBLE cmt. [2]	394 n.38
1.0(c)	247, 352, 382
1.0(f)	31, 120
1.0(k)	355

1.0(m)	376 n.8
1.1	182, 190, 192, 195, 232, 376, 382, 429, 450, 480, 481
1.1 cmt. [1]	183, 188, 189, 197
1.1 cmt. [2]	189, 191, 198
1.1 cmt. [3]	198
1.1 cmt. [6]	242
1.1 cmt. [8]	48 n.24, 194, 556
1.2	15, 33, 115, 118, 119, 120, 123, 145, 147, 193, 259, 429, 559
1.2(a)	116, 119, 204, 232, 333
1.2(b)	15, 175 n.77, 483
1.2(c)	93, 144, 145, 169 n.73
1.2(d)	16, 31, 33, 115, 120, 121, 123, 174, 179, 250, 410, 456
1.2 cmt. [1]	16, 115
1.2 cmt. [2]	116
1.2 cmt. [5]	15 n.25
1.3	197, 202, 232, 259, 394
1.3 cmt. [1]	394, 394 n.39
1.3 cmt. [2]	232
1.3 cmt. [3]	198
1.4	116, 119, 203, 204, 206, 223, 232, 242
1.4(b)	203
1.4 cmt. [2]	119, 204
1.4 cmt. [3]	48 n.24, 204
1.4 cmt. [4]	208
1.4 cmt. [5]	203
1.5	147, 148, 149, 156, 158, 179
1.5(a)	148, 149, 150, 155
1.5(b)	147
1.5(c)	148
1.6	47 n.23, 51, 73, 79, 132, 135, 245, 246, 247, 248, 249, 250, 252, 304, 305, 376, 377 n.10, 380, 383, 396, 409, 410, 429, 448, 457
1.6(a)	79, 246, 247, 250
1.6(b)	246, 248, 249, 250, 251, 251 n.3, 410
1.6(b)(1)-(7)	257, 340 n.46, 410
1.6(b)(1)	140
1.6(b)(2)	250, 251, 251 n.3, 257
1.6(b)(3)	250, 251, 257, 410
1.6(b)(4)	248
1.6(b)(5)	176 n.78, 248
1.6(b)(6)	176 n.78, 248, 380 n.12
1.6(b)(7)	248
1.6(c)	196, 247
1.6 cmt. [4]	246
1.6 cmt. [6]	256
1.6 cmt. [12]	380 n.12
1.6 cmt. [16]	257
1.6 cmt. [20]	247
1.7-1.12	310
1.7	130, 310, 311, 315, 324, 336 n.30, 338, 351, 354, 363, 496
1.7(a)	310, 318
1.7(b)	310, 310 n.1, 311, 312, 317, 338, 355
1.7(b)(1)-(4)	322
1.7 cmt. [8]	321, 322 n.9
1.7 cmt. [23]	321 n.5, 322 n.8
1.7 cmt. [24]	324
1.7 cmt. [28]	322 n.10, 323
1.7 cmt. [29]	318 n.3
1.8-1.12	310
1.8(a)-(i)	325
1.8(a)	310 n.1, 325, 325 n.14, 326, 327
1.8(a)(1)-(3)	326, 330
1.8(a) cmt. [1]	325 n.12
1.8(a) cmt. [2]	325 n.13
1.8(b)	247, 326, 327
1.8(c)	331
1.8(c) cmt. [6]	331 n.16
1.8(d)	331 n.17, 332
1.8(e)	332, 332 n.20, 333
1.8(e)(1)	332
1.8(e)(2)	332
1.8(e)(3)	332, 332 n.20
1.8(e)(3)(i)-(iii)	332 n.21
1.8(e) cmt. [10]	332 n.18, 332 n.19
1.8(g)	333, 333 n.23
1.8(g) cmt. [13]	334 n.24
1.8(h)	334
1.8(h)(1)	94, 334
1.8(h)(2)	94, 335
1.8(i)	335
1.8(j)	336, 336 n.30, 337 n.31, 352 n.50, 365
1.8(k)	352 n.50
1.9	245, 338, 341, 351, 354, 361, 363
1.9(a)	337 n.32, 340, 355 n.61
1.9(c)	247, 340 n.46, 355, 362
1.10	354, 355, 356
1.10(a)	351
1.10(a)(1)	352 n.49
1.10(a)(2)	354
1.10(a)(2)(i)	355
1.10(a)(2)(ii)	355
1.10(b)	360, 361
1.10(d)	356
1.10 cmt. [3]	352 n.49, 352 n.50
1.11	362, 363
1.11(a)	362
1.11(b)	356, 363
1.11(c)	356, 363
1.11(d)(1)	363
1.11(d)(2)	363
1.11 cmt. [2]	363

1.12	363	1.18(d)	114
1.12(a)	364	1.18 cmt. [2]	108, 109
1.13	43-44, 132, 136, 142	1.18 cmt. [6]	112
1.13(a)	125	2.1	15, 36, 37, 481
1.13(b)	134, 135, 136, 142	2.1 cmt. [1]	36, 38, 38 n.72
1.13(c)	135, 136, 142, 250 n.1	2.1 cmt. [2]	15
1.13(e)	135, 136	3.1	371, 371 n.2, 372, 375, 425
1.13(f)	131	3.1 cmt. [2]	371, 375 n.6
1.13(g)	129, 130	3.2	202, 392, 393
1.13 cmt. [6]	250 n.1	3.2 cmt. [1]	202
1.13 cmt. [7]	135	3.3	376, 376 n.8, 379, 381, 382,
1.13 cmt. [9]	142, 143		383, 454, 456, 457, 460, 463
1.13 cmt. [10]	132	3.3(a)	35 n.57, 376, 380, 383, 462, 463
1.13 cmt. [14]	130	3.3(a)(2)	381, 383
1.14	146, 146 n.44	3.3(a)(3)	377, 383, 383 n.16, 384, 388, 460,
1.14(b)	146		461, 463
1.14 cmt. [1]	146	3.3(a)(4)	456
1.14 cmt. [5]	146	3.3(b)	249, 396, 476
1.15(a)-(c)	159	3.3(c)	249
1.15(a)	159, 160 n.69, 167	3.3(d)	380
1.15(a) cmt. [4]	168 n.71	3.3(d) cmt. [14]	380 n.11
1.15(b)	160	3.3 cmt. [3]	381 n.15
1.15(c)	167	3.3 cmt. [7]	462
1.15(d)	159, 168	3.3 cmt. [8]	377 n.9, 384
1.15(e)	168	3.3 cmt. [9]	384 n.20
1.15 cmt. [1]	160, 167	3.3 cmt. [10]	377 n.10, 383 n.17, 387, 388
1.16	169, 173	3.4	446
1.16(a)	169, 174	3.4(a)	391, 391 n.22, 447, 447 n.18, 452 n.23
1.16(a)(1)	457	3.4(b)	388
1.16(a)(2)	174	3.4(d)	375, 392
1.16(b)	169	3.5	396
1.16(b)(1)	175	3.5(a)	396
1.16(b)(2)	175	3.5(b)	395
1.16(b)(3)	175	3.5(d)	393 n.29, 393 n.30, 396
1.16(b)(4)	16, 175	3.5 cmt. [4]	393 n.30
1.16(b)(5)	175	3.6	397, 398, 401, 445, 445 n.14
1.16(b)(6)	175	3.6(a)	397, 397 n.49
1.16(b)(7)	175	3.6(a) cmt. [6]	397 n.50
1.16(c)	169, 169 n.75	3.6(b)	397
1.16(d)	176, 176 n.80	3.6 cmt. [5]	445
1.16 cmt. [1]	169	3.7	338, 339 n.43, 339 n.44, 340, 397
1.16 cmt. [3]	175, 176	3.7(a)	339 n.41
1.16 cmt. [4]	169 n.74, 174	3.7 cmt. [1]	338 n.37
1.16 cmt. [5]	174	3.7 cmt. [2]	338 n.38
1.17	496	3.7 cmt. [6]	338 n.39
1.17(c)	497	3.8	420, 434, 445
1.17 cmt. [1]	496	3.8(a)	425
1.17 cmt. [2]	496	3.8(d)	433, 434, 435, 436
1.17 cmt. [5]	496 n.29	3.8(f)	445
1.17 cmt. [6]	496 n.30	3.8 cmt. [1]	420, 433
1.18	108, 109, 111, 112, 113, 114, 366, 531	4.1	250, 409, 410, 411
1.18(b)	247	4.1(a)	409, 413
1.18(c)	114, 337 n.32	4.1(b)	250, 251, 251 n.3, 409, 410

4.1 cmt. [2]	410
4.2	402, 403, 406, 407, 408, 408 n.59, 437, 439, 444, 470, 475
4.2 cmt. [7]	406 n.57
4.3	408
4.3 cmt. [2]	409 n.60
4.4(b)	393
5.1	475, 476
5.1(a)	474
5.1(c)	474
5.1(c)(1)	474
5.1 cmt. [2]	474
5.2	474, 475
5.2(a)	475, 480
5.2(b)	480
5.3	437, 474, 475 n.1, 476
5.3(c)	398, 475
5.4	485, 486, 492
5.4(a)	485
5.4(b)	485
5.4(c)	483
5.4(d)	491
5.5	501, 508, 508 n.44, 509
5.5(a)	497 n.31, 508
5.5(b)	508
5.5(c)	508
5.5(c)(3)	509
5.5(c)(4)	509
5.5 cmt. [1]-[2]	497 n.31
5.5 cmt. [2]	497 n.32
5.5 cmt. [14]	509 n.45
5.6	493, 496, 512
6.1	556, 556 n.27
6.2	16
6.2 cmt. [1]	16, 483 n.8
7.1	480, 514, 525, 528, 538
7.1 cmt. [3]	525
7.1 cmt. [5]	528
7.2	514, 528, 538
7.2(a)	529
7.2(b)	485, 486
7.2(b)(4)	486
7.2(b)(5)	485 n.17
7.2 cmt. [3]	524 n.16
7.2 cmt. [6]	485 n.18
7.2 cmt. [9]	527
7.2 cmt. [12]	528 n.29
7.3	514, 538
7.3(a)	514 n.3
7.3 cmt. [2]	538, 538 n.45
8	569
8.1	67
8.1(a)	51
8.1(b)	51, 51 n.37, 67 n.47

8.2	401
8.2(a)	401
8.2(b)	567
8.3	72, 73, 79
8.3(a)	72, 73, 481
8.3(b)	72
8.3(c)	79
8.3 cmt. [1]	73
8.3 cmt. [2]	73, 79 n.55
8.4	63, 64, 65, 407, 410, 411, 414, 415
8.4(a)	72, 398, 437
8.4(b)	64, 65
8.4(c)	65, 381, 392, 410, 413, 414, 415, 417, 438 n.11, 480
8.4(d)	65, 66, 394, 394 n.40
8.4(f)	567
8.4(g)	63-64, 63 n.43, 63 n.44
8.4(h)	65
8.5	70, 508 n.44
8.5(a)	70
8.5(b)(2)	70
8.5 cmt. [5]	48 n.24

FEDERAL RULES OF CIVIL PROCEDURE

Rule	Page(s)
Rule 8(a)	242
Rule 11	372, 374, 375
Rule 11(b)	372 n.3
Rule 11(c)	372
Rule 11(c)(2)	372 n.5
Rule 12(b)(6)	242
Rule 26(b)(3)	297, 300
Rule 37	392 n.27
Rule 60(b)	183, 183 n.2
Rule 60.02	21

FEDERAL RULES OF CRIMINAL PROCEDURE

Rule	Page(s)
Rule 16	430
Rule 44	320
Rule 44(c)	320

FEDERAL RULES OF EVIDENCE

Rule	Page(s)
Rule 501	259, 264, 265, 294
Rule 502	288, 289, 289 n.52
Rule 502(d)	289 n.54
Rule 502(e)	289, 289 n.55
Rule 503(d)(2)	291 n.56
Rule 503(d)(4)	291 n.56
Rule 612	390
Rule 801(d)(2)(D)	404

RESTATEMENT (THIRD) OF AGENCY

Section	Page(s)
§8.05	326 n.15

RESTATEMENT (SECOND) OF CONTRACTS

Section	Page(s)
§90	106 n.4

RESTATEMENT (THIRD) OF THE LAW GOVERNING LAWYERS

Section	Page(s)
§2	50, 51, 497 n.32
§3 cmt. e	509 n.45
§4 cmt. d	499 n.38
§48	81 n.57
§48 cmt. c	81, 81 n.56
§51	82
§52	83
§53	81 n.57
§54(4)(a)	94
§55 cmt. c	81
§59	247
§68	258
§69 cmt. d	280 nn.35-37
§69 cmt. g	260 n.9
§70	258 n.4
§71 cmt. b	261 n.15
§76	268 n.21
§78	279 n.33
§78(3)	280 n.37
§79	279 n.34
§79 cmt. b	279 n.32
§79 cmt. f	286 n.42, 287 nn.45-46
§79 cmt. h	288 n.48, 288 n.50
§81	291 n.56
§82(a)	291 n.58
§82(b) cmt. c	291 n.58
§87	78, 297 nn.70-74
§88 cmt. b	298 n.80, 298 n.82
§91	298 nn.83-84
§93	299 n.86
§100 cmt. g	407 n.58
§110 cmt. b	392 n.28
§110 cmt. e	392 n.26
§112 cmt. b	380 n.13
§116 cmt. b	390 n.21
§118 cmt. c	392 n.24
§121	309
§121 cmt. e(i)	318 n.3
§122(1)	337 n.34
§122 cmt. d	337 n.33
§122 cmt. g(iv)	323 n.11
§123 cmt. d(iv)	353 n.60
§123 cmt. d(v)	353 nn.56-57
§123 cmt. e	353 n.54
§128 cmt. c	317
§128 cmt. c(ii)	317 n.2
§128 cmt. e(i)	318 n.3
§131(g)	130
§134 cmt. f	144 n.42

FEDERAL STATUTES AND ADMINISTRATIVE REGULATIONS

Section	Page(s)
5 U.S.C. app'x §§1-16	574
8 U.S.C. §1229b(b)(1)(D)	199
15 U.S.C. §7245	7 n.10, 44 n.4, 134
16 U.S.C. §7602	264
18 U.S.C. §1503	446 n.16
18 U.S.C. §1512(c)	446 n.17
18 U.S.C. §1514A	141
18 U.S.C. §1519	446 n.16
18 U.S.C. §2340(A)	33
28 U.S.C. §455	568 n.2, 572, 572 n.42
28 U.S.C. §455(a)	572 n.42, 577, 580
28 U.S.C. §509	441
28 U.S.C. §515(a)	441
28 U.S.C. §515(c)	441
28 U.S.C. §516	441
28 U.S.C. §530B	444 n.13
28 U.S.C. §533	441
28 U.S.C. §547	441
28 U.S.C. §1927	374
29 U.S.C. §401	127 n.8
17 C.F.R. §205.3	134
17 C.F.R. §205.3(d)(2)	44 n.4
17 C.F.R. §205.3(d)(3)	250 n.1
45 C.F.R. pt. 1611 app'x A	552 n.11

Index

A

ABA. *See* American Bar Association
ABS (alternative business structures), 48, 492, 561-562
Access to justice, 4-6, 543-562. *See also* Right to counsel
  alternative business structures, 561-562
  court kiosks, 557-558
  court procedures, simplification of, 555-556
  document preparers, 560
  free legal services, 553
  IOLTA accounts and. *See* IOLTA (Interest on Lawyer's Trust Accounts)
  justice gap, 543-544, 552-555
  law school clinics, 553-554
  limited-scope representation, 559
  non-lawyers delivering legal services, 559-561
  non-recognition of need for legal services, 555
  possible solutions, 555-562
  pro bono services, 554, 556
  public interest organizations, 553
  regulatory changes, 559-562
  remote access to services, 557
  self-help centers, 558
  summary, 562
  technology and, 556-558
  unbundled legal services, 558-559
Accounting, 168. *See also* Client funds and property
Adams, John, 15, 483
Admission to bar, 48-62
  character and fitness, 50-62
  educational requirements, 49-50
Advance conflict waivers, 337-338
Advertising
  commercial speech, protection of, 513, 514
  constitutional limits on bar's power to restrict, 514-524
  direct mail, 516, 539
  electronic. *See* Electronic advertising
  Facebook, 513, 528
  false or misleading advertising, 525-528
  history of ban on, 514

  LinkedIn, 513, 528
  nicknames, use of, 526
  online advertising, 528-531
  past successes, 526
  ratings services, selection by, 526
  regulation of, 514-531
  required disclosures, 528
  specialization, 528
  summary, 539-540
  trade names, 528
  Twitter, 513, 528
  unsubstantiated comparison of services or fees, 525
Advising
  client to violate court order, 121
  communications for purpose of legal advice, 255, 259-261
  ethical advice, consultation exception for, 248
  financial advice to client, 261
  honest assessment, 38
  legal advice on social media network, 531
  outside checks of adversary system, 35-38
  responsibilities in, 35-38
  shaping client conduct, 31-35
Advocate, lawyer as. *See* Zealous advocacy
Advocate-witness rule, 338-340, 397
Affordable Care Act, 590
Agency relationship, 476
Aggravating factors for sanctions, 69
Aggregate settlement, 333-334
Alabama
  blackout periods, 523
  code of ethics for lawyers, 46
  judicial disqualification, 592
  judicial duties, performance of, 568-569
Alaska
  IOLTA, opting out, 160
  sexual relations with clients, 336-337
  writing testimonial bequests to self, prohibition against, 331
Albert, Linda, 238-239
Albrechtsen, Steven J., 193-194
Alcohol abuse, 64-65, 237-241
Alteration of evidence, 390-392

Alternative business structures (ABS), 48, 492,
    561-562
Alternative discipline program (ADP), 67
American Bar Association (ABA)
    Canons of Legal Ethics, 46
    Commission on Lawyer Assistance
        Programs, 238
    Commission on the Evaluation of
        Professional Standards (Kutak
        Commission), 46, 47
    Commission on the Future of Legal
        Services, 48
    Ethics 20/20 Commission, 47-48
    Ethics 2000 Commission, 47
    founding of, 45-46
    House of Delegates, 47
    Legal Technology Survey (2019), 528
    Model Code of Judicial Conduct, 567-568
    Model Code of Professional Responsibility, 47.
        See also Model Code of Professional
        Responsibility
    Model Rules for Lawyer Disciplinary
        Enforcement, 66
    Model Rules of Professional Conduct. *See*
        Model Rules of Professional Conduct
    Multidisciplinary Practice Commission
        (2000), 47
    Multijurisdictional Practice Commission
        (2002), 47, 508
    Standards for Imposing Lawyer Sanctions, 45
    Standards for the Administration of
        Criminal Justice, 469
    Standing Committee on Client
        Protection, 159
    Standing Committee on Ethics and
        Professional Responsibility, 47, 64, 436
American Civil Liberties Union (ACLU), 537
Antidiscrimination, 63
Appearance of impropriety
    judges, 572, 573
    lawyers, 316, 332
Arbitrators, 363-364
Arizona
    access to justice, 557-558
    advertising by lawyers, 514-516
    alternative business structures (ABS),
        492, 561
    Court Navigators program, 560
    document preparers, 560
    Legal Paraprofessionals, 560
    practice of law by non-lawyers, 499
Attorney-client privilege, 245, 246-279. *See also*
    Confidentiality
    defined, 258

adversarial proceedings, 280
agency relationship, 259
burden of proving applicability, 259
business advice not covered, 261
"circles of lawyer secrets," 303-304
"claw back" of inadvertent communication,
    286, 288
common interest doctrine. *See* Common
    interest doctrine
communications for purpose of legal advice,
    255, 259-261
communications not involving rendition of
    legal services, 261
confidential and privileged relationship, 259
confidentiality compared to, 246-247
control group test for entity clients, 264-265
crime-fraud exception, 255, 291-296
in digital age, 259, 261, 288-289
disciplinary claims, 280
discovery requests for large amounts of
    information, 288-289
duration of privilege, 259
elements defined, 258-259
entity clients, 262-267
exceptions, 291-296
ex parte proceedings, 380
fairness doctrine, 288, 296
government lawyers, 267-268
inadvertent disclosures, 286, 288-289
involuntary disclosure, 285
joint clients, 268, 296, 318
"joint defense" rule, 268
"last link" doctrine, 260
limited waiver, 280-286
malpractice claims, 280
mixed communications, 261
observations vs. communications, 260
overview, 258
partial disclosures, 286-288
preexisting client documents, 262
privilege holder's refusal to disclose
    evidence, 259
prospective clients, 247, 261
real evidence, 452
reasonable steps to prevent
    disclosure, 289
scope of privilege, 259-279
selective waiver, 280-286
self-defense exception, 248, 296, 304
subject matter waivers, 286-288
testimonial vs. non-testimonial settings,
    255, 287-288
third-party presence during
    communications, 260

voluntary disclosure, 279-280, 281, 285, 286-288
waivers, 279-291, 304
Attorney-client relationship, 101-179
abiding by client's wishes, 116-120
communication with. *See* Communication with clients
crime, counseling or assisting in, 31, 120-124
declination letter, use of, 107
exigent circumstances, formation in, 102
failure to inform client of settlement offer, 92
forming, 101-102
fraud, counseling or assisting in, 31, 120-124
implied, 102-108, 132-133
privilege. *See* Attorney-client privilege
pro bono representation, 30, 102, 554, 556
prospective clients, 108-115. *See also* Prospective clients
safeguarding client funds and property, 159-169. *See also* Client funds and property
scope of representation. *See* Scope of representation
summary, 177
termination of. *See* Termination of representation
Attorney's fees, 147-159
advance fees, 164, 166-167, 177
communicating fee to client, 147-148
competence and, 149
contingent fees, 148, 332, 333
customarily charged in locality for similar services, 149
double billing, 157-158
excessive, 91-92
failure of client to pay fees, refusal to turn over entire file, 176
failure of client to pay fees as cause for withdrawal, 175
failure to communicate rate and basis of fee, 150-156
fixed-fee limited-scope legal services referral programs, 486-491
fraudulent, 155, 156-159
inexperienced vs. experienced attorneys, 149
lodestar determination, 148
more than number of hours in a day, 157
non-contingent fee agreements, 147
padding a bill, 157
reasonableness of, 148-156
sharing fees with non-lawyers, 485-486
suits for, 92

withdrawal from representation, 101, 175
withholding file as security for payment of, 176 177
written fee agreement, 147-148
Autonomous self-interest, 11
Avvo Legal Services, 486, 491-492, 500, 528

B

Badgerow, J. Nick, 237
Bankruptcy petition preparers, 559
Bar associations, 45-48
integrated, 45
non-integrated, 45
non-unified, 45
unified, 45
"Beauty contest," client's search for representation deemed, 337
Billing. *See* Attorney's fees
Blogs, 513, 528
Boyle, William Anthony "Tony," 125-132
Brady obligations, 430-433, 436
Bribery, 396
Bundled services, 484, 485
"Buried Bodies Case," 257, 447-453
Business transactions with client, 325-330

C

Cady, Mark, 250-251
California
advertising and solicitation in, 529-530
apprenticeship for bar admission, 49
cloud computing services, use of, 194-195
document preparers, 560
future harms exception, 249
judges posting on social media, 571
"no-contact" rule, 438
practice of law by non-lawyers, 499, 560
pro bono services, 556
Public Records Act, 289-291
retaliatory discharge of in-house counsel, 141
social networking, 529-530
state-only accredited law schools, 50
threat to file disciplinary complaint, ban on, 72
unauthorized practice of law across jurisdictions, 501-510
undocumented immigrants, 53-54
Campaigns and other political activity by judges, 594-605
Candor, duty of, 23, 376-379. *See also* Truthful, obligation to be
Canons of Legal Ethics, 46
Carter, Jimmy, 544

CCJ (Conference of Chief Justices), 25
Character and fitness, 50-62
  deceitful conduct, 52-53, 63
  discrimination and harassment, 63
  dishonesty, 63, 65, 76-77, 410
  false statements, 51
  interviews of bar candidates, 52
  rehabilitation, 54-62
  undocumented immigrants, 53-54
Charging liens, 335-336
Charging power, 424-429. *See also* Prosecutors
Chat rooms, solicitation in, 538
Checklist for multiple/joint representation
  conflicts, 319
Cheney, Dick, 574-589
Child abuse or neglect proceedings, parent's
  right to counsel, 551
Children and minors, representation of,
  146-147, 551
Choice of law, 69-70
Churning, 158, 480
City Bar of New York, 45
Civil contempt, enforcement of child support
  orders, 545-551
"Civil Gideon" movement, 545
Civility, 394-395
Clark, Kathleen, 142-143
Class actions, 334
"Claw back" of inadvertent communication,
  286, 288
CLE (continuing legal education), 45
Client funds and property, 159-169
  accounting, 168
  bank service charges, 160
  client protection funds, 80, 159
  commingling forbidden, 159-160
  delivery, 168
  disputes over property held by attorney,
    168-169
  IOLTA programs and, 160
  misappropriation of funds, 71, 74-75,
    125-126, 159
  non-monetary property, 160
  notification of settlement, 168
  record keeping, 167
  segregation of, 159-167
  termination of representation, 176-177
  trust accounts, 159-160
Client intake, practical tip, 310
Clinton, Bill, 66
Cloud computing services, use of, 194-197
Cole, Martin, 207-208
Colorado
  advocate-witness rule, 338-340

materiality requirement, attorney
    disciplinary rules, 436
  misappropriation of client funds,
    disbarment for, 159
  proprietary interest in client matter, 335-336
Commercial speech, protection of, 513, 514.
  See also Advertising
Commissions (ABA). *See* American Bar
  Association
Common interest doctrine, 268-279
  expansion of, 278
  narrow approach to, 278
  requirements of, 268
  sample joint defense and common interest
    agreement, 269-273
  written agreements, 273
Communication with clients, 202-210
  categories of required communication,
    203-204
  criminal case, ineffective assistance of
    counsel in, 223-227
  declination letter, use of, 107
  disclosure by lawyers of their own mistakes
    to clients, 205-206
  failure to communicate, 150-156
  failure to return phone calls or emails,
    207-208
  false or misleading communication,
    525-528
  fee communications, 147-148, 150-156
  minimizing liability, 92, 208
  misunderstandings, 107
  promptness, 204
  requests for information, 206-208
  scope of representation, 147
Competence, 181-244. *See also* Diligence
  cloud computing services, use
    of, 194-197
  communication, 202-210
  criminal cases, 181
  excessive caseloads interfering with, 198,
    231-237
  fees and, 149
  incompetence that is not attorney's
    fault, 455
  indigent criminal defendants,
    representation of, 231-233
  ineffective assistance of criminal defense
    counsel. *See* Ineffective assistance of
    counsel
  inexperienced lawyers, 189-192
  legal knowledge and skill, 183-188
  mental health and, 237-241
  preparation, 192-194

procedural rules and requirements, knowledge of, 183, 188
substance abuse and, 64-65
summary, 241-242
technological, 194-197
thoroughness, 192-194
Concurrent client, 310, 313
Conference of Chief Justices (CCJ), 25
Confidentiality. *See also* Attorney-client privilege
"circles of lawyer secrets," 303-304
cloud computing services, use of, 196-197
compared with rule of privilege, 246-247
confidential material, definition of, 246
conflict checks, 248
duty of, 18-22, 246-258
ethical advice, consultation exception for, 248
exceptions, 248-249, 257
future harms exception, 249-258
implied authorization to disclose, 248
informed consent to disclosure, 247
misconduct, reporting of, 79
permissive exceptions, 255, 257, 410
receiving confidential information during consultation with prospective client, 109-114, 247
self-defense exception, 248, 296, 304
subpoena, disclosure pursuant to, 248
withdrawal from court proceeding, 175-176
witness false testimony in civil litigation, 383-384
Conflict shopping, 108-109
Conflicts of interest, 309-367
advance of living expenses to client, 332-333
advance waivers, prospective-clients, 337-338
advocate-witness rule, 338-340
aggregate settlements, 333-334
appearance of impropriety, 316, 332
business transactions with client, 325-330
client information, use of, 325-330
client intake tip, 310
concurrent client, 310, 313
current-client conflicts, 310-324. *See also* Current-client conflicts
directly adverse conflicts, 310
financial assistance to client, 332-333
former clients, 340-351
former government lawyers, 313, 362-363
former judges, 364
future conflicts that are not consentable, 313
gift solicitations, prohibition against, 330-331

gifts to client, 332-333
imputation of client conflicts, 313, 351-362
ineffective assistance of counsel, 231
judges, 363-364
literary rights, 331-333
material limitation conflicts, 310-318
media rights, 331-333
naming self as devisee in client's will, 331
opportunity to use client information for lawyer's own benefit, 326
personal-interest conflicts with clients, 325-340
proprietary interest in client matter, 335-336
prospective malpractice limitations, 334-335
screening, 114, 248, 353-356, 363
self-interest of lawyer, 29-30, 335-336
sexual relations with client, 336-337
standard commercial business transactions, 330
summary, 364-365
testimonial bequests to self, prohibition against writing into client's will, 331
types of, 309
unrepresented persons, communicating with, 335
waivers, 309, 321
Connecticut
blackout periods, 523
extrajudicial activities, 570-571
Consent. *See* Informed consent
Constitution, U.S.
First Amendment, 54, 63, 400-401, 479, 513, 516, 525, 595, 597
Fourth Amendment, 222, 437
Fifth Amendment, 67, 262, 320, 437, 553
Sixth Amendment, 181, 210-211, 212, 213, 321, 438, 453, 544-545, 547
Fourteenth Amendment, 211, 545-552
Due Process Clause, 211, 433, 436, 545-552
Privileges and Immunities Clause, 49
Supremacy Clause, 53, 499
Contempt
civil contempt proceedings, right to counsel, 545-551
counseling client to not comply with court order, 121
criminal contempt proceedings, right to counsel, 544
disruptive conduct, 394
threat of, 285
Contingent fees, 148, 332, 333
Continuing legal education (CLE), 45
"Control group" test, 264-265, 404-407

Convention Against Torture, 34-35, 37, 41

Corporate scandals, 7, 31-33, 36, 38, 134, 250

Court access. *See* Access to justice

Court costs, advance of, 332

Covenants not to compete, 493

Covert investigation to gather evidence of
  wrongdoing, 415

COVID-19 pandemic, effect on IOLTA
  funding, 553

Cramton, Roger, 10, 11, 142

Creativity, 35-36

Crime-fraud exception, 249-250, 291-296.
  See also Attorney-client privilege
  in camera review of evidence for
    applicability of, 295

Crime or fraud
  client's intent to commit crime,
    252-255, 291
  counseling or assisting in, 31, 120-124
  disclosure of client's crime or
    fraud, 250-251
  disclosure of future harms, exception to
    confidentiality duty, 249-258
  disclosure of material fact to prevent, 409
  withdrawing from case when client using
    lawyer to engage in, 16, 122-123,
    175, 250

Criminal defense lawyer, 446-469
  counseling or assisting another to obstruct
    access to evidence, 447
  cross-examining truthful witness, 463-469
  discrediting truthful testimony, 463
  lawyer's trilemma, 453, 462
  past crimes disclosed to, 448-451
  perjury by client, 453-461
  physical evidence, taking possession of,
    446-453
  putting client on stand, 453-463

Criminal practice, 419-470
  client's authority on entering a plea, waiving
    jury trial, or testifying, 204
  current-client conflicts, 320-322, 324
  defense lawyer, 446-469. *See also* Criminal
    defense lawyer
  failure to communicate plea offer, 223-228
  guilt beyond reasonable doubt, 5
  homicide cases, defense in, 221
  malpractice claims, 83
  plea bargaining, 448-451
  prosecutors, 419-445. *See also* Prosecutors
  summary, 469

Cross-border practice. *See also*
  Multijurisdictional practice
  imputation rule, 353

Cross-examination of truthful witness, 463-469

Current-client conflicts, 310-324
  appearance of impropriety, 316
  civil cases, 322-324
  client intake tip, 310
  concurrent client, 310, 313
  criminal cases, 320-322, 324
  directly adverse conflicts, 310-318
  former government lawyers, 313
  "general alignment of interests"
    doctrine, 323
  imputation of, 313
  informed consent, 311, 312, 322
  "issue" conflict, 324
  material limitation conflicts, 310-318
  multiple/joint representation conflicts,
    318-319
  "positional" conflict, 324
  reasonableness determination, 311
  roadmap for waiver of, 310, 317
  "significant risk of material limitation,"
    310, 324
  waivers, 310, 322-323

D

Defense lawyer. *See* Criminal defense lawyer

Deficient performance, 221-222. *See also*
  Competence

Delaware, positional conflict of interest in, 324

Delay in proceeding, 197-202. *See also* Diligence

Delivery of client funds and property, 168

Delivery of legal services. *See* Access to justice

Deportation consequences of a plea, 119, 204,
  228-229

Depression, 237-241

Derivative actions, joint representation in, 130

Dershowitz, Alan, 287-288

Destruction of evidence, 390-392

Diligence, 197-202
  unmanageable caseloads, 198, 231-237

Diminished capacity, clients with, 146-147

Diploma privilege, 49

Disbarment, 68, 123, 159

Disciplinary Rules (DRs), 46

Discipline, 62-80. *See also* Misconduct
  aggravating factors, 68-69
  alternative discipline program, 67
  choice of law, 69-70
  disbarment, 68, 123, 159
  misconduct, defined, 62-64
  mitigating factors, 68-69
  probation, 67
  process of, 66-68, 94
  reciprocal discipline, 70-71
  reprimand, public or private, 67
  sanctions, 68-69

standards of review, 68

suspension, 68

threat to file disciplinary complaint, 72

Discourteous behavior, 394-395

civility, 394-395

Discovery

abuse of, 392

delay, 172, 392-393

evasive or incomplete responses to requests, 392-393

failure to conduct, 222

frivolous requests, 375

inadvertent, 393

intentional or reckless failure to comply, 375-376

responsive and non-responsive documents, mixture of, 392-393

Discrediting truthful testimony, 463

Discriminatory behavior, 63

Disqualification

of judges, 572-590

of law firms, 363

Disruptive conduct, 393-394

District of Columbia

alternative business structures, 561

defense attorney receiving incriminating physical evidence, 452-453

lawyer's participation in preparation of witness's testimony, 389-390

perjury by client, 462

threat to file disciplinary complaint, ban on, 72

Document preparers (non-lawyers), 560

Document retention policies, 391-392

Double billing, 157-158

DRs (Disciplinary Rules), 46

Drug abuse, 64-65, 237-241

Dual representation, 316, 322-323

Due process of law

disclosure of exculpatory law, 433, 436

indigent's right to counsel, 545-551

lawyer's role as guardian of, 4-6, 15

recusal of judge, 591-594

Durable powers of attorney, 146

Duty of candor. *See* Candor, duty of

Duty of loyalty. *See* Loyalty, duty of

Duty to report another lawyer's misconduct, 71-80

E

Economic Policy Institute, 554

Educational requirements

admission to bar, 49-50

CLE (continuing legal education), 45

Effective assistance of counsel, 5, 7, 212. *See also* Ineffective assistance of counsel

Electronic advertising, 528-531

attorney-client relationship, formation of, 531

blogs, 513, 528

legal advice on social media network, 531

prospective client relationship, 531

third-party posts to social media, 531

unique dangers of social media and electronic advertising, 530-531

websites, 513, 528, 529

Electronically stored information, 393

Email and electronic communications

attorney-client privilege, 259, 261

cloud computing, 194

discovery requests for, 288-289

promptly responding to client via, 92

"real-time," 538

solicitation via, 538-539

web bugs to track, 63

Entity clients. *See* Organizational clients

Entity theory of organizational representation, 124-125

Entity warning, 132-133

Errors and omissions (E & O) insurance policies, 69, 93-94

Ethical considerations, 419-470

communications. *See* Communication with clients

competence. *See* Competence

confidentiality. *See* Confidentiality

conflicts of interest. *See* Conflicts of interest

core values and ideals of the profession, 28-29

fiduciary duties. *See* Fiduciary role

military commissions, 142

Ethics 20/20 Commission (ABA), 47-48, 492

Ethics 2000 Commission (ABA), 47

Evidence. *See also* Discovery

concealment and alteration in criminal investigations, 446

destruction of, 390-392

document retention policies, 391-392

exculpatory, 4-5. *See also* Exculpatory evidence

inculpatory, 430

spoliation of, 391

tampering with, 390-392

Exculpatory evidence, 4-5

constitutional and ethical duty to disclose, 429-433

hiding of, 4-5

inculpatory evidence vs., 430

"knew or should have known" standard, 436

materiality of evidence, 432

scope of disclosure obligation, 432

timely disclosure, 435

Ex parte communications, 395-396, 569
Ex parte proceedings
attorney-client privilege, 380
candor to tribunal, 380
duty to disclose material facts, 380
truthfulness, 380
Expediting litigation, 291, 371-372
Expert witnesses
compensation of, 396
on standard of reasonable care, 82-83
Extrajudicial activities, 570-571

F

FACA (Federal Advisory Committee Act), 574
Facebook, 513, 528, 571, 591
Fairness in adjudication, 6, 371-417
advocate-witness rule, 397
civility, 394-395
communicating with represented persons,
402-408. *See also* "No-contact" rule
communicating with unrepresented
persons, 408-409
discovery obligations. *See* Discovery
ex parte communications with judges or
jurors, 395
impartiality of the tribunal, 395-397
influencing or intimidating witnesses, 395
meritorious claims, 371-376
"no-contact" rule. *See* "No-contact" rule
obstruction of evidence, 390-392
to opposing party and counsel, 390-393
public comment on pending civil litigation,
397-401
statements to others, truthfulness in, 409-415
summary, 415-416
trial tactics, 393-395
truthfulness, 376-390. *See also* Truthful,
obligation to be
Falsehoods and misrepresentation, 65-66,
376-377
False or misleading advertising, 525-528
False statement of material fact, 409
False testimony in civil litigation, 383-390
Federal Advisory Committee Act (FACA), 574
Federal Rules of Civil Procedure
excusable neglect, 183
frivolous pleadings, 372
notice pleading, 242
work-product immunity, 297
Federal Rules of Criminal Procedure
inculpatory evidence, disclosure of, 430
joint representation, 320
Federal Trade Commission, 497-498
Fees. *See* Attorney's fees
Fiduciary role, 147-177

breach of. *See* Legal malpractice
client funds and property, duties owed as to,
159-169
fees charged. *See* Attorney's fees
obligations of, 245
"Fighting fire with fire" provision, 398
Financial advice to client, 261
Financial assistance to client, 332-333
Financial misconduct, 65
Fitness to practice law, 50-62. *See also*
Character and fitness
Florida
dual representation, 323
false or misleading advertising, 526
fundraising for judicial campaigns, 595
judges "friending" lawyers on Facebook, 591
judges on social media in, 591
marketing of legal services, 516-526
technology-related CLE requirements, 45
threat to file disciplinary complaint, ban on, 72
unauthorized practice of law, 499, 500
Floyd, Timothy, 23-24, 25
Former-client conflicts of interest, 340-351
substantial relationship test, application of,
340, 348-349
suit against former client on unrelated
matter, 341
Fox, Lawrence J., 583-589
Frankfurter, Felix, 51
Fraud, 63, 120-124
advertising, 513
counseling or assisting client in, 31, 120-124
duty to rectify client's fraud on tribunal, 249
fees charged by lawyer, 155, 156-159
prevention of financial fraud, 250-251, 257
Freedman, Monroe, 5, 192, 468
Free legal services, 553
Frivolous claims, 371-372
FTC. *See* Federal Trade Commission
Future harms exception, 249-258
financial harm, 250-251, 257
immediacy of harm, 256
Futures Commission (ABA Commission on the
Future of Legal Services), 48

G

GAAP (generally accepted accounting
practices), 167
Gag order, 397
Gallagher, John, 23-24, 25
Gambling, 237-241
Genego, William, 222
"General alignment of interests" doctrine, 323
Generally accepted accounting practices
(GAAP), 167

Gifts
    to clients, 332
    to judges, 571
    to lawyers, 330-331
Gillers, Stephen, 428-429
Ginsburg, Ruth Bader, 590
Globalization, 47, 310
Goldsmith, Jack, 34
Good character and fitness, 50-62
Government clients, 142-143
Government lawyers
    attorney-client privilege, 267-268
    conflicts of interest, 362-363
    current-client conflicts of former
        government lawyers, 313
Green, Bruce, 444, 482, 484
Group lawyering, 473-512
Guardianship
    diminished capacity, clients with, 146
    right to counsel, 551

H

Hamilton, Neil, 6-7, 25-30
Hand, Learned, 221
Harassment, 63
Hazelden Betty Ford Foundation, 238
Holmes, Oliver Wendell, 7-14, 22
Horton, James E., Jr., 212-213
House of Delegates (ABA), 47

I

Ibrahim, Darian M., 124
Identity of the client, 124-147
    diminished capacity, clients with, 146-147
    government clients, 142-143
    insureds, 143-145
    organizational clients, 124-141. *See also*
        Organizational clients
Illinois
    Legal Aid Online, 557
    legal malpractice, 84-88
    misconduct, reporting of, 74-79
    retaliatory discharge of in-house counsel,
        140-141
    threat to file disciplinary complaint,
        ban on, 72
Immigrants
    admission to practice, 53-54
    ban on entry under executive order, 102
    deportation and ineffective counsel, 198-202,
        228-229
    deportation consequences of a plea, 119,
        204, 228-229
    representation by non-lawyers, 560
Impartiality of the tribunal, 395-397

Impeachment of witness, 468
Implied attorney-client relationship, 102-108,
    132-133
Impropriety, appearance of, 316, 332
Imputation doctrine, 351-362
    screening to avoid, 114, 248, 353-356, 363
Inadvertent disclosure, 196-197, 247,
    288-291
Inadvertent discovery, 393
In camera review, 295
Inculpatory evidence, 430
Independence of judge, 597
Independence of lawyer, 481-497
    alternative business structures, 492
    fee sharing with non-lawyers, 485-486
    fixed-fee limited-scope legal services
        referral programs, 486-491
    lawyer independence, defined, 482
    legal services referral programs, 487
    multidisciplinary practice, 485
    from non-lawyers, 484-492
    from popular opinion, 483
    reciprocal referral agreement, 485-486
    restrictions on lawyer's practice, 492-496
    sale of law practice, 496-497
    third parties, pressure by, 483
Indigent persons, 332-333
    right to counsel in civil cases, 544-552
Ineffective assistance of counsel, 210-231
    conflict of interest, 231
    constitutional test for, 213-221
    deficient performance, 221-222
    deportation consequences of plea, 198-202,
        228-229
    failure to communicate, 223
    failure to investigate, 222-223
    incompetence that is not attorney's fault,
        231-237
    prejudice, 229-231
    public defenders, unmanageable caseloads
        for, 198, 231-237
    reasonableness under prevailing
        professional norms, 215-216, 220
Informed consent, 203-204, 223, 247
    defined, 247
    current-client conflicts, 311, 312, 322
Insurance
    errors and omissions policies, 69, 93-94
    malpractice, 93-94
Insureds
    letter from insurer's lawyer to, 145
    representation of, 143-145
    tripartite relationship, 144
Integrated bar, 45
Integrity, 51

Intent
  antidiscrimination standard of Model
    Rules, 64
  California PRA waiver provision, 290
  client's intent to commit crime, 252-255,
    291. *See also* Crime-fraud exception
  client's intent to commit perjury, 383,
    453-461
  E & O policies excluding intentional acts, 94
  lawyer's discipline, factor in determining, 68
  personal conscience, 26
  real evidence of, 446
  subject matter waivers, 286
Interactive legal-help websites, 501
Interest on Lawyer's Trust Accounts (IOLTA),
    160, 553
International jurisdictions, 508
Internet providers of legal information and
    services, 500-501
Involuntary commitment, right to counsel, 551
IOLTA (Interest on Lawyer's Trust Accounts),
    160, 553

J
Jackson, Andrew, 596
Jennings, Marianne M., 25
Joint client
  attorney-client privilege, 296, 318
  common interest doctrine distinguished, 268
Joint defense, 268
  common interest agreement (sample),
    269-273
  "pooled information" rule, 268
Joint representation, 130, 318-324
  checklist, 319
  civil cases, 322-324
  criminal cases, 320-322
  derivative actions, 130
  organizational clients, 125-129
Judge Advocate General military defense
    lawyers, 142
Judicial ethics, 567-607
  "announce" clause, 597-604
  campaigns and other political activity, 594-605
  conflicts of interest, 363-364
  disqualification, 572-590
  ex parte communications, 569
  extrajudicial activities, 570-571
  "friending" lawyers on Facebook, 591
  fundraising, 594-595
  gifts, 571
  impartiality, 572-590, 596
  impropriety, appearance of, 572, 573
  independence, 597

  independent investigation, 569
  judicial candidate's disclosure of party
    affiliation, 605
  Model Code of Judicial Conduct, 567-568
  partiality, appearance of, 573
  pecuniary stake in outcome of case, 592
  performance of judicial duties, 568-570
  "pledges and promises" ban, 570, 604
  recusal standard, 591-594, 595
  social media, use of, 569, 571, 590-591
  social relationships, 573
  summary, 605-606
Junior lawyers
  limited safe harbor for, 475
  misconduct of, 475
  responsibility of, 475-481
  unmanageable caseloads, 198
  vicarious liability of supervisory lawyers
    for, 474
Jurors, post-verdict contact with, 396
Justice Department (DOJ), 143
Justice gap, 543-544, 552-555
Justice system, role of lawyer in, 3-41. *See also*
    Role of lawyer
Juveniles in delinquency proceedings, right to
    counsel, 545

K
Kagan, Elena, 590
Kansas, opting out of IOLTA in, 160
Kentucky
  blackout periods, 523
  judicial candidate's disclosure of party
    affiliation, 605
  reciprocal discipline, 71
  social media, judge's use of, 591
Koniak, Susan, 31-32, 36-37, 38
Krill, Patrick, 238-239
Kutak Commission, 46, 47

L
Labor Management Reporting and Disclosure
    Act, 125
"Last link" doctrine, 260
Law clerks, 364
Law firms and associations, 474-481
  defined, 352
  disqualification of, 363
  imputation doctrine applicable to all firm
    members, 352
  junior lawyers. *See* Junior lawyers
  malpractice. *See* Legal malpractice
  marketing by. *See* Advertising
  mergers and acquisitions, 350-351

misleading names of, 528
multidisciplinary practices (MDPs), 485
solicitation of clients. *See* Solicitation
summary, 510
supervisory lawyers. *See* Supervisory
lawyers
Law school clinics, 553-554
Lawyer Assistance Programs, 240
Legal aid services, 543, 556
Legal malpractice, 80-94
breach of fiduciary duty and, 81, 88-92
case-within-a-case model, 83
criminal defendant suing for, 83
disclosure by lawyers of their own mistakes
to clients, 205-206
duty of reasonable care, failure to meet, 82
elements to prove, 81, 105
failure to protect confidentiality of client
communications, 248
minimizing liability for, 92-94
negligence and, 81-88, 106-107
non-clients, duty to, 82
pleading, 89, 91
privity defense, 82
prospective malpractice liability, agreements
to limit, 334-335
specialists, 81
statute of limitations, 81
third-party duty of care, 82
Legal realism, 9
Legal Services Corporation (LSC), 482, 552
Legal Technology Survey (ABA 2019), 528
LegalZoom, 500-501
Leibowitz, Samuel, 212
Lerman, Lisa, 157
License to practice law, 3
admission to bar, 48-62
apprenticeship for bar admission, 49
Limitations of actions, 81, 205
Limited liability companies (LLCs), 93
Limited liability partnerships (LLPs), 93
Limited License Legal Technician (LLLT), 48,
560-561
Limited-scope legal services referral programs
(fixed-fee), 486-491
Limited-scope representation, 169
LinkedIn, 513, 528, 591
Litigation, responsibilities in, 30-38. *See also*
Fairness in adjudication
Living expenses, advance to client for, 332-333
LLCs (limited liability companies), 93
LLLT (Limited License Legal Technician), 48,
560-561
LLPs (limited liability partnerships), 93

Lodestar determination of fee, 148
Louisiana
antidiscrimination provision, 63
blackout periods, 523
false or misleading advertising, 525, 526
misconduct, reporting of, 73
Loyalty, duty of, 124-125. *See also* Conflicts of
interest
fiduciary duty, 88, 246
self-interest interfering with, 335
Luban, David, 37

M
Maine, apprenticeship for bar admission in, 49
Mallen, Ronald E., 81
Malpractice. *See* Legal malpractice
Malpractice insurance, 93-94
Mandatory withdrawal, 169, 174, 250
Marketing legal services, 513-541. *See also*
Advertising; Solicitation
communications vs. solicitation, 514
social media, 513, 528
summary, 539-540
websites, 513, 528, 529
Markovic, Milan, 34
Marshall, Thurgood, 218-220
Martyn, Susan, 101
Maryland, blackout periods in, 523
Massachusetts
attorney-client privilege, 255
attorney disciplinary rules, 255-256
communication with represented person,
403-407
former-client conflict, 341-342
future harms exception, 252-256
materiality requirement, attorney
disciplinary rules, 436
misrepresentation by attorney to engage in
"testing," 411
perjury by client, 462
reasonableness of attorney's fee, 149
withdrawal from representation,
169-173
Material evidence, 377
Material misstatements by lawyer to third
party, 410
"puffing" exception, 410
McDade Amendment (1998), 444
MDP (multidisciplinary practice), 485
Media contact, 397-401
gag order, 397
prosecutor's statements to the media,
444-445
restriction on, 397

Media statements, 397

Meiklejohn, Alexander, 12, 13-14

Mental impairment
  of client, 146-147
  of lawyer, 174

Meritorious claims, 371-376
  pleadings, 371
  sanctions under FRCP 11, 372

Michigan, sanctioning judges in, 568

Minnesota
  judicial campaigning, 597-604
  multijurisdictional practice, 509

Misappropriation of funds, 71, 74-75,
  125-126, 159

Misconduct
  defined, 62-64
  catchall provisions, 63-64
  drug and alcohol abuse, 64-65
  duty to report another's misconduct, 71-80
  falsehoods, 65-66
  financial, 65

Mississippi
  former judge's conflict of interest, 364
  personal profit from representation of
    client, 332
  pro bono services, 556
  unauthorized practice of law, 500

Mitchell, John, 463-469

Mitigating factors for sanctions, 69

Mixed communications, 261

Model Code of Judicial Conduct, 567-568

Model Code of Professional Responsibility
  (ABA, predecessor to Model Rules), 46

Model Rules for Lawyer Disciplinary
  Enforcement (ABA), 66

Model Rules of Professional Conduct (ABA),
  6, 25, 46-47. *See also separate Table of Rules
  by number*

Moral character and implementation, 27-28

Moral dialogue, 15-24

Moral judgment, 27

Moral motivation and commitment, 27

Moral responsibility, 7-30
  bad man perspective, 7, 9-14
  moral dialogue, 15-24
  professional judgment, cultivation of, 24-30
  role morality, 15-24

Moral sensitivity, 27

Morgan, Thomas, 484, 492

MRPC. *See* Model Rules of Professional
  Conduct

Multidisciplinary practice (MDP), 485

Multidisciplinary Practice Commission (ABA), 47

Multijurisdictional practice (MJP), 501-510

Multijurisdictional Practice Commission
  (ABA), 47, 508

Multiple/joint representation conflicts. *See*
  Joint representation

N

National Association of IOLTA Programs
  (NAIP), 553

National Task Force on Lawyer Well-Being
  (2017 Report), 240

Nebraska, opting out of IOLTA in, 160

Negligence claims against lawyers. *See* Legal
  malpractice

Nevada
  document preparers, 560
  in-house counsel suing for wrongful
    discharge, 141
  public statements made by attorney with
    prejudicial effect, 445

New Hampshire, bar admission in, 49

New Jersey
  dual representation, 323
  future harms exception, 249
  real estate closing, 323, 498

New York
  apprenticeship for bar admission, 49
  blackout periods, 523
  Court Navigators program, 560
  judges on social media in, 591
  past crimes disclosed to lawyer, 448-451
  pro bono services, 556
  tape recording conducted surreptitiously,
    411-414
  unauthorized practice of law, 500

Nifong, Mike, 429, 445

"No-contact" rule, 402-408
  artificial persons, 403
  authorization by law or court order, 408
  business entities, 403
  "control group" test, 404-407
  former employees of corporation, 407
  post-indictment contact, 438
  pre-indictment context, 437-438
  prosecutor's contact with represented
    suspects, 437-444

Nonclients, fiduciary duties to, 82

Noncompetition agreements, 493

Non-integrated bar, 45

Non-lawyers
  delivering legal services, 559-561
  independence of lawyers in practice from,
    484-492
  ownership or direction of firm, 491-492
  unauthorized practice of law, 497-501

Non-unified bar, 45
North Carolina
    disclosure by lawyers of their own mistakes
        to clients, 205-206
    dual representation, 323
    unauthorized practice of law, 501

O

Obstruction of evidence, 390-392, 446
Obstruction of justice, 391
Obtaining clients
    advertising. *See* Advertising
    solicitation. *See* Solicitation
O'Connor, Sandra Day, 596, 607
Office of Legal Counsel (OLC), 33-34,
    37, 38, 41
Office-sharing arrangements, 353
Ohio
    cloud computing services, use of, 195-197
    Code of Professional Responsibility (1969)
        followed by, 47
    judicial impartiality, 592
    materiality requirement, attorney
        disciplinary rules, 436
    solicitation of clients, 532-538
    threat to file disciplinary complaint, ban
        on, 72-73
OLC (Office of Legal Counsel), 33-34,
    37, 38, 41
Online advertising, 528-531
Opinion work product, 298, 305
Ordinary work product, 298, 305
Organizational clients, 124-141
    attorney-client privilege, 132-133,
        262-267
    "control group" test, 264-265, 404-407
    corporate *Miranda* warning, 131-134
    derivative actions, 130
    discharge or withdrawal of attorney for
        reporting information, 135-141
    entity theory of organizational
        representation, 124-125
    entity warning, 132-133
    joint representation, 125-129
    reporting up and out, 134-141
    retaliatory discharge of attorney, 135
Outsourcing of legal work, 196

P

Padding a bill, 157
Paralegals
    imputation rule, 352
    "no-contact" rule, 475
    privileged communications, 260

Past crimes disclosed to defense lawyer,
    448-451
Patent agents, 499, 560
Pearce, Russell, 11
Peer-review, 29
Pemberton, Richard, 23
Pennsylvania
    cloud computing services, use of, 194
    fixed-fee limited-scope legal services
        referral programs, 486-491
    sharing fees with non-lawyers, 486
Perjury by client, 383-390, 453-461
Permissive disclosures, 410
Permissive withdrawal, 169, 175
"Perp walks," 445
Personal conscience, 26-28
Personal-interest conflicts with clients, 325-340
Pines, Daniel, 34
Pleas in criminal cases. *See* Criminal practice
Podgers, James, 238
Police departments
    public comments by police, 455
    undercover investigation, 411, 415, 437-438
Political activity by judges, 594-605
"Pooled information" rule, 268
Positivism, 9
Post-indictment contact, 438
Post-verdict contact with jurors, 396
Practice of law
    defined, 498-501
    admission to, 48-62
    law firms. *See* Law firms and associations
    unauthorized. *See* Unauthorized
        practice of law
"Predominant effects" standard, 48, 70
Prejudice, 445
Press. *See* Media contact
Privilege. *See* Attorney-client privilege
Privileges and Immunities Clause, 49
Probable cause, 425
Probation, 67
Pro bono services, 30, 102, 554
    mandatory, 556
    summary, 563
Procrastination, 198
Pro hac vice admission, 48
Promptness. *See* Diligence
Prosecutors, 419-445
    another's acts, responsibility for, 421
    charging power, 424-429
    exculpatory evidence, duty to disclose, 4-5,
        429-437
    ex parte communications with represented
        "persons," 437

Prosecutors (*continued*)
McDade Amendment, applicability of, 444
media, statements to, 444-445
minister of justice, 420-424
quantum of proof necessary for charging, 424-429
represented suspects, contact with, 437-444
self-executing duty, 431
statements to the media, 444-445
who is represented, 419-424
Prospective clients
defined, 108
advance waiver of conflict of interest, 337-338
attorney-client privilege, 261
confidential information during initial consultation, 109-114, 247, 337
conflict shopping, 108-109
electronic advertising, 531
forming relationship with, 108-115
solicitation, 538-539
Pryor, Ellen, 144
Public comment on pending civil litigation, 397-401
"fighting fire with fire" provision, 398
gag order, 397
prejudicial pretrial comments, 398-401
public records exception, 398
safe harbor provisions, 398
Public defenders
imputation of conflicts, 353
unmanageable caseloads, 198, 231-237
Public statements, 444-445
"Puffing" exception, 410
Purcell, Jeffrey W., 252-256

R

Real evidence, 446
attorney-client privilege, 452
Reasonable belief, 82
Reasonable remedial measures, 383
Reciprocal discipline, 70-71
Reciprocal referral agreements, 485-486
Recusal of judges, 591-594, 595
Regulation of lawyers, 43-97
admission to bar, 48-62. *See also* Admission to bar
bar associations, 45-48
conduct codes, 45-48
continuing legal education, 45
cross-border, 44, 48, 508
discipline, 62-80. *See also* Discipline
ethics codes, 45-48

malpractice, 80-94. *See also* Legal malpractice
state courts' powers, 44-45
summary, 94-95
Regulation of legal profession, 43-95
discipline of lawyer. *See* Discipline
lawyers. *See* Regulation of lawyers
malpractice. *See* Legal malpractice
misconduct. *See* Misconduct
Relational self-interest, 11
Representation
attorney-client relationship. *See* Attorney-client relationship
termination of. *See* Termination of representation
Reprimand, public or private, 67
Restatement (Third) of the Law Governing Lawyers
attorney-client privilege, 247, 258
bar admission, 50
breach of implied contract, 81
character and fitness requirement, 51
conflicts of interest, 309, 317
derivative actions, joint representation in, 130
dual representation, 323
multijurisdictional practice, 509
witness preparation, 390
work-product immunity, 297
Retainer, 67, 164-166
engagement, 166-167
general, 166
return of unearned portions upon withdrawal from case, 177
special, 164, 166, 167
Retaining liens, 176-177, 335
Rhode, Deborah, 17, 498, 544
Right to counsel, 5
civil cases, 543-544, 551
civil contempt proceedings for enforcement of child support orders, 545-551
criminal cases, 544, 547
guardianship proceedings, 551
indigent defendants, 544-552
involuntary commitment proceedings, 551
juveniles in delinquency proceedings, 545
summary, 562-563
termination of parental rights cases, 551
waiver, 438-444
Robot Lawyer app, 557
Roiphe, Rebecca, 482
Role morality, 15-24
Role of lawyer, 3-41
advising, responsibilities in, 35-38

guardians of due process, 4-6, 15
litigating, responsibilities in, 30-35
moral responsibility, 7-30
protection of public good, 6-7
self-regulation of legal profession, 6-7
shaping client conduct, 31-35
summary, 38-39
transactional planning, responsibilities
   in, 30-35
Rosin, Hanna, 61
Rossi, R.L., 335
Rude behavior, 394
civility, 394-395

S

Sale of law practice, 496-497
Sanctions, 68-69
aggravating and mitigating factors, 69
"conflict" prohibition, violation of, 309
disbarment, 68, 123, 159
probation, 67
public censure, 66
suspension, 65
Sandefur, Rebecca, 555
Sandoval-Moshenberg, Simon, 102
Sarbanes-Oxley Act, 7, 134, 141, 446
Scalia, Antonin, 574-589, 590
Scope of representation, 93
duty to communicate to client, 147
limited-scope representation, 169
"Scottsboro boys," 211-213
Screening, 114, 248, 353-356, 363
Searches and seizures, 222
Securities and Exchange Commission (SEC),
   43, 133-134, 143
Segal, David, 158
Segregation of client funds, 159-167
Selective waiver, 280-281
Self-defense exception
   to attorney-client privilege, 296, 304
   to duty of confidentiality, 248
Self-executing duty, 431
Self-incrimination, privilege against, 5
Self-regulation of legal profession, 6
Separation of powers doctrine, 437
Settlement
aggregate, 333-334
check, notification of receipt, 168
offers, 92, 94, 204
Sexual relations with clients, 336-337
Significant risk that conflict will materially
   limit, 310, 324
Silver, Charles, 144
Simon, William, 10

Sisk, Gregory, 250 251
Smartphones, 194
Smith, Abbe, 5, 192
Snitch rule, 480-481
Social media
advertising on, 528-529
judges' use of, 569, 571, 590-591
solicitation on, 538-539
unique dangers of, 530-531
Solicitation
chat rooms, 538
vs. communications, other types of, 514
constitutional limits on bar's power to limit,
   532-538
definition of person-to-person contact, 538
direct mailings, 537, 539
by email, 538
expression of personal political
   beliefs, 537
family members, 538
pro bono cases, 537
real-time electronic contact, 538
regulation of, 559
rules governing, 538-539
social media, use of, 538-539
summary, 539-540
South Carolina
antidiscrimination provision, 63
social media and electronic
   advertising, 531
solicitation by direct letter for pro bono
   representation, 537
Spaulding, David, 17-24
Specialists
advertising, 528
certification as, 45
standard of care, 82
Specialized knowledge and training, 182
Spoliation of evidence, 391
Standards for Imposing Lawyer Sanctions
   (ABA), 45
Standards for the Administration of Criminal
   Justice (ABA), 469
Standards of review of discipline, 68
Standing Committee on Client Protection
   (ABA), 159
Standing Committee on Ethics and Professional
   Responsibility (ABA), 47, 64, 436
State supreme courts, 6
discipline process, 68, 94
regulation of lawyers, 44-45, 94
Statutes of limitations, 205
malpractice, 81
Subin, Harry, 463-468

Subject matter waiver, 286-288
Subpoena, disclosure pursuant to
 attorney-client privilege, 285
 confidentiality, 248
 real evidence, 452
Substance abuse, 64-65
Supervisory lawyers, responsibility of, 474-475
Survey of Law Student Well-Being
 (SLSWB), 239
Suspension, 65

T

Tape recording conducted surreptitiously,
 411-414
Tarkington, Margaret, 15-16, 63
Task Force on Lawyer Business Ethics, 156
Tax cases, representation by non-lawyers
 in, 560
Technology
 access to justice and, 556-558
 competence in, 194-197
 Florida's technology-related CLE
  requirements, 45
 Legal Technology Survey (ABA 2019), 528
Tennessee
 antidiscrimination provision, 63
 failure to communicate fee and client
  charged unreasonable fee, 150-156
Termination of parental rights, right to
 counsel, 551
Termination of representation, 169-177
 duties owed to client after, 176-177
 firing by client, 135-141, 169
 withdrawal. *See* Withdrawal from
  representation
"Testing" (undercover investigations), 411,
 413, 415
Texas
 aggregate settlement, 333-334
 antidiscrimination provision, 63
 blackout periods, 523
 breach of fiduciary duty as legal
  malpractice, 88-92
 misconduct, reporting of, 72
 threat to file disciplinary complaint,
  ban on, 72
Texting to solicit business, 538
Third-party neutrals, 36
Thomas, Clarence, 590
Threat to file disciplinary complaint, 72
Token gifts, 331
Torture Memos (OLC), 33-35, 36, 37
Transactional planning
 honest assessment, 38

 responsibilities in, 30-38
 shaping client conduct, 31-35, 121
Trial tactics, 393-395
Trust accounts, 159-160
Truthful, obligation to be, 376-390
 ex parte proceedings, 380
 failure to disclose controlling legal
  authority, 380-383
 lawyer's trilemma, 376
 in statements to others, 409-415
Twitter, 513, 528

U

Unauthorized practice of law (UPL), 497-510
 defining practice of law, 498-501
 forms or information provided without
  advice, 499
 Internet providers of legal information and
  services, 500-501
 justifications for professional monopoly,
  497-498
 summary, 510
Unbundled legal services, 558-559
Undercover police investigations, 411, 415,
 437-438
Undocumented immigrants, 53-54
Undue influence, doctrine of, 331, 538
Unified bar, 45
Unrepresented persons, communicating with,
 408-409
Upjohn rule, 132
Utah
 disciplinary proceedings, 209
 legal malpractice, 183-188
 practice of law by non-lawyers, 499, 501
 reasonableness of attorney's fee, 149

V

Vermont, apprenticeship for bar
 admission in, 49
Vicarious responsibility, 474-475
Virginia
 apprenticeship for bar admission, 49
 IOLTA, opting out, 160
 materiality requirement, attorney
  disciplinary rules, 436
Vischer, Robert, 15
von Bülow, Claus, 287-288

W

Waivers
 advance conflict waivers, 337-338
 attorney-client privilege, 279-291, 304
 conflicts of interest, 309

current-client conflicts, 310, 322
   selective, 280-281
   subject matter waiver, 286-288
   work-product immunity, 289-291,
     298-304
Wald, Eli, 11, 202-203
Walker, Lawrence, 28
Washington
   apprenticeship for bar admission, 49
   Courthouse Facilitators, 560
   LLLTs (Triple LTs), 48, 560-561
Websites, 513, 528, 529
Weiser, Benjamin, 425-429
Wendel, W. Bradley, 32, 33-34, 36, 37, 38,
   311-313, 317
West Virginia, apprenticeship for bar
   admission in, 49
Wisconsin
   "diploma privilege," 49
   materiality requirement, attorney
     disciplinary rules, 436
   perjury by client, 462
Withdrawal from representation, 169-176
   crime or fraud, 16, 122-123, 175, 250
   duties to organizational client vs. individual
     constituents of organization, 125-131, 133
   fiduciary duty, 147
   fundamental disagreement with client, 116
   grounds for, 16, 169-173
   mitigation of harm from, 101
   permission to withdraw denied, 232
   reporting up duties, withdrawal to avoid,
     135-141

Witnesses
   advocate-witness rule, 338-340, 397
   experts. *See* Expert witnesses
   impeachment of, 468
   improperly influencing or intimidating, 395
   preparation, 388-390
   right to call and confront, 5
Woodshedding, 388
Work-product immunity, 245, 297-303
   anticipation of litigation, prepared in,
     299-302
   "circles of lawyer secrets," 303-304
   crime or fraud later accomplished, 299
   exceptions to, 298-304
   Federal Rule of Civil Procedure, 297
   opinion work product, 298, 305
   ordinary work product, 298, 305
   substantial need–undue hardship
     exception, 298
   types of work product, 297
   waivers, 289-291, 298-304
World Justice Project, 543
Wrongful discharge of attorney, 135-141
Wyoming, lodestar determination of fee in,
   148-149

Y

Yablonski, Joseph A., 125-132

Z

Zacharias, Fred, 420-425
Zealous advocacy, 29, 36, 118, 392, 394, 412,
   421, 446, 468